BLACKWELL'S
FIVE-MINUTE
VETERINARY
CONSULT
RUMINANT

BLACKWELL'S FIVE-MINUTE VETERINARY CONSULT RUMINANT

Scott R.R. Haskell, DVM, MPVM, PhD
Editor

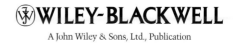
A John Wiley & Sons, Ltd., Publication

Edition first published 2008
© 2008 Wiley-Blackwell

Blackwell Publishing was acquired by John Wiley & Sons in February 2007. Blackwell's
publishing program has been merged with Wiley's global Scientific, Technical, and Medical
business to form Wiley-Blackwell.

Editorial Office
2121 State Avenue, Ames, Iowa 50014-8300, USA

For details of our global editorial offices, for customer services, and for information about how to
apply for permission to reuse the copyright material in this book, please see our website at
www.wiley.com/wiley-blackwell.

Library of Congress Cataloging-in-Publication Data

Blackwell's five-minute veterinary consult. Ruminant / [edited by] Scott R.R. Haskell. – 1st ed.
    p.   ;   cm.
  Includes bibliographical references and index.
  ISBN-13: 978-0-7817-5325-8 (alk. paper)
  ISBN-10: 0-7817-5325-2 (alk. paper)
  1. Ruminants–Diseases–Handbooks, manuals, etc.   I. Haskell, S. R. R. (Scott R. R.)
II. Title: Five-minute veterinary consult.   III. Title: Ruminant.
[DNLM: 1. Animal Diseases–Handbooks. 2. Ruminants–Handbooks. 3. Veterinary
Medicine–methods–Handbooks. SF 997.5.U5 B632 2008]
SF997.5.R86B532 2008
636.2′089–dc22

                                                                         2007040812

A catalogue record for this book is available from the U.S. Library of Congress.

Set in 9/10 AGaramond by Aptara, Inc.
Printed in Singapore by Markono Print Media Pte Ltd

Pharmaceutical Disclaimer

To *Dr. Bernard "Bernie" Feldman*, deceased Professor at Virginia Tech: mentor, friend, brilliant professor, and scholar. Bernie, your support in times of need to so many can never be repaid. You still remain my professional light. Thank you.

To *Dr. Charles "Charlie" Hjerpe*, Professor Emeritus at the University of California, Davis; feedlot antibiotic pioneer, mentor, gifted diagnostician, and friend. Charlie, you taught many of us through the years much more than bovine practice. Thank you.

To *Bette and Charles Haskell*, in memory of my loving parents who taught me perseverance, compassion, and fortitude. Thank you.

To *Parlin Gale*, my sister who consistently shows me warmth, intelligence, and support administered with humor. Thank you for your guidance on the journey.

To *Annie, Sydney, and Lilly Haskell*, my kindred spirits. You taught me compassion, unwavering devotion, and love. Thank you.

PREFACE

Keeping current is a difficult task for today's ruminant veterinary practitioner. The ability to stay current through veterinary literature and research is a daunting if not seemingly impossible task. Many of the research results and conclusions in the scientific literature are confusing and may be inconclusive to today's food animal practitioner. *Blackwell's Five-Minute Veterinary Consult: Ruminant* is designed to provide to the practicing veterinarian, veterinary student, animal scientist, extension specialist, and researcher a quick, concise, and practical review of many if not most of the important diseases and clinical problems facing ruminants and pseudoruminants in the new millennium. Our goal in creating this textbook in the Five-Minute format is to provide up-to-date information in an easy-to-use format. Emphasis has been placed on the diagnosis and treatment of problems and diseases commonly seen by the ruminant veterinarian.

Today's ruminant practitioners provide services that are not always taught at veterinary colleges. As reproductive specialists, they are asked to conduct breeding soundness examinations and give extensive reproductive support programs. Genetic evaluation and the selection of dams and sires are increasing in their importance. Vaccination and deworming program implementation and evaluation are daily encounters for the practicing veterinarian. Nutritional support and body condition scoring as well as foot care have become necessary tools for the competent practitioner. And finally, financial recommendations are becoming a common purview in ruminant practice. This text addresses these issues as well as leads the reader to suggested readings. Several good internal medicine and production medicine textbooks are available. The uniqueness and importance of *Blackwell's Five-Minute Veterinary Consult: Ruminant* are in its use as a quick reference guide.

Though this textbook is a treatise of ruminant production and diseases, camelids have been included due to their growing importance in domestic and international agriculture. Though camelids are technically pseudoruminants, their physiology and disease patterns are similar in many ways to true ruminants. The inclusion of selected camelid diseases here as a quick reference is important for the practicing veterinarian. Nondomesticated and semidomesticated ruminant species are more commonly found in multidimensional farming situations worldwide. Practitioners have little time to literature search the management and care of these species. In many cases, the information has not been readily available until this textbook. Research demands on practitioners have been increasing. Many practitioners now are called upon to design and implement field trials, on-farm vaccination evaluation programs, and independent epidemiologic evaluations as a necessary part of the busy practice.

Environmental issues will become the primary limitation to animal agriculture in many areas of the world in this millennium. Sections in this textbook alert the reader to important and practical considerations to the environmental concerns faced by animal agriculture today. Sustainability of animal agriculture for the future is being compromised. Emerging disease issues are also covered in the textbook. Today's events in agricultural biosecurity and disease introduction are an important component in veterinary medicine. Private practitioners are the frontline of defense and first responders in the protection against a large-scale disease outbreak.

I, the consulting editors, and the contributors are delighted, privileged, and honored to have been able to present this textbook. Over two hundred veterinary specialists have contributed. An expert wrote each chapter on the specified subject matter. I am indebted to the many contributors and the consulting editors, whose diligence and hard work allowed this textbook to be written and published. My goal is to revise this text every three years so that the contents will remain current, timely, and useful.

Scott R.R. Haskell
Davis, California

ACKNOWLEDGMENTS

I would like to thank the consulting editors and the contributors who by their knowledge and professional expertise have enhanced the quality of these writings. Without their exceptional writing capabilities and understandings of ruminant production medicine, this textbook would in no way reflect flare and topical issues. Their suggestions, input, and commitment made this text an exceptional diagnostic tool. Dr. Danelle Bickett-Weddle gave generously of her time and professional expertise in the foundation and progress to this text. Many thanks go to her and her tireless editing efforts.

CONSULTING EDITORS

DANELLE BICKETT-WEDDLE, DVM,
   MPH Dipl. ACVPM
Section Editor-Dairy
Center for Food Security and Public
   Health
Iowa State University
Ames, IA 50011

TERRY W. LEHENBAUER, DVM, MPVM,
   PhD, Dipl. ACVPM
Department of Veterinary Pathobiology
College of Veterinary Medicine
Oklahoma State University
Stillwater, OK 74078-2007

DAVID McKENZIE, DVM, PhD, Dipl.
   ACVIM
School of Veterinary Medicine
Tuskegee Institute
Tuskegee, AL 36088

CONTRIBUTORS

JOHN ADASKA
CAHFS
School of Veterinary Medicine
University of California
Davis, CA 95616

DANA ALLEN
Department of Animal Science
University of Minnesota
St. Paul, MN 55108

YESSENIA ALMEDIA
UT College of Veterinary Medicine
Dept. of Large Animal Clinical Sciences
Knoxville, TN 37996-4545

FREDERIC TRIPP ALMY
Department of Biomedical
Sciences and Pathobiology
Virginia-Maryland Regional
College of Veterinary Medicine
Blacksburg, VA 24061

KEVIN L. ANDERSON
Ruminant Medicine
Department of Farm Animal Health
and Resource Management
College of Veterinary Medicine,
North Carolina State University
Raleigh, NC 27606

BEAU BAMBERG
Roswell, NM 88201

NOAH BARKA
University of Minnesota
St. Paul, MN 55108

GEORGE BARRINGTON
Department of Veterinary
Clinical Sciences
Washington State University
Pullman, WA 99164-7060

PAUL BARROWS
Wimberley, TX 78676-2135

MICHELLE BARTON
College of Veterinary Medicine
University of Georgia
Athens, GA 30602

NEAL BATALLER
FDA/Center for Veterinary
Medicine (HFV-235)
Division of Compliance
Rockville, MD 20855-2773

RON BAYNES
College of Veterinary Medicine
North Carolina State University
Raleigh, NC 27606

JOHN ANDREW BEREZOWSKI
Alberta Agriculture, Food
and Rural Development
Food Safety Division
Agri-Food Systems Branch
Edmonton, AB T6H 4P2
Canada

STEVEN L. BERRY
Department of Animal Science
University of California
Davis, CA 95616-8521

MICHAEL D. BERNSTEIN
Israel Kimron Veterinary Institute
Bet Dagan, 20520, Israel

DANELLE BICKETT-WEDDLE
Center for Food Security
and Public Health
Iowa State University
Ames, IA 50011

CHRISTIAN BOEGEL
Animal & Veterinary Sciences
Cooperative Extension Diagnostic Lab
Orono, ME 04473

ROBERT BONDURANT
Population Health and Reproduction
School of Veterinary Medicine
University of California
Davis, CA 95616

EMILE BOUCHARD
Universite de Montreal-Quebec
Montreal, Quebec H3C 3T5
Canada

JOAN BOWEN
Wellington, CO 80549

DIPA PUSHKAR BRAHMBHATT
Texas A&M University
College Station, TX 77843

BEN BUCHANAN
UT College of Veterinary Medicine
Dept. of LACS
Knoxville, TN 37996-4545

BONNIE BUNTAIN
USDA/FSIS
Washington, DC 20002

CINDY BURNSTEEL
Division of Therapeutic
Drugs for Food Animals
Rockville, MD 20855

BARBARA BYRNE
Department of Pathology,
Microbiology and Immunology
School of Veterinary Medicine
University of California
Davis, CA 95616

CHRIS CALLOWAY
Department of Clinical Sciences
College of Veterinary Medicine
Kansas State University
Manhattan, KS 66506

JOHN CAMPBELL
Western College of Veterinary Medicine
University of Saskatchewan
Saskatoon, SK S7N 584
Canada

DAWN CAPUCILLE
College of Veterinary Medicine
North Carolina State University
Raleigh, NC 27606

CATHY CARLSON
College of Veterinary Medicine
University of Minnesota
St. Paul, MN 55108

MELISSA NADINE CARR
College of Veterinary Medicine
University of Minnesota
St. Paul, MN 55108

CHRISTOPHER CHASE
Department of Veterinary Science
South Dakota State University
Brookings, SD 57007

RICARDO C. CHEBEL
Caine Veterinary Teaching Center
University of Idaho
Caldwell, ID 83607

PETER CHENOWETH
Department of Clinical Sciences
Veterinary Medical Teaching Hospital
Charles Sturt University
Wagga Wagga, NSW 2678
Australia

MUNASHE CHIGERWE
College of Veterinary Medicine
University of Missouri
Columbia, MO 65211

CHRIS CLARK
Department of Large Animal
Clinical Sciences
Western College of Veterinary Medicine
University of Saskatchewan
Saskatoon, SK S7N 5B4
Canada

LUCAS CLOW
College of Veterinary Medicine
University of Minnesota
St. Paul, MN 55108

NATALIE COFFER
Dept. of LACS
College of Veterinary Medicine
University of Tennessee
Knoxville, TN 37996-4545

HEIDI COKER
School of Veterinary Medicine
University of California
Davis, CA 95616

KRISTY CORTRIGHT
College of Veterinary Medicine
University of California
Davis, CA 95616

PENELOPE COLLINS
Veterans Administration
Palo Alto, CA 94304-1290

VICTOR STUART COX
College of Veterinary Medicine
University of Minnesota
St. Paul, MN 55108

THOMAS M. CRAIG
Department of Veterinary Pathobiology
Texas A&M University
College Station, TX 77843-4467

JIM S. CULLOR
Dairy Food Safety Laboratory
University of California
Davis, CA 95616

ANGELA DANIELS
Circle H Animal Health LLC
CattleLac Services LLC
Dalhart, TX 79022

BENJAMIN DARIEN
Department of Medical Sciences
School of Veterinary Medicine
University of Wisconsin
Madison, WI 53706-1102

ANDRES DE LA CONCHA
Department of Veterinary Pathobiology
College of Veterinary Medicine
Texas A&M University
College Station, TX 77843-4467

AMANDA DENISEN
Farmington Veterinary Clinic
Farmington, MN 55024

GRANT A. DEWELL
Animal Population Health Institute
College of Veterinary Medicine
Colorado State University
Fort Collins, CO 80523

ALFREDO DICOSTANZO
Department of Animal Science
University of Minnesota
St. Paul, MN 55108

JESSICA DINHAM
College of Veterinary Medicine
University of Minnesota
St. Paul, MN 55108

*deceased

DOUGLAS DONOVAN
Food Animal Health and
Management Program
Department of Large Animal Medicine
College of Veterinary Medicine
University of Georgia
Athens, GA 30605

PATRICIA DOWLING
Department of Veterinary
Clinical Pharmacology
Western Centre Canadian GFARAD
Saskatoon, SK S7N 5B4
Canada

WILLIAM ROSSER DUBOIS
Circle H. Animal Health
Dalhart, TX 79022

GLENDA D. DVORAK
Center for Food Security
and Public Health
College of Veterinary Medicine
Iowa State University
Ames, IA 50011

MARCIA ENDRES
Department of Animal Science
University of Minnesota
St. Paul, MN 55108-6118

RICHARD W. ERMEL
Department of Comparative Medicine
Animal Resources Center
City of Hope
Duarte, CA 91010

ALEX ESTRADA
Department of Population Medicine
Ontario Veterinary College
University of Guelph
Guelph, ONT Canada N1G 2W1

TIM J. EVANS
Veterinary Medical Diagnostic Laboratory
Department of Veterinary Pathobiology
College of Veterinary Medicine
University of Missouri-Columbia
Columbia, MO 65211

JENNIFER EWOLDT (IVANY)
Scott County Animal Hospital
Eldridge, IA 52748

BERNIE FELDMAN*
Department of Biomedical
Sciences & Pathobiology
College of Veterinary Medicine
Virgiania Tech University
Blacksburg, VA 24061

ANN FITZPATRICK
Office of Regulatory Affairs
University of Minnesota
Minneapolis, MN 55455

DENNIS FRENCH
Department of Veterinary
Clinical Sciences
School of Veterinary Medicine
Louisiana State University
Baton Rouge, LA. 70803

CURTIS L. FRITZ
Vector-Borne Disease Section
Division of Communicable
Disease Control
California Department of Public Health
Sacramento, CA 94234-7320

JOHN GAY
Field Disease Investigation Unit
Washington State University
Pullman, WA 99164-6610

RONETTE GEHRING
Center for Chemical Toxicology
Research and Pharmacokinetics
College of Veterinary Medicine
North Carolina State University
Raleigh, NC 27606

JEREMY GESKE
Minnesota Lamb and
Wool Producers
New Prague, MN 56071

JOHN GIBBONS
Reproductive Physiology
Dept. of Animal and Veterinary
Sciences
Clemson University
Clemson, SC 29634-0311

MARGE GILL
Veterinary Clinical Sciences
School of Veterinary Medicine
Louisiana State University
Baton Rouge, LA 70803

JOHN GILLIAM
College of Veterinary Medicine
Oklahoma State University
Stillwater, OK 74078

MICHAEL GOEDKEN
Department of Pathobiology and
Veterinary Science
University of Connecticut
Storrs, Connecticut 06269-3089

KAREN GOH-CARBERRY
Department of Sciences
& Allied Health
Sacramento City College
Sacramento, CA 95822-1386

SERGIO GONZALES
Veterinary Teaching Hospital
University of Minnesota
St Paul, MN 55108

REUBEN N. GONZALEZ
Quality Milk Production Services
College of Veterinary Medicine
Cornell University
Ithaca, NY 14850-1263

SAGAR M. GOYAL
Department of Veterinary
Diagnostic Medicine
University of Minnesota
St. Paul, MN 55108

THOMAS GRAHAM
Veterinary Consulting Services
Davis, CA 95616

BETHANY GROHS
Environmental Protection Agency
Edison, NJ 08837

DAN GROOMS
College of Veterinary Medicine
Michigan State University
East Lansing, MI 48824

LEE KIRK GROSS
Monsanto
Beverly Hills, CA 90211

JERRY C. HAIGH
Department of Large Animal
Clinical Sciences
Western College of Veterinary
Medicine
Saskatoon, SK S7N 5B4
Canada

CAROLYN HAMMER
Center for Food Security
and Public Health
Iowa State University
Ames, IA 50011

KELSEY A. HART
Department of Large Animal Medicine
College of Veterinary Medicine
University of Georgia
Athens, GA 30602

SCOTT R.R. HASKELL
Graduate Group Comparative
Pathology
University of California
Davis, CA 95616

MARLENE HAUCK
College of Veterinary Medicine
North Carolina State University
Raleigh, NC 27606

DENNIS HERMESCH
Kansas State University
Manhattan, KS 66506

DONALD HOENIG
State Veterinarian
State Department of Agriculture
Food and Rural Resources
Augusta, ME 04333

TROY HOLDER
Dept. of LACS
College of Veterinary Medicine
University of Tennessee
Knoxville, TN 37996-4545

LARRY HOLLER
Department of Veterinary Science
South Dakota State University
Brookings, SD 57007

STACY HOLZBAUER
College of Veterinary Medicine
Iowa State University
Ames, IA 50011

HUSSEIN S. HUSSEIN
Department of Animal Biotechnology
School of Veterinary Medicine
University of Nevada-Reno
Reno, NV 89557

KENT JACKSON
Animal Medical Clinic of Auburn
Auburn, CA 95602

CARMELA JARAVATA
Dairy Food Safety Laboratory
Department of Population Health
and Reproduction
School of Veterinary Medicine
University of California
Davis, CA 95616

HEATHER JOHNSON
Dairy Food Safety Laboratory
Department of Population Health
and Reproduction
School of Veterinary Medicine
University of California
Davis, CA 95616

WALTER H. JOHNSON
Department of Population Medicine
Ontario Veterinary College
University of Guelph
Guelph, ON N1G 2W1
Canada

MEREDYTH JONES-RICHARDS
College of Veterinary Medicine
Oklahoma State University
Stillwater, OK 74078-2007

SERGIO DE OLIVEIRA JUCHEM
School of Veterinary Medicine
Animal Science Department
University of California
Davis, CA 95616

COLLIN KAMUNDE
Department of Biomedical Sciences
Atlantic Veterinary College
University of Prince Edward Island
Charlottetown , PEI C1A 4P3
Canada

J. JERRY KANEKO
Department of Pathology,
Microbiology & Immunology
School of Veterinary Medicine
University of California
Davis, CA 95616

RAY KAPLAN
Department of Infectious Diseases
College of Veterinary Medicine
University of Georgia
Athens, GA 30602

ANDREW KARTER
Epidemiology & Health
Services Research
Division of Research
Kaiser Permanente
Oakland, CA 94612

RAMANATHAN KASIMANICKAM
Food Animal Theriogenology
Virginia Maryland Regional College of
Veterinary Medicine
Virginia Polytechnic Institute
and State University
Blacksburg, VA 24061

PHILIP H. KASS
Department of Population
Health & Reproduction
School of Veterinary Medicine
University of California
Davis, CA 95616

BRENDA KENNEDY-WADE
Animal & Veterinary Sciences
Cooperative Extension Diagnostic Lab
Orono, ME 04473

LARRY KERR
Department of LACS
College of Veterinary Medicine
University of Tennessee
Knoxville, TN 37996-4545

GRACE KIM
Veterinary Service
School of Medicine
University of California
San Francisco, CA 94143-0410

ANNE M. KJEMTRUP
California Department of Health Services
Sacramento, CA 95899-7377

MICHELLE KOPCHA
Practice-based Ambulatory Program
Food Animal Medicine and Surgery
Department of Large Animal
Clinical Sciences
College of Veterinary Medicine
Michigan State University
East Lansing, MI 48824

MICHAELA KRISTULA
College of Veterinary Medicine
University of Pennsylvania
Kennet Square, PA

CARLA KUEHN
Department of Animal Science
University of Minnesota
St. Paul, MN 55108

JEFFREY LAKRTIZ
Department of Veterinary
Clinical Sciences
The Ohio State University
Columbus, OH 43210-1089

BOB L. LARSON
Department of Veterinary
Medicine and Surgery
College of Veterinary Medicine
University of Missouri
Columbia, MO 65211

STEPHEN LEBLANC
Department of Population Medicine
Ontario Veterinary College
University of Guelph
Guelph, ON N1G 2W1
Canada

TERRY W. LEHENBAUER
Department of Epidemiology
& Preventative Medcine
Center for Veterinary Sciences
Oklahoma State University
Stillwater, OK 74078-2007

JIM LINN
Department of Animal Science
University of Minnesota
St. Paul, MN 55108-6118

BONNIE LEE LOGHRY
Veterinary Technology Program
Yuba College
2088 North Beale Road
Marysville, CA 95901

CINDY LOVERN
Emergency Preparedness
and Response
American Veterinary Medical
Association
Schaumburg, IL 60173-4360

CHRISTOPHER LUBY
College of Veterinary Medicine
University of Missouri
Columbia, MO 65211

MARGO MACHEN
College of Veterinary Medicine
Western University of Health Sciences
Pomona, CA 91766-1854

SUSAN L. McCLANAHAN
College of Veterinary Medicine
University of Minnesota
St. Paul, MN 55108

SHEILA McGUIRK
School of Veterinary Medicine
University of Wisconsin
Madison, WI 53706

DAVID McKENZIE
School of Veterinary Medicine
Tuskegee University
Tuskegee, AL 36088

SANDY McLACHLAN
Department of Veterinary &
   Biomedical Sciences
Murdoch University
Murdoch, 6150
Western Australia

CHARLOTTE MEANS
ASPCA Animal Poison Control Center
Urbana IL 61802

RICHARD W. MEIRING
Department of Veterinary
   Preventative Medicine
College of Veterinary Medicine
The Ohio State University
Columbus, OH 43210

PAUL MENNICK
Pacific International Genetics
Los Molinos, CA 96055

PEDRO MELENDEZ
College of Veterinary Medicine
University of Florida
Gainesville, FL 32610

PAULA IRENE MENZIES
Department of Veterinary Medicine
Ontario Veterinary College
University of Guelph
Guelph, ON N1G 2W1
Canada

JAMES T. MERONEK
Dairy Forage Research Center
College of Agriculture & Life Sciences
University of Wisconsin
Madison, WI 53706

JOHN R. MIDDLETON
Department of Veterinary
   Medicine and Surgery
College of Veterinary Medicine
University of Missouri
Columbia, MO 65211

LOWELL T. MIDLA
OSU Large Animal Services
Marysville, OH 43040

JOSEPH MILLER
Rose Acre Farms
Seymour, IN 47274

ROBERT B. MOELLER
California Animal Health and
   Food Safety Laboratory
Tulare, CA 93274

HARRY MOMONT
School of Veterinary Medicine
University of Wisconsin
Madison, WI 53706

DALE MOORE
VMTRC
University of California
Tulare, CA 93274

KAREN MORIELLO
College of Veterinary Medicine
University of Wisconsin
Madison, WI 53706

DUSTY NAGY
College of Veterinary Medicine
University of Illinois
Urbana, IL 61802

LISA J. NASHOLD
Department of Comparative Biosciences
University of Wisconsin
Madison, WI 53706

DARYL V. NYDAM
Department of Population Medicine
   & Diagnostic Sciences
College of Veterinary Medicine
Cornell University
Ithaca, NY 14853

LARRY OCCHIPINTI
Tidewater, OR 97390

ERIK J. OLSON
Minnesota Veterinary Diagnostic
   Laboratory
College of Veterinary Medicine
University of Minnesota
St. Paul, MN 55108

VICTORIA M. OLSON
College of Veterinary Medicine
Iowa State University
Ames, IA 50011

MICHAEL W. OVERTON
School of Veterinary Medicine
University of California
Davis, CA 95616

LAUREN J. PALMER
Marine Mammal Care Center
   Fort MacArthur
San Pedro, CA 90275

JILL PARKER
Department of Clinical Sciences
College of Veterinary Medicine
Oregon State University
Corvallis, OR 97331

SIMON F. PEEK
School of Veterinary Medicine
University of Wisconsin
Madison, WI 53706

KEVIN D. PELZER
College of Veterinary Medicine
Virginia Tech University
Blacksburg, VA 24061

JOHN PERONI
Department of Large Animal Surgery
College of Veterinary Medicine
University of Georgia
Athens, GA 30606

MARKY PITTS
Laboratory Animal Services
University of California
La Jolla, CA 92093

PAUL J. PLUMMER
Veterinary Microbiology and
   Preventative Medicine
College of Veterinary Medicine
Iowa State University
Ames, Iowa 50011

TIM PORTILLO
Pacific International Genetics
Los Molinos, CA 96055

ED POWERS
Napa, CA 94558

BIRGIT PUSCHNER
CAHFS - Toxicology
School of Veterinary Medicine
University of California
Davis, CA 95616

RAVI KUMAR PUTLURU
Department of HNFAS
University of Hawaii - Manoa
Honolulu, HI 96822

MARY RAETH-KNIGHT
Department of Animal Science
University of Minnesota
St. Paul, MN 55108

PAUL RAPNICKI
Center for Dairy Health, Management
   & Food Quality
College of Veterinary Medicine
University of Minnesota
St. Paul, MN 55108

ALEJANDRO RAMIREZ
Center for Food Security & Public Health
College of Veterinary Medicine
Iowa State University
Ames, IA 50011

JAMES RASMUSSEN
Minnesota Zoological Gardens
Apple Valley, MN 55124

LARRY RAWSON
USDA/APHIS
Honolulu, HI 96822

GABE RENSEN
Dairy Food Safety Laboratory
Department of Population Health
   & Reproduction
School of Veterinary Medicine
University of California
Davis, CA 95616

JIM REYNOLDS
School of Veterinary Medicine
University of California
Davis, CA 95616

LAURA RIGGS
Department of Large Animal Medicine
Veterinary Teaching Hospital
University of Georgia
Athens, GA 30602

CARLOS RISCO
College of Veterinary Medicine
University of Florida
Gainesville, FL 32610

JERRY ROBERSON
Veterinary Medical Teaching
Hospital
Department of Clinical Sciences
Kansas State University
Manhattan, KS 66506-5606

JOSEPH DEEN RODER
Schering-Plough Corporation
Canyon, TX 79015

JOSEPH ROOK
Veterinary Clinical Center
College of Veterinary Medicine
Michigan State University
East Lansing, MI 48824

DAN RULE
Department of Animal Science
University of Wyoming
Laramie, WY 82070

GARY P. RUPP
Great Plains Veterinary
Educational Center
University of Nebraska
Clay Center, NE 68933

JULIANA M. RUZANTE
School of Veterinary Medicine
University of California
Davis, CA 95616

ABBY SAGE
College of Veterinary Medicine
University of Minnesota
St. Paul, MN 55108

JEREMY SCHEFERS
Minnesota Veterinary Diagnostic
Laboratory
College of Veterinary Medicine
University of Minnesota
St. Paul, MN 55108

YNTE H. SCHUKKEN
Schurman Hall College of
Veterinary Medicine
Cornell University
Ithaca, NY 14850

LOREN SCHULTZ
College of Veterinary Medicine
University of Missouri
Columbia, MO 65211

SUE SEMRAD
School of Veterinary Medicine
University of Wisconsin
Madison, WI 53706

BARRETT D. SLENNING
Department of Farm Animal Health &
Resource Management
College of Veterinary Medicine
North Carolina State University
Raleigh, NC 27606

BILLY I. SMITH
College of Veterinary Medicine
University of Pennsylvania
Kennet Square, PA

GREGORY STONER
Family Pet Hospital
Vacaville, CA 95616

CAROLYN STULL
Vet Med Extension
University of California
Davis, CA 95616

JAN SWANSON
Department of Animal Science
Kansas State University
Manhattan, KS 66506

PATRICIA ANN TALCOTT
College of Veterinary Medicine
Washington State University
Pullman, WA 99164-6520

JARED D. TAYLOR
Iowa State University
Ames, IA 50011

DEBBIE TERREL
College of Veterinary Medicine
Oklahoma State University
Stillwater, OK 74078

ROLAND ALEX THOMPSON
Global Disease Detection
Operations Center
Center for Disease Control
& Prevention
Atlanta, GA 30333

AHMED TIBARY
Department of Veterinary
Clinical Sciences
College of Veterinary Medicine
Washington State University
Pullman, WA 99164-6610

ASHEESH TIWARY
CAHFS-Toxicology
School of Veterinary Medicine
University of California
Davis, CA 95616

FERENC TOTH
Department of Large Animal
Clinical Sciences
College of Veterinary Medicine
University of Tennessee
Knoxville, TN 37996-4545

TORKILD TVERAA
Norwegian Institute for
Nature Research
Polarmiljosenteret
Tromso, N-9296
Norway

JEFF W. TYLER
College of Veterinary Medicine
University of Missouri
Columbia, MO 65211

STEVEN D. VAN CAMP
Lincoln, CA 95648

DEON VAN DER MERWE
College of Veterinary Medicine
North Carolina State University
Raleigh, NC 27606

ROBERT J. VAN SAUN
Department of Veterinary
& Biomedical Sciences
Pennsylvania State University
University Park, PA 16802-3500

KEVIN E. WASHBURN
College of Veterinary Medicine
Oklahoma State University
Stillwater, OK 74078-2007

ALISTAIR WEBB
Department of Physiological Sciences
College of Veterinary Medicine
University of Florida
Gainesville, FL 32610-0144

KIRSTEN WEGNER
College of Veterinary Medicine
VMTH
University of Florida
Gainesville, FL 32610-0136

MELISSA WEISMAN
Minnesota Zoological Garden
Apple Valley, MN 55124

MATT WELBORN
Department of Large Animal
Clinical Sciences
College of Veterinary Medicine
University of Tennessee
Knoxville, TN 37996-4545

JEFFREY JAY WICHTEL
Department of Health Management
Atlantic Veterinary College
University of Prince Edward Island
Charlottetown, PEI C1A 4P3
Canada

DAVID WILSON
Department of Clinical Sciences
Veterinary Medical Teaching Hospital
Kansas State University
Manhattan, KS 66506

PETER WILSON
Deer Health and Production
Institute of Veterinary, Animal
& Biomedical Sciences
Massey University
Palmerston North
New Zealand

TINA WISMER
Animal Poison Control Center
University of Illinois
Urbana, IL 61802

MAUREEN WITCHEL
Atlantic Veterinary College
University of Prince Edward Island
Charlottetown, PEI C1A 4P3
Canada

STEPHAN WITTE
Athens, GA 30606

KURT ZIMMERMAN
Department of Biomedical Sciences
& Pathobiology
Virginia Maryland Regional
College of Veterinary Medicine
Virginia Tech University
Blacksburg, VA 24061

JOSEPH ZINKL
Pathology, Microbiology & Immunology
School of Veterinary Medicine
University of California
Davis, CA 95616

Contents

TOPIC	

CONTENTS *by subject*

GASTROINTESTINAL DISEASE

NON-TRADITIONAL SPECIES

NUTRITIONAL DISEASES

PARASITOLOGY

RENAL-HEPATIC

REPRODUCTIVE DISEASES

TOPIC	

RESPIRATORY DISEASES

TOXICOLOGY

BLACKWELL'S FIVE-MINUTE VETERINARY CONSULT RUMINANT

ABOMASAL EMPTYING DEFECT (AED) IN SHEEP

BASICS

DEFINITION
Abomasal emptying defect (AED) is a syndrome of adult Suffolk sheep characterized by chronic, progressive weight loss and abomasal dilatation in the absence of mechanical obstruction.

PATHOPHYSIOLOGY
• The pathogenic mechanism for AED is unclear.
• The AED syndrome shares some characteristics of a human syndrome, chronic idiopathic intestinal pseudo-obstruction that affects children and adults. Affected individuals clinically appear to have a partial or complete gastric obstruction, but none is present.
• Morphologic investigations of human patients indicate degenerative changes in the smooth muscle or the tunica muscularis and/or neurons of the enteric plexus.

SYSTEMS AFFECTED
Gastrointestinal

GENETICS
Little information is available regarding genetic predisposition. A pedigree analysis performed on a flock in which 11 of 92 Suffolks were affected failed to show a hereditary pattern.

INCIDENCE/PREVALENCE
Unknown

GEOGRAPHIC DISTRIBUTION
None

SIGNALMENT
Species
Sheep

Breed Predilection
Suffolk is the predominant breed. The condition has also been reported in the Hampshire, Dorset, and Texel breeds.

Mean Age and Range
Adults that are at least 2 years of age.

Predominant Sex
This condition affects both males and females.

SIGNS

Historical Findings
• This condition usually occurs sporadically, affecting a single individual. Usually, affected flock management is excellent with the animals appearing healthy and in good body condition, except for the affected individual.
• The owners may report loss of weight in the individual, despite efforts to provide extra nutrition, anthelmintic treatment, and individual attention. Also, owners will report that animals appear "bloated" despite inappetence.

PHYSICAL FINDINGS
• Most typically body temperature is within normal limits unless there is concurrent disease present. Pulse and respiration rates may be normal to increased. Fecal consistency is usually normal, but fecal volume is often decreased.
• Careful examination of the abdomen is important and particular attention should be paid to the following:
  • Abdominal conformation—may be normal; bilateral, asymmetrical abdominal distention may be observed (distension high in the left paralumbar fossa and low on the right side when the animal is viewed from behind); unilateral distension may be present (low on the right ventrolateral aspect of the abdomen).
  • Rumen contractions—may be normal, increased, or decreased. Rumen hyperactivity is very dramatic to visually observe in AED sheep because the left paralumbar fossa appears to be in constant motion, reflective of the almost constant rumen activity.
  • Abdominal ballottement—Most AED sheep are in varying stages of cachexia and their abdominal wall feels "thin" or lacks tone due to muscle wasting. The gastrointestinal organs also may lack tone or give the impression of being fluid filled. In some instances, the caudal border of the abomasum may be outlined as it extends beyond the last rib on the ventrolateral aspect of the abdomen. The distended abomasum usually feels fluid filled rather than the doughy or firm consistency that is often associated with abomasal impaction in cattle.

RISK FACTORS
Unknown

DIAGNOSIS

DIFFERENTIAL DIAGNOSIS
• Differential diagnosis for chronic weight loss in adult sheep includes caseous lymphadenitis or other chronic infection, Johne's disease, malnutrition, dental problems, parasitism, and rarely neoplasia.
• The historical and physical findings, as described above, are fairly specific to AED.

CBC/BIOCHEMISTRY/URINALYSIS
• Hematological and serum chemistry analysis are usually normal.
• The typical metabolic alkalosis with hypochloremia and hypokalemia associated with proximal gastrointestinal obstruction (e.g., displaced abomasum in cattle) is not consistently noted with AED.
• Elevations in liver enzymes (SGOT/AST, SDH, GGT) may be noted; however, this can be misleading chemical data.
• Increased intra-abdominal pressure from a greatly distended abomasum may lead to secondary liver congestion and ischemia. This pressure can precipitate hepatic leakage of liver enzymes.
• Urinalysis is usually unremarkable.

OTHER LABORATORY TESTS
• An elevated rumen chloride concentration is probably the most useful test in supporting a diagnosis of AED.
• Normal rumen chloride in sheep is ≤ 15 mEq/L. Most often affected sheep will have at least a twofold increase. Rumen fluid samples are obtained most easily by percutaneous aspiration of the rumen from a site in the ventrolateral aspect of the left paralumbar fossa.

IMAGING
• Abdominal radiology may be helpful; however, unless the animal can be positioned for an oblique abdominal radiographic view, results will be difficult to interpret.
• Abdominal ultrasonography may be more useful than radiography in imaging the abomasum. A 3 to 5 MHz linear or sector scanner can provide adequate images of the abomasum. When placed on the lower right abdomen, the normal abomasum will not extend beyond the last rib. An animal's abomasum with AED will usually appear two to four times normal size.

ABOMASAL EMPTYING DEFECT (AED) IN SHEEP

DIAGNOSTIC PROCEDURES
N/A

PATHOLOGIC FINDINGS
• Gross necropsy finding: abomasum that is greatly distended with a patent pylorus.
• Abomasal contents are usually liquid but may be dry. Histopathologic changes in the abomasum include smooth-muscle degeneration, vacuolation, and varying degrees of necrosis. Degenerative changes have been reported in the celiacomesenteric ganglia.

TREATMENT

GENERAL CONSIDERATIONS
• The prognosis for recovery when intensive treatment is initiated is variable and dependant upon the duration of the abomasal dysfunction and distention. Medical therapy alone using various cathartics and laxatives and surgical therapy (abomasotomy) have had limited success.
• In animals that are good surgical candidates, abomasotomy followed by metoclopramide and supportive fluid therapy has provided some success.

SURGICAL CONSIDERATIONS
An abomasotomy is best performed under general anesthesia, although an anesthetic approach using a local line block can be used. The animal is placed in left-lateral recumbency and a right paracostal approach provides excellent access to the abomasum. Subsequently the abomasum is opened and its contents removed, and the organ is flushed and closed in a routine manner. Therapy with metoclopramide should be used as an adjunct to the surgery (see Medications section below). Also, fluid replacement and electrolyte correction therapy is critical to survival and success.

MEDICATIONS

DRUGS OF CHOICE
Metoclopramide (0.1 mg/kg, q 8 hrs, SQ) as an adjunct to abomasotomy has been reported to improve abomasal motility in selected cases. This medication should not be used if a gastrointestinal obstruction is suspected.

CONTRAINDICATIONS
• Neostigmine should not be used in affected animals.
• Appropriate milk and meat withdrawal times must be followed for all compounds administered to food-producing animals.

FOLLOW-UP

PATIENT MONITORING
• If intensive therapy is undertaken, the animal should be observed for attitude, appetite, volume of fecal production, and abdominal conformation. Positive signs of improvement following abomasotomy and during metoclopramide therapy may include improvement in attitude and an increased interest in eating.
• Fecal production should increase and abdominal distention should decrease if abomasal motility has returned.

PREVENTION/AVOIDANCE
Because the underlying cause of this condition is unknown, no recommendations can be made.

POSSIBLE COMPLICATIONS
• Complications related to abomasotomy: surgical dehiscence of the abomasal incision (especially if the abomasal wall has undergone degenerative changes) and dehiscence of the abdominal incision may occur (more likely to occur in a debilitated patient).
• Once the condition is recognized, if treatment is declined, euthanasia should be offered as a humane resolution.

EXPECTED COURSE AND PROGNOSIS
• The earlier the condition is recognized and treated, the better the prognosis; however, for long-term recovery, the prognosis is guarded.
• In certain circumstances such as a ram completing a breeding season, or a late gestation ewe completing her pregnancy, a fair to good prognosis may be offered if intensive treatment is provided early.

MISCELLANEOUS

ASSOCIATED CONDITIONS
Other concurrent conditions may occur with this disease. Pneumonia and other organ failures are viewed as secondary to any chronic debilitating diseases.

AGE-RELATED FACTORS
N/A

ZOONOTIC POTENTIAL
None

PREGNANCY
In spite of treatment, pregnant animals may abort. Pregnant animals (especially mid to late term) represent an increased surgical risk.

RUMINANT SPECIES AFFECTED
The condition has been reported in sheep only; however, the author has observed a similar syndrome in a geriatric crossbred dairy-type goat.

BIOSECURITY
N/A

PRODUCTION MANAGEMENT
This is usually observed in a single animal from a well-managed flock.

SYNONYMS
Abomasal dilatation and emptying defect
Abomasal impaction
Acquired dysautonomia
Functional pyloric stenosis
Ovine abomasal enlargement

SEE ALSO
N/A

ABBREVIATIONS
AED = abomasal emptying defect
AST = aspartate transaminase
GGT = gamma-glutamyltransferase
SDH = succinate dehydrogenase
SGOT = serum glutamic oxaloacetic transaminase

Suggested Reading
Kopcha, M. 1988. Abomasal dilatation and emptying defect in a ewe. *J Am Vet Med Assoc* 192:783–84.
Pruden, S. J., McAllister, M. M., Schultheiss, P. C., et al. 2004. Abomasal emptying defect of sheep may be an acquired form of dysautonomia *Vet Pathol*. 41:164–69.
Ruegg, P. L., George, L. W., East, N. E. 1988. Abomasal dilatation and emptying defect in a flock of Suffolk ewes. *J Am Vet Med Assoc* 193:1534–36.

Author: Michelle Kopcha

ABOMASAL IMPACTION

BASICS

OVERVIEW
• Blockage of fluid and ingesta from the abomasum through the pylorus by feed, sand, gravel, or neurological deficit.
• Pyloric obstruction from improper placement of percutaneous fixation of left-sided abomasum ("roll and toggle") can result in abomasal impaction.
• Signs can be acute or chronic and are characterized by loss of appetite, decreased or scant feces, distension of the abomasum, weakness, dehydration, metabolic alkalosis, and apparent abdominal pain.
• Found in cattle and sometimes sheep. Usually isolated cases but also may have low morbidity associated with low-quality forages. High mortality.
• Abomasal emptying defect (AED) is a disease syndrome that primarily affects Suffolk sheep and is characterized by distension and impaction of the abomasum.

PATHOPHYSIOLOGY
• Physical blockage of the outflow from the abomasum to the duodenum occurs. This may be due to the packing of straw or poor-quality roughages, sand, or gravel in the abomasum.
• Damage to branches of the vagus nerve from reticuloperitonitis or lymphoma can decrease the emptying ability of the abomasum. Failure of fluid to move from the abomasum to the intestines results in dehydration and starvation.
• Sequestration of hydrochloric acid in the abomasum can result in metabolic alkalosis.
• In sheep, no histologic lesion has been consistently associated with AED. There is no known etiology. In one study, histologic examination of celiacomesenteric ganglia from affected sheep revealed scattered chromatolytic or necrotic neurons, without inflammation. Chromatolytic neurons were observed more frequently in AED-affected sheep than in healthy Suffolk sheep. Neuronal necrosis was not observed in any of the healthy sheep. Neuronal lesions of AED resemble dysautonomic diseases of humans and other animals.

SYSTEMS AFFECTED
Gastrointestinal

GENETICS
N/A

INCIDENCE/PREVALENCE
Very low morbidity

GEOGRAPHIC DISTRIBUTION
Worldwide; seen more commonly where low-quality roughages or low-energy diets are fed.

Epidemiology
• Feeding chopped straw or low-quality forages has been associated with abomasal impaction. Excessive intake of such feeds in attempts to meet energy needs appears to predispose cattle.
• Feeding cattle on sand or gravel or including excessive dirt or gravel from feed storage areas into mixed feed.
• Late-gestation animals appear more frequently affected.

SIGNALMENT
Species Affected
Bovine, ovine

Breed Predilections
Suffolk sheep

Mean Age and Range
N/A

Predominant Sex
Commonly seen affecting pregnant females.

SIGNS
• Anorexia, weight loss, scant feces, dehydration, distension of the abomasum, decrease in rumen motility, recumbency
• Metabolic alkalosis in chronic cases
• In sheep, clinical signs consisted of chronic anorexia and weight loss. Also, laboratory analysis failed to show the hypochloremic, hypokalemic, metabolic alkalosis commonly found in cattle. Rumen chloride concentrations in sheep indicated reflux of abomasal contents into the rumen.

GENERAL COMMENTS
Reported most often in beef cattle fed low-energy, chopped forage diets in cold weather. Seen sporadically in dairy cattle.

HISTORICAL FINDINGS
• Cattle on poor pasture or fed chopped, low-quality forages with low dietary energy, especially in cold weather. Cattle eating on sand or gravel or excessive gravel from the feed storage area in the feed
• Pica

PHYSICAL EXAMINATION FINDINGS
Anorexia, depression, decreased rumen contractions. Distension of the abomasum may be determined by palpation or ballottement of the lower-right flank. Eventually, the animal has scant feces and becomes dehydrated.

CAUSES
• Physical blockage of the abomasum by low-quality chopped forages, sand or gravel, or "roll and toggle" sutures inadvertently placed in or near the pylorus.
• Damage to the vagus nerve

RISK FACTORS
• Cattle on low-energy diets being fed chopped forages, or fed on sand or gravel
• Certain lines of Suffolk sheep may be afflicted more than others.

DIAGNOSIS

DIFFERENTIAL DIAGNOSIS
Abomasal volvulus or torsion, reticuloperitonitis, lymphoma

CBC/BIOCHEMISTRY/URINALYSIS
• CBC usually normal
• Hypochloremic, hypokalemic metabolic alkalosis may be present in chronic cases.
• In sheep with AED, laboratory analyses failed to show the hypochloremic, hypokalemic, metabolic alkalosis commonly found in cattle. Rumen chloride concentrations in sheep indicated reflux of abomasal contents into the rumen.

OTHER LABORATORY TESTS
N/A

IMAGING
N/A

OTHER DIAGNOSTIC PROCEDURES
Laparotomy

GROSS AND HISTOPATHOLOGIC FINDINGS
Confirmation from laparotomy

 TREATMENT

Surgical correction by abomasotomy; possible softening of impacted material by per os mineral oil once daily for 2 to 4 days.

Inpatient Versus Outpatient
Inpatient treatment may include correction of metabolic alkalosis.

CLIENT EDUCATION
Feed cattle to energy requirements, especially cattle in cold weather. Do not feed chopped poor-quality forages with low-energy diets. Feed cattle on surfaces other than sand or gravel.

 MEDICATIONS

DRUGS OF CHOICE
Balanced electrolytes IV for 1 to 3 days to correct metabolic alkalosis.

CONTRAINDICATIONS
N/A

PRECAUTIONS
Lactated Ringer's solution should be used cautiously due to the possibility of metabolic alkalosis.

POSSIBLE INTERACTIONS
N/A

ALTERNATIVE DRUGS
N/A

 FOLLOW-UP

PATIENT MONITORING
Pain or suffering, fecal output, hydration status, electrolyte balance

PREVENTION/AVOIDANCE
Feed energy balance feeds with long fiber length. Avoid feeding on sand or gravel.

POSSIBLE COMPLICATIONS
Abomasal rupture and peritonitis

EXPECTED COURSE AND PROGNOSIS
Grave prognosis; death from dehydration, metabolic alkalosis, or peritonitis

 MISCELLANEOUS

PREVENTION
Feed good-quality, long forage with adequate energy supplementation. Avoid feeding on sand or gravel.

ASSOCIATED CONDITIONS
Reticuloperitonitis, lymphoma, displaced abomasum

AGE-RELATED FACTORS
More common in pregnant animals

ZOONOTIC POTENTIAL
N/A

PREGNANCY
Pregnancy predisposes due to increased energy needs and the possible effect of size and weight of the gravid uterus on abdominal organs

SYNONYMS
Abomasal emptying defect (AED) in Suffolk sheep

SEE ALSO
Abomasal emptying defect
Displaced abomasum, volvulus, or torsion
Fluid therapy
Lymphoma
Reticuloperitonitis

ABBREVIATIONS
AED = abomasal emptying defect
CBC = complete blood count
IV = intravenous

Suggested Reading
Belknap, E. B., Navarre, C. B. 2000, March. Differentiation of gastrointestinal diseases in adult cattle. In: *The veterinary clinics of north america, food animal practice, diagnosis of diseases of the digestive tract,* ed. R. G. Helman., vol. 16, no. 1. Philadelphia: W. B. Saunders.
Kline, E. E., Meyer, J. R., Nelson, D. R., Memon, M. A. 1983, Aug 20. Abomasal impaction in sheep. *Vet Rec.* 113(8): 177–79.
Pruden, S. J., McAllister, M. M., Schultheiss, P. C., O'Toole, D., Christensen, D. E. 2004, Mar. Abomasal emptying defect of sheep may be an acquired form of dysautonomia. *Vet Pathol.* 41(2):164–69.
Radostits, O. M., Gay, C. C., Blood, D. C., Hinchcliff, K. W., eds. 2000. *Veterinary medicine: a textbook of diseases of cattle, sheep, pigs, goats and horses.* 9th ed. London: W. B. Saunders.
Rings, D. M., Welker, F. H., Hull, B. L., Kersting, K. W., Hoffsis, G. F. 1984, Dec 15. Abomasal emptying defect in Suffolk sheep. *J Am Vet Med Assoc.* 185(12): 1520–22.
Ruegg, P. L., George, L. W., East, N. E. 1988, Dec 15. Abomasal dilatation and emptying defect in a flock of Suffolk ewes. *J Am Vet Med Assoc.* 193(12): 1534–36.

Author: James P. Reynolds

ABOMASAL ULCERS

BASICS

DEFINITION
• Damage to the abomasal mucosa continuing from erosion through complete perforation. Often subclinical but may be clinical.
• Classified as type I (nonperforating ulcers), type II (nonperforating with severe blood loss), type III (perforating with localized peritonitis), and type IV (perforating with diffuse peritonitis).
• Clinical signs associated with abdominal pain, blood loss, and peritonitis. Causes are not known, but may be associated with stress. Not associated with particular abomasal bacterial infections.

PATHOPHYSIOLOGY
• Injuries to the protective mucosal layer allow acid and pepsin to diffuse into the mucosa.
• Type I nonperforating ulcers have incomplete penetration, little local reaction, and minimal bleeding.
• Type II bleeding ulcers erode into a major blood vessel in the submucosa. There may be distension of the abomasum and reflux of abomasal contents into the rumen. There is usually melena.
• Type III ulcers completely perforate the wall with leakage of fluid and local peritonitis. Adhesions form to viscera localizing the peritonitis.
• Type IV ulcers perforate completely and the subsequent fluid leakage is not contained by adhesions, resulting in generalized peritonitis.

SYSTEMS AFFECTED
Gastrointestinal

GENETICS
N/A

INCIDENCE/PREVALENCE
Low, less than 1 or 2%. May be higher in some types of calf-raising systems.

GEOGRAPHIC DISTRIBUTION
N/A

Epidemiology
• Has been associated with physical irritation from straw in veal calves and high-grain diets in feedlot cattle
• May be related to postpartum conditions in dairy cattle; not definitively associated with bacteria such as clostridia, salmonella, or helicobacter
• No association with hairballs in veal calves

SIGNALMENT
Species Affected
Bovine

Breed Predilections
N/A

Mean Age and Range
Occurs in calves and adults

Predominant Sex
N/A

SIGNS
Anorexia, depression, pyrexia, abdominal pain, abdominal distension, melena, blanched mucous membranes. Peracute death common in adult cattle but not calves.

GENERAL COMMENTS
N/A

HISTORICAL FINDINGS
Changes in feeding, such as transition from milk to solid feed in calves or high roughage prepartum to high concentrate postpartum diets may be involved.

PHYSICAL EXAMINATION FINDINGS
• Melena or occult blood in feces; possible distension of abomasum detected by ballottement of ventral right abdomen; blanched mucous membranes (pallor) in cases with severe blood loss; painful abdomen
• Peritoneal emphysema may be detected during rectal exam.

CAUSES
Unknown in many cases, but can be related to feeds that irritate the abomasal mucosa, such as straw or almond hulls

RISK FACTORS
Sudden transition from milk diet to dry feed in calves, straw feeding in milk-fed calves, possibly high-concentrate diets

DIAGNOSIS

DIFFERENTIAL DIAGNOSIS
Lymphoma, left displaced abomasum, abomasal volvulus or torsion, duodenal ulcers, hemorrhagic bowel syndrome

CBC/BIOCHEMISTRY/URINALYSIS
Acute hemorrhagic anemia in cases of severe gastric hemorrhage

OTHER LABORATORY TESTS
Abdominocentesis may identify abomasal fluid in abdomen in some cases. Testing for occult blood in feces may detect blood in feces before melena is seen.

IMAGING
Ultrasonography may show free fluid in abdomen.

OTHER DIAGNOSTIC PROCEDURES
Exploratory surgery

GROSS AND HISTOPATHOLOGIC FINDINGS
• Ulcers are most commonly found along the greater curvature and usually in the fundic area. Ulcers can be a few millimeters to several centimeters in size. They are often filled with debris or clotted blood. Perforating ulcers are usually adhered to the omentum.
• Cattle with type IV ulcers have abomasal fluid in the abdominal cavity and may have fibrinous peritonitis.

TREATMENT

• Usually unrewarding. Antacids may protect the abomasal mucosa.
• Transfusions may be beneficial if bleeding stops or is controlled.
• Surgical correction of perforated ulcers for valuable cattle

Inpatient Versus Outpatient

The opportunity for successful surgical correction and adequate transfusion is greater in clinic than on farm.

CLIENT EDUCATION

Gradual introduction of dry feed to calves is preferred to abrupt exposure to dry feed during the milk-fed period.

MEDICATIONS

DRUGS OF CHOICE

• Antacids such as magnesium oxide (500 g/400 kg body weight daily for 2 to 4 days) has been suggested.
• Per os kaolin and pectin mixture (2 to 3 liters twice daily to mature cattle) has been suggested.

CONTRAINDICATIONS

NSAIDs that interfere with the production of prostaglandin E series via the arachadonic acid cascade are not recommended because the prostaglandins are important to the protective coating of the abomasal mucosa.

PRECAUTIONS

N/A

POSSIBLE INTERACTIONS

N/A

ALTERNATE DRUGS

N/A

FOLLOW-UP

PATIENT MONITORING

CBC, anemia, pain

PREVENTION/AVOIDANCE

Gradually introduce dry feed to calves

POSSIBLE COMPLICATIONS

Peritonitis

EXPECTED COURSE AND PROGNOSIS

Recovery for type I and type III ulcers; death from type II if severe hemorrhage; death from type IV

MISCELLANEOUS

PREVENTION

Avoid rapid change from liquid to dry feed in calves, avoid excessive concentrate diets in feedlot or dairy cattle.

ASSOCIATED CONDITIONS

Lymphoma

AGE-RELATED FACTORS

Affects all ages

ZOONOTIC POTENTIAL

N/A

PREGNANCY

N/A

SYNONYMS

N/A

SEE ALSO

Abomasal volvulus or torsion
Duodenal ulcers
Hemorrhagic bowel syndrome
Left displaced abomasum
Lymphoma

ABBREVIATIONS

NSAIDs = nonsteroidal anti-inflammatory drugs

Suggested Reading

Braun, U., Bretscher, R., Gerber, D. 1991. Bleeding abomasal ulcers in dairy cows. *Veterinary Record* 129(13): 279–84.

Jelinski, M. D., Ribble, C. S., Campbell, J. R., Janzen, E. D. 1996. Investigating the relationship between abomasal hairballs and perforating abomasal ulcers in unweaned calves. *Canadian Veterinarian Journal* 37(1): 23–26.

Jelinski, M. D., Ribble, C. S., Chirino-Trejo, M., Clark, E. G., Janzen, E. D. 1995. The relationship between the presence of *Helicobacter pylori*, *Clostridia perfringens* type A, *Campylobacter* spp., or fungi and fatal abomasal ulcers in unweaned beef calves. *Canadian Veterinarian Journal* 36(6):379–82.

Palmer, J. E., Whitlock, R. H. 1983. Bleeding abomasal ulcers in adult dairy cows. *Journal of the American Medical Association* 183(4): 448–51.

Palmer, J. E., Whitlock, R. H. 1984. Perforated abomasal ulcers in adult dairy cows. *Journal of the American Medical Association* 184(2): 171–74.

Radostits, O. M., Gay, C. C., Blood, D. C., Hinchcliff, K. W., eds. 2000. *Veterinary medicine: a textbook of diseases of cattle, sheep, pigs, goats and horses.* 9th ed. London: W. B. Saunders.

Author: James P. Reynolds

ABORTION

BASICS

DEFINITION
Loss of the fetus from 60 days to term. Prior to 60 days is considered embryonic mortality.

PATHOPHYSIOLOGY
• Camelids rely primarily on the corpus luteum for production of progesterone and maintenance of pregnancy for the entire gestation.
• Maintenance of the corpus luteum requires normal pregnancy recognition and establishment of placentation.
• Abortion is caused by any factor that acts directly or indirectly on the corpus luteum to cause luteolysis:
  • Treatment with prostaglandin F2 alpha
  • Inflammatory or febrile affection
  • Endotoxemia
  • Stress such as heat stress, transport
  • Debilitating diseases
• Abortion can be caused by factors that compromise fetal viability or placental integrity:
  • Placentitis
  • Placental insufficiency (endometrial fibrosis, uterine capacity in maiden females, twining)
  • Direct insult to the fetus (mechanical or infectious)
  • Fetal malformation/abnormal pregnancy
  • Hormonal insufficiency or unbalance

SYSTEMS AFFECTED
Reproductive—potentially all systems may be affected depending on the condition.

GENETICS
N/A

INCIDENCE/PREVALENCE
• Pregnancy loss ranges from 2% to 17%.
• Losses of up to 60% may be experienced in some leptospirosis outbreaks.
• Loss of 40–50% has been reported in maiden females under some management systems.

GEOGRAPHIC DISTRIBUTION
Potentially worldwide depending on camelid species and environment

SIGNALMENT
Species
Potentially all camelid species

Breed Predilections
N/A

Mean Age and Range
N/A

Predominant Sex
Female

SIGNS

Historical Findings
• Return to receptivity after confirmation of pregnancy
• Bloody or mucopurulent vaginal discharge
• Protrusion of the placenta or fetus
• Premature development of the mammary gland and lactation

PHYSICAL EXAMINATION FINDINGS
History
A complete history should be taken from each aborting case and include the following:
1. Age of the aborting animal
2. Breeding technique
3. Individual cases vs. outbreak
4. Reproductive history
5. Stage of pregnancy
6. Treatments and vaccination in the last 2 weeks
7. Animal movement in the last month
8. Feeding management
9. Layout of the facilities, proximity to stagnant waters, runoffs from dairy or swine operations
10. Contact with wildlife, feral cats

Clinical Examination of the Dam
Body condition score
Physical examination (TPR)
Demeanor
Transabdominal ultrasound
Vaginal examination
Uterine biopsy may be indicated in some cases.

Serology
Samples should be taken from:
  Fetus (cardiac blood)
  Aborting dam (paired samples) at abortion and 2 to 3 weeks later
  At-risk females in face of an outbreak

Bacteriology
Samples should be taken from:
  Fetus—stomach content, fetal fluids
  Dam—vaginal discharge, uterine swab
  Placenta

Necropsy/Histopathology
• Fetal necropsy
  Measurement of the crown-rump length
  External evaluation of the fetus for developmental abnormalities or lesions
  Internal evaluation of the fetus
  Samples from liver, brain, spleen, kidney, stomach and lungs should be submitted fresh or fixed
• Placenta
  External examination of the chorionic surface for signs suggesting insufficient development or lack of villi
  Examination for signs of placentitis
  Examination for developmental abnormalities or lesions of the umbilical cord

Hormone Assays
In habitual aborters, progesterone determination during pregnancy may be indicative of possible luteal insufficiency. Pregnant females with progesterone levels below 2 ng/ml should be considered suspicious. However, some females may be able to carry to term even if progesterone level is between 1.5 and 2 ng/ml.

CAUSES AND RISK FACTORS

DIAGNOSIS

DIFFERENTIAL DIAGNOSIS
Infectious Causes of Abortion
Brucellosis (*B. meletensis* in alpacas and llamas, *B. abortus* in camels)
Listeriosis
Chlamydiosis
Toxoplasmosis
Leptospirosis
Trypanosomiasis (in camels)
Hemorrhagic disease (*Bacillus cereus*, in camels)

Noninfectious Causes of Abortion
Administration of PGF2-alpha
Trauma: Breeding during pregnancy
Administration of corticosteroids (last trimester of pregnancy particularly, even topical corticosteroids may cause abortion)
Progesterone insufficiency
Hormonal imbalances, adrenal gland dysfunction particularly in fiber-producing animals
Some vaccines (Some vaccines have been associated with abortion)
Nutritional deficiencies
Toxic plants anecdotal; no precise information

CBC/BIOCHEMISTRY/URINALYSIS
May be indicated depending on disease condition

OTHER LABORATORY TESTS
See diagnosis above.

IMAGING
Ultrasound may be a helpful adjunct.

OTHER DIAGNOSTIC PROCEDURES

PATHOLOGIC FINDINGS

TREATMENT
• Abortion due to luteal insufficiency
Requires progesterone supplementation
Anecdotal reports of successful maintenance of pregnancy by administration of progestogens in oil (150 mg to 500 mg every week or every other week until 2 weeks before due date), Norgestomet implants weekly or biweekly
The author's observation is that natural progesterone (50 to 100 mg daily or long acting 500 to 1000 mg every week) is the most helpful in these cases if they can be diagnosed accurately. Fetal viability should be monitored regularly if these treatments are implemented.
• Placental insufficiency
Early diagnosis and termination of twins
Early diagnosis and treatment of uterine infection
Early diagnosis of uterine fibrosis (uterine biopsy) and sexual rest
Adequate breeding management of young females (should be at least 15 months old and 65% of adult weight)

• Drug induced
Avoid use in animals that may be pregnant: Prostaglandin F2 alpha or analogues, ecbolics, corticosteroids, multivalent clostridial vaccines
Cautious use in animals that may be pregnant: Anesthetics, organophosphates

ACTIVITY
N/A

DIET
N/A

CLIENT EDUCATION
N/A

MEDICATIONS
N/A

DRUGS OF CHOICE
N/A

CONTRAINDICATIONS
Appropriate milk and meat withdrawal times must be followed for all compounds administered to food-producing animals.

PREVENTION/AVOIDANCE
• Observe strict hygiene in breeding management and during parturition.
• Setup guideline for biosecurity—quarantine new animals; during movement of animals between shows and ranch, visiting animals for breeding.
• Vaccination for leptospirosis (four times a year in high risk areas)

POSSIBLE COMPLICATIONS
N/A

EXPECTED COURSE AND PROGNOSIS
See specific disease/condition.

MISCELLANEOUS

ASSOCIATED CONDITIONS
N/A

AGE-RELATED FACTORS
N/A

ZOONOTIC POTENTIAL
Brucellosis (*B. meletensis* in alpacas and llamas, *B. abortus* in camels)

BIOSECURITY
Set up guideline for biosecurity—quarantine new animals; during movement of animals between shows and ranch, visiting animals for breeding.

PRODUCTION MANAGEMENT
N/A

SYNONYMS
N/A

SEE ALSO
Brucellosis (*B. meletensis* in alpacas and llamas, *B. abortus* in camels)
Chlamydiosis
Hemorrhagic disease (*Bacillus cereus*, in camels)
Leptospirosis
Listeriosis
Nutritional deficiencies
Toxic plants anecdotal no precise information
Toxoplasmosis
Trypanosomiasis (in camels)

ABBREVIATIONS
• PGF2-alpha = prostaglandin F2 alpha
• TPR = temperature, pulse, and respiration

Suggested Reading
Gidlewski, T., Cheville, N. F., Rhyan, J. C., Miller, L. D., Gilsdorf, M. J. 2000, Jan. Experimental *Brucella abortus* induced abortion in a llama: pathologic effects. *Vet Pathol.* 37(1):77–82.
Gilsdorf, M. J., Thoen, C. O., Temple, R. M., Gidlewski, T., Ewalt, D., Martin, B., Henneger, S. B. 2001, July. Experimental exposure of llamas (*Lama glama*) to *Brucella abortus*: humoral antibody response. *Vet Microbiol. 3.* 81(1):85–91.
Johnson, L. W. 1993. Abortion in llamas. *Veterinary Clinics of North America Food Animal* 10(2): 541–44.
McLaughlin, B. G., Greer, S. C., Singh, S. 1993, Jan. Listerial abortion in a llama. *J Vet Diagn Invest*. 5(1):105–6.
Smith, B. B., Timm, K. I., Reed, P. J., Christensen, M. 2000, Aug. Use of cloprostenol as an abortifacient in the llama (*Lama glama*). *Theriogenology* 54(3): 497–505.
Tibary, A., Anouassi, A. Reproductive disorders in the female camelidae. In: *Theriogenology in Camelidae: anatomy, physiology, pathology and artificial breeding*, pp. 355–57. Actes Edition, Institut Agronomique et Veterinaire Hassan II, Morocco.

Author: Ahmed Tibary

ABORTION: BACTERIAL

BASICS

OVERVIEW
• Many species of bacteria may cause septicemia and/or localized lesions in adult cattle with a subsequent abortion. These agents usually cause sporadic abortions.
• The route of infection is usually hematogenous rather than ascending as interruption of the cervical seal occurs less often in cows than in mares. Often, cows may be predisposed to abortion by these bacteria by some immunosuppressive condition such as bovine virus diarrhea (BVD).
• Two categories of bacterial abortion: (1) ubiquitous environmental organisms: *A. pyogenes, E. coli, Bacillus* spp., *Streptococcus* spp.; (2) abortion secondary to specific disease: *Pasteurella* spp., *Salmonella* spp., *Haemophilus somnus*

SYSTEMS AFFECTED
Reproductive

GENETICS
N/A

INCIDENCE/PREVALENCE
Cattle
• In a 10-year survey, specimens from 8995 bovine abortions and stillbirths were evaluated for bacteria. Bacteria were determined to be the cause of 1299 (14.49%) of the presenting abortion cases.
• The five bacteria most commonly associated with bovine abortion or stillbirth were *Actinomyces pyogenes*, 378 (4.22%); *Bacillus* spp., 321 (3.58%); *Listeria* spp., 121 (1.35%); *Escherichia coli*, 98 (1.09%); and *Leptospira interrogans*, 79 (0.88%). Twelve other genera of bacteria were associated with > or = 10 abortions or stillbirths, and 12 more species were associated with < or = 10 abortions or stillbirths.
• The diagnostic success for determining the cause of abortions may be low (25%–40%).

Sheep
• In a similar 10-year study, 1799 accessions of ovine abortions and stillbirths were evaluated for bacteria. Etiologic diagnoses were made in 786 (44%) of the submitted cases.
• Infectious agents were found responsible in 702 accessions (39%), and noninfectious causes were involved in 84 (5%). No diagnosis was made in 998 accessions (56%).
• Together, *Toxoplasma gondii, Campylobacter* spp., and *Chlamydia psittaci* caused approximately 25% of all abortions and stillbirths examined.

Goats
• In an 8-year study of 217 caprine abortions, infectious agents as the cause were found in 37% of the cases: bacterial agents were identified in 30.5%, viral agents in 2%, fungal agents in 0.5%, and protozoal agents in 4% of the cases submitted.
• The most common causes of abortions were *Chlamydia psittaci* and *Coxiella burnetii* infection, which accounted for 23% of all goat abortions. Mineral deficiencies were observed in 4%, fetal anomalies accounted for 3%, and leukoencephalomalacia of the brain (probable oxygen deprivation) accounted for 3% of the submissions. No diagnosis was made in 112 of the 211 submissions (53%). No lesions were noted in 104 of the submissions (49%).

GEOGRAPHIC DISTRIBUTION
Worldwide depending on environment

Epidemiology
In a study of 58,048 pregnancies from 111 herds, the respective abortion density, proportion of aborted cows, and abortions per confirmed pregnancy were 4.2%, 5.9%, and 10.2%. Heifers had the lowest, and cows of second parity the greatest risk of fetal death. The greatest risk of fetal death was observed in the first, and the lowest in the second trimesters of pregnancy. Respective proportions of aborted cows with and without a previous abortion were 17.5% and 5.9%. Odds of aborting after twinning in multiparous cows in this study were 1.3 times greater than for those having a single calf. Risk of abortion in the autumn and early winter was greater than that in the summer months.

SIGNALMENT
Species
All ruminant species
Breed Predilections
N/A
Mean Age and Range
N/A
Predominant Sex
Female

DIAGNOSIS
See under specific microbial cause below.

TREATMENT
See under specific microbial cause below.

MEDICATIONS
See under specific microbial cause below.

CONTRAINDICATIONS
Appropriate milk and meat withdrawal times must be followed for all compounds administered to food-producing animals.

FOLLOW-UP
See under specific microbial cause below.

MISCELLANEOUS
Common microbial causes of abortion:

Arcanobacteriosis
• *Arcanobacterium pyogenes* (*A. pyogenes*, formerly *Actinomyces* or *Corynebacterium*) is the bacterium most frequently isolated from bovine abortions.
• It is a common inhabitant of the nasal, conjunctival, vaginal, and preputial mucosa of normal animals. The organism may reach the uterus by a hematogenous route, resulting in sporadic abortions.

Diagnosis
Culture of the organism from fetal tissue and placenta

Prevention and Treatment
None

Brucellosis
• Once considered the most important abortion disease of cattle, brucellosis has been nearly eradicated in North America, with the exception being some small local areas.
• *Brucella abortus* in cattle and *B. melitensis* in sheep and goats are gram-negative, intracellular coccobacilli able to survive in phagocytes.

Pathogenesis
The agent is transmitted by oral route. Aborted material contains large numbers of *Brucella* spp. organisms and contaminates the environment. Following ingestion, the organism locates in chorioallantois and results in fetal septicemia and abortion.

Clinical Signs
• Abortion occurring after the fifth month of gestation
• Thick, leathery placentitis, necrosis of the cotyledon
• Cows may have retained placenta and metritis.

Diagnosis
• Culture of the organism from fetal tissue and uterine fluids
• Infected animals identified by serology

Control
• Vaccination of calves between 4 and 12 months of age
• This is a reportable disease in most of North America; herds with positive testing animals are quarantined and an eradication program enforced.

Zoonosis
Human infection occurs from handling infected tissue and ingesting infected milk.

Campylobacteriosis
• Bovine campylobacteriosis is primarily a venereal disease resulting in early embryonic death, repeat breeders, an extended breeding season, a high percentage of open cows at the end of the breeding season, and an extended calving season. It causes occasional abortions, usually in midgestation.
• The primary cause of reproductive wastage is *C. fetus* ssp. *venerealis*. It infects the prepuce of bulls, and is transmitted to cows during breeding.
• Bulls may remain infected for life or recover spontaneously. The organism survives in frozen semen if not properly treated with antibiotics.
• *C. fetus* ssp. *fetus*, an inhabitant of the intestine, will occasionally spread to the uterus via a hematogenous route, resulting in abortion in cows. It is a more common cause of abortion in sheep.
• *C. jejuni* rarely causes bovine abortion but does so in sheep. Abortion due to *Campylobacter* spp. occurs between 4 and 8 months gestation.

Diagnosis
• Culture the organism from the prepuce of infected bulls and the anterior vagina of infected cows.
• Virgin heifer mating test: culture cervicovaginal mucus 18 to 30 days postcoitus.
• Culture the organism from aborted fetal tissues, abomasal contents, and placental fluids.

Treatment
Bulls—preputial lavage with antibiotics

Prevention
• Proper vaccination program
• Proper herd management
• Implement an artificial insemination program

Chlamydia
• *Chlamydia* are obligate, intracellular organisms that multiply in the cytoplasm of eukaryotic cells.

• *Chlamydia psittaci* is associated with reproductive wastage in cattle, sheep, and goats. In cattle it causes sporadic, late-term abortion and stillborn or weak-born calves.

Pathogenesis
• Transmission is by ingestion or inhalation of contaminated material.
• Persistent intestinal colonization results in sporadic placental infection.
• Possible venereal transmission

Diagnosis
• Necrotizing placentitis
• Identification of the organism in fetal liver or placenta
• Paired serum samples show a rising titer

Treatment
Antibiotics (tetracycline)

Zoonosis
Organisms are shed from the reproductive tract of infected animals. Pregnant women are susceptible to infection.

Epizootic Bovine Abortion (Foothills Abortion)
• EBA is limited to the foothills region of central California, coinciding with the range of the tick vector *Ornithodorus coriaceus*, the Pajahuello tick. The cause appears to be a spirochete-like agent.
• Abortion occurs in naïve cows in late gestation.
• The abortion rate may be 30% to 80% in susceptible cows.
• Native cows from enzootic areas do not abort.

Treatment and Control
• Chlortetracycline (2–5 g/day in feed) will reduce the abortion rate.
• Exposure of susceptible animals to the tick before breeding
• Fall calving to avoid exposure of pregnant cows to the tick

Haemophilosis
• The importance of *Haemophilus somnus* as a cause of abortion and infertility is controversial. It is a normal inhabitant of the male and female reproductive tract but may be a minor cause of pregnancy loss.
• Pure culture of *H. somnus*, in the absence of other organisms, may indicate this diagnosis.
• Treatment with antibiotics will reduce infection and a vaccination program may be beneficial.

Leptospirosis
• Leptospires are motile, helical spirochetes. Infection occurs by penetration of the nasal, ocular, genital, or intestinal mucosa. The organism can survive outside the host in moist, warm environments with a neutral to slightly basic pH.

• Direct transmission occurs by contact with infected urine, infected tissue, and fluids following abortion and sexual transmission.
• Indirect transmission occurs from contact with a contaminated environment.

Pathogenesis
• Leptospires localize in the proximal renal tubules and reproductive tract of cows and bulls.
• Organisms are shed in the urine and intermittent leptospiruria may persist for the lifetime of the animal.

Clinical Signs
• May include hemolytic anemia, hemoglobinuria, hepatorenal disease, abortion, and photosensitization.
• Abortion occurs 4 to 12 weeks following infection.
• Abortion due to *L. interrogans* serovar *hardjo* occurs throughout gestation due to serovar *pomona* usually in the last trimester.

Diagnosis
• Isolation of leptospires from fetal tissue such as kidney, urine, thoracic fluid, and aqueous humor. The organism does not survive well in the autolyzed fetus.
• Culture of the organism from cow's urine
• Immunofluorescent staining of fetal kidney
• Serologic testing

Control
• Vaccination programs
• Environmental cleanup, control population of wild animals and rodents that contaminate the environment

Treatment
Antibiotics (oxytetracycline or streptomycin)

Zoonosis
An important zoonotic potential

Listeriosis
• Listeria monocytogenes causes encephalitis, abortion, and neonatal septicemia.
• Infected cows often have fever and anorexia prior to aborting, with postparturient complications including retained placenta, pyometra septicemia, and occasionally death. Central nervous system signs seldom occur simultaneously with abortions.
• Organism ubiquitous in soil, vegetation, water, feces.
• Exposure often from spoiled silage
• More common in winter
• Usually sporadic, occasionally in outbreak form
• Organism has a predilection for fetoplacental tissues resulting in placentitis and fetal septicemia.

Abortion
• Usually last trimester
• Fetus autolyzed when expelled

ABORTION: BACTERIAL

Diagnosis
• Culture of organism from fetal tissues and stomach contents, placenta, uterine fluids
• Culture from feces of infected animals

Control
• Avoid feeding spoiled silage and other contaminated feed
• Aborted tissues source of contamination to herd mates

Zoonosis
Important zoonotic potential, especially in pregnant women

Neosporosis
• Neosporosis is caused by the protozoan *Neosporum caninum.* It has worldwide distribution. Dogs are identified as the intermediate host.
• Abortion usually occurs during the second trimester but may occur throughout gestation.

Clinical Signs
• Infected cows show no clinical signs.
• Infected calves may be born prematurely and exhibit neurological signs.

Pathophysiology
• The route of infection is vertical transmission with congenital infection occurring in 80% of seropositive cows.
• Seropositive cows are more likely to abort than seronegative herd mates.
• Repeat abortions occur following recrudescence of latent infections or following a new infection.

Diagnosis
• Observation of characteristic histological lesions or identification of the parasite in fetal tissue, especially brain, heart, liver, and skeletal muscle
• Fetal serology if abortion occurs after 5 months gestation
• Serologic testing of cows

Control and Prevention
• Prevention of postnatal transmission, possibly feed contamination by feces of infected dogs
• Removal of seropositive cows from the herd
• Embryo transfer to break the vertical transmission cycle
• A vaccine is available.

Trichomoniasis
• Trichomoniasis is a venereal disease caused by the protozoan *Tritrichomonas foetus.* Infection is demonstrated as early embryonic death, repeat breeders, an extended breeding season, a high percentage of open cows at the end of the breeding season, and an extended calving season.
• It causes occasional abortions, usually in the first half of gestation.

Diagnosis
• Bulls—identification and culture of the organism from preputial smegma
• Cows—identification and culture of the organism from cervicovaginal mucus and uterine contents in pyometra cases
• Virgin heifer mating test—culture cervicovaginal mucus 12 to 19 days postcoitus
• Culture the organism from aborted fetal tissues and fluids.

Prevention
• Proper vaccination program
• Proper herd management
• Implementation of artificial insemination program

Ureaplasmosis
• *Ureaplasma diversum* is a normal inhabitant of the reproductive tract of cows and bulls. In clinical conditions, it may result in granular vulvitis in cows.
• If artificial insemination does not include a guarded, double rod technique, the organism may be carried into the uterus, resulting in early embryonic death or abortion. Abortion is usually sporadic.

Diagnosis
Culture of the organism from fetal tissue

Treatment and Control
• Proper insemination technique
• Postbreeding infusion of tetracycline

ASSOCIATED CONDITIONS
N/A

AGE-RELATED FACTORS
Heifers had the lowest risk, and cows of second parity the greatest risk of fetal death.

ZOONOTIC POTENTIAL
Brucellosis, chlamydiosis, listeriosis, leptospirosis, and *Coxiella burnetii* are all potential zoonotic agents.

PREGNANCY
The greatest risk of fetal death was observed in the first, and the lowest in the second trimesters of pregnancy.

RUMINANT SPECIES AFFECTED
Potentially, all ruminant species are affected.

BIOSECURITY
N/A

PRODUCTION MANAGEMENT
N/A

SYNONYMS
N/A

SEE ALSO
• Diagnostic testing
• Reproductive pharmacology
• Serology
• Specific abortive disease agents

ABBREVIATIONS
• BVD = bovine viral diarrhea
• EBA = epizootic bovine abortion

Suggested Reading
Alexander, A. V., Walker, R. L., Johnson, B. J., Charlton, B. R., Woods, L. W. 1992, Mar 1. Bovine abortions attributable to *Listeria ivanovii*: four cases (1988–1990). *J Am Vet Med Assoc.* 200(5):711–14.
Barr, B. C., Anderson, M. L. 1993, Jul. Infectious diseases causing bovine abortion and fetal loss. *Vet Clin North Am Food Anim Pract.* 9(2):343–68.
Dubey, J. P., Lindsay, D. S. 1993, Dec. Neosporosis. *Parasitol Today* 9(12):452–58.
Ellis, W. A. 1994, Nov. Leptospirosis as a cause of reproductive failure. *Vet Clin North Am Food Anim Pract.* 10(3):463–78.
Hassig, M., Lubsen, J. 1998, Sep. Relationship between abortions and seroprevalences to selected infectious agents in dairy cows. *Zentralbl Veterinarmed B.* 45(7):435–41.
Kirkbride, C. A. 1993, Jul. Diagnoses in 1,784 ovine abortions and stillbirths. *J Vet Diagn Invest.* 5(3):398–402.
Kirkbride, C. A. 1993. Bacterial agents detected in a 10 year study of bovine abortions and stillbirths. *J. Vet Diagn Invest.* 5:63–68.
Mickelsen, W. D., Evermann, J. F. 1994, Mar. In utero infections responsible for abortion, stillbirth, and birth of weak calves in beef cows. *Vet Clin North Am Food Anim Pract.* 10(1):1–14.
Moeller, R. B., Jr. 2001, May. Causes of caprine abortion: diagnostic assessment of 211 cases (1991–1998). *J Vet Diagn Invest.* 13(3):265–70.
Seguin, B., Troedsson, M. 2002. Diseases of the reproductive system. In: *Large animal internal medicine*, ed. B. P. Smith. St. Louis: Mosby.
Smyth, J. A., Fitzpatrick, D. A., Ellis, W. A. 1999, Nov 6. Stillbirth/perinatal weak calf syndrome: a study of calves infected with Leptospira. *Vet Rec.* 145(19):539–42.

Authors: Walter Johnson and Alex Estrada

BASICS

DEFINITION
Loss of a fetus

Further Definitions
• Calf—cervid less than 1 year of age
• Hind—adult female cervid
• Stag—adult male cervid

PATHOPHYSIOLOGY
• The fetus may die due to a genetic or congenital abnormality.
• Infectious organisms may invade the fetus and lead to fetal death.
• Abnormalities or infections of the placenta or uterus may lead to placental separation, fetal death, and reabsorption or expulsion.
• Trauma, toxins, infections, malnutrition, metabolic disease, drugs, or other stress incurred by the hind may lead to fetal stress and abortion. Abnormalities of the hind's reproductive or endocrine system may lead to abortion.

SYSTEMS AFFECTED
Reproductive; other systems may be involved depending upon the underlying etiology of the abortion. The clinician may need to monitor other body systems for complications secondary to abortion.

GENETICS
N/A

INCIDENCE/PREVALANCE
The incidence of embryonic mortality in farmed deer is relatively low.
Insufficient data available for other species.

GEOGRAPHIC DISTRIBUTION
N/A

SIGNALMENT
Species
Depends upon underlying cause. Some cervids are more susceptible to infectious disease than others. When red deer hinds (*Cervus elaphus*) are crossbred with wapiti stags, there is a greater risk for dystocia and subsequent fetal death.

Mean Age and Range
First calving wapiti (*Cervus elaphus*) are more likely to deliver nonviable calves than are adults. Also, 2-year-old elk, fallow (*Dama dama*), and red deer have lower calving rates than mature animals.

Predominant Sex
Female only

SIGNS

HISTORICAL FINDINGS
• May be none evident, especially if the fetus is reabsorbed early in gestation
• Estrus detected on a hind previously diagnosed as pregnant
• Failure to produce an offspring (missed due date)
• Restlessness, solitude-seeking behavior, pacing, abdominal straining, and other signs of imminent parturition
• Discovery of expulsed fetus

PHYSICAL EXAMINATION FINDINGS
• May be none—fetal resorption early in gestation may have no visible signs. Hinds that were previously diagnosed as pregnant will later be found to be nonpregnant. If rectal palpation is done (in wapiti), the previously pregnant horn will cease to be enlarged. There will no longer be a fetal membrane slip.
• Late-term abortions in cervids living in large enclosures or parks may occur unobserved as the female usually eats the placenta and the dead fetus is consumed by predators.
• When clinical signs are present, they include:
  • Bloody or purulent vaginal discharge
  • Visibly expulsed fetus and/or placenta
  • Premature udder development and dripping
  • If abortion is due to systemic disease, may see other nonspecific signs of illness such as depression, dehydration, pyrexia, anorexia, and weight loss.
  • Brucellosis-induced abortion in female reindeer (*Rangifer tarandus*) is characterized by a retained placenta and metritis.

CAUSES

Degenerative
Anatomic/Congenital
Congenital abnormalities may lead to fetal death.

Metabolic
Febrile or severely stressed animals may abort.

Nutritional
• Inadequate nutrition—may cause a fetus to die or be born underweight and nonviable
• Iodine deficiency—may be caused by insufficient dietary intake, or be secondary to excessive calcium in the diet, overingestion of toxic plants such as *Brassica* spp., gross bacterial contamination of the feed, continuous intake of feeds containing cyanogenetic glucosides (i.e., white clover), or due to ingestion of canola (rapeseed and canola meal). An iodine deficiency can lead to goiter, prolonged gestation, and an increased incidence of stillbirth.

Infectious
Bacterial
• *Brucella abortus*
• *Brucella suis* type 4—most common cause of abortion in reindeer and caribou
• Leptospirosis—serovars found in North American cervids include *L. pomona*, *L. grippotyphosa*, *L. canicola*, and *L. pyogenes*. *Leptospira pomona* is believed to cause abortions in free-ranging white-tailed deer (*Odocoileus virginianus*) and red deer.
• Experimental infections in white-tailed deer have produced abortions, anorexia, fever, and death.
• Listeriosis—the septicemic form causes placentitis and endometritis leading to abortion in late-term pregnancy as well as the birth of weak, full-term young.

Fungal
Incidence of fungal infections in farmed wapiti and red deer is rare. However, fungal infections can cause abortions in other ruminant species. Therefore, it should not be excluded.

Parasitic
Toxoplasmosis—wapiti and red deer appear to be less susceptible to toxoplasmosis than other cervidae species.

Viral
• Bluetongue (orbivirus)—abortion and congenital deformities have been seen in white-tailed deer, but bluetongue has not been reported to cause serious clinical disease in wapiti or red deer.
• Bovine viral diarrhea virus—BVDV has not been reported as a clinical entity in wapiti or red deer, but virus has been isolated from red, fallow, and roe deer. Serological evidence of infection has been demonstrated in mule (*Odocoileus hemionus*), white-tailed deer, fallow deer, moose (*Alces alces*), and a Chinese water deer (*Hydroptes inermis*). Almost all of the reported BVD-related cervid cases involve a free-ranging animal, which makes it difficult to find aborted fetuses. Experimentally, BVDV isolated from a dead deer did cause stillborn fawns and mummified fetuses when injected into pregnant penned deer.

ABORTION: FARMED CERVIDAE

Traumatic
Congenital abnormalities, fetal oversize, or abnormalities of presentation at time of parturition may lead to dystocia and subsequent fetal death.

Toxic
Locoweed causes abortions in sheep and cattle and may be a problem for cervidae as well.

Drugs
Prostaglandin F2 alpha has been used to induce abortion in wapiti but is probably ineffective if given less than 10 days after breeding. Prostaglandins also can cause luteolysis in reindeer.

RISK FACTORS
Febrile or severely stressed animals may abort. The most common stressors for cervidae are severe weather, inadequate nutrition, recent capture or transport, and concurrent disease. It would also be wise to avoid the use of products that are known abortifacients in other ruminant species.

 DIAGNOSIS

DIFFERENTIAL DIAGNOSIS
• Other causes of vaginal discharge
  • Normal term parturition
  • Vaginitis
  • Pyometra
  • Metritis
  • Uterine trauma or hemorrhage
  • Uterine or vaginal neoplasia
• Other reasons for failure to deliver on due date
  • Infertility (animal never became pregnant)
  • Incorrect due date
  • Other causes of abdominal straining/discomfort such as colic

CBC/BIOCHEMISTRY/URINALYSIS
May be normal. It may also indicate systemic disease.

OTHER LABORATORY TESTS

Maternal Pregnancy Specific Protein B (PSPB)
Bovine pregnancy specific protein B antibody cross reacts with caribou, red, fallow, and white-tailed deer PSPB. Hence, the PSPB radioimmunoassay developed for domestic cattle can be used for pregnancy monitoring in some cervids. It is as effective as ultrasound in diagnosing the pregnant hind. In red and fallow deer, PSPB is present by 33 days after conception. It is nondetectable in open hinds.

Serum Progesterone Levels (P4)
Serum progesterone concentrations rise during pregnancy, but they also rise during the estrus cycle. Serial measurements can be done during the breeding season to determine if an animal is pregnant or in estrus. Otherwise, one can wait until the breeding season is over. A decrease in P4 levels in a previously pregnant animal suggests early embryonic loss.

Fecal Progesterone Levels
Reserved for use in free-ranging populations. This can be used for detecting pregnancy in elk during mid to late gestation. Several factors may influence fecal P4 excretion and therefore make this test less reliable.

Urinary PDG (pregnanediol-3alpha-glucuronide)
The simultaneous evaluation of urinary PdG and urinary estrogen conjugates was effective for estimating and tracking pregnancy stage in Pere David's deer. PdG excretions decreased to nadir concentrations between 1 and 2 weeks before abortion in the two hinds that aborted.

Paired Serology
To test for infectious disease

Testing Procedures for Specific Diseases
Bacterial
• Brucellosis—There are five serological tests available: complement fixation, tube agglutination, rapid card, buffered plate, and ELISA.
  • Leptospirosis
  • Paired serology
  • Dark field microscopy of the urine or aqueous humor on dead deer
  • ELISA test may become available.
• Listeriosis—Serological tests, but high number of false negatives occur

Viral
• Bluetongue serological tests include ELISA, immunodiffusion, radioimmunoassay, hemolysis-in-gel assay, and a genetic probe for detection of bluetongue viral DNA in fluids and tissues.
• Bovine viral diarrhea virus
  • Virus isolation from blood or nasal secretions
  • IFA or immunohistochemistry
  • ELISA
  • Paired serology (VN)

Protozoal: Toxoplasmosis
• Sabin-Feldman dye test (DT)
• Hemagglutination test (HA), may not be reliable for red deer.
• Direct agglutination

IMAGING

Transrectal Ultrasound
• Most practical method for diagnosing pregnancy in farmed deer
• Restraint in a crush is preferable, but manual restraint may work for some animals and handlers. In wapiti and red deer, the best time for pregnancy diagnosis is between 35 and 60 days gestation. This technique can be used as early as 33–35 days gestation in fallow deer.

Transabdominal Ultrasonography
To evaluate the fetus later in gestation

Radiographs
May be more practical for the smaller cervidae species

DIAGNOSTIC PROCEDURES
Bacterial culture and histological examination of the fetal, placental fluid and placental tissues. It may be difficult to obtain the placenta as the female usually ingests it. Also, secondary bacterial overgrowth is likely to occur prior to sample collection.

Bacterial
• Brucellosis
  • Bacterial isolation of *Brucella* spp. provides the only definitive diagnosis of this disease (caution: zoonotic risk, so wear gloves).
  • If index of suspicion is high, owner may elect to sacrifice the mother for culture of her major body lymph nodes and organs.
• Listeriosis—isolation of *Listeria* spp.
• Leptospirosis—can be isolated from urine or kidney cultures. If the hind has any swollen joints, these should also be cultured.

Fungal
Specific diagnosis may require culture of the organism.

PATHOLOGIC FINDINGS
Depends upon etiology

Bacterial
• Brucellosis—necrotizing placentitis characterized by a thickened placenta covered with a purulent exudate
• Listeriosis—in animals that abort, placentitis and endometritis occur.

Fungal
Gross pathology reveals discreet granulomas and raised circular areas on affected organs. Histopathology shows pyogenic inflammatory reaction, fungal hyphae.

TREATMENT

APPROPRIATE HEALTH CARE
• Depends upon underlying etiology—see specific disease chapter.
• None may be warranted
• Make appropriate changes in husbandry if condition was related to poor handling, sanitation, or malnutrition.

NURSING CARE
Supportive

ACTIVITY
N/A

DIET
If abortion was due to listeriosis or mycotoxins, make appropriate changes to silage feeding practices.

CLIENT EDUCATION
See Biosecurity and Production Management below.

SURGICAL CONSIDERATIONS
Reserved for dystocias when all else has failed

MEDICATIONS

DRUGS OF CHOICE
• Dependent upon underlying cause
• Antibiotics may be warranted for specific bacterial diseases, metritis, toxemia, and so on.

CONTRAINDICATIONS
Appropriate milk and meat withdrawal times must be followed for all compounds administered to food-producing animals.

PRECAUTIONS
N/A

POSSIBLE INTERACTIONS
N/A

ALTERNATIVE DRUGS
N/A

FOLLOW-UP

PATIENT MONITORING
Depends upon cause

PREVENTION/AVOIDANCE
Establish a good nutritional and preventative health program.

Brucellosis
A test and removal program is ideal for intensively managed deer farms. It may not be possible in game or wildlife parks to round up all animals in the herd at one time for testing. In the United States, vaccination is used in cattle under strict regulations, but it is not used in deer. There is a vaccination program in place for reindeer in Alaska. The program uses a killed, homologous vaccine in adjuvant, which provides protection for up to 4 years. Unfortunately, current testing methods cannot differentiate between vaccinated and infected animals. As such, special permission from the state veterinarian is required. A newer vaccine, strain RB51, is in use for bovidae. This vaccine does not cross-react with the test. Its efficacy in cervid species has yet to be determined. So far, experimental studies have shown that this vaccine failed to prevent abortion in elk. The best way to prevent brucellosis is to allow the introduction of only nonvaccinated, blood-test negative animals from known brucellosis-free herds.

Leptospirosis
Vaccine is available although its usage in cervidae species is extralabel in the United States.

Bluetongue
Use parasite control to decrease the number of arthropod vectors (e.g., *Culicoides* spp. or gnats). Vaccine is available for use in deer in affected areas, but its use would be extralabel in the United States. In endemic areas, young may obtain up to 3 months' protection from colostral antibodies.

BVDV
Isolation of virus from nasal swabs is evidence that deer via direct contact can transmit BVDV. Therefore, fencing of adequate height and double fencing are recommended in order to prevent direct contact and disease transmission between captive and wild cervids.

POSSIBLE COMPLICATIONS
Decreased fertility

EXPECTED COURSE AND PROGNOSIS
Dependent upon underlying cause

MISCELLANEOUS

ASSOCIATED CONDITIONS
Dystocia, reproduction management

AGE-RELATED FACTORS
In farmed deer herds—young females that are underweight for their age should not be subjected to the risks of pregnancy.

ZOONOTIC POTENTIAL
Brucellosis, toxoplasmosis, leptospirosis, listeriosis

PREGNANCY
N/A

ABORTION: FARMED CERVIDAE

RUMINANT SPECIES AFFECTED

Cervidae: wapiti (*Cervus elaphus*), fallow deer (*Dama dama*)

BIOSECURITY

• Newly acquired animals should always be quarantined for a minimum of 30 days before allowing entry into the herd.
• Preshipment testing for infectious diseases is advisable. Avoid purchasing animals from regions where brucellosis is endemic.
• Double fences may be warranted to prevent direct contact with wildlife species.
• Keeping cats and wild animals out of feed storage areas and animal enclosures will help lower the risks of infection with toxoplasmosis and leptospirosis. See specific chapters for additional measures.

PRODUCTION MANAGEMENT

• In farmed animals, it is important to monitor age, weight, and previous reproductive performance of hinds within a herd in order to maximize reproductive performance and overall production capability.
• Good nutrition management is mandatory. Young females that are small for their age should not be bred. If more than one animal aborts, testing of the herd for infectious diseases is advisable. Stress reduction also plays a major role in lowering the risk for disease and abortion.
• Habituating animals to gates and chutes makes handling during physical exams and other routine procedures less stressful on the animals. Avoid shipping animals during insect/vector season. Last, gross and histopathologic examination should always be performed on all dead fetuses and animals whenever possible.

SYNONYMS

N/A

SEE ALSO

• Brucellosis
• Dystocia

ABBREVIATIONS

• BVDV = bovine viral diarrhea virus
• DT = Sabin-Feldman dye test
• ELISA = enzyme-linked immunosorbent assay
• HA = hemagglutination test
• IFA = immunofluorescence antibody
• PDG = pregnanediol-3alpha-glucuronide
• PSPB = pregnancy specific protein B
• VN = virus neutralization test

Suggested Reading

Bingham, C. M., Wilson, P. R., Dives, A. S. 1990. Real time ultrasonography for pregnancy diagnosis and estimation of fetal age in farmed red deer. *Vet Rec.* 126(5): 102–6.

Cook, R. C., Garrot, R. A., Irwin, L. L., Monfort, S. L. 2002. Effects of diet and body condition on fecal progestagens (P4) for detecting pregnancy in elk (*Cervus elaphus*) during mid to late gestation. *J Wildl Dis.* 38(3): 558–65.

Dieterich, R. A., Morton, J. K. 1990. *Reindeer health aide manual*. 2nd ed. Agricultural and Forestry Experiment Station and Cooperative Extension Service, University of Alaska Fairbanks and U.S. Dept. of Agriculture Cooperating. AFES Misc. Pub. 90-4 CES 100H-00046.

Kreeger, T. J., Cook, W. E., Edwards, W. H., Elzer, P. H., Olsen, S. C. 2002. *Brucella abortus* strain RB51 vaccination in elk. II. Failure of high dosage to prevent abortion. *J Wildl Dis.* 38(1): 27–31.

Rowell, J. E., Russell, D. E., White, R. G., Sasser, R. G. 1998. Estrous synchronization and early pregnancy. *Rangifer* 2000;Special Issue (12).

Van Campen, H., Ridpath, J., Williams, E., Cavender, J., Edwards, J., Smith, S., Sawyer, H. 2001. Isolation of bovine viral diarrhea virus from a free-ranging mule deer in Wyoming. *J Wildl Dis.* 37(2): 306–11.

Author: Melissa Weisman

BASICS

DEFINITION
• Fetal loss, fetal wastage: loss of conceptus at anytime during pregnancy
• Most commonly observed in the last 2 months of pregnancy

PATHOPHYSIOLOGY
• Abortion results from
  • Fetal death from invasion by microorganisms
  • Fetal expulsion subsequent to placental disease, insufficiency
  • Fetal expulsion following maternal compromise
  • Premature parturition
  • Fetal reabsorption, maceration, autolysis
• Can be caused by a variety of infectious and noninfectious agents.
• Infectious causes of abortion are the most economically significant.
• Most common infectious causes are *Chlamydia psittaci, Toxoplasma gondii,* and *Campylobacter* spp., which may represent up to one-third of all cases of abortions.
• Chlamydiosis is more common in goats.
• Campylobacter is less common in goats in North America.

SYSTEMS AFFECTED
• Reproductive
• Others depending on the etiology

GENETICS
Angora goat may be a habitual aborter.

INCIDENCE/PREVALENCE
• Should be less than 5% on a flock basis (less than 2% ideal)
• Abortion storms may occur in the case of specific infectious diseases.

GEOGRAPHIC DISTRIBUTION
• Worldwide
• Some diseases processes may be regional (presence of vector).

SIGNALMENT
Nonspecific

SIGNS
• Early pregnancy loss may not be detected.
• Clinical signs in the aborting female vary depending on the cause.
• Complications depend on cause (deterioration of health, retained placenta, metritis).

Clinical Signs in Dam
• Bluetongue: febrile, swollen tongue, ear, or face; lameness; ulcerative lesions on mouth
• Akabane virus disease
• Campylobacteriosis: aborting goats may show diarrhea.

• Chlamydia: pneumonia, keratoconjunctivitis, epididymitis, and polyarthritis; anorexia, fever, bloody vaginal discharge 2 to 3 days before abortion
• Brucellosis: *B. melitensis* in goats causes abortion, weak kids, and mastitis. *B. ovis* in sheep is rarely a cause of abortion but is responsible for poor reproductive performance and in the ram contagious epididymitis.
• Aborting goats may experience fever, depression, weight loss, mastitis, and lameness.
• Leptospirosis: anorexia, fever, marked jaundice, hemoglobinuria, anemia, neurological signs, abortion, occasionally may be fatal
• Salmonellosis: abortion, retained placenta, metritis, and various systemic signs (fever, depression, diarrhea). Mostly in overcrowded flocks
• Toxoplasmosis: generally none, immunocompromised females may present a neurologic form of the disease.
• Leptospirosis: septicemia, fever, decreased appetite, reduced milk production, abortion, and meningoencephalitis
• Mycoplasmosis (goats): mastitis, arthritis, keratoconjunctivitis, vulvovaginitis, and abortion in the last third of pregnancy

HISTORICAL FINDINGS
• Introduction of new animals
• Vaginal discharges
• Premature udder development
• Presence of fetuses
• Premature/stillbirths
• Increased congenital abnormalities

PHYSICAL EXAMINATION FINDINGS
• Vaginal edema
• Vaginal discharge
• Anorexia
• Other signs in flock

CAUSES
• Viruses
• Bacteria
• Rickettsia
• Protozoa
• Fungi
• Toxins

RISK FACTORS
• Lack of biosecurity measures
• Vector population
• Overcrowding

 DIAGNOSIS

Brucellosis
• Isolation: best samples are vaginal discharges and milk, stomach contents.
• Indirect diagnosis: complement fixation, agglutination and precipitation tests may help identify carrier animals.

Chlamydiosis (Enzootic Abortion)
• *C. psittaci*, gram-negative intracellular organism
• Abortion and other signs
• Aborting females become immune
• Females infected after 100 days of pregnancy may not abort.
• Diagnosis
  • Generalized placentitis, abortion in the last month of pregnancy, high incidence in newly infected flocks
  • Demonstrations of characteristic inclusion bodies on smear from cotyledons, vaginal discharge, fetal stomach content
  • Culture from vaginal discharge, placenta, and fetal tissue
  • Serology: paired samples from dam and fetal serum
  • ELISA or Indirect Inclusion Fluorescence Antibody tests (IIFA)

Toxoplasmosis
• Goats more susceptible than sheep
• Diagnosis
  • Cotyledons are gray-white to yellow and present small, 1–3 mm focal area of necrosis and calcification. Intercotyledonary areas are generally normal. Macroscopic lesions: 2–3 mm necrotic foci on cotyledons, intercotyledonary allantochorion are generally normal. Fetus may be mummified or decomposed; chalky white necrotic brain lesions
  • Samples: placenta, fetal brain, fetal fluids, maternal blood, precolostral blood
  • Isolation from cotyledons, brain and fetal fluids, tissues (shipped packed in ice)
  • Histopathology: fixed cotyledons, fetal brain
  • Serology: presence of antibodies in fetal fluids or precolostral serum is the preferred diagnostic technique and indicate transplacental infection.

Q Fever (Coxiella burnetti)
• Placentitis, placental necrosis, thickening of the intercotyledonary areas, abortion, and stillbirth
• Isolation: placenta, vaginal discharges, fetal stomach content
• Demonstration of organism by Ziehl-Neelsen staining
• Complement fixation: need samples from several animals
• Fluorescent antibody test may be used to identify organism in frozen section of placenta.

Campylobacteriosis
• *Campylobacter jejuni* and *C. fetus*; most prevalent in sheep, rare in goats
• Gram-negative microaerophilic rods

Symptoms
• Abortion, stillbirths, and weak lambs, retained fetal membranes
• Placentitis, placental edema

ABORTION: SHEEP AND GOATS

- Fetus: hepatomegaly, hemorrhagic liver, necrotic foci of 1–3 cm
- Fetal subcutaneous edema, serosanguineous fluid in abdominal and thoracic cavity
- Fetus: bronchopneumonia

Isolation and Identification
- Samples: placenta and vaginal discharges, frozen fetal stomach content (-20°C)
- Transport medium required
- Isolation from placenta, vaginal discharge, fetal stomach contents
- Histopathology: necrotic areas of the chorionic villi, arterioles, and thrombosis of the hilus of the placentomes

Salmonellosis
- *Salmonella abortus-ovis, S. typhinurium, S. Dublin, S. Montevideo, S. arizonae*
- Direct diagnosis: culture from fetal tissues taken aseptically may be preserved at –20°C; placenta and uterine discharges
- Indirect diagnosis: seroagglutination

Listeriosis (Listeria monocytogenes)
- Gram-positive, non-acid-fast facultative microaerophilic organisms. *L. monocytogenes* affects sheep and goats; *L. ivanovii* affects sheep only.
- Direct diagnosis: placenta, fetal liver and spleen, fetal stomach content, vaginal discharge within 48 hours of abortion. Samples may be refrigerated if not cultured immediately.
- Indirect diagnosis: histopathology on placenta, fetal liver and spleen microabscesses (white pinpoint spots), and necrosis and macrophages and neutrophils infiltration. Gram stain reveals numerous gram-positive rods.

Leptospirosis
- Sheep and goats are generally less susceptible to leptospirosis than other species. Goats are more susceptible than sheep.
- Sheep: mostly *L. hardjo* sometime *L. pomona, L. ballum,* and *L. bratislava*; late-term abortion, stillbirths, and ill-thrift lambs
- Affected flocks are mostly reared indoors
- Agalactia
- Goat: *L. icterohaemorrhagiae, L. pomona, L. grippotyphosa*
- Clinical signs in case of acute infection
- Direct diagnosis: fetal tissue, fetal fluids, and placenta
  - Isolation is difficult
  - Demonstration by dark-filed microscopy, immunofluorescence and silver stain
- Indirect diagnosis: serology—macroscopic agglutination test

Border Disease
- Goats are fairly resistant.
- Virus isolation (buffy coat) and antigen demonstration—heparinized blood from dam or hairy shaker lambs, fetal tissue (thyroid, kidney, spleen, cerebellum, placenta), hairy shakers (thyroid, kidney, spleen, cerebellum, intestine, lymph nodes)

- Histopathology: cerebellum, spinal cord
- Serology: flood from dam and hairy shakers
- Clinical: small cotyledon with focal necrosis, hairy shakers,

Bluetongue
Viral isolation: blood, semen, fetal brain and spleen unlikely cause of abortion in goats

Akabane Disease
Fetal malformation, positive antibody titer in live-born and aborted fetuses

Cache Valley Virus
- Congenital abnormalities
- Detection of antibodies in fetal fluids or precolostral serum

Mycoplasmosis
- Mycoplasma abortions (*M. mycoides, M. agalactia*) are significant in goats.
- Diagnosis: culture and serotyping of the isolate from milk, fetal fluids, and placenta

Noninfectious Causes of Abortion
- Genetic (goat) may be a habitual aborter
  - Angora goats with fine mohair
  - Abortion at 100 days
  - Adrenal dysfunction
- Energy protein deficiency
- Phenothiazine and levamisole in the last 2 months of pregnancy; corticosteroids in late gestation
- Prostaglandin F 2 alpha or analogues (goats)
- Plants that accumulate nitrates

CBC/BIOCHEMISTRY/URINALYSIS
May be indicated if aborting dam is clinically sick

OTHER LABORATORY TESTS
- Sampling is critical for the proper diagnosis of abortion.
- Placenta
  - Ideal for the isolation of most abortion-causing agents
  - Ideal for identification using specific staining techniques on histological section or impression smears
  - For isolation: need five or six cotyledons and section of intercotyledonary spaces both from healthy appearing and diseased areas
  - If needed, this tissue may be rinsed with sterile saline.
  - For isolation: need a transport medium (i.e.,viruses; Campylobacter: FBP/glycerol; Leptospirosis 100 ml extender with 1% BSA)
  - For histopathology: 0.5 cm section of tissue in 10% formalin 1:10
  - For bacteriology: impression smears
- Vaginal discharges
  - Collect in sterile manner
  - Vaginal/uterine swabs
  - Use of specific transport medium is preferred if a specific germ is suspected.
- Fetal tissues
  - Tissue samples from all fetal organs (spleen, liver, kidneys, brain, lymph nodes, spinal cord) should be taken in an aseptic manner immediately after abortion or death.

- Handle in the same manner as for placenta.
- Fetal fluids
  - If fetus is not autolyzed
  - Stomach content
  - Peritoneal/thoracic fluids
  - Blood from the cardiac cavity
- Milk—Samples of milk are taken from both glands using aseptic techniques (clean the mammary gland, disinfect teats, and eliminate the first two jets).
- Blood
  - For isolation: immediately after/during abortion
  - For serology: paired samples immediately after abortion and 2 to 3 weeks later
  - In case of an outbreak, blood should be collected from aborting females as well as from lambs/kids before colostral intake.

IMAGING
N/A

OTHER DIAGNOSTIC PROCEDURES
N/A

PATHOLOGIC FINDINGS
Abortion Associated with Deformities
- Bluetongue: hydranencephaly
- Akabane disease: arthrogryposis (dystocia), hydranencephaly, and mummification
- Cache Valley: arthrogryposis, brachygnathia, hydranencephaly, microencephaly, spinal cord hypoplasia, and mummification
- Border disease: cerebellar hypoplasia, hydranencephaly, brachygnathia, arthrogryposis. dark pigmentation of the fleece, hairy shaker
- Toxic plants: lupine, skunk cabbage, locoweed, and Sudan grass
- Iodine, copper, manganese deficiency

Assessing Disease Risk
- Toxoplasmosis—cat population
- Leptospirosis
  - Rodent population
  - Humid hot environment
  - Proximity to dairy and swine operation
- Salmonellosis
  - Source of infection: bird, cattle, wildlife
  - Predisposing condition: overcrowding, shipping, climatic changes
- Chlamydia
  - Infection transmission: placenta, fetal fluids
  - Pigeon/sparrows are reservoirs, ticks or insects may play a role.
  - Vaginal discharge in goat up to 2 weeks before abortion
  - Reservoir: young maiden females
- Listeria
  - Organisms grow in poorly fermented silage.
  - Can survive in soil and feces for extended period of time
- Bluetongue: Culicoides gnat (cattle may be a reservoir)

• Akabane virus diseases: gnats and mosquito population
• Cache Valley virus: mosquitoes

Test Accuracy
• Diagnosis of a specific cause of abortion can be very challenging.
• Even if all samples are submitted adequately, the exact etiology will remain undiagnosed in half of the sporadic cases.
• Diagnosis of the cause of an outbreak is more rewarding.
• Most labs will run an abortion panel based on serology, histopathology, and culture tests described above.

TREATMENT

Treatment potential
• Campylobacter: penicillin or streptomycin or tetracycline in feed
• Chlamydia: tetracycline, tylosin
• Leptospirosis: tetracycline
• Toxoplasmosis: decoquinate, monensin
• Leptospirosis: tetracycline
• Mycoplasma: tetracycline and tylosin

CLIENT EDUCATION
• Establish good preventative program
  • Biosecurity measures
  • Vaccination
  • Good nutritional programs
• Consider every case of abortion as a possible outbreak.
• Act quickly and help collect appropriate samples to be examined by a veterinarian.

MEDICATIONS

Daily tetracycline treatment of the flock may help with some of the abortion-causing diseases.

DRUGS OF CHOICE
N/A

CONTRAINDICATIONS
N/A

PRECAUTIONS
Appropriate milk and meat withdrawal times must be followed for all compounds administered.

POSSIBLE INTERACTIONS
N/A

ALTERNATIVE DRUGS
N/A

FOLLOW-UP

PREVENTION/AVOIDANCE
• General prevention program for abortion
  • Quarantine new animals (4–6 weeks)
  • Nutrition
  • Vaccination: chlamydia, campylobacter (2 months and last month of pregnancy)
  • Feed chlortetracycline (200–400 mg/head/day), monensin (15 mg/head/day) during gestation
  • Keep feed, pasture, and water source free from contamination by runoff particularly from cattle and hogs.
  • Control rat, bird, cat population.
  • Act quickly on any abortion and assume it is an outbreak; submit complete samples.
  • Separate prepartum from postpartum females.
  • Keep good lambing/kidding facilities.
• Reduce stress due to poor nutrition, unsanitary environment, crowded conditions.

Vaccination
• Bluetongue: questionable
• Akabane virus: effective
• Cache Valley: effective
• Campylobacter: helpful
• Chlamydia: helpful
• Q fever: autogenous vaccines in conjunction with chlortetracycline may help.
• B. ovis: poor efficacy of killed vaccine
• B. melentensis: live attenuated good when permitted
• Salmonellosis: autogenous vaccine may be helpful
• Toxoplasmosis: may be helpful

POSSIBLE COMPLICATIONS
Dystocia, retained placenta, metritis, mastitis, male infertility (brucellosis, chlamydiosis), female infertility

EXPECTED COURSE AND PROGNOSIS
Depends on cause

MISCELLANEOUS

ASSOCIATED CONDITIONS
N/A

AGE-RELATED FACTORS
N/A

ZOONOTIC POTENTIAL
• *Campylobacter jejuni* (aborted fetus, stomach content, fetal membranes)
• *C. psittaci* (fetal membranes, vaginal discharges)
• Q fever (influenza-like symptoms, myalgia, endocarditis)
• Brucellosis (*B. melentensis*), Malta fever, undulating fever, joint pain
• Leptospirosis
• Toxoplasmosis (milk, fetal membranes)
• Listeriosis: aborted fetuses

PREGNANCY
N/A

RUMINANT SPECIES AFFECTED
Sheep/goat

BIOSECURITY

PRODUCTION MANAGEMENT

SYNONYMS
Specific disease condition

SEE ALSO
Specific disease condition

ABBREVIATIONS
• EED = early embryonic loss
• ELISA = enzyme-linked immunosorbent assay
• FA = fluorescent antibody
• RFM = retained fetal membrane
• IIFA = indirect inclusion fluorescence antibody

Suggested Reading
Kikbride, C. A. 1993. Diagnosis in 1784 ovine abortions and stillbirths. *J Vet Diagnon Invest*. 5: 398.
Menzies, P. I., Miller, R. 1986. Abortion in sheep: diagnosis and control. In: *Current therapy in theriogenology*, ed. R. S. Youngquist. 2nd ed. Philadelphia: Saunders.
Mobini, S. 2003. Investigation of abortion in sheep and goat. *Proceedings Annual Meeting of the Society for Theriogenology*, pp. 291–303.
Mobini, S., Heath, A., Pugh, D. 2002. Theriogenology in sheep and goats. In: *Sheep and goat medicine*, ed. D. Pugh. Philadelphia: Saunders.

Author: Ahmed Tibary

ABORTION: VIRAL, FUNGAL, AND NUTRITIONAL

BASICS

OVERVIEW
• Abortion is the expulsion of the fetus prior to the end of the normal gestation period. Besides bacterial etiology, viral, fungal, parasitic, and nutritional causes are not uncommon.
• Abortions may occur near normal delivery time and it is difficult to determine whether the dam has aborted or whether a premature birth has occurred.
• Diagnostic success rates for abortions of only 25%–30% attained by diagnostic laboratories are common.
• Abortion frequently results from an event that occurred weeks or even months prior to the event, making diagnosis difficult in many cases.
• Fungal abortions are normally sporadic, and occur from 4 months to term.
• The incidence of fungal abortions in temperate climates is highest in the winter months. Severe infection of the placenta, characterized by a leathery thickening of the areas in between the cotyledons, is a common finding.
• Toxic, pharmacologic, and genetic factors causing fetal death and/or abortion are many times not discernible in the specimens available for examination.

SYSTEMS AFFECTED
Reproductive

GENETICS
N/A

INCIDENCE/PREVALENCE
Viral
In a 10-year South Dakota abortion survey, viruses were associated with 10.58% of samples. Bovine herpesvirus-1 (IBR) was detected in 5.41%, and bovine viral diarrhea virus (BVDV) was detected in 4.54% of diagnostic submissions. Bovine herpesvirus-4 was isolated from 0.52%; parvovirus, enterovirus, adenovirus, parainfluenza virus, and pseudorabies virus were isolated in much smaller numbers. Malignant lymphoid neoplasia abortion was assumed to have been caused by the bovine leukosis virus.

Mycotic
In one study, mycotic infection was diagnosed in 6.8% of 6858 cases of bovine abortion and stillbirth examined during a 9-year period. Aspergilli were associated with approximately 5% of all abortion cases and 71% of 446 cases that were cultured for fungi and diagnosed as mycotic abortion. *Aspergillus fumigatus* was the most frequent isolate (62%), followed by *A. terreus* (6.7%), *Emericella (Aspergillus) nidulans* (3.0%), *A. flavus* (2.9%), and *E. rugulosus* (less than 1.0%). Zygomycetes (*Absidia, Mortierella, Rhizomucor, Rhizopus*) accounted for 21% of the cases. *Pseudallescheria boydii* and yeasts (*Candida, Torulopsis*) were each identified in 2% of the cases. Fungi that uncommonly cause infection accounted for 2% of the cases and included *Curvularia geniculata, Exophilia jeanselmei, Hendersonula toruloidea, Lecythosphora hoffmannii, Talaromyces flavus* var. *flavus* (*Penicillium vermiculatus*), *T. (Penicillium) thermophilus*, and *Wangiella dermatitidis*. About 10% of the mycotic cases were mixed fungal infections involving *A. fumigatus* (87%), *A. flavus* (12.5%), or *E. nidulans* (12.5%) coexisting with *Absidia corymbifera* (72%), *Rhizomucor pusillus* (4.3%), or *Rhizopus arrhizus* (4.3%). In each mixed infection, both septate and nonseptate hyphae were observed in placental tissues.

GEOGRAPHIC DISTRIBUTION
Worldwide, depending on species, agent, and environment

Epidemiology
In an Israeli study of 58,048 pregnancies from 111 herds, the respective abortion density, proportion of aborted cows, and abortions per confirmed pregnancy were 4.2%, 5.9%, and 10.2%. Among parities, heifers had the lowest risk, and cows of second parity the greatest risk of fetal death. The greatest risk of fetal death was observed in the first trimester, and the lowest in the second trimester of pregnancy. Respective proportions of aborted cows with and without a previous abortion were 17.5% and 5.9%. The potential of aborting after twinning in multiparous cows was found to be 1.3% greater than for those having a single calf. Risk of abortion was greater in the autumn and early winter than in the summer months.

SIGNALMENT
Species
All ruminant species
Breed Predilections
N/A
Mean Age and Range
Breeding-age females
Predominant Sex
Female

DIAGNOSIS
See also under specific cause of abortion below.

DIFFERENTIAL DIAGNOSIS
Nonbacterial

Bovine Abortion
• Bluetongue
• Bovine viral diarrhea virus (BVD)-mucosal disease
• Drug induced
• Fetal abnormalities
• Infectious bovine rhinotracheitis (IBR)
• Iodine deficiency
• Malnutrition
• Maternal stress
• Mycotic abortions
• Placenta abnormalities
• Q fever
• Twinning
• Vitamin A deficiency

Ovine Abortion
• Border disease (bovine viral diarrhea—BVD)
• Copper deficiency
• Maternal stress
• Mycotic
• Nutritional deficiency/excess
• Parasitic
• Selenium toxicity
• Starvation
• Toxic plant ingestion

Caprine Abortion, Early
• Drug induced/iatrogenic (diazepam, xylazine, Acepromazine)
• Nutrition
• Progesterone deficiency

ABORTION: VIRAL, FUNGAL, AND NUTRITIONAL

Caprine Abortion, Late
- Akabane
- Bovine viral diarrhea (BVD)
- Caprine herpesvirus
- Copper deficiency
- Corticosteroid administration
- Foot-and-mouth disease
- Malnutrition
- Selenium deficiency
- Stress
- Toxic plant ingestion
- Vitamin A deficiency

TREATMENT

MEDICATIONS

CONTRAINDICATIONS
Appropriate milk and meat withdrawal times must be followed for all compounds administered to food-producing animals.

FOLLOW-UP

MISCELLANEOUS

Bovine Virus Diarrhea
Caused by bovine virus diarrhea virus (BVDV)

Clinical Conditions
- Subclinical BVD—Most common form of infection
- Acute BVD—Generally mild with low mortality
- Persistently Infected (PI) Cattle—PI calves are infected in utero and are immunotolerant to the noncytopathic virus
- Mucosal Disease—PI calves become super-infected with a second, cytopathic biotype of BVDV resulting in a condition of low morbidity but high mortality
- Abortions
  - Fetal infection may result in either PI calves or abortion.
  - Abortion rates are higher in BVDV type II infections.
  - Infections near conception result in early embryonic death and infertility.

- Infections between 42 and 125 days gestation with noncytopathic biotypes result in PI calves, fetal death causing abortion or mummification, or congenital defects.
- Infection between 125 and 170 days gestation results in a lower incidence of abortion and congenital defects. Calves may have an antibody titer to BVDV.
- Infection after 170 days gestation has little effect on the fetus.

Diagnosis
- Good history relative to the health of the herd
- Virus isolation and antibody detection from herd mates
- Lesions in aborted fetus compatible with BVDV infection, virus isolation, and fetal antibody detection.
- Abortions prior to 4 months' gestation will have characteristic lesions and virus while those aborted after 4 months may have congenital defects, fetal antibodies, or virus.
- Calves born with congenital defects may have precolostral antibodies.
- PI calves will have no titer (except from colostrum) and may be identified by virus isolation

Prevention and Control
- Impeccable herd management
- Identification and removal of PI animals
- Proper vaccination program

Herpesviral Abortion
- In cattle, the alpha-herpesviruses, bovine herpesvirus-1 (infectious bovine rhinotracheitis virus), and bovine herpesvirus-5 (bovine encephalitis virus), and a gamma-herpesvirus, bovine herpesvirus-4, have all been implicated as causes of abortion.
- Caprine herpesvirus-1 causes abortion or neonatal deaths in goats.

Infectious Bovine Rhinotracheitis Virus (Bovine Herpesvirus 1)
- IBRV or BHV1 is the most frequently diagnosed viral abortion disease. In addition to abortion it causes rhinotracheitis, conjunctivitis, pustular vulvovaginitis, balanoposthitis, and enteritis.
- Herpesvirus may produce latent infection, localizing in the trigeminal and sacral ganglion, resulting in a source of persistent infection following stress.
- Transmission is by direct contact to respiratory, conjunctival, or genital mucous membranes. It may be spread in the semen of carrier bulls.

Abortions
- Most abortions occur in the second half of pregnancy.
- May occur 2 weeks to 4 months after infection; typically occurs about 20 to 45 days after infection.
- Abortion rate may be sporadic or in storms, depending upon the susceptibility of the herd.
- Vaccination of pregnant cattle with MLV may cause abortion.

Infertility
Infection near the time of breeding, from infected semen or other exposure routes, may cause endometritis and oophoritis, resulting in temporary infertility or early embryonic death.

Diagnosis
- The entire fetus and placenta should be submitted for postmortem.
- Fetus usually autolyzed, obscuring gross lesions.
- Microscopic lesions include intranuclear inclusions of liver, lung, thymus, or adrenal gland.
- Diagnosis is confirmed by virus isolation or antibody determination in fetal tissue, with cotyledons being the preferred tissue in severely autolyzed fetuses.
- Maternal antibody titer is of limited use as the abortion may occur several months following exposure and the nature of the virus is ubiquitous.

Prevention and Control
- Impeccable herd management
- Proper vaccination programs
- Use of semen from IBR-negative bulls

Bluetongue Virus
- BTV rarely causes abortion in cattle and sheep.
- Infection is transmitted by the insect *Culicoides* spp. Infection may result in early embryonic death, abortion, mummification, or cerebral malformation. It is shed in the semen of viremic bulls.
- Although the virus is widespread throughout the world, it is not considered a major cause of bovine abortion.

Mycotic Abortions
- The fungi responsible for mycotic abortion in cattle include *Aspergillus, Absidia, Mucor, Rhizopus, Candida,* and *Mortierella,* with *Aspergillus fumigatus* being the most common.
- Abortions are sporadic, of low incidence, and usually occur in late gestation.

ABORTION: VIRAL, FUNGAL, AND NUTRITIONAL

• Fungi seen in silver-impregnated sections of tissues could be placed into three categories designated Aspergillus, Phycomycete, and Atypical.
• Gross or microscopic examination or cultures of the placenta are valuable diagnostically but examination of the fetus is seldom of value as infection in most instances does not involve fetal tissues.
• Fertility following fungal abortion was apparently unimpaired.

Diagnosis
• A thick, leathery placentitis
• The fetus may be emaciated, with ringwormlike lesions on the skin.
• Identification of fungal hyphae in fetal tissues and placenta

Pathophysiology
• Route of infection is hematogenous spread from the respiratory or gastrointestinal tracts.
• Source of infection is often moldy feed.

Control
Reduction of exposure to fungal agents by proper stable environment and reduced consumption of spoiled feeds

Abortion Due to Nutritional Causes
• Several poisonous plants, including poison hemlock and locoweed, may cause sporadic abortion but more commonly cause a variety of congenital defects.
• Nutritional deficiencies have been implicated in embryo loss however a direct cause-and-effect relationship is difficult to establish. Beta-carotene, vitamin A, iodine, selenium, phosphorus, and copper deficiencies have been implicated.
• Usually, nutritional deficiencies will demonstrate primarily as reproductive problems other than abortion.

Pine Needle Poisoning
• Consumption of needles from ponderosa pine trees can cause abortion in the third trimester. Isocupressic and imbricatoloic acids have been identified as the probable abortifacient agent.
• Ingestion of pine needles causes a progressive reduction in uterine blood flow resulting in abortion or premature parturition within 3 days, although occasionally within 3 weeks. The problem may be prevented by providing an alternative feed source.

Nitrate Poisoning
• Ruminants are susceptible to nitrate poisoning because of the nitrate-reducing potential of rumen microbes.

• Plants that accumulate high levels of nitrates include Sudan grass, oats, wheat, corn, pigweed, and Johnson grass.
• Heavy fertilization and cool growing conditions are conducive to nitrate accumulation. The ingested nitrates are converted to nitrites, which converts hemoglobin to methemoglobin. Methemoglobin is unable to carry oxygen, resulting in a hypoxic state. The hypoxemia may result in fetal death and abortion, or a stress-induced increase in fetal cortisol resulting in induction of parturition.
• Severe methemoglobinemia may cause death of the cow.
• Treatment is methylene blue IV.

Sweet Clover Hay
• Moldy sweet clover hay will produce toxic levels of the anticoagulant dicoumarol. Ingestion of toxic levels will cause pregnancy loss as well as death of adult animals.
• Removal of the moldy feed from the diet will prevent or terminate the loss.

ASSOCIATED CONDITIONS
• Infertility and return to estrus
• Infection near the time of breeding, from infected semen or other exposure routes, may cause endometritis and oophoritis, resulting in temporary infertility or early embryonic death.

AGE-RELATED FACTORS
Among parities, heifers have the lowest risk, and cows of second parity the greatest risk of fetal death.

ZOONOTIC POTENTIAL
Mycotic agents can be zoonotic.

PREGNANCY
• Abortions may occur near normal delivery time and it is difficult to determine whether the dam has aborted or whether a premature birth has occurred.
• Abortion frequently results from an event that occurred weeks or even months prior to the event making diagnosis difficult in many cases.
• The greatest risk of fetal death is observed in the first trimester, and the lowest in the second trimester of pregnancy.

RUMINANT SPECIES AFFECTED
Potentially, all ruminant species are affected.

BIOSECURITY
• Test and isolate prior to herd/flock introduction.
• Impeccable herd management

PRODUCTION MANAGEMENT
• Vaccination is an important tool in disease prevention.
• Impeccable herd management

SYNONYMS
N/A

SEE ALSO
Bluetongue
Bovine viral diarrhea
Infectious bovine rhinotracheitis
Locoweed
Mycotic infections
Nitrate toxicity
Pine needle toxicity
Poison hemlock
Sweet clover

ABBREVIATIONS
BHV = bovine herpes virus
BTV = blue tongue virus
BVD = bovine viral diarrhea
BVDV = bovine viral diarrhea virus
IBR = infectious bovine rhinotracheitis
MLV = modified live vaccine

Suggested Reading
Johnson, C. T., Lupson, G. R., Lawrence, K. E. 1994, Mar 12. The bovine placentome in bacterial and mycotic abortions. *Vet Rec.* 134(11):263–66.
Kirkbride, C. A. 1992, Oct. Viral agents and associated lesions detected in a 10-year study of bovine abortions and stillbirths. *J Vet Diagn Invest.* 4(4):374–79.
Knudtson, W. U., Kirkbride, C. A. 1992, Apr. Fungi associated with bovine abortion in the northern plains states (USA). *J Vet Diagn Invest.* 4(2):181–85.
Markusfeld-Nir, O. 1997, Aug. Epidemiology of bovine abortions in Israeli dairy herds. *Prev Vet Med.* 31(3–4):245–55.
McCausland, I. P., Slee, K. J., Hirst, F. S. 1987, May. Mycotic abortion in cattle. *Aust Vet J.* 64(5):129–32.
Reuter, R., Bowden, M., Ellis, T., Carman, H. 1987, Mar. Abortion, stillbirth and ill thrift in cattle associated with mucosal disease virus. *Aust Vet J.* 64(3):92–93.
Seguin, B., Troedsson, M. 2002. Diseases of the reproductive system. In: *Large animal internal medicine*, ed. B. P. Smith. St. Louis: Mosby.
Smith, K. C. 1997, May. Herpesviral abortion in domestic animals. *Vet J.* 153(3):253–68.

Authors: Walter Johnson and Alex Estrada

BASICS

OVERVIEW

• Rumen acidosis is a pathological condition that can be acute (i.e., leading to death) or chronic (i.e., leading to short-term or long-term production inefficiencies and illnesses).

• Acidosis results from consumption of excessive amounts of readily fermentable carbohydrates (RFC) and, therefore, it can be a major problem for ruminants on high-concentrate diets (e.g., feedlot cattle).

• Rumen pH of 5.6 and 5.2 are used as benchmarks for chronic and acute acidosis, respectively.

• In the feedlot, acidosis occurs during adaptation of animals to high-concentrate diets and also in animals adapted to these diets due to engorgement of large amounts of RFC.

• Acidosis occurs in grazing animals when large amounts of high-starch supplements are fed.

• In dairy cows, the incidence of acidosis is highest during the first month postcalving. This is due to adaptation to high-concentrate diets containing more RFC than the cows are accustomed to utilizing during the dry period. It is important to note that the cow's body is also unable to handle acid loads during early lactation.

• Sources of RFC include immature/rapidly growing forages (i.e., high in intracellular carbohydrates), tubers/root crops (i.e., high in sugars), and cereal grains (i.e., high in starch).

• Cereal grains are considered the most important source of RFC in animals with acute or chronic acidosis.

• Cereal grains vary in their rate of ruminal starch fermentation (e.g., wheat is more fermentable than corn or milo, therefore, ruminants will be more susceptible to acidosis when fed wheat than corn).

• Sheep appear to be more susceptible to acidosis than cattle.

• Acidosis is of high economic significance because a large number of cattle and sheep are finished on high-concentrate diets.

• The economic losses include death and/or performance of animals at much less than their genetic potential.

• Many animals on high-concentrate diets experience chronic acidosis for extended periods of time without the condition being detected.

PATHOPHYSIOLOGY

• When the amount of RFC is increased abruptly, rapid rumen fermentation occurs and large amounts of volatile fatty acids (VFA; mainly acetate, propionate, and butyrate) are produced.

• These acids are continuously absorbed through the rumen wall without significant negative effects on the rumen environment. However, when large amounts of RFC are consumed, production of VFA is increased, and the rumen pH is decreased due to their accumulation.

• The decreased rumen pH causes significant changes in the ruminal microbial population, especially a rapid increase in numbers of the amylolytic or sugar-utilizing bacteria such as *Streptococcus bovis*.

• Under low pH conditions, lactate-producing bacteria (e.g., *Lactobacillus* spp.) also grow faster, increase in number, and produce increasing amounts of D- and L-lactate.

• Ruminants can utilize L-lactate, as it is an intermediary metabolite. They can also use D-lactate.

• In rumen environments not experiencing significant pH reductions, the lactate produced is absorbed in the rumen and small intestine or is immediately metabolized by lactate-utilizing bacterial species (e.g., *Megasphaera elsdenii*, *Propionibacterium shermanii*, and *Selenomonas ruminantium*). Thus, lactate either is not found in the rumen fluid or is detected at very low concentrations (< 5 ΦM).

• When large amounts of lactate are produced, the rumen ability to utilize it is exceeded and, as a result, it accumulates (up to 40 ΦM as is the case in severe acidosis) and causes significant reductions in rumen pH.

• Under these low pH conditions, lactate-producing bacterial species outnumber lactate-utilizing species, the number of *S. bovis* is decreased, and the number of *Lactobacillus* species is increased.

• The ability of lactate to decrease pH more drastically than a similar amount of other fermentation acids (e.g., acetate) is due to its lower pK (i.e., the point of maximum buffering) value (i.e., 3.8 vs. 4.8). It is important to note that total acid (VFA and lactate) load is responsible for acidosis and this acid load causes several ruminal and systemic effects.

SYSTEMS AFFECTED
Gastrointestinal, metabolic, musculoskeletal

GENETICS
N/A

INCIDENCE/PREVALENCE
N/A

GEOGRAPHIC DISTRIBUTION
Worldwide

SIGNALMENT

Species
Potentially all ruminant species

Breed Predilections
N/A

Mean Age and Range
N/A

Predominant Sex
N/A

SIGNS

HISTORICAL FINDINGS
• Marked reduction or cessation of feed intake (anorexia)
• Diarrhea or loose feces
• Lethargy

ACIDOSIS

- Laminitis or founder
- Vomiting
- Decreased rate of body weight gain
- Distressed appearance
- Polioencephalomalacia (cerebrocorticonecrosis). The thiamine deficiency is triggered by thiaminases produced by rumen bacteria under low pH conditions.
- Cessation of rumen motility
- In acute acidosis, dehydration occurs in response to the increase in ruminal osmotic pressure and the decrease in extracellular volume. The consequences of dehydration include decreased cardiac output, decreased peripheral perfusion, decreased renal blood flow, shock, and death.
- Symptoms detected in dead or slaughtered animals include rumenitis, inflammation of the small intestinal tissues, and high incidence of abscessed livers.

Rumen Effects
- A significant increase in numbers of amylolytic, sugar-utilizing, and lactate-producing bacterial species
- A continuous decrease in rumen pH to 6 and 5.2, which are lethal to major microbial populations such as the rumen protozoa and cellulolytic bacterial species, respectively.
- A decrease in the rumen motility and fermentation
- An increase in the rumen osmotic pressure (> 300 mOsm) due to accumulation of solutes such as VFA, lactate, glucose, and minerals
- When the rumen osmotic pressure exceeds that of the blood, a rapid influx of water from the blood occurs to neutralize the rumen osmotic pressure. This action results in significant rumen wall damage (i.e., swelling of the papillae and stripping of epithelium patches).
- The rumen microbes responsible for liver abscess (e.g., *Fusobacterium necrophorum*) can freely cross the damaged rumen wall and enter the blood.

- An increase in absorption of lactate
- In subclinical cases of acidosis (e.g., dairy cows in early lactation), the rumen pH drops daily to <5.5 for a given period of time. This has negative effects on fermentation and the subsequent utilization of nutrients by dairy cows.

Systemic Effects
- An increase in blood lactate concentration
- A decrease in blood bicarbonate concentration
- A decrease in blood pH below 7.35 (i.e., a life-threatening situation)
- A decrease in urine pH
- A decrease in blood concentration of minerals (e.g., calcium) and electrolytes
- An increase in blood histamine concentration
- An increase in blood osmolality due to loss of water to the rumen
- An increase in concentration of blood components (e.g., increased packed cell volume)
- Uncontrolled elevation of blood pressure
- Inflammation of the small intestine
- Coma and death (e.g., the sudden death in feedlots)

Promoting Factors
- Mismanagement of feeding RFC sources such as cereal grains
- Cold weather promotes consumption of large amounts of feed and, therefore, it may dispose feedlot cattle to acidosis.

 TREATMENT

Chronic Cases
- Increasing bicarbonate input from the diet and/or through salivation by increasing forage levels in the diet, especially long hay to stimulate rumination. Dietary or salivary bicarbonates increase pH and stimulate lactate utilization in the rumen.

- Increasing water intake causes dilution of rumen contents and reduction in rumen osmolality. This prevents water influx from the blood and helps maintain blood osmolality.
- Supplementation of B vitamins (i.e., B_{12} and thiamin) that are involved in VFA metabolism to decrease their blood levels
- Drenching with electrolytes

Acute Cases
- Evacuating the rumen after a stab incision in the paralumbar fossa area
- Use of antibiotics such as oral dosing of chlortetracycline and water
- Inoculation with rumen fluid from healthy animals
- Removing the RFC source from the diet
- Feeding good-quality forages
- Intravenous infusion of bicarbonate buffer to eliminate acidity but not to induce alkalosis
- Intravenous infusion of electrolytes
- Intravenous infusion of saline solution

 MEDICATIONS

CONTRAINDICATIONS
Appropriate milk and meat withdrawal times must be followed for all compounds administered to food-producing animals.

 FOLLOW-UP

PREVENTION/AVOIDANCE
- Gradual adaptation of animals to high-concentrate diets. A 4-week adaptation period was found to provide an opportunity to induce a gradual change and stabilization of a final ruminal microbial population that can handle the increased amounts of lactate produced when high-RFC diets are fed.

• Dietary inclusion of roughages (e.g., long forages or by-products containing fiber) at 10% to 15% of dry matter to enhance rumination and to increase salivation. The buffering capacity of ruminant saliva can help in reducing the negative effects of fermentation acids.
• Dietary exclusion of cereal grains that promote acidosis such as wheat
• Dietary exclusion of fermented feeds (e.g., silages) that are known to increase the acid load in the rumen
• Management and close monitoring of feeding processed grains such as steam-flaked corn. The gelatinization of starch during steam flaking increases its rate of fermentation.
• Modulating starch intake by restricting feeding (e.g., 90% of ad libitum intake) to eliminate excessive consumption of starch
• Restricting feeding after working cattle or during weather change
• Fat supplementation at levels up to 6% of the diet
• Feeding high-protein diets to increase production of rumen ammonia (i.e., alkaline) and to decrease rumen acidity
• Dietary inclusion of sodium bicarbonate at 1% or 2% of dry matter to increase the buffering capacity of the rumen and to ameliorate the acidic conditions during early feeding of high RFC levels.
• Allowing access to fresh feed and water at all times. Animals will eat smaller meals more often.
• Using feed additives with rumen effects such as the ionophores monensin and lasalocid. These additives alter rumen fermentation and allow adaptation to high-starch diets by inhibiting lactate-producing bacterial species and stimulating lactate-utilizing species. The actions of these ionophores are achieved by their interference with the normal transport of ions across bacterial cell membranes.

• Using feed additives with systemic effects such as the antibiotics chlortetracycline, tylosin, and virginiamycin to decrease the incidence of abscessed livers.
• Close monitoring of daily intake of diets containing high RFC levels

 MISCELLANEOUS

ASSOCIATED CONDITIONS
• Diarrhea, lethargy, laminitis, decreased rate of body weight gain
• Polioencephalomalacia
• Cessation of rumen motility
• Dehydration, decreased cardiac output, decreased peripheral perfusion, decreased renal blood flow, shock, and death

AGE-RELATED FACTORS
N/A

ZOONOTIC POTENTIAL
N/A

PREGNANCY
N/A

RUMINANT SPECIES AFFECTED
All ruminant species are affected.

BIOSECURITY
N/A

PRODUCTION MANAGEMENT
• Dietary inclusion of roughages
• Gradual adaptation of animals to high-concentrate diets
• Dietary exclusion of cereal grains that promote acidosis such as wheat
• Restricting feeding after working cattle or during weather change
• Dietary inclusion of sodium bicarbonate at 1% or 2% of dry matter to increase the buffering capacity of the rumen
• Allowing access to fresh feed and water at all times

SYNONYMS
Grain overload

SEE ALSO
Nutrition section
Polioencephalomalacia
Rumen dysfunction: alkalosis, transfaunation
Rumen fluid analysis

ABBREVIATIONS
RFC = readily fermentable carbohydrates
VFA = volatile fatty acids

Suggested Reading
Crichlow, E. C., Chaplin, R. K. 1985. Ruminal lactic acidosis: Relationship of forestomach motility to nondissociated volatile fatty acid levels. *Am J Vet Res.* 46:1908–11.
Huntington, G. B. 1988. Acidosis. In: *The ruminant animal: digestive physiology and nutrition*, ed. D. C. Church. Englewood Cliffs, NJ: Prentice Hall.
Newbold, C. J., Wallace, R. J. 1988. Effects of the ionophores monensin and tetronasin on simulated development of ruminal lactic acidosis in vitro. *Appl Environ Microbiol.* 54:2981–85.
Nocek, J. E. 1997. Bovine acidosis: implications on laminitis. *J Dairy Sci.* 80:1005–28.
Owens, F. N., Secrist, D. S., Hill, W. J., Gill, D. R. 1998. Acidosis in cattle: a review. *J Anim Sci.* 76:275–86.

Author: Hussein S. Hussein

ACTINOBACILLOSIS

 BASICS

DEFINITION
Actinobacillosis is caused by *Actinobacillus ligniersii* infection of the soft tissues, usually in the tongue.

PATHOPHYSIOLOGY
• *Actinobacillus ligniersii* is a gram-negative rod, which normally inhabits the mouth and rumen of domestic ruminants, and is also found on plant awns.
• Mucosal lesions anywhere on the body, typically in the mouth, can be invaded by these bacteria, causing a localized lesion. Bacteria can also spread to different parts of the body via lymphatic drainage.
• A typical site of bacterial invasion is through small ulcers in the sulcus lingualis at the base of the tongue, leading to hard, painful, diffuse lesions of the tongue interfering with prehension of food, hence the synonym "wooden tongue." The bacteria initially cause an acute diffuse myositis of the muscles of the tongue, followed by development of granules and fibrosis.

SYSTEMS AFFECTED
Alimentary, musculoskeletal

GENETICS
N/A

INCIDENCE/PREVALENCE
Seen in up to 3% of cattle tongues at slaughter

GEOGRAPHIC DISTRIBUTION
Worldwide

SIGNALMENT
Species
Mainly cattle and sheep, occasionally goats
Breed Predilections
N/A
Mean Age and Range
All ages
Predominant Sex
N/A

SIGNS
HISTORICAL FINDINGS
Abrasive feeds and crowded conditions in a herd outbreak; lesions outside the oral cavity may be associated with previous wounds or needle punctures.

PHYSICAL EXAM FINDINGS
Hard diffuse nodular swellings typically of the tongue in cattle and of the lips in sheep

CAUSES AND RISK FACTORS
Caused by infection of soft tissues by *Actinobacillus ligniersii*; abrasive feeds and crowded conditions may facilitate spread in a herd outbreak.

 DIAGNOSIS

DIFFERENTIAL DIAGNOSIS
• Dental disease
• Oral foreign bodies and generalized lesions
• Pharyngeal trauma
• Contagious ecthyma and caseous lymphadenitis in sheep

CBC/BIOCHEMISTRY/URINALYSIS
Chronic inflammatory profile

OTHER LABORATORY TESTS
• Biopsy/histopathology and culture of lesions
• Microscopic examination of pus compressed between two glass slides shows "sulfur granule" or clublike rosette appearance with a central mass of bacteria.

IMAGING
N/A

OTHER DIAGNOSTIC PROCEDURES
N/A

PATHOLOGIC FINDINGS
Firm, pale, gritty granulomatous abscesses with multifocal necrotic foci containing mononuclear cells, neutrophils, eosinophils, and plant fibers

 TREATMENT

ACTIVITY
N/A

DIET
Use of a soft feed will aid prehension during treatment.

CLIENT EDUCATION
See Diet above.

MEDICATIONS
• Sodium iodide
• Daily organic iodides orally in severe cases

DRUGS OF CHOICE
Sodium iodide 70 mg/kg IV as 10–20% solution; give once, repeat at least once at 7–10-day intervals.

CONTRAINDICATIONS
• Use sodium iodide with caution in pregnant cattle; see Precautions below.
• Appropriate milk and meat withdrawal times must be followed for all compounds administered to food-producing animals.

PRECAUTIONS
Anecdotal reports of association with abortion in cattle at high doses of sodium iodide

POSSIBLE INTERACTIONS
N/A

ALTERNATIVE DRUGS
Penicillin, tetracycline, ceftiofur

 FOLLOW-UP

May need surgical debulking of lesions in severe cases.

PATIENT MONITORING
If signs of iodism seen (dandruff, excessive lacrimation, inappetence, coughing, diarrhea), halt therapy until signs disappear.

PREVENTION/AVOIDANCE
Reduce access to abrasive feed and pastures with hard penetrating plant awns or thistles.

POSSIBLE COMPLICATIONS
Anecdotal reports of association with abortion in cattle at high doses of sodium iodide

EXPECTED COURSE AND PROGNOSIS
• Good prognosis if only the tongue is involved.
• Fair prognosis if atypical sites are involved.

 MISCELLANEOUS

ASSOCIATED CONDITIONS
N/A

AGE-RELATED FACTORS
N/A

ZOONOTIC POTENTIAL
Bite wounds from ruminants can contain *Actinobacillus ligniersii*, but rarely result in actinobacillosis.

PREGNANCY
See Precautions above.

RUMINANT SPECIES AFFECTED
Mainly cattle and sheep, rare in goats

BIOSECURITY
N/A

PRODUCTION MANAGEMENT
N/A

SYNONYMS
Wooden tongue

SEE ALSO
Caseous lymphadenitis
Contagious ecthyma
Dental disease
Oral foreign bodies
Pharyngeal trauma

ABBREVIATIONS
IV = intravenous

Suggested Reading

Pugh, D. G., ed. 2002. *Sheep and goat medicine.* Philadelphia: W. B. Saunders.
Radostits, O. M., Gay, C. C., Blood, D. C., Hinchcliff, K. W., eds. 2000. *Veterinary medicine.* 9th ed. London: W. B. Saunders.
Smith, B. P., ed. 2002. *Large animal internal medicine*, 3rd ed. St. Louis: Mosby.

Author: David McKenzie

ACTINOMYCOSIS: LUMPY JAW

 BASICS

OVERVIEW
Common, sporadic, chronic granulomatous osteomyelitis of cattle caused by non-spore-forming, filamentous, gram-positive, anaerobic bacterium *Actinomyces bovis*

PATHOPHYSIOLOGY
• *Actinomyces*
  • normal members of oral microbiota in cattle
  • same order as *Mycobacterium*
  • low virulence
  • only cause disease when mucosal barriers are compromised
  • gram-positive, branching/filamentous, nonencapsulated bacteria
• Trauma to oral mucosa from rough feed or foreign objects or dental alveoli permits entrance of *Actinomyces* into buccal tissues.
• Grows in anaerobic conditions associated with devitalized tissue, lack of phagocyte delivery.
• In mandible and maxillae, initially, painless, hard, *immovable* swellings. In weeks or months, swelling frequently develops along lower edge of bone and in intermandibular space.
• Abscess/granuloma formation, necrotic foci (mycetoma)
• Masses open through sinus tracts, lesions may become painful.
• Discharge of viscous, sticky, "honey- or whey-like," odorless, yellowish pus from openings.
• Pus contains sandlike, firm, yellowish granules, which do not contain sulfur. The granule contains microcolonies of *Actinomyces* in an eosinophilic, amorphous matrix made of calcium phosphate/antigen-antibody complexes.

• Occasional involvement of soft tissues, especially of esophageal groove with spread to lower esophagus, anterior wall of reticulum, may cause peritonitis.
• Rare hematogenous spread to other organs
• Local lymph nodes usually not involved
• Teeth may loosen.
• Swelling may cause dyspnea.
• Trauma to digestive tract could introduce *Actinomyces* into regions below oral cavity.

SYSTEMS AFFECTED
Musculoskeletal; rare hematogenous spread to other organs; oral cavity

GENETICS
N/A

GEOGRAPHIC DISTRIBUTION
Worldwide

INCIDENCE/PREVALENCE
Common, sporadic

SIGNALMENT
Species
Cattle; potentially all ruminant species
Breed Predilections
N/A
Mean Age and Range
Young cattle with erupting teeth, commonly
Predominant Sex
N/A

SIGNS
HISTORICAL FINDINGS
Hard, immovable swellings of maxillae/mandible
• Draining fistulous tracts—yellowish, sticky, odorless pus
• Misaligned teeth, difficulty masticating
• Weight loss, periodic diarrhea, chronic bloat
• Dyspnea
• Less frequently partial tracheal obstruction, orchitis, brain/lung abscesses

CAUSES AND RISK FACTORS
• Eruption of teeth in young cattle
• Rough feeds containing awns, foreign objects
• Procedures causing oral lacerations

SIGNALMENT
• Young cattle, erupting teeth
• Cattle fed awn-containing feeds or subjected to oral trauma
Source of Infections
• Endogenous infections; oral microbiota
• If noninfected cattle present with oral lacerations, *Actinomyces* may be spread from infected animals to noninfected animals via contaminated draining pus.
• Normally not contagious
Transmission
Endogenous; oral lacerations permit entry into devitalized buccal tissues and subsequent spread

 DIAGNOSIS

• Palpation of hard, immovable masses
• Draining tracts, odorless, sticky, yellowish pus with hard, small yellowish-white granules
• Microscopic exam of pus: mix with saline; crush granules between two glass slides; use Gram's stain. Rosettes of thin, filamentous, branching gram-positive rods seen at periphery of granule. May appear irregularly stained, "beaded." May be misidentified as fungi.
• Fastidious, slow-growing bacterium. Culture anaerobically 10–14 days or more.

DIFFERENTIAL DIAGNOSIS
• Cheek abscess, causes other than *Actinomyces* (movable, located in soft tissue)
• Impacted feed/foreign bodies between cheek and teeth

- Chronic peritonitis, causes other than *Actinomyces*
- Mandibular lymphosarcoma

CBC/BIOCHEMISTRY/URINALYSIS
N/A

OTHER LABORATORY TESTS
- Culture and sensitivity of the lesion is indicated.
- Microscopic exam of purulent debris: mix sample with saline and crush granules between glass slides; use Gram's stain.

IMAGING
Radiographs should reveal changes consistent with osteomyelitis of the affected mandible.

 TREATMENT

- Difficult to treat
- Surgical debridement/drainage. Pack wound with streptomycin or tincture of iodine soaked gauze.

DRUG(S) OF CHOICE
- Streptomycin, penicillin, sulfonamides
- Iodine therapy: (See Precautions below.) Some animals become distressed (restlessness, dyspnea, tachycardia). Stop when signs of iodism occur (lacrimation, anorexia, cough, scaling skin lesions). Subcutaneous iodine causes severe irritation and immediate swelling. Potassium iodine as drench. Sodium iodine IV as 10% solution.
- Isoniazid as adjunct to antibiotic/iodine therapy

CONTRAINDICATIONS
Appropriate milk and meat withdrawal times must be followed for all compounds administered to food-producing animals.

PRECAUTIONS
Caution: abortion has followed iodine therapy in some animals.

POSSIBLE INTERACTIONS
N/A

ALTERNATIVE DRUGS
N/A

 FOLLOW-UP

PREVENTION
- Avoid feeds/ procedures that could cause oral lacerations.
- Monitor young cattle for swelling of mandible especially following tooth eruptions.
- Isolate cattle with discharging lesions
- No vaccine

 MISCELLANEOUS

ASSOCIATED CONDITIONS
N/A

AGE-RELATED FACTORS
Young cattle with erupting teeth

ZOONOTIC POTENTIAL
No cattle-human transmission

PREGNANCY
N/A

RUMINANT SPECIES AFFECTED
Cattle; potentially all ruminant species

BIOSECURITY
N/A

PRODUCTION MANAGEMENT
N/A

SYNONYMS
Actinostreptothricosis
Cervicofacial actinomycosis
Lumpy jaw
Ray fungus disease

SEE ALSO
Cheek abscess, causes other than *Actinomyces* (movable, located in soft tissue)
Impacted feed/foreign bodies between cheek and teeth
Chronic peritonitis, causes other than *Actinomyces*

ABBREVIATIONS
IV = intravenous

Suggested Reading
Bertone, A. L., Rebhun, W. C. 1984, Jul 15. Tracheal actinomycosis in a cow. *J Am Vet Med Assoc.* 185(2): 221–22.
Radostits, O. M., Gay, C. C., Blood, D. C., Hinchcliff, K. W., eds. 2000. Actinomycosis. In: *Veterinary medicine.* 9th ed. Philadelphia: W. B. Saunders.
Seifi, H. A., Saifzadeh, S., Farshid, A. A., Rad, M., Farrokhi, F. 2003, May. Mandibular pyogranulomatous osteomyelitis in a Sannen goat. *J Vet Med A Physiol Pathol Clin Med.* 50(4): 219–21.
Smith, B. P. 2002. Actinomycosis (lumpy jaw). In: *Large animal internal medicine.* 3rd ed. St. Louis: Mosby.
Strohl, W. A., Harriet, R., Fisher, B. D., eds. 2001. *Lippincott's illustrated reviews: microbiology.* Philadelphia: Lippincott, Williams and Wilkins.
Watts, T. C., Olson, S. M., Rhodes, C. S. 1974, Feb. Letter: Use of isoniazid in cattle. *Can Vet J.* 15(2): 28.
Watts, T. C., Olson, S. M., Rhodes, C. S. 1973, Sep. Treatment of bovine actinomycosis with isoniazid. *Can Vet J.* 14(9): 223–24.

Author: Karen Carberry-Goh

ACUTE COLIC—ABDOMINAL PAIN

BASICS

DEFINITION
• Acute colic is abdominal pain of <48 hours duration.
• Once pain has exceeded 48 hours duration, it is considered chronic.

PATHOPHYSIOLOGY
• The gastrointestinal tract is the source of most acute abdominal pain, but any abdominal organ can be involved.
• Gastrointestinal pain can result from distension, displacement, torsion/volvulus, obstruction, smooth muscle spasm, and mesenteric tension, and may involve hypermotility, hypomotility, ischemia, and inflammation.
• Urinary tract pain can result from obstruction, inflammation, infection.
• Reproductive pain can result from parturition, abortion, dystocia, uterine torsion, inflammation, infection, or tumor.
• Peritoneal pain results from inflammation, infection, and penetrating metallic foreign bodies.
• Other abdominal organs are less likely sources of pain, but should be considered if the source of the pain cannot be identified.
• Gastrointestinal lesions can be strangulating or nonstrangulating.
• Strangulating lesions are by definition associated with reduced blood supply, which can result in necrosis.
• Nonstrangulating lesions result in less circulatory disturbance and as a result are not usually associated with necrosis unless chronic.
• Any interference with gastrointestinal function can result in endotoxemia due to the large volume of natural gastrointestinal flora.
• Lesions originating in one system or organ can eventually result in other organs being affected.

SYSTEMS AFFECTED
• Gastrointestinal
• Urinary
• Reproductive
• Cardiovascular
• Respiratory, if abdominal distension is severe

GENETICS
N/A

INCIDENCE/PREVALENCE
N/A

GEOGRAPHIC DISTRIBUTION
Worldwide distribution

SIGNALMENT
• All ages and sexes can be affected.
• Certain etiologies may be more common for specific groups.

SIGNS
• Abdominal pain may be mild to severe.
• Early signs may be subtle and easily missed, progressing in severity.
• Cause is often obvious from a careful physical examination including rectal examination.
• Ruminants are often stoic animals, bearing much pain without overt signs of colic as seen in the horse.
• The veterinarian should be familiar with the location of the gastrointestinal components in cattle, and with associated areas of tympany (pings), which indicate a gas-fluid interface under pressure.
• Sometimes diagnosis is made by presumption in early stages, based on a particular signalment and a few clinical symptoms.
• Mild colic—slight depression, reduced interest in feed, slight reduction in manure output, restlessness
• Moderate colic—reduced interest in feed, reduced manure output, restlessness, stretching abdomen (sawhorse stance), teeth grinding, posturing to urinate or defecate without producing much

• Severe colic—kicking at belly, recumbency (esp. lateral recumbency), severe depression, vocalization, straining to urinate or defecate, severe restlessness (getting up and down repeatedly), extended head and neck, rolling (very rare in ruminants)

PHYSICAL EXAM FINDINGS
• Depression
• Increased heart and respiratory rates
• Abdominal distension
• Change in body temperature above or below normal
• Reduced gastrointestinal sounds
• Gastrointestinal hypermotility
• The presence of pings in the abdomen
• Lack of urine or feces
• Discharge of uterine fluids
• Palpably distended or displaced viscus on rectal exam
• Grainy or constricted rectal palpation (peritonitis)
• Vomiting (rare)
• Dry prepuce (with urinary obstruction)

CAUSES

Forestomachs
• Ruminal acidosis (grain overload), vagal indigestion, traumatic reticuloperitonitis, omasal impaction, ruminal fermentation (calves), bloat (gas or frothy)
• Abomasum
• Ulcers, impaction, left displacement (LDA), right displacement (RDA), right abomasal volvulus (RAV), right omasal-abomasal volvulus (ROAV), abomasal rupture, vagal indigestion, abomasal stricture

Small intestine
Enteritis, ileus, impaction, stricture, entrapment, segmental torsion, jejunal flange torsion, jejunal hemorrhage syndrome, intussusception, adhesions, fat necrosis, tumor, hernia (inguinal, umbilical, diaphragmatic)

ACUTE COLIC—ABDOMINAL PAIN

Large intestine
Colitis, impaction, cecal tympany, displacement, torsion, volvulus, adhesions, fat necrosis, tumor, intussusception, atresia coli

Reproductive
Dystocia, parturition, abortion, tumor, peri-uterine abscess, testicular torsion, testicular trauma, penile/preputial trauma, vaginal prolapse, seminal vesiculitis, inguinal hernia

Urinary
Urolithiasis, cystitis, nephrolith, pyoureter, pyelonephritis

Other
Hernia, torsion of root of mesentery, peritonitis, hepatic inflammation, hepatitis, cholelith

RISK FACTORS
- Dietary change(s)
- Lack of access to water
- Pregnancy
- Stress
- Recent parturition

DIAGNOSIS

DIFFERENTIAL DIAGNOSIS
Many diseases can cause signs resembling abdominal pain, including choke, rabies, tetanus, myositis, hypocalcemia, septicemia, and obesity

CBC/CHEMISTRY/URINALYSIS
- Increased WBC count with peritonitis or other inflammation
- Increased PCV and TP with dehydration
- Decreased Cl, K, Na with most intestinal obstructive lesions in adult cattle
- Increased fibrinogen in inflammatory conditions

- Metabolic alkalosis in most gastrointestinal obstructive lesions in adult cattle
- Acidosis with grain overload or severe, long-standing obstructions
- Azotemia with urinary obstruction or severe dehydration
- Urinalysis shows increased WBC, RBC, bacteria, crystals in urinary tract

OTHER LAB TESTS
Abdominocentesis
- Increased WBC, TP, turbidity
- Serosanguineous color indicative of obstruction
- Foul smell indicative of GI rupture or enterocentesis
- Plant material indicative of rupture or enterocentesis
- Urine smell with uroabdomen
- Volume increased with pregnancy, inflammation
- Can be hard to obtain fluid in ruminants—try the flank region

Rumen Fluid Analysis
- Decreased protozoal activity with poor rumen function or obstruction
- Decreased pH with acidosis and abomasal reflux
- Increased Cl with abomasal reflux
- Abnormal color or smell with acidosis, ruminal fermentation, rumenitis

IMAGING
Ultrasound
- May be helpful in examination of urinary and reproductive tract
- Can identify fluid pockets in abdomen
- New publications suggest use transabdominal to detect abnormalities of the GI tract

Radiographs and contrast radiology
- Not usually useful in adult ruminants due to size
- May be useful in examination of the urinary tract

DIAGNOSTIC PROCEDURES
- *Liptak test*: Transabdominal paracentesis of a viscus on the left side of the adult cow to differentiate a LDA from rumen. Low pH = abomasum, high pH = rumen
- *Laparotomy*: Often used as diagnostic procedure in cows. The problem can be identified and repaired in many cases by flank laparotomy.
- *Laparoscopy*: Can be used as diagnostic procedure, but most abdominal problems require laparotomy to repair.

TREATMENT

APPROPRIATE HEALTH CARE
- Colic should be considered an emergency and diagnosis and treatment initiated immediately.
- Affected animals should not be fed until the cause is determined.
- Often the organ system involved is readily obvious following physical exam and the choice of medical treatment vs. surgery quickly made.
- Indications for immediate surgical treatment include severe abdominal pain, severe abdominal distension, HR >80 bpm, presence of pings, abnormal abdominocentesis, urinary obstruction, uterine torsion nonresponsive to rolling or manipulation, fetal oversize causing dystocia, confirmed gastrointestinal torsion, displacement, or obstruction.
- Surgical approach to the abdomen in adult bovines is made in a standing position by right flank laparotomy. If the desired lesion is located on the left side, a left flank approach can be made, but there can be limited exploration of the right side of the cow from this approach. In exploratory surgeries, the right flank is almost always chosen.
- In small ruminants, flank or middling approach can be used.

ACUTE COLIC—ABDOMINAL PAIN

NURSING CARE
• IV fluids will be necessary in most cases. As alkalosis is present in most adult cattle with GI problems, a neutral or acidifying fluid is recommended. In cattle with grain overload, and any other animals with confirmed acidosis, an alkalinizing fluid and/or bicarbonate are recommended.
• IV fluids should be supplemented to correct any electrolyte abnormalities.
• Oral fluids may be administered in certain cases, such as impaction, in order to provide a large volume of fluids to the GI tract.
• The use of oral fluids combined with hypertonic saline (1 ml/kg/min) has gained some favor as being cheaper than IV fluids, with similar effectiveness in restoring vascular volume.
• Caution should be used in supplementing calcium to endotoxemic cows, as endotoxin sensitizes the heart to potentially fatal arrhythmias.
• Animals with severe rumen bloat will require immediate ororuminal intubation to relieve the pressure.

ACTIVITY
N/A

DIET
• During the colic episode, feed should be withheld.
• Following resolution of the condition, refeeding should begin slowly to avoid recurrence or complications.

CLIENT EDUCATION
None

SURGICAL CONSIDERATIONS
None

MEDICATIONS

DRUGS OF CHOICE

Analgesics
• Flunixin meglumine: 1.1–2.2 mg/kg IV q24h or divided q12h
• Ketoprofen: 2 mg/kg IM q24h
• Phenylbutazone: 4 mg/kg IV or PO q24h
• The use of phenylbutazone is illegal in dairy animals and highly discouraged in all food animals.
• Butorphanol: 0.02–0.04 mg/kg IV

Laxatives
• Mineral oil: 10 ml/kg given by ororuminal tube
• Magnesium oxide: 0.5–1 kg for adult cow given by ororuminal tube
• Dactyl sodium succinate: 10–30 mg/kg of 10% solution given by ororuminal tube

Antibloat Agents
• Mineral oil: 10 ml/kg given by ororuminal tube
• Poloxalene: 30–60 mL per animal (can be repeated) by ororuminal tube
• Detergent soap can be used in emergency.

Prokinetics
• None are truly effective for promoting forestomach motility.
• Metoclopramide 0.1 mg/kg SQ q6–12h may provide some abomasal stimulation.
• Bethanechol: 0.07 mg/kg SQ q8h may provide some cecal stimulation.

Antibiotics
Necessary in infective conditions or following surgery

Transfaunation
• 4–8 L of fresh rumen juice for repopulation of rumen microbes
• Probiotic gels and yeast can be used for substitute.

Endotoxemia
Flunixin meglumine: 0.25–1.1 mg/kg IV q6–12h

CONTRAINDICATIONS
• Prokinetic drugs should not be used if obstruction present.
• Appropriate milk and meat withdrawal times must be followed for all compounds administered to food-producing animals.

PRECAUTIONS
• Prolonged use of NSAIDs can cause ulceration of abomasum and renal damage.
• Use of butorphanol or xylazine for pain control will cause ileus.

FOLLOW-UP

PATIENT MONITORING
• Once stable, refeeding should begin slowly and the animal monitored for passage of manure.
• If the urinary tract was involved, urination must be monitored.
• Patient should be monitored for recurrence of signs of abdominal pain or distension, or deteriorating cardiovascular status.

ACUTE COLIC—ABDOMINAL PAIN

PREVENTION/AVOIDANCE
• Avoid sudden feed changes.
• Ensure access to water in all weather and temperatures.
• Investigate signs of abdominal pain or distension early.
• Investigate cows not calving by their due date.

POSSIBLE COMPLICATIONS
• Peritonitis
• Adhesions
• Shock
• Endotoxemia
• Gastrointestinal or bladder rupture
• Fetal loss

EXPECTED COURSE AND PROGNOSIS
Varies with the condition

 MISCELLANEOUS

ASSOCIATED CONDITIONS
N/A

AGE-RELATED FACTORS
• Young animals more likely to have intussusception.
• Old animals more likely to have tumor, fat necrosis.
• Pregnant animals have indigestion of pregnancy/pseudo-obstruction.
• Peripartum animals predisposed to LDA, RDA <RAV, ROAV, abomasal ulcers
• Animals <18 months more likely to have urolithiasis

ZOONOTIC POTENTIAL
N/A

PREGNANCY
• Late gestation cows most likely to have indigestion of pregnancy/pseudo-obstruction, uterine torsion
• Parturition/abortion can resemble GI pain.

RUMINANT SPECIES AFFECTED
All

BIOSECURITY
N/A

PRODUCTION MANAGEMENT
N/A

SYNONYMS
Acute abdominal pain
Bloat
Colic

SEE ALSO
Individual diseases/diagnoses

ABBREVIATIONS
GI = gastrointestinal
HR = heart rate
IM = intramuscular
IV = intravenous
LDA = left displacement
NSAID = nonsteroidal anti-inflammatory drug
PCV = packed cell volume
RAV = right abomasal volvulus
RDA = right displacement
ROAV= right omasal-abomasal volvulus
SQ = subcutaneous
TP = total protein
WBC = white blood cell

Suggested Reading
Bickers, R. J., Templer, A., Cebra, C. K., Kaneps, A. J. 2000, Feb 1. Diagnosis and treatment of torsion of the spiral colon in an alpaca. *J Am Vet Med Assoc.* 216(3): 380–82.
Braun, U., Eicher, R., Hausammann, K. 1989, Sep 2. Clinical findings in cattle with dilatation and torsion of the caecum. *Vet Rec.* 125(10): 265–67.
Cable, C. S., Rebhun, W. C., Fortier, L. A. 1997, Oct 1. Cholelithiasis and cholecystitis in a dairy cow. *J Am Vet Med Assoc.* 211(7): 899–900.
Cebra, C. K., Cebra, M. L., Garry, F. B., Johnson, L. W. 1997, Sep 1. Surgical and nonsurgical correction of uterine torsion in New World camelids: 20 cases (1990–1996). *J Am Vet Med Assoc.* 211(5): 600–602.
Farrow, C. S. 1999, Jul. Reticular foreign bodies. Causative or coincidence? *Vet Clin North Am Food Anim Pract.* 15(2): 397–408.
Wikse, S. E., Craig, T. M., Hutcheson, D. P. 1991, Mar. Nutritional and dietary interrelationships with diseases of grazing beef cattle. *Vet Clin North Am Food Anim Pract.* 7(1): 143–52.

Author: Jennifer M. Ivany Ewoldt

ACUTE RENAL FAILURE

BASICS

OVERVIEW
• Acute renal failure (ARF) is caused by decline of renal function over a period of hours to days.
• This rapid onset of renal failure may result from prerenal, intrinsic renal, or postrenal causes.
• Intrinsic renal problems are usually due to ischemic or toxic insults resulting from injury, disease, or certain therapeutic agents.
• The kidneys are particularly susceptible to toxic injury.

PATHOPHYSIOLOGY
• The kidneys receive approximately 20% of cardiac output, which exposes them to a high proportion of toxicants present in the blood.
• The surface area of the large glomerular capillaries allows for a significant area of contact with toxic substances.
• The high metabolic rate of the epithelial cells in the proximal tubules and ascending loop of Henle makes them particularly susceptible to intoxication.
• Tubular epithelial cell resorption of toxins may cause excessive accumulation of toxins intracellularly.
• Tubule-concentrating ability may result in increased levels of toxicants in the distal portion of the nephron.

SIGNALMENT
All ruminants are susceptible to ARF if primary predisposing factors are present.

SIGNS
• Signs of acute renal failure are nonspecific in ruminants and may not be indicative of urinary dysfunction.
• Depending on the underlying cause, anuria, oliguria, or polyuria may be observed.
• Affected animals may present with depression, poor appetite, diarrhea, epistaxis.
• Saliva may have a strong ammonia odor.
• Severe cases develop muscular weakness and even recumbency due to electrolyte and acid-base abnormalities.
• Rectal palpation may not be remarkable although occasionally renal enlargement or perirenal edema may be detected.

CAUSES AND RISK FACTORS
• Risk of ARF is enhanced by dehydration, fever, sepsis, vasculitis, hypotension, electrolyte abnormalities, hypoalbuminemia, and exposure to nephrotoxic agents.
• Nephrotoxic agents include certain metals, antimicrobials, NSAIDs, toxic plants, hemoglobin, myoglobin, calcium oxalate, as well as other toxins.

DIAGNOSIS

DIFFERENTIAL DIAGNOSIS
• Development of a differential list is difficult due to the nonspecific clinical signs in cases of ARF and because of the variety of primary disease conditions that may predispose ruminants to ARF.
• Differentials include those diseases causing epistaxis (coagulopathies and pulmonary abscesses), diarrhea, and recumbency.

CBC/BIOCHEMISTRY/URINALYSIS
• Increased BUN and creatinine
• Isosthenuria on urinalysis indicates azotemia of renal origin.
• Proteinuria, hematuria, and granular casts may be present on UA.
• Metabolic alkalosis, hypochloremia, and hypocalcemia are common findings in ruminants with ARF.
• Hyponatremia, hyperphosphatemia, hypermagnesemia may also be seen.

OTHER LABORATORY TESTS
Fractional excretion of sodium may be evaluated but the test should be compared to a normal animal (e.g., herd mate) of similar age, physiologic state, and nutritional status.

IMAGING
Ultrasonographic evaluation may reveal enlargement of one or both kidneys or presence of perirenal edema.

DIAGNOSTIC PROCEDURES
Renal biopsy may provide diagnostic as well as prognostic information in cases of ARF.

PATHOLOGIC FINDINGS
Gross and microscopic findings depend on the initial cause of renal failure (ischemic, infectious, or toxic).

TREATMENT

• In cases of toxic nephrosis, the animal should be removed from the source of the toxin.
• If ARF is due to use of a nephrotoxic drug, treatment should be discontinued.
• Focus of treatment should be on IV fluid therapy for correction of acid-base and electrolyte abnormalities and encouragement of diuresis.
• Isotonic, sodium-containing fluids with added calcium and potassium, as indicated, should be utilized.
• Oral fluid therapy may be used if IV administration is impractical.
• IV or oral fluids should be administered at a rate of one-and-a-half to two times the adult maintenance rate of 60 ml/kg/day to encourage diuresis.
• Monitor hydration and plasma protein to avoid overhydration and edema formation.

• Once the animal begins to urinate, IV fluids should be maintained until the serum creatinine has returned to normal.
• Supportive care, which may be necessary for 2–3 weeks, includes rumen transfaunation and nutritional support.

MEDICATIONS

DRUGS OF CHOICE
• If fluid therapy does not promote diuresis, furosemide (1 mg/kg IV or IM, every 2–3 hours) may be beneficial.
• If anuria or oliguria persists, a dopamine drip (3–7 mcg/kg/min IV) should be considered.

CONTRAINDICATIONS
• With repeated use of furosemide, the patient's serum sodium and potassium must be monitored carefully.
• Drug withdrawal times need to be determined and maintained in food-producing animals.

FOLLOW-UP
N/A

MISCELLANEOUS
• ARF due to ischemic episodes generally results in a grave prognosis.
• Renal failure due to toxic causes may have a more favorable prognosis with early intervention and aggressive fluid therapy.

SEE ALSO
Diarrhea
Epistaxis (coagulopathies and pulmonary abscesses)
Recumbency

ABBREVIATIONS
ARF = acute renal failure
BUN = blood urea nitrogen
IM = intramuscular
IV = intravenous
NSAIDs = nonsteroidal anti-inflammatory drugs

Suggested Reading
Anderson, D. E., Constable, P. D., Yvorchuk, K. E., Anderson, N. V., St-Jean, G., Rock, L. 1994, May-Jun. Hyperlipemia and ketonuria in an alpaca and a llama. *J Vet Intern Med.* 8(3):207–11.
Pugh, D. G. 2002. *Sheep and goat medicine.* Philadelphia: W. B. Saunders.
Schlumbohm, C., Harmeyer, J. 2004 Feb. Hyperketonemia impairs glucose metabolism in pregnant and nonpregnant ewes. *J Dairy Sci.* 87(2):350–58.

Author: M. S. Gill

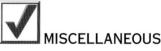

BASICS

OVERVIEW
• *Aesculus* is a toxic tree or shrub that may produce neurotoxicity in cattle or sheep. The tree is commonly observed in the eastern United States and in Europe in wooded areas or fencerows.
• Leaves are opposite palmately compound and consist of 5–7 leaflets.
• Fruit is a leathery capsule with or without spines (depending on species).
• Nuts are chocolate in color with a tan scar.
• Bark, leaves, and especially fruit are toxic, containing the glycosides aesculin and fraxin and neurotoxic saponins.

SIGNALMENT
Affects ruminant animals of all ages although cattle seem more often affected

SIGNS
• Onset of signs may be 12–16 hours after consuming buckeye.
• In calves, 0.5% body weight of nuts has produced poisoning.
• Initial signs in ruminants are staggering, weakness, muscle twitching, and an incoordinated gait.
• Recumbency may occur in severe cases followed by coma and death.
• Death is rare.

CAUSES AND RISK FACTORS
• Toxicosis may occur in the spring when young foliage is abundant.
• Toxicosis often occurs in the fall from ingestion of the nuts.
• Animals seldom eat the nuts if ample good-quality forage is available.

DIAGNOSIS

DIFFERENTIAL DIAGNOSIS
Other causes of CNS signs in cattle include hypomagnesemia, polio, *Claviceps paspali*, lead, arsenic, *Clostridium botulinum* type D, and insecticide poisonings.

CBC/BIOCHEMISTRY/URINALYSIS
• Blood glucose may be high.
• Glucosuria and proteinuria may be present in severe cases.

OTHER LABORATORY TESTS
N/A

IMAGING
N/A

DIAGNOSTIC PROCEDURES
N/A

PATHOLOGIC FINDINGS
No specific lesions are observed.

TREATMENT
No specific treatment

MEDICATIONS

DRUGS OF CHOICE
• Laxatives—mineral oil: 1/2–1 gallon for adult cow
• Activated charcoal—1/2–1 pound for adult cow
• IV calcium gluconate—500 ml/for adult cow
• IV 50% dextrose—500 ml/for adult cow
• If cases are found are found soon enough, stimulants and purgatives are indicated.

CONTRAINDICATIONS
• Appropriate milk and meat withdrawal times must be followed for all compounds administered to food-producing animals.
• Steroids should not be used in pregnant animals.

FOLLOW-UP

PATIENT MONITORING
N/A

PREVENTION/AVOIDANCE
• Provide ample good quality forage so that animals are not forced to ingest buckeye.
• Remove buckeye trees in areas where cattle graze.

POSSIBLE COMPLICATIONS
N/A

EXPECTED COURSE AND PROGNOSIS
• Mild cases of buckeye toxicosis respond without treatment if the source of the toxin is removed.
• More severe cases respond quickly following treatment and may be normal in 12–24 hours.
• Prognosis is poor for recumbent animals.

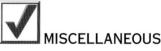
MISCELLANEOUS

ASSOCIATED CONDITIONS
• Initial signs in ruminants are staggering, weakness, muscle twitching, and an incoordinated gait.
• Recumbency may occur in severe cases followed by coma and death.
• Death is rare.

AGE-RELATED FACTOR
In calves, 0.5% body weight of nuts has produced poisoning.

ZOONOTIC POTENTIAL
N/A

PREGNANCY
N/A

RUMINANT SPECIES AFFECTED
Cattle, sheep; potentially all ruminant species

BIOSECURITY
N/A

PRODUCTION MANAGEMENT
N/A

SEE ALSO
Arsenic
Claviceps paspali
Clostridium botulinum type D
Hypomagnesemia
Insecticide poisonings
Lead
Polioencephalomalacia

ABBREVIATIONS
CNS = central nervous system

Suggested Reading
Burrows, G. E., Tyrl, R. S. 2001. *Toxic plants of North America*. Ames: Iowa State University Press.
Hulbert, L. C., Oehme, F. W. 1968. *Plants poisonous to livestock*. Manhattan: Kansas State University Printing Service.
Knight, A. P., Walter, R. G. 2001. *A guide to plant poisoning of animals in North America*. Jackson, WY: Teton New Media.

Author: Larry A. Kerr

AGRICULTURAL CHEMICAL TOXICITIES

BASICS

OVERVIEW
This chapter focuses on the ingestion, inhalation, and/or topical exposure to agricultural chemical compounds resulting in morbidity and/or mortality. Compounds include the following:
• Chlorinated hydrocarbons—a group of insecticides that incorporate a chlorine molecule and are also known as organochlorines. They are mostly known for their environmental persistence and bioaccumulation (concentration levels of compound increase in animals higher up in the food chain).
• Herbicides—compounds used for weed control. Many are selective against specific plants or types of plants.
• Fungicides—compounds used to treat or prevent fungal infections in plants or animals
• Polybrominated biphenyls (PBBs)—chemicals that were primarily used in industry as fire retardants in the 1970s
• Dinitro compounds—herbicides that are highly toxic to all animals

PATHOPHYSIOLOGY
• The mechanism of action in animals of most of these agricultural chemicals is unknown.
• Many of these chemicals, especially the herbicides, are frequently used in most agricultural crop enterprises today.
• Their widespread use can create opportunity for exposure.
• Toxicity typically occurs through oral or dermal exposure.
• The currently available fungicides appear to be some of the safest chemicals discussed here due to their inefficient digestive absorption as well as their low toxicity in mammals.
• Aerosol exposure to fungicides can cause irritation to the eyes and respiratory tract.
• Most of the highly toxic and environmentally persistent compounds are no longer available in the United States today, but can be found worldwide.
• Many of these compounds (especially many of the chlorinated hydrocarbons and all PBBs) are still present worldwide due to their previous extensive use and potential for bioaccumulation.
• Acute toxicities due to accidental exposures are the most common presentation.
• This exposure can occur either through contaminated feeds, access to stored chemicals or treated seeds for planting, or sometimes through exposure to fields or pastures recently treated with these chemicals.
• Fields treated with chemicals many times require livestock access to be limited for some period of time; always read and follow label directions.
• Acute toxicities will usually show up in the first 24 hours postexposure (ranging from a few hours up to a day or more).

• Systemic absorption will usually result in these compounds ending up in particular areas, especially the liver, brain, kidney, fat, and milk.
• Transplacental transmission can occur with some chemicals (especially the chlorinated hydrocarbons).
• Most toxicities will result in minimal or nonspecific manifestations.
• Carbamates are a type of herbicide with cholinesterase-inhibiting properties similar to organophosphates.
• Cerebral and spinal cord congestion are probably the most common presentation along with pulmonary congestion.
• Congestion of kidneys, liver, and spinal cord can also be seen.
• Liver injury can be common, especially with chronic exposure.

SYSTEMS AFFECTED
Systems affected vary with the different class of chemicals as well as a particular chemical within a class.
• Cardiovascular—methemoglobinemia (chlorate herbicides), cardiac arrest
• Endocrine/metabolic—pyrexia
• Gastrointestinal—anorexia, excess salivation, decreased rumen motility, bloat, digestive irritation and abdominal pain (especially some herbicides), diarrhea
• Hepatobiliary—congestion, hepatic lipidosis or amyloidosis
• Herd health—decreased milk production (PBBs), tainted milk (chlorinated hydrocarbons and PBBs), chronic poor performance
• Musculoskeletal—incoordination, recumbency, anorexia, extended hoof growth (PBBs)
• Nervous—stimulation or depression, ataxia, apprehension, hypersensitivity, muscle fasciculation, seizures, coma, death
• Ophthalmic—irritation (aerosol exposure), nystagmus
• Renal/urologic—congestion, nephritis (PBBs)
• Reproductive—early embryonic death (PBBs); cross placental barrier (chlorinated hydrocarbons)
• Respiratory—tachypnea, dyspnea, congestion
• Skin—alopecia (PBBs)

GENETICS
None

INCIDENCE/PREVALENCE
Rare

GEOGRAPHIC DISTRIBUTION
• Widespread use of many of these chemicals in today's agriculture.
• Many chlorinated hydrocarbons and all PBBs have been banned from use in many countries.

SIGNALMENT
Species
Susceptibility among compounds varies between ruminant species.

Breed Predilections
None

Mean Age and Range
None

Predominant Sex
None

SIGNS
Clinical signs or death are commonly seen within 24 hours of an acute exposure.

HISTORICAL FINDINGS
• Whole herd or a large percentage of the herd will usually be affected.
• Individual clinical signs may differ, but there usually will be a common system affected.
• Severe signs, including death, will be more common in the very young or old.
• Usually a new feed batch or pasture recently treated can be identified.
• Chronic exposures can be very difficult to identify.

PHYSICAL EXAMINATION FINDINGS
Elevated temperatures can be recorded due to seizuring or other excessive muscle movement.

CAUSES
• Exposure to significant amounts of these chemicals
• Toxicity levels vary for each compound as well as for the species involved.

RISK FACTORS
• Improper storage or labeling of chemicals
• Proper disposal of chemicals should have been followed especially for those products with bioaccumulation capabilities (chlorinated hydrocarbons, PBBs).
• Age of animals—very young or very old are at higher risk.
• Preexisting health and nutritional status
• Amount of exposure and time before first identified
• Dependent on chemical used, concentration, and formulation

DIAGNOSIS

History of possible exposure to chemicals directly to affected animal or to area/pasture where they were applied is suggestive.

DIFFERENTIAL DIAGNOSIS
• Neurologic signs—rabies, polioencephalomalacia, nervous ketosis, nervous coccidiosis, infectious thromboembolic meningoencephalitis, lead as well as other poisonings
• Digestive signs—poisonous plants, coccidiosis, grain overload, frothy or gas bloat
• Respiratory signs—infectious respiratory complex, nitrate toxicity (chlorate herbicides), bloat, acidosis, or other poisonings

CBC/BIOCHEMISTRY/URINALYSIS
- Increased SGOT (PBBs)
- Mostly unremarkable CBC and panels
- Urine can be analyzed in some instances for chemicals or their by-products.

OTHER LABORATORY TESTS
- Chromatography or other specialized tests can be run on frozen samples of brain, liver, kidney, fat, stomach contents, and suspected samples. These tests cannot be run on formalin-fixed tissues.
- Normal workup to rule out the more common infectious agents

IMAGING
N/A

DIAGNOSTIC PROCEDURES
Fat biopsies, urine, and milk samples sometimes can be used to determine possible exposure.

PATHOLOGIC FINDINGS
- Usually unremarkable
- Many times will have pulmonary, renal, hepatic, or brain and spinal congestion
- Petechial hemorrhages or blanching of the gastrointestinal tract
- Cardiac parenchymal petechial hemorrhages suggestive of sudden death

TREATMENT

APPROPRIATE HEALTH CARE
- Immediate removal of possible contaminated source
- Barbiturates, chloral hydrate, or diazepam for convulsing animals
- Activated charcoal (900 g/adult cow)
- Mineral oil drench
- For chloral hydrate herbicide poisoning and methemoglobinemia, use a 2%–4% solution of methylene blue at 10 mg/kg IV.
- Appropriate milk and meat withdrawal times must be followed for all compounds administered to food-producing animals.

NURSING CARE
Supportive care including IV fluids may be helpful.

ACTIVITY
Restrict activity and minimize stimulation.

DIET
Roughage diet may be needed if rumen motility was affected.

CLIENT EDUCATION
- Proper storage and disposal of chemicals as directed by labels
- Limit access of livestock to treated areas if indicated by label

SURGICAL CONSIDERATIONS
N/A

MEDICATIONS

DRUGS OF CHOICE
N/A

CONTRAINDICATIONS
Do not use corn oil or other type of digestible oil in drenching. These oils can increase the absorption of some chemicals. Only use mineral oil.

POSSIBLE INTERACTIONS
N/A

ALTERNATIVE DRUGS
N/A

FOLLOW-UP

PATIENT MONITORING
- Seizuring animals usually will do so only for the first 24 hours.
- Animal/milk testing may be needed to determine amount of contamination and expected time needed to clear their system based on half-life of chemical.

PREVENTION/AVOIDANCE
- Proper storage and disposal of all chemicals on farm
- Proper labeling of all chemicals
- Do not store chemicals next to feedstuffs.

POSSIBLE COMPLICATIONS
- Some animals may not recover.
- Some animals and/or their products (milk) may never be able to enter the human food chain.

EXPECTED COURSE AND PROGNOSIS
- Highly variable
- Severity of signs at any one point in time is not indicative of prognosis; must be able to monitor the progress before a better prognosis can be made.
- Poor future performance is possible.

MISCELLANEOUS

ASSOCIATED CONDITIONS
N/A

AGE-RELATED FACTORS
N/A

ZOONOTIC POTENTIAL
- There is potential for agricultural chemical exposure to animals from milk and meat of poisoned animals.
- In some states, there are restrictions on movement or marketing of cattle poisoned with agricultural chemicals.
- The veterinarian should consult the local diagnostic laboratory or department of public health for questions specific to their practice area.

PREGNANCY
Early embryonic deaths have been attributed to PBBs.

RUMINANT SPECIES AFFECTED
All ruminant species are susceptible to toxicosis.

BIOSECURITY
N/A

PRODUCTION MANAGEMENT
- Proper storage and disposal of all chemicals on farm
- Proper labeling of all chemicals
- Do not store chemicals next to feedstuffs.

SYNONYMS
Chlorinated hydrocarbons are also known as organochlorines.

SEE ALSO
FARAD
Specific toxicity chapters
Toxicology: herd outbreaks

ABBREVIATIONS
FARAD = Food Animal Residue Avoidance Databank
IV = intravenous
PBBs = polybrominated biphenyls
SGOT = serum glutamic oxaloacetic transaminase

Suggested Reading
Campagnolo, E. R., Kasten, S., Banerjee, M. 2002, Oct. Accidental ammonia exposure to county fair show livestock due to contaminated drinking water. *Vet Hum Toxicol.* 44(5): 282–85.
Coppock, R. W., Mostrom, M. S., Khan, A. A., Semalulu, S. S. 1995, Dec. Toxicology of oil field pollutants in cattle: a review. *Vet Hum Toxicol.* 37(6): 569–76.
Galey, F. D. 2000, Nov. Diagnostic toxicology for the food animal practitioner. *Vet Clin North Am Food Anim Pract.* 16(3): 409–21.
Hoff, B., Boermans, H. J., Baird, J. D. 1998, Jan. Retrospective study of toxic metal analyses requested at a veterinary diagnostic toxicology laboratory in Ontario (1990–1995). *Can Vet J.* 39(1): 39–43.
Reigart, J. R., Roberts, J. R. 1999. *Recognition and management of pesticide poisonings.* 5th ed. Washington, DC: U.S. Environmental Protection Agency. Also available online http://www.epa.gov/pesticides/safety/healthcare.
Smith, R. A. 2000, Nov. Toxicology. *Vet Clin North Am Food Anim Pract.* 16(3): 545–57.
Villar, D., Schwartz, K. J., Carson, T. L., Kinker, J. A., Barker, J. 2003, Mar. Acute poisoning of cattle by fertilizer-contaminated water. *Vet Hum Toxicol.* 45(2): 88–90.

Author: Alejandro Ramirez

AKABANE

 BASICS

DEFINITION
Akabane, also known as congenital arthrogryposis-hydranencephaly syndrome, is a viral disease of ruminants that has the potential for serious economic losses. It results in abortions, stillbirths, premature births, and deformities of the fetus or newborn with no clinical signs in the dam during pregnancy.

PATHOPHYSIOLOGY
• The Akabane virus is an arbovirus (transmitted by arthropods) in the family Bunyaviridae, genus *Orthobunyavirus*.
• The single-stranded RNA virus causes intrauterine infection of the fetus in pregnant cattle, sheep, and goats. After invading the endothelium of the placenta, the virus replicates in the trophoblastic cells and the fetus itself, resulting in death or deformities of the fetus or newborn.
• Akabane is similar to Cache Valley virus, which is found in the United States.
• The vector for Akabane virus has not been proven, however epidemiological evidence suggests that mosquitoes and gnats spread the virus.
• Akabane virus has been isolated from a number of mosquito species (*Aedes, Culex, Anopheles*) as well as *Culicoides* species (biting midges).
• Direct contact, infected tissues, exudates, body fluids, or fomites do not transmit Akabane.
• Ruminants do not appear to become long-term carriers of this virus.

SYSTEMS AFFECTED
• Reproductive—arthrogryposis-hydranencephaly syndrome, abortions, stillbirths
• Musculoskeletal—arthrogryposis (persistent flexion of joints)
• Neurological—hydranencephaly (absence of the cerebral hemisphere tissue, which becomes occupied by cerebrospinal fluid)

GENETICS
N/A

INCIDENCE/PREVALENCE
• Incidence for Akabane and the potential for epizootics is correlated with climatic factors, a distinct seasonal pattern (warm, moist summer and autumn months), the geographic distribution of competent vectors, and the availability of susceptible ruminant populations.
• In endemic areas, most animals are immune to Akabane virus by the time they reach sexual maturity.

• Surveys indicate that more then 80% of adult cattle in an endemic area are seropositive for the virus. However, following years of drought or times of reduced vector populations, native livestock may not be exposed prior to breeding age and therefore become susceptible.
• Data from Japanese and Australian outbreaks suggest that the virus subsequently may invade the fetus in approximately 30–40% of infected pregnant cows.

GEOGRAPHIC DISTRIBUTION
• Akabane is a foreign animal disease in the United States. It is, however, common in the tropics and subtropics. It is considered endemic in northern Australia, Japan, Israel, and Korea. Occasional outbreaks have occurred in southern Australia, Asia, the Middle East, and South Africa, when conditions are favorable for virus transmission.
• Outbreaks typically occur in areas where naïve and susceptible animals are located and when environmental conditions are favorable for the disease.
• Most epizootics occur at the northern and southern periphery of the endemic band or to susceptible animals introduced into endemic areas.
• Outbreaks usually occur in late winter, indicating that the peak of virus activity and fetal infections occurs during the previous late summer and early autumn periods.

SIGNALMENT

Species
Disease from Akabane virus only occurs in cattle, sheep and goats; however, antibodies to the virus have been found in horses, buffalo, deer, camels, dogs, monkeys, and most recently pigs.

Breed Predilections
N/A

Mean Age and Range
• The disease primarily affects fetal or newborn cattle, sheep, and goats.
• Adult animals do not typically show any sign of the disease. However, there has recently been documentation of five adult cattle in Korea that have developed neurological signs (encephalomyelitis) due to the virus.

Predominant Sex
N/A

SIGNS

GENERAL COMMENTS
• Adult ruminants with Akabane infection are typically asymptomatic.
• Viremia usually occurs 1–6 days after infection and lasts for 1–9 days. Only during this limited time are viral titers sufficient for potential vectors.
• Long-term carriers of the disease are not believed to occur.

HISTORICAL FINDINGS
Cases will most likely be noted in naïve pregnant animals that have been introduced into an endemic area or have had exposure to competent vectors.

PHYSICAL EXAMINATION FINDINGS
• Congenital abnormalities of the fetus or newborn are the hallmark of this disease. Effects on the young vary depending on the stage of gestation reached at the time of infection.
• When infected late in the first trimester, animals are usually born bright and alert but are unable to stand, are ataxic, and may have one or more paralyzed limbs.
• Muscle atrophy, limb rotation, exophthalmos (protruding eyes), and abnormal vocalization may also occur.
• Animals infected during the second trimester have arthrogryposis at birth; most cannot stand. The joints are rigid and fixed in flexion and muscles are severely atrophied.
• Torticollis, scoliosis, and kyphosis may also be seen.
• When infected late in pregnancy, animals can usually stand and walk, but have behavioral abnormalities, such as slow or absent suckle reflex, depression, dullness, periodic hyperexcitablility, incoordination, and blindness.
• Skull deformities can be common.
• Dystocia at parturition may occur due to the deformities of the fetus.

CAUSES
• Akabane virus is transmitted by arthropods (biting midges, mosquitoes) and the virus affects the developing fetus in ruminants.
• Outbreaks are typically related to seasonal conditions that enhance the vectors.

RISK FACTORS
The major risk factor for Akabane is exposure of pregnant ruminants (particularly naïve animals) to potential vectors in endemic areas.

 DIAGNOSIS

A presumptive diagnosis of Akabane disease can be made on the basis of clinical and postmortem examination. Diagnosis is typically confirmed by serology.

DIFFERENTIAL DIAGNOSIS
• Cache Valley virus
• Bluetongue
• Bovine viral diarrhea
• Border disease
• Wesselsbron virus
• Nutritional, genetic, or toxic causes of abortion and/or fetal deformities

CBC/BIOCHEMISTRY/URINALYSIS
N/A

OTHER LABORATORY TESTS
• Virus isolation should be done but is rarely successful unless the fetus and placenta were aborted before the fetus developed an immune response.
• Specimens to collect include the placenta, fetal muscle, cerebrospinal fluid, and fetal nervous tissue.
• Serology may be performed on fetal or precolostral serum and the serum from the dam.
• Histopathology of the spleen, liver, lung, kidney, heart, lymph nodes, affected muscle, spinal cord, and brain can also be done.

IMAGING
N/A

DIAGNOSTIC PROCEDURES
N/A

PATHOLOGIC FINDINGS
• Arthrogryposis and hydranencephaly are the most commonly noted lesions.
• Most of the affected joints are ankylosed and cannot be straightened.
• Other neurological lesions may include hydrocephalus, agenesis of the brain, microencephaly, proencephaly, and cerebellar cavitation.
• Additionally, fibrinous leptomeningitis or ependymitis, spinal cord agenesis or hypoplasia, torticollis, scoliosis, brachygnathism, cataracts, ophthalmia (severe inflammation of the eye), hypoplastic skeletal muscles and lungs, or fibrinous polyarticular synovitis may be seen.

TREATMENT

APPROPRIATE HEALTH CARE
• There is no effective treatment for Akabane virus.
• Most affected neonates die or must be euthanized soon after being born.
• Animals with mild symptoms may gradually become more mobile, but most die by 6 months.
• Subsequent pregnancies of the infected dam will not be affected.

NURSING CARE
N/A

ACTIVITY
N/A

DIET
N/A

CLIENT EDUCATION
In endemic areas, advise clients of the risks to newly introduced animals, especially during late summer and autumn months.

SURGICAL CONSIDERATIONS
N/A

MEDICATIONS

DRUGS OF CHOICE
N/A

CONTRAINDICATIONS
N/A

PRECAUTIONS
N/A

POSSIBLE INTERACTIONS
N/A

ALTERNATIVE DRUGS
N/A

FOLLOW-UP

PATIENT MONITORING
N/A

PREVENTION/AVOIDANCE
• Prevention of Akabane disease includes vector control measures and vaccination. Akabane virus does not appear to be transmitted between animals, except by arthropod vectors.
• Prevention efforts should include elimination of vector breeding sites, and repellants or screened housing for pregnant animals.
• Avoid breeding ruminants during the prime transmission season (late summer and autumn).
• An inactivated and an attenuated vaccine have been developed and used in Japan. An effective killed vaccine has been developed but not marketed in Australia. The vaccines must be used prior to exposure to the infected vectors. A vaccine is not currently available in the United States.

POSSIBLE COMPLICATIONS
N/A

EXPECTED COURSE AND PROGNOSIS
Most affected neonates die or must be euthanized soon after being born. Subsequent pregnancies of the infected dam will not be affected.

MISCELLANEOUS

ASSOCIATED CONDITIONS
N/A

AGE-RELATED FACTORS
Akabane affects fetal or newborn cattle, sheep, and goats.

ZOONOTIC POTENTIAL
There is no evidence that humans can be infected by Akabane virus.

PREGNANCY
Effects of Akabane virus are dependent on the stage of pregnancy when infected. However, most affected neonates die or must be euthanized soon after birth despite the time of infection.

RUMINANT SPECIES AFFECTED
Cattle, sheep, and goats

BIOSECURITY
Suspected cases or outbreaks of Akabane outside of its endemic area (see geographical distribution), should immediately be reported to the proper governmental veterinary authorities (e.g., state or federal veterinarian).

PRODUCTION MANAGEMENT
• In endemic areas, avoid introducing naïve pregnant animal in summer and autumn.
• Implement vector control measures to reduce the potential transmission of the virus.
• Consider vaccination protocols prior to breeding.

SYNONYMS
Acorn calves
Congenital arthrogryposis-hydranencephaly (A-H) syndrome
Congenital bovine epizootic A-H syndrome
Curly calf disease
Curly lamb disease
Dummy calf disease
Silly calves

SEE ALSO
Arthrogryposis
Bluetongue
Border disease
Bovine viral diarrhea
Cache Valley virus
Nutritional, genetic, or toxic causes of abortion and/or fetal deformities
Wesselsbron virus

ABBREVIATIONS
A-H = arthrogryposis-hydranencephaly

Suggested Reading
Charles, J. A. 1994. Akabane virus. *Vet Clin North Am Food Anim Pract.* 10(3): 525–46.
Foreign Animal Disease Gray Book. Akabane. Accessed at http://www.vet.uga.edu/vpp/gray_book/FAD/AKA.htm.
Kirkland, P. D. 2002. Akabane and bovine ephemeral fever virus infections. *Vet Clin North Am Food Anim Pract.* 18:501–14.

Author: Glenda Dvorak

ALOPECIA

 BASICS

DEFINITION
• Alopecia means partial or complete loss of hairs in an area where hairs are normally found.
• The terms "hair loss" and "alopecia" are often used interchangeably.
• The term "hypotrichosis" is a more accurate term for congenital or hereditary hair loss or alopecia because it refers to less than an expected amount of hair.

PATHOPHYSIOLOGY
• There are two major etiologies of alopecia or hair loss: *congenital or hereditary* and *acquired.*
• Acquired hair loss is the result of any disease that causes direct damage to the hair follicle or skin (e.g., dermatophytosis) or indirect damage (e.g., pruritus).
• Acquired hair loss may or may not be permanent depending upon the amount of follicular damage.
• Congenital alopecia may or may not be hereditary and it is caused by the lack of the development of hair follicles. These changes are permanent.

• Congenital alopecia is usually evident shortly after birth.
• Hereditary alopecia may be evident shortly after birth or may develop as the animal ages.

SYSTEMS AFFECTED
Skin

GENETICS
Hereditary and/or congenital alopecia are rare and several syndromes have been described (see Alopecia Table 1).

INCIDENCE/PREVALENCE
• Acquired alopecia is a common skin disease in ruminants.
• Hereditary and/or congenital alopecia is rare.

GEOGRAPHIC DISTRIBUTION
N/A

SIGNALMENT
• Congenital and/or hereditary alopecia may or may not be sex linked (Table 1).
• Congenital and/or hereditary alopecia is usually evident at birth or shortly thereafter (Table 1).
• The signalment of inflammatory causes of hair loss reflect those of the underlying disease.

SIGNS
• Alopecia may be focal, multifocal, symmetrical, or generalized.
• Alopecia may develop acutely or gradually depending upon the cause.
• Hyperpigmentation, lichenification, erythema, and pruritus are common findings in acquired alopecia.
• Acquired alopecia may also be complicated by bacterial infections and/or seborrhea.
• Congenital, hereditary, and endocrine alopecia is noninflammatory unless complicated by secondary infections or damage to the skin.

CAUSES
• Diseases that destroy or damage hairs/hair follicles include bacterial skin diseases, dermatophytosis, demodicosis, severe inflammatory diseases, trauma, burns, frostbite, poisonings, and parasites.
• Diseases that slow hair growth include poor nutrition and protein deficiencies.
• Pregnancy, lactation, severe illness, and/or fever can cause a temporary alopecia characterized by large amounts of shedding within a few days.
• Anagen defluxion occurs as a result of acute damage/cessation of growth in a growing hair shaft characterized by sudden massive hair loss.

• Telogen defluxion occurs as a result of stressful situations (fever, illness, shock, anesthesia, surgery, etc.) that cause cessation of anagen hairs and synchrony of hair follicles into telogen and loss of hairs 1–2 months post event.
• Any disease that causes pruritus (parasites, allergies, neoplasia) may result in hair loss.
• Friction can cause local hair loss.
• Alopecia areata is a rare disease that can cause focal noninflammatory alopecia in cattle.
• Follicular dysplasia can present as focal, regional, or diffuse adult onset slowly progressive noninflammatory hair loss.

RISK FACTORS
• Calves, kids, and lambs that develop severe illness and/or fevers are at risk for anagen defluxion.
• Animals undergoing stressful situations are at risk for development of telogen defluxion.
• Overcrowding, poor nutrition, and poor management may predispose animals to diseases associated with acquired hair loss.

DIAGNOSIS

DIFFERENTIAL DIAGNOSIS
• Focal, regional, or generalized hair loss in a neonate—congenital or hereditary hair loss

• Focal inflammatory alopecia: dermatophytosis, dermatophilosis, demodicosis, parasitic diseases, and staphylococcal folliculitis
• Focal noninflammatory hair loss: alopecia areata
• Generalized acute alopecia—telogen or anagen defluxion
• Excessive generalized hair loss in spring—abnormal spring shed
• Patchy hair loss in individual animals that have normal skin—abnormal shedding
• Adult onset slowly progressive alopecia-follicular dysplasia

CBC/BIOCHEMISTRY/URINALYSIS
Routine laboratory tests are not usually very helpful in the diagnosis of alopecia.

OTHER LABORATORY TESTS
N/A

IMAGING
N/A

DIAGNOSTIC PROCEDURES
• Skin scrapings to look for mites
• Flea combings to look for macroscopic parasites (lice, keds, fleas)
• Fungal culture for dermatophytosis
• Skin biopsy can help differentiate between acquired and congenital/hereditary causes of alopecia.

• Skin biopsy is the most cost effective diagnostic test.
• Hair trichogram for differentiation of anagen versus telogen defluxion

PATHOLOGICAL FINDINGS
• Anagen defluxion hairs have irregular and dysplastic hair shafts, hairs break easily.
• Telogen defluxion hairs have a normal, uniform shaft diameter, clubbed nonpigmented root lacking a root sheath.
• Small or absent hair follicles with little or no inflammatory changes are present in skin biopsies from congenital and hereditary alopecia.
• Inflammatory changes characterize acquired alopecia; special stains may identify infectious agents (e.g., dermatophytes).
• Atrophic, distorted hair follicles with melanin clumping are seen in follicular dysplasia.

TREATMENT
• Depends upon underlying cause
• No treatment for congenital or hereditary hair loss
• Successful treatment depends upon the underlying cause and diagnosis.

ALOPECIA

 MISCELLANEOUS

ASSOCIATED CONDITIONS
N/A

AGE-RELATED FACTORS
N/A

ZOONOTIC POTENTIAL
Some causes of acquired alopecia are of zoonotic importance.

PREGNANCY
N/A

RUMINANT SPECIES AFFECTED
Cattle, goats, sheep, llamas, camels; potentially all species

BIOSECURITY
Highly contagious parasitic diseases may require quarantine of specific animals or herds.

PRODUCTION MANAGEMENT
• Acquired causes of hair loss can cause decreased milk, meat, or reproduction depending upon the cause.
• Congenital and/or hereditary alopecia compromise the health of the animal because of the lack of normal protection.

SYNONYMS
Hair loss, hypotrichosis

SEE ALSO
Camelid dermatology
Dairy goat dermatology
Dermatologic pharmacology
Dermatophilosis
Hypothyroidism
Mange

ABBREVIATIONS
N/A

Suggested Reading
Drogemuller, C., Kuiper, H., Peters, M., Guionaud, S., Distl, O., Leeb, T. 2002. Congenital hypotrichosis with anodontia in cattle: a genetic, clinical and histological analysis. *Veterinary Dermatology* 13:307–13.
Howard, J. L., Smith, R. A. 1999. Skin diseases. In: *Current veterinary therapy 4: food animal practice*. Philadelphia: W. B. Saunders.
Martin, W. B., Aitken, I. D., eds. Skin diseases. In: *Diseases of sheep*. 3rd ed. Edinburgh: Blackwell Science.
Rebhun, W. C. 1995. Skin diseases. In: *Diseases of dairy cattle*. Baltimore: Williams and Wilkins.
Scott, D. W. 1988. Congenital and hereditary diseases. In: *Large animal dermatology*. Philadelphia: W. B. Saunders.
Steffen, D. J. 1993. Congenital skin abnormalities. *Veterinary Clinics of North America Food Animal Practice* 9(1): 105–14.

Authors: Karen A. Moriello and Susan D. Semrad

Table 1

Summary of Congenital and/or Hereditary Types of Hypotrichosis				
Name	Breeds Affected	Mode of Inheritance	Clinical Appearance	Other
Lethal hypotrichosis	Holstein-Friesians Japanese	Simple autosomal recessive	Calves die within hours, hair present only on muzzle, eyelids, ears, tail, pasterns	Hypoplasia of thyroid can occur.
Semihairlessness	Herefords and Polled Herefords	Simple autosomal recessive	Calves viable at birth but have thin, short, curly coat; coat is wiry and thin as animal matures and skin is wrinkled.	Calves do not grow well, can have "wild temperament."
Hypotrichosis and anodontia	Maine-Anjou Normandy mixed cattle	Sex-linked recessive	Affected calves born hairless and toothless, develop fine downy hair coat	Have long protruding tongue, defective horns, hypoplastic testicles
Viable hypotrichosis	Guernseys, Jerseys, Holsteins, Hereford	Simple autosomal recessive	Nearly hairless at birth, varying amounts of hair develop as animal ages	Some animals have dermal atriovenous anastomosis.
Variable hypotrichosis	Ayrshire, polled Herefords	Autosomal recessive	Animals born with fine, sparse, hair with thin epidermis, generalized but some regions (tail, distal limbs, eyelids, ears) may be less affected Affected calves cannot tolerate cold or extreme heat.	
Hypotrichosis and missing incisors	Holstein-Friesians, Maine-Anjou cross, Normandy	Trait linked and incompletely dominant	Patchy hypotrichosis on face and neck and lack 4–6 incisors Mild disease in cows with lusterless stubbly hypopigmented coats	
Streaked hypotrichosis	Female Holstein-Friesians	Sex-linked dominant, lethal to males	Animals lack hair in vertical streaks on hips, legs, sides.	
Tardive hypotrichosis	Female Holstein-Friesians	Sex-linked recessive	Animals normal at birth, develop hair loss at 6 weeks to 6 months of age	Hair loss is symmetrical, starts on face and neck, proceeds caudally.
Inherited congenital hypotrichosis	Polled Dorset sheep	Unknown	Hairs absent from face, ears, and lower legs, no eyelashes, skin is thickened, wrinkled, greasy, and scaly and erythematous	Excessive lacrimation
BVDV induced Hypotrichosis	Any	Viral Inutero infection with BVDV	Thin hair coat	
Badly calf syndrome	Female Holstein-Friesians	Autosomal recessive, homozygous state is usually lethal to males.	Affected calves normal at birth but live only 6–8 months; at 1–2 months they lose condition and develop generalized hair loss. Male Holstein calves may enter veal market. before clinical signs are seen.	Affected individuals have persistent salivation; clinical signs may resemble zinc deficiency. Ears may curl.
Viable hypotrichosis	Polled Dorset sheep	Simple autosomal recessive	Hypotrichotic at birth especially on face	
Cross-related hypotrichosis (rat tail)	Simmental-Angus and Simmental-Holstein	Unknown	Color dilution, sparse and short curly hair, tail switch is poor, hence rat tail name OR Color dilution, short curly hairs that are not sparse	Decreased growth

Source: Adapted from Scott, 1988.

ANALYTICAL TESTING

 BASICS

OVERVIEW
• Energy status, protein values, liver function, macromineral levels, micromineral levels, vitamin status of domestic livestock and wild ruminants are important in the animals' ability to maintain a healthy immune system.
• Measuring serum levels as a diagnostic/prognostic indicator of health is a crucial tool in maintaining healthy animal populations.

SYSTEMS AFFECTED
Potentially all systems can be affected.

GENETICS
N/A

INCIDENCE/PREVALENCE
N/A

GEOGRAPHIC DISTRIBUTION
N/A

SIGNALMENT
Species
All ruminant species

Breed Predilections
N/A

Mean Age and Range
N/A

Predominant Sex
N/A

 DIAGNOSIS

CBC/BIOCHEMISTRY/URINALYSIS
OTHER LABORATORY TESTS
Energy Status
Energy balance is by far one of the most critical nutritional factors in animal health, lactation, and reproductive performance. Traditionally we have monitored changes in energy balance via body weight and condition changes over time. This procedure, however, may not be a sensitive enough tool when dealing with the transition cow.
• NEFA—Nonesterified fatty acids
  • Serum NEFA concentration is directly associated with adipose tissue catabolism of triglycerides and is a measure of energy balance.
  • Feeding of dietary fats can slightly elevate serum NEFA, but not significantly to alter interpretation of energy balance.
  • Serum or plasma concentrations range from <0.1 to 2.5 mEq/L (<0.1–2.5 mmol/L).
  • Concentrations are higher prior to a major feeding bout and reduce significantly following feeding. There is less significant variation in total mixed ration fed farms.
  • Reasonably stable in serum or plasma, but concentration greatly affected by hemolysis (lowers value)

• BHB—β-hydroxybutyrate
  • One of three ketone bodies generated by partial oxidation of fatty acids
  • Can be elevated due to dietary sources (dietary ketosis), primarily poorly fermented silages high in butyric acid; butyric acid converted to BHB by rumen epithelium
  • Serum or plasma concentrations range from <1 mg/dL (0.1 mmol/L) to >40 mg/dL (0.38 mmol/L)
    1. Subclinical ketosis: >14.5 mg/dL (1.4 mmol/L)
    2. Clinical ketosis: >26 mg/dL (2.5 mmol/L)
  • Greatest blood concentrations found 3–5 hours after feeding
  • Very stable analyte, but hemolysis may artificially elevate value
• EXPECTED VALUES FOR METABOLIC PROFILING: Serum or plasma concentrations for NEFA and BHB in the periparturient dairy cow should remain below the concentrations shown (Table 1). Higher values are suggestive of potential energy balance problems.

Protein
There is no single measurable analyte that directly reflects protein status. As a result, a combination of metabolite parameters needs to be utilized, including serum or plasma UN, Cr, total protein, albumin, and Ck.
• Serum or Plasma UN
  • UN reflects dietary protein status and balance relative to rumen and animal needs and is intertwined with available dietary fermentable carbohydrate. Insufficient dietary protein or excessive fermentable carbohydrate relative to degradable protein will result in lower UN concentrations. Likewise, excessive dietary protein or insufficient fermentable carbohydrate results in high UN concentrations.
  • Cr is used to assess renal function and its impact on UN values.
  • Concentrations can range from near 0 to over 30 mg/dL (0 to 21.4 mmol/L) and vary with feeding. Highest values occur between 3 and 5 hours after a meal.
  • Very stable metabolite, not affected by hemolysis

• EXPECTED VALUES FOR METABOLIC PROFILING
  1. Dry cows should maintain a mean serum or plasma UN concentration between 10 and 12 mg/dL (7.14–8.57 mmol/L).
  2. Fresh cows should maintain a mean serum or plasma UN concentration between 12 and 14 mg/dL (8.57–10 mmol/L).
  3. Individual values below 8 mg/dL and above 16 mg/dL are of concern and should be investigated.
• Total protein
  • Concentration reflects dietary protein status, but due to half-life of protein molecules is not extremely sensitive to dietary changes.
  • Confounded by changes in gamma globulin in response to inflammatory conditions.
  • EXPECTED VALUES FOR METABOLIC PROFILING
    1. Early dry cows: 6.5– 8.3 g/dL
    2. Close-up dry cows: 5.8– 7.7 g/dL
    3. Fresh cows: 6.1– 8.8 g/dL
    4. Values below 6 g/dL and above 9.5 g/dL should be investigated.
• Albumin
  • Albumin has a relatively short half-life compared to other blood proteins and can reflect protein deficiency problems over a period of a month or two.
  • Physiologic concentrations range from 3.2 to 4.5 g/dL
  • Dehydration and protein-losing disease processes can confound interpretation of results.
  • Stable metabolite, even with hemolysis.
  • EXPECTED VALUES FOR METABOLIC PROFILING
    1. Early dry cows: 3.5–4.0 g/dL
    2. Close-up dry cows: 3.3–3.8 g/dL
    3. Fresh cows: 3.5– 4.2 g/dL
    4. Close-up dry and fresh cows with albumin concentration <3.25 g/dL and <3.5 g/dL, respectively, are at greater risk for periparturient disease problems.
• Ck (Creatine kinase)
  • Released from muscle when it is catabolized or injured

Table 1

Period	Sample	NEFA mEq/L (mmol/L)	BHB mg/dL	BHB mmol/L
Early dry	Individual	<0.325	<10.0	<0.96
	Group	<0.300	<6.6	<0.64
Close-up dry	Individual	<0.400	<10.0	<0.96
	Group	<0.350	<7.0	<0.67
Fresh (<30 DIM)	Individual	<0.700	<14.5	<1.40
	Group	<0.600	<10.0	<0.96

- Due to a tremendous range in values, provides little diagnostic value unless coupled with other parameters
- Concentrations between 400 and 1000 IU/L might suggest muscle breakdown and possible protein deficiency if coupled with corresponding changes in UN and albumin.

Liver Function
- Enzyme activities (GGT, AST, SDH) and total bilirubin concentrations
  - Elevations in any of these parameters suggest some insult has occurred to the liver but are not specific to liver.
  - SDH is liver specific for ruminants, but elevations cannot be directly attributed to fat infiltration of the liver.
  - Bilirubin values are most specific to bile flow problems than overt hepatocyte damage.
  - Enzyme activities have a wide potential range in values and need to be interpreted in conjunction with other measures of liver function.
  - Most enzymes are sensitive to freezing and thawing. Hemolysis will lower GGT, but increase AST activities.
  - EXPECTED VALUES FOR METABOLIC PROFILING
    1. AST: Dry cows: 46–83 U/L; fresh cows: 61–103 U/L
    2. GGT: Dry cows: 18–38 U/L; fresh cows: 20–49 U/L
    3. SDH: 6.4–58.5 U/L
    4. Total bilirubin: 0.1–0.3 mg/dL (1.71–5.13 mol/L)
    5. Enzyme activities exceeding the above ranges would be of concern and liver function should be further evaluated.
- Total cholesterol
  - Associated with various lipoprotein molecules in blood; provides an indicator for very low density lipoprotein (VLDL) production (fat export) by the liver
  - Serum or plasma concentrations are elevated with dietary fat feeding, which may confound interpretation.
  - Physiologic concentrations vary from <70 up to 300 mg/dL (<2.0 up to 8.7 mmol/L) with lowest values observed around the time of calving.
  - Very stable metabolite, but artificially increased with hemolysis
  - EXPECTED VALUES FOR METABOLIC PROFILING
    1. Early dry cows: >80 mg/dL (>2.28 mmol/L)
    2. Close-up dry cows: >75 mg/dL (>2.14 mmol/L)
    3. Fresh cows: >100 mg/dL (>2.86 mmol/L)
    4. Liver's capacity to export fat is of concern whenever fresh cow cholesterol concentrations are less than close-up dry cows.
- NEFA: Cholesterol ratio
  - The liver takes up NEFA in direct relationship with their concentration in blood. Once in the liver, NEFA can either

be partially metabolized to ketone bodies or they can be used to synthesize triglycerides.
- High NEFA associated with low cholesterol is suggestive of a situation where fat will accumulate in hepatocytes, inducing fatty liver condition.
- Ratio is calculated on a molar ratio (mmol NEFA/mmol cholesterol).
  1. mEq/L NEFA x 1 = mmol/L NEFA
  2. mg/dL cholesterol x 0.02856 = mmol/L cholesterol
- EXPECTED VALUES FOR METABOLIC PROFILING
  1. Calculated ratio ranges from 0.01 to 0.2 for healthy cows with increasing values from early dry to fresh period.
  2. Close-up dry cows with ratios >0.2 are at greater risk for experiencing one or more periparturient disease problems.
  3. Fresh cows with ratios >0.3 are at greater risk for having postpartum disease problems.

Macrominerals
- Macrominerals Ca, P, K, Mg, Na, Cl, and S are of extreme interest as to their status relative to their role in milk fever, alert downer cows, and weak cow syndrome.
- Most of these minerals are tightly regulated in the body through a variety of homeostatic processes.
- Blood concentrations of macrominerals are not reflective at all of dietary status when the homeostatic system is properly functioning.
- Phosphorus, K, Mg, and S are those macrominerals in which blood concentrations are somewhat sensitive to dietary intake.
- Macromineral concentrations need to be carefully interpreted in light of whether or not the homeostatic system is in proper operation.
- Mineral concentrations are very stable, but can be altered by prolonged exposure to the clot (serum sample) or hemolysis (P, Mg, K artificially elevated).
- EXPECTED VALUES FOR METABOLIC PROFILING (Table 2)

Microminerals
- Microminerals are of interest relative to their role in modulating immune function as well as other important metabolic roles.
- Cu, Fe, Se, and Zn are routinely assayed in blood as their concentrations are within detectable limits with current analytical diagnostics.
- Blood or serum micromineral concentrations are buffered from acute changes as a result of dietary problems through mobilization of storage minerals, usually from the liver; thus blood concentrations may not adequately reflect nutritional status.
- Liver trace mineral status may be a better indicator of dietary adequacy, whereas measurement of a mineral-specific enzyme activity better reflects presence of overt clinical deficiency disease compared to blood concentrations.
- Many trace mineral concentrations in blood are influenced by disease. Bacterial infections induce sequestering of iron and zinc and elevation of copper, thus confounding interpretation of blood mineral status.
- Physiologic state and age influence blood and liver micromineral concentrations and must be accounted for in interpretation of concentrations.
- Minerals are very stable in blood, serum, or plasma, but hemolysis can greatly distort serum Se and Zn concentrations.
- EXPECTED VALUES FOR METABOLIC PROFILING (ADULT VALUES ONLY) (Table 3)

Vitamins
- Vitamins A and E are of greatest potential interest for metabolic profiling relative to their role in immune function and association with mastitis, metritis, and retained placenta.
- Vitamin analyses are affected by hemolysis and are prone to oxidation (direct sunlight). Samples should be iced following collection and remain chilled or frozen until analysis.

Table 2

| Mineral | Adequate range | Concern Levels | |
		Individual	Group
Calcium	8.7–11.0 mg/dL (2.17–2.74 mmol/L)	<7 mg/dL (<1.75 mmol/L)	<8 mg/dL (<2.0 mmol/L)
Phosphorus	4.5–8.0 mg/dL (1.45–2.58 mmol/L)	<3.5 mg/dL (<1.13 mmol/L)	<3.8 mg/dL (<1.23 mmol/L)
Magnesium	2.0–3.5 mg/dL (0.82–1.43 mmol/L)	<1.5 mg/dL (<0.62 mmol/L)	<1.8 mg/dL (0.74 mmol/L)
Sodium	137–148 mEq/L[1]	<137 mEq/L	<139 mEq/L
Potassium	3.8–5.2 mEq/L[1]	<3.0 or >5.5 mEq/L	<3.5 or >4.8 mEq/L

[1] mEq/L = mmol/L.

ANALYTICAL TESTING

Table 3

Serum Mineral	Adequate Range		Concern Levels	
Copper	0.6–1.5 μg/mL	9.4–23.6 μmol/L	<0.45 μg/mL	<7.1 μmol/L
			>4 μg/mL	>63 μmol/L
Iron	130–250 μg/dL	23.3–44.8 μmol/L	<130 μg/mL	<23 μmol/L
			>1800 μg/mL	>322 μmol/L
Zinc	0.8–1.4 μg/mL	12.2–21.4 μmol/L	<0.5 μg/mL	<7.6 μmol/L
			>3 μg/mL	>45.9 μmol/L
Selenium, serum	70–100 μg/mL	0.89–1.3 μmol/L	<35 μg/mL	<0.44 μmol/L
			>800 μg/mL	>10.1 μmol/L
Selenium, whole blood	120–250 μg/mL	1.5–3.2 μmol/L	<50 μg/mL	<0.63 μmol/L
			>1900 μg/mL	>24 μmol/L

- Age and physiologic state influence serum and liver vitamin concentrations and reference values need to be adjusted accordingly.
- Vitamin A (total retinol)
  - Concentration of total retinol can be measured in serum (plasma) or liver tissue.
  - Serum concentration is less indicative of dietary status and can be influenced by Zn and protein status as they impact retinol-binding protein availability.
  - Serum concentration declines during late gestation.
  - Liver vitamin A concentration reflects the storage pool and is sensitive to dietary status.
  - Both serum and liver concentrations are diagnostic for disease problems.
  - EXPECTED VALUES FOR METABOLIC PROFILING (ADULTS ONLY) (Table 4)

- Liver vitamin E concentration is reflective of the storage pool and reflects nutritional status.
- Both serum and liver vitamin E concentrations are diagnostic for disease problems.
  - EXPECTED VALUES FOR METABOLIC PROFILING (ADULTS ONLY) (Table 5)

INTERPRETATION
- A complete understanding of underlying metabolic and physiologic mechanisms controlling blood metabolite concentrations is necessary to properly interpret metabolic profiles and their application.
- Unlike the interpretation of individual cow clinical chemistry profiles, interpretation of metabolic profiles requires appreciation of statistical probabilities and acceptable level of risk.

factors on analyte concentration and improve sensitivity of analyte to environmental (i.e., nutritional) influences.

REFERENCE VALUES
- Interpretation of metabolic profiles requires some standard reference values for comparison.
- Analyte reference values should represent the population mean and variation from a defined population of animals clinically evaluated to be free of disease and other health problems.
  - Each population mean needs to be statistically analyzed for a normal population distribution.
  - Median values should be used in place of means for metabolites not showing a normal distribution.
  - Abnormal metabolite values are defined as those outside of the predefined normal reference range.
- At present, few laboratories have specialized blood analyte reference criteria that are adjusted for age, physiologic state, and time relative to calving effects.
  - Research is currently under way to develop appropriate metabolic profiling reference criteria.

Table 4

Sample	Adequate Range	Deficient
Serum	225–500 μg/mL (0.79–1.74 μmol/L)	<150 μg/mL (<0.52 μmol/L)
Liver	300–1100 μg/g dry weight	<40 μg/g dry weight

- Vitamin E (α-tocopherol)
  - Concentration of α-tocopherol can be measured in either serum (plasma) or liver tissue.
  - Serum concentrations generally reflect dietary intake, but are influenced by variations in blood lipoprotein content.
  - Serum concentrations decline in late gestation.
  - Relating serum vitamin E to total cholesterol concentration reduces variation as vitamin E is carried on blood lipoproteins.
  - Vitamin E to cholesterol ratio is calculated on a molar basis (μmol vitamin E/μmol cholesterol) and is unitless.

Table 5

Sample	Adequate Range	Deficient
Serum	3–10 g/mL	<3.0 g/mL
Vitamin E : Cholesterol ratio	2.5–6.0	<1.5
Liver	20–40 μg/g dry weight	<10 μg/g dry weight

- Reference values for each metabolite need to be refined to minimize inherent variability due to effects of age, physiologic state, production level, and other cow-specific

- Until more specific criteria are developed, use of current reference ranges adjusted to α 1 or 1.3 standard deviation have been used for interpretation.

ASSESSMENT

- Metabolic profile results must be correlated with animal and dietary evaluations.
- Mean comparison to reference range
  - Individual samples within groupings
    1. Mean values and standard deviation for all analytes are calculated for each sampled individual within a defined group.
    2. Means and associated statistical variation are compared to reference range.
    3. Sampled populations where 10–25% of individuals are outside the reference range might be considered to be subclinical. If more than 40% are outside the range, then there is a greater risk of clinical disease.
  - Pooled samples within groupings
    1. Pooled analyte values are compared to reference range mean or median.
    2. Pooled values should be within α 0.5 standard deviations of reference mean to be considered normal.
    3. As pooled values deviate further from the reference mean, potential for subclinical and clinical disease will increase.
    4. More research is needed to better define pooled sample interpretation.
- Comparison across groups
  - Besides comparing individual group means to reference ranges, tracking metabolite concentrations across physiologic groups within a herd may provide useful information.
  - This assuming there have not been any major feed changes within group rations over a period of time.
  - This process is useful in evaluation of transition cow problems. Compare analyte values across early dry, close-up dry, and fresh cow groups.
  - Changes in group means are correlated with observed clinical signs, body condition changes, and ration evaluations to come up with some interpretation and recommendations.
- Mean comparison within groups over time
  - Statistical process control—statistical method used by industry to track quality control in manufacturing
  - Same concepts can be applied to repeated measures of analytes within a defined group over time.
  - Determine overall mean and statistical variation within and between time periods.
  - Track means graphically identifying individual tests outside of control limits or three or more consecutive means above or below overall average.
- Proportion comparison within groups
  - Compare individual samples to analyte reference value.
  - Identify all individuals that have values exceeding or below defined threshold value.
  - Determine proportion of individuals with abnormal values.
  - With increasing proportion of individuals with abnormal values, there is an increasing risk of subclinical to clinical disease problems.

 MISCELLANEOUS

ASSOCIATED CONDITIONS
N/A

AGE-RELATED FACTORS
N/A

ZOONOTIC POTENTIAL
N/A

PREGNANCY
N/A

RUMINANT SPECIES AFFECTED
All ruminant species are affected

BIOSECURITY
N/A

PRODUCTION MANAGEMENT
N/A

SEE ALSO
Bovine blood chemistry
Differential diagnosis: philosophy of test usage
Fatty liver
Ketosis
Rumen dysfunction: acidosis

ABBREVIATIONS
AST = aspartate aminotransferase
BHB = β-hydroxybutyrate
Ck = creatine kinase
Cr = creatinine
GGT = γ-glutamyltransferase
NEFA = nonesterified fatty acids
SDH = sorbitol dehydrogenase
UN = urea nitrogen

Suggested Reading
Herdt, T. H. 2000. Variability characteristics and test selection in herd-level nutritional and metabolic profile testing. *Vet Clinics NA: Food Anim Pract*. 16(2): 387–403.
Herdt, T. H., Dart, B., Neuder, L. 2001. Will large dairy herds lead to the revival of metabolic profile testing? *AABP Proceedings* 34:27–34.
Herdt, T. H., Rumbeiha, W., Braselton, W. E. 2000. The use of blood analyses to evaluate mineral status in livestock. *Vet Clinics NA: Food Anim Pract*. 16(3): 423–44.
Oetzel, G. R. 2003. Herd-based biologic testing for metabolic disorders. Available at: http://www.vetmed.wisc.edu/dms/fapm/ fapmtools/2nutr/herdtest.pdf, Accessed August 16, 2004.
Van Saun, R. J. 1997. Nutritional profiles: A new approach for dairy herds. *Bov Pract*. 31(2): 43–50.
Van Saun, R. J., Wustenberg, M. 1997. Metabolic profiling to evaluate nutritional and disease status. *Bov Pract*. 31(2): 37–42.

Author: Robert J. Van Saun

ANAPHYLAXIS

 BASICS

DEFINITION
• An anaphylactic reaction is a pathological immune response that occurs following exposure of a sensitized animal to a specific antigen. This exposure results in urticaria, pruritus, and angioedema, followed by vascular collapse, shock and often life-threatening respiratory distress.
• Anaphylaxis has now been included under type I (immediate) hypersensitivity.

PATHOPHYSIOLOGY
• Anaphylaxis is an acute systemic manifestation of the interaction of an antigen (allergen) binding to IgE antibodies, which are bound to mast cells and basophils. This binding of antigens to cell-bound IgE antibodies triggers the release of chemical substances from the mast cells and basophils.
• The major biologically active mediators produced by mast cells and basophils include histamine, leukotrienes, the eosinophilic chemotactic factor, platelet-activating factor, kinins, serotonins, and proteolytic enzymes. These chemicals directly affect both the vascular system, causing vasodilatation and increased vascular permeability, and smooth muscles, causing contraction of the bronchi and respiratory distress.

SYSTEMS AFFECTED
Cardiovascular, pulmonary, urinary, gastrointestinal, integument

GENETICS
There have been reports of higher incidence in certain lines and breeds of cattle.

INCIDENCE/PREVALANCE
Sporadic, dependent on exposure to inciting antigen

GEOGRAPHIC DISTRIBUTION
N/A

SIGNALMENT
Bovine, ovine; also reported in many other species of ruminants

SIGNS
• Sudden, severe dyspnea, muscle tremors, anxiety, occurs within a few to 10–15 minutes following exposure to the antigen; Muscle tremor may be severe and temperature may rise to 105°F
• History of injection in the previous hour
• Occasionally profuse salivation, mild bloat, diarrhea, urticaria, angioneurotic edema, and rhinitis
• Laminitis rarely occurs in ruminants.

PHYSICAL EXAMINATION FINDINGS
Auscultation of the chest—vesicular murmur, crackling if edema is present, and emphysema in the later stages if dyspnea was severe

CAUSES
• Common agents causing anaphylaxis include blood transfusions, vaccines, horse sera, insect bites, heterologous enzymes and hormones, and certain drugs, such as penicillin and lidocaine.
• Milk allergy occurs occasionally in cows. This can happen when there is increased intramammary pressure to a point that normally sequestered milk components, notably casein, gain access to the circulation; these "foreign" proteins induce a type I hypersensitivity.

RISK FACTORS
Previous exposure to antigens (i.e., previous treatment with blood or blood products or vaccines)

 DIAGNOSIS

DIFFERENTIAL DIAGNOSIS
Acute Bloat
A history of introduction to new forage and/or concentrate diet. Obvious distention of the rumen occurs suddenly, and the left flank may be so distended that the paralumbar fossa protrudes above the vertebral column; the entire abdomen is enlarged. Dyspnea and grunting are marked and are accompanied by mouth breathing, protrusion of the tongue, and extension of the head.

Acute Bronchopneumonia
A history of recent episodes of stress (i.e., weaning, transport, vaccination) within the last 2–7 days. Clinical signs of bacterial bronchopneumonia are often preceded by a viral infection of the respiratory tract. With the onset of secondary bacterial pneumonia, the severity of clinical signs increases and is characterized by depression and toxemia. There will be fever (104–106°F); serous to mucopurulent nasal discharge; moist cough; a rapid, shallow respiratory rate and dyspnea. Auscultation of the lung field reveals increased bronchial sounds, crackles, and wheezes. In severe cases, pleurisy may develop, which is characterized by an irregular breathing pattern and grunting on expiration.

CBC/BIOCHEMSTRY/URINALYSIS
Increase in PCV, high plasma K^+, neutropenia

OTHER LABORATORY TESTS
N/A

IMAGING
N/A

DIAGNOSTIC PROCEDURES
N/A

PATHOLOGIC FINDINGS
Lungs—severe pulmonary edema in calves and lambs; pulmonary edema and emphysema without blood engorgement

 TREATMENT

APPROPRIATE HEALTH CARE
• Ancillary support of blood pressure (IV fluids) and respiration may be necessary.

• In dairy cattle that have been recently dried off, recovery usually is prompt once the gland is emptied.

ACTIVITY
N/A

DIET
N/A

CLIENT EDUCATION
Clients may be instructed to have epinephrine on hand so it can be administered as soon as signs are noted.

SURGICAL CONSIDERATIONS
N/A

 MEDICATIONS

DRUGS OF CHOICE
• Anaphylactic shock is treated with an IV injection of epinephrine.
• Corticosteroids potentiate the effects of epinephrine and may be given following the administration of epinephrine.
• Antihistamines have no effect once signs are present.

CONTRAINDICATIONS
N/A

PRECAUTIONS
When treating food-producing animals, drug withdrawal times must be determined and maintained.

POSSIBLE INTERACTIONS
N/A

ALTERNATIVE DRUGS
N/A

 FOLLOW-UP

PATIENT MONITORING
Animals need to have their respiratory system monitored for the next 24 hours to detect any emphysema.

PREVENTION/AVOIDANCE
Discuss the situation associated with the onset with the producer. Certain products may need to be avoided.

POSSIBLE COMPLICATIONS
Emphysema may result from severe dyspnea and violent muscle spasms.

EXPECTED COURSE AND PROGNOSIS
Animals treated promptly usually return to normal within 12 to 24 hrs.

 MISCELLANEOUS

ASSOCIATED CONDITIONS
N/A

AGE-RELATED FACTORS
N/A

ZOONOTIC POTENTIAL
N/A

PREGNANCY
Following anaphylaxis, animals may spontaneously abort.

RUMINANT SPECIES AFFECTED
Bovine, ovine, other ruminants

BIOSECURITY
N/A

PRODUCTION MANAGEMENT
N/A

SYNONYMS
Type 1 hypersensitivity

SEE ALSO
Acute bloat
Acute bronchopneumonia

ABBREVIATIONS
IgE = immunoglobulin E
IV = intravenous
PCV = packed cell volume

Suggested Reading
Gershwin, L. J. 2001. Immunoglobulin E-mediated hypersensitivity in food-producing animals. *Vet Clin North Am Large Anim Pract*. 17(3): 599–619.
Meeusen, E. N. 1999, Aug 1. Immunology of helminth infections, with special reference to immunopathology. *Vet Parasitol*. 84(3–4):259–73.
Ruby, K. W., Griffith, R. W., Gershwin, L. J., Kaeberle, M. L. 2000, Oct 20. *Haemophilus somnus*-induced IgE in calves vaccinated with commercial monovalent *H. somnus* bacterins. *Vet Microbiol*. 76(4):373–83.
Ruby, K. W., Griffith, R. W., Kaeberle, M. L. 2002, Jan 25. Histamine production by *Haemophilus somnus*. *Comp Immunol Microbiol Infect Dis*. (1):13–20.
Schultz, K. T. 1982, Nov 15. Type I and type IV hypersensitivity in animals. *J Am Vet Med Assoc*. 181(10):1083–87.

ANAPLASMOSIS

BASICS

OVERVIEW
• Anaplasmosis is a hemoparasitic disease with a worldwide distribution, most common in tropical and subtropical areas.
• Upon infection, *Anaplasma* organisms double in number every 24 hours for the first several days.

PATHOPHYSIOLOGY
Infected red blood cells are destroyed by the reticuloendothelial system (spleen) leading to extravascular hemolysis and anemia.

SYSTEMS AFFECTED
Hemolymphatic

GENETICS
N/A

INCIDENCE/PREVALENCE
Unknown

GEOGRAPHIC DISTRIBUTION
Worldwide distribution

SIGNALMENT
Species
Primarily cattle but also sheep, goats, and many wild ruminants

Breed Predilections
N/A

Mean Age and Range
• Cattle under 6 months of age generally show no clinical signs.
• In cattle from 6 months to 3 years of age, signs are progressively more severe.
• Mature cattle (over 3 years of age) are the most susceptible to severe clinical manifestations of the disease. Mortality in this age group can be as high as 50% in naïve herds.

Predominant Sex
N/A

SIGNS
• In the early stages of the disease, cattle may appear lethargic, be anorexic, have decreased milk production, and develop fever.
• Pale or icteric mucous membranes will be present.
• Other signs include depressed rumination, constipation with dark brown mucous-covered feces, dry muzzle, and weight loss.
• Hemoglobinemia and hemoglobinuria are *not* seen with anaplasmosis.

• Infected cattle subsequently develop varying degrees of anemia, which can be fatal if untreated.
• Cattle exhibiting signs of anaplasmosis should be handled with caution.
  • Cerebral anoxia can cause aggressiveness.
  • Severe anemia coupled with stress may precipitate sudden death.
• If anemia is severe, abortions may occur due to fetal anoxia.
• If animals survive the initial infection, they generally become carriers, maintaining a low level of infection without overt clinical signs.

CAUSES AND RISK FACTORS
• Three species of *Anaplasma* have been identified.
  • *Anaplasma marginale* is the most common cause of disease in cattle.
  • *Anaplasma centrale* can cause mild disease in cattle.
  • *Anaplasma ovis* causes mild disease in sheep.
  • There is some cross-protection between species.
• Other species of *Anaplasma* are suspected but have not been definitely identified in ruminants.
• Strains of the organism vary in pathogenicity.
• The disease is spread biologically and mechanically.
  • Biological transmission occurs with *Dermacentor* spp. ticks.
  • Mechanical transmission occurs with tabanid flies and blood-contaminated instruments (such as needles, tattooers, dehorners, and castrating equipment).
• Transmission is highest during heavy tick and fly seasons.
• Moving naïve adults into an endemic area or carrier animals into a nonendemic area often results in outbreaks of the disease.
• Black-tailed deer are effective reservoirs of *A. marginale* and complicate control of the disease in some areas. White-tailed deer are uncommon reservoirs.

DIAGNOSIS

DIFFERENTIAL DIAGNOSES
• Babesiosis—presence of hemoglobinuria, identify typical piriform organisms on Giemsa-stained blood smear
• Leptospirosis—elevated titers, identification of organism in urine by dark-field microscopy

• Bacillary hemoglobinuria or *Clostridium novyi* infection—presence of hemoglobinuria, liver enzyme elevation; identify organisms on impression smear of liver on freshly dead specimen
• Hepatotoxic plants, for example: *Senecio* spp., *Crotalaria* spp., *Lantana camara*—evidence of plant ingestion, marked elevation of liver enzymes, histopathology of liver
• Severe intestinal parasitism—fecal examination
• Copper toxicity, most commonly in sheep—methemoglobinemia, hemoglobinuria, elevated serum, liver and kidney copper concentrations, elevated renal and hepatic enzymes

CBC/BIOCHEMISTRY/URINALYSIS
• Blood collected from animals showing clinical signs will appear thin and watery.
• The packed cell volume will be severely decreased (less than 30%).
• A regenerative response will appear leading to anisocytosis, basophilic stippling, poikilocytosis, polychromatophilia, and reticulocytosis.
• A blood smear stained with Wright's, new methylene blue, or Giemsa stain will definitively diagnose *Anaplasma* organisms. The organisms will appear darkly stained on red blood cells. *A. marginale* is typically at the periphery of the cell and *A. centrale* is at the center.
• A biochemical panel will generally show increased serum urea nitrogen, total and direct bilirubin (BILI), and aspartate aminotransferase (AST).
• Hemoglobinemia and hemoglobinuria are *not* seen in anaplasmosis.

IMAGING
N/A

DIAGNOSTIC PROCEDURES
• Cytology on a direct, Giemsa-stained blood smear is the most common method of diagnosis in animals showing clinical signs.
• Rapid card agglutination and complement fixation tests are commonly used to diagnose the carrier stage.
• Recent research suggests that a nested polymerase chain reaction (PCR) test is better at accurately detecting the carrier stage than complement fixation.

PATHOLOGIC FINDINGS

GROSS FINDINGS
- Tissues will have an anemic pallor.
- Icterus may be present later in the course of disease.
- Splenomegaly is common.
- Hepatomegaly is found in some cases.
- Petechiae are occasionally found in pericardial tissues.

HISTOPATHOLOGICAL FINDINGS
- Staining of tissues may reveal organisms infecting blood cells in capillaries.
- Hepatic changes may include swelling of parenchymal cells, centrilobular necrosis with bile retention and hemosiderosis
- Renal changes may include degeneration of tubular cells and protein infiltrates in tubular lumens and the capsular space.

TREATMENT
- Handle affected animals with caution, as anoxia can lead to aggressiveness or sudden death.
- Other than antibiotic therapy, only supportive care is needed.
- If PCV is below 12%, a blood transfusion may be warranted.

MEDICATIONS

DRUGS OF CHOICE
- Oxytetracycline is the treatment of choice for anaplasmosis infections and can be used according to labeled dosages.
- For treatment of acute disease, administer 11 mg/kg intravenously once daily for 3–5 days.
- A long-acting (or depot) form of oxytetracycline can also be used for treatment of acute disease at 20 mg/kg intramuscularly every 72 hours for one to two treatments.

- In endemic areas, control can be achieved with
  - 6.6–11mg/kg of the nondepot form or 20 mg/ml of the depot form of oxytetracycline every 21–28 days from the start of the vector season until 1–2 months after vector season ends.
  - Chlortetracycline in feed at 0.22–0.55 mg/kg daily year-round
  - Chlortetracycline in feed at 1.1 mg/kg daily during the vector season
- Clearance of the carrier state can be achieved with
  - Four treatments utilizing a depot form of oxytetracycline at 20 mg/kg intramuscularly or subcutaneously every 72 hours
  - Chlortetracycline in feed at 1.1 mg/kg daily for 120 days or 11 mg/kg daily for 60 days
- Observe appropriate meat and milk withdrawal times.

CONTRAINDICATIONS
- If the carrier state is cleared using antibiotic therapy, cattle will become susceptible to reinfection. In endemic areas, it may not be advisable to clear the carrier state.
- Drug withdrawal periods for meat and milk must be followed.

FOLLOW-UP

If cleanup of carriers is attempted, animals should be retested 6 months after treatment.

MISCELLANEOUS

There have been vaccines available at various times for use in controlling losses associated with anaplasmosis, however, their efficacy has generally been poor. A search of the Internet using the words "anaplasmosis vaccine" will enable you to find current products. Vaccines are not approved for use in all areas.
- Vaccination does not prevent disease but does decrease the severity of clinical signs when animals are infected.
- Some vaccines have been associated with the development of neonatal isoerythrolysis in calves so caution should be exercised when vaccinating late gestation females.

ASSOCIATED CONDITIONS
N/A

AGE-RELATED FACTORS
See Mean Age and Range above.

ZOONOTIC POTENTIAL
This disease does not have any zoonotic potential.

PREGNANCY
N/A

BIOSECURITY
N/A

PRODUCTION MANAGEMENT
N/A

SYNONYMS
N/A

SEE ALSO
Babesiosis
Bacillary hemoglobinuria
Clostridium novyi infection
Copper toxicity
Hepatotoxic plants
Leptospirosis

ABBREVIATIONS
AST = aspartate aminotransferase
BILI = direct bilirubin
PCR = polymerase chain reaction
PCV = packed cell volume

Suggested Reading
Kocan, K. M., Blouin, E. F., Barbet, A. F. 2000. Anaplasmosis control: past, present and future. *Ann of NY Acad Sci.* 916:501–09.
Kuttler, K. L. 1984. Anaplasma infections in wild and domestic ruminants: a review. *J Wildlf Dis.* 20:12–20.
Palmer, G. H., Lincoln, S. 2002. Anaplasmosis. In: *Large animal internal medicine*, ed. B. P. Smith. Philadelphia: Mosby.
Richey, E. J. 1999. Bovine Anaplasmosis. In: *Current veterinary therapy 4: food animal practice*, eds. J. L. Howard, R. A. Smith. Philadelphia: W. B. Saunders.

Author: Dawn J. Capucille

ANEMIA, NONREGENERATIVE: BOVINE

 BASICS

DEFINITION
• Anemia in adult cattle is indicated by a PCV (or Hct) of less than 23%.
• Beef cattle have higher hemoglobin, RBC, and PCV than dairy breeds.
• Anemias may be nonregenerative or regenerative. The lack of reticulocytes and polychromasia with normal red cell distribution width (RDW) is indicative of a nonregenerative response or erythropoietic depression.
• Lactating dairy cattle tend to have lower values than nonlactating cows.
• Bulls tend to have greater RBC counts than cows.
• Environmental, seasonal, and physiological differences may affect the hemogram.
• Diminished oxygen tension at elevated altitudes stimulates erythropoiesis resulting in increased RBC counts.

PATHOPHYSIOLOGY
• Anemia results from decreased production, or increased destruction (hemolysis) or loss (hemorrhage) of erythrocytes. Nonregenerative anemias are caused by decreased erythropoiesis.
• The onset of anemia and its related signs is insidious unless there is concurrent hemolysis or hemorrhage.

Anemia of Chronic Inflammation
• Established inflammation results in bone marrow depression due to alterations in iron metabolism, which results in sequestration of iron into the cells of the mononuclear phagocytic system. It is hypothesized that the iron sequestration is a nonspecific bacteriostatic process.
• This functional iron deficiency causes decreased erythropoiesis. However, the depression rarely results in the classic microcytic, hypochromic anemia of dietary iron deficiency or iron deficiency resulting from chronic hemorrhage.

Iron Deficiency
• Iron deficiency may be due to dietary iron deficiency or to chronic blood loss. Dietary iron deficiency is seldom recognized in cattle because soil contains a sufficient amount of iron to maintain hematopoiesis. It is possible that calves raised on concrete with a diet consisting exclusively of milk could have dietary iron deficiency.
• Chronic blood loss such as with certain intestinal helminth infections may result in enough loss of iron to cause iron deficiency. Other chronic bleeding conditions, such as intestinal tract ulcers or hemorrhaging tumors (e.g., lymphoma), can also cause iron deficiency.

• Classically, iron deficiency results in nonregenerative anemia (no reticulocytes or polychromasia) that has a microcytic, hypochromic erythrocyte profile.

Space Occupying Lesions of the Bone Marrow
• Myelophthisis is rare in cattle, perhaps because few cattle live to older age when an animal is more likely to develop tumors. Tumors that metastasize to the bone marrow would produce a depression anemia, which is most likely to have a normocytic, normochromic erythrocyte profile.
• Cancerous lymphocytes of lymphoma do not frequently multiply in the bone marrow, but occasionally this may occur. If sufficient amount of the marrow is involved, depression anemia can be an unusual secondary feature of bovine lymphoma.

Copper Deficiency
Copper deficiency causes nonregenerative anemia due to impaired absorption and utilization of iron. The majority of copper in the blood is bound to ceruloplasmin, an enzyme that is required for the binding of iron to the transport protein, transferrin. Copper deficiency may be either primary due to deficient intake or secondary due to high molybdenum content of soils and forage. Copper deficiency results in microcytic, hypochromic anemia for the reasons outlined above for iron deficiency.

Cobalt Deficiency
Cobalt is an essential component of Vitamin B_{12} (cyanocobalamins). Ruminant stomach microflora synthesizes vitamin B_{12}. Cobalt deficiency results in the depression of the vitamin B_{12}-containing enzyme 5-methyltetrahydrofolate homocysteine methyltransferase, which causes a reduction in folate metabolism and impeded DNA synthesis in developing erythrocytes. Anemia occurs late in the course of cobalt deficiency and may be normocytic or macrocytic.

Organ Dysfunction or Failure
• Nonregenerative anemia often occurs with chronic kidney diseases. This is due to decreased erythropoiesis as a result of decreased erythropoietin production. In addition, erythrocyte lifespan is decreased probably because uremic substances directly affect erythrocyte integrity (structural substances and/or metabolism).
• Nonregenerative anemia may occur with liver diseases. The processes that cause the anemia are unknown, but they may be the result of decreased absorption, distribution or use of elements necessary for erythropoiesis.

Peracute and Acute Hemorrhage or Hemolysis
• Apparent nonregenerative anemia may be suggested by hemogram findings for several days after rapid onset hemorrhage or hemolysis.

• Hypoxia stimulation of erythropoietin production occurs rapidly, but several days of increased erythropoiesis are required before evidence of increased erythropoiesis is evident in the hemogram.

Bracken Fern Toxicosis
• Chronic ingestion of bracken fern (*Pteridium aquilinum*) causes bladder hemorrhage and hematopoietic depression in cattle and sheep. The hemorrhage may be of sufficient magnitude and duration to cause severe anemia. Hemogram features often reveal a nonregenerative response, which is due to marrow hematopoietic suppression.
• Because of the bone marrow depression, thrombocytopenia and neutropenia may be evident. Moderate to severe thrombocytopenia likely contributes to the magnitude of the bladder hemorrhage and exacerbates the anemia due to bone marrow suppression.

SYSTEMS AFFECTED
• Hematopoietic: erythropoiesis is depressed. Bone marrow evaluation will reveal increased M:E (myeloid to erythroid ratio) because the myeloid activity is normal or increased, while the erythroid activity is depressed.
• Cardiovascular: hypoxia causes tachycardia. Decreased blood viscosity and turbulent blood flow may occasionally result in an auscultable heart murmur.
• Respiratory: hypoxia causes tachypnea.
• Central nervous system, liver, and kidney are particularly sensitive to hypoxia. Clinical and laboratory features suggestive of effects on these systems may be recognized.

GENETICS
N/A

INCIDENCE/PREVALENCE
N/A

GEOGRAPHIC DISTRIBUTION
• Potentially worldwide
• Chronic blood loss due to intestinal parasitism may have an increased prevalence in areas endemic to associated parasites.
• Copper and cobalt deficiencies are often associated with soil deficiency of these minerals. Functional copper deficiency may occur when there are excess amounts of molybdenum, zinc, and some compounds.

SIGNALMENT

Species
All cattle are susceptible to anemia.

Breed Predilections
N/A

Mean Age and Range
• Anemia due to chronic gastrointestinal blood loss secondary to abomasal ulcers or intestinal parasites may occur in cattle of all ages.
• Anemia due to other causes may affect any age animal.

Predominant Sex
There is no sex predilection.

SIGNS
N/A

HISTORICAL FINDINGS
Nonspecific signs of anemia include weakness, lethargy, anorexia, dyspnea, tachypnea, dark feces (melena), pica (especially with mineral deficiencies). Decreased growth and productivity may occur in iron-, copper-, or cobalt-deficient animals; diarrhea may be found in copper- and cobalt-deficient animals; and faded hair coat occurs in copper-deficient animals.

PHYSICAL EXAMINATION FINDINGS
Pale mucous membranes, tachycardia, tachypnea, melena occasionally observed in animals with gastric ulcers, unthrifty appearance. Faded hair coat may be seen with copper deficiency.

CAUSES AND RISK FACTORS
Anemia of Chronic Inflammation
Inflammation of any cause may result in anemia provided that the inflammatory condition is present for sufficient time. The degree of anemia will depend upon the duration of inflammation. Generally, mild anemia can be recognized by laboratory evaluation within 1 to 2 weeks after onset of inflammation.

Iron Deficiency Anemia
Any form of chronic external blood loss; blood loss in cattle most commonly results from loss through the gastrointestinal tract. Gastric ulcers and trichostrongylosis are frequent causes of GI blood loss. Neonates on all-milk diets without access to soil may develop anemia relatively rapidly because their erythrocyte mass is expanding as they grow.

Copper Deficiency Anemia
• Primary copper deficiency may occur in milk-fed animals or in animals pastured on copper-deficient soils.
• Secondary copper deficiency can occur with excess dietary molybdenum, sulfates, or zinc.

Cobalt Deficiency
• Primary cobalt deficiency occurs in areas of cobalt-deficient soils or on pastures heavily fertilized with limestone, which reduces cobalt availability.
• Secondary cobalt deficiency may occur with excess manganese, zinc, or iodine, which apparently antagonizes use of cobalt.

Anemia Secondary to Organ Dysfunction
• Chronic renal failure and hepatic dysfunction may result in depression anemia.
• Peracute and acute hemorrhage or hemolysis
• Early (approximately the first 3 to 5 days) in any hemolytic crisis of hemorrhagic condition, hemogram often suggests erythropoietic depression because several days are required before hypoxic stimulation of erythropoiesis is manifested as recognizable features of polychromasia, reticulocytosis, etc., in the blood.

DIAGNOSIS

DIFFERENTIAL DIAGNOSIS
• On the hemogram, nonregenerative anemia is distinguished from regenerative anemia in the lack of reticulocytosis and polychromasia. Hemogram features in the early stages of hemolysis or hemorrhage may be similar to those of depression anemia (see above, Peracute and Acute Hemorrhage or Hemolysis).
• In iron deficiency, microcytosis and hypochromasia are usually evident.
• In cobalt deficiency, macrocytosis may be evident.

CBC/BIOCHEMISTRY/URINALYSIS
Anemia Due to Chronic Inflammation
CBC
• Generally there are mild decreases in RBC, Hgb, and PCV (anemia is rarely severe).
• The hemogram reveals normocytic, normochromic, nonregenerative anemia (no reticulocytes or polychromasia with normal RDW).
• Often an inflammatory leukogram consisting of neutrophilia, ± left shift, ± toxic change (often indicates bacterial etiology), ± monocytosis (presence indicates inflammation of some duration or tissue damage/necrosis is present).
• Lymphopenia may indicate stress (endogenous corticosteroid release).
• Thrombocytosis may be found.
• Hyperfibrinogenemia is often found with active inflammation.

Serum Biochemistry
• Hyperglobulinemia is often found in chronic inflammation, particularly when infectious agents such as bacteria cause the inflammation.
• Hypoalbuminemia may be present with active inflammation especially if there is marked hyperglobulinemia.

Anemia Due to Iron or Copper Deficiency
CBC
• There are mild to marked decreases in RBC, Hgb and PCV.
• Microcytosis (low MCV) is often found
• Hypochromasia (low MCHC) also occurs.
• There may be either regenerative or nonregenerative response to the anemia; the latter is more common.
• Characteristic changes in erythrocytes observed on blood films include increased central pallor (hypochromasia), anisocytosis and moderate to marked poikilocytosis such as dacrocytes (tear-drop shape).
• Thrombocytosis is common; this may be extreme.

Serum Biochemistry
Hypoproteinemia with both hypoalbuminemia and hypoglobulinemia is a

consistent finding if iron deficiency is due to sustained gastrointestinal blood loss.

Anemia Due to Cobalt Deficiency
CBC
• There are mild decreases in RBC, Hgb, and PCV.
• Usually the RBCs are normocytic (MCV in reference range) to occasionally macrocytic (increased MCV), normochromic (reference range MCHC), and nonregenerative anemia.
• There may be a stress (corticosteroid) leukogram.

Serum Biochemistry
• If ketosis develops secondary to anorexia, ketone bodies may be detected in the serum.
• There may be increased liver enzyme activity— AST, SDH, GGT.

Urinalysis
If ketosis develops secondary to anorexia, ketone bodies are detectable by urine dipstick.

Anemia Due to Secondary Organ Failure/Dysfunction—Chronic Renal Failure
CBC
• There are mild to moderate decreases in RBC, Hgb, and PCV.
• The anemia is normocytic, normochromic, nonregenerative.

Serum Biochemistry
With kidney failure there will be increased BUN (not as striking as in monogastric animals), creatinine, and possibly phosphorus with variably low bicarbonate, sodium, and chloride.

Urinalysis
Isosthenuria (Sp. Gr. 1.008—1.012) with variable proteinuria is found.

Anemia Due to Secondary Organ Failure/Dysfunction—Liver Disease
CBC
• There are mild to moderate decreases in RBC, Hgb, and PCV.
• The anemia is normocytic, normochromic, nonregenerative.

Serum Biochemistry
Increased SDH, LDH, AST, GGT; variably high bilirubin; occasionally low BUN; decreased total protein with decreased albumin are some features of liver damage.

OTHER LABORATORY TESTS
Chronic Blood Loss/Iron Deficiency
• Hypoferremia (serum iron $<30\ \mu g/dL$) is consistently found.
• Transferrin saturation is decreased.
• Total iron binding capacity is increased.
• Fecal flotation may suggest intestinal parasites (*Trichostrongylus* spp.) as the cause of blood loss.
• Fecal occult blood test may reveal location of blood loss (*caution:* some plant peroxidases can result in a false positive).

ANEMIA, NONREGENERATIVE: BOVINE

- Space occupying lesions of the bone marrow
- Examination of the bone marrow may reveal neoplastic lymphocytes.

Copper Deficiency
Plasma copper levels are decreased.

Cobalt Deficiency
Low serum cobalamin (vitamin B_{12}) concentration. (Cobalt concentration is not reliable.)

OTHER DIAGNOSTIC PROCEDURES
Chronic Blood Loss/Iron Deficiency
Cytological evaluation of bone marrow specimen stained with Prussian blue for iron particles should reveal the absence of hemosiderin. Marrow evaluation for iron is only recommended when documentation of iron deficiency by other means is difficult.

PATHOLOGIC FINDINGS
Chronic Blood Loss/Iron Deficiency
Intestinal parasitism with mucosal petechiation; abomasal ulcers.

TREATMENT

- Successful treatment of nonregenerative anemia usually revolves around correction of the underlying cause(s).
- Treat with appropriate antimicrobials, anthelmintics, or correct dietary insufficiencies.

ACTIVITY
Restrict activity until the animal(s) can exert themselves without developing significant dyspnea.

DIET
Treat with appropriate antimicrobials, anthelmintics, or correct dietary insufficiences. (Refer to specific chapters for types, dosages, and amounts.)

Chronic Inflammation
Determine source of inflammation and treat with appropriate antimicrobials if bacterial or fungal etiology. Hot pack external abscesses.

Chronic Blood Loss/Iron Deficiency
- Identify and correct the cause of external blood loss.
- Treat with appropriate anthelmintic based on specific parasite(s) detected by fecal evaluation.
- Iron may be provided as an oral supplement or as a feed additive. Iron dextran injections should be avoided in cattle because it can cause anaphylaxis, especially if used repeatedly. Injected iron may cause acute iron overload resulting in massive hepatic necrosis leading to death in cattle. Injectable iron should be used with caution in cattle.

Copper and Cobalt Deficiencies
Addition of copper or cobalt to diet by feeding free-choice trace mineral/salt mix is effective, but the animals consume the mix frequently.

Renal Failure
If possible, stabilize the animal and rehydrate with fluids.

Early Peracute and Acute Hemorrhage or Hemolysis
- Treat the specific condition.
- In valuable animals, transfusions may be used to maintain oxygen carrying capacity until effective erythropoiesis contributes to increased oxygen-carrying capacity of the blood.

MEDICATIONS

- See specific chapters on infectious diseases, parasitism for appropriate drugs and dosages.
- See specific chapters on mineral deficiencies for supplementation and dosages.

DRUGS OF CHOICE
- Appropriate antibiotics for inflammatory conditions with infectious etiologies
- Appropriate anthelmintics for parasitism

CONTRAINDICATIONS
Appropriate milk and meat withdrawal times must be followed for all compounds administered to food-producing animals.

FOLLOW-UP

PATIENT MONITORING
- Respiration and heart rates and mucous membrane color are useful for recognizing the success of therapy.
- In patients with severe anemia, CBC or PCV with a blood smear examination should be performed every 1–2 days until a significant erythropoietic response is recognized.

PREVENTION/AVOIDANCE
See specific chapters for nutritional deficiencies, intestinal parasites, etc.

POSSIBLE COMPLICATIONS
- Appropriate milk and meat withdrawal times must be followed for all compounds administered to food-producing animals.
- Injected iron can cause anaphylaxis (iron dextran) or liver necrosis.

EXPECTED COURSE AND PROGNOSIS
Clinical course and prognosis vary and are associated with the underlying disease condition causing the nonregenerative anemia.

MISCELLANEOUS

ASSOCIATED CONDITIONS
N/A

AGE-RELATED FACTORS
Young animals on milk diets are susceptible to iron deficiency.

ZOONOTIC POTENTIAL
N/A

PREGNANCY
A mild anemia may be observed in some pregnant animals due to dilution of RBC mass by a high blood volume.

RUMINANT SPECIES AFFECTED
Potentially, all ruminant species are affected.

BIOSECURITY
N/A

PRODUCTION MANAGEMENT
- In areas of mineral-deficient soils, feed should be appropriately supplemented or it should contain commodities (grain, hay, etc.) grown on properly supplemented land.
- Preventative anthelmintic therapy should be practiced in areas of endemic parasitism.

SYNONYMS
Depression anemia
Nonresponsive anemia

SEE ALSO
Chronic renal failure
Cobalt deficiency
Copper deficiency
Iron deficiency
Liver diseases
Parasitism
Regenerative anemia

ABBREVIATIONS
AST = aspartate aminotransferase
GGT = gamma glutamyltransferase
Hgb = hemoglobin
LDH = lactate dehydrogenase
MCHC = mean cell hemoglobin concentration
MCV = mean cell volume
RDW = red cell distribution width
SDH = sorbitol dehydrogenase

Suggested Reading
Feldman, B. F., Zinkl, J. G., Jain, N. C., eds. 2000. *Schalm's veterinary hematology*. 5th ed. Baltimore: Lippincott Williams and Wilkins.
Jain, N. C. 1986. *Schalm's veterinary hematology*. 4th ed. Philadelphia: Lea and Febiger.
Smith, B. P., ed. 2001. *Large animal internal medicine*. 3d ed. Philadelphia: Mosby.

Authors: Joseph G. Zinkl and Bernard F. Feldman

ANEMIA, NONREGENERATIVE: CAMELIDS

 BASICS

DEFINITION
• Anemia in adult llamas and alpacas is indicated by a PCV of less than 25%. A PCV of ≤28% in camels is indicative of anemia.
• High concentrations of erythrocytes are observed in healthy camelids, but because the cells have a small mean cell volume, the PCV, or Hct, is relatively low.
• Anemias may be nonregenerative or regenerative. The lack of polychromasia, reticulocytes, and nucleated erythrocytes is indicative of depression or a nonregenerative response.

PATHOPHYSIOLOGY
Anemia may result from either decreased production or increased destruction of erythrocytes. Nonregenerative anemias are most often associated with decreased erythropoiesis. The onset of anemia and its related signs is insidious unless there is concurrent RBC destruction or loss.

Anemia of Chronic Inflammation
• Decreased production of erythrocytes is often associated with established or chronic inflammation in camelids, but iron or copper deficiency may also cause nonregenerative anemia. A mature neutrophilia (>25,000 neutrophils/μL) ± hyperfibrinogenemia (>400 mg/dL) is consistent with inflammatory disease. The presence of immature neutrophils (e.g., left shift) is supportive of active inflammation. Inflammatory disease results in cytokine-mediated disturbances in iron metabolism and decreased availability for erythropoiesis. Lack of polychromasia and reticulocytes indicates nonregenerative anemia.
• Mild, normocytic, normochromic, nonregenerative anemia has been reported in juvenile llamas affected with juvenile llama immunodeficiency syndrome (JLIDS). Anemia is probably a result of chronic and repeated infections resulting in decreased iron availability.

Iron Deficiency Anemia
Iron deficiency may be primary or secondary. In either case, iron deficiency results in moderate nonregenerative anemia due to insufficient iron for hemoglobin synthesis. Erythrocytes are microcytic (decreased MCV) due to an additional cell division during development. Hypochromasia (decreased MCHC) results from decreased hemoglobin concentration in the erythrocytes. Chronic blood loss can result in iron deficiency and nonregenerative anemia. Trichostrongylus infection causes a mildly regenerative, normocytic, normochromic blood loss anemia. Bleeding gastric ulcers can result in chronic blood loss.

Copper Deficiency Anemia
Copper deficiency causes nonregenerative anemia due to impaired absorption and utilization of iron. The majority of copper in the blood is bound to ceruloplasmin, an enzyme that is required for the binding of iron to the transport protein, transferrin. Copper deficiency may be either primary due to deficient intake or secondary due to high molybdenum content of soils and forage. Copper deficiency results in microcytic, hypochromic anemia for the reasons outlined above for iron deficiency.

Cobalt Deficiency
Cobalt is an essential component of vitamin B_{12} (cyanocobalamins). Camelid stomach microflora are presumed to synthesize vitamin B_{12}. Cobalt deficiency results in the depression of the vitamin B_{12}-containing enzyme 5-methyltetrahydrofolate homocysteine methyltransferase, which causes a reduction in folate metabolism and impedes DNA synthesis in developing erythrocytes. Anemia occurs late in the course of cobalt deficiency and may be normocytic or macrocytic.

Secondary Organ Failure
• Renal failure results in decreased production of erythropoietin necessary for erythropoiesis. RBC lifespan is decreased. Uremic acids inhibit hemostasis.
• Hepatic failure may result in decreased absorption, distribution, or utilization of elements necessary for erythropoiesis.
• Hypothyroidism leads to decreased erythropoiesis probably through decreased tissue O_2 requirements as well as a direct effect on erythrocyte production.

SYSTEMS AFFECTED
• Hemic/Lymphatic/Immune
• Hepatobiliary—chronic hypoxia due to marked anemia results in centrilobular necrosis. Mild hyperbilirubinemia may occur due to decreased hepatic function and mass.
• Cardiovascular—hypoxia causes tachycardia; decreased blood viscosity and turbulent blood flow may occasionally result in an auscultable heart murmur.
• Respiratory—hypoxia results in tachypnea.
• Renal/urologic—chronic hypoxia may lead to renal tubular necrosis.
• Gastrointestinal—colic may occur secondary to gastric ulcers.

GENETICS
Young llamas affected with JLIDS are often anemic. Although there are apparent familial links in affected llamas, reliable genealogical information is not available and a definitive genetic basis has not been established.

INCIDENCE/PREVALENCE
Unknown

GEOGRAPHIC DISTRIBUTION
Chronic blood loss due to intestinal parasitism may have an increased prevalence in areas endemic to associated parasites.

SIGNALMENT
Species
All camelids are susceptible to anemia. Llamas and alpacas may be more susceptible to iron and copper deficiency anemias than camels, but the condition is uncommon in all species.

Breed Predilections
N/A

Mean Age and Range
• Anemia due to chronic gastrointestinal blood loss secondary to gastric ulcers may occur in llamas and alpacas of all ages including nursing animals.
• Median age of llamas affected with JLIDS and that are anemic, 13.8 months; range 6 months–4 years.
• Anemia due to other causes may affect any age animal.

Predominant Sex
No sex predilection

SIGNS

HISTORICAL FINDINGS
Nonspecific signs of anemia include weakness, lethargy, anorexia, dyspnea, tachypnea; reddish-brown urine (hemoglobinuria) if anemia is severe; dark feces (melena); pica, decreased growth and productivity may occur in iron-, copper-, or cobalt-deficient animals; diarrhea in cobalt-deficient animals.

PHYSICAL EXAM FINDINGS
Pale mucous membranes, tachycardia, tachypnea, icterus if anemia is severe; melena occasionally observed in llamas with gastric ulcers; unthrifty appearance and poor hair coat reported with cobalt deficiency.

CAUSES AND RISK FACTORS
Anemia of Chronic Inflammation
• Any cause of inflammatory disease including internal or cutaneous infections, infectious diseases, traumatic tissue damage, or fractures
• Active malignant neoplasia—lymphosarcoma, squamous cell carcinoma, mammary and uterine adenocarcinoma
• Juvenile llama immunodeficiency syndrome (JLIDS)

Iron Deficiency Anemia
• Any form of chronic external blood loss
• Blood loss in adult camelids most commonly results from loss through the gastrointestinal tract
• Gastric ulcers and trichostrongylosis are frequent causes of GI blood loss
• Copper deficiency can lead to secondary iron deficiency
• Neonates on all-milk diets without access to soil
• Hemostatic defects

Copper Deficiency Anemia
• Primary copper deficiency—milk-fed animals, pastured animals on copper-deficient soils, pregnancy may exacerbate deficiency.
• Secondary copper deficiency—dietary molybdenum, sulfates or zinc excess (inhibits copper absorption).

ANEMIA, NONREGENERATIVE: CAMELIDS

Cobalt Deficiency
• Primary cobalt deficiency—cobalt-deficient soils or pastures heavily fertilized with limestone reduces cobalt available to plants and animals.
• Secondary cobalt deficiency—manganese, zinc, and iodine may antagonize utilization of cobalt.

Anemia Secondary to Organ Dysfunction
Chronic renal failure; hepatic dysfunction—hepatic lipidosis, ketosis, infectious hepatitis; endocrine disorders—hypothyroidism

 DIAGNOSIS

DIFFERENTIAL DIAGNOSIS
Specific features in the erythrogram are used to identify not only nonregenerative (depression) anemias from regenerative anemias, but also some specific causes of the anemia such as iron deficiency.

CBC/BIOCHEMISTRY/URINALYSIS
Anemia Due to Chronic Inflammation
CBC
• Normocytic, normochromic, nonregenerative anemia
• Mild decreases in RBC, Hgb, and PCV (anemia is rarely severe)
• Inflammatory leukogram—neutrophilia, ± left shift, ± toxic change (indicates bacterial etiology), ± monocytosis (presence indicates inflammation of some duration or tissue damage/necrosis)
• Lymphopenia may indicate effects of stress (endogenous corticosteroid release)
• ± Thrombocytosis (reactive)
• Hyperfibrinogenemia often observed with more acute or active inflammatory conditions

Serum Biochemistry
• Hypoalbuminemia if active inflammation
• Hyperglobulinemia if chronic inflammation
• Hypoglobulinemia often observed in llamas with JLIDS, especially in the face of chronic and repeated infections

Anemia Due to Iron or Copper Deficiency
CBC
• Microcytosis indicated by a low mean cell volume.
• Hypochromia indicated by low mean corpuscular hemoglobin concentration.

• Mild to moderate decreases in RBC, Hgb, and PCV
• Anemia, either regenerative or nonregenerative; the latter is more common.
• Characteristic changes in erythrocytes observed on blood films include increased central pallor (hypochromia), anisocytosis, and moderate to marked poikilocytosis such as dacrocytes (teardrop shape).
• ± Thrombocytosis

Serum Biochemistry
Hypoproteinemia is a consistent finding if iron deficiency is due to sustained gastrointestinal blood loss. Hypoalbuminemia and hypoglobulinemia.

Anemia Due to Cobalt Deficiency
CBC
• Normocytic to occasionally macrocytic, normochromic, nonregenerative anemia
• Mild decreases in RBC, Hgb, and PCV
• Stress (corticosteroid) leukogram

Serum Biochemistry
• If ketosis develops secondary to anorexia, ketone bodies may be detected in the serum.
• Increased liver enzyme activity—AST, SDH, GGT.

Urinalysis
If ketosis develops secondary to anorexia, ketone bodies (primarily acetoacetate) are detectable by urine dipstick.

Anemia Due to Secondary Organ Failure/Dysfunction—Chronic Renal Failure
CBC
• Normocytic, normochromic, nonregenerative anemia
• Mild decreases in RBC, Hgb, and PCV
• Inflammatory leukogram if suppurative nephritis present

Serum Biochemistry
High BUN, creatinine, ± phosphorus; variably low bicarbonate, sodium, and chloride

Urinalysis
Isosthenuria (Sp. Gr. 1.008—1.012); variable proteinuria and active sediment

Anemia Due to Secondary Organ Failure/Dysfunction, e.g., Hepatic Lipidosis
CBC
• Normocytic, normochromic nonregenerative anemia
• Mild to moderate decreases in RBC, Hgb, and PCV

• Inflammatory leukogram if suppurative hepatitis present

Serum Biochemistry
High glucose, ketone bodies, SDH, LDH, AST, GGT, triglycerides, creatinine; variably high bilirubin; variable high or low BUN; low potassium, total protein, albumin, ± phosphorus; variably low bicarbonate, sodium, and chloride.

Urinalysis
• Ketone bodies (note: acetoacetate and acetone are normally present in urine from pregnant alpacas, trace amount present in llama urine)
• Variable specific gravity variable proteinuria and active sediment

OTHER LABORATORY TESTS
Chronic Blood Loss/Iron Deficiency
• Hypoferremia (serum iron $\leq$60 μg/dL)
• Decreased transferrin saturation
• Fecal flotation to rule out intestinal parasites (*Trichostrongylus*) as cause of blood loss
• Fecal occult blood test (caution: some plant peroxidases can result in a false positive.)

Copper Deficiency
Plasma copper levels

Cobalt Deficiency
Low serum cobalamin (vitamin B$_{12}$) concentration (cobalt concentration is not reliable).

Hepatic Lipidosis
High serum bile acids, nonesterified fatty acids (NEFA), beta-hydroxybutyrate

IMAGING
Chronic Blood Loss/Iron Deficiency
Radiographic or ultrasonographic imaging may reveal evidence of gastrointestinal disease accounting for blood loss.

OTHER DIAGNOSTIC PROCEDURES
Chronic Blood Loss/Iron Deficiency
• Gastric endoscopy may reveal evidence for gastric ulceration.
• Cytologic evaluation of bone marrow specimen stained with Prussian blue for iron particles should reveal the absence of hemosiderin. Marrow evaluation for iron is only recommended when documentation of iron deficiency by other means is difficult.

PATHOLOGIC FINDINGS
Chronic Blood Loss/Iron Deficiency
Intestinal parasitism with mucosal petechiation; gastric ulcers

TREATMENT

The successful treatment of nonregenerative anemia usually revolves around correction of the underlying cause. General treatment and supportive care recommendations follow. See specific disease chapters for detailed treatment information.

ACTIVITY
Restrict

DIET
Correct dietary insufficiencies as described below and within specific nutritional deficiency chapters.

Chronic Inflammation
Determine source of inflammation and treat with appropriate antimicrobials if bacterial or fungal etiology. Hot pack external abscesses.

Chronic Blood Loss/Iron Deficiency
• Identify and correct the cause of external blood loss.
• Oral supplementation of iron is less effective than parenteral administration if anemia is severe, but a safe and effective dose for injectable iron dextran has not been established in camelids.
• Incorporation of ferrous sulfate into a mineral mix advised for prevention.

Copper and Cobalt Deficiencies
Addition of copper or cobalt to diet by feeding free-choice trace mineral/salt mix—effective only if animals consume the mix daily.

Renal Failure
• Increase RBC mass (blood transfusion) if patient is symptomatic for anemia (PCV ≤15%).
• Stabilize azotemia and carefully rehydrate with appropriate fluids.
• Correct electrolyte and acid-base imbalances with appropriate fluid therapy and supplementation when necessary.

CLIENT EDUCATION
Conditions associated with severe nonregenerative anemia or pancytopenia generally carry a guarded to poor prognosis and may require long-term therapy without complete resolution.

MEDICATIONS

DRUGS OF CHOICE
Specific therapy for increasing RBC mass:
• If anemia is unusually severe (PCV ≤15%), transfusion may be required to treat life-threatening anemia. Whole blood, 0.1 ml/kg at a rate of 5–20 ml/kg/hr.
• Numerous blood types are present in the llama and alpaca. However, incompatibility reactions are very rare with the first transfusion. Subsequent transfusions increase the risk for an adverse reaction. Blood cross matching is advised for repeated transfusions.

CONTRAINDICATIONS
Appropriate milk and meat withdrawal times must be followed for all compounds administered to food-producing animals.

PRECAUTIONS
N/A

POSSIBLE INTERACTIONS
N/A

ALTERNATIVE DRUGS
Oxyglobin has been used successfully in dogs, cats, and horses. If packed RBCs or whole blood is not available, Oxyglobin may be a suitable alternative in cases of severe anemia or until whole blood products are available.

FOLLOW-UP

PATIENT MONITORING
• Respiration and heart rate, mucous membrane color
• In patients with severe anemia, CBC or PCV with blood smear examination every 1–2 days
• In stabilized animals with a chronic disease or slowly improving disease course, reevaluation every 7–10 days

PREVENTION/AVOIDANCE
See specific chapters for nutritional deficiencies, intestinal parasites, etc.

POSSIBLE COMPLICATIONS
N/A

EXPECTED COURSE AND PROGNOSIS
Clinical course and prognosis vary and are associated with the underlying disease condition causing the nonregenerative anemia. Other cytopenias in addition to the anemia typically warrant a guarded to poor prognosis.

MISCELLANEOUS

ASSOCIATED CONDITIONS
N/A

AGE-RELATED FACTORS
The mean age of llamas affected with JLIDS is 13.8 months.

ZOONOTIC POTENTIAL
N/A

PREGNANCY
A mild anemia may be observed in some pregnant animals due to dilution of RBC mass by a high blood volume.

RUMINANT SPECIES AFFECTED
Alpaca, camel, guanaco, llama, vicuña

BIOSECURITY
N/A

PRODUCTION MANAGEMENT
N/A

SYNONYMS
Depression anemia
Nonresponsive anemia

SEE ALSO
Chronic renal failure
Cobalt deficiency
Copper deficiency
Hepatic lipidosis
Iron deficiency

ABBREVIATIONS
AST = aspartate aminotransferase
GGT = gamma glutamyltransferase
Hgb = hemoglobin
JLIDS = juvenile llama immunodeficiency syndrome
LDH = lactate dehydrogenase
MCHC = mean cell hemoglobin concentration
MCV = mean cell volume
SDH = sorbitol dehydrogenase

Suggested Reading
Fowler, M. E. 1998. *Medicine and surgery of South American camelids.* 2d ed. Ames: Iowa State University Press.
Garry, F., Weiser, M. G., Belknap, E. 1994. Clinical pathology of llamas. *Vet Clin North Am Food Anim Pract.* 10:201–9.
Wernery, U., Fowler, M. E., Wernery, R. 1999. *Color atlas of camelid hematology.* Berlin: Blackwell Wissenschafts-Verlag,

Author: Frederic S. Almy

ANEMIA, REGENERATIVE: BOVINE

BASICS

DEFINITION
• Anemia in adult cattle is indicated by a PCV (or Hct) of less than 23%.
• Beef cattle have higher hemoglobin, RBC, and PCV than diary breeds.
• Anemias may be nonregenerative or regenerative. The presence of reticulocytes, polychromasia, and increased red cell distribution width (RDW) is indicative of a regenerative response.
• Lactating dairy cattle tend to have lower values than nonlactating cows.
• Bulls tend to have greater RBC counts than cows.
• Environmental, seasonal, and physiological differences may affect the hemogram.
• Diminished oxygen tension at elevated altitudes stimulates erythropoiesis resulting in increased RBC counts.

PATHOPHYSIOLOGY
• Anemia results from decreased production or increased destruction (hemolysis) or loss (hemorrhage) of erythrocytes. Regenerative anemias are caused by hemolysis or hemorrhage.
• Anemia caused by hemolysis or hemorrhage and the related signs may be insidious or acute.
• Recognition of the indicators of erythropoietic response (reticulocytosis, polychromasia, and increased RDW) to hemorrhage- or hemolysis-induced hypoxia will not be evident for 3 to 6 days after the onset of anemia because the proliferation and differentiation of precursor cells of the erythropoietic series must occur. These events require several mitotic events and considerable protein, especially hemoglobin, synthesis. A single precursor cell may give rise to 16 to 32 mature RBCs.

Hemorrhagic Anemia
Hemorrhage is caused by vessel injury or disease. It may be internal (within the body) or external. With external hemorrhage, blood cells and their iron are lost from the system. Thus, the regenerative response is typically mild to moderate. Chronic external blood loss (e.g., GI bleeding) often leads to a nonregenerative anemia due to iron depletion. In peracute and acute hemorrhage, response to anemia-induced hypoxia will not be recognized by CBC parameters for 3 to 6 days after the initial hemorrhage.

Hemolytic Anemia
Hemolysis results from intravascular, extravascular (primarily in the spleen and/or liver), or a combination of both intravascular and extravascular destruction of RBCs. In contrast to hemorrhagic anemia, the regenerative response to hemolytic anemia is quite vigorous since iron is retained and is readily utilized for erythropoiesis. Extravascular hemolysis occurs as a result of erythrocyte sequestration in the spleen or liver where they are phagocytosed or lysed by the mononuclear phagocytic system. Hemolysis may be antibody and/or complement mediated, associated with infectious agents, drugs, or alterations in the immune system. Infectious agents may alter membrane antigens, form immune complexes that adsorb to the RBCs and fix complement, or cross-reacting antibody may be formed in response to the infectious agent. Less frequently, alterations in immune function may be secondary to some lymphoid malignancies. Intravascular hemolysis may be secondary to complement-mediated lysis such as with IgM-involved immune mediated anemia, neonatal isoerythrolysis or incompatible transfusions. Traumatic injury to the RBCs from intravascular fibrin deposition due to DIC or vasculitis can cause intravascular hemolysis. Oxidative injury to hemoglobin results in Heinz body formation that may cause RBC membrane damage sufficient to cause hemoglobin leakage and hemoglobinemia

SYSTEMS AFFECTED
• Hemic/lymphatic/immune—moderate to marked erythrocyte hyperplasia in the bone marrow. Splenomegaly can be a feature of extravascular hemolysis.
• Hepatobiliary—hypoxia due to marked anemia results in centrilobular necrosis. Hyperbilirubinemia may occur due to hypoxic hepatic injury and decreased hepatic functional mass, but icterus in patients with hemolytic anemia is primarily prehepatic.
• Cardiovascular—hypoxia causes tachycardia; decreased blood viscosity and turbulent blood flow may occasionally result in an auscultable heart murmur.
• Respiratory—hypoxia results in dyspnea and tachypnea.
• Renal/urologic—chronic hypoxia may lead to renal tubular necrosis. Additionally, free hemoglobin may precipitate in tubules and lead to renal failure.
• Central nervous system, liver, and kidney are particularly susceptible to hypoxia.

GENETICS
• Congenital erythropoietic porphyria is inherited in an autosomal recessive manner in Holstein cattle. It has also been recognized in shorthorn and Jamaican cattle.
• Coagulation factor VIII deficiency is inherited in a sex-linked recessive manner in Hereford cattle.
• Coagulation factor XI deficiency is inherited in an autosomal recessive manner in Holstein cattle.
• *Bos indicus* breeds exhibit resistance to babesiosis.

INCIDENCE/PREVALENCE
Anaplasmosis and babesiosis are endemic to locales with the proper tick vectors.

GEOGRAPHIC DISTRIBUTION
• Hemorrhagic and hemolytic conditions occur worldwide.
• Certain toxicosis and deficiencies are confined to specific regions depending upon geological origin, ecological features, or agricultural practices.
• Hemolytic anemia due to infectious organisms such as *Babesia* and *Anaplasma* species occur in areas endemic for the vectors associated with these organisms.

SIGNALMENT
Breed Predilections
• Hemorrhage and hemolysis may occur with cattle of all types.
• Cattle on range in endemic areas for some infectious agents that cause anemia are more likely to be affected than confined cattle in the same geographic area.
• Coagulation factor VIII deficiency is inherited in a sex-linked recessive manner in Hereford cattle.
• Coagulation factor XI deficiency and erythropoietic porphyria are inherited as autosomal recessives in Holstein cattle.

Mean Age and Range
• Anaplasmosis and babesiosis occur most frequently in adult cattle.
• Neonatal isoerythrolysis occurs within 24 to 48 hours after birth.
• Erythropoietic porphyria is usually recognized during the first 10 days after birth.
• Inherited coagulopathies are recognized in very young cattle. They may first be manifested after castration or minor trauma.
• Anemia due to other causes may affect any age animal.

Predominant Sex
Factor VIII deficiency is sex-linked. Therefore, it is a disease of newborn males.

ANEMIA, REGENERATIVE: BOVINE

SIGNS

HISTORICAL FINDINGS

• Signs of anemia include weakness, lethargy, depression, inability and reluctance to exercise, decreased milk production, and anorexia.
• With anaplasmosis, there may be a history of recent movement of cattle from a nonendemic area.

PHYSICAL EXAMINATION FINDINGS

• Pale or icteric mucous membranes, tachycardia, tachypnea, melena in animals with intestinal bleeding, frank external bleeding, petechia, ecchymosis, icterus, hemoglobinuria
• Frank, extreme, external bleeding is obvious, but intestinal or internal bleeding may be difficult to recognize.
• Icterus is often seen with intravascular and extravascular hemolytic anemia, but hemoglobinuria occurs only with intravascular hemolysis. Icterus may not be recognized with some cases of hemolytic anemia.

CAUSES AND RISK FACTORS

Anaplasmosis

• Anaplasmosis is a hemolytic disease caused by the rickettsial organisms *Anaplasma marginale* and *Anaplasma centrale*. Transmission between animals is generally by ticks (*Dermacentor andersoni* in western North America), but mechanical transmission by biting flies, mosquitoes, hypodermic needles, dehorning, castrating, and ear tagging can occur.
• *A. marginale* are small (0.5–1 μm diameter) inclusions along the margin of mature erythrocytes. *A. centrale* are of similar size but are found near the center of the erythrocytes. Generally, a single organism is found, but two or more organisms can be found occasionally especially in severe cases.
• *A. marginale* causes extravascular hemolytic anemia in adult cattle 3 years old or older. Animals less than 1 year old are resistant. Anemia develops through an immune reaction wherein antibody binds to infected erythrocytes, which are subsequently removed by mononuclear phagocytes of the spleen, liver, etc.
• Major clinical features are those of hemolytic anemia including pale mucous membranes, icterus, dyspnea, tachypnea, tachycardia, fever, lethargy, and reluctance to move.
• Diagnosis is based on finding organisms associated with erythrocytes or by card agglutination test.

• Laboratory features include moderate to severe anemia with evidence of response including reticulocytosis, polychromasia, microcytosis (increased MCV), hypochromasia (decreased MCHC), and increased RDW along with hyperbilirubinemia.
• Two vaccines are currently used to produce immunity in cattle. One consists of modified-live organisms and the other contains killed organisms. The live vaccine is only available in California. It should only be given to calves under 11 months of age. The killed vaccine can be given to cattle of any age. Two doses must be given in order to obtain full immunity. A killed vaccine that is no longer on the market has been implicated in producing neonatal isoerythrolysis (NI) in calves born to cows that were vaccinated in the last trimester. Apparently neither of the current vaccines has been evaluated for the potential for producing NI. (It is unlikely that the live vaccine would do so since it should not be used in animals of reproductive age.)
• Affected cattle are typically treated with tetracycline antibiotics.
• Also, tetracyclines can clear carrier cattle of *A. marginale*. From two to five treatments with LA-200 (long-acting tetracycline injectable product) given at 7-day intervals will clear the anaplasmosis organism from infected carrier cattle. However, cattle that are cleared will be susceptible and can be re-infected.

Babesiosis

• Babesiosis is a hemolytic disease caused by the protozoan organisms *Bebesia bovis* and *Babesia bigemina*.
• *B. bovis* and *B. bigemina* are piroplasm (piriform, teardrop shaped) bodies found in erythrocytes that are approximately 2 μm (*B. bovis*) or 4 μm (*B. bigemina*) in diameter. Usually there are pairs of organisms, but greater numbers (usually multiples of 2) can be found occasionally.
• *Babesia* species cause intravascular hemolysis, which may cause visually detectable hemoglobinuria and hemoglobinemia.
• Major clinical features are those of hemolytic anemia including pale mucous membranes, icterus, hemoglobinuria, hemoglobinemia dyspnea, tachypnea, tachycardia, fever, lethargy, and reluctance to move.

• Diagnosis is based on finding piriform organisms in erythrocytes. Capillary blood has higher numbers of organisms than does large vessel blood. Additionally, the infected erythrocytes are in greater numbers at the edge of blood smears than they are in the central, monolayer area. Thick blood smears improve the likeliness of finding organisms.
• Laboratory features include moderate to severe anemia with evidence of response including reticulocytosis, polychromasia, microcytosis (increased MCV), hypochromasia (decreased MCHC), increased RDW, hyperbilirubinemia, hemoglobinuria, and hemoglobinemia.
• Imidocarb has been used for therapy.
• An attenuated vaccine has been produced and successfully used in Australia for the prevention of *B. bovis*.
• *Bos indicus* breeds exhibit resistance.

Eperythrozoonosis

• *Mycoplasma wenyonii* (basonym *Eperythrozoon wenyonii*) occurs worldwide as a latent infection in healthy cattle. It causes hemolytic anemia only in critically ill cattle.
• Significant parasitemia without anemia but with hind limb edema and lymphadenopathy has been reported in cattle.
• On blood smears, *E. wenyonii* are small (0.5 μm diameter) basophilic, pleomorphic organisms. They vary from ring forms to cocci to rods.
• General signs of anemia may accompany those of other diseases that allowed the organisms to cause hemolysis.

Theileriosis

• *Theileria parva* and *Theileria annulata* are pathogenic for cattle. *T. parva* causes East Coast fever in Africa, and *T. annulata* causes tropical theileriosis in the Mediterranean area, the Middle East, and Asia.
• *T. annulata* causes hemolytic anemia with hemoglobinuria.
• Pleomorphic merozoites of approximately 1 μm diameter and varying from ring- to comma-shaped are found within erythrocytes.

Trypanosomiasis

Several trypanosomes cause hemolytic and/or nonregenerative anemia in cattle.

Bacillary Hemoglobinuria

• Bacillary hemoglobinuria is a highly fatal disease caused by *Clostridium haemolyticum* in damaged liver tissue.

ANEMIA, REGENERATIVE: BOVINE

• Often there is an association with massive liver fluke (*Fasciola hepatica*) migration, but liver damage from toxins, inflammation, and biopsy can cause the development of hypoxic areas that allow the anaerobic organisms to grow and produce toxins (including β toxin) that cause hemolysis.

• Generally, the disease is rapidly fatal and diagnosis is made from history of sudden death and postmortem lesions. Postmortem lesions include pale and icteric mucous membranes, large volumes of red-tinged fluid in abdominal and thoracic cavities, hemoglobinuria, hemoglobin casts, and liver lesions that may include the presence of liver flukes, necrotic biopsy site, or other indicators of liver damage.

Other Bacterial Diseases That Cause Anemia

• Many bacterial infections may cause anemia. Generally, the anemia is due to the erythropoietic depression that occurs with inflammation (see Anemia, Nonregenerative).

• Infection with *Leptospira* species may cause hemolytic anemia in calves.

Postparturient Hemoglobinuria

• Sporadic cases of anemia accompanied by hemoglobinuria occur throughout the world in dairy cows during the first month after calving. The anemia is often severe and may be regenerative if the cow has been anemic for several days.

• Although it is not completely understood, hypophosphatemia due to loss in milk is thought to disrupt erythrocyte energy metabolism, which results in erythrocyte lysis.

• Treatment is with sodium phosphate solution or transfusions (if economically reasonable).

Copper Toxicosis

• Copper toxicosis most commonly causes hemolytic anemia in sheep. However, calves may develop massive hemolytic anemia when copper accumulated through long-term ingestion is released from liver storage. Copper interacts with membrane proteins leading to lysis of the cells.

• Massive hemolysis leads to sudden death. Hematological features suggesting response to anemia are not found because the extreme peracute hemolysis does not allow sufficient time for the hypoxic stimulus to produce new erythrocytes.

Heinz Body Anemia Toxicosis

• Heinz bodies form through oxidation of sulfur containing amino acids of hemoglobin and other proteins of erythrocytes, which denatures the proteins and results in inclusion bodies in erythrocytes. These inclusion bodies are called Heinz bodies, and they are most readily detected by microscopic examination of smears of blood that have been incubated with new methylene blue.

• Erythrocytes containing Heinz bodies are removed from the blood by the mononuclear phagocyte system. This extravascular hemolysis can result in severe, rapidly developing anemia.

• Numerous oxidative substances have been implicated in the production of Heinz bodies. Some oxidants include wild or domestic onions and members of the Brassica family (turnips, kale, and rape). The cause of anemia of copper toxicosis is oxidation of erythrocytes.

• Animals from selenium-deficient areas are of increased risk to develop Heinz body anemia because selenium is a vital component of the erythrocyte enzyme glutathione peroxidase, which participates in the antioxidant activity of erythrocytes. Blood glutathione peroxidase activity has been used as an indicator of selenium deficiency in cattle, but this method has been replaced by trace mineral analysis.

• Heinz body formation may cause massive hemolysis leading to sudden death. Hematological features suggesting response to anemia are not found because the extreme, peracute hemolysis does not allow sufficient time for the hypoxic stimulus to produce new erythrocytes.

• Animals with Heinz-body-mediated anemia may be icteric and have hyperbilirubinemia provided they live long enough for hemoglobin to be catabolized to bilirubin.

Water Intoxication Toxicosis

• Intake of large amounts of water can result in intravascular erythrocyte lysis due to extreme, rapidly developing blood hypotonicity.

• Milk-fed calves may develop severe anemia when first given access to unlimited amounts of water.

• Cattle given sudden access to water after being deprived of water such as with extreme cold when all supplies are frozen may suddenly develop severe anemia.

• Features of severe water toxicosis include severe anemia, hypoproteinemia, hemoglobinuria, hypotonicity with decreased electrolyte concentrations.

Congenital Erythropoietic Porphyria

• Congenital erythropoietic porphyria (CEP) is an inherited disease of cattle, particularly Holsteins.

• CEP is caused by a defect in production of the heme portion of hemoglobin. In addition to decreased erythrocyte production, toxic porphyrin products are present in high concentrations in erythrocytes.

• The abnormal porphyrins in high concentrations are toxic to the erythrocytes resulting in hemolysis. In addition, hemoglobin production is decreased, which results in decreased erythrocyte production.

• Affected calves develop severe photosensitivity in the light parts of their hair coat. Teeth are dark and fluoresce under ultraviolet light. Urine is often dark and also fluorescent.

Traumatic or Ulceration Induced Hemorrhage

• Bleeding is generally obvious with external hemorrhage, but internal hemorrhage into cavities or the intestines may be difficult to recognize.

• Dark-colored feces may indicate bleeding in the upper gastrointestinal tract; red-stained feces suggest bleeding in the lower GI tract.

• Red urine may be due to hemoglobin, which is suggestive of intravascular hemolysis, or hematuria (erythrocytes in urine), which is suggestive of hemorrhage into either the urinary tract or the genital system.

• Chronic ingestion of bracken fern (*Pteridium aquilinum*) causes urinary bladder hemorrhage in cattle and sheep. (See Anemia, Nonregenerative: Bovine.)

Inherited Coagulopathies

• Factor VIII deficiency (hemophilia A) has been described in Hereford cattle in Australia. Hemophilia A is inherited in a sex-linked recessive manner; therefore, it is essentially a condition of males. Clinical features include profuse bleeding and death after surgery such as castration. Diagnosis depends upon determination of prothrombin time (normal), partial thromboplastin time (markedly prolonged), and factor VIII levels (markedly decreased).

• Factor XI deficiency has been described in Holstein cattle. It is inherited as a simple autosomal recessive. Spontaneous bleeding is rare, and delayed (12–14 hours), often severe hemorrhage occurs following surgery or trauma. Diagnosis depends upon determination of prothrombin time (normal), partial thromboplastin time (markedly prolonged). Specific diagnosis requires determination of factor XI levels.

Vitamin K Antagonist Rodenticide Toxicity Coagulopathies

• Damaged or moldy sweet clover hay and coumarin and indandione anticoagulant rodenticides and pharmaceuticals cause bleeding by inhibiting the production of functional coagulation factors II (prothrombin), VII, IX, and X. Hemorrhages may occur in the cerebral vasculature, abdominal cavity, pericardial sac, mediastinum, thorax, subcutaneously, or into joints. Outward signs of hemorrhage may not exist.

• Diagnosis depends upon determination of prothrombin time (prolonged) and partial thromboplastin time (prolonged) along with history, laboratory analysis for detection of specific anticoagulants in biological fluids, or analysis of suspect hay or silage for dicumarol content.

• Therapy consists of injectable vitamin K_1 (1–3 mg/kg BW). Because there is great variation in the duration of activity of the various rodenticides, it may be necessary to maintain therapy for several weeks. In small animals and humans, the coagulation test PIVKA (proteins induced by vitamin K absence or antagonism) has been successfully used to determine when vitamin K therapy can be stopped.

DIAGNOSIS

DIFFERENTIAL DIAGNOSIS

• On the hemogram, regenerative anemia is distinguished from nonregenerative anemia by the presence of reticulocytosis, polychromasia, increased RDW, microcytosis, and hypochromasia.

• Anemia due to either hemolysis or hemorrhage may be distinguished by evaluation of bilirubin and protein concentration. Frequently, hyperbilirubinemia occurs in hemolytic anemia. Hypoproteinemia is a common finding in external hemorrhage. However, internal hemorrhage may not cause significant decrease in plasma protein concentration.

• Specific etiologic diagnosis requires evaluation of blood smears for organisms, culture of tissues, immunology-based testing, and possibly PCR for specific gene sequences.

CBC/BIOCHEMISTRY/URINALYSIS

Anaplasmosis
CBC
• Moderate to marked decreases in RBC, Hgb, and PCV

• Regenerative anemia with numerous typical inclusion bodies on RBCs
• Inflammatory leukogram—neutrophilia, ± left shift
• Lymphopenia may indicate effects of stress (endogenous corticosteroid release).

Serum Biochemistry
• Hyperbilirubinemia
• Normal plasma protein
• Increased liver enzyme activity—AST, SDH, GGT

Babesiosis
CBC
• Moderate to marked decreases in RBC, Hgb and PCV
• Regenerative anemia with occasional, typical inclusion bodies in RBCs
• Inflammatory leukogram—neutrophilia, ± left shift
• Lymphopenia may indicate effects of stress (endogenous corticosteroid release)

Serum Biochemistry
• Hyperbilirubinemia
• Normal plasma protein
• Increased liver enzyme activity—AST, SDH, GGT

Urinalysis
Hemoglobinuria

Heinz Body Anemia
CBC
• Moderate to marked decreases in RBC, Hgb, and PCV
• Either nonregenerative or regenerative anemia depending upon the duration of the condition.
• Many typical inclusion bodies in RBCs that are best revealed with new methylene blue staining.

Serum Biochemistry
• Hyperbilirubinemia depending on the duration of the condition
• Normal plasma protein

Postparturient Hemoglobinuria
Serum Biochemistry
Hypophosphatemia in affected cows and in other cows of the dairy

Water Toxicosis
CBC
Nonregenerative anemia

Serum Biochemistry
• Decreased plasma protein concentrations
• Hyponatremia, hypochloremia, decreased osmolarity

Hemorrhage
CBC
• Regenerative anemia but generally not as robust as in hemolytic anemia

• Variable decreases in RBC, Hgb, and PCV

Serum Biochemistry
• Hypoproteinemia especially with external bleeding
• Increased liver enzyme activity—AST, SDH, GGT

Urinalysis
Hematuria (intact erythrocytes in urine) if bleeding is urogenital

OTHER LABORATORY TESTS

Anaplasmosis
In addition to recognizing organisms on erythrocytes, diagnosis is through the CF (complement fixation) or RCA (rapid card agglutination) tests.

Babesiosis
• Complement fixation and indirect fluorescent antibody tests are available from National Veterinary Services Laboratories (USDA: APHIS).
• A PCR method has been developed for detecting *B. bovis* carrier cattle. Its sensitivity is significantly improved over that of current methods.

Heinz Body Anemia
Possible low blood selenium concentrations

Bacillary Hemoglobinuria
Culture of liver; however, caution must be used when interpreting the results because *Clostridium* species often proliferate in tissues after death.

Copper Toxicosis and Selenium Deficiency
Trace metal analysis

Congenital Erythropoietic Porphyria
Blood or urine porphyrin analysis in animals of proper breed and with skin and teeth lesions

OTHER DIAGNOSTIC PROCEDURES

Bone Marrow Evaluation
Cytological evaluation of bone marrow specimen is not indicated when response to anemia-driven hypoxia is recognized by hematological features (reticulocytosis, polychromasia, macrocytosis, hypochromasia, and increased RDW).

PATHOLOGIC FINDINGS

Hemolytic Anemias
• Enlarged spleen and liver may be found with many hemolytic anemias especially those of extravascular pathogenesis.
• Tissues may be pale or have a red appearance. In massive hemolytic anemias (e.g., copper toxicosis), the kidneys may be dark and have a "gun metal" appearance.
• Hemoglobinuria indicates extravascular hemolysis.

ANEMIA, REGENERATIVE: BOVINE

• Liver lesions including liver flukes, biopsy site necrosis may be suggestive of bacillary hemoglobinuria.

• Discolored bone and teeth in congenital erythropoietic porphyria

Hemorrhage

Large amounts of blood in intestines, thorax, abdomen, joints, etc.; petechia and ecchymosis of skin, sclera, urinary tract, mucous membrane; and ulcers of the intestinal tract may be found with various causes of hemorrhage.

TREATMENT

• Successful treatment depends upon specific therapy for the underlying cause of the anemia. Appropriate milk and meat withdrawal times must be followed for all compounds administered to food-producing animals.

• Transfusion may be used with animals that are of sufficient value to make the procedure economically feasible. Generally, it is unlikely that a recipient that has never received a transfusion will experience a transfusion reaction. Therefore, almost any adult bovine can be used as a donor. Occasionally, transfusion reactions may occur because of J antigen incompatibilities.

ACTIVITY

Restrict activity until the animal(s) can exert themselves without developing significant dyspnea.

DIET

Correct dietary insufficiencies such as selenium deficiency or excess copper in the diet.

CLIENT EDUCATION

• Advise clients in anaplasmosis-endemic areas to purchase replacement cows from anaplasmosis-endemic areas or purchase heifers that were vaccinated for anaplasmosis as calves.

• Advise clients to use proper anthelmintic therapy for liver flukes.

MEDICATIONS

DRUGS OF CHOICE

• Cattle with anaplasmosis are typically treated with tetracycline antibiotics.

• Also, tetracyclines can clear carrier cattle of *A. marginale*. From two to five treatments with LA-200 (long-acting tetracycline injectable product) given at 7-day intervals will clear the anaplasmosis organism from infected carrier cattle. However, cattle that are cleared will become susceptible and can be reinfected.

• Imidocarb has been used for therapy for babesiosis.

• If economically feasible, anticoagulant rodenticide toxicity can be treated with injectable vitamin K_1 (1–3 mg/kg BW). PIVKA can be used to determine when therapy can be discontinued.

CONTRAINDICATIONS

Appropriate milk and meat withdrawal times must be followed for all compounds administered to food-producing animals.

PRECAUTIONS

Cattle treated with tetracycline antibiotics at dosages that clear *Anaplasma* organisms are susceptible to reinfection.

FOLLOW-UP

PATIENT MONITORING

• Respiration and heart rates and mucous membrane color are useful for recognizing the success of therapy.

• In patients with severe anemia, CBC or PCV with a blood smear examination should be performed every 1–2 days until a significant erythropoietic response is recognized.

PREVENTION/AVOIDANCE

• If animals are to be pastured on range endemic for anaplasmosis, they should be vaccinated or purchased from an endemic area. Modified-live vaccine should be used only in calves less than 11 months old.

• An attenuated vaccine has been produced and successfully used in Australia for the prevention of *B. bovis*. *Bos indicus* breeds exhibit resistance to *Babesia* species.

• Appropriate anthelmintic therapy should be used in order to prevent liver fluke parasitism.

• Possibly initiate phosphorus supplementation if soil or feed is deficient especially in high producing dairy cows.

• Possibly provide selenium supplementation if soil or feed is deficient.

POSSIBLE COMPLICATIONS

N/A

EXPECTED COURSE AND PROGNOSIS

Clinical course and prognosis vary and are associated with the underlying disease condition causing the anemia.

MISCELLANEOUS

ASSOCIATED CONDITIONS

N/A

AGE-RELATED FACTORS

• Adult cattle that have neither been vaccinated nor raised in endemic areas are highly susceptible to anaplasmosis, but calves develop resistance.

• Adult cattle are more susceptible to babesiosis than calves.

ZOONOTIC POTENTIAL

N/A

PREGNANCY

N/A

RUMINANT SPECIES AFFECTED

Potentially, all ruminant species are affected by many of these conditions.

BIOSECURITY

N/A

SYNONYMS

Responsive anemia

SEE ALSO

Specific diseases and conditions

ABBREVIATIONS

AST = aspartate aminotransferase
CEP = Congenital erythropoietic porphyria
GGT = gamma glutamyltransferase
Hgb = hemoglobin
LDH = lactate dehydrogenase
MCHC = mean cell hemoglobin concentration
MCV = mean cell volume
RDW = red cell distribution width
SDH = sorbitol dehydrogenase

Suggested Reading
Feldman, B. F., Zinkl, J. G., Jain, N. C. 2000. *Schalm's veterinary hematology.* 5th ed. Baltimore: Lippincott Williams and Wilkins.
Smith, B. P. 2001. *Large animal internal medicine.* 3rd ed. Philadelphia: Mosby.

Authors: Joseph G. Zinkl and Bernard F. Feldman

BASICS

DEFINITION
• A syndrome characterized by decreased circulating RBC mass (anemia in adult llamas and alpacas indicated by a PCV ≤25%; in camels a PCV ≤28% indicates anemia), together with an appropriate compensatory increase in RBC production by the bone marrow.
• The presence of polychromasia, reticulocytes ± nucleated erythrocytes are indicative of an appropriate regenerative response.
• Because it takes the bone marrow 3–5 days for a maximum response, evidence for regeneration may not be apparent until several days after the onset of anemia.
• High concentrations of erythrocytes are observed in healthy camelids, but because the cells have a small mean cell volume, the PCV, or Hct, is relatively low.

PATHOPHYSIOLOGY
• Anemia may result from either decreased production or increased destruction of erythrocytes. Regenerative anemias are most often associated with two general mechanisms: blood loss (hemorrhage) or hemolysis. Chronic blood loss can result in iron deficiency and nonregenerative anemia. Trichostrongyle infection causes a mildly regenerative, normocytic, normochromic blood loss anemia.
• Hemolysis in camelids most commonly occurs secondary to anti-RBC antibodies formed against altered erythrocyte membrane antigens. Infectious organisms (e.g., *Leptospira interrogans*, *Trypanosoma*, hemotrophic *Mycoplasma*), exposure of previously unexposed antigens, or adsorption of antigen-antibody complexes to the erythrocyte membrane can alter RBC membrane antigens and render RBCs susceptible to accelerated destruction or removal by the mononuclear phagocytic system of the spleen and/or liver (extravascular hemolysis). Certain bacterial infections (i.e., *Clostridium perfringens* type A) cause direct erythrocyte damage due to hydrolysis of membrane phospholipids. The result is marked intravascular hemolysis.
• RBC parasites such as *Candidatus Mycoplasma haemolamae* (formerly *Eperythrozoon* spp.) adhere to the surface of RBC membranes. Affected erythrocytes are removed by the mononuclear-phagocytic system of the spleen and/or liver. Young llamas and alpacas are more susceptible to

acute infection and severe parasitemia with clinically significant extravascular hemolysis. Anemia may be nonregenerative or regenerative depending on the presence or lack of other clinical problems.

Hemorrhagic Anemia
RBCs are lost from the vasculature due to vascular injury or disease. Hemorrhage may be internal (within the body) or external. RBC lifespan is unaltered in this condition. Both blood cells and iron are lost from the body with external hemorrhagic anemia. Thus, the regenerative response is typically mild to moderate. Chronic external blood loss (e.g., GI bleeding) often leads to a nonregenerative anemia due to iron depletion.

Hemolytic Anemia
In patients with hemolytic anemia, the vasculature is typically intact. Hemolysis results from intravascular, extravascular (primarily in the spleen and/or liver) or a combination of both intravascular and extravascular destruction of RBCs. In contrast to hemorrhagic anemia, the regenerative response to hemolytic anemia is quite vigorous since iron is retained and is readily utilized for erythropoiesis. Extravascular hemolysis occurs as a result of erythrocyte sequestration in the spleen or liver where they are phagocytosed or lysed by the mononuclear phagocytic system. Hemolysis may be antibody and/or complement mediated, associated with infectious agents, drugs, or alterations in the immune system. Infectious agents may alter membrane antigens, form immune complexes that adsorb to the RBC and fix complement, or cross-reacting antibody may be formed in response to the infectious agent. Less frequently, alterations in immune function occur secondary to some lymphoid malignancies. Intravascular hemolysis may occur secondary to complement-mediated lysis such as with IgM-involved immune-mediated anemia, neonatal isoerythrolysis, or incompatible transfusions. Traumatic injury to the RBCs from intravascular fibrin deposition due to DIC or vasculitis can cause intravascular hemolysis. Oxidative injury to hemoglobin results in Heinz body formation that may cause RBC membrane damage sufficient to cause hemoglobin leakage and hemoglobinemia. The unique shape and low osmotic fragility of camelid RBCs probably render a protective effect against hemolysis from oxidative injury, unless severe.

SYSTEMS AFFECTED
• Hemic/Lymphatic/Immune—moderate to marked erythrocyte hyperplasia in the bone marrow. Splenomegaly can be a feature of extravascular hemolysis.
• Hepatobiliary—hypoxia due to marked anemia results in centrilobular necrosis. Hyperbilirubinemia may occur due to hypoxic hepatic injury and decreased hepatic functional mass, but icterus in patients with hemolytic anemia is primarily prehepatic.
• Cardiovascular—hypoxia causes tachycardia; decreased blood viscosity and turbulent blood flow may occasionally result in an auscultable heart murmur.
• Respiratory—hypoxia results in tachypnea.
• Renal/urologic—chronic hypoxia may lead to renal tubular necrosis. Free hemoglobin is also nephrotoxic and can lead to renal failure.

GENETICS
Young llamas affected with juvenile llama immunodeficiency syndrome (JLIDS) are often anemic. Although there are apparent familial links in affected llamas, reliable genealogical information is not available and a definitive genetic basis has not been established.

INCIDENCE/PREVALENCE
Unknown

GEOGRAPHIC DISTRIBUTION
Chronic blood loss due to intestinal parasitism may have an increased prevalence in areas endemic to associated parasites.

SIGNALMENT
Species
All camelids are susceptible to anemia. Llamas and alpacas may be more susceptible to RBC parasitism than camels are.

Mean Age and Range
• Anemia due to infection with *Candidatus Mycoplasma haemolamae* generally affects llamas and alpacas ≤1 year; range neonate to adult.
• Median age of llamas affected with JLIDS and that are anemic 13.8 months; range 6 months–4 years.
• Anemia due to other causes may affect any age animal.

Predominant Sex
No sex predilection

SIGNS

HISTORICAL FINDINGS
Nonspecific signs of anemia include weakness, lethargy, anorexia, dyspnea, tachypnea; reddish-brown urine (hemoglobinuria) if hemolysis is severe; dark feces (melena).

ANEMIA, REGENERATIVE: CAMELIDS

PHYSICAL EXAMINATION FINDINGS
Clinical signs of hemorrhage with blood loss; pale or icteric mucous membranes; tachycardia; tachypnea; melena occasionally observed in llamas with gastric ulcers

CAUSES AND RISK FACTORS
Blood Loss/Hemorrhagic Anemia
Blood loss may be subdivided into acute and chronic causes of hemorrhage.

Acute Hemorrhage
Trauma, lacerations, GI ulcers, and hemostatic defects such as DIC, spoiled sweet clover hay poisoning, anticoagulant rodenticides, and bracken fern poisoning.

Chronic Hemorrhage
Intestinal parasites, GI ulcers or tumors, hematuria, vascular neoplasm, vitamin K deficiency, and thrombocytopenia

Hemolytic Anemia
Many of the causes listed below have both intravascular and extravascular components, but are listed where the majority of the hemolysis occurs.

Intravascular Hemolysis
Leptospirosis, bacillary hemoglobinemia/ hemoglobinuria, copper toxicity, molybdenum deficiency, propylene glycol, vitamin K_3, incompatible transfusions, hypophosphatemia.

Extravascular Hemolysis
Mycoplasma haemolamae (formerly *Eperythrozoon*), *Trypanosoma* spp., occasionally drugs such as penicillin, hemangiosarcoma, autoimmune mediated hemolytic anemia (uncommon in camelids).

 DIAGNOSIS

DIFFERENTIAL DIAGNOSIS
Regenerative anemia is differentiated from nonregenerative anemia by increased reticulocyte count, polychromasia and ± nucleated RBCs. Specific features of the erythrogram, biochemical profile, and urinalysis are used to differentiate among blood loss anemia and intravascular and extravascular hemolysis.

CBC/BIOCHEMISTRY/URINALYSIS
• Anemia in adult llamas and alpacas is indicated by a PCV of less than 25%. A PCV of ≤28% in camels is indicative of anemia.
• High concentrations of erythrocytes are observed in healthy camelids, but because the cells have a small mean cell volume, the PCV, or hematocrit, is relatively low.

Anemia Due to Blood Loss/Hemorrhage
CBC
• If blood loss is chronic, one may observe normocytic to microcytic, normochromic to hypochromic anemia with mild reticulocytosis. Higher reticulocyte counts may be observed with internal hemorrhage compared to external blood loss.
• Acute blood loss may result in normocytic, normochromic, nonregenerative anemia if the bone marrow has not had adequate time to respond (usually 3–5 days).
• Mild to marked decreases in RBC, Hgb, and PCV (degree of anemia based upon severity and duration of blood loss). Internal hemorrhage is usually associated with less-severe anemia.
• Anisocytosis, polychromasia, poikilocytosis.
• Inflammatory leukogram—neutrophilia, ± monocytosis (tissue damage/necrosis due to trauma).
• Lymphopenia may indicate effects of stress (endogenous corticosteroid release).
• ±Thrombocytosis (reactive)

Serum Biochemistry
Hypoproteinemia is associated with chronic blood loss (e.g., GI bleeding).

Urinalysis
Hematuria due to urinary tract hemorrhage. (Rarely is urinary tract hemorrhage alone severe enough to cause clinical signs of anemia.)

Intravascular Hemolytic Anemia
CBC
• MCV is normal to increased. MCHC is typically low, but a falsely increased MCHC may occur due to hemoglobinemia.
• Moderate reticulocytosis (counts are higher in hemolytic anemia than external hemorrhagic anemia).
• Moderate to marked decreases in RBC, Hgb, and PCV.
• Anisocytosis, polychromasia, abnormal erythrocyte morphology (e.g., Heinz bodies, RBC parasites, schistocytes, keratocytes)
• Inflammatory leukogram (neutrophilia with left shift, ± monocytosis)
• ±Thrombocytosis
• Normal to increased plasma protein concentration

Serum Biochemistry
• Hyperbilirubinemia
• Hyperproteinemia due to hyperglobulinemia

Urinalysis
Hemoglobinuria

Extravascular Hemolytic Anemia
CBC
• MCV is normal to increased. MCHC is typically low.
• Moderate reticulocytosis (counts are higher in hemolytic anemia than external hemorrhagic anemia).
• Moderate to marked decreases in RBC, Hgb, and PCV
• Inflammatory leukogram (neutrophilia with left shift, ± monocytosis)
• ±Thrombocytosis

Serum Biochemistry
Hyperbilirubinemia if magnitude of hemolysis exceeds liver capacity to process

Urinalysis
Hemoglobinuria is absent.

OTHER LABORATORY TESTS
Blood Loss/Hemorrhage
• Fecal flotation to rule out intestinal parasites (*Trichostrongylus*) as cause of blood loss
• Fecal occult blood test (Caution: Some plant peroxidases as part of the normal diet can result in a false positive.)
• Coagulation profile to rule out hemostatic defects

Hemolytic Anemia
• PCR analysis to confirm *Mycoplasma haemolamae* RBC parasitism
• Copper levels to confirm copper toxicosis
• New methylene blue stained blood smear to confirm presence of Heinz bodies

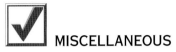

IMAGING

Blood Loss/Hemorrhage
Radiographic or ultrasonographic imaging may reveal evidence of gastrointestinal disease accounting for blood loss.

OTHER DIAGNOSTIC PROCEDURES

Blood Loss/Hemorrhage
• Gastric endoscopy may reveal evidence for gastric ulceration.
• Bone marrow evaluation reveals erythroid hyperplasia. Cytologic evaluation of bone marrow is only needed when there is not evidence of RBC responsiveness in the peripheral blood, but regenerative anemia is still suspected.

TREATMENT

• An emergency situation exists if anemia is severe or develops rapidly. Massive hemorrhage results in hypovolemic shock and hypoxia/anoxia.
• The successful treatment of regenerative anemia usually revolves around correction of the underlying cause.
• General treatment and supportive care recommendations follow. See specific disease chapters for detailed treatment information.

ACTIVITY
Restrict

DIET
Correct any dietary insufficiencies as described within specific nutritional deficiency chapters.

CLIENT EDUCATION
N/A

MEDICATIONS

DRUGS OF CHOICE
Specific therapy for increasing RBC mass:
• If anemia is unusually severe (PCV ≤15%), transfusion may be required to treat life-threatening anemia: whole blood, 0.1 ml/kg at a rate of 5–20 ml/kg/hr.
• Numerous blood types are present in the llama and alpaca. However, incompatibility reactions are very rare with the first transfusion. Subsequent transfusions increase the risk for an adverse reaction. Blood cross matching is advised for repeated transfusions.
• Fluid therapy to correct hypovolemia may be indicated early in the course of traumatic hemorrhagic anemia.
• Oral or parenteral iron supplementation may be of benefit in patients with external blood loss anemia.

CONTRAINDICATIONS
Appropriate milk and meat withdrawal times must be followed for all compounds administered to food-producing animals.

PRECAUTIONS
N/A

POSSIBLE INTERACTIONS
N/A

ALTERNATIVE DRUGS
Oxyglobin has been used successfully in dogs, cats, and horses. If packed RBCs or whole blood is not available for transfusion, Oxyglobin may be a suitable alternative in cases of severe anemia or until whole blood products are available.

FOLLOW-UP

PATIENT MONITORING
• Respiration and heart rate, mucous membrane color
• Initially, in patients with severe anemia, CBC or PCV with blood smear examination every 24 hours. As regeneration increases RBC mass and polychromasia is apparent on blood smear evaluation, rechecks recommended at 3–5 day intervals.

PREVENTION/AVOIDANCE
See specific chapters for toxicants, nutritional deficiencies, RBC and intestinal parasites, etc.

POSSIBLE COMPLICATIONS
N/A

EXPECTED COURSE AND PROGNOSIS
• Clinical course and prognosis vary and are associated with the underlying disease condition causing the anemia.
• Return to normal values is expected within 10 to 14 days following the initial insult if the underlying cause has been corrected.

MISCELLANEOUS

ASSOCIATED CONDITIONS
None

AGE-RELATED FACTORS
None

ZOONOTIC POTENTIAL
None

PREGNANCY
N/A

RUMINANT SPECIES AFFECTED
Alpaca, camel, guanaco, llama, vicuña

BIOSECURITY
N/A

PRODUCTION MANAGEMENT
N/A

SYNONYMS
Responsive anemia

SEE ALSO
Bacillary hemoglobinuria
Bracken fern
Copper toxicity
DIC
Leptospirosis
Mycoplasma
Rodenticide toxicity
Trypanosomiasis

ABBREVIATIONS
Hct = hematocrit
Hgb = hemoglobin
MCHC = mean cell hemoglobin concentration
MCV = mean cell volume
PCV = packed cell volume
RBC = red blood cells

Suggested Reading
Fowler, M. E. 1998. *Medicine and surgery of South American camelids*. 2d ed. Ames: Iowa State University Press.
Garry, F., Weiser, M. G., Belknap, E. 1994. Clinical pathology of llamas. *Vet Clin North Am Food Anim Pract*. 10:201–9.
Wernery, U., Fowler, M. E., Wernery, R. 1999. *Color atlas of camelid hematology*. Berlin: Blackwell Wissenschafts-Verlag.

Authors: Frederic S. Almy and Tripp Almy

ANESTHESIA AND ANALGESIA

BASICS

OVERVIEW
• Anesthesia: local, regional (epidural, intrathecal), or general; local and regional methods most commonly employed in ruminants
• Analgesia: local, regional, systemic, multimodal, short-term, long-term
• Pain: an unpleasant sensory and emotional experience associated with actual or potential tissue damage or described in terms of such damage
• Types: acute, chronic, visceral, and somatic
• Suffering: a reaction to the physical or emotional components of pain with a feeling of uncontrollability, helplessness, hopelessness, intolerability, and interminableness. Suffering implies a threat to the wholeness of patient comfort within the environment.
• Virtually all anesthetics and analgesics are *off-label use* in any ruminant species. Please see Suggested Reading below for guidelines on off-label use of analgesic and anesthetic drugs in ruminants. The relief of pain and suffering in ruminants can and should be accomplished within these guidelines.

SYSTEMS AFFECTED
CNS, musculoskeletal, respiratory

GENETICS
N/A

INCIDENCE/PREVALENCE
N/A

GEOGRAPHIC DISTRIBUTION
Worldwide

SIGNALMENT
Species
Potentially, all ruminant species
Breed Predilections
N/A
Mean Age and Range
N/A
Predominant Sex
N/A

SIGNS
Pain Behaviors in Ruminants: vacant stare, loss of mobility, guarding or splinting of affected limb, altered avoidance patterns, vocalization, tachypnea, repetitive motor activities, loss of socialization, repeated attempts at lateral recumbency, inappetence, reduced grooming behavior, bruxism. Behaviors and degree of distress depend on species, breed, temperament, rearing, and housing.

CAUSES AND RISK FACTORS
• Acute pain: trauma, surgery, GI accident, urogenital injury/obstruction, pneumonia/pleuritis, husbandry practices
• Chronic pain: osteoarthritis including CAE-related arthritis in goats, neoplasia, chronic osteomyelitis, chronic hoof rot, husbandry practices

DIAGNOSIS

DIFFERENTIAL DIAGNOSIS
Some pain behaviors are not pain-specific. However, for a given species, a behavior indicates pain if it is seen during and/or after a specific tissue-damaging injury, disease, or procedure, but is not seen in healthy or nondamaged animals, and not seen when local anesthesia or effective analgesics are delivered.

CBC/BIOCHEMISTRY/URINALYSIS
May be indicated as routine preoperative workup

OTHER LABORATORY TESTS
N/A

IMAGING
N/A

DIAGNOSTIC PROCEDURES
N/A

TREATMENT

MEDICATIONS

DRUGS OF CHOICE
Anesthetics Used in Ruminants: General Anesthesia
• Often not necessary for some procedures with adequate local or regional anesthesia and sedation due to ruminant temperament
• Protecting the airway is essential whether inhalant or injectable anesthetics are used; an endotracheal tube with cuff is always recommended. Proper positioning of the head during recumbency allows regurgitation to flow from the mouth. Techniques for inhalant anesthesia and monitoring are covered in depth elsewhere.
• Injectable anesthesia may be administered as a single or repeated bolus, or by continuous infusion.
• An IV catheter (jugular v., cephalic v., ear v.) is advised for continuous infusion; 5% guaifenesin and thiopental must be administered via jugular catheter only. Although not necessary for many ruminants, use of a preanesthetic sedative and analgesic will smooth induction and recovery.
• Doses for commonly used agents are listed in Table 1.
• Acepromazine is not an analgesic or a potent sedative, and has several adverse side effects in ruminants.

Analgesics Used in Ruminants
Choice of analgesic is defined by type of pain, location of pain, duration of pain, species, breed, husbandry, meat and milk withdrawal times, and other federal and state drug use restrictions. Combinations of analgesics allows lower dosing of individual drugs and better pain control. See Table 2 for individual drugs.

Opioids
Inhibit pain transmission peripherally and in the spinal cord by binding mu or kappa receptors. All opioids are controlled substances in the United States. Cardiopulmonary, GI, sedative, and excitatory side effects are possible and dose- and drug-dependent.
Indications: acute pain, moderate to severe, visceral or somatic. May be given parenterally or regionally; fentanyl may be given topically in patch form. Opioids and alpha-2 agonists are synergistic; combining these drugs gives greater analgesia at lower doses for both drugs.

Alpha-2 Agonists
Produce central analgesia, sedation, and muscle relaxation by binding alpha-2 receptors in the brain and spinal cord. Cardiopulmonary, GI, and other side effects are dose dependent and can be severe. May cause abortion in late-term gestation. Use in sheep can cause severe arterial hypoxemia.
Indications: acute pain, moderate to severe, visceral, may be given parenterally or regionally, commonly used premedication for anesthesia. Opioids and alpha-2 agonists are synergistic; combining these drugs gives greater analgesia at lower doses for both drugs.

Steroids
Not analgesics but potent anti-inflammatory agents. Pain due to inflammation may be treated in part with steroids. Concurrent use of both steroids and NSAIDs should be avoided due to additive adverse renal and gastric side effects. Steroids should not be used in pregnant ruminants.
Indications: Short-term adjunct therapy in nonseptic inflammatory conditions

NSAIDs
Weak organic acids, which inhibit cyclooxygenase (COX) and reduce release of prostaglandins and thromboxanes. Anti-inflammatory, central and peripheral analgesic, and antipyretic effects, as well as adverse GI and renal effects are possible, and may relate to the COX1 and COX2 selectivity of the drug.
Indications: acute and chronic pain, mild to moderate, visceral and somatic, and for pain and concurrent sepsis or fever, may be given parenterally or orally.

Local Anesthetics
Block sodium channels and inhibit nerve transmission. Motor as well as sensory transmission is blocked. Produce anesthesia at and distal to the site of application, may be analgesic when given parenterally by infusion. Cardiovascular and CNS side effects are possible with high doses.

Table 1

Anesthetic Induction Protocols			
Drug	Dose (mg/kg)	Route	Species
Xylazine, then	0.05–0.2	IV/IM	B
Ketamine	2	IV	
Xylazine, then	0.03–0.2	IV/IM	O, C
Ketamine	5	IV	(See *Caution*)[1]
Xylazine, then	0.25–0.44	IV/IM	L
Ketamine	5	IV	
Xylazine, then	0.05–0.1	IV/IM	B, L, O, C
Telazol	2–4	IV (IM)	
Diazepam, then	0.1	IV	B, L, O, C
Ketamine	4.5	IV	
Diazepam, then	0.25	IV	O, C
Ketamine	7.5	IV	
Medetomidine, then	0.02	IV	B (calf), O, C
Ketamine	0.5–1	IV	
GKX: 1L 5% guaifenesin +	0.5–1.0 mL/kg to effect	IV	B, O, C
1000 mg ketamine +	1.5–2 ml/kg/hr to effect for	IV	L: increase xylazine to
50 mg xylazine	maintenance		100 mg
1 L 5% guaifenesin +	(Following sedation)	IV	B, L, O, C
2000–4000 mg thiopental	2 mL/kg to effect		
Detomidine, then	0.01	IM	O, C
Propofol	3–5	IV	

Note: IV = intravenous; IM = intramuscular; IV/IM = via both routes, LOWER dose IV; B = bovine; L = llama/alpaca; O = ovine; C = caprine.

[1]*Caution*: xylazine and other alpha-2 agonists can cause severe hypoxemia and pulmonary edema in sheep.

Indications: acute pain, mild to severe, visceral and somatic, and for regional anesthesia, administered subcutaneously, over peripheral nerves, and epidurally or intrathecally.

Other Agents
DMSO
Free-radical scavenger with anti-inflammatory, diuretic, vasodilatory, and anticholinesterase properties. Acts as a carrier agent for other drugs when applied topically as it readily crosses skin. DMSO is only labeled for topical use and not labeled for use in food animals.

Hyaluronic Acid and Polysulfated Glycosaminoglycans
Reported effects include inhibition of inflammatory mediators in joints and analgesia and improved range of motion for osteoarthritis pain; not licensed in food animals; oral and parenteral formulations.
Author's note: parenteral hyaluronic acid and polysulfated glycosaminoglycans at one-fourth the equine dose improve the comfort and mobility of small ruminants (which are not intended for food) suffering from osteoarthritis.

Ketamine
NMDA receptor antagonist that can prevent or reverse wind-up pain at subanesthetic doses. Subanesthetic use of ketamine is still largely experimental in food animals; ketamine is not labeled for use in food animals. *Author's note:* ketamine administered

IM at 0.25–0.5 mg/kg q 6–8 hours, along with opioids and NSAIDs may be helpful for severe pain such as burn injury, or for severe polyarthritis or osteomyelitis in small ruminants.

LOCAL AND REGIONAL ANESTHETIC TECHNIQUES
Note: IV = intravenous; IM = intramuscular; IV/IM = via both routes, LOWER dose IV; PO = oral; SQ = subcutaneous; B = bovine; L = llama/alpaca; O = ovine; C = caprine.

Local
- *Infiltration*: wound edges, incision line, inverted L block, ring block
- *Drugs*: lidocaine, mepivacaine, bupivacaine. Epinephrine, 0.1 mL of the 1 mg/mL (1:1000) solution to 20 mL of local anesthetic prolongs the duration of lidocaine and mepivacaine. Do not use epinephrine in limb blocks or wound edges as ischemia and tissue necrosis can occur.
- *Dosing*
  - B: 5 mg/kg lidocaine (125 mL of 2% solution for adult cattle), similar for mepivacaine, 2 mg/kg bupivacaine. *Toxic doses:* >10 mg/kg lidocaine or mepivacaine, >4 mg/kg bupivacaine.
  - O, C: 2–5 mg/kg lidocaine or mepivacaine, diluting to 1% with saline extends volume without increasing dose, 1 mg/kg bupivacaine. *Toxic doses:* >5 mg/kg

lidocaine, mepivacaine, >1 mg/mg bupivacaine. Combining lidocaine and bupivacaine 1:1 or 2:1 allows a long-term block with less bupivacaine volume. Toxic signs include excitation, sedation, recumbency, tonic-clonic convulsions, cardiopulmonary depression, and death.

Specific Nerve Blocks
- *Ocular, periocular*: ocular exam, topical treatment, enucleation, periorbital surgery.
- *Topical:* proparacaine 0.5%, 2–10 drops.
- *Auriculopalpebral block*: B, O, C—20–24 G 2.5 cm needle placed subcutaneously over the nerve (palpable in a notch of the zygomatic arch), 2–10 mL lidocaine for aknesia of eyelids (no analgesia).
- *Retrobulbar*
  - B: 15 cm 18G slightly curved needle passed through the dorsal or ventral lateral or medial eyelid behind the globe, 10–15 mL 2% lidocaine (with epinephrine) or 5–6 mL lidocaine and 5–6 mL bupivacaine injected following aspiration as the needle is advanced.
  - O, C: 3.75 cm 22G slightly curved needle, 3–5 mL 2% lidocaine (with epinephrine) (or equal volumes of lidocaine and bupivacane as for B) injected following aspiration. *Risks:* bleeding, subarachnoid deposition of local anesthetic with possible severe neurologic side effects.

ANESTHESIA AND ANALGESIA

Table 2

		Common Analgesics Used in Ruminants			
Class	Drug	Dose (mg/kg)	Route	Interval (hour)	Species
Opioid	Morphine	0.1–0.5	IM	4	O, C
Opioid	Butorphanol	0.05–0.5	IV/IM	2–4	B, L, O, C
Opioid	Buprenorphine	0.005–0.01	IV/IM	8–12	O, C
Opioid	Fentanyl patch	10 mg and 5 mg patch/70 kg	Trans-dermal	3–4 days	O
Opioid antagonist (reversal)	Naloxone	0.01–0.02 (dilute and titrate to effect)	IV		
Alpha-2 agonist	Xylazine (See *Caution*)[1]	0.01–0.02	IV	2–4	B, O, C
		0.05–0.1	IM	(Once)	B, O, C
		0.1–0.5	IV/IM		L
Alpha-2 agonist	Detomidine	0.005–0.05	IV/IM	3–6 (Once)	B, L, O, C
Alpha-2 agonist	Medetomidine	0.005–0.04	IV/IM	3–6 (Once)	B, L, O, C
Alpha-2 antagonist (reversal)	Tolazoline	0.5–2 (Dilute and titrate to effect)	IV		B, L, O, C
Alpha-2 antagonist (reversal)	Yohimbine	0.1–1 (Dilute and titrate to effect)	IV		B, L, O, C
Alpha-2 antagonist (reversal)	Atipamezole	0.02–0.1 (Titrate to effect)	IV		B, L, O, C
NSAID	Acetylsalicylic acid	50–100	PO	12–24	B, O, C
NSAID	Phenylbutazone	2–4	PO	24	B
		10	PO	24	O
NSAID	Flunixin	1–2.2	IV, SQ, PO	24	B, L, O, C
NSAID	Ketoprofen	3	IV, IM	24	B, O, C
NSAID	Carprofen	1–2	IV, SQ, PO	24	B, C
		4	SQ	24	O
NSAID	Meloxicam	0.5	IV, SQ	72	B

Note: IV = intravenous; IM = intramuscular; IV/IM = via both routes, LOWER dose IV; PO = oral; SQ = subcutaneous; B = bovine; L = llama/alpaca; O = ovine; C = caprine.

[1]*Caution* xylazine and other alpha-2 agonists can cause severe hypoxemia and pulmonary edema in sheep, and may cause abortion in ruminants.

• *Peterson Eye Block:* B—20–25 mL lidocaine subcutaneously and at the orbitorotundum foramen for immobilization of the globe and anesthesia of the globe and orbit.

Dehorning
• B: 2.5 cm 22G or 25G needle, 5–10 mL lidocaine injected subcutaneously over the palpable cornual branch of the zygomaticotemporal (lacrimal) nerve between the temporalis and frontalis muscles midway between the lateral canthus of the eye and the lateral base of the horn.
• C: 2.5 cm 22G or 25 G needle, 1–3 mL lidocaine injected subcutaneously over BOTH the zygomaticotemporal nerve midway between the lateral canthus and the base of the horn, and the infratrochlear nerve between the medial canthus and medial base of the horn at the dorsomedian margin of the orbit. *For kids:* 0.5 mL 2% lidocaine diluted for a ring block at the base of the horn to reduce possible toxicity.

Proximal and Distal Paravertebral Block
Anesthesia of skin, musculature, and peritoneum of the flank on the side treated, spinal nerves T13, L1, L2 for standing abdominal procedures.
• *Proximal*
  • B: 2.5–5 cm from midline immediately in front of the transverse process of L1, L2, and L3. After desensitizing the skin, an 18G 4.25–15 cm spinal needle is walked off the cranial edge of the transverse process while aspirating then infusing 1–2 mL lidocaine. Following aspiration, 15 mL lidocaine are injected ventral to the intertransverse ligament, 5 mL are injected proximally with minimal resistance.
  • O, C: 1.5–3 cm off midline, 20G 4.25 cm spinal needle, 2–3 mL lidocaine per site. *Risks:* penetration of aorta, vena cava, or other vessels, caudal migration of lidocaine to L3 causing ataxia or recumbency.
• *Distal*
  • B: 18G 3–7.5 cm needle inserted ventral and dorsal to the tip of the transverse

process of L1, L2, and L4. Up to 20 mL lidocaine is infused in a fanned-out pattern ventrally at each site, 5 mL injected dorsally.
• O, C: 20G 3 cm needle, 1–3 mL lidocaine at each site

Regional
Caudal Epidural Anesthesia:
Obstetric and surgical procedures of the tail, perineum, anus, rectum, vulva, vagina, prepuce, and skin of the scrotum
• B: 18G 3 cm needle or 5 cm spinal needle midline at the S5-Co1 or Co1-Co2 junction following sterile prep and skin desensitization. After contact with the floor of the neural canal, withdraw needle slightly. Place lidocaine in the hub of the needle and slowly withdraw the needle until the lidocaine is aspirated from the hub by the negative pressure of the epidural space. Alternatively, 1 mL of air may be slowly injected as the needle is withdrawn until no resistance is felt. Inject 5–6 mL lidocaine slowly for a 450 kg animal.
• O, C: 20G 1.5–3 cm needle midline at the S4-Co1 or Co1-Co2 space. Administer 0.5–1 mL lidocaine/50 kg of body weight.

• L: 20 G 1.5–3 cm needle midline at the S5-Co1 space. Administer 0.22 mg/kg lidocaine.
• *Risks:* ataxia due to cranial spread of lidocaine, infection due to nonsterile technique
• Other epidural drugs
  • B: bupivacaine mixed with lidocaine 1:2 to extend the block duration, xylazine 0.03–0.07 mg/kg diluted to 5–7 mL with saline, xylazine 0.03 mg/kg plus lidocaine to a total volume of 5 mL. Morphine alone, 0.1 mg/kg diluted to 5–8 mL or combined with xylazine 0.01 mg/kg or detomidine, 0.01 mg/kg, may be useful for longer term analgesia.
  • O, C: bupivacaine as for cattle, xylazine as for cattle, but diluted to 1–2 mL, xylazine plus lidocaine as for cattle, but diluted to 1–2 mL
  • L: bupivacaine as for cattle, xylazine 0.17 mg/kg diluted with 2 mL/150 kg sterile water, xylazine 0.17 mg/kg plus lidocaine 0.22 mg/kg

Lumbosacral Epidural Anesthesia
Procedures performed caudal to the diaphragm in calves, sheep, and goats. The technique may be performed in cattle, but anatomic considerations and loss of sensory and motor function of the hind limbs preclude its routine utility. Cardiovascular depression can occur from sympathetic blockade.
• O, C: 20 G 5–7 cm spinal needle with the bevel pointing craniad inserted midline between L6 and S1, midway between the wings of the ileum and just caudal to the dorsal spinous process of L6, following sterile prep and skin desensitization. Advance slowly until the needle pops through the interarcuate ligament to lie in the epidural space. The absence of blood or CSF in the needle hub, aspiration of saline from the needle hub, and no resistance to injection of 1 mL air all indicate correct placement. If CSF is observed (intrathecal position), reduce the dose of drug(s) to one-fourth that for epidural administration.
• *Drugs:* lidocaine 1 mL/5–7 kg body weight, bupivacaine 0.75% 1 mL/10 kg, morphine 0.1 mg/kg diluted with saline or local anesthetic to 0.1–0.2 mL/kg. All drugs must be administered slowly.
• *Risks:* prolonged caudal paralysis, cardiovascular effects from segmental sympathetic blockade, caudal pruritus (morphine), and infection

Adjunct Therapy
Bandages, splints, physical therapy, heat therapy, cold therapy, hydrotherapy, massage, acupuncture, topical therapy (local anesthetics, DMSO, capsaicin, diclofenac, etc.), confinement, housing (deep bedding, padding for recumbent animals, slinging, temperature-controlled environments), social and environmental enrichment

CONTRAINDICATIONS
POSSIBLE INTERACTIONS
• Regulatory restrictions: See Web sites below for links to FDACVM and the AMDUCA flowchart for recommendations on the use of analgesics and anesthetics in food animals.
• Meat and milk withholding: See Web sites below for the link to FARAD for recommendations on meat and milk withholding times for analgesics and anesthetics in food-producing animals.

 FOLLOW-UP

PATIENT MONITORING
See Alpha-2 agonists and Local Anesthetics above

PREVENTION/AVOIDANCE
See Alpha-2 agonists and Local Anesthetics above

POSSIBLE COMPLICATIONS
See Alpha-2 agonists and Local Anesthetics above

EXPECTED COURSE AND PROGNOSIS
N/A

 MISCELLANEOUS

Web Sites
American Association of Bovine Practitioners—http://www.aabp.org/
American Association of Small Ruminant Practitioners—http://www.aasrp.org/
American Veterinary Medical Association AMDUCA Guide and Flowsheet—http://www.avma.org/scienact/amduca/amduca1.asp (This document is in the member center and may be accessed only by American Veterinary Medical Association members.)
FDA Center for Veterinary Medicine (FDACVM)—http://www.fda.gov/cvm/default.html
FDA-approved Animal Drug Products Online Database System—http://dil.vetmed.vt.edu/
Food Animal Residue Avoidance Databank (FARAD)—http://www.farad.org
International Veterinary Academy of Pain Management—http://www.animalanalgesia.com
Minor Use Animal Drug Program—http://www.nrsp-7.org

ASSOCIATED CONDITIONS
N/A

AGE-RELATED FACTORS
See Local Anesthetics: Dehorning above

ZOONOTIC POTENTIAL
N/A

PREGNANCY
Alpha-2 agonist drugs may cause abortion in late-term gestation.

RUMINANT SPECIES AFFECTED
Potentially, all ruminant species are affected.

BIOSECURITY
N/A

PRODUCTION MANAGEMENT
N/A

SYNONYMS
N/A

SEE ALSO
FARAD
NSAIDs

ABBREVIATIONS
AMDUCA = Animal Medicinal Drug Use Classification Act
CAE = caprine arthritis encephalitis
CNS = central nervous system
Co1-Co2 = first and second coccygeal space
COX = cyclooxygenase
DMSO = dimethyl sulfoxide
FARAD = Food Animal Residue Avoidance Databank
FDACVM = Food and Drug Administration Center for Veterinary Medicine
GI = gastrointestinal
IM = intramuscular
IV = intravenous
NMDA = N-methyl-D-asparate
S5-Co1 = sacrococcygeal space

Suggested Reading
Ewing, K. K. 1990, Nov. Anesthesia techniques in sheep and goats. *Vet Clin North Am Food Anim Pract.* 6(3): 759–78.
Fajt, V. R. 2001. Label and extralabel drug use in small ruminants. *Vet Clin North Am Food Anim Pract.* 17(2): 403–20.
Greene, S. A. 2003. Protocols for anesthesia in cattle. *Vet Clin North Am Food Anim Pract.* 19:680–93.
Jorgensen, J. S., Cannedy, A. L. 1996, Nov. Physiologic and pathophysiologic considerations for ruminant and swine anesthesia. *Vet Clin North Am Food Anim Pract.* 12(3): 481–500.
Papich, M. G. 2003. Drug residue considerations for anesthetics and adjunctive drugs in food-producing animals. *Vet Clin North Am Food Anim Pract.* 12(3): 693–706.
Skarda, R. T. 1996, Nov. Local and regional anesthesia in ruminants and swine. *Vet Clin North Am Food Anim Pract.* 12(3): 579–626.
Tobin, E., Hunt, E. 1996, Nov. Supplies and technical considerations for ruminant and swine anesthesia. *Vet Clin North Am Food Anim Pract.* 12(3): 531–62.
Tranquilli, W. J., Grimm, K. A. 2003. Pharmacology of drugs used for anesthesia and sedation. *Vet Clin North Am Food Anim Pract.* 12(3): 501–29.

Author: Kirsten Wegner

ANESTRUS

BASICS

OVERVIEW
Anestrus is the absence of behavioral signs of estrus activity or behavior, although follicular waves are generally still present.

PATHOPHYSIOLOGY
Cattle are polyestrus, but cyclicity may be influenced by factors such as:
- Nutrition
- Environment
- Physiological conditions
- Breed
- Management

Anestrus in cattle can be a response to aberrant release patterns at the level of the hypothalamus (GnRH) or the pituitary (LH and FSH).

SYSTEMS AFFECTED
Endocrine/metabolic, reproductive

SIGNALMENT
Breed differences are related to
- Lactational status
- Nutritional intake
- Estrus intensity and duration

SIGNS
History of female estrous cyclicity and hormonal patterns may increase estrus detection efficiencies.

CAUSES AND RISK FACTORS
Other causes may include
- Anestrus females may actually be pregnant.
- Systemic disease
- Lameness
- Utero-ovarian disorders
- Postpartum anestrus period (1–3 months) is common.

DIAGNOSIS

Estrus behavior (and lack thereof) and observations can be supported by
- Estrus cyclicity records
- Lack of palpable CL
- No vaginal mucus discharge
- No mounting activity when placed with other estrous females or males
- Unresponsive to estrus synchronization treatments

DIFFERENTIAL DIAGNOSIS
General health/reproductive history

CBC/BIOCHEMISTRY/URINALYSIS
N/A

OTHER LABORATORY TESTS
Serum progesterone concentration > 2 ng/ml may confirm ovulation activity and presence of functional CL, < 2 ng/ml may confirm anestrus.

IMAGING
Ultrasonic imaging in an anestrous female should reveal:
- Small inactive ovaries
- Small dominant follicle (10–15 mm) or evidence of follicular activity may be present.

DIAGNOSTIC PROCEDURES
- Serum progesterone analysis
- Transrectal ultrasonography
- Rectal palpation
- Visual observation

TREATMENT
- Correct nutritional intake.
- House anestrus females with actively cycling females.

MEDICATIONS

DRUGS OF CHOICE
- GnRH (200 μg) followed by PGF2alpha (according to label) treatment (7 days apart) may initiate cyclicity.
- CIDR treatment (7 days) followed by estrus detection (1–7 days)
- MGA (0.5–1.0 mg/head /day) for 10–14 days followed by estrus detection (1–7 days)

CONTRAINDICATIONS
N/A

PRECAUTIONS
PGF2alpha is a vasoconstrictor known to cause abortions and respiratory complications (cattle and humans).

POSSIBLE INTERACTIONS
N/A

FOLLOW-UP

PATIENT MONITORING
- Behavioral activity
- Transrectal ultrasonography
- Palpation
- Serum progesterone levels

POSSIBLE COMPLICATIONS
- Pyometra
- Endometritis
- Systemic disease
- Freemartin

EXPECTED COURSE AND PROGNOSIS
Anestrus females usually regain estrus cyclicity once nutritional, reproductive, and management issues are addressed.

MISCELLANEOUS

ASSOCIATED CONDITIONS
N/A

AGE-RELATED FACTORS
Older females may exhibit reduced fertility and estrus cyclicity patterns.

ZOONOTIC POTENTIAL
N/A

PREGNANCY
Many females considered to be anestrus may be pregnant (with a viable on nonviable fetus) and may abort with PGF2alpha treatment.

RUMINANT SPECIES
Cattle; other ruminants may be seasonally polyestrus.

BIOSECURITY
N/A

PRODUCTION MANAGEMENT
Consistently anestrus females in well-monitored operations with strong management and husbandry protocols should be considered for culling.

SEE ALSO
Economics of beef cattle reproductive decisions
Endometritis
Estrus behavior
Estrus detection
Estrus synchronization
Freemartinism
Pyometra

ABBREVIATIONS
AI = artificial insemination
CIDR = vaginal progesterone inserts
CL = corpus luteum
FSH = follicle stimulating hormone
GnRH = gonadotropic releasing hormone
LH = luteinizing hormone
MGA = melengestrol acetate
PGF2alpha = prostaglandin F-2alpha

Suggested Reading
Beardon, H. J., Fuquay, J. W., Wilard, S. T. 2004. *Applied animal reproduction.* 6th ed. Upper Saddle River, NJ: Pearson-Prentice Hall.
Day, M. L. 2004. Hormonal induction of estrous cycles in anestrous *Bos taurus* beef cattle. *Animal Reproduction Science* 82–83: 487–94.
Ginther, O. J., Wiltbank, M. C., Fricke, P. M., Gibbons, J. R., Kot, K. 1996. Selection of the dominant follicle in cattle. *Biology of Reproduction* 55:1187–94.

Author: John Gibbons

ANGULAR LIMB DEFORMITY

 BASICS

DEFINITION
• Angular limb deformity (ALD) is a deviation from the normal axis of a limb (in the frontal plane) and is defined by the joint involved and the direction that the distal aspect of the limb is deviated.
   • Valgus deformity: the limb distal to the lesion deviates *laterally.*
   • Varus deformity: the limb distal to the lesion deviates *medially.*
   • ALDs are further described by the location of the pivot point (axis of deviation) and by the location of the site of defective growth.
• Related conditions include flexural deformities, tendon injuries, joint luxations, and rotational deformities.
• Spider lamb syndrome (SLS) or hereditary chondrodysplasia (HC) is a hereditary condition in young lambs characterized by a number of skeletal deformities, including angular limb deformities.

PATHOPHYSIOLOGY
• ALDs are considered multifactorial in origin and have congenital/perinatal and developmental predisposing factors.
• Cattle and llamas have a complete osseous ulna. In llamas, the distal ulnar epiphysis fuses with the distal radial epiphysis. This unique development of the distal portion of the ulna is associated with forelimb valgus deformities in crias. The ulnar epiphysis extends distally, crosses the radial physis, and fuses with the radial epiphysis. This early fusion demands synchronous growth to ensure normal limb development.
• Most calves have a mild carpal valgus deformity of approximately 7 degrees, which does not require treatment. Varus deformities in cattle are abnormal and often need treatment.

SYSTEMS AFFECTED
Musculoskeletal, involving the tibia, radius, ulna, carpus/tarsus, and metacarpus/metatarsus

GENETICS
• The questions of heritability in angular limb deformities have not been definitively answered.

• ALDs in Jersey calves are genetically transmitted as a simple autosomal recessive trait.
• Hereditary chondrodysplasia, or "spider-lamb syndrome" (SLS), of Suffolk and Suffolk-cross sheep is inherited as a single, autosomal recessive gene that has been localized to the distal end of chromosome 6. A defect in the gene encoding fibroblast growth factor receptor 3 (FGFR3) is suspected. DNA tests (blood or semen) are available to identify homozygous and heterozygous animals.

INCIDENCE/PREVALENCE
Valgus and varus angular limb deformities (ALD) are common and well documented in horses but rare in ruminants.

GEOGRAPHIC DISTRIBUTION
ALDs are thought to occur worldwide.

SIGNALMENT

Species
Bovine (cattle), ovine (sheep), goats (caprine), South American camelids (especially llama crias), cervids—including fallow deer (*Dama dama*), red deer (*Cervus elaphus*), white-tailed deer (*Odocoileus virginianus*)—and a single case report of ALD in a giraffe calf (*Giraffa camelopardalis*).

Breed Predilections
ALDs have been described in many different beef and dairy cattle breeds. SLS primarily affects black-faced breeds of sheep (Suffolk, Hampshire, Southdown, Shropshire, and Oxford).

Mean Age and Range
ALDs primarily affect young growing animals up to 7 months of age, but can be seen in older animals (e.g., trauma-induced ALD). SLS has two distinct clinical entities: lambs are either grossly abnormal at birth or develop the abnormal conformation at 4–6 weeks of age. Radiographic changes at birth are similar for both.

Predominant Sex
No apparent gender predisposition

SIGNS

HISTORICAL FINDINGS
A complete history including current age, birthing details, age at which the deformity was noticed, course and progression of deformity, and diets of affected animal and dam should be obtained.

PHYSICAL EXAMINATION FINDINGS
• The animal's conformation should be assessed first by having the animal stand in a symmetrical manner on a firm, flat surface and observing it from multiple angles. Affected animals may appear to be knock-kneed or bowlegged. All limbs should be palpated and affected limbs should be manually manipulated. Clinical signs such as abnormal bending of the affected limb, increased laxity, muscle atrophy, swelling, heat, pain on manual pressure, abrasions on lateral or medial side of hoof wall, presence of orthopedic injury, and abnormal gait and locomotion are indicative of ALD.
• Compensatory deviation (opposite that of the affected limb) is relatively common in the contralateral limb.
• If varus deformity is found unilaterally, the contralateral limb should be examined for a significant orthopedic injury as a cause of excessive weight bearing in the deformed limb/joint.
• Since cattle are considered to have a "normal" degree of medial deviation at the level of the carpus and hock, as well as normal external rotation of the lower limb, ALDs tend to be missed in the early stages of development.

SLS
In sheep affected with SLS, various degrees of angular limb deformities of fore- and/or hind limbs will be noted. Other physical exam findings include severe scoliosis/kyphosis of the thoracic spine, pectus excavatum, retarded growth rates, facial deformities such as angular deviation and/or shortening of maxilla, rounding of the dorsal silhouette, and Roman-shaped noses.

CAUSES AND RISK FACTORS
ALDs are often related to asymmetrical growth of the physis, ligament rupture, or orthopedic injuries.

Congenital Predisposing Factors
• Incomplete cuboidal bone ossification (carpal and/or tarsal)
• Physiological immaturity at birth
• Uterine malpositioning
• In utero bending stress and bone remodeling early in gestation
• Twin (or triplet) pregnancy
• Laxity of periarticular supporting structures
• Disproportionate osseous growth of medial and lateral aspects of long bones (e.g., distal radius, tibia, metatarsus)

- Nutritional imbalance during gestation
- Genetic causes

Developmental Predisposing Factors
- Conformational defects (causing abnormal weight distribution across a joint)
- Nutritional disorders (e.g., improper dietary calcium and phosphorus ratios; copper, zinc, manganese, iron, and molybdenum concentrations)
- External trauma (e.g., compression of or trauma to growth plate, malunion of fractures)
- Iatrogenic (e.g., assisted delivery)
- Excessive exercise
- Hematogenous osteomyelitis involving the physeal region
- Rapid weight gain in heavy breeds
- Often, no specific cause is identified.

Camelids
- May see ALDs (usually carpal valgus) in growing camelids with hypophosphatemic rickets syndrome.
- Ill-thrift syndrome in llamas may be associated with ALDs as well as anemia, low serum iron concentrations, and metabolic disorders (hypothyroidism). Underlying cause not established.

DIAGNOSIS

DIFFERENTIAL DIAGNOSIS
SLS
- May be confused with arthrogryposis-hydranencephaly syndrome (AHS) in lambs, in which there is characteristic hyperflexion of forelimbs, cranial overextension of hind limbs, with a corkscrew deviation of the spine.
- In lambs with AHS, severe deformities result from primary abnormalities of the CNS (including hydranencephaly, micromyelia, hydrocephalus, and cerebellar hypoplasia) and not of the skeleton.

Camelids
True ALDs in llamas must be differentiated from valgus deformities of the forelimbs in newborn crias that self correct without surgical treatment.

CBC/BIOCHEMISTRY/URINALYSIS
There are usually no associated laboratory abnormalities with ALD.

SLS
May see slightly elevated serum alkaline phosphatase activity; insufficient for diagnostic purposes.

Camelids
- Ill-thrift syndrome: serum vitamin D (25-hydroxycholecalciferol) concentrations are often diagnostic.
- May also see hypothyroidism, anemia, erythrocyte dyscrasias, hypophosphatemia, and low serum iron concentrations.

OTHER LABORATORY TESTS
N/A

IMAGING
- Radiographs are critical in diagnosing ALDs—at least two views, 90 degrees apart, should be taken of the affected joint, including joints immediately proximal and distal to the affected joint.
- The dorsopalmar/dorsoplantar (DP) view is needed for examination of the anatomical location of the deformity and for measurements. The pivot point is defined as the intersection between lines drawn through the long axis at the center of the proximal and distal long bone using the dorsopalmar view. Location of the pivot point identifies the type of deformity. Measure the angle of deviation with a protractor.
- SLS: most consistent lesions include multiple islands of ossification of the anconeal process and malformed, displaced sternebrae. The anconeal lesions of HC are progressive, whereas similar lesions in other skeletal conditions of lambs regress.

DIAGNOSTIC PROCEDURES
- Bacterial cultures may be indicated in cases of septicemia, arthritis, or osteomyelitis.
- Toxicology (heavy metal and mineral analysis) and feed analysis may assist in diagnosis.

PATHOLOGIC FINDINGS
SLS
Histology (vertebrae and long bones): increase in width of the zone of proliferation and hypertrophy and unevenness of growth cartilage; failure to form or maintain orderly columns of chondrocytes.

TREATMENT

APPROPRIATE HEALTH CARE
Treatment of neonatal animals with incomplete ossification involves the application of tube casts or splints to the affected limb(s) until ossification is complete (based on repeated radiographs).

NURSING CARE
- Severely affected animals may be unable to rise to nurse and require additional supportive care. Protect limbs with thick, soft bandages that fit well.
- Care should be taken to maintain a soft (padding), clean, and dry environment and to minimize decubital/pressure sores, open arthritis, muscle atrophy, umbilical infections, and septicemia.

ACTIVITY
Physical confinement (stall) is recommended for the management of ALDs to limit stresses placed on affected limbs.

DIET
- Nutritional imbalances have been implicated, such as ill-thrift in llamas. Treatment for this condition includes appropriate vitamin D supplementation.
- Other dietary imbalances should be corrected while treating cases of ALD.

CLIENT EDUCATION
- Examination and intervention of young animals with congenital angular limb deformities should be done as early as possible.
- Due to the possible hereditary link with ALDs, breeding of affected animals is not recommended.

ANGULAR LIMB DEFORMITY

NONSURGICAL CONSIDERATIONS/ CONSERVATIVE TREATMENT

• Many cases of ALD will resolve without surgery if the underlying cause(s) can be identified and addressed and if the animal does not damage the affected physis or joints with vigorous exercise.
• Specific treatment methods are selected on the basis of age, degree of angulation, remaining growth potential of the involved physis, and experience of the veterinarian.
• Minor limb deviations may be conservatively treated by manual alignment and external support of the limb (e.g., rigid splinting, bandaging, or casting/tube casts) and/or hoof (claw) trimming.
• Hoof manipulations create growth-plate response to stress applied opposite the deformity, and self correction occurs. The hoof tends to turn in the direction of the longer claw or toward the side of the wider wall, resulting in straightening and derotation of the limb.
• Medial (varus) deformities can be treated by trimming the medial claw shorter than the lateral claw and by placing an acrylic (methyl methacrylate) wing on the weight-bearing surface of the lateral claw (to increase lateral contact with the ground).
• Treatment should be directed at the orthopedic injury when varus deformity is present secondary to a contralateral limb injury.

SURGICAL CONSIDERATIONS

• Surgery is recommended for older animals (near the end of active physeal growth), for those that do not respond to conservative treatments, and for animals with bone malformations that require realignment (via osteotomy).
• The choice of surgical technique should take into consideration the economic value and age of the animal, severity of the deformity, and the joint involved.

Treatment Strategies Include the Following:

Growth Acceleration (Periosteal Stripping/Elevation)

In young calves and lambs with early cases of ALD, surgical growth stimulation via periosteal stripping on the concave aspect (shorter side) of the deformity has been used successfully. Based on the remaining growth potential in the physis, allow the animal to correct the deviation by physeal growth.

Growth Retardation (Transphyseal Bridging)

• Transphyseal bridging is indicated for severe cases of ALD or in animals past the rapid growth phase of the radius and ulna (often recommended for animals older than 5 months of age).
• By creating a temporary transphyseal bridge on the convex side of the deformity using staples or screws and wires, limb growth is slowed by restricting growth and allows the other side to continue growing, resulting in limb straightening.
• The surgical implants must be removed when the limb achieves normal conformation to prevent overcorrection. This can be used in combination with periosteal stripping to increase the likelihood of full correction in animals with severe deviations.

Corrective Wedge Osteotomy

• This procedure is indicated in mature animals with ALD and in neonates with congenital fracture malunion. If the growth plates are closed or if the growth plate is not involved in an ALD, a corrective osteotomy is recommended. This requires more experience and equipment and often is reserved for valuable animals when response to other therapies has failed.
• The site and orientation of the wedge should be determined by clinical and radiographic examination.
• The limb needs to be stabilized by internal fixation with a plate and screws for an extended postoperative period.

Camelids

An ulnar osteotomy must be done in conjunction with the periosteal transection because the ulna spans the radial physis.

 MEDICATIONS

DRUGS OF CHOICE

Nonsteroidal anti-inflammatory agents (NSAIDs) are recommended to reduce inflammation in some cases of ALD, especially those associated with physitis.

CONTRAINDICATIONS

• Prolonged NSAID administration has been associated with gastrointestinal (abomasal) ulcers.
• Appropriate milk and meat withdrawal times must be followed for all compounds administered to food-producing animals.

PRECAUTIONS

Many of these affected animals are young; precautions regarding drug choices must take age into consideration.

POSSIBLE INTERACTIONS

N/A

ALTERNATIVE DRUGS

N/A

 FOLLOW-UP

PATIENT MONITORING

• Frequent physical monitoring and repeated radiographs should be done to assess the efficacy of corrective measures and to monitor progress.
• In cases of transphyseal bridging surgery, owner cooperation is required to determine when the limb has regained its normal conformation, at which time the implants must be removed to prevent overcorrection.

PREVENTION/AVOIDANCE
Avoid breeding affected animals.

POSSIBLE COMPLICATIONS
• In cases of valgus deformity, efforts should be taken to prevent compensatory varus in the contralateral limb. Persistence of hoof distortion is possible if the angular deformity is not corrected.
• Surgical: transphyseal bridging—overcorrection of the physis is possible. Owner cooperation is required to determine when limb has regained its normal conformation.
• Possible ALD surgical complications include muscle, tendon, and ligament atrophy/laxity, hyperextension of limbs, fibrous scar tissue development, and postoperative infection.

EXPECTED COURSE AND PROGNOSIS
• Prognosis is guarded, yet reasonable for ALDs associated with growth plate imbalances, such as most valgus deformities.
• The prognosis for ALDs secondary to contralateral orthopedic injury (such as most varus deformities) is generally poor because it is usually centered over a joint and is dependent on the prognosis of the primary orthopedic injury.
• SLS-affected individuals rarely survive the neonatal period.
• Camelids: the prognosis for ill-thrift syndrome in llamas is poor; etiologic agent often not identified.

 MISCELLANEOUS

ASSOCIATED CONDITIONS
• Conditions associated with ALDs include osteochondrosis of the physis, epiphysitis, and incomplete ossification of the cuboidal carpal bones.

• Hyena disease (premature physeal closure) has been reported in calves due to overdose of vitamins A, D_3, and E.
• Congenital lethal chondrodysplasia in Australian Dexter cattle = "Dexter bulldog calves."
• Congenital chondrodysplastic dwarfism in Holstein calves
• Complex vertebral malformation is a familial syndrome of Holstein calves.
• Syndrome known as "bentleg" or "bowie" associated with ingestion of *Trachymene glaucifolia* (wild parsnip) by pregnant ewes in Australia and New Zealand

AGE-RELATED FACTORS
The majority of ALDs occurs during the active growth phase of the affected bone/joint.

ZOONOTIC POTENTIAL
N/A

PREGNANCY
• Many of the causes of ALDs are congenital diseases in which the in utero environment is somehow disturbed (hormones, vascular supply, teratogens, mechanical factors, or prenatal virus infections).
• Cases of ALDs in goats pregnant with triplets have been reported.
• Contributing factors likely include stress and in utero malpositioning.

RUMINANT SPECIES AFFECTED
Bovine, ovine, caprine, cervid, camelid

BIOSECURITY
N/A

PRODUCTION MANAGEMENT
N/A

SYNONYMS
Hereditary chondrodysplasia (spider lamb syndrome)

SEE ALSO
Arthrogryposis
Cleft palate
CNS anomalies
CNS: brain lesions
CNS: nerve
Crooked calf syndrome
Lameness: muscle/tendon—contracted tendons
Spider lamb disease

ABBREVIATIONS
AHS = arthrogryposis-hydranencephaly syndrome
ALD = angular limb deformity
CNS = central nervous system
HC = ovine hereditary chondrodysplasia
NSAIDs = nonsteroidal anti-inflammatory drugs
SLS = spider lamb syndrome

Suggested Reading
Duchame, N. G. 2004. Angular deformities. In: *Farm animal surgery*, ed. S. L. Fubini, N. G. Ducharme. Philadelphia: W. B. Saunders.
Ferguson, J. G. 1997. Angular deformity of radiocarpal and tibiotarsal joints. In: *Lameness in cattle*, ed. P. R. Greenough. 3rd ed. Philadelphia: W. B. Saunders.
Kaneps, A. J. 1996. Orthopedic conditions of small ruminants, llama, sheep, goat, and deer. Advances in ruminant orthopedics. *Veterinary Clinics of North America: Food Animal Practice* 12(1):211–31.
Paul-Murphy, J. R., Morgan, J. P., Snyder, J. R., Fowler, M. E. 1991. Radiographic findings in young llamas with forelimb valgus deformities: 28 cases (1980–1988). *JAVMA* 12(15):21107–11.

Authors: Erik J. Olson and Cathy S. Carlson

ANTHRAX

BASICS

DEFINITION
Anthrax is an almost invariably fatal septicemic disease caused by a large, gram-positive spore-forming bacterial rod *Bacillus anthracis*, which is part of the normal soil flora in most geographic areas, particularly those with alkaline soils.

PATHOPHYSIOLOGY
• Spores of the causal agent gain entry to the host by ingestion, by inhalation, or through skin lesions.
• Once the bacillus enters the body, it is ingested by macrophages and enters into lymphatic vessels and lymph nodes to cause lymphangitis and lymphadenitis.
• The spores germinate to a vegetative form, multiply extracellularly, and are disseminated throughout the host.
• The organisms produce toxins (lethal factor, edema factor, and protective antigen) that cause widespread damage of the vasculature and reticuloendothelial system to result in edema, tissue damage, shock, renal failure, anoxia, and ultimately death.

INCIDENCE/PREVALENCE
• In the United States, the disease is usually seen in one or only a few animals at a time and is sporadic.
• Both sporadic cases and outbreaks are often associated with disruption of the soil. This disruption brings bacterial spores to the soil surface where they are ingested. Similarly, animals grazing short grasses during drought periods may ingest spores.
• Outbreaks can occur over large areas if animals are fed contaminated feeds, such as meat and bone meal.
• Pastures can be contaminated by effluent from textile mills that were using animal products, such as wool, in the manufacturing process.
• Morbidity varies widely but case mortality is 90%–95%.
• Control efforts are successful in domestic species but wildlife can suffer large outbreaks.

GEOGRAPHIC DISTRIBUTION
The anthrax bacillus has a worldwide distribution but some areas have a higher rate of disease.

SIGNALMENT
• Anthrax can affect all livestock species but the major ruminant species—cattle, goats, and sheep—are more susceptible than horses and pigs.

• There are some reports of males being more susceptible than females and older animals being more susceptible than young animals but these probably reflect differences in stress and grazing habits rather than inherent differences in susceptibility.

SIGNS
• Many animals die suddenly and there are no clinical signs noted.
• Animals develop fever, depression, muscle tremors, dyspnea, diarrhea, and other signs related to septicemia. A smaller number of more chronic cases may develop subcutaneous edema, hematuria, rumen stasis, and decreased milk production with blood-tinged milk.

GENERAL COMMENTS
N/A

HISTORICAL FINDINGS
N/A

PHYSICAL EXAMINATION FINDINGS
N/A

CAUSES
• Anthrax is caused by *Bacillus anthracis*, a large, gram-positive, spore-forming bacterial rod.
• Infection can occur by ingestion, which is the most common route, by inhalation, or by contamination of skin wounds.
• Primary cases are usually due to ingestion but secondary cases on the same premises may be due to contact with infectious discharges from the primary cases or by ingestion of tissues from the primary case.

RISK FACTORS
• Anthrax cases are more common in years when there have been major climate changes (e.g., wet spring followed by a drought or a drought followed by heavy rains).
• Disruption of the soil can bring infectious spores to the surface where they are more easily ingested or inhaled.
• Close grazing of poor-quality, coarse feed can lead to oral trauma and predispose animals to infection.

DIAGNOSIS

DIFFERENTIAL DIAGNOSIS
Because the signs of anthrax are not specific, almost any disease can be considered in the differential diagnosis. Some that merit specific mention include acute toxicity, anaplasmosis, vena cava syndrome with exsanguination from the respiratory tract, blackleg, malignant edema, and bacillary hemoglobinuria.

CBC/CHEMISTRY/URINALYSIS
N/A

OTHER LABORATORY TESTS
N/A

IMAGING
N/A

DIAGNOSTIC PROCEDURES
• Because of the zoonotic risk of anthrax and the poor response to treatment, a full clinical workup is generally not warranted.
• Diagnosis is based on the demonstration of the causal organism in body fluids, and laboratory professionals best perform this testing function.
• Blood from an ear tip or jugular vein in the live animal (or one dead less than 12 hours) or aqueous humor or an entire eyeball from a dead animal are all acceptable samples for finding the organism.
• Bacteremia may not occur until just before death, and demonstration of the agent may be difficult in the live animal particularly if antibiotic therapy has begun.
• The organism on Giemsa or Wright stain is typically seen as a square-ended bacterial rod that occurs singly or in short chains and resembles "railroad boxcars."

PATHOLOGIC FINDINGS
• Because of the danger of environmental contamination, if anthrax is suspected, a full necropsy is contraindicated.
• Animals that die from anthrax undergo rapid decomposition and generally do not develop full rigor.
• The carcass will be gas distended and have a "saw-horse" appearance.
• Natural body orifices may have an exudate consisting of dark, unclotted, tarry blood.
• On necropsy, there will be marked splenic enlargement (two to three times normal size), serosal and mucosal edema and hemorrhage, edema and hemorrhage in lymph nodes, unclotted blood, intramuscular edema, and possibly enteritis.
• In sheep and goats, the disease progresses very rapidly and there may not be localized lesions in the carcass.

TREATMENT
• The prognosis for animals with anthrax is poor but there are reports of animals that have survived.
• The anthrax bacillus is susceptible to a wide range of antibiotics but treatment will make demonstration of the organism in body fluids more difficult.

- Streptomycin (8–10 g/day in 2 doses) or oxytetracycline (5 mg/kg/day) are recommended by some texts.
- Antibiotic treatment should be for a minimum of 5 days and preferably 10 days, and the first dose should be given IV if this is a possible route with the antibiotic chosen.
- An antiserum is available in some areas but is often quite expensive.
- Appropriate milk and meat withdrawal times must be followed for all compounds administered to food-producing animals.

CLIENT EDUCATION
- The client must be made aware of the potential of the organism to infect a variety of species, including humans, via skin wounds, ingestion, or inhalation.
- Carcass disposal can be problematic.
- The anthrax bacillus is generally destroyed during putrefaction of the carcass and if the carcass is not opened and if discharge of fluids into the environment does not occur, there will not be significant contamination of the site.
- Since treatment is typically not successful, prevention and control should be emphasized.

 MEDICATIONS
N/A

 FOLLOW-UP

PATIENT MONITORING
N/A

PREVENTION/AVOIDANCE
- Hygiene and carcass disposal are of paramount importance.
- Autolysis of the carcass destroys the vegetative forms of *B. anthracis* and, therefore, if carcasses are not opened up, the potential for contamination of the environment is minimized.
- Carcasses should be disposed of by burning or deep (>6 feet) burial that occurs well away from water sources.
- Burning may release spores into the rising heat column and disperse them, and therefore hot fires that take hold quickly are best. The risk from burning carcasses is probably less than not burning the carcass, however.

- Livestock can be vaccinated with Stern-strain spore vaccine. Booster vaccination is given 4–5 weeks following the initial vaccination, and then annually thereafter.
- The vaccine is a live nonencapsulated organism and therefore antibiotics should not be given within 7 to 10 days of vaccine administration.
- Following vaccination, there is a 60-day withdrawal time for the carcass, and milk should be discarded for at least 72 hours.
- There may be a localized reaction at the vaccination site and this can be quite severe in some animals.
- Spores are very resistant and can survive in contaminated soils for 15–30 years. Therefore, anthrax is still a potential danger in areas with historic cases.

 MISCELLANEOUS

ASSOCIATED CONDITIONS
Animals develop fever, depression, muscle tremors, dyspnea, diarrhea, and other signs related to septicemia. A smaller number of more chronic cases may develop subcutaneous edema, hematuria, rumen stasis, and decreased milk production with blood-tinged milk.

AGE-RELATED FACTORS
There are some reports of males being more susceptible than females and older animals being more susceptible than young animals, but these probably reflect differences in stress and grazing habits rather than inherent differences in susceptibility.

ZOONOTIC POTENTIAL
Anthrax is primarily a disease of herbivores, but all mammals, including humans, are susceptible and therefore care must be exercised when working in areas where spores are potentially present.

PREGNANCY
N/A

RUMINANT SPECIES AFFECTED
All ruminant species are affected.

BIOSECURITY
- Anthrax is a reportable disease.
- Once anthrax is diagnosed, the farm will be quarantined, all carcasses and fluids will be destroyed, survivors will be vaccinated, and the farm will be isolated for at least 2 weeks.

- Because of the association between anthrax and disturbed soils and/or localized areas, animals surviving an outbreak may be moved to different pastures or holding pens in order to reduce the possibility of additional cases.
- Scavenger control is important to prevent the spread of the disease.
- Because of recent concerns about bioterrorism, the Federal Bureau of Investigation will likely become involved in any cases of anthrax in the United States.

PRODUCTION MANAGEMENT
- Hygiene and carcass disposal are of paramount importance.
- Autolysis of the carcass destroys the vegetative forms of *B. anthracis* and, therefore, if carcasses are not opened up, the potential for contamination of the environment is minimized.
- Carcasses should be disposed of by burning or deep (>6 feet) burial that occurs well away from water sources.
- Livestock can be vaccinated with Stern-strain spore vaccine. Booster vaccination is given 4–5 weeks following the initial vaccination, and then annually thereafter.
- Close grazing of poor-quality, coarse feed can lead to oral trauma and predispose animals to infection.

SYNONYMS
N/A

SEE ALSO
Acute toxicity
Anaplasmosis
Bacillary hemoglobinuria
Blackleg
Malignant edema
Vena cava syndrome with exsanguination from the respiratory tract

ABBREVIATIONS
N/A

Suggested Reading
Anthrax. 2000. In: *Veterinary medicine*, ed. O. M. Radostits, C. C. Gay, D. C. Blood, K. W. Hinchcliff. 9th ed. Philadelphia: W. B. Saunders.
Mosier, D. A., Chengappa, M. M. 1999. Anthrax. In: *Current veterinary therapy 4: food animal practice*, ed. J. L. Howard, R. A. Smith. Philadelphia: W. B. Saunders.
Pipkin, A. B. 2002. Anthrax. In: *Large animal internal medicine*, ed. B. P. Smith. 3rd ed. St. Louis: Mosby.

Author: John M. Adaska

ARSENIC TOXICOSIS

BASICS

OVERVIEW
• Arsenic has been reported to be the second most common heavy metal intoxication of cattle after lead.
• Arsenic is still used in herbicides, defoliants, and wood preservatives.
• The use of arsenic-containing products has decreased in the recent past as other insecticides and herbicides become available.

SYSTEMS AFFECTED
• Gastrointestinal
• Renal
• Nervous (phenylarsonic compounds)

Sources
• Inorganic arsenic
   • Arsenate—natural, pentavalent form of arsenic
   • Trivalvent forms are manufactured inorganic arsenic: arsenic trioxide (insecticide and herbicide); trivalent arsenic (arsenite)
   • Pressure-treated woods (green in color): chromated copper arsenate (CCA). Cattle have been poisoned by consumption of ashes from burnt pressure-treated wood.
   • Inorganic arsenic is more commonly associated with intoxication in cattle.
• Organic arsenic
   • 3-nitro, 4-hydroxyphenylarsonic acid (3 nitro)—a feed additive
   • Thiacertarsaminde—heartworm therapy
   • Monosodium methanearsonate (MSMA)—herbicide
   • Disodium methanearsonate (DSMA)—herbicide

Toxic Dose
• Toxicity depends upon the formulation, route of exposure, and duration of exposure.
• Trivalent forms are 5–10 times more toxic than pentavalent forms.
• For most species, the toxic oral dose of sodium arsenite is 1 to 25 mg/kg of body weight.

GENETICS
N/A

INCIDENCE/PREVALENCE
Unknown

GEOGRAPHIC DISTRIBUTION
Worldwide

SIGNALMENT

Species
N/A

Breed Predilections
N/A

Mean Age and Range
N/A

Predominant Sex
N/A

SIGNS
• Sudden death (peracute toxicosis)
• Acute to subacute toxicosis
   • Diarrhea +/− hemorrhagic
   • Anorexia
   • Dehydration
   • Weakness
   • Ruminal atony
   • Colic

CAUSES AND RISK FACTORS
N/A

DIAGNOSIS
• Clinical signs
• Possible history of exposure
• Chemical determination of arsenic in tissues
• Liver or kidney arsenic concentrations greater than 3 ppm
• Stomach content or urinary arsenic greater than 2 ppm
• Chemical determination of arsenic in water or feedstuffs

DIFFERENTIAL DIAGNOSIS
• Bovine viral enteritis (BVD)
• Bacterial enteritis (*Salmonella* spp.)
• Organophosphorus insecticides
• Other heavy metals (lead)
• Urea toxicosis

CBC/BIOCHEMISTRY/URINALYSIS
None specific to arsenic toxicosis

OTHER LABORATORY TESTS
N/A

PATHOLOGIC FINDINGS

GROSS FINDINGS
• Gastrointestinal: generalized or localized reddening of the gastrointestinal mucosa; hemorrhage; erosions; submucosal edema
• Kidneys: pale, swollen

HISTOPATHOLOGICAL FINDINGS
• Multifocal hepatic and renal necrosis
• Dilation of intestinal capillaries
• Submucosal congestion and edema
• Intestinal epithelial necrosis
• Renal tubular necrosis

ARSENIC TOXICOSIS

TREATMENT

Symptomatic and Supportive Therapy
• Very important, as animals may present late in the clinical course
• Fluid therapy
• Blood transfusion +/−

Antidotal Therapy—Chelation
• Thioctic acid (lipoic acid or alpha lipoic acid)
  • More effective in cattle than dimercaprol
  • No commercially available source
  • 50 mg/kg divided into two to three injection sites
  • Administer q 8 hours
• 2, 3-dimercaptosuccinic acid (DMSA)
  • Also known as CHEMET or Succimer
  • Water-soluble analog of British Anti Lewisite (BAL)
  • Given orally
  • Commercially available product (humans)
  • 10 mg/kg per os q 8 hours (human and small animal dose)

MEDICATIONS

CONTRAINDICATIONS
Appropriate milk and meat withdrawal times must be followed for all compounds administered to food-producing animals.

FOLLOW-UP

MISCELLANEOUS

ASSOCIATED CONDITIONS
• Gastrointestinal: intestinal epithelial necrosis
• Kidneys: renal tubular necrosis

AGE-RELATED FACTORS
N/A

ZOONOTIC POTENTIAL
N/A

PREGNANCY
N/A

RUMINANT SPECIES AFFECTED
Potentially all ruminant species

BIOSECURITY
N/A

PRODUCTION MANAGEMENT
Keep agricultural chemicals away from livestock at all times.

SYNONYMS
N/A

SEE ALSO
Toxicology: herd outbreaks

ABBREVIATIONS
• BAL = British Anti Lewisite
• BVD = bovine viral diarrhea
• CCA = chromated copper arsenate
• DMSA = 2, 3-dimercaptosuccinic acid
• DSMA = disodium methanearsonate
• MSMA = monosodium methanearsonate

Suggested Reading
Faires, M. C. 2004. Inorganic arsenic toxicosis in a beef herd. *Can Vet J.* 45(4): 329–31.
Hullinger, G., Sangster, L., Colvin, B., Frazier, K. 1998. Bovine arsenic toxicosis from ingestion of ashed copper-chrome-arsenate treated timber. *Vet Hum Toxicol.* 40(3): 147–48.
Stair, E. L., Kirkpatrick, J. G., Whitenack, D. L. 1995. Lead arsenate poisoning in a herd of beef cattle. *J Am Vet Med Assoc.* 207(3): 341–43.
Thatcher, C. D., Meldrum, J. B., Wikse, S. E., Whittier, W. D. 1985. Arsenic toxicosis and suspected chromium toxicosis in a herd of cattle. *J Am Vet Med Assoc.* 187(2): 179–82.
U.S. EPA. *Chromated copper arsenate (CCA) and its use as a wood preservative.* Web site visited October 8, 2004.http://www.epa.gov/pesticides/factsheets/chemicals/1file.htm.

Author: Joe Roder

ARTHROGRYPOSIS

 BASICS

DEFINITION
• Congenital arthrogryposis is defined as a syndrome of persistent joint contracture (bilateral rigidity) present at birth and may involve one or multiple limbs (forelimbs and/or hind limbs).
• Arthrogryposis is often associated with cleft palate and primary CNS lesions such as hydranencephaly and syringomyelia.
• The arthrogryposis-hydranencephaly syndrome (AHS) is usually associated with flexural contracture of the limbs rather than angular limb deformities (ALDs).
• Crooked calf syndrome (CCD) is a congenital deformity condition widely recognized in western North America, characterized by arthrogryposis, scoliosis, torticollis, and cleft palate. CCD is observed in calves after maternal ingestion of lupines containing the quinolizidine alkaloid anagyrine during gestation days 40–100.
• Congenital arthrogryposis may be associated with denervation muscle atrophy.

PATHOPHYSIOLOGY
• Congenital arthrogryposis is considered multifactorial in origin and has multiple predisposing factors and etiologies.
• It can be caused by a number of etiologic agents including: plant teratogens (e.g., lupines), spinal dysraphism, prenatal viral infections (e.g., Akabane virus), and in utero hormonal and vascular defects.
• It may also be attributed to a decrease or lack of motion of the fetus during critical stages of development, such as malpositioning and overcrowding caused by the size of the fetus relative to the dam.
• Ingestion of teratogenic plants (e.g., *Astragalus* or *Oxytropis* spp. = locoweed; *Veratrum californicum* = skunk cabbage; piperidine alkaloid-containing plants such as *Lupinus, Conium,* and *Nicotiana* species).
 • Repeated dosing or continuous low-level ingestion over time may result in cumulative intoxication and/or teratogenesis.
 • Teratogenic plant alkaloids may be transferred to the placenta and induce a sedative or anesthetic effect in the fetus.

• In CCD, there is often a lesion in the CNS that may result in reduced or complete absence of movement of the affected body parts in the developing fetus, especially during the period of rapid growth. Studies have demonstrated a significant reduction in number of α-motorneurons in the cervical spinal cord. May cause disruption in normal innervation of muscles leading to paresis and instability of the limb, or may result in hypotonic condition of extensor muscle and dysfunction of the radial nerve.

SYSTEMS AFFECTED
Musculoskeletal—involving forelimbs, hind limbs, or both. The carpal and phalangeal joints are most commonly affected, followed by metacarpophalangeal and metatarsophalangeal joints.

GENETICS
The questions of heritability in arthrogryposis have not been definitively answered.

Lambs
A congenital arthrogryposis exists in pedigree Suffolk and Australian Merino lambs as an inherited limb deformity.

INCIDENCE/PREVALENCE
• For CCD, there are reports of up to 40% of calves from a single herd being affected. The incidence of disease varies with year, area, and herd.
• Cattle records reveal that the disease usually affects <10% of a herd.

GEOGRAPHIC DISTRIBUTION
• Arthrogryposis is thought to occur worldwide. Depending on the etiologic cause, the geographic distribution may vary (e.g., crooked calf syndrome is most common in western North America).
• Calf arthrogryposis has been reported from most parts of the world and in many breeds of cattle.

SIGNALMENT
Species
Bovine, ovine, caprine, camelids

Breed Predilections
• Arthrogryposis has been described in many different beef and dairy cattle breeds. Certain syndromes are predominantly reported to occur in certain breeds (e.g., congenital arthrogryposis in Charolais cattle). CCD has

been observed in most dairy breeds and in all breeds of beef cattle common to western North America.
• No breed predilection or genetic susceptibility in cattle to the lupine-induced condition has been determined.

Mean Age and Range
• Arthrogryposis tends to affect young, growing animals. The incidence of CCD is highest in heifers at first calving, but the disease has been observed in calves from cows of all ages.
• For each species (cattle, sheep, and goats), there are specific periods of gestation when the fetus is susceptible to plant teratogens. The critical gestational period for exposure of cattle to lupines is 40–70 days with susceptible periods extending to 100 days.

Predominant Sex
No apparent gender predisposition

SIGNS

HISTORICAL FINDINGS
A complete history including age, birthing details, age at which the deformity was noticed, course and progression of deformity, diets of affected animal and dam should be obtained. The animal may be normal at birth and develop the flexural deformity within hours or days.

PHYSICAL EXAMINATION FINDINGS
• The animal's conformation should be assessed first by having the animal stand in a symmetrical manner on a firm, flat surface and observing it from multiple angles.
• Arthrogryposis in CCD is characterized by deformities of the limbs (rigid flexion of elbows and carpal joints), and spinal column (scoliosis, lordosis, kyphosis), and rib cage abnormalities. Affected calves occasionally have torticollis and cleft palate.
• The joints are often flexed and cannot be extended even after the flexor tendons are cut—distinguishing the disease from contracted tendons.

CAUSES
A number of etiological agents such as intrauterine infection with border disease virus (a pestivirus), Akabane virus, Cache Valley virus, and bluetongue virus, as well as teratogenic plant ingestion have been implicated in the pathogenesis of arthrogryposis (crooked limbs) in small ruminants.

Congenital Predisposing Factors
• Uterine malpositioning
• Genetic causes
• Ingestion of teratogenic plants by pregnant dam (e.g., *Astragalus* or *Oxytropis* spp. = locoweed; *Verratrum californicum* = skunk cabbage; piperidine alkaloid-containing plants such as *Lupinus, Conium,* and *Nicotiana* species).
• Conditions associated with arthrogryposis include crooked calf syndrome/congenital arthrogryposis, spider lamb syndrome (hereditary chondrodysplasia), ill-thrift syndrome in llamas, metabolic, and neurovascular disorders.
• Leg deformities in young calves are most commonly associated with congenital contraction of the tendons. Flexural deformities involving contracted tendons and ligaments may be seen in many breeds of cattle and small ruminants.

RISK FACTORS
Predisposing factors for congenital arthrogryposis include male gender, posterior intrauterine presentation, and double muscling.

DIAGNOSIS

DIFFERENTIAL DIAGNOSIS
• Arthrogryposis and CCD differ from contracted tendons; in animals with contracted tendons, the joints are usually properly aligned and the legs are not rotated. In calves with arthrogryposis, the articular and osseous changes are usually permanent and worsen as the calf grows.
• Congenital arthrogryposis rule-outs: BVD, IBR, bluetongue virus, Akabane virus, and Cache Valley virus
• Arthrogryposis-hydranencephaly syndrome (AHS) in lambs may be confused with spider lamb syndrome (SLS), in which there is characteristic hyperflexion of forelimbs, cranial overextension of hind limbs, with a corkscrew deviation of the spine. In lambs with AHS, severe deformities result from primary abnormalities of the CNS and not of the skeleton. Hydranencephaly, micromyelia, hydrocephalus, and cerebellar hypoplasia are also seen with AHS.

CBC/BIOCHEMISTRY/URINALYSIS
N/A

OTHER LABORATORY TESTS
N/A

IMAGING
• Radiographs can be used to diagnose angular limb deformities; at least two views, 90 degrees apart, should be taken of the affected joint.
• The dorsopalmar/dorsoplantar (DP) view is needed for examination of the anatomical location of the deformity and for measurements. Shoot with radiographic beam in line with the claws.

DIAGNOSTIC PROCEDURES
• Serology and virological diagnostic assays may aid in ruling out in utero viral infections (e.g., Cache Valley virus).
• Feed analysis and assessment of the availability of potentially toxic plants in the environment (pasture) may assist in diagnosis.

PATHOLOGIC FINDINGS
CCD
• No consistent primary lesion, rather a number of varied tissue responses are observed. It is likely that these findings are at least in part due to the animal's inability to stand.
• Histology: few lesions, restricted to muscles of the forelimb, external intercostalis muscle, or radial and femoral nerves—myositis, myodegeneration, muscle necrosis and atrophy, cellulitis, and perineuritis.

TREATMENT

APPROPRIATE HEALTH CARE
N/A

NURSING CARE
• Severely affected animals may be unable to rise to nurse and require additional supportive care.

• Protect limbs with thick, soft bandages that fit well.
• Provide good footing and allow for stretching of flexor tendons.
• Care should be taken to maintain a soft (padding), clean, and dry environment and to minimize decubital/pressure sores, open arthritis, muscle atrophy, umbilical infections, and septicemia.

ACTIVITY
Activity should be restricted until it is certain that the deformity is improving; however, some degree of exercise allows for stretching and lengthening of affected limb structures.

DIET
Correction of any dietary imbalances should be addressed while treating cases of arthrogryposis.

CLIENT EDUCATION
• Examination of young animals with congenital arthrogryposis should be done as early as possible to assess the degree of manual correction possible.
• Because of a possible hereditary component associated with some forms of arthrogryposis, breeding of affected animals is not recommended.

NONSURGICAL CONSIDERATIONS/ CONSERVATIVE TREATMENT
• Mildly affected animals may recover spontaneously.
• Weight bearing provides the necessary physical exercise to strengthen and lengthen affected tendons and musculature.
• Minor deformities may be corrected by manual alignment and external support of the limb (e.g., rigid splinting, bandaging, or casting/tube casts).

SURGICAL CONSIDERATIONS
• Surgery may be required for animals with severe deformities and for animals that do not improve with age or conservative management.
• Treatment of arthrogryposis includes surgery to improve the animal's posture sufficient for it to obtain slaughter weight (a salvage procedure).

ARTHROGRYPOSIS

• Surgical procedures include: transection of flexor tendon and suspensory ligament, joint capsule release, flexor tendon lengthening procedures, and joint arthrodesis.
• May require postoperative splinting or casting for support

MEDICATIONS

DRUGS OF CHOICE
N/A

CONTRAINDICATIONS
N/A

PRECAUTIONS
N/A

POSSIBLE INTERACTIONS
N/A

ALTERNATIVE DRUGS
N/A

FOLLOW-UP

PATIENT MONITORING
Frequent physical examinations and assessing the efficacy of corrective measures should be done to monitor progress.

PREVENTION/AVOIDANCE
• CCD: Avoid breeding affected animals.
• Coordinate grazing times and alter breeding dates to minimize exposure. Avoid grazing the potentially teratogenic plants when pregnant cows are at the susceptible stage of pregnancy.
• Control teratogenic plant populations with herbicide treatment.

POSSIBLE COMPLICATIONS
Some severe cases of arthrogryposis cannot be corrected and full extension may not be possible postoperatively.

EXPECTED COURSE AND PROGNOSIS
• The prognosis is guarded for arthrogryposis, depending on the severity of the flexural deformity. Severe deformities requiring surgery often have a poor prognosis.

• For arthrogryposis in cattle, approximately 80% of surgically treated animals can be kept until they reach normal slaughter weight.
• If untreated, arthrogryposis is usually lethal in cattle, resulting in skin necrosis over the carpus, arthritis, and septicemia.

MISCELLANEOUS

ASSOCIATED CONDITIONS
A syndrome known as "bentleg" or "bowie" has been associated with ingestion of *Trachymene glaucifolia* (wild parsnip) by pregnant ewes in Australia and New Zealand.

AGE-RELATED FACTORS
The majority of arthrogryposis cases occurs during the active growth phase of the affected bone/joint.

ZOONOTIC POTENTIAL
N/A

PREGNANCY
In cases of congenital arthrogryposis, the teratogenic plants are ingested by the pregnant dam and the compounds are passed to the fetus through the placenta.

RUMINANT SPECIES AFFECTED
Bovine, ovine, caprine, camelid

BIOSECURITY
N/A

PRODUCTION MANAGEMENT
• Producers should be aware of the association between certain toxic plants (e.g., lupines) and angular limb deformities such as CCD.
• To reduce the incidence of crooked calf syndrome, graze lupines during their least hazardous growth period and reduce exposure of pregnant cows. Lupines are most hazardous when they are young or in the mature seed stage.
• Fence off heavily infested pasture areas and use intermittent, short-term grazing of lupine pastures.

SYNONYMS
N/A

SEE ALSO
Akabane virus
Cache Valley virus/disease
Cleft palate
CNS anomalies
CNS: brain lesions
Lameness: muscle/tendon—contracted tendons
Lupine toxicity

ABBREVIATIONS
AHS = arthrogryposis-hydranencephaly syndrome
ALD = angular limb deformity
BVD = bovine viral diarrhea virus
CCD = crooked calf disease/syndrome
CNS = central nervous system
IBR = infectious bovine rhinotracheitis virus
SLS = spider-lamb syndrome

Suggested Reading
Anderson, D. E., St. Jean, G. 1996. Diagnosis and management of tendon disorders in cattle. Advances in ruminant orthopedics. *Veterinary Clinics of North America: Food Animal Practice* 12(1): 89–93.
Kaneps, A. J. 1996. Orthopedic conditions of small ruminants, llama, sheep, goat, and deer. Advances in ruminant orthopedics. *Veterinary Clinics of North America: Food Animal Practice* 12(1): 225–26.
Panter, K. E., James, L. F., Gardner, D. R. 1999. Lupines, poison-hemlock and *Nicotiana* spp: toxicity and teratogenicity in livestock. *Journal of Natural Toxins* 8(1): 117–34.
Panter, K. E., Keeler, R. F., Bunch, T. D., Callan, R. J. 1990. Congenital skeletal malformations and cleft palate induced in goats by ingestion of *Lupinus, Conium,* and *Nicotiana* species. *Toxicon* 28(12): 1377–85.
Van Huffel, X., De Moor, A. 1987. Congenital multiple arthrogryposis of the forelimbs in calves. *Compendium-Food Animal* 9(10): F333–F339.

Authors: Erik J. Olson and Cathy S. Carlson

BASICS

OVERVIEW
• *Aspergillus* spp. are ubiquitous environmental organisms that can cause disease in many mammalian species. This saprophytic fungus is present in the soil and other decaying matter.
• *Aspergillus* is an opportunistic pathogen and usually occurs secondary to chronic disease, immunosuppression, stress, or metabolic disturbances. It can also occur with chronic antibiotic or steroid use.
• In ruminants, *A. fumigatus* is the most common isolate involved in clinical disease.
• The disease can manifest in ruminants as one of several forms including pulmonary, intestinal, systemic, and/or as a cause of abortion or mastitis.

SIGNALMENT
• In cattle, aspergillosis is a major cause of mycotic abortion. Primary pulmonary infections are rare but can be caused by inhalation of spores from contaminated feedstuffs. It can occur secondary to concurrent disease in a pulmonary or intestinal form. Mastitis caused by *Aspergillus* has also occasionally been seen in cattle.
• Once infected, cattle may then develop a systemic aspergillosis due to invasion of blood vessels and dissemination of the organism throughout the body.
• Housed calves may be more susceptible to pulmonary infection.
• In sheep and goats, *Aspergillus* spp. may cause a primary mastitis. Disseminated aspergillosis may occur in conjunction with mastitis. Primary pulmonary infections are rare in sheep and goats.
• Pulmonary and disseminated aspergillosis have also been reported in llamas and alpacas, camels, American bison, and cervidae.

SIGNS
Pulmonary
• May cause few clinical signs. Mild respiratory disease and/or weight loss may be the only symptoms.
• Other respiratory signs may include fever, anorexia, cough, nasal discharge, tachypnea, dyspnea, and recumbency.
• Development of pneumonia may be acute.

Mastitis
Sheep and goats may have purulent mammary secretions, slight fever, and weight loss. The affected quarter becomes swollen and firm. Clinical signs from disseminated infection include depression, fever, and weight loss.

Abortion
• Bovine abortions due to *Aspergillus* spp. usually occur in the third trimester.

• Retained placenta and placentitis are seen.
• Fetal lesions may consist of bronchopneumonia and dermatitis.

CAUSES AND RISK FACTORS
• Chronic disease, immunosuppression, concurrent disease
• Viral erosive diseases, intestinal disease, metabolic disturbances
• Chronic stress, postpartum stress
• Antimicrobial therapy, chronic steroid or antibiotic use
• Unsanitary administration of intramammary antibiotics (dry cow treatment)
• Moldy feedstuffs

DIAGNOSIS

DIFFERENTIAL DIAGNOSIS
• Calves: enzootic pneumonia, tuberculosis, lungworms
• Cattle
  • Pulmonary form: shipping fever, mycoplasma bovis, tuberculosis, lungworms
  • Intestinal form: displaced abomasums, traumatic reticuloperitonitis, abomasal ulcers
• Sheep/Goats
  • Pulmonary form: caseous lymphadenitis, lungworms, pasteurellosis, tuberculosis, caprine arthritis/encephalitis virus (CAEV), ovine progressive pneumonia (OPP)
  • Mastitis form: bacterial mastitis
• Llamas/alpacas: third compartmental ulcers, bacterial pneumonia, intestinal impaction

CBC/BIOCHEMISTRY/URINALYSIS
• No specific findings for aspergillosis
• May aid in diagnosis of underlying disease

OTHER LABORATORY TESTS
• Fungal culture—identify organism; because of presence in environment, may be a contaminant.
• Transtracheal wash—identify organism; also potential to be a contaminant.
• Histopathology of lesions—demonstration of invasion into tissue
• Immunohistochemistry—along with clinical signs and other diagnostics

IMAGING
Thoracic radiographs may show evidence of multiple densities throughout all lung fields.

PATHOLOGIC FINDINGS
Pulmonary
• Severe fibrinous pneumonia (in calves) and multiple, small, white, discrete granulomas surrounded by necrotic tissue or with necrotic centers on gross pathology (ruminants)
• Alpacas infected with the pulmonary form of *Aspergillus niger* may demonstrate severe pyogranulomatous bronchopneumonia with bronchiectasis and the presence of calcium oxalate crystals.

Mastitis
• Nonspecific signs of mastitis
• Demonstration of septate branched fungal hyphae on histopathology

Intestinal
• Focal hemorrhagic and necrotic lesions in the omasum, rumen, reticulum, or small intestine
• Demonstration of fungal elements in the tissues

TREATMENT

MEDICATIONS

• Surgical resection of lesions
• Antifungal drugs, including intramammary application
• Antifungal drugs have not been approved for use in food-producing animals.
• Dosages for these agents have not been established in camelids.
• Prevention would involve avoiding moldy feed, and proper administration of intramammary antibiotics.

MISCELLANEOUS

ASSOCIATED CONDITIONS
N/A

AGE-RELATED FACTORS
N/A

ZOONOTIC POTENTIAL
Can affect humans due to similar environmental exposure; is not passed from animals to humans or between individual animals or humans.

ABBREVIATIONS
CAEV = caprine arthritis/encephalitis virus
OPP = ovine progressive pneumonia

Suggested Reading
Jensen, H. E., Olsen, S. N., Albaek, B. A. 1994. Gastrointestinal aspergillosis and zygomycosis in cattle. *Vet Pathol.* 31:28–36.
Wiske, S. E. 2002. Mycotic pneumonias. In: *Large animal internal medicine*, ed. B. P. Smith. 3rd ed. St. Louis: Mosby.

Authors: Susan L. McClanahan and Ann M. Fitzpatrick

ASPIRATION PNEUMONIA

 BASICS

DEFINITION
Inhalation or accidental administration of large volumes of foreign liquids, aspiration of solids (foreign bodies, plant debris, dirt) resulting in gangrenous pneumonia, or, in the case of oils, lipid pneumonia.

PATHOPHYSIOLOGY
Gangrenous pneumonia develops due to either infectious or chemical irritants damaging the airways and lung parenchyma.

SYSTEMS AFFECTED
Primarily the respiratory system; secondarily, multiple organ system dysfunction/failure

GENETICS
N/A

INCIDENCE/PREVALENCE
Uncommon, usually accidental or due to inadvertent exposure to risk factors

GEOGRAPHIC DISTRIBUTION
Potentially worldwide, depending on species and environment

SIGNALMENT
• Calves, lambs, and kids receive accidental orotracheal intubation when feeding colostrum, or inhalation of meconium containing fetal fluids during difficult parturition.
• Necrotic laryngitis in calves resulting in altered (turbulent) airflow through larynx and subsequent aspiration of pharyngeal secretions
• Adult cattle, sheep, goats: esophageal obstruction, oropharyngeal trauma, abscesses, consumption of raw turnips, beets, oranges, or other by-product type feeds
• Parturient paresis associated with recumbency in recently fresh dairy cows
• Lead-poisoning-induced dysphagia
• Crude oil, fuel oil, or natural gas condensate ingestion by livestock
• Listeriosis or botulism resulting in cranial nerve dysfunction, regurgitation or dysphagia and aspiration of gut/pharyngeal contents

Species
Potentially all ruminant species

Breed Predilections
N/A

Mean Age and Range
N/A

Predominant Sex
N/A

SIGNS
• Acute onset of depression, tachypnea, dyspnea, coughing, fever, foul breath odor.
• Adventitious lung sounds, pleural friction rubs auscultable. In severe cases or when associated with specific conditions, recumbency, shock, and sudden death may be observed.

HISTORICAL FINDINGS

RISK FACTORS
Improper administration of oral medications, dystocia, exposure to viral (IBR), bacterial agents or their products (listeria, *Clostridium botulinum*), using by-product feed supplements, toxin exposures, use of dips on livestock (submerged dips)

 DIAGNOSIS

DIFFERENTIAL DIAGNOSIS
Acute bronchopneumonia, septicemia, toxic ingestion

CBC/BIOCHEMISTRY/URINALYSIS
Complete blood count may demonstrate leukocytosis, leukopenia with left shift, elevated total plasma protein, hyperglobulinemia, hyperfibrinogenemia, dehydration, and azotemia.

OTHER LABORATORY TESTS
N/A

IMAGING
N/A

OTHER DIAGNOSTIC PROCEDURES
N/A

PATHOLOGIC FINDINGS

 TREATMENT

• Treatment is aimed at both gram-positive and gram-negative bacterial agents, removal (if possible) of primary problem (foreign body esophagitis/choke). Protection of airway from further injury.
• Prognosis often grave in cases where significant contamination of lungs with liquids has occurred.
• Nonsteroidal and steroidal anti-inflammatory agents should be administered to prevent mediator-induced inflammation and shocklike sequelae.

MEDICATIONS

CONTRAINDICATIONS
Appropriate milk and meat withdrawal times must be followed for all compounds administered to food-producing animals.

FOLLOW-UP

EXPECTED COURSE AND PROGNOSIS
Prognosis is often grave in cases where significant contamination of lungs with liquids has occurred.

MISCELLANEOUS

ASSOCIATED CONDITIONS
N/A

AGE-RELATED FACTORS
N/A

ZOONOTIC POTENTIAL
N/A

PREGNANCY
N/A

RUMINANT SPECIES AFFECTED
Potentially, all ruminant species are affected.

BIOSECURITY
N/A

PRODUCTION MANAGEMENT
N/A

SYNONYMS
N/A

SEE ALSO
• Crude oil, fuel oil, or natural gas condensate ingestion by livestock
• Esophageal obstruction, oropharyngeal trauma, abscesses, consumption of raw turnips, beets, oranges or other by-product type feeds.
• Lead-poisoning-induced dysphagia
• Listeriosis or botulism resulting in cranial nerve dysfunction, regurgitation or dysphagia, and aspiration of gut/pharyngeal contents
• Necrotic laryngitis
• Parturient paresis associated with recumbency in recently fresh dairy cows

ABBREVIATIONS
IBR = infectious bovine rhinotracheitis

Suggested Reading
Adler, R., Boermans, H. J., Moulton, J. E., Moore, D. A. 1992. Toxicosis in sheep following ingestion of natural gas condensate. *Vet Pathol*. 29:11–20.
Davidson, H. P., Rebhun, W. C., Habel, R. E. 1981. Pharyngeal trauma in cattle. *Cornell Vet*. 71:15–25.
Lopcz, A., Bildfcll, R. 1992. Pulmonary inflammation associated with aspirated meconium and epithelial cells in calves. *Vet Pathol*. 29:104–11.
Lopez, A., Lofstedt, J., Bildfell, R., Horney, B., Burton, S. 1994. Pulmonary histopathologic findings, acid-base status, and absorption of colostral immunoglobulins in newborn calves. *Am J Vet Res*. 55:1303–7.
Toofanian, F., Aliakbari, S., Ivoghli, B. 1979. Acute diesel fuel poisoning in goats. *Trop Anim Health Prod*. 2:98–101.

Author: Jeff Lakritz

ATYPICAL INTERSTITIAL PNEUMONIA

BASICS

DEFINITION
Atypical interstitial pneumonia is defined as disease(s) presenting with sudden onset of dyspnea (severe respiratory distress or difficulty breathing) due to congestion or edema, hyaline membranes, alveolar epithelial hyperplasia, and interstitial emphysema. This definition is limited for the purposes of this discussion to intoxication of cattle with L-tryptophan, 4-Ipomeanol, perilla ketones.

PATHOPHYSIOLOGY
3-Methylindole
Ruminal conversion of L-tryptophan to 3-methylindole, which is absorbed from the rumen and is metabolized in the lung resulting in bronchiolar, alveolar epithelial, and endothelial damage; pulmonary edema; hyaline membranes; lung cell hyperplasia; and interstitial emphysema (see Table 1).

4-Ipomeanol
• Formation of pneumotoxic 3-substituted furans (ipomeanine, 4-ipomeanol, 1-ipomeanol, and 1,4-ipomeadiol by *Fusarium solani*–infected sweet potatoes.
• These compounds are absorbed from rumen, and further metabolism of 4-ipomeanol and its analogs in the lung produces bronchiolar, alveolar epithelial, and endothelial injury by irreversible (covalent) binding to proteins within the cells.
• The loss of cellular function results in cell death, edema, and clinical signs associated with toxicity.

Perilla Ketones (Perilla frutescens)
• Cattle grazing dry grasses on sparse pastures in late summer in the southeastern United States and New Zealand (*Perilla maculatta*). The tall, green plant is found along the edge of wooded areas in pastures and grows well in later summer when other plants are dry. Intoxication commonly occurs in drought years.
• Consumption of the plant results in absorption of perilla ketone and two related compounds causing lung injury associated with dyspnea and acute death.

SYSTEMS AFFECTED
Production management, nutrition, respiration

GENETICS
No breed predilection

INCIDENCE/PREVALENCE
• Descriptions from the United Kingdom, Canada, and the western United States (3-methylindole toxicity)
• Moldy sweet potato toxicity observed in southeastern United States.
• Perilla ketone toxicity observed in southeastern United States.

GEOGRAPHIC DISTRIBUTION
Worldwide, depending on plant species and environment

SIGNALMENT
Species
Potentially all ruminant species

Breed Predilections
N/A

Mean Age and Range
Adult ruminants. Generally, adult brood cows or bulls (> 2 years of age). Suckling calves generally not affected and yearlings less susceptible.

Predominant Sex
N/A

SIGNS
• Adult cattle moved from dry summer forage to irrigated or fertilized pastures in fall.
• Herd outbreak of severe expiratory dyspnea, open-mouth breathing, excessive salivation, head and neck extension, distress and anxiousness, with quiet lung sounds
• Affected animals do not generally cough. Animals forced to walk or move through alleys may collapse and die (see Table 1).

RISK FACTORS
Typical management conditions predispose to toxicity.

DIAGNOSIS

DIFFERENTIAL DIAGNOSIS
• Parasitic bronchitis
• Aspiration syndrome
• Atelectasis
• Pneumonia
• Pulmonary hemorrhage
• Congestive heart failure
• Endotoxemia/sepsis
• Metabolic (acidosis, hypoglycemia)
• Persistent pulmonary hypertension
• Severe anemia
• Tracheal collapse
• Anaphylaxis/allergy
• Postparturient hemoglobinuria
• Anaplasmosis

CBC/BIOCHEMISTRY/URINALYSIS
Stress leukogram, not generally helpful

IMAGING
N/A

OTHER DIAGNOSTIC PROCEDURES
Necropsy, demonstration of appropriate feedstuffs in rumen (perilla mint, moldy sweet potatoes), primarily lung lesions with lack of other organs affected.

PATHOLOGIC FINDINGS
• Typical lesions are confined to respiratory system. Lungs are heavy and wet and have rubbery consistency (do not float). Lungs may fail to collapse and maintain rib impressions after thorax is opened.

• Petechial hemorrhages in upper respiratory tract, foamy fluid in large airways, congestion, edema and hyaline membranes, hepatization of lung, interstitial emphysema, large bullae with marked accumulation of edema in interlobular septae, proliferation of alveolar epithelial cells.

TREATMENT
• Management practices that prevent abrupt exposure of animals to lush green forage. Provision of feed and minerals during latter parts of summer to limit consumption of toxic plants.
• Do not feed moldy sweet potatoes to livestock.
• In animals that are exposed to such management conditions routinely, prior treatment with monensin or lasalocid (200 mg/head/day) for 1 day (monensin) or 6 days (lasalocid) prior to placing them on suspect pasture. Maintain access to ionophore for at least 10 days after introduction to feed.

MEDICATIONS

CONTRAINDICATIONS
• Appropriate milk and meat withdrawal times must be followed for all compounds administered to food-producing animals.
• Steroids should not be used in pregnant animals.

FOLLOW-UP

MISCELLANEOUS

ASSOCIATED CONDITIONS
• Endothelial damage, pulmonary edema, hyaline membranes, lung cell hyperplasia, and interstitial emphysema
• Bronchiolar, alveolar epithelial and endothelial injury
• The loss of cellular function results in cell death, edema, and clinical signs associated with toxicity.
• Lung injury associated with dyspnea and acute death

AGE-RELATED FACTORS
Adult ruminants—generally adult brood cows or bulls (> 2 years of age); suckling calves generally not affected and yearlings less susceptible.

ZOONOTIC POTENTIAL
N/A

PREGNANCY
N/A

ATYPICAL INTERSTITIAL PNEUMONIA

Table 1

Intoxication with Perilla Ketone, 4-Ipomeanol, Parasitic Bronchitis					
Toxin	Signalment	History	Clinical signs	Pathology	Treatment/Prevention
3-methylindole	Adult	Moved from dry, sparse feed, to lush green pasture, irrigated/fertilized aftermath	Open-mouth breathing, head and neck extension, frothing, sudden death. Multiple animals affected. Little coughing	Heavy, wet lungs, upper airway edema and hemorrhage, lung epithelial necrosis, hyaline membranes, epithelial proliferation, interlobular and subpleural emphysema	Ionophore in feed prior to changing diet. Aspirin, flunixin meglumine, furosemide.
4-ipomeanol	Adult	Provision or access to moldy sweet potatoes.	Open-mouth breathing, head and neck extension, frothing, sudden death. Multiple animals affected. Little coughing	Heavy, wet lungs, upper airway edema and hemorrhage, lung epithelial necrosis, hyaline membranes, epithelial proliferation, interlobular and subpleural emphysema	No effective treatment. Prevent access to moldy sweet potatoes.
Perilla ketone	Adult, older calves	Late summer/fall. Limited feed, access to open, wooded areas	Open-mouth breathing, head and neck extension, frothing, sudden death. Multiple animals affected. Little coughing	Heavy, wet lungs, upper airway edema and hemorrhage, lung epithelial necrosis, hyaline membranes, epithelial proliferation, interlobular and subpleural emphysema	No effective treatment. Prevent consumption of toxic plant by provision of quality feed and minerals in late summer/fall.

RUMINANT SPECIES AFFECTED

Potentially all ruminant species can be affected.

BIOSECURITY

N/A

PRODUCTION MANAGEMENT

• Management practices that prevent abrupt exposure of animals to lush green forage. Provision of feed and minerals during latter parts of summer to limit consumption of toxic plants.
• Do not feed moldy sweet potatoes to livestock.

SYNONYMS

Fog fever

SEE ALSO

• 3-Methylindole toxicity
• Moldy sweet potato toxicity
• Perilla toxicity
• Plants associated with respiratory disease
• Toxicology herd outbreak
• Toxic plant chapters

ABBREVIATIONS

Suggested Reading

Breeze, R. 1985. Respiratory disease in adult cattle. *Vet Clin North Amer: Food Animal Practice* 1:311–46.
Kerr, L. A., Johnson, B. J., Burrows, G. E. 1986, Oct. Intoxication of cattle by *Perilla frutescens* (purple mint). *Vet Hum Toxicol.* 28(5):412–16.
Kerr, L. A., Linnabary, R. D. 1989, Jun. A review of interstitial pneumonia in cattle.

Vet Hum Toxicol. 31(3):247–54.
Loneragan, G. H., Gould, D. H., Mason, G. L., Garry, F. B., Yost, G. S., Lanza, D. L., Miles, D. G., Hoffman, B. W., Mills, L. J. 2001, Oct. Association of 3-methyleneindolenine, a toxic metabolite of 3-methylindole, with acute interstitial pneumonia in feedlot cattle. *Am J Vet Res.* 62(10):1525–30.
Medeiros, R. M., Simoes, S. V., Tabosa, I. M., Nobrega, W. D., Riet-Correa, F. 2001, Aug. Bovine atypical interstitial pneumonia associated with the ingestion of damaged sweet potatoes (*Ipomoea batatas*) in northeastern Brazil. *Vet Hum Toxicol.* 43(4):205–7.

Author: Jeff Lakritz

AVOCADO TOXICOSIS

 BASICS

OVERVIEW
Lactating animals that consume avocado leaves may develop noninfectious mastitis and agalactia.

Source
• Avocado plant (*Persea americana*)
• Leaves, fruit, bark, and seeds reported to cause toxicosis
• Drying the leaves does not reduce toxic potential.

Toxin
• Thought to be due to a "persin," which has been identified as (Z,Z)-1-(acetyloxy)-2-hydroxy-12,15-heneicosadien-4—one that can be isolated from the leaves of the avocado plant.
• The exact mechanism of action of this toxin on target is not known.

Toxic Dose
Symptoms of noninfectious mastitis and agalactia have been noted with 60–100 mg/kg of the toxin in an experimental setting.

SYSTEMS AFFECTED
Mammary glands, cardiovascular (mouse model) at doses higher than those that cause agalactia

INCIDENCE/PREVALENCE
N/A

GEOGRAPHIC DISTRIBUTION
N/A

SIGNALMENT
Species
Cattle, goats, sheep
Predominant Sex
Female

SIGNS
• Noninfectious mastitis
• Agalactia

CAUSES AND RISK FACTORS
N/A

 DIAGNOSIS

• Mastitis that is not explained by an infectious agent
• History of exposure to the plant

CBC/BIOCHEMISTRY/URINALYSIS
N/A

PATHOLOGIC FINDINGS
Histopathology
• Agalactia/mastitis
  • Extensive coagulative necrosis of the secretory acinar epithelium
  • Interstitial edema
  • Congestion
  • Edema
• Cardiotoxicity (described in a mouse model)
  • Necrosis of myocardial fibers
  • Myocardial fibrosis if animals survive

 TREATMENT

• No specific antidote or treatment
• Symptomatic and supportive therapy is indicated.

 MEDICATIONS

None

 FOLLOW-UP

PREVENTION/ AVOIDANCE
• Prevent exposure of lactating animals to these plants.
• Ideally, animals should not be exposed to this plant.

EXPECTED COURSE AND PROGNOSIS
• Mastitis should resolve within 1 week to 10 days.
• Agalactia requires a longer period of time for resolution.
• Milk production may not reach original levels.

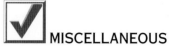 **MISCELLANEOUS**

ASSOCIATED CONDITIONS
Mastitis

AGE-RELATED FACTORS
N/A

ZOONOTIC POTENTIAL
N/A

PREGNANCY
N/A

RUMINANT SPECIES AFFECTED
Potentially all ruminant species are affected

BIOSECURITY
N/A

PRODUCTION MANAGEMENT
Restrict grazing of livestock from avocado groves.

SYNONYMS
N/A

SEE ALSO
Mastitis: noninfectious
Toxicology: herd outbreaks

ABBREVIATIONS
N/A

Suggested Reading
Craigmill, A. L., Eide, R. N., Shultz, T. A., Hedrick, K. 1984. Toxicity of avocado (*Persea americana* (Guatamalan var)) leaves: review and preliminary report. *Vet Hum Toxicol*. 26(5): 381–83.
Craigmill, A. L., Seawright, A. A., Mattila, T., Frost, A. J. 1989. Pathological changes in the mammary gland and biochemical changes in milk of the goat following oral dosing with leaf of the avocado (*Persea americana*). *Aust Vet J*. 66(7): 206–11.
Oelrichs, P. B., Ng, J. C., Seawright, A. A., Ward, A., Schaffeler, L., MacLeod, J. K. 1995. Isolation and identification of a compound from avocado (*Persea americana*) leaves which causes necrosis of the acinar epithelium of the lactating mammary gland and the myocardium. *Nat Toxins*. 3(5): 344–49.

Author: Joe Roder

B VITAMINS

BASICS

OVERVIEW

• The B vitamins are a family of water-soluble micronutrients, which act primarily as coenzymes, and are essential to normal metabolism.
• The B vitamins are thiamine (B_1), riboflavin (B_2), niacin (B_3), pyridoxine (B_6), the cobalamins (B_{12}), biotin, folic acid, pantothenic acid, and inositol.
• Common feedstuffs usually contain substantial amounts of several of the B vitamins.
• Ruminal microorganisms synthesize B vitamins in quantities that, under most conditions, meet metabolic needs; therefore, there are no specific dietary requirements for B vitamins in animals possessing a functioning rumen.
• Preruminants are susceptible to deficiencies, but these are rare when the principle feed is milk.
• Under certain nutritional, management, or disease conditions, deficiencies may result in disease, the most clinically significant being polioencephalomalacia (PEM) associated with vitamin B_1 deficiency.
• The trace element cobalt (Co) is required for the synthesis of vitamin B_{12} and a lack of this vitamin is responsible for the ill thrift associated with Co deficiency.

SIGNALMENT

B-vitamin deficiencies are noted in all ruminants, with growing animals most at risk. Sheep are most susceptible to vitamin B_{12} deficiency.

SIGNS

• Vitamin B_1 deficiency—a history of acute neurologic disease in growing ruminants fed highly fermentable carbohydrate is suggestive. Clinical signs include excitability, circling behavior, abnormal vision, head pressing, followed by depression, convulsions and coma.
• Vitamin B_{12} deficiency—often accompanied by a history of ill thrift in animals offered what would appear to be an adequate ration. Animals may have been fed a ration grown in a region known to possess Co-deficient soils. Clinical signs include retarded growth, muscular weakness, anemia, ketosis and general poor condition. In sheep, a syndrome termed ovine white liver disease has been identified that is characterized by ill thrift together with serous ocular discharge, fatty degeneration of the liver and sometimes photosensitization.
• Other B vitamin deficiencies—are extremely rare or unknown in ruminants under typical management conditions, but are most likely to result in nonspecific signs of ill thrift, poor growth, skin lesions, poor coat condition, and central nervous system abnormalities.

CAUSES AND RISK FACTORS

• Deficiencies of vitamin B_1 can occur when there is production or ingestion of inactive B vitamin analogs, or excessive destruction of B vitamins in the rumen. This occurs most commonly under conditions of ruminal lactic acidosis, induced by diets containing a high proportion of concentrate or other source of highly fermentable carbohydrate such as very lush pasture. A diet of highly fermentable carbohydrate can induce changes in ruminal flora so that rumen bacteria produce excessive amounts of thiaminase, reducing the amount of thiamine available for intestinal absorption. Some plants, such as bracken fern (*Pteridium aquilinum*) contain thiaminase.
• In vitamin B_{12} deficiency, ruminal microorganisms are incapable of producing sufficient cobalamins due to a lack of Co. The concentration of Co in crops and forages depends on a variety of factors including Co concentration of the soil, plant species, rate of plant growth, and soil pH, drainage, and fertilization. Soils are generally considered Co deficient if they contain less than 2 ppm Co. Such soils are widely distributed throughout the world.

B VITAMINS

DIAGNOSIS

DIFFERENTIAL DIAGNOSIS

• Vitamin B_1 deficiency—clinical signs are nonspecific and may be confused with PEM associated with water deprivation and toxicosis due to sulfur, salt, lead, amprolium, lasalocid, and some anthelmintics. Differential diagnoses should include the following causes of encephalitis or meningoencephalitis: focal symmetric encephalomalacia (*Clostridium perfringens* type D); thrombotic meningoencephalitis (*Hemophilus somnus*); nervous coccidiosis; listeriosis; rabies, and herpes virus. Toxicoses due to ethylene glycol, lead and selenium, and deficiencies of vitamin A and magnesium should also be considered.
• Vitamin B_{12} deficiency—differential diagnoses that should be considered are gross malnutrition; intestinal parasitism; paratuberculosis; and deficiencies of vitamin D, selenium, and copper. Diagnosis may be complicated by the fact that cattle are more susceptible to intestinal parasitism under conditions of vitamin B_{12} deficiency.

CBC/BIOCHEMISTRY/URINALYSIS

No consistent abnormalities are observed.

OTHER LABORATORY TESTS

• Vitamin B_1 deficiency—antemortem diagnostic aids for thiamine deficiency include the following: blood concentrations of thiamine, lactate, and pyruvate; erythrocyte transketolase activity, and fecal thiaminase activity. Many laboratories do not offer these tests routinely and, due to the acute nature of the condition, postmortem diagnosis is more commonly performed (see below).
• Vitamin B_{12} deficiency—diagnosis may be made by measuring serum or liver vitamin B_{12} concentrations or serum methylmalonic acid concentration.

PATHOLOGIC FINDINGS

Gross pathologic signs of vitamin B_1 deficiency are symmetric and include cortical swelling and flattened gyri with thinning and yellowing of the cortex. Necrotic areas of the brain may autofluoresce under ultraviolet light. A diagnosis of PEM can be confirmed by histopathology.

TREATMENT

If clinical signs are noted in one or more animals, it is likely that a large proportion of the herd or flock is subclinically affected.
• Vitamin B_1 deficiency—provide good quality roughage and/or remove thiaminase-containing forage. Cease treatment with any medications that might be associated with PEM.
• Vitamin B_{12} deficiency—supplementation is usually applied on a flock or herd basis.

MEDICATIONS

• Vitamin B_1 deficiency—thiamine hydrochloride solution 10–20 mg/kg IM or SC three times daily. The same dose can be given IV if diluted in isotonic intravenous fluids and administered slowly. Corticosteroids and diuretics to reduce cortical swelling may be useful.
• Vitamin B_{12} deficiency— injection of vitamin B_{12} solution SC at a dose of 100–300 μg weekly or 2000–3000 μg weekly for small and large ruminants, respectively, is effective.
• Weekly oral treatment with a dilute cobalt sulfate solution at 7 mg Co per animal (small ruminants), or 35–70 mg Co per head (large ruminants) is also effective.

CONTRAINDICATIONS

Appropriate milk and meat withdrawal times must be followed for all compounds administered to food-producing animals.

FOLLOW-UP

PREVENTION/AVOIDANCE

• Vitamin B_1 deficiency—provide adequate roughage in the diet to avoid lactic acidosis. Avoid feeding plants containing thiaminase. Add thiamine mononitrate to the ration at 125 g per tonne. Ruminants should be introduced to high-grain diets gradually and large variations in intake should be avoided.

• Vitamin B_{12} deficiency—ensure Co is supplied at a rate of at least 0.1 mg/kg DM in the total ration. Rations supplemented at this level, or salt licks containing 0.1% Co (as cobalt carbonate), should prevent the disease. Oral administration of intraruminal boluses made of metal oxides or soluble glass, where available, provides supplementary Co for periods in excess of 1 year. Cobalt sulfate applied to pasture (1.5 kg/ha every 3–4 years) can be effective also. An injectable product containing microencapsulated vitamin B_{12} has been developed in New Zealand for supplementation of sheep and is effective for up to 8 months after treatment.

EXPECTED COURSE AND PROGNOSIS

• Vitamin B_1 deficiency—response to treatment should be noted within minutes. Individuals that are recumbent and showing severe neurologic signs at the time of treatment have a poorer prognosis. Recovered individuals may be left with residual neurologic deficits.
• Vitamin B_{12} deficiency— response to Co or vitamin B_{12} supplementation is usually good and improvement is noted within days of treatment, however affected growing animals may never attain full mature weight.

 MISCELLANEOUS

ASSOCIATED CONDITIONS
• Ruminal lactic acidosis in vitamin B_1 deficiency
• Intestinal parasitism in vitamin B_{12} deficiency

RUMINANT SPECIES AFFECTED
All ruminant species are affected.

PRODUCTION MANAGEMENT
There is some evidence that the health and production of high-producing dairy cattle may be enhanced by supplementation of some B vitamins (niacin, biotin, and folic acid) and Co even though these cattle are not at risk of overt deficiency. Most researched is the effect of biotin on the incidence of lameness in dairy cattle.

SEE ALSO
Chapters on nutrition, vitamins, PEM, lameness

ABBREVIATIONS
Co = cobalt
DM = dry matter
PEM = polioencephalomalacia

Suggested Reading
Lee, J., Knowles, S. O., Judson, G. J., Freer, M., Dove, H. 2002. Trace element and vitamin nutrition of grazing sheep. In: *Sheep nutrition.* Wallingford, UK: CABI Publishing.
Loneragan, G. H., Gould, D. H. 2002. Polioencephalomalacia. In: *Large animal internal medicine,* ed. B. P. Smith. 3rd ed. St. Louis, MO: Mosby.
Maas, J. 2002. Cobalt deficiency in ruminants. In: *Large animal internal medicine,* ed. B. P. Smith. 3rd ed. St. Louis, MO: Mosby.
National Research Council. 2001. *Nutrient requirements of dairy cattle.* 7th rev ed. Washington, DC: National Academy of Sciences.

Author: Jeff Wichtel

BABESIOSIS

 BASICS

DEFINITION
• Although it has been eradicated in the United States for 60 years, babesiosis remains an important disease in cattle throughout the world where the tick vector is prevalent.
• The causative agent is an intraerythrocytic protozoan that produces intravascular hemolysis in the ruminant host.

PATHOPHYSIOLOGY
• Babesiosis is contractible via inoculation of infected blood.
• Ticks are considered to be the principal vectors (see Table 1), although transmission may also occur via blood-contaminated needles or instruments.
• The organism is transmitted by several one-host ticks; the genus *Boophilus* is particularly important.
• Female ticks become infected during blood engorgement on infected cattle, with subsequent replication of the *Babesia* in the tick's embryos. As the tick embryos develop into larvae, nymphs, and adults, the *Babesia* persist and can be transmitted to new mammalian hosts during tick feeding. For *B. bigemina*, only nymph or adult ticks are capable of transmitting the disease. The infection does not persist beyond the larval stage in *B. bovis*.
• Although considered rare, vertical transmission within the mammalian host has been reported.
• Once inoculated, the incubation period is 2 to 3 weeks.
• In endemic areas, wherein passive humoral immunity is transferred from dam to offspring, clinical signs of disease are uncommon in cattle less than 6 months of age.
• Immunosuppressed or immunologically naïve individuals are susceptible to parasitemia, and clinical signs of disease develop. If an animal survives the initial episode of infection, active immunity rapidly ensues, thereby controlling parasitemia.
• Immunity to the disease after natural exposure may be as long as 1 to 2 years, however, the development of immunity may be insufficient to completely eliminate the organism, allowing for the persistence of the organism without clinical signs of disease (premunition).
• These subclinical "carriers" of *Babesia* serve as a silent reservoir for persistent infection within a herd.
• Carriers also may experience episodic clinical signs of recrudescence as protective immunity and the extent of parasitemia wax and wane.
• Although some individuals may eventually eliminate the infection, other chronic carriers eventually succumb to the disease.

• Upon inoculation, infective sporozoites enter red blood cells wherein binary fission occurs within 14 days of inoculation. When replication is complete, the organisms are released by erythrolysis to propagate infection in new red blood cells.
• Thus the predominant clinical signs of disease are fever and intravascular hemolysis. Other factors that may contribute to hemolysis include increased red blood cell fragility, removal of infected cells by the mononuclear phagocytic system, and the development of secondary autoimmune hemolytic anemia.
• Anemia develops, and in severe cases (typically immunosuppressed or immunologically naïve adults), death from hypoxemia may ensue.
• With *B. bovis* infection, the release of inflammatory mediators in response to infection may also lead to intense hypotension, cardiovascular shock, and disseminated intravascular coagulation.
• *B. bigemina* may also replicate within the endothelium of the cerebrum, causing local hypoxemia and the development of "cerebral babesiosis," characterized by acute onset of signs of cerebral disease.

SYSTEMS AFFECTED
• Hemic: regenerative anemia, intravascular hemolysis, disseminated intravascular coagulation, hemoglobinemia, hemoglobinuria, icterus
• Cardiovascular: hypoxemia, hypotension
• Cerebral: ataxia, blindness, maniacal behavior

GENETICS
Zebu, Afrikaner, and Santa Gertrudis cattle are less susceptible to babesiosis than are other breeds of cattle.

INCIDENCE/PREVALENCE
• The disease is widespread in endemic areas.
• The existence of asystematic carriers obscures accurate estimate of the true prevalence of infection.
• Wide application of sensitive PCR testing will be necessary to establish the actual rate and distribution of infection.

GEOGRAPHIC DISTRIBUTION
• Cases have been reported throughout the world. The disease is endemic in tropical climates where the tick vectors flourish (see Table 1).
• Rigid measures to control the *Boophilus* tick population were primarily responsible for eradication of babesiosis from the United States.

SIGNALMENT
Species
Cattle and small ruminants are the principal hosts, but cases have been reported in other ruminants, such as water buffalo, reindeer, and the American bison.

Breed Predilections
N/A

Mean Age and Range
• Any age may be affected, but younger calves in endemic areas, wherein infected dams have provided passive immunity to their offspring, rarely develop infection prior to 6 months of age.
• Immunosuppressed, debilitated, stressed, or immunologically naïve adult ruminants are more susceptible to infection and often are more severely affected by the disease.

Predominant Sex
N/A

SIGNS

GENERAL COMMENTS
• Severely debilitated, immunosuppressed, or immunologically naïve individuals in endemic areas are most susceptible to disease.
• Seasonality of the disease is mostly dependent on the peak occurrence of the tick vector population.

HISTORICAL FINDINGS
Concurrent illness; progressive depression, weakness, and lethargy; poor growth; poor coat quality; separation from the herd; anorexia; tick infestation; hemoglobinuria; fever; and icterus

PHYSICAL EXAMINATION FINDINGS
• The onset of clinical signs depends on the size of the inoculum.
• Signs of disease can develop within 1 week of inoculation of infected blood, but may not be apparent for 2 to 3 weeks.
• High fever, depression, anorexia, and progressive weakness occur first.
• The predominant clinical signs develop with the onset of intravascular hemolysis that occurs as reproducing merozoites destroy erythrocytes in the circulation.
• Tachycardia and tachypnea may be profound and depend on the degree and rate at which the anemia develops. A low-grade systolic murmur may be present over the heart base as the viscosity of the blood decreases.
• Hemoglobinemia and pallor of the mucous membranes precede hemoglobinuria and the development of icterus. Pregnant cows often abort their fetuses.
• In severe cases, death occurs as a result of anoxic shock. If the infected animal survives the initial episode of hemolysis, convalescence is prolonged until anemia has regenerated (weeks to months).
• Emaciation, poor condition, and failure to thrive, and the existence of the carrier stage are common developments during convalescence.
• Infection of the endothelium of the central nervous system in cattle with *B. bigemina* may result in clinical signs of cerebral disease, including maniacal behavior, hyperexcitability, seizures, bruxism, opisthotonus, blindness, ataxia, and coma.
• The prognosis for this form of the disease typically is grave.
• A unique phenomenon of anal sphincter spasm in cattle infected with *B. divergens* may

produce the additional clinical sign of pipe stream feces.

CAUSES
• Babesiosis is caused by infection with protozoa from the phylum Apicomplexa, order Piroplasmida, genus *Babesia*.
• There are at least six species of *Babesia* that affect cattle and two species that affect small ruminants (see Table 1). *B. bovis* is frequently considered to be the most pathogenic of the *Babesia* species; *B. major* and *B. ovate* are less pathogenic to nonpathogenic.

RISK FACTORS
Immunologically naïve (typically mature cattle) or immunosuppressed or otherwise debilitated individuals in endemic areas wherein the tick vectors reside are most at risk for contracting the infection.

DIAGNOSIS

DIFFERENTIAL DIAGNOSIS
• Any cause of intravascular hemolysis in cattle would result in similar signs including leptospirosis, bacillary hemoglobinuria, Heinz body anemias (onion, rape, kale toxicity), theileriosis, postparturient hemoglobinuria, and autoimmune hemolytic anemia.
• Differentials for extravascular hemolysis should also be considered.
• Copper toxicity should be considered as differential diagnoses in sheep.

CBC/BIOCHEMISTRY/URINALYSIS
• Anemia
• Regenerative anemia 5 to 7 days after onset (signs of regeneration include an increased MCV, anisocytosis, polychromasia, basophilic stippling, reticulocytes, Howell Jolly bodies, nucleated red blood cells)
• Hemoglobinemia (pink plasma, MCH, and MCHC increased)
• Hemoglobinuria (red-brown urine, urine dipstick positive for blood; positive for hemoglobin with saturated ammonium sulfate test)
• Hyperbilirubinemia (unconjugated)
• Hypokalemia
• Thrombocytopenia
• Metabolic acidosis

OTHER LABORATORY TESTS
• *Babesia* species may be seen within erythrocytes in a peripheral Wright- or Giemsa-stained blood smear. *B. bovis* is often difficult to find in the peripheral blood.
• The protozoa appear as nonpigmented, pyriform to irregular, round or amoeba-shaped organisms.
• Often, the protozoa appear in groups of two, with the "tops" of the pear-shaped organisms joined at an angle to form a "v."
• Parasitemia is often low, or affected cells are removed from the circulation, therefore absence of visible protozoa does not preclude the diagnosis.

• The humoral response to *Babesia* can usually be detected within a week of infection.
• Numerous serologic assays have been developed to detect *Babesia*, but the complement fixation, ELISA, and the indirect fluorescent antibody tests are most commonly used.
• Because humoral immunity postinfection is long lived, it may be difficult to distinguish active infection from previous exposure.
• Highly sensitive and specific PCR assays recently have been developed as extremely useful tools in the diagnosis and surveillance of active infection in both ticks and cattle.

IMAGING
N/A

DIAGNOSTIC PROCEDURES
N/A

PATHOLOGIC FINDINGS
• Sudden death is not uncommon. Depending on the stage of the disease, diffuse pallor of the tissues or icterus is present.
• Splenomegaly, hepatomegaly, edema, body cavity effusion, petechial and ecchymotic hemorrhages on the heart and gastrointestinal tract, thin blood, thrombi, gallbladder distension, and the presence of red-brown urine in the urinary bladder are common findings.
• In chronically infected cattle, emaciation is an additional expected feature. *B. bigemina* tends to proliferate in peripheral vessels, whereas *B. bovis* multiplies in visceral blood vessels.
• Direct fluorescent antibody staining and PCR assay of blood or tissues are the most specific tests used to confirm the diagnosis postmortem.

TREATMENT

APPROPRIATE HEALTH CARE
Inpatient or outpatient care

NURSING CARE
• If anemia is severe and clinical or laboratory evidence of hypoxemia is evident (intense lethargy or weakness, profound tachycardia or tachypnea, severe anemia, acidosis, increased anion gap), a whole blood transfusion is indicated.
• The normal total blood volume is approximately 8% of the body weight (i.e., 0.08 x body weight in kilograms equals the total blood volume in liters). Typically, transfusing one-fourth to one-third of the total blood volume is adequate.

ACTIVITY
Confined

DIET
N/A

CLIENT EDUCATION
• See Prevention/Avoidance below.

• Immunologically naïve cattle moving into endemic areas should be vaccinated prior to movement.

SURGICAL CONSIDERATIONS
N/A

MEDICATIONS

DRUGS OF CHOICE
• Numerous drugs have been used for the treatment of babesiosis.
• The most commonly used drugs include diminazene diaceturate (Berenil; 3–5 mg/kg IM), phenamidine diisethionate (Lomadine; 8–13 mg/kg, SQ or IM), imidocarb dipropionate (Imizol; 1–3 mg/kg, SQ or IM), and amicarbalide diisethionate (Diampron; 5–10 mg/kg IM). Imidocarb therapy may prevent reinfection for up to 2 months.
• Overzealous use of babesiocidal drugs may abruptly reduce parasitemia to a level that is inadequate for establishment of protective immunity.

CONTRAINDICATIONS
Meat and milk withdrawal periods must be maintained.

PRECAUTIONS
N/A

POSSIBLE INTERACTIONS
N/A

ALTERNATIVE DRUGS
N/A

FOLLOW-UP

PATIENT MONITORING
Heart rate, respiratory rate, attitude, appetite, PCV, body weight

PREVENTION/AVOIDANCE
• Most control programs are tailored to the particular circumstances of infection in the herd.
• Complete eradication in a herd within an endemic area leaves that herd susceptible to future reinfection from surrounding herds.
• Thus most control programs are aimed at balancing the degree of infection with an appropriate level of immunity. This is most effectively achieved by reducing the tick population with acaricides and vaccination with live or live-attenuated organisms to establish a state of premunition.
• As older animals are more sensitive to the effects of infection, vaccination with live organisms is often followed with babesiostatic drugs.
• Newer vaccines using cell culture or recombinant proteins are promising, but are not currently widely available. There is little cross protection between species of *Babesia*.

BABESIOSIS

Table 1

	Distribution and Vectors for *Babesia* in Ruminants		
Species	Geographic location	Reported vectors	Infective stage of tick vector
B. bigemina	South America, Europe, Africa, Australia, Middle East, Asia, West Indies	*Boophilus annulatus, B. decoloratus, B. microplus, B. calcaratus, Rhipicephalus evertsi, R. bursa, R. appendiculatus, Haemaphysalis punctata*	Nymphs and adults
B. bovis (also includes *B. berbera*, or *B. argentina*)	South America, Europe, Russia, Africa, Asia, Australia	*B. annulatus, B. microplus, Ixodes spp., Rhipicephalus bursa*	Larvae
B. divergens	Europe, Africa	*Ixodes ricinus*	Larvae
B. major	Europe, Russia, North Africa, Middle East	*Haemaphysalis punctata*	Adults
B. jakimovi	Siberia, Asia	*Ixodes ricinus*	
B. ovata	Japan	*Haemaphysalis longicornis*	
B. motasi (sheep and goats)	Europe, South America, Africa	*Dermacentor silvarum, Haemaphysalis, Rhipicephalus bursa*	Adults
B. ovis (sheep and goats)	Europe, Russia, Asia, Middle East	*Ixodes ricinus, Rhipicephalus bursa, Dermacentor reticulatis*	Adults

POSSIBLE COMPLICATIONS

Death from hypoxemic anemia or cerebral babesiosis is not uncommon. Treatment frequently does not eliminate the carrier state.

EXPECTED COURSE AND PROGNOSIS

• Carriers and recrudesce are common in endemic areas. Infection with *B. bovis* is generally more severe than infection with other species.
• The presence of cerebral babesiosis warrants a grave prognosis.
• The mortality rate is high in adult immunologically naïve or immunosuppressed individuals.

MISCELLANEOUS

ASSOCIATED CONDITIONS
N/A

AGE-RELATED FACTORS
Younger cattle in endemic areas are rarely infected.

ZOONOTIC POTENTIAL
Although rare, immunosuppressed humans may be susceptible to infection.

PREGNANCY
Immunization of pregnant cows with live or live-attenuated vaccines may induce neonatal isoerythrolysis.

RUMINANT SPECIES AFFECTED
• Cases of babesiosis have been reported in cattle, small ruminants, white-tailed deer, American bison, water buffalo, reindeer, Asian elk, Tartarean roe deer, and African buffalo.

• Recent application of PCR techniques revealed that 16% of the cottontail rabbit population on Nantucket Island, Massachusetts, were carriers for *B. divergens*.
• The significance of this finding has not been fully determined, but widespread use of PCR assays may unveil a wider range of distribution of the organism.

BIOSECURITY
N/A

PRODUCTION MANAGEMENT
N/A

SYNONYMS
Bovine malaria
Piroplasmosis
Redwater
Texas fever
Tick fever
Tristeza

SEE ALSO
Autoimmune hemolytic anemia
Bacillary hemoglobinuria
Copper toxicity
Heinz body anemias (onion, rape, kale toxicity)
Intravascular hemolysis
Leptospirosis
Postparturient hemoglobinuria
Theileriosis

ABBREVIATIONS
ELISA = enzyme-linked immunosorbent assay
IM = intramuscular
MCH = mean corpuscular hemoglobin
MCHC = mean corpuscular hemoglobin concentration
MCV = mean corpuscular volume
PCR = polymerase chain reaction
SQ = subcutaneous

Suggested Reading
Goethert, H. K., Telford, S. R. 2003. Enzootic transmission of *Babesia divergens* among cottontail rabbits on Nantucket Island, Massachusetts. *Am J Trop Med Hyg.* 69(5):455–60.
Goff, W. L., McElwain, T. F., Suarez, C. E., Johnson, W. C., Brown, W. C., Norimine, J., Knowles, D. P. 2003. Competitive enzyme linked immunosorbent assay based on a rhoptry associated protein 1 epitope specifically identifies *Babesia bovis* infected cattle. *Clin Diagn La Immunol.* 10(1):38–43.
Regassa, A., Penzhorn, B. L., Bryson, N. R. 2003. Attainment of endemic stability to *Babesia bigemina* in cattle on a South African ranch where nonintensive tick control was applied. *Vet Parasitol.* 116(4):267–74.
Vos, A. J., Bock, R. E. 2000. Vaccination against *Babesia*. *Annals of the New York Academy of Sciences.* 916:540–45.
Yeruham, I., Avidar, Y., Aroch, I., Hadani, A. 2003. Intrauterine infection with *Babesia bovis* in a 2-day-old calf. *J Vet Med B Infect Dis Vet Public Health* 50(2):60–62.

Author: Michelle Henry Barton

BASICS

DEFINITION
Peracute, highly fatal, anaerobic infection of cattle and other ruminants caused by rapid proliferation of *Clostridium haemolyticum* (*Clostridium novyi* type D) after hepatic insult and resulting in sudden death or fulminant disease with characteristic necrotic hepatic infarct, hemolysis, hemoglobinuria, and toxemia.

OVERVIEW
• Disease primarily of cattle and sheep caused by proliferation of and toxin(s) released by *Clostridium haemolyticum* (*Clostridium novyi* type D)
• Spores of *Cl. haemolyticum* are normally found in the soil and GIT (liver, feces) and urine of healthy cattle and sheep grazing on contaminated pastures.
• Disease results when a hepatic insult or damage creates an area of anaerobiosis in the liver appropriate for spore germination and resulting vegetative cell multiplication and toxin production.
• Hepatic insult often results from migration of liver flukes (*Fasciola hepatica, Dicrocoelium dendriticum,* or *Cysticercus cellulosae*) or trauma (iatrogenic or spontaneous).
• Disease causes sudden death or fulminant toxemia.
• Clinical signs and pathologic lesions primarily due to toxin(s) produced by organism
• Organism produces at least three exotoxins.
  • Principle toxin, β-toxin, is a phospholipase C with lethal necrotizing (hydrolyzes lecithin and sphingomyelin) and hemolytic (hemolyzes erythrocytes) activity.
  • Tropomyosinase
  • θ-toxin: a lipase
• Toxins induce localized hepatic necrosis, toxemia, and intravascular hemolysis.
• Seasonal disease occurring mostly in summer and fall

• Outbreaks in feedlot cattle fed hay from infected fields
• Disease is spread from contaminated pasture to uninfected area by carrier animals, flooding or natural water drainage, or feeding of contaminated hay or bones of infected animals.

PATHOPHYSIOLOGY
• *Clostridium haemolyticum* is endemic in moist or swampy areas with a high soil pH (~8).
• Organism spores survive in soil and bones from affected animal carcasses for years.
• Once ingested by animal during grazing, spores are transported via lymphatic and blood to liver and tissue where they remain dormant.
• Asymptomatic but infected cattle harbor the organism in their GIT, liver, and tissues and may shed it in feces and urine.
• Any liver insult or damage that results in suitable anaerobic conditions fosters conversion of spores to vegetative organisms and bacterial proliferation.
• Vegetative growth associated with production and release of potent exotoxins, which induce hepatic necrosis, hemolysis, and severe toxemia
• A single ischemic pale hepatic infarct is highly suggestive of the disease.

SIGNALMENT
• Occurs in western United States, along the Gulf of Mexico, Wisconsin, Florida, New Zealand, Australia, Mexico, Venezuela, Chile, Great Britain, Ireland, Middle East
• High incidence in animals grazing irrigated or poorly draining alkaline pastures
• Usually affects mature cattle
• Highly conditioned cattle seem most susceptible.
• Mature sheep affected sporadically
• No sex or breed predilection

SIGNS
• Sudden death with no premonitory signs
• Duration of symptoms usually ranges from 12 hours to 4 days

• Peracute toxemia
  • High fever (103°F –106°F; 39.5°C–41°C)
  • Severe depression
  • Tachycardia
  • Abdominal pain
  • Ileus
  • Hypolactia/agalactia
  • Anorexia
  • Dark feces
  • Dysentery with blood and mucus
  • Arched-back stance
  • Grunting
  • ±Brisket edema
  • Abortion in pregnant cows
  • Recumbency
  • Shock
  • Death within 12 to 48 hours
• Intravascular hemolysis
  • Dyspnea
  • Progressive tachycardia
  • Hemoglobinuria
  • Red stain to perineal wool
  • Progressive anemia
  • Icterus
  • ±Tachypnea
• Immune carriers: animals exposed to subclinical infections

Pathologic Lesions
• Rapid onset of rigor mortis
• Anemic (pale) infarct of liver is virtually pathognomonic.
  • Usually a single infarct but occasionally multiple of varying size
  • Dark-red zone of hyperemia around infarcts
• Red urine in kidney and bladder
• Dehydration
• Icterus
• Anemia
• Subcutaneous gelatinous edema
• Petechial or diffuse subcutaneous hemorrhage
• Bloody fluid in abdominal, pericardial, and thoracic cavities
• Trachea has bloody exudate and mucosal hemorrhages

BACILLARY HEMOGLOBINURIA

- Intestinal tract is hemorrhagic and may contain free or clotted blood.
- ±Subcutaneous edema
- ±Hemorrhages in renal parenchyma

CAUSES AND RISK FACTORS
- Pasturing of cattle in areas where liver flukes reside
- Geographic areas with wet or swampy conditions and high soil pH
- Irrigated pastures
- Hepatic insult(s) in cattle, which creates an appropriate anaerobic environment for germination of spores include migration of liver flukes, liver abscesses, septicemia, metabolic anoxia of liver, hepatotoxins, trauma, biopsy, and high nitrate diets.
- In sheep, telangiectasis, necrobacillosis, and *Cysticercus tenuicollis* are also precipitating factors.
- Unvaccinated cattle, sheep

DIAGNOSIS
- History of grazing cattle in pasture containing liver flukes or of a known insult to the liver
- Gross necropsy lesions
- Identification of large, gram-positive rods on impression smear from liver lesion
- Culturing of *Cl. haemolyticum* from tissue from the edge of liver infarct fresh carcass
- Demonstrate organism in liver by clostridial fluorescent antibody test (FAT) or immunohistochemistry
- Toxin identification
  - Demonstration of only β lecithinase in peritoneal effusion
  - Saline extract of liver infarct
- Definitive diagnosis by culture and GLC confirmation that isolate is *Cl. haemolyticum*
- Complete blood count
  - Evidence of hemolysis in plasma or serum
  - Anemia

- Primarily leukocytosis ± left shift
- May have leukopenia with left shift
- ±Anaerobic blood cultures (acute stage)
- Serum chemistry panel often reflects severe insult to liver and accompanying changes in other organ systems, hydration status, or hypophagia
  - Elevated liver enzymes (SDH, GGT, AST)
  - Hyperbilirubinemia
  - Azotemia
  - Elevated creatine kinase, if recumbent
  - Electrolyte abnormalities
  - Metabolic acidosis

DIFFERENTIAL DIAGNOSIS
- Leptospirosis
- Postparturient hemoglobinuria
- Hemolytic anemia from cruciferous plants
- Enzootic hematuria (bracken fern toxicosis)
- Anaplasmosis
- Chronic copper poisoning
- Black disease
- Acute pyelonephritis
- Hemorrhagic cystitis

CBC/BIOCHEMICAL/URINALYSIS
- Progressive anemia
- Leukocytosis with neutrophilia
- Hemoglobinuria

OTHER LABORATORY TESTING

IMAGING
Hepatic Ultrasound
- Infarct
- Disruption of normal parenchyma
- Vascular changes

DIAGNOSTIC PROCEDURES
- Caution interpreting Gram stains, culture, or FAT of liver
  - *Cl. haemolyticum* is a normal inhabitant of the liver
  - Cross reacts with *Cl. novyi* type B on FAT
- Ultrasound of liver
- Blood culture

TREATMENT
- Seldom successful
- High doses of aqueous potassium or sodium penicillin, intravenously (44,000 IU/kg QID) preferred
- High doses of procaine penicillin IM
- Tetracycline has also been recommended.
- Blood transfusion(s) as indicated; minimum of 4–6 liters for adult cattle
- Antitoxic serum, if available
- Intravenous fluids to maintain normovolemia, and electrolyte and acid-base balance
- Appropriate treatment of secondary organ disease or dysfunction
- If recovery, treat for liver flukes

MEDICATIONS

DRUGS OF CHOICE
- High doses of penicillin or tetracycline
- Blood transfusion
- Antitoxic serum
- Polyionic fluids

CONTRAINDICATIONS
- Monitor for blood transfusion reaction
- Appropriate milk and meat withdrawal times must be followed for all compounds administered to food-producing animals.

FOLLOW-UP

EXPECTED COURSE AND PROGROSIS
- Mortality in untreated animals is 95%.
- Mortality in treated animals is high.
- On endemic farms, death losses may be as high as 25%.

• Heavy mortalities when naïve, unvaccinated cattle brought onto infected pastures
• Recovered animals may become poor doers: chronic weight loss, poor production
• Cattle surviving subclinical attacks of disease may act as immune carriers.

 MISCELLANEOUS

ASSOCIATED CONDITIONS
• Toxemia, hypovolemia, and severe anemia may result in damage to other organs.
• Renal or pulmonary emboli
• Renal infarcts
• Cardiac arrhythmias
• Pigment nephropathy

ZOONOTIC POTENTIAL
N/A

RUMINANT SPECIES AFFECTED
• Cattle
• Adult sheep primarily
• Uncommonly elk, other ruminants

BIOSECURITY
N/A

PRODUCTION MANAGEMENT
• Cattle should not be grazed on liver fluke infested pastures.
• Treat cattle with anthelmintics effective against liver flukes.

• Aquatic snails are intermediate hosts and needed for the flukes to complete their life cycle; use muskicide to remove snails, or fence cattle away from areas with standing water.
• Avoid feeding practices that induce ruminal acidosis or rumenitis to decrease liver abscess formation.
• In United States, vaccination recommended in spring; do not vaccinate within 21 days before slaughter.
• Calf vaccination
  • Commercial bacterin-toxoids *Cl. haemolyticum*
  • Vaccinate calves twice 3– 4 weeks apart at 3–4 months of age
  • Booster annually or every 6 months in endemic areas
  • Deworm sheepdogs to reduce *C. tenuicollis* infection.
• Avoid pasture contamination by removing contaminated feces or properly disposing (burn, deep burial, remove from premises) of decomposing carcasses of affected animals.

SYNONYMS
Icterohemoglobinuria
Infectious icterohemoglobinuria
Red water

SEE ALSO
Acute pyelonephritis
Anaplasmosis
Black disease
Chronic copper poisoning
Enzootic hematuria (bracken fern toxicosis)

Hemolytic anemia from cruciferous plants
Hemorrhagic cystitis
Leptospirosis
Liver flukes
Postparturient hemoglobinuria

ABBREVIATIONS
AST = aspartate transaminase
FAT = fluorescent antibody test
GGT = gamma-glutamyltransferase
GIT = gastrointestinal tract
GLC = gas-liquid chromatography
IM = intramuscular
QID = four times daily
SDH = sorbitol dehydrogenase

Suggested Reading
Dennis, S. 1998. Clostridial diseases. In: *Merck veterinary manual*, ed. S. E. Aiello. 8th ed. Whitehouse Station, NJ: Merck & Co.
Hoyt, J., Snyder, J., Snyder, S. 2002. Bacillary hemoglobinuria. In: *Large animal internal medicine*, ed. B. Smith. St. Louis: Mosby.
Lewis, C. J. 2000. Clostridial diseases. In: *Diseases of sheep*, ed. W. B. Martin, I. D. Aitken. 3rd ed. Oxford: Blackwell Science.
Pugh, D. G. 2002. Diseases of the integumentary system. In: *Sheep and goat medicine*. Philadelphia: W. B. Saunders.
Rebhum, W. C. 1995. Miscellaneous infectious diseases. In: *Diseases of dairy cattle*. Media, PA: Williams and Wilkins.

Authors: Susan Semrad and Sheila McGuirk

BACKGROUNDING BEEF CALVES

BASICS

OVERVIEW
- The term "backgrounding" is used to describe many different systems in which cattle are grown after weaning but before being placed into a feedlot.
- Some people may use backgrounding and preconditioning interchangeably but backgrounding can include much more than just a preconditioning period.
- Backgrounding programs are often called stocker programs in the southern and southwestern United States.
- The ultimate goal of a backgrounding program is to enable calves to gain frame and muscle mass without gaining excessive condition.
- Most backgrounding programs rely on forage-based diets and may take advantage of inexpensive regional feeds such as grain by-products or crop residues.
- Backgrounding programs may provide more flexibility and market opportunity for producers and may give producers a good way to use available forages and/or feeds.
- Numerous backgrounding systems exist, and one system is not appropriate for all producers or all types of cattle.
- Backgrounding programs may be used for home-raised calves, or calves may be purchased from other producers and placed into a backgrounding program. Some producers provide custom backgrounding services for other producers.

Types of Backgrounding Systems: Preconditioning, Wintering, Growing, Grazing Wheat Pasture, Fast-Track Systems, Calf-Fed Finishing Systems
Preconditioning
- Preconditioning is a 30–45-day period occurring immediately after weaning in which calves are weaned, taught to eat dry feed from a bunk, and taught to drink from a water tank.
- Numerous health management practices such as vaccination, dehorning, implants, and castration can occur during this time.
- Efforts should be made to reduce stress as much as possible during this period so it is beneficial to perform the health management factors described above at least a few weeks prior to weaning.

- Preconditioning may be part of a larger backgrounding program or it may occur alone with calves being placed directly in the feedlot after the preconditioning period.
- Gains during this period are usually minimal.
Wintering
- This system focuses on using large quantities of forage (e.g., crop residues, hay, and dormant pastures) to carry calves through the winter.
- Targeted gains range between 0.5 and 1.5 lbs/hd/day.
- The overall goal is to minimize winter-feed cost and keep cattle healthy.
- Calves may be sold in the spring when prices are favorable or grazed through the summer to take advantage of additional cheap gains.
- Smaller framed British or British-cross cattle tend to fit this system well.
  - These cattle tend to have excess finish and light carcass weights if placed directly on feed after weaning.
  - Overwintering coupled with summer grazing allows these cattle to gain adequate frame and muscle prior to finishing so that their finished carcass weights better meet the industry standards.
- Large-framed exotic or exotic-cross cattle do not fit this system well because they become too large and finish with carcass weights that exceed the industry standards.
Growing
- This system targets higher rates of gain (1.5–2.5 lbs/hd/day) over a shorter period of time.
- This system utilizes a mixture of forage and grains and is a good way to utilize forages or grains grown on the farm.
- The cattle best suited to this system include moderate framed exotic and British breed cattle that may become too large in an overwintering system but become too fleshy if grown at a faster rate.
Grazing Wheat Pasture
- This system is the most common backgrounding system in the U. S. southern plains states.
- Calves are placed on wheat pasture around the middle of November and removed around the middle of March if wheat is to be harvested. If the producer elects not to harvest wheat grain, the pasture can be "grazed out" usually until the middle of May.
- The rates of gain and type of cattle are similar to those for other growing systems.

Fast-Track Systems
- These systems involve feeding rations that are quite similar to those fed in a finishing program.
- The goal is to get cattle to gain as fast as possible and gains should be 3 lbs/hd/day or more.
- The fast-track systems are best suited to large-framed exotic or exotic-cross cattle with genetic potential for rapid gains.
- They require a much higher level of management and have an increased risk of digestive problems.
Calf-Fed Finishing Systems
- These systems involve placing calves directly on feed after weaning or after a preconditioning program.
- Calf-fed finishing systems are better suited to commercial feedlots and are best suited for large-framed exotic cattle.
- This production system may get cattle finished earlier and allow the producer to take advantage of seasonal variations in price.

Backgrounding Facilities
Pens
- Pens should be designed to provide adequate space, protection from cold winds, adequate bunk space, adequate water supply, ease of handling, and safety.
- Calves in backgrounding systems generally require 150–300 square feet of space per calf.
- Pens should slope away from the feed bunk and have adequate drainage to reduce mud.
- Concrete aprons should be provided around feed bunks and waterers to reduce mud.
- Properly designed mounds should be included to provide calves a dry place to rest.
- Pen size should be no greater than 150 head per pen.
Feed and Water
- Calves fed once daily should have 18–26 inches of bunk space per calf.
- Calves fed twice daily should have 8–11 inches of bunk space per calf.
- If self-feeders are used, 3–4 inches of trough space per calf is required.
- Bunks should be easy to clean.
- Feeding on the ground should be avoided due to increased wastage and disease transmission.
- Placing waterers along fence lines will help new calves find the water.

Handling Facilities
• Handling facilities should be designed to promote smooth flow of calves through the system.
• Numerous publications are available describing facilities design.

Advantages of Backgrounding
• Calves can be grown to optimum size to increase feeding efficiency and maximize returns.
• Homegrown feed resources can be marketed through backgrounded calves.
• Backgrounding gives producers more flexibility and allows marketing of calves at times when demand and prices may be higher.
• Calves may be healthier and enter the feedlot with less stress when they have been backgrounded.

PATHOPHYSIOLOGY
• Stress is a major contributor to disease in weaning-age calves. Reducing the stress of weaning by performing health management practices prior to weaning should help reduce disease in these calves.
• Stress is also a major contributor to disease in cattle entering a feedlot.
  • Backgrounding programs may reduce the stress of feedlot placement by giving the calves the opportunity to learn to eat from a bunk and drink from a water tank. Getting calves used to eating dry feeds is also a benefit.
  • Properly backgrounded calves should have greater resistance to disease because of proper vaccination during the backgrounding period.
  • Increasing the age and maturity of calves through backgrounding prior to feedlot placement also should increase disease resistance.

SYSTEMS AFFECTED
The respiratory and gastrointestinal systems are most commonly affected by disease in weaned calves and cattle placed in the feedlot; production management

GENETICS
• Calf genetics play a very important role in deciding if and how to background calves.
• Numerous backgrounding systems exist and the system should be carefully matched to the type of cattle in order to take maximum advantage of the system.

INCIDENCE/PREVALENCE
N/A

GEOGRAPHIC DISTRIBUTION
• Most cattle are shipped to the Great Plains states for finishing and slaughter.
• Backgrounding programs may be performed on the farm or ranch of origin or calves may be purchased from several producers and shipped to a backgrounding program.
• Preconditioning calves on the farm or ranch of origin provides the best health benefits because stress and commingling are reduced at the time of weaning.

SIGNALMENT
• The type of cattle best suited for a particular backgrounding program depends on the genetics of the calf.
• See Types of Backgrounding Systems above for a description of the types of cattle best suited to each program.

SIGNS
• Calves should be watched very closely for signs of disease throughout a backgrounding period, especially during the preconditioning and early backgrounding phase.
• The most common diseases affecting calves at this time are respiratory and gastrointestinal diseases.

CAUSES
The causes of disease during the backgrounding period are numerous and most commonly include diseases of the respiratory and gastrointestinal tract.

RISK FACTORS
Stress and commingling with calves from other farms are two of most important risk factors for disease in calves during a backgrounding program.

 DIAGNOSIS

DIFFERENTIAL DIAGNOSIS
N/A

CBC/BIOCHEMISTRY/URINALYSIS
N/A

OTHER LABORATORY TESTS
N/A

IMAGING
N/A

DIAGNOSTIC PROCEDURES
N/A

PATHOLOGIC FINDINGS
Postmortem examinations should be performed on all cattle that die during a backgrounding program in order to make appropriate management decisions about disease prevention and treatment.

 TREATMENT

APPROPRIATE HEALTH CARE
• If possible, management practices such as castration, dehorning, implants, and vaccination should occur prior to weaning.
• If necessary, these practices can be performed during the backgrounding, or preconditioning, period.
• These practices should not be performed at the time of weaning because of the increased stress to the calves. If performed during the preconditioning period, they should be performed after the calves have had some time to recover from the stress of weaning.

NURSING CARE
N/A

ACTIVITY
N/A

DIET
• Much of the advantage of a backgrounding program is gained from feeding forage-based diets to achieve moderate rates of gain.
• Depending on the type of backgrounding system and the type of cattle being fed, the diet will vary from mostly forage to diets that may be similar to those used in a feedlot.
• Adequate nutrition is very important to the success of a backgrounding system.
  • Calves must be provided adequate protein and energy to provide for maintenance needs as well as to provide the desired amount of gain.
  • A balanced mineral supplement should be available at all times because proper trace mineral nutrition is essential for optimum immune system function.
• Calves should have constant access to a clean water source and should be watched closely to make sure they are drinking adequately during the initial phase of the backgrounding period.
• Feeding management

BACKGROUNDING BEEF CALVES

• Calves should be fed long-stemmed grass hay from the bunks for 4–7 days to help get them accustomed to the bunks. Once calves are eating from the bunks, a starter ration can be top dressed over the hay to get calves started on the ration.

• Allowing waterers to run over for a few days will help calves find the waterers. The sound of running water will attract the calves.

• Bunks should be kept clean and any old or moldy feed should be removed.

• See the Suggested Reading list below for more information on feeding management.

CLIENT EDUCATION
N/A

SURGICAL CONSIDERATIONS
N/A

MEDICATIONS

DRUGS OF CHOICE
• Calves should receive respiratory virus and clostridial vaccines prior to weaning or as part of the preconditioning program.

• Several antibiotics are labeled for metaphylactic (mass medication) use and may be beneficial in high-risk calves.

• Treatment protocols should be established to provide adequate and consistent treatment.

CONTRAINDICATIONS
Appropriate milk and meat withdrawal times must be followed for all compounds administered to food producing animals.

MISCELLANEOUS

ASSOCIATED CONDITIONS
N/A

AGE-RELATED FACTORS
• Young calves may be at increased risk of developing disease during the backgrounding period.

• Younger calves may also be less likely to respond to vaccines due to the interference of colostral antibodies.

ZOONOTIC POTENTIAL
N/A

PREGNANCY
• Calves should not be exposed to bulls during the backgrounding period due to the risks associated with pregnancy in feeder heifers.

• Many heifers will reach puberty during the backgrounding period and should not be pastured with intact bulls.

RUMINANT SPECIES AFFECTED
Cattle

BIOSECURITY
• Biosecurity should be considered in order to protect calves from as much disease exposure as possible.

• If calves from other sources are being backgrounded, they should be maintained separately, if possible, to prevent the introduction of disease in the home-raised calves.

PRODUCTION MANAGEMENT
Backgrounding systems should have a production management plan in order to provide and monitor production, nutrition, and disease occurrence.

SYNONYMS
Growing programs
Preconditioning programs
Stocker programs

SEE ALSO
Beef nutrition
Bovine respiratory disease complex

Coccidiosis
Feed bunk management
Vaccination and deworming programs for beef cattle

ABBREVIATIONS
Lbs/hd/day = pounds of gain per head per day

Suggested Reading
Avent, R. K., Ward, C. E., Lalman, D. L. *Economic value of preconditioning feeder calves*. Oklahoma State University Extension Publication F-583. 2003.
Lalman, D., Smith, R. *Effects of preconditioning on health, performance and prices of weaned calves*. Oklahoma State University Extension Publication F3529. 2003.
Lardy, G. 1999, Jan. *Feeding management for backgrounders*. North Dakota State University Extension Publication AS-1158. Available at: http://.ext.nodak.edu/extpubs/ansci/beef/as1158w.htm
Peel, D. S. 2003, July. Beef cattle growing and backgrounding programs. *Veterinary Clinics of North America Food Animal Practice*, pp. 365–85.
Stoltenow, C., Lardy, G. 1999, Jan. *Preconditioning programs: vaccination, nutrition, and management*. North Dakota State University Extension Publication AS-1160. Available at: http://.ext.nodak.edu/extpubs/ansci/beef/as1160w.htm

Authors: John Gilliam and Alfredo DiCostanzo

BASICS

DEFINITION
An acute, subacute, or chronic infection involving one or more of the heart valves or parietal endocardium resulting in variably sized masslike lesions on or near the valves, valvular insufficiency or stenosis, and progression to heart failure.

OVERVIEW
• Most common valvular or endocardial disease in adult cattle but often unrecognized or misdiagnosed
• Vegetative lesions result from hematogenous infection of valvular or mural (parietal) endocardium
• Gram-positive organisms, *Arcanobacterium pyogenes*, α-streptococci, most commonly cultured from blood of affected cattle
• Tricuspid valve most frequently and severely affected in cattle
• Often more than one valve involved
• Initial clinical signs are vague and variable; later signs relate to cardiac insufficiency or septic thromboembolism
• Long-term antimicrobial and supportive therapy required
• General prognosis is guarded to poor for productivity and long-term survival

PATHOPHYSIOLOGY
• Unclear whether bacteria in bloodstream directly adhere to endocardium or valvular surfaces or enter hematogenously through capillaries at base of valve.
• Circulating bacteria enter endocardial surface(s) and initiate infection.
• Local proliferation of bacteria (bacterial colonies grow in laminar fashion).
• Endothelial damage exposes collagen and enhances platelets and fibrin; fibrin is a major component of the vegetative lesion.
• Certain bacteria synthesize polysaccharides (dextrans) and fibronectin, which enhance their ability to adhere to and colonize endothelial surfaces (vascular walls, heart valves) and thrombi.
• Bacteria adhering to valve surface activates coagulation cascade via release of tissue thromboplastin and extrinsic pathway.
• Reseeding of endothelial surface with continued bacteremia.
• Preexisting structural damage to endothelium (valvular or mural) and nonbacterial thrombi may or may not be required to initiate disease.

• Heart failure, right-sided more commonly than left-sided, may subsequently develop.
• In cattle, tricuspid valve is most frequently affected followed by mitral, pulmonary, and aortic valve, and endocardium adjacent to valves.
• Multiple valve involvement reported.
• Bacterial embolism to secondary organs is common.
• Lesions may be small to large enough to occupy most of adjacent heart chamber.
• Three histologic zones in lesions: (1) inner zone composed of fibrous tissue, (2) intermediate zone contains fibrin and bacterial colonies, and (3) superficial zone of fibrin and blood cells.
• Gross necropsy findings: (1) valvular lesions, often vegetative or fibrotic, thickening and distortion of valve leaflet, (2) embolic lesions to other organs, (3) signs of right-sided or congestive heart failure (e.g., hydrothorax, hydroperitoneum, passive congestion of liver, subcutaneous edema).

SIGNALMENT
• Seen worldwide
• Primarily in mature cattle
• More common in adult, small ruminants than in young
• No sex or breed predilection

SIGNS
• Frequently animal has history of temporary remission of clinical signs during antibiotic therapy.
• Clinical signs are often variable and vague.
• Tachycardia is the most consistent finding.
• Decreased appetite
• Weight loss
• Intermittent or constant fever
• Lameness, septic arthritis
• Hypolactia
• Heart murmur noted in ~50% of cattle cases
  • Primarily holosystolic or pansystolic on right side because of propensity for tricuspid valve to be affected
  • Diastolic and continuous also reported
  • Location, timing, and point of maximum intensity of murmur depends on valve(s) affected
  • ±Thrill
• Cardiac arrhythmias in ~10% of affected cattle
• ±Variable intensity of heart sounds
• ±Painful on palpation over heart region
• Less common signs: weakness, diarrhea, abdominal pain, pale mucous membranes

• As disease progresses, signs of heart failure, primarily right-sided, develop
  • Right-sided heart failure: ventral, mandibular, or brisket edema, jugular or mammary vein distention ± vein pulsation, tachycardia, hepatomegaly
  • Left-sided heart failure: tachycardia, tachypnea, dyspnea, coughing, abnormal lung sounds on auscultation
• Occasionally, affected cattle die suddenly without observed clinical signs
• Signs of secondary organ (lung, kidney) involvement (infection, infarction) or embolic disease

CAUSES AND RISK FACTORS
• At least eight bacterial species have been isolated from cattle with bacterial endocarditis.
• *Arcanobacterium (Actinomyces) pyogenes*, α-hemolytic streptococci are most commonly isolated.
• Other common isolates: *Escherichia coli, Micrococcus* spp., *Staphylococcus aureus, Pseudomonas* spp., *Klebsiella pneumoniae, Proteus mirabilis, Clostridium* spp. *Bacterioides* spp., *Fusobacterium necrophorum.*
• Uncommon isolates: *Mycoplasma mycoides, Erysipelothrix rhusipathia, Helcococcus ovis.*
• Predisposing factors include chronic infection, chronic bacteremia, and underlying damage to valvular or endocardial surface.
• Risk factors include ruminal acidosis (acute, subacute, chronic), thrombophlebitis, infection site (mastitis, metritis, septic arthritis, tail infection, pneumonia, omphalophlebitis, abscesses, etc.), traumatic reticulopericarditis, decubital ulcers, traumatic myocarditis, indwelling intravenous catheter, iatrogenic lesions.

DIAGNOSIS

• Based on compatible history and clinical findings (murmur, persistent tachycardia), positive blood cultures, and confirmed by echocardiographic identification of consistent lesions
• History and physical examination
  • Tachycardia
  • ±Cardiac murmur
  • ±Fever
  • ±Obvious sites of infection
• Hyperfibrinogenemia
• Hypergammaglobulinemia due to infectious or inflammatory process

BACTERIAL ENDOCARDITIS

- Aerobic and anaerobic blood cultures and sensitivity
  - Blood sample(s) obtained before antimicrobial therapy is initiated
  - Minimum of 10 ml of blood collected aseptically
  - Two to three cultures drawn 1–2 hours apart from separate venipuncture sites preferred but not often obtained
  - Culture in broth medium
  - Antimicrobial removal device (ARD) used if animal previously received antimicrobial drugs
  - Alternatively, if animal's condition permits, withdraw antimicrobial therapy for 24 to 48 hours before obtaining blood samples for culture
  - Failure to obtain a positive blood culture does not rule out the presence of bacterial endocarditis
- Examination of buffy-coat smears or leukocyte monolayer preparation stained with gram or Giemsa stain
- Echocardiography
  - Visualize and measure size of vegetative lesion on or around heart valve leaflets.
  - Lesions appear as echogenic shaggy, smooth, or cystic masses.
  - Valve thickening with ventricular hyperkinesis.
  - ±Enlargement of chambers on affected side.
  - ±Acoustic reverberation and production of microbubbles.

CBC/BLOOD SERUM CHEMISTRY/URINALYSIS
- Complete blood count
  - ±Nonregenerative anemia
  - Most commonly leukocytosis ± left shift; monocytosis
  - May have normal leukogram or leukopenia with left shift
  - Cattle have less consistent leukocyte response compared to other species
- Serum chemistry panel often reflects accompanying changes in other organ systems, hydration status, or hypophagia
  - Azotemia
  - Elevated GGT
  - Elevated creatine kinase if recumbent
  - Electrolyte abnormalities from anorexia
- Urinalysis if renal infection or infarct suspected

OTHER LABORATORY TESTING
- Electrocardiogram if arrhythmia present
- Transtracheal wash for cytology and microbiologic cultures if signs of pulmonic disease
- Thoracic radiographs of limited value in evaluating cardiac disease in cattle
- Arterial blood gas to evaluate oxygenation status
- Venous blood gas to evaluate metabolic status

IMAGING
- Echocardiogram: vegetative lesion on or near one or more heart valves, most commonly tricuspid valve, ± secondary chamber enlargement (right atrial).
- Negative study does not rule out diagnosis of bacterial endocarditis.

DIAGNOSTIC PROCEDURES
- Thorough history and physical examination
- Blood cultures
- Echocardiogram
  - Adult cattle: sector scanners, 3.5 mHz (or smaller) transducer
  - Young calf or small ruminant: 5.0 mHz
  - May need to scan adult cattle from both sides

DIFFERENTIAL DIAGNOSIS
Bacterial, viral, or protozoal myocarditis
Brisket disease
Cardiac lymphosarcoma or other neoplasm
Congenital cardiac abnormalities
Congestive heart failure
Cor pulmonale
Dilative cardiomyopathy
Endocardiosis
Nutritional myodegeneration
Parasitic endocarditis
Septic pericarditis
Toxic myocardial necrosis (ionophore toxicity, gossypol toxicity, plant toxicosis)

TREATMENT
- Long term and often costly
- Often palliative rather than curative
- Aimed at (1) sterilizing lesion and stopping spread of infection and (2) controlling signs of heart failure

- Ideally, antimicrobial therapy based on sensitivity of bacteria isolated from blood culture or other site of infection
- Parenteral administration of bactericidal antimicrobials required for a minimum of 4 to 6 weeks and often as long as 8 to 12 weeks
- Ideally, initial therapy includes broad spectrum antimicrobials given intravenously (IV) to provide maximum blood levels
- In cattle, penicillin and beta-lactam drugs are frequently first-choice therapy due to high percentage of gram-positive organisms isolated from affected animals
- Early withdrawal of therapy may result in relapse
- Often, extralabel use of antimicrobial is required because few are labeled for long-term therapy
- Anti-inflammatory/antipyretic agents: aspirin, flunixin meglumine
- Anticoagulants to limit enlargement of vegetative lesions and thromboembolic disease; bovine platelets respond poorly to antithrombotic effects of aspirin
- If signs of heart failure are present, diuretics and dietary sodium restriction are added to therapy
- Maintenance of normal blood electrolyte concentrations, acid-base status, and hydration
- Appropriate treatment of secondary organ disease or dysfunction
- Correct hypokalemia (± hypocalcemia) associated with anorexia and diuretic therapy
- Oxygen supplementation if hypoxemic

MEDICATIONS

DRUGS
- Penicillin: 22,000 IU/kg: Aqueous potassium penicillin IV QID or procaine penicillin IM BID
- Amoxicillin: 10 mg/kg IM BID
- Ampicillin: 20 mg/kg IV TID; 10 to 20 mg/kg IM BID
- Rifampin: 5 mg/kg PO BID, as adjunct therapy to enhance antibiotic penetration into lesion
- Anti-inflammatories: flunixin meglumine, aspirin

BACTERIAL ENDOCARDITIS

• Anticoagulants: aspirin, 30 to 100 mg/kg PO every 12 to 24 hours; heparin, 30 U/kg SC every 12 hours (of questionable value)
• Furosemide: 0.5 to 1 mg/kg IV every 12 to 24 hours
• Potassium supplement (50 to 200 g/day PO) if on potassium-wasting diuretics

CONTRAINDICATIONS/POSSIBLE INTERACTIONS

Appropriate milk and meat withdrawal times must be followed for all compounds administered to food producing animals.

 FOLLOW-UP

EXPECTED COURSE AND PROGNOSIS

• Most cases die or are culled due to poor prognosis and expense of therapy.
• One study reported 29% of affected cattle survived until discharge.
• Long-term survival rate and productivity level is not known.
• Prognosis is generally guarded to poor for recovery and productivity.
• Animals diagnosed early and treated aggressively with small or single lesions have a fair to good prognosis.
• Monitoring resolution of disease or lesion.
  • Regression of clinical signs
  • Return of fibrinogen and serum protein concentrations to normal
  • Echocardiogram to measure size of lesion(s)
  • Repeat blood culture 3–4 days after discontinuing antimicrobial therapy
• Reasons for therapeutic failure.
  • Advanced stage of disease at initiation of therapy
  • Premature withdrawal of therapy
  • Ongoing valvular thrombosis due to endothelial damage
  • Bacterial recolonization of valve
  • Change in sensitivity or type of infecting bacteria

 MISCELLANEOUS

ASSOCIATED CONDITIONS

• Cardiac arrhythmias including sinus tachycardia, premature ventricular contractions, and atrial fibrillation
• Septic arthritis
• Passive hepatic congestion
• Congestive heart failure
• Myocardial disease
• Most common sequelae include embolic pneumonia, renal infarction, suppurative arthritis, hepatic emboli
• Less common sequelae: cerebral and adrenal emboli, epididymitis, pleural effusion

ZOONOTIC POTENTIAL

N/A

RUMINANT SPECIES AFFECTED

• Mostly mature cattle
• Goats, sheep

BIOSECURITY

N/A

PRODUCTION MANAGEMENT

• Observe appropriate milk and meat withdrawal times for drugs administered.
• Treatment of unregistered animals with bacterial endocarditis is often not undertaken due to costs.
• Genetically valuable animals often treated to enhance options for genetic salvage procedures (e.g., semen collection, embryo collection, cloning).
• Infection results in decreased milk and meat production.

SEE ALSO

Bacterial, viral, or protozoal myocarditis
Brisket disease
Cardiac lymphosarcoma or other neoplasm
Congenital cardiac abnormalities
Congestive heart failure
Cor pulmonale
Dilative cardiomyopathy
Endocardiosis
Nutritional myodegeneration
Parasitic endocarditis
Septic pericarditis
Toxic myocardial necrosis (ionophore toxicity, gossypol toxicity, plant toxicosis)

ABBREVIATIONS

ARD = antimicrobial removal device
BID = twice daily
IM = intramuscular
IV = intravenous
PO = per os, by mouth
QID = four times daily
SC = subcutaneous
TID = three times daily

Suggested Reading

Diseases of the heart. 1999. In: Radostits, Gay, Blood, Hinchcliff, ed., *Veterinary medicine: a textbook of diseases of cattle, sheep, pigs, goats, and horses*, 9th ed., pp. 387–89. New York: WS Saunders.

Dowling, M. P., Tyler, J. W. 1994. Diagnosis and treatment of bacterial endocarditis in cattle. *JAMA* 204(7):1013–16.

Kasari, T. R., Roussel, A. J. 1989. Bacterial endocarditis: Part I. Pathophysiologic, diagnostic, and therapeutic considerations. *Compendium Continuing Education* 11 (5):259–64.

Reef, V. B., McGuirk, S. 2002. Diseases of the cardiovascular system. In: Smith, B., ed., *Large animal internal medicine*, 3d ed, pp. 454–58. St. Louis: Mosby.

Roussel, A. J., Kasari, T. R. 1989. Bacterial endocarditis in large animals: Part II. Incidence, causes, clinical signs and pathologic findings. *Compendium Continuing Education* 11:769–73.

Tyler, J. W., George, L., Bartram, P. A. 1991. Endocarditis in a cow. *JAMA* 198(8): 1410–12.

Authors: Susan Semrad and Sheila McGuirk

BACTERIAL MENINGITIS

BASICS

DEFINITION
• Meningitis is defined as a bacteria-associated inflammatory process that involves the meninges of the brain and/or spinal cord.
• Disease is most commonly seen in neonates but may also occur in older animals as a result of osteonecrosis induced by thermal cauterization during dehorning, extension of localized infection from skull fractures or coccygeal vertebrae (poor docking hygiene), or secondary to left-sided bacterial endocarditis.

PATHOPHYSIOLOGY
• Bacterial meningitis occurs by direct extension of an infectious agent into the calvarium or by hematogenous spread to the CNS from a distant site.
• The relative lack of bactericidal and opsonic activities in the CNS predisposes animals to meningeal infection.
• The inflammatory response resulting from bacterial invasion of the subarachnoid space is due in large part to the activity of host-derived mediators (cytokines), and it is this inflammatory response that is responsible for the long-term neurological sequelae and death associated with bacterial meningitis.
• Defects of cerebrospinal fluid (CSF) drainage occurring secondary to meningeal inflammation lead to hypertensive hydrocephalus.

SYSTEMS AFFECTED
Nervous system

GENETICS
None reported

INCIDENCE/PREVALENCE
The disease is common in neonatal farm animals. One survey reported a 43% prevalence of septic meningitis in necropsied calves (Green and Smith, 1992).

GEOGRAPHIC DISTRIBUTION
Worldwide occurrence

SIGNALMENT
Neonates of all species, especially calves

SIGNS

HISTORICAL FINDINGS
• There may be a history of prematurity, dystocia, or lack of colostral intake.
• There may be a history of hyperesthesia, stiff neck, depression, seizures, or blindness, with or without a history of another illness, such as enteritis or polyarthritis.
• There may be a history of trauma, recent dehorning, or tail docking, or there may be information relating to the presence of a wound near the calvarium or vertebrae (usually older ruminants), or an infection of the sinuses, middle ear, or inner ear.

PHYSICAL EXAMINATION FINDINGS
Acute meningitis may or may not be accompanied by fever in the neonate.

Depression, anorexia, omphalophlebitis, polyarthritis, and ophthalmitis are frequent concurrent findings.

Neurological Examination Findings
• Ataxia, with or without spasticity and mild tetraparesis, hyperesthesia, neck pain, depression, wandering, star-gazing, and abnormal vocalization, may be seen.
• Lethargy, recumbency, anorexia, loss of suckle reflex, coma, opisthotonus, convulsions, tremors, and hyperesthesia are the most common clinical signs in calves.

CAUSES
• Meningitis most commonly results from hematogenous extension of a preexisting bacterial infection, or results from traumatic penetration of the CNS.
• Failure of passive transfer of maternal antibodies predisposes to hematogenous meningitis.
• The bacteria involved most commonly are those associated with neonatal sepsis.
• Gram-negative bacteria are the predominant cause of infection in large animal neonates although polymicrobial infections also occur.
• *Escherichia coli* is the most common bacterium isolated. Other isolates include *Klebsiella pneumonia*, *Salmonella* spp. (*S. dublin* and *S. typhimurium*), *Staphylococcus* spp., *Streptococcus* spp., and *Bacillus* spp. in calves; *Klebsiella pneumonia*, *Salmonella* spp., *Streptococcus* spp., *Arcanobacterium pyogenes*, *Erysipelothrix rhusiopathiae*, and occasionally *Leptospira interrogans*, *Listeria monocytogenes*, *Mycoplasma* spp., and *Fusobacterium necrophorum* in sheep and goats in North America.

RISK FACTORS
Both maternal and neonatal factors contribute to the development of sepsis in the neonate. They include bacterial placentitis, perinatal stress, prematurity, dystocia, birth asphyxia, unsanitary or adverse environmental conditions, overcrowding, failure of passive transfer of maternal antibodies, contamination of the environment with pathogenic bacteria, and the presence of enteritis, omphalitis, or respiratory infections in the neonate.

DIAGNOSIS

DIFFERENTIAL DIAGNOSIS
• Metabolic disease (e.g., hypoglycemia, hypomagnesemia)
• Cerebral edema
• Hydrocephalus
• Encephalitis (e.g., viral)
• Toxicity

CBC/BIOCHEMISTRY/URINALYSIS
• Leukocytosis with a left shift is common in calves.
• Respiratory acidosis, hypernatremia, hyponatremia, hyperkalemia,

hypomagnesemia, and hypoglycemia may be observed also.

OTHER LABORATORY TESTS
• Low serum immunoglobulin concentrations may be observed.
• In the presence of neurological signs, a positive blood culture supports a diagnosis of bacterial meningitis secondary to neonatal infection. Other samples, such as synovial fluid, also may culture positive.

IMAGING
Radiographs and/or ultrasound may be indicated when trauma or extension of a localized infection is suspected.

DIAGNOSTIC PROCEDURES
Definitive diagnosis is based on the presence of a neutrophilic pleocytosis, xanthochromia, turbidity, high total protein concentration in the CSF, and, ideally, positive culture from the CSF. Although often unrewarding, Gram stain and culture should be attempted.

TREATMENT

APPROPRIATE HEALTH CARE
• Early diagnosis and aggressive treatment are imperative for a successful outcome. By the time clinical signs are present, treatment is often unrewarding.
• Within the herd, minimize perinatal stress, ensure passive transfer of maternal antibodies, and employ proper dehorning technique and hygiene during tail docking.

NURSING CARE
Provision of adequate nutritional support and a clean, comfortable environment; protection from self-inflicted trauma; and maintenance of body temperature, fluid, and acid-base balance are critical for a successful outcome.

ACTIVITY
N/A

DIET
N/A

CLIENT EDUCATION
Treatment may be expensive and mortality rate high despite appropriate therapy.

SURGICAL CONSIDERATIONS
N/A

MEDICATIONS

DRUGS OF CHOICE

Antimicrobials
NOTE: ∗ = Not approved for use in food animals in the United States; ∗∗ = Approved for use in cattle, except lactating cows, in the United States; extralabel dose
• Antimicrobial therapy is the hallmark of treatment.
• Drugs that penetrate the blood-CSF barrier are lipid soluble, nonionized at physiologic

pH, not extensively protein bound, and of low molecular weight. Drugs that satisfy these criteria and that are approved for use in food animals are limited, but include trimethoprim sulfa and sulfonamides (except lactating dairy animals). Inflammation markedly enhances CSF concentrations of penicillins, particularly cephalosporins, which normally penetrate poorly. Other drugs, such as aminoglycosides, do not penetrate CSF even in the presence of inflammation.
• Selection of an antimicrobial drug in ruminants should also be based on the pharmacokinetics and pharmacodynamics of the drug in neonates, the likelihood of antimicrobial resistance, and the potential for violative antimicrobial tissue residues.
• Bacteriocidal drugs are superior to bacteriostatic drugs.
• Where possible, the selection of antimicrobial drugs should be based on either smears stained by Gram stain or culture from infected areas. Treatment should not be delayed, however, until results of sensitivity testing are known. Empiric antimicrobial therapy should include gram-negative and gram-positive spectrum.
• Antibiotics should be administered by intravenous routes in order to attain maximum peak blood and CSF concentrations.
• The efficacy of specific antimicrobial therapy for treatment of meningitis in food animals is unknown because of the lack of CSF pharmacokinetic data in ruminants. Specific antimicrobial therapy could include, but is not limited to trimethoprim sulfa (30 mg/kg, IV, q 12 h)*; cefazolin (20 mg/kg, IV, q 6 h)*; florfenicol (20 mg/kg, IV, q 12 h)**.
• Relapses may occur as meningeal inflammation subsides and CNS concentrations of (nonlipophilic) antimicrobial drug(s) fall.
• Antimicrobial drug therapy should continue for at least 7 days after resolution of all clinical signs.

Anticonvulsants
The following drug doses have been extrapolated from recommended doses for equine neonates.
• Diazepam (5–10 mg/45 kg, slowly IV, repeated if necessary) is used for short-term control.
• If two to three doses of diazepam fail to control convulsions, a loading dose of phenobarbital (10–20 mg/kg diluted in 30 ml saline, IV over 15 minutes) should be given. Oral therapy (5–10 mg/kg, q 8 h to q 12 h) is then used for maintenance for long-term control.
• Pentobarbital (2–4 mg/kg, IV, slowly) has been advocated, but depth of anesthesia must be monitored to prevent respiratory arrest.

Other Treatments
• Consider DMSO (1 gm/kg, IV as a 10% solution in 5% dextrose or saline), corticosteroids (dexamethasone at 0.15 mg/kg

15–20 minutes before the first dose of antibiotic, then every 6 hours for 4 days), or a combination of both if progression is rapid.
• Following rehydration, nonsteroidal anti-inflammatory drugs may be beneficial (flunixin meglumine, 0.5–1.0 mg/kg, IV, q 12 h to q 24 h; ketoprofen, 2.2 mg/kg, IV, q 24 h; or aspirin, 100 mg/kg, PO, q 24 h in neonates)
• A plasma transfusion may be required.
• Additional therapy may be required to resolve secondary complications (i.e., antiulcer medications, ophthalmic drugs, etc.).

CONTRAINDICATIONS
• Acepromazine should not be used as a sedative due to its ability to lower the seizure threshold.
• Drug withdrawal times must be determined for all drugs used to treat food-producing animals.

PRECAUTIONS
Care should be exercised when dosing anticonvulsant drugs in neonates because of the increased permeability of their blood brain barrier.

POSSIBLE INTERACTIONS
N/A

ALTERNATIVE DRUGS
N/A

 FOLLOW-UP

PATIENT MONITORING
Close monitoring of vital parameters and metabolic indices is warranted during antimicrobial therapy, especially in animals showing seizure activity.

PREVENTION/AVOIDANCE
• The key to prevention of meningitis in neonates is paying attention to the events leading up to and including parturition, and ensuring adequate colostral intake.
• Proper dehorning technique and hygiene during tail docking will decrease the incidence of meningitis in older animals.

POSSIBLE COMPLICATIONS
N/A

EXPECTED COURSE AND PROGNOSIS
Prognosis in neonatal ruminants with septic meningitis is poor, despite treatment. The key to a successful outcome relies on early recognition of CNS involvement and institution of aggressive, appropriate therapy.

 MISCELLANEOUS

ASSOCIATED CONDITIONS
Generalized sepsis typically accompanies septic meningitis in neonates.

AGE-RELATED FACTORS
Neonates are most commonly affected.

ZOONOTIC POTENTIAL
N/A

PREGNANCY
Diseases affecting the dam during gestation may predispose the neonate to partial or complete failure of passive transfer after birth.

RUMINANT SPECIES AFFECTED
All species are susceptible.

BIOSECURITY
N/A

PRODUCTION MANAGEMENT
• Measures taken that reduce perinatal stress will reduce the incidence of septic meningitis in the neonate.
• Proper dehorning technique and hygiene during tail docking will reduce the incidence of septic meningitis in older animals.

SYNONYMS
• Meningoencephalitis
• Meningomyeloencephalitis
• Suppurative meningitis

SEE ALSO
Neonatal sepsis

ABBREVIATIONS
CNS = central nervous system
CSF = cerebrospinal fluid
DMSO = dimethyl sulfoxide
IV = intravenous
PO = per os, by mouth
q = for

Suggested Reading
Aldridge, B. M., Garry, F. B., Adams, R. 1993. Neonatal septicemia in calves: 25 cases (1985–1990). *J Amer Vet Med Assoc.* 203:1324–29.
Cebra, C., Cebra, M. 2002. Diseases of the hematologic, immunologic, and lymphatic systems (multisystem diseases). In: *Sheep and goat medicine*, ed. D. G. Pugh. Philadelphia: W. B. Saunders.
Fecteau, G and George, L. 2004. Bacterial meningitis and encephalitis in ruminants. *Veterinary Clinics of North America: Food Animal Practice.* 20(2):363–77.
Fecteau, G., Van Metre, D. C., Paré, J., Smith, B. P., Higgins, R., Holmberg, C. A., Jang, S., Guterbock, W. 1997. Bacteriological culture of blood from critically ill neonatal calves. *Can Vet J.* 38:95–100.
Green, S. L., Smith, L. L. 1992. Meningitis in neonatal calves: 32 cases (1983–1990). *J Am Vet Med Assoc.* 201:125–28.
Prescott, J. F. 2000. Infections of the nervous system: meningitis and encephalitis. In: *Antimicrobial therapy in veterinary medicine*, ed. J. G. Prescott, J. D. Baggot, R. D. Walker. 3rd ed. Ames: Iowa State University Press.

Author: Maureen E. G. Wichtel

BEEF BULL MANAGEMENT

 BASICS

OVERVIEW

• It is well known that the reproductive program in each herd has a major influence on productivity and is directly linked to profitability.

• Good reproductive performance requires diligent management of many important and interrelated factors.

• The performance of herd bulls during natural service is dependent upon not only their health and proper management but also the health of the females they will be breeding.

• To be successful, programs should start with good planning and genetic selection considerations for the important traits necessary for each herd and continue through the implementation stages of the breeding season.

• At the end of the production cycle, success is measured by overall reproductive efficiency and the performance of the offspring.

SYSTEMS AFFECTED

Male reproductive, production management, nutrition

GENETICS

N/A

INCIDENCE/PREVALENCE

N/A

GEOGRAPHIC DISTRIBUTION

Worldwide distribution

SIGNALMENT

Species

Beef cattle

Breed Predilections

All breeds

BULL MANAGEMENT PROGRAMS

• Bull management programs begin with the purchase of new herd sire prospects.

• The genetic direction of the herd is of obvious importance.

• In addition to inherent genetic traits, bulls must be healthy, fertile, and capable of expressing the desirable traits.

• Bulls should be purchased from seed-stock breeders that have documented herd health programs that minimize the likelihood of infectious diseases.

• The bulls should be immunized against common diseases and, if necessary, treated for parasites or tested for diseases indicated from a biosecurity standpoint.

• All bulls should undergo a complete breeding soundness evaluation (BSE) performed by a competent veterinarian to assess their general physical and reproductive soundness. This includes newly purchased bulls and a yearly reexamination of herd bulls.

• In addition to the general physical examination, it is important to collect semen and evaluate the sample for spermatozoal motility and morphology.

• Bulls should meet the minimum standards established by the Society for Theriogenology (BIF).

• Each component of the BSE such as scrotal circumference (SC) should be accurately measured and utilized within the context of age, weight, nutritional status, and contemporary group.

• SC is a good indicator trait for age at puberty in offspring; it is highly correlated with daily sperm production and is mildly correlated with the percentage of normal spermatozoa.

• Body condition, structural correctness of feet and legs, and general soundness are also important factors for new sire prospects.

BULL TO FEMALE RATIO

The number of bulls required to adequately cover a given number of breeding females is related to a variety of factors. An arbitrary classification of some considerations follows:

Factors Influencing Bull to Female Ratio (BFR)

• Pasture or range conditions and cattle distribution
    1. Terrain
    2. Water availability and location(s)
    3. Carrying capacity
    4. Pasture adaptation
    5. Pasture size

• Individual bull variation
    1. Age
    2. Condition
    3. Fertility
    4. Mating ability
    5. Social behavior
    6. Injury

• Operation and management
    1. Length of breeding season
    2. Animal breeding and selection

    3. Reproductive disease
    4. Nutrition and body condition
    5. Management observation

• Defining the optimum BFR is difficult because certain factors influencing each set of circumstances are unpredictable.

• The expected number of estral females available to the bull(s) on any given day is an important point that must be considered.

• Anecdotal reports indicate that smaller breeding pastures with fewer animals are more efficient and provide more uniform distribution of bulls and females. This obviously limits the total number of females exposed to dominant bulls when compared to large multisire pastures where females congregate in a sexually active group. This is a group of estral females that band together from preestrus through standing estrus.

• The bull(s) join this group and are constantly moving throughout the pasture. This is of most concern in very large groups of females because the bulls tend to run together.

• It is possible for single bulls to cover 60 breeding females in limited breeding seasons and produce comparable reproductive rates to a much lower BFR.

• Generally, BFRs of 1:25 or 1:30 for mature bulls and BFRs of 1:15 or 1:20 for yearling bulls have been utilized for range areas with minimal observation and little breeding season management.

• This may be an important area of management consideration if optimizing efficiency and reducing expenditures is desirable.

Other Considerations

• The time each cow settles in relation to the start of the breeding season influences the weaning weight of her offspring and the ability to select replacement heifers with adequate age in a yearly production cycle.

• In limited breeding seasons, efficient management requires early conception and higher overall pregnancy rates.

• It is important to identify and optimize the use of bulls with preferred genetic traits, especially as producers move toward value-based marketing through vertically coordinated programs.

• The use of frequent observation of breeding pastures and immediate detection and correction of problems is important.

Molecular Evaluation
- More recent technology utilizing a commercially available set of DNA microsatellite markers to identify each sire's progeny from multisire breeding pastures has been developed.
- Proteomics shows promise in terms of accurately identifying progeny. As new technology advances, it may reach an economic level that could permit its use in commercial herds.
- The identification of progeny in multisire breeding pastures will permit an accurate genetic evaluation system for a greater number of young sires.
- This potential could rapidly revolutionize bull selection programs and permit the ability to select and optimize the use of bulls with superior reproductive and genetic traits.

SELECTION GUIDELINES
- Select superior bulls from a genetic standpoint.
- Carefully screen the health of all new bulls.
- Conduct a breeding soundness evaluation on all bulls and select bulls that are above average in scrotal circumference, motility, and percent normal sperm morphology.
- Conduct breeding soundness evaluations on bulls yearly, preferably just before breeding season begins.
- Develop a method to identify some progeny of each sire.
- Observe mating ability of bulls during breeding at the start and several times during the breeding season.
- Utilize knowledge of social behavior, terrain, calving pattern, bull performance, and other factors to determine the number of bulls, bull to female ratio, and grouping of bulls.

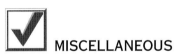 **MISCELLANEOUS**

ASSOCIATED CONDITIONS
Lameness, infertility, nutritional deficiencies

AGE-RELATED FACTORS
N/A

ZOONOTIC POTENTIAL
N/A

PREGNANCY
- It is possible for single bulls to cover 60 breeding females in limited breeding seasons and produce comparable reproductive rates to a much lower BFR.
- Generally, BFRs of 1:25 or 1:30 for mature bulls and BFRs of 1:15 or 1:20 for yearling bulls have been utilized for range areas with minimal observation and little breeding season management. This may be an important area of management consideration if optimizing efficiency and reducing expenditures are desirable.
- The time each cow settles in relation to the start of the breeding season influences the weaning weight of her offspring and the ability to select replacement heifers with adequate age in a yearly production cycle.
- Therefore, in limited breeding seasons, efficient management requires early conception and higher overall pregnancy rates.

RUMINANT SPECIES AFFECTED
Beef bulls

BIOSECURITY
N/A

PRODUCTION MANAGEMENT
- The performance of herd bulls during natural service is dependent not only upon their health and proper management but also upon the health of the females they will be breeding.
- To be successful, programs should start with good planning and genetic selection considerations for the important traits necessary for each herd and continue through the implementation stages of the breeding season.

SYNONYMS
N/A

SEE ALSO
Animal identification
Beef bull behavior
Beef cattle nutrition
Body condition scoring
Record keeping
Reproductive disease chapters
Semen evaluation

ABBREVIATIONS
BFR = bull to female ratio
BSE = breeding soundness evaluation
DNA = deoxyribonucleic acid
SC = scrotal circumference

Suggested Reading
Blockey, M. A. deB. 1989. Relationship between serving capacity of beef bulls as predicted by the yeard test and their fertility during paddock mating. *Australian Vet J.* 66(11): 348–51.
Chenoweth, P. J. 2000. Rationale for using bull breeding soundness evaluations. *Comp Cont Ed, Food Anim Suppl.* 22(2): s48–s55.
Lunstra, D. D., Laster, D. B. 1982. Influence of single-sire and multiple-sire natural mating on pregnancy rate of beef heifers. *Theriogenology* 18(4): 373–80.
McGrann, J. M., Leachman, L. 1995, Jul. Seedstock beef cattle: SPA. *Vet Clin North Am Food Anim Pract.* 11(2): 375–88.
Rupp, G. P., Ball, L., Shoop, M. C., Chenoweth, P. J. 1977. Reproductive efficiency of bulls in natural service: Effects of male to female ratio and single- vs multiple-sire breeding groups. *JAVMA* 171(7): 639–42.
Sanderson, M. W., Gay, J. M. 1996, Feb 15. Veterinary involvement in management practices of beef cow-calf producers. *J Am Vet Med Assoc.* 208(4): 488–91.
Wiltbank, J. N., Parish, N. R. 1986. Pregnancy rate in cows and heifers bred to bulls selected for semen quality. *Theriogenology* 30:779–83.

Author: Gary P. Rupp

BERSERK MALE SYNDROME/ABERRANT BEHAVIOR SYNDROME

 BASICS

OVERVIEW

- Berserk syndrome or berserk male syndrome (BMS), aberrant behavior syndrome (ABS)
- As with any behavioral difficulty, there is a wide range in the severity of syndrome expression.
- A berserk male is a male camelid who has been improperly imprinted on humans, is extremely aggressive, and is very territorial. The extreme case is possibly incurable. However, most ABS camelids are not this severe and a more favorable prognosis is accorded.
- Territorial males typically direct their aggression toward other male llamas and their aggressiveness is misdirected at humans. In a domestic camelid, this syndrome is unacceptable for caretaker safety.
- Symptoms that indicate a camelid is at significant risk for developing ABS generally begin between 12 and 18 months of age; severe ABS begins between 2 and 3 years of age.
- Behavioral signs include: screaming, excessive spitting, attacking humans and other animals, charging, biting, butting, and lying on people.
- BMS/ABS is the result of a male llama being abnormally socialized to people at an early age. Common causes include bottle feeding, excessive handling, limited discipline of poor behaviors, removal from mother/peers, and isolation from the rest of the herd.

- Male crias are imprinted upon people and essentially see them as another llama in the herd.
- ABS crias communicate with people through behaviors like spitting, chest butting, and wrestling.
- Territoriality of males increases over time.

SYSTEMS AFFECTED
Behavioral

GENETICS
N/A

INCIDENCE/PREVALENCE
N/A

GEOGRAPHIC DISTRIBUTION
Worldwide in camelids

SIGNALMENT

Species
Camelids

Breed Predilections
N/A

Mean Age and Range
Symptoms that indicate a camelid is at significant risk for developing ABS generally begin between 12 and 18 months of age; severe ABS begins between 2 and 3 years of age.

Predominant Sex
Males

SIGNS

Clinical Signs
ABS camelids may have the following history:
- Bottle or tube fed/supplemented
- Separated from mother, generally early in life

- Separated from other camelid peers
- Early veterinary treatment, sometimes extensive
- Handled by numerous inexperienced people with the exclusion of camelid peers

Behavioral Signs
- Does not respond to training
- ABS camelids are usually under 4 years old.
- Regularly follow people within a 2-foot distance.
- Orgle at humans
- Quite human aggressive
- Drop to a U-neck position near humans
- Flip tail over back into an aggressive positioning
- Aggressively pursue people and run up to people on sight

 TREATMENT

- Castration is mandatory. Early castration is preferred. Castration generally helps and may in fact alleviate the syndrome in some cases. Once the syndrome is diagnosed, castration should be accomplished.
- Postcastration, remove the camelid completely from his territory. He should be moved into an established pasture of an aggressive older male. This should be done as soon as possible postsurgery. The new pasture should be out of the visual territory of the previous pasture. The animal should be maintained in this mixed pasture for several months prior to a training program.

BERSERK MALE SYNDROME/ABERRANT BEHAVIOR SYNDROME

• Training program with a qualified camelid trainer/behaviorist is necessary if a poor postsurgical/mature peer response occurs.
• In severe cases, euthanasia is indicated.

 FOLLOW-UP

PREVENTION/AVOIDANCE
• Raise young males with one or more assertive adult males/geldings. These animals will teach the young crias needed socialization and "manners."
• Young intact males should be raised within the territory of an established male.
• Pushiness or aggressiveness should be firmly/positively corrected early on.
• Begin behavior training at an early age.
• Regular brushing/grooming while haltered allows socialization to humans.
• Do not allow crias to invade personal human space (2-foot distance rule).
• Halter training can begin around 2 months of age and is done slowly allowing camelid acceptance. All training should be directed toward eliminating cria aggression.
• Early camelid training must establish you as the alpha leader and the cria should learn to follow instructions.
• Do not allow attention at people's feet by crias.

Genetic Selection
• Don't breed from aggressive camelid stock; select less-aggressive dams and sires.
• Select against territorial instincts.
• Select away from guarding instincts, if possible.
• Keeping geldings away from females early on. Mixing can encourage possessive behavior and territoriality in ABS crias.
• Do not breed males before 4–5 years of age.
• Castrate all young males that show excessive fear, aggression, or territoriality or challenge adult animals/humans.

 MISCELLANEOUS

ASSOCIATED CONDITIONS
N/A

AGE-RELATED FACTORS
Camelids are at significant risk for developing ABS symptoms generally between 12 and 18 months of age; severe ABS begins between 2 and 3 years of age.

ZOONOTIC POTENTIAL
N/A

PREGNANCY
N/A

RUMINANT SPECIES AFFECTED
Camelids

BIOSECURITY
N/A

PRODUCTION MANAGEMENT
See above

SYNONYMS
Berserk male syndrome or aberrant behavior syndrome

SEE ALSO
Body condition scoring
Camelid nutrition
Euthanasia and disposal
Tooth root abscess

ABBREVIATIONS
ABS = aberrant behavior syndrome
BMS = berserk male syndrome

Suggested Reading
Ebel, S. 1989, Mar. The llama industry in the United States. *Vet Clin North Am Food Anim Pract.* 5(1):1–20.
Fowler, M. 1989, Mar. Llama medicine. Physical examination, restraint and handling. *Vet Clin North Am Food Anim Pract.* 5(1):27–35.
Fowler, M. E. 1996, Mar. Husbandry and diseases of camelids. *Rev Sci Tech.* 15(1):155–69.
McGee, M. 1994, Jul. Llama handling and training. *Vet Clin North Am Food Anim Pract.* 10(2):421–34.

Author: Scott R. R. Haskell

BESNOITIOSIS

 BASICS

DEFINITION
• Infection with a coccidian protozoa of genus *Besnoitia,* family Sarcocystidae, which primarily affects the skin, subcutis, blood vessels, mucous membranes, and tissues of cattle, horses, goats, and other herbivores
• Organism is closely related to genus *Toxoplasma.*

OVERVIEW
• Chronic debilitating disease primarily of cattle, goats, and rarely horses
• Affects antelope, blue duiker, and blue wildebeest in Africa, caribou in Canada, and wildlife in Australia
• Endemic disease in some tropical and subtropical areas, sporadic elsewhere
• High morbidity, significant economic loss, and low mortality in endemic areas
• Reported in cattle in southwest Europe (France, Portugal), Africa, South America (Venezuela), Israel, Kazakhstan, South Korea, Asia, and Soviet Union
• Reported in goats in Iran, New Zealand, Africa
• Reported sporadically in horses in Africa, southern Europe, Mexico, and in two imported burros in the United States
• Not reported in cattle in North America
• Reported in North America in wildlife including opossum, caribou, reindeer, and mule deer; other wildlife that prey upon definitive host (i.e., cats) may also be affected.
• Three of the seven classified species occur in domestic livestock and four in wildlife.
• Life cycle involves a definitive host and an intermediate host.
• *Besnoitia* are host specific for intermediate hosts.
  • *Besnoitia besnoiti* in cattle
  • *B. bennetti* infects horses, donkeys, mules
  • *B. caprae* in goats (not sheep)
  • *B. tarandi* in reindeer, mule deer, and caribou
  • *B. jellisoni* and *B. wallacei* infect rodents
  • *B. darlingi* from lizards, opossums, and snakes
  • *B. sauriana* in lizards
• Cats are the definitive host for some *Besnoitia* spp. infecting wildlife; sexual reproduction occurs in the intestines of the definitive host.
• Transmission to wildlife may be fecal-oral route by ingestion of oocysts (contaminated feeds or water) shed in cat (final host) feces.

• Definitive host and mechanism of transmission for species affecting domestic livestock is unknown.
• Mechanical transmission via biting insects/flies (tabanids, tsetse, ticks) possible in cattle and goat; ingestion of feedstuffs or water contaminated with cat feces
• Transmission via semen suspected.
• Experimentally, can transmit some *Besnoitia* spp. by needle inoculation of cyst-containing tissues into suitable host.
• Organism localizes in thick-walled cyst(s) in the skin, blood vessels, mucous membranes of upper respiratory tract and subcutaneous and other tissues.
• Anasarca gives way to sclerodermatitis with loss of hair and epidermis and development of severe dermatitis.
• Condition may become generalized and disseminated

PATHOPHYSIOLOGY
• Upon entrance into a susceptible intermediate host, sporulated oocysts release sporozoites that produce tachyzoites via endodyogeny.
• Parasitemia is associated with tachyzoites (endozoites) replicating in the host's macrophages, fibroblasts, and endothelial cells.
• Tachyzoites are released from endothelial cells and reinvade other endothelial cells causing vasculitis, increased permeability, anasarca, and thrombosis in capillaries and small veins of the dermis, subcutis, and testes (known as anasarca stage).
• Tachyzoites migrate into connective tissues and initiate cyst formation within endothelium and fibroblasts. They mature here to form bradyzoite cysts (cystozoites).
• Cellular destruction and release of inflammatory mediators during replication of organisms in endothelial, histiocytic, and other cells result in clinical signs and formation of large thick-walled cysts filled with bradyzoites.
• Connective tissue reaction around the cysts produces a thickening of the skin and resulting circulation disturbances, alopecia, and necrosis (scleroderma stage).
• Cysts are most commonly within the dermis, subcutaneous connective tissues, conjunctiva, sclera, scrotum, and mesentery.
• Location of cyst formation and size help determine which clinical signs predominate in any given case.

SIGNALMENT
No age, sex, or breed predilection

SIGNS
• Many affected animals are asymptomatic except for cysts in scleral conjunctiva.
• Cattle commonly have two stages of the disease: an acute stage associated with endozoite proliferation and a chronic stage with scleroderma and cyst formation.
• Incubation period in cattle is 6 to 10 days.

Cattle: Signs Seen During Acute Phase
• Fever
• Warm, painful ventral swellings and reluctance to move
• Anasarca (generalized edema of skin)
• Tachypnea
• Tachycardia
• Hypophagia
• Swollen lymph nodes
• Nasal discharge (rhinitis)
• Lacrimation
• ±Diarrhea
• Loss of condition
• Hypolactia
• Photophobia
• ±Orchitis
• ±Abortion
• Small whitish to clear pinpoint nodules on scleral conjunctiva and nasal, pharyngeal, and laryngeal mucosa

Cattle: Signs Seen During Chronic Phase
• Skin lesions progress to severe dermatitis over most of body
• Sclerodermatitis
• Infected cysts in the skin and subcutaneous tissue
• Subcutaneous lumps
• Variable alopecia
• Hyperpigmentation
• Skin thickens, wrinkles, and cracks
• Thickened folds of skin around neck, shoulders, rump
• Inspiratory dyspnea
• Secondary bacterial infection or myiasis of skin
• Bulls frequently become sterile: scrotal skin affected, and orchitis, epididymitis, periorchitis, vascular lesions in testes
• Teat lesions
• Mouth lesions in suckling calves
• Loss of hair, especially on face and lower legs in wildlife

Other Lesions That May Be Seen with Generalization of Disease
• ±Focal or disseminated myositis, keratitis, periostitis, endostitis, lymphadenitis, pneumonia, arteritis, perineuritis
• Severe weight loss

In Goats
- Rarely see acute stage
- Animals present in chronic stage with dermatitis and respiratory dyspnea
- Thickening, lichenification, alopecia, fissures, and oozing serum of legs (carpus/tarsus) and ventral abdomen
- Lesions severe on scrotum and fetlocks
- ± Subcutaneous papules over hindquarters

Postmortem Lesions
- Parasitic cysts in dermis, subcutaneous and other fascia
- Pharyngitis, laryngitis, tracheitis
- Cysts present in scrotum and testes of males
- Sandlike granules and cysts in nostrils and turbinates
- Sandlike granules in vascular endothelium
- Widespread vascular lesions
- Dermatitis
- Secondary lesions in skeletal and heart muscle, and lungs
- Histology: parasite evident in cystic lesions

CAUSES AND RISK FACTORS
- Endemic area
- Disease outbreaks in cattle and goats occur during fly/insect season
- Contamination of feedstuffs with cat feces
- High feral cat population

DIAGNOSIS
- Diagnosis is based upon history and geographical area.
- Appearance of cyst in scleral conjunctivas or nasal mucosa
- Identification of crescent-shaped bradyzoites surrounded by a collagen capsule in skin or scleral conjunctival scrapings or skin biopsy
- Ear-tip biopsy commonly used in goats
- Affected animals are often asymptomatic.

DIFFERENTIAL DIAGNOSIS
- Lumpy skin disease
- Sweating sickness
- Ectoparasites: ticks, fungi, mites

CBC/BIOCHEMISTRY/URINALYSIS
- No characteristic changes
- ±Hyperproteinemia, hypergammaglobulinemia

OTHER LABORATORY TESTS
- Serum antibodies by indirect immunofluorescence or ELISA
- Tests have only moderate sensitivity

IMAGING
N/A

DIAGNOSTIC PROCEDURES
- Scleral conjunctival or skin scrapings
- Skin biopsy

TREATMENT
- Isolate affected animals.
- No specific treatment; treat symptomatically.
- Supportive therapy; dermatitis, enteritis, fever.
- Reported clinical cure in donkey after prolonged administration of trimethoprim-sulfamethoxazole.
- Reportedly in rabbits, antimony and sulfanilamide complex prevented cyst formation.
- Oxytetracycline may have some value if given early in the course of the disease.

MEDICATIONS
N/A

DRUGS OF CHOICE
N/A

CONTRAINDICATIONS
Appropriate milk and meat withdrawal times must be followed for all compounds administered to food-producing animals.

FOLLOW-UP
- Case fatality about 10%
- Long convalescence period (many months)
- Sterility and infertility may be transient or permanent

MISCELLANEOUS

PREVENTION
- Reduce exposure to biting insects and ticks.
- Avoid exposure of wildlife to feces of infected cats.
- Avoid feed contamination with cat feces.
- Control feral cat population.
- Vaccine produced using *B. besnoiti* isolated from wildebeest and grown on tissue culture is effective.
  - Durable immunity in all vaccinates
  - Subclinical infection occurred at low level.

ASSOCIATED CONDITIONS
- Secondary bacterial or myiasis
- ±Focal or disseminated myositis, keratitis, periostitis, endostitis, lymphadenitis, pneumonia, arteritis, perineuritis

ZOONOTIC POTENTIAL
N/A

RUMINANT SPECIES AFFECTED
- Cattle
- Goat
- Wild ruminants: antelope, wildebeest

BIOSECURITY
N/A

PRODUCTION MANAGEMENT
- Affected animals remain carriers for life.
- Chronic cystic stage results in severe production loss.
- Economic losses in endemic areas due to mortality (<10%), sterility (temporary or permanent), loss of condition, and lower market value, and damage to hide.
- Carcasses approved if localized lesions only, no systemic involvement
- Carcass condemned if disseminated lesions with emaciation

SYNONYMS
"Dimple" in goats
Globidiosis

SEE ALSO
Ectoparasites: ticks, fungi, mites
Lumpy skin disease
Sweating sickness

ABBREVIATIONS
ELISA = enzyme-linked immunosorbent assay

Suggested Reading

Besnoitiosis. 1998. In: *The Merck veterinary manual*, eds. S. E. Aiello, A. May, 8th ed. Whitehouse Station, NJ: Merck & Co., Inc.

Diseases caused by protozoa. 1999. In: *Veterinary medicine: a textbook of diseases of cattle, sheep, pigs, goats, and horses*, ed. O. M. Radostits *et al.*, 9th ed. London: W. B. Saunders.

Lloyd, J. E. 1999. Dermatologic diseases. In: *Current veterinary therapy 4, food animal practice*, eds. J. L. Howard, R. A. Smith. Philadelphia: W. B. Saunders.

Parasitic diseases. *Manual on meat inspection for developing countries.* http://www.fao.org/docrep/003/t0756e/T0756E04.htm; accessed August 25, 2007.

Smith, M. C., Sherman, D. M. 1994. Skin. In: *Goat medicine*. Philadelphia: Lea & Febiger.

Authors: Susan Semrad and Karen A. Moriello

BLACK LOCUST TOXICITY

 BASICS

OVERVIEW
• There are two lectins present in the bark of the *Robinia pseudoacacia* (black locust) tree. They are the major lectin RPbAI and the minor lectin RPbAII. The seeds and leaves are also toxic.
• Plants from this family are in the same family as the *Abrus precatorius* (rosary pea) and the *Ricinus communis* (castor bean), as well as the *Phoradendron* (mistletoe) and *Phytolacca americana* (pokeweed).
• The lectins act as hemagglutinins and bind to mucous membranes, where they impair nutrient absorption and inactivate rRNA—particularly within the crypt epithelium. Also, due to the inhibition of protein synthesis, they impair the immune system and put the animal at risk for secondary bacterial infection.

GEOGRAPHIC DISTRIBUTION
These trees are typically found in the woods of the eastern United States but are also used as landscape trees throughout the United States.

SIGNALMENT
• Toxicity from the black locust is more prevalent in the summer and fall, when there is less forage available to grazing animals.
• Any ruminant on pasture can be potentially exposed to this toxin.

SIGNS
• Clinical signs can be acute or chronic and can consist of inappetance, bloody diarrhea, and salivation. Weakness and incoordination can be present due to posterior paralysis. There can be dyspnea, dehydration, laminitis, and recumbency. A weak pulse may be present due to systemic shock.
• Death is infrequent.

CAUSES AND RISK FACTORS
The major risk factor is animals grazing on sparse pasture in the late summer and fall.

 DIAGNOSIS

DIFFERENTIAL DIAGNOSIS
Vomitoxin from moldy concentrates or arsenic toxicity as well as other causes of gastroenteritis

CBC/BIOCHEMISTRY/URINALYSIS
There will be increased hepatic enzymes—AST, ALT, LDH, GOT, and GGT. There can be increased BUN and creatinine. Decreased serum total protein, specifically albumin, can be present. There can be hemoconcentration (increased PCV and TP) due to the dehydration.

OTHER LABORATORY TESTS
RBC agglutination, precipitin test

IMAGING
N/A

DIAGNOSTIC PROCEDURES
Presence of black locust seeds or plant materials in the forage or rumen contents upon necropsy is most diagnostic.

PATHOLOGIC FINDINGS

GROSS FINDINGS
• Postmortem lesions are generally restricted to the GI tract.
• There can be fatty hepatic change and erosions of abomasal and intestinal epithelium.
• There can be pulmonary hemorrhage, edema, and emphysema.

HISTOPATHOLOGICAL FINDINGS
• You may find central lobular hepatic necrosis, lymphoid necrosis, and crypt cell epithelial necrosis.
• Histopathological evidence of pulmonary hemorrhage, edema, and emphysema may be evident.
• There may be necrosis of the renal convoluted tubules.

 TREATMENT

Treatment consists of antiserum for ricinus toxicity, sedatives for convulsions, arecoline hydrobromide and saline cathartics.

MEDICATIONS
N/A

CONTRAINDICATIONS
Appropriate milk and meat withdrawal times must be followed for all compounds administered to food-producing animals.

FOLLOW-UP

PATIENT MONITORING
The recovery period can be extensive.

PREVENTION/AVOIDANCE
Control black locust plants in pastures.

POSSIBLE COMPLICATIONS
Secondary bacterial infections due to impairment of the immune system.

EXPECTED COURSE AND PROGNOSIS
Prognosis is usually good once the forage is removed from the diet, but recovery can be prolonged.

MISCELLANEOUS

ASSOCIATED CONDITIONS
• Inappetance, bloody diarrhea, and salivation
• Weakness and incoordination due to posterior paralysis
• There can be dyspnea, dehydration, laminitis, and recumbency.
• Death is infrequent.

AGE-RELATED FACTORS
N/A

ZOONOTIC POTENTIAL
N/A

PREGNANCY
N/A

RUMINANT SPECIES AFFECTED
Potentially, all ruminant species can be affected.

BIOSECURITY
N/A

PRODUCTION MANAGEMENT
Control black locust plants in pastures.

SYNONYMS

SEE ALSO
Arsenic toxicity
Other causes of gastroenteritis
Toxicology: herd outbreaks
Vomitoxin

ABBREVIATIONS
ALT = alanine transferase
AST = aspartate transferase
BUN = blood urea nitrogen
GGT = gamma-glutamyl transferase
GOT = glutamyl oxaloacetic transaminase
LDH = lactate dehydrogenase
PCV= packed cell volume
RBC = red blood cell
TP = total protein

Suggested Reading
Aiello, S. E., ed. 1998. *Merck veterinary manual*. 8th ed. Whitehouse Station, NJ: Merck and Co.
Barri, M. E., El Dirdiri, N. I., Abu Danir, H., Idris, O. F. 1990, Dec. Toxicity of *Abrus precatorius* in Nubian Goats. *Veterinary and Human Toxicology* 32(6): 541–45.
Van Damme, E. J., et al. 1995, Mar. The bark of *Robinia pseudoacacia* contains a complex mixture of lectins. Characterization of the proteins and the cDNA clones. *American Society of Plant Physiologists, Plant Physiology*. 107(3): 833–43.

Author: Heidi Coker

BLINDNESS

 BASICS

DEFINITION
Loss of vision in one or both eyes

PATHOPHYSIOLOGY
Can be due to the blocking of light from entering the eye correctly (cataracts), retinal disease, optic nerve lesions, or brain lesions

SYSTEMS AFFECTED
Ophthalmic, CNS

GENETICS
• Congenital cataracts reported in cattle, sheep, rare in goats. Autosomal recessive in several breeds of cattle: Jersey, Hereford, Holstein-Friesian
• Albinism/subalbinism primarily in cattle and sheep, optic disc with dominant form of incomplete albinism in Hereford cattle
• Retinal degeneration of Toggenburg goats

INCIDENCE/PREVALENCE
N/A

GEOGRAPHIC DISTRIBUTION
Worldwide

SIGNALMENT

Species
Cattle, sheep, goats, camelids; potentially all ruminant species

Breed Predilections
• Congenital cataracts have been reported in cattle, sheep, rare in goats.
• Autosomal recessive in several breeds of cattle: Jersey, Hereford, Holstein-Friesian cattle
• Albinism/subalbinism in cattle and sheep; dominant form of incomplete albinism in Hereford cattle
• Retinal degeneration of Toggenburg goats

Mean Age and Range
N/A

Predominant Sex
N/A

SIGNS

HISTORICAL FINDINGS
• Inability to see, bumping into objects, unwilling or hesitant to move, eyes wide open, startles easily or overreacts when touched or when bumps an object
• Eyes may show an abnormal sheen due to degeneration of the retina. Determine if the disease is in a specific individual or multiple members of the herd/flock.

• Young animals may lack a menace response yet not be blind; need to watch them navigate an obstacle course.

PHYSICAL EXAMINATION FINDINGS

CAUSES AND RISK FACTORS
• Congenital cataracts can be associated with microphthalmia and retinal lesions from in utero exposure to BVD during days 76–150 of gestation, secondary to inflammation, toxins, and metabolic disease. In cattle can be secondary to IBK, malignant catarrhal fever, IBR, or retinal dysplasia of cattle. In sheep, bluetongue is often associated with retinal detachment.
• Chorioretinitis: in cattle, it can be associated with neonatal septicemia, TEME, rabies, toxoplasmosis, tuberculosis, and listeriosis. In sheep, this can be associated with mycoplasmosis, listeriosis, elaeophorosis, toxoplasmosis, bluetongue, and scrapie.
• Retinal degenerations are more commonly acquired vitamin A deficiency in cattle.
• Bracken fern (*Pteris aquiline*) toxicity and PEM are common in sheep.

 DIAGNOSIS

DIFFERENTIAL DIAGNOSIS
Causes:

Toxins
There are many plant and fungal toxins, the most common are listed here.
• *Stypandra glauca* (blind grass)—causes retinal degeneration and optic nerve neuropathy
• *Astragalus mollisimus* (locoweed)—causes dry eye and retinal degeneration
• Bracken fern (*Pteris aquiline*)—causes polioencephalomalacia and degeneration of outer retinal layers
• Sweet clover—coumarin causing intraocular hemorrhaging
• Lead toxicity
• Sulfur—see edema and decreased pupillary light response.
• Trauma to the brain
• Neoplasia—in the occipital cortices, lateral geniculate bodies, or optic radiations

Systemic Disease
• Meningitis/encephalitis—see pale swollen optic disc with hazy margins.
• Bluetongue in sheep—causes retinal dysplasia
• Listeriosis
• Neonatal septicemia
• Equine herpes type 1 virus in llamas—optic nerve and retinal degeneration

• Mycoplasmas—in goats can cause corneal opacification
• Diabetes mellitus in ram lambs can cause cataracts.

Parasitic
• Elaeophorosis, toxoplasmosis, trypanosomiasis—cause inflammation of fundus; elaeophorosis can cause cataracts.
• *Echinococcus granulosis*—hydatid cysts in the brain
• *Paraelaphostrongylus tenuis* (meningeal worm) in llamas

Deficiencies
• Thiamine
• Vitamin A
• Water deprivation
• CNS hypoxia—postanesthesia or other prolonged hypoxia

Congenital/Degenerative
• Retinal degeneration of Toggenburg goats
• Hydrocephalus
• Congenital malformations
• Glaucoma
• Cataracts
• Wool blindness of sheep

CBC/BIOCHEMISTRY/URINALYSIS
• Consistent with an underlying cause
• Ram lambs with diabetes mellitus–induced cataracts will have elevated glucose.

OTHER LABORATORY TESTS
• Practitioners use direct ophthalmoscopy more frequently than indirect ophthalmoscopy. It is important to view the tapetal fundus several inches from the patient and then move to 1–2 inches from the patient's eye when the optimum focus is achieved and the animal has adapted to the restraint. The diopter setting is usually started at "0" and adjusted to between +3 to −3 diopters to provide the sharpest image possible.
• Indirect ophthalmoscopy complements direct ophthalmoscopy.

IMAGING
Ultrasound evaluation of the corneal surfaces, the anterior and posterior lens surfaces, the retina, and any abnormal intraocular material will aid intraocular diagnosis. This is especially useful when dense corneal opacity or mature cataract obscures the view of the fundus.

OTHER DIAGNOSTIC PROCEDURES
• Examination of the cornea is incomplete without utilization of topical ophthalmic stains.

• Fluorescein is used to demonstrate the presence or absence of corneal ulcers. For topical use, fluorescein-impregnated paper strips are preferred to fluorescein solution to insure sterility.

PATHOLOGIC FINDINGS

TREATMENT
• Ensure nutrition and management are adequate, remove from toxin sources.
• Remove objects that can cause ocular trauma.
• Affected animals will need to be hand-fed and watered separately due to inability to compete with the rest of the herd.

CLIENT EDUCATION

MEDICATIONS

DRUGS OF CHOICE
• Pharmaceutical choice depends on the specific etiology.
• Trauma—corticosteroids and IV DMSO may help decrease swelling.
• Polioencephalomalacia—thiamine HCl 6–10 mg/kg IM or IV, antibiotics

CONTRAINDICATIONS
• Appropriate milk and meat withdrawal times must be followed for all compounds administered to food-producing animals.
• Topical corticosteroids and anesthetics are contraindicated when the cornea retains fluorescein stain.

PRECAUTIONS
N/A

POSSIBLE INTERACTIONS
N/A

ALTERNATIVE DRUGS

FOLLOW-UP

PATIENT MONITORING
With optic nerve lesions, on initial exam the fundus may appear normal. It can take 4 weeks for the optic disc to become pale and the retinal vessels to start regression.

PREVENTION/AVOIDANCE

POSSIBLE COMPLICATIONS
Permanent vision loss

EXPECTED COURSE AND PROGNOSIS
Prognosis for the return of sight is very guarded, but depends on the degree of damage and the etiology.

MISCELLANEOUS

ASSOCIATED CONDITIONS
Note: animals with a disease causing mental dullness or vestibular signs may appear blind.

AGE-RELATED FACTORS
• Young animals may lack a menace response yet not be blind; need to evaluate them while navigating an obstacle course.
• Diabetes mellitus will induce cataracts in ram lambs

ZOONOTIC POTENTIAL
N/A

PREGNANCY
Many diseases that cause blindness may also induce abortion.

RUMINANT SPECIES AFFECTED
Potentially, all ruminant species are affected.

BIOSECURITY
Quarantine new animals, isolate affected animals.

PRODUCTION MANAGEMENT
• Ensure nutrition and management are adequate; remove from toxin sources.
• Remove objects that can cause ocular trauma.
• Fence off toxic plants to prevent grazing.
• Minimize the incidence of nutritional PEM.

SYNONYMS
Bright blind
Glass eyed
Moon blind

SEE ALSO
Corneal ulceration
Ectropion
Entropion

Enucleation
FARAD
Keratoconjunctivitis
Microphthalmia
Ocular surgery

ABBREVIATIONS
BVD = bovine viral diarrhea
CNS = central nervous system
DMSO = dimethyl sulfoxide
FARAD = Food Animal Residue Avoidance Databank
IBK = infectious bovine keratoconjunctivitis
IBR = infectious bovine rhinotracheitis
IM = intramuscular
IV = intravenous
PEM = polioencephalomalacia
TEME = thromboembolic meningoencephalitis

Suggested Reading
Gelatt, K. N. 2000. *Essentials of veterinary ophthalmology*. Baltimore: Lipincott, Williams and Wilkins.
Hirono, I., Ito, M., Yagyu, S., Haga, M., Wakamatsu, K., Kishikawa, T., Nishikawa, O., Yamada, K., Ojika, M., Kigoshi, H. 1993, Dec. Reproduction of progressive retinal degeneration (bright blindness) in sheep by administration of ptaquiloside contained in bracken. *J Vet Med Sci.* 55(6):979–83.
Moore, C. P. 1996. Signs of ocular disease. In: *Large animal internal medicine*, ed. B. P. Smith. 2nd ed. St. Louis: Mosby.
Niles, G. A., Morgan, S. E., Edwards, W. C. 2000, Oct. Sulfur-induced polioencephalomalacia in stocker calves. *Vet Hum Toxicol.* 42(5):290–91.
O'Toole, D., Raisbeck, M., Case, J. C., Whitson, T. D. 1996, Jan. Selenium-induced "blind staggers" and related myths. A commentary on the extent of historical livestock losses attributed to selenosis on western US rangelands. *Vet Pathol.* 33(1):109–16.
Whitley, R. D., Moore, C. P. 1984, Nov. Ocular diagnostic and therapeutic techniques in food animals. *Vet Clin North Am Large Anim Pract.* 6(3):553–75.

Author: Melissa N. Carr

BLOAT

BASICS

DEFINITION
Gas distension of the rumen and reticulum. Primary, or frothy, bloat occurs when rumen gas is trapped in bubbles/froth, and cannot be eructated. Secondary, or free gas, bloat occurs because of physical blockage of the esophagus or from decreased vagal nerve function.

PATHOPHYSIOLOGY
• Normal rumen bacterial fermentation produces gases that are eructated from the rumen.
• Primary, or frothy, bloat occurs when the gas is trapped in bubbles/froth, and cannot be eructated. Immature legumes and clovers are rapidly fermented by rumen microflora, resulting in release of chloroplast particles that trap gas bubbles and prevent their coalescence.
• Additionally, liquid is trapped in the foam, reducing the passage of liquid from the rumen. This serves to enhance bacterial growth and increase gas and foam production. Feeding finely ground grains can also cause frothy bloat.
• Secondary, or free gas, bloat occurs because of physical blockage of the esophagus or from decreased vagal nerve function. Expansion of the rumen within the abdominal cavity eventually compresses the diaphragm decreasing lung volume and oxygenation and the venous return to the post cava causing hypovolemia.
• Young calves can bloat from fermentation of milk or milk replacer in the rumen.

SYSTEMS AFFECTED
Gastrointestinal, cardiovascular

GENETICS
N/A

INCIDENCE/PREVALENCE
• Normally very low incidence, generally less than 1%

• Incidence of primary bloat may be over 25% if animals are grazed on immature legumes/clover or fed excessive amounts of highly fermentable carbohydrates, such as finely ground grains.

GEOGRAPHIC DISTRIBUTION
Worldwide

Epidemiology
• Primary bloat is associated with grazing or feeding immature legumes/clover. Finely ground grain diets are also associated with frothy bloat.
• Secondary bloat is associated with feeds that can block the esophagus such as potatoes/beets and with masses that either block the esophagus or interfere with the vagus nerve in the mediastinum.
• Examples are tumors from lymphoma, enlarged lymph nodes from tuberculosis, and chronic bacterial pneumonia.

SIGNALMENT
Species Affected
Ruminants, especially cattle

Breed Predilections
N/A

Mean Age and Range
N/A

Predominant Sex
N/A

SIGNS
• Distension of the left flank from gas accumulation, tachycardia from hypoxia. Rumen contractions may decrease but often remain normal. Abdominal discomfort is evident.
• Severe cases may show open mouth breathing and staggering. Animal may become recumbent from hypoxia.

GENERAL COMMENTS
Bloat should be considered a medical emergency due to potential death from hypoxia and hypovolemia.

HISTORICAL FINDINGS
Sheep and cattle grazing on lush pastures, especially young legumes or clovers; high-concentrate diets with finely ground grains; history of chronic pneumonia

PHYSICAL EXAMINATION FINDINGS
• Distension of the dorsal left flank. Cattle with chronic vagal indigestion may have concurrent distension of ventral right flank due to rumen emptying defect ("papple-shape").
• Tachycardia often present

CAUSES
• Ingestion of immature legumes and clovers or finely ground grains
• Blockage of the esophagus or interference with the vagus nerve

RISK FACTORS
• Grazing or feeding early legumes or clovers; feeding finely ground grains or rapidly fermented carbohydrates
• Factors associated with the spread of tuberculosis or bovine leukemia virus; chronic bacterial pneumonia

DIAGNOSIS

DIFFERENTIAL DIAGNOSIS
• Ruminants often bloat postmortem. Necropsy signs of antemortem bloat include compression of blood and lymph flow in the neck and thorax, resulting in enlarged cervical vessels and lymph nodes. There is often a visible "white line" demarcation in the esophagus near the thoracic inlet from compression of the distal esophagus and congestion in the proximal esophagus.
• Lymphoma, enlarged lymph nodes from tuberculosis, and chronic bacterial pneumonia

CBC/BIOCHEMISTRY/URINALYSIS
N/A

BLOAT

OTHER LABORATORY TESTS
N/A

IMAGING
N/A

OTHER DIAGNOSTIC PROCEDURES
Passing a stomach tube differentiates primary (frothy) from secondary (free gas) bloat. Esophageal blockages may often be detected while passing the stomach tube.

GROSS AND HISTOPATHOLOGIC FINDINGS
Distension of the rumen and reticulum with gas; congestion of cervical lymph nodes and vessels; "white line" demarcation in esophagus at interface of compressed and congested tissue

TREATMENT
• Depends on the cause and degree of hypoxia. Severely hypoxic animals should be intubated to relieve the free gas. The tube often plugs with froth or dips below the fluid level in the rumen, requiring clearing the tube by blowing into it or moving the end within the rumen.
• It may be necessary to place a rumen trocar in the dorsal left flank. Mild to moderate cases of frothy bloat often respond to surfactants such as poloxalene (25–50 g per animal).

Inpatient Versus Outpatient
N/A

CLIENT EDUCATION
• Advise clients about the danger of grazing or feeding immature legumes/clovers especially to hungry animals.
• Discuss the importance of a functional rumen mat in cattle on high-concentrate diets.
• Discuss early recognition of bloat and treatments such as poloxalene and stomach tubing.

MEDICATIONS

DRUGS OF CHOICE
Poloxalene (25–50 g per animal) for primary bloat

CONTRAINDICATIONS
N/A

PRECAUTIONS
N/A

POSSIBLE INTERACTIONS
N/A

ALTERNATE DRUGS
Mineral oil or vegetable oils may act as antifoaming agents.

FOLLOW-UP

PATIENT MONITORING
Watch for recurrence.

PREVENTION/AVOIDANCE
• Avoid feeding or grazing risk plants such as legumes or clovers. Do not overfeed finely ground grain or other highly fermentable carbohydrates.
• Prevent infections with bovine leukemia virus and tuberculosis.

POSSIBLE COMPLICATIONS
• Physical damage to the vagus nerve or branches of the vagus from excessive rumen distension may result in rumen dysfunction and possibly recurrence.
• Trocarization may result in localized or diffuse peritonitis.

EXPECTED COURSE AND PROGNOSIS
• Spontaneous recovery in mild cases and those patients sufficiently relieved by stomach tube/trocar or treated with poloxalene
• Death from hypoxia in severe cases

MISCELLANEOUS

PREVENTION
N/A

ASSOCIATED CONDITIONS
Lymphoma, vagal indigestion, tuberculosis

AGE-RELATED FACTORS
Young calves may bloat from fermentation of milk or milk replacer in the rumen.

ZOONOTIC POTENTIAL
N/A

PREGNANCY
N/A

SYNONYMS
Bloat, ruminal tympany

SEE ALSO
Chronic bacterial pneumonia
Enlarged lymph nodes from tuberculosis
Lymphoma
Vagal indigestion

ABBREVIATIONS
N/A

Suggested Reading
Majak, W., Hall, J. W., McCaughey, W. P. 1995. Pasture management strategies for reducing the risk of legume bloat in cattle. *Journal of Animal Science* 73:1493–98.
Radostits, O. M., Gay, C. C., Blood, D. C., Hinchcliff, K. W., eds. 2000. *Veterinary medicine: a textbook of diseases of cattle, sheep, pigs, goats and horses.* 9th ed. London: W. B. Saunders.

Author: James P. Reynolds

BLUE-GREEN ALGAE POISONING

BASICS

OVERVIEW
- Over 50 genera of freshwater blue-green algae (also referred to as cyanophytes or cyanobacteria) exist worldwide that produce two major types of toxins: neurotoxic alkaloids, such as anatoxins, and hepatotoxic peptides, such as microcystins.
- Very few cases of anatoxin poisoning (often produced by *Anabaena flos-aquae*) have been reported in cattle with clinical signs resembling organophosphorus insecticide poisoning (depolarizing neuromuscular blocking agent), such as muscle weakness and paralysis.
- Microcystin toxicosis is much more common than anatoxin poisoning and numerous cases have been reported in cattle and sheep worldwide. Therefore, microcystin toxicosis is discussed in detail.
- Microcystins are primarily produced by *Microcystis aeruginosa*, but many other cyanobacteria produce these peptides such as other *Microcystis* spp., *Anabaena* spp., *Oscillatoria* spp., and *Nostoc* spp.
- Microcystins are usually confined within the algal cells and are released only when cells are damaged (e.g., when cells encounter the acidic environment of the stomach).
- Microcystins enter the hepatocytes through a carrier-mediated transport system and cause inhibition of protein phosphatase (1 and 2A) in the hepatocytes. Dissociation and necrosis of hepatocytes lead to intrahepatic hemorrhage and diffuse centrilobular hepatocellular degeneration.
- Sudden death is possible as a result of hemorrhagic shock.
- Death in animals usually occurs within hours to days postexposure.
- Animals that survive the acute phase of poisoning can recover, but may develop clinical signs related to liver disease (e.g., hepatogenous photosensitization; drop in production).
- Respiratory—pulmonary edema and congestion have been reported in acute cases.

GENETICS
N/A

INCIDENCE/PREVALENCE
- Blue-green algae poisoning occurs seasonally during warm weather conditions. The blooms are most common in the summer and fall when bodies of water are stagnant and warm and contain ample nutrients.
- A breeze blowing across the water may help concentrate the organisms near a shore.

GEOGRAPHIC DISTRIBUTION
Worldwide

Epidemiology
- Not all animals in a herd may be affected. Several important factors are related to occurrence of poisoning. Favorable algae growth conditions are usually required to produce sufficiently high concentrations of algae in water. Nutrient pollution of lakes and ponds with phosphorus and nitrogen leads to eutrophication and accelerated algae growth.
- Long periods of sustained sunshine, which produce warm water temperatures, are usually necessary. A breeze blowing across the water has also been identified as critical in some situations for concentrating algae near a shore where cattle congregate on the leeward side during hot weather.
- Microcystins are the most prevalent hepatotoxins and are produced by several cyanobacteria genera including *Microcystis*, *Planktothrix*, *Anabaena*, and *Oscillatoria*. Anatoxins are produced mainly by *Anabaena* spp. in addition to *Aphanizomenon*, *Microcystis*, and *Oscillatoria* spp. Saxitoxin production is associated with a few specific freshwater cyanobacteria species found in the genera of *Anabaena*, *Aphanizomenon*, *Cylindrospermopsis*, *Lyngbya*, and *Planktothrix*.

SIGNALMENT
- All ruminant species are susceptible to blue-green algae toxins. Microcystin poisoning has been reported in cattle and sheep.
- Dead animals are often found close to water bodies that have a "painted green" or "scumlike" bloom.

SIGNS
- Animals exposed to blue-green algae toxins are often found dead near water that has a thick algal bloom. Cattle may have algae on their limbs.
- Abrupt onset of apprehension and distress occurs within hours of microcystin exposure.
- This is quickly followed by pale mucous membranes, ruminal atony, diarrhea, weakness, nervousness, ataxia, and anorexia. In severe cases, the animals become recumbent and comatose.

- Death may occur within 24 hours of exposure, but may be delayed several days.
- Animals that survive the initial toxicosis may develop hepatogenous photosensitization.

CAUSES AND RISK FACTORS
- Exposure to water contaminated with toxin-producing cyanobacteria
- Warm, dry weather and stagnant water and a breeze that blows across water, allowing the organisms to concentrate near a shore
- High concentrations of nutrients in the water, such as nitrates and phosphates from sewage, detergents, industrial pollution, and fertilizers increase the risk for a blue-green algae bloom.

DIAGNOSIS

DIFFERENTIAL DIAGNOSIS
- Other hepatotoxicants—metals (detection in liver and kidney, histopathological lesions), aflatoxins (detection in feed, often chronic), pyrrolizidine alkaloids (evidence of plant consumption, histopathologic lesions, chronic disease)
- Hepatopathy—serum clinical chemistry and liver biopsy
- Nitrate toxicosis—chocolate-colored blood, exposure to nitrate-accumulating plants
- Cyanide poisoning—mucous membranes are initially bright cherry red, evidence of exposure to cyanogenic plants, chemical analysis for cyanide in gastrointestinal contents, liver, or muscle
- Larkspur poisoning—mainly found in the western states; bloat is a common finding, evidence of exposure to *Delphinium* spp.
- Grass tetany—hypomagnesemia
- Electrocution or lightning strike
- Organophosphorus or carbamate insecticide exposure—commonly associated with gastrointestinal irritation and neurological signs, evaluation of cholinesterase activity, detection of pesticides in gastrointestinal contents
- Lead poisoning—determination of blood lead concentration
- Exposure to neurotoxic plants, such as poison hemlock, water hemlock, tree tobacco, lupine—chemical analysis for plant toxins in gastrointestinal contents, history of presence of plants in the environment
- Exposure to cardiotoxic plants, such as oleander, milkweed, and azalea—chemical analysis for plant toxins in gastrointestinal contents, history of presence of plants in the environment

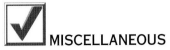

BLUE-GREEN ALGAE POISONING

CBC/BIOCHEMISTRY/URINALYSIS
Increased GGT, AST, SDH, and GLDH

OTHER LABORATORY TESTS
• Direct microscopic examination of water and gastrointestinal contents
• Mouse bioassay
• Detection of microcystins in water or rumen contents by high-performance liquid chromatography/mass spectrometry
• Analysis of suspect water by direct competitive ELISA

IMAGING
N/A

DIAGNOSTIC PROCEDURES
N/A

PATHOLOGIC FINDINGS
• Postmortem lesions in animals that died of exposure to microcystins include hepatomegaly, congested and hemorrhagic liver.
• Histopathologically, microcystin toxicosis results in centrilobular hepatocellular degeneration and necrosis; dilatation and engorgement of sinusoids; and loss of hepatic cords.
• Postmortem lesions are generally nonspecific in animals that died of exposure to neurotoxic blue-green algae toxins (e.g., anatoxins).

TREATMENT
• Treatment of animals exposed to blue-green algae toxins is primarily supportive and symptomatic. Supportive therapy should include administration of intravenous fluids, corticosteroids, and calcium.
• Poisoned animals should be removed immediately from the source.
• Adsorption of toxins with activated charcoal has been suggested.
• Rumenotomy or a rumen lavage may be considered in valuable animals.

CLIENT EDUCATION
• Create awareness for potential of blue-green algae toxicity, especially during sunny, warm weather and other favorable environmental conditions.
• A heavy water bloom of algae producing a surface scum is usually necessary for poisonings to occur.

MEDICATIONS

DRUGS OF CHOICE
• No antidote is available.
• Activated charcoal, mineral oil, or saline cathartics
• Corticosteroids
• Vitamin E and selenium supplementation

CONTRAINDICATIONS
N/A

POSSIBLE INTERACTIONS
N/A

ALTERNATIVE DRUGS
Hepatic uptake blockers, such as rifampicin and cyclosporin A, may be helpful, but their usefulness in the treatment of cardiac glycoside-poisoned ruminants has not been evaluated.

FOLLOW-UP

PATIENT MONITORING
• Monitoring of liver enzymes is helpful.
• Monitor serum electrolytes.

PREVENTION/AVOIDANCE
• Keep animals away from water bodies with visible algal blooms.
• Precipitation of algal cells:
• Lime (100–250 mg/l) to precipitate cells without rupturing them
• Suspend ferric alum block (1 kg/10,000 L)
• Suspend gypsum block (50 kg/1000 L)
• Algaecide (lysis of algal cells): copper sulfate at 20–40 g/50,000 L (target concentration: 0.2–0.4 ppm). After treatment with copper sulfate, animals must be removed from the water source for approximately 7 days.
• Use of straw bales (100 g/1000 L) to control algal blooms has also been reported. Barley straw seems to be more effective when compared to wheat or other straws.

POSSIBLE COMPLICATIONS
Hepatogenous photosensitization

EXPECTED COURSE AND PROGNOSIS
• Animals poisoned with microcystins are often found dead.
• Microcystin poisoning progresses rapidly, and treatment is often too late. If animals exhibit clinical signs of liver failure, the prognosis is poor.
• Animals that survive 24 to 72 hours after exposure usually survive but may develop clinical signs associated with hepatic failure.

MISCELLANEOUS

ASSOCIATED CONDITIONS
Hepatopathy

AGE-RELATED FACTORS
N/A

ZOONOTIC POTENTIAL
N/A

PREGNANCY
N/A

BIOSECURITY
N/A

PRODUCTION MANAGEMENT
N/A

SYNONYMS
N/A

SEE ALSO
• Aflatoxins and pyrrolizidine alkaloids
• Cardiotoxic plants (i.e., oleander, milkweed, azalea)
• Cyanide poisoning
• Grass tetany—hypomagnesemia
• Larkspur poisoning
• Lead poisoning
• Neurotoxic plants (i.e., poison hemlock, water hemlock, tree tobacco, lupine)
• Nitrate toxicosis
• Organophosphorus or carbamate insecticide exposure

ABBREVIATIONS
• AST = aspartate aminotransferase
• ELISA = enzyme linked immunosorbent assay
• GGT = gamma-glutamyl transferase
• GLDH = glutamate dehydrogenase
• SDH = sorbitol dehydrogenase

Suggested Reading
Dawson, R. M. 1998. The toxicology of microcystins. *Toxicon.* 36:953–62.
Puschner, B., Galey, F. D., Johnson, B., et al. 1998. Blue-green algae toxicosis in cattle. *J Am Vet Med Assoc.* 213:1605–7.
Roder, J. D. 2004. Blue-green algae. In: *Clinical veterinary toxicology*, ed. K. H. Plumlee. St. Louis: Mosby.

Authors: Asheesh Tiwary, Birgit Puschner, Terry W. Lehenbauer

BLUETONGUE

 BASICS

OVERVIEW

Bluetongue (BT) is an arthropod-borne, noncontagious viral infection of ruminants caused by BT virus (BTV), of the genus *Orbivirus* within the Reoviridae family.
• Transmission of BTV among susceptible hosts occurs through the bite of certain species of infected *Culicoides* or biting midges.
• The main vector of BTV in North America is *Culicoides sonorensis* (*C. sonorensis*; previously known as *C. varipennis*); in Australia, *C. brevitarsis;* and in Africa, Asia, and Europe, *C. imicola.*
• In the absence of a competent vector, transmission of BTV to cattle occurs occasionally by insemination with infected semen and transplacentally.
• Due to its potential for rapid spread across borders, and its capability to produce serious economic losses, the Office International des Epizooties (OIE) includes BT in their A list of diseases.

PATHOPHYSIOLOGY

Bluetongue virus infection presents initially with dyspnea and increased respirations followed by fever, hyperemia of the ears, lips, and muzzle, and ulceration of the oral mucosa. The tongue can become cyanotic and swollen, hence the disease name, bluetongue. Lameness and widespread muscle necrosis are additional sequellae.

SYSTEMS AFFECTED

• Cardiovascular—vascular injury leading to hemorrhages, congestion, heart failure.
• Musculoskeletal—intramuscular edema, hemorrhages, coronitis.
• Reproductive—infection during pregnancy can cause fetal loss or malformations.
• Gastrointestinal—vascular damage causes ulcerations and hemorrhages in the oral cavity, fore stomachs, and intestine.
• Respiratory—vascular damage leads to congestion and edema.

GENETICS

N/A

INCIDENCE/PREVALENCE

N/A

GEOGRAPHIC DISTRIBUTION

• Twenty-four BTV serotypes (BTV-1 to -24) have been found worldwide. Four of them are endemic in the United States (BTV-10, BTV-11, BTV-13, BTV-17). BTV-2, although not prevalent in the United States, has been isolated sporadically in the past.
• BTV infection occurs in tropical and temperate regions of Africa, Asia, Australia, and the Americas. Periodic incursions of the infection also occur in southern Europe.

• The distribution of BTV is limited by the distribution of the vector. BTV is considered to be present between approximate latitudes 35°S and 40°N. In some regions the presence of BTV may extend to 50°N. BTV transmission occurs only when weather conditions are favorable and adult vectors are active.
• In the United States, BTV infection is more prevalent in the southern and western parts of the country, and most infections occur in late summer and fall. Variations in weather patterns may affect the distribution of the vector and BTV transmission.

SIGNALMENT

• BTV infects a wide range of domestic and wild ruminants. Severe disease occurs almost exclusively in sheep and some species of deer, most notably the white-tailed deer of North America. Cattle commonly have inapparent infections.
• Mortality rates and severity of disease in sheep may vary, with fine-wool breeds and older sheep considered to be more susceptible.

SIGNS

• BTV infection can cause inapparent infection or acute fulminant disease.
• Clinical disease is largely restricted to sheep and white-tailed deer; in cattle and goats, infection is usually asymptomatic. Infected bulls may shed BTV in their semen.
• The incubation period ranges from 2–15 days.
• The acute fulminant form is characterized by fever of up to 107.6°F (42°C), leukopenia, anorexia, weight loss, depression, with edema and swelling of the face, lips, muzzle, and ears, reddening of the oral mucosa, and salivation.
• Crusting and accumulation of mucopurulent discharge in the muzzle and nostrils are common. In a small percentage of cases, the tongue appears edematous and purplish-blue (hence the name of the disease) as a result of cyanosis.
• Hemorrhages, erosions, and ulcers in gums, cheeks, tongue, and nostrils are often present.
• Lameness, stiffness, and prostration may develop as a result of muscle degeneration and laminitis. Laminitis may manifest as swelling, hyperemia, and hemorrhage of the hoof laminae and coronary band. Lameness may progress to "knee walking" or recumbency.
• Death due to bronchopneumonia or secondary bacterial infections may occur 8 to 10 days after the initial signs appear. Some severely affected sheep may recover.
• BTV infection of pregnant sheep or cattle may result in abortion, stillbirths, fetal malformation, or the birth of live but weak offspring (dummy lambs/calves). These negative effects have been linked to the use of modified-live vaccines (MLV) rather than to natural infection with wild-type BTV. Ovine

fetuses are more susceptible to the teratogenic effects when infection occurs during the fifth and sixth weeks of gestation.
• Pregnant sheep may abort during the acute phase of BT disease in the absence of fetal infection as a result of maternal stress.

CAUSES AND RISK FACTORS

Ruminants living in areas where the vector, *Culicoides,* and bluetongue virus coexist

 DIAGNOSIS

DIFFERENTIAL DIAGNOSIS

• Differential diagnosis includes other ulcerative diseases of the respiratory and digestive tracts of ruminants such as foot-and-mouth disease, orf, sheep pox, peste des petits ruminants, photosensitization, and diseases that cause stiffness and lameness including polyarthritis, and foot rot.
• In white-tailed deer, BT needs to be differentiated from epizootic hemorrhagic disease (EHD).
• The differential diagnosis of BTV fetal infection, malformations, and abortions includes infection with Cache Valley, Akabane, border disease, Rift Valley fever, Nairobi sheep disease, Wesselsbron disease, genetic defects, and ingestion of teratogenic plants.

CBC/BIOCHEMISTRY/URINALYSIS

N/A

DIAGNOSTIC PROCEDURES

• Serological assays available for the demonstration of BTV antibodies include complement fixation, virus neutralization, the agar gel immunodiffusion (AGID) test, and several ELISA formats.
• Only the AGID and competitive ELISA (cELISA) are recommended by the OIE as prescribed tests for international movement of ruminants.
• Virus isolation can be done by inoculation of susceptible sheep or embryonated chicken eggs with heparinized blood or homogenized lymph nodes, spleen, or lung of infected animals. Subsequent adaptation to cell culture and serotyping of the virus may be necessary. Blood and tissue samples for diagnosis need to be preserved at 4°C, and not frozen.
• BTV can be isolated from blood of infected sheep and cattle for up to 11 and 49 days postinfection, respectively. BTV nucleic acids can be detected by reverse transcription-polymerase chain reaction (RT-PCR) for up to 222 days postinfection. However, blood from sheep and cattle is infectious for *C. sonorensis* for only 21 days after infection of the ruminant host.

• Sheep and cattle whose blood contains BTV nucleic acid as detected by RT-PCR, but not infectious virus as determined by virus isolation, are unlikely to play an important role in the epidemiology of BTV infection.
• BTV antibodies can be demonstrated in precolostral serum samples of lambs infected in utero. BTV virus also can be isolated in some of these lambs due to immune tolerance and persistent infection.

PATHOLOGIC FINDINGS

GROSS FINDINGS
• BTV infection in sheep and white-tailed deer may result in extensive vascular injury that leads to congestion, edema, hemorrhage, disseminated intravascular coagulation, and tissue necrosis.
• The vascular damage results in ulcerations and hemorrhage of the tongue, oral mucosa, hard palate, dental pad, and sometimes fore stomachs and intestine.
• The lips, gums, and tongue may be edematous, congested, or cyanotic.
• There is subcutaneous and intramuscular edema and hemorrhages.
• The superficial lymph nodes may be enlarged and edematous.
• The most consistent lesion in sheep is hemorrhages in the tunica media at the base of the pulmonary artery. Hemorrhages are also present in the aorta, epicardium, endocardium, and myocardium.
• Pale areas as a result of necrosis may be found in skeletal and cardiac muscles.
• Pulmonary congestion and edema as a result of heart failure, and pneumonia due to secondary bacterial infections, may be present.
• Fetal lesions consist of hydranencephaly, poroencephaly, and arthrogryposis.

HISTOPATHOLOGIC FINDINGS
The characteristic lesion consists of microvascular thrombosis resulting in congestion, edema, hemorrhage, and tissue necrosis.

TREATMENT
There are no specific treatments for BT.

NURSING CARE/ACTIVITY/DIET
Secondary infections may be treated with broad-spectrum antibiotics. Anti-inflammatory and pain relief medications can be used to limit the symptoms. Affected animals should be placed in shaded pens protected from the environment and provided with clean water and good-quality hay or feed.

MEDICATIONS

DRUGS OF CHOICE
N/A

CONTRAINDICATIONS
N/A

POSSIBLE INTERACTIONS
N/A

ALTERNATIVE DRUGS
N/A

FOLLOW-UP

PATIENT MONITORING
N/A

PREVENTION/AVOIDANCE
• Modified live virus vaccines are available in some parts of the world.
• In the United States, MLV containing serotype 10 is available. In addition, MLV vaccines containing serotypes 10, 11, or 17 can be obtained for use only in California. Lambs can be vaccinated close to weaning and the breeding stock at least 3 weeks before breeding or after lambing. Pregnant animals should not be vaccinated because of the potential teratogenic effects.
• To induce protection, the BTV serotype of the vaccine must correspond to the serotype of the virus in the region.
• Limiting vector exposure by housing sheep during peak feeding times (from dusk to dawn) may reduce the risk of exposure, but vectors may be active during daytime when overcast.
• Reduction of the vector population through the use of insecticides or by making vector habitat unsuitable can aid in BT control.
• Many countries impose restrictions to the movement of livestock and germ plasm from infected areas.

MISCELLANEOUS

AGE-RELATED FACTORS
N/A

ZOONOTIC POTENTIAL
There is no evidence to indicate that BTV is infectious to humans.

PREGNANCY
Modified live BTV vaccines may cause pregnancy loss and teratogenesis.

RUMINANT SPECIES AFFECTED
Sheep, cattle, white-tailed deer

BIOSECURITY/PRODUCTION MANAGEMENT:
N/A

SYNONYMS
Muzzle disease
Pseudo foot-and-mouth disease
Sore muzzle

SEE ALSO
Epizootic hemorrhagic disease

ABBREVIATIONS
BT = bluetongue
BTV = bluetongue virus
EHD = epizootic hemorrhagic disease
ELISA = enzyme-linked immunosorbent assay
MLV = modified live vaccine
OIE = Office International des Epizooties
RT-PCR = reverse transcription-polymerase chain reaction

Suggested Reading
Aradaib, I. E., Smith, W. L., Osburn, B. I., Cullor, J. S. 2003. A multiplex PCR for simultaneous detection and differentiation of North American serotypes of bluetongue and epizootic hemorrhagic disease viruses. *Comp Immunol Microbiol Infect Dis.* 26:77–87.
Bonneau, K. R., DeMaula, C. D., Mullens, B. A., MacLachlan, N. J. 2002. Duration of viremia infectious to *Culicoides sonorensis* in bluetongue virus-infected cattle and sheep. *Vet Microbiol.* 88: 115–25.
Breard, E., Hamblin, C., Hammoumi, S., Sailleau, C., Dauphin, G., Zientara, S. 2004, Aug. The epidemiology and diagnosis of bluetongue with particular reference to Corsica. *Res Vet Sci.* 77(1):1–8.
Clavijo, A., Heckert, R. A., Dulac, G. C., Afshar, A. 2000. Isolation and identification of bluetongue virus. *J Virol Methd.* 87:13–23.
MacLachlan, N. J., Conley, A. J., Kennedy, P. C. 2000. Bluetongue and equine arteritis viruses as models of virus-induced fetal injury and abortion. *Anim Reprod Sci.* 60–61:643–51.
Mellor, P. S., Wittmann, E. J. 2002. Bluetongue virus in the Mediterranean basin, 1998–2001. *Vet J.* 164:20–37.

Author: Andrés de la Concha-Bermejillo

BODY CONDITION SCORE: CAMELIDS AND CAMELS

 BASICS

DEFINITION
Body condition score is a subjective technique of categorizing animals based on the amount of adipose tissue stores.

SYSTEMS AFFECTED
• Musculoskeletal
• Nutritional
• Production management

GENETICS
N/A

INCIDENCE/PREVALENCE
N/A

GEOGRAPHIC DISTRIBUTION
Worldwide

SIGNALMENT
Species
Camelids and Camels

Breed Predilections
N/A

Mean Age and Range
N/A

Predominant Sex
N/A

SIGNS

HISTORICAL FINDINGS

PHYSICAL EXAMINATION FINDINGS
Body Areas to Be Assessed
• Dorsal aspect of the thorax, just caudal to the withers
• Fiberless area behind the elbows
• Region between the hind legs
• Brisket area
NOTE: Palpation of the pelvis is less than ideal due to the inherent thin skin, light muscling, and minimal fat cover in this area.

BODY CONDITION SCORES: GENERAL CONSIDERATIONS AND CAUTION
• Camelids have a great variability of body type and conformation even within the same species. Therefore weight alone is not a good indicator of body condition.
• Body condition scoring (BCS) does not replace actual weighing. Both should be considered if possible.
• A single score is usually not helpful. It is the variation of the BCS that needs to be stressed.
• Fiber coat may be misleading. Animals require direct palpation.
• Accumulations of adipose tissue characteristics are essential in assessing BCS. Evaluating adipose cover over the rib cage and the axilla region is important to the overall scoring process. It should be understood that body condition scoring is a subjective measure of a herd nutrition and care program.
• Pelvic area is always bony.
• Neck is not a good indicator of body condition score.
• Characteristic regions of fat deposition in camelids: Shoulders; briskets; cranial ribs; inner thighs; perineum; camel: hump (or humps).
• Body condition scoring is a good management tool to evaluate if the nutritional demands required by specific physiologic situations (particularly lactation and late pregnancy) are being met.
• In addition, body condition scores allow monitoring animals through a change in feed or feeding systems.
• In range animals' changes in body conditions, scores are important in the evaluation of the nutritive value of pastures.

BCS Technique
BCS should be assessed at least four times and ideally six times a year.
Best times for assessment of body condition scores for the herd in general are
• Before winter
• In the middle of winter
• In spring
• In summer
• In fall
Best times for assessment of body conditions scores for breeding females are
• Early pregnancy
• Midpregnancy
• At parturition
• Six weeks after parturition (corresponds in general with the early pregnancy in rebred females)
• At weaning (corresponds in general to midpregnancy in rebred females)
Technique for evaluation
• General appreciation from a distance for camels and camelids and if animals are sheared (llamoids).
• Depending on the body area, palpation evaluates fat deposit or both muscle mass and fat deposit.
• Palpate over the lumbar (loin) areas to feel the spinous and transverse processes and evaluate presence or absence of depression and its depth or roundness. Evaluating the angle from between the thumb on one side of the spinous process and the other fingers on the other side.
• Inspect and palpate the paralumbar fossa and evaluate the depth of the shelf created by the transverse process of the lumbar vertebrae.
• Palpate over the ribs to feel the fat cover in that region.
• Raise the tail and inspect the perineal area and the inguinal area for shape (curvature and fat deposition).
• Palpate the brisket for roundness and shape.
• Palpate the shoulders for fat deposit.
• In camels, inspect the size and shape of the hump.

Body Condition Scores
• Scores are given from 1 (emaciated animals) to 5 or 9 (obese animals) depending on preference.
• Generally, people using the 5-point system use intermediate scores in increments of 0.25 to 0.5.

BODY CONDITION SCORE: CAMELIDS AND CAMELS

- The ideal BCS

  Males: 3 to 3.25 before the breeding season. Males will lose 0.5 to 1.0 points during the breeding season. Camels in free mating systems may lose up to 2 points during rutting season.

  Females: 2.5 to 3.25 for open or lactating females; 3.25 to 3.5 in the last trimester of pregnancy. Lactating females should not loose more than 0.5 to 0.75 points.

Score 1: Emaciated Animal

Extreme loss of muscle mass
Thin face
Deep depression over the lumbar area
Gaunt, visible, tucked-in paralumbar fossa
No perineal fat, sharp visible ischial tuberii
Inverted "V" inner thighs shape
Narrow prominent V-shaped brisket
Ribs easily identified, depressed intercostals area
Camels: flat back or flopped-over hump

Score 2: Thin

Muscle mass is minimal.
Lumbar area depression slightly filled in but easily palpable
Lumbar fossa prominent
Some fat deposition in the perineal area
Gradual filling of the inner thighs
Gradual filling on the brisket and loss of sharp edges of the sternum
Camels: moderate hump

Score 3: Moderate

Normal muscle mass and smooth appearance
Lumbar area depression palpable with slight pressure
Lumbar fossa not evident
Perineum filled in
Inner thighs rounded
Brisket: sternum still palpable but starting to become round

Ribs can still be palpated with some pressure.
Camels: shoulder and rump muscles can still be delineated, hump normal size with angular dorsal edge

Score 4: Fat

Musculature not well defined —"buried in fat"
Lumbar area rounded to nearly flat
No shelf formed by the transverse process of the lumbar vertebrae
Perineum filled in, no depression under the tail
Inguinal area filled in
Brisket flat
Ribs can only be palpated with firm pressure.
Camel: hump round and wide at the base, shoulders very thick

Score 5: Obese

Smooth, rounded appearance due to excessive fat deposition
Lumbar area completely rounded
Bony structures difficult to palpate
Bulging perineum
Thick tail-head
Convex inguinal appearance
Rounded brisket
Camels: obviously fat on shoulders, hump very large and round

 MISCELLANEOUS

ASSOCIATED CONDITIONS
N/A

AGE-RELATED FACTORS
N/A

ZOONOTIC POTENTIAL
N/A

PREGNANCY
Pregnancy may affect body condition scoring.

RUMINANT SPECIES AFFECTED
Camelids and camels

BIOSECURITY
N/A

PRODUCTION MANAGEMENT
Body condition scoring should be performed on all animals within the herd at minimum on a quarterly basis.

SYNONYMS
N/A

SEE ALSO
Body condition scoring by species

ABBREVIATIONS
BCS = body condition score

Suggested Reading
Fowler, M. E. 1989. *Medicine and surgery of South American camelids.* Ames: Iowa State University Press.
Johnson, L. W. 1994. Update on llama medicine. *Veterinary Clinics of North America Food Animal Practice* 10:198–99.
Tibary, A., Anouassi, A. 1997. Management of reproduction in camelidae. In: Theriogenology in *camelidae*, pp. 453–79. Rabat, Morocco: Actes Edition.
Van Saun, R. J. 2003. Feeding alpacas. In: Hoffman, E. (ed), *The complete alpaca book*, pp. 179–232. Santa Cruz, CA: Bonny Doon Press.

Authors: Ahmed Tibary and Debbie Terrel

BORDER DISEASE

BASICS

OVERVIEW
• Neonatal condition of lambs as a result of a viral infection of the dam during pregnancy. The virus crosses the placenta and infects the lamb.
• The border disease virus (BDV) is closely related to other pestiviruses such as hog cholera virus (HCV), which causes classical swine fever, and bovine viral diarrhea virus (BVDV).
• Also called hairy shaker and fuzzy lamb disease

SYSTEMS AFFECTED
Reproductive, musculoskeletal, central nervous system

GENETICS
N/A

INCIDENCE/PREVALENCE
Unknown

GEOGRAPHIC DISTRIBUTION
Worldwide

SIGNALMENT
• Sheep
• Goats
• Pregnant cattle inoculated early in gestation with border disease virus frequently abort and develop antibodies to bovine viral diarrhea. Swine may possibly be affected.

Species
Sheep and goats

Breed Predilections
N/A

Mean Age and Range
Clinical manifestations in the fetus depend on the stage of gestation when infection occurs.

Predominant Sex
N/A

SIGNS
Clinical signs are determined by the animal's age when infected.
• Animals infected as adults are subclinical. However, when the ewe is infected during pregnancy, the virus crosses the placenta and infects the fetus. Disease is suspected with increased numbers of barren ewes or ewes bearing mummified or malformed lambs.
• Clinical manifestations in the fetus depend on the stage of gestation when infection occurs.
• Placentitis occurs 10–30 days postinfection and may cause fetal expulsion, resorption, or mummification.
• Early gestational infections may result in immune tolerance in the lamb. These lambs are permanent carriers and shedders of the virus, but do not develop clinical signs of disease.
• Other surviving fetuses infected <90 days gestation may not develop immune tolerance. These lambs develop the characteristic signs of border disease.
• Affected lambs are of small size with possible skeletal defects such as dropped pasterns or mandibular brachygnathia
• Involuntary tonic/clonic muscular tremors and ataxia
• Hypertrophy of primary hair follicles results in a long, coarse, and straight birth coat. It is sometimes described as "hairy." The coat may also be pigmented.
• Kids and some rough-coated breeds of sheep do not demonstrate the characteristic hair changes.

CAUSES AND RISK FACTORS
The main sources of infection are the asymptomatic, persistently infected sheep. These animals shed the virus in saliva, respiratory secretions, urine, feces, or semen. Transmission occurs across mucous membranes.

DIAGNOSIS

DIFFERENTIAL DIAGNOSIS
• Other causes of abortion such as *Salmonella* spp., *Campylobacter* spp., *Chlamydia* spp., *Toxoplasma gondii*, and *Rickettsia* spp.
• In lambs other neurological conditions such as enzootic ataxia (swayback), bacterial meningoencephalitis, focal symmetrical encephalomalacia, and "daft lamb" disease

CBC/BIOCHEMISTRY/URINALYSIS
N/A

OTHER LABORATORY FINDINGS
Possibility of decreased levels of thyroid hormones contributing to growth retardation

IMAGING
N/A

DIAGNOSTIC PROCEDURES
• Fluorescent antibody tests for viral antigens performed on tissues of affected lambs. Tissues for collection include: abomasum, pancreas, kidneys, thyroid, testicles, and skin biopsies.
• Serology includes serum neutralization, agar gel immunodiffusion (AGID), and complement fixation tests of ewes. Ewes infected as adults develop serum neutralization (SN) titers ranging from 1:20 to 1:320. Animals with congenital infection may have negative SN titers or titers <1:10.
• Precolostral blood cultures: colostral antibody can mask virus for up to 2 months.
• RT-PCR

PATHOLOGIC FINDINGS

GROSS FINDINGS
• Hydranencephaly
• Undersized cerebral cortex
• Severe cases may have cavitations or cysts of the cerebrum and/or spinal cord.
• Doming of the frontal bones of the skull

- Abnormal curvature of the ribs
- Brachygnathia
- Abnormal "hairy" appearance of birth coat due to increased proportion of primary hair follicles
- Abnormal skin pigmentation
- Placentitis and placental necrosis can occur.

HISTOPATHOLOGICAL FINDINGS
- White matter lesions in the CNS
- Increase in intrafascicular glial cells with myelinlike lipid droplet accumulation
- CNS and spinal cord hypomyelinogenesis
- Endothelial swelling and thrombotic occlusion of the vessels in the placenta

TREATMENT
No effective treatment

MEDICATIONS
None

CONTRAINDICATIONS
N/A

FOLLOW-UP

PATIENT MONITORING
N/A

PREVENTION/AVOIDANCE
- Serology should be performed. Most dams of affected lambs should have high levels of antibody and be immune to further challenge by the same strain of the virus in subsequent pregnancies. Ewes with negative antibody titers may be persistently infected. Blood cultures and examination of skin biopsies by fluorescent antibody tests should be performed on these animals to identify carriers.
- Pregnant noninfected ewes should be kept separated from the rest of the flock for the first 60 days of gestation.
- Infected lambs should be culled from the flock before breeding season.
- There are no approved vaccines for use against border disease virus in the United States. Bovine viral diarrhea vaccines for cattle are not recommended for use in sheep.

POSSIBLE COMPLICATIONS
N/A

EXPECTED COURSE AND PROGNOSIS
Affected lambs that survive the first few months will gradually resolve neurologic signs and fleece abnormalities.

MISCELLANEOUS

ASSOCIATED CONDITIONS
Bovine viral diarrhea (BVD) and hog cholera virus (HCV) are very closely related pestiviruses.

AGE-RELATED FACTORS
Age at time of infection determines clinical signs in the individual.

ZOONOTIC POTENTIAL
N/A

PREGNANCY
Clinical disease or death in lambs is the result of infection of the dam during gestation.

SYNONYMS
Also called hairy shaker and fuzzy lamb disease.

SEE ALSO
Other causes of abortion such as *Salmonella* spp., *Campylobacter* spp., *Chlamydia* spp., *Toxoplasma gondii,* and *Rickettsia* spp. Other neurological conditions such as enzootic ataxia (swayback), bacterial meningoencephalitis, focal symmetrical encephalomalacia, and "daft lamb" disease

ABBREVIATIONS
BDV = bovine diarrhea virus
HCV = hog cholera virus
SN = serum neutralization
RT-PCR = reverse transcription polymerase chain reaction

Suggested Reading
Jones, T. C., Hunt, R. D., King, N. W. 1997. *Border disease of sheep, veterinary pathology.* 6th ed. Baltimore, Maryland: Williams & Wilkins.
Loken, T. 1995, Nov. Border disease in sheep. *Vet Clin North Am Food Anim Pract.* 11(3): 579–95.
Nettleton, P. F., Gilray, J. A., Russo, P., Dlissi, E. 1998, May-Aug. Border disease of sheep and goats. *Vet Res.* 29(3–4): 327–40.
Pratelli, A., Bollo, E., Martella, V., Guarda, F., Chiocco, D., Buonavoglia, C. 1999, Oct. Pestivirus infection in small ruminants: virological and histopathological findings. *New Microbiol.* 22(4): 351–56.
Thur, B., Hilbe, M., Strasser, M., Ehrensperger, F. 1997, Dec. Immunohistochemical diagnosis of pestivirus infection associated with bovine and ovine abortion and perinatal death. *Am J Vet Res.* 58(12): 1371–75.
Vilbek, S., Paton, D. J. 2000, Jul-Aug. A RT-PCR assay for the rapid recognition of border disease virus. *Vet Res.* 31(4): 437–45.

Author: Lisa Nashold

BORNA DISEASE

BASICS

OVERVIEW
• Borna disease is a sporadic, transmissible, progressive encephalitis.
• The virus does not have a direct cytopathic effect.
• Virally infected cells initiate a T cell immune response, which leads to tissue destruction.

SYSTEMS AFFECTED
CNS

GENETICS
N/A

INCIDENCE/PREVALENCE
Unknown

GEOGRAPHIC DISTRIBUTION
• Borna disease was historically endemic to areas of Germany and Switzerland. Confirmed outbreaks of the disease have generally been in middle and eastern Europe and in horses in the Middle East.
• Clinically normal animals have tested positive for the RNA virus responsible for the disease in many areas of the world including the United States.

SIGNALMENT
• Natural infections occur in sheep and horses. Goats and cattle can also be affected.
• BDV has been experimentally transmitted to a wide range of animals including chickens, rabbits, rats, guinea pigs, and monkeys.
• Antibodies have been identified in monkeys, humans, and birds.

SIGNS
• Borna disease is a progressive neurologic disease.
• Initial signs are generally nonspecific and include anorexia, fever, excessive salivation, yawning, and chewing movements.

• Early neurologic signs include hyperesthesia, ataxia, head pressing, head tremors, muscle contractions, and depression.
• Transient signs of irritability, kicking, biting or compulsive movements may occur.
• In later stages of disease, animals may lean against objects or maintain a sawhorse stance. Convulsion or coma is possible.
• Nystagmus is observed in terminal cases.

CAUSES AND RISK FACTORS
• Borna disease virus (BDV) is an enveloped RNA virus from the Flaviviridae family.
• Actively infected, convalescent, and immune carrier animals shed the virus in nasal secretions, saliva, urine, or milk.
• Infection often occurs due to contaminated food and water.
• The virus moves to the CNS by intra-axonal transport via nerves in the nose and throat area.
• Disease outbreaks are more commonly seen in spring and early summer.
• The virus is transmitted between birds by the tick *Hyalomma anatolicum*. An arthropod vector is not necessary for transmission in other species.
• An outbreak of disease in horses in the Middle East was associated with a dense population of infected wild birds.
• Rodents have also been suspected as a source of infection.

DIAGNOSIS

DIFFERENTIAL DIAGNOSIS
• Other encephalopathies such as St. Louis encephalitis or West Nile virus
• Scrapie, bovine spongiform encephalopathy, chronic wasting disease in elk and deer
• Rabies
• Metabolic or digestive disorders—milk fever, nervous ketosis
• CNS tumor
• *Oestrus ovis* infestations in sheep
• Pseudorabies

CBC/BIOCHEMISTRY/URINALYSIS
N/A

OTHER LABORATORY FINDINGS
In some cases, serum and CSF may contain antibodies to BDV.

IMAGING
N/A

DIAGNOSTIC PROCEDURES
Polymerase chain reaction (PCR) viral amplification and in situ hybridization have been used to demonstrate viral RNA in neurons, astrocytes, Schwann cells, and ependymal cells.

PATHOLOGIC FINDINGS

GROSS FINDINGS
No characteristic gross lesions

HISTOPATHOLOGICAL FINDINGS
• Inclusion bodies in neuronal nucleus known as Joest or Joest-Degen bodies are found in ganglion cells of the hippocampus and olfactory lobes of the cerebral cortex. They are considered pathognomonic for Borna disease.
• Other lesions are characteristic of encephalitis including perivascular cuffing, ganglion cell degeneration, and gliosis.
• Neuronophagic nodules may be found.
• Lesions are typically found in gray matter of the cerebral hemispheres and brain stem. The most severe lesions are found in the olfactory bulbs, caudate nucleus, and hippocampus.
• Cerebellum is spared.

TREATMENT

• No specific treatment is available.
• Supportive therapy with mannitol may temporarily relieve cerebral edema. Anti-inflammatory medications may reduce discomfort.

MEDICATIONS
No specific medications

CONTRAINDICATIONS
Appropriate milk and meat withdrawal times must be followed for all compounds administered to food-producing animals.

FOLLOW-UP

PATIENT MONITORING
Surviving animals may have permanent neurological deficits.

PREVENTION/AVOIDANCE
• Animals should not be fed and watered together in large numbers and should be kept separate from horses and cattle.
• Insect and tick control may be helpful.
• Incoming animals should be quarantined for 2 months due to the long incubation period of the disease, and tested twice during this period for the presence of antibodies.
• BDV is resistant to drying and other adverse environmental conditions.

POSSIBLE COMPLICATIONS
N/A

EXPECTED COURSE AND PROGNOSIS
• Unlike other viral encephalitides, the incubation period can vary from 3 weeks to months or possibly years. The average incubation period is usually from 2 to 3 months.
• Duration of clinical illness is normally 1–3 weeks.

• Mortality rates can range from 60% to 95% in animals exhibiting clinical signs.
• Surviving animals may remain permanently neurologically impaired.

MISCELLANEOUS

ASSOCIATED CONDITIONS
• The viruses of Borna disease and near eastern encephalitis are indistinguishable.
• Serologically distinct from the viruses that cause West Nile virus (WNV), eastern equine encephalitis (EEE), western equine encephalitis (WEE), Venezuelan encephalitis (VE)

AGE-RELATED FACTORS
N/A

ZOONOTIC POTENTIAL
BDV antibodies have been found in humans with various neuropsychiatric disorders such as schizophrenia. The actual significance of BDV in these disorders has yet to be determined.

PREGNANCY
N/A

SEE ALSO
Bovine spongiform encephalopathy
Chronic wasting disease in elk and deer
Metabolic or digestive disorders: milk fever, nervous ketosis
Oestrus ovis infestations in sheep
Other encephalopathies such as St. Louis encephalitis or West Nile virus
Pseudorabies
Rabies
Scrapie

ABBREVIATIONS
APHIS = Animal and Plant Health Inspection Service
BDV = Borna disease virus
CNS = central nervous system
CSF = cerebral spinal fluid
EEE = eastern equine encephalitis
PCR = polymerase chain reaction
VEE = Venezuelan equine encephalitis
WEE = western equine encephalitis
WNV = West Nile virus

Suggested Reading
Jones, T. C., Hunt, R. D., King, N.W. 1997. *Borna disease, veterinary pathology.* 6th ed. Baltimore, Maryland: Williams & Wilkins.
Smith, B. 2002. *Borna disease (near eastern encephalitis), large animal internal medicine.* 3rd ed. St. Louis: Mosby.
Timoney, J. F., Gillespie, J. H., Scott, F.W., Barlough, J. E., ed. 1992. Borna disease. In: *Hagan and Bruner's microbiology and infectious diseases of domestic animals.* 8th ed. Cornell University, Ithaca, NY: Comstock Publishing Associates a division of Cornell University Press.
USDA. 2002. Sept. *Borna disease, factsheet.* Riverdale, Maryland: APHIS, Veterinary Services.

Author: Lisa Nashold

BOTULISM

BASICS

OVERVIEW
• Toxins produced by the bacteria *Clostridium botulinum* cause botulism.
• There are eight botulinum toxins produced by the bacteria. These toxins are antigenically distinct toxins and identified as types A, B, C_1, C_2, D, E, F, and G. Each of these toxins is found in different environments and affect different species of animals.
• Botulinum toxin types B, C, and D are the most common toxins to cause toxicity in cattle.

PATHOPHYSIOLOGY
• Intoxication by *Clostridium botulinum* is primarily by ingestion of the preformed toxin in a contaminated feed source. Spoiled oat, rye, and barley silage and hay are common sources for type B botulinum intoxication.
• The ingestion of poultry litter containing bird parts or the ingestion of other forages contaminated with toxin-ladened animal parts is a source for type C botulinum toxin.
• Type D botulinum intoxication is common in phosphorus-deficient areas where toxin-contaminated bones are ingested. The ingestion of contaminated water (usually type C and D botulinum toxin) from nutrient-rich ponds has also been a source of intoxication.
• Wound infections can also lead to botulinum intoxication but is rare in ruminants.

SYSTEMS AFFECTED
• Ingestion of preformed toxin is the usual means of intoxication of ruminates.
• The toxin is absorbed by the intestines and distributed to the nerves that innervate the muscles (neuromuscular junction).
• The toxin attaches to the nerve and is incorporated into the cytoplasm where it acts as a metaloprotease that inactivates proteins needed to release the neurotransmitter acetylcholine.

INCIDENCE/PREVALENCE
• With modern production processes, the potential for animals ingesting toxin-laden food sources can occur, resulting in catastrophic consequences to the affected herd.

• Areas of the world where intoxication is a fairly common occurrence and is considered an endemic problem include Australia, South Africa, and South America.

GEOGRAPHIC DISTRIBUTION
The various botulinum toxins tend to have a unique geographical area of the world. *Clostridium botulinum* type B is commonly found in Europe and the eastern United States. *Clostridium botulinum* type C is commonly found in the western United States. *Clostridium botulinum* type D is commonly found in South Africa, South America, and Australia.

SIGNALMENT
• Most cases involve adult or young growing animals.
• Cattle are extremely sensitive to the toxins. Cattle have been determined to be 12.88 times more sensitive to botulinum toxin type C on a kilogram basis than the mouse. The median toxic dose for botulinum toxin type C in lactating dairy cows is 0.38 ng/kg.

SIGNS
• The rapidity of development of clinical signs depends on the amount of toxin ingested.
• Clinical signs develop usually between 48 and 72 hours after ingestion, but may appear as early as 24 hours and as late as 10–14 days after ingestion.
• Animals first appear to be constipated with dry feces and may seem uneasy on their feet. Over the next 24 to 48 hours, the animals become weaker with staggering and muscle fasciculation of large muscle groups. Animals will lean against fences and walls for support. When lying down they will remain in sternal recumbency.
• On clinical examination, the animals will usually lose tail tone with the tail easily handled and elevated. Animals lose tongue tone. An animal will remain alert and actively try to eat but cannot chew properly resulting in food being dropped from the mouth. The lack of tongue control causes the animal to be unable to clean its nose resulting in a dirty dry nose. Some animals will drool. When drinking water, the animal may stick its nose down deep into the water trough to get a drink.
• Labored abdominal breathing is usually seen in animals late in the course of the intoxication.

CAUSES AND RISK FACTORS
• Ingestion of spoiled hay or silage made from oats, barley, or rye is a common cause of intoxication for botulinum toxin type B.
• Ingestion of contaminated animal parts in hay, silage, or poultry litter is a common cause in botulinum toxin type C intoxication.
• In phosphorus-deficient areas of the world, ingestion of toxin-contaminated bones are a common source of intoxication particularly for type D botulinum toxin.
• Ingestion of water from shallow, warm, nutrient-rich ponds has been implicated in the intoxication of some animals.

DIAGNOSIS

DIFFERENTIAL DIAGNOSIS
Diagnosis of botulism can be difficult and is usually one of exclusion of other causes.
• Hypocalcemia, hypomagnesemia, and hypokalemia should be ruled out. However, there is a decreased chance of an acute outbreak involving multiple animals with a deficiency of calcium, magnesium, or potassium.
• Monensin and other ionophore toxicities can cause cardiac and skeletal muscle lesions leading to weakness in the animals.
• Gossypol toxicity can cause cardiac problems leading to weakness in the animals.
• Organophosphate and carbamate toxicity due to interference with neurotransmitters
• Chlorinated hydrocarbon (organochlorine insecticides) interferes with sodium and potassium channels leading to weakness, tremors, ataxia, and salivation.

CBC/BIOCHEMISTRY/ URINALYSIS
CBC and blood chemistries should be normal in affected animals.

DIAGNOSTIC PROCEDURES
• Confirmation of a positive case of botulinum intoxication can be difficult.
• Feed samples from the previous 2 to 5 days should be immediately evaluated for botulinum toxin contamination.
• Animal samples to submit for botulinum toxin testing are serum, liver, rumen content, and cecal content. The testing procedure usually performed is the mouse protection bioassay. However, agar immunodiffusion testing and ELISA testing for the toxin can also be performed.

• Bacterial culturing of fresh rumen and cecal content from animals immediately euthanized or freshly dead for *Clostridium botulinum* organism can also aid in a diagnosis.
• The finding of preformed toxin in any of the feed or tissues submitted and/or the finding of *Clostridium botulinum* organisms present in the fresh rumen or cecal content suggests that the animal was intoxicated by botulinum toxin.

PATHOLOGIC FINDINGS

GROSS FINDINGS
• Gross lesions are few. No histopathologic lesions are noted.
• The rumen may have a decreased fill of forage and forage in the rumen may be dry due to the animal's inability to swallow and drink water.

 TREATMENT

APPROPRIATE HEALTH CARE
• The toxin is long acting and can affect the animal for several weeks, which makes treatment difficult.
• Treatment is mainly supportive with the animal receiving fluids for dehydration and hand-feeding to maintain the animal's caloric intake. Animals must remain in sternal recumbency or bloat will occur. Animals should be made to move and rise to prevent crush injuries to large muscle groups.
• The treatment of cattle with a pentavalent antitoxin has been of little success and is expensive.
• Avoid antimicrobials that potentiate muscle weakness (aminoglycosides, tetracycline, procaine penicillin)
• In some areas of the world, vaccination of cattle with a toxoid for types B, C, and D botulinum toxin has been successful in preventing outbreaks.

CLIENT EDUCATION
• The most common source of intoxication is through feed.
• Insure ensiled feed (e.g., rye, oat, and barley silage and hay) has been fermented correctly. No animal parts are present in the feed.

 MEDICATIONS

CONTRAINDICATIONS
• Avoid aminoglycosides, tetracycline, and procaine penicillin for treatment of wounds since these can potentiate muscle weakness.
• Appropriate milk and meat withdrawal times must be followed for all compounds administered to food-producing animals.

 FOLLOW-UP

PATIENT MONITORING
• Monitor cattle for dehydration and bloating. Keep animals in sternal recumbency so that bloat will not occur.
• Watch for muscle damage in recumbent animals.

PREVENTION/AVOIDANCE
Clients need to insure that silage is properly fermented and no animal parts are inadvertently incorporated into hay or feed.

EXPECTED COURSE AND PROGNOSIS
The prognosis is poor in most affected animals. Prolonged and intense supportive care is often needed lasting several weeks to months.

 MISCELLANEOUS

ASSOCIATED CONDITIONS
N/A

AGE-RELATED FACTORS
Most cases involve adult or young growing animals.

ZOONOTIC POTENTIAL
• Since this is an intracellular toxin bound to the nerves, the chance of individuals working with affected animals becoming intoxicated is minimal. Affected animals should be disposed of by burial or rendering.
• Animals should not be sent to slaughter for human consumption.
• No evidence of milk contamination with the toxin from intoxicated cows has been identified.

PREGNANCY
N/A

RUMINANT SPECIES AFFECTED
Cattle, sheep, and goats are most commonly affected.

BIOSECURITY
N/A

PRODUCTION MANAGEMENT
Insure ensiled feed (e.g., rye, oat, and barley silage and hay) has been fermented correctly. No animal parts are present in the feed.

SYNONYMS
Bulbar paralysis
Lamziekte
Loin disease

SEE ALSO
Chlorinated hydrocarbon (organochlorine insecticides)
Gossypol toxicity
Hypocalcemia
Hypokalemia
Hypomagnesemia
Monensin and other ionophore organophosphate and carbamate toxicity

ABBREVIATIONS
N/A

Suggested Reading
Galey, F. D., Terra, R., Walker, R., Adaska, J., Etchebarne, M. A., Puschner, B., Fisher, E., Whitlock, R. H., Rocke, T., Willoughby, D., Tor, E. 2000. Type C botulism in dairy cattle from feed contaminated with a dead cat. *J Vet Diagn Invest*. 12(3):204–9.
Kelch, W. J., Kerr, L. A., Pringle, J. K., Rohrbach, B. W., Whitlock, R. H. 2000. Fatal *Clostridium botulinum* toxicosis in eleven Holstein cattle fed round bale barley haylage. *J Vet Diagn Invest*. 12(5):453–55
Martin, S. 2003. *Clostridium botulinum* type D intoxication in a dairy herd in Ontario. *Can Vet J*. 44(6):493–95.
Moeller, R. B., Jr., Puschner, B., Walker, R. L., Rocke, T., Galey, F. D., Cullor, J. S., Ardans, A. A. 2003. Determination of the median toxic dose of type C botulinum toxin in lactating dairy cows. *J Vet Diagn Invest*. 15(6):523–26.

Author: Robert B. Moeller, Jr.

BOVINE EPHEMERAL FEVER

BASICS

OVERVIEW
Bovine ephemeral fever (BEF) is a seasonal, arthropod-transmitted, viral disease of cattle and water buffalo that occurs in the subtropics or temperate regions of Africa, Australia, and Asia.

SIGNALMENT
• BEF is a seasonal disease whose severity varies from year to year and region to region. Epidemics may occur periodically and are characterized by rapid onset within days or a few weeks of many animals in a region.
• Ephemeral fever is most prevalent in the wet season in the tropics and in summer to early autumn in the subtropics or temperate regions when conditions favor the presence of biting arthropods. BEF disappears abruptly in winter.
• Morbidity may be as high as 80%; overall mortality is usually 1–2%, although it is higher in well-conditioned cattle (10–20%).

SIGNS
• The clinical signs occur suddenly and vary in severity. They include biphasic or polyphasic fever, shivering, inappetence, lacrimation, serous nasal discharge, drooling, dyspnea, atony of the fore stomachs, depression, stiffness and lameness, and a sudden decrease in milk yield. Cattle may also become recumbent and paralyzed for 8 hr to > 1 wk.
• After recovery, milk production often fails to return to normal levels until the next lactation.
• Abortion, with total loss of the season's lactation, occurs in ~5% of cows pregnant in months 8 and 9 of the last trimester.

• Bulls, market cattle, and heavily producing dairy cows are the most severely affected, but even so, spontaneous recovery usually occurs within a few days.

CAUSES AND RISK FACTORS
• The disease is caused by ephemeral fever virus, a Rhabdovirus (single-stranded, negative sense RNA in the same family as rabies virus).
• The virus can be mechanically transmitted by IV inoculation of blood from infected viremic cattle to susceptible cattle. The virus has been recovered from some *Culicoides* (biting midge) and mosquito species (*Anopheles* and *Culicine* spp.) collected in the field and has been shown to multiply in *Culicoides* and *Culex* mosquitoes in the laboratory. The role of the insect in mechanical transmission has not been established.
• Transmission by contact or fomites does not occur, and the virus does not appear to persist in recovered cattle.

DIAGNOSIS

DIFFERENTIAL DIAGNOSIS
Parturient paresis (milk fever, hypocalcemia) is an afebrile disease of mature dairy cows that occurs most commonly within 72 hours of parturition. The clinical signs progress through three stages: Stage 1, changes in attitude (i.e., hypersensitivity and excitability); Stage 2, generalized paresis; Stage 3, circulatory collapse, coma, and death.

CBC/BIOCHEMISTRY/URINALYSIS
Clinical cases have a neutrophilia with bands.

OTHER LABORATORY TESTS
Viral serum neutralization, complement fixation, and the blocking ELISA tests are used for serology. Virus isolation can also be done but isolation usually requires mouse inoculation.

IMAGING
N/A

DIAGNOSTIC PROCEDURES
• Diagnosis of BEF is usually based on history and clinical signs (rapid onset of febrile signs for 2–5 days with spontaneous recovery).
• The clinical outbreak is confirmed by serology in paired serum samples collected during illness and 2–3 weeks later with a fourfold rise in antibodies.

PATHOLOGIC FINDINGS
• The gross lesions of BEF include polyserositis affecting joint, pleural, and peritoneal surfaces. Some lung edema is evident, atelectasis, cellulitis, and focal necrosis of skeletal muscle. The lymph nodes are edematous.
• The histological findings include neutrophilia, leukocytosis, and high fibrinogen deposition.
• Hemosiderosis of the lymph nodes and spleen from loss of erythrocytes early in infection has been observed.
• The venules and capillaries of the tendon sheath, synovial membranes, muscle, and fascia have perivascular neutrophilic infiltration, focal or complete necrosis of vessel walls, thrombosis, and perivascular fibrosis.

BOVINE EPHEMERAL FEVER

TREATMENT

• Complete rest is the most effective treatment, and recovering animals should not be stressed or worked because relapse is likely.
• Isotonic fluids can be administered IV to treat dehydration. Oral dosing should be avoided unless the swallowing reflex is functional.

MEDICATIONS

DRUGS OF CHOICE

• Anti-inflammatory drugs can be given early and in repeated doses for 2–3 days.
• IV or subcutaneous administration of calcium borogluconate has been found to be beneficial in some animals.
• Antibiotics can be administered to prevent secondary bacterial infections.

CONTRAINDICATIONS

During acute illness, no oral therapy should be given to avoid inhalation pneumonia due to the inability of the animal to swallow.

PRECAUTIONS/POSSIBLE INTERACTIONS

Appropriate milk and meat withdrawal times must be followed for all compounds administered.

ALTERNATIVE DRUGS

N/A

FOLLOW-UP

PATIENT MONITORING

• Animals should be encouraged to stand within 2–5 days. The animals should be rolled over several times a day to help avoid loss of circulation to the underside limbs, which will result in permanent muscle damage.

• The heavier the animal is, the more critical it is to get it back on its feet as quickly as possible.

PREVENTION/AVOIDANCE

A modified live vaccine is available that confers good protection. An inactivated vaccine is also available but it gives only 6 months of protection.

POSSIBLE COMPLICATIONS

Pneumonia, mastitis, hind limb paralysis, abnormal gait, abortion in late pregnancy, and temporary (up to 6 months) infertility in bulls

EXPECTED COURSE AND PROGNOSIS

A complete recovery occurs in 95–97% of cases. BEF virus infection confers life-long immunity to cattle.

MISCELLANEOUS

ASSOCIATED CONDITIONS

Pneumonia, mastitis, hind limb paralysis, abnormal gait, abortion in late pregnancy

AGE-RELATED FACTORS

N/A

ZOONOTIC POTENTIAL

N/A

PREGNANCY

Infection in the last trimester can result in abortion.

RUMINANT SPECIES AFFECTED

Bovine and water buffalo

BIOSECURITY

The virus cannot be spread by direct animal-to-animal contact. However, it can be spread from infected animals to susceptible animals by injection, so single-use needles should be used.

PRODUCTION MANAGEMENT

N/A

SYNONYMS

Bovine epizootic fever
Dengue fever of cattle
Lazy man's disease
Stiff sickness
Three day fever
Three day sickness

SEE ALSO

Abnormal gait and abortion in late pregnancy
Hind limb paralysis
Mastitis
Parturient paresis
Pneumonia

ABBREVIATIONS

BEF = bovine ephemeral fever
ELISA = enzyme-linked immunosorbent assay
IV = intravenous

Suggested Reading
Kirkland, P. D. 2002, Nov. Akabane and bovine ephemeral fever virus infections. *Vet Clin North Am Food Anim Pract*. 18(3): 501–14.
Nandi, S., Negi, B. S. 1999, Apr. Bovine ephemeral fever: a review. *Comp Immunol Microbiol Infect Dis*. 22(2): 81–91.
NSW Department of Primary Industries/Agriculture. Bovine ephemeral fever: three-day fever. May 18, 2001. Agfact A0.9.50 (first edition) http://www.agric.nsw. gov.au/reader/cattlehealth/a0950.htm

Author: Christopher C. L. Chase

BOVINE LAMENESS

BASICS

DEFINITION
Lameness is an alteration of gait. Clinically affected cattle are reluctant to move and may spend a great proportion of the day lying down. The affected limb typically has reduced contact time. Cattle will preferentially stand in such a manner that the affected limb bears little weight.

SYSTEMS AFFECTED
Musculoskeletal

GENETICS
N/A

INCIDENCE/PREVALENCE
N/A

GEOGRAPHIC DISTRIBUTION
Potentially worldwide depending on environment

SIGNALMENT
Species
Bovine

Breed Predilections
N/A

Mean Age and Range
N/A

Predominant Sex
N/A

General Considerations
• Lameness is one of the most costly diseases of dairy cattle. Only mastitis and reproductive failure have greater economic impact.
• The vast majority of lameness can be localized to the hind limb.
• The vast majority of lameness in cattle is associated with hoof lesions.
• The vast majority of hoof lesions in the hind limb are located in the lateral claw.
• Hoof lesions are typically bilaterally symmetrical. Similar lesions are present in the right and left hoof.
• With the exception of interdigital cellulitis, parenteral antibiotics have little benefit in most lame cows.

DIAGNOSIS

DIFFERENTIAL DIAGNOSES
• Laminitis: acute laminitis, chronic laminitis, septic white line disease, horizontal hoof cracks, thimbles
• Sole ulcers

• Sole abscesses
• Corkscrew claw
• Interdigital cellulitis (foot rot)
• Digital dermatitis (heel warts)
• Heel erosions
• Vertical hoof cracks, sand cracks
• Interdigital fibroma

LAMINITIS
Definition
An inflammatory process that disrupts the junction of sensitive and insensitive lamina of the hoof. Acute disease will often cause permanent changes in hoof structure, which predispose to other hoof lameness.
• *Acute laminitis*—Clinical signs include hemorrhage at the white line, warm foot, softening of the coronary band, and prominent digital pulses. It is often difficult to localize the lesion to a specific hoof and most patients are lame in multiple hooves. Concrete floors accentuate gait abnormality. Hind limbs may be drawn under the body in an attempt to shift weight off the front feet
• *Chronic laminitis*—Loss of normal white line structure permits widening of white line and altered hoof angle and a loss of parallelism with P3. The toe becomes abnormally long. Weight is shifted onto heel and off of toe, potentiating abnormal hoof growth. The hoof wall often has raised horizontal ridges or rings; in severe cases horizontal fissures or thimbles may be present
• *Septic white line disease*—junction of sensitive and insensitive lamina is compromised and may separate permitting debris and infection to dissect along white line. Severe cases may have draining tracts erupt from coronary band.
• Diagnosis based on physical examination, radiographs rarely performed to document rotation of P3 and altered hoof angle

Cause
• Subclinical or clinical grain engorgement—a single episode can permanently disrupt laminar growth and integrity; grain engorgement is typically occult/subclinical in dairy and feedlot cattle; repetitive episodes will potentiate lesions and abnormalities; cattle with grossly abnormal hoof growth usually do not have clinical signs of acute laminitis; specific dietary causes include high proportions of easily fermented carbohydrates and short dietary fiber length.
• Septicemia—common primary causes include metritis, mastitis, peritonitis, and pneumonia.
• Trauma—heat (use of power sander on hooves), concrete floors

Treatment
• *Acute laminitis*—treat underlying diseases (septicemia or grain engorgement), place cows on softer surface (dirt vs. concrete) for 5 to 7 days, and administer nonsteroidal anti-inflammatory agents (flunixin meglumine).
• *Chronic laminitis*—perform corrective hoof trimming. Preferentially shorten the toe, altering the hoof angle. Remove all infected, underrun or unattached hoof.

Prevention/Management
• Dairy—limit concentrates to a maximum of 60% of diet. Insure adequate long-stem fiber in the diet. Screen total mixed rations on a routine basis to assess proportionate fiber length of feed. Monitor rumen pH to screen for subclinical grain engorgement. Consider inclusion of buffers in diet. Increase frequency of feeding. Eliminate component feeding. Provide routine hoof trimming. Recognize that a degree of laminitis is "normal" in dairy cows.
• Beef—attempt to limit frequency of severe disease. If possible and economical, adopt slow transition to high (>90%) concentrate diets. Consider inclusion of dietary ionophores and provide access to more comfortable footing.

SOLE ABSCESSES
Definition
Abscesses located at the junction of sensitive and insensitive lamina.

Cause
This disease occurs when sensitive (living) tissues are exposed by a penetrating wound or separation of the white line (laminitis). Lesions are most common on the lateral claw of the hind foot. Structure of hoof wall limits drainage and host's ability to clear infections.

Clinical Signs and Diagnosis
Infection dissects along the junction of sensitive and insensitive tissues forming a circumscribed abscess covered by a "false sole." The history often includes fluctuating degree of lameness. Enclosed abscesses produce pressure and severe lameness. Drainage to the exterior will often cause short-term dramatic improvement in gait. Untreated infection may eventually involve deeper tissue (P3, navicular bone, flexor tendons, coffin joint, etc.), and cause irreparable damage.

Treatment
Pare out abscesses and underrun areas completely. If deep, sensitive tissues need to be debrided, consider a Baer block (distal intravenous anesthesia). Affix a wooden block

to the unaffected digit making the lesion non–weight bearing. Lesions are typically not bandaged. If deep tissues are infected, consider soaking the foot one to two times a day for 10–15 minutes. Soak solutions typically contain betadine and Epsom salts ($MgSO_4$). Simple uncomplicated lesions do not require antibiotic therapy.

Prevention
Prevention of laminitis and trauma, routine hoof trimming

SOLE ULCERS (RUSTERHOLTZ ULCER, PODODERMATITIS CIRCUMSCRIPTA)

Clinical Signs and Diagnosis
• Sole ulcers are typically located at the juncture of the sole and heel on the lateral claw of the hind foot.
• Lesions typically consist of a circular defect in the sensitive layers of the sole with a mass of proliferative granulation tissue protruding through the defect. An intact sheet of insensitive sole typically covers early lesions. Later lesions may have a defect in the wall of the sole.
• The cause, origin, and pathogenesis of this disease are unknown. Postulated causes include laminitis, frostbite, and conformational defects.

Treatment
Excise sole wall overlying the defect in sensitive hoof wall and expose the defect in sensitive hoof wall. Remove the proliferative granulation tissue. Apply mild cautery or administer local treatment of lesions with compounds that kill living tissue (10% formaldehyde). Affix a wooden block to the unaffected digit making the lesion non–weight bearing.

Prevention
Design of specific preventative programs is difficult given unknown etiology. Routine hoof trimming recommended in dairy cattle.

CORKSCREW CLAW (SCREWCLAW)

Definition/Clinical Description
Corkscrew claw is an excessive growth of the abaxial wall of either the lateral hoof of the hind foot (most common) or medial claw of the front foot, which curves under the ventral surface of hoof. This growth pattern causes the toe to not bear weight. Long toes and an altered hoof angle usually accompany the rolling of the hoof wall.
Additionally, infected heel cracks and sole ulcers are commonly seen in cattle with screwclaw.

Cause
The conformation of cattle seems to predispose some beef cattle to this disorder. Affected beef cattle are usually heavily muscled with a wide rump. These cattle stand with their hind limbs abnormally close together and preferentially bear weight on the abaxial aspect of the lateral claw. Laminitis and preexisting damage to the hoof wall or coronary band are probably important predisposing causes.

Treatment
Corrective hoof trimming is the most appropriate treatment. Aggressive shortening of the affected abaxial hoof wall. Hoof trimming should provide a flat solar surface, which is perpendicular to abaxial hoof wall.

Prevention
Farmers should consider selection of breeding stock (especially bulls) for proper hoof conformation. The practitioner may consider aggressive corrective hoof trimming of young actively growing animals (less than 18 months of age). This procedure will force proper placement of feet, permitting animals to grow into a structure or conformation, which permits flat placement of hoof. Although this procedure may improve the health and survival of individual animals, it may mask conformational defects, which may have a genetic component.

INTERDIGITAL CELLULITIS (FOOT ROT, INTERDIGITAL PHLEGMON)

Definition
Infection of the skin and subcutaneous tissues of the interdigital cleft

Cause
Primary etiologic agent is *Fusobacterium necrophorum*, a gram-negative anaerobe. Trauma and abrasions of the interdigital skin are important predisposing factors.

Clinical Signs and Diagnosis
• Has the appearance of a wound with gray, devitalized edges. Lesion has a foul, necrotic odor characteristic of anaerobic infections. The foot dorsal to the coronary band is often swollen, warm, and erythematous.
• Untreated disease or delayed treatment may result in deeper tissues being affected and cause irreparable damage.

Treatment
• Optimal treatment is systemic antibiotics. Common treatments include long-acting oxytetracycline (20 mg/kg IM) and procaine penicillin G (20,000 IU/kg IM). Some dairy clients will treat with ceftiofur (1–2 mg/kg) because this does not necessitate milk withholding. The author finds this treatment less efficacious.
• Topical therapy is less effective and unreliable.

Contraindications
Appropriate milk and meat withdrawal times must be followed for all compounds administered to food-producing animals.

Prevention
Avoid traumatic footing and irregular flooring surfaces like frozen mud, gravel, or grain stubble. Consider use of trace-mineralized salt containing organic iodine compounds.

DIGITAL DERMATITIS (HEEL WARTS, HAIRY HEEL WARTS)

Definition
A warty to verrucous lesion located on the bulbs of the heels or the caudal interdigital cleft

Cause
Disease appears to be caused by an as yet unnamed spirochete bacterium. Organism functions as a contagious pathogen and is readily passed among cattle in a herd. This disease is very common in dairy cattle and seen occasionally in beef cattle.

Clinical Signs and Diagnosis
• Lesions vary in appearance from warty and verrucous lesions to a raw, circumscribed granulation bed surrounded by a white to gray skin edge. Long hairlike fibrils often protrude from lesions.
• Lesions are confined to areas of haired skin and typically spare the hoof wall. These lesions are very painful when palpated.

Treatment
Large lesions should be debrided. Application of topical tetracycline or lincocin with or without bandages is effective. Dairy herds often spray the bulbs of the heel with topical antibiotic to either treat lesions or limit their severity.

Contraindications
Appropriate milk and meat withdrawal times must be followed for all compounds administered to food-producing animals.

BOVINE LAMENESS

Prevention
• Herds free of digital dermatitis should practice strict biosecurity to prevent introduction of the agent.
• Providing dry environment seems to limit the spread and severity of lesions. In endemically infected herds farmers may spray the bulbs of the heel with topical antibiotics to limit lesion severity. A vaccine is available; however, its efficacy has not been documented in controlled clinical trials.
• Farriers and hoof trimmers should disinfect hoof tools after treating affected cattle.

HEEL EROSIONS (SLURRY HEEL, HEEL CRACKS)

Clinical Signs and Diagnosis
• Deep erosive cracks that originate from the junction of heel and sole on the axial surface of hoof and extend caudally through the heel at a 45-degree angle.
• These lesions may extend as deep as the sensitive tissue and may become infected, dissecting cranial and caudal under the surface of the sole and heel.
• Lesions typically are present on both the medial and lateral claw of both hind feet. Lesions are predisposed by wet conditions and preexisting chronic laminitis.

Treatment
Completely pare out lesions. Consider corrective hoof trimming with particular emphasis on shortening the toe, which will shift weight off the heels and onto the toes. Affix a wooden block to the normal digit if only one claw is affected.

Prevention
Implement routine hoof trimming in dairy cattle. Avoid excessively wet conditions. Management of the diet to prevent laminitis.

VERTICAL HOOF CRACKS (SAND CRACKS)

Clinical Signs and Diagnosis
• Vertical cracks are typically located on the anterior to anterior-lateral surface of the hoof. They are most common on the front feet.
• Lesions are more common in beef cattle than dairy cattle. The underlying hoof wall is greatly thickened.
• Cracks that do not extend to the coronary band rarely cause lameness. Hoof wall adjacent to the crack may become underrun. In some instances, granulation tissue may protrude through the crack.
• Dry conditions and firm, hard footing may predispose, but the exact cause is unknown.

Treatment
• Pare out fissure (crack) completely. Thin (grind) hoof wall over and to either side of the fissure. This procedure will make that portion of the hoof non–weight bearing and shift weight onto the sole of the hoof. This procedure will limit flexing of hoof wall and coronary band, providing nearly immediate pain relief in many cattle.
• Normal hoof wall will grow out at a rate of approximately one-fourth inch/month. Replacement of entire edge of the hoof will require a minimum of 1 year. Repetitive hoof trimming may be needed to insure the affected portion of the hoof remains non–weight bearing.
• Protruding granulation tissue should be removed and its regrowth limited by topical application of 10% formaldehyde.

Prevention
Unknown

INTERDIGITAL FIBROMA (CORNS)
Proliferation of fibrous connective tissue and skin in the interdigital space. Most corns do not cause lameness. Corns that are not infected and not in contact with the ground rarely cause gait abnormalities. One should be careful not to attribute lameness to corns and miss other problems, which may cause irreversible damage if not treated. Laxity of intercornual ligaments probably predisposes.

Treatment
Surgical resection of corn

MISCELLANEOUS

ASSOCIATED CONDITIONS
N/A

AGE-RELATED FACTORS
N/A

ZOONOTIC POTENTIAL
N/A

PREGNANCY
N/A

RUMINANT SPECIES AFFECTED
Potentially, all ruminant species are affected.

BIOSECURITY
N/A

PRODUCTION MANAGEMENT
N/A

SYNONYMS
Corkscrew claw (screwclaw)
Digital dermatitis (heel warts, hairy heel warts)
Heel erosions (slurry heel, heel cracks)
Interdigital cellulitis (foot rot, interdigital phlegmon)
Interdigital fibroma (corns)
Sole ulcers (Rusterholtz ulcer, pododermatitis circumscripta)
Vertical hoof cracks (sand cracks)

SEE ALSO
Acute laminitis
Chronic laminitis
Corkscrew claw
Digital dermatitis (heel warts)
Heel erosions
Horizontal hoof cracks
Interdigital cellulitis (foot rot)
Interdigital fibroma
Laminitis
Sand cracks
Septic white line disease
Sole abscesses
Sole ulcers
Thimbles
Vertical hoof cracks

ABBREVIATIONS
IM = intramuscular

Suggested Reading
Blowey, R. 1992, Mar. Diseases of the bovine digit. Part 1: Description of common lesions. *Practice*. 14(2):85–90.
Leach, K. A., Logue, D. N., Randall, J. M., Kempson, S. A. 1998, Jan. Claw lesions in dairy cattle: methods for assessment of sole and white line lesions. *Vet J*. 155(1): 91–102.
Offer, J. E., Logue, D. N., Offer, N. W., Marsden, M. 2004, Jan. The effect of concentrate composition on lameness and hoof health in dairy cows. *Vet J*. 167(1): 111–13.
Raber, M., Lischer, Ch. J., Geyer, H., Ossent, P. 2004, May. The bovine digital cushion—a descriptive anatomical study. *Vet J*. 167(3): 258–64.
van Amstel, S. R., Shearer, J. K., Palin, F. L. 2004, Mar. Moisture content, thickness, and lesions of sole horn associated with thin soles in dairy cattle. *J Dairy Sci*. 87(3): 757–63.

Author: Jeffrey W. Tyler

BASICS

DEFINITION
Bovine leukemia is a term used for two hematopoietic oncogenic diseases: sporadic bovine leukosis (SBL), which does not have an infectious cause, and enzootic bovine leukemia (EBL), a disease caused by a retrovirus, bovine leukemia virus (BLV).

PATHOPHYSIOLOGY
• Four clinical syndromes are recognized: calf, thymic, skin, and adult. The first three syndromes are called sporadic bovine leukosis because there is no evidence for the etiology.
• The adult form, enzootic bovine leukosis (EBL), is caused by infection of B cells with the bovine leukosis virus (BLV).
• BLV infections are lifelong infections. Thirty percent of the animals develop elevated lymphocyte counts (lymphocytosis). The development of solid tumors (lymphomas) from BLV occurs in a small percentage of animals.
• There is no relationship between lymphocytosis and the progression to lymphomas.
• Over 50% of the lymphomas contain a mutation in the p53 tumor suppression gene. These lymphomas develop most frequently in the lymph nodes, abomasum, heart, spleen, kidneys, uterus, spine, and retrobulbar lymphatic tissue.

SYSTEMS AFFECTED
Lymphoreticular system, skin

GENETICS
• There is a genetic component to BLV susceptibility.
• Cattle with the major histocompatibility complex allotype, BoLA-w8, have been shown at higher risk of being seropositive.
• The BoLA-DA12.3 allotype is prone to increased persistent lymphocytosis (increased numbers of B cells), while the BoLA DA7 allotype is resistant to lymphocytosis.

INCIDENCE/PREVALANCE
• The three syndromes of sporadic bovine leukosis are very rare and usually occur in animals less than 2 years of age.
• Seroprevalence to BLV, the causative agent of EBL, varies from 0%–100% by herd. In 1996, 89% of dairy herds and 43.5% of dairy cows in the United States were BLV seropositive. In 1997, a survey of beef herds showed that 38% of all beef operations and 10.3% of all beef cows were BLV seropositive.
• The development of EBL following a BLV infection is a rare event.
• The incidence of animals developing EBL (leukemia/lymphosarcoma) varies among herds with the average annual incidence in infected cattle estimated to be 0.3%–1.0%.
• Most animals that develop EBL are >2 years of age with peak incidence at 5–8 years of age.

GEOGRAPHIC DISTRIBUTION
• Sporadic bovine leukosis occurs worldwide.
• The geographic distribution of enzootic bovine leukosis is also worldwide but is dependent on the distribution of BLV. North and South America, Eastern Europe, Russia, and portions of Australia are BLV-endemic areas.

SIGNALMENT
• SBL is a disease mainly of young cattle.
• Three SBL syndromes are recognized: calf, thymic, and skin. The calf form usually appears in animals <6 months old and results in generalized proliferation of lymph nodes, liver, spleen, and bone marrow and in lymphoblastic leukemia in about 50% of the animals. The thymic form occurs at 6–30 months of age and the primary neoplasm involves the thymus although lymph nodes and other organs can be affected also. Skin lymphosarcoma form is extremely rare. This syndrome has cutaneous tumors that spontaneously disappear and the animal appears healthy. The syndrome is usually only temporary and the skin tumors reappear along with lymphoid tumors in other tissues. All three SBL syndromes are usually fatal.

• BLV infections are asymptomatic and can be recognized only by a serological test that detects BLV antibody. Animals become seropositive 4–12 weeks after exposure.
• Persistent lymphocytosis develops in ~30% of infected cattle, but this lymphocytosis is not associated with any clinical signs of disease.
• EBL occurs in 0.3–1.0% of BLV-infected animals. These animals will have enlarged superficial lymph nodes (retropharyngeal, mandibular, prescapular, subiliac, mammary) that are two to three times larger than normal size with no signs of inflammation. Lymphomas will infiltrate and affect the function of the abomasum, heart, spleen, kidneys, uterus, spine, and eyes [retrobulbar lymphatic tumor (exophthalmia)].
• The clinical signs may include weight loss, decreased milk production, loss of appetite, rear-limb weakness, fever, protruding eyeballs, gastrointestinal obstruction, and heart failure. These animals frequently suffer from anemia.
• Pregnant animals develop more rapid symptoms probably due to the immunosuppression associated with pregnancy.
• The lymphoma form of EBL is always fatal.

CAUSES
• There are no known etiological agents for SBL.
• Bovine leukemia virus, a C-type retrovirus, causes EBL. Retroviruses are enveloped, single-stranded RNA viruses. They integrate their genes into the B lymphocytes and the cattle are infected for life. This virus is highly cell associated and does not survive well outside the host.

RISK FACTORS
• Transmission of BLV occurs primarily by transfer of blood lymphocytes between animals. The use of common bleeding needles and surgical equipment (tattoo pliers, dehorners, castration knives, etc.) without proper disinfection are the most common mechanisms of transmission.

BOVINE LEUKEMIA

• Rectal palpation with a common sleeve is another high-risk practice.
• Virus is rarely present in nasal secretions, saliva, urine, or semen, except when those fluids are contaminated by blood or cellular exudate.
• Insects may act as mechanical vectors of blood. BLV can be transmitted to fetuses in utero, but usually <10% of calves from infected dams carry the virus at birth.
• When embryos from cows infected with BLV are transferred to BLV-negative cows, the calves produced are routinely free of infection.
• Transmission of BLV to calves through colostrum or milk can occur but is rare because of the presence of BLV colostral antibody.

DIAGNOSIS

DIFFERENTIAL DIAGNOSIS
• Other tumors can be differentiated only by histology.
• Lumpy jaw caused by *Actinomyces bovis* causes hard swellings on the jaw and neck. These infections usually have some areas filled with purulent material and some of the abscesses may have already drained and may not have purulent material.

CBC/BIOCHEMISTRY/URINALYSIS
• Persistent lymphocytosis (PL), identified as absolute lymphocytosis in two consecutive complete blood counts obtained 3 months apart, occurs in approximately 30% of BLV-infected cattle.
• Circulating lymphocytes can be morphologically normal or exhibit morphologic features of "reactive" B cells.
• When bone marrow becomes lymphomatous in cattle with BLV-induced malignant lymphoma (ML), leukemia with lymphocyte counts as high as $100,000/\mu l$ can occur. In leukemic cattle, circulating lymphoid cells can appear "immature or blastic."

• Some cattle with BLV-induced ML have lymphopenia, probably because circulating lymphoid cells are "trapped" in lymphomatous tissues.
• Lymphocytosis, usually in the 8000 to 20,000/ul range can also occur with other chronic infectious diseases, like tuberculosis, trypanosomiasis, or brucellosis.

OTHER LABORATORY TESTS
N/A

IMAGING
N/A

DIAGNOSTIC PROCEDURES
• Two commercial serology tests for the detection of BLV antibody are available: the agar gel immunodiffusion (AGID) and the antibody capture ELISA. These two tests have similar sensitivity and specificities. However, they fail to detect between 35% and 39% of BLV serologically positive animals.
• Reverse transcriptase–polymerase chain reaction (RT-PCR) assays for the detection of the virus in milk and blood are available and are more sensitive and less likely to have false negatives seen with the serological tests. RT-PCR can also detect the infection prior to the presence of antibody.

PATHOLOGIC FINDINGS
• Grossly, EBL can be suspected when tumors of the visceral lymph nodes, uterus, abomasum, heart (especially right atrium), liver, spleen, and kidneys are found. These tumors are usually soft and gray-white, and can include friable areas of necrosis.
• Microscopically, massive lymphoid cell infiltration is observed in the affected organs as they replace normal cells.

TREATMENT

APPROPRIATE HEALTH CARE
Supportive treatment but prognosis is poor

ACTIVITY
N/A

DIET
N/A

CLIENT EDUCATION
Essential practices for controlling BLV infections are
• using hypodermic needles that are designed to be discarded after one injection
• using a different obstetrical sleeve to palpate each cow
• washing and then disinfecting any instruments that may be contaminated with blood. The use of two sets of instruments with one soaking in disinfectant while the other is being used should be encouraged.
• using electric dehorners rather than gouges or saws. The latter cause profuse hemorrhage and are difficult to sanitize.

SURGICAL CONSIDERATIONS
N/A

MEDICATIONS

DRUGS OF CHOICE
N/A

CONTRAINDICATIONS
N/A

PRECAUTIONS
N/A

POSSIBLE INTERACTIONS
N/A

ALTERNATIVE DRUGS
N/A

FOLLOW-UP

PATIENT MONITORING
N/A

PREVENTION/AVOIDANCE
• BLV-infected animals are a source of infection to all other animals.
• The low occurrence of clinical disease in herds with high seroprevalence to BLV frequently makes the priority of culling BLV seropositive animals low.

- Four essential practices for controlling BLV infections are listed above under Client Education.
- BLV eradication programs have been developed in Europe and in New York. The New York State Bovine Leukosis Virus Eradication and Certification Program (NYSBLVECP) was designed to help producers in establishing a BLV-free herd. The NYSBLVECP guidelines include the four practices outlined above along with many other steps for separation and rearing of infected animals and young stock.
- Although BLV-seropositive animals pose a risk to the herd, using only serology will lengthen the time to identify and eradicate BLV from a herd.
- BLV-positive animals with lymphocytosis are a larger risk because of their higher concentrations of BLV-infected lymphocytes. Removing these animals will have a faster impact on reducing the BLV risk in the herd.
- There are no commercial BLV vaccines available. Two experimental BLV vaccines, a modified-live gene deleted and a DNA vaccine, have been developed and prevented BLV infection in over 85% of the animals.

POSSIBLE COMPLICATIONS
N/A

EXPECTED COURSE AND PROGNOSIS
- With SBL, the prognosis is poor and the course of the disease from the first appearance of tumors will be only weeks to months.
- The vast majority of BLV infections are inapparent. Although 30% of BLV-seropositive animals will develop lymphocytosis, these animals are not at a greater risk for developing EBL.
- Animals with clinical signs of EBL have a poor prognosis and the course of the disease from the first appearance of tumors is short similar to SBL.

MISCELLANEOUS

ASSOCIATED CONDITIONS
N/A

AGE-RELATED FACTORS
Animals <2 years of age develop SBL. Most animals that develop EBL are >2 years of age with peak incidence at 5–8 years of age.

ZOONOTIC POTENTIAL
No risk

PREGNANCY
The immunosuppression of pregnancy appears to accelerate the development of BLV lymphomas.

RUMINANT SPECIES AFFECTED
Bovine and ovine

BIOSECURITY
- BLV-infected animals have the potential of producing infectious BLV for life.
- BLV-seropositive animals need to be considered a reservoir of the virus.
- New arrivals should be tested prior to introduction for BLV antibodies.
- In a BLV-positive herd, testing for lymphocytosis also may be advisable to identify animals with higher numbers of BLV-infected lymphocytes that would pose a higher risk to the herd.
- The use of single-use materials (needles, gloves, etc.), as described above, along with proper disinfection of surgical instruments are essential components of a BLV biosecurity plan.
- Depending on the level of control desired, BLV seropositive and seronegative animals should be housed separately.
- Seronegative animals should always be processed before seronegative animals.

PRODUCTION MANAGEMENT
- The economic impact of BLV on dairy cows is $59 per year per cow resulting from a ~3% decrease in milk production per cow.
- The overall economic impact of BLV on milk production for the United States is $525 million per year.

SYNONYMS
Bovine leukemia
Bovine leukosis
Enzootic bovine leukosis

SEE ALSO
Differential diagnosis
Laboratory diagnosis
Lumpy jaw caused by *Actinomyces bovis*
Sampling techniques

ABBREVIATIONS
AGID = agar gel immunodiffusion
BLV = bovine leukemia virus
EBL = enzootic bovine leukemia
ELISA = enzyme-linked immunosorbent assay
ML = malignant lymphoma
NYSBLVECP = New York State Bovine Leukosis Virus Eradication and Certification Program
PL = persistent lymphocytosis
RT-PCR = reverse transcriptase–polymerase chain reaction
SBL = spontaneous bovine leukemia

Suggested Reading
Choi, K. Y., Liu, R. B., Buehring, G. C. 2002. Relative sensitivity and specificity of agar gel immunodiffusion, enzyme immunosorbent assay, and immunoblotting for detection of anti-bovine leukemia virus antibodies in cattle. *J Virol Meth*. 104:33–39.
Evermann, J. F., Jackson, M. K. 1997. Laboratory diagnostic tests for retroviral infections in dairy and beef cattle. *Vet Clin North Am Food Animal Pract*. 13:87–106.
Hopkins, S. G., DiGiacomo, R. F. 1997. Natural transmission of bovine leukemia virus in dairy and beef cattle. *Vet Clin North Am Food Animal Pract*. 13:107–28.
Kabeya, H., Ohashi, K., Onuma, M. 2001. Host immune responses in the course of bovine leukemia virus infection. *J Vet Med Sci*. 63:703–708.

Author: Christopher C. L. Chase

BOVINE PAPULAR STOMATITIS

 BASICS

DEFINITION
• A mild viral disease of calves characterized by proliferative lesions around the mouth caused by a parapoxvirus.
• Infections are usually asymptomatic, but raised papules may be observed on nasal planum, hard palate, nares, and occasionally on the esophageal or ruminal mucosa.
• There are no lesions at the coronary band.

SYSTEMS AFFECTED
Epithelium of nares, oral cavity, esophagus, and rumen

GENETICS
No association with breed or genetics observed; commonly observed in dairy calves and recent arrivals in feedlots

INCIDENCE/PREVALENCE
Worldwide distribution

SIGNALMENT
• Young dairy calves, feedlot calves shortly after arrival. Commonly observed in calves from 1 to 12 months of age
• Rare in adult cattle

SIGNS
• Acute lesions consist of 2–4 mm macules on the nares and muzzle that progress rapidly to papules with raised periphery and depressed center. Lesions later develop in the oral cavity.
• Lesion size may increase to 1 cm in diameter or greater (coalescence of multiple lesions) and regress within several days to weeks.
• Most animals are afebrile, eat normally, and have no clinicopathologic alterations associated with viral infection.

PATHOPHYSIOLOGY
• Viral infection results in early hyperemia and inflammation in focal regions of the nares and mouth. Secondary lesions may occur for up to 4 months.
• Histopathological evaluation of lesions demonstrates degeneration of epithelial cells and eosinophilic inclusions in degenerated cells.
• Hyperplasia of the papillae of the lamina propria is observed.
• Ulceration of lesions is accompanied by bacterial infection and sloughing of the epithelium.
• A chronic form of BPS has been described associated with more severe clinical signs (salivation, diarrhea, anorexia, and fever). The ulcers in chronic cases become encrusted with exudates.
• Similar to contagious ecthyma and pseudocowpox in sheep and goats, bovine papular stomatitis is zoonotic and common in veterinary personnel.

RISK FACTORS
• Calves born to cows affected by BPS when young
• Adult cows may serve as reservoir for future calf infection.
• Recent introduction of naïve animals to feedlot

 DIAGNOSIS

DIFFERENTIAL DIAGNOSIS
Foot-and-mouth disease, vesicular stomatitis, and bovine virus diarrhea/MD, pseudocowpox viruses. Lesions are not found at coronary band, and generally are asymptomatic.

CBC/BIOCHEMISTRY/URINALYSIS
No abnormalities consistently associated with viral lesions

IMAGING
N/A

DIAGNOSTIC PROCEDURES
• Polymerase chain reaction, electron microscopy and histopathology are useful in the diagnosis of BPS.
• Histopathological evaluation of lesions demonstrates degeneration of epithelial cells and eosinophilic inclusions in degenerated cells.
• Confirmation of BPS in a new area requires virus isolation and identification.
• Typical parapoxvirus virions can be seen using transmission electron microscopy of biopsy samples.

 TREATMENT

 MISCELLANEOUS

PREVENTION
• Symptomatic treatment of severely affected animals.
• Prevention can focus on biosecurity and production of vaccines using locally obtained viral strains.

ASSOCIATED CONDITIONS
N/A

AGE-RELATED FACTORS
• Young dairy calves, feedlot calves shortly after arrival; commonly observed in calves from 1 to 12 months of age
• Rare in adult cattle

ZOONOTIC POTENTIAL
Similar to contagious ecthyma and pseudocowpox in sheep and goats, bovine papular stomatitis is zoonotic and common in veterinary personnel. The mild clinical manifestations make the condition relatively minor; however, the occasional case may have more severe lesions.

PREGNANCY
N/A

BIOSECURITY

PRODUCTION MANAGEMENT
N/A

SYNONYMS
N/A

SEE ALSO
Bovine virus diarrhea/MD
Foot-and-mouth disease,
Pseudocowpox viruses
Vesicular stomatitis

ABBREVIATIONS
BPS = bovine papular stomatitis
MD = mucosal disease

Suggested Reading
Buttner, M., Rziha, H. J. 2002. Parapoxviruses: from the lesion to the viral genome. *Journal Veterinary Medicine B* 49:7–16.
Delhon, G., Tulman, E. R., Afonso, C. L., Lu, Z., de la Concha-Bermejillo, A., Lehmkuhl, H. D., Piccone, M. E., Kutish, G. F., Rock, D. L. 2004. Genomes of the parapoxviruses Orf virus and bovine papular stomatitis virus. *Journal of Virology* 78:168–77.
Guo, J., Rasmussen, J., Wunschmann, A., de la Concha-Bermejillo, A. 2004. Genetic characterization of orf viruses isolated from various ruminant species of a zoo. *Veterinary Microbiology* 99: 81–92.
Inoshima, Y., Morooka, A., Sentsui, H. 2000. Detection and diagnosis of parapoxvirus by the polymerase chain reaction. *Journal of Virological Methods* 84: 201–8.
Stroebel, J. C., Gerdes, G. H. 1996. Bovine papular stomatitis-an incidental finding. *Journal of the South African Veterinary Association* 67: 104.
Yeruham, I., Abraham, A., Nyska, A. 1994. Clinical and pathological description of a chronic form of bovine papular stomatitis. *Journal of Comparative Pathology* 111: 279–86.

Author: Jeff Lakritz

BASICS

DEFINITION
- Bovine petechial fever is an infectious disease of cattle characterized by petechial and echymotic hemorrhages on mucosal membranes. The disease is also known as Ondiri disease.
- Bovine petechial fever is endemic in some parts of East Africa (Kenya and possibly Tanzania). The disease has not been reported in North America.

SIGNALMENT
- There is no sex or age predisposition. *Bos taurus* breeds are more susceptible than *Bos indicus*.
- The disease also has been reported in sheep, goats, and wild ruminants following experimental infection, but natural infection has been reported only in cattle.

SIGNS
- Affected animals have a fluctuating fever.
- The most consistent signs are petechiation and echymosis of mucous membranes. Unilateral conjuctival edema, hyphema, epistaxis, and anemia are present in some severe cases.
- Dairy cattle imported into endemic areas often exhibit a profound drop in milk production.

CAUSES
- The cause is *Ehrlichia (Cytoecetes) ondiri*. The organism is endemic in wild animals particularly the bushbuck (*Tragelaphus scriptus*) of highlands above 5000 feet in East Africa. Cattle acquire the disease when grazing on edges of thick, humid forests particularly when they are grazed in these areas at the end of the dry season.
- Bovine petechial fever is common in cattle that have been recently introduced to these areas while indigenous cattle appear to acquire resistance.
- The disease is thought to be transmitted by an arthropod vector. The vector has yet to be identified, but epidemiological findings suggest a tick vector.

RISK FACTORS
Grazing in or adjacent to thick, high elevation East African forests and the presence of the bushbuck, the reservoir of the organism, are important risk factors. Recently introduced animals are more susceptible.

DIAGNOSIS

Ehrlichia ondiri is diagnosed on demonstration of the organism in peripheral blood monocytes and granulocytes after Giemsa staining but cannot be cultured.

DIFFERENTIAL DIAGNOSIS
- Differential diagnosis includes bracken fern poisoning and tropical diseases including acute trypanosomiasis and theileriosis.
- Bracken fern poisoning is associated with pastures containing the plant and affected animals have hematuria.
- Trypanosomiasis occurs in the tropics where the vector, the tsetse (*Glossina* sp.) fly is found.
- Theileriosis is also common in areas where the tick vector *Rhipicephalus* sp. is present. Trypanosomiasis causes lymphadenopathy and the organism can be demonstrated in blood smears. Theileriosis causes lymphadenopathy and can be demonstrated in blood smears and lymph node aspirates.

TREATMENT

Tetracyclines are effective as a treatment. Recovered animals are immune to reinfection for at least 2 years.

MEDICATIONS

CONTRAINDICATIONS
Appropriate milk and meat withdrawal times must be followed for all compounds administered to food-producing animals.

FOLLOW-UP

PROGNOSIS
- Prognosis is guarded. The mortality is up to 50% in affected animals.
- The disease is important in imported animals introduced into risk areas where significant losses are recorded.

MISCELLANEOUS

ASSOCIATED CONDITIONS
N/A

AGE-RELATED FACTORS
N/A

ZOONOTIC POTENTIAL
N/A

PREGNANCY
N/A

RUMINANT SPECIES AFFECTED
The disease also has been reported in sheep, goats, and wild ruminants following experimental infection, but natural infection has been reported only in cattle.

BIOSECURITY
N/A

PRODUCTION MANAGEMENT
- Bovine petechial fever is common in cattle that have been recently introduced to infected areas while indigenous cattle appear to acquire resistance.
- Grazing in or adjacent to thick, high elevation East African forests and the presence of the bushbuck, the reservoir of the organism, are important risk factors. Recently introduced animals are more susceptible.

SYNONYMS
Ondiri disease

SEE ALSO
Bracken fern poisoning
Theileriosis
Trypanosomiasis

ABBREVIATIONS
N/A

Suggested Reading
Davies, G. 1993. Bovine petechial fever (Ondiri disease). *Vet Microbio.* 34:103–21.
Radostits, O. M., Gay, C. C., Blood, D. C., Hinchcliff, K. W. 2000. *Veterinary medicine*, 9th ed. New York: W. B. Saunders.

Author: Munashe Chigerwe

BOVINE RESPIRATORY DISEASE COMPLEX (BRD)

BASICS

OVERVIEW
• Bovine respiratory disease (BRD) complex refers to the general development of respiratory disease in cattle. In most cases, it specifically refers to respiratory disease outbreaks among multiple animals. BRD most commonly occurs in cattle fed for slaughter, although it can also occur in cattle raised for milk production.
• BRD is commonly called "shipping fever."
• It is estimated that over $3 billion are spent annually on prevention, treatment, and production losses related to BRD in the United States fed cattle industry.
• The etiology of BRD is very often multifactorial, and may include viruses, bacteria, parasites, nutrition, environmental stressors, and host susceptibility. The severity of BRD outbreaks is often influenced by the relative combination of these factors.

SIGNALMENT
• BRD can occur in any age and class of cattle.
• Younger animals under stressful conditions are most at risk.

SIGNS
• Clinical signs may vary depending on the agents involved and the severity of infection.
• The first sign often recognized is a reduction in appetite. Cattle may not show typical enthusiasm for coming to the feed bunk when fed.
• Cattle off feed may have a sunken appearance in the left para lumbar fossa as a result of decreased rumen fill.
• Affected animals often separate from their herd mates.
• Movement of affected animals is typically slower than nonaffected herd mates. They may show a reluctance to rise.
• A general appearance of depression is often appreciated.

• Affected cattle often stand with their heads down and extended.
• Cattle may have a serous to mucopurulent nasal discharge.
• Serous ocular discharge is often present.
• Coughing is often evident, especially when cattle are forced to move.
• Depending on the severity, shallow to labored and rapid breathing may be evident.
• Cattle affected with BRD typically have a fever ranging from 103.5°F to 105.5°F.
• A cranial ventral distribution of lung sounds consistent with bronchopneumonia and lung consolidation is found on auscultation. Moist crackles are heard with bronchopneumonia when the bronchi contain watery secretion or exudation. As the exudate thickens, the sound changes to a dry crackle. Consolidated areas of lung associated with bronchopneumonia (or large abscesses) contain no air and are completely silent.

CAUSES AND RISK FACTORS
• Viruses commonly implicated in BRD include bovine herpesvirus 1 (BHV-1), bovine viral diarrhea virus (BVDV), bovine respiratory syncytial virus (BRSV), parainfluenza-3 (PI-3), bovine respiratory corona virus (BRCV), and adenoviruses.
• Bacteria commonly involved in BRD include *Mannheimia haemolytica* (formerly *Pasteurella haemolytica*), *Pasteurella multocida*, *Mycoplasma bovis*, *Haemophilus somnus,* and *Actinomyces pyogenes.*
• Environmental factors that increase the risk of BRD include poor sanitation, poor ventilation, overcrowding, lack of adequate feed bunk space, lack of adequate water availability.
• Stressful events such as transportation, mixing of cattle from multiple sources, castration, dehorning, vaccination, starvation, and weaning increase the risk of BRD developing.

DIAGNOSIS

DIFFERENTIAL DIAGNOSIS
• Allergic interstitial pneumonia
• Pulmonary edema
• Pleuritis
• Pulmonary fibrosis
• Lungworms

CBC/BIOCHEMISTRY/URINALYSIS
N/A

OTHER LABORATORY TESTS
Culture and antimicrobial sensitivity are often done on lung samples collected at necropsy or following transtracheal bronchial alveolar lavage.

DIAGNOSTIC PROCEDURES
• Nasal swabs are of limited value, as many of the pathogens involved in BRD inhabit the nasal passages normally.
• Transtracheal bronchial alveolar lavage will identify pathogens most likely involved with pneumonic process.
• Necropsy provides the most useful information on the etiological agents and pathological processes involved. Necropsies on cases early in the course of the disease and prior to antibiotic therapy yield the best results.

GROSS FINDINGS
• Gross lesions will depend on the pathological agents involved in the BRD outbreak and the chronicity of the disease process.
• Necrotizing lesions of the upper respiratory tract and trachea may be present.
• Pneumonic lesions are typically distributed in a bilateral cranial ventral pattern, often with a sharp line of demarcation between the normal and abnormal lung.
• There may be varying degrees of pleural adhesion between lung lobes and to the chest wall.

• The lung parenchyma typically has a lobulated pattern that imparts a marbled appearance both on the pleural and cut surface.
• Affected parenchyma is firm in palpation and may range in color from pink to tan to red to red-black depending on the amount of necrosis present.
• Necrotic tissue may progress to abscessation.

HISTOPATHOLOGICAL FINDINGS
N/A

TREATMENT

• Antimicrobials directed against common BRD bacteria.
• Moving sick cattle to separate pens may be indicated to reduce the stress of competing with healthy cattle.

MEDICATIONS

• Common antimicrobial classes used for treatment of BRD include penicillins, cephalosporins, oxytetracyclines, floroquinalones, macrolides.
• Ancillary treatments such as nonsteroidal anti-inflammatory drugs, corticosteroids, antihistamines, and vitamin injections may be of value on a case-by-case basis, but in general have limited application in treatment of BRD.

CONTRAINDICATIONS
• Some antibiotics are not approved for certain classes of cattle, such as lactating dairy cattle.
• Meat and milk withhold times must be considered before administrating any medication to food-producing cattle.

POSSIBLE INTERACTIONS
N/A

FOLLOW-UP

PATIENT MONITORING
• Daily observation of attitude and appetite will provide a good indication of treatment success.
• Gaining of weight is associated with a good prognosis while continued weight loss is a poor sign.
• Reduction of rectal temperature in 24–48 hours posttreatment is associated with a good prognosis.

PREVENTION/AVOIDANCE
• Immunization against common pathogens associated with BRD
• Minimizing stressful events
• Maintaining well-ventilated and sanitary environments with plenty of bunk space and water availability

POSSIBLE COMPLICATIONS
• Pericarditis
• Endocarditis
• Pleuritis
• Polyarthritis is often a sequela of *Mycoplasma bovis* and *Haemophilus somnus* pneumonia.

EXPECTED COURSE AND PROGNOSIS
• Prognosis is generally favorable if intervention occurs early.
• If intervention is started early, most cattle respond to treatment in 24–72 hours.
• Failure to respond to initial treatments generally indicates advanced disease and the prognosis should be guarded.

MISCELLANEOUS

ASSOCIATED CONDITIONS
N/A

AGE-RELATED FACTORS
N/A

ZOONOTIC POTENTIAL
Agents commonly involved in BRD are not zoonotic.

PREGNANCY
N/A

SEE ALSO
Bovine respiratory syncytial virus
Bovine viral diarrhea virus
Haemophilosis
Infectious bovine rhinotracheitis virus
Mannheimiosis
Mycoplasma bovis
Parainfluenza-3 virus

ABBREVIATIONS
BHV-1 = bovine heresvirus 1
BRCV = bovine respiratory corona virus
BRD = bovine respiratory disease
BRSV = bovine respiratory syncytial virus
BVDV = bovine viral diarrhea virus
PI-3 = parainfluenza-3

Suggested Reading
Bovine respiratory disease: sourcebook for the veterinary professional. 1996. Chatham, NJ: Veterinary Learning Systems.
Chirase, N. K., Greene, L. W., Purdy, C. W., Loan, R. W., Auvermann, B. W., Parker, D. B., Walborg, E. F., Jr., Stevenson, D. E., Xu, Y., Klaunig, J. E. 2004, Jun. Effect of transport stress on respiratory disease, serum antioxidant status, and serum concentrations of lipid peroxidation biomarkers in beef cattle. *Am J Vet Res.* 65(6):860–64.
Martin SW, Nagy E, Armstrong D, Rosendal S. 1999, Aug. The associations of viral and mycoplasmal antibody titers with respiratory disease and weight gain in feedlot calves. *Can Vet J.* 40(8):560–67, 570.
Woolums, A. R., Mason, G. L., Hawkins, L. L., Brown, C. C., Williams, S. M., Gould, J. A., Fox, J. J., Sturgeon, S. D., Anderson, J. L., Duggan, F. E., Sanchez, S., Barrett, P. B., Chitwood, S.W. 2004, Nov. Microbiologic findings in feedlot cattle with acute interstitial pneumonia. *Am J Vet Res.* 65(11):1525–32.

Author: Daniel L. Grooms

BOVINE RESPIRATORY SYNCYTIAL VIRUS

 BASICS

DEFINITION

Bovine respiratory syncytial virus (BRSV) induces a mild to severe lower respiratory disease in cattle. This infection is one of the viral factors associated with bovine respiratory disease complex.

PATHOPHYSIOLOGY

• BRSV induces damage to the respiratory epithelium with a concomitant influx of inflammatory cells (neutrophils and cytotoxic lymphocytes) and cytokines (tumor necrosis factor). This lowers arterial oxygen by 30%–40%.
• The damage to epithelium coupled with inflammatory changes increases the susceptibility of the lung to secondary bacterial infection.
• Severe BRSV infections can cause severe damage to bronchiolar and alveolar epithelial tissue resulting in the formation of bullae and interstitial emphysema.

SYSTEMS AFFECTED

Respiratory

GENETICS

N/A

INCIDENCE/PREVALANCE

• BRSV is endemic in cattle.
• BRSV is seldom seen in calves less than 2 weeks of age, and is most prevalent and severe in animals between 1 month and 8 months of age.
• BRSV disease is rarely seen in cattle >9 months of age. Adult cattle can occasionally experience severe disease.
• Seroprevalence in herds is often >90%.

GEOGRAPHIC DISTRIBUTION

Worldwide

SIGNALMENT

• BRSV infection results in respiratory signs. These respiratory signs can be mild, with increased respiratory rate and increased harshness in respiratory sounds, to severe, with dyspnea, forced expiration, and open-mouth breathing.
• Spontaneous cough can be easily induced and can vary from dry and nonproductive to moist.

• Nasal discharge can vary from none to serous to mucopurulent.
• Conjunctivitis and lacrimal discharge are seen infrequently. There is an increased rectal temperature (104–108°F [40–42°C]), depression, and decreased feed intake.
• Secondary pneumonia with bacterial pathogens (*Mannheimia haemolytica*, *Pasteurella multocida*, *Haemophilus somnus*) or *Mycoplasma bovis* is a frequent sequela.

CAUSES

BRSV is an enveloped, negative, single-stranded RNA virus in the pneumovirus group of the paramyxovirus family. The virus is easily inactivated by desiccation, heat, and disinfectants.

RISK FACTORS

• Stress (weaning, shipping, etc.) will increase the risk. Excessive levels of dust have been reported to increase clinical BRSV.
• Maternal antibody will inhibit vaccine response but will not prevent infection. However, it will lessen the clinical course of disease.
• Concurrent infection with other viral agents, particularly bovine viral diarrhea virus (BVDV), exacerbates BRSV clinical disease.

 DIAGNOSIS

DIFFERENTIAL DIAGNOSIS

• Three other bovine viruses—BVDV, bovine parainfluenza-3 virus (PI-3), and bovine herpesvirus 1 (BHV-1)—commonly cause similar respiratory disease.
• BHV-1 is associated with rhinotracheitis and upper respiratory disease. BHV-1–infected calves frequently have mucopurulent discharge and conjunctivitis.
• BVDV is associated with oral ulcers, mucopurulent discharge, and upper respiratory disease.
• PI-3 infection is usually a mild lower respiratory disease.
• Bovine coronavirus (BCV) has also been associated with respiratory disease. In younger calves, it is seen in calves suffering from enteritis and diarrhea. BCV in 5–13-month-old cattle causes symptoms of dyspnea, nasal discharge, and increased respiratory rate.

• Atypical interstitial pneumonia (AIP) is characterized by sudden onset of disease with subsequent death. AIP animals have labored breathing with loud expiration, frothing at the mouth, and open-mouth breathing. They have harsh respiratory sounds with crackles and rhonchi. These animals usually have a recent history of grazing lush pastures or having a ration change in a feedyard.

CBC/BIOCHEMISTRY/URINALYSIS

BRSV causes a slight lymphopenia 3–10 days postinfection.

OTHER LABORATORY TESTS

N/A

IMAGING

N/A

DIAGNOSTIC PROCEDURES

• BRSV is a very difficult virus to detect by virus isolation. Animals need to be sampled in the incubation or acute phase of infection (3–7 days).
• Transtracheal washes have been used to detect BRSV using polymerase chain reaction (PCR). Antigen detection kits have been developed and can detect BRSV antigen.
• Other procedures that have proved useful in detection of BRSV antigen are fluorescent antibody tests of fresh tissue and immunohistochemistry staining of cell cultures or formalin-fixed paraffin embedded tissues.
• Paired serum samples can be used in the diagnosis of BRSV infection. However, the antibody titer of animals with well-developed clinical disease may be higher in acute samples than the samples taken 2–3 weeks later.
• BRSV antibody response often develops rapidly, and clinical signs follow virus infection by up to 7–10 days.
• Single serum samples showing high antibody titers from a number of animals in a respiratory outbreak may be useful in making a diagnosis if coupled with clinical signs.
• Younger calves infected with BRSV in the presence of maternally acquired antibody may not seroconvert.

PATHOLOGIC FINDINGS

• Gross lesions include a diffuse interstitial pneumonia with subpleural and interstitial emphysema along with interstitial edema. These lesions are similar to and must be differentiated from AIP.

BOVINE RESPIRATORY SYNCYTIAL VIRUS

• Regional suppurative bronchopneumonia of bacterial origin is usually present.
• Histologic examination reveals necrotizing and proliferative bronchiolitis with alveolitis that is sometimes proliferative along with hyaline membrane formation and edema.
• Syncytial cells are present in bronchiolar epithelium and lung parenchyma.

TREATMENT

APPROPRIATE HEALTH CARE
The therapy for BRSV is supportive. Severely diseased animals that are dehydrated may receive oral and/or intravenous fluids.

ACTIVITY
Handling of BRSV-infected animals should be minimized to decrease the risk of secondary bacterial infections.

DIET
Concentrate and silage should not be fed to severely diseased animals.

CLIENT EDUCATION
Minimize handling of animals, decrease animal exposure to high levels of dust, and use preventative vaccines.

SURGICAL CONSIDERATIONS
N/A

MEDICATIONS

DRUGS OF CHOICE
• Corticosteroids or nonsteroidal anti-inflammatory drugs (NSAIDs) may have some benefit to lessen the severity of BRSV disease.
• Antimicrobial treatment is utilized to reduce secondary bacterial infections.

CONTRAINDICATIONS
Appropriate milk and meat withdrawal times must be followed for all compounds administered to food-producing animals.

PRECAUTIONS
N/A

POSSIBLE INTERACTIONS
N/A

ALTERNATIVE DRUGS
N/A

FOLLOW-UP

PATIENT MONITORING
Respiratory characteristics along with rectal body temperatures should be frequently monitored to assess BRSV clinical progression and also the development of secondary bacterial infections that would result in bovine respiratory disease complex (BRDC).

PREVENTION/AVOIDANCE
• Both modified-live-virus (MLV) and inactivated-virus BRSV vaccines are available.
• Vaccination is an important part of a BRSV control program.

POSSIBLE COMPLICATIONS
• Some formaldehyde-inactivated BRSV vaccines have been shown to increase the severity of BRSV disease. This method of inactivation is not currently used for commercial vaccines.
• Maternal antibodies in calves interfere with development of an effective BRSV immune response with MLV vaccines.

EXPECTED COURSE AND PROGNOSIS
• Uncomplicated BRSV infections will resolve in 10–14 days.
• Animals that have secondary infections usually will develop bronchopneumonia with varying levels of morbidity and mortality.

MISCELLANEOUS

ASSOCIATED CONDITIONS
BRDC is a frequent sequela to BRSV infections.

AGE-RELATED FACTORS
Younger animals (between 1and 8 months of age) are usually affected.

ZOONOTIC POTENTIAL
N/A

PREGNANCY
N/A

RUMINANT SPECIES AFFECTED
Bovine, ovine

BIOSECURITY
• BRSV survives very poorly in the environment and is susceptible to UV light, desiccation, heat, and disinfectants. The virus will survive better in the winter.
• Animals exhibiting clinical signs of BRSV should be isolated from other cattle as transmission of BRSV occurs by the oronasal route.
• In pens of animals that have had a BRSV outbreak, it would be prudent to clean the water sources.

PRODUCTION MANAGEMENT
In herds with a history of BRSV in their calves, a BRSV vaccine program should be implemented.

SYNONYMS
N/A

SEE ALSO
Atypical interstitial pneumonia
Bovine coronavirus
Bovine herpesvirus 1
Bovine parainfluenza-3 virus
Bovine viral diarrhea virus

ABBREVIATIONS
AIP = atypical interstitial pneumonia
BCV = bovine coronavirus
BHV-1 = bovine herpesvirus 1
BRDC = bovine respiratory disease complex
BRSV = bovine respiratory syncytial virus
BVDV = bovine viral diarrhea virus
MLV = modified-live virus
NSAIDs = nonsteroidal anti-inflammatory drugs
PCR = polymerase chain reaction
PI-3 = bovine parainfluenza-3 virus

Suggested Reading
Larsen, L. E. 2000. Bovine respiratory syncytial virus (BRSV) review article. *Acta Vet Scand*. 41:1–24.
Woolums, A. R., Anderson, M. L., Gunther, R. A., Schelegle, E. S., LaRochelle, D. R., Singer, R. S., Boyle, G. A., Frieberthauser, K. E., Gershwin, L. J. 1999. Evaluation of severe disease induced by aerosol inoculation of calves with bovine respiratory syncytial virus. *AJVR* 60:473–80.

Author: Christopher C. L. Chase

BOVINE SPONGIFORM ENCEPHALOPATHY

BASICS

DEFINITION
Bovine spongiform encephalopathy (BSE) is a progressively fatal, neurodegenerative disease of cattle and is a type of transmissible spongiform encephalopathy.

PATHOPHYSIOLOGY
• Since its first diagnosis in the United Kingdom in 1986, different theories about the origin of BSE have been proposed.
• The most common theory is that BSE mutated from the scrapie agent found in sheep, and changes in the rendering processes for livestock feed allowed this prion to survive and be fed to cattle. Then further rendering of infected cattle carcasses to make meat and bone meal amplified the agent.
• Another theory is that BSE has always existed in cattle but went virtually unrecognized until 1986 when the outbreaks occurred in the UK.

SYSTEMS AFFECTED
Nervous

GENETICS
• Offspring of BSE-infected cattle seem to have an increased risk of developing BSE but exact etiology is unknown at this time.
• Vertical or venereal transmission has not been proven.

INCIDENCE/PREVALENCE
• Annual incidence data are only available for the countries in which BSE has been diagnosed and in cattle over 24 months of age because the incubation period is thought to be more than one year.
• The 2003 data range from as low as 0.16 cases per million bovines over 24 months of age in Canada to 137.19 cases per million bovines over 24 months of age in Portugal.

GEOGRAPHIC DISTRIBUTION
Infected indigenous cattle have been found in Austria, Belgium, Canada, Czech Republic, Denmark, Finland, France, Germany, Greece, Ireland, Israel, Italy, Japan, Lichtenstein, Luxembourg, Netherlands, Poland, Portugal, Slovakia, Slovenia, Spain, Switzerland, United Kingdom, and the United States. Imported cattle with BSE have been reported in the Falkland Islands and Oman.

SIGNALMENT

Species
Cattle, bison

Breed Predilections
NA

Mean Age and Range
Generally affects cattle between 3 and 6 years of age and the incubation period ranges from 2 to 8 years.

Predominant Sex
NA

SIGNS

HISTORICAL FINDINGS
Usually an insidious onset of neurologic signs in cattle older than 3 years of age.

PHYSICAL EXAMINATION FINDINGS
Slowly progressive, degenerative neurological disease. Cattle will often be ataxic, primarily on the hind limbs with hypermetria. They will also have hyper-reflexia, muscle fasciculation and tremors, fall down, and behavior changes such as nervousness and frenzy. Over time, the animal will become anorexic and lose weight and body condition; dairy animals will have decreased milk production.

CAUSES
• The agent that causes BSE is smaller than most viruses and highly resistant to common disinfectants, heat, UV light, and ionizing radiation.
• While it has not been observed microscopically, there are three main theories as to the causative agent. First is that it is just an unconventional virus. Second is that it is an incomplete virus or virino. Third, and the most widely accepted theory, is that small prions, or proteinaceous infectious particles, cause normal prion proteins to change to an abnormal form and cause degenerative changes in the brain of infected cattle.

RISK FACTORS
Cattle consuming scrapie-infected meat and bone meal or other ruminant by-products that may be contaminated with the BSE agent

DIAGNOSIS

DIFFERENTIAL DIAGNOSIS
Rabies, lead poisoning, nervous ketosis, listeriosis, polioencephalomalacia, hypomagnesemia, intracranial tumors, and spinal cord trauma

CBC/BIOCHEMISTRY/URINALYSIS
There is no antemortem test for BSE as the host does not mount an immune response to the agent.

OTHER LABORATORY TESTS

IMAGING

DIAGNOSTIC PROCEDURES
N/A

PATHOLOGIC FINDINGS
• Gross lesions are restricted to carcass changes such as emaciation and damage to the hide from ataxia and nervousness.
• Histopathologic detection of neurodegeneration lesions in the brain (bilaterally symmetrical spongiform changes in the grey matter) will help confirm the diagnosis. Immunohistochemistry, immunoblotting, and ELISA to demonstrate accumulations of the prion (PrP^{res}) protein are needed for definitive diagnosis.

TREATMENT

APPROPRIATE HEALTH CARE, NURSING CARE, ACTIVITY
There is no treatment for this disease.

DIET, CLIENT EDUCATION
Restrictions have been put in place in many countries that preclude the feeding of ruminant products back to ruminants, but clients should be made aware of this as a risk factor and prevent contamination of any cattle feed on their farms.

SURGICAL CONSIDERATIONS
N/A

 MEDICATIONS

DRUGS OF CHOICE
N/A

CONTRAINDICATIONS
N/A

POSSIBLE INTERACTIONS
N/A

ALTERNATIVE DRUGS
N/A

 FOLLOW-UP

PATIENT MONITORING
N/A

PREVENTION/AVOIDANCE
Do not feed ruminant products to ruminants.

POSSIBLE COMPLICATIONS
N/A

EXPECTED COURSE AND PROGNOSIS
This is a progressively fatal neurodegenerative disease and 100% of the cases will die.

 MISCELLANEOUS

ASSOCIATED CONDITIONS
N/A

AGE-RELATED FACTORS
Most often seen in cattle between 3 and 6 years of age.

ZOONOTIC POTENTIAL
• There is evidence to suggest that persons consuming BSE-contaminated products may develop a disease called variant Creutzfeldt-Jakob disease.
• The exact incubation period for this disease is unknown but it is thought to be decades. It too is a progressively fatal neurologic disease with 28 years of age being the mean age at death of those affected with vCJD.
• Since the first discovery of vCJD in 1996 through November 2006, there have been 200 cases worldwide, with the majority of cases in the UK (164) and France (21). The United States has reported 3 cases, but the patients had resided in the UK (2) and Saudi Arabia (1) the majority of their lives.
• There are recommendations regarding blood donations, surgical equipment, and organ transplants from countries where vCJD has been diagnosed to prevent further spread of this disease.

PREGNANCY
Vertical transmission of BSE has not been documented but offspring of BSE-infected cattle are at higher risk for developing the disease; offspring are usually culled.

RUMINANT SPECIES AFFECTED
Bovine, bison

BIOSECURITY, PRODUCTION MANAGEMENT
N/A

SYNONYMS
Mad cow disease

SEE ALSO
Chronic wasting disease
Hypomagnesemia
Intracranial tumors

Lead poisoning
Listeriosis
Nervous ketosis
Polioencephalomalacia
Rabies
Scrapie
Spinal cord trauma.
Variant Creutzfeldt-Jakob disease

ABBREVIATIONS
BSE = bovine spongiform encephalopathy
ELISA = enzyme linked immunosorbent assay
PrP^{res} = abnormal prion protein
vCJD = variant Creutzfeldt-Jakob disease

Suggested Reading
Aiello, S. E., ed. 1998. *Merck veterinary manual*, 8th ed. Whitehouse Station, NJ : Merck and Co.
Bovine Spongiform Encephalopathy disease card from the OIE website accessed May 9, 2004, at http://www.oie.int/eng/maladies/fiches/a_B115.htm.
Bovine Spongiform Encephalopathy from the United States Department of Agriculture, Animal and Plant Inspection Service website accessed May 9, 2004, at http://www.aphis.usda.gov/lpa/issues/bse/bse.html.
Bovine Spongiform Encephalopathy in the *Manual of Standards for Diagnostic Tests and Vaccines*. Paris, Office International des Epizooties, 2000, Chapter 2. 3. 13.
Centers for Disease Control and Prevention. BSE and vCJD Infectious Disease information websites accessed May 9, 2004, and January 16, 2007, at http://www.cdc.gov/ncidod/diseases/submenus/sub_bse.htm.

Authors: Danelle Bickett-Weddle and Neal Bataller

BOVINE VIRAL DIARRHEA VIRUS

 BASICS

OVERVIEW
• Bovine viral diarrhea (BVD) is a multifaceted disease with complicated pathogenesis and one of the most significant viral infections of cattle.
• Bovine viral diarrhea virus (BVDV) is capable of infecting and causing pathology in many different organ systems.
• Cattle can become acutely infected with BVDV at any age. This is also referred to as primary infection or transient infection.
• Fetal infection prior to day 125 of gestation can result in the development of immunotolerance to the BVDV and the development of a persistent infection (PI) with the virus.
• Cattle persistently infected with BVDV shed large amounts of virus during their lifetime. They are the major source of virus spread within and between farms.

SIGNALMENT
All ages and classes of cattle are susceptible to infection with BVDV.

INCIDENCE/PREVALENCE
BVDV is a ubiquitous pathogen of ruminants with high seroprevalence worldwide (up to 60% of adult cattle have antibodies). Infections with BVDV are endemic in many countries and are often associated with severe economic losses for the cattle industry.

GEOGRAPHIC DISTRIBUTION
Worldwide

Species
BVDV was thought to be species-specific but is now known to cause infection in species other than cattle including llama, alpaca, pigs, sheep, goats, white-tail deer, and mule deer.

Breed Predilections
N/A

Mean Age and Range
N/A

Predominant Sex
N/A

SIGNS
• Infections are mostly subclinical in nature. However, there has been an emergence of new virulent BVD viruses that cause thrombocytopenia and hemorrhagic disease.
• BVDV infection may result in subclinical acute infections; severe acute infections characterized by fever, leukopenia, and thrombocytopenia; persistent infections; reproductive disease presenting as congenital defects, repeat breeding, abortion, or mummification; enteric disease, respiratory disease; and immunosuppression. The severity of disease depends upon host and viral factors.
• Acute infection may be defined as the infection of an immunocompetent animal with BVDV.
• Following infection with BVDV, a short incubation period of 5–7 days is followed by viremia, which generally lasts for 1–2 days but may persist for 15 days.
• A mild, biphasic elevation in body temperature and leukopenia may be evident.
• Lactating cattle may have an associated decrease in milk production.
• Some strains are pneumotropic and may cause severe fibrinopurulent bronchopneumonia in the presence of *Mannheimia hemolytica*.
• Mucosal disease is characterized by fever, anorexia, depression, profuse salivation, nasal discharge, severe diarrhea, hemorrhages and erosions in gastrointestinal tract, and a very high case fatality rate (see Mucosal Disease in this volume).
• BVDV subtype 2 is usually involved in severe acute BVD characterized by severe thrombocytopenia with hemorrhages (prolonged bleeding from venipuncture sites; hemorrhages on sclera of eye and inner surface of eyelids; hemorrhages on mucosal surfaces of cheeks, lower gingiva, tongue, and soft palate), fever, pneumonia, diarrhea, and sudden death in 10–100% of infected animals.
• BVDV can result in immunosuppression following acute infection resulting in secondary infections caused by opportunistic pathogens. BVDV has been implicated most often as an immunosuppressive component of the bovine respiratory disease complex.

• In calves: diphasic pyrexia, leukopenia, anorexia, diarrhea, immunosuppression
• In pregnant animals: early embryonic death, abortion, congenital infection (if infected within 45 to 125 days of gestation). At 12 days of gestation, infection usually results in the birth of PI animals. Signs may include cerebral hypoplasia, retinal atrophy, cataract, growth retardation, arrested bone development, and pulmonary hypoplasia.

CAUSES AND RISK FACTORS
• BVDV is an RNA virus and a member of the genus *Pestivirus* in the family Flaviviridae.
• The BVDV is antigenically related to classical swine fever virus (CSFV) of pigs and border diseases virus (BDV) of sheep. All pestiviruses are antigenically cross reactive.
• The subtypes of BVDV include BVDV 1a, BVDV 1b, BVDV 2a, and BVDV 2b. All of these viruses can be either cytopathic (cp) or noncytopathic (ncp); the cp strains have an additional nonstructural protein. Both virulent and nonvirulent strains have been reported. Virulence does not depend on biotype (cp or ncp) or genotype.
• The major risk factor for BVDV being introduced into a farm is the acquisition of new cattle. Other risk factors include sharing of pastures with other cattle (direct or fence line) and lack of a BVDV vaccination program.

Transmission
• The virus is shed in most secretions and excretions of infected animals including tears, milk, saliva, urine, feces, nasal secretions, and semen.
• Two main methods of virus transmission include postnatal horizontal transmission and gestational vertical transmission from a viremic dam to her fetus. Transmission may occur by aerosols, nose-to-nose contact, and via semen, rectal palpation, and embryo transfer. PI animals are much more efficient transmitters of BVDV than transiently infected animals because they shed large amounts of virus for a long period of time.
• Infection at 120–150 days of gestation may result in abortion, resorption, stillbirths, or PI animals.

• After 120 days, infection results in abortion, stillbirth, congenital defects, and normal appearing calves.
• Virus can survive for several days or even weeks in a cool, protected environment and hence fomites (nose tongs, halters, etc.) play a role in virus transmission.
• Flies can also transmit the virus.
• The virus can be present in milk and colostrums.

DIAGNOSIS

DIFFERENTIAL DIAGNOSIS
• Differential diagnosis for calves with diarrhea as the result of BVDV includes any pathogen known to cause diarrhea in neonatal calves. In adult cattle, differential diagnoses would include winter dysentery and salmonella.
• Differential diagnosis for abortions caused by BVDV includes BHV-1, neospora, leptospirosis, and brucellosis.
• Differential diagnosis for thrombocytopenia induced by BVDV includes sweet clover poisoning, coumarol poisoning, and vitamin K deficiency.

CBC/BIOCHEMISTRY/URINALYSIS
• Severe leukopenia is characteristic in the early stages of acute BVD, with total leukocyte count in the range of 1000–5000/μl being common.
• Isolates of BVDV associated with hemorrhagic BVDV can result in severe thrombocytopenia and subsequently anemia.

IMAGING
N/A

DIAGNOSTIC PROCEDURES
• Virus isolation from serum, whole blood, nasal swabs, or lymphoid tissue
• PCR on serum, whole blood, nasal swabs, or lymphoid tissue
• Identification of a fourfold increase in virus-neutralizing antibody titers in acute and convalescent serum samples

• Persistent infection with BVDV can be diagnosed by identification of virus from serial samples taken 3 weeks apart using virus isolation, antigen detection ELISA, or PCR, or identification of BVDV antigen in skin samples by immunohistochemistry.

Virus/Viral Antigen Detection
• Viral antigen can be found in brain, spinal cord, kidney, spleen, lymph nodes, testicular tubules, and endothelial cells of PI animals.
• High throughput methods are now available for whole-herd screening to identify and remove PI animals.
• For direct detection of viral antigen, cryostat sections of fresh tissues are stained with fluorescein-conjugated anti-BVDV antibody and then examined under a fluorescent microscope. The presence of apple-green fluorescence indicates a positive test.
• Immunohistological staining of formalin-fixed, paraffin-embedded skin biopsies (ear notch samples) using 15C5 monoclonal antibody has been used to detect PI animals and is often considered better than histopathology and direct immunofluorescence (DFA) of tissues.
• Antigen-capture ELISA (AC-ELISA) can be used for the detection of BVDV antigen in buffy coat cells, serum, and ear notch samples. Monoclonal antibody directed against a conserved antigenic domain of a nonstructural protein (NS2/3) of pestiviruses is used as a capture antigen followed by detection of antigen-antibody complex with enzyme-conjugated antibody. Serum can be used for the detection of PI animals by AC-ELISA. Acute animals are rarely detected by this test because the virus is present in the blood of acutely infected animal for only a short time.
• Bovine turbinate (BT) cells, primary bovine embryo kidney (pBEK) cells, and cell lines originating from bovine embryonic trachea (EBTr) and buffalo lung (IMR-31) can be used for the isolation of BVDV from nasal discharge, peripheral blood leukocytes (PBL), lungs, semen, blood, serum, fetus, and feces. The isolated virus can be confirmed/identified

by DFA, immunoperoxidase monolayer assay (IPMA), monolayer enzyme-linked immunosorbent assay (M-ELISA), AC-ELISA, or RT-PCR. The presence of anti-BVDV antibody in serum and buffy coat samples may interfere with virus isolation.

Antibody Detection
• An indirect measure of virus infection is the detection of virus-specific antibodies in the sera of animals. Unfortunately, it is often difficult to differentiate among antibodies produced in response to acute infection, vaccination, or transfer of maternal antibodies from dam to offspring. In cattle, calves are usually born without antibody but seroconvert after colostrum consumption. These passive antibodies wane after 3–8 months. Hence, the presence of antibody in colostrum-deprived calves can be due only to active infection (either in utero or postnatal) or vaccination.
• Seroconversion of sentinel animals can be used as an evidence for possible exposure to PI animals. Many tests are available for the detection of anti-BVDV antibodies, namely, virus-neutralization (VN), indirect immunofluorescence (IIF) assay, indirect immunoperoxidase (IIP) assay, and ELISA tests.
• The virus neutralization (VN), also known as serum neutralization (SN), is considered to be the gold standard test for the detection of anti-BVDV antibodies and is used worldwide. The test can be used for the detection of antibodies against BVDV 1 or BVDV 2 depending upon the virus used in the test. In most situations, cp strains of BVDV are used in the test so that the presence of neutralizing antibodies can be detected by inhibition of viral infectivity as detected by the absence of viral cytopathology. Titers due to active infection can be differentiated from vaccination titers by demonstrating a fourfold rise in antibody titers using paired (acute and convalescent) serum samples. Virus neutralizing antibodies usually appear 3–4 weeks after infection and persist for years. Titers induced by vaccination may also persist for a long time. Passive antibodies decline at 105–230 days (but may persist for more than a year).

BOVINE VIRAL DIARRHEA VIRUS

• ELISA tests have been developed for the detection of anti-BVDV antibodies in serum samples. The antigens used in ELISA tests include whole-virus antigen, nonstructural protein (p125/80), monoclonal antibodies, and peptides. The advantages of the ELISA test include its sensitivity, ease, and objectivity in reading results, nondependability on cell cultures.
• Indirect immunoperoxidase and indirect immunofluorescence tests also have been used for the detection of anti-BVDV antibodies.

Nucleic Acid Detection
• Detection by reverse transcription–polymerase chain reaction (RT-PCR) has been found to be more sensitive and rapid than virus isolation. In addition, contrary to virus isolation, RT-PCR is not affected by the presence of antibodies in serum samples.
• Due to its high sensitivity, RT-PCR is considered as an alternative to current standard methods for detecting BVDV, especially in pooled samples such as bulk tank milk. However, RT-PCR does not differentiate between nucleic acid from live or inactivated virus and may yield false positive results.
• The prolonged stability of viral nucleic acid as compared to the virus itself has led to a simple method for the collection, storage, transport, and testing of blood samples. In this procedure, 10 μl of blood or serum is applied to a Whatman No. 1 paper, the sample is air dried and then tested.
• Several single- and two-tube RT-PCR assays have been described for the detection of BVDV RNA in serum, buffy coat cells, and fresh and formalin-fixed tissues (including ear notches).

Diagnosis by Testing Bulk Milk
• Screening of bulk milk for antibody or antigen has been used to detect BVDV infection in cattle herds. The milk is centrifuged to remove fat and undiluted skim milk is tested for antibodies using an ELISA test. There is an excellent correlation between the level of antibodies in the bulk-tank milk and the prevalence of BVDV-antibody-positive cows.
• RT-PCR assay to screen bulk milk samples for BVDV is also a sensitive and economic method for the detection of PI animals within a group because virus titers are usually higher in milk than in serum samples.

GROSS FINDINGS
• In most cases, acute BVDV presents with no gross lesions that are specific.
• Cattle may have lesions similar to those found with mucosal disease including erosions in the oral cavity, esophagus, rumen, abomasums, and small intestine, especially over areas of the Peyer's patches.
• Widespread petechial and ecchymotic hemorrhages may be present in cattle suffering from hemorrhagic syndrome.
• No specific lesions are seen in aborted fetuses.
• Cerebellar hypoplasia can be seen grossly in congenitally affected calves.

HISTOPATHOLOGICAL FINDINGS
Lymphoid depletion of the Peyer's patches, lymph nodes, spleen, and thymus are common with acute BVDV infections.

TREATMENT
• Cattle acutely infected with BVDV typically recover over time.
• In severe cases, supportive therapy is indicated.
• There is no treatment for cattle persistently infected with BVDV.

CLIENT EDUCATION
Eradication
• Sweden was one of the first countries to introduce a national BVDV control program in 1993, which now forms the basis for control programs in many other countries.
• The eradication programs are based mostly on detection and elimination of PI animals and immunization of breeding females prior to first gestation.
• Vaccination is not allowed in Denmark. Therefore, it is easy in that country to detect infected animals by testing for the presence of antibodies.
• The primary aims of eradication programs are the establishment of BVDV-free herds and prevention of reinfection of these herds so that there is a gradual decrease in the number of infected herds. This model works well in countries where cattle density is low and vaccination is not allowed but may not work in countries where both virus prevalence and cattle densities are high and where vaccination is permitted.

MEDICATIONS
N/A

CONTRAINDICATIONS
N/A

FOLLOW-UP
PATIENT MONITORING
N/A

PREVENTION/AVOIDANCE
• Implementation of a whole-herd vaccination program against BVDV is recommended.
• Vaccinations should include antigens against both type 1 and type 2 BVDV.
• Newly acquired cattle should be screened for persistent infection.
• Newly acquired cattle should be quarantined for a minimum of 3 weeks.

Vaccination

- Vaccination to prevent fetal infections is likely the most important measure to control the occurrence of PI calves.
- Effective vaccines against infectious agents must account for both antigenic and genetic diversity, and they should provide fetal protection.
- It should be remembered that colostral antibodies, which may last for 6 months, may interfere with vaccination.
- Both modified-live (MLV) and killed vaccines are available. Most vaccines in the United States include BVDV 1a cp strains, although some vaccines do contain BVDV 2 cp strains.
- Only a single dose of MLV vaccine is needed for initial immunization as opposed to killed vaccine that may require 2 or more doses. However, MLV vaccines are susceptible to inactivation by chemicals and/or exposure to higher temperatures. The MLV may also lead to mucosal disease when an animal persistently infected with an ncp strain is exposed to a closely related cp strain included in MLV.
- Because of multiple doses needed and the added cost of adjuvants, killed vaccines turn out to be more expensive. However, they are recommended for dairy herds where pregnant animals are always likely to be present. Killed vaccines are also recommended for bulls in AI centers.

POSSIBLE COMPLICATIONS

- The use of modified-live vaccines against BVDV in pregnant cattle is contraindicated unless specified by the product manufacturer.
- Modified-live vaccines may be immunosuppressive and therefore should be used with caution.

EXPECTED COURSE AND PROGNOSIS

Most cattle recover within 10 to 14 days.

MISCELLANEOUS

ASSOCIATED CONDITIONS

- Mucosal disease occurs in cattle persistently infected with BVDV following a superinfection with an antigenically related cytopathic BVDV strain.
- Cytopathic BVDV may also arise by mutation of the infecting ncp virus.

AGE-RELATED FACTORS

Colostral antibodies can protect newborn calves for 2–4 months.

ZOONOTIC POTENTIAL

BVDV is not considered a zoonotic agent.

PREGNANCY

- Fetal infection with BVDV can result in abortion, congenital defects, persistent infection, or seroconversion. The result of fetal infection is dependent on the virus strain and biotype and the stage of gestation when fetal infection occurs.
- In utero infection of the fetus with ncp BVDV prior to 120 days of gestation leads to immune tolerance and the birth of persistently infected (PI) calves that are unthrifty and poor doers and act as a source of virus for the rest of the herd. PI families can arise by breeding PI animals.

SEE ALSO

BHV-1
Brucellosis
Coumarol poisoning
Leptospirosis
Mucosal disease
Neospora
Salmonella
Sweet clover poisoning
Vitamin K deficiency
Winter dysentery

ABBREVIATIONS

BDV = border diseases virus of sheep
BHV = bovine herpes virus

BT = bovine turbinate
BVD = bovine viral diarrhea
BVDV = bovine viral diarrhea virus
CP = cytopathic
CSFV = classical swine fever virus
DFA = direct immunofluorescence
ELISA = enzyme-linked immunosorbent assay
IIF = indirect immunofluorescence assay
IIP = indirect immunoperoxidase assay
IPMA = immunoperoxidase monolayer assay
mAbs = monoclonal antibodies
M-ELISA = monolayer enzyme-linked immunosorbent assay
NCP = noncytopathic
PBL = peripheral blood leukocytes
PCR = polymerase chain reaction
PI = persistent infection
RT-PCR = reverse transcription–polymerase chain reaction
SN = serum neutralization
VN = virus neutralization

Suggested Reading

Baker, J. C., Houe, H., eds. 1995, Nov. Bovine viral diarrhea virus. *Vet Clin North Am Food Anim Pract.* 11(3):521–47.

Bitsch, V., Ronsholt, L. 1995, Nov. Control of bovine viral diarrhea virus infection without vaccines. *Vet Clin North Am Food Anim Pract.* 11(3):627–40.

Campbell, J. R. 2004, Mar. Effect of bovine viral diarrhea virus in the feedlot. *Vet Clin North Am Food Anim Pract.* 20(1):39–50.

Fray, M. D., Paton, D. J., Alenius, S. 2000, Jul 2. The effects of bovine viral diarrhoea virus on cattle reproduction in relation to disease control. *Anim Reprod Sci.* 60–61:615–27.

Grooms, D. L. 2004, Mar. Reproductive consequences of infection with bovine viral diarrhea virus. *Vet Clin North Am Food Anim Pract.* 20(1):5–19.

Kelling, C. L. 2004, Mar. Evolution of bovine viral diarrhea virus vaccines. *Vet Clin North Am Food Anim Pract.* 20(1):115–29.

Authors: Daniel L. Grooms and Sagar Goyal

BRACKEN FERN TOXICITY

 BASICS

OVERVIEW
• All ruminant species are at risk of developing toxicosis. Most cases of poisonings have been reported in cattle.
• Bracken fern, or brake fern (*Pteridium aquilinum*), is a native perennial fern, 1 to 6 feet tall, with triangular, coarse, pinnately compound fronds. It has a deep-seated, black, elongate, branched, hairy, horizontal rhizome. Spores develop late in the summer and are found rolled under the blade edges. This is the only *Pteridium* species that is considered toxic in the United States. Other *Pteridium* species have been shown to contain the toxic principle in other parts of the world.
• The plant prefers moist to dry woods and open slopes, with good drainage. It tends to occur naturally in very dense stands.
• The young plants and rhizomes are the most toxic part of the plant, green or dried.
• Disease in ruminants is generally seen following chronic exposures of variable concentrations of the plant in the diet.
• Poisonings with this plant are relatively uncommon.
• Diseases reported in ruminants include bone marrow suppression, enzootic hematuria, bladder and gastrointestinal carcinomas, and progressive retinal degeneration.
• Key to controlling the disease is prevention. Bracken fern is susceptible to a wide variety of herbicides.

PATHOPHYSIOLOGY
• Ptaquiloside is thought to be the main toxic principle. Other agents reported to be toxic include quercetin and shikimic acid. The species of animal exposed, and the dose and duration of exposure, are thought to be the limiting factors in determining which disease the animal succumbs to.

• Bone marrow suppression has been observed in clinically affected animals; there is suppression of all cell lines (radiomimetic effect).
• Clinically affected animals generally present with signs associated with thrombocytopenia and neutropenia; anemia may occur as a result of blood loss or later as the red cells disappear from circulation (long life span).
• Bovine enzootic hematuria ("red water") has been reported in cattle chronically exposed to bracken fern. This syndrome is linked to the development of bladder lesions, some of which are neoplastic. Hematuria and bladder neoplasms predominate in cattle, but papillomas, sarcomas, and carcinomas of the jaw and gastrointestinal tract can occur in sheep. Exposures of months or years are required to cause these types of changes. It has been speculated that viruses (bovine papillomavirus type 2 and type 4) may play a role in the development of neoplastic lesions.
• Experimentally, bracken fern exposure for 4 to 12 months has been associated with progressive retinal degeneration in sheep.
• Polioencephalomalacia has been reported in sheep chronically exposed to the plant (rare).

SYSTEMS AFFECTED
Bone marrow, urinary tract, gastrointestinal tract, and eye

GENETICS
N/A

INCIDENCE/PREVALENCE
Unpredictable and uncommon

GEOGRAPHIC DISTRIBUTION
Worldwide

SIGNALMENT
Cattle are most commonly affected.

Species
All ruminants appear susceptible; most poisonings have been reported to occur in cattle.

Breed Predilections
N/A

Mean Age and Range
Enzootic hematuria and tumors are generally observed in older animals, following months or years of exposure.

Predominant Sex
N/A

SIGNS
• Cattle afflicted with bone marrow suppression generally present with bloody nasal discharge, petechiation and ecchymoses, and weakness. Secondary bacterial infections are common (e.g., lung), and signs of dyspnea, decreased appetite, and hyperthermia can be observed.
• Red to brown urine is a common change in those cattle suffering from enzootic hematuria.
• Signs can be varied depending on the tumor site.
• Sheep suffering from retinal degeneration show bilateral pupil dilatation and have a glassy-eyed appearance ("bright blindness").

CAUSES AND RISK FACTORS
• Poisonings can occur as a result of grazing the fresh plant (thought to be unpalatable) or following chronic consumption of contaminated hay.
• The plant is toxic green or dry; the most toxic parts of the plant are the young developing fronds (fiddleheads or crosiers) and rhizomes.
• Clinical disease is generally seen when animals consume significant amounts of plant material (up to 20% of their diet) for 30 days or more.

 DIAGNOSIS

DIFFERENTIAL DIAGNOSIS
Thrombocytopenia has been reported with BVD virus infection.

CBC/BIOCHEMISTRY/URINALYSIS
• Thrombocytopenia and neutropenia; anemia is observed later on.
• Inflammatory leukogram, hyperproteinemia, elevated fibrinogen can be due to secondary infectious processes.
• Hematuria

OTHER LABORATORY TESTS
Prolonged bleeding times

IMAGING
N/A

DIAGNOSTIC PROCEDURES
Examination of the bone marrow may reveal pancytopenia—risky procedure in compromised patients.

PATHOLOGIC FINDINGS
• Petechiation and ecchymoses, multiple hemorrhages throughout the tissues, pale bone marrow, edematous and ulcerated GIT
• Numerous neoplastic conditions of the GIT and urinary tract—papillomas, transitional cell carcinomas, squamous cell carcinomas, adenocarcinomas, hemangiomas
• Retinal degeneration and atrophy of the outer layers

TREATMENT
• Find and remove the suspect source or remove animals from the contaminated environment.
• Most animals respond poorly to treatment.
• Broad-spectrum antibiotic use, animal stress reduction, and good nursing care can be utilized.
• Appropriate milk and meat withdrawal times must be followed for all compounds administered to food-producing animals.

MEDICATIONS
N/A

CONTRAINDICATIONS
Appropriate milk and meat withdrawal times must be followed for all compounds administered to food-producing animals.

FOLLOW-UP
N/A

PATIENT MONITORING
• Monitor platelet, neutrophil, and red blood cell values.
• Check for onset of secondary infections.

PREVENTION/AVOIDANCE
• Be able to recognize bracken fern in the field or in hay, and avoid excessive grazing.
• Herbicide application can be successful in eliminating the plant.

POSSIBLE COMPLICATIONS
N/A

EXPECTED COURSE AND PROGNOSIS
Animals suffering from bone marrow suppression almost never recover.

MISCELLANEOUS

ASSOCIATED CONDITIONS
Monogastrics exposed to bracken fern suffer from neurologic disease that is thought to be related to a thiamine deficiency.

AGE-RELATED FACTORS

ZOONOTIC POTENTIAL
Since ptaquiloside is a direct-acting carcinogen, people conceivably can be affected through direct consumption of the plant or ingesting meat or milk from exposed animals.

PREGNANCY
N/A

RUMINANT SPECIES AFFECTED
Cattle are most commonly reported to be affected; but there are reports of sheep, llamas, and other ruminants being affected.

BIOSECURITY
N/A

PRODUCTION MANAGEMENT
• Avoid feeding "weedy" hay.
• Avoid grazing in bracken dense areas, provide adequate forage, and instill appropriate stocking densities.

SYNONYMS
Bracken fern, brake fern
Bright blindness

SEE ALSO
BVD
Toxicology: herd outbreaks

ABBREVIATIONS
BVD = bovine viral diarrhea
GIT = gastrointestinal tract

Suggested Reading
Plumlee, K. H., Nicholson, S. S. 2004. Ptaquiloside. In: *Clinical veterinary toxicology*, ed. K. H. Plumlee. St. Louis: Mosby.
Pteridium. 2001. In: *Toxic plants of North America*, ed. G. E. Burrows, R. J. Tyrl. Ames: Iowa State University Press.

Author: Patricia Talcott

BRASSICA SPP. TOXICITY

BASICS

OVERVIEW
- Ingestion of *Brassica* spp. can cause various diseases including goiter, enteritis, and Heinz body anemia in ruminant animals.
- Forages or roots of the genus *Brassica* include kale, rape, turnips, mustards, cabbage, brussels sprouts, and others. *Brassica* spp. contain glucosinolates, which have goitrogenic effects and induce gastrointestinal irritation.
- These plants also contain S-methylcysteine sulphoxide (SMCO), which causes Heinz body anemia.
- Other diseases associated with *Brassica* spp. ingestion include polioencephalomalacia, photosensitization, and acute bovine pulmonary emphysema and edema.
- There are three groups of glucosinolates, which can be enyzmatically broken down into different metabolites: isothiocyanates, thiocyanate ion, and thiones.
- Isothiocyanates are found in mustard oils contained in plant seeds. These are irritants to the gastrointestinal mucosa causing enteritis and diarrhea.
- Thiocyanate ion can cause goiter when ingested in small amounts over extended periods of time, particularly if the dietary content of iodine is low. Thiocyanate ion reduces iodine uptake by the thyroid and can be treated with exogenous iodine.
- Thiones are a potent goitrogen, which interferes with the formation of thryoxine. Treatment with iodine does not alleviate clinical signs.
- "Rape blindness" has been observed in cattle and sheep grazing on rape. Other neurological signs such as head pressing and behavioral changes have been noted. These signs may be as a result of a mild degree of polioencephalomalacia or hepatotoxicity.
- Acute bovine pulmonary emphysema and edema have been observed in cattle on *Brassica* spp. plants. *Brassica* spp. forage may precipitate 3-methylindole–associated disease.

PATHOPHYSIOLOGY
- Thiocyanate ion can cause goiter when ingested in small amounts over extended periods of time, particularly if the dietary content of iodine is low.
- Thiocyanate ion reduces iodine uptake by the thyroid and can be treated with exogenous iodine. Thiones are a potent goitrogen, which interferes with the formation of thryoxine.
- Another toxin is S-methylcysteine sulphoxide (SMCO), which is converted to dimethyl disulphide (DMDS) by the rumen or gut organisms.
- DMDS interferes with disulphide exchange reactions, which results in changes in red blood cell membranes and hemoglobin. This can lead to Heinz body formation and anemia.
- *Brassica* spp. have also been associated with primary and secondary or hepatogenous photosensitization.

SYSTEMS AFFECTED
- Hemic
- Lymphoreticular
- Gastrointestinal
- Nervous
- Respiratory
- Integumentary

GENETICS
N/A

INCIDENCE/PREVALENCE
N/A

GEOGRAPHIC DISTRIBUTION
Potentially worldwide depending on species and environment

SIGNALMENT
- *Brassica* spp. poisoning has been reported in cattle, sheep, goats, and pigs. Goiter may be seen in animals of any age. Feeding *Brassica* spp. to pregnant dams may result in neonates with goiter.
- Hemolytic anemia occurs after 1–3 weeks of ingestion of a diet consisting mainly of *Brassica* spp. plants. Enteritis can occur after ingestion of large amounts of rapeseed and *Brassica* spp. seeds containing mustard oils.
- Pulmonary emphysema has been reported only in cattle.

Species
Potentially all ruminant species

Breed Predilections
N/A

Mean Age and Range
Any age

Predominant Sex
N/A

SIGNS

HISTORICAL FINDINGS
- Clinical signs for goiter include thyroid enlargement, weakness, lethargy, and recumbency. Animals with goiter may show signs of weight loss or failure to gain weight.
- Animals in hemolytic anemia crisis may show signs of lethargy, anorexia, dyspnea, coffee-colored urine and mucous membranes, icterus, hypoxic abortion, and cardiovascular shock. Death results from respiratory failure secondary to anemia.
- Clinical signs associated with enteritis include diarrhea, dysentery, abdominal pain, salivation, and occasionally vomiting. Anorexia, ruminal stasis, and scant, sticky feces may also be noted with gastrointestinal disturbances.
- Signs of photosensitization include erythema and blistering of affected areas, particularly areas of light-pigmented skin.

PHYSICAL EXAMINATION FINDINGS

CAUSES AND RISK FACTORS
- *Brassica* poisoning can be found in any commercial operation that provides *Brassica* plants or seeds as feed.
- Glucosinolate concentration can vary between *Brassica* plant species and can vary with season. The highest concentration of glucosinolates can be found in seeds, but are present in all parts of the plants. Plants become more toxic as they mature.
- The SMCO content of *Brassica* plants also increases with maturity and the flowers and seeds are particularly toxic.

DIAGNOSIS

DIFFERENTIAL DIAGNOSIS

• A nutritional deficiency of iodine can cause goiter. Goiter may also be caused by the ingestion of couch grasses (*Cynodon aethiopicus, C. nlemfuensis*) and white clover (*Trifolium repens*).
• Differential diagnoses for signs of hemolytic anemia include onion toxicity, red maple toxicity as well as leptospirosis, hypophosphatemia in postparturient cows, babesiosis, anaplasmosis, chronic copper poisoning, as well as immune-mediated and drug-induced hemolytic anemias.
• Differential diagnoses for *Brassica* spp.–induced signs of gastritis are numerous including ingestion of oak species, *Nerium* spp. (oleander), *Geigeria* spp., *Eupatorium rugosum,* and others, as well as parasitic, viral, and bacterial etiologies.
• Many species of plants, grasses, and blue-green algae can cause primary and secondary photosensitization.

CBC/BIOCHEMISTRY/URINALYSIS

• Assays of serum glucosinolate levels are available.
• Heinz bodies and decreased serum hemoglobin levels can be observed on complete blood counts.

TREATMENT

• There is no specific treatment for *Brassica* spp. poisoning. Removal of *Brassica* spp. feedstuffs and relocating animals away from pastures populated with *Brassica* spp. are recommended.
• Administration of iodine may be beneficial in cases of iodine deficiency. Blood transfusions may be necessary in cases of severe hemolytic anemia.

MEDICATIONS

DRUGS OF CHOICE

CONTRAINDICATIONS

Appropriate milk and meat withdrawal times must be followed for all compounds administered to food-producing animals.

PRECAUTIONS

N/A

POSSIBLE INTERACTIONS

N/A

FOLLOW-UP

PREVENTION/AVOIDANCE

Removal of *Brassica* spp. feedstuffs and relocating animals away from pastures populated with *Brassica* spp. are recommended.

EXPECTED COURSE AND PROGNOSIS

Fair to guarded if removed from plant

MISCELLANEOUS

ASSOCIATED CONDITIONS

N/A

AGE-RELATED FACTORS

N/A

ZOONOTIC POTENTIAL

N/A

PREGNANCY

Feeding *Brassica* spp. to pregnant dams may result in neonates with goiter.

RUMINANT SPECIES AFFECTED

Potentially all ruminant species are affected.

BIOSECURITY

N/A

PRODUCTION MANAGEMENT

Removal of *Brassica* spp. feedstuffs and relocating animals away from pastures populated with *Brassica* spp. are recommended.

SYNONYMS

N/A

SEE ALSO

Anaplasmosis
Babesiosis
Blue-green algae
Chronic copper poisoning
Ingestion of oak species
Leptospirosis
Nutritional deficiency of iodine
Oleander
Onion toxicity
Primary photosensitization
Red maple toxicity

ABBREVIATIONS

DMDS = dimethyl disulphide
SMCO = S-methylcysteine sulphoxide

Suggested Reading

Bell, J. M. 1984, Apr. Nutrients and toxicants in rapeseed meal: a review. *J Anim Sci.* 58(4): 996–1010.
Bray, T. M., Kirkland, J. B. 1990. The metabolic basis of 3-methylindole-induced pneumotoxicity. *Pharmacol Ther.* 46(1): 105–18.
Gonzalez, J. M., Yusta, B., Garcia, C., Carpio, M. 1986, Oct. Pulmonary and hepatic lesions in experimental 3-hydroxymethylindole intoxication. *Vet Hum Toxicol.* 28(5): 418–20.
Morton, J. M., Campbell, P. H. 1997, Feb. Disease signs reported in south-eastern Australian dairy cattle while grazing *Brassica* species. *Aust Vet J.* 75(2): 109–13.
Stoewsand, G. S. 1995, Jun. Bioactive organosulfur phytochemicals in *Brassica oleracea* vegetables—a review. *Food Chem Toxicol.* 33(6): 537–43.
Taljaard, T. L. 1993, Jun. Cabbage poisoning in ruminants. *J S Afr Vet Assoc.* 64(2): 96–100.

Author: Natalie Coffer

BASICS

DEFINITION
• Breeding soundness examination of the male camelid is becoming an integral part of many prepurchase examinations requested by breeders. This examination is not intended to measure fertility but to help identify males with reproductive problems.
• The reproductive system of the male camelid presents several anatomical and physiological peculiarities (see Camelid Reproduction). The practitioner should be familiar with these peculiarities in order to complete a thorough examination of a male.

SYSTEMS AFFECTED
Reproductive

GENETICS
N/A

INCIDENCE/PREVALENCE
N/A

GEOGRAPHIC DISTRIBUTION
Worldwide

SIGNALMENT
Species
Camelids
Breed Predilections
N/A
Mean Age and Range
N/A
Predominant Sex
Male

SIGNS

HISTORY AND PHYSICAL EXAMINATION
History and Signalment
• Age of the animal is important. Problems such as inability to mount or exteriorize the penis or even substandard fertility can be due to sexual immaturity
• Origin and type of management
• Breeding records
• Previous health problems
• Reason for examination

Physical Examination
• Reproductive performance of the male can be affected by diseases of other systems.
• Prolonged febrile condition or debilitating diseases can affect testicular function and spermatogenesis.

• A complete health history, including previous illnesses, vaccination, and recent treatments, should be taken.
• A general physical examination should be performed including general appearance and body condition of the animal. During the sire-selection process, particular attention should be given to the presence of congenital or potentially heritable conditions.

Reason for Examination
• Reasons for examination can be generally divided into two categories: prepurchase examination of a herd sire and examination for infertility or obvious genital lesions.
• It is very important to define exactly the problem(s) to be addressed: existence of visible lesions, suspicion of infertility due to many unsuccessful breedings, or a change in the reproductive behavior (reduced libido).
• An approximate date of the onset of the problem should be obtained as well as conditions: did the problem appear suddenly or was it a slow, progressive process?

Examination of the Prepuce and Penis
• Examination should be done when there is an obvious problem at this level, such as an abnormally pendulous prepuce, presence of edema, or laceration.
• Examination of the prepuce may require sedation of the animal.
• Ability to exteriorize the penis is best observed during a live cover.
• The penis is normally extended when the male assumes the breeding position but full erection is completed intravaginally.
• Penile attachment to the prepuce is normal in young, prepuberal animals but can signal the presence of adhesions in the mature male. In llamoids, the penis should be completely free at 3 years of age.

Examination of the Testicles and Scrotal Content
• The scrotal region is examined from a distance to evaluate testicular descent and integrity of the skin in the area.
• Both testes should be present and visible within the scrotum in the perineal region.
• In older males, the scrotum may sometimes be pendulous.
• One of the testicles is usually situated slightly more ventral than the other, but both should be nearly equal in size (difference less than 15%).
• Testicles are predisposed to traumatic lesions including bites by other males.

• Palpation of the scrotum and its contents is necessary to appreciate the regularity of the contour of the testes as well as their consistency.
• The surface of the testes should be smooth and regular.
• The testes are normally resilient. They become hard and fibrotic or very soft in the case of degenerative changes.
• The scrotal sac should be free from fluid.
• The tail of the epididymis is palpable as a small hard nodule.
• Testicular size is an important indicator of sperm production capacity. Size of the testis can be evaluated by measuring its length and width using precision calipers or ultrasonography. In the llama, the long axis should measure at least 1.1 cm in a yearling and 3.2 cm by 2 to 3 years of age. In alpacas, the testes' long axis should be at least 3.5 cm in order to achieve good fertility in a herd. The length and width of the testicle in adult males should be 5–7 cm and 3–4 cm in llamas and 4–5 cm and 2.5–3 cm in alpacas.
• Ultrasound of the testicle should be part of the routine breeding soundness examination. It is preferably done with a linear 7.5 MHz transducer (see Camelid Reproduction).

Examination of the Accessory Sex Glands
• When examination of the accessory sex glands is required, transrectal ultrasonography is the best method to accomplish this.
• The bulbourethral glands are found just cranial and on each side of the anal sphincter.
• Following the pelvic portion of the penis cranially images the prostate.

Evaluation of Mating Behavior
• Mating ability of the male is best observed in the presence of a receptive female.
• During this evaluation, the succession of normal behavioral patterns is recorded as well as the times needed for each step: chasing, forcing down, mating, intromission, and duration of copulation.
• Behavioral problems at mating can be due to shyness, inexperience, or lack of libido.

Semen Collection
• Semen collection presents many difficulties due mainly to the nature of copulatory behavior and the slow (dribbling) process of ejaculation in camelids.
• Semen collection using an artificial vagina is possible but requires training and the use of a specially designed dummy mount fitted with

BREEDING SOUNDNESS EXAMINATION AND INFERTILITY IN MALE CAMELIDS

a collection apparatus. The average duration of collection is about 30 minutes in llamas and 22 minutes in alpacas.

• Electroejaculation, using ram probes in llamoids and bovine probes in camels, has been accomplished under various degrees of sedation or anesthesia.

• Response to the electrical stimulus varies greatly from one individual to the other.

• Erection is possible during electroejaculation but failure to obtain an ejaculate or only a few sperm cells is common.

• The ejaculate obtained by electroejaculation is often of poor quality and contaminated with urine and cellular debris.

• In practice, the techniques most commonly used are vaginal aspiration and electroejaculation.

• Vaginal aspiration is accomplished by allowing a male to complete breeding with a receptive female. Upon completion of the mating an infusion pipette is introduced vaginally and the seminal fluid is aspirated using a 12 ml syringe.

Semen Evaluation

The major problem in interpreting semen analysis in the camelid is the lack of standard methods for collection and for examination.

Volume

• Ejaculate volume varies greatly depending on the method of collection used, duration of copulation, and male variation.

• Ejaculate volume ranges from 0.4 to 12.5 ml.

• Vaginal aspiration yields volumes ranging from 0.25 ml to 5 ml.

Color

• The color of semen varies according to sperm concentration.

• It is predominately milky white whether it is collected by electroejaculation or by other methodology, but can sometimes be creamy white.

• Ejaculate may be heterogeneous with some translucent material mixed with cloudy areas.

• Ejaculates collected by vaginal aspiration may be pink or red because of contamination with blood from the cervix.

Consistency and Liquefaction

• Camelid semen is viscous and requires some time to liquefy.

• The degree of viscosity depends on the individual male and on the proportion of seminal gelatinous fluid and tends to decrease with number of ejaculates.

• The time required for liquefaction varies from one male to another and from one ejaculate to another.

• Viscosity is attributed to the presence of mucopolysaccharides from secretions of the bulbourethral glands or the prostate.

• Liquefaction of camelid semen can be obtained by addition of trypsin or collagenase to the ejaculate.

Sperm Concentration

• Concentration of semen is best estimated using a hemocytometer technique after liquefaction.

• Sperm concentration is highly variable (82,000 to 250,000/mm^3) and is affected by age, method of collection, and ejaculate rank.

pH

• The pH of semen varies between 7.5 and 8.1.

• Semen pH is affected by method of collection and rank of ejaculate.

Semen Motility

• Motility of semen is appreciated on nondiluted samples (mass activity) and on diluted samples (individual sperm motility).

• Mass activity is generally poor in camelidae semen unless the ejaculate is constituted exclusively by the sperm-rich fraction.

• In fresh nondiluted samples, only oscillatory movements are observed.

• Initial motility is very low (5%) and increases as the ejaculate liquefies.

• Progressive motility can only be estimated after liquefaction and dilution with a suitable extender.

Semen Morphology

• The head of camelidae spermatozoa is described as elliptical as opposed to ovoid in other species.

• Lengths of the head and middle piece are shorter than those of other animals.

• Morphology of the spermatozoa can be evaluated on smears stained with eosine-Nigrosin Hancock stain or Diff Quick (Giemsa) stains.

• A total of at least two hundred sperm cells from different fields should be evaluated from each sample.

• Morphological evaluation is done under phase contrast microscopy as for other species.

• The morphological abnormalities should be reported according to type and location.

• Effect of various types of abnormalities on fertility has not yet been determined.

• Total abnormalities should not exceed 50%.

• The most common abnormalities are proximal droplets, knobbed or swollen acrosome and tail, and midpiece reflex.

Endocrine Evaluation

• Information on endocrinological evaluation of the infertile male camelid is completely lacking. The only practical use of endocrine evaluation is in the differential diagnosis between cryptorchidism and castration.

• Presence of testicular tissue can be ascertained if there is at least a twofold increase in serum testosterone level within 8 to 24 hours after IV administration of hCG (3000 IU for alpacas, 5000 IU in llamas, 10,000 IU in camels).

Testicular Biopsy

Indications

• Testicular biopsy is not a routine procedure for the evaluation of the breeding soundness in the male.

• Testicular biopsy should be considered in males that have low fertility, testicular asymmetry, and abnormal testicular ultrasonography that is not consistent with hematoma or orchitis.

• This technique is useful for diagnosis of spermatogenic arrest, oligospermatogenesis, hypogonadism, inflammations, and neoplasm.

Techniques

• *Wedge biopsy*: an incisional or open biopsy requires general anesthesia. After surgical preparation of the scrotum, an incision (0.5 cm) is made over the skin, parietal vaginal tunic, and the exposed tunica albuginea avoiding vascular areas. Testicular tissue allowed to protrude from the rent in the tunica albuginea is ablated using a scalpel blade. The tunica albuginea, parietal vaginal tunic, and scrotal skin are closed with absorbable suture.

• *Trucut*: use under sedation or anesthesia. After surgical preparation of the testicles, the scrotum is incised using a sterile #10 surgical blade (alpacas) or #11 scalpel (llamas). The trucut (14-gauge self-firing) biopsy needle is inserted in the testicle through the tunica albuginea. The scrotum is closed with two skin sutures using 2-0 Vetafil. Results obtained with this technique are more reliable but hemorrhage at the biopsy site is more frequent.

• "Core" biopsy: A needle "core" biopsy can be performed using a 1 1/2 in., 16-gauge needle after heavy sedation of the animal. After surgical preparation of the scrotal skin,

BREEDING SOUNDNESS EXAMINATION AND INFERTILITY IN MALE CAMELIDS

the needle is introduced into the testicular parenchyma and redirected by a gentle push-pull movement into two different sites. The needle is retracted from the tissue while a finder is placed over the hub to maintain the core sampled. A direct smear is prepared from the sample obtained.
• *Fine needles aspirate*: Fine needle aspirate cytology is a commonly used technique for the evaluation of azoospermia and testicular neoplasm in humans. It is rapid, simple, and inexpensive. Testicular tissue is aspirated with a 20-gauge needle and 12 ml syringe. A puncture is made and aspirates are taken in three to four directions making sure not to include the epididymis. Cytological smears stained with Diff Quick are interpreted based on the different types of spermatogenic cells.

Interpretations
• Interpretation should be done by an individual familiar with the technique and histology of camelid testes.
• Fine-needle aspirates are very difficult to interpret. The relative frequency of cell types provides a differential diagnosis between hypospermatogenesis, spermatogenic arrest, and normal spermatogenesis. A fine-needle aspirate from azoospermic animals consists of Sertoli cells alone, a few mature spermatozoa, and scant cell material or spermatid but no spermatozoa.
• "Core" biopsy provides more cellular material than fine-needle biopsy.
• Trucut or self-firing biopsy instruments are safe and provide a good amount of tissue for examination of seminiferous tubule spermatogenic activity.
• Presence of normal spermatogenic activity in cases of azoospermia may suggest the presence of segmental aplasia or other forms of obstructive azoospermia.
• Atypical spermatogenic cells are usually associated with testicular neoplasm (seminoma).
• No spermatogenic cells are obtained from atrophic testicles.

Complications
• Hematoma or hemorrhage
• Adhesions and inflammation
• Autoimmune reactions (development of antisperm antibodies)
• Degeneration of germinal epithelium and tubules

• Transient decrease in sperm output that lasts for several months
• Wedge biopsy is the most unsafe of all methods
• Complication risk increases if the technique is not performed correctly and quickly

Reproductive Disorders in the Male Camelid
Inpotentia Cuendi
• Inability to complete mating may be due to poor libido, erection or ejaculation failure.
• Poor libido may be associated with endocrinological disorders, systemic diseases or diseases of other organs (including megaesophagus!) and high ambient temperature.
• Young male may be too shy to perform particularly in clinic setting.
• Erection failure may be due to neurological disorders, painful conditions, or preputial stenosis.
• Incomplete mating may be due to obesity or abdominal pain.

Impotentia Gerandi
• Inability to achieve fertilization
• May be due to azoospermia or severe oligospermia of testicular (hypoplasia, degeneration) or epididymal (stenosis, segmental aplasia) origin
• Asthenozoospermia (lack of motility)
• Teratospermia (increased rate of abnormalities)

Diseases of the Penis and Prepuce
• Infections of the prepuce and the penis are relatively rare in camelidae because they are well protected due to their anatomic position.
• Preputial swelling is due to local inflammation caused by contact with chemical or physical irritants, parasitic infestation, or rupture of the urethra.
• Preputial swelling can also be part of a large ventral edema in some animals suffering from heat stress.
• Preputial prolapse is often seen in alpacas. It may require surgical correction.
• Paraphymosis can become complicated by the presence of dirt in the preputial opening and lead to a balanoposthitis, sometimes with necrosis of the tip of the penis.
• Early detection of paraphymosis and treatment will avoid these complications.
• In llamas, paraphymosis and balanoposthitis can be due to the presence of "hair rings" if the females are not clipped before breeding.

• Urolithiasis: most calculi occur at the level of the distal part of the urethra or at the level of the sigmoid flexure. Relief of the condition can be attempted via urethrostomy. Recurrence of obstruction is common even after urethrostomy.

Diseases of the Testis
• Scrotal trauma
  • Bites from other males are a common complaint in the male camelid.
  • Prognosis for the reproductive life of the individual male depends on the extent of the injury and the time elapsed until detection.
  • The affliction should be differentiated from orchitis or hydrocele.
  • Deep lacerations are frequently complicated by testicular hemorrhage, infection, and development of schirrous cord and require urgent surgical intervention (castration).
• Hydrocele
  • Due to an inflammatory or noninflammatory process.
  • The scrotal sac becomes pendulous and increased in size.
  • Initial diagnosis is based on palpation of the scrotum and its content.
  • The scrotum is not painful and the testes are usually free within the scrotal sac and fluid can be isolated in one area.
  • Confirmation is done by visualization of the fluid by ultrasonography.
  • Moderate hydrocele is sometimes observed in summer. The condition resolves progressively with decreasing ambient temperature.
  • Hydrocele can develop following obstruction of the normal blood flow in the spermatic cord.
  • Hydrocele may be due to the presence of an abscess at the level of the external inguinal ring.
  • Long-standing hydrocele affects the thermoregulation of the testes and decreases the quality and quantity of semen.
• Orchitis
  • Usually caused by hematogenous route.
  • Systemic antimicrobial therapy is indicated but is generally not efficacious.
  • Castration of the affected testicle in valuable males may increase the chance of salvaging the nonaffected testicle and the reproductive life of the animal.

BREEDING SOUNDNESS EXAMINATION AND INFERTILITY IN MALE CAMELIDS

- Testicular degeneration
  - The most common cause of infertility in camelids.
  - The degenerated testicles are smaller than normal and either soft or hard and fibrous.
  - Semen shows increased abnormalities and the presence of spheroid (round) germinal cells.
- Partial or total testicular hypoplasia or atrophy
  - Testicular hypoplasia is common in camelids.
  - Differential diagnosis between hypoplasia and atrophy requires histopathological techniques.
  - Semen may show increased abnormalities and poor concentration.
- Cryptorchidism
  - Relatively rare in camelids.
  - Can be unilateral or bilateral and is suspected when inspection of the perineal region shows a flat or absent scrotum.
  - The undescended testicles are usually found close to the internal inguinal opening but could also be found intra-abdominally, caudal to the kidney, or within the inguinal canal.
  - Cryptorchidism was reported in related vicuñas, which suggests that the affliction may be hereditary.
  - Should be differentiated from anorchism (absence of a testicle), which is generally accompanied by absence of the kidney on the same side.
  - Differential diagnosis: endocrinology, laparoscopy, laparotomy.
- Testicular tumors
  - Rare
  - Seminomas are the most common
  - Sertoli cell tumors and teratomas are possible
- Testicular cysts
  - Found in 15% of all males examined by the author.
  - Can be detected ultrasonographically.
  - They can be located in the rete testis, seminiferous tubules, head or tail of the epididymis.
  - The effect on fertility varies from complete sterility (azoospermia) to subfertility depending on the size and location of the cysts.
  - Some males with small testicular cysts have normal fertility.

Diseases of the Epididymis
- Epididymitis is usually associated with orchitis.
- Epididymal cysts are common in alpacas and llamas.
- Cysts are found on the anterior aspect of the head of the epididymis and near the ventral border of the testis.
- Cysts vary in size between 1 mm and 50 mm.
- Large cysts may be due to segmental aplasia of the epididymal duct.

Subfertility or Infertility of Unexplained Origin
- Decreased fertility may be due to overuse or senile changes.
- The author has seen cases of infertility/sterility with normal seminal parameters and behavior.
- Molecular factors (immunologic or genetic) may be involved in males with unexplained infertility.
- Males have different abilities to induce ovulation (lack or reduced activity of the ovulation inducing agent present in seminal plasma).

 MISCELLANEOUS

ASSOCIATED CONDITIONS
It is very important to define exactly the problem(s) to be addressed: existence of visible lesions, suspicion of infertility due to many unsuccessful breeding attempts, or a change in the reproductive behavior (reduced libido).

AGE-RELATED FACTORS
Penile attachment to the prepuce is normal in young, prepuberal animals but can signal the presence of adhesions in the mature male. In llamoids, the penis should be completely free at 3 years of age.

ZOONOTIC POTENTIAL
Brucellosis, though not common in camelids, is a zoonotic disease worth concern.

PREGNANCY
N/A

RUMINANT SPECIES AFFECTED
Camelids and camels

BIOSECURITY
N/A

PRODUCTION MANAGEMENT
N/A

SYNONYMS
N/A

SEE ALSO
BSE: Bovine, Ultrasound

ABBREVIATIONS
BSE = breeding soundness exam
HCG = human chorionic gonadotropin
IU = international units
IV = intravenous

Suggested Reading
Bravo, P. W., Flores, D., Ordonez, C. 1997. Effect of repeated collection on semen characteristics of alpacas. *Biol Reprod.* 57:520–24.

Flores, P., Garcia-Huidobro, J., Munoz, C., Bustos-Obregon, E., Urquita, B. 2002. Alpaca semen characteristics previous to a mating period. *Animal Reproduction Science* 72: 259–66.

Heath, A. M., Pugh, D. G., Sartin, E. A., Navarre B., Purohit, R. C. 2002. Evaluation of the safety and efficacy of testicular biopsies in llamas. *Theriogenology* 58(6):1125–30.

Tibary, A., Anouassi, A. 1997. Pathology and surgery of the reproductive tract and associated organs in the male camelidae. In: *Theriogenology in Camelidae: anatomy, physiology, BSE, pathology and artificial breeding*, ed. A. Tibary. Actes Edition, Institut Agronomique et Veterinaire Hassan II, Morocco.

Tibary, A., Anouassi, A., Memon, A. M. 2001. Approach to infertility diagnosis in camelids: retrospective study in alpacas, llamas and camels. *Journal of Camel Practice and Research.* 8:167–79.

Author: Ahmed Tibary

BREEDING SOUNDNESS EXAM: BEEF BULL

 BASICS

DEFINITION
• A breeding soundness exam (BSE) is an evaluation of a bull's reproductive soundness based on a physical examination of the reproductive tract and semen evaluation.
• The primary focus is on the reproductive system but the musculoskeletal system and ophthalmic systems must be evaluated as well.
• Some examiners will include libido or serving capacity tests as part of a BSE.
• The BSE is not meant to be a general health exam.

PATHOPHYSIOLOGY
N/A

SYSTEMS AFFECTED
Reproductive, musculoskeletal, ophthalmic, behavioral

GENETICS
• Genetics play an important role in the onset of puberty.
• Large breed differences exist in age and weight at puberty and testicular size (scrotal circumference).

INCIDENCE/PREVALENCE
N/A

GEOGRAPHIC DISTRIBUTION
Worldwide

SIGNALMENT
• All bulls should receive a BSE prior to the breeding season.
• A BSE is particularly important in young bulls prior to their first breeding season.

SIGNS
N/A

CAUSES
The causes of poor fertility that can be detected during a BSE are numerous and include:
• Late maturation
• Small testicles
• Poor semen quality
• Injuries to the penis, prepuce, or testes
• Lameness
• Poor or excessive body condition
• Infectious processes involving the testes or accessory sex glands
• Eye injuries
• Congenital reproductive anomalies

RISK FACTORS
N/A

 DIAGNOSIS

DIFFERENTIAL DIAGNOSIS
Infertility
• Deficiencies: iodine, manganese, vitamin A, zinc
• Environment: cold weather infertility, heat stroke
• Hereditary: Bulls cotwin with freemartin heifer, chromosomal abnormalities, inbreeding, segmental aplasia of reproductive tract
• Lameness
• Malnutrition
• Penis/prepuce: balanoposthitis; bovine herpes virus-1; dermatophilosis; hematoma, hematocele; loss of penile sensation; micropenis, hypoplasia; papillomatosis, warts; paraphimosis; penile deviation; penile hair ring; penile preputial adhesion; persistent penile frenulum; prolapsed prepuce; trauma
• Psychologic impotency
• Scrotum: abscess, dermatophilosis, frostbite, inguinal scrotal hernia
• Seminal vesiculitis
• Sperm: abnormalities of spermatogenesis, hemospermia, infectious bovine rhinotracheitis (IBR), bovine viral diarrhea (BVD) contaminated semen, sperm granuloma
• Testicles: cryptorchidism, degeneration, hypoplasia/atrophy, orchitis, trauma, tumors
• Urethra and erectile tissue: corpus cavernosum vascular shunts, urethral fistula, urolithiasis
• Varicocele
• Vertebral spondylosis

Lack of Libido
• Epididymitis
• Iodine deficiency
• Lameness
• Malnutrition
• Orchitis
• Penis/prepuce problems: trauma-hematoma, prolapsed penis, loss of penile sensation, corpus cavernosum vascular shunts, persistent penile frenulum, posthitis
• Psychogenic impotency
• Vertebral osteophytosis/spondylosis
• Zinc deficiency

Sexual Malfunction
• Penile/preputial problems: balanoposthitis; deviation; herpes vulvovaginitis; infectious bovine pustular vulvovaginitis; papillomatosis; paraphimosis; penile/preputial adhesions; penile hair ring; persistent penile frenulum; phimosis; ruptured urethra; trauma, hematoma, abscesses; urethral calculi

• Prepuce: abscess/cellulitis, foreign body, preputial stenosis, prolapsed prepuce, trauma
• Testicles, spermatic cord, and scrotum: brucellosis; cryptorchidism; epididymitis; segmental aplasia; sperm granuloma; spermatocele; testicular degeneration, hypoplasia, atrophy; testicular trauma; testicular tumors; varicocele; zinc deficiency

CBC/BIOCHEMISTRY/URINALYSIS
N/A

OTHER LABORATORY TESTS
Culture and sensitivity may be indicated when disease is suspected.

IMAGING
Ultrasound examination may be a helpful adjunct.

DIAGNOSTIC PROCEDURES
Physical Soundness
• Careful attention must be paid to the structural correctness of the feet and legs of a potential breeding bull.
• A bull must be able to cover large distances to search out and find cows in estrus.
• Pain in the limbs and/or back may prevent a bull from successfully servicing cows.
• Breeding bulls should be free of heritable abnormalities such as post-leggedness, sickle hocks, and corkscrew claw.
• The eyes should be examined since a bull primarily uses eyesight to detect cows in estrus.

Evaluation of the Scrotum and Testes
• Visual inspection of the scrotum reveals information about the symmetry, size, and shape of the scrotum.
• The scrotum should have a distinct neck above the testicles to allow adequate thermoregulation.
• Appraisal of the scrotal skin allows detection of scrotal dermatitis or frostbite, which may affect semen quality.
• The testicles should be equal in size, shape, and consistency and be freely moveable within the scrotum.
• Palpation of lumps, soft spots, or any other abnormality of the testicles should alert the examiner to the possibility of an abnormality that may affect semen quality.
• Scrotal circumference (SC) should be measured.
  • Changes in SC from year to year may be evidence of problems within the testes.
  • Most breed associations have established minimum SC measurements in order for yearling bulls to pass a BSE.
  • Some variability exists between breed associations but most have a minimum SC of at least 32 cm for bulls 12–15 months of age.

• SC is measured by grasping the neck of the scrotum and firmly pulling the testes down into the scrotum. The thumb and fingers should be on the sides of the scrotum rather than between the testicles. The measuring tape should be looped around the greatest diameter of the scrotum.
• Each epididymis should be evaluated by palpation.
• The head of the epididymis can usually be palpated on the craniodorsal aspect of the testicle.
 • The body of the epididymis can be palpated on the medial aspect of the testicles. Abnormalities of the body are rare.
 • The tail of the epididymis can be palpated at the base, or ventral aspect, of the scrotum.
 • Each epididymis should be evaluated for side-to-side differences, swellings or masses, firmness, warmth, or pain.

Palpation of the Penis and Prepuce
Palpation of the penis and prepuce should be performed.
• The penis should be palpated through the skin from the base of the scrotum to the glans. Detection of any swellings along the penis should alert the examiner to the possibility of an injury that may affect the bull's ability to service cows.
• The prepuce should be palpated from the preputial orifice to the reflection onto the glans. Special attention should be paid to the reflection of the prepuce onto the glans, as this is a very common site of preputial injury.

Transrectal Examination of Accessory Sex Glands and Inguinal Rings
Transrectal examination of the accessory sex glands and inguinal rings should be performed.
• The urethra is usually the first structure palpated. It is a firm tubular structure and usually becomes pulsatile upon palpation.
• The prostate is usually encountered next and can be palpated as a firm transverse ridge at the cranial aspect of the urethra.
• The vesicular glands, or seminal vesicles, can be palpated craniolateral to the prostate. These glands vary in size between bulls but should be uniform in size, lobulated, turgid, and moveable.
• The ampullae may be difficult to identify by palpation but they lie on the pelvic floor cranial to the prostate. Disease of the ampullae is rare.

• The ampullae can be followed to the ductus deferens, which enters the abdominal cavity through the internal inguinal rings.
• The internal inguinal rings can usually be palpated 15–20 cm ventral to the brim of the pelvis and 5–15 cm lateral to midline. One to three fingers can usually be inserted into the internal rings. Enlarged rings may predispose a bull to scrotal hernia.
• The bulbourethral glands are imbedded in the urethralis muscle and cannot be palpated.
• The most common abnormality found on rectal examination is enlargement, excessive firmness, or loss of lobulation of the vesicular glands.
 • Seminal vesiculitis occurs most commonly in young bulls.
 • Adhesions, abscessation, and development of a draining tract may occur in chronic cases.
 • Purulent material may be grossly evident in a semen sample or neutrophils may be seen upon microscopic examination of specially stained smears.
 • Samples for culture and sensitivity may be obtained by passing a long, sterile catheter up the urethra and massaging the vesicular glands per rectum.
• After completion of the rectal exam, the pelvic urethra should be massaged to prepare the bull for semen collection.

Collection and Evaluation of Semen Sample
Collection and evaluation of a semen sample is an integral part of a BSE.
• The nature of the bull, available facilities, response of the bull to previous collection attempts, and examiner preference should all be considered when attempting to collect a semen sample.
• Semen may be collected by transrectal massage of the pelvic urethra, by electroejaculation, or by use of an artificial vagina.
• Transrectal massage usually works well in calm bulls but requires at least two people, often does not result in protrusion of the penis, and is tiring to the person performing the massage.
• Numerous types of electroejaculation equipment are available.
 • When using electroejaculation, a bull must be properly restrained.
 • The amount of stimulation should be determined by the bull's response.

• Stimulation should be low at first and gradually increased until the bull gains an erection and ejaculates. If maximal stimulation is reached without ejaculation, the bull should be allowed to rest for a few minutes and the collection attempted again. If collection is unsuccessful after two to three attempts, the bull should be retested on another day or by another means.
• Some bulls will not ejaculate in response to electroejaculation and other means must be used.
• A caudal epidural prior to collection attempts may reduce discomfort for the bull.
• The semen sample should be obtained when the ejaculate becomes cloudy.
• Semen collection by use of an artificial vagina (AV) is primarily used in artificial insemination centers.
 • Safety for the bull, the mount animal, and the collection personnel must be considered.
 • Collection of semen using an AV may be useful for bulls that fail to ejaculate in response to electroejaculation.
• It is important that a bull achieve erection and protrusion of the penis so that the penis and prepuce can be carefully evaluated.

Semen Sample Examination
The semen sample should be examined microscopically as soon as possible after collection.
• Equipment used in semen evaluation should be kept clean and warm in order to prevent a reduction in sperm motility.
• Contamination of a semen sample with urine, blood, pus, or chemicals may reduce sperm motility.
• The semen sample should be evaluated for both gross and individual motility.
 • Gross motility is evaluated according to the following:
  Very good—rapid dark swirls
  Good—slower swirls and eddies
  Fair—no swirls but prominent individual cell motion
  Poor—little or no individual cell motion
• Individual motility is evaluated by preparing a wet mount by placing a drop of semen on a warm slide and placing a warm cover slip over it.

BREEDING SOUNDNESS EXAM: BEEF BULL

• Individual motility is determined based on an estimate of the percentage of progressively motile cells.
  Very good—80–100%
  Good—60–79%
  Fair—40–59%
  Poor—< 40%
  Sperm morphology is evaluated by mixing a drop of semen and a drop of stain on a slide and preparing a smear.
• Live-dead stains are most commonly used. With these stains, live cells appear clear while dead cells are stained pink.
• Sperm cell morphology has historically been evaluated based on the percentage of normal cells versus the percentages of primary and secondary abnormalities.
• Primary abnormalities have their origin in the testes during spermatogenesis while secondary abnormalities originate in the epididymis.
• Some variability exists in the classification of primary versus secondary abnormalities. Generally speaking, abnormalities of the head or midpiece are considered primary while those of the tail are considered secondary. There are exceptions to this rule of thumb and the reader is referred to the Suggested Reading list at the end of the chapter for a more detailed description of these abnormalities.
• Some authors question the validity of this classification system and propose a differential count of all abnormalities instead.
• Primary abnormalities are not more important than secondary abnormalities as both types will reduce the viability of the cell.
• Under most circumstances, a minimum of 30% progressively motile sperm and 70% morphologically normal cells are adequate to pass a BSE.
  • Bulls are classified as satisfactory potential breeders or unsatisfactory potential breeders, or classification may be deferred.
  • Bulls with poor semen quality but without obvious physical abnormalities should be deferred and retested.
  • Detection of a heparin binding protein known as fertility-associated antigen in bull semen may be an indicator of fertility. This test may be useful in further identifying subfertile bulls among bulls that pass a standard BSE.

Serving Capacity/Libido Test
A serving capacity/libido test may be included as part of a BSE.
• Bulls are exposed to restrained, estrus cows for specified time periods and are observed for sexual behavior and mating activity.

• Bulls may also be exposed to a small number of estrous cows in a small pen and be observed for mating activity.
• Most standard BSEs do not include a serving capacity/libido test.
• A rough estimation of serving capacity/libido can be obtained by observing the activity of bulls in a natural mating situation.

Classification Systems and Evaluation Forms
Different classification systems and evaluation forms are available but the most commonly used evaluation form is produced by the Society for Theriogenology.

PATHOLOGIC FINDINGS
N/A

TREATMENT

CLIENT EDUCATION
• Reproductive efficiency is the most economically important aspect of beef production.
• Scrotal circumference is closely related to age of puberty and fertility in daughter progeny.
• Each gram of testicular tissue produces roughly the same number of sperm cells so bulls with larger testicles produce a larger volume of semen.

MEDICATIONS

FOLLOW-UP

MISCELLANEOUS

ASSOCIATED CONDITIONS
N/A

AGE-RELATED FACTORS
N/A

ZOONOTIC POTENTIAL
• Infectious orchitis caused by *Brucella* spp. poses some zoonotic risk to humans.
• Animals diagnosed with infections caused by these organisms should be culled.
• Brucellosis is a reportable disease.

PREGNANCY
N/A

RUMINANT SPECIES AFFECTED
Beef bulls

BIOSECURITY
Quarantine all new bulls and those returning from shows for a determined period of time to protect herd health.

PRODUCTION MANAGEMENT
• All bulls should receive a BSE prior to the breeding season.
• A BSE is particularly important in young bulls prior to their first breeding season.

SYNONYMS
N/A

SEE ALSO
• Beef bull behavior
• Beef bull management
• Body condition score bovine
• Testicular anomalies
• Ultrasounding bovine reproductive tract

ABBREVIATIONS
• AV = artificial vagina
• BSE = breeding soundness exam
• BVD = bovine viral diarrhea
• cm = centimeter
• IBR = infectious bovine rhinotracheitis
• SC = scrotal circumference

Suggested Reading
Bellin, M. E., Oyarzo, J. N., et al. 1998. Fertility associated antigen on bull sperm indicates fertility potential. *Journal of Animal Science* 76:2032–39.
Morrow, D. A. 1986. *Current therapy in theriogenology 2*. Philadelphia: W. B. Saunders.
Van Camp, S. D., ed. 1997, July. Bull infertility. In: *Veterinary clinics of North America, food animal practice*. Philadelphia: W. B. Saunders.
Youngquist, R. S. 1997. *Current therapy in large animal theriogenology*. Philadelphia: W. B. Saunders.

Author: John Gilliam

BASICS

DEFINITION
Brucellosis is a reproductive disease of cattle, bison, elk, yaks, sheep, and goats caused by a gram-negative, facultative, intracellular bacterium.

PATHOPHYSIOLOGY
• *Brucella abortus, B. melitensis,* and *B. ovis* can be shed in the blood, urine, milk, semen, placenta, fetus, and vaginal discharges of infected animals.
• Susceptible animals that come in contact with these fluids, either through ingestion, contact with mucous membranes, or skin abrasions, can develop a septicemia and abort if pregnant, deliver weak-born animals, and/or become a chronic carrier.

SYSTEMS AFFECTED
Reproductive in all ruminants, musculoskeletal (arthritis) in cattle affected with *B. abortus.*

GENETICS
N/A

INCIDENCE/PREVALENCE
• Incidence of brucellosis varies between countries.
• In the United States, since the implementation of the Bovine Brucellosis Eradication Plan in 1934, infection rate is less than 0.25% in two states (Class A status) as of May 2004.
• More than 50% of the bison and elk herd in Yellowstone National Park and Grand Teton National Park have tested positive for brucellosis.

GEOGRAPHIC DISTRIBUTION
• Can be found worldwide
• *B. abortus* has been eradicated from Japan, Canada, Northern Europe, Australia, and New Zealand.
• *B. melitensis* does not occur in northern Europe, southeast Asia, Australia, or New Zealand and is rare in the United States.
• *B. ovis* is seen in Australia, New Zealand, and the United States and is endemic in other sheep-raising regions of the world.

SIGNALMENT
Species
• Cattle, bison, water buffalo, sheep, goats—*B. abortus*
• Sheep—*B. melitensis, B. ovis*
• Goats—*B. melitensis*

Breed Predilections
N/A

Mean Age and Range
Reproductively active animals are susceptible, so age can vary depending on species.

Predominant Sex
N/A

SIGNS

HISTORICAL FINDINGS
• In cattle, weak or stillborn calves, abortions during the second half of gestation, and decreased milk production may be the only clinical signs.
• In sheep, late-term abortions and retained placenta. Rams may develop orchitis, epididymitis, and impaired fertility.
• In goats, abortions can be noted during the fourth month, as well as mastitis and lameness. Bucks may develop orchitis and epididymitis.

PHYSICAL EXAMINATION FINDINGS
• Most often, systemic signs are rare with brucellosis infection.
• Upon physical exam, retained placenta, decreased milk production may be noted in females.
• Male sheep may have decreased sperm counts and swollen testicles.

CAUSES
Susceptible animals that come in contact with contaminated blood, urine, milk, semen, placenta, fetus, and vaginal discharges from infected animals, either through ingestion, contact with mucous membranes, or skin abrasions, can develop brucellosis infection.

RISK FACTORS
Contact with infected herd mates or wildlife.

DIAGNOSIS

DIFFERENTIAL DIAGNOSIS
• In cattle, BVD, IBR, leptospirosis, listeriosis, neosporosis, mycotic abortion, trichomoniasis, campylobacteriosis, chlamydiosis, epizootic bovine abortion (in California), bluetongue, parainfluenza-3, *Ureaplasma, Mycoplasma, Haemophilus somnus, Salmonella,* and *Arcanobacter pyogenes.*
• Noninfectious causes include heat stress, ponderosa pine needle ingestion, locoweed, broomweed, and mycotoxins.
• In sheep and goats, vibriosis (primarily sheep), enzootic abortion (*Chlamydia psittaci*), toxoplasmosis, listeriosis, salmonellosis, and leptospirosis in goats.
• Noninfectious causes are similar to those of cattle.

BRUCELLOSIS

CBC/BIOCHEMISTRY/URINALYSIS
N/A

OTHER LABORATORY TESTS
• Serology can be used to diagnose brucellosis infection (*B. abortus*, *B. melitensis*) by card and plate agglutination (buffered *Brucella* antigen tests).
• ELISA tests can be used to detect *B. abortus* in milk and *B. abortus* and *B. ovis* in serum.
• The milk ring test can be used to detect *B. abortus* in bulk milk samples in cattle but not in small ruminants.
• Complement fixation can be used to identify *B. abortus* and *B. ovis*.

IMAGING
N/A

DIAGNOSTIC PROCEDURES
Brucella abortus can often be cultured from fetal membranes, vaginal discharge, milk, semen, or aborted fetuses.

PATHOLOGIC FINDINGS
• Aborted fetuses can be normal or autolyzed with evidence of bronchopneumonia.
• Placentitis in cattle and sheep consists of edema and necrotic cotyledons.
• In cattle, the cotyledons could also be normal, red, or yellow in color. The intercotyledonary area is leathery and thickened and has a wet appearance in cattle and sheep.
• Goats have a normal placenta.
• In the case of joint involvement, inflammatory lesions may be seen.
• Granulomatous lesions may be found upon slaughter in the reproductive tract, supramammary lymph nodes, and the mammary gland.

TREATMENT

APPROPRIATE HEALTH CARE
• All cases of brucellosis need to be reported to the state or federal veterinarian and the animals need to be eliminated from the herd.
• No treatment is effective.

ACTIVITY

DIET
N/A

CLIENT EDUCATION
Veterinarians should educate cattle owners regarding their state's recommendations regarding vaccinating young stock in keeping with the eradication program in the United States.

SURGICAL CONSIDERATIONS
N/A

MEDICATIONS

DRUGS OF CHOICE
• No treatment is recommended for cattle.
• In the case of valuable breeding rams, prolonged antibiotic therapy based upon culture and sensitivity can be used. However, fertility may never return to normal.

CONTRAINDICATIONS
N/A

POSSIBLE INTERACTIONS
N/A

ALTERNATIVE DRUGS
N/A

FOLLOW-UP

PATIENT MONITORING:
N/A

PREVENTION/AVOIDANCE
• Vaccination of female calves against *B. abortus* with RB-51 from 4 to 12 months of age in endemic areas increases resistance to infection.
• Adult cattle can also be vaccinated but only with permission of the state, provincial, or federal veterinarian. RB-51 is currently being used experimentally in bison, and disease status is being monitored to assess efficacy.
• Goats and sheep can be vaccinated with live, attenuated Rev-1 *B. melitensis* in various parts of the world, but it is not available in the United States.
• Rams have been immunized against *B. ovis* in New Zealand with some success; not available in the United States.

POSSIBLE COMPLICATIONS
• Brucellosis leads to abortions in ruminant species with fertility ramifications in sheep and goats.
• Contact with fetal fluids in infectious and carrier animals can spread the disease to all susceptible animals in a given herd/flock or geographic location.

EXPECTED COURSE AND PROGNOSIS
• Ruminants typically abort only during their first gestation, 80% in late gestation.
• Fertility can be permanently impaired in rams and bucks.
• Death is uncommon in adult animals.

MISCELLANEOUS

ASSOCIATED CONDITIONS
Arthritis in goats

AGE-RELATED FACTORS
Breeding-age animals most susceptible

ZOONOTIC POTENTIAL
• Humans are susceptible to *B. melitensis* and *B. abortus* infection through direct contact with infectious fluids from animals and absorption across mucous membranes or breaks in the skin.
• Brucellosis infection can also result from consumption of unpasteurized milk or cheese products from endemic areas.
• There is concern with aerosolized particles being used as a bioterrorism agent and causing widespread disease in humans.
• Disease can range from asymptomatic infection to chronic complications such as arthritis, endocarditis, orchitis, osteomyelitis, and other bone lesions.

PREGNANCY
Naïve animals abort late gestation in cattle and sheep and fourth month in goats.

RUMINANT SPECIES AFFECTED
Cattle, bison, elk, camels, water buffalo, yaks, sheep, goats

BIOSECURITY
• Ensure newly purchased cattle have been vaccinated against brucellosis if they are coming from endemic areas. Do not introduce animals directly into the herd for at least 3 weeks.
• Perform breeding soundness examinations on all sexually active males to make sure they are clear of disease and abnormalities.

PRODUCTION MANAGEMENT
• Vaccination of female calves against *B. abortus* with RB-51 from 4 to 12 months of age in endemic areas increases resistance to infection.
• Adult cattle can also be vaccinated but only with permission of the state, provincial, or federal veterinarian. RB-51 is currently being used experimentally in bison, and disease status is being monitored to assess efficacy.
• Goats and sheep can be vaccinated with live, attenuated Rev-1 *B. melitensis* in various parts of the world, but it is not available in the United States.

SYNONYMS
Bang's disease
Contagious abortion
Enzootic abortion

SEE ALSO
Arcanobacter pyogenes
Bluetongue
Broomweed
BVD
Campylobacteriosis
Chlamydiosis
Enzootic abortion (*Chlamydia psittaci*)
Epizootic bovine abortion
Haemophilus somnus
Heat stress
IBR
Leptospirosis
Listeriosis
Locoweed
Mycoplasma
Mycotic abortion
Mycotoxins
Neosporosis
Parainfluenza-3
Ponderosa pine needle ingestion
Salmonella
Salmonellosis
Serology
Toxoplasmosis
Trichomoniasis
Ureaplasma
Vibriosis (primarily sheep)

ABBREVIATIONS
BVD = bovine viral diarrhea
ELISA = enzyme-linked immunosorbent assay
IBR = infectious bovine rhinotracheitis

Suggested Reading
Aiello, S. E., Mays, A., ed. 1998. *Merck veterinary manual*. 8th ed. Whitehouse Station, NJ: Merck & Co.
Animal and Plant Health Inspection Services, Veterinary Services Division, United States Department of Agriculture. *Brucellosis in cattle and bison*. Accessed at http://www.aphis.usda.gov/vs/nahps/brucellosis/cattle.htm on May 8, 2004.
Corbel, M. J. 1997, Apr-June. Brucellosis: an overview. *Emerging Infectious Disease* 3(2):213–21.
Cutler, S., Whatmore, A. 2003, Nov 22. Progress in understanding brucellosis. *Vet Rec.* 153(21): 641–42.
Development of new/improved brucellosis vaccines: report of WHO meeting with participation of FAO and OIE, Geneva, Switzerland, December 11–12, 1997. Accessed at http://www.who.int/emc-documents/zoonoses/docs/whoemczdi9814.pdf on May 11, 2004.
Fosgate, G. T., Adesiyun, A. A., Hird, D. W., Johnson, W. O., Hietala, S. K., Schurig, G. G., Ryan, J. 2002, Nov. Comparison of serologic tests for detection of *Brucella* infections in cattle and water buffalo (*Bubalus bubalis*). *Am J Vet Res.* 63(11): 1598–605.
Metcalf, H. E., Luchsinger, D. W., Ray, W. C. 1994. Brucellosis. In: *Handbook of zoonoses: section A, bacterial, rickettsial, chlamydial, and mycotic zoonosis*, ed. G. Beran, J. Steele. 2nd ed. Boca Raton, FL: CRC Press.

Author: Danelle Bickett-Weddle

BURN MANAGEMENT

 BASICS

OVERVIEW
• Burns in livestock are not common but may occur by several mechanisms:
  • Thermal—fire (barn, brush, forest), heat (heat lamps, heating pads), hot solutions
  • Electrical—lightning, electrocution
  • Frictional—rope burns, abrasions
  • Chemical—caustic agents, topical medications
  • Ultraviolet—sunburn
  • Radiation
  • Freeze "burns"
• Burns in livestock commonly occur over back, face, udder, and teats, and over ventrum with brush fires.
• Classification of burns is based on depth to which burn penetrates skin and extent of body surface involved.
  • First-degree burn: involves superficial layers of epidermis; characterized by erythema, transient edema, and pain, and generally heals without complication or extensive scarring, prognosis good
  • Second-degree burn: partial-thickness burns involving all epidermal layers but spare hair follicles and sweat glands; characterized by erythema, pain, and vesicles (blisters), necrosis, and sloughing with superficial and eschar with deep second-degree burns; usually re-epithelialized with proper care, some scarring
  • Third-degree burn: full thickness burns involving entire epidermis, dermis, and appendages and exposing deeper structures, local blood vessels and hair follicles destroyed; characterized by necrosis, ulceration, anesthesia, eschar, and extensive scarring, require extensive wound care ± skin grafting

• Fourth-degree burn: involve entire skin, subcutis, underlying fascia, muscle, and tendon
• The full extent of the thermal burn is difficult to predict immediately after injury.
• Burns are usually complex with body areas being affected to different degrees.
• The development of blisters, fluid separation of epidermis and dermis and eschars may not appear for several days.
• Thermal injuries caused by fire associated with more than skin pathology
  • Fluid shifts, hypovolemia
  • Electrolyte abnormalities
  • Hypoproteinemia (loss of plasma is maximal in first 12 to 24 hours)
  • Extreme stress
  • Smoke inhalation
  • Immune suppression
• Extracutaneous complications of burns may be cardiopulmonary, ocular, hematologic, renal
• Animals suffering burns and/or smoke inhalation need to be closely monitored and repeatedly examined as signs and lesion development may be delayed.
• Wound or burn infection is common in cattle and *Pseudomonas aeruginosa* is the most common organism to establish infection.
• Infection under eschars is a common problem.
• Animals with second-degree and third-degree burns over 50% of their body usually die.
• Poor prognosis if second-degree and third-degree burns affect more than 10% to 15% of body surface
• Sequelae to burn injuries
  • Hypoproteinemia from protein exudate from wounds
  • Progressive edema
  • Hyperkalemia
  • Burn-induced immunosuppression

• Progressive anemia
• Secondary infections; pneumonia, skin infections
• Multiple system involvement, i.e., renal shut down, eye damage
• Scarring
• Damage to eyelids, conjunctiva, cornea, anterior uveitis, exfoliation of lens capsule
• Sunburn
  • White and light-skinned animals, lateral aspects of teats, ears, nose, areas covered with little hair are most susceptible to ultraviolet light, 290–320 nm.
  • White-faced sheep, especially ears and face
  • Exposure to sunlight is associated with skin tumor development especially on udder of white goats.
  • Erythema, pain, swelling, blisters, erosions
• Complications of teat burns include obstruction of teat orifice, distorted teats, mastitis

SIGNALMENT
• No age, sex, or breed predilection
• Sunburn: light-skinned or white animals, white-faced sheep

SIGNS
• Severity of burn determines signs present, maybe mild erythema and superficial scabbing to extensive tissue damage and necrosis with severe protein exudation
• Wool is fire-retardant; burns on sheep most commonly found on legs and around face
• Goats and cattle are likely to have burns on any part of body.
• Signs of sunburn
  • Erythema, swelling, crusting of skin
  • Headshaking, pruritus
  • Discomfort during milking or nursing if udder or teats burned
• Teat burns
  • Mild burns: erythema, sloughing of outer, white, paper-thin tissue; areas of sloughing, crusting, and discoloration of tissue; milk is apparently normal; teat pliable on palpation

- Severe burns: teats tend to be dull brown or black, dry, and often corrugated; thick layer of tissue is sloughed, underneath is red hemorrhagic tissue; teat is leatherlike and lacks pliability ± distorted.
- Healing lesions may be very pruritic causing animals to scratch or lick at affected sites.

CAUSES AND RISK FACTORS
- Symptoms can be acute or subacute
- Nondermatological signs occur about 7 days prior to onset of skin lesions: pyrexia.

DIAGNOSIS
Diagnosis is based upon history and clinical signs.

DIFFERENTIAL DIAGNOSIS
Differentiate sunburn from photosensitivity.

CBC/BIOCHEMISTRY/URINALYSIS
N/A

OTHER LABORATORY TESTING

IMAGING
N/A

DIAGNOSTIC PROCEDURES
N/A

TREATMENT
- Initial overall assessment of survivors—recumbent, obviously badly burned, suffering animals should be euthanized.
- Evaluation of animal's systemic and local injuries is essential.
- Repeat examination is necessary to determine response to therapy and development of delayed signs and lesions.
- Treatment is aimed at care of initial injuries, cardiovascular support, respiratory support, and prevention of secondary infection

- Goal of treatment is epithelialization of wound.
  - First- and mild second-degree burns should heal well by epithelialization.
  - Severe second-degree and most third-degree burns require skin grafts.
- Cool affected body areas to reduce heat retention and limit necrosis.
  - Hosing with cool water for 15 minutes
  - Wet cool towels
- Hosing also removes burnt hairs, crust, and debris.
- Blisters allowed to remain in place for 1–2 days on second-degree burns
- Burn wound care
  - Thorough cleaning with irrigation or dilute chlorhexidine solution (controversial); repeat two to three times daily
  - Daily hydrotherapy
  - Topical antimicrobial; use water-soluble emollient antimicrobial cream, silver sulfadiazine (Silvadene)
  - Use of hydrogel and nonadherent, absorbent dressings, which are not constrictive, may be indicated in some cases, must be kept clean and changed at appropriate intervals.
  - Avoid occlusive dressings, which produce closed wound with bacterial proliferation and delayed healing.
  - Eschar over large second- or third-degree burns should be left undisturbed until natural sloughing occurs or if infection develops under eschar.
  - Wound debridement after 24 to 36 hours if necessary
  - Wound allowed to heal by granulation
- Systemic antimicrobials fail to penetrate local burn wound infections, may permit growth of resistant organisms.
- Systemic antimicrobials reserved for use when documented site of infection (i.e., pneumonia)

- Analgesia as needed—nonsteroidal anti-inflammatory drugs (concern these may delay healing)
- Correct hypovolemia: rule of thumb—give 3 to 4 ml/kg of body weight for each percentage body surface involved.
- Maintenance of electrolyte and acid-base balance
- Plasma administration if severe hypoproteinemia
- Keep animal in clean environment.
- Provide adequate nutrition.
- Tetanus booster if indicated
- Prevent delayed healing and self-mutilation from scratching and licking as lesions heal (pruritus), sedation may be required.
- Eye damage
  - Cornea and eyelid damage are of particular concern.
  - With burns on face, cornea should be treated with artificial tears.
  - Gently remove debris from eye with saline-soaked cotton swab.
  - Inspect and fluorescein stain eye for ulcers.
  - Apply topical antibiotics with atropine.
  - Third eyelid flap if necessary to protect eye
- Teat burns
  - Soothing, softening burn ointments, lanolin ointments, aloe vera
  - Antimicrobial ointment if skin surface sloughs
  - Maintain open teat orifice.
  - Healing is slow, takes many weeks to months.
- Sunburn
  - Remove from exposure to sunlight.
  - Provide shelter.
  - Soothing burn ointments, topical human sunburn medications, or aloe vera, topical steroids
  - Application of pigmented teat dips
  - Contamination of milk should be avoided.
  - For secondary bacterial infection, use topical or systemic antimicrobial agents.
  - Prevention recommendations: see Production Management

BURN MANAGEMENT

 MEDICATIONS

N/A

DRUGS OF CHOICE

N/A

CONTRAINDICATIONS/POSSIBLE INTERACTIONS

Appropriate milk and meat withdrawal times must be followed for all compounds administered to food-producing animals.

 FOLLOW-UP

• Lesions can persist for up to 12 weeks.
• Recovered cattle have immunity for months.

 MISCELLANEOUS

ASSOCIATED CONDITIONS

Smoke Inhalation

Involves carbon monoxide toxicity and smoke toxicity

Three Mechanisms of Injury to Respiratory System

• First stage: heat damage to upper respiratory tract, injury from toxic chemicals in smoke and carbon monoxide toxicity; usually signs within first 6 hours
  • Inflammation, edema, and necrosis of nasal passages, pharynx, and larynx lead to airway obstruction ± laryngospasm

• Bronchoconstriction of lungs; inhalation of soot, noxious gases
• Carbon monoxide toxicity: hypoxemia and tissue hypoxia in all organs, especially brain; level above 10% carbon monoxide is consistent with toxicity
• Shock
• Second stage: formation of pulmonary edema
  • Within 12 to 72 hours after exposure
  • Damage due to inflammatory mediators (cytokines, proteolytic enzymes, oxygen free radicals)
  • Obstruction of small airway from deposition of smoke material and inflammatory debris
• Third stage: bronchopneumonia
  • Result of impaired immune system and exposure to pathogens
  • May occur within 24 to 48 hours or 1 to 3 weeks after initial injury

Clinical Signs

• Many signs may not be apparent for 1 to 2 days after fire.
• Oral burns, nasal mucosal swelling, pharyngeal swelling, laryngospasm, conjunctivitis
• Hoarseness, expiratory wheezes, cough, stridor, tachypnea
• Tachycardia
• Bright mucous membranes with carbon monoxide toxicity may mask cyanosis.
• ±Cyanosis
• Signs of hypovolemia
• Signs of shock
• Depression, disorientation, irritability, ataxia, or even comatose
• ±Signs of septicemia or pneumonia

Treatment

• Depends on stage and severity of injury
• Oxygen support
• Maintenance of airway
  • Tracheotomy if upper airway obstruction
• Keep airways clean.
• Bronchodilators to counteract bronchoconstriction
• Diuretics and anti-inflammatory agents (nonsteroidal anti-inflammatory drugs) to reduce edema and inflammation
  • Use of corticosteroids is controversial.
• Analgesics
• Fluid therapy if hypovolemic, electrolyte imbalances, or acid-base derangements
  • Caution not to fluid overload if ongoing protein loss through burns or from vasculature
• Plasmas therapy if hyperproteinemia
• Strict hygiene, nursing care, and optimal nutritional support
• Prophylactic antimicrobials are not recommended.
• Appropriate antimicrobials based on culture and sensitivity from documented site of infection

ZOONOTIC POTENTIAL

N/A

RUMINANT SPECIES AFFECTED

• Cattle
• Goats
• Sheep
• Camelids
• Wild ruminants

BIOSECURITY

N/A

PRODUCTION MANAGEMENT
• Recovery time is prolonged with teat burns and extensive burns.
• Need to determine which animals to be euthanized or culled due to poor prognosis for successful recovery
  • Animals with second- and third-degree burns over extensive area
  • Burnt teats that will not withstand milking; mastitis is inevitable.
  • Badly burned feet may slough claws.
  • Facial burns involving cornea may lead to permanent stromal opacities.
• Teat burns
  • Mild lesions have good prognosis.
  • Severe lesions prognosis variable; may have mastitis, occlude, or heal distorted
  • Mature adult cows are more likely to return to full function than heifers.

• Prevention of sunburn
  • Gradual acclimation to exposure to sunlight
  • Provide shade
  • Application of sun blocking screens or ointments; use sunblocks with highest SPF available and those that are suitable for use in children; avoid PABA as it is not recommended as safe in children and little is known about its safety in animals.
  • Iodophor teat dips
  • Pet animals may wear fly nets on ears, hats, or bonnets.

SYNONYMS
N/A

SEE ALSO
Frostbite
Lightening strike
Wound care, euthanasia

ABBREVIATIONS
PABA = para-aminobenzoic acid

Suggested Reading
Knottenbelt, D. C. 2003. Management of burn injuries. In: *Current therapy in equine medicine 5*, ed. N. E. Robinson. Philadelphia: W. B. Saunders.
Marsh, P. 2002. Smoke inhalation. In: *Large animal internal medicine*, ed. B. P. Smith, 3rd ed. St. Louis: Mosby.
Pugh, D. 2002. Diseases of the integumentary system. In: *Sheep and goat medicine*. Philadelphia: W. B. Saunders.
Rebhun, W. C. 1995. Skin diseases. In: *Diseases of dairy cattle*. Baltimore: Williams and Wilkins.
Scott, D. W. 1999. Environmental skin diseases. In: *Current veterinary therapy 4: food animal practice*, ed. J. L. Howard, R. A. Smith. Philadelphia: W. B. Saunders.
Smith, M. C., Sherman, D. M. 1994. Environmental insults. In: *Goat medicine*. Philadelphia: Lea & Febiger.

Authors: Susan Semrad and Karen A. Moriello

CACHE VALLEY VIRUS

BASICS

OVERVIEW
• Cache Valley (CV) is a viral infection afflicting a wide variety of domestic and wild ruminants as well as humans.
• Cache Valley virus (CVV) belongs to the genus *Bunyavirus* in the family Bunyaviridae, the latter being the largest single family of animal viruses with more than 350 members.
• CV is endemic throughout the United States, Canada, and Mexico. Several CVV subtypes, such as E4-3484, CbaAr 426, and Fort Sherman, that are indistinguishable by neutralization tests from CVV, have been isolated in Central and South America.
• CVV transmission to vertebrates occurs through bites of infected mosquitoes, including several species of *Aedes, Psorophora, Anopheles, Coquillettidia, Culex*, and from *Culiseta inornata.*
• The majority of infections are subclinical, but embryonic mortality, fetal teratogenesis, and stillbirth may be common in sheep.
• In the southwestern United States, lambs born in December, January, and February are more likely to show CVV-induced teratogenesis. This period coincides with increased rainfall and mosquito activity.
• Fetal susceptibility to CVV-induced pathology is higher during the first 2 months of pregnancy.

SIGNALMENT
• Infection by CVV has been reported in humans, sheep, goats, cattle, horses, pigs, deer, mouflon, caribou, raccoons, foxes, black-tailed jackrabbit, woodchuck, and turtles.
• In sheep there is a positive relationship between seropositivity to CVV and age. This reflects the likelihood of exposure as the age of sheep increases.
• In pregnant ewes, the CVV can cross the placenta causing embryonic death, mummification, or fetal malformation.

SIGNS
• In most animals, CVV infection is subclinical.
• In pregnant ewes, CVV infection may result in embryonic mortality, fetal mummification, and various degrees of musculoskeletal or central nervous system (CNS) abnormalities.
• Experimentally, CVV-induced fetal malformation occurs when the virus infects the fetus between days 27 and 54 of pregnancy.
• After the second month of pregnancy, fetal infection results in the production of fetal neutralizing antibodies that control and eliminate CVV without apparent consequences to the fetus.
• Dystocia may be a sequela in ewes that deliver full-term malformed offspring.
• Ewes that are CVV seropositive at the time of breeding are resistant to reinfection with CVV.
• There is no cross-protection against other related bunyaviruses.

DIAGNOSIS

DIFFERENTIAL DIAGNOSIS
• Main Drain, La Crosse, and San Angelo bunyaviruses induce similar fetal pathology.
• Bluetongue virus of vaccine origin and border disease virus also may result in fetal infection and CNS malformations in sheep.
• Akabane, Rift Valley fever, Nairobi sheep disease, and Wesselsbron viruses are exotic to North America but may cause similar fetal pathology in sheep.
• Other causes of teratogenesis and pregnancy loss, such as genetic defects and teratogenic plants, need to be included in the differential diagnosis of CV.

DIAGNOSTIC PROCEDURES
• CVV can be isolated from blood during the acute viremic phase by intracranial inoculation of suckling mice or infection of susceptible cell lines such as Vero cells. Because viremia is short-lived, in most cases results are negative.

• CVV serum antibodies are more often demonstrated by serum neutralization, but ELISA, complement fixation, and hemagglutination-inhibition tests also have been used. In adult animals, serum antibodies are indication of previous exposure, but do not provide information regarding the infectious status of individuals.
• Malformed fetuses that survive in utero for some time develop neutralizing antibodies and eliminate the virus. In these cases, assaying precolostral fetal serum for the presence of CVV neutralizing antibodies does the diagnosis.
• In full-term malformed fetuses or newborns, virus isolation is always unsuccessful.
• Lack of CV antibodies in sera of ewes lambing malformed fetuses rules out CVV as the cause.

PATHOLOGIC FINDINGS
Macroscopic
• In sheep, CVV intrauterine infection during pregnancy may result in embryonic mortality, fetal teratogenesis, stillbirth, and/or oligohydroamnion.
• Congenital abnormalities include arthrogryposis, hydranencephaly, hydrocephalous, microcephalous, porencephalia, cerebellar hypoplasia, scoliosis, torticollis, and lordosis.
• In multiple pregnancies, the degree and type of fetal pathology may be different in each fetus. In some cases, one fetus may be normal while the others may show malformations.
• In other ruminants, fetal abnormalities as a result of natural CVV infection during pregnancy happen sporadically.

Microscopic
• Histologic lesions are more frequently observed in the brain, spinal cord, and skeletal muscle of malformed fetuses. In the CNS, microscopic lesions are consistent with the gross lesions. Some of the brain cavities contain blood, and evidence of neutrophil rarefaction and malacia may be present. In moderately affected lambs, muscle fibers are small, but in more severe cases, fibers are narrow and short with few nuclei and no cross striations.

- Affected lambs often have meconium in pulmonary alveoli as a result of intrauterine stress.
- Perivascular infiltration of neutrophils in placentas of affected ewes has been observed in some cases, but this is more likely an incidental finding and not a hallmark of CVV infection.

TREATMENT
There is no treatment for CVV infections.

MEDICATIONS
N/A

CONTRAINDICATIONS
N/A

POSSIBLE INTERACTIONS
N/A

FOLLOW-UP
N/A

PATIENT MONITORING
N/A

PREVENTION /AVOIDANCE
- There are no vaccines available to protect animals against CVV infection.
- Ewes that are seropositive to CVV at the time of breeding are protected from subsequent infection with CVV and its adverse effects on pregnancy, but they are susceptible to infection by bunyaviruses of different serogroups, some of which may induce similar fetal pathology.
- Insect control is difficult because of the wide range of mosquito vectors and vertebrate hosts. Application of insecticides may not be ecologically admissible. Other insect control methods such as tire removal may greatly reduce the abundance of the vector.
- Breeding ewes after the first frost of the fall reduces the risk of fetal infection.

MISCELLANEOUS
ASSOCIATED CONDITIONS
The majority of infections are subclinical, but embryonic mortality, fetal teratogenesis, and stillbirth may be common in sheep.

AGE-RELATED FACTORS
The prevalence or CVV antibodies in sera of animals increases with age. This is a reflection of the likelihood of exposure in older sheep and not related to increased susceptibility of this particular age group.

ZOONOTIC POTENTIAL
- CV is an indirect zoonotic in which humans may get infected through the bite of infected mosquitoes but not directly from infected vertebrate animals. Infection also can occur through accidental puncture with infected needles.
- The great majority of CVV infections in humans are subclinical. However, fever, myalgia, chills, headache, vomiting and death have been reported in a few cases.
- There is no conclusive evidence that CV virus in humans causes fetal malformation or pregnancy loss.
- Further research is necessary to determine the role of CVV in human disease, particularly in human immunodeficiency virus (HIV)-infected individuals and those affected by other types of immune deficiencies.

PREGNANCY
- Pregnancy loss and/or fetal malformation are common in CVV-infected sheep.
- In pregnant ewes, CVV infection may result in embryonic mortality, fetal mummification, and various degrees of musculoskeletal or central nervous system (CNS) abnormalities.

SYNONYMS
N/A

SEE ALSO
Akabane
Bluetongue virus
Border disease virus
Nairobi sheep disease
Rift Valley fever
Teratogenic plant consumption.
Wesselsbron disease

ABBREVIATIONS
- CNS = central nervous system
- CVV = Cache Valley virus
- ELISA = enzyme-linked immunosorbent assay

Suggested Reading
Chung, S. I., Livingston, C. W., Jr., Edwards, J. F., Crandell, R. W., Shope, R. E., Shelton, M. J., Collisson, E. W. 1990. Evidence that Cache Valley virus induces congenital malformations in sheep. *Vet Microbiol*. 21: 297–307.
Chung, S. I., Livingston, C. W., Jr., Edwards, J. F., Gauer, B. B., Collisson, E. W. 1990. Congenital malformations in sheep resulting from in utero inoculation of Cache Valley virus. *Am J Vet Res*. 51: 1645–48.
Chung, S. I., Livingston, C. W., Jr., Jones, C. W., Collisson, E. W. 1991. Cache Valley virus infection in Texas sheep flocks. *J Am Vet Med Assoc*. 199: 337–40.
de la Concha-Bermejillo, A. 2003. Cache Valley virus is a cause of fetal malformation and pregnancy loss in sheep. *Small Rum Res*. 49:1–9.
Edwards, J. F. 1994. Cache Valley virus. *Vet Clin North Am-Food Anim Pract*. 10: 515–24.
Edwards, J. F., Karabatsos, N., Collisson, E.W., de la Concha-Bermejillo, A. 1996. Ovine fetal malformations induced by in utero inoculation with Main Drain, San Angelo, and LaCrosse viruses. *Am J Trop Med Hyg*. 56: 171–76.

Author: Andrés de la Concha-Bermejillo

BASICS

DEFINITION
• *Fusobacterium necrophorum* infection of the larynx and pharynx of calves
• The organism is an opportunistic pathogen that causes numerous necrotic conditions (necrobacillosis), such as bovine hepatic abscesses, ruminant foot abscesses, and oral infections.
• Because of the unavailability of suitable immunoprophylaxis, the control of *F. necrophorum* infection has depended mainly on the use of antimicrobial compounds.

PATHOPHYSIOLOGY
• Injury to the mucosa of the pharynx and larynx allows *Fusobacterium necrophorum*, an oral commensal bacteria, to invade and infect the tissues. Inflammation can constrict the larynx, causing dyspnea.
• *Fusobacterium necrophorum* is a gram-negative, non-spore-forming anaerobe and is a normal inhabitant of the respiratory and alimentary tracts of animals.
• Two types of *F. necrophorum*, subspecies *necrophorum* (biotype A) and *funduliforme* (biotype B), have been recognized. These two biotypes differ morphologically, biochemically, and biologically.
• The pathogenic mechanism of *F. necrophorum* is complex and not well defined.
• Several toxins, such as leukotoxin, endotoxin, haemolysin, haemagglutinin, and adhesin, have been implicated as virulence factors. Among these, leukotoxin and endotoxin are believed to be more important than other toxins in overcoming the host's defense mechanisms to establish the infection.

• *F. necrophorum* is encountered frequently in mixed infections and, therefore, synergisms between *F. necrophorum* and other pathogens may play an important role in infection.

SYSTEMS AFFECTED
GI/respiratory

GENETICS
N/A

INCIDENCE/PREVALENCE
Low incidence

GEOGRAPHIC DISTRIBUTION
Worldwide

Epidemiology
• Occurs most commonly in calves up to 18 months of age, but can occur in older animals.
• Abrasive feed, trauma to mucosa during oral medication, or other damage to the mucosa allows infection by the bacteria. Housed cattle and feedlot cattle are at higher risk.

SIGNALMENT
Species
Bovine

Breed Predilections
N/A

Mean Age and Range
Three to 18 months.

Predominant Sex
N/A

SIGNS

GENERAL COMMENTS
Clinical signs are associated with edema and inflammation of the pharynx and larynx, making swallowing difficult and painful. Obstruction of the larynx causes dyspnea and may lead to death.

HISTORICAL FINDINGS
Rough or abrasive feeds, unsanitary feeding areas, recent oral bolus medication

PHYSICAL EXAMINATION FINDINGS
• High fever (106°F); inspiratory dyspnea; difficulty swallowing; salivation; moist cough; anorexia; depression; swollen, painful pharynx
• Visual observation of the pharynx and larynx reveal inflamed and necrotic mucosa.

CAUSES
Fusobacterium necrophorum infection through abraded or damaged mucosa in the larynx and pharynx

RISK FACTORS
Rough or abrasive feeds, unskilled workers giving oral medications

DIAGNOSIS

DIFFERENTIAL DIAGNOSIS
• Foreign bodies or traumatic pharyngitis
• Aspiration

CBC/BIOCHEMISTRY/URINALYSIS
N/A

OTHER LABORATORY TESTS
• Culture and sensitivity are indicated in economically valuable animals. The most common sites or conditions from which members of this genus are isolated are abscesses, the respiratory tract, and pleural and peritoneal cavities.
• Most specimen cultures contain a single *Fusobacterium* species. The most commonly isolated species is *Fusobacterium necrophorum*. Almost all of the specimens contain other obligate anaerobes together with facultative and obligate aerobes.

IMAGING
N/A

OTHER DIAGNOSTIC PROCEDURES
Bacterial culture of lesions

GROSS AND HISTOPATHOLOGIC FINDINGS
Swelling and edema of laryngeal-pharynx area, sometimes with necrosis of the mucosal tissue

TREATMENT
Cases with severe swelling and dyspnea may require tracheostomy.

CLIENT EDUCATION
Minimize abrasive materials such as sticks and cockleburs in hays and pastures. Keep feed areas, mangers, and feed equipment clean.

MEDICATIONS

DRUGS OF CHOICE
• Broad-spectrum systemic antimicrobial therapy for several days. Early recognition is essential for successful therapy.
• Anti-inflammatory drugs such as corticosteroids or NSAIDs may be useful to reduce the swelling and dyspnea.

CONTRAINDICATIONS
• Oral bolus medications
• Appropriate milk and meat withdrawal times must be followed for all compounds administered to food-producing animals.

PRECAUTIONS
N/A

POSSIBLE INTERACTIONS
N/A

ALTERNATE DRUGS
N/A

FOLLOW-UP

PATIENT MONITORING
Ability to breath and swallow without difficulty should be monitored.

PREVENTION/AVOIDANCE
Sanitary feed areas and equipment; avoid rough feeds.

POSSIBLE COMPLICATIONS
Toxemia

EXPECTED COURSE AND PROGNOSIS
Recovery if treated early before chronic damage to epiglottis occurs.

MISCELLANEOUS

PREVENTION
Avoid rough feeds and maintain clean feed areas.

ASSOCIATED CONDITIONS
Necrotic stomatitis

AGE-RELATED FACTORS
Appears most commonly in calves 3 to 18 months old, but can occur in older animals.

ZOONOTIC POTENTIAL
N/A

PREGNANCY
N/A

SYNONYMS
Necrotic laryngitis
Oral necrobacillosis

SEE ALSO
Necrotic stomatitis

ABBREVIATIONS
NSAIDs = nonsteroidal anti-inflammatory drugs

Suggested Reading
Jang, S. S., Hirsh, D. C. 1994, Feb. Characterization, distribution, and microbiological associations of *Fusobacterium* spp. in clinical specimens of animal origin. *J Clin Microbiol.* 32(2): 384–87.
Langworth, B. F. 1977, Jun. *Fusobacterium necrophorum*: its characteristics and role as an animal pathogen. *Bacteriol Rev.* 41(2): 373–90.
Radostits, O. M., Gay, C. C., Blood, D. C., Hinchcliff, K. W., eds. 2000. *Veterinary medicine: a textbook of diseases of cattle, sheep, pigs, goats and horses.* 9th ed. London: W. B. Saunders.
Smith, G. R., Barton, S. A., Wallace, L. M. 1991, Apr. Further observations on enhancement of the infectivity of *Fusobacterium necrophorum* by other bacteria. *Epidemiol Infect.* 106(2): 305–10.
Tan, Z. L., Nagaraja, T. G., Chengappa, M. M. 1996. *Fusobacterium necrophorum* infections: virulence factors, pathogenic mechanism and control measures. *Vet Res Commun.* 20(2): 113–40.

Author: James P. Reynolds

CALVING-RELATED DISORDERS

 BASICS

DEFINITION
• Calving-related disorders (CRD) occur during the transition period of dairy cows (21 days before expected parturition to 21 days postpartum).
• The most important CRDs are hypocalcemia, retained fetal membranes (RFM), metritis, displacement of abomasums (DA), ketosis, fatty liver, and udder edema.
• Other conditions such as lameness and mastitis are also related to the transition period but they can occur at any time during the production cycle.

PATHOPHYSIOLOGY
• The transition period is a very dynamic stage in the production cycle of the cow.
• During the prepartum, the fetus grows exponentially and cows start to decrease dry matter intake (DMI), especially during the last week of gestation. As a response, cows start to mobilize fat from body reserves. The result is an increase of nonesterified fatty acids (NEFA) in the blood. This is especially true in obese cows, and fatty liver may occur.
• Calving is a stressful process that results in metabolic and hormonal changes that contribute to immunosuppression and a subsequent decrease of host resistance to diseases. Mammary gland tissue starts to extract elevated levels of calcium from the blood supply. Therefore, there is a more intense negative calcium balance with development with a concomitant hypocalcemia.
• If calving is complicated, hypocalcemia worsens affecting uterine and gastrointestinal motility.
• Retained fetal membranes may occur, with consequent metritis if preventive measures are not considered.
• Displacement of abomasums may be also a consequence.

• When lactation advances, energy requirements increase dramatically and DMI recovers slowly. This creates a typical negative energy balance during the first weeks of lactation. In addition, mammary glands extract large amounts of glucose from the blood for lactose synthesis. Hypoglycemia may develop and ketosis may be established.

SYSTEMS AFFECTED
Systems affected will depend on the calving-related disorder: mammary, hepatic, cardiovascular, gastrointestinal, respiratory, reproductive, nutritional, and production management

GENETICS
Some CRDs may have a hereditary component (ketosis and somatic cell count).

INCIDENCE/PREVALENCE
• Incidences of CRDs are extremely variable and depend on factors such as season, geographical location, breed, type of housing, environment, and management.
• Reported incidences for some CRDs include clinical hypocalcemia 0.2%–2%, retained fetal membranes 8%–14%, metritis 6%–12%, ketosis 2%–6%, displacement of abomasums 2%–6%.

GEOGRAPHIC DISTRIBUTION
Worldwide where dairy farming occurs

SIGNALMENT
Related to the periparturient period of dairy cows; there may be breed predispositions for some CRD (Jersey cows and hypocalcemia).

SIGNS
Retained fetal membranes (visible membranes after 24 h postpartum), metritis (fever, foul-smelling discharge), hypocalcemia (musculoskeletal compromise), ketosis (decrease in milk yield, high ketones in blood, urine, or milk), displacement of abomasums (high-pitch sound at auscultation on left flank, last two rib spaces).

CAUSES
Inadequate management of the prepartum, calving, and postpartum period; improper nutrition, environment, and management

RISK FACTORS
Management, breed, genetic potential, nutrition, season, herd size, geographical location

 DIAGNOSIS

DIFFERENTIAL DIAGNOSIS
• Hypocalcemia
• Retained fetal membranes (RFM)
• Metritis
• Displacement of abomasums (DA)
• Ketosis
• Fatty liver
• Udder edema
• Lameness
• Mastitis

CBC/BIOCHEMISTRY/URINALYSIS
• Important tools for ketosis diagnosis (ketones in urine, blood, or milk). CBC/biochemistry can be useful in determining hydration, calcium and potassium levels, liver function, and infection level.
• Urine pH should be monitored to evaluate anionic salts during prepartum period for the prevention of hypocalcemia. Urine pH should be between 6.5 and 7.0.
• Serum Ca, Mg, P, nonesterified fatty acids (NEFA), beta hydroxy butyrate (BHBA), glucose, insulin, T3 and T4, liver enzymes, and urea nitrogen all can be monitored depending on differential diagnosis.

OTHER LABORATORY TESTS
Liver biopsy can be helpful with the diagnosis of hepatic lipidosis.

IMAGING
Ultrasound imaging can be a useful adjunctive tool.

DIAGNOSTIC PROCEDURES
N/A

PATHOLOGIC FINDINGS
N/A

TREATMENT

APPROPRIATE HEALTH CARE
N/A

NURSING CARE
N/A

ACTIVITY
N/A

DIET
• Proper transition diet. Moderate energy and protein levels. Prepartum diet with a negative cation-anion difference. Appropriate amount and particle size of fiber.
• Fresh cow rations should be intermediate between the close-up and the high group rations.
• Cows should be fed ad libitum—that means a 5% to 10% feed refusal. If concentration of energy and protein are somewhat low in the ration fed right after calving, it is important not to leave the cows in this group for too long of a time.
• Rations should have at least 21% neutral detergent fiber (NDF) from forage and enough particle size to support good chewing activity and rumen fill.
• Diets should have 8% to 10% of particles on the top screen of the Penn State Particle Size Separator for both prefresh and fresh cows. Researchers suggest feeding 3 to 5 lb of high-quality long forage to maintain rumen function.
• Forage quality is very important in the transition period.
• As for the close up group, it is important to feed adequate levels of copper, zinc, manganese, selenium, and vitamin E.
• Researchers suggest 2000 IU of vitamin E per day for fresh cows.

CLIENT EDUCATION
Proper nutrition and general management in transition cows is important.

SURGICAL CONSIDERATIONS
Considered important for displaced abomasum

MEDICATIONS

DRUGS OF CHOICE
N/A

CONTRAINDICATIONS
N/A

PRECAUTIONS
N/A

POSSIBLE INTERACTIONS
N/A

ALTERNATIVE DRUGS
Feed additives to improve energy and mineral balance such as propylene glycol, niacin, calcium propionate, vitamin E, selenium

FOLLOW-UP

PATIENT MONITORING
• Monitoring of body condition score during dry period; cows should not lose condition or gain excessive weight during the transition period.
• Urine pH should be monitored to evaluate anionic salts during prepartum period for the prevention of hypocalcemia. Urine pH should be between 6.5 and 7.0.

PREVENTION/AVOIDANCE
Proper general and nutritional management

POSSIBLE COMPLICATIONS
Decreased milk production, infertility, and death

EXPECTED COURSE AND PROGNOSIS
N/A

MISCELLANEOUS

ASSOCIATED CONDITIONS
Calving-related disorders are intimately related to each other. Cows with hypocalcemia are more likely to develop retained fetal membranes. Cows with RFM are more likely to develop metritis. Cows with metritis are more likely to develop ketosis and cows with ketosis are more likely to develop displacement of abomasums.

AGE-RELATED FACTORS
Older cows are more likely to develop clinical hypocalcemia, ketosis, and displacement of abomasum.

ZOONOTIC POTENTIAL
N/A

PREGNANCY
Prepartum management is critical for prevention of calving-related disorders. Enough feed bunk space, adequate shade, and comfortable environment are essential for prepartum dairy cows.

RUMINANT SPECIES AFFECTED
Dairy cattle

BIOSECURITY
N/A

PRODUCTION MANAGEMENT
Nutrition and feeding, housing, management
• Dry cows (7 to 9 month pregnant nonlactating cows) need adaptation to their next lactation diet. Preparation for parturition and avoidance of calving-related disorders is an important component of this program.
• Consequently, dry cows need to be moved to a prepartum transition pen (close-up pen).
• Three weeks prior to freshening is sufficient for adult mature cows. However, 5 weeks should be considered for pregnant heifers because they are still growing and they have not experienced the challenges of calving and lactation before.
• Close-up heifers and cows should be handled in different pens.
• Prepartum transition animals need a comfortable environment with adequate shade, bunk space, and good-quality water.

CALVING-RELATED DISORDERS

• Prepartum transition pens must be situated in a strategic location of the farm, with easy labor access and planned handling.
• Transition pens must be monitored twice daily for cows showing signs of udder edema development and signs of impending parturition.
• Calving may occur either in the same prepartum transition pen or in the maternity pen, depending on management criteria.
• The calving environment must be quiet, clean, and easy to access if calving assistance is needed.
• Major concerns of the prepartum transition period and calving are udder edema, dystocia, and hypocalcemia.
• Udder edema must be addressed through proper nutritional management. Excess nutritional sodium and potassium are related to this metabolic condition.
• Dystocia is a multifactorial problem where proper assistance is the key. Good knowledge of parturition physiology and obstetric intervention are basic and needed.
• For the postpartum transition cow, the same recommendation of a good environment applies. The postpartum pen also should be in a strategic location.

• Cows need to be monitored for retained fetal membranes, metritis, ketosis, and abomasal displacement.
• A strategic plan should include monitoring cows during the first 10 days postpartum for fever development and ketone bodies either in urine or milk.
• If cows are either febrile, positive to ketones, or both, they should be separated and evaluated through a complete physical examination.
• Body condition of cows is important. On a scale of 1 to 5, they should be between 3.25 and 3.75.
• Overconditioned animals are more likely to experience dystocia and calving-related disorders. Therefore, energy density of dry cow diets must be consistent and adequate.
• Mineral content is important to the prevention of hypocalcemia and other related disorders.
• Typical prepartum diets are rich in cations (sodium and potassium). Therefore, the difference in mEq/kg between (Na+K) − (Cl+S) should be positive ($\sim$ +150 to +350 mEq/kg). This diet institutes an alkaline environment, which favors the development of hypocalcemia.

• Receptors for parathormone and vitamin D are altered structurally by alkaline environments.
• If the cow's acid-base status has shifted to a more acidic level, these receptors work more efficiently with a better bioavailability and absorption of calcium.
• A goal should be a urine pH between 6.0 and 7.0. This pH level has been associated with a lowered incidence of hypocalcemia.
• Dietary ingredients of the prepartum diet should be exactly the same as the postpartum lactation diet to insure a better rumen microbial adaptation.
• The diet should contain a higher level of effective fiber (NDF, neutral detergent fiber) with adequate particle size to stimulate rumination, avoid acidosis, improve rumen fermentation, and avoid abomasal displacement.

Close-up Cows
Feeding strategies needed during the close-up period to achieve these goals are:
• Condition should be maintained during the dry period. Excessive body condition at calving can increase incidence of ketosis and fatty liver.

CALVING-RELATED DISORDERS

- Increase grain feeding to 0.5%–0.75% of body weight.
- Target 35%–40% nonfiber carbohydrates as a % of DM.
- Feed high-quality forages with sufficient effective fiber.
- Limit fat to 1/4–1/3 lb per day.
- Feed low-potassium forages; balance for potassium concentration less than 1.5% of diet DM (get as close to 1% as possible).
- Provide adequate magnesium (0.4% of diet DM) and calcium (1%–1.2% of diet DM).
- Feed adequate selenium (0.3 ppm) and vitamin E (2000 IU per day).
- Supply extra trace minerals such as copper, manganese, and zinc to account for decline in feed intake.
- Feed adequate crude protein (cows need 12%–13%, heifers 15% of diet DM).

Fresh Cows

- Calving and the change to lactating status are very stressful in the life of a cow. They need a lot of care. Assign your best employee/ person to monitor this group of cows.
- Maternity facilities must be clean, dry, well lit, well ventilated, and comfortable. After leaving the maternity pens, cows should ideally be moved to a fresh cow group. There is also benefit in having a separate heifer group, because heifers are smaller and do not compete as well at the feed bunk.

- The first 1 to 2 weeks after calving set the stage for the entire lactation. Studies have shown that for each 1 lb increase in peak milk, there is a 220 lb milk production increase for the entire lactation.

Monitoring Progress

- After calving, it is important to optimize dry-matter intake as soon as possible.
- Monitor feed intake by rating how the cow consumes fresh feed on a scale of 1 to 4 (1 = 0%–33% consumed; 2 = 33%–66% consumed; 3 = 66%–90% consumed; 4 = all consumed). Cows off feed require special treatment. Observe chewing and rumination activity.
- Rumen movements should be monitored using a stethoscope—healthy cows have about 1.5 to 2 rumen movements per minute.
- Body temperatures should be recorded daily. The goal is to be below 103°F for mature cows and 102.5°F for heifers.
- Uterine discharges should be checked and a ketone test on the cow's urine or milk is recommended.

SYNONYMS

Diseases of peripartum
Periparturient disorders

SEE ALSO

Body condition scoring: dairy cattle
Displacement of abomasums
Hypocalcemia
Ketosis

Lameness
Mastitis
Metritis
Milk fever
Postparturient paresis
Retained fetal membranes
Transition management

ABBREVIATIONS

CRD = calving-related disorder
DA = displacement of abomasums
DMI = dry matter intake
NDF = neutral detergent fiber
NEFA = nonesterified fatty acids
RFM = retained fetal membranes
WBCs = white blood cells

Suggested Reading
Melendez, P., Donovan, A., Risco, C. A., Littell, R., Goff, J. 2003. Effect of calcium-energy supplements on calving-related disorders, fertility and milk yield during the transition period in cows fed anionic diets. *Theriogenology* 60:843–54.
Metabolic disorders of ruminants. 2000. In: *Veterinary clinics of North America, food animal practice.* Philadelphia: W. B. Saunders.
National Research Council. 2001. *Nutrient requirements of dairy cattle.* 7th ed. Washington, DC: National Academy Press.
Risco, C. A., Melendez, P. 2003. Periparturient disorders. In: *Encyclopedia of dairy science.* H. Roginski, J. Fuquay, P. Fox(ed). Burlington, MA: Academic Press.

Author: Pedro Melendez

CAMELID TOOTH ROOT ABSCESSES

BASICS

DEFINITION
Tooth root abscess is a localized osteitis, pulpitis, and/or alveolar periostitis around one or more tooth roots, often draining purulent exudates by a fistulous tract through the skin overlying the abscess.

PATHOPHYSIOLOGY
• The adult camelid dental formula is: (I 1/3, C 1/1, PM 1-2/1-2, M 3/3) × 2 for 30 to 32 teeth.
• The upper incisors are actually found caudally in the region of the canine teeth.
• Cheek teeth can be numbered from 1 to 5 (rostral to caudal), or labeled according to the dental chart (PM 1 & PM 2, M 1 to M3).
• The upper premolars have three roots each; lower have two roots each.
• The upper molars have four roots each; lower M1 and M2 have two roots, M3 has three roots, but two are fused.
• Tooth fracture, gingival penetration, or infundibular decay and infection can result in tooth root abscess. Often the source is unknown.
• Periostitis and osteitis of the mandible secondary to tooth root abscess can spread along the mandibular canal.

SYSTEMS AFFECTED
• Gastrointestinal
• Musculoskeletal

GENETICS
None

INCIDENCE/PREVALENCE
• Unknown
• Mandibular molars 1 and 2 are most often affected
• Maxillary teeth are rarely affected
• Canine teeth may be affected: incidence appears to be decreasing with change in methods for trimming fighting teeth.

GEOGRAPHIC DISTRIBUTION
Worldwide

SIGNALMENT
• All camelids can be affected.
• Rarely seen in very young animals, usually >12 months of age
• Median of 5 years

SIGNS
• Firm swelling of the jaw
• Drainage of exudates from mandible or maxilla
• Reluctance to eat
• Dropping food
• Strange chewing habits
• Nasal discharge if sinus affected.
• Quidding

CAUSES
• Gingival penetration along alveolus
• Infundibular decay
• Tooth fracture or trauma
• Mandibular/maxillary fracture

DIAGNOSIS

DIFFERENTIAL DIAGNOSIS
• Mandibular osteitis
• Subcutaneous abscess/cellulites
• Fracture
• Sinusitis
• Tumor
• Actinomycosis
• Osteomyelitis
• Salivary gland disease

CBC/CHEMISTRY/URINALYSIS
• Not usually useful
• May see slight elevation in WBC count in chronic periostitis/osteitis

OTHER LABORATORY TESTS
Culture of exudates may sometimes indicate the bacteria involved, but is rarely necessary as tooth removal and flushing resolves the problem in most cases.

IMAGING
• Radiology is essential for diagnosis of tooth root(s) involved.
• Multiple oblique open-mouth views are often necessary, so sedation or anesthesia is usually required.
• Mandibular abscesses are easier to image than maxillary abscess.
• Contrast agent may be injected into a draining tract if the affected root is not obvious.
• Extent of osteitis/periostitis can be determined from radiographs also
• Bone lysis
• Loss of lamina dura
• Periodontal sclerosis
• Periosteal reaction
• Fistulous tracts

DIAGNOSTIC PROCEDURES
None

PATHOLOGIC FINDINGS
If seen at necropsy, localized purulent exudates, necrotic bone and alveolus, fistulous tract, loose teeth, and bony proliferation may be seen around the affected tooth roots.

TREATMENT

APPROPRIATE HEALTH CARE
• Tooth root abscesses require surgical care (nonemergency) and subsequent medical treatment.
• Extraction is generally required.
• Teeth can be removed by several methods in the anesthetized camelid.
• Oral extraction may be appropriate for premolars, canines, and incisors.
  • Elevation from the alveolus may be difficult by oral approach due to the limited excursion of the jaws in these species.
  • Ensure all roots are removed.
• Some curettage of alveolus will help remove necrotic bone.
• Repulsion of the cheek teeth has been recommended by some.
• Extreme care must be taken due to the fragility of the mandible and maxilla, which can be easily fractured.
• Trephine openings are made as in horses—landmarks are described in references.
• Motorized burr has been very successful for removal of an affected tooth, especially mandibular teeth.
• Incision is made along the ventral or ventrolateral aspect of the mandible, resecting draining fistula if possible.
• Periosteum and overlying musculature are elevated along the lateral aspect of the mandible to the level of the gingival attachment.
• If a draining tract is present, it can be followed to the tooth using the burr to remove the overlying bone on the lateral aspect.
• If no draining tract is present, the affected tooth is identified by oral palpation and an approach is made through the lateral alveolar plate to the tooth.
• Following removal of the overlying bone, the tooth and roots are carefully elevated and removed.
• Care must be taken not to damage adjacent normal tooth roots. Knowledge of anatomy and study of radiographs are essential.
• In some cases, resection of the single affected root using the burr can be effective in resolving the problem without complete extraction.
• A ventral opening in the incision is left for drainage, closing the remainder of the incision.
• The empty alveolus can be packed with gauze or acrylic if desired, and may be necessary in the maxilla. In the mandible, it is not deemed to be necessary.

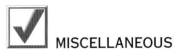
CAMELID TOOTH ROOT ABSCESSES

NURSING CARE
• Following surgery, daily or twice daily flushing of the tract with dilute chlorhexidine solution to remove food particles
• Flush until closed completely.

ACTIVITY
No restriction

DIET
• No change required
• Animals will usually begin eating within hours of anesthetic recovery.

CLIENT EDUCATION
• Early signs of dental disease should be investigated immediately.
• Subcutaneous infection can occur.
• Osteitis prolongs treatment.
• Packing of cavity with food will promote infection and prolong healing.
• Proliferative bone may remain present for the life of the animal.
• Animals are often chronic at the time of presentation because the masses are difficult to detect if heavy face fleece is present.
• Palpation or close observation of jaw lines when handling may allow for earlier recognition.

SURGICAL CONSIDERATIONS
None

MEDICATIONS

DRUGS OF CHOICE
• Flunixin meglumine 1.1 mg/kg IV q24h for postsurgical pain; rarely required for more than 48 hours
• Procaine penicillin G 20,000 U/kg IM q12h for 7–10 days or longer if required by infection severity
• Other antibiotics can be used if cultures indicate.
• Oxytetracycline—18 mg/kg SC q 48 hours
  • Postoperatively—5–10 days of treatment
  • Medical treatment—14–30 days treatment
• Ampicillin—2.5 mg/kg IM q 12 hours
  • Postoperatively—5–10 days of treatment
  • Medical treatment—14–30 days treatment

CONTRAINDICATIONS
None of the drugs listed are approved for use in camelids and do not have established withdrawal times associated with their use.

PRECAUTIONS
None

POSSIBLE INTERACTIONS
None

ALTERNATIVE DRUGS
Any broad-spectrum antibiotics effective against *A. pyogenes* and common oral bacterial inhabitants

FOLLOW-UP

PATIENT MONITORING
• Daily monitoring for cavity flushing will be required.
• Further follow-up care is rarely required unless another abscess occurs.

PREVENTION/AVOIDANCE
• Not much can be done
• Avoiding stemmy hay and foxtail may be helpful.

POSSIBLE COMPLICATIONS
• Ongoing osteitis and drainage
• Damage to adjacent tooth roots
• Infection of alveolar packing material
• Electrolyte loss and/or dehydration if salivary drainage through ventral drainage opening is excessive

EXPECTED COURSE/PROGNOSIS
• Healing will occur over several weeks, preferably healing from the inside out.
• Prognosis is excellent; good if bony infection is severe.
• Bony proliferation may be permanent.

Surgical Tooth Removal —Excellent
• Short term (<30 days)
  • Decreased size of facial swelling within 1 week postoperatively
• Long term (>30 days)
  • Resolution of facial swelling
  • Additional abscesses at adjacent teeth possible if extent of disease not identified at initial exam

Medical Treatment —Excellent-Good
• Short term (<30 days)
  • Decreased size of facial swelling
  • Progression of disease possible in minor number of patients
• Long term (>30 days)
  • Resolution of disease in most
  • Recrudescence possible: may respond to additional round of medical therapy

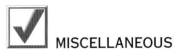
MISCELLANEOUS

ASSOCIATED CONDITIONS
• Retained tooth root
• Fracture
• Recurrence at adjacent teeth

Medical Treatment
• Failure to respond
• Recurrence

AGE-RELATED FACTORS
Rarely seen in animals <12 months of age

ZOONOTIC POTENTIAL
None

PREGNANCY
N/A

RUMINANT SPECIES AFFECTED
All camelids

BIOSECURITY
N/A

PRODUCTION MANAGEMENT
N/A

SYNONYMS
None

SEE ALSO
Body condition scoring: camelids, anesthesia and analgesia

ABBREVIATIONS
C = canine teeth
I = incisor teeth
IM = intramuscular
M = molar teeth
PM = premolar teeth
SC = subcutaneous
WBC = white blood cell

Suggested Reading
Cebra, M. L., Cebra, C. K., Garry, F. B. 1996. Tooth root abscesses in New World camelids: 23 cases (1972–1994). *J Am Vet Med Assoc.* 209:819–22.
Fowler, M. E. 1998. Digestive system. In: Fowler, M. E., ed., *Medicine and surgery of South American camelids*, 2d ed., pp. 305–59. Ames: Iowa State University Press.
Fowler, M. E. 1998. Surgery. In: Fowler, M. E., ed., *Medicine and surgery of South American camelids*, 2d ed., pp. 108–47. Ames: Iowa State University Press.
Kock, M. D. 1984. Canine tooth extraction and pulpotomy in the adult male llama. *J Am Vet Med Assoc.* 185(11): 1304–6.
Long, P. 1989. Llama herd health. *Vet Clin Food Anim.* 5(1): 227–32.

Authors: Jennifer M. Ivany Ewoldt and Dusty W. Nagy

CAMPYLOBACTER

 BASICS

DEFINITION
• Campylobacter is a group of small, curved or spiral-shaped, gram-negative bacterial rods that can cause significant reproductive disease and loss in ruminant species.
• *Campylobacter fetus* subspecies *fetus* is responsible for abortions in sheep. Bovine venereal campylobacteriosis is due to *C. fetus* subspecies *venerealis* and results in decreased fertility, early embryonic death and less often, midterm abortions.
• In addition, *Campylobacter jejuni* and *C. coli* can cause minor, self-limiting enteritis and diarrhea in ruminants.

PATHOPHYSIOLOGY
Campylobacter Fetus subsp. Fetus
• Between outbreaks of abortion, the agent is present in the gallbladder and intestine of apparently normal sheep and then spreads to susceptible ewes via contamination of feed and water.
• Bacteremia in the ewe allows the agent to reach the fetus via the circulation where it results in systemic infection of the fetus with hepatitis.
• Ultimately, *C. fetus* subsp. *fetus* can cause late-term abortions, stillbirths, and birth of premature lambs.
• *C. fetus* subsp. *fetus* can also cause abortions in cattle due to localization of a systemic infection in the dam in the pregnant uterus with the production of endotoxins.

Campylobacter Fetus subsp. Venerealis
• Cattle are the primary host and main reservoir of *C. fetus* subsp. *venerealis,* which is an obligate parasite of the bovine reproductive tract that cannot survive outside the host for any extended time.
• Transmission is via the venereal route and can approach 100% from an infected bull to an uninfected cow.
• Transmission between cows can also occur via unsanitary artificial insemination and cows can be infected with contaminated semen.
• In cows, the bacteria initially infect the vagina and cervix and then spread to the uterus and oviducts.
• The embryo is not directly affected but instead the agent results in endometritis and salpingitis that in turn causes early embryonic death.
• *C. fetus* subsp. *venerealis* establishes itself in the prepuce of the male but does not interfere with semen quality or breeding ability.

SYSTEMS AFFECTED
In ruminants, *Campylobacter* causes disease primarily in the reproductive system but can, much less commonly and with only minor significance, cause disease in the gastrointestinal system that results in mild diarrhea.

INCIDENCE/PREVALENCE
• *Campylobacter fetus* subsp. *fetus* and *C. fetus* subsp. *venerealis* are both widely distributed but the incidence and prevalence of reproductive disease within a geographical region is widely variable depending primarily on management factors such as vaccination and herd dynamics.
• *Campylobacter jejuni* and *C. coli* often can be isolated from healthy ruminants but the underlying factors that lead some animals to develop enteritis and diarrhea are not certain.
• Tend to see the diarrhea cases due to *C. jejuni* and *C. coli* in herds with better hygiene and this probably reflects lack of prior exposure and immunologic experience

GEOGRAPHIC DISTRIBUTION
Worldwide

SIGNALMENT
Species, Breed Predilections, Mean Age and Range, Predominant Sex
• *Campylobacter* diarrhea can occur in ruminants of any age but young animals are more commonly involved.
• Reproductive disease due to *Campylobacter* is encountered as abortions or poor reproductive performance in females but males are not clinically affected.
• With *C. fetus* subsp. *venerealis*, bulls are not clinically affected but serve as an important reservoir and vector for spreading the agent among cows.

SIGNS
GENERAL COMMENTS
• Calves experimentally infected with *C. jejuni* and *C. coli* had thick mucoid feces with flecks of blood; sheep had feces of normal consistency but also with flecks of blood. Animals may develop a minor fever.
• Ewes that abort with *C. fetus* subsp. *fetus* only rarely have systemic disease (diarrhea, depression, fever, vaginal discharge) but they may develop endometritis due to the retention of fetal membranes and secondary bacterial infections.
• Cows infected with *C. fetus* subsp. *venerealis* may develop a mucoid to mucopurulent vaginal discharge.

HISTORICAL FINDINGS
Campylobacter Fetus subsp. Fetus
• Outbreaks of *C. fetus* subsp. *fetus* abortion in ewes generally start with only a few affected animals but progressively larger numbers are affected.
• If the flock consists of large numbers of young or maiden ewes, the abortion rate may approach 70%.

Campylobacter Fetus subsp. Venerealis
• In cows infected with *C. fetus* subsp. *venerealis,* the main historical sign is infertility with longer interestrus intervals, increased numbers of repeat breedings, and late calvings.
• Infected herds have low fertility and early in the process this may be as low as 15–20%.

• In more chronically infected herds, newly introduced animals will have very poor reproductive rates.
• Cows with chronic infection have minimal clinical signs and these may only consist of a mucopurulent vaginal discharge in a small percentage of cows.
• Abortions due to *C. fetus* subsp. *venerealis* are unusual and may occur in less than 10% of affected cows and are typically mid- to late-gestation abortions.

PHYSICAL EXAMINATION FINDINGS
N/A

CAUSES
N/A

RISK FACTORS
• There is not significant venereal transmission of *C. fetus* subsp. *fetus* and the major risk factor for an abortion outbreak in sheep due to this agent is widespread pasture contamination.
• The major risk factor for the introduction and maintenance of *C. fetus* subsp. *venerealis* in a cattle herd is the frequent purchase of adult bulls and cows from herds of uncertain health status.

 DIAGNOSIS

DIFFERENTIAL DIAGNOSIS
• In sheep, agents other than *C. fetus* subsp. *fetus* that need to be considered in abortion storms include *Chlamydia*, *Coxiella*, and *Toxoplasma*.
• In cattle, the major differential for the herd-level reproductive problems with Campylobacteriosis is *Tritrichomonas foetus*.
• In both sheep and cattle, *Campylobacter jejuni* causes sporadic abortions rather than outbreaks.

CBC/BIOCHEMISTRY/URINALYSIS
N/A

OTHER LABORATORY TESTS
N/A

IMAGING
N/A

DIAGNOSTIC PROCEDURES
• For both *C. fetus* subsp. *fetus* and *C. fetus* subsp. *venerealis,* the definitive diagnosis is by culturing the causal organism.
• With *C. fetus* subsp. *fetus,* the aborted fetus is the most likely source from which to isolate the agent.
• With *C. fetus* subsp. *venerealis,* the aborted fetus and preputial washes from infected bulls are the most likely sources from which to isolate the agent. The agent can sometimes be isolated from infected cows if the animal is early in the course of the disease.

PATHOLOGIC FINDINGS

On postmortem examination, animals with *Campylobacter enteritis* will have an ileum and perhaps jejunum with a thickened somewhat reddened mucosa.

Campylobacter Fetus subsp. *Fetus*

• Aborted lambs are generally in the last 6 weeks of gestation.
• About 20–30% of fetuses will have multifocal areas of hepatic necrosis, which consist of pale areas up to 2–3 cm in diameter with a reddened margin. There is also fibrinous polyserositis in some fetuses.
• Cotyledons will have necrosis and edema and intercotyledonary areas will appear edematous.

Campylobacter Fetus subsp. *Venerealis*

• Cows will develop a mucopurulent endometritis with lymphocytic infiltrates; salpingitis and cervicitis may also occur. Bulls do not have significant lesions.
• Aborted fetuses will often have fibrinous pericarditis, pleuritis, and peritonitis on gross necropsy. Histologically, the fetus often has hepatitis and suppurative bronchopneumonia.
• The cotyledons are often edematous and have a tan/brown discoloration. Histologically, these areas have necrosis, vasculitis with fibrinoid degeneration of blood vessels, and mixed inflammatory infiltrates with a predominance of neutrophils.

TREATMENT

N/A

APPROPRIATE HEALTH CARE
N/A

NURSING CARE
N/A

ACTIVITY
N/A

DIET
N/A

CLIENT EDUCATION
N/A

MEDICATIONS

DRUGS OF CHOICE
• Ovine abortion storms due to *C. fetus* subsp. *fetus* can be treated with streptomycin, penicillin, and/or oral chlortetracycline.
• Treatment of individual cattle for *C. fetus* subsp. *venerealis* with antibiotics is often extralabel and is not warranted on a herdwide basis if adequate control measures are instituted.

CONTRAINDICATIONS

Appropriate milk and meat withdrawal times must be followed for all compounds administered to food-producing animals.

FOLLOW-UP

EXPECTED COURSE AND PROGNOSIS
• Convalescent immunity may occur in sheep flocks with *C. fetus* subsp. *fetus* and prevent infection and abortions for the next 2 to 3 years resulting in cyclical abortions.
• Cows infected with *C. fetus* subsp. *venerealis* develop immunity and generally clear the infection over 3 to 6 months, although a long-term carrier state is possible.
• Bulls infected with *C. fetus* subsp. *venerealis* develop a long-term carrier state with the organisms surviving in the deep crypts of the preputial epithelium. Because younger bulls have shallower crypts, they are less likely to develop persistent infection than are older bulls.
• Over time, the reproductive efficiency of the herd infected with *C. fetus* subsp. *venerealis* will improve and approach a normal rate as cows develop immunity and clear the infection.

MISCELLANEOUS

RELATED CONDITIONS
• Campylobacter is a group of small, curved or spiral-shaped, gram-negative bacterial rods that can cause significant reproductive disease and loss in ruminant species.
• *Campylobacter fetus* subspecies *fetus* is responsible for abortions in sheep. Bovine venereal campylobacteriosis is due to *C. fetus* subspecies *venerealis* and results in decreased fertility, early embryonic death, and, less often, midterm abortions.
• *Campylobacter jejuni* and *C. coli* can cause minor, self-limiting enteritis and diarrhea in ruminants.

AGE-RELATED FACTORS
N/A

ZOONOTIC POTENTIAL
C. jejuni is the most frequent cause of food-borne enteritis and diarrheal disease in humans in the United States. Raw milk and contaminated meat are the primary sources.

PREGNANCY
See Related Conditions above.

RUMINANT SPECIES AFFECTED
Potentially all ruminant species

BIOSECURITY
N/A

PRODUCTION MANAGEMENT

• Vaccines exist but to be most effective against *C. fetus* subsp. *fetus* abortion storms they need to be given before the outbreak. If the abortion outbreak has already begun, then animals that have not yet been exposed can be vaccinated.
• Control of *C. fetus* subsp. *venerealis* involves elimination of carrier bulls with two or more years of artificial insemination (since cows can be chronically infected) followed by use of young bulls that have previously been tested for *Campylobacter* and *Tritrichomonas*.
• Semen used in artificial insemination must be free of *C. fetus* subsp. *venerealis,* and extenders that include antibiotics are recommended.
• Vaccination is effective and is the best method of prevention and control of *C. fetus* subsp. *venerealis* in bull-bred herds. Vaccination is initially given prior to the breeding season and boosted 2–4 weeks later so that the series is completed about 2–4 weeks prior to the start of the breeding season. Vaccination is then given annually.

SYNONYMS
Vibrio
Vibriosis

SEE ALSO
Bovine abortion
Campylobacter jejuni
Chlamydia
Coxiella
Toxoplasma
Tritrichomonas foetus

ABBREVIATIONS
N/A

Suggested Reading
Drost, M., Thomas, P. G. A., Seguin, B., Troedsson, M. H. T. 2002. Female reproductive disorders. In: *Large animal internal medicine*, ed. B. P. Smith. 3rd ed. St. Louis: Mosby.
Marshall, R. 1999. Nonvenereal campylobacteriosis. In: *Current veterinary therapy 4: food animal practice*, ed. J. L. Howard, R. A. Smith. Philadelphia: W. B. Saunders.
Walker, R. L. 1999. Bovine Venereal Campylobacteriosis. In: *Current veterinary therapy 4: food animal practice*, ed. J. L. Howard, R. A. Smith. Philadelphia: W. B. Saunders.
Yaeger, M., Holler, L. 1997. Bacterial causes of bovine infertility and abortion. In: *Current therapy in large animal theriogenology*, ed. R. E. Youngquist. Philadelphia: W. B. Saunders.

Author: John M. Adaska

CANDIDIASIS

 BASICS

DEFINITION

Yeast infection of mammals most commonly caused by *Candida albicans* and primarily involving the intestinal, reproductive, and respiratory tracts of compromised animals

OVERVIEW

- Organism is found worldwide.
- Yeasts are not highly pathogenic and rarely cause disease in healthy animals.
- Considered normal microflora of intestinal, oral, upper respiratory, and reproductive tracts of mammals especially *Candida albicans*
- Commonly found in the feces of animals
- Opportunistic invader of skin, mucocutaneous areas, and external ear canal
- Superficial infection of the oral mucomembranes is the most common form of candidiasis in mammals having been reported in humans, dogs, cats, horses, cattle, swine, and nonhuman primates.
- In susceptible animals (immunocompromised, malnourished), *Candida* spp. may cause systemic disease affecting one or multiple organ systems.
- Primary causal agent is *Candida albicans*; most infections are endogenous.
- *C. tropicalis, C. pseudotropicalis, C. krusei, C. parakrusei, C. parapsilosis, C. guilliermondii,* and *C. stellatoidea* may also cause disease.
- Candidal dermatitis is uncommon in large animals.
  - Reported in goats, cattle, feeder pigs, horses
  - Commonly, animals are immunocompromised or malnourished.
  - Chronic moisture and skin maceration predispose to yeast invasion.
- Goats: generalized exfoliative dermatitis
  - Reported in protein-deficient goats
  - Evaluate affected goat(s) for chronic wasting disease or for trace-mineral deficiency.
  - Yeast may represent secondary opportunist.
- Cattle: ulceration, erosion, scaling, crusting, papules, pustules, and secondary alopecia
- Feeder pigs: *C. albicans* caused exudative dermatitis.
- Horse
  - *C. guilliermondii* caused generalized nodular skin disease with mastitis reported in mare.
  - *C. albicans* caused oral candidiasis in immunodeficient foals.
  - Generalized candidiasis in debilitated and immunocompromised foal undergoing intensive care
- Systemic mycotic disease due to *Candida* spp. occurs less frequently.

- In cattle, systemic disease may affect gastrointestinal tract, lungs, liver, kidney, brain, udder, or reproductive tract.
- Peracute septicemic infections reported in newborn calves.
- Calves
  - Diarrhea in young calves following prolonged use of antimicrobials
  - Oral candidiasis
  - Mycotic pharyngitis and gastroenteritis in calves result in white pseudomembranes at back of pharynx and extending down to stomach and diarrhea.
- Mycotic omasitis, rumentitis, and enteritis reported in adult ruminants; forestomach lesions include acute hemorrhagic mucosal necrosis.
- Mycotic pneumonia in young calves and lamb raised indoors in intensive housing units
- Mycotic pneumonia and pulmonary abscess in ruminants; pulmonary candidiasis reported as outbreak in feedlot cattle.
- *C. parapsilosis* most commonly reported in bovine mycotic abortion.
- Yeast mastitis in cattle and goats due to *Candida* spp.

PATHOPHYSIOLOGY

- *Candida* spp. are yeasts that propagate by budding.
- Prominent cell shape is oval and buds are single or multiple.
- Form blastoconidia, pseudohyphae, and true hyphae in culture and in tissues
- Following nutritional or atmospheric alterations in habitant environment, *Candida* spp. on mucus-containing membranes or in the invasive phase of infection (when actively invading tissue) undergo spore germination to form mycelium or form pseudomycelium by cellular elongation and filament formation.
- *Candida* spp. produce acid proteinases and keratinases, which degrade the stratum corneum, and phospholipases, which aid in penetration of tissues.
- *Candida* spp. may induce serious local or systemic infections.
- In systemic mycosis, the alimentary tract is most common route of entry of the organism, which then spreads hematogenously to other tissues.

SIGNALMENT

- Most common in young or debilitated animals
- Neonates are most prone to develop candidiasis of oral mucous membranes.
- Commonly occurs as complication of antimicrobial therapy
- Can complicate any open wound near oral mucosa, genital, or respiratory tract

SIGNS

- Depends on which organ(s) is (are) affected
- Fever (104–107°F, 40–40.5°C)
- Abortion
- Mastitis: transient and self-limiting to severe; udder spongy and swollen

- Dermatitis
  - Goats: nonpruritic dermatitis with alopecia, scales, crusting, greasiness, and lichenification; lesions were fairly symmetrical.
  - Feeder pigs: exudative dermatitis of distal limbs, thighs, abdomen; surface exudate was gray, skin was lichenified and bluish.
- Oral candidiasis characterized by white pseudomembranous plaque and ulcer over tongue and gingiva
- Calves: chronic diarrhea
- Cattle with omasitis, rumenitis, and enteritis may show nonspecific signs including lethargy, hypophagia, decreased milk production, decreased ruminal and intestinal motility, ± fever, ± low-grade abdominal pain.
- Feedlot cattle with chronic pneumonia, dyspnea, moderate fever, brown-streaked nasal discharge, diarrhea, and lacrimation

CAUSES AND RISK FACTORS

- Disruption of normal cutaneous or mucosal barriers
- Exposure to chronic moisture and skin maceration
- Compromised immune system: inherent or disease-induced
- Prolonged antibiotic therapy or heavy oral dosing
- Glucocorticoid or immunosuppressive therapy
- Feeding of poorly formulated or administered artificial diets to newborns
- Malnutrition
- Use of intramammary infusion tube may be risk for development of candida mastitis

 DIAGNOSIS

- Diagnosis is based upon history, clinical signs, and lesions.
- Isolation of organism from infected material
- Identification of mycelial and pseudomycelial yeast forms in Gram-stained smears of infected material
- Direct smears stained with new methylene blue or Diff-Quik reveal budding cells and pseudohyphae.
- Periodic acid-Schiff or Gidley and Gomori methenamine silver techniques make organisms easily discernible.
- Skin scraping cytology or impression smears: budding yeast or pseudohyphae on cytology best taken from edge of lesion
- Culture of skin biopsy: Sabouraud's dextrose agar incubated at 30°C
- Skin biopsy: superficial perivascular dermatitis and/or folliculitis; identify form of organism and demonstrate it is invading tissue.
- Fecal smears and cultures in calves with chronic diarrhea and history of antimicrobial therapy

Lesions
- Superficial form
  - White pseudomembrane overlying skin or mucous membranes
  - Pseudohyphae, septate, hyphae, and budding yeast organisms in membrane
  - Invades epithelium but rarely beyond basal layer
  - Neutrophilic, lymphocytic infiltrate beneath epidermis
- Systemic form: lesions depend on organ(s) infected

DIFFERENTIAL DIAGNOSIS
- Other fungal skin infections
- Other systemic mycoses
- Common causes of diarrhea, mastitis, pneumonia in ruminants

CBC/BIOCHEMISTRY/URINALYSIS
N/A

OTHER LABORATORY TESTS
In systemic mycosis to identify pathogen
- Polymerase chain reaction
- Murine monoclonal rabbit polyclonal antibodies in histochemistry
- Immunoblotting
- ELISA of antibodies in serology

IMAGING
N/A

DIAGNOSTIC PROCEDURES
- Direct smear: cytology of lesion exudate
- Culture of infected material or lesion exudate
- Skin biopsy

TREATMENT
- Treatment of underlying condition
  - Remove from excessive moisture
  - Provide adequate and balanced nutrition
  - Treat underlying disease process if present
  - Withdrawal of immunosuppressive drugs
  - Withdrawal of antimicrobial drugs, if possible
- Focal lesions: clip, dry, and apply topical antifungal agents.
- Topical therapy for mild dermatitis
  - Only use approved drugs in food animal.
  - Apply two to three times a day until lesions are healed.
  - Nystatin (100,000 U/gm)
  - 2% Miconazole (topical small animal products)
  - 1% Clotrimazole (Over-the-counter vaginal creams can be used.)
  - Potassium permanganate (1:3000 in water)
  - Enilconazole

- Treatment for severe dermatitis: may require administration of oral or parenteral antifungal agents
- Systemic antifungal agents not approved for use in food animals
- Efficacy of oral antifungal agents in ruminants is not well known
- Treatment of systemic mycosis is often unrewarding.
  - Amphotericin B has been the primary drug previously used but is no longer advocated, as there are less toxic and more efficacious products available.
  - Enilconazole (topical agent, not available in United States)
  - Fluconazole
  - Itraconazole
  - Ketoconazole (generic drug available, therefore most cost-effective systemic agent, 5–10 mg/kg PO once daily)
- No specific treatment for young calves with enteric (diarrheal) candidiasis
  - Supportive care
  - Withdrawal of antimicrobial therapy
  - Depending on age, probiotics or transfaunation with normal rumen flora

MEDICATIONS
N/A

DRUGS OF CHOICE
N/A

CONTRAINDICATIONS
- Many of the suggested drugs for therapy are not approved and therefore should not be used in food animals.
- Confirm safety of drugs in species to be treated before initiating therapy.
- Appropriate milk and meat withdrawal times must be followed for all compounds administered to food-producing animals.

FOLLOW-UP
- If underlying condition is an inherent immunodeficiency, prognosis may be guarded to poor.
- Systemic mycosis may not respond well to therapy.

MISCELLANEOUS

ASSOCIATED CONDITIONS
- Immunocompromise: inherent or disease-induced
- Malnutrition

- Exposure to excessive moisture
- Intensive care therapy including prolonged antimicrobials

ZOONOTIC POTENTIAL
N/A

RUMINANT SPECIES AFFECTED
- Cattle
- Goats
- Potentially, all species of ruminants may become affected.

BIOSECURITY
N/A

PRODUCTION MANAGEMENT
- Keep animals in dry, clean environment.
- Provide adequate and appropriate nutrition.
- Avoid prolonged use or inappropriate use of antimicrobial agents and corticosteroids.
- Use appropriate hygiene and technique when infusing intramammary medications into udder.

SYNONYMS
Candidosis
Moniliasis
Thrush

SEE ALSO
Abortion
Fungal pneumonia
Fungal reproductive infections
Yeast or fungal mastitis

ABBREVIATIONS
ELISA = enzyme-linked immunosorbent assay
PO = per os, by mouth

Suggested Reading
Diseases caused by fungi. 1997. In: *Veterinary pathology*, ed. T. C. Jones, R. D. Hunt, N. W. King. 6th ed. Philadelphia: Lippincott Williams & Wilkins.
Prescott, J. F. 1999. Systemic mycoses. In: *Current veterinary therapy 4: food animal practice*, ed. J. L. Howard, R. A. Smith. Philadelphia: W. B. Saunders.
Pugh, D. 2002. Diseases of the integumentary system. In: *Sheep and goat medicine*. Philadelphia: W. B. Saunders.
Radostits, O. M., Gay, C. C., Blood, D. C., Hinchcliff, K. W., eds. 1999. *Veterinary medicine: textbook of diseases of cattle, sheep, pigs, goats, and horses*. 9th ed. New York: W. B. Saunders.
Scott, D. W. 1988. Fungal infections. In: *Large animal dermatology*. Philadelphia: W. B. Saunders.
Scott, D. W., Miller, W. H. 2003. *Equine dermatology*. St. Louis: W. B. Saunders.

Authors: Susan Semrad and Karen A. Moriello

CAPRINE ARTHRITIS ENCEPHALITIS

BASICS

OVERVIEW
• Caprine arthritis encephalitis (CAE) is a disease characterized by signs of chronic degenerative polyarthritis, chronic indurative mastitis, and/or chronic pneumonia in adult goats and less frequently by acute paralysis in young kids.
• CAE is one of the most important diseases affecting dairy goats in industrialized countries.
• In the United States, seroprevalence of CAEV antibodies ranges from 38% to 81% in dairy goatherds.
• The disease is caused by caprine arthritis-encephalitis virus (CAEV), a species of the ovine/caprine lentivirus group in the *Lentivirus* genus of the family Retroviridae.
• CAEV is closely related to other human and animal lentiviruses, particularly visna maedi virus (VMV) of sheep.
• CAEV replication cycle includes the reverse transcription of the viral RNA genome into a DNA copy called the provirus. During cell division the provirus integrates into, and becomes part of, the host cellular DNA. As a result, once infected with CAEV, goats remain infected for life.
• Ingestion of CAEV-contaminated colostrum or milk by newborns is the most common form of disease transmission.
• Feeding pooled colostrum or unpasteurized milk and bad hygiene practices during milking increase the risk of CAEV transmission.
• Transmission by close contact between infected and noninfected goats particularly during lactation and parturition also may occur.
• CAEV-PCR–positive cells have been found in oviductal flushing media samples from CAEV-positive goats and shedding of CAEV in semen has been reported. Therefore for control purposes, the venereal and transplacental routes of transmission should be considered as potential sources of CAEV.
• Economic losses are associated with decreased productivity as a result of clinical disease. Diminished production is related to secondary infections, animal deaths, and the potential loss of international markets due to trade barriers.

SIGNALMENT
• Goats are the natural host of CAEV infection. Sheep can be infected experimentally with CAEV. Phylogenetic analyses indicate that cross-species transmission of small ruminant lentiviruses (CAEV and VMV) occurs regularly under natural conditions.
• Infection by CAEV is more common in dairy goats. Host genetics may influence the clinical outcome of CAEV infection. Goats of the Saanen breed that carry the CLA Be7 specificity are less likely to develop arthritis

after CAEV infection than goats missing this specificity.
• CAE infection rates among meat and hair goat breeds in North America seem to be low. This may reflect differences in management practices between dairy and meat/hair goats that prevent transmission rather than differences in breed susceptibility.
• Mouflon-domestic sheep hybrids are susceptible to experimental infection with CAEV.
• Clinical signs of CAE-associated arthritis, mastitis, and/or pneumonia are manifested more often in goats 2 years of age or older. Chronic progressive paralysis has been described occasionally in adult goats. Paralysis that follows a rapid clinical course in kids 2 to 6 months of age also has been reported.

SIGNS
• Differences in virus strain, individual host susceptibility factors, and the presence of concurrent infections may influence the clinical outcome of CAEV infections.
• In the majority of CAEV-infected goats, the infection is subclinical.
• In approximately 25% of seropositive goats, arthritis, mastitis, and/or pneumonia are manifested only several years after CAEV primary infection (clinical latency). More than one clinical manifestation may be observed in the same animal.
• Chronic, proliferative arthritis ("big knee") in mature goats is the most common clinical manifestation of CAE. Goats with CAE-associated arthritis show swelling of the joints, particularly the carpi and less frequently the stifle, hock, hip, and atlantooccipital joints. The onset of arthritis is insidious, with short periods of swelling followed by periods of remission. Eventually, affected animals show pain, decreased range of articular motion, stiff gate, "knee walking," and chronic weight loss.
• The majority of CAE arthritic goats also show chronic indurative mastitis ("hard bag"). In these cases, the mammary gland is firm on palpation and symmetrically enlarged. Although normal in appearance, milk production may be reduced. In more severe cases, there is agalactia that occurs at the time of parturition.
• Some CAEV-infected goats develop chronic nonsuppurative pneumonia with signs of dyspnea and weight loss.
• Although unusual, neurological involvement in adult goats can occur. Initially, these goats show slight aberration in gait. Over the course of several months, the clinical course progresses to complete paralysis.
• Once CAEV-infected goats show clinical signs of the disease, death months or years after primary infection is the end result, usually as a consequence of secondary infections.
• A different clinical presentation of CAE, characterized by a rapid clinical course and afebrile paralysis in kids 2 to 6 months of age

has been described. The paralysis starts in the rear legs and progresses toward the front of the animal. Affected kids continue to be alert and eat if hand-fed, but often develop bloating and urinary retention as a result of recumbency. A few affected kids show blindness or circling. During the acute stages of the disease, affected kids develop severe pleocytosis with up to 100,000 mononuclear inflammatory cells per cubic millimeter.

DIAGNOSIS

DIFFERENTIAL DIAGNOSIS
• CAE needs to be differentiated from other causes of chronic weight loss, such as caseous lymphadenitis, paratuberculosis (Johne's disease), internal abscesses, scrapie, chronic parasite infestations, and malnutrition.
• In goats with arthritis, bacterial, chlamydial, and mycoplasmal polyarthritis (contagious agalactia) need to be included in the differential diagnosis of CAE.
• The differential diagnosis of the chronic respiratory form of CAE should include chronic bacterial and verminous pneumonia and lung abscesses.
• The neurologic form of CAE needs to be distinguished from trauma of or abscesses in the brain or spinal cord, meningitis, parelaphostrongylosis, vitamin E and Se deficiency, copper deficiency, listeriosis, scrapie, rabies, and bacterial polyarthritis.

DIAGNOSTIC PROCEDURES
• CAEV replicates in the presence of antiviral immune responses and persists for life in cells of infected goats. For this reason, determination of anti-CAEV antibodies in sera is the method most commonly used to identify infected goats.
• Serum antibodies can be detected as early as 3 to 6 weeks after exposure, but some infected goats may remain seronegative for 8 months or more in spite of being virus and PCR positive.
• The agar gel immunodiffusion (AGID) test and the enzyme-linked immunosorbent assay (ELISA) are the two most commonly used assays to detect CAEV-infected goats. None of these tests is standardized across diagnostic laboratories, and their sensitivity and specificity may vary widely. Consequently, unnecessary culling of false positive goats from, or the retention of false negative goats in herds during eradication programs may occur.
• A competitive ELISA (cELISA) with high sensitivity and specificity is commercially available.
• Because of the high cost of cELISA, it is recommended that the AGID test be used for the first round of testing, after which all positive reactors should be segregated from the herd. Then, the more sensitive cELISA can be used for subsequent testing at 3- to 6-month intervals. Once all animals in the

CAPRINE ARTHRITIS ENCEPHALITIS

herd give a negative result in at least two consecutive tests, annual retesting and the purchase of replacement animals from CAEV-free flocks should be implemented.
• Virus isolation from "buffy coats" is the most definite way to confirm CAE. However, this method is expensive, cumbersome, and often unsuccessful. For these reasons, this technique is not recommended as a routine diagnostic test for CAE.
• Although PCR is a highly sensitive technique, its usefulness for the detection of CAEV in clinical samples from naturally infected goats still needs validation.

PATHOLOGIC FINDINGS

GROSS FINDINGS
• Affected goats may be thin to emaciated and have long, coarse, dull hair coats.
• Swelling of carpi and less frequently the stifle, hock, hip, and atlantooccipital joints are present in goats affected with arthritis. The swelling also affects associated tendons, bursa, and adjacent periarticular tissues. In early stages, the synovial fluid is increased but remains translucid. Mineralization of periarticular tissues and erosion of articular cartilage are found in more advanced cases.
• The mammary gland in goats affected with mastitis is symmetrically enlarged and firm on palpation.
• In most CAEV goats with pulmonary involvement, lung lesions are imperceptible.
• The lymph nodes draining affected joints, mammary gland, or lung may be enlarged.

Microscopic Findings
• Histologic lesions in joints of goats with CAE-induced arthritis are characterized by various degrees of infiltration of lymphocytes, plasma cells, and macrophages in the synovium. and proliferation of villi. As the disease progresses, degeneration of the articular cartilage, fibrosis, mineralization of the joint capsule, and periosteal replacement growth become evident.
• In the mammary gland of CAE goats with mastitis, there is interstitial infiltration of lymphocytes, and plasma cells in the interstitium surrounding lobular ducts. Often, macrophages can be seen in the luminal epithelium.
• Pulmonary lesions are typical of lymphoid interstitial pneumonia and are characterized by the presence of numerous mononuclear cell aggregates and lymph follicles adjacent to bronchioles and small blood vessels. In more severe cases, there is thickening of the interalveolar septa due to infiltration of mononuclear cells and fibrosis.
• In goat kids affected by the neurological form of CAE, there is chronic, nonsuppurative inflammation of the brain accompanied by destruction of myelin and proliferation of glial cells.

TREATMENT

There are no specific treatments available for CAE.

MEDICATIONS

CONTRAINDICATIONS
N/A

FOLLOW-UP

N/A

PREVENTION/AVOIDANCE
• There are no commercial vaccines available to prevent CAEV infection.
• Serological testing and segregation of positive reactors can achieve eradication of CAE from a herd.
• Some CAEV-infected goats may remain seronegative for weeks or months after infection. These goats may shed the virus in milk and other body secretions at irregular intervals, thus representing a major problem in CAE control and eradication programs.
• For these reasons, retesting every 3 to 6 months with elimination of new positive reactors is necessary until three to five consecutive tests result in 100% of the goats being seronegative. Then, yearly testing and acquisition of replacements from CAE-free flocks are recommended.
• Separation of offspring from their mothers before the ingestion of colostrum and the use of heat-inactivated colostrum (56°C for 60 min) and milk substitutes have been used in the past with limited success. The method is labor intensive and not always effective.

MISCELLANEOUS

ASSOCIATED CONDITIONS
N/A

AGE-RELATED FACTORS
• Clinical signs of arthritis, mastitis, and pneumonia are seen more often in goats 2 to 3 years old or older.
• Acute leukoencephalomyelitis, although uncommon, is seen in 2- to 6-month-old kids.

ZOONOTIC POTENTIAL
There is no evidence to indicate that CAEV is infectious to humans.

PREGNANCY
Vertical transmission from mother to fetus does not seem to be an important event in the epidemiology of CAE.

SYNONYMS
"Big knee"

SEE ALSO
Abscesses in the brain or spinal cord
Bacterial polyarthritis
Bacterial, chlamydial, and mycoplasmal polyarthritis (contagious agalactia)
Caseous lymphadenitis
Chronic parasite infestations and malnutrition
Copper deficiency
Internal abscesses
Listeriosis
Lung abscesses
Meningitis
Paratuberculosis (Johne's disease)
Parelaphostrongylosis
Rabies
Scrapie
Verminous pneumonia
Visna maedi virus
Vitamin E and Se deficiency

ABBREVIATIONS
AGID = agar gel immunodiffusion
CAE = caprine arthritis encephalitis
CAEV = caprine arthritis-encephalitis virus
ELISA = enzyme-linked immunosorbent assay
PCR = polymerase chain reaction
VMV = visna maedi virus

Suggested Reading
de la Concha-Bermejillo, A. 2003. Caprine arthritis encephalitis: an update. *Sheep Goat Res J.* 18:69–78.
Knowles, D. P., Jr. 1997. Laboratory diagnostic tests for retrovirus infections of small ruminants. *Vet Clin North Amer-Food Anim Pract.* 13:1–11.
Rowe, J. D., East, N. E. 1997. Risk factors for transmission and methods for control of caprine arthritis-encephalitis virus infection. *Vet Clin North Amer -Food Anim Pract.* 13:35–53.
Shah, C., Böni, J., Huder, J. B., Vogt, H.-R., Mühlerr, J., Zanoni, R., Miserez, R., Lutz, H., Schüpbach, J. 2004. Phylogenetic analysis and reclassification of caprine and ovine lentiviruses based on 104 new isolates: evidence of regular sheep-to-goat transmission and worldwide propagation through livestock trade. *Virol.* 319(1): 12–26.

Author: Andrés de la Concha-Bermejillo

CAPTURE MYOPATHY

 BASICS

OVERVIEW
• Capture myopathy (CM) is also known as postcapture myopathy, overstraining disease, transport myopathy, exertional rhabdomyolisis, exertional myopathy, and leg paralysis.
• Has been reported in numerous species of mammals and birds, often associated with capture and or restraint.
• Has been reported in animals captured by a variety of methods, including short or long-distance chases, chemical immobilization, drop netting, net gunning, boma capture, handling, and restraint in chutes
• Rarely reported in carnivores
• Appropriate capture method of wild species governs outcome and development (or not) of CM.
• Habituation of captive animals to handling is an important tool in prevention.
• CM can be broadly divided into four categories according its physical manifestation. These are peracute, acute, subacute, and chronic. It should be remembered that these are phases in a continuum, and that the borders are not rigid.

SYSTEMS AFFECTED
Musculoskeletal

GENETICS
N/A

INCIDENCE/PREVALENCE
N/A

GEOGRAPHIC DISTRIBUTION
Worldwide, depending on production management and species

SIGNALMENT
Sudden death, collapse, lameness, torticollis, recumbency—vary according to syndrome

Species
Cervidae

Breed Predilections
N/A

Mean Age and Range
N/A

Predominant Sex
N/A

CAUSES AND RISK FACTORS
• Several factors can act alone or, more commonly, in combination, to lead to the development of CM.
• These factors include restraint methodology, overexertion, hyperthermia, isometric exercise, drug effects, alterations in the muscle pump activity.
• Species predisposition and individual variation
• Season and effects upon dietary intake and ambient temperature
• Physical fitness (training)
• Fear, habituation, and familiarity with events, environment, and personnel

 DIAGNOSIS

• Clinical signs and history are important components in the diagnosis; in peracute and acute cases, there will be little or no opportunity for laboratory tests before death supervenes, although serum potassium and lactic acid are elevated.
• Acute or subacute cases may show lameness or be recumbent.
• In long-term chronic cases, wasting and debility may occur.

DIFFERENTIAL DIAGNOSIS
• If the precipitating factors are known, there may be little that should be confused with CM, but the clinical picture may be similar to conditions such as enzootic ataxia or acute central nervous system disease.
• In areas where selenium deficiency is recognized, CM can closely resemble white muscle disease, which may occur in calves born to selenium-deficient mothers, or in other age groups taking sudden exercise.
• Fracture or other traumatic injuries
• In long-term chronic cases, wasting and debility may occur.

CBC/BIOCHEMISTRY/URINALYSIS
• Early in acute phase serum pH, lactic acid and serum potassium are elevated.
• Once muscle and organ damage becomes evident, serum enzymes such as aspartate aminotransferase and creatine kinase are elevated, but serum pH, lactic acid, and serum potassium may have returned to normal. Myoglobinuria is often evident.
• Little information exists about effects of long-term chronic CM or repeated low-level stimuli that can lead to kidney damage. However, severe damage could lead to impaired renal function, which could include azotemia and inappropriate urine-specific gravity.

OTHER LABORATORY TESTS
N/A

IMAGING
N/A

DIAGNOSTIC PROCEDURES
History, clinical signs, serum chemistry, urinalysis

PATHOLOGIC FINDINGS

GROSS FINDINGS
• Peracute—few postmortem signs
• Acute—include pulmonary edema, severe congestion of the small intestine and liver, muscle hemorrhage or rupture, often in the gastrocnemius muscle.
• Subacute to chronic —areas of pale muscle or muscle groups. The muscle lesions are usually bilateral, but not necessarily symmetrical and may involve almost any muscle or even part of a muscle. Kidney damage and dark brown urine containing myoglobin may be seen in the bladder.
• Chronic—kidney and widespread muscle damage

HISTOPATHOLOGICAL FINDINGS
Varying degrees of damage and loss of striation in skeletal muscle may be seen. Deposition of hemoglobin and myoglobin in the glomeruli may occur.

TREATMENT

- Seldom effective in acute cases or those severely affected
- Prevention is important.
- In affected animals, a considerable variety of treatments including vitamins and anti-inflammatory and pain relieving drugs have been tried, usually with little success.
- Their success is dependent upon both the type of CM that is involved and the extent to which treatments can be administered without exacerbating existing conditions.
- Vitamin E/Se injections are used routinely to treat cattle and sheep with white muscle disease. White muscle disease has some similarities to certain forms of CM.

MEDICATIONS

Prophylactic use of taming or sedative drugs has been employed to prevent the development of capture myopathy syndromes, especially in African species captured from the wild and destined for game ranches. Combinations of a variety of these products, collectively known as long-acting neuroleptics (LANs), have been shown to greatly reduce morbidity and enhance the capture and translocation of several species.

CONTRAINDICATIONS

- If wild animals are to be released after capture, the use of LANs may be contraindicated as reduced perceptiveness may lead to an increased risk of predation.
- LANs are not licensed for use in food-producing animals.
- Appropriate milk and meat withdrawal times must be followed for all compounds administered to food-producing animals.

FOLLOW-UP

PATIENT MONITORING

PREVENTION/AVOIDANCE

- Choice of the most suitable method of restraint is vital. This will depend upon the needs of the situation.
- One of the simplest forms of prevention is to ensure that the animals are dealt with in the training, taming, & tempo (TT&T) methods of handling.
- Training means that all the animals can be trained to use the corrals and handling systems to the point where they feel little or no stress.
- Taming involves acclimatization to humans by regular feeding from a vehicle, or by the use of special calls at feeding time. Animals should not be handled when strangers are present.
- Tempo—animals should never be rushed; handlers must be alert to animal responses, and working in unsuitable conditions should be avoided (windy days, high temperatures).
- LANs where appropriate

POSSIBLE COMPLICATIONS

Animals can apparently recover from a handling incident, but have long-term muscle damage (e.g., cardiac) and can succumb to subsequent adverse stimuli.

EXPECTED COURSE AND PROGNOSIS

Usually fatal in all but chronic forms. When chronic, slow debility and decline leads to loss of productivity or failure to breed.

MISCELLANEOUS

ASSOCIATED CONDITIONS

White muscle disease (cattle), March myoglobinuria (humans), rhabdomyolisis (humans), delayed acute capture myopathy (deer)

AGE-RELATED FACTORS

All ages may be affected.

ZOONOTIC POTENTIAL
N/A

PREGNANCY
N/A

SYNONYMS
N/A

SEE ALSO
Acute central nervous system disease
Enzootic ataxia
Malignant hyperthermia
Porcine stress syndrome
White muscle disease

ABBREVIATIONS
CM = capture myopathy
LANs = long-acting neuroleptic agents
TT&T = training, taming, and tempo

Suggested Reading
Chalmers, G. A. and M. W. Barrett. 1977. Capture myopathy in elk in Alberta, Canada: a report of three cases. *J Amer Vet Med Assoc.* 171: 927–32.
Harthoorn, A. M. 1982. Mechanical capture as a preliminary to chemical immobilization and the use of taming and training to prevent post capture stress. In: *Chemical immobilization of North American wildlife*, ed. L. Nielsen, J. C. Haigh, M. E. Fowler. Milwaukee: Wisconsin Humane Society Inc.
Montane, J., Marco, I., Manteca, X., Lopez, J., Lavin, S. 2002, Mar. Delayed acute capture myopathy in three roe deer. *J Vet Med A Physiol Pathol Clin Med.* 49(2): 93–98.
Spraker, T. R. 1982. An overview of the pathophysiology of capture myopathy and related conditions that occur at the time of capture of wild animals. In: *Chemical immobilization of North American wildlife*, ed. L. Nielsen, J. C. Haigh, M. E. Fowler. Milwaukee: Wisconsin Humane Society Inc.
Williams, E. S., Thorne, E.T. 1996. Exertional myopathy (capture myopathy). In: *Non-infectious diseases of wildlife*, ed. A. Fairbrother, L. N. Locke, G. L. Hoff. 2nd ed. Ames: Iowa State University Press.

Author: Jerry Haigh and Peter Wilson

CARBAMATE TOXICITY

 BASICS

OVERVIEW
• Carbamates are anticholinesterase insecticides commonly found in crop insecticides.
• The binding of carbamates is reversible and temporary, unlike the mechanism of another class of anticholinesterase insecticide, the organophosphates, which is irreversible.

PATHOPHYSIOLOGY
Anticholinesterase insecticides bind with and inhibit acetylcholinesterase, the enzyme that breaks down the neurotransmitter acetylcholine. These compounds cause acetylcholine to accumulate at nerve junctions and cause excessive synaptic activity. The effects are in the parasympathetic nervous system and at neuromuscular sites.

SYSTEMS AFFECTED
CNS, production management

GENETICS
N/A

INCIDENCE/PREVALENCE
Unknown

GEOGRAPHIC DISTRIBUTION
Worldwide distribution

SIGNALMENT
Any domestic animal can be exposed to toxic levels of carbamate insecticides.

Species
All species of ruminants

Breed Predilections
N/A

Mean Age and Range
N/A

Predominant Sex
N/A

SIGNS

Muscarinic Symptoms
Result from stimulation of the parasympathetic nervous system and are described by the acronym SLUD:
• Salivation
• Lacrimation
• Urination
• Defecation

Other Possible Muscarinic Signs
• Vomiting
• Myosis
• Bradycardia
• Dyspnea

Nicotinic (Neuromuscular) Signs
• Muscle tremors
• Ataxia
• Progressive paresis to paralysis

Central Nervous System (CNS) Signs
• Depression
• Seizures
• Behavioral changes

CAUSES AND RISK FACTORS
• Domestic animals are usually exposed to carbamate insecticides due to drift, accidental ingestion, or improper treatment by owners. Carbamate insecticides are used primarily on crops and other plants. They were previously commonly used for ectoparasite control.
• Carbamates are anticholinesterase insecticides commonly found in crop insecticides.
  • Carbaryl—LD50 in rats is 307 mg/kg orally and >500 mg/kg dermally.
  • Carbofuran—Minimum toxic dose in sheep and cattle is 4.5 mg/kg, becoming lethal for sheep at 9 mg/kg and for cattle at 18 mg/kg.
  • Methomyl—LD50 in rats is 17 mg/kg orally.
  • Propoxur—LD50 in rats is 95 mg/kg orally and in goats is >800 mg/kg orally.

 DIAGNOSIS

DIFFERENTIAL DIAGNOSIS
• Rabies
• Other pesticides including organophosphates, rodenticides, metaldehyde (snail bait), haloxon anthelmintic
• Other toxins such as strychnine or lead
• Numerous plant toxicities cause tremor or ataxia.
• Metabolic disturbances such as nervous ketosis
• Gastrointestinal causes of diarrhea

CBC/BIOCHEMISTRY/URINALYSIS
N/A

OTHER LABORATORY TESTS
N/A

IMAGING
N/A

DIAGNOSTIC PROCEDURES
• Diagnosis is often based on known exposure to carbamate and response to treatment with atropine.
• Prompt testing is necessary due to the temporary binding of carbamate toxins. Cholinesterase activity may return to normal before or during laboratory testing.
• Cholinesterase activity in whole blood, retina, or brain that is 25%–50% of normal for the species being tested indicates cholinesterase inhibitor toxicosis. If less than 25% of normal, clinical correlation of symptoms is required for diagnosis.
• Check with the laboratory before submitting blood samples because some testing methods may require serum instead of whole blood samples.
• Half of the brain should be submitted for homogenization, as cholinesterase activity varies in different brain regions.

CARBAMATE TOXICITY

PATHOLOGIC FINDINGS

GROSS FINDINGS
None

HISTOPATHOLOGICAL FINDINGS
None

TREATMENT

• Provide supportive care for SLUD or secondary clinical signs such as dehydration.
• Wash the animal with soap and water if dermal exposure occurs to decrease absorption. Clipping may be advisable in long-haired animals.
• Administer activated charcoal at a dose of 1–2 lb PO per 500 kg animal.
• Atropine should be given at a dose of 0.1–0.5 mg/kg to competitively bind acetylcholine. Give one-fourth of the initial dose IV and the rest subcutaneously or intramuscularly. Dosage can be repeated in 6 hours if clinical signs recur.

MEDICATIONS

• Activated charcoal
• Atropine

CONTRAINDICATIONS
• Oximes such as pralidoxime chloride (2-PAM) that are used to release the acetylcholinesterase-organophosphate bond are *not* used due to the reversible nature of carbamate binding to acetylcholinesterase.
• Appropriate milk and meat withdrawal times must be followed for all compounds administered to food-producing animals.

POSSIBLE INTERACTIONS
N/A

FOLLOW-UP

PATIENT MONITORING
• Heart rate
• Respiration
• Fluid and feed intake

PREVENTION/AVOIDANCE
• Closely follow instructions for dilution and application found on carbamate insecticide label.
• Premises should be washed and contaminated soil removed. Runoff can poison fish and aquatic animals.
• Avoid use of carbamate insecticides for ectoparasite control especially on sick or debilitated animals.

POSSIBLE COMPLICATIONS
N/A

EXPECTED COURSE AND PROGNOSIS
Good prognosis if treated promptly

MISCELLANEOUS

ASSOCIATED CONDITIONS
N/A

AGE-RELATED FACTORS
N/A

ZOONOTIC POTENTIAL
• Carbamate toxicity is not a transmissible disease; however, humans are also susceptible to toxic exposures.
• Follow labeled instructions and precautions when handling carbamate insecticides.
• Use caution when washing poisoned animals.

PREGNANCY
N/A

SEE ALSO
Gastrointestinal causes of diarrhea
Metabolic disturbances such as nervous ketosis
Numerous plant toxicities cause tremor or ataxia
Other pesticides including organophosphates, rodenticides, metaldehyde (snail bait), haloxon anthelmintic
Other toxins such as strychnine or lead
Rabies

ABBREVIATIONS
2-PAM = pralidoxime chloride
SLUD = salivation, lacrimation, urination, defecation

Suggested Reading

Aiello, S. E., ed. 1998. Carbamate insecticides. In: *Merck veterinary manual*. 8th ed. Whitehouse Station, NJ: Merck and Co.

Lloyd, W. E. 1978, May. Chemical detection techniques for diagnosing dairy herd health problems. *J Dairy Sci.* 61(5): 676–78.

Osweiler, G. D. 1996. Organophosphorus and carbamate insecticides. In: *Toxicology*. Baltimore: Williams and Wilkins.

Smith, B. P., ed., 2002. Toxicology of organic compounds. In: *Large animal internal medicine*. 3rd ed. St. Louis: Mosby.

Tilley, L. P., Smith, F.W. K., Jr., ed. 2004. Organophosphate and carbamate toxicity. In: *The 5-minute veterinary consult—canine and feline*. 3rd ed. Philadelphia: Lippincott, Williams & Wilkins.

Author: Lisa Nashold

CARDIOMYOPATHY

 BASICS

DEFINITION
• Diseases of the heart resulting from primary myocardial dysfunction of unknown etiology and are characterized by dilation and/or hypertrophy
• Secondary cardiomyopathies include myocardial disease of known cause and other cardiovascular disorders which lead to dilation and/or hypertrophy of the heart

OVERVIEW
• Uncommon condition in large animals
• Sporadic occurrence
• Holstein cattle seem most sensitive
• Three forms of cardiomyopathy
• Dilated or congestive cardiomyopathy is characterized by
  • Cardiomegaly
  • Dilatation of all chambers and atrioventricular rings
  • Increased ventricular mass
  • Reduced myocardial contractility
  • Decreased systolic function
  • Outcome is heart failure.
  • Dilated cardiomyopathy described in Canadian black and white Holstein
  • Etiology: idiopathic, familial, secondary
• Hypertrophic cardiomyopathy
  • Diastolic disorder resulting from decreased ventricular myocardial compliance
  • Hypertrophy of left ventricular free wall and septum results in reduced distensibility, impaired relaxation of ventricle, and decreased diastolic flow from and dilation of left atrium
  • Symmetrical or asymmetrical chamber or septal hypertrophy
• Restrictive cardiomyopathy is characterized by impeded diastolic relaxation and reduced left ventricular filling.
• In cattle, inherited myocardial disease is a primary dilated cardiomyopathy.
• Two cases of hypertrophic cardiomyopathy have been reported in Holstein cattle.
• Disease in sheep and goats is due primarily to secondary cardiomyopathies.

PATHOPHYSIOLOGY
General
• Progressive loss of myocardial contractility
• Decrease in cardiac output
• Blood volume and pressure increases within chambers causing them to dilate
• Constant sympathetic stimulation of the heart leads to arrhythmias and myocytes death
• Renin-angiotensin-aldosterone release causes vasoconstriction and sodium and water retention
• Signs of congestive heart failure develop

SIGNALMENT/ INHERITED SYNDROMES
Holstein-Friesian Cattle
• Reported in Holstein-Friesian cattle in Canada, Great Britain, Japan, Austria, Germany
• Reported in Simmental-Red Holstein crosses and black spotted Friesians in Switzerland
• Autosomal-recessive trait
• Cattle may be genetically linked by presence of red Holstein gene.
• Affected cattle range from 1.5–6 to 7 years old
• Most affected have clinical signs by 3 to 4 years of age.
• Stress (late pregnancy, early lactation) often precipitates onset of clinical signs.
• No sex predilection
• Initially, left ventricle fails to compensate leading to pulmonary hypertension, hypertrophy of right ventricle, and right heart failure.
• Lesions: cardiomyopathy, ventricular and atrial dilatation, variable hypertrophy, necrosis, and fibrosis, ± hepatomegaly (congestion and fibrosis), systemic cardiac edema, interstitial nephritis

Japanese Black Cattle
• Inherited: autosomal-recessive trait
• Affected calves usually die by 30 days of age; may survive 120 days
• Lesions: extensive myocardial necrosis with cardiomegaly and marked left ventricular dilation leading to congestive heart failure (pulmonary edema, ascites, hydrothorax)

Australian Polled Herefords
• Inherited; single autosomal recessive gene
• Associated with dense, tight, curly (wooly) haircoat
• Survival time reported as up to 3 months or 6 months of age
• Calves often die by 7 days of age.
• Arrhythmias noted included multifocal ventricular premature contractions, ventricular tachycardia, bigeminal rhythms.
• Lesions: myocardial necrosis; fibrosis and mineralization; vascular congestion of liver, spleen and lung; diffuse streaking of myocardium
• Also reported in horned Herefords

SIGNS
Holstein-Friesian Cattle
• Initially, clinical signs are indistinct and slowly progressive: cows are weak, unable to track with herd, and low-milk producers.
• Once cardiac signs are evident, disease progresses rapidly with cattle dying or culled within days or weeks.

• Signs of right heart failure:
  • Submandibular, brisket, and ventral edema
  • Muffled heart sounds
  • Tachycardia, gallop rhythm
  • Jugular and mammary vein distention and pulsation
  • Hepatomegaly
  • Pleural or pericardial effusion

Japanese Black Cattle
• Signs of progressive heart failure
• Severe dyspnea prior to death

Australian Polled Hereford Calves
• Rapid growth rate
• Short curly coat
• Moderate bilateral exophthalmia
• Exercise intolerance
• Sudden death, usually precipitated by stress
• Dyspnea
• Blood froth from nose
• Congestive heart failure

Pathologic Lesions
• See above under each syndrome.
• Lesions of congestive heart failure

CAUSES AND RISK FACTORS
• Etiology— unknown
• Genetic predisposition in some cattle breeds
• Stress may precipitate clinical signs

 DIAGNOSIS

• History and clinical signs of heart failure
• Echocardiography
  • To rule out other causes of cardiac disease
  • To document heart chamber dilatation ± hypertrophy
• Electrocardiogram if arrhythmias are present.
• Thoracic radiographs in calves to document cardiomegaly
• Arterial blood gas

DIFFERENTIAL DIAGNOSIS
• Ionophore toxicity
• Gossypol toxicosis
• Selenium- vitamin E deficiency
• Plant toxicosis: *Cassia occidentalis, Phalaris* spp.
• Viral-induced
• Myocarditis
• Endocarditis
• Primary or secondary copper deficiency
• Cardiac neoplasia: lymphosarcoma, fibrosarcoma
• Generalized glycogenosis type II

CBC/BIOCHEMISTRY/URINALYSIS
- CBC: normal or stress leukogram
- Serum electrolytes: normal or hyponatremia, hypokalemia, hypochloremia due to anorexia or retention of fluid in vascular space
- Serum chemistry changes reflect secondary organ involvement
  - Elevated GGT due to passive congestion of liver
  - Elevated creatine due to renal hypoperfusion

OTHER LABORATORY TESTS
- Hepatic ultrasound: ± hepatomegaly
- Transferrin: serum and urinary concentrations increased in cattle with bovine dilated cardiomyopathy

IMAGING
- Echocardiography
- Thoracic radiographs
- Ultrasound of abdomen or chest

TREATMENT
- Short-term management only
- Cardioglycosides: Digoxin
- Diuretic: Furosemide, if pulmonary edema present
- Dietary restriction of sodium
- Dietary supplementation of potassium chloride (KCl)
- Monitor blood acid-base, electrolyte, and hydration status

MEDICATIONS

DRUGS OF CHOICE
- Furosemide: 0.5–1.0 mg/kg IV, IM BID
- Digoxin
  - 0.86 μg/kg per hour IV (valuable hospitalized animals) or 3.4 μg/kg IV every 4 hours; greater risk of inducing digoxin toxicity
  - Supplement with KCl if animal is inappetent.
- Dietary restriction of sodium in older calves
- KCl: 5 to 10 g per day PO in older calves; 50–200 g daily PO for adult cow/bull
- Appropriate milk and meat withdrawal times must be followed for all compounds administered to food-producing animals.

FOLLOW-UP
- Plasma/serum digoxin concentrations to monitor for toxicity
- Monitoring of blood electrolyte and acid-base status
- Monitoring of hydration status
- Monitoring of weight gain or loss

EXPECTED COURSE AND PROGROSIS
- 100% mortality in long term
- Holstein-Friesian and Simmental-Red Holstein may survive up to 6 to 7 years.
- Japanese black cattle often die by 1 month but may survive to 4 months of age.
- Australian polled Hereford calves usually succumb by 3 months but may live until 6 months of age.

MISCELLANEOUS

ASSOCIATED CONDITIONS
- Cardiac arrhythmias
- ±Hepatomegaly
- Hypovolemic nephropathy
- Interstitial nephritis

ZOONOTIC POTENTIAL
N/A

RUMINANT SPECIES AFFECTED
Cattle, sheep, goats

BIOSECURITY
N/A

PRODUCTION MANAGEMENT
- Holstein-Friesian cattle: 3%–5% incidence in inbred cattle
- Do not breed suspected carriers of traits

SEE ALSO
Cardiac neoplasia: lymphosarcoma, fibrosarcoma
Endocarditis
Generalized glycogenosis type II
Gossypol toxicosis

Ionophore toxicity
Ionophore toxicosis, gossypol toxicity, toxic plants
Myocarditis
Plant toxicosis: *Cassia occidentalis, Phalaris* spp.
Primary or secondary copper deficiency
Selenium-vitamin E deficiency
Virus-induced
White muscle disease, selenium deficiency

ABBREVIATIONS
BID = twice daily
CBC = complete blood count
GGT = gamma-glutamyltransferase
IM = intramuscular
IV = intravenous
KCl = potassium chloride
PO = per os, by mouth

Suggested Reading
Borsberry, S., Colloff, A. 1999. Cardiomyopathy in adult Holstein Friesian cattle. *Vet Rec.* 144(26):735–36.
Dolf, G., et al. 1998. Evidence for autosomal recessive inheritance of a major gene for bovine dilated cardiomyopathy. *J Animal Sci.* 76:1824–29.
Graber, H. U., Pfister, H., Martig, J. 1995. Increased concentrations of transferrin in urine and serum of cattle with cardiomyopathy. *Res Vet Sci.* 59(2):160–63.
Jones, T. C., Hung, R. C., King, N. W. 1997. Cardiovascular disease. In: *Veterinary pathology*, 6th ed., pp. 985–86. Philadelphia: Lippincott Williams and Wilkin.
Rebhum, W. C. 1995. The cardiovascular diseases. In: *Diseases of dairy cattle*. Lippincott Williams & Wilkins.

Authors: Susan Semrad and Sheila McGuirk

CARDIOTOXIC PLANTS

 BASICS

OVERVIEW

A large group of unrelated plants can be cardiotoxic to livestock; the majority contains cardiac glycosides. Other cardiotoxic plants that have resulted in livestock poisoning include yew (*Taxus* spp.), grayanotoxin-containing plants, death camas (*Zigadenus* spp.), and avocado (*Persea* spp.).

Cardiac Glycoside–Containing Plants

• Plants containing cardiac glycosides include oleander (*Nerium oleander*), summer pheasant's eye (*Adonis aestivalis*), foxglove (*Digitalis purpurea*), lily-of-the-valley (*Convallaria majalis*), dogbane (*Apocynum* spp.), and some species of milkweed (*Asclepias* spp.).
• Oleander is cultivated widely in the southern United States and is most commonly associated with plant poisonings in livestock. Therefore, oleander is discussed in detail as a representative of plants containing cardiac glycosides.
• Cardiac glycosides cause poisoning by inhibiting the cellular membrane Na^+/K^+-ATPase, which results in an indirect increase in intracellular Ca^{2+} concentrations and a subsequent positive inotropic effect. In addition, direct effects on the sympathetic nervous system are seen.
• All parts of oleander are extremely toxic, whether the plant is fresh or dried. Ingestion of dried oleander clippings is a common source of poisoning in livestock.
• The median toxic dose of oleander leaves in cattle is 45 mg of plant material per kg body weight or approximately 12 averaged-sized leaves.

Yews

• Yews are popular shrubbery used as a hedge or foundation planting. Several *Taxus* species are found in the United States with *T. baccata* (English yew) and *T. cuspidata* (Japanese yew) most commonly reported in poisonings. However, all species of *Taxus*, including *T. brevifolia* (Pacific or western yew) should be considered toxic.

• Yews contain taxine alkaloids (major alkaloids are taxine A and taxine B) that cause an increase in cytoplasmic calcium by interfering with both the calcium and the sodium ion channel conductance across the myocardial cells. This results in the depression of cardiac depolarization and conduction of the heart.
• All parts of the plant, green or dried, with the exception of the red fleshy part surrounding the seed (aril portion), are toxic. Ingestion of yew clippings is most often the cause of poisonings.
• The minimum lethal dose in adult cattle is estimated to be approximately 200 g of dried leaves.

Grayanotoxin-Containing Plants

• Plants containing grayanotoxins include *Rhododendron* spp. (rhododendron, azalea, rosebay), *Kalmia* spp. (mountain laurel, sheep laurel, lambkill, sheepkill, dwarf laurel, calico bush), *Pieris* spp. (Japanese pieris, mountain pieris), *Leucothoe* spp. (dog hobble, dog laurel, fetter bush, black laurel), and *Lyonia* spp. (fetter bush, maleberry, staggerbush).
• Grayanotoxins are diterpenes that exert their toxic effect by binding to sodium channels in excitable cell membranes. The resulting increase in membrane permeability to sodium ions maintains excitable cells in a state of depolarization. Accumulation of intracellular sodium results in an exchange with extracellular calcium and plays an important role in the control of transmitter release. The membrane effects caused by grayanotoxins account for the observed responses of skeletal and myocardial muscle, nerves, and central nervous system.
• Toxicosis usually occurs when animals are offered plant trimmings or stray into wooded areas during adverse weather conditions and little else is available to eat.
• In cattle and sheep, ingestion of 0.2%–0.6% of an animal's body weight is considered toxic. Goats can be poisoned by the ingestion of fresh foliage in the amount of 0.1% of the animal's body weight.

Death Camas

• Many species of death camas occur across the United States and are seasonal with the greatest abundance being in the spring.
• Death camas contains steroidal alkaloids, such as zygacine and zygadenine. The alkaloids decrease blood pressure, slow the heart rate, and lead to respiratory depression.
• Leaves during the early stages of growth pose the greatest risk for poisoning. Seeds and fruits as well as the dried plant in hay are also toxic.
• The minimum lethal dose of the green plant in sheep is approximately 1% of the animal's body weight, but serious illness may be seen with as little as ingestion of 0.2% of an animal's body weight. Cattle are equally or possibly more susceptible than sheep.

Avocado

• Avocado is extensively cultivated in California and Florida, but can also be found as an ornamental in the gulf coast areas.
• The Guatemalan race and its hybrid ("Fuerte") are reportedly toxic to livestock. The Mexican race has low toxicity and no reports of poisoning in livestock exist.
• The toxic compound is called persin, but the exact mechanism of action remains unclear.
• The leaves are especially toxic, but ingestion of fruit and seeds can also result in poisoning.
• In goats, ingestion of 30 g/kg body weight of fresh leaves can result in cardiac effects. At exposures greater than 20 g/kg body weight of fresh leaves, lactating goats can develop severe mastitis. Even though goats seem to be particularly sensitive to avocado poisoning, cattle and sheep are also affected.

SIGNALMENT

Cardiac Glycoside–Containing Plants

All species are susceptible to cardiac glycoside-containing plants. Oleander poisoning is commonly seen in llamas and alpacas. Severe losses have also been reported in cattle.

Yew

Most poisonings with yew have involved cattle, but sheep, goats, and wild ruminants are also susceptible. Deer are able to tolerate considerable amounts of yew during the winter months, probably because of lower concentrations of taxine alkaloids in newly grown shoots.

Grayanotoxin-Containing Plants
Grayanotoxin poisoning has been reported in cattle and sheep, but most reports of poisoning involve goats.

Death Camas
Sheep are at highest risk, especially when hungry, because they are most likely to eat the death camas in early spring when little alternative forage is available. However, cattle have also been poisoned.

Avocado
Goats are highly susceptible to the mammary-induced effects of avocado poisoning, although all lactating animals can develop noninfectious mastitis and agalactia. With respect to cardiotoxic effects of avocado, all animal species are considered susceptible.

SIGNS
• Animals exposed to cardiotoxic plants are often found dead.
• If animals are presented alive, clinical signs of colic (abdominal pain) are often seen within hours of exposure. Progression of disease is rapid and animals develop weakness, tremors, excessive salivation, incoordination, dyspnea, and sometimes convulsions.
• In cardiac glycoside poisonings, animals often have an irregular, fast pulse with tachycardia, ventricular arrhythmias, or gallop rhythms.
• Animals exposed to avocado develop subcutaneous edema of the neck and brisket, submandibular edema, respiratory dyspnea, and cardiac arrhythmias. Lactating animals exposed to a low dose of avocado develop noninfectious mastitis and agalactia within 24 hours of exposure.

CAUSES AND RISK FACTORS
• Ingestion of cardiotoxic plants presents a great risk to ruminants. Plants most commonly associated with acute poisoning are oleander, yew, and rhododendron.
• Hungry animals are most likely to receive toxic exposures.
• Young and rapidly growing plants often contain highest concentrations of toxins.
• Fresh plant material of cardiotoxic plants is often considered to be of low palatability. However, animals frequently eat the leaves readily, if no other forage is available.
• Plant trimmings present the most common source for oleander and yew poisoning.
• Plant trimmings of cardiac glycoside-containing plants and yews remain toxic.

 DIAGNOSIS

DIFFERENTIAL DIAGNOSIS
• Nitrate toxicosis—chocolate-colored blood, exposure to nitrate-accumulating plants
• Cyanide poisoning—mucous membranes are initially bright cherry red; evidence of exposure to cyanogenic plants, chemical analysis for cyanide in gastrointestinal contents, liver, or muscle
• Larkspur poisoning—mainly found in the western states; bloat is common finding, evidence of exposure to *Delphinium* spp.
• Grass tetany—hypomagnesemia
• Organophosphorus or carbamate insecticide exposure—commonly associated with gastrointestinal irritation and neurological signs, evaluation of cholinesterase activity, detection of pesticides in gastrointestinal contents
• Lead poisoning—determination of blood lead concentration
• Exposure to neurotoxic plants, such as poison hemlock, water hemlock, tree tobacco, lupine—chemical analysis for plant toxins in gastrointestinal contents, history of presence of plants in the environment
• Exposure to the plant "fly poison" (*Amianthium muscaetoxicum*)— found only in the eastern United States, most commonly seen in the spring, history of presence of plants in the environment
• Exposure to star-of-Bethlehem (*Ornithogalum* spp.)—mainly found in the Northeast and Midwest, severe diarrhea, history of presence of plants in the environment
• Nonprotein nitrogen (NPN) toxicosis—history of NPN supplements in the feed ration, detection of toxic levels of ammonia in rumen content and blood
• Ionophore antibiotics—history of ionophores (e.g., monensin) in the feed ration, detection of toxic concentrations of ionophores in the feed, histologic lesions

CBC/BIOCHEMISTRY/URINALYSIS
• Serum chemistry changes are limited.
• Myocardial damage may result in hyperkalemia, and elevated LDH, CK, and AST activities.

OTHER LABORATORY TESTS
• Detection of oleandrin, gitoxin, digitoxin, grayanotoxins, strophanthidin, or other cardiac glycosides or aglycones in blood, rumen, cecal, or colon contents, and liver
• Detection of taxine alkaloids in rumen contents
• Visual and microscopic examination of rumen or intestinal contents for plant fragments

IMAGING
N/A

DIAGNOSTIC PROCEDURES
N/A

PATHOLOGIC FINDINGS
• In peracute cases, no lesions are found.
• Postmortem lesions are generally nonspecific in animals that died of exposure to cardiotoxic plants. Lesions include reddening of the mucosa of the gastrointestinal tract and congestion of organs.
• Cattle with oleander poisoning have evidence of fluid in the bowel and thrombosis and hemorrhage in the heart.
• There are no or very few lesions in cases of yew, grayanotoxin, or death camas poisoning.
• Avocado poisoning can result in fluid accumulation in the pericardial sac and in the thoracic and abdominal cavities. Edema of the gallbladder and perirenal tissues and a flabby, pale heart have been observed. Mammary glands are edematous with clots in the large ducts.

 TREATMENT

• Immediate removal of the toxic plant material to prevent further exposure. Provide the animals with good-quality feed.
• Treatment of animals exposed to cardiotoxic plants is primarily supportive and symptomatic. Supportive therapy should include administration of intravenous fluids, antiarrhythmics, and antibiotics if indicated.
• Adsorption of toxins with activated charcoal has been suggested.

CARDIOTOXIC PLANTS

• Rumenotomy may be considered in a valuable individual animal if ingestion is known and clinical signs have not yet developed.
• Passing a stomach tube, if necessary, should relieve bloat.
• Any possible stress or trauma should be avoided.
• If edema is present in avocado poisoning, administration of diuretics is recommended.
• Atropine should be considered in cases of severe bradycardia. Additionally, it may be warranted in severely poisoned animals that do not respond to decontamination procedures and fluid therapy alone.

 MEDICATIONS

DRUGS OF CHOICE
• Lidocaine, phenytoin, or propranolol to treat tachyarrhythmias
• Atropine to treat bradyarrhythmias
• Activated charcoal

CONTRAINDICATIONS
• Do not administer potassium in fluids if hyperkalemia is present.
• Avoid calcium-containing solutions and quinidine.
• Appropriate milk and meat withdrawal times must be followed for all compounds administered to food-producing animals.

ALTERNATIVE DRUGS
Anticardiac glycoside Fab antibodies have been used in humans and small animals, but their usefulness in the treatment of cardiac glycoside-poisoned ruminants has not been evaluated.

 FOLLOW-UP

PATIENT MONITORING
Monitor progression of clinical signs.

PREVENTION/AVOIDANCE
• Prevent hungry animals from accessing new pasture, especially in the spring when only limited (and often toxic) forage is available.
• Animals should be denied access to landscaped yards and discarded clippings.
• Suspect forage should be inspected for the presence of cardiotoxic plants before allowing ruminants to graze.
• Hay should be inspected carefully for weeds, as many cardiotoxic plants remain toxic when dried (oleander, death camas, yew).

POSSIBLE COMPLICATIONS
N/A

EXPECTED COURSE AND PROGNOSIS
• Animals poisoned with cardiotoxic plants are often found dead.
• Cardiotoxic plant exposure progresses so rapidly that treatment is often too late. In most cases, the affected animals have a poor-to-grave prognosis.
• If treatment is initiated promptly after the onset of clinical signs, the prognosis is fair.
• Animals that survive the acute poisoning may suffer from myocardial damage and may be more prone to stress.

 MISCELLANEOUS

ASSOCIATED CONDITIONS
N/A

AGE-RELATED FACTORS
N/A

ZOONOTIC POTENTIAL
N/A

PREGNANCY
N/A

RUMINANT SPECIES AFFECTED
Cattle, sheep, goats, llamas, alpacas, deer

BIOSECURITY
N/A

PRODUCTION MANAGEMENT
In lactating animals poisoned with avocado, the milk production remains reduced even after the mastitis has been controlled.

SEE ALSO
Cyanide poisoning
Grass tetany
Ionophore antibiotics
Larkspur poisoning
Lead poisoning
Neurotoxic plants, such as poison hemlock, water hemlock, tree tobacco, lupine
Nitrate toxicosis
Nonprotein nitrogen (NPN) toxicosis
Organophosphorus or carbamate insecticide
Specific plant toxicity chapters
Star-of-Bethlehem (*Ornithogalum* spp.)
Toxicologic outbreak management

ABBREVIATIONS
N/A

Suggested Reading
Burrows, G. E., Tyrl, R. J. 2001. Zigadenus. In: *Toxic plants of North America*, ed. G. E. Burrows, R. J. Tyrl. Ames: Iowa State University Press.
Casteel, S. W. Taxine alkaloids. 2004. In: *Clinical veterinary toxicology*, ed. K. H. Plumlee. St. Louis: Mosby.
Galey, F. G. Cardiac glycosides. 2004. In: *Clinical veterinary toxicology*, ed. K. H. Plumlee. St. Louis: Mosby.
Oelrichs, P. B., Ng, J. C., Seawright, A. A., et al. 1995. Isolation and identification of a compound from avocado (*Persea americana*) leaves which causes necrosis of the acinar epithelium of the lactating mammary gland and the myocardium. *Nat Toxins* 3:344–49.
Puschner, B. 2004. Grayanotoxins. In: *Clinical veterinary toxicology*, ed. K. H. Plumlee. St. Louis: Mosby.

Author: Birgit Puschner

CASEOUS LYMPHADENITIS (CLA)

 BASICS

DEFINITION
An endemic, infectious contagious disease caused by *Corynebacterium pseudotuberculosis*, characterized by caseous abscessation of the internal and external lymph nodes and internal visceral organs of sheep, goats, and rarely camelids.

PATHOPHYSIOLOGY
• Bacteria invade through wounds, unbroken or abraded skin, or mucous membranes.
• Animal may contract bacteria through contaminated fomites (particularly water, feed, soil, or housing) or directly from animals with draining abscesses, or from pulmonary abscesses from coughing.
• The bacteria then travel through lymphatic system or blood stream to local lymph nodes and organs.
• Phospholipase D (PLD) exotoxin, secreted by the bacteria, causes the breakdown of the endothelium and is leukotoxic. This enables the spread of the bacteria through tissues.
• The cell wall is thick with a high lipid content, which enables the bacteria to resist phagocytosis.
• Thus, abscesses form generally first in the lymph node(s) draining the site of initial infection, but may form anywhere in the body.
• Abscesses may rupture (through skin or into bronchi) or regress. New abscesses may form months later in the same or different location.

SYSTEMS AFFECTED
• Most commonly affects the lymphatic system (lymph nodes) in any location and lung parenchyma (respiratory system)
• In North American and European housed sheep and goats, most commonly affects parotid, submandibular, and cervical lymph nodes as well as the respiratory system
• In range flocks in Australia, mostly affects the respiratory system (parenchyma and mediastinal lymph nodes) and popliteal lymph nodes.
• Less commonly but not rare, abscesses are formed: externally in the prescapular, prefemoral, or mammary lymph nodes; internally in the liver, kidney, adrenal glands, pituitary gland, or vertebrae.

GENETICS
NA

INCIDENCE / PREVALENCE
• Common in all sheep- and goat-raising countries in the world
• Flock / herd prevalence likely greater than 75% in adult animals if no control program
• Flock / herd incidence varies depending on management and level of surveillance, but likely > 15%
• Prevalence of abscesses found at abattoirs estimated at 17% to 24% in adult sheep
• Recognized as an important cause of carcass condemnation and trim

GEOGRAPHIC DISTRIBUTION
• Widely distributed in North America.
• Mostly in terminal sire flocks in the UK

SIGNALMENT
Species
• Sheep (domestic and wild)
• Goats (domestic and wild)
• Camelids (llamas and alpacas)

Breed Predilections
None reported

Mean Age and Range
• Can affect lambs and kids as young as 6 weeks of age but mostly a disease of animals > 3 months
• Generally found in higher prevalence in adults than in young stock

Predominant Sex
None reported

HISTORICAL FINDINGS
• Most commonly, producers will report finding a lump under the skin or a ruptured abscess.
• Many abscesses may be missed because of long wool or hair coat.
• Occasionally, an adult may present with chronic weight loss with no external evidence of disease.
• Less commonly, an affected animal may present with respiratory difficulty from either an enlarged retropharyngeal lymph node or from extensive involvement of the respiratory system.
• Rarely an animal may present acutely off-feed and with cellulitis at the site of primary infection.
• Occasionally, an animal is found dead with no previous signs of disease, although there is usually a history of disease in the flock or herd.

• Although most cases of the disease do not adversely affect the general health of the animal, owners may be very concerned with the negative aesthetics of the sight of draining abscesses, particularly in purebred show sheep.

PHYSICAL EXAMINATION FINDINGS
• Affected animals are generally bright, alert, afebrile, and have a good appetite.
• The external abscess is initially discreet, cool, and firm to the touch, but as it matures it becomes soft.
• Prior to rupture, the hair is lost from the center of the lesion and the overlying skin thins.
• The purulent matter expressed from the abscess is thick, cream colored to slightly green, and has no discernable odor.
• Abscesses in sheep often have several concentric layers like an onion skin, but in goats, this feature is absent.
• When the abscesses affect the internal organs, physical findings are nonspecific. Often even with severe pulmonary involvement, there are no signs referable to the respiratory system.
• Animals with chronic wasting due to CLA will often be afebrile but have unexplained weight loss. Appetite is variable.
• Rarely animals experience acute swelling and pain with a high fever (>40°C) when initially infected. It is believed that this is due to the affects of the PLD exotoxin.
• At the flock level, decreased weight gains and wool growth have been reported.

CAUSES
• The bacteria *Corynebacterium pseudotuberculosis,* a small gram-positive rod, is the only etiology of CLA.
• *C. pseudotuberculosis* is a facultative intracellular parasite and produces PLD exotoxin.
• There are two biotypes classified on nitrate requirements: those isolates that are nitrate negative are responsible for CLA, as well as some cases of ulcerative lymphangitis in cattle; those that are nitrate positive are the etiologic agent of ulcerative lymphangitis of horses. Nitrate positive isolates do not cause disease in sheep and goats.
• The bacteria can survive several days in water, several weeks on fomites such as wooden feeders, and several months in soil. Cool moist conditions improve its survival.

CASEOUS LYMPHADENITIS (CLA)

RISK FACTORS
• Gathering the flock for shearing allows transmission of the bacteria by coughing (pulmonary abscesses).
• Nicking an abscess during shearing contaminates the shears, thus allowing transmission to others shorn later. Shearers that do not clean their equipment or clothing between flocks have been shown to bring the disease to unaffected flocks.
• Broken or abraded skin, which can occur during shearing, increases the risk of transmission, although the bacteria can penetrate unbroken skin.
• Draining abscesses that contaminate feed, water, and feeders are an important source of infection.
• Fighting between rams or bucks has also been shown to transmit the bacteria.

DIAGNOSIS

DIFFERENTIAL DIAGNOSIS
• External abscesses
  • Many bacteria cause abscesses that may or may not be associated with a lymph node.
  • Most common in sheep and goats are abscesses of the cheek or jaw associated with trauma from feed, although any trauma may result in an abscess. A wide variety of bacteria has been isolated from these including anaerobes (e.g., *Fusobacterium necrophorum*), *Mannheimia haemolytica*, *Staphylococcus aureus*, many species of streptococci, and *Escherichia coli*. They may have a watery content, with or without gas, and a foul odor and often do not involve a lymph node.
  • Sterile abscesses are found in about one-third of animals recently vaccinated with a multiway clostridial vaccine.
  • Abscesses on the back of the neck are often caused by sheep crawling under wooden feeders that then become infected secondarily with *S. aureus*.
• Chronic wasting
  • Diseases in which a few individuals in the flock are clinically affected: dental disease; competition; paratuberculosis; ovine progressive pneumonia (OPP), also known as maedi visna (sheep); caprine arthritis; encephalitis (goats); and scrapie
  • Diseases in which a large proportion of the flock is clinically affected: gastrointestinal parasitism, nutritional deficiency

• Respiratory disease: Bacterial pneumonia, lung worm (*Dictyocaulus viviparus* or *Muellerius capillaris* in goats only), sheep pulmonary adenomatosis, transmissible nasal carcinoma
• Lymphosarcoma may present as external and /or internal masses, cause chronic wasting, and /or be space occupying in the thorax.

CBC / BIOCHEMISTRY / URINALYSIS
Generally, no specific abnormalities are seen.

OTHER LABORATORY TESTS
• Culture of abscess prior to rupture. This is best done by using a sterile needle and syringe to aspirate, or by lancing the abscess with a sterile scalpel and collecting abscess material in a sterile container. Submit for routine culture.
• Serology. A variety of serological tests has been developed to detect antibodies to important antigens. Most commonly the tests detect antibody to PLD, for example, the synergistic hemolysin inhibition (SHI) test and many different ELISA tests. Sensitivity on a flock basis is good but only fair on an individual animal level, likely because the bacteria are walled off after initial infection. Titers may be higher and more persistent in goats than in sheep. Vaccines that contain PLD toxoid interfere with interpretation, (i.e., reduce specificity).
• IFN gamma ELISA. Using whole blood, this assay detects CMI. Response does not appear to decrease with time postinfection and vaccination will not interfere with interpretation.

IMAGING
In cases of chronic wasting or respiratory disease: ultrasound or radiograph of the thorax will reveal number and size of abscesses affecting the respiratory system.

DIAGNOSTIC PROCEDURES
N/A

PATHOLOGIC FINDINGS
• Abscesses may occur in any lymph node or visceral organ. Routine culture will determine if *C. pseudotuberculosis* is the causative agent.
• In cases of sudden death, cut down the trachea and bronchial tree to check for evidence of an abscess rupturing into and occluding an airway.

TREATMENT

APPROPRIATE HEALTH CARE
• No treatment regime has been shown to influence the course of disease.
• Many months or years may pass between abscess events in an animal, but once an animal exhibits an abscess, it should be considered to be infected for life.
• Although the bacterium is sensitive to many antibiotics, including penicillin, abscess formation prevents effective therapy.
• To hasten recovery and prevent contamination of the environment, isolate animals with abscesses until healed.
• Isolation facility should have the following features:
  • No shared waterer or feeder with other animals
  • Ideally, in a separate air space
  • Pen must be dedicated to housing animals with abscesses (e.g., not used for lambing or for housing animals sick with another disease)
• Lance abscess with sterile scalpel blade when it becomes soft. Wear disposable gloves. Catch all material in a container (e.g. rectal sleeve) to prevent environmental contamination. Clean abscess wound with iodine or chlorhexidine. Repeat twice per day until wound is scabbed and dry. In cases of chronic and /or repeated episodes of abscess development, strongly consider culling so as to reduce the risk of infection of the rest of the flock or herd.

NURSING CARE
Keep in isolation pen until abscess is healed

ACTIVITY
N/A

DIET
N/A

CLIENT EDUCATION
CE needs to focus on what a diagnosis means to the flock/herd so that control measures can be instituted as quickly as possible. See Prevention /Avoidance section below.

SURGICAL CONSIDERATIONS
• Retropharyngeal abscesses may be surgically drained under anesthesia if animal value warrants it.
• Surgical removal of an external lymph node has been done in selected cases.

CASEOUS LYMPHADENITIS (CLA)

MEDICATIONS

DRUGS OF CHOICE
N/A

CONTRAINDICATIONS
N/A

PRECAUTIONS
N/A

POSSIBLE INTERACTIONS
N/A

ALTERNATIVE DRUGS
N/A

FOLLOW-UP

PATIENT MONITORING
If the owner elects not to cull, the animals should be checked at least once / month for new abscesses.

PREVENTION /AVOIDANCE
A control program is based on:
• Reduction of environmental contamination with the bacteria:
  • Routine palpation of external lymph nodes whenever sheep and goats are handled
  • Isolation of affected animals and appropriate treatment
  • Disinfection of shearing blades and pieces whenever an abscess is nicked
  • Routine washing of hands with chlorhexidine soap when handling infected animals
  • Use feeders that reduce contact of the head and neck with the feeder (e.g., bars or keyhole feeders).
  • Cull all affected animals if economics allow.
  • Cull all repeat offenders.
• Reduction of risk of transmission to uninfected animals:
  • Rear young stock away from adults (e.g., remove at birth and rear artificially in another barn).
  • Shear young sheep first and older and infected sheep last.
  • Milk affected does last and wash down parlor with disinfectant afterward.
  • Limit purchases of breeding stock from flocks of unknown health status.
  • Shearers should wear clean clothing (including footwear) that has not been worn to another flock without laundering. For best biosecurity, producers should purchase their own shearing equipment.
  • Treat all shearing wounds immediately with iodine or other topical disinfectant.

• Improve the immune status of uninfected animals:
  • Commercial vaccines that contain PLD toxoid and some cell components are licensed for use in sheep but not goats. The vaccines are marketed as a combined clostridial-CLA vaccine.
  • The vaccine works best if administered before chance of infection and after colostral immunity has waned (around 3 months of age).
  • A vaccination program involves vaccination of young stock with a primary series (e.g., vaccinate at 3 and 4 months of age) and an annual booster.
  • For breeding ewes, this annual booster can be administered 1 month prior to lambing, so as to optimize transfer of colostral immunity to offspring.
  • The vaccine will not cure existing infections and works best when combined with other control measures as it will reduce risk of infection but will not totally prevent. Routine vaccination, when combined with culling of affected sheep, can reduce flock prevalence to < 2% (cull animals at the abattoir).
  • Vaccine efficacy may be improved by increasing the frequency of vaccination to every 3 to 6 months, particularly if sheep and goats are housed all or part of the year.
  • No vaccine is licensed for use in goats and some cause adverse reactions in goats that are already infected, so extreme caution should be used when vaccinating this species.
  • Autogenous vaccines have been employed in the past, but if the PLD toxin is not totally inactivated, severe illness and death may occur.

POSSIBLE COMPLICATIONS
N/A

EXPECTED COURSE AND PROGNOSIS
• Most infected animals do not experience severe disease.
• The disease is more important at the herd level where it can cause chronic wasting, sudden death, premature culling, and carcass condemnation and trim.

MISCELLANEOUS

ASSOCIATED CONDITIONS
N/A

AGE-RELATED FACTORS
N/A

ZOONOTIC POTENTIAL
C. pseudotuberculosis infection of humans has been reported but is not common. Suppurative granulomatous lymphadenitis may occur secondary to wound contamination when treating or handling infected animals or contaminated materials. It is important to wear gloves when lancing abscesses and wash hands with chlorhexidine soap after treating this disease.

PREGNANCY
N/A

RUMINANT SPECIES AFFECTED
Primarily sheep and goats and less common camelids; llamas are most often reported as they are used frequently as guard animals with sheep.

BIOSECURITY
Outlined under Prevention/Avoidance above

PRODUCTION MANAGEMENT
Outlined under Prevention/Avoidance above

SYNONYMS
Cheesy gland
CL
CLA

SEE ALSO
Caprine arthritis encephalitis (goats)
Competition
Dental disease
Maedi visna (sheep)
Ovine progressive pneumonia (opp)
Paratuberculosis
Scrapie

ABBREVIATIONS
CLA = caseous lymphadenitis
CMI = cell-mediated immunity
ELISA = enzyme-linked immunosorbent assay
IFN = interferon
PLD = phospholipase D exotoxin

Suggested Reading
Arsenault, J., Girard, D., Dubreuil, P., et al. 2003. Prevalence of and carcass condemnation from maedi-visna, paratuberculosis and caseous lymphadenitis in culled sheep from Quebec, Canada. *Prev Vet Med*. 59:67–81.
Baird, G., Synge, B., Dercksen, D. 2004. Survey of cascous lymphadenitis seroprevalence in British terminal sire sheep breeds. *Vet Rec*. 154:505–506.
Paton, M. W., Walker, S. B., Rose, I. R., Watt, G. F. 2003. Prevalence of caseous lymphadenitis and usage of caseous lymphadenitis vaccines in sheep flocks. *Aust Vet J*. 81:91–95.
Prescott, J. F., Menzies, P. I., Hwang, Y. T. 2002. An interferon-gamma assay for the diagnosis of *Corynebacterium pseudotuberculosis* infection in adult sheep from a research flock. *Vet Microbiol*. 88: 287–97.

Author: Paula I. Menzies

CASTOR BEAN TOXICITY

BASICS

OVERVIEW
• Castor bean, or palma christi (*Ricinus communis*), is grown for the commercial production of castor oil.
• The leaves are large, mottled, and usually a light brown; seeds resemble engorged ticks and weigh approximately 0.3 g each.
• The castor bean is a semiwoody plant with large, alternate, starlike leaves that grows as a tree in tropical regions and as an annual in temperate regions. Its flowers are very small and inconspicuous. Its fruits grow in clusters at the tops of the plants.
• All parts of the plant are very poisonous to eat.
• The poisonous principle of castor beans is ricin, a water-soluble, proteinaceous material that is concentrated in the seeds.
• This plant is found in all tropical regions and has been introduced to temperate regions.
• The plant can be found in any location in North America.

SYSTEMS AFFECTED
Gastrointestinal, CNS, cardiovascular

GENETICS
N/A

INCIDENCE/PREVALENCE
N/A

GEOGRAPHIC DISTRIBUTION
Potentially worldwide, depending on the environment

SIGNALMENT

Species
• All animals
• Sheep and cattle are more resistant to its effects.
• Humans and horses are most susceptible.

Breed Predilections
N/A

Mean Age and Range
N/A

Predominant Sex
N/A

SIGNS
• There is a characteristic latent period from ingestion to onset of clinical signs, which can be as long as 2–3 days.
• Acute signs are seen when large quantities are ingested.
• Profuse catarrhal to hemorrhagic diarrhea (cattle)
• Neuromuscular signs may be observed and include a swaying gait, recumbency after brief exercise, and muscle tremors. Increased salivation and exaggerated chewing may be observed.
• Depression
• Seizures can occur.
• Increased thirst (polydipsia)
• Colic
• Elevated heart rate and/or temperature
• Clinical signs are progressive and may increase in severity with time.

CAUSES AND RISK FACTORS
• The seed is one source of toxicity. It has a hard capsule and has little taste unless the coat is broken.
• Ricin, the active principle of the seed, belongs to the group of plant toxins known as phytotoxins and is absorbed from the intestine.
• Phytotoxins are found in all parts of the plant but seeds are especially toxic.
• Heat reduces but does not eliminate the toxicity.

DIAGNOSIS

DIFFERENTIAL DIAGNOSIS
Other causes of enteritis

CBC/BIOCHEMISTRY/URINALYSIS
Leukopenia with a marked left shift and an elevated PCV has been detected approximately 10 hours postingestion.

OTHER LABORATORY TESTS
• Microscopic examination for castor seeds
• Hemagglutination test
• Precipitin test on extracts of excreta or intestinal contents

IMAGING
N/A

DIAGNOSTIC PROCEDURES
N/A

PATHOLOGIC FINDINGS
• Gut contents are fluid or semifluid.
• Hemorrhages on the serosal and mucosal surfaces of the stomach, intestines, and bladder
• Hepatic necrosis
• Enlarged mesenteric lymph nodes
• Liver, lung, and spleen are all affected—may appear edematous upon postmortem examination.

TREATMENT
• Specific antiserum is the ideal antidote.
• GI decontamination may be useful.
• Symptomatic treatment
• Adequate nursing care for recumbent animals

MEDICATIONS
• Maintain body fluid and electrolyte balance
• Sedatives
• Arecoline hydrobromide followed by saline cathartics may be helpful.

CONTRAINDICATIONS
Appropriate milk and meat withdrawal times must be followed for all compounds administered.

FOLLOW-UP

PATIENT MONITORING
N/A

MISCELLANEOUS

ASSOCIATED CONDITIONS
N/A

AGE-RELATED FACTORS
N/A

PREGNANCY
N/A

RUMINANT SPECIES AFFECTED
Potentially all ruminant species are affected

SEE ALSO
N/A

ABBREVIATIONS
CNS = central nervous system
GI = gastrointestinal
PCV = packed cell volume

Suggested Reading
Christiansen, V. J., Hsu, C. H., Dormer, K. J., Robinson, C. P. 1994, Mar. The cardiovascular effects of ricin in rabbits. *Pharmacol Toxicol.* 74(3): 148–52.
Fodstad, O., Johannessen, J. V., Schjerven, L., Pihl, A. 1979, Nov. Toxicity of abrin and ricin in mice and dogs. *J Toxicol Environ Health* 5(6): 1073–84.
Rauber, A. 1999. Plantlore revisited. *J Toxicol Clin Toxicol.* 37(4): 521–24.
Rauber, A., Heard, J. 1985, Dec. Castor bean toxicity reexamined: a new perspective. *Vet Hum Toxicol.* 27(6): 498–502.
Wedin, G. P., Neal, J. S., Everson, G. W., Krenzelok, E. P. 1986, May. Castor bean poisoning. *Am J Emerg Med.* 4(3): 259–61.

Author: Troy Holder

CECAL DILATION AND VOLVULUS

BASICS

DEFINITION
• Cecal dilation is primarily a disease of high-producing adult dairy cattle occurring within the first 1–2 months postpartum.
• It is believed to share similar epidemiologic and physiologic characteristics as abomasal dilation and displacement, however research may challenge this relationship.
• Cecal dilation is also reported in calves less than 6 months of age, the majority of which are fed high-concentrate diets for purposes of early slaughter.

PATHOPHYSIOLOGY
Cecal Dilation
• The presence of excess gas from the digestion of fermentable substrates and decreased intestinal motility
• When animals are fed diets high in concentrates and containing inadequate roughage, high levels of fermentable carbohydrates pass beyond the forestomachs into the lower intestine. Lower intestinal flora digest the excess carbohydrates into volatile fatty acids (VFAs), methane, and carbon dioxide. Increased VFAs present in the cecum and ascending colon are believed to cause a reduction in intestinal motility.
• Decreased intestinal motility may also result from decreased levels of ionized calcium.

Cecal Volvulus
The exact cause of cecal volvulus is unknown, however it is believed to be predisposed by, and therefore be a sequela to, the occurrence of cecal dilation.

SYSTEMS AFFECTED
Gastrointestinal

GENETICS
N/A

INCIDENCE/PREVALENCE
N/A

GEOGRAPHIC DISTRIBUTION
Worldwide

SIGNALMENT
Species
Cattle

Breed Predilections
N/A

Mean Age and Range
Adult cattle within 2 months postpartum

Predominant Sex
Female

SIGNS

HISTORICAL FINDINGS
• Cattle suffering cecal dilation typically present with mild to moderate anorexia and decreased milk production.
• Cattle suffering cecal volvulus typically demonstrate abrupt anorexia, rumen stasis, and significantly decreased milk production.

PHYSICAL EXAMINATION FINDINGS
• Cattle with cecal dilation have an area of increased resonance ("ping") that is auscultated over the right paralumbar fossa. The right paralumbar fossa may be distended, and cattle may exhibit mild to moderate signs of abdominal pain.
• Fecal output is normal to decreased and fecal consistency is typically more fluid.
• During rectal examination, a gas distended cecum is usually palpable with the apex located in or near the pelvic inlet.
• Cattle with cecal volvulus have moderate to severe abdominal pain (colic).
• Animals are often tachycardic and tachypnic, and produce little to no feces.
• Rectal examination usually reveals a markedly distended cecum containing both gas and fluid. The apex of the cecum is often not palpable as it is positioned cranially. The area of resonance in the right paralumbar fossa is generally much larger than that noted with simple cecal dilation. Increased resonance may even be noted over the caudal dorsal left paralumbar fossa.
• Mild to moderate anorexia and decreased milk production are commonly seen.

CAUSES/RISK FACTORS
Postpartum cattle fed low-roughage, high-concentrate diets are predisposed, also, those suffering from hypocalcemia, metritis, mastitis, or indigestion that could result in gastrointestinal ileus.

DIAGNOSIS

DIFFERENTIAL DIAGNOSIS
Right displaced abomasum or abomasal volvulus, small intestinal obstructions, intussusception

CBC/BIOCHEMISTRY/URINALYSIS
• Serum biochemical profile, blood gas analysis, and complete blood count are typically unremarkable, though a stress leukogram may be observed in cecal dilation cases.

• Depending on the severity and duration of cecal volvulus, cattle may present with moderate to severe acid-base and electrolyte derangements. Hypochloremic, hypokalemic metabolic alkalosis is most commonly observed, however, mixed acid-base abnormalities (concurrent metabolic acidosis and alkalosis) can also occur.

OTHER LABORATORY TESTS
N/A

IMAGING
Ultrasonography via the right abdominal wall at the level of the tuber coxae may be useful in the diagnosis.

DIAGNOSTIC PROCEDURES
Rectal palpation

PATHOLOGIC FINDINGS
N/A

TREATMENT

APPROPRIATE HEALTH CARE
• Cecal dilation is usually treated successfully via medical management. Large volumes (20 liters) of oral fluids containing electrolytes (8 oz NaCl, 2 oz KCl), calcium (12 oz calcium propionate), and cathartics (12 oz Mg-hydroxide, Mg-sulfate) can be given one to two times daily. Intravenous fluids can also be administered.
• Transfaunation with rumen liquor (10–20 liters) can be used to stimulate rumen motility and appetite. Finally, intravenous or subcutaneous calcium borogluconate solutions (20 grams in 500 ml) can be useful in lactating cows.

ACTIVITY
N/A

DIET
Animals should be provided access to a palatable, coarse, high-fiber diet.

CLIENT EDUCATION
Warranted in cases that are induced by inappropriate diet

SURGICAL CONSIDERATIONS
• In cattle with recurrent cecal dilation, preventative typhlectomy may be indicated.
• Cattle with cecal volvulus typically require surgical intervention along with appropriate fluid therapy to correct fluid, acid-base, and electrolyte abnormalities. A right paralumbar approach is typically used. Decompression via typhlotomy may be necessary to remove excess fluid and gas and to facilitate correction of a volvulus. In the event that ischemic necrosis is severe, a typhlectomy may be required.

MEDICATIONS

DRUGS OF CHOICE

CONTRAINDICATIONS

POSSIBLE INTERACTIONS

ALTERNATIVE DRUGS
N/A

FOLLOW-UP

PATIENT MONITORING
Increased appetite and milk production with manure production are all good signs that treatment is working.

PREVENTION/AVOIDANCE
Pre- and postpartum management of dairy cattle to maximize adequate intake of a forage-based diet, minimize infections of the uterus and vagina by calving in a clean environment, and minimizing the risk of gastrointestinal upset

POSSIBLE COMPLICATIONS
Cecal torsion leading to rupture and peritonitis in severe untreated cases

EXPECTED COURSE AND PROGNOSIS
• For patients with normal heart rate, some manure production, a small appetite, no dehydration, and minimal abdominal distension, medical treatment is usually successful.
• Patients with elevated heart rates, no appetite or manure production, dehydration, and a distended abdomen with colic signs, surgery is indicated. Prognosis depends upon the degree of ischemic compromise to the cecum and adjacent bowel, successful correction of acid-base and electrolyte derangements, and appropriate surgical technique.

• Postsurgical prognosis is dependent on the degree of ischemic compromise to the cecum and adjacent bowel, successful corrections of acid-base and electrolyte derangements, and appropriate surgical technique.

MISCELLANEOUS

ASSOCIATED CONDITIONS
Mastitis, metritis, hypocalcemia, inappetence

AGE-RELATED FACTORS

ZOONOTIC POTENTIAL
N/A

PREGNANCY
Generally, a postpartum condition

RUMINANT SPECIES AFFECTED
Bovine

BIOSECURITY
N/A

PRODUCTION MANAGEMENT
Pre- and postpartum management of dairy cattle to maximize adequate intake of a forage-based diet, minimize infections of the uterus and vagina by calving in a clean environment, and minimize the risk of gastrointestinal upset.

SYNONYMS
N/A

SEE ALSO
Gastrointestinal pharmacology
Intussusception
Right displaced abomasum or abomasal volvulus
Rumen displacement
Small intestinal obstructions
Ultrasounding: bovine

ABBREVIATIONS
VFA = volatile fatty acid

Suggested Reading
Abegg, R., Eicher, R., Lis, J., Lischer, C. J., Scholtysik, G., Steiner, A. 1999. Concentration of volatile fatty acids in digesta samples obtained from healthy cows and cows with cecal dilation or dislocation. *Am J Vet Res.* 60:1540–45.
Braun, U., Amrein, E., Koller, U., Lischer, C. 2002. Ultrasonographic findings in cows with dilation, torsion and retroflexion of the caecum. *Vet Rec.* 150:75–79.
Braun, U., Hermann, M., Pabst, B. 1989. Haematological and biochemical findings in cattle with dilation and torsion of the caecum. *Vet Rec.* 125:396–98.
Eicher, R., Audige, L., Braun, U., Blum, J., Meylan, M., Steiner, A. 1999. Epidemiology and risk factors of cecal dilation/dislocation and abomasal displacement in dairy cows. *Schweiz Arch Tierheilkd.* 141:423–29.
Guard, C. 2002. Obstructive intestinal diseases. In: *Large animal internal medicine*, ed. B. P. Smith. 3rd ed. St. Louis, MO: Mosby.

Author: George Barrington

CERVIDAE TUBERCULOSIS (*MYCOBACTERIUM BOVIS*)

BASICS

OVERVIEW
• A common problem that affects the captive and wildlife deer population is the presence of *Mycobacterium bovis*, otherwise known as tuberculosis.
• Deer seem to show an increased sensitivity to mycobacterial infections compared to other animals; thus, the ramifications of this disease are higher.
• In the United States, most notably in the northern parts of Michigan, the deer serve as a reservoir host of *M. bovis*. This makes eradication of this disease among domestic livestock and other wildlife impossible since the tuberculosis cannot be controlled among the wildlife population.
• *M. bovis* is also a zoonotic disease that can affect humans, so a correct diagnosis is critical when tuberculosis is suspected.
• The most common lesions are found in the medial retropharyngeal lymph nodes and the thorax. In many situations, hunters submit the head of the deer for a tuberculosis diagnosis so that the medial retropharyngeal lymph nodes may be inspected (among other cranial lymph nodes).

SYSTEMS AFFECTED
Production management, respiratory, immune

GENETICS
N/A

INCIDENCE/PREVALENCE
N/A

GEOGRAPHIC DISTRIBUTION
Worldwide, depending on species and environment

SIGNALMENT
Species
Cervidae

Breed Predilections
N/A

Mean Age and Range
N/A

Predominant Sex
N/A

SIGNS
N/A

HISTORICAL FINDINGS
• There are differences in host response to *M. bovis*.
• The New Zealand red deer tends to produce external draining sinuses from the infected lymph nodes. This fluid is most likely responsible for the transmission of the disease. In contrast, white-tailed deer were not found to have draining lesions, thus they lack this mode of transmission. Other bodily fluids, such as saliva, nasal secretions, urine, and feces, were found to be contaminated with *M. bovis* in white-tailed deer.

PHYSICAL EXAMINATION FINDINGS

CAUSES AND RISK FACTORS
• *M. bovis* is a gram-positive rod-shaped bacterium.
• Tuberculosis in deer can be seen as a pulmonary disease, where the bacteria are inhaled and proliferate into a focal region.
• The bacteria may also seed into a lymph node and spread via the lymphatic system. This infection can cause rapidly disseminated tuberculosis, which causes an acute disease.
• *M. bovis* may lie dormant and become reactivated in the face of an immunocompromised state. Once it becomes reactivated, it progresses to the disseminated form.
• Its modes of transmission include inhalation or ingestion.
• One study suggests that *M. bovis* persists in the tonsilar crypts for prolonged periods of time. Thus, *M. bovis* may be shed into the saliva and nasal secretions. These secretions serve as sources of transmission to other animals and humans.

DIAGNOSIS

DIFFERENTIAL DIAGNOSIS
• Progressive pneumonia
• Caseous lymphadenitis lesions
• Other causes of chronic respiratory disease—chronic lung abscesses, aspiration pneumonia
• Other causes of chronic weight loss and ill thrift—Johne's disease, parasitism

CBC/BIOCHEMISTRY/URINALYSIS
There are no specific clinical pathology data typical for this disease in cervidae.

OTHER LABORATORY TESTS

IMAGING
Depending on the location of the suspected lesion, radiography and ultrasonography may demonstrate the presence of tubercles within the body and are used to evaluate the extent of the infection.

OTHER DIAGNOSTIC PROCEDURES
• If tuberculosis is suspected in deer, there are several ways to diagnose the disease.
• The intradermal tuberculin test is widely used to diagnose tuberculosis among cattle; the injection is normally placed in the caudal tail fold. This location is not reliable in the deer, whereas the single cervical tuberculin test (SCT) has proven to be more diagnostic. If the deer responds positively to the injection, then it is retested with the comparative cervical tuberculin test (CCT).
• The CCT consists of injecting both bovine purified protein derivative and avian purified protein derivative. The response to both injection sites is compared.
• Another option besides the CCT is the blood tuberculosis test (BTB), a test that has been reported with > 95% sensitivity and > 98% specificity.
• Other immunodiagnostic tests include the lymphocyte transformation test, ELISA, gamma interferon assay, and the Ag85 blot immunoassay.
• If there is a positive reaction to either the CCT or BTB, then that animal is classified as a reactor.
• All herds that contain a reactor are immediately quarantined and/or depopulated.

PATHOLOGIC FINDINGS
• A Michigan study on tuberculosis lesions in white-tailed deer counted 58 positive cultures for *M. bovis* out of 19,500 total samples. In the majority of the samples, only the head was submitted. The rest of the samples consisted of the extracranial portions of the deer carcass.
• The cranial gross lesions were mostly found in the medial retropharyngeal lymph nodes. In addition, solitary unilateral parotid lymph node lesions were found. Extracranially, most of the lesions were in the thoracic region.
• Other sites included the liver, spleen, rumen, and mammary gland.
• In another study conducted in New Zealand, *M. bovis* was isolated from 14 of 116 deer. Nine out of the 14 had lesions consistent with tuberculosis (medial retropharyngeal lymph node and lung were mostly affected). However, 5 out of the 14 had no gross lesions, yet *M. bovis* was cultured. This study indicated that examination of only the lymph nodes and the lungs could significantly underestimate the prevalence of tuberculosis among the deer population.

CERVIDAE TUBERCULOSIS (*MYCOBACTERIUM BOVIS*)

• Disease manifestation varies by the cervid species involved. One study compared lesions from cattle, fallow deer, Sitka deer, and elk (red deer). Elk lesions showed scattered peripheral mineralization rather than central mineralization. These lesions also contained more neutrophils and fewer giant cells than the bovine lesions. The fallow deer lesions showed more giant cells; otherwise, the lesions were similar to the elk/red deer lesions. The Sitka deer lesions had more giant cells, but fewer neutrophils than the bovine lesions. The giant cells were also larger and contained more nuclei than the giant cells of other species. These histopathological differences could perhaps serve as aids in diagnosis.

TREATMENT

• Since tuberculosis is a contagious disease of both animals and humans, the most effective and recommended way of handling this disease is by control and eradication (test and slaughter).
• There have been only isolated incidents where treatment was attempted on exotic herds. The treatment consisted of a three-drug regimen of isoniazid, rifampin, and ethambutol.

ACTIVITY
N/A

DIET
N/A

CLIENT EDUCATION
The most effective and recommended way of handling this disease is by control and eradication (test and slaughter).

MEDICATIONS
N/A

DRUGS OF CHOICE
N/A

CONTRAINDICATIONS
Appropriate milk and meat withdrawal times must be followed for all compounds administered to food-producing animals.

PRECAUTIONS
N/A

POSSIBLE INTERACTIONS
N/A

ALTERNATIVE DRUGS

FOLLOW-UP

PATIENT MONITORING

PREVENTION/AVOIDANCE
• Usually, treatment is not warranted. The only practical steps to take are control and prevention.
• A vaccine for tuberculosis has not been produced.
• A test and slaughter method could be used for captive deer, but this would not be possible among free-roaming deer.
• One management goal is to decrease deer density, which would in effect also decrease the amount of deer-to-deer transmission.
• Decreasing the amount of supplemental feeding that occurs during the winter months could greatly decrease the deer density. Supplemental feeding causes an increase in the number of deer that tend to congregate in one area.
• Transmission through aerosol or contaminated feed could easily occur, thus eliminating supplemental feedings should help decrease transmission.

POSSIBLE COMPLICATIONS
N/A

EXPECTED COURSE AND PROGNOSIS
Grave

MISCELLANEOUS

ASSOCIATED CONDITIONS
• Tuberculosis in deer can be seen as a pulmonary disease, where the bacteria are inhaled and proliferate into a focal region.
• The bacteria may also seed into a lymph node and spread via the lymphatic system. This infection can cause rapidly disseminated tuberculosis, which causes an acute disease.

AGE-RELATED FACTORS
N/A

ZOONOTIC POTENTIAL
• Cervidae tuberculosis is zoonotic. Care must be taken in the collection of laboratory samples and the diagnosis of affected animals.
• The presence of tuberculosis within the deer population, wild and captive, poses a major health concern.

PREGNANCY
N/A

RUMINANT SPECIES AFFECTED
All cervid species can be affected.

BIOSECURITY
• Isolation and quarantine of new stock entering the herd/flock
• Test and cull reactor animals prior to herd introduction.

PRODUCTION MANAGEMENT
• When cleaning a facility after the elimination of positive reactors, the facility can be decontaminated using 2% cresylic compounds or phenol derivatives. Before repopulating the facility, it is recommended to disinfect twice at 14- to 21-day intervals.
• All personnel involved with the facility and deer handling should wear respirator masks and be properly tested for tuberculosis.

SYNONYMS
TB

SEE ALSO
Bovine tuberculosis
Caseous lymphadenitis lesions
Other causes of chronic respiratory disease (chronic lung abscesses, aspiration pneumonia)
Other causes of chronic weight loss and ill thrift (Johne's disease, parasitism)
Progressive pneumonia
Small ruminant tuberculosis

ABBREVIATIONS
BTB = blood tuberculosis test
CCT = comparative cervical tuberculin test
ELISA = enzyme linked immunosorbent assay
SCT = single cervical tuberculin test

Suggested Reading
McCarty, C. W., Miller, M. W. 1998. A versatile model of disease transmission applied to forecasting bovine tuberculosis dynamics in white tailed deer populations. *Journal of Wildlife Diseases* 34(4): 722–30.
O'Brien, D. J., Fitzgerald, S. D., Lyon, T. J. 2001. Tuberculosis lesions in free-ranging white tailed deer in Michigan. *Journal of Wildlife Diseases* 37(3): 608–13.
Palmer, M. V., Waters, W. R., Whipple, D. L. 2004, Nov. Investigation of the transmission of *Mycobacterium bovis* from deer to cattle through indirect contact. *Am J Vet Res.* 65(11):1483–89.
Palmer, M. V., Whipple, D. L. 2000. Reemergence of tuberculosis in animals in the U.S. In: *Emerging disease of animals*. Washington, DC: ASM Press.
Palmer, M. V., Whipple, D. L., Olsen, S. C. 1999. Development of a model of natural infection with *M. bovis* in white-tailed deer. *Journal of Wildlife Diseases* 35(3): 450–57.
Rhyan, J. C., Saari, D. A. 1995. A comparative study of the histologic features of bovine tuberculosis in cattle, fallow deer (*Dama dama*), sika deer (*Cervus nippon*), and red deer and elk (*Cervus elaphus*). *Veterinary Pathology* 32: 215–20.

Author: Grace Kim

CESAREAN SURGERY: INDICATIONS

BASICS

DEFINITION
• A cesarean operation is a surgical procedure whereby the fetus is removed from the uterus through an abdominal and uterine incision in the dam.
• The operation is indicated when vaginal delivery is impossible or cannot be done without causing fetal death or damage to the maternal reproductive tract.

PATHOPHYSIOLOGY
• The indications for a cesarean operation for cattle are similar to other species.
• There is an inability to deliver the fetus vaginaly due to a fetopelvic disproportion, dead or emphysematous fetus, failure of the cervix to dilate, fetal malposture, fetal monster, or uterine torsion that cannot be corrected manually.
• An elective cesarean operation can be undertaken when severe preparturient conditions exist, such as ketosis, fetal dropsy, prolapse of the vagina, or to deliver valuable fetuses from small recipients in cases of embryo transfer.
• The operation can be performed in dams that carry a live or dead fetus. However, when the fetus is dead, the clinician must weigh the risk of complications such as peritonitis in comparison to performing a fetotomy. In the author's experience, a fetotomy is indicated in the case of a decomposed or emphysematous fetus.

SYSTEMS AFFECTED
• Endocrine/metabolic
• Herd health
• Musculoskeletal
• Reproductive

GENETICS
• Bulls whose daughters have too small a pelvis to deliver calves of normal size or those whose offspring are oversized in comparison to the breed average.
• Small breeds of goats such as the French Alpine.

INCIDENCE /PREVALENCE
• The incidence varies according to clinician preference in performing a fetotomy versus a cesarean in cases where the fetus is dead.
• About 5%–7% of dystocia cases in dairy cattle and goats are delivered via a cesarean. In beef cattle, the figure is slightly higher.

GEOGRAPHIC DISTRIBUTION
Worldwide

SIGNALMENT

Species
Bovine, ovine, caprine

Breed Predilection
• The overall incidence of dystocia varies with the species and with breeds within species.
• The bovine species is most often affected but ewes and does when carrying twins may show a high incidence.

• In the Belgian blue cattle breed, 80% of parturitions are delivered by cesarean.

Mean Age and Range
Similar to dystocia the incidence of cesarean operation is higher in primiparous than in multiparous animals.

SIGNS

GENERAL COMMENTS
• Defects in the components of the parturition process, the expulsive forces, the birth canal, fetus, and torsion of the uterus must be considered when assisting a case of dystocia.
• Before proceeding with a cesarean section, the clinician must be comfortable that the fetus cannot be delivered manually or by forced extraction after following the guidelines to determine whether or not the fetus can be delivered vaginally.

HISTORICAL FINDINGS
• Lack of progress after initiation of parturition
• Continuous violent abdominal contractions without visualization of fetal parts.
• Unsuccessful attempts by either an owner or herdsman to deliver the calf.

PHYSICAL EXAMINATION
First, a vaginal exam must be performed to determine the presentation, position, and posture of the calf within the birth canal. Second, malposition or malpresentation is corrected and calf viability is determined. Last, the clinician should attempt to deliver the calf and determine whether or not a vaginal delivery is possible after applying the appropriate guidelines for either an anterior or posterior presentation.

RISK FACTORS
• Obesity
• Twins
• Hypocalcemia
• Small frame size
• Small pelvic diameter
• Large calf

DIAGNOSIS

DIFFERENTIAL DIAGNOSIS
N/A

CBC/BIOCHEMISTRY/URINALYSIS
N/A

OTHER LABORATORY TESTS
N/A

IMAGING
N/A

DIAGNOSTIC PROCEDURES
N/A

PATHOLOGICAL FINDINGS
In cases of dystocia caused by hydroallantois, adventitial placentation is commonly found.

TREATMENT

APPROPRIATE HEALTH CARE
A cesarean procedure is a surgical case that may require hospitalization. However, most procedures are performed on-farm provided that there are suitable restraining or handling facilities and that appropriate care can be given to the patient.

NURSING CARE
Administration of postsurgical treatments such as antibiotics, ecbolic agents, energy and calcium supplements. Appetite, vaginal discharge, and temperature should be assessed regularly.

ACTIVITY
No restrictions

DIET
No restrictions

CLIENT EDUCATION
• Management practices to prevent risk factors for dystocia
• Training in observation strategies and techniques for prompt and correct diagnosis of dystocia

SURGICAL CONSIDERATIONS
• The surgical approach for a cesarean depends on the experience of the clinician, facilities, cause of the dystocia, and condition of the dam and fetus.
• The surgical risk is greatly increased when the patient is recumbent in mud or other inconvenient situations. Preferably, the surgery should be performed in a location of the farm or stable that offers less risk for complications.
• The surgical instruments listed below are recommended:
  • 4 to 12 towel clips
  • A scalpel
  • 6 to 10 hemostats
  • A needle driver
  • 2 pairs of Glock's uterine forceps
  • Blunt-point scissors
  • 2 pairs of Allis peritoneal forceps
  • Rat-toothed forceps
  • 2 short obstetrical chains and handles
  • No. 3 or 4 chromic catgut or polyglycolic acid suture material
  • Size 4 silk nonabsorbable suture
  • Suture needles
  • Iodine-based solution for surgical scrub
  • Alcohol
  • 4 × 4 cotton gauzes (30)
  • Bucket with antiseptic for the chains and handles
• There are three main approaches for the cesarean operation in the cow: left flank, ventrolateral, and ventral midline.
• Routine surgical procedures should be followed when incising the flank or abdomen and entering into the peritoneal cavity. In addition, the following surgical considerations are important:

• Epidural anesthesia with 2% lidocaine hydrochloride can be used to obviate abdominal contractions that are usually present.
• The skin incision in the flank or abdomen should be located in a site where the uterus is accessible, and should be long enough to remove the fetus through it.
• Exteriorize the gravid uterine horn into the incision site as much as possible.
• Make the uterine incision in the greater curvature, avoiding incising a placentome, and make it large enough to extract the fetus without causing tearing.
• Close the uterus using an absorbable suture with a continuous inverting pattern such as the Cushing and the Lembert patterns or the Utrecht uterine suture pattern, which is a modified Cushing.
• A single layer is sufficient if the uterine wall is healthy and not septic.
• Placental tissue should not be included in the suture.
• The muscle layers and skin are sutured in a routine fashion.
• Administer 2–40 U/kg of oxytocin postoperatively to help expel the placenta.
• Cesarean procedures in sheep and goats can be done with general anesthesia. However, most clinicians prefer to position the ewe/doe in right lateral recumbency with rope restraint and perform the incision through a left flank approach and a local anesthesia similar to that in cows. The incision is made in vertical direction in the left flank paralumbar fossa.
• Multiple births are common in sheep and goats and they can be delivered through the same uterine incision. However, an incision in the contralateral horn is often necessary.
• Keep in mind: goats are more sensitive to lidocaine and xylazine than are cows.
• The same surgical considerations and postoperative care given to cows should be followed for sheep and goats.
• Paravertebral anesthesia can be used to desensitize the paralumbar fossa if a left flank approach is selected.
• Local anesthetic solution can also be injected subcutaneously and deep into the abdominal musculature dorsal and cranial to the proposed incision site in the shape of an inverted L.
• In addition, a line block can also be used in a similar fashion desensitizing the proposed incision site. As much as 50 ml of lidocaine may be required in the mature cow depending on the incision length.

MEDICATIONS

DRUGS OF CHOICE
• The drug of choice for desensitization of the incision site is lidocaine. A balance anesthetic plane can be achieved by using xylazine at a dose of 0.02 mg/kg (bovine dose) in conjunction with the lidocaine blocks.

• A variety of broad-spectrum antibiotics are recommended postsurgically to prevent peritonitis and septic conditions. Label recommendations to avoid antibiotic residues in saleable milk should be followed when systemic antibiotics are used.
• Penicillin or a synthetic analog: 20,000 to 30,000 U/kg bid
• Ceftiofur: 1–2.2 mg/kg bid
• Some cases may require supportive treatment with fluids, electrolytes, and anti-inflammatory agents.

CONTRAINDICATIONS
• Xylazine may induce uterine contractions and make exteriorization of the gravid uterine horn difficult.
• Appropriate milk and meat withdrawal times must be followed for all compounds administered to food-producing animals.

PRECAUTIONS
If the operation is performed on a standing animal, care must be taken not to overdose with lidocaine in the epidural or xylazine for sedation, to prevent the animal from becoming recumbent.

POSSIBLE INTERACTIONS
N/A

ALTERNATIVE DRUGS
Acetylpromazine maleate at a dose of 0.044–0.088 mg/kg IM or IV can be used to achieve sedation. However, acetylpromazine is generally not recommended in ruminant species due to its negative effect on rumen motility and subsequent bloat.

FOLLOW-UP

PATIENT MONITORING
Animals should be monitored for signs of septicemia and peritonitis.

PREVENTIVE AVOIDANCE
• Proper management of the prepartum cow
• Genetic considerations to help reduce fetal size
• Training of farm personnel in proper observation of preparturient animals.

POSSIBLE COMPLICATIONS
• Peritonitis
• Wound dehiscence
• Retained fetal membranes
• Toxic metritis
• Incision site abscess
• Uterine adhesions

EXPECTED COURSE AND PROGNOSIS
• Survival depends on the degree of uterine-content contamination of the peritoneum, closure of the uterine wall, and overall surgical technique. In addition, cows placed on systemic antibiotics have a more favorable prognosis.
• A recovery rate of 70% should be expected in uncomplicated cases. However, the majority of cows that have a cesarean

operation experienced reduced fertility postpartum.

MISCELLANEOUS

ASSOCIATED CONDITIONS
N/A

AGE-RELATED FACTORS
Cesarean operations may be more common in primiparous than multiparous animals.

ZOONOTIC POTENTIAL
N/A

PREGNANCY
N/A

RUMINANT SPECIES AFFECTED
Bovine, caprine, ovine

BIOSECURITY
N/A

PRODUCTION MANAGEMENT
Attention to appropriate management of the periparturient animal

SYNONYMS
Cesarian section
C-section

SEE ALSO
Anesthesia and analgesia
Calving difficulties
Cesarean section techniques
Species-specific reproductive chapters

ABBREVIATIONS
IM = intramuscular
IV = intravenous
U = international units

Suggested Reading
Oehme, F. 1967. The ventro lateral cesarean section in the cow. *Veterinary Medicine/Small Animal Clinician.* 62: 889–893.
Roberts, S. J. 1985. Dystocia. In: *Veterinary obstetrics and genital diseases (theriogenology),* ed. S. J. Roberts. Woodstock, VT: Published by the author.
Schuijt, G., Ball, L. 1980. Delivery by forced extraction and other aspects of bovine obstetrics. In: *Current therapy in theriogenology,* ed. D. A. Morrow. Philadelphia: W. B. Saunders.
Sloss, V., And Dufty, J.H. 1980. *Handbook of bovine obstetrics.* 2nd edition. Baltimore, MD: Williams and Wilkins Company.
Vandeplassche, M. 1974. Embryotomy and cesarotomy. In: *Large animal surgery,* ed. F. W. Oehme, J. E. Prier. Baltimore, MD: Williams and Wilkins.
Younquist, R. S., Shore, M. D. 1997. Postpartum uterine infections. In: *Current therapy in large animal theriogenology,* ed. R. S. Youngquist. Philadelphia: W. B. Saunders.

Author: Carlos A. Risco

CHLAMYDIOSIS

 BASICS

DEFINITION

Chlamydia are intracellular bacteria that constitute one of the most important causes of small ruminant abortion in most parts of the world (also denoted enzootic abortion of ewes) as well as a number of other disease syndromes in sheep, goats, cattle, and llamas.

OVERVIEW

- Chlamydiosis may occur as a variety of disease syndromes, depending on the strain of *Chlamydia* and the animal species involved.
- The most important of these are reproductive diseases
  - Third-term abortion, endometritis, and infertility in females
  - Orchitis and seminal vesiculitis in males
- Other diseases include pneumonia, enteritis, encephalomyelitis, polyarthritis, and conjunctivitis.
- Infection may be unapparent or present with severe clinical disease affecting most of the herd or flock.
- Two distinct *Chlamydia* species have been implicated in ruminant disease: *Chlamydophila abortus* (previously *Chlamydia psittaci* biotype I) and *Chlamydophila pecorum* (previously *Chlamydia pecorum*).
- Aborted fetuses, placentas, and uterine discharges are the main sources of *C. abortus* infections.
- In-utero infection may lead to fetal death or perinatal disease.
- Although cattle strains may infect sheep and goats and vice versa, avian *Chlamydia psittaci*, strains from humans, cats, and other mammals are not generally associated with disease in ruminants.
- *C. abortus* is zoonotic and has been reported to cause abortion in women.

PATHOPHYSIOLOGY

- *Chlamydophila abortus* strains are invasive as opposed to *C. pecorum*, which tends to colonize mucosal surfaces causing clinically inapparent or mild local infections.
- Both strains may be harbored in the alimentary tract and transmitted through feces, although the main source of *C. abortus* is aborted infected tissues and fluids.
- Infection is usually oral-nasally after which proliferation in the lymphoid tissues and the gastrointestinal mucosa leads to *Chlamydia* that are usually cleared after 7–10 days.

- Inhibition of chlamydial replication by the immune system may keep the disease quiescent until past midpregnancy when hormonal changes or immunosuppression are thought to permit replication in the placental trophoblasts.
- The production of proinflammatory chemokines, cytokines, and other modulators by the infected cells seems to be the cause of increased chlamydial proliferation and the intense tissue reactions that lead to necrotizing lesions.
- Migration of the bacteria from the placenta to the fetus induces fetal pathology that may culminate in abortion or the premature birth of weak lambs.
- Chlamydial invasion of the endometrial epithelium results in endometritis characterized by necrosis and mucosal sloughing.
- In cases of polyarthritis, the inflammatory reaction in the synovium, tendon sheaths, and subsynovial tissues induces fibrosis and both articular and periarticular damage.
- In young calves and lambs, diffuse interstitial bronchopneumonia may be seen with thickened alveolar septae and focal neutrophilic bronchiolitis and alveolitis. Disease is often concurrent with other pathogens, which exacerbate the syndrome.
- Sporadic bovine encephalitis (SBE) results from generalized chlamydial infection. Inflammation of the vascular endothelium, mesenchymal tissue, and most serosal membranes leads to organ damage, while nervous signs are a result of brain edema and hyperemia.

SIGNALMENT

- Chlamydiosis in ruminants has been reported in most parts of the world. In New Zealand, the disease has not been described, and in Australia, abortion from this agent is rare.
- *C. abortus* causes sporadic third-term abortion in cattle or abortion storms after 90 days gestation in sheep and goats.
- All naïve animals are susceptible, but the strong immunity that develops after abortion will prevent further fetal loss.
- In a newly infected sheep flock, between 30% and 60% of the pregnant animals may abort. Storms of 60%–90% abortions in goats have been reported.

Mean Age and Range

- In an endemic herd or flock, the animals in their first gestation are of highest risk to abort.
- Enteritis, pneumonia, and polyarthritis are generally limited to young stock below 6 months of age with a morbidity ranging from 2% to 75%.

Predominant Sex

N/A

SIGNS

- Third-term abortion storms in sheep and goats; dark red or clay-colored placental cotyledons
- Sporadic abortions in cattle
- Inflammation of the seminal vesicles, epididymitis, or testicles, which may become atrophic
- Stillbirth, perinatal weakness, or death
- Coughing, depression, dyspnea, mucoid or mucopurulent nasal discharge in young stock; may be fever
- Shifting lameness, stiffness, pyrexia, and anorexia; painful joints, which may or may not be swollen but contain grayish-yellow synovial fluid with fibrin clots. Stiffness often seems to improve with forced exercise.
- Hyperemia of the conjunctiva and sclera, serous discharge that may become purulent due to secondary infection; small corneal ulcers may develop.
- SBE is characterized by depression, anorexia, pyrexia, dyspnea, and nasal discharge. Increased salivation and diarrhea may be seen; stiff gait, circling, staggering, and paralysis; up to 60% mortality. Survivors perform poorly.

CAUSES AND RISK FACTORS

- The main sources of *C. abortus* are the fetal membranes, tissues, and uterine discharges of animals that have aborted.
- Both *C. abortus* and *C. pecorum* may be harbored in the alimentary tract and transmitted through feces.
- Venereal spread may be due to infected semen from males with seminal vesiculitis or orchitis.
- Vertical transmission may lead to infected offspring.

DIAGNOSIS

DIFFERENTIAL DIAGNOSIS
• Causes of third-term or late gestation abortion associated with placentitis: toxoplasmosis, Q fever, *Campylobacter jejuni* or *C. fetus fetus*, brucellosis, listeriosis, salmonellosis, aspergillosis, leptospirosis
• Generalized stiffness and lameness: Lyme disease, mycoplasmosis, caseous lymphadenitis, infectious or septic tenosynovitis, tendonitis, synovitis, *Histophilus somnii*, louping ill (UK), monensin, lasalocid or ionophore toxicity, white muscle disease, foot-and-mouth, bluetongue
• Diarrheic syndrome in calves: feed related, BVD, salmonellosis, rotavirus, coronavirus, coccidiosis, nematodes
• Keratoconjuctivitis: *Mycoplasma* spp., *Moraxella bovis*, IBR, environmental irritants

CBC/BIOCHEMISTRY/URINALYSIS
N/A

OTHER LABORATORY TESTS
N/A

IMAGING
N/A

DIAGNOSTIC PROCEDURES
Serology
• Generally, complement fixation (CF), but also ELISA or other methods
• Most labs use MOMP (major outer membrane protein) antigens, which produce serological titers that do not discern between *C. abortus* and *C. pecorum*.
• A large proportion of the ruminant population will exhibit titers without clinical disease
• Newer synthetic or soluble antigens have been developed that can identify *C. abortus* or *C. pecorum*; not commonly used by most laboratories.
• In most labs, CF titers of 1:16 to 1:32 are considered positive.
• Most animals that have aborted from chlamydiosis will have a titer of 1:80 or higher that peaks 2–3 weeks after abortion.
• Serology is generally not useful for individual animal diagnosis.

• It cannot be used to detect infection in rams or latently infected animals.
• High titers in a group that aborted as opposed to negative or low titers in a parallel group that had normal parturition is indicative of *C. abortus*.
• Serological titers due to vaccination cannot be distinguished from those due to infection.
• Fetal serology, although less sensitive than detection of chlamydial LPS antigen, may be of particular use when placenta is not available.

Culture
Not generally performed for veterinary diagnostic purposes as is only possible in cell culture or embryonated hen's eggs.

Microscopy
Staining by modified Ziehl-Neelsen (Stamp, Gimenez, or Macchiavello) or Giemsa may give a tentative indication but is not specific.

Immunofluorescence/Antigen ELISA
Diagnostic when positive on placentas or other pathological material

PCR
• This test is becoming more common in regional and central laboratories.
• Due to its high sensitivity and the prevalence of fecal and environmental *Chlamydia* species, samples must be taken and processed extremely carefully.
• False negative results may occur due to inhibitors in the samples.

PATHOLOGIC FINDINGS
GROSS FINDINGS
• Placenta: raspberry or clay-colored cotyledons, leathery intercotyledonary areas
• Fetus: usually fresh but may be autolyzed. Often excess fluid is seen in the abdominal cavity, as are small necrotic foci in the liver.
• Joints may be swollen due to periarticular fibrosis and subcutaneous edema, but even in nonenlarged joints, excessive grayish-yellow turbid synovial fluid with fibrin plaques may be present.

HISTOPATHOLOGICAL FINDINGS
Abortions
• Grossly, there is thickening and yellow to red-brown discoloration of the placenta, especially in the intercotyledonary areas; necrotizing vasculitis and thrombosis with mononuclear and neutrophillic infiltration.

• Microscopically, necrotizing placentitis is accompanied by nonsuppurative vasculitis. There are no specific gross postmortem lesions in the fetus, but nonsuppurative meningoencephalitis, necrotizing hepatitis, and proliferation of mononuclear cells in spleen and lymph nodes may occur.

Polyarthritis
Synovial joint fluid is nonpurulent and may be off-color with flakes of fibrin. There is no change to the cartilage, and mononuclear cells predominate in the synovial fluid. The tendon sheaths and subsynovial tissues exhibit primarily an inflammatory reaction, which extends to involve the synovial membranes.

Pneumonia
• Bronchopneumonia is characterized by edematous septae and thickened bronchioles that produce turbid exudate on compression. There may be consolidation of cranial lung lobes with interstitial changes and intracytoplasmic elementary bodies within alveolar macrophages.
• Lungs: peribronchiolar lymphocytic cuffing, bronchiolitis, and alveolitis.

Keratoconjunctivitis
• Conjunctival hyperemia can progress to lymphoid follicle formation, and corneal vascularization and corneal edema may be present. Conjunctival epithelial cells are often necrotic.
• Conjunctival smears show numerous neutrophils and some lymphocytes; as the disease progresses there are more neutrophils and fewer mononuclear cells.

Placenta
Fetus: often few lesions seen but occasionally multifocal necrosis in the liver or spleen or mild interstitial pneumonia in the lungs. Chlamydial inclusions may be seen in the abomasal mucosa.

Brain
Perivascular cuffing and inflammatory cell infiltration evenly distributed through most parts of the brain.

TREATMENT
• Abortions—various protocols suggested
  • Long-acting oxytetracycline (OTC) (20 mg/kg) at 10–14-day intervals from midgestation until parturition.

CHLAMYDIOSIS

• 400–450 mg OTC /head/day orally (abortions in goats)
• 200 mg tylosin/head/day orally (abortions in goats)
• General chlamydiosis
  • Single long-acting OTC (20 mg/kg)
  • Three treatments at 3-day intervals suggested
  • 150–200 mg tetracycline /head/day orally for lambs or kids

MEDICATIONS

CONTRAINDICATIONS
Appropriate milk and meat withdrawal times must be followed for all compounds administered to food-producing animals.

FOLLOW-UP

PREVENTION/AVOIDANCE

Vaccination
• Killed whole cell bacterins given prior to breeding will significantly reduce the level of abortion but do not eliminate the carrier state or excretion.
• In the midst of an abortion storm, antibiotic treatment is the only course available, as most vaccines are not licensed for use during gestation.
• A temperature-sensitive avirulent vaccine for use in sheep is produced and marketed in Europe. It is claimed to prevent both abortions and shedding.

Management
• Closed flock management is advised.
• Stud males should be screened or treated prior to breeding.
• All aborting animals should be segregated from the flock to prevent transmission to other stock. Aborted fetuses, placental membranes, bedding, and other contaminated materials should be removed and destroyed.
• In cases of synchronized breeding, the flock should be divided into small groups that have close parturition dates.

• Judicious use of disinfectants should be geared toward preventing manual transmission of the disease through boots, clothing, and instruments from aborting or lambing animals to those still pregnant. Newborn lambs may be infected.
• As animals that aborted may continue to excrete the organism, breeding rams that have been with them should not have access to other clean stock.
• Antibiotics and vaccines should be incorporated into a flock-management program.

POSSIBLE COMPLICATIONS
The avirulent live vaccine for use in sheep may have zoonotic implications.

EXPECTED COURSE AND PROGNOSIS
• After the initial outbreak, good management techniques combined with judicial use of antibiotics and/or vaccines should reduce the rate of abortion to negligible levels.
• Animals that have aborted are immune from further abortions.

MISCELLANEOUS

ZOONOTIC POTENTIAL
• *C. abortus* may cause abortion in pregnant woman who should, therefore, not work in a flock with this disease.
• The avirulent live vaccine for use in sheep may have zoonotic implications.

SEE ALSO
Aspergillosis
Bluetongue
Brucellosis
BVD
Campylobacter jejuni or *C. fetus fetus*
Caseous lymphadenitis
Coronavirus
Foot and mouth
Histophilus somnii
IBR
Infectious or septic tenosynovitis
Lasalocid or ionophore toxicity
Leptospirosis
Listeriosis
Louping ill (UK)
Lyme disease
Monensin
Moraxella bovis
Mycoplasma spp.
Mycoplasmosis
Q fever
Rotavirus
Salmonellosis
Synovitis
Tendonitis
Toxoplasmosis
White muscle disease

ABBREVIATIONS
CF = complement fixation
ELISA = enzyme-linked immunosorbent assay
FA = fluorescent antibody
OTC = oxytetracycline
PCR = polymerase chain reaction
SBE = sporadic bovine encephalitis

Suggested Reading
Chalmers, W. S., Simpson, J., Lee, S. J., Baxendale, W. 1997, Jul 19. Use of a live chlamydial vaccine to prevent ovine enzootic abortion. *Vet Rec.* 141(3): 63–67.
DeGraves, F. J., Gao, D., Hehnen, H. R., Schlapp, T., Kaltenboeck, B. 2003, Apr. Quantitative detection of *Chlamydia psittaci* and *C. pecorum* by high-sensitivity real-time PCR reveals high prevalence of vaginal infection in cattle. *J Clin Microbiol.* 41(4): 1726–29.
Nietfeld, J. C. 2001, Jul. Chlamydial infections in small ruminants. *Vet Clin North Am Food Anim Pract.* 17(2): 301–14, vi.
Papp, J. R., Shewen, P. E. 1996, Apr. Pregnancy failure following vaginal infection of sheep with *Chlamydia psittaci* prior to breeding. *Infect Immun.* 64(4): 1116–25.
Reggiardo, C., Fuhrmann, T. J., Meerdink, G. L., Bicknell, E. J. 1989, Oct. Diagnostic features of chlamydia infection in dairy calves. *J Vet Diagn Invest.* 1(4): 305–8.
Rodolakis, A., Salinas, J., Papp, J. 1998, May–Aug. Recent advances on ovine chlamydial abortion. *Vet Res.* 29(3–4): 275–88. Review.

Authors: Michael D. Bernstein and Tina Wismer

CHRONIC WASTING DISEASE

BASICS

OVERVIEW
• Chronic wasting disease (CWD) is a transmissible spongiform encephalopathy (TSE) that affects free-ranging and captive cervids including mule deer, white-tailed deer, and Rocky Mountain elk.
• CWD was first recognized in captive mule deer in Colorado in the 1960s and later identified as a TSE in 1978.
• TSEs are a group of diseases characterized by the accumulation of a misfolded normal host prion protein in the brain.
• Additional TSEs in other species include BSE in cattle, scrapie in sheep, kuru, CJD, and vCJD in humans, and feline spongiform encephalopathy.
• CWD has been detected in wild populations in Wisconsin, Nebraska, South Dakota, New Mexico, western Colorado, and Saskatchewan, Canada. CWD has been diagnosed in captive populations in numerous other states.
• Horizontal spread of the disease by oral exposure to infected carcasses, excretions, secretions, or other tissue source has been proven by epidemiological studies.
• Clinical signs of CWD include changes in behavior, weight loss, loss of muscle mass, and salivation. The average age of affected animals ranges from 3 to 5 years.

PATHOPHYSIOLOGY
• Transmission of CWD within wild populations appears to be via exposure to infected carcasses, secretions, and excretions.
• Dead and decaying carcasses, placenta, and placental fluids are suspected to be common sources of infection.
• Analysis by immunohistochemical studies of the tissue distribution of prions in CWD-infected cervids identified the agent in the brain, spinal cord, eyes, peripheral nerves, and lymphoreticular tissues.
• Distribution of the CWD agent outside of the brain seems to be less widespread in elk than in deer.

• Involvement of the tonsils and peripheral nerves early in the course of experimental and natural prion infection suggests the possible involvement of the lymphoreticular and peripheral nervous systems in the pathogenesis and transmission of the disease.
• A unifying feature of all the prionoses is their neuropathology. CWD affects the grey matter of the central nervous system (CNS), producing neuronal loss, gliosis, and characteristic spongiform change. In addition, plaques with the typical staining properties of amyloid (e.g., apple-green birefringence after Congo red staining when viewed under polarized light) are observed. These amyloid plaques are immunoreactive with antibodies to the prion protein and do not immunoreact with antibodies to other amyloidogenic proteins, such as the amyloid-beta.
• CWD and other TSEs are believed to be caused by a pathogenic effect on neurons of an abnormal isoform of a host-encoded glycoprotein, the prion protein.
• The pathogenic form of this protein appears to be devoid of nucleic acids and supports its own amplification in the host. TSEs in animals primarily occur by transmitting the etiologic agent within a species, either naturally or through domestic husbandry practices. A notable exception among the human TSEs is the variant form of Creutzfeldt-Jakob disease (vCJD), which is believed to have resulted from the foodborne transmission of bovine spongiform encephalopathy (BSE) to humans.
• Although CWD does not appear to occur naturally outside the cervid family, it has been transmitted experimentally by intracerebral injection to a number of animals, including laboratory mice, ferrets, mink, squirrel monkeys, and goats.
• In an experimental study, the CWD agent was transmitted to 3 of 13 intracerebrally injected cattle after an incubation period of 22 to 27 months. In ongoing experimental studies, after > 6 years of observation, no prion disease has developed in 11 cattle orally challenged with the CWD agent or 24 cattle living with infected deer herds.

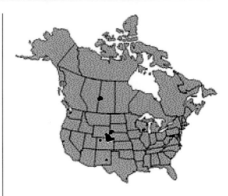

Figure 1.

The geographical distribution of CWD in free-ranging deer in the United States and Canada.

• In addition, domestic cattle, sheep, and goats residing in research facilities in close contact with infected cervids did not develop a prion disease.

SYSTEMS AFFECTED
CNS, musculoskeletal

GENETICS
N/A

INCIDENCE/PREVALENCE
• The low prevalence and lack of large-scale surveys has hampered identifying genetic profiles of susceptible populations and the use of genotyping to identify susceptible populations.
• Epidemiologic modeling suggested that chronic wasting disease might have been present among free-ranging animals in some portions of the disease-endemic area several decades before it was initially recognized.
• This disease can be highly transmissible within captive deer and elk populations. A prevalence of > 90% was reported among mule deer in facilities where the disease has been endemic for > 2 years.

GEOGRAPHIC DISTRIBUTION
North America, potentially worldwide (see Figure 1)
• Chronic wasting disease appears to have been introduced into Canada through the importation of infected farmed elk from the United States in the late 1980s and early 1990s, at a time when little was known about the disease.

CHRONIC WASTING DISEASE

• Eradication efforts in Canada have led to the control of the spread of CWD in the farmed elk industry.

• Immunohistochemical (IHC) staining of the retropharyngeal lymph nodes and obex with a monoclonal antibody is considered the gold standard for postmortem diagnosis of CWD. Lymph node staining has been approved as a valid diagnostic procedure. There is currently no antemortem diagnostic test.

• CWD appears host specific and will not readily transmit to humans, sheep, swine, cattle, or other wildlife.

• Increasing spread of CWD has raised concerns about the potential for increasing human exposure to the CWD agent. The foodborne transmission of bovine spongiform encephalopathy to humans indicates that the species barrier may not completely protect humans from animal prion diseases.

• Conversion of human prion protein by CWD-associated prions has been demonstrated in an in vitro cell-free experiment, but limited investigations have not identified strong evidence for CWD transmission to humans.

National Programs

• State and national programs have been implemented to reduce the spread of CWD.

• Many states have mandatory identification and postmortem testing of all captive cervids. In addition to testing, some states have restricted movement of deer and elk across state boundaries.

• Captive herds with a CWD-positive animal are typically eliminated.

• CWD, like other prion proteins, can survive in contaminated environments for many years.

• In Canada, CWD was first detected in free-ranging cervids (two mule deer) in 2001 in Saskatchewan; a few additional deer tested positive in 2002 and 2003. Saskatchewan Environment has implemented a herd-reduction program using "control permits" to prevent further spread of the disease among free-ranging cervids.

SIGNALMENT

Species

Both free-ranging and captive white-tailed deer (*O. virginianus*), Rocky Mountain elk (*Cervus elaphus nelsoni*), mule deer (*Odocoileus hemionus*) have all been diagnosed with CWD.

Breed Predilections

N/A

Mean Age and Range

• Most affected cervids are greater than 2 years of age and many are 3 to 5 years old.

• In captive cervids, most cases occur in animals 2–7 years of age; however, the disease has been reported in cervids as young as 17 months and as old as > 15 years of age.

Predominant Sex

N/A

SIGNS

HISTORICAL FINDINGS

• Many cervids diagnosed with CWD are asymptomatic. The more chronically affected animals have progressive fat and muscle loss over a period of weeks or months.

• Additional clinical signs include changes in behavior, which can include loss of fear to humans, increased salivation, and atrophy of muscles around the head leading to droopy ears.

• There are no gross pathognomonic changes in cervids with CWD. Gross exam of the brain is unremarkable in cervids with CWD. Additional postmortem changes in chronically affected animals are nonspecific, but can include emaciation, serous atrophy of fat, abomasal ulcers, and aspiration pneumonia.

PHYSICAL EXAMINATION FINDINGS

• Clinical manifestations of CWD include weight loss over weeks or months, behavioral changes, excessive salivation, difficulty swallowing, polydipsia, and polyuria. In some animals, ataxia and head tremors may occur.

• Most animals with the disease die within several months of illness onset, sometimes from aspiration pneumonia. In rare cases, illness may last for ≥ 1 year.

• The mode of transmission among deer and elk is not fully understood; however, evidence supports lateral transmission through direct animal-to-animal contact or as a result of indirect exposure to the causative agent in the environment, including contaminated feed and water sources.

 DIAGNOSIS

• Histopathological lesions of chronic wasting disease include spongiform change of the grey matter; neuronal intracytoplasmic vacuolation, degeneration, and loss; and astrocytosis in the absence of a host inflammatory response.

• Immunohistochemical (IHC) staining of the retropharyngeal lymph nodes and obex with a monoclonal antibody is considered the gold standard for postmortem diagnosis of CWD. The recent development of an ELISA-based diagnostic test on fresh retropharyngeal lymph has been used to test large numbers of wild cervids in a short time frame.

• There is currently no approved antemortem test for CWD.

OTHER DIAGNOSTIC PROCEDURES

• Two major types of the proteinase-K–resistant prion protein fragment have been identified on the basis of their molecular size by one-dimensional immunoblot analysis: type 1 migrating at 21 kDa and type 2 at 19 kDa. N-terminal protein sequencing indicated that the cleavage site of the type 1 fragment is generally at residue 82 and that of type 2 is at residue 97.

• Prion strain diversity is believed to be encoded in the three-dimensional conformation of the protein, which determines the cleavage site and molecular size of proteinase-K–treated prion fragment, indicating that the difference in molecular size may correlate with strain differences. However, one-dimensional immunoblot analysis may not identify more subtle differences that may influence the conformation of different prion strains.

• Analysis of the glycoform ratios of prion fragments and application of a two-dimensional immunoblot may help further identify these subtle differences.

• On one-dimensional immunoblot analysis, the prion fragment from several CWD-infected deer and elk migrated to 21 kDa, corresponding to the type 1 pattern. This specific type has been identified in most cases of sporadic CJD in the United States. However, the deer and elk prion fragment differs from that in sporadic CJD cases in the glycoform ratio.

• In the CWD-associated prion fragment, the diglycosylated form was predominant, but in the CJD-associated prions, the monoglycosylated form was predominant.

• Preliminary analysis using two-dimensional immunoblot indicates that the CWD-associated prion fragment exhibited patterns different from that of the CJD-associated prion fragment from a human patient with the type 1 pattern.

PATHOLOGIC FINDINGS

Histopathological lesions of chronic wasting disease include spongiform change of the grey matter; neuronal intracytoplasmic vacuolation, degeneration, and loss; and astrocytosis in the absence of a host inflammatory response.

MISCELLANEOUS

ASSOCIATED CONDITIONS
N/A

AGE-RELATED FACTORS
In captive cervids, most cases occur in animals 2–7 years of age; however, the disease has been reported in cervids as young as 17 months and as old as > 15 years of age.

ZOONOTIC POTENTIAL
There is no plausible link between CWD and BSE in cattle and scrapie in sheep. No known human has been infected with CWD.

PREGNANCY
N/A

RUMINANT SPECIES AFFECTED
Cervidae

BIOSECURITY
See Pathophysiology above

PRODUCTION MANAGEMENT
• Mandatory identification and postmortem testing of all captive cervids
• Captive herds with a CWD-positive animal are typically eliminated.
• CWD, like other prion proteins, can survive in contaminated environments for many years.

SYNONYMS
N/A

SEE ALSO
Body condition scoring: cervidae
BSE
Cervidae management
Scrapie
Wildlife diseases

ABBREVIATIONS
BSE = bovine spongiform encephalopathy
CJD = Creutzfeldt-Jakob disease
CNS = central nervous system
CWD = chronic wasting disease
ELISA = enzyme-linked immunosorbent assay
IHC = immunohistochemical staining
TSE = transmissible spongiform encephalopathy
vCJD = variant form of Creutzfeldt-Jakob disease

Suggested Reading
Gross, J. E., Miller, M. W. 2001. Chronic wasting disease in mule deer: disease dynamics and control. *J Wildl Manag.* 65: 205–15.
Hamir, A. N., et al. 2001. Preliminary findings on the experimental transmission of chronic wasting disease agent of mule deer to cattle. *J Vet Diagn Invest.* 13: 91–96.
Miller, M. W., et al. 2000. Epizootiology of chronic wasting disease in free-ranging cervids in Colorado and Wyoming. *J Wildl Dis.* 36: 676–90.
Miller, M. W., Wild, M. A., Williams, E. S. 1998. Epidemiology of chronic wasting disease in captive Rocky Mountain elk. *J Wildl Dis.* 34: 532–38.
Williams, E. S., Miller, M. W. 2002. Chronic wasting disease in deer and elk in North America. *Rev Sci Tech.* 21: 305–16.
Williams, E. S., Young, S. 1993. Neuropathology of chronic wasting disease of mule deer (*Odocoileus hemionus*) and elk (*Cervus elaphus nelsoni*). *Vet Pathol.* 30: 36–45.
Wolfe, L. L., et al. 2002. Evaluation of antemortem sampling to estimate chronic wasting disease prevalence in free-ranging mule deer. *J Wildl Manag.* 66: 564–73.

Authors: Jeremy Schefers and Dennis Hermesch

CICUTA SPP. (WATER HEMLOCK) TOXICITY

BASICS

OVERVIEW
• Water hemlock poisoning in ruminants, particularly cattle, is not an uncommon occurrence.
• Four species (*C. bulbifera, C. douglassi, C. maculata, C. virosa*) can be encountered in North America.
• These plants are members of the Apicacea family and all have similar physical characteristics—perennials with tall (3–10 feet), erect, stout, hollow stems (except at the nodes). The leaflets are lance shaped, with the majority of the secondary veins terminating at the small notch at the leaf edge. The small white cluster of umbrella-shaped flowers is located at the tips of the branches. The root is bulbous (similar to a potato with sprouts) and is often located very close to the surface.
• Cicuta plants are always found in wet areas, along streams, ditches, and in marshy areas.
• The lower stem, tuber, and roots ooze a yellow resinous liquid between hollowed out chambers.
• The toxin present in the resin can cause acute onset of salivation, tachypnea, muscle tremors, and convulsions.
• Death is typically within a few hours of ingestion.

PATHOPHYSIOLOGY
• Cicutoxin is the primary toxin concentrated in the yellow resin of the tubers, roots, young shoots, and green seeds.
• Definitive mechanism of action is yet unclear; possibilities include interference with sodium and potassium channels, interference with GABA, and effects on the brain stem.

SYSTEMS AFFECTED
Nervous and cardiopulmonary systems

GENETICS
N/A

INCIDENCE/PREVALENCE
Not uncommon in many areas of the United States and Canada, more prevalent in wet areas

GEOGRAPHIC DISTRIBUTION
Throughout North America

SIGNALMENT
All ruminants, particularly cattle

Species
All ruminants appear to be susceptible; most cases seem to be reported in cattle.

Breed Predilections
N/A

Mean Age and Range
N/A

Predominant Sex
N/A

SIGNS
• Animals found dead
• Muscle twitching, excessive salivation, tachycardia, dilated pupils, and tachypnea are some of the earlier signs seen within 30–90 minutes of ingestion, depending on dose.
• Rapidly followed by recumbency, excessive chewing movements, and violent convulsions; death may quickly follow due to respiratory paralysis.

CAUSES AND RISK FACTORS
• Most poisonings occur in animals ingesting the tuber, roots, and very young shoots. This can occur any time of year; however, most cases occur in the early spring when the tubers are sprouting. The roots are very near the surface and are easily accessible.
• Reported lethal doses of tuber are greater than 1.2 g fresh tuber/kg BW in sheep, and 0.1% in cattle. Lethal doses of fresh green plant material have been reported to be 2 ounces for sheep and 10–12 ounces for adult cattle; field cases indicate that fatal doses may be much less than this.

• Animals grazing the immature seeds can be susceptible to poisoning.
• It is possible that animals can be poisoned by drinking out of water puddles where the green seeds have concentrated or plant material has been trampled.
• The remainder of the plant is low in toxicity, and drying the plant greatly reduces the toxicity.

DIAGNOSIS

DIFFERENTIAL DIAGNOSIS
Bacterial or viral meningitis or encephalitis, lead poisoning, Dicentra poisoning, nitrate toxicity, hypomagnesemia, rabies, nervous coccidiosis

CBC/BIOCHEMISTRY/URINALYSIS
• No specific or diagnostic changes have been reported.
• Elevation of AST, LDH, and CK may be indicative of muscle pathology.

OTHER LABORATORY TESTS
N/A

IMAGING
N/A

DIAGNOSTIC PROCEDURES
• One can often readily identify pieces or whole tubers/roots within the rumen or reticulum during necropsy.
• Rumen/reticulum contents can be tested for the presence of cicutoxin (not very stable; samples need to be collected within 24 hours of death). This analysis can be extremely difficult to perform on other tissues due to the short half-life of the toxin.

PATHOLOGIC FINDINGS
• Nonspecific evidence of generalized congestion, and signs of a terminal convulsion
• Myocardial degeneration and necrosis of the heart and skeletal muscle may be observed in those animals with severe and prolonged seizure activity.

CICUTA SPP. (WATER HEMLOCK) TOXICITY

TREATMENT

• Treatment is generally not possible due to the short time course of clinical signs.
• Can attempt oral activated charcoal and saline cathartic (magnesium sulfate).

MEDICATIONS

• Control the muscle tremors or seizures with valium or phenobarbital/pentobarbital.
• Barbiturate-induced anesthesia prior to the onset of seizures can lead to complete recovery.

CONTRAINDICATIONS

N/A

FOLLOW-UP

Recovery is potentially possible if the animal is still alive 2–4 hours following ingestion.

PATIENT MONITORING

Monitor respiratory function, and control seizure activity.

PREVENTION/AVOIDANCE

• Avoid access to the plant. This is unlikely to be hay-related poisoning.
• Dig up and remove the roots, or control chemically with appropriate herbicides.

POSSIBLE COMPLICATIONS

N/A

EXPECTED COURSE AND PROGNOSIS

Most clinically affected animals are expected to die.

MISCELLANEOUS

ASSOCIATED CONDITIONS

N/A

AGE-RELATED FACTORS

N/A

ZOONOTIC POTENTIAL

N/A

PREGNANCY

N/A

RUMINANT SPECIES AFFECTED

All ruminants are susceptible.

BIOSECURITY

N/A

PRODUCTION MANAGEMENT

Prevent access to the plant.

SYNONYMS

Beaver poison
Children's bane
Cowbane
Death-of-man
False parsley
Poison parsnip
Snakeweed

SEE ALSO

Bacterial or viral meningitis or encephalitis
Dicentra poisoning
Hypomagnesemia
Lead poisoning
Nervous coccidiosis
Nitrate toxicity
Rabies
Toxicology by species
Toxicosis herd outbreak

ABBREVIATIONS

• AST = aspartate aminotransferase
• BW = body weight
• CK = creatinine phosphokinase
• GABA = gamma aminobutyric acid
• LDH = lactate dehydrogenase

Suggested Reading

Burrows, G. E., Tyrl, R. J. 2001. Cicuta. In: *Toxic plants of North America*, ed. G. E. Burrows, R. J. Tyrl. Ames: Iowa State University Press.
Panter, K. E., Baker, D. C., Kechele, P. O. 1996. Water hemlock (*Cicuta douglasii*) toxicosis in sheep: pathologic description and prevention of lesions and death. *J Vet Diagn Invest* 8:474–80.

Author: Patricia Talcott

CIRCULATORY SHOCK

BASICS

DEFINITION
Circulatory shock is defined as severe insufficiency in capillary perfusion. Shock begins with a hormone-mediated *hyperdynamic phase* that is characterized by bounding pulses, tachycardia, and decreased capillary refill time of mucous membranes. This phase is transient and is quickly followed by the *hypodynamic phase* of circulatory failure. Usual causes of circulatory shock are marked depletion of extracellular fluid volume (*hypovolemic*), loss of effective cardiac pumping action (*cardiogenic*), and dysfunction of the small vessels (*vasulogenic*). In the most severe cases, it is often fatal if left untreated.

PATHOPHYSIOLOGY
The effective circulatory blood volume may be diminished by actual loss or sequestration of blood or plasma. Shock may result from diverse causes such as vascular and myocardial effects of circulating endotoxins from enteric organisms.

Hypovolemic Shock (Due to Reduction in Blood Volume)
• Loss of whole blood by external or internal hemorrhage
• Loss of plasma by exudation (e.g., burns) or into body cavities
• Loss of water and electrolytes by excessive sweating, diarrhea, diuresis, regurgitation, and transudation

Cardiogenic Shock (Due to Acute Changes in Cardiac Pumping Effectiveness)
• Interference with effective cardiac filling such as cardiac tamponade, constrictive pericarditis, and hydropericardium
• Restricted ventricular emptying such as acute cor pulmonale, increased vascular resistance, toxic myocardial depression, and cardiac dysrhythmias

Vasogenic Shock (Due to Changes in Venous Dysfunction or Peripheral Resistance).
• Endotoxins and vasoactive agents of anaphylaxis
• Vasomotor paralysis from CNS trauma or infection

SYSTEMS AFFECTED
• Cardiovascular—inability to provide sufficient circulating fluid volume leads to ischemia in other organs.
• GI—decrease in urine volume and mucosal necrosis as a result of microvascular thrombosis
• Lymphatic/immune—tendency toward thrombosis in the early stages, then hemorrhagic

GENETICS
N/A

INCIDENCE/PREVALENCE
N/A

SIGNALMENT
N/A

SIGNS

Clinical Signs
General Comments: Large varieties of clinical signs are associated with infection and include central depression, and altered cardiovascular status.

HISTORICAL FINDINGS
• Morbidity and mortality due to enterotoxemia or diarrhea
• Exposure to cardiotoxic plants, such as oleander (*Nerium oleander*), foxglove (*Digitalis purpurea*), lily of the valley (*Convallaria majalis*), yew (*Taxus* spp.), Indian hemp (*Apocynum cannabinum*), false hellebore (*Veratrum* spp.), milkweed (*Asclepias* spp.), avocado (*Persea americana*), oleander, caltrops (*Calotropis procera*), and red cotton (*Asclepia curassavica*)
• Exposure to calcium salts and ionophore coccidiostats

PHYSICAL EXAMINATION FINDINGS
• Visible weakness, obtundation, cold extremities, tachycardia with a weak pulse, decreased urination and defecation, cyanotic or pale mucus membranes, shallow breathing and prolonged capillary refill time.

CAUSES
• Sepsis, localized bacterial infection, myocarditis, dehydration, electrolyte and acid-base disturbances and cardiovascular anomalies
• Yew and false hellebore contain toxic alkaloids.
• Ionophore toxicity is known to occur in sheep and the use of ionophores for control of coccidiosis in goats is increasing.

DIAGNOSIS

DIFFERENTIAL DIAGNOSIS
Diagnosis is by recognition of characteristic clinical signs and clinicopathologic abnormalities.

CBC/BIOCHEMISTRY/URINALYSIS
• Depending on the organ system affected, laboratory evidence of hepatic, renal, or metabolic dysfunction, coagulopathy, and electrolyte imbalances may exist.
• Leukopenias with neutropenia, lymphopenia, or thrombocytopenia are often associated with severe sepsis and shock.

OTHER LABORATORY TESTS
• Arterial and venous blood gas analysis is helpful to evaluate pulmonary and metabolic function, respectively.
• Blood cultures are indicated when sepsis is suspected.

IMAGING
• Transabdominal, transrectal, or thoracic ultrasonography for assessment of fluid distribution
• Renal ultrasonography for assessment of cortical and or medullary sclerosis
• Echocardiography to assess cardiac function

DIAGNOSTIC PROCEDURES
• Thoracic radiographs help in recognition pulmonary edema.
• Direct or indirect blood pressure monitoring to assess hypotension

PATHOLOGIC FINDINGS
Generally reflect the primary underlying disease process

TREATMENT

APPROPRIATE HEALTH CARE
General Comments
This life threatening condition always warrants intensive care. Therapy should target the underlying infection and/or disease process and provide hemodynamic and pulmonary (oxygen) support and anti-inflammatory therapy.

Herd Management
Address historical problems resulting in shock

Individual Patient Care
Urgent repletion of circulating volume is of utmost importance
• Necessary volume of IV fluids should be calculated based on central venous pressure monitoring, but levels should be increased to supranormal values as demands following clinical shock are markedly elevated.
• A shock dose of 8% of the animal's body weight should be administered as initial bolus. Homologous blood may be of value if significant hemorrhaging has occurred and should be administered with two to six times the volume of a balanced electrolyte solution.
• Arterial blood oxygen levels need to be at least 60% concentration. Oxygen can be administered by endotracheal tube, mask, bag, or nasal cannula.

ACTIVITY
Strictly limited

DIET
Total or partial parenteral may be required to meet increased energy and metabolic demands due to shock.

CLIENT EDUCATION
Generally positive, but if the condition deteriorates, the prognosis becomes progressively worse.

MEDICATIONS

DRUGS OF CHOICE

• Supportive tissue perfusion with polyionic IV fluids is mandatory.
• Amount of fluid administered over 24 hours should = excess fluid loss + maintenance (starting at 100 mL/kg per 24 hours for first 10 kg + 50 mL/kg per 24 hours for second 10 kg + 25 mL/kg per 24 hours for weight > 20 kg).
• IV glucose is administered to meet the metabolic demands induced by shock.
• Dextrose can be administered in a 5 or 10% solution and should achieve 0.1–0.2 gm/kg per hour (5–10 gm/hour for 50 kg patient).
• Flunixin meglumine (0.25 mg/kg IV BID or TID)
• Whole plasma transfusion (15–30 mL/kg) to restore low oncotic pressure in cases of hypoalbuminemia. If available, hyperimmune plasma with a higher titer of antiendotoxin antibody may be beneficial.
• When indicated, treat all cases aggressively with IV antibiotics approved for food animal use, which can be reviewed on the Internet: (www.farad.org).
• Pressor or ionotrope therapy to increase effective circulatory fluid pressure. These drugs must be delivered by an IV pump to control their effect.
• Dopamine (5–20 μg/kg per min; usual starting dosage is 10 μg/kg per min)
• Dobutamine (5–40 μg/kg per min; usual starting dosage is 10 μg/kg per min)
• Epinephrine (0.1–3 μg/kg per min; usual starting dosage is 0.5 μg/kg per min)
• Norepinephrine (0.05–2 μg/kg per min; usual starting dosage is 0.5 μg/kg per min)
• Corticosteroid use is widely successful but only after circulatory volume has increased to a safe level because of their anti-inflammatory and membrane-stabilizing effects.
• Heparin may be used to prevent DIC in cases with acquired coagulopathies.
• Mannitol may be administered to increase urine flow and reduce cerebral edema.

CONTRAINDICATIONS

• Adrenergic drugs, especially catecholamines, are limited in success because they are vasoconstrictive, arrhythmogenic, and generally enhance tissue oxygen demands. The exception to this is anaphylactic shock in which they are critical for maintaining cardiac function.
• Drugs that cause or may exacerbate preexisting hypotension (e.g., acepromazine) should be avoided.
• Avoid potentially nephrotoxic drugs and those requiring hepatic metabolism.

FOLLOW-UP

PATIENT MONITORING

• Constant close attention during administration of therapeutic fluids and cardiac inotropic drugs until the animal has reached a stable condition is required.
• Physical examination every 2–4 hours with particular attention to heart and respiratory rate, temperature, urine output, presence of arrhythmias, pulse intensity, and mucous membrane coloration.
• Check PCV and TP every 12 hours during the initial treatment with IV fluid to expand the intravascular fluid volume and during equilibration with the extravascular pool.

PREVENTION/AVOIDANCE

Herd Management

Identify the primary disorder(s) and make necessary management changes and initiate specific therapies

Individual

Early detection and aggressive treatment of primary disease(s)
Aggressive treatment of sepsis and localized bacterial infections that have progressed to the stage where fluid intake of the animal has been compromised

POSSIBLE COMPLICATIONS

Multiple organ dysfunction (MOD) such as heart and renal failure, respiratory distress syndrome, and DIC

EXPECTED COURSE AND PROGNOSIS

If treatment is early enough, the prognosis is very good; as the condition progresses, prognosis becomes increasingly worse.

MISCELLANEOUS

AGE-RELATED FACTORS

Immune system response time and effectiveness decreases from peak capability with age. The urgency of treatment is compounded with increasing age.

ZOONOTIC POTENTIAL

Depends on the pathogen involved. Infectious contagious enteritis, such as salmonellosis, has zoonotic implications.

Suggested Reading
Cardiovascular system. 1994. In: *Goat medicine*, ed. M. C. Smith and D. M. Sherman. Philadelphia: Lea & Febiger
Cebra, C., and Cebra, M. 2002. Diseases of the cardiovascular system. In: *Sheep and goat medicine*, ed. D. G. Pugh. Philadelphia: W. B. Saunders.
Clark, D. R. 1986. Diseases of the cardiovascular and hemolymphatic systems. In: *Current veterinary therapy food animal practice 2*, ed. J. L. Howard. Philadelphia: W. B. Saunders.

Author: Benjamin J. Darien

CLEFT PALATE (PALATOSCHISIS)

 BASICS

DEFINITION
• Cleft palate (palatoschisis) is a common congenital anomaly characterized by a midline fissure of the hard and soft palate.
• Bilateral cleft palate is most common. The lesion is symmetrical and the ventral edge of the nasal septum can be seen from an open mouth view.
• Cleft palate is an occasional congenital anomaly affecting ruminants and camelids.
• Unilateral cleft palate is asymmetrical; the ventral edge of the nasal septum (vomer) is not visible because it is fused with the palatal shelf of the normal side.
• Cleft lip is not usually associated with cleft palate in ruminants. The majority of cases of cleft palate in cattle are thought to be genetic but the mode of inheritance is uncertain and other environmental factors may be implicated.
• Cleft palate has been documented to occur in association with consumption of piperidine alkaloids contained in plants of the lupine, hemlock, and tobacco families in cattle, sheep, and goats during early gestation.

PATHOPHYSIOLOGY
• The hard palate is formed by fusion of symmetrical palatal "shelves" that divide the primitive stomadeum into nasal cavity and oral cavity. Caudally, the same is true for the soft palate, which divides the nasal pharynx from the oral cavity and oropharynx.
• Experimental work indicates that cleft palate results from mechanical blockage by the tongue preventing fusion of the palatal "shelves."
• Any substance that inhibits normal fetal movement of the tongue during the critical period of palatal fusion will result in cleft palate.
• The critical period for palatal fusion is 35–40 days gestation in goats and sheep and 40–50 days in cattle.
• After the critical period, the edges of the palatal shelves are covered by epithelium that prevents fusion of the palatal edges with each other and the ventral edge of the nasal septum.

SYSTEMS AFFECTED
Potentially all depending on condition

GENETICS
• Cleft palate is a component of the inherited congenital neuromuscular syndrome of Charolais cattle.
• A familial history of progeny from dam or sire; having cleft palate may be present.

INCIDENCE/PREVALENCE
N/A

GEOGRAPHIC DISTRIBUTION
Worldwide

SIGNALMENT
Species
Potentially all ruminant species

Breed Predilections
• Cleft palate is a component of the inherited congenital neuromuscular syndrome of Charolais cattle.
• The condition has a higher prevalence in the Saanen breed compared to other breeds of goat.

Mean Age and Range
• The condition is usually diagnosed in neonates when the defect involves the hard palate or hard and soft palates.
• Small soft palate defects may be clinically inapparent and go undiagnosed.

Predominant Sex
N/A

SIGNS
• Nasal discharge of milk while nursing.
• Periodic sneezing and occasional coughing during and after nursing
• Respiratory distress (if aspiration of milk occurs); complications including rhinitis and aspiration pneumonia are common.
• Failure to thrive with poor weight gains is a consequence of cleft palate.
• Reluctance to nurse or bottle-feed.
• General unthriftiness (if aspiration occurs)

CAUSES AND RISK FACTORS
Plants containing alkaloids have been shown to produce cleft palate when fed to ruminant dams during the critical period for palate fusion. These plants include poison hemlock (*Conium maculatum*), burley tobacco (*Nicotiana tabacum*), and wild tree tobacco (*Nicotiana glauca*). *Lupinus* spp. also have been associated with cleft palate when ingested by pregnant ruminants.
• In humans, genetic factors and certain environmental teratogens such as cigarette smoke and ethanol have been implicated as causes of cleft palate.
• Cleft palate occurs due to developmental errors of the facial embryonic segments with subsequent craniofacial skeletal and soft tissue abnormalities in the roof, wall, and floor of the nasal cavity and the boundary between the nasal and oral cavities.
• Genetic and environmental factors are proposed.
• Risk factors include forage or pasture access to piperine-containing oleoresin and alkaloids by dam during early to mid gestation
• Goats are more sensitive to these teratogens than sheep and tailcup lupine (*L. caudatus*) only affects cattle.

 DIAGNOSIS

DIFFERENTIAL DIAGNOSIS
• Other causes of nasal regurgitation of milk and dysphagia in neonates
• Dysphagia in neonates due to white muscle disease (selenium deficiency)
• Oropharyngeal foreign body, esophageal obstruction, esophageal stricture, megaesophagus, pharyngeal trauma
• Neurologic causes of dysphagia and nasal regurgitation of feed (listeriosis, meningitis, cervical vagus injury) and retropharyngeal trauma
• Neuromuscular causes of dysphagia and nasal regurgitation of feed—botulism
• Nonpaltischisic congenital oropharynx malformations, esophageal stricture due to persistent right aortic arch
• Toxicities causing dysphagia—organophosphates, oral irritants

CBC/BIOCHEMISTRY/URINALYSIS
• CBC, if aspiration pneumonia is suspected
• Laboratory diagnostics are generally not useful, affected neonates with aspiration pneumonia will have an inflammatory leukogram.

OTHER LABORATORY TESTS
• Generally unnecessary; cleft palate is a clinical diagnosis.
• Whole blood selenium levels to rule out white muscle disease
• Tracheal lavage cytology if pneumonia is suspected

IMAGING
• Radiographs may demonstrate foreshortening of the palatal tissues on lateral, dorsoventral, and intraoral films.
• Contrast radiography to demonstrate nasal access by oral contents may be performed in equivocal cases or those with very small, hard to visualize defects.

DIAGNOSTIC PROCEDURES
• The condition is easily diagnosed by visual inspection and palpation of the dorsocaudal oral cavity and oropharynx.
• Endoscopy of the oral cavity, oropharynx, and nasopharynx may be diagnostic with small defects.

TREATMENT

• While surgical repair is frequent in humans and occasionally done for foals, there is little or no justification for it in ruminants. Treatment for the main secondary problem, pneumonia, is covered elsewhere in this text.
• Attempts at surgical repair in calves have a very high rate of surgical dehiscence.
• Most affected animals are euthanized.
• Contrary to "conventional wisdom," some young ruminants can thrive with cleft palate after early conversion to pail feeding or even when bottle-fed with a long nipple.

MEDICATIONS

Medical management of pneumonia is covered elsewhere in this text.

FOLLOW UP

PATIENT MONITORING
• Owners who elect to raise a young ruminant with cleft palate must always maintain a vigil for aspiration pneumonia. Second, weight should be monitored before weaning to ensure that adequate milk is being consumed.
• Calves should get fluid milk equivalent to 10%–15% body weight/day and kids need 15%–20%.

PREVENTION/AVOIDANCE
• Care should be taken to avoid ingestion of known teratogenic plants mentioned above, especially during the first trimester of gestation.
• Eradication of poisonous plants with herbicides may be helpful.
• Until genetic factors are better understood, breeding of animals with cleft palate should be avoided.

POSSIBLE COMPLICATIONS
The main complication is aspiration. Careful feeding should minimize this risk. Leaky nipples should be avoided when bottle-feeding.

MISCELLANEOUS

ASSOCIATED CONDITIONS
• Since cleft palate has been shown to be associated with decreased fetal movement, it is often associated with multiple congenital contractions of the limbs but these may resolve during the postnatal period.
• Occasional cases may be associated with other congenital defects such as arthrogryposis (cattle, goats, and sheep), micrognathia (sheep), or the absence of ears (sheep).

AGE-RELATED FACTORS
Condition is congenital, only seen in neonates.

ZOONOTIC POTENTIAL
N/A

PREGNANCY
• The dam/sire combination should not be repeated with subsequent breedings.
• Assess pasture type and forage consumption during early gestation for evidence of exposure to piperine-containing oleoresin and alkaloids.

RUMINANT SPECIES AFFECTED
Both ruminants and pseudoruminants (camelids) can be affected.

BIOSECURITY
N/A

PRODUCTION MANAGEMENT
N/A

SEE ALSO
Other causes of nasal regurgitation of milk and dysphagia in neonates
Dysphagia in neonates due to white muscle disease (selenium deficiency)

Oropharyngeal foreign body, esophageal obstruction, esophageal stricture, megaesophagus, pharyngeal trauma
Neurologic causes of dysphagia and nasal regurgitation of feed (listeriosis, meningitis, cervical vagus injury) and retropharyngeal trauma.
Neuromuscular causes of dysphagia and nasal regurgitation of feed—botulism
Non-palatoschisis congenital oropharynx malformations, esophageal stricture due to persistent right aortic arch
Toxicities causing dysphagia—organophosphates, oral irritants

ABBREVIATIONS
CBC = complete blood count

Suggested Reading
Bowman, K. F., Tate, L. P., Jr., Evans, L. H., Donawick, W. J. 1982, Mar 15. Complications of cleft palate repair in large animals. *J Am Vet Med Assoc*. 180(6): 652–57.
Griffith, J. W., Hobbs, B. A., Manders, E. K. 1987, Jan. Cleft palate, brachygnathia inferior, and mandibular oligodontia in a Holstein calf. *J Comp Pathol*. 97(1): 95–99.
Mulvihill, J. J., Mulvihill, C. G., Priester, W. A. 1980. Cleft palate in domestic animals: epidemiologic features. *Teratology* 21:109–12.
Panter, K. E., Keeler, R. F. 1993. Quinolizidine and piperidine alkaloid teratogens from poisonous plants and their mechanism of action in animals. *Vet Clin North Am: Food Animal Prac*. 9: 33–40.
Panter, K. E., Weinzweig, J., Gardner, D. R., Stegelmeier, B. L., James, L. F. 2000. Comparison of cleft palate induction by *Nicotiana glauca* in goats and sheep. *Teratology* 61, 203–10

Authors: Victor S. Cox and Simon F. Peek

CLOSTRIDIAL DISEASE: GI

BASICS

DEFINTION
Clostridial gastroenteritis is an acute inflammatory noncontagious disease of young ruminants that usually results in death.

PATHOPHYSIOLOGY
• Clostridial bacteria are ingested as spores from the environment or carrier animals and are considered normal bacterial flora.
• Factors favoring intestinal clostridial bacteria overgrowth, such as high-carbohydrate diets, result in rapid toxin production with subsequent clinical signs and death.
• Clinical signs depend on the predominate type of toxin produced although there is considerable crossover.
• There are four major lethal toxins (alpha, beta, epsilon, and iota) and five types (A–E). Alpha toxin (types A–E) usually results in an intravenous hemolytic crisis of the abdominal and thoracic cavities with or without subsequent icterus. Beta toxin (types B and C) results in necrosis and hemorrhage of affected tissues, especially the intestine. Epsilon toxin (types B and D) causes intestinal necrosis, and increases vascular permeability with subsequent hemorrhage and edema. Iota toxin (type E) causes increased vascular permeability.

SYSTEMS AFFECTED
The gastrointestinal tract is primarily affected with systemic involvement of most other systems especially cardiovascular and neurologic.

GENETICS
No genetic predisposition known

INCIDENCE/PREVALENCE
• The disease incidence has been reported to range from 0% to as high as 50% of calves (unsubstantiated) in the herd.
• *Clostridium perfringens* was diagnosed in 9.2% of calves with gastrointestinal disease or septicemia in a German study. On routine culture, type A is the most common type isolated from cattle. In a Montana study, type C was more common in clinical cases than type A. Type D may still occur in vaccinated feedlot lambs with an incidence up to 1%, whereas the incidence in unvaccinated feedlot lambs may approach 10%. As a disease syndrome, type D is probably the most common, especially in unvaccinated herds/flocks.

GEOGRAPHIC DISTRIBUTION
• Clostridial bacteria are common worldwide.
• *Clostridium perfringens* A, C, and D are considered problems in the United States. Type B (Europe, Africa, and Asia) is not considered a problem in the United States. Type E tends to be rarer but has been reported in calves in the United States.

SIGNALMENT
Acute onset of clinical signs followed by rapid death or sudden death in a healthy, rapidly growing young ruminant is classic. Type A typically affects calves and lambs less then 3 months of age. Type C is most typical in calves and lambs less than 2 weeks old, especially those with high-producing dams. Type D is more common in feedlot lambs and occasionally calves.

SIGNS
• Because there is considerable overlap in the clinical signs among *Clostridium perfringens* types, clinical signs are suggestive but not definitive in differentiating the type.
• Type A is most commonly associated with depression, abomasal bloat, and abomasitis. Early signs may present as abdominal pain with the patient kicking at the abdomen. The animal becomes increasingly depressed and uncomfortable as abdominal distension progresses. Eventually the young ruminant becomes recumbent and semicomatose.
• Type C has commonly been associated with acute fatal hemorrhagic enteritis in young calves and lambs. This bloody, mucoid diarrhea has also been a consistent finding in goat kids.
• Type D, the agent of enterotoxemia also known as "overeating disease," primarily affects young ruminants undergoing nutritional changes.
• Regardless of the type, many cases are simply found dead. If affected animals are found alive, most cases present with colic and/or neurologic signs such as convulsions and opisthotonus prior to death.
• Young ruminants surviving more than 4–5 hours may develop hemorrhagic diarrhea.

CAUSES
Clostridium perfringens types A, B, C, and D

RISK FACTORS
• Risk factors usually include a change of diet (usually from milk/forage to grain), feedlot animals on a high-grain diet, or offspring of dams that produce an abundance of milk. In addition, lush pastures may also predispose to the disease.
• Singles are more likely to be affected than twins. The healthy, rapidly growing young ruminant is most at risk.
• Copper deficiency may contribute to type pathology.

DIAGNOSIS

DIFFERENTIAL DIAGNOSIS
• Anything causing acute death: anthrax, various poisonings, other clostridial diseases
• Right displacement and torsion of the abomasum
• Salmonellosis
• Sarcina bacteria may be involved in abomasal bloat cases.
• Ruminal acidosis
• Leptospira
• Polioencephalomalacia

CBC/BIOCHEMISTRY/URINALYSIS
In sheep afflicted with type D, hyperglycemia (more than five times normal) and glucosuria may be present but are inconsistent findings.

OTHER LABORATORY TESTS
Culture and impression smears may be useful. Toxin identification is essential for control and prevention recommendations.

IMAGING
N/A

DIAGNOSTIC PROCEDURES
• Intestinal contents may be stained and examined for large gram-positive rods. Culture and toxin typing would be necessary for definitive identification. It is important to note that *C. perfringens* is a normal inhabitant of the GI system, especially type A.
• Because clostridial organisms proliferate rapidly after death, intestinal contents should be collected immediately after death. Intestinal fluid for toxin evaluation should be placed in a cool environment or frozen until testing because the toxins, especially beta toxin, are fragile.
• ELISA and counter-immunoelectrophoresis tests are now offered and have proven comparable to the traditional mouse lethality tests.

PATHOLOGIC FINDINGS
• Type A (alpha toxin) necropsy findings show watery blood, icterus, hemoglobinuria, excessive fluid in abdominal and thoracic cavities, and evidence of hemorrhages on thoracic and abdominal viscera, yet these findings are not consistent among calves.
• Type B (alpha, beta, and epsilon toxins) necropsy findings tend to be restricted to the intestinal tract, liver, and adjacent lymphatics in which inflammation, ulceration, and necrosis are evident.
• Type C (alpha and beta toxins) presents with an acute hemorrhagic enteritis in which bloody diarrhea may or may not be present at death. An additional finding in type C disease is swollen and hemorrhagic mesenteric lymph nodes.

• Paintbrush hemorrhages of the subendocardium of the left ventricle are most typical of type D (alpha and epsilon toxins). Additionally, hydropericardium is considered one of the most significant lesions of type D.

TREATMENT

APPROPRIATE HEALTH CARE
• The response to treatment is usually poor. However, if right-sided bloat is evident, relieving the distention in the abomasum may benefit some patients.
• Intravenous or subcutaneous infusion of clostridium C and D antitoxin may be beneficial at doses ranging from 3 ml in lambs to over 30 ml in adult cattle. Dosages can be repeated every 3–4 hours provided improvement is seen. Anaphylactoid reactions may occur.
• Activated charcoal and mineral oil have also been suggested but have not been scientifically evaluated. Chelating agents, such as EDTA, have been reported to influence the disease outcome if given early in the disease.

NURSING CARE
Maintenance: alkalinizing IV fluids

ACTIVITY
N/A

DIET
If at all possible, eliminate oral nutrition during treatment to decrease bacterial substrate.

CLIENT EDUCATION
N/A

SURGICAL CONSIDERATIONS
N/A

MEDICATIONS

DRUGS OF CHOICE
Procaine penicillin G (300,000 IU/ml) at 1 ml/11 kg (1 ml/25 lb) orally, IM, or subcutaneously is the drug of choice.

CONTRAINDICATIONS
Appropriate milk and meat withdrawal times must be followed for all compounds administered to food-producing animals.

PRECAUTIONS
N/A

POSSIBLE INTERACTIONS
N/A

ALTERNATIVE DRUGS
Oral sulfadimethoxine has been recommended.

FOLLOW-UP

PATIENT MONITORING
N/A

PREVENTION/AVOIDANCE
• Passive antibodies to *Clostridium perfringens* C & D can be protective.
• The C & D toxoid may be given to dams in late gestation or to neonates beginning at 10 days of age and 2 weeks later. Young stock should be revaccinated at weaning and prior to feed changes.
• Antitoxin may be given to neonates at birth during outbreak situations. In a reported outbreak, 5 ml of *C. perfringens* type C & D were administered subcutaneously to neonatal calves and no more cases occurred. Decreasing concentrate and increasing roughage may reduce feedlot deaths.
• Additionally, chlortetracycline may be added to concentrates to help decrease the incidence of type D. Type A is poorly antigenic; effective vaccines have not been developed, although autogenous vaccines have been used with mixed results. Suggested methods to prevent type A disease include proper animal husbandry, sanitation, and feeding.
• There has been some suggestion that when young ruminants ingest large amounts of milk, the milk backflows to the rumen leading to *Clostridium perfringens* type A overgrowth and subsequent disease. Therefore, avoiding excessive intake may be helpful in disease prevention of type A. Vaccines for type B have been developed and appear useful in countries in which the disease occurs.

POSSIBLE COMPLICATIONS
N/A

EXPECTED COURSE AND PROGNOSIS
If the patient is still ambulatory when treatment is initiated, the prognosis is fair at best. If the patient is recumbent, the prognosis is guarded to grave. Mortality approaches 100% regardless of type.

MISCELLANEOUS

ASSOCIATED CONDITIONS
N/A

AGE-RELATED FACTORS
This is a disease of young, healthy ruminants although adults have been reported to be sporadically affected.

ZOONOTIC POTENTIAL
No known zoonotic potential

PREGNANCY
N/A

RUMINANT SPECIES AFFECTED
All ruminant species may be affected but best documentation is in sheep and cattle.

BIOSECURITY
The organism is widespread in the environment and within the gastrointestinal tract, thus biosecurity measures are of little benefit; however, carcasses should be disposed of properly by burial or incineration. A high concentration of bacterial spores may contaminate the area.

PRODUCTION MANAGEMENT
N/A

SYNONYMS
Enterotoxemia
Lamb dysentery (type B)
Overeating disease (type D)
Pulpy kidney disease (type D)
Struck (type C)
Yellow lamb disease (type A)

SEE ALSO
Anything causing acute death: anthrax, various poisonings, other clostridial diseases
Leptospira
Polioencephalomalacia
Right displacement and torsion of the abomasum
Ruminal acidosis
Salmonellosis
Sarcina bacteria

ABBREVIATIONS
ELISA = enzyme-linked immunosorbent assay
IM = intramuscular
IV = intravenous

Suggested Reading
Dennison, A. C., VanMetre, D. C., Callan, R. J., Dinsmore, P., Mason, G. L., Ellis, R. P. 2002, Sep 1. Hemorrhagic bowel syndrome in dairy cattle: 22 cases (1997–2000). *J Am Vet Med Assoc.* 221(5): 686–89.
Herrmann, J. A. 2002, Nov 1. Thoughts on bowel treatment in cattle. *J Am Vet Med Assoc.* 221(9): 1250.
Marks, S. L., Kather, E. J. 2003, Jun 24. Antimicrobial susceptibilities of canine *Clostridium difficile* and *Clostridium perfringens* isolates to commonly utilized antimicrobial drugs. *Vet Microbiol.* 94(1): 39–45.
Sato, Y., Matsuura, S. 1998, Aug. Gastric mucormycosis in a sika deer (*Cervus nippon*) associated with proliferation of *Clostridium perfringens*. *J Vet Med Sci.* 60(8): 981–83.
Silvera, M., Finn, B., Reynolds, K. M., Taylor, D. J. 2003, Jul 12. *Clostridium tertium* as a cause of enteritis in cattle. *Vet Rec.* 153(2): 60.
Sugimoto, N., Horiguchi, Y., Matsuda, M. 1996. Mechanism of action of *Clostridium perfringens* enterotoxin. *Adv Exp Med Biol.* 391:257–69.

Author: Jerry R. Roberson

CLOSTRIDIAL MYOSITIS

BASICS

DEFINITION
Clostridial myositis is a term used to describe a group of acute diseases characterized by a rapid course of myonecrosis and high mortality.

PATHOPHYSIOLOGY
• Any muscle or muscle groups may be involved such as rear and forelimb muscle systems, abaxial muscles, the diaphragm, and the heart. When an area of muscle becomes anaerobic (such as a bruise or injury), the spore may convert to a bacterial toxin-producing state.
• The organisms then produce powerful exotoxins, which are responsible for the local necrotizing myositis and systemic toxemia.
• The predominant signs that develop depend on the predominant clostridial organism.

SYSTEMS AFFECTED
Musculoskeletal

GENETICS
None

INCIDENCE/PREVALENCE
• The incidence will rarely be more than 10% and only during outbreaks. The prevalence will be virtually zero because affected livestock usually die within hours of the disease onset.
• Some herds may go for many years without clostridial myositis cases.
• Most cases are seen in the late summer to early winter.

GEOGRAPHIC DISTRIBUTION
Worldwide

SIGNALMENT
• Clostridial myositis is typically a disease of young cattle and is relatively rare in other ruminants.
• Cattle over 2 years old appear to develop a natural resistance to the disease.

SIGNS
• Sudden death common
• If blackleg, there will be areas of subcutaneous emphysema.
• Affected cattle are usually downers or extremely lame.
• Affected areas may be cold to the touch and will appear be swollen and edematous (if malignant edema).
• Other common nonspecific signs are depression, anorexia, and lethargy.

CAUSES
• *Clostridium chauvoei* is the agent of classic blackleg.
• *Clostridium septicum* is the agent of malignant edema.
• The organisms exist as spores in the environment. Cattle are thought to eat these spores in the process of grazing. The spores then find their way to various locations within the bovine (exact mechanism not known but may be via tissue macrophages). The spores are also normal in bovine feces. Conditions causing anaerobic muscle allow the spores to convert to the bacterial toxin-producing state.

RISK FACTORS
• Animals on high planes of nutrition and in excellent body condition are most likely to develop the disease, the assumption being a larger muscle mass.
• Herds that are not vaccinated are most at risk.

DIAGNOSIS

DIFFERENTIAL DIAGNOSIS
Conditions that result in sudden death in young, well-muscled ruminants should be considered as differentials. These include but are not limited to gunshot, anthrax, snakebite, *Clostridium perfringens*, taxus (Japanese yew), various toxicants (lead, arsenic), nitrate and cyanide poisoning.

CBC/BIOCHEMISTRY/URINALYSIS
Of little benefit

OTHER LABORATORY TESTS
Of little benefit

IMAGING
Of little benefit

DIAGNOSTIC PROCEDURES
• Diagnosis is usually based on characteristic signs and gross lesions; impression smears showing large gram-positive rods may be helpful.
• Aspirates from the affected tissue can be submitted for fluorescent antibody testing and anaerobic bacterial culture.

PATHOLOGIC FINDINGS
Necropsy should reveal an area of "black" muscle necrosis and subcutaneous gas (hence the name blackleg). The affected muscle may have an odor of rancid butter. Malignant edema tends to have more edema than subcutaneous gas.

TREATMENT

APPROPRIATE HEALTH CARE
If treatment is considered appropriate, supplying the animal with feed and water would be a necessity. Antitoxin for these clostridial organisms is not readily available.

NURSING CARE
As above

ACTIVITY
The animal would limit its own activity.

DIET
N/A

CLIENT EDUCATION
The most important client education is to convey the need to protect unaffected herd mates.

SURGICAL CONSIDERATIONS
None, short of serial fasciotomy of affected areas to allow aeration and drainage.

MEDICATIONS

DRUGS OF CHOICE
• Procaine penicillin G at high doses (24,000 IU/kg) IM; injecting PPG around the affected tissue may help stop the advancement of the clostridial organisms.
• Anti-inflammatory drugs may be administered for pain, shock, and inflammation.
• With blackleg, it has been recommended to place skin incisions within the affected area to allow oxygen to the area.
• Treatment is usually a moot point because most are found dead.

CONTRAINDICATIONS
• Because of the poor prognosis, humane euthanasia should be considered. Slaughter is usually not an option.
• Drug withdrawal time must be determined and maintained for the treated animal.

PRECAUTIONS
None

POSSIBLE INTERACTIONS
None

ALTERNATIVE DRUGS
Many other antimicrobials may be effective, but penicillin is the drug of choice.

FOLLOW-UP

PATIENT MONITORING
N/A

PREVENTION/AVOIDANCE
• Vaccinate all young stock (< 2 years of age) at least twice a year. Valuable and purebred stock should be vaccinated 3–4 times a year. Protective immunity should occur by 2 weeks postvaccine.
• Vaccinate cows in late gestation to boost colostral immunity for neonates that won't be vaccinated until the next cattle working period.
• When faced with an outbreak, vaccinate all susceptible stock and administer PPG at the same time in an attempt to prevent further cases while you're waiting for protective titers to develop.
• Vaccines are economical and efficacious.
• One vaccine to a calf that is 1 or 2 months old will usually not lend protective immunity because of interference with passive immunity.
• Carcasses should be burnt or buried deeply and covered with lime, as they represent concentrated areas of clostridial spores.

POSSIBLE COMPLICATIONS
None

EXPECTED COURSE AND PROGNOSIS
Prognosis is guarded to grave at best. Even if the animal survives, it may be permanently disabled.

MISCELLANEOUS

ASSOCIATED CONDITIONS
None

AGE-RELATED FACTORS
The disease appears to be most common among young ruminants between 3 months and 2 years of age.

ZOONOTIC POTENTIAL
None

PREGNANCY
N/A

RUMINANT SPECIES AFFECTED
Predominantly bovine, however goats, sheep, and camelids may be affected.

BIOSECURITY
N/A

PRODUCTION MANAGEMENT
Vaccination should help prevent clinical disease.

SYNONYMS
Black leg
Malignant edema

SEE ALSO
Anthrax
Clostridium perfringens
Gunshot
Nitrate and cyanide poisoning
Snakebite
Taxus (Japanese yew)
Various toxicants (lead, arsenic)

ABBREVIATIONS
IM = intramuscularly
PPG = procaine penicillin G

Suggested Reading
De Groot, B., Dewey, C. E., Griffin, D. D., Perino, L. J., Moxley, R. A., Hahn, G. L. 1997, Sep 15. Effect of booster vaccination with a multivalent clostridial bacterin-toxoid on sudden death syndrome mortality rate among feedlot cattle. *J Am Vet Med Assoc.* 211(6): 749–53.
Farrow, C. S. 1999, Jul. Gas. Radiographic indicator of infection. *Vet Clin North Am Food Anim Pract.* 15(2): 253–64, vi.
Troxel, T. R., Burke, G. L., Wallace, W. T., Keaton, L. W., McPeake, S. R., Smith, D., Nicholson, I. 1997, Jan. Clostridial vaccination efficacy on stimulating and maintaining an immune response in beef cows and calves. *J Anim Sci.* 75(1): 19–25.
Troxel, T. R., Gadberry, M. S., Wallace, W. T., Kreider, D. L., Shockey, J. D., Colburn, E. A., Widel, P., Nicholson, I. 2001, Oct. Clostridial antibody response from injection-site lesions in beef cattle, long-term response to single or multiple doses, and response in newborn beef calves. *J Anim Sci.* 79(10): 2558–64.
Useh, N. M., Nok, A. J., Esievo, K. A. 2003, Dec. Pathogenesis and pathology of blackleg in ruminants: the role of toxins and neuraminidase. A short review. *Vet Q.* 25(4): 155–59.

Author: Jerry R. Roberson

CLUB LAMB DISEASE

 ## BASICS

OVERVIEW
• Club lamb disease or club lamb fungus is another name for ringworm or fungal skin infection in lambs.
• Ringworm is a common problem in show lambs but is uncommon in commercial sheep and goat herds.

SIGNALMENT
• Round, raised skin lesions are most commonly noticed on the face and ears of show lambs but lesions may develop under the wool anywhere on the body.
• There is no age, breed, or sex predilection for ringworm, but the condition most commonly occurs during the summer show season when market lambs less than 125 pounds (60+ kg) are repeatedly shorn, washed, and transported to shows.

SIGNS
• Round, raised skin lesions appear on the face, ears, and neck.
• The wool over affected skin is raised above the surrounding fleece.
• Some lesions appear mildly pruritic.
• Alopecia develops from fungal invasion of the keratinized hair shafts.
• Crusts form from accumulation of fungal hyphae and epithelial debris.
• The underlying skin appears reddened, thick, and abraded.

CAUSES AND RISK FACTORS
• The more common fungal species involved are *Trichophyton verrucosum* and *T. mentagrophytes.*
• Ringworm is transmitted by direct contact with infected animals or indirect contact from contaminated equipment such as clippers, shears, hoof trimmers, hoses, and buckets.
• Repeated bathing and excessively short shearing of show lambs irritates the skin and makes the epidermis more susceptible to fungal infection.

 ## DIAGNOSIS

DIFFERENTIAL DIAGNOSIS
• Soremouth, also known as contagious ecthyma or orf
• Chemical burns
• Parasitic skin disease
• Photosensitivity

CBC/BIOCHEMISTRY/URINALYSIS
N/A

OTHER LABORATORY TESTS
• Fungal culture on Sabourad's dextrose agar.
• Microscopic examination of wet mounts prepared with 20% potassium or sodium hydroxide from skin scrapings or hair shafts. *Trichophyton* spores appear as round or polyhedral, highly refractive bodies in chains.
• *Trichophyton* species do not fluoresce under Wood's lamp examination.

IMAGING
N/A

DIAGNOSTIC PROCEDURES
N/A

PATHOLOGIC FINDINGS
N/A

 ## TREATMENT

• Ringworm is highly contagious and affected animals should be isolated and confined separately until after the wool has grown back and the lesions have healed.
• Health certificates should not be written and travel should not be allowed for affected animals until after the lesions have healed.
• Ringworm is zoonotic.
• Ringworm is a self-limiting infection and most lesions heal within 4 to 5 weeks.
• Segregation and treatment of affected lambs may decrease spread to other animals and contamination of the environment.

 ## MEDICATIONS

• Crusts and debris should be removed by scraping or brushing.
• Medication should be vigorously rubbed or brushed into the lesions.
• Medications used for daily local treatment of a few distinctly separate lesions (adapted from Pugh, 2002):
    (1) Dilute topical iodine compounds (2–5%)
    (2) 2% chlorhexidine solution
    (3) 2 to 5% lime sulfur
    (4) 3% captan
• Sprays and washes can be applied to the entire body surface daily for treatment of widespread infections or when prophylactic treatment of contacts may be desirable.
    (5) 5% lime sulfur
    (6) 3% captan
    (7) 0.5% sodium hypochlorite
• Systemic treatment with oral griseofulvin produces variable results.

CONTRAINDICATIONS
• Ringworm is a self-limiting disease of animals that are used for food. An adequate withdrawal time must be established and followed for any medication applied topically or administered orally.
• Griseofulvin should not be used in animals intended for food in the United States.
• Captan should not be used in animals intended for food in the United States.

CLUB LAMB DISEASE

FOLLOW-UP

PATIENT MONITORING
N/A

PREVENTION/AVOIDANCE
• Animals with club lamb disease should not travel to shows and should be segregated to prevent transmission to unaffected stock.
• Equipment such as trimmers and shears should be thoroughly cleaned between flocks to prevent the spread of ringworm.
• Housing facilities should be thoroughly cleaned and sprayed with 2.5 to 5% phenolic disinfectant, dilute iodine, 2% chlorhexidine, 5% lime sulfur, 5% formalin, 5% sodium hypochlorite, or 3% captan after the lesions have healed.

POSSIBLE COMPLICATIONS
Lambs in poor physical condition/BCS or with low nutritional status are susceptible to secondary bacterial infection of ringworm lesions. Poor physical condition or inadequate nutrition should be corrected with improved management.

EXPECTED COURSE AND PROGNOSIS
Club lamb disease is self-limiting and usually resolves in individuals within 4 to 5 weeks. The course of disease through the entire flock may run several months.

MISCELLANEOUS

ASSOCIATED CONDITIONS
N/A

AGE-RELATED FACTORS
Club lamb disease is usually limited to market lambs.

ZOONOTIC POTENTIAL
Trichophyton species are readily transmitted to humans. Persons examining or treating affected animals should wear protective gloves and wash thoroughly after handling affected animals.

PREGNANCY
N/A

RUMINANT SPECIES AFFECTED
Sheep; occasionally goats housed with sheep

BIOSECURITY
• Club lamb disease is highly contagious and is easily spread through direct contact and indirect contact with contaminated equipment and facilities.
• Show lambs should be housed separately from the main flock for 4 to 5 weeks following return to the flock.

PRODUCTION MANAGEMENT
Lambs in poor body condition and low nutritional status are more susceptible to ringworm.

SYNONYMS
Club lamb fungus

SEE ALSO
Chemical burns
Contagious ecthyma, or orf
Parasitic skin disease
Soremouth

ABBREVIATIONS
BCS = body condition score

Suggested Reading
McKellar, Q., Fishwick, G., Rycroft, A. 1987, Aug 22. Ringworm in housed sheep. *Vet Rec.* 121(8): 168–69.
Mullowney, P. C. 1984, Mar. Skin diseases of sheep. *Vet Clin North Am Large Anim Pract.* 6(1): 131–42.
Pier, A. C., Smith, J. M., Alexiou, H., Ellis, D. H., Lund, A., Pritchard, R. C. 1994. Animal ringworm—its etiology, public health significance and control. *J Med Vet Mycol.* 32 Suppl 1:133–50.
Pugh, D. G. 2002. *Sheep and goat medicine.* Philadelphia: W. B. Saunders.
Radostits, O. M., Gay, C. C., Blood, D. C., Hinchcliff, K. W. 2000. *Veterinary medicine*, 9th ed. Philadelphia: W. B. Saunders.
Sargison, N. D., Thomson, J. R., Scott, P. R., Hopkins, G. 2002, Jun 15. Ringworm caused by *Trichophyton verrucosum*—an emerging problem in sheep flocks. *Vet Rec.* 150(24): 755–56.

Author: Joan S. Bowen

CNS: BRAIN LESIONS

BASICS

OVERVIEW
• Brain diseases often affect only one portion of the brain; however, multifocal lesions are possible.
• Disorders can be due to infectious, congenital, nutritional, toxic, metabolic, immune-mediated, neoplastic, and traumatic causes among other causes.

PATHOPHYSIOLOGY

Brain Abscess
Abscesses can be caused by direct spread of infection or septic embolism to cerebral vessels.

Meningitis
• Inflammation of the meninges
• Often due to infectious agents such as bacteria, viruses, fungi, protozoa, or parasites
• Other causes include chemical agents and immune-mediated diseases

Cerebellar Hypoplasia
Lack of development or loss of one or more layers of the cerebellar cortex usually occurs due to in utero viral infections.

Hydrocephalus
Accumulation of excess CSF within the ventricular system of the brain

SYSTEMS AFFECTED
CNS

GENETICS
N/A

INCIDENCE/PREVALENCE
Unknown

GEOGRAPHIC DISTRIBUTION
Worldwide in distribution

SIGNALMENT
• All species
• Bacterial causes of meningitis are more common in ruminants.
• Viral infections in cattle, sheep, and goats can result in hydranencephaly syndrome.

Species
All ruminant species

Breed Predilections
N/A

Mean Age and Range
N/A

Predominant Sex
There is no predominant sex.

SIGNS
Signs of CNS disease in the brain depend on the location of the lesions (see Table 1).

Meningitis
• Earliest signs include anorexia, diarrhea, fever, stiff neck, and hyperesthesia.
• Signs progress to decreased sensation, propulsive walking, status epilepticus, and coma.

Brain Abscess
Signs are those of a steadily progressive mass lesion and can occur in any part of the brain.

Hydrocephalus and Cerebellar Hypoplasia
• Dome-shaped calvarium
• Often open fontanelle in neonates
• Congenital causes usually result in symmetric, nonprogressive signs.
• Degenerative causes of disorder such as demyelination diseases and spongiform encephalopathies have progressive signs.

CAUSES AND RISK FACTORS

Meningitis
• Neonatal ruminants
  • Sequela of septicemia caused by *E. coli, Salmonella* spp., or *Streptococci* spp.
  • Failure of passive transfer predisposes to oomphlophlebitis or enteritis, with hematogenous spread to the CNS.
• Adult animals
  • Thrombotic meningoencephalitis (TMS) in cattle due to *Haemophilus somnus* and septicemia in feeder lambs by *H. agni* spread to CNS via hematogenous route.
  • *Pseudomonas aeruginosa* mastitis of cattle and goats
  • *Pasteurella haemolytica* and *P. multocida* pneumonia or hemorrhagic septicemia.
  • *Listeria monocytogenes* infection ascends to the CNS via transaxonal migration in cranial nerves.

Brain Abscess
There is usually a history of concurrent infection such as inner ear or respiratory infection. Otitis interna infections may spread by extension to the brain stem. Respiratory and other infections spread hematogenously to any part of the brain.

Hydrocephalus and Cerebellar Hypoplasia
• Occasional idiopathic congenital malformation
• Prenatal viral infections with such viruses as akabane virus, bluetongue virus, bovine virus diarrhea virus are possible causes of hydrocephalus in ruminants.

• The akabane virus is spread by mosquitoes and the midge.
• Degenerative causes include demyelinating diseases, spongiform encephalopathies, and abiotrophies.

DIAGNOSIS

DIFFERENTIAL DIAGNOSIS

Meningitis
• Hypomagnesemia and hypoglycemia signs resemble meningitis. Neonates may have these conditions concurrently in cases of septic meningitis.
• Cervical vertebral fractures and luxations can result in similar neck stiffness and pain.

Brain Abscess
Other space-occupying masses in the CNS such as tumors

Hydrocephalus and Cerebellar Hypoplasia
Spongiform encephalopathies, demyelinating diseases, and abiotrophies

CBC/BIOCHEMISTRY/URINALYSIS

Meningitis
• Findings are inconsistent and are usually related to concurrent conditions such as septicemia, diarrhea, or overaggressive fluid therapy.
• Possible leukocytosis, left shift, toxic changes
• Hyperkalemia, respiratory acidosis, hypoglycemia, hyponatremia, or hypernatremia

Hydrocephalus and Cerebellar Hypoplasia
Normal findings

OTHER LABORATORY FINDINGS

Meningitis (Bacterial) and Brain Abscesses
CSF findings can include:
• Turbid and white-to-amber in color
• May foam when shaken
• May clot
• Increased protein concentrations (20–270 mg/dl)
• Xanthochromia
• Increased WBC count (avg. 4000 WBC/ml)
• CSF concentration of glucose often < 50% of the corresponding blood concentration
• Possible positive culture or using Gram stain may show high bacterial titers.

IMAGING
Advanced imaging with CT or MRI can identify many neurologic defects, but is of limited availability for large animals.

Table 1

Symptoms Associated with Neurological Lesions.	
Brain stem lesions	Altered mentation—depression, stupor, coma Circling Ataxia, falling Hemiparesis or tetraparesis Cranial nerves III–XII—deficits Visual deficits (normal pupils)
Vestibular lesions	Loss of balance Head tilt Falling or rolling Circling Nystagmus Strabismus Cranial nerve deficits (possible V, VI, VII in central lesions and possible VII in peripheral lesions) Horner's syndrome possible in peripheral lesions Cerebellar signs of mental depression and hemiparesis with ipsilateral postural reaction deficits (ataxic) possible in central lesions.
Cerebellar lesions	Dysmetria, spastic, stiff-limbed gait with normal strength Truncal ataxia Intention tremors Broad-based stance Postural reactions delayed with exaggerated responses +/− Menace deficit with normal PLR +/− Anisocoria (pupil dilated contralateral to side of lesion) +/− Opisthotonus (rare) +/− Vestibular signs (rare)
Cerebral lesions	Altered mental status—most commonly depression, lethargy Occasional hyperexcitability Change in behavior Normal gait on level surface with postural defects (delayed) Circling, twisted head and trunk (pleurothotonus), head pressing Abnormal gait going up or down hill CP deficits Menace decreased or absent with normal PLR Seizures Coma

Hydrocephalus
• Some neonates with hydrocephalus have an open fontanelle, which can allow ultrasound examination of the lateral ventricles for dilation and increased fluid accumulation.
• Radiographs of the skull may indicate a thin and possibly dome-shaped calvarium.

DIAGNOSTIC PROCEDURES

Hydrocephalus and Cerebellar Hypoplasia
• Blood for virus isolation, serologic testing, and quantitative immunoglobulin determination can be useful in cases due to in utero viral infection.
• Presuckle serum samples may be seropositive for akabane or bluetongue virus.

PATHOLOGIC FINDINGS

GROSS FINDINGS

Meningitis
• Meningeal vessels are congested.
• Meninges are swollen, opalescent, and petechiated.

Hydrocephalus and Cerebellar Hypoplasia
• Domed skull
• Dilated lateral ventricles
• Thinning of cerebellar cortices
• Secondary skeletal changes may occur in viral diseases such as arthrogryposis, abnormally curved ribs, kyphosis, and brachygnathia.

HISTOPATHOLOGICAL FINDINGS

Meningitis
• Meninges infiltrated by neutrophils and lymphocytes
• Endarteritis of meningeal vessels
• Choroiditis
• Leptomeningeal hemorrhages
• Bacterial colonies around blood vessels, meninges, and brain parenchyma

Brain Abscesses
In chronic abscesses, fibrinous leptomeningitis may develop adjacent to the abscess.

CNS: BRAIN LESIONS

Hydrocephalus and Cerebellar Hypoplasia

• If disease is a result of akabane virus infection in the neonate, there may be additional neurologic pathology such as nonsuppurative encephalomyelitis, necrosis, and endothelial proliferation.
• Thinning of periventricular white matter

TREATMENT

Treatment of brain disorders involves treatment of the specific disease if possible and supportive care and prevention of life-threatening complications such as brain edema.

Meningitis (Bacterial) and Brain Abscesses

Early recognition and treatment with appropriate antibiotic therapy are essential.

Cerebellar Hypoplasia and Hydrocephalus

No specific treatment is available.

MEDICATIONS

Meningitis (Bacterial)

• Appropriate antibiotic therapy based on Gram stain characteristics of sedimented bacteria and the initial 24-hour cultures to begin treatment as soon as possible
• CSF antibiotic concentrations should range from 10 to 30 times the MIC of the infecting bacteria. Note that some antibiotics more effectively cross the blood-brain barrier (BBB) than others. Bactericidal antibiotics are preferable to bacteriostatic antibiotics.

Meningitis (Protozoal)

May respond to sulfa/pyrimethamine combination or clindamycin therapy

CONTRAINDICATIONS

• In cases of infectious meningitis, glucocorticoids are usually contraindicated; however, a single high-dose short-term course of dexamethasone or methylprednisolone may control complications such as acute cerebral edema.
• Appropriate milk and meat withdrawal times must be followed for all compounds administered to food-producing animals.
• Steroids should not be used in pregnant animals.

FOLLOW-UP

PATIENT MONITORING

Monitor for progression of neurologic signs

PREVENTION/AVOIDANCE

Meningitis (Bacterial)

• Ensure appropriate colostrum intake by neonates
• Appropriate environmental sanitation
• Quarantine of new animals brought to farm to prevent spread of infectious disease

POSSIBLE COMPLICATIONS

Depends on underlying cause of disease

EXPECTED COURSE AND PROGNOSIS

Meningitis (Bacterial)

Ensure appropriate colostrum intake by neonates

Hydrocephalus

Neonates often die of secondary conditions such as malnutrition and septicemia due to inability to suckle. Animals that survive have permanent neurologic deficits.

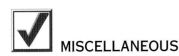

MISCELLANEOUS

ASSOCIATED CONDITIONS
Spinal cord lesions and peripheral nerve disorders

AGE-RELATED FACTORS
• Congenital hydrocephalus and cerebellar hypoplasia occur during fetal development.
• Secondary obstructive (adult onset) hydrocephalus is generally due to obstruction of CSF flow due to such causes as intracranial masses or impaired CSF resorption at arachnoid villi due to inflammation.

ZOONOTIC POTENTIAL
E. coli, Salmonella spp., and *Streptococci* spp. can be zoonotic. Care should be included in the handling of laboratory samples.

PREGNANCY

Cerebellar Hypoplasia and Hydrocephalus
Most commonly occur in neonates due to in utero viral infections

SEE ALSO
Cervical vertebral fractures and luxations
Demyelinating diseases
Hypoglycemia
Hypomagnesemia
Septic meningitis
Spongiform encephalopathies

ABBREVIATIONS
BBB = blood brain barrier
CNS = central nervous system
CP deficits = conscious proprioceptive deficits
CSF = cerebral spinal fluid
CT = computed tomography
MIC = minimum inhibitory concentration
MRI = magnetic resonance imaging
TMS = thrombotic meningoencephalitis
WBC = white blood cell

Suggested Reading
Aiello, S. E., ed. 1998. Meningitis and encephalitis. In: *Merck veterinary manual*. 8th ed. Whitehouse Station, NJ: Merck & Co.

Braund, K. G., ed. *Clinical neurology in small animals—localization, diagnosis, and treatment*. Ithaca, NY: International Veterinary Information Service (last updated 7 Feb 2003).
Jones, T. C., Hunt, R. D., King, N. W., ed. 1996. Akabane disease (congenital arthrogryposis, hydranencephaly syndrome). *Veterinary Pathology*, 6th edition, p. 358.
Oliver, J. E., Jr., Lorenz, M.D., Kornegay, J. N., ed. 1997. Localization of lesions in the nervous system. In: *Handbook of veterinary neurology*. 3rd ed. Philadelphia: W. B. Saunders.
Smith, B. P. 2002. Hydrocephalus and hydranencephaly of cattle. In: *Large animal internal medicine*. 3rd ed. St. Louis: Mosby.
Smith, B. P. 2002. Meningitis (suppurative meningitis). In: *Large animal internal medicine*. 3rd ed. St. Louis: Mosby.

Author: Lisa Nashold

CNS: NERVE LESIONS

 BASICS

OVERVIEW
Peripheral nerve lesions are commonly due to traumatic injuries. The following conditions often occur in small ruminants and other large animals:
- Brachial plexus avulsion
- Suprascapular nerve (sweeney)
- Spastic paresis (elso heel)
- Radial nerve trauma
- Femoral nerve trauma
- Peroneal nerve trauma

PATHOPHYSIOLOGY
Depends on the specific condition

SYSTEMS AFFECTED
CNS

GENETICS
N/A

INCIDENCE/PREVALENCE
Unknown

GEOGRAPHIC DISTRIBUTION
Worldwide distribution

SIGNALMENT
Species
All ruminant species are affected

Breed Predilections
N/A

Mean Age and Range
N/A

Predominant Sex
N/A

 DIAGNOSIS

DIFFERENTIAL DIAGNOSIS
CNS lesions such as demyelination, encephalitis, parasitic visceral migrans, or other lesions

CBC/BIOCHEMISTRY/URINALYSIS
Usually normal

OTHER LABORATORY FINDINGS
Electrolyte abnormalities may occur and exacerbate muscular weakness:
- Hypocalcemia
- Hypokalemia
- Hypomagnesimia

IMAGING
- Radiographs may show bony changes that can occur with chronic disorders.
- Changes in chronic spastic paresis include osteoporosis, lipping of dorsal aspect of tibial epiphysis, excessive straightening of the tuber calcis, and plantar displacement proximal portion of the tibial diaphysis and epiphysis

DIAGNOSTIC PROCEDURES
Thorough neurologic evaluation

PATHOLOGIC FINDINGS

GROSS FINDINGS
Depends on underlying cause

HISTOPATHOLOGICAL FINDINGS
Depends on underlying cause

 TREATMENT

- Reduce inflammation
  - Dexamethasone (0.05 mg/kg IV daily for 3 to 5 days)
  - Apply cold packs to the affected area during the first day after injury.
- Treat electrolyte abnormalities if present.
  - Calcium gluconate (500 ml SC daily)
  - Potassium chloride can be given in water via stomach tube.
- Relieve musculoskeletal pain.
  - NSAIDs such as banamine, phenylbutazone, or aspirin may be indicated.
  - Morphine
- Prevent secondary medical complications such as dehydration and malnutrition.
- Turn recumbent animals six to eight times daily to prevent decubital ulcers and pressure sores.
- Goats often tolerate dog slings to assist them to stand.
- Provide adequate dry bedding to allow traction and prevent further injury.
- Spastic paresis can potentially be treated surgically with tibial nerve neurectomy or superficial digital flexor tenotomy proximal to the tuber calcis. It is often not treated due to familial nature of the disorder.

 MEDICATIONS

See Treatment above.

CONTRAINDICATIONS
- Do not use NSAIDs and steroids concurrently.
- Monitor drug withdrawal times for meat and milk.
- Appropriate milk and meat withdrawal times must be followed for all compounds administered to food-producing animals.
- Do not use steroidal drugs with pregnant animals.

 FOLLOW-UP

PATIENT MONITORING
Monitor for progression of neurologic disorder and secondary conditions such as dehydration, malnutrition, electrolyte abnormalities, or pressure sores in recumbent animals.

PREVENTION AVOIDANCE
- Prevent traumatic injuries using appropriate management, housing, and equipment.
- Use care when assisting with dystocia.

POSSIBLE COMPLICATIONS
Depends on cause of disease

EXPECTED COURSE AND PROGNOSIS
Depends on severity of injuries and neurologic impairment

 MISCELLANEOUS

ASSOCIATED CONDITIONS
See Table 1.

AGE-RELATED FACTORS
Spastic paresis can occur in calves or as an adult-onset condition.

ZOONOTIC POTENTIAL
N/A

PREGNANCY
Dystocia or trauma in assisted parturition can result in nerve damage.

BIOSECURITY
N/A

PRODUCTION MANAGEMENT
N/A

SYNONYMS
Elso heel
Spastic paresis
Sweeney

SEE ALSO
Demyelination
Encephalitis
Parasitic visceral migrans or other CNS lesions

ABBREVIATIONS
CNS = central nervous system
NSAIDs = nonsteroidal anti-inflammatory drugs

Suggested Reading
Aiello, S. E., ed. 1998a. Diseases of the peripheral nerve and neuromuscular junction. In: *Merck veterinary manual*. 8th ed. Whitehouse Station, NJ: Merck & Co.

Aiello, S. E., ed. 1998b. Diseases of the spinal column and cord. In: *Merck veterinary manual*. 8th ed. Whitehouse Station, NJ: Merck & Co.

Braund, K. G., ed. *Clinical neurology in small animals—localization, diagnosis, and treatment*. Ithaca, NY: International Veterinary Information Service (last updated 7 Feb 2003).

Smith, B. P. 2002a. Peripheral nerve disorders. In: *Large animal internal medicine*. 3rd ed. St. Louis: Mosby.

Smith, B.P. 2002b. Spastic paresis. In: *Large animal internal medicine*. 3rd ed. St. Louis: Mosby.

Author: Lisa Nashold

CNS: NERVE LESIONS

Table 1

Symptoms and Causes Associated with Neurological Lesions.		
Nerve/Condition	**Common Causes of Injury**	**Signs**
Brachial plexus avulsion	Traumatic injury Severe extension or abduction of thoracic limb causes stretching or tearing of the nerve roots from their spinal cord attachment.	Complete flaccidity and desensitization of the thoracic limb Unable to bear weight Triceps and biceps reflexes are absent Abduction of the elbow due to loss of pectoral nerve function Dropped shoulder Hyperextension of the elbow at rest and inability to flex the elbow due to musculocutaneous nerve paralysis Complete desensitization of thoracic
Radial nerve	Traumatic injury Direct trauma at lateral aspect of the elbow joint Prolonged anesthesia or restraint in lateral recumbency on hard surface	Signs depend of location of injury High radial nerve paralysis occurs with lesions near the elbow joint. Signs include dropped elbow, foot knuckled over at rest, scuffing of the toes, and flexion of joints distal to injury. The animal is unable to bear weight on thoracic limb. Low radial nerve paralysis results in knuckling of the carpus, fetlock, and pastern joints. The animal can bear weight if the metacarpus and elbow can extend. Triceps reflex is decreased or absent.
Femoral nerve	Traumatic injury Overextension of the hip and stifle joint commonly due to a fall or forced posterior delivery of calf	Inability to extend or fix the stifle Reciprocal apparatus cannot fix the hock causing collapse of the limb when attempting to bear weight. Metatarsal and tarsal joints remain in flexion. There is loss of sensation on medial aspect of the limb from the proximal thigh to medial malleolus of the tibia.
Peroneal nerve	Direct trauma as nerve crosses over the lateral condyle of the fibula Commonly seen after recumbency due to hypocalcemia or other causes	Extension of hock joint Flexion of the digits Decreased sensation of craniodorsal surface of foot, hock, and stifle Some animals can bear weight only if the limb is manually placed in the proper position.
Suprascapular nerve (sweeney)	Trauma to the shoulder region	Instability of the scapulohumeral joint with outward bowing of the joint Neurogenic atrophy results in prominent appearance of scapular spine.
Spastic paresis (elso heel)	Etiology is undetermined. Not a result of insult to a single peripheral nerve and may be due to CNS lesions. Two syndromes—both are considered familial conditions and have been found in several breeds of cattle. In calves, clinical signs of lumbar lordosis and caudal extension of limbs are seen between 1 week and 1 year of age. In adults, clinical onset usually occurs between 3 and 7 years of age.	Extension of stifle and tarsus Spastic contracture of gastrocnemius and superficial flexor muscles as animal attempts to walk. Other muscles in pelvic limbs can also be affected. Limb is circumducted when walking to prevent dragging the foot. If untreated, the disease will progress. Often responds favorably to tibial nerve neurectomy.

CNS: SPINAL COLUMN AND CORD ANOMALIES

BASICS

OVERVIEW
Spinal cord anomalies can be the result of many disease processes including trauma, infection or inflammation, nutritional diseases, congenital disorders, degenerative diseases, toxins, and vascular diseases.

PATHOPHYSIOLOGY
• Vertebral body fractures
  • In large animals, vertebral fractures are a common cause of spinal cord injury.
  • Fractures can be due to trauma, nutritional deficiencies, or other pathologic causes.
• *Hypoderma bovis* (heel flies)
  • *Hypoderma bovis* are long, hairy, beelike flies. The female flies attach their eggs to the hair on the legs and lower body of cattle and bison.
  • The migration of the first stage larvae through the epidural fat along the spinal cord can result in inflammation and clinical signs of spinal cord disease.
• Vertebral spondylosis
  • Spondylosis is a disease of the intervertebral joints. There is ossification in the joint space between bone and ligament or tendon. There can be complete bridging (ankylosis) between vertebral discs. It can be due to progressive development of vertebral enthosophytes or secondary to degenerative joint disease.
  • Ankylosing spondylitis is a progressive inflammatory disease affecting joint tissue that can result in fusion of lumbar vertebrae in bulls and rams.

SYSTEMS AFFECTED
Musculoskeletal, CNS, skin, nutritional

GENETICS
N/A

INCIDENCE/PREVALENCE
Unknown

GEOGRAPHIC DISTRIBUTION
Worldwide distribution

SIGNALMENT
• Due to differences in management, temperament, and anatomy affecting regional strength of the spine, the common locations of spinal injury sites differ among species.
• Breeding injuries occur more commonly in cattle.
• Cattle and sheep incur pathologic fractures due to nutritional deficiencies or vertebral osteomyelitis.
• Vertebral spondylosis occurs in bulls and rams. Spondylosis results in culling of approximately 4% of Holstein bulls used for artificial insemination.
• All species of domestic livestock are susceptible to CNS disease resulting from nematode and insect larvae migration through the CNS. *Hypoderma bovis* infest cattle and bison. *Parelaphostrongylus tenuis* infestations occur in sheep, goats, and llamas.

Species
• All species
• Breeding injuries occur more commonly in cattle.
• Vertebral spondylosis occurs in bulls and rams.

Breed Predilections
Spondylosis results in culling of approximately 4% of Holstein bulls used for artificial insemination.

Mean Age and Range
N/A

Predominant Sex
Vertebral spondylosis occurs in bulls and rams.

SIGNS
The signs of any spinal cord injury are related to the level of the spinal cord segment(s) involved. Clinical signs can help localize the site of damage in the majority of cases with neurologic problems. (See Table 1.)

Vertebral Fracture
• Acute signs may progress in unstable fractures or luxations. Progression to respiratory muscles results in death.
• Spondylosis most frequently affects the lumbosacral region.

Hypodermiasis
• The majority of *Hypodermis bovis* first-stage larvae lodges in the lumbosacral region of the spinal cord. However, larvae can potentially migrate to other parts of the spinal cord or even brain stem.
• Inflammatory process results in acute, often asymmetric, and progressive signs.
• Cattle may exhibit a stampeding behavior described as "gadding" when chased by the female *Hypoderma bovis* flies. This behavior can result in injury or decreased feeding.

CAUSES AND RISK FACTORS
Vertebral Fractures
• Abnormal bone mineralization may predispose to fractures. Common sites in calves are the C2–C4, T10–T13, and L3–L6 vertebrae.
• Nutritional deficiencies of copper, vitamin D, or calcium in 3–6- month-old ruminants can result in vertebral fractures.
• Traumatic cervical fractures may be caused by injuries sustained in falls, roadway accidents, butting of other animals, predation, or squeeze chutes.
• Pygmy goats may have traumatic luxations or fractures of the atlantooccipital and atlantoaxial joints when the horns are held during restraint.
• Chronic ankylosing spondylosis in mature bulls and rams can result in traumatic lumbar vertebral fractures.

DIAGNOSIS

DIFFERENTIAL DIAGNOSIS
• Meningitis can result in stiffness and resistance to passive flexion of the neck as seen in cervical fractures.
• Osteoarthritis or degenerative joint disease (DJD)
• Nematodes other than *Hypoderma bovis* can migrate through the CNS. In cattle, *Setaria* spp. causes pathology. Small ruminants may become infected with *Parelaphostrongylus tenuis* when pastured where white-tailed deer also feed.

CBC/BIOCHEMISTRY/URINALYSIS
Normal

OTHER LABORATORY FINDINGS
• CSF findings in vertebral fracture—acute changes (< 1 day after injury) include high RBCs, normal to high WBCs, and high protein concentration.
• CSF findings in vertebral fracture—chronic changes (> 1 day) include normal to slightly increased WBCs, possible xanthochromia.
• CSF findings in hypodermiasis are variable. Increased eosinophils are suggestive but may not be present because the larvae infestations are extradural. The CSF changes reflect increased pressure. Mild xanthochromia and normal to increased WBCs may be present if there is vascular damage due to pressure changes.

IMAGING
Fractures
Survey and contrast radiography often identify vertebral fractures and luxations.

DIAGNOSTIC PROCEDURES
• Complete and accurate history
• Thorough physical examination with fullest neurologic examination possible including evaluation of cutaneous desensitization to pinprick can help localize the lesion.
• Evaluation of gait is very valuable for large animals. Ambulation while blindfolded and while walking up and down a grade may accentuate subtle gait defects.
• Evaluate neck and limbs for pain, muscle atrophy, and cutaneous trunci reflex.
• Electrodiagnostic testing for neuromuscular conduction abnormalities

PATHOLOGIC FINDINGS

GROSS FINDINGS
• Vertebral fracture with possible evidence of spinal cord hemorrhage or necrosis
• Bridging of vertebral bodies in cases of ankylosing spondylosis

CNS: SPINAL COLUMN AND CORD ANOMALIES

Table 1

Symptoms Associated with Neurological Lesions.	
Spinal Cord Segments	Principal Signs
C1–C5	Weakness or paralysis in all limbs or in limbs on one side of the body
	UMN signs of normal or increased reflexes and muscle tone in all limbs and extensor rigidity on the same side as the lesion in all limbs
	Conscious proprioceptive deficits on the same side as the lesion in all limbs
	Hyperesthesia at the level of the lesion
	The neck is held stiff. Affected animals resist passive flexion of the head. May refuse to lower the head and may kneel when trying to eat from the ground.
	Thoracic limb held in partial flexion or repetitive stamping
	Urinary incontinence
	Persistent scratching at the neck
	Possible Horner's syndrome
	Possible dyspnea
	Possible torticollis/scoliosis
C6–T2 brachial plexus (thoracic limb)	Weakness or paralysis in all limbs, limbs on one side of the body, or a single limb
	LMN signs of decreased reflexes and flaccid muscle tone in thoracic limbs
	UMN signs of normal or increased reflexes and increased extensor muscle tone in pelvic limbs
	CP deficits in one thoracic limb, limbs on one side of the body, or all limbs
	Hyperesthesia at level of lesion
	Cutaneous trunci reflex reduced or absent behind the level of the lesion (unilateral or bilateral)
	Persistent scratching at one side of the neck or shoulder region
	Horner's syndrome
T3–L3	Weakness or paralysis of pelvic limbs
	UMN signs of normal or increased reflexes and increased extensor muscle tone in pelvic limbs. Initially, there is no muscle atrophy in pelvic limbs.
	Hyperesthesia at the level of the lesion
	Cutaneous trunci reflex reduced or absent behind the level of the lesion
	Urinary incontinence
	Thoracolumbar kyphosis
	Possible dyspnea or respiratory paralysis in cases with descending myelomalacia
	Possible Schiff-Sherrington posture[1]
L4–S2 lumbosacral plexus (pelvic limb)	Weakness or paralysis of pelvic limbs
	Hyperesthesia at the level of lesion
	LMN signs of muscle atrophy in pelvic limbs, and decreased anal sphincter tone.
	CP deficits in one or both pelvic limbs
	Reduced sensitivity in perineal region, pelvic limbs, or tail
	Urinary or fecal incontinence
S1–Cd5	Urinary or fecal incontinence
	Reduced sensitivity in perineal region or tail

[1] Schiff-Sherrington phenomenon is paraplegia with increased extensor tone in the thoracic limbs.

CNS: SPINAL COLUMN AND CORD ANOMALIES

HISTOPATHOLOGICAL FINDINGS
• Vertebral fractures can result in spinal cord demyelination with secondary changes of ascending and descending necrosis of the spinal cord (myelomalacia) with possible evidence of compromised blood flow (hematomyelia).
• Parasite migration results in inflammation and tissue necrosis.

TREATMENT

FRACTURES
• Recovery after 4–6 weeks of stall rest is often possible if neurologic deficits are mild and the fracture or luxation is not unstable.
• Small ruminants with cervical fractures and luxations may be stabilized by casting. A fiberglass cast should extend from the middle part of the thorax to the tip of the nose.
• Raise feed and water sources to allow animals with cervical fractures to eat and drink without bending the neck.
• Dietary intake of copper, molybdenum, and calcium should be evaluated and measured if possible. Supplementation may be necessary to avoid additional pathologic fractures.
• Avoid restraint of animals with metabolic bone disease to avoid additional pathologic fractures.

HYPODERMA BOVIS
Parasitides should be administered to prevent further parasite migration in the CNS. This treatment can cause severe reactions associated with the death of the parasites, so concurrent heavy anti-inflammatory therapy is required.

MEDICATIONS

VERTEBRAL FRACTURES
• Spinal cord contusions generally recover spontaneously without medication.
• Acutely affected animals can be treated with
  • Dimethyl sulfoxide (DMSO) (0.25–1 g/kg IV in 5% dextrose as a 40% DMSO solution); do not use DMSO in concentrations > 20% in horses.
  • Dexamethasone (0.1–0.2 mg/kg given 4 times daily for 2–4 days)
• If extremely painful, narcotic agents such as morphine (0.2–0.4 mg/kg) may be administered. Another analgesic option is lumbar epidural injection of morphine (0.1 mg/kg in 10–20 ml of normal saline).
• Instead of dexamethasone, treatment with methylprednisolone within the first hours of injury may be helpful (30 mg/kg IV, followed 2 hours later by 15 mg/kg IV, followed 6 hours later by 15 mg/kg IV, every 6 hours for a total of 24 hours of treatment). Do not use NSAIDs in conjunction with corticosteroids.
• Meat and milk drug withdrawal times must be strictly enforced. Consult FARAD when possible.

HYPODERMA BOVIS
• Systemic organophosphates or other insecticides are the only way to eliminate migrating larvae. Avoid treatment with systemic insecticides when larvae are in the epidural space.
• Topical insecticides can be used to kill eggs and larvae on the hair and skin of the lower body and legs.
• Organophosphates must be used in strict accordance with label instructions to prevent toxicity to the host animal.

• Organophosphates are not permitted for use on lactating dairy animals.
• The following insecticides are available for use:
  • Crufomate (75 mg/kg as 13.5% Ruelene)
  • Trichlorfon (40 mg/kg PO)
  • Famphur (13.2% 1 fluid ounce 90 kg of body weight, not to exceed a total dosage of 4 oz for cattle)
  • Ronnel (100 mg/kg PO for cattle)
  • Ivermectin 0.5% (1 ml/10 kg, max 10 ml / injection site): recommend treatment immediately after the adult fly season
  • Fenbendazole and thiabendazole have been reported to be used but are not labeled for use against *Hypoderma* spp.
• If systemic treatment must be given when the larvae are in the epidural space, the potential adverse effects must be addressed with concomitant heavy anti-inflammatory treatment with corticosteroids or NSAIDs. Do not use steroids and NSAIDs concurrently.
  • Dexamethasone (0.1–0.25 mg/kg IV every 6 hours) or
  • Phenylbutazone (10 mg/kg once every 36 hours IV or PO in cattle)
  • Aspirin (100 mg/kg PO 2–3 times daily for cattle)
  • Flunixin meglumine (1–2.2 mg/kg IV given 2 times daily for cattle)

CONTRAINDICATIONS
• Avoid treatment with systemic insecticides when the larvae are located in the epidural space (October 1–March 1 in the northern United States). Dying worms can directly release toxic factors and can cause local immunologic responses. Neurologic disturbances are aggravated and can be potentially fatal.

CNS: SPINAL COLUMN AND CORD ANOMALIES

• Tranquilizers should be administered with care to ambulatory patients because ataxia may result in a fall and worsen spinal cord damage.
• Appropriate milk and meat withdrawal times must be followed for all compounds administered to food-producing animals.
• Do not use steroidal drugs in pregnant animals.

 FOLLOW-UP

PATIENT MONITORING
Monitor for progression of neurologic signs.

PREVENTION/AVOIDANCE
• Efforts should be made to differentiate nutritional deficiencies from traumatic causes to allow proper preventive measures for other animals.
• Treat with appropriate anthelminthics before larval migration of *Hypoderma bovis*.

POSSIBLE COMPLICATIONS
Treatment complications are possible. See Treatment section above.

EXPECTED COURSE AND PROGNOSIS
Fractures
• Guarded prognosis in recumbent animals
• Poor prognosis if deep pain perception is lost caudal to the lesion.

Hypoderma bovis
• The life cycle of the fly is complete in 1 year.
• Eggs are deposited by the female fly in May–July in the northern United States.
• The first-stage larvae travel down the hair shaft and penetrate the skin within 3–7 days.
• Then they migrate through fascial planes between muscles, along connective tissue, or along nerve pathways to the region of the epidural fat between the dura mater and periosteum along the spinal canal where they accumulate for 2–4 months.

• In early winter, the larvae begin to arrive in subdermal tissue of the back of the host. They make breathing holes through the skin and the "warbles" form around the first-stage larvae. The larvae go through the second and third stages within these cysts. The warble stage lasts 1–3 months.
• The third stage larvae emerge through the breathing holes in the skin, drop to the ground, and pupate.
• Adult flies do not feed and live only 1 week.
• The prognosis is guarded because treatment results in potentially life-threatening complications. Dying worms release toxic factors and there is a local inflammatory response to dying worms, which aggravates neurologic conditions. Anti-inflammatory medications must be given at the time of treatment for the parasites.

 MISCELLANEOUS

ASSOCIATED CONDITIONS
Brain disorders and peripheral nerve disorders.

AGE-RELATED FACTORS
Immature animals (3–6 months of age) more frequently suffer pathologic fractures due to nutritional deficiencies.

ZOONOTIC POTENTIAL
N/A

PREGNANCY
Nutritional deficiencies in the dam can affect skeletal development of the fetus.

SEE ALSO
Hypoderma
Meningitis
Osteoarthritis or degenerative joint disease (DJD)
Parelaphostrongylus tenuis

ABBREVIATIONS
CNS = central nervous system
CSF = cerebral spinal fluid high
DJD = degenerative joint disease
DMSO = dimethyl sulfoxide
FARAD = Food Animal Residue Avoidance Databank
IV = intravenous
NSAIDs = nonsteroidal anti-inflammatory drugs
PO = per os, by mouth
RBCs = red blood cells
WBCs = white blood cells

Suggested Reading

Braund, K. G., ed. *Clinical neurology in small animals—localization, diagnosis, and treatment*. Ithaca, NY: International Veterinary Information Service (last updated 7 Feb 2003).
McAllister, M. M., O'Toole, D., Griggs, K. J. 1995, Oct 1. Myositis, lameness, and paraparesis associated with use of an oil-adjuvant bacterin in beef cows. *J Am Vet Med Assoc.* 207(7): 936–38.
Oliver, J. E., Jr., Lorenz, M.D., Kornegay, J. N., ed. 1997. Localization of lesions in the nervous system. In: *Handbook of veterinary neurology*. 3rd ed. Philadelphia: W. B. Saunders.
O'Toole, D., McAllister, M. M., Griggs, K. 1995, Apr. Iatrogenic compressive lumbar myelopathy and radiculopathy in adult cattle following injection of an adjuvanted bacterin into loin muscle: histopathology and ultrastructure. *J Vet Diagn Invest.* 7(2): 237–44.

Author: Lisa Nashold

COCCIDIOIDOMYCOSIS

BASICS

OVERVIEW
• The dimorphic soil fungus, *Coccidioides immitis*, causes coccidioidomycosis.
• Inhalation of arthrospores frequently leads to asymptomatic infection.
• Mild respiratory disease may rarely lead to disseminated disease in some animals.

PATHOPHYSIOLOGY
• Soil mycelial phase release arthrospores, which can survive for many years in environment
• Arthrospores are inhaled and reach alveoli.
• Arthrospores form endospore-producing spherules.
• Spherules rupture, releasing endospores that form additional spherules.
• Spherules destroy tissue as they are formed and rupture.
• Frequently, infection is confined to respiratory tract and results in asymptomatic infection. In human studies, 60% of infected patients exhibit asymptomatic respiratory infection within 10–14 days of spore inhalation.
• Some animals develop mild respiratory disease with diffuse pulmonary infiltrates. In human studies, 40% of infected patients developed symptoms of mild or, infrequently, more severe flulike respiratory disease (primary pulmonary disease). Fibrotic/ cavernous lesions of lungs may be sequelae of primary pulmonary infection.
• Rarely will *Coccidioides* spread hematogenously.
• Phagocytic cells play crucial role in defense against *Coccidioides immitis*.
• Granulomatous lesions/abscesses may be found in lungs, bronchial and mediastinal lymph nodes; infrequently in submaxillary/ retropharyngeal lymph nodes. In most cattle, carcass quality is not affected.

• Lesions may contain a creamy purulent material or be calcified.
• In disseminated disease, lesions may be found in other tissues including CNS, bone, joints.

INCIDENCE/PREVALENCE
• Of feedlot cattle, 5%–20% at slaughter exhibited lesions of coccidioidomycosis in one study (Arizona).
• Of human population, 3% converts to positive *Coccidioides* skin test annually in endemic regions.

GEOGRAPHIC DISTRIBUTION
• Lower Sonoran zones of the southwest United States, Mexico, Central and South America
• Arid/semiarid climates, low-elevation deserts, alkaline soils

SIGNALMENT
• All species of mammals, including humans, dogs, cattle, sheep, goats, swine, rodents, may be infected.
• In endemic areas, infection of cattle, humans, and dogs is common.
• Coccidioidomycosis should be part of differential diagnosis of chronically ill animals in endemic areas.

SIGNS
• Commonly causes asymptomatic infections
• Animals may exhibit chronic weight loss, persistent cough, fever.
• Granulomatous lesions/abscesses most commonly found in lungs and bronchial and mediastinal lymph nodes.

Source of Infection
• Soil reservoir
• Although zoonotic potential, no transmission reported between animals or between animals and humans.

Transmission
• Inhalation of spores, especially following dust storms
• Possible infection via ingestion (if devitalized tissue present)/skin abrasions

RISK FACTORS
• Exposure to spore-contaminated dust (spores resistant to heat, drying, salinity)
• Presence of devitalized tissue from preexisting disease
• Overuse of corticosteroids
• Granulocyte abnormalities
• Not contagious from animal to animal
• Highly infectious from environmental, laboratory culture mycelial phase

DIAGNOSIS

• Direct microscopic examination and culture of transtracheal wash, pus, pleural fluid, necropsy sample
• Samples should be placed in sterile containers and prevented from drying (small amount sterile water or 0.85% saline for biopsy/necropsy samples, no preservatives, antibiotics may be added to inhibit bacterial overgrowth).
• Formalin-fixed specimens cannot be used for culture but can be used for histological examination.
• Examine/culture within 1 hour or refrigerate
• Presence of spherules upon microscopic exam of tissues
• Spherules: round, nonbudding, thick-walled, 20–200 micrometer in diameter, endosporulating
• Serum: complement fixation/precipitin/FA inhibition tests
• Intradermal sensitivity tests use coccidiodin extract (nonspecific). Inject 0.1 ml in flank skin fold intradermally. Positive test if after 48 hours, 5 mm edema/induration. Nonspecific cross-reactions with histoplasmin.

DIFFERENTIAL DIAGNOSIS
• Tuberculosis
• Caseous lymphadenitis (sheep/goats)
• Actinomycosis
• Actinobacillosis
• Nocardiosis
• Histoplasmosis
• Blastomycosis

TREATMENT
• No effective treatment
• Eukaryotic fungi are not inhibited by antibiotics.
• Amphotericin B and azoles used to treat human cases.
• In human cases, prognosis for primary pulmonary disease is good.
• Disseminated disease is usually fatal.

MEDICATIONS
CONTRAINDICATIONS
Appropriate milk and meat withdrawal times must be followed for all compounds administered to food-producing animals.

FOLLOW-UP
PREVENTION/AVOIDANCE
• Reduce dust by planting grass/installing water sprinklers. In one study, 90% of visible particles collected from stable air studies were fungal spores/actinomycetes.
• Avoid clearing brush while animals are present.
• No vaccine is available.

MISCELLANEOUS
ASSOCIATED CONDITIONS
N/A
AGE-RELATED FACTORS
N/A
ZOONOTIC POTENTIAL
Does not spread from animals to humans, although it is highly infectious when grown under lab conditions.
PREGNANCY
N/A
RUMINANT SPECIES AFFECTED
Potentially, all ruminant species are affected.
BIOSECURITY
N/A
PRODUCTION MANAGEMENT
N/A
SYNONYMS
Desert fever
Posada's disease
San Joaquin Valley fever
SEE ALSO
Actinobacillosis
Actinomycosis
Blastomycosis
Caseous lymphadenitis (sheep/goats)
Histoplasmosis
Nocardiosis
Tuberculosis

ABBREVIATIONS
FA = fluorescent antibody test
Suggested Reading
Centers for Disease Control and Prevention. 2003, Mar 26. Increase in coccidioidomycosis—Arizona, 1998–2001. *JAMA*. 289(12): 1500–1502.
Diseases caused by algae and fungi. 2000. In: *Veterinary medicine*, ed. O. M. Radostits, C. C. Gay, D. C. Blood, K. W. Hinchcliff. 9th ed. Philadelphia: W. B. Saunders.
Kern, M. E., Blevins, K. S. 1997. *Medical mycology*. 2nd ed. Philadelphia: F. A. Davis Co.
Smith, J.A. 2002. Mycotic pneumonias. In: *Large animal internal medicine*, ed. B. P. Smith. 3rd ed. St. Louis: C. V. Mosby.
Sweeney, C. 2002. Fungal pneumonias. In: *Large animal internal medicine*, ed. B. P. Smith. 3rd ed. St. Louis: C. V. Mosby.
Winn, W. A. 1960, Oct. Coccidioidomycosis. The need for careful evaluation of the clinical pattern and anatomical lesions. *Arch Intern Med*. 106:463–66.

Author: Karen Carberry-Goh

234   BLACKWELL'S FIVE-MINUTE VETERINARY CONSULT

COCCIDIOSIS

 BASICS

DEFINITION
Coccidiosis refers to the clinical symptoms that result from an infection with one of several *Eimeria* species.

OVERVIEW
• Most ruminants are exposed to and infected with coccidia. Infection is usually asymptomatic and self-limiting with the development of species-specific immunity.
• Clinical signs develop when large numbers of oocytes are ingested or the host's immune system is suppressed.

Causative Agent
Eimeria species infect ruminants. Coccidia are species specific. The most common coccidia in cattle are *E. bovis* and *E. zuernii*, in sheep *E. ovina*, and in goats *E. arloingi*.

PATHOPHYSIOLOGY
• Oocysts are shed in the feces of infected animals, either those with clinical signs or older carrier animals. The oocysts sporulate in moist warm environments and become infective.
• During the developmental stages of the parasite's life cycle, intestinal cells are damaged. The number of infective oocysts ingested is related to the severity of clinical signs.
• Healthy nonimmune animals ingesting few oocysts may not show any clinical signs as intestinal damage is not significant and is quickly repaired. If a healthy nonimmune animal is exposed to many oocysts, widespread intestinal damage occurs with disruption of the intestinal mucosa.
• Mucosal damage results in alterations in gut function, loss of blood, fluid, protein, and electrolytes into the intestinal lumen resulting in diarrhea. Fecal material may contain pieces of sloughed mucosa and blood. Mucosal damage allows for bacterial invasion into and through the gut wall.
• Animals experiencing stress are more likely to exhibit clinical signs. Animals acquire active immunity to the species to which they are exposed.
• The pathophysiology of nervous coccidiosis is not fully elucidated but a neurotoxin is suspected to be involved.

SYSTEMS AFFECTED
• Gastrointestinal
• Nervous

GENETICS
N/A

INCIDENCE/PREVALENCE
Incidence of nervous coccidiosis is highest in the winter. Incidence of diarrhea is related to the buildup of infective oocysts within the animal's environment.

SIGNALMENT
Species
Bovine, caprine, and ovine
Breed Predilections
N/A
Mean Age and Range
• There is no specific age range for infection but clinical signs appear in animals as young as 16 days of age.
• Clinical signs are often associated with the stress of weaning and movement into a feed yard.
Predominant Sex
N/A

SIGNS
GENERAL COMMENTS
• The disease is primarily of young animals managed as groups in unsanitary conditions. Most animals in a group become infected but only a minority exhibits signs.
• Animals exhibiting clinical signs often have suppressed appetites and poor weight gains for several weeks after enteric signs resolve.

HISTORICAL FINDINGS
• Animals were recently weaned, moved from individual to group housing, housed in a crowded area that has a buildup of fecal material, and/or the housing environment has become wet or muddy.
• Owners may report poor feed intakes and weight gains.
• Cases of nervous coccidiosis—animal has recently exhibited signs of diarrhea, tenesmus, or hematochezia along with cold environmental temperatures.

PHYSICAL EXAMINATION FINDINGS
• Rough hair coat, poor body condition, and feces-stained perineum are common in young animals. Animals have varying degrees of dehydration, anorexia, and weakness.
• Depending on the severity of the infection, feces may contain mucus, strands of mucosa, and blood. Feces may be dark in small ruminants but hematochezia is rarely observed.
• Tenesmus is common with slight rectal prolapse.
• Nervous coccidiosis—initial signs of depression and incoordination are noted, progressing to muscle tremors, hyperesthesia, clonic-tonic convulsions, nystagmus, and blindness.
• The case fatality rate is high.

CAUSES
Eimeria species infect ruminants. Coccidia are species specific. The most common coccidia in cattle are *E. bovis* and *E. zuernii*, in sheep *E. ovina*, and in goats *E. arloingi*.

RISK FACTORS
• Changes in feed, weaning, and transport increase the development of clinical signs of disease.
• Housing that encourages buildup of fecal material such as crowded conditions and group housing
• Exposure to moist environments such as areas around leaking waterers or poorly drained feeding stations

 DIAGNOSIS

DIFFERENTIAL DIAGNOSIS
Enteric Coccidiosis
Salmonellosis, BVDV infection, abomasal or intestinal nematode parasitism, cryptosporidiosis
Nervous Coccidiosis
Polioencephalomalacia, lead intoxication, thromboembolic meningitis

CBC/BIOCHEMISTRY/URINALYSIS
Nothing particularly significant

CBC/BIOCHEMISTRY/URINALYSIS
• Hemoconcentration, although a slight anemia may exist but is masked by dehydration; a mild inflammatory leukogram if mucosal damage is severe.
• Plasma proteins are increased initially due to dehydration; however, plasma protein levels decrease due to leaking into gut and depressed feed consumption.

OTHER LABORATORY TESTS
• Fecal flotation
• Diarrhea may be present for 3 or 4 days prior to the presence of oocysts in the feces.
• Checking multiple individuals increases the chances of finding oocysts, as stages of oocyst development will vary among individual animals.
• Presence or absence of oocysts in a single fecal exam is neither diagnostic nor confirmatory for coccidiosis. An animal can shed large numbers of oocysts; yet show no clinical disease because of immune status.

PATHOLOGIC FINDINGS
Mucosa of the ileum, cecum, colon, and rectum may be congested, hemorrhagic, and thickened. The mucosa may be sloughing and ulcerated in severe cases. Lumen contents may contain blood and pieces of the mucosa.

TREATMENT

APPROPRIATE HEALTH CARE
N/A

NURSING CARE
Fluid therapy, consisting of commercial oral or intravenous polyionic fluids may be needed to correct dehydration and restore electrolytes.

ACTIVITY
N/A

DIET
Because animals tend to be thin, feeding an appropriate amount of grain for that animal may be helpful.

CLIENT EDUCATION
• Clients should be made aware of the potential shedding of oocysts in feces and contamination of the environment.
• A preventive program, including coccidiostats, should be discussed and implemented as soon as possible to prevent future infections.

 MEDICATIONS

DRUGS OF CHOICE
• Sulfamethazine 110 mg/kg for 5 days—cattle (may help control bacterial invasion and pneumonia). Resistance to sulfamethazine has been observed.
• Amprolium 10 mg/kg for 5 days—cattle
• Amprolium 50 mg/kg for 5 days—goats and sheep, extralabel

CONTRAINDICATIONS
• Use of amprolium may increase the risk of polioencephalomalacia.
• With the use of medications, the meat and milk withdrawal times must be maintained appropriately.

 FOLLOW-UP

PATIENT MONITORING
Monitor attitude, appetite, fecal color and consistency, and hydration status.

PREVENTION/AVOIDANCE
• Cleanliness is the basis of prevention. Clean and disinfect animal holding facilities between groups of animals. Drying and exposure to sunlight increases die off of oocysts.
• Do not overcrowd animals. Reduce manure buildup. Eliminate muddy areas in the animal's environment. Feed up off the ground.
• Do not allow animals to defecate in water or feed. Feeding of coccidiostats in feed or in salt mixes:
  • Amprolium—5 mg/kg for 30 days cattle
  • Decoquinate —0.5 mg/kg for 30 days, cattle, goats, and sheep
  • Lasalocid —20–30 g /ton of feed, cattle and sheep, or 1 mg/kg per head per day
  • Monensin— 20 g/ton of feed, cattle and goats, or 1 mg/kg per head per day

POSSIBLE COMPLICATIONS
• Pneumonia has been associated with outbreaks of coccidiosis.
• Bacterial invasion through damaged gut wall may lead to septicemia.

EXPECTED COURSE AND PROGNOSIS
• Course of diarrhea is dependent on severity of infection. Feces begin to firm after several days of treatment with antimicrobials or amprolium.
• Prognosis is based on how debilitated the animal is at the time of presentation.
• Animals that are severely affected may have long-term reduction in weight gains, especially kids, as a result of damage to the intestinal lining.

 MISCELLANEOUS

AGE- RELATED FACTORS
• Clinical signs of disease can occur anytime after 16 days of age.
• All ages are susceptible until immunity is developed.

ZOONOTIC POTENTIAL
None

RUMINANT SPECIES AFFECTED
Bovine, caprine, ovine

PRODUCTION MANAGEMENT
Do not overcrowd animals. Reduce manure buildup. Eliminate muddy areas in the animal's environment. Feed up off the ground.

SYNONYMS
N/A

SEE ALSO
Abomasal or intestinal nematode parasitism
BVDV infection
Cryptosporidiosis
Lead intoxication
Polioencephalomalacia
Salmonellosis
Thromboembolic meningitis

ABBREVIATIONS
BVDV = bovine viral diarrhea virus
CBC = complete blood count

Suggested Reading
Foreyt, W. 1990. Coccidiosis and cryptosporidiosis in sheep and goats. In: *The veterinary clinics of North America, food animal practice.* Philadelphia: W. B. Saunders.
Uhlinger, C. 2002. Coccidiosis in food animals. In: *Large animal internal medicine,* ed. B. P. Smith, 3rd ed. St. Louis: Mosby

Author: Kevin D Pelzer

COENUROSIS

 BASICS

DEFINITION
Coenurosis is a condition in sheep caused by invasion of the central nervous system (CNS) by *Coenurus cerebralis* in its cystic larval stage, or metacestode stage of the tapeworm *Taenia multiceps* (bladder worm). This parasite normally inhabits the intestinal tract of carnivores when they eat infected sheep's brain (raw) or cyst-contaminated offal.

PATHOPHYSIOLOGY
Sheep become infected when they eat forage contaminated with tapeworm or *Taenia* eggs and then the embryos pass from the blood to the CNS. Lesions of the CNS may result from:
- The large numbers of immature/migrating worms entering and causing encephalitis
- Interference with cerebrospinal fluid drainage
- Large cerebral cysts compressing surrounding nervous tissue

Most signs are caused by the mature *Coenurus cerebralis,* which may be up to 5 cm in diameter after 6–7 months of development.

SYSTEMS AFFECTED
CNS

SIGNALMENT

Species
Most common in sheep (can also affect cattle, goats, and wild ruminants)

Breed Predilection
N/A

Mean Age and Range
N/A

Predominant Sex
N/A

GENETICS

SIGNS
- Acute conditions may occur due to migrating larvae approximately 10 days after ingestion. This is most common in young lambs (6–8 weeks of age). Signs may include:
  - Blindness
  - Ataxia
  - Muscle tremors
  - Nystagmus
- Chronically infected animals with mature *Coenurus cerebralis* that have hatched, migrated, and grown over 2–6 months may show signs of:
  - Solitude
  - Partial or complete unilateral blindness
  - Depression
  - Head pressing and incoordination
  - Gradual development of paresis/paralysis and recumbency if the spinal cord is involved

CAUSES AND RISK FACTORS
Ingestion of forage contaminated with *Taenia* eggs

 DIAGNOSIS

- Presumptive diagnosis can be based on clinical signs and knowledge of *Taenia* presence in the area.
- Localization of metacestode in the brain or spinal cord is necessary for definitive diagnosis.

DIFFERENTIAL DIAGNOSIS
Coenurosis should be differentiated from other local space-occupying lesions in the CNS, including abscesses, hemorrhage, and neoplasia as well as listeriosis and bluetongue.

CBC/BIOCHEMISTRY/URINALYSIS

OTHER LABORATORY TESTS
N/A

IMAGING
Skull radiographs may be helpful in localizing the cyst.

PATHOLOGIC FINDINGS
- Thin-walled cysts are most commonly found on the external surfaces of the cerebral hemispheres.
- Local pressure atrophy of nervous tissue is usually apparent.
- Spinal cord lesions usually occur in the lumbar region.

TREATMENT

• Surgical drainage of the cyst may prolong life.
• Surgical removal of the cyst may lead to complete recovery.

MEDICATIONS

N/A

CONTRAINDICATIONS
N/A

FOLLOW-UP

PATIENT MONITORING
N/A

PREVENTION/AVOIDANCE
• The spread of infection with *Taenia multiceps* is best prevented by controlling the mature worms in dogs through effective periodic deworming.
• Carnivores should not be given access to carcasses of animals infested with the intermediate stage of *Taenia multiceps*.
• Carnivores should be prevented from defecating in areas where ruminants graze to minimize exposure to *Taenia* eggs.

EXPECTED COURSE AND PROGNOSIS
Prognosis is poor without surgery, although surgery can be difficult depending on the location of the cyst.

MISCELLANEOUS

ZOONOTIC POTENTIAL
Human infection can occur but it is very rare. Proper hygiene (washing hands or wearing gloves) after handling dog feces or infected sheep carcasses helps prevent infection.

PREGNANCY
N/A

RUMINANT SPECIES AFFECTED
Sheep, goats, cattle, and wild ruminants

BIOSECURITY
Not allowing dogs to defecate on forages to be consumed by ruminants will help decrease exposure to *Taenia* eggs.

SYNONYMS
Sheep gid
Staggers
Sturdy
Vertigo
Water brain

SEE ALSO
N/A

ABBREVIATIONS
CNS = central nervous system

Suggested Reading
Coenurosis. 1998. In: *Merck veterinary manual*, ed. S. E. Aiello and A. Mays. 8th ed. Whitehouse Station, NJ: Merck and Co.
Hansen, J., Perry, B. 1994. Coenurosis. In: *The epidemiology, diagnosis and control of helminth parasites of ruminants*. Nairobi: Kenya International Laboratory for Research on Animal Diseases.
Leontides, S., Psychas, V., Argyroudis, S., Giannati-Stefanou, A., Paschaleri-Papadopoulou, E., Manousis, T., Sklaviadis, T. 2000. A survey of more than 11 years of neurologic diseases of ruminants with special reference to transmissible spongiform encephalopathies (TSEs) in Greece. *J Vet Med B Infect Dis Vet Public Health* 47(4):303–9.

Authors: Ferenc Toth and Danelle Bickett-Weddle

CONGESTIVE HEART FAILURE

BASICS

DEFINITION
Congestive heart failure is a syndrome, not a specific disease, resulting from a number of causes and occurring when the heart becomes weak and is unable to effectively contract and pump blood to organs and peripheral tissues resulting in congestion of the lungs and other tissues.

OVERVIEW
• Heart failure can involve the heart's left side, right side, or both sides.
• Occurs when any of the heart chambers lose their ability to efficiently pump the amount of blood flow returning to the heart
• May result from primary cardiovascular disease or secondary to disease in other organ(s) or systemic disease
• Left-sided or left-ventricular failure
   • Left ventricle loses ability to contract (systolic failure) and force blood into the circulation. Ventricle becomes dilated.
   • Left ventricle loses its ability to relax (diastolic failure) because muscles are stiff and the ventricle cannot fill properly with blood during the resting period. Ventricular wall thickens.
   • Congestion in pulmonary circuit (pulmonary edema)
   • Systemic blood pressure falls.
   • Fluid builds up in tissues of body (edema).
• Right-sided or right-ventricular failure
   • Occurs as result of left-sided failure or alone
   • Right ventricle cannot pump the volume of blood returned to it.
   • Congestion of systemic venous system, decreased output to lungs causes venous distention, hepatomegaly, splenomegaly, edema of the intestinal tract, and peripheral edema.
• Congestive heart failure is usually a chronic event, occasionally acute.
• Heart tries to compensate for changes occurring with heart failure by enlarging, developing more muscle mass, and/or pumping faster.
• Body tries to compensate for heart failure by vasoconstriction, diverting blood from less important organs to maintain flow to most important organs.

PATHOPHYSIOLOGY
• Cardiac contractility is compromised resulting in inefficient heart contraction and movement of blood through the heart and circulatory beds.
• As blood flowing out of the heart slows, blood returning to the heart via the veins backs up causing congestion in the tissues and frequently edema.
• Pulmonary edema may develop resulting in dyspnea and coughing.
• Secondary compromise of renal function results in retention of fluid and edema.

SIGNALMENT
• Uncommon, sporadic disease
• Cattle
• Goats, sheep

SIGNS
• Most affected animals presented for signs of heart failure
• Exercise intolerance
• Weight loss
• Hypophagia
• Tachycardia
• Muffled heart sounds
• Signs of left-heart failure: tachypnea, coughing, dyspnea
• Signs of right-heart failure: submandibular, brisket, or ventral edema, jugular and mammary vein distention, and pulsation with right-heart failure
• Heart sounds may vary in intensity.
• Fast and weak peripheral pulses
• Pulse deficit
• ±Heart murmur
• ±Arrhythmia
• ±Hepatomegaly
• ±Diarrhea

PATHOLOGIC LESIONS
• Right-sided heart failure: subcutaneous edema, ascites, hydrothorax, hydropericardium, hepatic congestion, hepatomegaly
• Left-sided heart failure: pulmonary congestion and edema
• Heart enlargement and dilation

CAUSES AND RISK FACTORS
• CHF may result from previous heart disease (e.g., myocardial degeneration, myocarditis, cardiomyopathy, endocarditis, valvular defect, ruptured valve or chordae), pericarditis, pericardial tamponade, congenital heart defects, hypertension, disease of the arteries supplying the heart muscle, or cardiac neoplasia.
• Pressure load (e.g., aortic or pulmonic stenosis, pulmonary hypertension)
• Left-heart failure: myocardial disease, aortic insufficiency, hypertension, cardiomyopathy
• Right-heart failure: left-heart failure, obstructive lung disease, congenital heart defects, neoplasia (lymphosarcoma) in right atria
• Arrhythmias
• Nutritional muscular dystrophy
• Ionophore toxicosis
• Ingestion of cardiotoxic plants (e.g., oleander, lily of the valley, yew, Indian hemp, false hellebore, milkweed, avocardo, caltrops, coffee weed, senna, etc.)
• In goats, CHF due to cor pulmonale secondary to pneumonia, mediastinal thyoma, and ventricular septal defect
• Gousiekte or "quick disease" in South Africa due to ingestion of plants in Rubiaceae family

DIAGNOSIS

• History and clinical signs of heart failure
• Auscultation: tachycardia, crackles over the lung fields
• Echocardiography
   • Assess valve function, heart wall and septum motion and contraction, overall heart size, presence of pericardial effusion
   • Document ventricular hypertrophy and dilatation
• Thoracic radiography: ± cardiomegaly, ± pulmonary edema
• Electrocardiogram for arrhythmias
• Cardiac catheterization to document increased pulmonary artery pressure
• Arterial blood gas

DIFFERENTIAL DIAGNOSIS
• Brisket disease or mountain sickness
• Cardiomyopathy
• Endocarditis
• Myocarditis
• Pericarditis
• Cardiac lymphosarcoma
• Cardiotoxic plants
• Ionophore toxicosis
• Selenium deficiency
• Gossypol toxicosis
• Parasitism

CBC/BIOCHEMICAL/URINALYSIS
• Normal or variable CBC changes depending on underlying causes
• Hyponatremia, hypochloremia due to dilutional effect following retention of fluid and anorexia
• Hypokalemia ± hypocalcemia from anorexia
• Hypoproteinemia, hypoalbuminemia due to retained fluid or loss of protein into interstitial space, ascites, or intestinal tract
• Elevated γ glutamyl transferase (GGT) indicating biliary stasis due to passive congestion of the liver.

OTHER LABORATORY TESTING
Hepatic ultrasound
• Infract
• Disruption of normal parenchyma
• Vascular changes

IMAGING
• Echocardiography
• Radiography

DIAGNOSTIC PROCEDURES
As above

CONGESTIVE HEART FAILURE

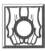

TREATMENT

- Treat specific underlying causes of CHF, if known
- Aimed at increasing the pumping ability of the heart, reducing the blood volume that must be pumped, reducing fluid retention, and management of vascular tone
- Short-term management only
- Stall rest
- Inotropics-digoxin: improve cardiac contractility; dobutamine
- Diuretic: furosemide, to aid elimination of excess fluid and salt from body
- Drugs to expand blood vessels and decrease resistance in vessels (efficacy in ruminants is unknown)
  - Vasodilators
  - ACE (angiotensin-converting enzyme) inhibitors
  - Calcium channel blockers
- ± Beta blockers: improve contractility of left ventricle
- Antiarrhythmic: if arrhythmia present and serum electrolytes and calcium and acid-base and hydration status are normal
- Dietary restriction of sodium
- Dietary supplementation of potassium chloride (KCl) if needed
- Monitor and supplement calcium as needed
- Monitor blood acid-base and electrolyte status every other day
- Other supplements recommended when appropriate for specific conditions associated with heart impairment: vitamin E, selenium, thiamin, magnesium, L-carnitine
- Surgical therapy (pacemakers, heart valve replacement, transplant); not reported in ruminants

MEDICATIONS

DRUGS
- Furosemide: 0.5–2.0 mg/kg IV, IM BID, SID
- Digoxin
  - Initial loading dose of 2.2 mg/100 kg IV followed by 0.34 mg /100 kg every 4 hours
  - 0.86 μg/kg per hour IV (valuable hospitalized animals) or

- 3.4 μg/kg IV every 4 hours; greater risk of inducing digoxin toxicity
- supplement with KCl if animal is inappetent
- KCl: 50 to 150 g per day for adult cattle on potassium-wasting diuretics
- Appropriate milk and meat withdrawal times must be followed for all compounds administered to food-producing animals.

FOLLOW-UP

EXPECTED COURSE AND PROGNOSIS
100% mortality in long term

MISCELLANEOUS

ASSOCIATED CONDITIONS
- Hypovolemia may result in damage to other organs.
- Renal or pulmonary emboli
- Renal infarcts
- Cardiac arrhythmias

ZOONOTIC POTENTIAL
N/A

RUMINANT SPECIES AFFECTED
Cattle, goat, sheep

BIOSECURITY
N/A

PRODUCTION MANAGEMENT
- Proper treatment of primary cardiovascular and pulmonary diseases
- Clean pastures of potentially cardiotoxic plants
- Selenium/vitamin E supplement in deficient areas or for animals fed feeds deficient in selenium

SEE ALSO
Brisket disease or mountain sickness
Cardiac lymphosarcoma
Cardiomyopathy
Cardiotoxic plants
Cor pulmonale
Endocarditis
Gossypol toxicosis
Ionophore toxicosis
Myocarditis
Parasitism
Pericarditis
Selenium deficiency

ABBREVIATIONS
BID = twice daily
CHF = congestive heart failure
GGT = gamma-glutamyltransferase
IM = intramuscular
IV = intravenous
KCl = potassium chloride
SID = once daily

Suggested Reading
Cardiovascular system. 1994. In: *Goat medicine*, ed. M. C. Smith and D. M. Sherman. Philadelphia: Lea & Febiger.
Cardiovascular system. 1997. In: *Veterinary pathology*, ed. R. C. Jones, R. D. Hunt, and N. W. King, 6th ed. Philadelphia: Lippincott Williams and Wilkins.
Constable, P. D. Therapeutic management of cardiovascular disease. 1999. In: *Current veterinary therapy 4*, ed. J. Howard and R. Smith, 4th ed. Philadelphia: W. B. Saunders and Co.
Diseases of the heart. 1999. In: *Veterinary medicine: a textbook of the diseases of cattle, sheep, pigs, goats, and horses*, ed. O. M. Radostits. et al., 9th ed. New York: W. B. Saunders and Co.
Reef, V. B., and McGuirk, S. M. 2002. Diseases of the cardiovascular system. In: *Large animal internal medicine*, ed. G. Smith, 3rd ed. St. Louis: Mosby.

Authors. Susan Semrad and Sheila McGuirk

CONIUM SPP. (POISON HEMLOCK) TOXICITY

 BASICS

OVERVIEW
• Poison hemlock (*Conium maculatum*) toxicity in ruminants is an uncommon occurrence.
• Poison hemlock is a member of the Apiaceae family. It is a biennial. The first-year seedling plant contains leaves that are fernlike in appearance—three to four times pinnately divided, and the leaflets are 1/4 in. long and segmented. The foliage has a strong mousy, parsniplike odor.
• The mature plant is erect, 3–8 feet tall, with a stout hollow stem (except at the nodes) that is smooth and often purple splotched. The plant has a long white/yellow taproot, which resembles a carrot or parsnip.
• Small, white flowers are arranged in umbrella-shaped clusters at the tips of the uppermost stems.
• It is a commonly encountered weed throughout North America, sometimes forming heavy dense stands that are difficult to control.
• Two types of clinical conditions can be encountered—acute toxicities (nicotinic effects) and malformations in young exposed in utero ("crooked calf disease").
• Treatment is nonspecific in nature, and emphasis should be placed on identification of the plant and preventing access to it.

PATHOPHYSIOLOGY
• The piperidine alkaloids have nicotinic-like effects—stimulate, then paralyze the nicotinic receptors. Large exposures cause neuromuscular block, hypotension, and bradycardia.
• Gamma-coniceine is thought to be the agent responsible for the malformations; inhibits fetal movement.

SYSTEMS AFFECTED
Nervous and musculoskeletal systems

GENETICS
N/A

INCIDENCE/PREVALENCE
Not very common; the plant is not generally considered palatable (particularly the mature plant) and animals don't readily graze it unless forced to do so. Animals may acquire a taste for the plant.

GEOGRAPHIC DISTRIBUTION
Throughout North America

SIGNALMENT
All ruminants, particularly cattle (considered more susceptible)

Species
Cattle, sheep, and goats appear to be susceptible.

Breed Predilections
N/A

Mean Age and Range
N/A

Predominant Sex
N/A

SIGNS
• Abrupt onset (within a few hours of ingestion) of muscle tremors, ataxia, muscle weakness, excessive salivation and lacrimation, mydriasis, and frequent urination and defecation
• This can progress to recumbency, depression, abdominal pain, respiratory distress, and death from respiratory arrest.
• Skeletal deformations observed when pregnant animals are exposed include arthrogryposis, cleft palate, microphthalmia, and spinal column deformities.

CAUSES AND RISK FACTORS
• Concentrations of the toxic alkaloids vary between parts of the plant and stage of maturity.
• All parts of the plant are potentially toxic, and toxicity is thought to increase as the plant matures.
• Approximate toxic and lethal dose for poison hemlock: cattle > 1.0 g fresh plant/kg BW; sheep > 5.4 g fresh plant/kg BW; goats > 7.8 g fresh plant/kg BW
• Some toxicity is lost in drying; but there have been cases where cattle have been poisoned as a result of ingesting contaminated hay.
• Contaminated grain by the seeds can be a problem as well.

 DIAGNOSIS

DIFFERENTIAL DIAGNOSIS
Organophosphate or carbamate poisoning, poisoning with *Lupinus* or *Nicotiana* spp.

CBC/BIOCHEMISTRY/URINALYSIS
No specific diagnostic changes have been reported.

OTHER LABORATORY TESTS
N/A

IMAGING
N/A

DIAGNOSTIC PROCEDURES
• One can attempt to confirm exposure through feed microscopy of the rumen contents.
• Alkaloids can be detected in the rumen contents or urine, also in liver, kidney, and blood.

CONIUM SPP. (POISON HEMLOCK) TOXICITY

PATHOLOGIC FINDINGS
• Renal tubule necrosis and skeletal muscle degeneration has been reported in fatal cases involving people.
• A mousy, parsnip odor can be detected from the freshly open rumen.
• Skeletal malformations include cleft palate, arthrogryposis, scoliosis, kyphosis, and torticollis.

TREATMENT
• Symptomatic and supportive in nature. Decontaminate the gastrointestinal tract with activated charcoal and saline cathartic.
• Providing adequate respiratory support would be next to impossible in the field.

MEDICATIONS
Atropine should be used with caution.

CONTRAINDICATIONS
Appropriate milk and meat withdrawal times must be followed for all compounds administered to food-producing animals.

FOLLOW-UP
N/A

PATIENT MONITORING
Monitor respiratory function.

PREVENTION/AVOIDANCE
• Avoid access to the plant.
• Control chemically with appropriate herbicides.

POSSIBLE COMPLICATIONS
N/A

EXPECTED COURSE AND PROGNOSIS
Highly dependent on the exposure dose or the severity of the malformations.

MISCELLANEOUS

ASSOCIATED CONDITIONS
• Depression, abdominal pain, respiratory distress, and death from respiratory arrest
• Skeletal deformations observed when pregnant animals are exposed include arthrogryposis, cleft palate, microphthalmia, and spinal column deformities.

AGE-RELATED FACTORS
N/A

ZOONOTIC POTENTIAL
N/A

PREGNANCY
Attempts should be made to prevent pregnant animals' access to the plant during susceptible periods (cattle days 40–100 of gestation; sheep and goats—30–60 days of gestation).

RUMINANT SPECIES AFFECTED
All ruminants considered susceptible; most commonly reported in cattle.

BIOSECURITY
N/A

PRODUCTION MANAGEMENT
• Prevent animals from accessing the plant.
• Some toxicity is lost in drying; but there have been cases where cattle have been poisoned as a result of ingesting contaminated hay.
• Contaminated grain by the seeds can be a problem as well.

SYNONYMS
Fool's parsley
Poison carrot
Poison parsley
Spotted hemlock
St. Bennett's weed
Stinkweed

SEE ALSO
Crooked calf disease
Organophosphate or carbamate poisoning, poisoning with Lupinus or Nicotiana spp.

ABBREVIATIONS
BW = body weight

Suggested Reading
Burrows, G. E., Tyrl, R. J. 2001. Conium. In: *Toxic plants of North America*, ed. G. E. Burrows, R. J. Tyrl. Ames: Iowa State University Press.
Galey, F. D., Holstege, D. M., Fisher, E. G. 1992, Jan. Toxicosis in dairy cattle exposed to poison hemlock (*Conium maculatum*) in hay: isolation of *Conium* alkaloids in plants, hay, and urine. *J Vet Diagn Invest*. 4(1):60–64.
Lopez, T. A., Cid, M. S., Bianchini, M. L. 1999, Jun. Biochemistry of hemlock (*Conium maculatum L.*) alkaloids and their acute and chronic toxicity in livestock. A review. *Toxicon*. 37(6):841–65.
Panter, K. E. 2004. Piperidine alklaloids. In: *Clinical veterinary toxicology*, ed. K. H. Plumlee. St. Louis: Mosby.
Vetter J. 2004, Sep. Poison hemlock (*Conium maculatum L.*). *Food Chem Toxicol*. 42(9):1373–82.

Author: Patricia Talcott

CONTAGIOUS BOVINE PLEUROPNEUMONIA

BASICS

DEFINITION
• Contagious bovine pleuropneumonia (CBPP) is a highly contagious bacterial disease of primarily cattle resulting in severe, acute pneumonia and occasionally a polyarthritis with high mortality.
• CBPP can be acute, subacute, or chronic in nature. It is caused by *Mycoplasma mycoides mycoides*.

PATHOPHYSIOLOGY
• Carrier animals of the bacterial agent *M. mycoides mycoides* small-colony type (SC type) shed the organism in respiratory secretions during periods of stress to susceptible cattle, resulting in severe respiratory disease and mortality in a herd. Secondary infections with other viral and bacterial pneumonias complicate disease presentation and diagnosis.
• *M. mycoides mycoides* large-colony type (LC type) is pathogenic for goats and sheep but does not affect cattle. *M. mycoides mycoides* (SC type) survives well in vivo, but is quickly inactivated by external environmental conditions.
• CBPP is often unilateral.

SYSTEMS AFFECTED
Respiratory and occasionally musculoskeletal

GENETICS
• Predominantly a disease of the genus *Bos*.
• Anecdotal reports suggest breed differences affecting susceptibility.
• European cattle breeds tend to be more susceptible than indigenous African breeds.
• The infection has been recorded in yak, bison, and the domestic buffalo (*Bubalus bubalis*).

INCIDENCE/PREVALENCE
• Incidence for CBPP varies worldwide.
• Morbidity often reaches 100% and mortality may be 10–70%.
• Mortality may depend on other herd-management decisions and concurrent disease processes.

GEOGRAPHIC DISTRIBUTION
• Endemic in most regions of Africa
• Regions of Asia, particularly India and China
• Europe (Spain, Portugal, and Italy)
• North America and the western hemisphere are currently free of contagious bovine pleuropneumonia.
• Reported in 25 countries during the years 2001–2004.

SIGNALMENT
Species
• Bovine: *Bos indicus* and *Bos taurus*
• Other susceptible species: yak, bison, antelope
• Water buffalo in Italy
• Sheep and goats in Africa and Portugal

Mean Age and Range, Predominant Sex
Some age resistance does appear evident. Cattle less than 3 years of age have been shown to be less resistant to experimental challenge.

SIGNS

HISTORICAL FINDINGS
• Severe respiratory disease in cattle with high morbidity and mortality within 7–10 days after clinical disease onset. Contagious bovine pleuropneumonia is spread by inhalation of aerosolized droplets from a moribund coughing animal.
• The time from disease exposure to overt symptomatology varies but generally is quite prolonged. Animals introduced into a CBPP-infected herd may show signs of disease in 20 to 123 days.
• CBPP has been implicated in MAKEPS syndrome (mastitis, arthritis, keratitis, pneumonia, and septicemia)

PHYSICAL EXAMINATION FINDINGS
• Depression, inappetence, and pyrexia
• Coughing with concomitant thoracic pain, dyspnea, and increased respiratory rate
• Animals classically position themselves with elbows abducted to increase chest capacity.
• Thoracic auscultation reveals rales, crepitation, and pleuritic friction rubs; labored respiration attempts and open-mouthed breathing
• Occasionally in calves polyarthritis is evident.
• Frothy nasal discharge and continuous stringy salivation appear shortly before death. Chronic cases can recover and become carrier animals.

CAUSES
• The bacterial agent *M. mycoides mycoides* small-colony type (SC type)
• Disease spread is through direct contact and inhalation of infective aerosols.

RISK FACTORS
• Exposure to carrier animals shedding organisms after periods of stress, such as sudden climatic changes (heavy rains or cold spells), especially in close confinement or overcrowded conditions can predispose CCBP outbreaks.
• Introduction of carrier animals into previously uninfected herds
• Herd outbreaks usually occur as the result of animal importation/movement patterns into a naïve herd.
• Persistent carriers may develop after chronic infection and may harbor infectious organisms within a pulmonary sequestrum.
• Fomite transmission may be possible.

DIAGNOSIS

DIFFERENTIAL DIAGNOSIS
Pasteurellosis, other *Mycoplasma* spp. pneumonias, *Haemophilus* spp., and *Salmonella* spp., BVD, BRSV, IBR, PI3, East Coast Fever, hydatid cyst, TRP, *Mycobacterium bovis*, *Mannheimia hemolytica*

CBC/BIOCHEMISTRY/URINALYSIS
N/A

OTHER LABORATORY TESTS
• Serological tests such as complement fixation (detects 99% of active cases and 70% of chronic cases), passive hemagglutination, and ELISA can be used on a herd basis to detect antibodies to CBPP.
• Polymerase chain reaction on lung, pleural fluid, urine, and cultured colonies
• Histopathology
• Immunohistochemistry

Diagnostic Specimens for Laboratory
Live animal samples
Nasal swabs, tracheal wash, thoracocentesis fluid, serum

Postmortem sample
Fresh lung, Pleural fluid, tracheobronchial lymph nodes, and synovial fluid

IMAGING
Although not commonly done, radiographs would reveal evidence of fluid in the thoracic cavity, pulmonary consolidation, and nodules.

DIAGNOSTIC PROCEDURES
Confirmatory diagnosis is made by culturing the agent from lung, pleuritic fluid, swabs of major bronchi, and tracheobronchial or mediastinal lymph nodes and identified by complement fixation or by growth or metabolic inhibition tests.

PATHOLOGIC FINDINGS
• Acute lesions: alveolar spaces infiltrated by edema fluid and accumulations of leukocytes. Fibrin thrombi are evident with intense inflammatory infiltration and concomitant necrosis of alveolar septae.
• Chronic lesions: lymphocytic infiltration with thickening along interlobular septae, fibrosis of interlobular septae and coagulative necrosis of lobules.
• Unilateral pleuritis and pneumonia. There is a decided "marbling" effect of lung tissue due to distended interlobular septae. Sequestra in pulmonary tissue are encapsulated with fibrosis.
• Acute through chronic stages are common in the same animal.
• There will be straw-colored fluid in the thorax. The lungs themselves will have a fibrinous pneumonia and pea-sized, yellow-colored nodules appear in early infection.

CONTAGIOUS BOVINE PLEUROPNEUMONIA

TREATMENT

- *Mycoplasma mycoides mycoides* (SC type) is susceptible to a variety of antimicrobials. These may include tetracycline, streptomycin, and chloramphenicol (where legal).
- Antimicrobial therapy may favor the formation of sequestra and create a carrier state.

APPROPRIATE HEALTH CARE, NURSING CARE

Due to the contagious nature of this disease, affected animals should be isolated and the entire herd placed under quarantine.

ACTIVITY

Animals should be isolated and activity restricted because of the exercise intolerance due to the severe respiratory disease.

DIET

Maintain a good plane of nutrition with fresh food and water daily.

CLIENT EDUCATION

Clients should be made aware of the seriousness of CBPP and the contagious aspects so as to protect their nonexposed susceptible animals on their facility.

SURGICAL CONSIDERATIONS

N/A

MEDICATIONS

DRUGS OF CHOICE

- Broad-spectrum antibiotics EARLY in the course of disease
- Macrolides, tetracyclines, and quinolones are active against *M. mycoides mycoides* (SC type) but do not always clear an animal of carrier status.
- Tylosin and oxytetracycline appear effective. Drug withdrawal periods for meat and milk are important to monitor when using antibiotic agents.

CONTRAINDICATIONS

POSSIBLE INTERACTIONS

ALTERNATIVE DRUGS

N/A

FOLLOW-UP

PATIENT MONITORING

Respiratory distress is a large component of this disease, so monitor animals for signs of labored breathing and nasal discharge to ensure they have a patent airway.

PREVENTION/AVOIDANCE

- In Africa, routine vaccination against CBPP remains the primary control option.
- Current live attenuated vaccine performance is suboptimal. Low efficacy (33–67%) and a short duration of immunity (6–12 months) are recurring problems with this vaccine. Vaccination of animals with a live attenuated and inactivated vaccines have had varying degrees of success in parts of the world.
- Two vaccine strain types are currently used in Africa: strain T1 44 and T1 SR.
- Vaccination often generates a local quite extensive tissue reaction. Therefore, it is often given in the tail tip, which may become necrotic and slough.
- Quarantine of farms with testing and slaughtering of animals has been proven effective as a control plan in the event of an outbreak.
- Serologic testing of herds for importation is recommended.

POSSIBLE COMPLICATIONS

Cattle that recover maintain a long-term carrier status, leading to exposure of susceptible animals during periods of stress.

EXPECTED COURSE AND PROGNOSIS

Recovered animals can become long-term carriers of mycoplasma.

MISCELLANEOUS

ASSOCIATED CONDITIONS

N/A

AGE-RELATED FACTORS

N/A

ZOONOTIC POTENTIAL

CBPP is not a zoonotic disease.

PREGNANCY

N/A

RUMINANT SPECIES AFFECTED

- Bovine: *Bos indicus* and *Bos taurus*
- Other susceptible species: yak, bison, antelope
- Water buffalo in Italy
- Sheep and goats in Africa and Portugal

BIOSECURITY

Isolating infected animals is imperative to the control of this disease.

PRODUCTION MANAGEMENT

- *M. mycoides mycoides* does not survive in meat or meat products.
- Many of the routinely used disinfectants will effectively inactivate the organism.

SYNONYMS

Mycoplasma

SEE ALSO

BRSV
BVD
East coast fever
Hemophilus spp.
Hydatid cyst
IBR
Mannheimia hemolytica
Mycobacterium bovis
Other *Mycoplasma* spp. pneumonias
Pasteurellosis
Pi3
Salmonella spp.
TRP

ABBREVIATIONS

CBPP = contagious bovine pleuropneumonia
ELISA = enzyme-linked immunosorbent assay

Suggested Reading

Contagious bovine pleuropneumonia. 1991. *Tech. Off. Int. Epizoot.* 6:565–624.
Cottew, G. S. 1979. Pathogenicity of the subspecies mycoides of *Mycoplasma mycoides* for cattle, sheep and goats. *Zbl. Bakt. Hyg.*, 1. Abst, Orig, A,. 245:164.
FAO Animal Health Disease Cards, Contagious Bovine Pleuropneumonia accessed at http://www.fao.org/ag/againfo/subjects/en/health/diseases-cards/ccpp.html on May 16, 2004.
Provost, A., Perreau, P., Breard, A., Legoff, C., Martel, J. L., and Cottew, G. S. 1987. Contagious bovine pleuropneumonia. *Rev. Sci. Tech. Off. Int. Epizoot.* 6:625–79.
United States Animal Health Association, Foreign Animal Diseases book website, Contagious Bovine Pleuropneumonia accessed at http://www.vet.uga.edu/vpp/gray_book/FAD/CCP.htm on May 30, 2004.

Authors: Scott R.R. Haskell and Danelle Bickett-Weddle

CONTAGIOUS CAPRINE PLEUROPNEUMONIA

BASICS

DEFINITION
Contagious caprine pleuropneumonia (CCPP) is an extremely contagious bacterial disease of goats resulting in severe, acute pneumonia with high mortality. CCPP is considered to be the most devastating disease of goats worldwide.

PATHOPHYSIOLOGY
Carrier animals of the bacterial agent *Mycoplasma capricolum capripneumoniae* (mycoplasma biotype F-38) shed the organism in respiratory secretions during periods of stress to susceptible goats, resulting in severe respiratory disease and mortality in a herd. Infection with *Mycoplasma mycoides capri* (type strain PG-3) can occur but less commonly. Secondary infections with other viral pneumonias complicate disease presentation and diagnosis.

SYSTEMS AFFECTED
Respiratory

GENETICS
N/A

INCIDENCE/PREVALENCE
• Incidence for CCPP varies worldwide but infection with *Mycoplasma capricolum capripneumoniae* (mycoplasma biotype F-38) is more common and severe than *Mycoplasma mycoides capri* (type strain PG-3).
• Morbidity often reaches 100% and mortality may be 70–100%.

GEOGRAPHIC DISTRIBUTION
• While not found in the United States, CCPP has been reported in over 40 countries including Africa, Asia, Eastern Europe, the Middle East, and the former Soviet Union.
• Isolating the mycoplasma organism proves difficult in some countries and has been done only in Africa (Eritrea, Ethiopia, Kenya, Mali, Niger, Sudan, Chad, Tunisia, Tanzania, Uganda), Asia, and the Mediterranean (United Arab Emirates, Oman, Yemen).

SIGNALMENT
Species
Caprine

Breed Predilections, Mean Age and Range, Predominant Sex
N/A

SIGNS

HISTORICAL FINDINGS
Severe respiratory disease in goats with high morbidity and mortality within 7–10 days after clinical disease onset.

PHYSICAL EXAMINATION FINDINGS
• Infection with mycoplasma F-38 is respiratory in nature with a fever (106°F), cough, labored breathing, weakness, anorexia, leading to exercise intolerance and respiratory distress. Goats will stand with legs spread, neck extended downward, and tongue protruded.
• Frothy nasal discharge and continuous stringy salivation appear shortly before death. Chronic cases can recover and become carrier animals.
• Infection with type strain PG-3 results in a more generalized infection with respiratory signs (although less severe), reproductive signs, and gastrointestinal signs due to acute or peracute septicemia.

CAUSES
• The bacterial agent *Mycoplasma capricolum capripneumoniae* (mycoplasma biotype F-38) is the most common cause of CCPP. It is also the most contagious and virulent.
• *Mycoplasma mycoides capri* (type strain PG-3) also causes CCPP in goats but less commonly and with a different clinical presentation.
• Disease spread is through direct contact and inhalation of infective aerosols.

RISK FACTORS
• Exposure to carrier animals shedding organisms after periods of stress, such as sudden climatic changes (heavy rains or cold spells), especially in close confinement or overcrowded conditions can predispose CCPP outbreaks.
• Introduction of carrier animals into previously uninfected herds

DIAGNOSIS

DIFFERENTIAL DIAGNOSIS
Peste des petits ruminants, pasteurellosis, other *Mycoplasma* spp. pneumonias, *Haemophilus* spp., and *Salmonella* spp.

CBC/BIOCHEMISTRY/URINALYSIS
N/A

OTHER LABORATORY TESTS
• Serological tests such as complement fixation, passive hemagglutination, and ELISA can be used on a herd basis to detect antibodies to mycoplasma F-38.
• Whole blood or serum can be used for the latex agglutination test (most commonly done in Africa).

IMAGING
Although not commonly done, radiographs would reveal evidence of fluid in the thoracic cavity, pulmonary consolidation, and nodules.

DIAGNOSTIC PROCEDURES
Confirmatory diagnosis is made by culturing the agent from lung, pleuritic fluid, swabs of major bronchi, and tracheobronchial or mediastinal lymph nodes and identified by immunofluorescence or by growth or metabolic inhibition tests.

PATHOLOGIC FINDINGS
• With *M. capricolum capripneumoniae* infection, one or both lungs may be affected and may be adhered to the thoracic cavity due to thickened pleura. There will be straw-colored fluid in the thorax. The lungs themselves will have a fibrinous pneumonia and pea-sized, yellow-colored nodules appear in early infection.
• More advanced cases will have congestion surrounding the nodules. An entire lobe may become solidified or develop massive hepatization (appearance of liver). There is no thickening of the interlobular septa as in bovine pleuropneumonia.
• Histopathology reveals serofibrinous to fibrinonecrotic pleuropneumonia with infiltrates in the alveoli, bronchioles, interstitial septae, and subpleural connective tissue.
• Peribronchial lymphoid hyperplasia with mononuclear cell infiltration can also be seen.
• In the case of infection with *M. mycoides capri*, lung lesions are more likely unilateral with extensive pleuritis, fibrinous pneumonia with hepatization, most commonly of the cardiac and diaphragmatic lobes.
• The interlobular septa are dilated.
• Since this form of CCPP causes a more generalized infection, other lesions such as encephalitis/meningitis, lymphadenitis, splenitis, and genitourinary tract and intestinal changes will be seen.

TREATMENT

APPROPRIATE HEALTH CARE, NURSING CARE
• Due to the contagious nature of this disease, affected animals should be isolated and the entire herd placed under quarantine.
• Early in the course of disease, antibiotics may be warranted.

ACTIVITY
Animals should be isolated and activity restricted because of the exercise intolerance due to the severe respiratory disease.

DIET
Maintain a good plane of nutrition with fresh food and water daily.

CLIENT EDUCATION
Clients should be made aware of the seriousness of CCPP and the contagious aspects so as to protect their nonexposed susceptible animals on their facility.

SURGICAL CONSIDERATIONS
N/A

CONTAGIOUS CAPRINE PLEUROPNEUMONIA

MEDICATIONS

DRUGS OF CHOICE
• Broad-spectrum antibiotics EARLY in the course of disease
• Macrolides, tetracyclines, and quinolones are active against *M. capricolum* subsp. *capripneumoniae* but do not always clear an animal of carrier status.
• Tylosin and oxytetracycline appear effective.

CONTRAINDICATIONS, POSSIBLE INTERACTIONS, ALTERNATIVE DRUGS
Drug withdrawal periods for meat and milk are important to monitor when using antibiotic agents.

FOLLOW-UP

PATIENT MONITORING
Respiratory distress is a large component of this disease, so monitor animals for signs of labored breathing and nasal discharge to ensure they have a patent airway.

PREVENTION/AVOIDANCE
• Vaccination of animals with a live attenuated and inactivated F-38 vaccines has had varying degrees of success in parts of the world.
• A lyophilized saponin-inactivated F-38 vaccine had 100% effectiveness in preventing contact exposure in field tests in Kenya. It is used in goat kids older than 10 weeks and is effective for approximately 1 year.
• Quarantine of farms with testing and slaughtering of animals has been proven effective as a control plan in the event of an outbreak.

POSSIBLE COMPLICATIONS
Goats that recover maintain a long-term carrier status, leading to exposure of susceptible animals during periods of stress.

EXPECTED COURSE AND PROGNOSIS
Acute disease has a morbidity of 70–100% with mortality reaching 100% in some goat herds. Recovered animals can become long-term carriers of mycoplasma.

MISCELLANEOUS

ASSOCIATED CONDITIONS
N/A

AGE-RELATED FACTORS
N/A

ZOONOTIC POTENTIAL
CCPP is not a zoonotic disease.

PREGNANCY
N/A

RUMINANT SPECIES AFFECTED
Goats

BIOSECURITY
Isolating infected animals is imperative to the control of this disease.

PRODUCTION MANAGEMENT
N/A

SYNONYMS
Mycoplasma strain F-38

SEE ALSO
Haemophilus spp.
Other *Mycoplasma* spp. pneumonias
Pasteurellosis
Peste des petits ruminants
Salmonella spp.

ABBREVIATIONS
CCPP = contagious caprine pleuropneumonia
ELISA = enzyme-linked immunosorbent assay

Suggested Reading
Aiello, S. E., ed. 1998. *Merck veterinary manual*, 8th ed. Whitehouse Station, NJ: Merck and Co.
Contagious caprine pleuropneumonia. 2002. In: *Recent advances in goat diseases*, ed. M. Tempesta. International Veterinary Information Service, Ithaca, NY (www.ivis.org), A0907.0802 accessed at http://www.ivis.org/advances/Disease_Tempesta/nicholas/chapter_frm.asp?LA1 on May 16, 2004.
FAO Animal Health Disease Cards, Contagious Caprine Pleuropneumonia accessed at http://www.fao.org/ag/againfo/subjects/en/health/diseases-cards/ccpp.html on May 16, 2004.
Office International des Epizooties. 2000. *Manual of Standards Diagnostic Tests and Vaccines* chapter 2.4.6. information about Contagious Caprine Pleuropneumonia website accessed at http://www.oie.int/eng/normes/mmanual/A_00066.htm on May 16, 2004.
United States Animal Health Association, Foreign Animal Diseases book website, Contagious Caprine Pleuropneumonia accessed at http://www.vet.uga.edu/vpp/gray_book/FAD/CCP.htm on May 15, 2004.

Author: Danelle Bickett-Weddle

COPPER DEFICIENCY OF SHEEP AND GOATS

 BASICS

DEFINITION
A disease condition caused by either primary or secondary copper deficiency that is manifested in the neonate by congenital posterior paresis or paralysis and occasionally more severe neurological disease, and in the growing lamb/kid or adult with reduced growth or chronic wasting, anemia, lameness, changes to the wool/hair coat, and occasionally diarrhea.

PATHOPHYSIOLOGY
• Primary copper (Cu) deficiency occurs because of insufficient copper in the diet of the pregnant ewe/doe (congenital) and/or the diet of the growing lamb/kid. Plant copper levels of < 5 mg/kg DM are dangerous and < 3 mg/kg DM are likely to result in primary Cu deficiency. Cu-deficient soils are generally sandy and poor quality.
• Secondary Cu deficiency occurs when levels of molybdenum (Mo) (most commonly), sulphur (S) (occasionally), or iron (Fe) or zinc (Zn) (rarely) are high in the diet. These minerals compete with Cu uptake and cause increased excretion of Cu. Forage levels of Mo > 10 mg/kg are associated with secondary Cu deficiency. Peaty soils are more often associated with excess Mo. S-containing fertilizers may exacerbate Cu deficiency.
• Cu is a necessary component of ceruloplasmin, an enzyme involved in the cytochrome oxidase system, and of other enzymes such as erythrocyte superoxide dismutase. Failure of these enzyme systems may cause poor tissue oxidation, which then interferes with cell growth and function.

SYSTEMS AFFECTED
Congenital Form
Present at birth in kids and lambs. White matter of the cerebrum is affected. Areas of fluid-filled cavities may be grossly evident in the most severely affected cases.

Delayed Form
• In kids and lambs within 2 to 4 months of age: affects the spinal cord and brain stem. Lesions are found in the large neurons of the red and vestibular nuclei, the reticular formation, and the ventral horns of the spinal cortex. In kids, may also affect cerebellum. Altered or reduced myelination is the primary feature.
• Acute delayed Cu deficiency has been reported in the UK, where lambs 2 to 4 weeks of age are suddenly affected with incoordination, tremors, frothing at the mouth, grinding of the teeth, and finally opisthotonus and death due to cerebral edema and herniation of the medulla and cerebellum through the foramen magnum.
• The delayed form may be caused by marginally low Cu in the pregnant adult, poor transfer of Cu stores to the fetus, and continued deficiency in the neonatal period. Severity and length of the deficiency dictates the severity of the disease in the young lamb/kid.

Young Stock and Adults
• Hemoglobin production for red blood cells is inhibited by the lack of Cu to aid in recycling of iron. This results in hypochromic anemia without hemolysis.
• Wool lacks keratinization and becomes straight and brittle (steely wool) and colored fleeces lack color. This impairment of keratinization also affects skin.

• With primary Cu deficiency: bone is affected with osteoporosis, widening of the long bones, and overgrowth of epiphyseal cartilage most notably at the costochondral junction. Osteoblastic activity is impaired. With Mo excess: most of the effect is at the epiphyses.
• Both humoral and cell-mediated immunity are impaired, as well as the nonspecific immune system. Resistance to parasites is decreased with Cu deficiency.

GENETICS
• There is a strong breed component to the susceptibility of sheep to Cu deficiency. Breeds such as the Scottish blackface and Finnish Landrace, are poor utilizers of Cu, very susceptible to Cu deficiency, and, conversely, resistant to Cu toxicity. Texel sheep require little Cu and are resistant to Cu deficiency but are very susceptible to Cu toxicity.
• This is not as well studied in goats but genetic variability is suspected between breeds.

INCIDENCE/PREVALENCE
• Overall not a common disease, but one that is generally associated with a specific geographic region.
• Excess supplementation of S, either on pasture or as a mineral supplement or water high in S, may cause an "outbreak" in a specific flock that was not noted previously to be at risk.
• Water high in iron may also contribute if Cu availability is marginal.

GEOGRAPHIC DISTRIBUTION
• Soil type determines the likelihood of Cu deficiency in the plants (e.g., sandy and limestone soils and soils that are washed out may have low Cu levels). A specific geographic area may be known to be risky. Many areas in the United States and Canada are known to be Cu deficient although there may be tremendous variation in Cu soil content within a small region, even on a given farm.
• Reclaimed swamps or peat bogs often are high in Mo.

COPPER DEFICIENCY OF SHEEP AND GOATS

SIGNALMENT

Species
Sheep and goat

Breed Predilections
See Genetics above

Mean Age and Range
• Congenital is present at birth.
• Delayed generally occurs between 2 and 4 months of age.
• Adult can occur at any age.

Predominant Sex
N/A

GENERAL COMMENTS
N/A

HISTORICAL FINDINGS
• A particular farm may have chronic problems due to Cu or Mo levels in the forages or S or Fe levels in the water.
• There may be a history of a change in feeding practices (e.g., addition of S to ration or to pasture).

PHYSICAL EXAMINATION FINDINGS

Congenital
Lambs or kids are born small, weak, and ataxic or unable to stand. Severe cases may be blind or show tremors. If not fed colostrum, they often die of septicemia secondary to failure of passive transfer.

Delayed
• Lambs or kids are born normally but may develop ataxia (paresis) or paralysis of the hind end or lameness.

• They are more prone to parasitic infections such as coccidiosis and haemonchosis.
• They may be found down in the pasture, but if they are still alert, the owner may note that the ewe/doe will still be nursing them.
• Fractures may occur secondary to osteoporosis. Fractures may be minute and may present as angular deformities.
• Lameness due to inflammation of the epiphyses

Adult
• Mildly to profoundly anemic
• Lame due to minute fractures of the trabeculae, epiphysitis, or long bone fractures.
• The wool is straight, without crimp, may exhibit wool-break due to weakness of the fiber, and in colored fleeces and hair may lack color.
• Growth of young stock is reduced and in severe cases, animals may show weight loss.
• If Cu is secondary to Mo access, diarrhea may develop (peat scours) although this is more common in cattle.
• Infertility may be linked to Cu deficiency but this is not well proven.
• New work shows an association between Cu metabolism and conformational changes in the scrapie prion protein in susceptible sheep but the clinical significance of this is not well understood at this point.

CAUSES
• Forages deficient in Cu
• Forages containing excess Mo or S
• Water containing excess S or Fe (less common)

RISK FACTORS
• Susceptibility of breed (i.e., ability of breed to absorb Cu)
• Heavy parasitism will reduce Cu liver levels.
• Cu does not accumulate in the ovine fetal liver as well as in other species (e.g., cattle).

 DIAGNOSIS

DIFFERENTIAL DIAGNOSIS

Congenital Form
Any disease that causes birth of weak lambs or kids (e.g., enzootic abortion, iodine deficiency)

Delayed Form
Tail docking abscess, traumatic fracture of a vertebra or long bone, CAE/MV (OPP), rickets due to vitamin D deficiency, down due to vitamin E selenium deficiency

Adult
• Poor growth due to parasitism, poor nutrition
• Anemia due to parasitism, chronic disease, blood loss
• Poor wool due to sulphur deficiency, external parasites

CBC/BIOCHEMISTRY/URINALYSIS
Anemia in lambs is hypochromic and microcytic, in adults is hypochromic and macrocytic.

OTHER LABORATORY TESTS

Sheep
• Serum Cu
  • Deficient—0.10–1.00 ppm
  • Marginal—0.40–1.00 ppm

COPPER DEFICIENCY OF SHEEP AND GOATS

- Plasma Cu: deficient— < 0.60 ppm
- Erythrocyte superoxide dismutase activity
  - Short-duration deficiency—youngstock > 0.5 and adult > 0.3 mg/g hemoglobin
  - Prolonged deficiency—youngstock < 0.3 and adult < 0.2 mg/g hemoglobin
- Tissue Cu
  - Liver—deficient 0.5–4.0 ppm WW
  - Liver—marginal 5.0–20.0 ppm WW
  - Fetal liver—deficient 1.0–10 ppm WW
  - Wool—deficient 0.5–2.5 ppm DW

Goat
- Serum Cu
  - Deficient—0.04–0.40 ppm
  - Marginal—0.40–0.80 ppm
- Tissue Cu
  - Liver—deficient 0.4–10.0 ppm WW
  - Fetal liver—deficient 1.6–20.0 ppm WW
  - Hair—deficient < 3.0 ppm DW

IMAGING
N/A

DIAGNOSTIC PROCEDURES
N/A

PATHOLOGIC FINDINGS
See Systems Affected above.

TREATMENT

APPROPRIATE HEALTH CARE

NURSING CARE
Lambs and kids that are severely affected with either the congenital or delayed form should be humanely euthanized.

ACTIVITY
N/A

DIET

Sheep
- If Mo 0.05–1.0 ppm, then Cu 5.0–10.0 ppm DW
- Cu:Mo ratio > 2:1 and < 20:1 (~ 6:1)
- Maximum safe level of Mo 8.0–10.0 ppm DW

Goats
Copper levels should be 10–23 ppm DW.

CLIENT EDUCATION
Inform client of balancing dietary needs with respect to Cu, particularly if secondary Cu deficiency.

SURGICAL CONSIDERATIONS
NA

MEDICATIONS

DRUGS OF CHOICE
- Oral treatment: 1.5 g Cu sulphate for ewes and 35 mg for lambs as a single dose
- Dosing ewes 8 and 4 weeks prior to lambing with 200 mg Cu sulphate can prevent the congenital form.
- 5 mg Cu methionate injection in lambs at 3 to 10 days of age to prevent delayed form
- Some injectable forms may be recommended (Cu calcium edetate or Cu methionate) but may cause tissue reaction.

CONTRAINDICATIONS
- If diagnosis is not correct, (i.e., not supported by analysis of Cu levels in the animal), then supplementation of Cu may result in toxicity.
- Appropriate milk and meat withdrawal times must be followed for all compounds administered to food-producing animals.

PRECAUTIONS
Excessive treatment with Cu may cause toxicity.

POSSIBLE INTERACTIONS

ALTERNATIVE DRUGS

FOLLOW-UP

PATIENT MONITORING
To monitor effectiveness of control program, may wish to monitor Cu liver levels or, in ewes, serum Cu levels.

PREVENTION/AVOIDANCE

Copper Supplement for Sheep
- Copper oxide wire particles or rods orally (1.25 g Cu to weaned lambs and 2.5 g Cu to adults) generally administered in a gelatin capsule, which dissolves in the abomasum. The Cu oxide rods or wires dissolve slowly.
- Copper heptonate as an intramuscular injection (25 mg Cu to weaned lambs and 37.5 mg Cu to adults) once every 3 to 9 months, respectively.
- Copper sulphate spread on pasture at 2.0 kg/ha.

Copper Supplements for Goats
Oral—2 g copper oxide needles to kids at 5 weeks of age and 4 g copper oxide needles to does in early pregnancy

POSSIBLE COMPLICATIONS
Diagnosis should be confirmed before preventive therapy is commenced.

EXPECTED COURSE AND PROGNOSIS
- Lambs and kids born with the congenital form will not respond to therapy.
- Lambs and kids that develop the delayed form may respond if clinical signs are mild. Certainly supplementation of the animals at risk may prevent additional animals from developing the delayed form.

COPPER DEFICIENCY OF SHEEP AND GOATS

• Adults will respond rapidly to supplementation, particularly wool growth will improve within days of supplementation and anemia will become less severe. Lameness may not improve or only improve marginally, however.

 MISCELLANEOUS

ASSOCIATED CONDITIONS
N/A

AGE-RELATED FACTORS
N/A

ZOONOTIC POTENTIAL
If Mo is present at a high level in the diet, it may accumulate in the liver and kidneys. If this is the case, then animals intended for slaughter should have kidneys and liver discarded as unfit for human consumption.

PREGNANCY
Supplementation of pregnant ewes and does is critical to preventing the congenital and delayed form of this disease.

RUMINANT SPECIES AFFECTED
Primarily sheep but also goats and cattle

BIOSECURITY
N/A

PRODUCTION MANAGEMENT
See under Prevention/Avoidance above.

SYNONYMS
Enzootic swayback
Neonatal ataxia
Peat scours (secondary Cu deficiency due to high Mo)
Steely wool
Swayback

SEE ALSO
CAE/MV (OPP)
Enzootic abortion
Iodine deficiency
Sulphur deficiency
Vitamin D deficiency
Vitamin E selenium deficiency

ABBREVIATIONS
CAE = caprine arthritis encephalitis
Cu = copper
DM = dry matter
DW = dry weight
Fe = iron
Mo = molybdenum
MV = maedi visna
OPP = ovine progressive pneumonia
ppm = parts per million
S = sulphur
WW = weight/weight

Suggested Reading
Donoghue, S., Kronfeld, D. S. 1990. Clinical nutrition of sheep and goats. *Vet Clin North Am Food Anim Pract*. 6: 563–76.
Judson, G. J., Babidge, P. J. 2004. An assessment of the safety of copper heptonate for parenteral therapy in sheep. *Aust Vet J*. 82:75–78.
Puls, R. 1994. *Mineral levels in animal health*. 2nd ed. Clearbrook BC, Canada: Sherpa International.
Suttle, N. F. 1986. Copper deficiency in ruminants; recent developments. *Vet Rec*. 119:519–22.
Suttle, N. F., Jones, D. G. 1989. Recent developments in trace element metabolism and function: trace elements, disease resistance and immune responsiveness in ruminants. *J Nutr*. 119:1055–61.

Author: Paula I. Menzies

COPPER TOXICITY

 BASICS

OVERVIEW
• Copper (Cu) is an essential trace element that is a component of several enzyme systems. The Cu-dependent enzymes are involved in critical metabolic and physiological functions such as iron (Fe) metabolism, elastin and collagen formation, melanin production, and integrity of the central nervous system (CNS).
• Cu is also a toxic element if consumed in excess amounts.
• The liver is considered the key organ in Cu metabolism, storage, and excretion.
• Ruminants store Cu in the liver during excess intake and deplete when Cu intake is low.
• Several elements have a negative impact on Cu absorption and its metabolism. These include molybdenum (Mo) and sulfur (S). The negative interactions between Cu and these elements significantly affect Cu availability and animal requirements. Consumption of high-Mo forages results in molybdenosis or hypocuprosis in grazing ruminants.

PATHOPHYSIOLOGY
• High concentrations of other minerals, especially Mo and S, have negative effects on Cu absorption and its metabolism. In the rumen, sulfate is reduced to sulfide that reacts with Mo to form thiomolybdate (MoS_4^{2-}). The thiomolybdate possesses a high affinity for Cu and is capable of rendering it insoluble and nonabsorbable by forming Cu thiomolybdate ($CuMoS_4$).
• Some of thiomolybdates are absorbed and affect systemic metabolism of Cu negatively. The absorbed thiomolybdates result in Cu being tightly bound to albumin in plasma and not available for biochemical functions.
• S alone at high levels affects Cu absorption negatively. This is due to formation of insoluble nonabsorbable Cu sulfide.
• High levels of Fe and Zn also decrease Cu absorption.
• Interference of Fe with Cu absorption is not well understood. This negative interaction was suggested to involve formation of ferrous sulfide complexes in the rumen that become soluble in the abomasum where the sulfide may dissociate and form insoluble complex with Cu.

SYSTEMS AFFECTED
Production management, skin, central nervous system, musculoskeletal, cardiovascular

GENETICS
N/A

INCIDENCE/PREVALENCE
N/A

GEOGRAPHIC DISTRIBUTION
• Worldwide depending on species and environment
• Cu deficiency in ruminants is common under natural grazing conditions in many countries, especially Australia, New Zealand, the Netherlands the UK, and the United States.

SIGNALMENT
Species
Potentially all ruminant species

Breed Predilections
• Sheep breeds appear to vary in their tolerance to high Cu levels (Merino sheep are known to be more tolerant than other sheep breeds).
• Chronic toxicity of Cu has been reported in dairy cows fed diets containing 37.5 mg/kg DM during lactation and 22.6 mg/kg DM dry cows.
• Simmental and Charolais cattle appear to have higher Cu requirements than Angus cattle.

Mean Age and Range
• In general, Cu is poorly absorbed by ruminants and the absorption rate is higher in suckling than in adult animals (i.e., 5%–10% vs. 1%–3%).
• Adult cattle are more resistant to toxicity than younger cattle.

Predominant Sex
N/A

SIGNS
HISTORICAL FINDINGS
Copper Deficiency
• Ruminants, especially sheep, are more susceptible to Cu deficiency than nonruminants.
• Cu deficiency is considered a severe limitation to grazing ruminants throughout the world. Cu deficiency is more frequent on pastures than in feedlots.

• Cu deficiency in ruminants can result from low Cu concentration in feeds (i.e., <3 mg/kg DM) but most commonly occurs when Cu concentrations in forages are normal (i.e., 6 to 16 mg/kg DM) but unavailable due to high concentrations of Mo or S.
• With regard to Mo, Cu deficiency occurs when forage Mo concentration exceeds 3 mg/kg DM and Cu concentration is less than 5 mg/kg DM.
• Cu deficiency can occur under different dietary conditions such as low Cu (i.e., <5 mg/kg DM), low Cu and high Mo (i.e., ratio 2:1), higher Mo (i.e., >20 mg/kg DM), normal Cu and low Mo but with high levels of soluble proteins from lush pastures.
• Anemia results from the delay in maturation and shortening of the life span of red blood cells. Anemic ruminants have a hemoglobin level of 5.9 g/100 mL vs. 13.7 g/100 mL after Cu administration.
• The impaired keratinization of hair and wool
• The CNS disorders are attributed to the demyelination of the nerves.
• The symptoms of reproductive failure include low fertility, delayed or depressed estrus, fetal death and resorption, calving difficulties, retained placenta, and calves born with congenital rickets.
• Achromotrichia is a lack of tyrosinase (i.e., polyphenyl oxidase) activity. This results in breakdown in the conversion of L-tyrosine to melanin and the subsequent loss of pigments in hair and wool. Examples include lightening of hair coat in black or red animals, showing reddish tinge in the case of black animals behind the shoulder and on the lower quarters, and finally rough hair coat.
• Bone problems include development of fragile bones, especially long bones that break easily without an apparent cause. Cattle can have swelling or enlargement of the ends of the leg bones and, therefore, move like a pacing horse (i.e., pacing gait).
• Falling disease or sudden death in cattle is attributed to heart lesions.
• Negative effects of Cu deficiency on immune function
• Severe diarrhea is also a common symptom of Cu deficiency; however, diarrhea is less common in sheep than in cattle.
• Poor growth and/or loss of body weight are also common symptoms of Cu deficiency.

PHYSICAL EXAMINATION FINDINGS

Symptoms
• The symptoms of Cu toxicity include nausea, vomiting, salivation, abdominal pain, convulsions, paralysis, collapse, hemolysis, methemoglobinemia, hemoglobinuria, jaundice, icterus, widespread necrosis, and death.
• Additional symptoms include anemia, muscular dystrophy, decreased growth, and impaired reproduction.

CAUSES AND RISK FACTORS

Functions
• Cu is needed for several metabolic functions such as cellular respiration, bone formation, normal cardiac function, connective tissue development, myelination of the spinal cord keratinization, and tissue pigmentation.
• Additionally, Cu serves as a catalyst for hemoglobin synthesis. Cu also is needed for normal reproduction and immune function.

Sources
• Cu is distributed in feeds at various levels ranging from 1 to 50 mg/kg of dry matter (DM).
• The Cu content of feeds depends on geographical location, soil pH, climate, crop management, and plant species, maturity, and yield. Cu concentrations were reported to be highest for legumes (i.e., 15 mg/kg DM), lowest for grasses (i.e., 5 mg/kg DM), and intermediate for grains (i.e., 4–8 mg/kg DM).
• Several Cu salts (inorganic forms) are commonly used in ruminant diets to meet the requirements. These include (from highest to lowest in biological availability) cupric sulfate ($CuSO_4$), cupric carbonate ($CuCO_3$), and cupric oxide (CuO).
• Inorganic Cu sources such as CuO are used in a bolus form that provides long-term supplementation through the slow release of Cu in the rumen over an extended period of time.
• Chelated forms (organic complexes) of Cu have higher bioavailability than do inorganic sources.

Toxicity
• An extended period of time (i.e., weeks or months) is needed for development of Cu toxicity.
• Ruminants are more susceptible to Cu toxicity than nonruminants. This is due to the very narrow range between adequate and toxic Cu levels.

• Sheep are considered the most sensitive domestic animal species to Cu toxicity. This was illustrated in the marked elevation of hepatic Cu when sheep were fed diets containing Cu at 26–38 mg/kg DM, whereas rats tolerated diets containing Cu levels as high as 500 mg/kg DM.
• Significant differences were also shown between sheep and cattle in dietary Cu tolerance (i.e., 25 vs. 100 mg/kg DM). The sensitivity of sheep to Cu could be explained by comparing the adequate (i.e., 5–8 mg/kg DM) to the toxic (i.e., >8 mg/ kg DM) levels of their diets.

DIAGNOSIS

DIFFERENTIAL DIAGNOSIS
• Iodine deficiency
• Rickets due to vitamin D deficiency
• Vitamin E selenium deficiency
• Parasitism (internal and external)
• Poor nutrition
• Anemia due to parasitism, chronic disease, blood loss
• Sulfur deficiency

CBC/BIOCHEMISTRY/URINALYSIS
Anemia—in young, hypochromic and microcytic; in adults, hypochromic and macrocytic

OTHER LABORATORY TESTS

IMAGING

OTHER DIAGNOSTIC PROCEDURES

Deficiency Diagnosis
• Analysis of feed for Cu, Mo, S, and Fe to assess the Cu status and possible availability. Forage containing <8–10 mg/kg DM are Cu deficient. Forages containing Mo at >1–3 mg/kg DM or having Cu:Mo ratios >3.1 or 4:1 usually have low levels of available Cu.
• Measuring Cu concentration in plasma or serum. The normal range (i.e., 0.6–1.5 $\gamma g/ml$) is wide for cattle, sheep, and goats.
• Cu deficiency is commonly associated with decreased number of mineral elements in the liver and other organs (e.g., kidney and brain).
• Liver biopsies to assess the storage status of Cu. Normal concentrations range from 100 to 400 mg/kg liver DM.

Toxicity Diagnosis
• Increased serum glutamate oxaloacetate transaminase activity before death
• Increased serum arginase in liver damage

TREATMENT

Deficiency Treatment
• Cu deficiency is corrected by supplementation of Cu in the diet. This is possible through Cu inclusion in the concentrate mixture of feedlot diets. Grazing ruminants are supplemented with Cu compounds through dosing or drenching at intervals (e.g., monthly). The boluses used are usually slow-release forms of Cu compounds that provide the required amounts over time.
• Another method of Cu delivery is through subcutaneous or intramuscular injection of organic forms. Injectable forms of Cu (e.g., Cu glycinate and Cu EDTA) were suggested to be given at 3- to 6-month intervals to prevent deficiency.
• Cu also can be offered in a free-choice mineral mix containing 0.1%–0.2% Cu sulfate. Under severe deficiency, Cu sulfate could be increased in the mineral mix to 0.5%.

Toxicity Treatment
• For treatment of sheep, administration of Mo and S (e.g., 100 mg of ammonium molybdate and 1 g of sodium sulfate in 20 mL of water or in feed daily for 5 to 6 weeks) is recommended.
• Because high levels of Zn can protect against Cu toxicity, administration of Zn at 100 mg/kg DM will decrease liver Cu storage.

MEDICATIONS

CONTRAINDICATIONS
• Appropriate milk and meat withdrawal times must be followed for all compounds administered to food-producing animals.
• Injectable copper can be highly toxic in sheep and goats.

PRECAUTIONS
Ionophores (e.g., monensin and lasalocid) can increase Cu accumulation in the liver of ruminants with monensin having the greatest effect.

COPPER TOXICITY

POSSIBLE INTERACTIONS
N/A

ALTERNATIVE DRUGS
N/A

FOLLOW-UP

PATIENT MONITORING

PREVENTION/AVOIDANCE
Under certain conditions, the forages that cause Cu deficiency when they are grazed will not do so when harvested and fed as hay.

POSSIBLE COMPLICATIONS
N/A

EXPECTED COURSE AND PROGNOSIS
.

MISCELLANEOUS

ASSOCIATED CONDITIONS
The Cu deficiency symptoms include anemia, severe diarrhea, bone disorders, neonatal ataxia, reproductive failure (e.g., temporary infertility), cardiovascular disorders (e.g., heart failure), achromotrichia (i.e., loss of pigmentation), nerve disorders, depressed immune function, poor growth, reduced appetite, keratinization failure in hair and wool, and weak, fragile long bones that break easily.

AGE-RELATED FACTORS
In general, young and growing ruminants have higher Cu requirements than older animals and both the requirements and tolerance are affected by the genetic makeup.

ZOONOTIC POTENTIAL
N/A

PREGNANCY
Abortion secondary to copper deficiency

RUMINANT SPECIES AFFECTED
Potentially, all ruminant species can be affected.

BIOSECURITY
N/A

PRODUCTION MANAGEMENT
Nutritional Requirements
• It is difficult to provide the exact dietary Cu requirements or to predict potential toxic levels of Cu for ruminants under different feeding programs. This is because Cu concentrations and availability vary significantly among feeds and even for the same feed (e.g., a forage species grown in different environmental conditions). Absorption rates of Cu are also affected by homeostatic controls and many dietary factors.
• Dietary Mo concentrations have the greatest impact on Cu requirements. Increasing dietary Mo, as is the case under certain grazing conditions, significantly increases Cu requirements.
• Although Mo is less of a problem in the feedlot, Cu requirements of cattle on high-concentrate diets are still not well defined.
• A Cu:Mo ratio of 4:1 was suggested to ensure meeting Cu requirements.
• Cu requirements are increased when intakes of Zn or Fe are high due to decreased Cu absorption.
• Dietary Cu levels of 8, 10, and 7–11 mg/kg DM were recommended to meet the requirements of beef cattle, dairy cattle, and sheep, respectively.
• Cu availability in feeds is a limiting factor, especially under grazing conditions. Thus, more supplemental Cu is required for grazing cattle than for those on high-concentrate diets.
• Because Cu availability in lush pastures is low and its level decreases with forage maturity, Cu supplementation should be increased at early and late maturity stages of forages to prevent deficiency.

SYNONYMS
Neonatal ataxia
Ovine enzootic ataxia
Swayback

SEE ALSO
Copper deficiency in small ruminants
Herd toxicity management
Molybdenum
Zinc deficiency

ABBREVIATIONS
CNS = central nervous system
Cu = copper
DM = dry matter
Fe = iron
Mo = molybdenum
S = sulfur
Zn = zinc

Suggested Reading
Corah, L. 1996. Trace mineral requirements of grazing cattle. *Anim Feed Sci Technol*. 59:61–70.
McDowell, L. R. 1992. *Minerals in animal and human nutrition*. San Diego: Academic Press.
Solaiman, S. G., Maloney, M. A., Qureshi, M. A., Davis, G., D'Andrea, G. 2001, Aug. Effects of high copper supplements on performance, health, plasma copper and enzymes in goats. *Small Rumin Res*. 41(2):127–39.
Ward, J. D., Spears, J. W., Gengelbach, G. P. 1995. Differences in copper status and copper metabolism among Angus, Simmental, and Charolais cattle. *J Anim Sci*. 73:571–77.
Xin, Z., Waterman, D. F., Hemken, R. W., Harmon, R. J. 1991. Effects of copper status on neutrophil function, superoxide dismutase, and copper distribution in steers. *J Dairy Sci*. 74:3078–85.

Author: Hussein S. Hussein

BASICS

DEFINITION
• An alteration in the structure and function of the right ventricle caused by a primary disorder of the respiratory system
• Collectively refers to conditions of right-heart hypertrophy, dilatation, and subsequent failure caused by pulmonary hypertension and increased pulmonary vascular resistance

OVERVIEW
• Sporadic disease that occurs most commonly in animals with chronic lung disease and ongoing lung pathology
• May develop secondary to a variety of cardiopulmonary diseases
• Regardless of cause, pulmonary hypertension is the common link between lung dysfunction and the heart in cor pulmonale.
• Pulmonary hypertension leads to right ventricular hypertrophy, dilatation, or failure.
• Most common cause for pulmonary hypertension is chronic alveolar hypoxia and hypoxic vasoconstriction.
• Commonly has a chronic progressive course but may have an acute onset

PATHOPHYSIOLOGY
• Pathophysiologic mechanisms that lead to pulmonary hypertension and cor pulmonale include
  • Pulmonary vasoconstriction due to alveolar hypoxia or acidemia

• Lung disorders (e.g., emphysema, thromboembolism, interstitial disease) resulting in anatomic compromise of pulmonary vasculature
  • Increased blood viscosity
  • Idiopathic primary pulmonary hypertension
• Pulmonary hypertrophy of medial smooth musculature within pulmonary arteries and arterioles results in increased work for the right ventricle.
• Right-ventricular hypertrophy predominates in chronic cor pulmonale.
• Right-ventricular dilatation occurs predominately in acute cor pulmonale.

SIGNALMENT
• Uncommon, sporadic disease
• No age or sex predelection
• Cattle: highly susceptible to brisket disease due to well-developed smooth muscle in pulmonary circulation
• Holstein dairy cattle may be particularly sensitive.
• Goats
• Sheep

SIGNS
• Signs generally are nonspecific.
• Early signs: subtle respiratory signs or exercise intolerance
• Exercise intolerance on exertion
• Fatigue
• Dyspnea
• Tachycardia
• Cough
• Syncope with exercise
• Later stages: signs of right-heart failure—ventral edema, mammary and jugular vein distension, jugular vein pulsation, passive hepatic congestion

• Heart sounds are normal or increased in intensity.
• ±Cyanosis
• ±Heart murmur: tricuspid valve insufficiency or pulmonic valve ejection
• ±Gallop rhythm
• ±Atrial fibrillation (especially in goats)
• ±Splitting of second heart sound
• ±Hemoptysis
• Respiratory signs and thoracic auscultation reflect chronic and ongoing lung pathology

PATHOLOGIC LESIONS
• Lesions of underlying respiratory or cardiovascular disease
• Right-ventricular hypertrophy or dilation
• Enlargement of and wall thickening of pulmonary arteries and arterioles
• Lesions of right-heart failure (peripheral edema, hydrothorax, ascites, hepatic congestion)
• Lesions of locoweed toxicity in other organs

CAUSES AND RISK FACTORS
• Any condition that leads to prolonged high blood pressure in the arteries or veins of the lungs (pulmonary hypertension)
• Occurs most commonly in animals with chronic pneumonia, bronchiectasis, pulmonary abscesses, consolidated anterioventral lung lobes from previous pneumonia or chronic lung worm
• Mountain sickness (high-altitude disease); cattle exposed to high altitudes (elevation of 1600 m above sea level)
• Concurrent ingestion of locoweed (*Astragalus* spp. and *Oxytropis* spp.) enhances brisket disease in animals at high elevations
• *Pimelea* spp. toxicosis
• Hypoxia in neonatal calves

COR PULMONALE

- Pulmonary hypertension secondary to pulmonary and bronchial arteritis and periarteriolar sclerosis reported in dairy calves presumably exposed to monocrotaline, a pyrrolizidine alkaloid
- Chronic interstitial pneumonia and emphysema
- Chronic obstructive pneumonia, chronic bronchitis, pulmonary interstitial fibrosis
- Obesity in feedlot cattle
- Primary pulmonary hypertension
- Pulmonary embolism
- Pulmonary vascular disease
- Smoke inhalation
- Air pollution
- Silicosis
- Chest wall disease
- Abnormal ventilatory drive
- Surgical resection of lung tissue

 DIAGNOSIS

- History of chronic pulmonary disease or exposure to high altitude in animal with signs of right-heart failure
- Echocardiography
  - Rule out primary cardiac disease.
  - Document right-ventricular hypertrophy or dilatation.
  - Paradoxical interventricular septal movement during systole
  - ±Thickening of interventricular septum
  - Tricuspid valve insufficiency or pulmonic valve ejection jet
  - Dilation of pulmonary artery
  - Doppler echocardiography to measure pulmonary artery pressure

- Cardiac catheterization to document increased pressure in pulmonary artery, right ventricle, and right atrium
- Thoracic radiographs
  - Pulmonary disease
  - Evidence of pulmonary artery enlargement or right-heart enlargement
- Characterization of underlying pulmonary disease
  - Transtracheal wash—cytology, gram stain, culture, and sensitivity
  - Bronchoalveolar lavage—cell count and cytology
  - Thoracic ultrasound
  - Thoracic radiographs
- Baermann's technique to rule out lung worm
- Arterial blood gas: hypoxemia, ± hypercapnia

DIFFERENTIAL DIAGNOSIS
- Brisket disease or mountain sickness
- Farmer's lung
- Parasitic pneumonitis
- Allergic pneumonitis
- Cardiomyopathy
- Endocarditis
- Myocarditis
- Pericarditis
- Congestive heart failure
- Cardiac lymphosarcoma

CBC/BIOCHEMISTRY/URINALYSIS
- Variable: Normal or reflect chronic inflammatory/infectious disease
- ± Polycythemia
- ±Monocytosis or hyperproteinemia from chronic infection

OTHER LABORATORY TESTS
- Hepatic ultrasound
  - Infract
  - Disruption of normal parenchyma
  - Vascular changes
- Electrocardiogram
- Pulmonary function tests

IMAGING
- Echocardiography
- Radiography
- Thoracic CT scan
- Pulmonary angiography
- Cardiac catheterization
- Magnetic resonance imaging

DIAGNOSTIC PROCEDURES
- Echocardiography
- Doppler echocardiography
- Thoracic radiography
- Cardiac catheterization
- Lung biopsy to determine underlying etiology

 TREATMENT

- Treat primary lung disease when present
  - Antimicrobial agents for bacterial infections
  - Anthelmintics for lungworm infestations
  - Anti-inflammatories as needed
- Diuretics: furosemide
- ±Vasodilators; calcium channel blockers, prostaglandins; efficacy unknown in ruminants
- ±Digoxin: use controversial
- Oxygen therapy

• Animals with brisket disease: treat with oxygen, move to lower altitude; ± phlebotomy recommended by some authors for polycythemia
• Bronchodilators if underlying obstructive pulmonary disease
• Anticoagulant therapy if underlying thromboembolism
• Dietary salt restriction
• Appropriate milk and meat withdrawal times must be followed for all compounds administered to food producing animals.

MEDICATIONS

DRUGS OF CHOICE
• Furosemide: 0.5–1.0 mg/kg IV, IM Bid
• Digoxin: 0.86 μg/kg per hour IV (valuable hospitalized animals)

FOLLOW-UP

• Serum digoxin levels should be monitored to avoid toxicity.
• Monitoring of serum electrolytes and calcium, acid-base balance, and hydration status, if on diuretics

EXPECTED COURSE AND PROGNOSIS
• Guarded to poor prognosis depending on underlying cause
• Recovered animals may become poor doers: chronic weight loss, poor production.

MISCELLANEOUS

ASSOCIATED CONDITIONS
• Right-heart failure
• Hypoperfusion of vital organs (e.g., kidney, liver, gut)

ZOONOTIC POTENTIAL
N/A

RUMINANT SPECIES AFFECTED
Cattle, goat, sheep

BIOSECURITY
N/A

PRODUCTION MANAGEMENT
• Careful adaptation of animals when moving them to higher altitudes
• Routine deworming of cattle on pastures known to be contaminated with lung worms
• Avoid confining cattle in dusty barns and exposure to fungal allergens

SYNONYMS

SEE ALSO
Allergic pneumonitis
Brisket disease or mountain sickness
Cardiac lymphosarcoma
Cardiomyopathy
Congestive heart failure
Congestive heart failure, myocarditis, endocarditis, cardiomyopathy
Endocarditis
Farmer's lung
High-mountain disease/brisket disease and lung diseases
Myocarditis
Parasitic pneumonitis
Parasitic pneumonitis (lung worm infestation)
Pericarditis

ABBREVIATIONS
Bid = twice daily
CT = Computed tomography imaging
IM = intramuscular
IV = intravenous

Suggested Reading

Cardiovascular system. 1997. In: *Veterinary pathology*, ed. R. C. Jones, R. D. Hunt, and N. W. King, 6th ed., pp. 982–84. Philadelphia: Lippincott Williams and Wilkins.
Diseases of the heart. 1999. In: *Veterinary medicine: a textbook of the diseases of cattle, sheep, pigs, goats, and horses*, ed., O. M. Radostits et al., 9th ed. New York: W. B. Saunders and Co.
Lemler, M. A., et al., 2000. Myocyte cytoskeletal disorganization and right heart failure in hypoxia-induced neonatal pulmonary hypertension. *Am J Physiol Heart Circ Physiol*. 279: H1365–76.
Reef, V. B., and McGuirk, S. M. 2002. Diseases of the cardiovascular system. In: *Large animal internal medicine*, ed. G. Smith., 3rd ed. St. Louis: Mosby.
Yunis, N. A., and Crausman, R. S. *Cor pulmonale*. www.emedicine.com/med/topic449.htm

Authors: Susan Semrad and Sheila McGuirk

CORKSCREW CLAW IN CATTLE

BASICS

DEFINITION
Corkscrew claw is an abnormal growth of the abaxial wall of the hoof, usually the lateral rear claw with concurrent misalignment of the phalanges. The abaxial wall grows beneath the claw and causes the sole to be displaced axially. The condition is thought to be hereditary.

PATHOPHYSIOLOGY
• The second and third phalanges are misaligned with the third phalanx becoming long and narrow.
• The abaxial wall grows longer than normal and curves under the claw to become the weight-bearing surface, displacing the sole axially.
• An exostosis may form at the abaxial border of the distal interphalangeal joint and may cause excess growth of the abaxial wall.

SYSTEMS AFFECTED
Musculoskeletal and dermatologic

GENETICS
• Condition is considered heritable and bulls exhibiting this condition should not be used for breeding.
• Cows with this condition should not be used for replacement heifers.
• Heritability is about 0.05.

INCIDENCE/PREVALENCE
Incidence is reported to be from about 3% to 18%.

GEOGRAPHIC DISTRIBUTION
Worldwide

SIGNALMENT
Species
Bovine

Breed Predilections
Reported mostly in dairy cattle

Mean Age and Range
Cattle older than 3.5 years

Predominant Sex
Both cows and bulls, but seen most often in cows

SIGNS

HISTORICAL FINDINGS
Lameness can be a feature of this disease due to overburdening of the lateral, rear claws.

PHYSICAL EXAMINATION FINDINGS
• Overgrowth of the abaxial walls on lateral rear claws causing the sole to be displaced axially.
• The claw looks like a "corkscrew."
• There is often a palpable exostosis at the coronary band.
• Hemorrhage of the sole and white line, white line separation, and sole ulcers are commonly observed secondary lesions due to the increased weight bearing on the lateral claws.

CAUSES

RISK FACTORS
Poor hoof health management and improper or infrequent hoof trimming may play a role in incidence.

DIAGNOSIS

DIFFERENTIAL DIAGNOSIS
Chronic laminitis, "slipper foot," "hooking" or "scissor claws" on the front claws, rotation of the medial claw in heifers

CBC/BIOCHEMISTRY/URINALYSIS
N/A

OTHER LABORATORY TESTS
N/A

IMAGING
N/A

DIAGNOSTIC PROCEDURES
Visual observation, characteristic appearance.

PATHOLOGIC FINDINGS
• Abnormal angulation of the second and third phalanges with the plantar surface of the third phalanx rotated axially.
• Exostosis of the abaxial distal phalangeal joint
• A groove may develop on the inside of the hoof capsule due to rotation of third phalanx, causing the abaxial sole to be thin. The third phalanx may be long and thin.

TREATMENT

APPROPRIATE HEALTH CARE
• Functional hoof trimming; however, trimming is a challenge due to the rotation of the third phalanx and thinning of the sole near the abaxial white line. It may be necessary to trim the lateral claw first to allow more weight bearing on the medial claw.
• The dorsal wall of the corkscrew claw should be straightened with a rasp or angle grinder and hoof-trimming wheel.
• If the lateral claw cannot be trimmed to match the medial claw, it may be helpful to apply an orthopedic block to the medial claw to help stimulate growth on the medial claw and take some of the weight off of the lateral claw.
• Cattle with this condition will need to be trimmed every 3–4 months.

NURSING CARE
If secondary conditions such as sole ulcer occur, they must be treated and reexamined after 1–2 weeks to determine if healing is occurring normally.

ACTIVITY
Cows that are lame should be moved closer to the milking parlor.

DIET
If incidence is high, diet and feeding management should be investigated, but if nutrition is a problem, we would expect to see an increased incidence of laminitis.

CLIENT EDUCATION
Clients should be educated about the possible heritability of this condition, and progeny from affected cows should not be kept for breeding stock.

SURGICAL CONSIDERATIONS
N/A

CORKSCREW CLAW IN CATTLE

MEDICATIONS

DRUGS OF CHOICE
N/A

CONTRAINDICATIONS
N/A

PRECAUTIONS
N/A

POSSIBLE INTERACTIONS
N/A

ALTERNATIVE DRUGS
N/A

FOLLOW-UP

PATIENT MONITORING
Monitor for lameness and occurrence of secondary laminitis lesions.

PREVENTION/AVOIDANCE
• Perform functional hoof trimming on all cows at dry-off and midlactation.
• Perform functional hoof trimming on heifers before they calve.
• Cows with corkscrew claw will have to be trimmed more often than other cows.

POSSIBLE COMPLICATIONS
Sole hemorrhage, sole ulcer, white line separation

EXPECTED COURSE AND PROGNOSIS
Corkscrew claw is irreversible, but proper trimming may prolong the cow's useful life.

MISCELLANEOUS

ASSOCIATED CONDITIONS
Sole hemorrhage, sole ulcer, white line separation

AGE-RELATED FACTORS
Most common in cows over 3.5 years old.

ZOONOTIC POTENTIAL
N/A

PREGNANCY
N/A

RUMINANT SPECIES AFFECTED
Bovine

BIOSECURITY
N/A

PRODUCTION MANAGEMENT
• Proper preventive hoof trimming, not using bulls with abnormal curvature of the dorsal wall of the lateral, rear claws
• Frequent trimming of affected cows

SYNONYMS
N/A

SEE ALSO
Laminitis
Scissor claw
Slipper foot

ABBREVIATIONS
N/A

Suggested Reading
Greenough, P. R., Schugel, L. M., Johnson, A. B. 1997. *Zinpro corporation's illustrated handbook on cattle lameness.* Eden Prairie, MN: Zinpro Corporation.
Kloosterman, P. 1997. Claw care. In: *Lameness in cattle,* ed. P. R. Greenough, A. D. Weaver. Philadelphia: W. B. Saunders.
Pijl, R. 2000. Rotation of the medial claw of the hind feet. *Proc. XI Intl. Symp. on Disorders of the Ruminant Digit & III Intl. Conf. on Bovine Lameness.* Parma, Italy.
van Amstel, S. R., Palin, F. L., Shearer, J. K. 2002. Application of functional trimming procedures to corkscrew claws. *Proc. 12th Intl. Symp. on Lameness in Ruminants.* Orlando, FL.
van Amstel, S. R., Shearer, J. K. 2001. Abnormalities of hoof growth and development. *Vet Clin N Amer Food Anim Pr.* 17(1): 73–91.

Author: Steven L. Berry

CORNEAL ULCERATION

BASICS

DEFINITION
• Corneal ulcers can be caused by primary infections, can occur as secondary manifestations of system disease, or can be traumatic in origin.
• The vast majority of corneal ulcers in cattle are caused by infectious bovine keratoconjunctivitis (IBK), a specific disease caused by infection with *Moraxella bovis*.
• Debate exists regarding the role of several ancillary or potential pathogens in the development of corneal ulcers.

SIGNALMENT
• Infectious bovine keratoconjunctivitis occurs worldwide.
• The disease is most common in late spring, summer, and early fall. The seasonal pattern is probably associated with populations of the face fly, which serves as a mechanical vector.
• Young animals are most susceptible; however, cattle of all ages may be affected.

SIGNS
• The earliest clinical signs of corneal ulcers are epiphora and blephrospasm. Either one or both eyes may be affected. As lesions progress and mature, clouding of the cornea becomes apparent and vascular in-growth from the corneal scleral junction becomes visible.
• In cattle with *Moraxella bovis* infections, the ulcer is situated central in the cornea and later replaced by a raised white papilla, which includes inflammatory exudates.
• In severe cases, the integrity of the corneal lesions may be lost and a descemetocoele may be observed.
• Untreated, the clinical course may be as long as one month. A significant percentage of affected eyes will become nonfunctional with severe, permanent corneal opacity. Residual central corneal opacities are common.
• *Chlamydophila* sp., *Mycoplasma* sp., and *Branhamella* sp. in small ruminant species produce similar lesions.
• Viral keratitis generally produces multifocal to diffuse corneal lesions, the exception being malignant catarrhal fever (MCF) in which a zone of limbal or peripheral edema is the most consistent ocular sign.

CAUSES
• The most common cause of corneal ulcers in cattle is infectious bovine keratoconjunctivitis (IBK) caused by *Moraxella bovis*. Isolates of *M. bovis* vary greatly in their virulence. Virulence appears to be linked to the production of pilus adhesins, leukotoxins, hemolysins, and proteases.
• Occasionally, herd outbreaks of corneal ulcers have been associated with alternative pathogens. The virulence of these organisms is a subject of ongoing debate. At the very least, these organisms appear to increase the severity of IBK and under unique circumstances may serve as primary pathogens.
• Common infectious causes of corneal ulcers in sheep and goats include *Mycoplasma* sp., *Chlamydophila* sp. (formerly *Chlamydia* sp.), and infectious bovine rhinotracheitis virus (IBR, goats only).
• Other causes of corneal ulcers are usually JUST sporadic observations in single individuals.

RISK FACTORS
• Common risk factors for IBK include exposure to insect vectors (particularly face flies), ultraviolet light, dust, tall pasture grasses, recent additions to the herd, and carrier animals. *Moraxella bovis* will overwinter in the eyes of carrier cattle.
• Atypical herd outbreaks of corneal ulcers of non-IBK etiology often occur in the fall of the year. These atypical outbreaks often involve closely confined, recently weaned calves in open-herd settings in which feeder calves are continually added to a group. These groups often have a history of recurrent respiratory disease and/or polyarthritis. The author has identified a high prevalence of *Mycoplasma* sp. ocular infections in these outbreaks. Mature cows and neonatal calves in close proximity to these open source groups occasionally experience continual flare-ups.

DIAGNOSIS

DIFFERENTIAL DIAGNOSIS
• Infectious bovine keratoconjunctivitis (*Moraxella bovis*, pinkeye)
• *Branhamella* sp. (small ruminants)
• Grass awns
• *Mycoplasma* sp.
• *Chlamydophila* sp.
• Viral keratitis (IBR, MCF, BVD, rinderpest)
• *Pasteurella multocida* (capsular type A)
• Trauma
• Exposure
• Neurogenic, loss of palpebral function (e.g., listeriosis, otitis interna, etc.)
• Exophthalmos, retrobulbar masses (e.g., lymphosarcoma, abscess, etc.)
• Parasitic (e.g., *Thelazia* sp., *Onchocerca* sp., *Elaeophora* sp.)
• Entropion

CBC/BIOCHEMISTRY/URINALYSIS
N/A

OTHER LABORATORY TESTS
• Clinical exam is typically sufficient to permit a diagnosis. Application of a fluorescein stain will increase the sensitivity of ocular examinations.
• In the face of atypical or unresponsive outbreaks, microbiologic culture, virus isolation, and polymerase chain reaction assays (PCR) on ocular swabs may be considered.

TREATMENT

• Accepted treatments include subcutaneous long-acting oxytetracycline, topical therapy using ophthalmic ointments, or dry cow intramammary infusions and subconjunctival injections of penicillin with or without dexamethasone. Two treatments with long-acting oxytetracycline at 72-hr intervals have been reported to eliminate carrier states and demonstrated promise in terminating outbreaks.

• A number of other antibiotics including fluorphenicol have been demonstrated efficacious in the treatment of IBK; however, *M. bovis* is often resistant to tylosin, erythromycin, and lincomycin.

• In cattle, early recognition and treatment will typically limit the severity of disease and the degree of corneal scarring.

• Infectious corneal ulceration in sheep and goats appears more aggressive and less responsive to treatment.

• Treatment in sheep and goats typically consists of systemic administration of long-acting oxytetracycline because the vast majority of potential pathogens are at least nominally sensitive to this antibiotic.

• Anecdotal reports have suggested that aqueous ceftiofur is efficacious as a subconjunctival injection, and this approach is particularly appealing in lactating dairy cattle because milk withholding is avoided; however, the author is aware of no documentary evidence supporting this approach.

• When topical treatment is used, appropriate hygienic precautions should be employed to prevent transmission to additional animals.

• Adjuncts to treatment, which are occasionally used, include an eye patch covering the affected eye, third eyelid flaps to prevent impending corneal perforation, and use of topical or systemic anti-inflammatory agents.

MEDICATIONS

CONTRAINDICATIONS

Appropriate milk and meat withdrawal times must be followed for all compounds administered to food-producing animals.

FOLLOW-UP

PREVENTION

• Prevention should include control of face flies (insecticide impregnated ear tags or residual fly sprays), clipping tall pastures, elimination of dusty environments, elimination of carrier cattle and vaccines.

• Animals with active clinical disease should be isolated from unaffected herd mates.

• Vaccine efficacy appears highly variable and difficult to predict due to the variation in the strain of IBK responsible for a given outbreak.

• Mass medication with oxytetracycline using either subcutaneous injections or the addition of antibiotics to salt or concentrates also will limit the severity of outbreaks and ameliorate the presence of carrier animals.

• It should be noted that mass antibiotic therapy may cure asymptomatic anaplasmosis carriers, rendering these cattle susceptible to clinical anaplasmosis if the disease is reintroduced.

• In herds with atypical fall or winter pinkeye, efforts should be made to reduce the severity of endemic respiratory disease (*Mycoplasma* sp.). These efforts should include preconditioning programs and restricting the continual addition of susceptible cattle to groups experiencing corneal ulceration.

MISCELLANEOUS

ASSOCIATED CONDITIONS

• These groups often have a history of recurrent respiratory disease and/or polyarthritis.

• Mass antibiotic therapy may cure asymptomatic anaplasmosis carriers, rendering these cattle susceptible to clinical anaplasmosis if the disease is reintroduced.

AGE-RELATED FACTORS

Young animals are most susceptible; however, cattle of all ages may be affected.

ZOONOTIC POTENTIAL

The *Chlamydophila* sp. associated with ocular disease in small ruminants may be zoonotic.

PREGNANCY

Chlamydial and mycoplasmal species can cause abortion.

RUMINANT SPECIES AFFECTED

Potentially all ruminant species are affected.

BIOSECURITY

• Prevention should include control of face flies (insecticide impregnated ear tags or residual fly sprays), clipping tall pastures, elimination of dusty environments, elimination of carrier cattle and vaccines.

• Animals with active clinical disease should be isolated from unaffected herd mates.

• Restrict the continual addition of susceptible cattle to groups experiencing corneal ulceration.

PRODUCTION MANAGEMENT

• Reduce exposure to insect vectors, particularly face flies, exposure to ultraviolet light, dust, tall pasture grasses, recent additions to the herd, and carrier animals.

• Prevention efforts should include preconditioning programs and restricting the continual addition of susceptible cattle to groups experiencing corneal ulceration.

SYNONYMS

Pinkeye

SEE ALSO

Chlamydiophila sp.
Entropion
Infectious bovine keratoconjunctivitis (*Moraxella bovis*, pinkeye)
Listeriosis
Lymphosarcoma
Mycoplasma sp.
Otitis interna
Parasitic (*Thelazia* sp., *Onchocerca* sp., *Elaeophora* sp.)
Pasteurella multocida (capsular type A)
Viral keratitis (IBR, MCF, BVD, rinderpest)

ABBREVIATIONS

BVD = bovine viral diarrhea
IBK = infectious bovine keratoconjunctivitis
IBR = infectious bovine rhinotracheitis
MCF = malignant catarrhal fever
PCR = polymerase chain reaction

Suggested Reading

Brown, M. H., Brightman, A. H., Fenwick, B. W., Rider, M. A. 1998. Infectious bovine keratoconjunctivitis: a review. *J Vet Intern Med.* 12:259–66.

George, L. W. 1990. Antibiotic treatment of infectious bovine keratoconjunctivitis. *Cornell Vet.* 80:229–35.

Miller, R. B., Fales, W. H. 1984. Infectious bovine keratoconjunctivitis: an update. *Vet Clin NA: Large Animal* 6:597–608.

Radostits, O. M., Gay, C. C., Blood, D. C., Hinchcliff, K. W. 2000. *Veterinary medicine.* 9th ed. London: W. B. Saunders.

Author: Jeff Tyler

CORONAVIRUS

BASICS

OVERVIEW
- Disease of neonatal ruminants
- The causative agent is a coronavirus. All coronaviruses are of the same serotype.
- Pathogenicity is related to load of exposure, level of immunity to the virus, concurrent infection with other neonatal pathogens, and stress. Most infections are concurrent with other neonatal pathogens.
- The virus is ubiquitous with seroprevalence in the adult herd of 80–90%.
- Morbidity of coronavirus is estimated to be 15–25%. Mortality rate in uncomplicated cases is 5–10% but may reach 50% with concurrent bacterial or parasitic infections.

PATHOPHYSIOLOGY
- The virus is acquired either through the ingestion of feces-contaminated material or inhalation. Initially, villous epithelial cells are infected in the proximal small intestine with infection progressing caudally with time. The crypt cells of the small intestine are not affected.
- The infection extends into the colon resulting in infection of the epithelial cells of the ridges as well as the crypts.
- The virus is cytocidal resulting in sloughing of epithelial cells. Coronavirus may also infect undifferentiated epithelial cells, fibroblasts, and endothelial cells of the lamina propria resulting in significant damage to the colon. Infected cells contain large numbers of virus and are desquamated into the lumen. Immature crypt cells replace the absorptive epithelium of the small intestine but denuded areas within the colon may take several days to heal.
- The loss of epithelial cells results in a maldigestive as well as a malabsorptive type of diarrhea.
- Undigested carbohydrates undergo bacterial fermentation resulting in an increase in osmotic pressure and water being drawn into the intestinal lumen. The crypt cells of the small intestine are not affected and continue to secrete fluid resulting in net secretion exceeding absorptive capacity.
- Diarrhea results due to increased osmotic pressure and decreased absorption. The physical loss of the epithelial cells results in increased susceptibility to other pathogens because of loss of the villous integrity and decreased secretion of lactoferrin and lysozymes as well as the release of inflammatory mediators.
- Damage predisposes the attachment of ETEC and attaching and effacing *E. coli* to the intestinal villi.
- The loss of electrolytes, bicarbonate, and water leads to dehydration and metabolic acidosis.
- The virus can also infect the respiratory epithelium resulting in a mild respiratory or subclinical respiratory infection.

SYSTEMS AFFECTED
Gastrointestinal, respiratory

GENETICS
N/A

INCIDENCE/PREVALENCE
Prevalence of coronavirus infections ranges from 15% to 25% with a great variation in mortality, 5–50% depending on concurrent bacterial and parasitic infections. Seroprevalence in the adult herd may be close to 100%.

SIGNALMENT
Species
Bovine, ovine, caprine; potentially, all ruminant species can be infected.

Breed Predilections
N/A

Mean Age and Range
- Most infections occur during the second week of life. Range is 3 days to 3 weeks.
- Calves as old as 3 months of age may be affected.

Predominant Sex
N/A

SIGNS

GENERAL COMMENTS
- Clinical signs are more severe than rotavirus-induced diarrhea.
- Acute onset of diarrhea varying from mild to severe, depression, and reluctance to nurse; feces may contain mucus, milk curds, and occasionally flecks of blood.

• Clinical signs last 3–5 days during which calves become progressively depressed, weak, and experience weight loss.
• Some calves may exhibit signs of abdominal pain. In the case of uncomplicated cases, diarrhea may exist for 2 to 3 days. In cases of secondary bacterial infection, diarrhea may last 3–5 days.

HISTORICAL FINDINGS
• Sudden onset of diarrhea that spreads rapidly through the neonatal population
• A few cases may have been noticed initially but the frequency of cases increases as the calving season progresses due to buildup of pathogen load.
• Increased number of cases observed following periods of stress such as a snowstorm or cold wet weather.

PHYSICAL EXAMINATION FINDINGS
• Mild to severe watery diarrhea with pieces of milk curd and flecks of blood; color, consistency, and composition will vary with coexisting infections.
• Dehydration and depression with degrees of inappetence or reluctance to nurse. Some animals may be weak to the point of recumbency.
• Bruxism and nasal discharge

CAUSES
Coronavirus. All cattle coronaviruses are of the same serotype.

RISK FACTORS
• Inadequate colostral transfer of immunoglobulins resulting in agammaglobulinemia or hypogammaglobulinemia. Lack of local colostral immunity in calves 5 days postpartum or in calves raised on milk replacers.
• Birthing areas contaminated with fecal material containing coronavirus
• Neonatal housing in which buildup of pathogen load occurs
• Neonates housed or maintained in a cold, wet environment.

DIAGNOSIS

DIFFERENTIAL DIAGNOSIS
• Diarrhea may be caused by a variety of infectious agents as well as nutritional causes.
• *Clostridium perfringens* type C—acute death and hemorrhagic enteritis. *E. coli* infections are usually seen in calves less than 7 days of age. Cryptosporidia and rotavirus are hard to differentiate from coronavirus. Salmonellosis animals are usually febrile; coronaviral infections temperature will be variable.
• Nutritional causes of diarrhea may be differentiated from coronavirus diarrhea if history contains a dietary change or examination of the feedstuffs and identification of deficiencies or excesses.

CBC/BIOCHEMISTRY/URINALYSIS
• CBC: hemoconcentration, increased plasma proteins
• Serum chemistry: metabolic acidosis with low plasma bicarbonate. Glucose and electrolyte values will be low depending on severity of diarrhea.
• Urinalysis: depending on state of dehydration, urine will be concentrated resulting in an increased specific gravity.

OTHER LABORATORY TESTS

DIAGNOSTIC PROCEDURES
• Feces should be collected as soon as diarrhea is noted because exfoliation of virus-laden enterocytes is short-lived and occurs early in the disease process.
• Feces can be submitted for electron microscopy and identification of virus. A few drops of formalin can be added to 10 cc of feces, or feces can be frozen.
• Serology can detect seroconversion or a fourfold increase in serum immunoglobulin levels.
• Fresh sections of the small intestine, preferably mid ileum, and colon tied at the cut ends to contain intestinal contents can be submitted on ice for immunofluorescent microscopy.

PATHOLOGIC FINDINGS
• No specific gross lesions; distended bowel containing undigested milk and fluid. The mucosa may be congested and there may be petechial hemorrhages throughout the intestinal tract.

CORONAVIRUS

• Histologically, the villi will be shortened, covered with squamous to cuboidal epithelial cells.

TREATMENT

APPROPRIATE HEALTH CARE
N/A

NURSING CARE
• Fluid therapy is needed to correct dehydration, circulatory impairment, and electrolyte and metabolic imbalances.
• Fluid deficit should be calculated as well as maintenance requirement, 80–100 ml/kg, to determine volume of fluids needed during a 24-hour period. Fluid may be administered orally or intravenously. Commercial oral electrolyte solutions containing glucose and an alkalinizing agent are recommended if the neonate is still nursing. Although oral electrolytes are less likely to be absorbed due to enterocyte pathology, not all enterocytes are affected so some absorption may occur.
• Neonates without a suckle response need IV fluids. IV administration of lactated Ringer's solution is adequate. With severe acidosis, isotonic sodium bicarbonate solution (1.3%, 13 of sodium bicarbonate to 1 l of distilled water) may be used. Dextrose solutions (2.5–5%) are indicated in cases of hypoglycemia.
• With hypoglycemia and an unknown electrolyte and acid-base status, a 2.5% dextrose and 0.45% saline solution has been recommended.

ACTIVITY
N/A

DIET
• Neonates with a suckle response should be left with the dam and allowed to nurse.
• Animals being reared artificially should remain on their diet or switch to whole milk or colostrum. If the diarrhea becomes worse or the calf becomes depressed, removal from the dam or milk is warranted. In case of hand-fed neonates that are depressed and not interested in sucking, or neonates not nursing the dam, neonates should receive a high-energy electrolyte solution at a rate of 10% of body weight divided into a minimum of four feedings.
• Once neonates are suckling, feed milk at a rate of 5% of body weight in four feedings a day, increasing the amount per feeding gradually so calf is back on full feed within 2 to 3 days.
• Calves should also receive 5% of their body weight in electrolyte solutions spacing 2 hours before or after milk feedings. Milk should not be withheld longer than 24 hours and can be given via an esophageal feeder. No more than 1 liter should be tubed at a time.
• Milk and electrolyte solutions can be altered as described previously with a minimum of 10% body weight of fluid per day.
• Oral electrolytes containing an alkalinizing agent, other than acetate, should not be fed when calves are receiving milk as milk digestion maybe disrupted.

CLIENT EDUCATION
• Clients need to ensure the calves acquire an adequate amount of colostrum. Neonates should be kept dry and in a draft-free environment.
• Animals should be moved and fed in such a way as to reduce the buildup of mud and fecal material in the neonate's environment. Diarrheic animals should be isolated from healthy neonates as they are sources for large numbers of pathogens.
• Owners should work with healthy calves before working with sick calves and should clean equipment, bottles, and nipples adequately between calf usage.
• Owners should be advised as to how to reduce pathogen transfer between calves in regard to clothing and shoes.

MEDICATIONS

DRUGS OF CHOICE
• Broad-spectrum antibiotics may be considered because of the potential for mixed infections as well as the loss of mucosal integrity. Oral amoxicillin trihydrate 10 mg/kg PO q 12h for nonruminating calves, 20-day slaughter withdrawal (extralabel in small ruminants). Amoxicillin trihydrate-clavulanate potassium 12.5 mg combined drug/kg PO q 12 h (extralabel usage) for 3 days.
• Parenteral ceftiofur 2.2 mg/kg IM/SC q 24 h for 3 days (extralabel usage) for 3 days.

Plasma Transfusion

Although not specific for corona viral infections, in cases of failure of passive transfer and depending on value of the animal, plasma transfusion may be warranted.

CONTRAINDICATIONS

• Do not use kaolin and pectin as use may increase electrolyte loss.
• Meat and milk withdrawal time periods must be maintained.

 FOLLOW-UP

PATIENT MONITORING

• Monitor attitude, suckling response, appetite, fecal color and consistency, and hydration status.
• Monitor age cohorts for signs of diarrhea.

POSSIBLE COMPLICATIONS

Hypovolemic shock and death

PREVENTION/AVOIDANCE

• Reduce exposure, clean maternity areas, move to a clean area after birth. Those handling sick neonates should practice biosecurity measures to reduce exposure to healthy neonates, wash hands and disinfect boots, maintain clothes free of fecal material.
• Vaccination of dams prepartum according to manufacturer's recommendations with a coronavirus vaccine may increase colostral antibody; results are variable.

• Oral vaccination of neonate with a modified-live oral vaccine will produce IgA and IgM. This vaccine is cumbersome for management as it is to be given prior to colostrum consumption and colostrum must be withheld for several hours after vaccination. This may increase the opportunity for bacterial infections and failure of passive transfer.
• In the case of dairy animals, feed neonates colostrum for 30 days if coronavirus is an endemic problem.
• Eliminate areas of fecal buildup.
• Keep environment dry and draft free.

EXPECTED COURSE AND PROGNOSIS

• In uncomplicated infections, diarrhea is present for 2 to 3 days. Prognosis is good, as this infection tends to be self-limiting and generally requires minor supportive care.
• Duration of diarrhea may be 4–6 days with secondary bacterial infections. Prognosis is dependent on the degree of pathology produced by the secondary bacteria.
• Prognosis is good to fair with supportive care. It may take a couple of weeks for animals to fully recover.

 MISCELLANEOUS

ASSOCIATED CONDITIONS

A mild respiratory infection may occur simultaneously.

AGE-RELATED FACTORS

• Most cases occur at 7 to 14 days of age.
• Range is 1 day to 3 weeks.

ZOONOTIC POTENTIAL

None

PREGNANCY

N/A

RUMINANT SPECIES AFFECTED

Bovine, ovine, caprine; potentially, all ruminant species can be infected.

SYNONYMS

N/A

SEE ALSO

Clostridium perfringens type C
Cryptosporidiosis
E. coli
Rotaviruses
Salmonellosis
Toxic ingestion

ABBREVIATIONS

CBC = complete blood count
ETEC = enterotoxigenic *E. coli*
IM = intramuscular
IV = intravenous
PO = per os, by mouth
SC = subcutaneous

Suggested Reading

Constable, P. D. 2004. Antimicrobial use in the treatment of calf diarrhea. *J Vet Intern Med.* 18:8–17.
Hirsh, D. C., Zee, Y. C. 1999. *Veterinary microbiology*. Malden, MA: Blackwell Science.
Naylor, J. M. 2002. Neonatal ruminant diarrhea. In: *Large animal internal medicine*, ed. B. P. Smith. 3rd ed. St. Louis: Mosby.
Torres-Medina, A., Schlafer, D., Medus, C. 1985. Rotaviral and coronaviral diarrhea. In: *The veterinary clinics of North America, food animal practice*. Philadelphia: W. B. Saunders.

Author: Kevin D. Pelzer

COWPOX

 BASICS

OVERVIEW
• Cowpox is caused by an orthopoxvirus that is closely related to but distinguishable from the human orthopoxviruses vaccinia and variola.
• Animals develop poxlike lesions commonly on the teat and udder.

SIGNALMENT
• The virus tends to spread through a naïve herd rapidly particularly during times of the year when the teats and udders are likely to have abrasions on the surface.
• Heifers as they are introduced to the milking string are more likely to become involved in endemic herds.

SIGNS
• Incubation period is between 3 and 10 days.
• Typical pox lesions are usually noted only on the teats and udder. However, in severe cases, the pox lesions can be identified on the thin skin of the inside of the inguinal region and occasionally on the perineum.
• Bulls can get lesions on the scrotum.
• Nursing calves can get oral lesions similar to bovine papular stomatitis.
• Lesions usually progress from circular raised reddened areas of erythema and edema to firm 1–2 cm nodules that form a central vesicle. The vesicle eventually ruptures or collapses forming a central crater in the raised circumscribed area. The central area undergoes further necrosis and scab formation if the animal is not being milked.
• Milked animals develop a raised circumscribed lesion with a central umbilicated ulcer that is slow to heal.

CAUSES AND RISK FACTORS
Disease is endemic in rodents of Europe and Asia with the virus occasionally infecting cattle.
• Voles are a common rodent that is infected with the virus.
• Domestic cats are commonly infected in endemic areas by hunting and eating infected rodents and are believed to act as a means of spreading the disease to humans and cattle.
• Being milked by infected hands of herdsmen or by inoculation with contaminated fomites such as teat dipping cups and milking equipment can infect cattle.
• Insects are also suspected of transferring the virus from cow to cow.

 DIAGNOSIS

DIFFERENTIAL DIAGNOSIS
• Pseudocowpox (milkers nodules): Pseudocowpox is a parapoxvirus with lesions similar to cowpox. Virus is similar to bovine papular stomatitis.
• Herpes mammillitis: Small ulcers develop on teats and udders that are slow healing. Viral culturing will assist in differentiating poxviruses from herpesviruses.
• Vesicular stomatitis: Lesions are often also prevalent in the mouth and feet.
• Foot-and-mouth disease: Lesions in the mouth and on the feet are also present in infected animals.
• Caustic substances that are placed on the teat
• *Staphylococcus aureus* infections on the teats can cause vesicles, which may spread to the udder resulting in furunculitis and boils.

CBC/ BIOCHEMISTRY / URINALYSIS
N/A

OTHER LABORATORY FINDINGS
N/A

IMAGING
N/A

DIAGNOSTIC PROCEDURES
• Biopsies of the lesions will identify typical poxvirus intracytoplasmic inclusions on the epithelium.
• Electron microscopy of the infected epithelium identifies characteristic poxvirus present in infected keratinocytes.

PATHOLOGIC FINDINGS

GROSS FINDINGS
• The pox lesions are circumscribed raised firm nodules that are blanched usually with a circular area of hyperemia around the base. These raised nodules eventually form a vesicle and then a pustule in the center of the raised nodules. Lesions eventually undergo necrosis and collapse causing a cavitary depression in the center of the nodules. A scab will form over the necrotic tissue, which, once removed, identifies an ulcerated surface that is slow to heal.
• Lesions are seen primarily on the teats and udder but can also be seen in the peritoneal region and on the scrotum of bulls.
• Suckling calves can have similar lesions in the oral cavity.

HISTOPATHOLOGIC FINDINGS
• The pox lesions consist of edema, congestion, and lymphocytic infiltration of the superficial dermis.
• The associated epithelium becomes hyperplasic with ballooning degeneration and necrosis of the affected epithelium in the stratum spinosum.
• Eosinophilic intracytoplasmic inclusion bodies are seen in the swollen keratinocytes in the stratum spinosum.
• Epithelial cells of the stratum spinosum separate forming small vesicles that fill with neutrophils forming a pustule. Later, the associate epithelium beneath the pustules becomes necrotic forming an ulcerated epidermis with serocellular debris overlying the lesion.
• Variable numbers of neutrophils are present in the dermal connective tissues.

 TREATMENT

• There is no treatment for the pox-associated lesions.
• One needs to keep the lesions clean and free of secondary bacterial infections.
• Debris or scabs from wounds should be picked up and disposed of to insure that contaminated materials do not contact other animals.
• Antibacterial ointments may assist in healing.

 MEDICATIONS

N/A

CONTRAINDICATIONS/POSSIBLE INTERACTIONS
Appropriate milk and meat withdrawal times must be followed for all compounds administered to food-producing animals.

FOLLOW-UP

PATIENT MONITORING
• Lesions are usually self-limiting.
• Keeping the lesions clean and free of contamination is important in preventing bacterial infections.

PREVENTION/AVOIDANCE
• Herdsmen with lesions should limit involvement in milking since this is a major method of spreading the disease.
• Cleaning cloths, teat dipping cups, and milking machines should be disinfected thoroughly before use on noninfected animals.
• Quaternary ammonia compounds and other teat-dipping compounds with viricidal activity should be adequate for preventing the spread of the disease.
• Currently, no vaccine is available for use in outbreaks.

POSSIBLE COMPLICATIONS
Secondary bacterial infections of the lesions can occur with the development of mastitis in affected quarters or a severe dermatitis involving the skin of the affected udder.

EXPECTED COURSE AND PROGNOSIS
Cowpox is considered a mild disease and should cause little discomfort to affected cattle. Most cases resolve without complications.

MISCELLANEOUS

ASSOCIATED CONDITIONS
N/A

AGE-RELATED FACTORS
Young animals, particularly naïve heifers coming into an endemic herd, are most susceptible.

ZOONOTIC POTENTIAL
People handing infected material can get lesions on their hands and face. The lesions are usually mild and self-limiting.

PREGNANCY
N/A

SYNOMYNS
N/A

SEE ALSO
Pseudocowpox (Milkers nodules)
Herpes mammillitis
Vesicular stomatitis
Foot-and-mouth disease
Teat trauma
Frost bite
Staphylococcus aureus

ABBREVIATIONS
N/A

Suggested Reading
Bennett, M., Baxby, D. 1996. Cowpox. *J Med Microbiol*. 45(3):157–58.
Cavanagh, R. D., Lambin, X., Ergon, T., Bennett, M., Graham, I. M., van Soolingen, D., Begon, M. 2004, Apr 22. Disease dynamics in cyclic populations of field voles (*Microtus agrestis*): cowpox virus and vole tuberculosis (*Mycobacterium microti*). *Proc R Soc Lond B Biol Sci*. 271(1541):859–67.
Feuerstein-Kadgien, B., Korn, K. 2003, Jan 30. Images in clinical medicine. Cowpox infection. *N Engl J Med*. 348(5):415.
Hazel, S. M., Bennett, M., Chantrey, J., Bown, K., Cavanagh, R., Jones, T. R., Baxby, D., Begon, M. 2000, Jun. A longitudinal study of an endemic disease in its wildlife reservoir: cowpox and wild rodents. *Epidemiol Infect*. 124(3):551–62.
Pastoret, P. P., Bennett, M., Brochier, B., Akakpo, A. J. 2000, Apr. Animals, public health and the example of cowpox. *Rev Sci Tech*. 19(1):23–32.

Author: Robert B. Moeller, Jr.

CRYPTOCOCCOSIS

 BASICS

OVERVIEW
• Cryptococcosis is a mycotic infection caused by the basidiomycete *Cryptococcus (Filobasidiella) neoformans*.
• Usually rare, sporadic cases of respiratory disease and/or meningitis or mastitis
• Worldwide distribution
• Important risk factor is exposure to soil/dust enriched with pigeon excreta.

PATHOPHYSIOLOGY
• Animals infected by inhaling dust carrying basidiospores/yeast forms
• Contaminated udder infusions can cause outbreaks of mastitis.
• Thick polysaccharide capsule of *Cryptococcus neoformans* inhibits phagocytosis
• Most infections are mild, subclinical lung infections.
• May cause formation of lung abscess/nodule or diffuse pulmonary infiltrates
• Nodules, or "cryptococcoma," vary in size and have a gummy, gelatinous consistency
• Solitary pulmonary nodules may be confused with carcinoma.
• Occasional hematogenous spread of *Cryptococcus neoformans* from lungs/udder
• Most frequent secondary site of colonization is meninges, leading to meningitis.
• Lymph nodes, skin, bone, liver, kidneys, and other organs may also be involved.

INCIDENCE/PREVALENCE
• Rare, sporadic
• Outbreaks of mastitis may occur in a herd if contaminated udder infusions are used.
• True prevalence is unknown, as infections normally are subclinical and lack a reliable skin test.

GEOGRAPHIC DISTRIBUTION
Worldwide

SIGNALMENT
• *Cryptococcus neoformans* can infect most animals, especially debilitated or immunocompromised animals.
• Host species include cattle, sheep, goats, horses, dogs, cats, zoo animals, and humans.
• Debilitated/immunocompromised animals are at higher risk for disseminated disease.
• Birds may carry *Cryptococcus neoformans* in the intestinal tract but do not suffer clinical disease.

SIGNS
• Upper or lower respiratory disease
• Fever
• Weight loss
• Neurological changes: stiffness, hyperesthesia, blindness, incoordination
• Skin lesions
• Lymphadenitis
• Mastitis

CAUSES AND RISK FACTORS
• *Cryptococcus neoformans* can survive in dry, nitrogen/creatinine-enriched, alkaline environments.
• Contaminated soil is the reservoir for *Cryptococcus neoformans*.
• Exposure to soil/dust enriched with pigeon excreta increases risk of inhalation of *Cryptococcus neoformans*.
• Debilitated/immunocompromised animals may be at higher risk for disseminated disease.
• No known animal-to-animal transmission
• No known animal-to-human transmission

 DIAGNOSIS

DIFFERENTIAL DIAGNOSIS
• Respiratory disease: viral, bacterial or other fungal respiratory pathogens
• Bacterial mastitis
• Neurological disease: viral (e.g., rabies, arboviruses), bacterial pathogens

CBC/BIOCHEMISTRY/URINALYSIS
N/A

OTHER LABORATORY TESTS
N/A

IMAGING
N/A

OTHER DIAGNOSTIC PROCEDURES
• Serological tests; latex agglutination tests to detect cryptococcal antigens in serum/CSF
• Culture of tissues/fluids
• Identification of thickly encapsulated yeast forms via India ink wet mounts and microscopic exam

TREATMENT
- Frequently self-limiting
- Surgical removal of lung nodules
- Disseminated disease frequently fatal if not treated
- In humans, combination therapy of amphotericin B and 5-flucytosine for 6–10 weeks has been successful.
- Drug withdrawal periods must be determined and maintained.
- Mortality rates in humans with treated disseminated cryptococcosis is approximately 30%.

MEDICATIONS
CONTRAINDICATIONS
Appropriate milk and meat withdrawal times must be followed for all compounds administered to food producing animals.

PRECAUTIONS
N/A

FOLLOW-UP
PREVENTION/AVOIDANCE
- Avoid exposure of animals to pigeon excreta.
- Avoid contamination of udder infusions.

MISCELLANEOUS
ASSOCIATED CONDITIONS
- Weight loss
- Neurological changes: stiffness, hyperesthesia, blindness, incoordination
- Skin lesions
- Lymphadenitis
- Mastitis

AGE-RELATED FACTORS
N/A

ZOONOTIC POTENTIAL
- No known cases of animal-to-human transmission
- Humans can become infected by inhaling *Cryptococcus neoformans* basidiospores/yeast from soil/pigeon excreta-enriched dust.
- Care should be taken while handling infected tissues, as zoonotic potential may exist.

PREGNANCY
N/A

RUMINANT SPECIES AFFECTED
Potentially, all ruminant species are affected.

BIOSECURITY
N/A

PRODUCTION MANAGEMENT
Contaminated udder infusions can cause outbreaks of mastitis.

SYNONYMS
Pigeon fanciers disease

SEE ALSO
Fungal mastitis
Other fungal diseases

ABBREVIATIONS
CSF = cerebral spinal fluid

Suggested Reading
Cryptococcossis. 1980. In: *Manual of clinical microbiology*, ed. E. H. Lennette, A. Balows, W. J. Hausler, J. P. Truant. Washington, DC: American Society for Microbiology.
Kielstein, P., Hotzel, H., Schmalreck, A., Khaschabi, D., Glawischnig, W. 2000. Occurrence of *Cryptococcus* spp. in excreta of pigeons and pet birds. *Mycoses* 43(1–2):7–15.
Pal, M., Mehrotra, B. S. 1983, Dec. Cryptococcal mastitis in dairy animals. *Mykosen* 26(12):615–16.
Singh, M., Gupta, P. P., Rana, J. S., Jand, S. K. 1994, Jun. Clinico-pathological studies on experimental cryptococcal mastitis in goats. *Mycopathologia* 126(3):147–55.
Van de Wetering, J. K., Coenjaerts, F. E. J., Vandrager, A. B., Van Golds, L. M. G., Batenburg, J. J. 2004. Aggregation of *Cryptococcus neoformans* by surfactant protein D is inhibited by its capsular component glucuronoxylomannan. *Infection and Immunity* 72: 145–53.

Author: Karen Carberry-Goh

CRYPTOSPORIDIOSIS

BASICS

OVERVIEW
• Cryptosporidiosis is caused by a nonhost-specific and widely distributed coccidian parasite *Cryptosporidium parvum*.
• *C. parvum* is an important cause of neonatal diarrhea that is clinically similar to other causes of calfhood scours.

PATHOPHYSIOLOGY
• Shed oocysts are sporulated and immediately infective.
• The primary route of transmission is typically fecal-oral; however, environmental contamination can spread the pathogen.
• Sporozoites from the oocysts primarily infect the brush border of the distal small intestine and large intestine.
• A vacuole is formed between the cytoplasm and cell membrane that causes villous atrophy, villous fusion, and, later, inflammatory changes of the mucosa.
• Clinical diarrhea develops on average 4 days after infection as a result of a combination of malabsorption and maldigestion.

SYSTEMS AFFECTED
Gastrointestinal

GENETICS
N/A

INCIDENCE/PREVALENCE
C. parvum was found in 22.4% of calves in one nationwide survey of dairy farms.

GEOGRAPHICAL DISTRIBUTION
Worldwide distribution

SIGNALMENT

Species
Cryptosporidiosis causes diarrhea in mammals (including cattle, sheep, goats, and humans) but it can also affect birds and reptiles.

Breed Predilections
N/A

Mean Age and Range
Highest frequency of infection is seen in calves aged 0–3 weeks.

Predominant Sex
N/A

SIGNS

GENERAL COMMENTS
• Diarrhea, dehydration, anorexia, and tenesmus are nonspecific findings for enteric infections in calves, including cryptosporidiosis.
• Diarrhea in uncomplicated cryptosporidiosis in immunocompetent individuals usually resolves in one week without anorexia.
• Infection without clinical signs can occur.

PHYSICAL EXAMINATION FINDINGS
• Diarrhea, dehydration, anorexia, and tenesmus are evident on physical examination.
• Mixed bacterial or viral etiologies should be considered in severe presentations with acid-base abnormalities, electrolyte disturbances, hypothermia, and weight loss.

CAUSES
• Cryptosporidiosis is caused by coccidian parasites of the phylum Apicomplexa called *Cryptosporidium* spp.
• The pathology in most domestic mammals is due to *Cryptosporidium parvum*.
• Recent evidence has shown some strain or genotype variability in *C. parvum*.

RISK FACTORS
• Poor hygiene in calf management can increase pathogen exposure from the environment and calf to calf.
• Immunocompromised calves are at greater risk for severe infections.

DIAGNOSIS

DIFFERENTIAL DIAGNOSIS
• Bovine viral diarrhea (BVD)
• *Clostridium perfringens* infection
• Coccidiosis
• Coronaviral infection
• *Escherichia coli* infection
• Feeding error (incorrect formulation of milk replacer, over/under feeding, etc.)
• Giardiasis
• Rotaviral infection
• Salmonellosis

CBC/BIOCHEMISTRY/URINALYSIS
• The CBC may show evidence of dehydration, hyperkalemia, and hypoglycemia.
• Blood gas analysis may show acidosis.

OTHER LABORATORY TESTS
High-power magnification with acid fast staining can be used on mucosal scrapings or after fecal flotation for identification of the organism.

IMAGING
N/A

GROSS AND HISTOPATHOLOGICAL FINDINGS
• Gross necropsy findings reveal hyperemic intestinal mucosa with yellow degraded intestinal contents.
• Histology reveals atrophy, fusion, and inflammation of the intestinal villi with circular, intramembranous, extracytoplasmic organism in the brush border.

TREATMENT

• There is no specific therapy for cryptosporidiosis but the diarrhea is usually self-limiting (7 day course in uncomplicated cases).
• Treatment is supportive including nutritional support, fluid and electrolyte replacement, and correction of acidosis and hypothermia.
• Antimicrobial therapy may be indicated in cases with secondary bacterial infections.
• Appropriate milk and meat withdrawal times must be followed for all compounds administered to food-producing animals.

ACTIVITY
N/A

DIET
• Electrolyte and rehydration therapy do not provide nutritional support so milk replacer needs to be fed.
• Electrolyte/fluid product may inhibit milk clot formation in the abomasum so it should be administered 1–2 hours after milk feedings.
• Decreasing the volume but increasing the number of feedings may help reduce the osmotic effects in the gut.

CLIENT EDUCATION
Cryptosporidiosis is a zoonotic pathogen so appropriate hygiene precautions should be taken when dealing with infected individuals.

MEDICATIONS

• Antimicrobial therapy if there is evidence of secondary bacterial infection
• Nonsteroidal anti-inflammatory therapy may be used to reduce pain and discomfort in some cases.

CONTRAINDICATIONS
N/A

PRECAUTIONS
N/A

POSSIBLE INTERACTIONS
N/A

FOLLOW-UP

CONTROL
• *Cryptosporidium* organisms are very resistant to temperature and chemical disinfection. Ammonia products (5%) and desiccation have been demonstrated to help disinfect the environment.
• Individual housing and sanitation of feeding equipment between calves can help control exposure.
• Adherence to hygienic practices in maternity area and in cleaning manure from calf areas can also help decrease environmental exposure.

MISCELLANEOUS

Gastric cryptosporidiosis: *Cryptosporidium andersoni* (formerly categorized as *C. muris*) causes nonzoonotic gastric cryptosporidiosis by infecting the glands of the abomasum in a small percentage of adult cattle. Animals appear clinically normal but inhibition of acid production in the abomasum can lead to decreased milk production in chronically affected cattle. Histopathology, fecal floatation, and acid fast staining can be utilized for identification of the organism.

SEE ALSO
Bovine viral diarrhea (BVD)
Clostridium perfringens infection
Coccidiosis
Coronavirus infection
Escherichia coli infection
Feeding error (incorrect formulation of milk replacer, over/under feeding, etc.)
Giardiasis
Rotavirus infection
Salmonellosis

ABBREVIATIONS
BVD = bovine viral diarrhea
CBC = complete blood count

Suggested Reading
Aiello, S. E., ed. 1998. Cryptosporidiosis. *The Merck veterinary manual*. 8th ed. Merck and Co. Inc. [online] Available at: http://www.merckvetmanual.com/mvm/index.jsp?cfile=htm/bc/21007.htm; accessed September 30, 2004.
Harp, J. A., Goff, J. P. 1998. Strategies for control of *Cryptosporidium parvum* infection in calves. *J Dairy Sci*, 81;289–94.
Naylor, J. M. 2002. Neonatal ruminant diarrhea. In: *Large animal internal medicine*, ed. B. P. Smith. 3rd ed. St. Louis: Mosby.
Rebhun, W. C. 1995. *Diseases of dairy cattle*. Philadelphia: Lippincott Williams and Wilkins.

Author: Noah Barka

CULLING STRATEGIES

 BASICS

DEFINITION
For the purpose of this discussion, the culling rate will be the number of animals removed divided by the average number of animals at risk for removal. This is really a proportion as it does not have time in the denominator, but it is a commonly used term of herd improvement associations.

OVERVIEW
Successful replacement strategies focus on removing animals because newly arriving animals allow for a higher economic return to the enterprise than the animal leaving (expected average profit of the new animal exceeds the remaining average profit of the animal replaced). Primary variables in replacement strategies are:
• Value of replaced animal (e.g., for meat or sale to another herd)
• Potential production (milk, meat, wool, offspring) and stage of production (lactation, pregnancy status, rate of gain, and weight for age)
• Expected fertility
• Health/expected survivorship (age)
• Cost of treatment or intervention
• Genetic value, phenotype, or conformation (i.e., udder, feet and legs, reproductive efficiency, milk/meat/wool production)
• Cost, availability, and quality of replacements
• Capacity of facility or ability to expand
• Operating goals of the owner/management team

SYSTEMS AFFECTED
Any, depending on condition

GENETICS
Dependent on herd needs and goals:
• Milk production or milk components
• Specific proteins (as cloned into transgenic animals)
• Mastitis or other disease resistance
• Conformation (head length or width, feet and leg conformation, vulvar conformation, udder conformation, teat size, rumen capacity, top line, etc.)
• Color, wool quality, fiber length or crimp, etc.
• Production trait (frame size, pelvic size, muscling, etc).

INCIDENCE/PREVALENCE
• Highly variable depending on herd, markets, value of products, disease incidence, etc. Incidence will vary from the high teens to an excess of 100%.
• Herds with excellent management that control disease well will have low cull rates when expanding, but can approach 50% if they are stable in size and have an excellent heifer or purchasing ability.
• It can make sense to sell the entire herd when the value of animals is high and the

replacement costs are low or expected to be low in the near future. For example, cows bought inexpensively in the sale ring or from herds with poorly conditioned, low-producing cows can be managed in another facility in a way that cows can gain weight and produce modest levels of milk at a low cost. Not many managers can accomplish this, but after cows increase their body condition, their value can increase from a low $0.15–$0.20/pound live weight to $0.35–$0.45/pound live weight, and they may gain weight (200–300 pounds) as well. Milk production can pay for a cow's feed and profit is generated from her sale for meat. In such herds, the cull rate can exceed 100% with cows being replaced within 6 or 7 months of purchase.

GEOGRAPHIC DISTRIBUTION
Worldwide, depending on species and management

SIGNALMENT

Species
All ruminant species

Breed Predilections
Only if the herd is changing from one breed to another because of specific production traits or costs of production.

Mean Age and Range
All ages are susceptible, but older animals are usually more likely than younger. This is because as animals age, their productive potential decreases and/or the probability of disease increases over time.

Predominant Sex
• Dependent on the facility's business priorities. For example, herds with high genetic merit will have bulls, heifers, and cows removed depending on their value to supply genetics to the herd compared to their value for sale to other herds.
• Commercial herds may keep a few bull calves for replacing their herd bulls in low production strings, but herds that use all-bull breeding will often buy seedstock from high genetic value herds. Other bull calves will be sold immediately after birth for meat production.
• Herds with a reputation for high genetic merit (usually measured as milk production, wool, or weaning weights) can sell their less-desirable animals to commercial herds at a value above sale for meat, but often close to their cost of rearing their own heifer. In these high genetic merit herds, owners will often calve out all their heifers, keeping all female offspring. These herds often have a large excess of heifers available to replace animals that are least desirable for their production and management goals.

SIGNS

PHYSICAL EXAMINATION FINDINGS
Animals can be healthy, but replacements have higher value compared to animals currently in the herd.

CAUSES AND RISK FACTORS
• Several models examining factors influencing decision making by managers for replacing animals have been developed.
• Dairy cows will be used in several examples of factors identified as important to predicting reasons and mechanisms for culling.

Value of Replaced Animal
This will vary depending on market effects, proximity to markets, transportation costs, breed, genetic value, and condition/production at sale. For example, a heifer can be purchased for $1500 and is expected to produce 22,000 pounds of milk. A third lactation cow that is 35 days pregnant, 300 days in milk, and 60 pounds of milk using rBST has a value of $600 if sold for meat; the milk price is $9/cwt and the cost of making that milk is $5.85/cwt. The dairy is losing $2/cwt milking this dairy cow. Compare this cow to a second lactation cow that is 210 days pregnant, has produced 25,000 pounds of milk, but can be fed in the dry lot for $1.25 per day. Assuming the dairy is full and the milk price is likely to rise to $12/cwt in the next 3 months, the first cow should be sold for meat, the second cow dried, and the fresh heifer should replace the first cow.

Potential Production
The likelihood of an animal to produce at age adjusted herd average or better, including conceiving within accepted goals (i.e., a 13-month calving interval), what stage of production they are in (i.e., days lactating), and, in the case of dairy animals, whether they conceived a heifer or bull calf (ultrasound diagnosis). For example: compare a first lactation dairy cow who is 200 days in milk, carrying a 120-day heifer, and producing 100 pounds of milk without use of rBST to a herd mate that is 35 days pregnant, 200 days in milk, and 80 pounds of milk using rBST. The second cow can be sold to a neighbor for $1200 and the cost of raising replacement heifers on the dairy is $1200. If the herd were expanding, all these animals would likely be kept. If the herd is not expanding, then the second cow is sold and the cost of rearing the heifer is paid for by the sale of the second cow.

Expected Fertility
In general, younger animals have a higher likelihood of conceiving than an older cow, and as age increases, the likelihood of fetal loss increases. In pregnant cows, culling is highly associated with inflammatory disease. As a cow's age increases, and the age at conception increases, her likelihood of culling also increases. Fetal loss, cystic ovarian disease, dystocia, metritis, retained placenta, lack of expression of estrus or anestrus will increase likelihood of a cow being culled, because of their effect on fertility.

Health/Expected Survivorship (Age/Stage of Lactation)
Unhealthy cows make less milk than healthy cows and are at an increased risk for removal

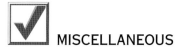

because of their low milk production. However, a cow with severe perimetritis leading to infertility may remain in the herd until her production drops below her costs of production, while a cow with an uncomplicated left displaced abomasum 1 week after calving may have no change in her likelihood of staying in the herd compared to healthy herd mates, as long as she has a good production potential. In other words, a cow's milk production potential is still the largest determinant for risk of replacement, and a cow that becomes low producing and unhealthy or fails to conceive is much more likely to be replaced.

Cost of Treatment or Intervention

As cost of treatment/intervention exceeds the potential profitability of the cow, the more likely she is to be sold. Using decision tree analysis for a specific disease, the likelihood of treatment success and failure and the cost of intervention allow for better decision making.

Genetic Value, Phenotype, or Conformation (e.g., Udder, Feet, and Legs, Reproductive Efficiency, Milk/Meat/Wool Production)

Decisions for genetic improvement are quite varied, but principally focus on production traits. Selection on a single trait (i.e., milk production) is often at the expense of fertility, mastitis control, feet and leg conformation, or other traits related to longevity in the herd. Arguably, the current genetic value for milk production in today's bull studs is sufficient to maintain or increase milk production in most commercial dairies. Selection on other important traits is probably more critical to increasing longevity. Although disease per se may not be associated with an increase in culling, it will limit choices as to which animals must remain in the herd.

Cost, Availability, and Quality of Replacements

Keeping replacement costs low is principally achieved by reducing feed cost/unit of gain. Animals entering the herd at a younger age can reduce costs of heifer production and reduce total animal units on the facility (lower generation time). Cost and success at raising replacement heifers is directly related to the ability of a dairy to supply heifers for replacement. Several approaches to acquiring replacements for a dairy are taken. One end of the spectrum is the sale of all calves born with the subsequent purchase of primiparous

heifers just before calving. This reduces the number of animals on a facility, which can be important for facilities with limited land facing environmental constraints. Alternatively, dairies with high conception rates using high-quality bulls, good success in delivering live calves, low calf mortality rates, and low to modest rearing costs will have an excess of young stock to replace animals of lower value in their milking herd. However, a milking herd with high losses (death, disease, infertility) can exceed the heifer replacement capacity of the dairy, requiring purchase of replacements if the herd is to remain at current herd capacity.

Capacity of Facility or Ability to Expand

Simply, this is the desire or ability of the management to add cows to the herd. Environmental constraints can be one factor limiting growth, but availability of affordable land, willingness to relocate, quality of available land, or the desire to add more cows are decisions that management must consider when deciding whether to raise their heifers, sell cows, retain cows, or purchase replacements.

Operating Goals of the Owner/Management Team

It is critical that members of management set goals for themselves and their employees and advisors. Without this, decision making can be unfocused or capricious. Whether the goal is the highest milk production, maximum profitability, highest quality genetics, more time off, maximum use of the facility, or something else, defining replacement strategies for the production goals is critical.

TREATMENT

DIET
Appropriate for the maintenance of body condition and health

CLIENT EDUCATION
Teaching your clients the value of their replacement animals and the value of keeping cows healthy is critical for understanding costs involved in maintaining a profitable business.

MEDICATIONS

Appropriate milk and meat withdrawal times must be followed for all compounds administered to food-producing animals.

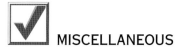

MISCELLANEOUS

PREGNANCY
Typically, nonpregnant cows are culled.

RUMINANT SPECIES AFFECTED
All ruminant species are affected.

BIOSECURITY
Lack of disease control can greatly affect culling risk.

PRODUCTION MANAGEMENT
N/A

SYNONYMS
N/A

SEE ALSO
Heifer rearing
Species-specific sections on biosecurity
Species-specific sections on body condition scoring

ABBREVIATIONS
BCS — body condition score
rBST = recombinant bovine somatotropin

Suggested Reading
Bascom, S. S., Young, A. J. 1998. A summary of the reasons why farmers cull cows. *J Dairy Sci.* 81(8):2299–2305.
Dohoo, I. R., Martin, S.W. 1984. Disease, production and culling in Holstein-Friesian dairy cows. *Prev Vet Med.* 2:771–84.
Faust, M. A., Kinsel, M. L., Kirkpatrick, M. A. 2001. Characterizing biosecurity, health, and culling during dairy herd expansions. *J Dairy Sci.* 84(4): 955–65.
Graham, T. W., Thurmond, M. C., Keen, C. L. 1994. Serum zinc and copper concentrations predict culling in pregnant Holstein dairy cows. *J Anim Sci.* 72(S1):345.
Grohn, Y. T., Ducrocq, V., Hertl, J. A. 1997. Modeling the effect of a disease on culling: an illustration of the use of time dependent covariates for survival analysis. *J Dairy Sci.* 80(8): 1755–66.
Grohn, Y. T., Rajala-Schultz, P. J., Allore, H. G., DeLorenzo, M. A., Hertl, J. A., Galligan, D. T. 2003. Optimizing replacement of dairy cows: modeling the effects of diseases. *Prev Vet Med.* 61:27–43.
Tozer, P. R., Heinrichs, A. J. 2001. What affects the cost of raising replacement heifers: a multiple component analysis. *J Dairy Sci.* 84(8): 1836–44.

Author: Thomas W. Graham

CUTANEOUS MYIASIS OF SHEEP AND GOATS

BASICS

OVERVIEW
- Myiasis is parasitism of living animals by the larvae of dipteran flies.
- Blowfly strike is facultative cutaneous myiasis caused by members of the family Calliphoridae (blowflies).
- Sheep worldwide are affected by blowfly strike, but the causative species of blowfly vary by region.
- Goats are rarely affected by blowfly strike.
- Blowfly strike is seasonal, with peak occurrence during warm, humid periods.
- Primary flies can initiate fly-strike on intact skin. First instar larvae must have a protein meal on the skin surface; second and third instar larvae penetrate intact skin.
- Secondary flies extend already struck areas, and initiate strike in wounds.
- Three distinct forms of fly-strike occur: breech strike, body strike, and wound strike.

SYSTEMS AFFECTED
Skin and musculoskeletal

GENETICS
N/A

INCIDENCE/PREVALENCE
Unknown

GEOGRAPHIC DISTRIBUTION
- Blowfly strike is the most economically significant animal health issue in the main sheep raising areas of the Southern Hemisphere.
- Screwworm infestation is a form of wound myiasis. *Chrysomya bezziana* "Old World screw-worm" is distributed throughout Sub-Saharan Africa, and across South and East Asia to Melanesia. *Cochliomyia homnivorax* "New World screw-worm" is distributed from southern Mexico to the southern subtropical Americas, having been eradicated from the southern USA and most of Mexico.
- Both screwworm species are obligate parasites.

SIGNALMENT

Species
Sheep of all ages can be affected, but weaned lambs are particularly susceptible to blowfly strike.

Breed Predilections
N/A

Mean Age and Range
Sheep of all ages can be affected, but weaned lambs are particularly susceptible to blowfly strike.

Predominant Sex
N/A

CAUSES AND RISK FACTORS

Blowfly Strike
Primary Flies
Green bottles *Lucilia sericata* (worldwide), *Lucilia cuprina* (Southern Africa and Australasia), *Lucilia illustris* (North America); black blowflies *Phormia regina* and *Phormia terrae-novae* (Northern Hemisphere); and the brown blowfly *Calliphora stygia* (New Zealand).

Secondary Flies
- Many *Chrysomya* species, particularly *Chrysomya rufifacies*, and *Sarcophaga* species where they occur
- The primary risk factor for fly-strike is the size and activity level of the blowfly population, which depends on high ambient temperature, high humidity, and availability of susceptible sheep and carrion.
- Susceptibility to primary strike depends on bacterial dermatitis of water-macerated skin providing serous exudate for the first instar larvae to have a protein meal, and shaded areas for oviposition.
- Breech strike is facilitated by soiling of the wool and perineal skin by urine and wet feces.
- Body strike is facilitated by constant fleece wetness, and especially by fleece-rot or dermatophilosis.
- The fetid odor of struck sheep attracts secondary flies.

- Fetid exudate from foot rot smeared on the body when the sheep lie down attracts flies.
- Open wounds oozing serous exudate are attractive to flies as a source of moisture and protein. Rams with head lacerations from fighting are prone to poll strike.
- Balanoposthitis predisposes to prepuce strike.

DIAGNOSIS

- Breech strike is the most common, but body strike has more severe consequences because detection is delayed.
- Initially, struck sheep twitch the tail, stamp their feet, attempt to bite at the affected part, and are generally distracted.
- The wool about the struck area is wet, discolored grey, and malodorous.
- Many maggots infest the affected area, and there maybe covert strikes elsewhere populated by a few maggots.
- As the strike progresses, affected animals separate from the mob, reduce feed intake, and tend to lie down for extended periods.
- The body temperature rises to around 41°C. Pulse and respiratory rates increase in concert with the development of toxemia.

DIFFERENTIAL DIAGNOSIS
N/A

CBC/BIOCHEMISTRY/URINALYSIS
N/A

OTHER LABORATORY TESTS
N/A

IMAGING
N/A

DIAGNOSTIC PROCEDURES
N/A

PATHOLOGIC FINDINGS
N/A

CUTANEOUS MYIASIS OF SHEEP AND GOATS

TREATMENT

MEDICATIONS

DRUGS OF CHOICE
• Apply liquid larvicidal insecticide to the struck area, and thoroughly saturate a wide margin of surrounding wool.
• Wet but do not remove the wool covering the wound. The wool takes up insecticide and dries out once the maggots are dead. Thus, the treated wool provides a protective covering against further strike, and against sunburn.

CONTRAINDICATIONS / POSSIBLE INTERACTIONS
Insure that meat and milk withdrawal periods are monitored for treatment programs.

FOLLOW-UP

PATIENT MONITORING
Frequent careful monitoring of sheep at pasture is critical during the fly challenge period to identify and treat struck animals before they succumb.

PREVENTION/AVOIDANCE
• Dock tails to the correct length to avoid fecal soiling of the perineal wool. When the animal defecates, the stump of tail should lift the wool clear, but should not be so long that it becomes soiled. The tail should reach beyond the tip of the vulva, and this length is achieved by docking at the third joint, which is located at the distal extremity of the ventral caudal folds.
• Dock early in the season before the fly challenge period.
• Control gastrointestinal parasitism to prevent diarrhea.
• Clip the wool around the breech short, or if necessary shear the sheep.
• Topically apply chemoprophylactic insecticide or insect growth regulator. At docking, apply to the wool around tail docking / castration wounds / rings, and the wool around the breach.

• Older animals can be treated either by jetting targeted at the tail and breech, or by saturation dipping.
• Pesticide categories marketed for fly-strike prevention include organophosphates, pyrethroids, macrocyclic lactones (topical and intraruminal), benzoyl ureas, triazine, and pyrimidine carbonitrile.
• Great care must be taken to match: the pesticide formulation, the application method, the wool type and length, the anticipated period of protection, withholding period, operator safety, and cost.
• Control fleece-rot and dermatophilosis by saturation dipping with zinc sulphate added at 0.5% w/v.
• In Australia, the Mules operation is performed to remove skin folds from the perineum of Merino and Merino-derived breeds of sheep.

POSSIBLE COMPLICATIONS
• Failure to prevent flystrike
• Reasons are any one or a combination of factors including: an inappropriate formulation of pesticide was used, insufficient volume of chemoprophylactic was applied, constant rain leached pesticide from the wool resulting in an abbreviated period of protection, the fly population was resistant to the pesticide (diazinon), climatic conditions favored an intense fly challenge of susceptible sheep, or fecal soiling of the breech was not prevented.

EXPECTED COURSE AND PROGNOSIS
• With treatment: full recovery
• Without treatment: some animals may self-cure mild blowfly strikes especially early in the season, severe infestations are invariably fatal.

MISCELLANEOUS

ASSOCIATED CONDITIONS
N/A

AGE-RELATED FACTORS
Young animals with gastrointestinal parasite burdens are more prone to diarrhea, and therefore fecal soiling of the breech.

ZOONOTIC POTENTIAL
N/A

PREGNANCY
N/A

BIOSECURITY
Screwworms are of regulatory importance.

PRODUCTION MANAGEMENT
N/A

RUMINANT SPECIES AFFECTED
Potentially all ruminant species

SYNONYMS
Blowfly strike
Screwworm infestation

SEE ALSO
External parasites of sheep
Myiasis
Sheep keds
Wound management

ABBREVIATIONS
N/A

Suggested Reading
Arundel, J. H., Sutherland, A. K. 1988 Animal health in Australia, Volume 10, *Ectoparasitic diseases of sheep, cattle, goats and horses.* Bureau of Rural Resources, Department of Primary Industries and Energy, Canberra, Australian Government Publishing Service.
Charleston, W. A. G., ed. 1985. *Ectoparasites of sheep in New Zealand and their control.* Palmerston North: New Zealand Veterinary Association Sheep and Beef Cattle Society.
Heath, A., Cole, D., Bishop, D. 1999. AgFact No. 29: Flystrike awareness, management and control. ISSN 1172-2088 http://www.agresearch.co.nz/agr/pubs/agfact/pdf/029flystrike.pdf (03/28/04).
Kaufmann, J. 1996. *Parasitic infections of domestic animals, a diagnostic manual.* Basel; Boston; Berlin: Birkhäuser Verlag.
Urquhart, G. M., Armour, J., Duncan, J. L., Dunn, A. M., Jennings, F. W. 1996. *Veterinary parasitology.* 2nd ed. Oxford: Blackwell Sciences Ltd.
Williams, R. E., Hall, R. D., Broce, A. B., Scholl, P. J., eds. 1985. *Livestock entomology.* New York; Toronto: John Wiley & Sons.

Author: A. D. (Sandy) McLachlan

CYANIDE TOXICOSIS

BASICS

OVERVIEW
• Cyanide poisoning is characterized by the abrupt onset of severe neurologic signs.
• Cyanogenic glycosides are commonly known as amygdalin, prunasin, dhurrin, linamarin, and triglocinin.
• Many *Prunus* spp. are cyanogenic, but only a few present a serious risk to livestock: choke cherry (*P. virginiana*), black cherry (*P. serotina*), and cherry laurel (*P. laurocerasus*).
• Other cyanide-containing plants associated with livestock toxicosis are Sudan grass and Johnson grass (*Sorghum* spp.), arrow grass (*Triglocin* spp.), vetch (*Vicia* spp.), corn (*Zea mays*), clover (*Trifolium* spp.), California holly (*Heteromeles arbutifolia*), June berry (*Amelanchior* spp.) and eucalyptus (*Eucalyptus* spp.).
• Hydrogen cyanide is readily absorbed from the gastrointestinal tract and acts by inhibiting cytochrome oxidase.
• Ruminants are more susceptible to the toxic effects than monogastric animals because rumen microorganisms produce enzymes that facilitate rapid hydrolysis of cyanogenic glycosides.
• All parts of the plants have cyanogenic potential. The highest concentrations of cyanogenic glycosides are found in the leaves, but concentrations are subject to many influences and may vary considerably.

SIGNALMENT
• All ruminant species are very susceptible. Most reported cases involve goats and cattle.
• Losses in sheep and deer have also been reported.

SIGNS
• Abrupt onset of apprehension and distress occurs within 10 to 15 minutes of ingestion.
• This is quickly followed by weakness, ataxia, hyperventilation, and hypotension. In severe cases, the animals become recumbent and develop cardiac arrhythmias and tetanic-type seizures.

• Death may occur within 15 to 60 minutes of exposure.
• Mucous membranes are initially bright cherry red due to the well-oxygenated venous blood.
• Cyanosis may be observed at a later stage of poisoning.

CAUSES AND RISK FACTORS
• Young and rapidly growing plants have the highest concentration of cyanide.
• Plant trimmings remain toxic as long as the leaves are green and have not completely dried.
• Insect-, frost-, and drought-damaged cyanogenic plants have been associated with a greater risk for cyanide poisoning.
• Concentrations of greater than 200 μg/g of cyanide in plant material are considered potentially toxic.
• Cyanide in mill tailing ponds at gold mines can present a risk to wild ruminants.

DIAGNOSIS

DIFFERENTIAL DIAGNOSIS
• Nitrate/nitrite toxicosis—chocolate-colored blood
• Nonprotein nitrogen toxicosis—exposure to NPN supplements, toxic levels of ammonia in rumen content and blood
• Organophosphorus or carbamate insecticide exposure—gastrointestinal irritation and neurological signs, evaluation of cholinesterase activity, detection of pesticides
• Lead poisoning—determination of blood lead concentration
• Neurotoxic plants (poison hemlock, water hemlock, tree tobacco, lupine)—analysis for plant toxins in gastrointestinal contents, history of exposure
• Cardiotoxic plants (oleander, milkweeds, and azaleas)—analysis for plant toxins in gastrointestinal contents, history of exposure
• Neurotoxic blue-green algae—identification of algae material in rumen contents
• ABPE—onset of clinical signs usually 1–4 days after an abrupt change to lush pasture, pathological evaluation of lung

CBC/BIOCHEMISTRY/URINALYSIS
No specific changes occur.

OTHER LABORATORY TESTS
• Detection of cyanide in blood, rumen content, liver, and skeletal muscle
• Samples must be collected promptly and stored frozen in airtight containers until analysis.
• Concentrations in tissues from lethal exposures may be reduced to one-third of the initial values within 1 hour of death.
• If liver is not collected within 4 hours of death, skeletal muscle is the preferred sample for analysis.
• Because of the volatility of hydrogen cyanide in biological samples, "toxic" thresholds are not established.

IMAGING
N/A

DIAGNOSTIC PROCEDURES
N/A

PATHOLOGIC FINDINGS
• There are no clearly distinctive changes.
• Cherry red blood immediately after death, but the color of blood darkens as postmortem time increases
• Hemorrhages may occur in the subendocardium, subepicardium, and abomasums.
• There may be mild congestion and edema of the lungs.

TREATMENT
• Immediate removal of the cyanogenic plant material
• Avoid stress
• General supportive care in nonsevere cases
• Administration of antidotes as soon as possible in severe cases

MEDICATIONS

DRUGS OF CHOICE
• The primary antidote for ruminants is thiosulfate. Thiosulfate (20%–40% solution) administered IV at a dose of 25–50 mg/100 kg bodyweight
• Sodium nitrite can be given concurrently, but may not be of additional benefit in ruminants. If given, the recommended dose is 10–20 mg/kg bodyweight IV.
• Cobalt compounds, such as cobalt chloride or hydroxycobalamin, have been used successfully in the treatment of cyanide poisoning in Europe, but have not been approved for use in animals in the United States.

CONTRAINDICATIONS
• Do not administer methylene blue, as it is ineffective as a producer of methemoglobinemia.
• If there is suspicion that cyanide poisoning is combined with nitrate poisoning, administration of sodium nitrite is contraindicated.
• Meat and milk withdrawal periods for drugs given must be determined.

FOLLOW-UP

PATIENT MONITORING
Clinical signs

PREVENTION/AVOIDANCE
• Delaying grazing until cyanogenic forage has matured.
• Slow and thorough drying of forage reduces the cyanide concentration.
• Avoid exposure of animals to frost- or insect- damaged cyanogenic plants. After a killing frost, wait for at least 4 to 6 days before grazing.

• Do not allow hungry cattle to graze cyanogenic plants.
• Feeding material as silage will reduce the risk of poisoning, as correct ensilage for 3 weeks reduces levels of toxin by approximately 50%.
• Suspect forage should be analyzed for cyanide concentrations.

POSSIBLE COMPLICATIONS
N/A

EXPECTED COURSE AND PROGNOSIS
• Animals poisoned with cyanide are often found dead.
• Cyanide poisoning progresses so rapidly that treatment is often too late. In most cases, the affected animals have a poor-to-grave prognosis.
• If treatment is initiated promptly, the prognosis is fair.
• Animals that live beyond 1 hour following intake are likely to survive.

MISCELLANEOUS

ASSOCIATED CONDITIONS
Sorghum spp. often contain toxic nitrate concentrations.

AGE-RELATED FACTORS
N/A

ZOONOTIC POTENTIAL
N/A

PREGNANCY
N/A

RUMINANT SPECIES AFFECTED
Cattle, sheep, goats, deer

BIOSECURITY
N/A

PRODUCTION MANAGEMENT
• Delay grazing until cyanogenic forage has matured.
• Slow and thorough drying of forage reduces the cyanide concentration

• Avoid exposure of animals to frost- or insect- damaged cyanogenic plants. After a killing frost, wait for at least 4 to 6 days before grazing.
• Do not allow hungry cattle to graze cyanogenic plants.
• Ruminants are more susceptible to the toxic effects than monogastric animals because rumen microorganisms produce enzymes that facilitate rapid hydrolysis of cyanogenic glycosides.

SEE ALSO
Cardiotoxic plants (oleander, milkweeds, azaleas)
Lead poisoning
Neurotoxic blue-green algae
Neurotoxic plants (poison hemlock, water hemlock, tree tobacco, lupine)
Nitrate/nitrite toxicosis
Nonprotein nitrogen toxicosis
Organophosphorus or carbamate insecticide exposure

ABBREVIATIONS
• ABPE = acute bovine pulmonary edema and emphysema
• IV = intravenous
• NPN = nonprotein nitrogen

Suggested Reading
Burrows, G. E., Tyrl, R. J. 2001. Rosaceae. In: *Toxic plants of North America*, ed. G. E. Burrows, R. J. Tyrl. Ames: Iowa State University Press.
Pickrell, J. A., Oehme, F. 2004. Cyanogenic glycosides. In: *Clinical veterinary toxicology*, ed. K. H. Plumlee. St. Louis: Mosby.
Tegzes, J. H., Puschner, B., Melton, L. A. 2003. Cyanide toxicosis in goats after ingestion of California holly (*Heteromeles arbutifolia*). *J Vet Diagn Invest*. 15:478–80.
Terblanche, M., Minne, J. A., Adelaar, T. F. 1964. Hydrocyanic acid poisoning. *J S Afr Vet Med Assoc*. 35:503–06.

Author: Birgit Puschner

DAIRY BUCK MANAGEMENT

BASICS

OVERVIEW
• Buck management is the most overlooked program in goat production worldwide.
• Body-condition scoring of breeding bucks on a regular basis is important to the reproductive health of the herd.
• The performance of herd bucks is dependent upon their health, nutrition, and proper management.
• Buck-management programs should start with breed-specific genetic selection considerations for the important traits necessary for each herd.
• Bucks should be housed separately from does and brought together for breeding only.
• Buck success is measured by overall reproductive efficiency and the performance of the offspring.
• A buck must be prepared for the breeding season with good nutrition, vaccination, and parasite control as well as foot trimming/care.
• Breeding soundness examination should be carried out annually prior to the breeding season.
• A 1 to 2 year old buck should make 25–50 services in a year. More services are common for older bucks.
• Body condition, structural correctness of feet and legs, and general soundness are also important factors for new breeding buck prospects.

SYSTEMS AFFECTED
Production management, nutrition, musculoskeletal, immune, gastrointestinal, reproductive, skin

GENETICS
• Intersex condition is linked to the polled gene in many breeds of goats and the use of phenotypically polled bucks should be discouraged.
• Selection and progeny test programs should be developed for the buck herd. Important traits include: multiple birth numbers, milk production, carcass quality, environmental adaptability, and feet and leg scores.
• Testicular diameter is directly correlated with fertility.
• Meat breeds generally require growth rate, carcass quality, and feed conversion traits to be superior.

INCIDENCE/PREVALENCE
N/A

GEOGRAPHIC DISTRIBUTION
• Worldwide; over 90% of the world's goats are in developing countries.
• Goats are important in developing countries as subsistence food producers.

SIGNALMENT
Species
Meat and dairy goats

Breed Predilections
• Specific meat and dairy goat breeds

• Angora and pygmy goats have been reported to be sensitive to copper supplementation.

Mean Age and Range
N/A

Predominant Sex
Male

MEDICATIONS

DRUGS OF CHOICE

CONTRAINDICATIONS
Appropriate milk and meat withdrawal times must be followed for all compounds administered to food-producing animals.

MISCELLANEOUS

MANAGEMENT EVALUATION
• Producers should be concerned with the body condition of their breeding bucks especially during breeding season. Goats should not be allowed to become too thin or too fat. Body condition score directly affects libido.
• The buck pasture should be far enough from the breeding doe herd that scent emitted by glands located behind the base of the buck's horns will not induce estrus in does. This allows the "buck effect" to occur. Does will come into estrus approximately 7–10 days after the introduction of the buck (buck effect).
• Trimming the hooves of breeding animals is extremely important to buck health and reproductive performance. Bucks with poor hoof health may breed only sporadically or even not at all.

BUCK MANAGEMENT PROGRAMS
• Buck management programs begin with the purchase of new herd sire(s).
• The genetic direction of the herd is of obvious importance in trait/sire selection.
• In addition to inherent genetic traits, bucks must be healthy, fertile, and capable of expressing their desirable traits.
• Bucks tend to lose weight during the progression of the breeding season. Breeding soundness exams should be performed monthly and energy deficiencies rectified. Bucks should enter the breeding season with a body condition score (BCS) of 3.0. It should be remembered that high levels of concentrates fed to bucks may stimulate urolithiasis and ruminal acidosis.
• Foot care is essential in breeding bucks. Though it is often overlooked due to buck hygiene, it is imperative that the feet and legs be cared for on a scheduled regular basis.
• Bucks should be purchased from seed-stock breeders that have documented herd health programs that minimize the likelihood of infectious diseases.

• Herd bucks should be immunized against common diseases and, if necessary, treated for parasites or tested for diseases indicated from a biosecurity standpoint.
• All bucks should undergo a complete breeding soundness evaluation (BSE) to assess their general physical and reproductive soundness. Important components include: physical examination, libido check, examination of genitalia, and a semen evaluation.
• Each component of the BSE such as scrotal circumference (SC) should be accurately measured and utilized within the context of age, weight, nutritional status, and contemporary group. It should be noted that semen quality and testicle size fluctuates seasonally.

Behavior
• Goats are natural climbers and jumpers. Bucks are intelligent animals and are quick to learn and like attention.
• Bucks commonly spray urine on their forequarters during the breeding season as an attractant. Clipping beards and coat hair prior to the breeding season can reduce the overall offensiveness of smell for the handler.
• Bucks can also acquire annoying habits and owners should be careful how goats are handled, especially kids (e.g., pushing on a kid's head will encourage it to butt). Treat all bucks with the respect necessary to maintain social order.
• Bucks are oftentimes housed in groups and a social order develops. Introduction of new bucks into this hierarchy can be dangerous. This is especially true with younger, smaller, or more timid animals.

Reproduction
• Goats are seasonally polyestrous (seasonal anestrus) breeders. Gestation length is 5 months.
• The breeding season typically runs from August through January (in the Northern Hemisphere), with an 18–23-day estrous cycle.
• The typical buck to doe ratio is 1 buck to 20–30 does. A 1:50 ratio is not uncommon in mature bucks.
• A buck should not be expected to breed more than 50 does in a 6-week period.
• Does usually remain in heat for 1 to 2 days. Puberty occurs at 6–8 months of age with breeding at 7–10 months of age or when doelings reach 60%–75% of mature body weight.
• Conception is highest from the middle to the latter part of the heat period. Therefore, if estrus is detected in the afternoon, goats should be bred late the following morning.
• Individual buck breeding variation:
  1. Age
  2. Body condition
  3. Fertility
  4. Libido
  5. Social behavior
  6. Injury

- Pheromonal communication plays an important role in goat behavior. Bucks have a strong odor during the breeding season. Pheromones are air-borne chemical substances released in the urine or secreted from cutaneous glands that are perceived by the olfactory system and elicit both behavioral and endocrine responses in females.
- The buck has a strong characteristic seasonal odor and a buck jar containing the odor of the buck can be used as an aid in the detection of estrus in does.
- In goats, exposure of seasonally anestrous females to sexually active males results in activation of luteinizing hormone (LH) secretion and synchronized ovulation. This phenomenon is named "the buck effect" and constitutes the major control of reproductive events. The sudden introduction of bucks to a group of anestrous does will stimulate them to naturally synchronize (assuming the does have not heard or smelled a buck prior). The does generally cycle within 3 days.
- Keeping bucks apart from does for the first 2 days will stimulate buck semen production. Does bred to bucks that are "warmed-up" will have increased fertility rates and may breed successfully the first cycle.
- Conduct a breeding soundness evaluation on all bucks. Select bucks that are above average in scrotal circumference, motility, and percent normal sperm morphology.
- Breeding soundness evaluations should be done yearly, preferably just before breeding season begins.
- Develop a method to identify some progeny of each sire for sire trait evaluation.

Disease Control
- Obstructive urolithiasis is a major concern in breeding bucks. Nutritional management is important in its prevention (see Urolithiasis in Small Ruminants).
- Urine scald can be common secondary to the males' tendency to chronically urinate on themselves during the breeding season. Secondary bacterial dermatitis is a common sequela on the caudal aspect of the forelimbs.
- Horn scur trauma is common in group-housed males. These animals can bleed extensively and owners should become concerned with wound myiasis in warmer climates.
- Parasites can be a substantial problem in some breeding schemes. Fecal examination should be performed twice yearly.
- In certain parts of the world, venereal disease can be an important impediment to fertility (e.g., brucellosis, Q-fever, *Chlamydia* sp.).
- Lameness and foot disease can be sequelae to poorly managed and trimmed feet.
- Arthritis can be common in older bucks.
- Breeding bucks should be found negative for CAE and Johne's disease.

Facilities
- Escape-proof fences are important due to the goat's climbing capabilities.
- Goats should be provided with dry, clean bedding in a draft-free enclosure (15 sq ft/goat). Buck barns/sheds should be well ventilated.
- A well-drained outside pen large enough for the bucks to get ample exercise should be provided.
- Placement of large objects such as tree stumps, rocks, and wooden spools in the pen provides goats with climbing exercise and social diversion.
- Buck fences should be at least 42 inches in height and predator proof. When using woven (net) wire fence, use a 12 inch by 6 inch wide opening to prevent goats from getting their heads caught in the fence.
- Place feeders at least 6 inches off the ground.
- To help reduce disease transmission, raise hay and mineral feeders off the ground.
- Feed troughs should be designed so that goats cannot stand in them (they may defecate or urinate on the feed).
- Fresh water is essential. Check water availability on a daily basis and regularly drain and clean water troughs.
- Keep water cool during warm weather and, if possible, locate water source in the shade.
- Goats may drink large amounts of water during hot weather. It is very important to encourage water intake to help prevent formation of urinary calculi.

Dehorning
- It is preferable to dehorn (disbud) kids when they are a few days old. Dehorning animals becomes more stressful as horn size increases.
- Dehorning mature bucks is a SUBSTANTIAL venture requiring general and local anesthesia and the removal of the cornual tissue into the sinuses. The healing process takes 6–8 weeks and myasis is a common sequela in warmer months.
- Horned bucks can be extremely dangerous and require constant observation. Always exercise caution around breeding bucks.

Hoof Trimming
- Rough terrain generally will wear down a goat's hooves in pastured animals.
- Goats kept in pens or on smooth terrain require regular hoof trimming/care approximately every 6 weeks.

ASSOCIATED CONDITIONS
- Obstructive urolithiasis
- Urine scald
- Horn scur trauma
- Wound myiasis
- Parasites can be a substantial problem
- Lameness, infertility, nutritional deficiencies, behavioral issues

AGE-RELATED FACTORS
Bucks are often housed in groups and a social order is developed. Introduction of new bucks into this hierarchy can be dangerous. This is especially true with younger, smaller, or more timid animals.

ZOONOTIC POTENTIAL
Several goat diseases are zoonotic. Care must be taken in the collection of laboratory samples and the diagnosis/treatment of affected animals.

PREGNANCY
N/A

RUMINANT SPECIES AFFECTED
Dairy and meat goats

BIOSECURITY
- Isolation and quarantine of new stock entering the herd
- Treat and/or cull new animals for disease conditions prior to herd introduction.
- Herd bucks should be immunized against common diseases and, if necessary, treated for parasites or tested for diseases indicated from a biosecurity standpoint.

PRODUCTION MANAGEMENT
Production systems:
- Monitor body condition of bucks and supplement feed if necessary.
- Evaluate bucklings and cull unsound or inferior animals.
- Monitor internal parasites through regular fecal samples.
- Treat for internal and external parasites as indicated.
- Replacement bucks should have good conformation, good constitution, muscling, and increased weight for their age.
- Buck breeding ratio of 1 buck per 20–30 does is dependent on management and on pasture size/conditions.
- After the breeding season, remove bucks and feed to regain body condition.

SYNONYMS
Buck effect

SEE ALSO
Body condition scoring goats
Goat nutrition
Myasis
Small ruminant reproduction
Small ruminant urolithiasis

ABBREVIATIONS
BCS = body condition score
BSE = breeding soundness evaluation
CAE = caprine arthritis encephalitis

Suggested Reading
Erasmus, J. A. 2000, May 1. Adaptation to various environments and resistance to disease of the improved Boer goat. *Small Rumin Res.* 36(2):179–87.
Gelez, H., Fabre-Nys, C. 2004, Sep. The "male effect" in sheep and goats: a review of the respective roles of the two olfactory systems. *Horm Behav.* 46(3):257–71.
Glimp, H. A. 1995, Jan. Meat goat production and marketing. *J Anim Sci.* 73(1):291–95.
Malan, S. W. 2000, May 1. The improved Boer goat. *Small Rumin Res.* 36(2):165–70.
Rekwot, P. I., Ogwu, D., Oyedipe, E. O., Sekoni, V. O. 2001, Mar 30. The role of pheromones and biostimulation in animal reproduction. *Anim Reprod Sci.* 65(3–4):157–70.

Author: Scott R. R. Haskell

DAIRY BULL MANAGEMENT

 BASICS

OVERVIEW
• Efficient reproductive performance is a critical element in the profitability and ultimately the survival of any dairy operation.
• The performance of any natural-service breeding program depends on the fertility of the bulls and cows and the influences of the management system that we create for them to work in.
• These management systems range from a health-conducive environment with clean, dry pasture to free-stall housing with slippery concrete floors and poor sight lines.
• Ideally, bulls used for natural service would be physically sound, highly fertile transmitters of desirable genetic traits and would not create a safety hazard for people or other cattle of the dairy.
• In the real world, natural-service sires usually fall far short of this ideal.
• The breeding soundness examination (BSE) of bulls as recommended by the Society for Theriogenology is a valuable tool for preventing breeding problems or solving them once they have occurred.
• A BSE should be conducted on every sexually mature dairy bull before purchase, every 6 months during his service life, and whenever a problem with his performance is suspected.

SYSTEMS AFFECTED
Reproductive

GENETICS
N/A

INCIDENCE/PREVALENCE
More than half of dairy producers use natural-service sires either as their primary breeding method or for "clean-up" after a variable number of AI services or days postcalving have elapsed.

GEOGRAPHICAL DISTRIBUTION
Worldwide distribution

SIGNALMENT
Species
Dairy cattle

Breed Predilections
All breeds

 TREATMENT

BULL MANAGEMENT PROGRAMS
Sire Selection
• Dairy farmers will often select bull calves from "superior" cows to serve as natural-service sires.
• This approach is almost certain to fail as a means of improving either milk production or other inherited aspects of cow performance or conformation.
• The reality is that the AI industry has access to highly selected bull calves from the elite cows in the national dairy herd and even these bulls routinely fail to transmit genetic superiority to their offspring.
• Calving ease is also a desirable trait in bulls used for natural service, especially those used to breed heifers.
• No reliable calving ease information is available for dairy bulls used in natural service.

• Small bulls may be the result of poor nutrition and may have associated problems with fertility while offering no real advantage in calving ease for the cows or heifers that do become pregnant when bred by them.
• Only healthy, fertile bulls from dairy herds with a high health status should be considered as natural-service sires.

Sire Evaluation
• The breeding soundness examination (BSE) consists of a thorough physical examination of the bull with a special focus on the systems that most dramatically influence reproduction.
• Bulls rely on many cues to detect estrus in cows but visual identification of the sexually active group is probably the most critical so the eyes should be carefully examined.
• The physical ability to mate is primarily a function of the musculoskeletal system.
• Sound feet and legs are essential with special attention paid to conformational problems in the hooves and hind legs.
• Physical examination of the genital tract should follow the guidelines as set forth by the Society for Theriogenology.
• Scrotal circumference, sperm motility, and sperm morphology are critical elements of the BSE and a bull must meet minimal standards for all three criteria to be considered a satisfactory potential breeder.
• In addition, the bull must be free of physical defects that would interfere with his ability to breed cows. More than half the bulls rejected by a BSE are rejected because of problems detected during the physical examination before semen is collected and evaluated.

DAIRY BULL MANAGEMENT

- Libido, or desire to breed, is also important but is difficult to predict or evaluate as part of the BSE.
- Dairy clients should be advised to monitor bulls carefully during use to ascertain that they are aggressively seeking out cows in estrus and mating with them.

Bull to Female Ratio (BFR)
- Serving capacity, or the ability to provide a fertile mating for every cow eligible to be bred, is an important consideration when evaluating a natural breeding system.
- Serving capacity is a function of the bull's libido, physical mating ability, and fertility and all three of these factors play a role in determining the number of bulls required to breed a group of cows or heifers.
- Breeding efficiency is a function of the bull's age or breeding experience, his fertility, and the fertility of the cows he is bred to, as well as the breeding environment.
- Selecting the correct BFR is often a matter of trial and error.
- A 1:20 BFR is a reasonable starting point and can be adjusted up or down based on herd reproductive performance.
- A BFR of 1:10 or 1:15 may be more realistic for yearling bulls.
- More bulls will be required if estrus synchronization programs that result in concentrated breeding activity are used on the farm.
- Adding more bulls during warm weather may help with fertility problems caused by heat stress but supplementing the bulls with AI is probably more efficient.
- Rotating groups of bulls through strings of open cows or heifers on a 7–14-day schedule will minimize the impact of a group of subfertile bulls.

Monitoring Performance
- Palpation per rectum or ultrasonographic diagnosis of pregnancy in cows and heifers exposed to the bull is the most timely and effective method for monitoring reproductive performance.
- Typical 21-day pregnancy rates for bull-bred dairy cows range from 12% to 17%.
- Special attention to performance is required during hot, humid weather.
- For most dairy producers who are using bulls, there is little economic justification for treating the infertile bull.
- The usual solution is to identify him, cull him, and replace him with another more fertile bull.

CLIENT EDUCATION
Clients should be made aware that the reproductive performance of natural-service bulls is usually poorer than AI and generates additional costs associated with loss of genetic progress, feed consumption, and the creation of health and safety hazards.

 MISCELLANEOUS

AGE-RELATED FACTORS
- Older, sexually experienced bulls are more likely to harbor and transmit venereal diseases.
- Older bulls are also larger and therefore more likely to injure cows or themselves during copulation.
- Older bulls are more aggressive and are more likely to cause aggression-related injuries to other bulls or people.

RUMINANT SPECIES AFFECTED
Dairy bulls

BIOSECURITY
- All males to be used as breeding animals should be subject to the same parasite control and vaccination procedures as the cows and heifers in the herd except that bulls should not be vaccinated for brucellosis.
- All bulls entering a herd should undergo a breeding soundness examination and an appropriate period of quarantine followed by reexamination.
- Specific testing for venereal diseases (campylobacteriosis and trichomoniasis) should be conducted as necessary.

SYNONYMS
N/A

SEE ALSO
Beef bull management
Breeding soundness exam
Body condition score: bovine

ABBREVIATIONS
AI = artificial insemination
BFR = bull to female ratio
BSE = breeding soundness examination

Suggested Reading
Barth, A. D., Oko, J. 1989. *Abnormal morphology of bovine spermatozoa*. Ames: Iowa State University Press.
Fricke, P., Niles, D. 2003. Don't fall for the bulls-are-cheaper, more fertile myth. In: *Bulls are no bargain. Hoard's Dairyman* (Suppl.), pp. 8–9.
Geary, T. W., Reeves, J. J. 1992. Relative importance of vision and olfaction for detection of estrus by bulls. *J Anim Sci.* 70:2726–31.
Hopkins, F. M., Spitzer, J. C. 1997. The new Society for Theriogenology breeding soundness evaluation system. *Vet Clin North Am: Food Anim Pract.* 13:283–93.
Niles, D., Risco, C. A. 2002, April. Seasonal evaluation of artificial insemination and natural service pregnancy rates in dairy herds. *Comp Contin Educ.*, pp. S44–S48.

Author: Harry Momont

DAIRY GOAT DERMATOLOGY

 BASICS

OVERVIEW
• Many of the same skin diseases found in cows and sheep also affect dairy goats.
• The most important skin diseases of dairy goats are those that are contagious, zoonotic, and/or affect production.
• The most common skin diseases of dairy goats are dermatophytosis, tick and mange infestations, lice, keds, screwworm infestations, contagious ecthyma, caprine herpes virus, and staphylococcal infections.

SYSTEMS AFFECTED
Skin

GENETICS
N/A

INCIDENCE/PREVALENCE
N/A

GEOGRAPHIC DISTRIBUTION
Worldwide depending on environment

SIGNALMENT
Species
Caprine

Breed Predilections
N/A

Mean Age and Range
N/A

Predominant Sex
N/A

 DIAGNOSIS

DIFFERENTIAL DIAGNOSIS (BASED UPON BODY REGION)
Lips, Face, and Neck
• Contagious ecthyma
• Capripox
• Staphylococcal folliculitis
• Dermatophytosis
• Dermatophilosis
• Peste des petits ruminants (morbillivirus)
• Sarcoptic mange
• Zinc deficiency
• Selenium deficiency
• Pemphigus foliaceus

Ears
• Dermatophytosis
• Dermatophilosis
• Sarcoptic mange
• Ear mites
• Photodermatitis
• Frostbite
• Pemphigus foliaceus

Feet
• Contagious ecthyma
• Foot and mouth disease
• Staphylococcus folliculitis
• Interdigital fusiform infection
• Dermatophilosis
• Sarcoptic mange
• Chorioptic mange
• Pelodera dermatitis
• Besnoitia dermatitis
• Zinc deficiency
• Contact dermatitis
• Pemphigus foliaceus

Udder
• Contagious ecthyma
• Staphylococcal folliculitis
• Zinc deficiency
• Hyperpigmentation from exposure to sun
• Cutaneous papillomas in white Saanens

Perineum
• Contagious ecthyma
• Caprine herpes virus
• Staphylococcal dermatitis
• Ticks
• Neoplasia
• Ectopic mammary gland

DIFFERENTIAL DIAGNOSIS (BASED UPON DERMATOLOGIC PROBLEM)
Pruritus
• Lice
• Sheep keds
• Fleas
• Ticks
• Mites: Psoroptes (ear mange), Sarcoptes, Chorioptes
• Migrating helminthes (*Metastrongylus* and *Parelaphostrongylus tenuis*)
• Flies: *Musca* (bush fly), *Stomoxys calcitrans* (stable fly), *Culicoides* (no-see-ums), *Tabanus* (March flies)

Pustular/Papular/Vesicular Lesions
• Impetigo caused by *Staphylococcus*
• Contagious ecthyma
• Pemphigus foliaceus
• Capripox
• Foot and mouth disease
• *Pelodera*
• Caprine herpesvirus

Crusting and Scaling
• Dermatophytosis
• Dermatophilosis
• Malassezia dermatitis
• Protozoal: *Toxoplasma* sp., *Besnoitia* sp.
• Hypothyroidism
• Contagious ecthyma
• Zinc deficiency
• Selenium deficiency and undetermined vitamin E uptake
• Pemphigus foliaceus
• Capripox
• Mites
• *Pelodera*

Hair Loss
• Hypothyroidism
• Dermatophytosis
• Contact dermatitis
• Mites
• *Pelodera*
• Selenium deficiency and undetermined vitamin E uptake

Nodules With or Without Ulcers
• Demodicosis
• Staphylococcal dermatitis
• Mycetoma (fungal tumors)
• Abscesses (caseous lymphadenitis)
• Cutaneous papillomas
• Squamous cell carcinoma
• Melanoma
• Tuberculosis

Erythema
Sunburn: erythema of skin

Sloughing of Affected Area
Frostbite

CBC/BIOCHEMISTRY/URINALYSIS
N/A

OTHER LABORATORY TESTS
N/A

IMAGING
N/A

DIAGNOSTIC PROCEDURES
• Mite infestations and *Pelodera* can be diagnosed based upon positive skin scrapings and/or response to miticidal therapy (e.g., ivermectin).
• Bacterial skin infections can be diagnosed based upon skin cytology, impression smears of intact pustules, and/or bacterial culture and sensitivity testing.
• Dermatophytosis can be definitively diagnosed by dermatophyte culture or skin biopsy.
• Dermatophilosis can be diagnosed based upon biopsy, impression smears of skin beneath an avulsed crust, culture, or cytological exam of avulsed crusts.
• Skin biopsy is the most cost effective diagnostic aid for skin diseases where the diagnosis cannot be made clinically or with the above diagnostic tests.

SELECTED SKIN DISEASES
Most diseases listed above are discussed in detail elsewhere in this book. Selected diseases are discussed below.

Interdigital Fusiform Infection
• Benign interdigital dermatitis due to *Fusiformis* infection
• Clinically presents as mildly malodorous condition
• Readily responds to single injection of penicillin/streptomycin or to topical application of antibacterials such as copper sulfate or sulfonamide powder

DAIRY GOAT DERMATOLOGY

Ectopic Mammary Gland
- Affects individual animals
- Ectopic mammary glands are extra teats.
- These should be removed from kids before they develop.
- If not removed, they are problematic because they interfere with normal milking procedures and, although somewhat developed, are not productive.

Pelodera
- Parasitic disease caused by invasion of the skin by larvae of a free-living nematode, *Pelodera strongyloides*.
- Larvae live in decaying organic material and exposure occurs from contact with damp, filthy bedding.
- Larvae cannot invade healthy skin; moisture and microtrauma to the skin are predisposing factors.
- Lesions are confined to areas in contact with bedding.
- Affected skin has any combination of erythema, alopecia, pustules/papules, crusts, erosions, or ulceration.
- Pruritus is common.
- Larvae are easily found on skin scrapings and are large 600 × 38 μm.
- *Pelodera* is a disease of poor management.
- Treatment: clean environment, move animals to clean dry bedding, disease is self-limiting but ivermectin may speed resolution.

Parelaphostrongylus Tenuis
- Pruritic parasitic infection
- Clinically presents as vertically oriented pruritic excoriations over body wall or shoulders
- It is proposed that migrating larvae irritate dorsal nerve roots causing pruritus in the dermatome.
- Treatment includes corticosteroids and anthelmintics.

Selenium Deficiency
- Selenium deficiency and undetermined vitamin E intake in young goats causes periocular hair loss and generalized scaling and brittle hair coat.
- Affected animals respond in 2–4 weeks to vitamin E/selenium injections.
- Continued supplementation is needed if diet is not corrected.

Mycetoma
- Caused by fungi or actinomycetes bacteria
- Classic clinical presentation is a painless, slowly developing mass with draining tracts and "tissue grains."
- Skin biopsy and special stains will demonstrate organisms; nodular to diffuse pyogranulomatous inflammation is classic.
- Surgical excision is the treatment of choice, if possible.
- Affected animals acquire lesion via traumatic inoculation of skin.

Pemphigus Foliaceus
- Affects individual animals
- Can occur at any age but most common in goats less than 3 years of age
- PF is a rare immune-mediated skin disease caused by the production of autoantibodies against the intercellular bridges and cell-cell detachment (acantholysis).
- Clinically characterized by pustules, scales, crusting, and patchy alopecia.
- Presumptive diagnosis can be made via clinical signs and acantholytic cells and neutrophils on cytological examination of pustule contents.
- Definitive diagnosis is made by skin biopsy revealing intraepidermal and subcorneal vesiculopustules, neutrophils, and acantholytic cells.
- Affected animals require lifelong immunosuppressive therapy with oral prednisone (2–3 mg/kg divided q 12 hrs), aurothioglucose (1 mg/kg IM q 48 hrs) until clinical remission and then weekly or biweekly as needed.
- Immunosuppressive therapy will predispose affected animals to mastitis, secondary infections, and mite infestations.

Caprine Herpesvirus
- Cutaneous viral skin disease caused by a herpesvirus.
- Clinical signs include vesicles, ulcers, and crusts on the muzzle, feet, oral mucosa.
- Similar lesions can be found in the esophagus, rumen, and intestines.
- Can be the cause of abortions in pregnant does; high fevers accompany these infections
- Diagnosis is based upon history, clinical signs, and virus isolation.
- Skin biopsy reveals acidophilic intranuclear inclusion bodies in epithelial cells; these findings are typical of all herpesvirus infections.
- There is no treatment; disease must run its course.

Cutaneous Aspects of Peste Des Petits Ruminants
- This disease is caused by a morbillivirus and is an important disease of sheep and goats especially in Africa.
- It is also known as pseudorinderpest, pest of small ruminants, goat plague, pest of sheep and goats, Kata, stomatitis-pneumoenteritis syndrome, contagious pustular stomatitis, and pneumoenteritis.
- Cutaneous symptoms include dry hair coat, dry muzzle, edema, and brown crusts on lips; lesions may ulcerate and become crusted.
- Systemic symptoms of respiratory disease rapidly develop.
- This disease is discussed in detail in the Peste Des Petits Ruminants chapter.

CONTRAINDICATIONS
- Appropriate milk and meat withdrawal times must be followed for all compounds administered to food-producing animals.
- Steroids should not be used in pregnant animals.

 MISCELLANEOUS

ASSOCIATED CONDITIONS
The most common skin diseases of dairy goats are dermatophytosis, tick and mange infestations, lice, keds, screwworm infestations, contagious ecthyma, caprine herpesvirus, and staphylococcal infections.

AGE-RELATED FACTORS
N/A

ZOONOTIC POTENTIAL
Several of these pathogenic conditions are caused by zoonotic agents. Care should be exercised in the collection and evaluation of samples.

PREGNANCY
Steroids should not be used in pregnant animals.

RUMINANT SPECIES AFFECTED
Caprine

BIOSECURITY
Quarantine new animal arrivals to prevent ectoparasitic infestation in a herd.

PRODUCTION MANAGEMENT
Ectopic mammary glands, if not removed, are problematic because they interfere with normal milking procedures and, although somewhat developed, are not productive.

SYNONYMS
- Orf
- Sore mouth

SEE ALSO
Frostbite
Specific disease chapters
Toxic plant ingestion

ABBREVIATIONS

Suggested Reading
Mullowney, P. C., Baldwin, E. W. 1984. Skin diseases of goats. *Symposium on Large Animal Dermatology, Veterinary Clinics of North America* 6:131–42.
Pappalarado, E., Abramo, F., Noli, C. 2002. Pemphigus foliaceus in a goat. *Veterinary Dermatology* 13: 331–35.
Scott, D. W. 1984. *Large animal dermatology.* Philadelphia: W. B. Saunders.
Smith, M. C., Sherman, D. M. 1994. Skin diseases. In: *Goat medicine.* Philadelphia: Lea & Febiger.

Authors: Karen A. Moriello and Susan Semrad

DEATH CAMAS (ZYGADENUS)

BASICS

OVERVIEW
• *Zygadenus* spp., or death camas, has a steroidal veratrum-type alkaloid, zygacine or zygadenine, which causes arteriolar dilatation and hypotension. It is similar to the toxin in *Veratrum californicum* and *Schoenocaulon* spp.
• Alkaloids occur as glycosides, aglycones or in the form of esters with various acids.
• The entire death camas plant is toxic but the seeds are the most toxic followed by the bulb. The leaves and stems lose toxicity as the plant matures.
• The mechanism of action of the toxin is that it increases cell permeability to sodium ions. There is increased reflex activity and repetitive discharge in response to stimuli of the afferent nerve pathways.

GEOGRAPHIC DISTRIBUTION
Death camas grows in the western United States in wet meadows and along streams.

SIGNALMENT
• Sheep are the most susceptible ruminant species, then cattle.
• Zygadenus is most toxic in spring when other forage is not available.

SIGNS
• High fatality in sheep
• Signs include profuse, frothy salivation, GI upset, hypotension, and death.
• There can be muscle weakness, depression, ataxia, recumbency, and coma.
• Hypotension is experienced due to arteriolar dilation, venous constriction, and bradycardia from A-V dissociation.
• Death occurs from central respiratory depression.

CAUSES AND RISK FACTORS
The major risk factor is grazing on pastures containing *Zygadenus* in the spring.

DIAGNOSIS

DIFFERENTIAL DIAGNOSIS
Toxicity from *Asclepias* spp. (milkweed) and other cardiac glycoside-containing plants such as *Apocynum* (dogbane), *Adonis* (summer pheasant eye), *Digitalis* (foxglove), *Taxus* (yew), and *Rhododendron* (azalea). *Gossypium* (cotton seed meal) can cause similar signs. Also consider pulmonary toxicants such as *Medicago* (alfalfa), *Perilla* (purple mint), Brassicaceae, and *Fusarium*.

CBC/BIOCHEMISTRY/URINALYSIS
NA

OTHER LABORATORY TESTS
N/A

IMAGING
N/A

DIAGNOSTIC PROCEDURES
Presence of *Zygadenus* seeds or plant materials in the forage or rumen upon necropsy is most diagnostic.

PATHOLOGIC FINDINGS
GROSS FINDINGS
• There are no distinctive lesions.
• There may be gross severe pulmonary congestion and subcutaneous hemorrhage.

HISTOPATHOLOGICAL FINDINGS
Minimal lesions consisting of GI tract and liver congestion

TREATMENT

Atropine sulfate (2 mg) can be administered to sheep.

MEDICATIONS

N/A

CONTRAINDICATIONS
Appropriate milk and meat withdrawal times must be followed for all compounds administered to food-producing animals.

FOLLOW-UP

PATIENT MONITORING
Monitor and treat symptomatically.

PREVENTION/AVOIDANCE
Control *Zygadenus* in pastures through spraying as burning does not eliminate the plant; it regrows from the roots.

POSSIBLE COMPLICATIONS
N/A

EXPECTED COURSE AND PROGNOSIS
High fatality in sheep

MISCELLANEOUS

ASSOCIATED CONDITIONS
• Frothy salivation, GI upset, hypotension, and death
• Muscle weakness, depression, ataxia, recumbency, and coma
• Hypotension is experienced due to arteriolar dilation, venous constriction, and bradycardia from A-V dissociation.
• Death occurs from central respiratory depression.

AGE-RELATED FACTORS
N/A

ZOONOTIC POTENTIAL
N/A

PREGNANCY
N/A

RUMINANT SPECIES AFFECTED
• Potentially, all ruminant species can be affected.
• Sheep are the most susceptible ruminant species, then cattle.

BIOSECURITY
N/A

PRODUCTION MANAGEMENT
Control *Zygadenus* in pastures through spraying as burning does not eliminate the plant; it regrows from the roots.

SYNONYMS
N/A

SEE ALSO
Adonis (summer pheasant eye) toxicity
Apocynum (dogbane) toxicity
Asclepias spp. (milkweed) toxicity
Digitalis (foxglove) toxicity
Gossypium (cotton seed meal) toxicity
Pulmonary toxicants (*Medicago* alfalfa, *Perilla* purple mint, Brassicaceae, *Fusarium*)
Rhododendron (azalea) toxicity
Taxus (yew) toxicity

ABBREVIATIONS
A-V = atrioventricular
GI = gastrointestinal

Suggested Reading
Aiello, S. E., ed. 1998. *Merck veterinary manual*. 8th ed. Whitehouse Station, NJ: Merck and Co.
Champion, M. 2000. *Zygadenus venenosus*: Meadow death camas, poison sego lily, death camas, lobelia-Fact Sheets For Some Common Plants On Rangelands In Western Canada (Plant Ecology 434.3)http://www.usask.ca/agriculture/plantsci/classes/range/zygadenus.html. Accessed April 15, 2008.
Festa, M., Andreetto, B., Ballaris, M. A., Panio, A., Piervittori, R. 1996, May. A case of veratrum poisoning. *Minerval Anesthesiology* 62(5):195–96.
Osweiler, G. D. 1996. Plants causing cardiotoxicity. In: *Toxicology*. Media, PA: Williams and Wilkins.
Panter, K. E., Ralphs, M. H., Smart, R. A., Duelke, B. 1987, Feb. Death camas poisoning in sheep: a case report. *Veterinary Human Toxicology* 29(1): 45–48.

Author: Heidi Coker

DERMATOLOGIC MICROBIOLOGY

BASICS

OVERVIEW
• Diseases of the skin may be categorized as primary in which the lesions are primarily on the skin and may then spread to organ systems. Disease of the skin may be secondary in which the organ systems are initially infected and then cutaneous lesions will appear on the skin.
• In order to distinguish if the skin disease is primary or secondary, a complete clinical examination is necessary. Careful examination and knowledge of the patient's history can lead to accurate diagnosis.
• Normal microbial flora of the skin includes but is not limited to:
  • Some *Staphylococcus* spp.
  • *Dermatophilus congolensis* (can be pathogenic)
• Some of the most common skin diseases include but are not limited to:
  • Dermatitis (*Staphylococcus aureus*, *Strongyloides* spp., protozoan *Besnoitia* spp.)
  • Fibropapillomas (warts) (Bovine papilloma virus—BPV)
  • Impetigo (*Staphylococcus* spp.)
  • Ringworm (*Trichophyton verrucosum*)
  • Bluetongue (*Orbivirus*)

SIGNALMENT
N/A

SIGNS
• Dermatitis: increased warmth and erythema, diffuse weeping or discrete vesicular lesions, and may lead to more serious symptoms that include: edema, necrosis, gangrene, cellulites, lesions, shock, and toxemia
• Fibropapillomas: pedunculated or sessile epidermis outgrowths; in cattle, the warts can be > 1 cm in size and are found on the head, near the eyes, and on the shoulders and neck; warts are dry and crusty, and are white to gray in color; may lead to urinary bladder tumors
• Impetigo: A zone of erythema surrounds 3–6 mm lesions, small vesicles; pustules develop due to the eruption of vesicles and form scabs; acne and more extensive lesions develop in areas of hair.
• Ringworm: exudation, alopecia, and crusted lesions
• Bluetongue: fever, mucosal lesions, swelling of lips and gums, alopecia, diarrhea

CAUSES AND RISK FACTORS
• Dermatitis: in calves, bacteria can be excreted in the dam's milk.
• Fibropapillomas: direct contact with infected animals, virus enters through minor abrasions, use of contaminated instruments.

• Impetigo: bacteria enter through minor abrasions; spread to other animals can easily occur.
• Ringworm: use of contaminated instruments, contaminated environment
• Bluetongue: vector-borne disease transmitted by *Culicoides*

DIAGNOSIS

DIFFERENTIAL DIAGNOSIS
• Dermatitis: culture on swab or skin scraping
• Fibropapillomas: biopsy of a lesion, ELISA, histological examination
• Impetigo: culture of vesicular fluid
• Ringworm: culture of hair from the lesion, scrapings of lesions, skin biopsies
• Bluetongue: serological examination

CBC/BIOCHEMISTRY/URINALYSIS
N/A

OTHER LABORATORY TESTS
N/A

IMAGING
N/A

DIAGNOSTIC PROCEDURES
N/A

TREATMENT
• Dermatitis: if possible, decrease bacteria levels in the immediate environment and add protein supplement for efficient skin repair.
• Fibropapillomas: surgical removal of warts may be indicated in valuable stock.
• Impetigo: daily bath 2x/day with germicidal skin wash
• Ringworm: brush off infective crusts; use topical antifungal and disinfective agents to improve dermatophyte contact.

MEDICATIONS

DRUGS OF CHOICE
• Dermatitis: antihistamines may be useful if there are allergies present or if there is tissue destruction; topical antibiotics or antifungals, autogenous vaccine
• Fibropapillomas: intradermal injected vaccine made from warts from infected animal 1–2 weeks apart; commercial wart vaccines are available.
• Impetigo: erythromycin or dicloxacillin may be helpful; suggest culture and sensitivity to determine effective treatment options

• Ringworm: griseofulvin (7.5 to 60.0 mg/kg orally for 7 or more days) or topical treatment:—2–5% lime sulfur, 1% iodophor, 0.5% sodium hypochlorite, 3% orthocide
• Bluetongue—no treatment
• It is important in choosing treatment options that appropriate drug withdrawal periods be determined and maintained for treated animals.

CONTRAINDICATIONS
Appropriate milk and meat withdrawal times must be followed for all compounds administered to food-producing animals.

FOLLOW-UP
• Local anesthetic ointments to prevent further pruritus may be helpful.
• Use absorptive dressing when large areas are affected.
• Addition of protein to marginal diets may augment skin repair.
• Use sterile or disinfected instruments when working herd or flock.
• Make sure living quarters are clean, disinfected; sunlight is helpful with dermatophytes.

MISCELLANEOUS
N/A

SEE ALSO
Specific dermatologic disease

ABBREVIATIONS
ELISA = enzyme-linked immunosorbent assay

Suggested Reading
Blank, H., Haines, H. 1976, Jul. Viral diseases of the skin, 1975: a 25-year perspective. *J Invest Dermatol*. 67(1): 169–76.
Moriello, K. A., Cooley, J. 2001, Jan 1. Difficult dermatologic diagnosis. Contagious viral pustular dermatitis (orf), goatpox, dermatophilosis, dermatophytosis, bacterial pyoderma, and mange. *J Am Vet Med Assoc*. 218(1): 19–20.
Radostits, O. M., Blood, D. C., Gay, C. C. 1994. *Veterinary medicine*. 8th ed. London: Baillere Tindall.
Rebhun, W. C., Guard, C., Richards, C. M. 1995. *Diseases of dairy cattle*. Baltimore: Williams & Wilkins.

Authors: Carmela Jaravata and Heather Johnson

DERMATOPHILOSIS

 BASICS

DEFINITION
Common pustular/crusting disease of ruminants caused by *Dermatophilus congolensis*

PATHOPHYSIOLOGY
• Caused by aerobic, gram-positive filamentous bacteria *Dermatophilus congolensis*
• Moisture and damage to the skin cause organism to be attracted to stratum corneum where it germinates and bacterial filaments proliferate and invade the epidermis.
• Damage to the skin via shearing, insect bites, or ticks may predispose animal to microtrauma.
• Neutrophilic infiltrate creates serous/crusting exudation resulting in matting of wool or hair.
• Rewetting of the skin results in release of packets of zoospores that escape to the surface of the skin and start the cycle over again of invasion of tissue, exudating, and further matting.
• Incubation can be as short as two weeks.

SYSTEMS AFFECTED
Skin

GENETICS
• Breed variability with respect to susceptibility
• Zebu cattle are considered more resistant than *Bos taurus.*
• West African N'dama, and Muturu breeds are highly resistant.
• Fine wool breeds of sheep are more susceptible.

INCIDENCE/PREVALENCE
• Disease most common in regions with wet weather
• Morbidity can reach 100%.
• Subclinical infections can be present in endemic areas.
• Lambs less than 5 weeks of age are most susceptible.
• Mature animals and males are more commonly affected in Africa.
• Young animals are more commonly infected in South America.

GEOGRAPHIC DISTRIBUTION
• Worldwide distribution
• The disease is of particular importance in Africa, the Americas, the Middle East, and Mediterranean Europe.

SIGNALMENT
• All ruminants are susceptible.
• Can occur in any age, but more often in young animals

SIGNS
• Clinical signs correspond to the predisposing factors: moisture and microtrauma of the skin.
• Hallmark clinical sign is crusting and matting of hair/wool.
• Cattle: paintbrush-like lesions, crusts, or scabs, and/or marked accumulations of "wart-like lesions" on the head, dorsum, upper lateral surface of neck and chest. Lesions are found on legs of cattle that stand in water, mud, or lush pasture; lesions may be localized to udder in dairy cow and to the scrotum in bulls.
• Sheep: early lesions start as serous exudate at base of wool that results in matting of fleece, lumpy masses of wool may result (i.e., "lumpy wool disease"), lameness and proliferative inflammation on feet (strawberry foot rot), crusts in areas where fleece has been shorn, chronic lesions can persist as crusts on face, nose, ears.
• Lambs can rapidly develop generalized infection on back and dorsum, severe serous exudate can make movement difficult; lambs can die from severe secondary bacterial infections or fly-strike.
• Goats: ears first affected with wartlike scabs on inner pinnae; nose, muzzle, feet, scrotum, and tail may be affected; areas most commonly affected are those exposed to trauma.
• Buffaloes and bulls can develop erosive and/or granulomatous lesions on palate, lips, and tongue.
• Subcutaneous and lymph node abscesses can be seen in cattle, sheep, goats.
• "Strawberry foot rot" is an infection of distal extremities in sheep in which large crust formation around carpus, tarsus, and coronary bands is seen. Clinical cases in flocks are most severe in young stock (less than 1 year old). Lesions heal by granulation, which is observed with forced removal of crusts (hence, the strawberry appearance).

CAUSES AND RISK FACTORS
• Most important predisposing factors are chronic wetting (rain, snow) and maceration of the skin and microtrauma to the skin as organism is thought not to be able to invade healthy skin.
• Outbreaks most common after periods of heavy rain and/or high humidity
• Long hair may predispose animals to infection.
• Ectoparasites are important causes of microtrauma.
• Mechanical transmission of the organism can occur via flies and ectoparasites, in animal to animal contact, and during dipping practices.
• Pastures can be contaminated.

• Dried scabs from infected animals are important potential sources of infection for susceptible animals and for reinfection.
• Sheep may carry the infection subclinically and serve as carriers of the disease.
• Infective stage is a motile zoospore that can remain viable in crusts at temperatures of 28 to 31°C for up to 42 months.
• Zoospores in crusts can remain viable when dried and after being heated to temperatures of 100°C.

 DIAGNOSIS

Most commonly diagnosed based upon seasonality, history of chronic wetting, and clinical signs

DIFFERENTIAL DIAGNOSIS
• Dermatophytosis, staphylococcal infections, zinc responsive skin disease, pemphigus foliaceus
• Fleece rot, crusted mange lesions
• Muzzle lesions can resemble *peste des petits ruminants* in sheep or contagious ecthyma in goats.
• Malignant catarrh or mucosal lesions in cattle

CBC/BIOCHEMISTRY/URINALYSIS
N/A

OTHER LABORATORY TESTING
N/A

IMAGING
N/A

DIAGNOSTIC PROCEDURES
• Cutaneous impression smears of underside of moist scabs—Giemsa, Gram stain, or Diff Quik will demonstrate coccoid and branching filamentous organisms (use oil immersion magnification).
• Cytologic examination of the deep layer of the crusts (adjacent to the granulation tissue) reveals coccoid bacteria branching into the formation similar to "railroad tracks."
• Mince preparations of crusts: mince crusts in sterile water on glass microscope slide; allow to dry; stain and examine oil immersion; may be helpful when only older crusts are available.
• Skin biopsy: folliculitis, intraepidermal pustular dermatitis, intracellular edema, surface crusting characterized by alternating layers of ortho and/or parakeratotic hyperkeratosis and neutrophilic exudate; organism seen within keratinous debris.
• Bacterial culture: organism can be grown on blood agar in increased carbon dioxide atmosphere; organism can be grown from crusts or skin biopsy.
• Indirect fluorescent antibody and ELISA tests are available for herd investigations.

PATHOLOGICAL FINDINGS

Skin biopsy: folliculitis, intraepidermal pustular dermatitis, intracellular edema, surface crusting characterized by alternating layers of ortho and/or parakeratotic hyperkeratosis and neutrophilic exudate; organism seen within keratinous debris.

TREATMENT

• Separate clinically affected animals from normal animals.
• Provide shelter from rain.
• Improve nutrition (protein, energy, mineral) and ectoparasite control.
• Remove infected crusts from skin.
• Protect animals from fly-strike.
• Infections often resolve spontaneously over several weeks if affected animals can be kept dry. Remove tufts of crusted hair or clip matted hair to reduce number of organisms present.
• Tick control is very important in preventing the disease.

MEDICATIONS

• Procaine penicillin G (20,000 to 70,000 units/kg body weight) every 12 to 24 hours
• Oxytetracycline 20 mg/kg SQ or IM q 72 hrs
• Copper sulfate (0.2%), zinc sulfate (0.2% to 0.5%), or potassium aluminum sulfate (1%) can be used as topical dips or sprays.

CONTRAINDICATIONS

Appropriate milk and meat withdrawal times must be followed for all compounds administered to food-producing animals.

FOLLOW-UP

• Disease usually self-cures in 2–4 weeks when animals are removed from wet, moist conditions.
• Key preventative measures: provide shelter from excessive moisture and minimize ectoparasite infestations.
• Other preventive measures: isolate infective animals, cull chronically infected animals, and disinfect environments.

MISCELLANEOUS

ASSOCIATED CONDITIONS

• Lameness in sheep
• Mastitis in dairy cows, sheep, and goats

AGE-RELATED FACTORS

Disease more prevalent in young and debilitated animals

ZOONOTIC POTENTIAL

• Possible zoonotic disease, handle infected animals with care.
• Wear gloves when handling infected animals or hair/wool or crusts.
• Dispose of all infected materials (hair, wool, crusts) properly and disinfect all items in contact with affected areas (grooming materials, clippers, etc.).
• Wear gloves and wash hands with disinfectant soaps.

PREGNANCY

N/A

RUMINANT SPECIES AFFECTED

Cattle, sheep, goats, llamas, buffalo, camels

BIOSECURITY

N/A

PRODUCTION MANAGEMENT

• Can cause decreased milk production in dairy cows and goats
• Severe infections may result in decreased fertility.
• Severely infected animals may die from cachexia.
• Can impair heat resistance in camels
• Hides and skin from infected animals are often unsuitable for leather.
• Fleece with scabs is often downgraded.
• May predispose animals to fly-strike

SYNONYMS

Cakey wool
Kirchi (Nigeria)
Lumpy wool
Mycotic dermatitis
Rain scald
Saria (Malawi)
Senkobo skin disease (central Africa)
Strawberry foot rot
Streptothricosis

SEE ALSO

Contagious ecthyma
Crusted mange lesions
Dermatophytosis
Fleece rot
Malignant catarrh
Mucosal disease
Pemphigus foliaceus
Peste des petits ruminants
Staphylococcal infections
Zinc responsive skin disease

ABBREVIATIONS

ELISA = enzyme-linked immunosorbent assay
IM = intramuscular
SQ = subcutaneous

Suggested Reading
Anderson, D. E., Rings, D. M., Pugh, D. G. 2002. Diseases of the integumentary system. In: *Sheep and goat medicine*, ed. D. G. Pugh. Philadelphia: W. B. Saunders.
Dermatophilosis. 1998. *The Merck veterinary manual.*, ed. S. E. Aiello., 8th ed. Philadelphia: National Publishing, Inc.
Lloyd, D. H. 1999. Dermatophilosis. In: *Current veterinary therapy 4, food animal practice*. Philadelphia: W. B. Saunders.
Rebhum, W. C. 1995. Skin diseases. In: *Diseases of dairy cattle*. Baltimore: Williams & Wilkins.
Scott, D. W. 1984. *Bacterial diseases. Large animal dermatology*. Philadelphia: W. B. Saunders.
Smith, M. C., Sherman, D. M. 1994. Skin diseases. In: *Goat medicine*. Philadelphia: Lea & Febiger.

Authors: Karen A. Moriello and Susan Semrad

DERMATOPHYTOSIS

 BASICS

DEFINITION
• Superficial infection of the cornified regions of hair, nails, and stratum corneum.
• The most commonly involved organisms are *Trichophyton* spp. and *Microsporum* spp.

PATHOPHYSIOLOGY
• The naturally infective state is an arthrospore.
• Exposure to infective spores occurs from direct contact with an infected animal and/or exposure to a contaminated environment. Contaminated environments are overlooked sources of exposure.
• Rodents may be reservoirs of infection for *Trichophyton* spp.
• Exposure does not guarantee infection as the organism must evade natural host defenses; infective spores may be brushed off or fall off; organism may trigger inflammation, which will eliminate the infection.
• Moisture and microtrauma to the skin allow for the organism to gain entry and germinate; organism invades actively growing hairs (keratin) making them fragile.
• Incubation takes 1–3 weeks.
• Recovery from infection occurs when the host develops a cell-mediated immune response.
• Animals will generally self cure.
• Duration of immunity is unknown.

SYSTEMS AFFECTED
Skin

GENETICS
No evidence of a genetic predisposition to infection has been shown in large animals, but there is evidence of this in small animals.

INCIDENCE/PREVALENCE
• In the United States, this is not a reportable disease; prevalence is unknown.
• Dermatophytosis is one of the most common infectious/contagious skin diseases of large animals.

GEOGRAPHIC DISTRIBUTION
• Worldwide distribution
• More common in warm subtropical/tropical geographic regions

SIGNALMENT
• Can occur in any age, sex, or breed
• Most common in young, old, or debilitated animals

SIGNS
• Clinical signs are highly variable in presentation and may be affected by palliative treatments administered by the owner.
• Classic lesions include any combination of the following:
  • Variable pruritus: none to severe
  • Variably sized annular rings of hair loss
  • Erythema
  • Scaling, crusting, to mounded thick adherent crusts
• Cattle: lesions are well demarcated, tightly adherent, grayish crusts that may develop into severe areas of alopecia, crusting, exudation, and ulceration. Lesions in calves are most common around the eyes and on the head and neck. In cows and heifers, lesions are most common on the udder. Bulls commonly have lesions on the dewlap and intermaxillary spaces.
• Goats: lesions are common on the face, ears, neck, udder, and limbs. Lesions are circular to diffuse areas of alopecia with scaling, crusting, and erythema.
• Sheep: lesions are most common on face, neck, thorax, and back and appear as circular areas of alopecia and thick, gray crusts.
• Lesions around coronary band may lead to lameness.
• Kerion reactions are inflammatory reactions, particularly to *M. gypseum*, that can look like an abscess.

CAUSES
• *Trichophyton* spp.: *T. verrucosum, T. mentagrophytes, T. equinum*
• *Microsporum* spp.: *M. canis, M. gypseum*

RISK FACTORS
• Age extremes, preexisting illness and debilitation, immunocompromised hosts
• Poor nutrition
• Overcrowding and lack of exposure to sunlight
• Exposure to excessive moisture and warmth leading to maceration and damage of skin.
• Adult animals become infected/reinfected when new animals are introduced to herd.
• Parasitic infestations may predispose animals to infection.

 DIAGNOSIS

DIFFERENTIAL DIAGNOSIS
• Dermatophilosis
• Staphylococcal infection
• Demodicosis
• Zinc responsive skin diseases
• Pemphigus foliaceus

CBC/BIOCHEMISTRY/URINALYSIS
N/A

OTHER LABORATORY TESTS
N/A

IMAGING
N/A

DIAGNOSTIC PROCEDURES
• Wood lamp examination is not useful in large animals as *M. canis* is the only pathogen that regularly fluoresces and this is an uncommon cause of dermatophytosis.
• KOH examination of hair and scale may reveal ectothrix spores. This is not cost effective and many artifacts can occur; invasion of hair shafts is most easily seen with *M. canis*.
• Dermatophyte culture—suspect lesions should be wiped with alcohol and allowed to dry. Remove crusts or pluck infected hairs/scale. Gently embed in fungal culture media. Microscopic examination of fungal culture colony is mandatory.
  • Sab-Duets fungal culture plates are recommended.
  • Easy to inoculate
  • Dual plate has plain Sabouraud's dextrose agar and Dermatophyte Test Medium.
  • Color change (red) on DTM does NOT indicate that there is a pathogen present, only that the rapidly growing colony is suspect.
  • Potential pathogens: pale to cream colonies that develop red color change as they grow; *Microsporum* spp. colonies usually grow within 7 to 10 days but *Trichophyton* spp. may take up to 21 days.
  • Pathogens are never grossly or microscopically pigmented.
  • Use lactophenol cotton blue stain and clear cellophane tape to identify colonies.
• Skin biopsy is the most cost-effective diagnostic tool. Do not scrub or prep the lesion prior to biopsy. Be sure to include the crust.
• In many cases, dermatophytosis, especially in cattle, is diagnosed based upon history and clinical signs; it may not be cost-effective to make a definitive diagnosis in all cases.

PATHOLOGIC FINDINGS
• Folliculitis, furunculosis, hyperkeratosis, intraepidermal pustules, nodular to diffuse pyogranulomatous infiltrates
• Definitive diagnosis requires finding fungal hyphae in nodular reactions, in hair shafts, or in hair follicles. Fungal elements may be seen with H&E stain, but special stains may allow for easier identification.
• Skin biopsy is recommended in any animal in which lesions are atypical and/or where the animal does not respond to appropriate therapy.

DERMATOPHYTOSIS

TREATMENT

• Infected animals should be isolated from other animals.
• Crusts and scales should be removed from lesions and burned.
• Ideally, infected hairs should be clipped from the lesions.
• Nutrition and housing should be improved; allow animals to go outside, decrease crowding.
• Infective spores will contaminate the environment; debris should be removed from the environment and burned.
• Areas that can be scrubbed should be cleaned with soap and water and copiously rinsed. Bleach 1:10 is the most cost-effective disinfectant; enilconazole is an alternative but is expensive and appropriate drug withdrawal periods may not be determined. Consult FARAD.
  • Enilconazole spray (Clinafarm EG)
  • Enilconazole smoke bombs (Clinafarm EG)
  Gross cleaning and disinfection needs to be done repeatedly as infective spores are hard to kill and eradicate.

MEDICATIONS

• Topical treatments are the most cost-effective in large animals.
• First remove crusts and scales, and then wash the animal in an inexpensive shampoo. Towel dry.
• Three weekly topical application of an antifungal solution
• The entire animal must be treated either as vat dip or via a sprayer that thoroughly soaks the hair coat/wool. The solution is not rinsed off. Recommended treatments include
  • Lime sulfur, 8 oz/gal twice weekly
  • Enilconazole 0.2% (Imaverol emulsion) twice weekly (not licensed in United States)
  • Enilconazole (Clinafarm EC in United States ONLY) 55.6 ml/gal twice weekly; off label use
• Ineffective products that should not be used: thiabendazole, betadine, captan, chlorhexidine. Treat infected animals until cured; clinical cure will occur before mycological cure is obtained. Minimum treatment period is 4–6 weeks or 8–12 topical applications.

ALTERNATIVE DRUGS

Systemic Antifungal Drugs
• Efficacy of systemic antifungal drugs is unknown, but based upon what is known, in small animals they are likely to be effective.
• Griseofulvin 50 mg/kg orally once daily until cure
• Itraconazole 5–10 mg/kg orally once daily until cured, or use as pulse therapy (week on-week off)
• Systemic therapy is cost prohibitive in most animals.
• Prior to use of antifungal agents, appropriate withdrawal periods for meat and milk should be determined.

FOLLOW-UP

PREVENTION/AVOIDANCE

Antifungal Vaccines
• Antifungal vaccines are not available in the United States.
• Live antifungal vaccines in eastern Europe and Scandinavia have been shown to decrease clinical symptoms.
• Use of vaccines is controversial and there is no evidence that they are protective against challenge exposure.

POSSIBLE COMPLICATIONS (CONTRAINDICATIONS)
• Lime sulfur will discolor white hair coats.
• Systemic antifungals (especially griseofulvin) are teratogenic and should not be used in pregnant animals.
• Appropriate milk and meat withdrawal times must be followed for all compounds administered to food producing animals.

EXPECTED COURSE AND PROGNOSIS
• All animals need to be treated to prevent reinfection and/or spread of the disease.
• Infected animals will generally self-cure within 70 to 100 days.
• New animals should be isolated before being added to the herd. Prophylactic dipping with lime sulfur may be useful in preventing introduction of organism in "clean" herd.
• Provide good nutrition, good housing, and adequate exposure to dry, well-ventilated housing.

MISCELLANEOUS

ASSOCIATED CONDITIONS
N/A

AGE-RELATED FACTORS
N/A

ZOONOTIC POTENTIAL
This is a zoonotic disease.

RUMINANT SPECIES AFFECTED
Cattle, sheep, goats, llamas

BIOSECURITY
N/A

PRODUCTION MANAGEMENT
• Economic losses due to infection are unknown with respect to meat and milk production.
• Infections will decrease hide value.

SYNONYMS
Ringworm

SEE ALSO
Alopecia
Differential diagnosis of scaling and crusting
FARAD
Pruritus

ABBREVIATIONS
DTM = dermatophyte test medium
FARAD = Food Animal Residue Avoidance Databank
H&E = hematoxylin and eosin stain
KOH = potassium hydroxide

Suggested Reading
Anderson, D. E., Rings, D. M., Pugh, D. G. 2002. Diseases of the integumentary system. In: Sheep and goat medicine, ed. D. G. Pugh. Philadelphia: W. B. Saunders.
Scott, D. W. 1984. Fungal diseases. Large animal dermatology. Philadelphia: W. B. Saunders.
Semrad, S. D., Moriello, K. A. 1999. Dermatophytosis (ringworm). In: Current veterinary therapy 4, food animal practice. Philadelphia: W. B. Saunders.
Smith, M. C., Sherman, D. M. 1994. Skin diseases. In: Goat medicine. Philadelphia: Lea & Febiger.

Authors: Karen A. Moriello and Susan D. Semrad

DIFFERENTIAL DIAGNOSIS OF LUMPS AND SWELLINGS

BASICS

OVERVIEW
• Lumps and swellings are common dermatological problems.
• These lesions can be a cause of great anxiety because they may be due to neoplasia.
• Causes include: infections, trauma, foreign bodies, allergic reactions, parasitic migration, granulomas, and tumors.

SYSTEMS AFFECTED
Production management, skin

GENETICS
N/A

INCIDENCE/PREVALENCE
N/A

GEOGRAPHIC DISTRIBUTION
Worldwide depending on species and environment

SIGNALMENT
Species
All ruminant species

Breed Predilections
N/A

Mean Age and Range
N/A

Predominant Sex
N/A

SIGNS
• Lumps and swellings can be described by any number of the following terms:
  • Papule—small red mass less than 1 cm in diameter
  • Nodule—firm mass up to > 1 cm in diameter caused by infiltration of inflammatory or neoplastic cells
  • Tumor—solid mass of tissue caused by infiltration or expansion of neoplastic cells

• Abscess—firm to fluctuant cavity in the skin filled with exudate
• Hematoma—a blood-filled cavity in the skin, usually caused by trauma
• Seroma—a serum-filled cavity in the skin
• Cyst—epithelial lined cavity in the skin filled with keratin, corneocytes, hair, sebum, or clear fluid
• Urticaria or wheal—well-circumscribed raised area of skin caused by edema in the dermis

DIAGNOSIS

DIFFERENTIAL DIAGNOSIS
Table 1 summarizes the common causes of lumps and swellings by contents.
Table 2 summarizes common causes of infectious, granulomatous, or neoplastic masses.

CBC/BIOCHEMISTRY/URINALYSIS
N/A

OTHER LABORATORY TESTS
N/A

IMAGING
N/A

DIAGNOSTIC PROCEDURES
• Cytology and biopsy are the two most useful diagnostic tests.
• Cytology
  • Fine-needle aspirate of the mass
  • Impression smear of cut surface of a biopsy or from surface of the mass
• Biopsy
  • Excisional diagnostic biopsies should be performed, if possible.
  • Deep-wedge biopsies with scalpel blade should be performed if excisional biopsy cannot be done.
  • Do not use punch biopsy instrument, as this will obtain a superficial sample.

• Blot blood from surface of specimen before placing in 10% neutral buffered formalin.
• Special stains for infectious agents should be requested.
• Culture and sensitivity should be performed if either cytology and/or biopsy samples reveal infectious agent.
  • Wedges of tissue in sterile saline are more useful for culture in the case of firm, hard masses or if a culture swab is negative for growth.
  • Sterile culture swabs can be used to obtain cultures, if pus is present culture.
  • Cultures cannot be performed on formalinized samples.

TREATMENT
• Specific treatment depends upon definitive diagnosis.
• Surgical treatment is the most cost-effective approach to the management of tumors in ruminants.

CONTRAINDICATIONS
• Appropriate milk and meat withdrawal times must be followed for all compounds administered to food-producing animals.
• Steroids should not be used in pregnant animals.

MISCELLANEOUS

ASSOCIATED CONDITIONS
See Tables 1 and 2.

AGE-RELATED FACTORS
N/A

Table 1

Differential Diagnosis of Lumps and Swellings		
Contents of Lump/Swelling	Diagnosis	Comments
Edema	Urticaria/angioedema	Allergic reactions, milk allergy, drug allergy; trypanosomiasis
Serum	Seroma	Common cause, tissue reaction to foreign body
Pus	Infection	Subcutaneous infection with or without draining tracts; see Table 2
Blood	Hematoma, vascular tumor parafilariasis	Trauma most common cause of hematoma; seasonal hemorrhagic nodules
Anuclear proteinaceous debris	Cutaneous cyst	
Fat	Lipoma	
Hyperplastic tissue	Nevus, dermatofibroma, scar tissue	
Inflammatory cells		See Table 2
Neoplastic epithelial, spindle or round cells		See Table 2
Melanocytes	Melanoma	
Demodex mites	Demodicosis	Can occur in any animal, most common in goats

DIFFERENTIAL DIAGNOSIS OF LUMPS AND SWELLINGS

Table 2

| Differential Diagnosis of Lumps and Swellings Containing Pus, Inflammatory Cells, and/or Neoplastic Cells | | | |

PUS

Disease	Common Name	Major Dermatological Sign	Species
Corynebacterium pseudotuberculosis	Caseous lymphadenitis	Abscesses of lymph nodes	Sheep and goats
Clostridial infections	Gas gangrene	Pitting edema with erythema	All ruminants
Fungal kerion	Subcutaneous dermatophyte	Nonhealing wound	All
Trichophyton spp.			
Microsporum spp.			
Mycetoma	"Fungal tumor"	Cold swelling with draining tracts and "tissue grains"	All
			All
Actinomycosis	Lumpy jaw		
Nocardiosis			
Actinobacillosis	"Big head," "wooden tongue"		
Phaeohyphomycosis			
Dermatiaceous fungi		Chronic, subcutaneous painless swelling	All
Abscesses			

INFLAMMATORY CELLS/GRANULOMA

Disease	Common Name	Major Dermatological Sign	Species
Follicular cyst		Single or multiple, firm or hard, containing hair, sebum, cells; frequently rupture	All
Wattle cyst		Round, smooth fluctuant masses, at neck	Goat
Panniculitis	Fat necrosis	Firm to fluctuant mass, may drain yellow-brown fluid	
Eosinophilic granuloma		Hard pruritic mass	Cattle
Theileria parva	East coast fever	Firm, pruritic nodules	Cattle in Africa
Hypoderma	Cattle grub	Firm mass with breathing pore	Cattle

NEOPLASIA

Disease	Common Name	Major Dermatological Sign	Species
Papillomatosis	Warts	Hyperkeratotic proliferative, cauliflower-like lesions	Cattle, sheep, goats
Squamous cell carcinoma		Ulcerative to proliferative masses	Cattle, sheep, goats
Hemagioma		Purple plaques progressing to verrucous masses that bleed	Cattle
Mast cell tumor		Multiple firm to fluctuant masses; in young cattle 6–7 months of age	Cattle
Lymphosarcoma		Multiple lesions, anywhere but especially over trunk, young 1–4 years of age.	Cattle
Melanoma		Single to multiple lesions pigmented	All species

ZOONOTIC POTENTIAL
Several of these diseases are zoonotic. Care must be taken in the collection of laboratory samples and the diagnosis/treatment of affected animals.

PREGNANCY
N/A

RUMINANT SPECIES AFFECTED
All ruminant species are affected.

BIOSECURITY
Several of these diseases are reportable foreign animal diseases.

PRODUCTION MANAGEMENT
N/A

SYNONYMS
N/A

SEE ALSO
Specific disease chapters
Serology
Zoonosis

ABBREVIATIONS
N/A

Suggested Reading
Aiello, S. E., ed. 1998. *The Merck veterinary manual*. 8th ed. Philadelphia: National Publishing, Inc.
Anderson, D. E., Rings, D. M., Pugh, D. G. 2002. Diseases of the integumentary system. In: *Sheep and goat medicine*, ed. D. G. Pugh. Philadelphia: W. B. Saunders.
Hill, P. B. 2002. *Small animal dermatology—a practical guide to diagnosis and management of skin diseases*. Edinburgh: Elsevier Science.
Howard, J. L., Smith, R. A., eds. 1999. *Current veterinary therapy 4, food animal practice*. Philadelphia: W. B. Saunders.
Scott, D. W. 1984. *Large animal dermatology*. Philadelphia: W. B. Saunders.
Smith, M. C., Sherman, D. M. 1994. Skin diseases. In: *Goat medicine*. Philadelphia: Lea & Febiger.

Authors: Karen A. Moriello and Susan D. Semrad

DIFFERENTIAL DIAGNOSIS OF PRURITUS

BASICS

OVERVIEW
- Pruritus is an unpleasant sensation that triggers the host to scratch.
- A specific end organ of itch has not been found.
- The sensation of itch is carried from nerve endings to the spinal cord via the ventrolateral spinothalamic tract via the thalamus to the cortex.
- Pruritus is not a disease, but rather a clinical sign.
- The most common causes of pruritus in ruminants include parasites, infections, and allergies.
- Mediators of pruritus include histamine and proteolytic enzymes (proteases).

SYSTEMS AFFECTED
Skin and adnexa

GENETICS
N/A

INCIDENCE/PREVALENCE
Unknown

GEOGRAPHIC DISTRIBUTION
Worldwide distribution

SIGNALMENT
Species
All ruminant species
Breed Predilections
Varies by specific disease entity
Mean Age and Range
Varies by specific disease entity
Predominant Sex
Varies by specific disease entity

SIGNALMENT
- Highly variable, depending upon the cause
- History is very important. Multiple animals affected suggests infectious or contagious agent. Single animal involved suggests allergy, neoplasia, or other cause.

SIGNS
- Symptoms of pruritus can include any combination of the following:
  - Scratching
  - Biting
  - Rubbing
  - Restlessness
  - Excoriations
  - Hair loss characterized by broken hairs
  - Inflammation of the skin, erythema, scaling, crusting
- Decreased production commonly accompanies pruritic skin diseases.
- Evidence of pruritus can be obtained via the history and physical examination.
- Owners may or may not be aware the animal is pruritic; part of the exam should include visual observation of the animal's behavior for a period of time.

CAUSES AND RISK FACTORS
- The most common causes include ectoparasites, superficial skin infections, and allergies.
- Crowding and poor management will enhance the spread of parasites and contagious skin infections.
- Poor management may also predispose animals to irritant reactions and secondary infections, which are often pruritic.
- Contact allergies from fly sprays, wipes, powders, or shampoos can also cause pruritus.
- Ectoparasites and superficial skin infections usually involve more than one animal.
- Allergic causes do not involve multiple animals.

DIAGNOSIS

DIFFERENTIAL DIAGNOSIS
- See Tables 1, 2, 3, and 4 for differential diagnoses.
- Also see specific chapters for detailed information on clinical signs, diagnosis, and treatment.

CBC/BIOCHEMISTRY/URINALYSIS
N/A

OTHER LABORATORY TESTS
N/A

IMAGING
N/A

DIAGNOSTIC PROCEDURES
- Visual examination with handheld magnifying lens and flashlight aids in locating fleas, ticks, lice, etc.
- Skin scrapings for finding mites
- Superficial fungal cultures for identification of dermatophytosis
- Impression smears of exudate or open wounds may reveal eosinophilia, which suggests allergic or parasitic skin disease.
- Skin biopsy is useful when lesions are abnormal or a cause cannot be identified.
- Response to treatment is a common diagnostic test.

TREATMENT
- Specific treatment for pruritus depends upon the definitive diagnosis.
- Palliative topical treatment for pruritus may include cool water soaks, bathing in a mild cleansing shampoo (i.e., grooming shampoo), and topical oatmeal soaks.
- Topical lime sulfur is antibacterial, antifungal, antiparasitical, and antipruritic.

MEDICATIONS

DRUGS OF CHOICE
- Glucocorticoids block all the pathways that cause itch.
- Systemic glucocorticoids can be used for palliative relief; use short term.
- Palliative systemic treatment is best done with glucocorticoids (i.e., prednisone 0.5 mg/kg PO q 24 hrs).
- Glucocorticoid-containing topical ointments are practical for focal application but not if the pruritus is widespread.
- Antihistamines are of limited use as a sole agent for relief of pruritus.

CONTRAINDICATIONS
- Appropriate milk and meat withdrawal times must be followed for all compounds administered to food-producing animals.
- Steroids should not be used in pregnant animals.

MISCELLANEOUS

ASSOCIATED CONDITIONS
N/A

AGE-RELATED FACTORS
N/A

ZOONOTIC POTENTIAL
Several of these diseases are zoonotic. Care must be taken in the collection of laboratory samples and the diagnosis/treatment of affected animals.

PREGNANCY
N/A

RUMINANT SPECIES AFFECTED
Potentially, all ruminant species

BIOSECURITY
- Isolation and quarantine of new stock entering the herd/flock
- Treat and/or cull new animals for disease conditions prior to herd introduction.

PRODUCTION MANAGEMENT
N/A

SYNONYMS
N/A

SEE ALSO
Species-specific dermatologic disease, differential diagnosis by condition

ABBREVIATIONS
PO = per os, by mouth

Suggested Reading
Aiello, S. E., ed. 1998. *The Merck veterinary manual*. 8th ed. Philadelphia: National Publishing, Inc.
Anderson, D. E., Rings, D. M., Pugh, D. G. 2002. Diseases of the integumentary system. In: *Sheep and goat medicine*, ed. D. G. Pugh. Philadelphia: W. B. Saunders.
Howard, J. L., Smith, R. A., eds. 1999. *Current veterinary therapy 4, food animal practice*. Philadelphia: W. B. Saunders.
Scott, D. W. 1984. *Large animal dermatology*. Philadelphia: W. B. Saunders.
Smith, M. C., Sherman, D. M. 1994. Skin diseases. In: *Goat medicine*. Philadelphia: Lea & Febiger.

Authors: Karen A. Moriello and Susan D. Semrad

DIFFERENTIAL DIAGNOSIS OF PRURITUS

Table 1

Differential Diagnosis of Common Causes of Pruritus in Ruminants: Parasites			
Disease	Etiology	Clinical Signs	Diagnosis
Lice*	Hamatopinus (sucking) Linognathus (sucking) Solenopotes (sucking) Damilina (biting)	Location of lice depends upon species, sucking lice produce anemia; irritability, poor hair coat, selftrauma	Visual identification, response to treatment
Mange mites*	Sarcoptes scabiei (all) Psoroptes (C, S, G) Chorioptes (all) Psorobia ovis (S, C) Demodex (all) Trombiculiasis (all)	All mange mites cause moderate to severe pruritus, scaling, papular eruptions. Chorioptes starts on legs and becomes generalized.	History and clinical signs, skin scrapings, and/or response to treatment
Fleas	Many species, not host specific, can affect all ruminants	Varying pruritus, rubbing, chewing, scratching, self-trauma, broken wool, crusts, anemia in heavy infestations	Visual exam
Rhabditic dermatitis	Pelodera strongyloides (all)	Papular, pustular, ulcerative, alopecic pruritic lesions on skin in contact with moist, filthy environment, most common in fall and winter	History, clinical signs, skin scrapings, and skin biopsy
Migrating helminths	Metastronglus and Parelaphostrongylus tenuis	Focal linear, vertically oriented lesions, unilateral, pruritic, neurological symptoms common	History, clinical signs, skin biopsy, CFS analysis
Ticks	Otobius Dermatocentor Amblyomma Boophilus Ixodes	Most commonly problem in spring, extent of discomfort related to species and severity of infestation: crusts, erosions, alopecia, nodule formation.	Visual identification
Stephanofilariasis	Stephanofilaria (C, G)	Nonseasonal dermatitis, papules, crusts, ulcers, alopecia, variable pruritus on distribution of clinical signs depends upon geographic region	History, clinical signs, skin scrapings, and skin biopsy
Elaeophoriasis	Elaeophora schneideri (S)	Usually first noticed in winter, unilateral lesions on poll, forehead, face most commonly, hair loss, ulceration, crusting, and intense pruritus	History, clinical signs, and biopsy
Keds	Melophagus ovinus (S)	Severe pruritus, broken wool, excrement-stained wool, alopecia, excoriations	Visual examination
Flies*	Mosquitoes, Culicoides, Simulans, Tabanus, Chrysops, Stomoxys, Hematobia, Musca, Hydrotaea	Small biting insects cause pruritus and papular eruption; large biting flies cause painful pruritic nodules.	Clinical history and physical examination findings

Note: C-cattle, S-sheep, G-goats, L-llama.
* Most common.

Table 2

Differential Diagnosis of Common Causes of Pruritus in Ruminants: Infectious Diseases			
Disease	Etiology	Clinical Signs	Diagnosis
Dermatophytosis	Trichophyton spp. Microsporum spp.	Variable pruritus, focal to multifocal to severe alopecia and crusting	History, clinical signs, fungal culture, possibly skin biopsy
Dermatophilosis	Dermatophilosis congolensis	Paintbrushlike matting of hair coat in areas of chronic wetting; lesions most common on dorsum but may be found on any area where there is chronic moisture and maceration of tissue	History, clinical signs, cytological demonstration of organisms, skin biopsy
Staphylococcal infections	Staphylococcus spp.	Variable pruritus, intact pustules, papules, epidermal collarettes, scaling	History, clinical signs, cytological demonstration of cocci, culture and sensitivity
Pseudorabies	Herpesvirus	Intense, localized, unilateral pruritus, violent licking, biting, and chewing, severe excoriations	History, clinical signs, exposure to infected pigs, necropsy
Scrapie	Slow virus (S)	Most common in 2–5-year-old sheep, intermittent, bilaterally symmetrical severe pruritus that often begins on tail head and progresses cranially; chronic rubbing and biting lead to severe hair loss and excoriations, serpentine tongue movements.	History, clinical signs, necropsy

Note: Diseases can occur in all ruminants unless otherwise indicated.

DIFFERENTIAL DIAGNOSIS OF PRURITUS

Table 3

Differential Diagnosis of Common Causes of Pruritus in Ruminants: Allergic Diseases and Miscellaneous Causes			
Disease	Etiology	Clinical Signs	Diagnosis
Urticaria and angioedema	Immune-mediated reaction, type 1	Acute or chronic, localized or generalized wheals and bumps that "pit" with dermal pressure, may ooze serum; Jerseys and Guernseys can become sensitized to their own casein (milk allergy).	History and clinical signs, biopsy usually not necessary
Allergic contact dermatitis	Immune-mediated type 4 reaction	Pruritic lesions in area where offending allergen contacts skin, disease of individual animals; moisture is a predisposing factor as it allows allergens to penetrate skin.	History, clinical signs, skin biopsy, provocative challenge with suspect compound
Atopic dermatitis	Immune-mediated type 1 and type 4 reactions to environmental allergens (rare in ruminants)	Recurrent, seasonal or nonseasonal pruritus on face, ears, ventrum, and legs	History, clinical signs, biopsy, and intradermal skin test
Erythema multiforme	Immune-mediated disease (C)	Maculopapular eruptions, urticarial plaques with central depression; annular to polycyclic shapes, unlike urticaria lesions, persist for days to weeks; scaling and crusting may occur.	History, clinical signs, and skin biopsy that shows hydropic interface degeneration

Table 4

Differential Diagnosis Based Upon Predominant Clinical Signs

SEVERE PRURITUS
   Mange mites
   Pseudorabies
   Scrapie
   Keds
   Elaeophoriasis

PRURITUS WITH SCALING/CRUSTING
   Dermatophytosis
   Dermatophilosis
   Staphylococcal infections
   Urticaria/angioedema (individual animal)
   Erythema multiforme (individual animal)
   Atopy, contact allergy (individual animal)

**VARIABLE PRURITUS WITH PAPULES OR
   NODULES**
   Fly-strike
   Stephanofilariasis
   Ticks
   Rhabditic dermatitis
   Fleas
   Ticks
   Lice

**VARIABLE PRURITUS WITH ANEMIA,
   HAIRLOSS**
   Fleas
   Ticks
   Lice

DIFFERENTIAL DIAGNOSIS OF SCALING AND CRUSTING

BASICS

OVERVIEW
• Scaling and crusting are common presenting dermatological problems.
• There are two major types of scaling and crusting diseases: primary and secondary.
• "Primary" diseases are caused by a genetic or heritable defect in the production of the stratum corneum and/or skin lipids. This is commonly referred to as "primary seborrhea."
• Primary seborrhea (primary disorder of keratinization) is rare in ruminants.
• "Secondary" diseases are caused by any skin or metabolic disease and are more common in ruminants. Ectoparasites, infections, allergies, neoplasia, nutritional diseases, immune-mediated disorders, metabolic disorders, and other environmental factors may cause secondary skin disease.
• Secondary seborrhea is common.

SYSTEMS AFFECTED
Skin and adnexa

GENETICS
N/A

INCIDENCE/PREVALENCE
Unknown

GEOGRAPHIC DISTRIBUTION
Worldwide distribution

SIGNALMENT
Species
All ruminant species

Breed Predilections
Varies by specific disease entity

Mean Age and Range
Varies by specific disease entity

Predominant Sex
Varies by specific disease entity

SIGNS
Scaling and crusting diseases may present with any combination of the following signs:
• Scale—gross visible accumulation of corneocytes (dandruff)
• Oily seborrhea—excessively greasy skin
• Epidermal collarette—circular ring of scale with central area of alopecia and/or hyperpigmentation; erythema may be present.
• Exfoliation—shedding of large amounts of scale over the body
• Matting/exudate—pustular diseases can cause exudate that results in matting of the hair coat.
• Hyperkeratosis—thick, adherent keratin
• Comedome—accumulation in hair follicle; "blackhead"
• Follicular adherent sheath of scales surrounding a hair shaft just above the hair follicle opening
• Lichenification—marked thickening of the skin over large areas with exaggerated skin ridges "elephantlike skin"
• Plaque—localized patch of thickened skin that is raised with a flat surface
• Callus—focal, alopecic, lichenifed plaque over pressure point

DIAGNOSIS

DIFFERENTIAL DIAGNOSIS
• See Table 1.
• The most common dermatological problem of ruminants is pruritus; pursue pruritic causes of skin disease first.

CBC/CHEMISTRY/URINALYSIS
Laboratory tests are rarely helpful in identifying underlying cause except in cases where the cause is suspected to be metabolic (e.g., malnutrition, toxicity, etc.).

OTHER LABORATORY TESTS
N/A

IMAGING
N/A

DIAGNOSTIC PROCEDURES
• Skin scrapings to look for mites, lice, and other ectoparasites
• Dermatophyte culture to rule in or out superficial fungal disease
• Bacterial culture and sensitivity in patients with primarily pustular diseases
• Skin biopsy—most useful diagnostic test; do not prep or scrub skin. Submit full thickness biopsy with crust adhered to surface. Submit multiple biopsy specimens.

PATHOLOGIC FINDINGS
Skin biopsy findings depend upon the underlying causes.

DIFFERENTIAL DIAGNOSIS OF SCALING AND CRUSTING

Table 1

Differential Diagnosis of the More Common Causes of Crusting and Scaling in Ruminants					
Disease	Etiology	Signs	Diagnostic Tests	Treatment	Miscellaneous
Dermatophytosis	Superficial fungal infection caused by *Trichophyton* spp. and *Microsporum*.	Any combination of hair loss, crusting, scaling, with or without pruritus	Fungal culture Skin biopsy	Isolate infected animals Remove crusts Twice weekly topical sponge-or dips to entire body with lime sulfur or enilconazole See chapter "Dermatophytosis"	All species Zoonotic Highly contagious
Dermatophilosis	Bacterial infection of skin caused by *Dermatophilosis congolensis*	Paintbrushlike matting of hair coat with moist erythematous skin beneath avulsed crust	Impression smear Mince prep of crust Skin biopsy	Isolate infected animals Move to dry area Gently remove crusts and scales via warm water soaks. Bathe in antibacterial shampoo (benzoyl peroxide, chlorhexidine) Systemic antibiotics for 3–10 days See chapter "Dermatophilosis"	All species
Staphylococcal infections	*S. aureus* is primary pathogen, others possible.	Impetigo (pustules) and/or epidermal collarettes	Cytology Culture and sensitivity Biopsy	Topical antibacterial therapy with benzoyl peroxide or chlorhexidine shampoo, iodine shampoos least effective	All species
Malassezia dermatitis	Superficial yeast infection caused by overgrowth of Malassezia	Oily seborrhea and/or dry seborrhea, pruritus common	Impression smear Biopsy	Topical therapy twice weekly with lime sulfur, chlorhexidine/ketoconazole shampoo, miconazole shampoo, selenium disulfide shampoo	Goats and cows
Malnutrition/ malabsorption	Any disease that causes loss of protein or body condition	Signs of systemic debilitation, scaling, poor hair coat	Rule out other causes Clinical signs Evidence of underlying metabolic disease	Identify underlying disease and treat Wash hair coat to remove excessive scales and crusts	All species
Irritant reactions	Most common feces, urine, wound secretions, caustic agents, inappropriately applied insecticides	Crusting and scaling are late findings, early findings include erythema, pain, vesicles.	History, clinical signs, biopsy sometimes helpful	Identification and removal of the offending agent is key. Residual material is removed via copious amounts of water and mild cleansing soap. Topical antibiotic creams/ointments may be helpful.	All species, true irritants cause reactions in all in-contact animals
Mite infestations	Sarcoptes, Chorioptes, Psoroptes,	Pruritus and scaling	Skin scrapings, response to treatment	Ivermectin, doramectin, amitraz See chapter mite infestation	All species
Zinc responsive skin disease	Primary deficiency or related to poor nutrition	Mild to marked scaling that can be localized to face and pressure points or generalized	Skin biopsy AND response to treatment	Oral zinc supplementation See chapters on nutritional supplementation.	All species, but especially goats, sheep, llamas
Bovine exfoliative erythroderma	Suspect immune-mediated etiology	Early lesions start as erythema and vesicles on muzzle and progress to generalized erythema and crusting, easily epilated hair.	Biopsy	Affected animals recover without treatment	Rare disease in cattle Reported in cattle
Epitheliotropic lymphoma	Cutaneous lymphoma	Erythema, scaling, pruritus, nodules in late stages	Skin biopsy	Cull animal, no successful treatment	
Pemphigus foliaceus	Immune-mediated disease	Primary lesion is pustule; pustules coalesce to thick adherent scaling and crusting on head, neck, face, ears, and eventually whole body.	Skin biopsy	Treatment practical only in single animals or pet goats Systemic glucocorticoids or gold salts Lifelong therapy required; quality of life can be good. Treatment is expensive.	Goats
Chemical toxins	Arsenic Chlorinated naphthalene Polybrominated and polychlorinated biphenyl Iodism	Varying degrees of scaling and crusting	Identification can be difficult and may require multiple samplings of serum, hair, skin biopsy, feed samples, etc.	Treatment depends upon individual agent. See chapters on specific toxicities.	
Photosensitization	UV light induced inflammation of the skin Exposure may be primary or secondary.	Symptoms occur in light skin areas; scaling and crusting are late-stage findings after initial erythema and inflammation.	History, clinical signs	Remove animal from sunlight. Supportive care for lesions to prevent infection; treatment may include glucocorticoids. See chapter "Photosensitization."	

DIFFERENTIAL DIAGNOSIS OF SCALING AND CRUSTING

TREATMENT

• Treatment depends upon identification of the underlying cause.
• Removal of crusting and scaling may be necessary for recovery of animal.
  • Collect all diagnostic specimens before initiating topical therapy.
  • Topical hydrotherapy with warm water and a mild antimicrobial shampoo is recommended.
  • Shampoos containing tar should be limited to cases where the scaling and crusting are primarily greasy.
  • Sulfur- and salicylic-acid-containing shampoos will remove crusts and scales but require 10–15 minutes of contact time.
  • Topical antibiotic ointment (e.g., triple antibiotic, Nolvasan cream/ointment) should be applied to areas where the removal of crusts results in denuded, eroded, or ulcerative skin.

CONTRAINDICATIONS

• Appropriate milk and meat withdrawal times must be followed for all compounds administered to food-producing animals.
• Steroids should not be used in pregnant animals.

FOLLOW-UP

Appropriate follow-up depends upon underlying skin disease.

MISCELLANEOUS

ASSOCIATED CONDITIONS
N/A

AGE-RELATED FACTORS
Species-specific dermatologic disease

ZOONOTIC POTENTIAL
Several of these diseases are zoonotic. Care must be taken in the collection of laboratory samples and the diagnosis/treatment of affected animals.

PREGNANCY
N/A

RUMINANT SPECIES AFFECTED
Potentially, all ruminant species can be affected

BIOSECURITY
• Isolation and quarantine of new stock entering the herd/flock
• Treat and/or cull new animals for disease conditions prior to herd introduction.

PRODUCTION MANAGEMENT
N/A

SYNONYMS
Species-specific dermatologic disease

SEE ALSO
Differential diagnosis by symptom
Species-specific dermatologic disease

ABBREVIATIONS
N/A

Suggested Reading

Aiello, S. E., ed. 1998. *The Merck veterinary manual*. 8th ed. Philadelphia: National Publishing, Inc.
Anderson, D. E., Rings, D. M., Pugh, D. G. 2002. Diseases of the integumentary system. In: *Sheep and goat medicine*, ed. D. G. Pugh. Philadelphia: W. B. Saunders.
Howard, J. L., Smith, R. A., eds. 1999. *Current veterinary therapy 4, food animal practice*. Philadelphia: W. B. Saunders.
Scott, D. W. 1984. *Large animal dermatology*. Philadelphia: W. B. Saunders.
Smith, M. C., Sherman, D. M. 1994. Skin diseases. In: *Goat medicine*. Philadelphia: Lea & Febiger.

Authors: Karen A. Moriello and Susan D. Semrad

DIFFERENTIAL DIAGNOSIS OF SKIN DISEASES OF THE UDDER

BASICS

OVERVIEW
• Skin diseases of the udder are common and causes include parasitic, infectious, and/or opportunistic agents; poor management and milking practices; milking machines; exposure to environmental factors; and trauma.
• Skin diseases can occur in any species, but are most common in lactating animals.
• Skin diseases of the udder can predispose animals to mastitis and result in decreased milk production.

SYSTEMS AFFECTED
Skin and adnexa

GENETICS
N/A

INCIDENCE/PREVALENCE
Unknown

GEOGRAPHIC DISTRIBUTION
Worldwide distribution in ruminants

SIGNALMENT
Species
Potentially, all ruminant species are affected.

Breed Predilections
Varies by disease

Mean Age and Range
Varies by disease

Predominant Sex
Varies by disease

DIAGNOSIS

DIFFERENTIAL DIAGNOSIS
The differential diagnoses of skin diseases that affect the udder are summarized in Table 1.

CBC/BIOCHEMISTRY/URINALYSIS
N/A

OTHER LABORATORY TESTS
N/A

IMAGING
N/A

DIAGNOSTIC PROCEDURES

TREATMENT
• Treatment depends upon the underlying cause.
• See specific chapters on the various diseases listed in Table 1.

CONTRAINDICATIONS
• Appropriate milk and meat withdrawal times must be followed for all compounds administered to food producing animals.
• Steroids should not be used in pregnant animals.

FOLLOW-UP
N/A

MISCELLANEOUS

ASSOCIATED CONDITIONS
N/A

AGE-RELATED FACTORS
N/A

ZOONOTIC POTENTIAL
Several of these diseases are zoonotic. Care must be taken in the collection of laboratory samples and the diagnosis/treatment of affected animals.

PREGNANCY
N/A

RUMINANT SPECIES AFFECTED
Potentially all ruminant species can be affected

BIOSECURITY
• Isolation and quarantine of new stock entering the herd/flock
• Treat and or cull new animals for disease conditions prior to herd introduction.

PRODUCTION MANAGEMENT
N/A

SYNONYMS
N/A

SEE ALSO
Specific dermatologic disease, differential diagnosis by symptom

ABBREVIATIONS
N/A

Suggested Reading
Aiello, S. E., ed. 1998. *The Merck veterinary manual*. 8th ed. Philadelphia: National Publishing, Inc.
Anderson, D. E., Rings, D. M., Pugh, D. G. 2002. Diseases of the integumentary system. In: *Sheep and goat medicine*, ed. D. G. Pugh. Philadelphia: W. B. Saunders.
Howard, J. L., Smith, R. A., eds. 1999. *Current veterinary therapy 4, food animal practice*. Philadelphia: W. B. Saunders.
Scott, D. W. 1984. *Large animal dermatology*. Philadelphia: W. B. Saunders.
Smith, M. C., Sherman, D. M. 1994. Skin diseases. In: *Goat medicine*. Philadelphia: Lea & Febiger.
Warnick, L. D., Nydam, D., Maciel, A., Guard, C. L., Wade, S. 2002. Udder cleft dermatitis and sarcoptic mange in a dairy herd. *JAVMA* 221:273–76.

Authors: Karen A. Moriello and Susan D. Semrad

DIFFERENTIAL DIAGNOSIS OF SKIN DISEASES OF THE UDDER

Table 1

Skin Diseases That Affect the Udder				
Disease	Etiology/Predisposing Factors	Lesions	Diagnosis	Treatment/Miscellaneous
Impetigo	Staphylococcal infection (*S. areus*) Predisposing factors include stress, poor housing, wet environment, trauma.	Pustules, circular brown-crusted lesions, may become ulcerative.	Culture Cytology	Topical washes with chlorhexidine or betadine; systemic therapy not usually needed. Milk affected animals last. Mechanical transmission via milkers is common.
Conditions Associated with Swelling of Udder				
Udder edema	High milk production, low blood protein at calving, related to feed intake	Diffuse swelling of udder	Clinical signs	Frequent milkings, massage, diuretics, anti-inflammatory drugs
Necrotic dermatitis	Udder edema causes ischemia and necrosis of opposing skin sites.	Pain, fold pyoderma necrosis located between wall of udder and medial thigh	Occurs several weeks postcalving and udder edema episode, first-calf heifers most commonly affected	Reduce edema with diuretics, topical antibiotics, pain medications, and glucocorticoids.
Udder intertrigo	Fold pyoderma caused by moisture and chronic maceration of udder wall against another skin surface	Moist exudative, painful dermatitis	Clinical signs; cytological exam of exudate will help determine if bacteria and/or yeast are present. Impression smears	Treat topically using antibacterial/antifungal shampoo.
Udder cleft dermatitis	Most common in older cows; sarcoptic mites believed to be part of the etiology	Lesions most common on cranial edge of cleft between two cranial quarters; moist exudative; malodorous dermatitis	Clinical signs Skin scrapings	Topical antibiotics; improve milking procedures; hydrotherapy to remove exudate; treat herd for mites to minimize outbreaks.
Nodular Lesions				
Contusion or hematoma	Trauma: milking machines and/or poor milking practices	Painful swelling	Clinical signs Needle aspirate Biopsy	Cold compresses for acute lesions, followed by warm compresses and massage. Gentle milking. **Do not incise hematoma unless infected**
Disease	Etiology/Predisposing Factors	Lesions	Diagnosis	Treatment/Miscellaneous
Abscesses	Secondary to trauma, wounds, mastitis, infected hematoma, contusion	Painful mass with or without exudate	Clinical signs Needle aspirate	Incise and drain lesions, flush with antiseptic solution (e.g., dilute betadine or chlorhexidine)
Teat spiders	Occurs during dry period caused by accumulations of butterfat, minerals, and/or tissue	Small masses in skin of teat	Clinical signs	Forced manual expression via teat canal or removal by forceps of mass through teat canal
Demodex mites	*Demodex* mites	Small haired sub cutaneous nodular lesions in skin	Examine exudate; all ruminants, especially goats	Lance nodule
Urticaria	Immunologic or allergic trigger	Multifocal soft swelling, "hives"	Clinical signs	Identify underlying trigger, antihistamines corticosteroids
Scar tissue	Common posttrauma	Hard irregular swellings	Biopsy	None needed unless scar tissue interferes with milkings
Macular, Vesicular/Bullous, and or Ulcerative Lesions				
Poxvirus	*Orthopoxvirus* cowpox, vaccine *Capripoxvirus* sheep pox, goat pox *Parapoxvirus* pseudocowpox, orf	Macular-papular-vesicular lesions that crust and leave a raised "pock" lesion	Clinical signs and biopsy Virus isolation	Supportive care to prevent secondary infections
Bovine herpesvirus	Herpesvirus 2	Usually on teats; vesicular to ulcerated lesions on teats; linear to ulcerative plaques, sloughing of skin	Clinical signs Biopsy Virus isolation Paired viral titers	Worldwide distributions. Predisposes animal to mastitis, causes marked production drop. Mammillitis. Isolate infected cows, supportive care to prevent secondary infections and mastitis
Bovine herpesvirus	Herpesvirus 4	1–10-mm vesicles and pustules on lateral and ventral udder	See above	See above
Bovine malignant catarrhal fever	Herpesvirus	Scaling crusting of udder; ulcerative lesions on coronary band, may have udder lesions	See above	No treatment; disease highly contagious; disease is usually fatal.
Foot-and-mouth disease	Picorna virus	Vesicles and bulla, lesions may occur on udder.	See above	No treatment; disease highly contagious; disease is usually fatal.
Vesicular exanthema	Picorna virus	Vesicles and bulla, lesions on udder may be seen.	See above	

DIGITAL (PAPILLOMATOUS) DERMATITIS

BASICS

OVERVIEW
- Digital (papillomatous) dermatitis [(P)DD, footwarts] is a relatively recently described condition seen almost exclusively in dairy cattle. It is an extremely painful condition resulting in severe lameness and reduced milk production.
- It is highly contagious and can rapidly spread through a dairy herd. Fortunately, the disease can be easily treated.
- Discussion of the condition is hampered by the great variety of names that are used to describe the condition including:
  - Hairy heel wart
  - Mortellaro's disease
  - Spirochetal dermatitis
  - Strawberry foot rot
- Affected cattle will often have lameness and will tend to walk on the toes of the feet with lesions. Lesions occur most commonly on the palmar surface of the rear feet near the interdigital ridge.
- Most commonly found in confined dairy cattle, although it has been reported in grazing dairy cattle and beef cattle.
- It is an animal welfare concern.

PATHOPHYSIOLOGY
- Transmission of (P)DD requires constant moisture (hydropic maceration) and low oxygen tension.
- Early lesions are erosive and clearly circumscribed. More chronic lesions can be proliferative and papillomatous.
- Most commonly, lesions are 2–6 cm in diameter, are circular to oval, and have clearly demarcated, raised borders.
- Lesion borders are often surrounded by true hairs that are 2–3 times the length of normal hairs.
- Lesion surfaces may have filiform papillae varying in length from 1 mm to longer than 2 cm (hence, the name "hairy footwarts"). Lesions without the filiform papillae can have a granular appearance.
- Washed lesions are varied in color from bright red to gray or brown and are generally very painful to the touch or spray from a water jet.
- Histopathologically, lesions are characterized by ulcerative and proliferative changes consisting of ulceration of the tips of dermal papillae, epidermal hyperplasia with parakeratosis and hyperkeratosis, colonization by profuse numbers of spirochetes (*Treponema* spp.), and inflammation.

SYSTEMS AFFECTED
Skin, production management and musculoskeletal

GENETICS
N/A

INCIDENCE/PREVALENCE
- Infection spreads rapidly in susceptible cows, once introduced into a naïve herd.
- (P)DD will often affect the majority of cows within the first year of infection. When established in a herd, lesions and lameness are more common in lactation 1 and 2 cows. Prevalence in endemic herds can vary from low (< 5%) to very high (>70%) depending on conditions and control programs on the dairy.

GEOGRAPHIC DISTRIBUTION
Worldwide distribution; mostly found in cows on confinement dairies but has been reported on pasture-based dairies and in beef cattle.

SIGNALMENT
- Although digital dermatitis is a disease that is predominately seen in dairy cattle, it has also been described in beef cattle and sheep.
- The disease commonly occurs in herd outbreaks.

Species
Dairy cattle, occasionally beef cattle, and rarely sheep

Breed Predilections
Most often reported in Holstein dairy cattle, less often in Jersey cattle, other dairy, and beef breeds

Mean Age and Range
- Anecdotal evidence suggests that older animals may develop immunity to the condition, consequently in herds, which are endemically affected with digital dermatitis the disease is most commonly seen in heifers when they are introduced to the milking group.
- Younger cows, lactation 1 and 2, are seen with lesions more often than older cows.

Predominant Sex
Cows are seen most often; bulls are susceptible but not seen as often, possibly due to their low numbers on most dairies.

SIGNS

HISTORICAL FINDINGS
- Lameness is a common herd sign with cows walking on their toes. Affected cows may have "club feet" (i.e., heels will grow longer than nonlame cows since cows are reticent to put weight on their heels).
- The main sign of digital dermatitis is extremely severe lameness in one or more limbs; affected animals are extremely reluctant to bear weight on an affected limb. Such animals are prone to recumbency and often also show a precipitous drop in milk production. The disease is highly contagious and outbreaks are common.

- Lesions have a characteristic "sour" smell and many producers with experience of the disease may detect the disease in the early stages by identifying the smell while milking the herd.
- Diagnosis of digital dermatitis should always be made on close examination of the foot.
- The classical lesion is found on the caudal aspect of the skin above the heel.
- Lesions are typically on the midline between the heel bulbs and below the accessory digits (dew claws) and are covered in a friable layer of grey fibrinlike material.
- The area should be carefully cleaned to remove any debris so that the lesion can be clearly seen.
- Cleaning should be attempted with great care, as the lesion is extremely painful. In some cases an intravenous and/or regional anesthetic may be necessary.
- Two distinct forms of the disease have been described:
  - Erosive form: a reddened raw area of granulation tissue with a "strawberry" appearance
  - Proliferative form: in some chronic cases there may be proliferation of the epithelial tissue to form hairy, frondlike projections.
- Although the majority of cases is seen affecting the heels, lesions may on occasion be found on the skin in the interdigital cleft and on the coronary band on the abaxial aspect of the foot.
- Regardless of the position of the lesion, the severe pain associated with what appears to be a mild lesion is almost diagnostic for digital dermatitis.

CAUSES AND RISK FACTORS
- The causative agent for digital dermatitis has been recently identified as the spirochete bacteria *Treponema brennaborense* sp. *nov.*
- The disease is highly contagious between housed dairy cattle. It is typically brought into a herd through the purchase of an affected animal. However, the veterinarian or lay foot trimmers may also transmit it through contaminated hoof trimming equipment.
- Once the disease is in the herd it is thought to spread through unsanitary conditions in the barn.
- The disease is less common in cattle housed in stanchion barns as the animals do not move around and the disease cannot spread.
- The disease is most common in free stall barns particularly when there is freestanding water and fecal material in the passageways.
- On occasion, digital dermatitis may be diagnosed in beef cattle. This is a rare occurrence and is only seen when animals are kept in wet conditions.
- Muddy or wet conditions and purchasing animals from off premises are the two most common risk factors.

• Poor freestall and bedding management will exacerbate the problems since cows will spend more time standing in the manure slurry for longer periods of time, not allowing the feet to dry out periodically.

DIAGNOSIS

DIFFERENTIAL DIAGNOSIS
• There are few conditions that can be confused with digital dermatitis, as there is really nothing else that is as contagious or as painful.
• Laminitis, foot rot, interdigital dermatitis and heel horn erosion, interdigital fibroma, traumatic injury, and thin soles from excessive wear or improper hoof trimming
• The following may be confused with the condition:
  • Slurry heel
  • Interdigital fibroma
  • Traumatic injury to the distal limb
  • Foot rot—interdigital necrobacillosis

CBC/BIOCHEMISTRY/URINALYSIS
N/A

OTHER LABORATORY TESTS
• Serology may be helpful but not necessary and is not readily available.
• Culture and sensitivity may be indicated if the lesions appear to be infectious.

IMAGING
N/A

DIAGNOSTIC PROCEDURES
• In most cases, the clinical signs of digital dermatitis are all that is required to make a diagnosis.
• If a definitive diagnosis is required, this is best achieved by taking a skin biopsy using a biopsy punch.
• Histopathology using an appropriate stain can demonstrate the presence of spirochete bacteria within the tissue.
• Culture of the proposed etiological agent *Treponema brennaborense* sp. *nov* is extremely difficult and not recommended.

PATHOLOGIC FINDINGS
Histopathology is helpful but not necessary for diagnosis. Histopathological findings include a combination of ulcerative and proliferative changes consisting of ulceration of tips of dermal papillae, epidermal hyperplasia with parakeratosis and hyperkeratosis, colonization and invasion by profuse numbers of spirochetes, and inflammation.

TREATMENT
One should approach the treatment of digital dermatitis from two different standpoints: (1) treatment of the individual animals that are clinically affected and showing signs of severe discomfort, and (2) treatment of the entire herd, which is probably subclinically affected.

Individual Animal Treatment
• The affected area should be thoroughly cleaned with a suitable disinfectant scrub solution and any underrun heel horn should be removed.
• The area should then be treated with topical oxytetracycline (either 3cc injectable oxytetracycline or a small volume of oxytetracycline water additive powder) and a light dressing applied to keep the antibiotic in contact with the lesion.

Herd Treatment.
There are essentially two ways to mass treat a group of animals with digital dermatitis:
• A solution of either 5 g/L oxytetracycline (made using water additive powder) or 1.5 g/L lincomycin/spectinomycin (Linco-spectin water additive powder) may be prepared and applied to the heel of all cattle using a "garden sprayer." To be effective, the feet should first be cleaned using a high-pressure hose. Many producers like to treat the feet in conjunction with milking.
• A footbath may be prepared using either 4–6 g/L oxytetracycline or 0.75–1g/L Linco-spectin and cattle forced to walk through the solution. In order to be effective, it is preferable that cattle have their feet cleaned with either a hose or a primary foot bath containing free-flowing water prior to the medicated footbath. Costs may be kept lower by using a minimum solution footbath (MSFB) with a sponge base that keeps the volume of solution required to a minimum.

CLIENT EDUCATION
Clients should be educated regarding diagnosis, risk factors, and treatment strategies.

MEDICATIONS

DRUGS OF CHOICE
• The most effective treatments are oxytetracycline HCl or lincomycin HCl, applied as a paste under a bandage, or as an aqueous spray applied to the lesions after washing the feet with clear water.

• If applied as an aqueous spray, lesions should be treated once per day for 7 to 14 days. Common dosages for bandage treatments are 10 g of oxytetracycline or lincomycin mixed with approximately 3 ml water to form a paste. Cows must be restrained on a hoof-trimming chute. Common concentrations for the aqueous sprays are 25 g/L for oxytetracycline or 8 g/L for lincomycin, mixed with deionized or distilled water.
• Recurrence is common, so control must be ongoing. Monitoring herd prevalence will help to determine how aggressive the control program needs to be.
• Footbaths are also used as treatment/prevention.
• Most common footbath products are copper or zinc sulfate or formalin (5%–10%).
• Footbaths must be maintained to keep the treatment solution clean and active.
• They should be drained, cleaned, and refilled every 100–300 cow passages depending on the dairy.
• Copper and zinc are problematic due to their heavy metal content and formalin is a carcinogen and respiratory irritant.
• Some commercial companies are developing automated footbaths and proprietary treatment solutions, which may overcome some of the present limitations.

Drugs
• Anecdotal reports indicate that in animals that are not lactating and may be hard to handle, systemic treatment with a long-acting oxytetracycline preparation may be indicated.
• In severe cases, clinicians may consider the use of systemic NSAIDs due to the level of discomfort shown by the animals.

CONTRAINDICATIONS
• The drugs used for treating digital dermatitis are not licensed for this use and great care must be taken to avoid contaminating the udder or the milking machine with the antibiotic aerosol and causing violative residues in the milk. Drug withdrawal times for meat and milk must be maintained.
• Great care must also be taken to ensure that cattle do not drink the footbath solutions as this will also result in residue violation and in the case of Linco-spectin possible toxicity.

PRECAUTIONS
When using aqueous antibiotic sprays in the parlor, care must be taken to avoid spraying the udder or milking machine. Antibiotic residues have not been reported from treatment.

DIGITAL (PAPILLOMATOUS) DERMATITIS

ALTERNATIVE DRUGS
• Various proprietary products are available but have not been demonstrated to be as consistent or efficacious as antibiotics.
• Vaccination: A vaccine for the condition has been developed but its efficacy has been questioned.

FOLLOW-UP

PATIENT MONITORING
• The dressings should be removed within 24 hours of their application. Otherwise, bandage material becomes contaminated and the bandage then creates a good environment to incubate reinfection.
• Most animals will show rapid recovery. Animals that still have significant lameness after 72 hours should be reexamined for an additional cause of lameness.
• Cows should be monitored for recurrence and retreated as necessary.

PREVENTION/AVOIDANCE
• Vaccination: A vaccine for the condition has been developed but its efficacy has been questioned.
• Due to the high costs associated with the disease, prevention is the goal (see Biosecurity below).
• Once digital dermatitis has become endemic within a herd, good hygiene within the barn (regular scraping of passageways and maintaining clean dry stalls) will minimize the spread of the condition.
• It may also be necessary to use prophylactic footbath treatments every 4–6 weeks.

POSSIBLE COMPLICATIONS
Some (P)DD lesions will undermine the horn of the heel or wall, which will necessitate removing the horn overlying the active lesion and treating it with topical antibiotics.

EXPECTED COURSE AND PROGNOSIS
• Animals typically show increased discomfort immediately after treatment but lameness should resolve almost fully within 48 hours.
• Most animals do not require any further treatment and the disease has no long-lasting effects.
• In rare cases where the disease affects the coronary band, it appears that the coronary band may be disrupted and there may be a failure of normal horn production resulting in a full thickness vertical fissure that grows down from the coronary band causing great pain.

• This lesion should not be confused with the classical vertical fissure (sand crack) and treatment is rarely successful.

MISCELLANEOUS

ASSOCIATED CONDITIONS
• Lameness, decreased milk production, decreased life in the herd
• Erosive form: a reddened raw area of granulation tissue with a "strawberry" appearance.
• Proliferative form: in some chronic cases, there may be proliferation of the epithelial tissue to form hairy, frondlike projections.

AGE-RELATED FACTORS
More common in younger cows (lactation 1–2).

ZOONOTIC POTENTIAL
The (P)DD-associated spirochetes are similar to those that cause periodontal disease in humans but zoonotic potential is unknown.

PREGNANCY
N/A

RUMINANT SPECIES AFFECTED
Bovine; potentially all ruminant species can be affected.

BIOSECURITY
• All new animals to the dairy herd should be quarantined and have their feet prophylactically treated, especially if there is any suspicion that they come from a herd that is affected with digital dermatitis.
• Any individual involved in foot care should take great care to ensure that equipment is suitably disinfected between farm visits.
• (P)DD-free herds should not buy replacements from off premises.
• Herds with endemic (P)DD should isolate and treat new animals before introducing them to the herd.

PRODUCTION MANAGEMENT
• Recommendations that pertain to cow comfort, including well-designed and bedded freestalls or open housing
• Prompt and aggressive treatment of active lesions will help control (P)DD.

SYNONYMS
Hairy heel wart
Mortellaro's disease
Spirochetal dermatitis
Strawberry foot rot

SEE ALSO
Interdigital fibroma
Interdigital necrobacillosis
Slurry heel
Specific lameness chapters
Traumatic injury to the distal limb

ABBREVIATIONS
MSFB = minimum solution footbath
NSAIDs = nonsteroidal anti-inflammatory drugs
(P)DD = (papillomatous) digital dermatitis

Suggested Reading
Berry, S. L. 2001. Diseases of the digital soft tissues. *Vet Clin N Amer Food Anim Pr.* 17:129–142.
Demirkan, I., Murray R. D., and Carter, S. D. 2000. Skin diseases of the bovine digit associated with lameness. *Vet Bull.* 70:149–71.
Hernandez, J., Shearer, J. K., Webb, D. W. 2002, Mar 1. Effect of lameness on milk yield in dairy cows. *J Am Vet Med Assoc.* 220(5):640–4.
Milinovich, G. J., Turner, S. A., McLennan, M. W., Trott, D. J. 2004, Apr. Survey for papillomatous digital dermatitis in Australian dairy cattle. *Aust Vet J.* 82(4):223–7.
Shearer, J. K., Elliott, J. B. 1998. Papillomatous digital dermatitis: treatment and control strategies—part I. *Compend Cont Educ Pract Vet.* 20:S158–73.
Shearer, J. K., Hernandez, J., Elliott, J. B. 1998. Papillomatous digital dermatitis: treatment and control strategies—part II. *Compend Cont Educ Pract Vet.* 20:S213–23.
Trott, D. J., Moeller, M. R., Zuerner, R. L., Goff, J. P., Waters, W. R., Alt, D. P., Walker, R. L., Wannemuehler, M. J. 2003, Jun. Characterization of *Treponema phagedenis*-like spirochetes isolated from papillomatous digital dermatitis lesions in dairy cattle. *J Clin Microbiol.* 41(6):2522–29.

Authors: Chris Clark and Steven L. Berry

BASICS

OVERVIEW
• Displacement of the abomasum (DA) is very common in lactating dairy cattle, but has also been reported in sheep, goats, beef cattle, and calves.
• The abomasum is the fourth or "true" stomach in the cow and normally lies in a ventral position in the right cranial quadrant of the abdomen between the 7th and 11th ribs.
• Displacement may occur when the muscular stomach wall loses tone, fills with gas, and is displaced dorsally along the left side (~90% of the time) or to the right side (~10% of displacements).
• In right side displacements, a life-threatening volvulus or torsion may develop in some cases. Much has been written regarding the cause, effects, and treatment of both left and right side displacement.
• This chapter will assist veterinarians in the investigation of increased incidence or risk of displaced abomasums on dairies.

SYSTEMS AFFECTED
Production management, gastrointestinal

GENETICS
There appears to be a genetic component, with some cow lines showing an increased risk.

INCIDENCE/PREVALENCE
• In high-producing, well-managed herds, risk for abomasal displacement should be less than 3%, where risk is calculated as # of cases/ # of calvings. In most dairy herds, over 85% of the cases of LDA occur within the first 6 weeks of calving.
• Prevalence varies depending upon herd and nutritional management practices, geographical location, and climate.

GEOGRAPHIC DISTRIBUTION
Worldwide in dairy cattle

SIGNALMENT
Species
Bovine

Breed Predilections
Dairy breeds

Mean Age and Range
N/A

Predominant Sex
Female

SIGNS
Most common clinical signs: abrupt decrease in feed intake and a concurrent drop in milk production or a failure of postparturient cows to increase in feed intake and milk production

PHYSICAL EXAMINATION FINDINGS
• High-pitched ping during simultaneous percussion and auscultation over the ipsilateral paracostal area
• Mild to moderate tachycardia
• Ketonuria
• Scant, pasty manure, but at times may see diarrhea, constipation, or even normal manure consistency depending on duration of the displacement and the presence of concurrent disease
• Dehydration may be present but is usually mild unless the displacement is to the right side. Cows experiencing a right side displacement with a volvulus may demonstrate tachycardia, rapid dehydration, and metabolic alkalosis due to the tapping of hydrogen ions in the abomasums.
• +/− abdominal distension, especially in the paralumbar fossa corresponding to the side of displacement
• In some cases, a hollow viscus may be palpable during a routine rectal examination depending upon the size of the cow and the amount of gaseous distention.

CAUSES
• The precise cause of abomasal displacement is unknown, but most will agree that it is a multifactorial syndrome, with the highest risk period for abomasal displacement being the immediate postparturient period.
• Feed intake normally drops during last 2 weeks of the dry period and the lower intake carries over into early lactation.
• In addition, hypocalcemia, a known risk factor, is also common during this period of time, especially in multiparous cows.
• This period of altered feed intake leads to three major changes that occur in the GI tract:
  • Decrease in ruminal fill
  • Altered gastrointestinal motility and abomasal distention
  • Gas production within the abomasum

• A partially empty rumen creates a void in the abdominal cavity and if the abomasum fills with gas, it may float up and fill the empty space. Escape of either fermentation end products or the raw substrates (starch, sugars, silage acids) from the forestomachs may lead to an alteration in pH, additional bacterial fermentation, altered motility, and gas production.
• Most DAs occur early in lactation, but it is possible to see mid- to late-lactation occurrences as well. Typically, the ones that occur past the periparturient period are associated with alterations in feed quality, feed intake, fermentation within the cow, or combinations of these problems and are most common in high corn-silage-based rations.

RISK FACTORS
• Reduced feed intake is normally found during the periparturient period (3 weeks before and after calving).
• Cows calving with either clinical or subclinical hypocalcemia are at increased risk for abomasal displacement due to the altered GI motility and reduced feed intake.
• Reduction in intake is greater in fat cows or in cows that experience periparturient conditions, such as milk fever, dystocia, metritis, ruminal acidosis, mastitis, or that deliver twin calves. These cows are also at greater risk for primary or secondary ketosis and endotoxemia, which may potentiate the development of abomasal displacement.
• Stress has also been suggested as a risk factor, especially during the immediate periparturient period when feed intake is already reduced. Stress may be caused by excessive pen changes; mixing of primiparous and multiparous cows; overcrowded housing and feeding systems; prolonged confinement in individual maternity pens; environmental problems such as heat, mud, or extreme cold; and inappropriate calving assistance or general cow handling.
• There appears to be a genetic component, with some cow lines showing an increased risk.
• Ration-based risk factors:
  • Inadequate effective fiber levels
  • Overabundance of rapidly fermentable feeds
  • Easily sortable rations that allow cows to pick through the ration
  • Silages that contain abnormal levels of butyric or propionic acid

DISPLACED ABOMASUM

- Weather-related risk factors:
  - Periods of rainfall: (1) Forages exposed to rain will change in dry-matter content; (2) certain feed bunk designs may not allow water to properly drain and may lead to ration problems such as molds, yeasts, and lower total intakes; (3) resulting mud may decrease willingness of cows to approach bunk to eat.
  - Heat stress: (1) Lower total dry-matter intake per day; (2) higher risk of large swings in dry-matter intake.

DIAGNOSIS

- Diagnosis of a displaced abomasum involves simultaneous percussion and auscultation of the thoracic and abdominal walls above and below an imaginary line extending from the hip to the elbow on each side of the animal.
- Cattle with an abomasal displacement will have gas trapped within the hollow viscus that yields a "pinging" sound from the gas/fluid interface that can be heard with a stethoscope.
- The size of the ping may vary from only 3–4 inches to over 24 inches in diameter and can be located over the 10th, 11th, and 12th rib. In some cases, larger distensions will result in the sound extending past the 13th rib and into the paralumbar fossa on the side of the displacement. As there are other causes of pings, the clinician should be careful to distinguish a DA ping from gas in the spiral colon, rumen gas cap, or collapsed rumen and other causes of gas-fluid interfaces that may be less commonly found.

CBC/BIOCHEMISTRY/URINALYSIS

- Clinical findings are consistent with other intestinal flow abnormalities and may include hypochloremia, hypokalemia, hypocalcemia, metabolic alkalosis, ketonemia, and elevated levels of betahydroxybuturate and nonesterified fatty acids.
- These changes are due to a combination of depressed feed intake and sequestration of hydrochloric acid within the abomasum

TREATMENT

- There is a variety of treatments. The most common and successful strategies include replacing and securing the abomasum in its normal position using surgical abomasopexy or omentopexy via laparotomy, or casting and rolling the cow before applying 1–2 toggle-pin sutures via an external ventral approach.
- The results of surgery are usually good for survival immediately postsurgery and most cows that survive return to a similar production level as before, regardless of approach; however, follow-up studies have shown that cows with DAs have a higher risk for culling during the current and following lactation, even after a successful short-term recovery and that surgically corrected cows, on average, produce less milk.
- Laparotomy approaches have traditionally been the treatment of choice and complete recovery from surgery (including a return to normal production levels) has been reported to range from approximately 60% to 90%.
- More recently, the roll and toggle technique is reported to have similar or slightly less successful recoveries, but with a greater risk of culling in the follow-up period.
- Supportive therapies are used to correct underlying metabolic changes and more promptly return cows to production. They include IV calcium and dextrose, oral fluids containing electrolytes and glucose precursors, anti-inflammatories such as flunixin meglumine for pain management and preexisting fever, systemic antibiotics for 3–5 days, and IV fluids, depending on the cow's acid-base status and whether fluid was removed from the abomasum during surgical correction.
- Due to costs associated with surgical correction and differences in survival and production following surgical correction, treatment is not recommended for every case when examined economically.

- Each case should be evaluated independently and the decision based on the surgeon's skill and experience, probability of successful recovery and return to lactation, cost of the procedure, and repayment potential (current lactation number, previous/predicted production level, and milk price).
- Younger animals that are average or above in production are predicted to have the best opportunity for economic payback from the surgical intervention, while older animals with a shorter expected future productive life, or lower producing animals, have a lower predicted return and are often culled instead.

MEDICATIONS

CONTRAINDICATIONS

- Appropriate milk and meat withdrawal times must be followed for all compounds administered to food producing animals.
- Steroids should not be used in pregnant animals.

FOLLOW-UP

PREVENTION/AVOIDANCE

- While the precise cause for LDA is unknown, high-producing dairy cows that experience some type of abnormal periparturient event are most commonly affected.
- Management of LDA problems in herds typically centers on decreasing the known predisposing factors by improving periparturient nutritional management and decreasing the risk for additional declines in feed intake.

• A variety of factors including excessive body condition; stressful housing conditions such as overcrowding, heat, cold, or mud; and improperly balanced or managed rations can increase the risk of larger than normal declines in intake prior to calving and predispose cattle to ketosis. From calving until approximately 4 weeks in lactation, the high-producing dairy cow is susceptible to hypocalcemia, ketosis, and negative energy balance, metritis, and acidosis.

• Management should be addressed to (1) limiting the risk for development of these problems and (2) providing prompt, appropriate therapy as soon as they are diagnosed.

 MISCELLANEOUS

ASSOCIATED CONDITIONS
Most common clinical signs: abrupt decrease in feed intake and concurrent drop in milk production or failure of periparturient cow to increase in feed intake and milk production

AGE-RELATED FACTORS
Younger animals that are average or above in production are predicted to have the best opportunity for economic payback from surgical intervention; older animals with a shorter expected future productive life, or lower producing animals, have a lower predicted return and are often culled instead.

ZOONOTIC POTENTIAL
N/A

PREGNANCY
N/A

RUMINANT SPECIES AFFECTED
High-producing lactating dairy cattle

BIOSECURITY
N/A

PRODUCTION MANAGEMENT
A variety of factors including excessive body condition; stressful housing conditions such as overcrowding, heat, cold, or mud; and improperly balanced or managed rations can increase the risk of larger than normal declines in intake prior to calving and predispose cattle to ketosis. From calving until approximately 4 weeks in lactation, the high-producing dairy cow is susceptible to hypocalcemia, ketosis, and negative energy balance, metritis, and acidosis.

SYNONYMS
DA

SEE ALSO
Abdominal surgery
Acidosis
Dairy cattle nutrition
Heat stress in dairy cattle
Hypocalcemia
Ketosis
Metritis
TRP

ABBREVATIONS
DA = displaced abomasum
GI = gastrointestinal
IV = intravenous
LDA = left displaced abomasum

Suggested Reading
Bartlett, P. C., Kopcha, M., Coe, P. H., Ames, N. K., Ruegg, P. L., Erskine, R. J. 1995. Economic comparison of the pyloro-omentopexy vs. the roll-and-toggle procedure for treatment of left displacement of the abomasum in dairy cattle. *JAVMA* 206:1156–62.
Geishauser, T., Shoukri, M., Kelton, D., Leslie, K. 1998. Analysis of survivorship after displaced abomasum is diagnosed in dairy cows. *J Dairy Sci.* 81:2346–53.
Kelton, D. F., Garcia, J., Guard, C. L., Dinsmore, R. P., Powers, P. M., Smith, M. C., Stehman, S., Ralston, N., White, M. E. 1988. Bar suture (toggle pin) vs open surgical abomasopexy for treatment of left displaced abomasum in dairy-cattle. *JAVMA* 193:557–59.
Raizman, E. A., Santos, J. E. P. 2002. The effect of left displacement of abomasum corrected by toggle-pin suture on lactation, reproduction, and health of Holstein dairy cows. *J Dairy Sci.* 85:1157–64.
Shaver, R. D. 1997. Nutritional risk factors in the etiology of left displaced abomasum in dairy cows: a review. *J Dairy Sci.* 80:2449–53.
Sterner, K. E., Grymer, J. 1982. Closed suturing techniques using a bar-suture for correction of left displaced abomasum—a review of 100 cases. *Bov Pract.*, 80–84.
Van Winden, S. C. L., Jorritsma, R., Muller, K. E., Noordhuizen, J. P. T. M. 2003. Feed intake, milk yield, and metabolic parameters prior to left displaced abomasum in dairy cows. *J Dairy Sci.* 86:1465–71.

Author: Michael W. Overton

DISSEMINATED INTRAVASCULAR COAGULOPATHY (DIC)

BASICS

DEFINITION
A syndrome characterized by hemorrhage and thrombosis, which results from the systemic activation and consumption of coagulation and fibrinolytic proteins, consumption of platelets and vascular injury.

PATHOPHYSIOLOGY
• Any primary disease or disorder that activates the coagulation system and circulating platelets and causes vascular injury has the potential to result in coagulopathies.
• If not treated or corrected, the acquired coagulopathy may proceed to DIC. Clots forming within the small vessels and microvasculature result in ischemic injury, which may become irreversible.
• As the naturally circulating anticoagulants ATIII and proteins C & S are consumed in response to the hypercoagulable coagulopathy, the patient advances to a prothrombotic state.
• As clotting factors are consumed in the diffuse microvascular thrombotic process, hemorrhagic diathesis ensues.

SYSTEMS AFFECTED
All body systems can become affected by microvascular thrombosis initially and subsequently by hemorrhaging as the condition progresses. The severity and duration of the underlying disease or disorder influences the procoagulant stimulus and the associated clinical manifestation(s).
• Cardiovascular—early stages appear as thrombosis, as condition progresses hemorrhaging predominates.
• Pulmonary—thrombosis of the pulmonary vessels can result on hypoxia and respiratory distress.
• GI—microvascular thrombosis results in ischemic condition and irreversible mucosal injury or hepatobiliary dysfunction.
• Lymphatic/immune—thrombosis in early stages progressing to uncontrolled hemorrhaging as condition worsens
• Renal/urologic—microvascular thrombosis may result in acute renal ischemia, hematuria, oliguria, and failure.

GENETICS
N/A

INCIDENCE/PREVALENCE
N/A

SIGNALMENT
N/A

SIGNS

General Comments
• DIC is secondary to a primary underlying disease process or syndrome.
• Almost any body system is prone to microvascular thrombosis and consequently a wide variety of clinical signs are described.

Historical Findings
Depends on the underlying disease process or condition

Physical Examination Findings
• Microvascular thrombosis and hemorrhage may cause colic, oliguria, dyspnea, respiratory distress, or altered mentation.
• Large vessel thrombosis is commonly associated with catheter sites and venipuncture.
• Petechial or ecchymotic hemorrhaging, prolonged bleeding following venipuncture, may be noticed, but this is relatively uncommon.

CAUSES
• Most commonly, DIC occurs secondary to inflammatory or ischemic GI disorders and gram-negative infections, resulting in circulating endotoxemia.
• Less commonly associated with viral, rickettsial, protozoal, or parasitic diseases; heat stroke; burns; neoplasia; or severe trauma.

RISK FACTORS
Any disease or event that activates coagulation or causes significant blood loss can result in DIC if left untreated.

DIAGNOSIS

DIFFERENTIAL DIAGNOSIS
• Early detection in the hypercoagulable phase is a diagnostic challenge but important with respect to prognosis.
• Patients with primary disorders that have the potential to progress into DIC should be monitored closely.
• Hypercoagulation or DIC should be suspected in patients who fail to respond to appropriate therapy of the primary disease or develop diminished renal, hepatic, or cardiopulmonary function.
• Decreased tissue perfusion as a result of microthrombosis is evidence of specific organ failure.

CBC/BIOCHEMISTRY/URINALYSIS
• Laboratory examination is crucial for determining the systemic hematologic and biochemical alterations but is not pathognomonic for diagnosing altered hemostasis.
• Leukopenias with neutropenia, lymphopenia, or thrombocytopenia are common CBC abnormalities associated with severe sepsis and shock.
• Hypofibrinogenemia is uncommon because most DIC-associated disorders are associated with severe inflammation.
• Altered electrolytes or biochemical parameters may reflect renal azotemia or hepatobiliary injury.

OTHER LABORATORY TESTS
• Laboratory tests of hemostasis are most beneficial when performed serially and should always be interpreted with respect to patient clinical assessments.
• Proper venipuncture technique and sample handling are important to avoid spurious laboratory results.
• Increased fibrin degradation products (> 40 μg/mL) and decreased antithrombin III activity (>60% of control)
• Prolongation of the clotting time tests [prothrombin time (PT) and activated partial thromboplastin time (APTT)] occurs as a late event in DIC and are not sensitive enough to diagnose the preceding phase of hypercoagulation.

IMAGING
Arterial thrombosis can be imaged by vascular digital subtraction contrast angiography.

DIAGNOSTIC PROCEDURES
N/A

PATHOLOGIC FINDINGS
Generally reflect the primary disease process and focal to diffuse thrombosis, and petechial and ecchymotic hemorrhages may be evident grossly or histologically.

TREATMENT
Hospitalization and intensive care are required to address the needs of this life-threatening condition.

DISSEMINATED INTRAVASCULAR COAGULOPATHY (DIC)

SUPPORTIVE CARE
• Constant monitoring of coagulation parameters is necessary to avoid a recurrent event.
• Frequent patient assessment and monitoring catheter and venipuncture sites are imperative.

ACTIVITY
Limited

DIET
Total or partial parenteral may be required to meet increased energy and metabolic demands due to shock.

CLIENT EDUCATION
DIC is associated with a poor prognosis.

SURGICAL CONSIDERATIONS
If the primary disorder is a surgical lesion, compounded with DIC the prognosis is grave.

MEDICATIONS

DRUGS OF CHOICE
• Treatment of the underlying disease process, which is driving the coagulopathy, is the primary concern.
• Immediate and aggressive fluid administration to maintain tissue perfusion and correct balance of acid-base and electrolyte levels
• Fresh whole plasma transfusion (15–30 mL/kg) to restore the consumed coagulation proteins and platelets. If available, hyperimmune plasma with a higher titer of antiendotoxin antibody may be beneficial.
• The use of heparin is controversial and, if used, should be administered in combination with plasma to assure adequate activity of coagulation proteins.

CONTRAINDICATIONS
• Drugs that cause or may exacerbate preexisting hypotension (e.g., acepromazine) should be avoided.
• Avoid potentially nephrotoxic drugs and those requiring hepatic metabolism.

POSSIBLE INTERACTIONS
N/A

ALTERNATIVE DRUGS
N/A

FOLLOW-UP

PATIENT MONITORING
• Physical examination every 2 to 4 hours with particular attention to heart and respiratory rate, temperature, urine output, presence of arrhythmias, pulse intensity, and mucous membrane coloration.
• Laboratory tests of hemostasis (platelet count, PT, APTT, FDPs, and ATIII) are most beneficial when performed serially and should always be interpreted with respect to patient clinical assessments.
• Check PCV and TP every 12 hours during the initial treatment with IV fluid to expand the intravascular fluid volume and during equilibration with the extravascular pool.

PREVENTION/AVOIDANCE
Early detection, treatment, and monitoring patients with disorders known to result in DIC are critical.

POSSIBLE COMPLICATIONS
Multiple organ failure and cardiovascular shock

EXPECTED COURSE AND PROGNOSIS
The diagnosis of DIC is based on a prolongation of the clotting times, decreased platelet count and ATIII activity, and increased fibrinogen degradation products, which are not normally present until the condition has progressed to a terminal stage when life threatening hemorrhage and multiple organ and circulatory failure are present.

MISCELLANEOUS

ASSOCIATED CONDITIONS
• Large and small-vessel thrombosis
• Ecchymotic and petechial hemorrhage, epistaxis
• Multiple organ failure, death

AGE-RELATED FACTORS
Only if associated with the underlying primary disorder

ZOONOTIC POTENTIAL
N/A

PREGNANCY
N/A

SYNONYMS
• Consumptive coagulopathy
• Death is coming.
• Intravascular coagulation or fibrinolysis
• Defibrination syndrome

SEE ALSO
Circulatory and hemorrhagic shock
Sepsis

ABBREVIATIONS
APTT = activated partial thromboplastin time
ATIII = antithrombin III
FDPs = fibrinogen degradation products
GI = gastrointestinal
PCV = packed cell volume
PT = partial thromboplastin time
TP = total protein

Suggested Reading
Cardiovascular system. 1994. In: *Goat medicine*, ed. M. C. Smith and D. M. Sherman. Philadelphia: Lea & Febiger.
Cebra, C., and Cebra, M. 2002. Diseases of the cardiovascular system. In: *Sheep and goat medicine*, ed. D. G. Pugh. Philadelphia: W. B. Saunders.
Clark, D. R. 1986. Diseases of the cardiovascular and hemolymphatic systems. In: *Current veterinary therapy food animal practice 2*, ed. J. L. Howard. Philadelphia: W. B. Saunders.

Author: Benjamin J. Darien

DOWN CAMELID

 BASICS

DEFINITION
Inability to stand and/or remain standing without assistance

SYSTEMS AFFECTED
• Musculoskeletal
• CNS

GENETICS
N/A

INCIDENCE/PREVALENCE
Worldwide; can occur wherever camelids are raised

GEOGRAPHIC DISTRIBUTION
• Depends on cause.
• Meningeal worm occurs in warmer climates wherever white-tailed deer are in contact with camelids.
• GI parasitism is more common in subtropical and tropical climates.

SIGNALMENT
Species
Camelid

Breed Predilections
N/A

Mean Age and Range
N/A

Predominant Sex
N/A

General Considerations
Llamas and alpacas will sit in sternal recumbency ("cush") and resist standing when agitated or stressed. The clinician needs to distinguish between refusal to stand and inability to stand.

 DIAGNOSIS

DIFFERENTIAL DIAGNOSIS
Neurologic Disease
• *Parelaphostrongylus tenuis*
• Listeriosis
• Polioencephalomyelacia
• EHV-1
• Tick paralysis
• Rabies
• Trauma
• Neoplasia of CNS or spinal cord
• Abscess of CNS or spinal cord

Alimentary Disease
• Debilitation due to severe gastrointestinal parasitism: Coccidiosis; *Haemonchus contortus*
• Debilitation due to social starvation

Musculoskeletal Disease
• Peripheral nerve damage
• Trauma

Hematologic
Mycoplasma haemolama (formerly Eperythrozoonosis)

Parelaphostrongylus tenuis (meningeal worm)
• Nematode found in white-tailed deer and carried by snails and slugs.
• Llama ingests snail or slug carrying larvae.
• Larvae are released in stomach and migrate to spinal cord and mature in gray matter; migrate to brain through the spinal subdural space.

Clinical Signs
• The parasite does not cause clinical signs in white-tailed deer.
• Infection in camelids can cause signs of neurologic disease including ataxia, paresis, lameness, circling, blindness, and recumbency.

Diagnosis
• There is no reliable antemortem diagnostic test.
• A peripheral eosinophilia may be seen or an eosinophilia in CSF.

Treatment
• Ivermectin (2.5 ml/75 lbs SQ) for 3 days followed by fenbendazole at a dose rate of 30 mg/kg PO for 3 days
• Supportive care is indicated including intravenous fluids and/or parenteral nutrition, as necessary, in addition to anti-inflammatory medication such as flunixin meglumine or corticosteroids or DMSO.
• Flotation therapy and/or physical therapy may be beneficial.

Prevention
Monthly deworming with ivermectin (1 ml/75 lb body weight SQ) to eliminate parasite larvae as they migrate through the body.

Listeriosis
Acute meningoencephalitis caused by gram-positive bacterium *Listeria monocytogenes*

Clinical Signs
Listeriosis can cause a wide range of neurologic signs including cranial nerve deficits, circling, ataxia, paresis, fever, depression, recumbency, and death.

Diagnosis
• Diagnosis is based on clinical signs and elimination of other differential diagnoses.
• Additionally, analysis of CSF may reveal elevated protein (>40 mg/dl) and >12 mononuclear cells/μl.

Treatment
• Oxytetracycline (10 mg/kg IV twice daily) or high doses of penicillin (40,000 U/kg three to four times daily or 60,000 U/kg twice daily) in addition to supportive care.

Polioencephalomyelacia
Necrosis of cortical gray matter associated with thiamine deficiency

Clinical Signs
Neurologic signs are variable depending on which area of the brain is affected including blindness, depression, muscle tremors, anorexia, opisthotonus, recumbency, and seizures.

Diagnosis
A range of laboratory diagnostic tests are available (Smith, 1969); however, diagnosis is usually based on history, signalment, and clinical signs.

Treatment
Administration of thiamine (10 mg/kg) once daily intramuscularly or intravenously for 3–5 days is recommended. Thiamine hydrochloride can cause anaphylaxis if given intravenously, therefore it is recommended that the thiamine dose be diluted and administered slowly.

Equine Herpes Virus-1
• A virus similar to EHV-1 has been identified in camelids and may be associated with blindness and encephalitis, which may lead to recumbency.
• Treatment includes NSAIDs and supportive care.

Tick Paralysis
Caused by a neurotoxin from female *Dermacentor variabilis* or *D. andersoni*. The condition is observed more commonly in western states.

Clinical Signs
• Ataxia, paresis, and paralysis can progress over a few hours or more slowly over 24–48 hours.
• Ascending paralysis can result in dysphagia and death due to asphyxia due to respiratory paralysis.

Treatment
• Resolution of signs will not occur until the tick is removed.
• Recommended treatment includes topical administration of pyrethrin insecticides and ivermectin (0.2 mg/kg). Signs can reverse within 2–12 hours of removing the tick.

Rabies
Invariably fatal neurologic disease caused by rabies virus

Clinical Signs

• Neurologic signs are variable and include depression, ataxia, and anorexia, and can progress to recumbency, salivation, coma, and convulsions among many other signs.
• Rabies should be considered in any case of nonresponsive central nervous system disease.

Diagnosis

• No clinical diagnostic test is available.
• Postmortem diagnosis is confirmed by histopathology of brain tissue and indirect fluorescent antibody testing of brain sections.

Trauma

• Differential diagnoses to be considered include musculoskeletal or peripheral nerve injury or head trauma.
• A complete physical exam should include palpation of extremities for crepitus and/or muscle atrophy, testing of reflexes, and palpation and manipulation of joints.

Neoplasia or Abscess of CNS or Spinal Cord

• A neurologic exam should be performed to attempt to localize the lesion.
• Diagnosis can be achieved in some cases with head or spinal radiographs, magnetic resonance imaging, or computed tomography.

Coccidiosis

A heavy gastrointestinal burden of coccidia, specifically the pathogenic species *Eimeria macusansiensis*, can be debilitating in camelids.

Clinical Signs

Camelids with heavy infections can present in poor body condition with diarrhea, weight loss, poor hair coat, weakness, and recumbency in severe cases.

Diagnosis

• Diagnosis is based on clinical signs and presence of large numbers of coccidia on fecal floats.
• Camelids can carry nonpathogenic species of coccidia, therefore speciation of oocysts is recommended.

Treatment

• *E. macusansiensis* can be difficult to treat. Ponazuril at 10–20 mg/kg PO can be effective.
• Daily oral doses of amprolium until fecal floats are clear have also been effective.
• In severe cases, supportive care including intravenous fluids and/or parenteral nutrition may also be indicated.

Prevention

Effective preventative measures include addition of coccidiostats to feed or water for camelid herds, reducing stocking densities, regular doses of coccidiostats such as amprolium or sulfadimethoxine, prevention of fecal contamination of feed and water, and proper manure disposal.

Haemonchus Contortus

A blood-sucking gastrointestinal strongyle parasite

Clinical Signs

Camelids infected with this parasite can present with generalized weakness, anemia, depression, anorexia, and diarrhea.

Diagnosis

Diagnosis is based on clinical signs and presence of large numbers of strongyle eggs on fecal float.

Treatment

• Elimination of *Haemonchus contortus* burdens can be difficult due to widespread resistance to commonly used dewormers.
• Ivermectin has been effective against the adult and hypobiotic larval stages, but resistance is occurring.
• Combinations of ivermectin and fenbendazole or ivermectin and pyrantel can be effective.
• Fecal egg count reduction tests are recommended to determine the effectiveness of treatment.
• Moxidectin has been used in salvage situations, but widespread use is leading to development of resistance in some populations.
• Blood transfusions may also be necessary depending on the degree of anemia.

Mycoplasma Haemolamae

A hemoparasite that can cause clinical disease in immunosuppressed or stressed camelids. It can also be found in low numbers in healthy camelids.

Clinical Signs

Infected camelids can present with anemia, depression, acute recumbency, weight loss, and death.

Diagnosis

• The presence of *M. haemolamae* on blood smears with concurrent clinical signs supports diagnosis.
• A PCR-based assay is available from Oregon State University for definitive diagnosis.

Treatment

• Various regimens of tetracycline have been recommended including oxytetracycline at a rate of 10 mg/kg intravenously once or twice a day.
• Supportive care and blood transfusions may also be necessary depending on the degree of anemia.

Other Differential Diagnoses to Consider

• C3 ulcers
• Rickets
• Toxoplasmosis
• Sarcocystosis
• Bacterial, viral bacterial or fungal encephalitis or meningitis
• Intervertebral disk extrusion
• Vertebral osteomyelitis
• Myelitis

CONTRAINDICATIONS

Appropriate milk and meat withdrawal times must be followed for all compounds administered to food producing animals.

 MISCELLANEOUS

ASSOCIATED CONDITIONS
C3 ulceration

AGE-RELATED FACTORS
N/A

ZOONOTIC POTENTIAL
Rabies is a zoonotic disease.

PREGNANCY
N/A

RUMINANT SPECIES AFFECTED
Camelids

BIOSECURITY
N/A

PRODUCTION MANAGEMENT
N/A

SYNONYMS

SEE ALSO
Bacterial, viral bacterial or fungal encephalitis or meningitis
C3 ulcers
Intervertebral disk extrusion
Myelitis
Rickets
Sarcocystosis
Toxoplasmosis
Vertebral osteomyelitis

ABBREVIATIONS
CNS= central nervous system
CSF= cerebral spinal fluid
DMSO=dimethyl sulfoxide
EHV-1= equine herpes virus-1
IV= intravenous
NSAIDs= nonsteroidal anti-inflammatory drugs
PCR= polymerase chain reaction
PO= per os, by mouth
SQ= subcutaneous

Suggested Reading
Baum, K. H. 1994, July. Neurologic diseases of llamas. *Veterinary Clinics of North America: Food Animal Practice—Update on Llama Medicine.* 10(2): 383–90.
Fowler, M. E. 1998. *Medicine and surgery of South American camelids.* 2nd ed. Ames: Iowa State University Press.
Smith, B. P. 1996. *Large animal internal medicine.* 2nd ed. St. Louis, MO: Mosby.

Author: Natalie Coffer

DOWNER COW

BASICS

DEFINITION
• Persistent sternal recumbency with no apparent cause
• Usually associated with the periparturient period and often follows parturient paresis
• Some animals may crawl ("creepers").
• Two forms: alert and nonalert

PATHOPHYSIOLOGY
• Primary recumbency may be due to muscle weakness resulting from metabolic disturbances such as parturient paresis or hypokalemia.
• Nerve damage due to intrapelvic trauma during calving may be a factor contributing to primary recumbency.
• Other causes are toxic substances from metritis or mastitis.
• Primary recumbency not associated with calving may be due to sepsis from peritonitis or pneumonia.
• Regardless of the cause of primary recumbency, pressure damage of muscle and nerves leads to secondary recumbency. Experimentally, this can occur within 6 hours.
• Tertiary recumbency due to muscle tearing occurs in some cases as a result of struggling to move. The hamstring muscles are most often affected.
• Muscle damage can cause severe myoglobinemia leading to renal damage.
• Hip luxation and fractures of the pelvis and femoral head or neck are additional, contributing secondary or tertiary factors in some cases.
• Pain due to muscle damage is another contributing factor. Dermatitis due to urine scalding leads to more pain and hence reluctance to move.
• Massive tissue destruction can lead to DIC.

SYSTEMS AFFECTED
Musculoskeletal, CNS, production management

GENETICS
N/A

INCIDENCE/PREVALENCE
N/A

GEOGRAPHIC DISTRIBUTION
N/A

SIGNALMENT
Usually a periparturient cow and typically a mature, high-producing dairy animal housed on concrete

SIGNS
• Inability to stand. Typical downers maintain sternal recumbency. Those in lateral recumbency are dying animals rather than typical downers.
• Appetite of alert downers is better than that of nonalert downers.
• Movement decreases as the duration of recumbency increases. Alert downers are more active.
• Dry stools are common. Dark urine, especially brown urine, is a grave sign.
• Knuckling (digital flexion) of hind limbs when attempting to stand

CAUSES AND RISK FACTORS
• Metabolic problems such as parturient paresis
• Intrapelvic trauma as a result of dystocia
• Toxic metritis and mastitis
• Wet, slippery concrete
• Large size and excessive weight

DIAGNOSIS

HISTORY
• What is the age, parity, and production level of the cow?
• How long has the cow been down and has it been moved to present location?
• Did calving occur recently? If so, when and was there dystocia? What was the duration of dystocia and how was it managed? Was the calf dead or alive? What was the size?
• Did retained placenta occur and how was it managed?
• Did parturient paresis occur and how was it treated? What was the response to treatment?
• How has recumbency been managed? Has the patient been lifted?

DIFFERENTIAL DIAGNOSIS
• The goal is to identify specific causes of recumbency in order to determine whether treatment is justified and what the management plan should be (see Figure 1).
• Alert downers commonly suffer from local nerve and/or musculoskeletal damage.
  • Pressure damage to peripheral nerves such as the sciatic, obturator, and common peroneal, will have broad locomotor consequences. Less commonly, vertebral lymphoma can cause local nerve damage.
  • Muscle damage can be due to compression or rupture. Most often the hamstring muscles are involved but pressure damage of the crural region and gastrocnemius rupture may occur also. When massive, muscle damage can have severe systemic effects that may lead to a nonalert downer.
  • Fracture of the pelvis or proximal femur. Less commonly, vertebral fracture
  • Hip luxation or less commonly vertebral or sacroiliac luxation

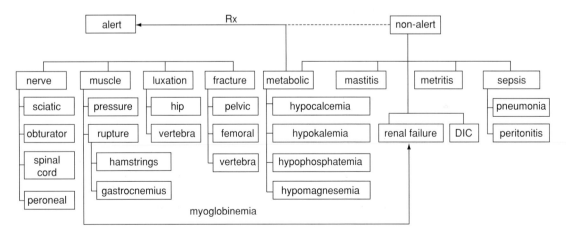

Figure 1.

Diagnostic algorithm for downer cattle. Only the most common causes are shown. In any particular case, multiple causes may be involved and may change with time.

DOWNER COW

• Nonalert downers usually suffer from systemic problems, which broadly include metabolic, toxic, and septic problems. As mentioned above, massive muscle damage can cause systemic failure. Kidney damage and a cascade leading to DIC may be involved.
  • Toxic metritis or mastitis
  • Unresolved hypocalcemia, hypophosphatemia, and hypokalemia
  • Sepsis due to pneumonia or peritonitis. These can be the result of many things such as "hardware disease," rupture of lung or liver abscess, or perforation of an abomasal ulcer.

LABORATORY TESTS
• CBC and chemistry panel may reveal signs of underlying disease.
• Serum creatinine kinase (CK), a marker for muscle damage, is elevated significantly in the early stages but has a short half-life and is not reliable for prognosis in clinical cases.
• Serum calcium and potassium levels may point to metabolic problems
• Urine should be examined for color and if possible for myoglobin levels, specific gravity evaluated

IMAGING
Impractical in most cases; radiology could be used to confirm pelvic fracture or hip luxation.

DIAGNOSTIC PROCEDURES
• TPR, examination of the udder and uterus for signs of mastitis and metritis
• Cutaneous testing of hind limbs for evidence of sensory reflexes
• Palpation of limbs for luxation or fractures
• Rectal palpation for pelvic fractures or hip luxation, evidence of crepitus
• Lifting with hip clamps is useful for musculoskeletal and neurologic examination but should be very brief to avoid pressure damage of muscles in the tuber coxae region. The clamps should be well padded to minimize tissue damage.
• Some cows may be able to stand unassisted once lifted but most will not. As support of the hip clamps is released, muscle strength can be determined.
• Response to treatment in a floatation tank is useful but labor intensive.

TREATMENT
• The first goal is to prevent further muscle and nerve damage due to recumbency.
• Provision of soft, clean, and dry bedding is essential. Sand is easier to keep clean than straw bedding. Hard, slippery concrete should be avoided.
• Frequent repositioning will reduce pressure damage.
• Floatation therapy is the best way to reduce pressure damage and enhance vascular supply to compressed tissues. Hot water (body temperature) is essential for hydrotherapy to

be beneficial. A side effect is to cleanse the skin and reduce dermatitis.
• Hobbles on the hind limb pasterns have been used to prevent limb abduction into the so-called spread-eagle (splay-legged) position but the practice can be dangerous and is unnecessary on good nonslip bedding.
• Hind limb knuckling (digital flexion) can be managed with a cast on the affected lower limb.
• Surgical amputation or hemiamputation of a toxic udder by ligation of one or both external pudendal arteries.

MEDICATIONS
• Antibiotic treatment is indicated in the case of metritis, mastitis or generalized sepsis.
• Pain medication will make the patient more willing to attempt to move and improve appetite.
• Topical ointments for dermatitis and pressure sores
• Appropriate milk and meat withdrawal times must be followed for all compounds administered to food-producing animals.

FOLLOW-UP

PATIENT MONITORING
• Successful treatment of downer cows is labor intensive and requires frequent monitoring of the patient.
• Keeping the bedding clean and dry is important.
• Providing a constant supply of fresh drinking water is important but difficult when animals move continually. A large rubber tub that is not easily turned over works best.
• Frequent skin cleansing is important to prevent urine scalding.
• Frequent repositioning is helpful to minimize pressure damage.
• Floatation therapy requires frequent monitoring to prevent drowning. Keep the water close to body temperature.

POSSIBLE COMPLICATIONS
• Hamstring or gastrocnemius muscle tearing due to struggling to stand
• Hip luxation during ataxic attempts to move, especially when hind limbs are abducted in the so-called "spread eagle" or "splay-legged" position.
• Muscle damage due to excessive use of hip clamps by owners. Some owners may use hip clamps to facilitate milking. They should be advised that it is better to dry the cow off and save the cow rather than lose the cow while trying to save the lactation.
• Drowning or chilling due to improper use of a floatation tank.
• Rope burns of the udder or pasterns due to improper use of hobbles

MISCELLANEOUS
• Prevention is more important than therapy.
• Dry cow feeding should be aimed at prevention of parturient paresis.
• Provision of clean, well-bedded calving stalls is essential.
• Periparturient cows should be monitored frequently so that problems can be treated before they get worse.
• Owners should know that a down cow is an emergency case because irreversible pressure damage can occur in as short as 6 hours of recumbency.

ASSOCIATED CONDITIONS
N/A

AGE-RELATED FACTORS
N/A

ZOONOTIC POTENTIAL
N/A

SYNONYMS
N/A

SEE ALSO
Cattle physical examination
Dystocia
Lameness

ABBREVIATIONS
CBC = complete blood count
CK = serum creatinine kinase
CNS = central nervous system
DIC = disseminated intravascular coagulopathy
TPR = temperature/pulse/respirations

Suggested Reading
Cox, V. S. 1999. Downer cow syndrome. In: *Current Veterinary Therapy 4: Food Animal Practice*, ed. J. L. Howard, R. A. Smith. Philadelphia: W. B. Saunders.
Sielman, E. S., Sweeney, R. W., Whitlock, R. H., Reams, R. Y. 1997. Hypokalemia syndrome in dairy cows: 10 cases (1992–1996). *J Am Vet Med Assoc.* 210:240–43.
Smith, B. P., Angelos, J., George, L. W., Fecteau, G., Angelos, S., et al. 1997. Down cows: causes and treatments. *Proc Ann Conf Am Assoc Bovine Practitioners* 30:43–45.
Van Metre, D. C., Callan, R. J., Garry, F. B. 2001. Examination of the musculoskeletal system in recumbent cattle. *Compen Cont Ed Prac Vet.* 23:S5–S13.

Author: Victor S. Cox

DRUG INTERACTIONS

 BASICS

DEFINITION
A drug interaction can be defined as the influence of one drug on the biological activity of another drug administered to the same animal simultaneously.

OVERVIEW
• Drug interactions lead to drug(s) producing unexpected effects that may be harmful, inconsequential, or even beneficial.
• Can occur in vitro due to physical or chemical incompatibilities or in vivo as a result of pharmacokinetic or pharmacodynamic interactions.
• Drug interactions may result in a fatal outcome.
• Employment of relatively large doses, using multiple-drug therapy, and a debilitated state of the patient can increase the probability of severe drug interactions.
• Consider the possibility of drug interaction, evaluate laboratory testing parameters, evaluate and notify pharmaceutical companies of adverse reactions.

SYSTEMS AFFECTED
Production management, metabolic, immune

GENETICS
N/A

INCIDENCE/PREVALENCE
N/A

GEOGRAPHIC DISTRIBUTION
Worldwide depending on species and drugs utilized

SIGNALMENT
• All animals susceptible if more than one drug is administered simultaneously.
• Possibility of higher prevalence in young animals or animals kept under intensive conditions due to higher level of drug use.

Species
Potentially all ruminant species

Breed Predilections
N/A

Mean Age and Range
N/A

Predominant Sex
N/A

SIGNS
• Drug toxicity
• Augmented or decreased drug effect
• Changes in onset or duration of drugs' effect(s)
• Unexpected effects or side effects

CAUSES AND RISK FACTORS
• Can occur whenever two or more drugs are administered concurrently.
• Likelihood of interactions increases as number of drugs administered concurrently increases.

In Vitro Incompatibilities
Combination of two or more drugs in solution may lead to physical or chemical changes in one of the active ingredients with resultant inactivation.

Semisynthetic penicillins, barbiturates, benzylpenicillin, diazepam, promethazine hydrochloride, sulfonamides, and vitamin B complex should not be mixed with other drugs, as they have many incompatibilities.

In Vivo Interactions
• Interactions that affect drug absorption
  • Increased solubility of lipophilic drugs when coadministered orally with surfactants
  • Decreased oral availability of drugs due to adsorption or chelation (divalent ions and tetracyclines, kaolin and lincomycin, activated charcoal)
  • Changes in gut motility (e.g., coadministered cholinergic drugs)
• Interactions that affect drug distribution: displacement of highly plasma-protein-bound drugs when coadministered (e.g., sulfonamides, phenylbutazone, other NSAIDs, and warfarin)
• Interactions that affect drug metabolism
  • Induction of metabolizing (e.g., phenobarbitone, diphenhydramine, griseofulvin, phenylbutazone, cortisol, and some inhalation anesthetics).
  • Inhibition of metabolizing enzymes (e.g., chloramphenicol).
• Interactions that affect renal excretion of drugs
  • Competition for nonspecific carrier proteins affects the excretion of weak organic acids or bases by tubular secretion (e.g., probenecid prolongs the action of penicillins).

• Urinary acidification or alkalinization will affect the tubular reabsorption of drugs that are either weak organic acids or weak organic bases (e.g., alkalinization of urine promotes the excretion of sulfonamides).
• Effects at receptor sites
  • Two drugs acting at the same effector site or different sites but with related effects (e.g., organophosphates and carbamates, neuromuscular blockade caused by anesthetics and aminoglycosides)
  • Decreased efficacy of bactericidal antibiotics when coadministered with bacteriostatic antibiotics
  • Synergistic effects of tranquillizers, sedatives, and anesthetics for balanced anesthesia

 DIAGNOSIS

• The signs of a drug interaction are highly variable and dependent on the dose and types of drugs administered as well as the type of interaction.
• Be aware of potential interactions when administering more than one drug simultaneously, particularly if the effect is not acute/obvious.

 TREATMENT

• Discontinue treatment
• Use alternatives if available
• Adjust doses according to effect
• Avoid coadministering drugs with known interactions
• Keep number of drugs administered to a minimum
• Supportive therapy as needed

 MEDICATIONS

CONTRAINDICATIONS
• Appropriate milk and meat withdrawal times must be followed for all compounds administered to food-producing animals.
• Steroids should not be used in pregnant animals.

Table 1

	Acetylpromazine	Calcium gluconate	Chlorpromazine hydrochloride	Lincomycin	Streptomycin	Tetracyclines
Important Incompatibilities in Drugs for Parenteral Administration						
Atropine sulfate			X			
Calcium gluconate					X	X
Cephalosporins						X
Penicillins				X		X
Phenylbutazone	X		X			
Sodium bicarbonate					X	X
Tetracyclines		X	X			
Tylosin					X	X
Vitamins B and C			X			

FOLLOW-UP

MISCELLANEOUS

ASSOCIATED CONDITIONS
N/A

AGE-RELATED FACTORS
Depends on agent utilized

ZOONOTIC POTENTIAL
N/A

PREGNANCY
• Depends on agent utilized
• Steroids should not be used in pregnant animals.

RUMINANT SPECIES AFFECTED
Potentially, all ruminant species are affected.

BIOSECURITY
N/A

PRODUCTION MANAGEMENT
N/A

SYNONYMS
N/A

SEE ALSO
Additional pharmacology chapters
Extralabel drug use
Pharmacokinetics

ABBREVIATIONS
NSAIDs = nonsteroidal anti-inflammatory drugs

Suggested Reading
Avoiding drug interactions. 2004, Jun. *Prescrire Int.* 13(71): 99–102.
Eckhoff, G. A. 1980, May 15. Mechanisms of adverse drug reactions and interactions in veterinary medicine. *J Am Vet Med Assoc.* 176(10 Spec No):1131–33.
Paul, J. W. 1987, Apr. Drug interactions and incompatibilities. *Vet Clin North Am Equine Pract.* 3(1):145–51.
Reilly, P. E. B., Isaacs, J. P. 1983. Adverse drug interactions of importance in veterinary practice. *The Veterinary Record* 112:29–33.
Roos, T. C., Merk, H. F. 2000, Feb. Important drug interactions in dermatology. *Drugs* 59(2):181–92.

Authors: Ronette Gehring and Deon van der Merwe

DYSTOCIA

 BASICS

DEFINITION
• Dystocia occurs when the first or second stage in the parturition process is interrupted or prolonged, necessitating artificial assistance for delivery of the fetus.
• The main objective when assisting a dystocia case is to deliver the fetus without causing trauma to the dam, and if possible to deliver a live fetus.

PATHOPHYSIOLOGY
• Expulsive forces may be weakened in cases of hypocalcemia.
• The most common causes for dystocia are related to fetal/maternal size disproportions, as well as malposition, malpresentation and malposture of the calf.

SYSTEMS AFFECTED
Reproductive, musculoskeletal, production management, endocrine/metabolic

GENETICS
• Sires whose daughters have reduced pelvic diameter
• Those animals whose offspring are oversized in comparison to the breed average

INCIDENCE/PREVALENCE
The incidence of dystocia is about 15% of all parturitions with a reported range from 3% to 25%.

GEOGRAPHIC DISTRIBUTION
Worldwide distribution

SIGNALMENT

Species
Potentially all ruminant species

Mean Age and Range
The incidence of dystocia is higher in primiparous than multiparous animals.

Predominant Sex
Female

Breed Predilection
• The overall incidence of dystocia varies by species and breed.
• The bovine is most often affected but ewes and does when carrying twins may show a high incidence of dystocia.

SIGNS

GENERAL COMMENTS
Defects in the components of the parturition process such as expulsive force, birth canal diameter, fetal size, and uterine torsion must be considered when assessing a dystocia case.

HISTORICAL FINDINGS
• Lack of delivery progress after initiation of parturition
• Continuous violent abdominal contractions without visualization of fetal parts
• Unsuccessful attempts by either an owner or herdsman to deliver the calf

PHYSICAL EXAMINATION FINDINGS
In cattle:
• Prior to assisting a dystocia, the minimal requirements are an ample supply of clean warm water, disinfectant, buckets, lubricants (petroleum jelly or methylcellulose-derived products), two obstetrical chains with handles, and the hormone oxytocin.
• When there has been little progress for 2 hours after the amnionic sac is presented at the vulva, the animal should be examined manually to determine the cause of the dystocia and assess the most appropriate route of delivery.
• The calf can live up to 10 hours within the birth canal after the amnionic sac is ruptured.
• The purpose of the vaginal exam is to determine the presentation, position, and posture of the calf within the birth canal.
• If the calf is in an anterior presentation (cranial), it must first be determined if the head, neck, and front legs are extended.
• In a posterior presentation, it must be determined if the hind legs are extended. At the same time, calf viability must be ascertained.
• If the head is accessible in an anterior presentation, the swallowing reflex may be elicited by inserting a finger into the mouth; if the calf is alive, swallowing will occur.
• The pedal reflex may be applied by putting pressure on the hooves in an anterior or posterior presentation; a responsive calf will retract its leg.
• During the evaluation process, the position and posture must also be considered.

• The position is related to the dorsum of the calf in relation to the maternal sacrum, pubis, and ileal shafts.
• The posture is related to the fetal extremities (neck and legs) and can be either extended or flexed. These considerations are important because prior to extraction, the calf must be in normal position and posture to prevent trauma to the dam.
• If the fetal head or neck is flexed backward or to a side, this abnormal fetal posture must be corrected prior to extraction.
• Before attempting to extract the calf, it must be ascertained that the presentation, position, and posture are normal.
• The position of the calf must be dorsosacral with a normal posture prior to extraction.
• The final step is to determine whether or not there is sufficient space and lubrication to deliver the calf vaginally.

Anterior Presentation (Cattle)
• The head of the calf should rest on both knees of the front limbs with the legs fully presented in the birth canal.
• There will be sufficient room to pull the calf, if one person can pull the first leg presented until the pastern is 6 inches (12 cm) outside the vulva and, if next while holding the first leg in this position, again one person can pull the second leg equally far outside the vulva.
• At these distances, both shoulders of the calf will have passed the bony entrance of the maternal pelvis.

Posterior Presentation (Cattle)
• About 10%–15% of parturitions occur when the calf is in a posterior presentation.
• Again after applying chains below the dewclaws of the calf and having two persons pull, if both hocks can be presented at the vulva, it indicates that the fetal pelvis has passed through the maternal pelvis and there is sufficient room to deliver the calf vaginally.

RISK FACTORS
• Obesity
• Twins
• Hypocalcemia
• Small frame size
• Large calf

DIAGNOSIS

DIFFERENTIAL DIAGNOSIS
N/A

CBC/BIOCHEMISTRY/URINALYSIS
N/A

OTHER LABORATORY TESTS
N/A

IMAGING
N/A

DIAGNOSTIC PROCEDURES
N/A

PATHOLOGIC FINDINGS
N/A

 TREATMENT

APPROPRIATE HEALTH CARE
• Observation for appetite, vaginal discharge, and temperature
• Certain cases may require systemic antibiotic treatments if they develop metritis.

NURSING CARE
Administration of antibiotics, NSAIDs, and energy and calcium supplements may be indicated.

ACTIVITY
Walking or movement should be limited in those animals that are weak after parturition.

DIET
No limitations

CLIENT EDUCATION
• Management practices to prevent risk factors for dystocia.
• Training in observational strategies and techniques for prompt and correct diagnosis of dystocia.

SURGICAL CONSIDERATION
• Cesarean section may be indicated if a live calf cannot be delivered vaginally.
• Conversely, dead emphysematous calves may require a fetotomy.

 MEDICATIONS

DRUGS OF CHOICE
• Oxytocin 2–3 times/day after parturition. Reassess in 24 hours.
• Systemic antibiotics in prolonged cases may be indicated.

CONTRAINDICATIONS
• Sedatives are contraindicated because they may cause recumbency.
• Appropriate milk and meat withdrawal times must be followed for all compounds administered to food-producing animals.

PRECAUTIONS
Care should be taken that the dam is handled safely.

POSSIBLE INTERACTIONS
N/A

ALTERNATIVE DRUGS
N/A

 FOLLOW-UP

PATIENT MONITORING
Cows should be monitored for signs of toxic metritis.

PREVENTION/ AVOIDANCE
• Proper management of the prepartum cow
• Genetic considerations to help reduce fetal size
• Training of farm personnel in proper observation of preparturient animals.

POSSIBLE COMPLICATIONS
• Trauma and lacerations to the genital tract
• Downer cow (nerve damage)
• Toxic metritis

EXPECTED COURSE AND PROGNOSIS
The majority of assisted dystocia cases properly recover.

 MISCELLANEOUS

ASSOCIATED CONDITIONS
N/A

AGE-RELATED FACTORS
• Obese primiparous animals
• The incidence of dystocia is higher in primiparous than multiparous animals.

ZOONOTIC POTENTIAL
N/A

PREGNANCY
Complicated cases may experience lower fertility.

RUMINANT SPECIES AFFECTED
All ruminant species

BIOSECURITY
N/A

PRODUCTION MANAGEMENT
Attention to appropriate management of the transition period and peripartal animal.

SYNONYMS
Calving problem

SEE ALSO
• Cesarean
• Downer cow
• Reproductive pharmacology
• Toxic metritis

ABBREVIATIONS
NSAIDs = nonsteroidal anti-inflammatory drugs

Suggested Reading
Dargatz, D. A., Dewell, G. A., Mortimer, R. G. 2004, Apr 15. Calving and calving management of beef cows and heifers on cow-calf operations in the United States. *Theriogenology* 61(6):997–1007.
Drost, M. 1992. Management of obstetrics. In: *Large dairy herd management*, ed. H. H. VanHorn, C. J. Wilcox. Champaign, IL: American Science Association.
Larson, R. L., Tyler, J. W., Schultz, L. G., Tessman, R. K., Hostetler, D. E. 2004, Jan 1. Management strategies to decrease calf death losses in beef herds. *J Am Vet Med Assoc.* 224(1):42–48.
Noakes, D. E. 1997, Mar. Dystocia in cattle. *Vet J.* 153(2):123–24.
Roberts, S. J. 1985. Dystocia. In: *Veterinary obstetrics and genital diseases (theriogenology)*, ed. S. J. Roberts. Woodstock, VT: Published by the author.

Author: Carlos A. Risco

ECONOMICS OF BEEF CATTLE REPRODUCTIVE DECISIONS

BASICS

OVERVIEW
Economics is the management of "material wealth." Beef cattle "material wealth" is difficult to quantify, and the return on investment (ROI) varies and depends upon many factors including:
• Ranch business dynamics (family vs. cooperate)
• Geography—United States beef cattle operations are divided roughly by the Mississippi River. Western states have a higher percentage of ranches (27.4%) with ≥50 animals than eastern states (13.8%).
• Goals—Financial gain from beef cattle production may be diluted by "off-farm" income, which can account for over half of total income in small- and medium-sized operations.
• Philosophy—Economic decisions should be followed and reviewed consistently in order to realize progress and goal accomplishment.
• Level of investment—A variety of reproductive tools is available, which range from low to high management intensity and financial involvement. Independent analysis and ROI should be evaluated for each.

PATHOPHYSIOLOGY
N/A

SYSTEMS AFFECTED
Endocrine/metabolic, reproductive, gastrointestinal/nutritional

SIGNALMENT
Some breeds may be more productive in specific geographic locations and require special consideration of:
• Heat tolerance
• Parasite resistance
• Disease resistance
• Native forage availability
• Water availability
• Cattle growth dynamics

SIGNS
Knowledge of beef markets essential

CAUSES AND RISK FACTORS
Financial risks associated with economics of beef cattle reproductive decisions are considerable and are based on:
• Labor—Labor is the single largest cost associated with beef cattle reproductive decisions. Even low-input reproductive decisions such as estrus synchronization requires gathering and handling of cattle, which may be difficult or cost-prohibitive depending upon the geography and dynamics of the operation.
• Record keeping—Although considerable genetic gain can be accomplished using AI or superovulation and ET, this gain may not be readily recognized and, therefore, may be undervalued. Keeping consistent and valid records is an invaluable tool that can help the producer make the appropriate decision about

the future and understand the impact of the reproductive decisions made over the last few years.
• Culling of nonproductive beef cattle—The primary consideration to cull cattle should be lack of productivity. Although the scope of this decision is broader than reproduction, focusing reproductive decisions on cattle that have strong opportunities to become pregnant, rather than on cattle that are available only as a result of inconsistent culling patterns, will reflect a more legitimate view of the reproductive status of the herd (See Table 1).

Table 1

Costs-Benefits Analysis of Some Reproductive Decisions in Beef Cattle

Technique—Estrus Detection
• Costs = $15–50/cow
• Benefits = ↓ calving season
• Other = ↑ labor intensity during breeding and calving

Technique—AI
• Costs = $10–75/cow
• Benefits = ↑ genetic gain, ↑ pounds weaned, ↑ calf value, ↓ bull maintenance
• Other = ↑ semen costs and specialized labor

Technique—ET (donors)
• Costs = $200–350/cow
• Benefits = ↑ visibility, and market scope, international sales
• Other = Few cattle (< 10%) have marketable genetics

Technique—ET (recipients)
• Costs = $50–100/cow
• Benefits = Promotes partnerships, ↑ visibility, market potential
• Other = ↑ facility costs, ↑ labor intensity (calving)

Technique—IVP embryos
• Costs = $2000–3000/calf
• Benefits = Niche market for genetics of geriatric or dying cattle
• Other = Sex ratio skewed to produce more males, large calves, ↑ labor, ↑ lab fees

Technique—Cloning
• Costs = $20,000/calf
• Benefits = Genetic preservation, ↑ market potential
• Other = ↑ labor, ↑ death loss, ↑ maintenance costs

Note: ↓ = decrease; ↑ = increase; AI = artificial insemination; ET = embryo transfer; IVP = in vitro embryo production.

• Miscellaneous (needles, syringes, palpation sleeves, lube, etc.)
• Vaccines, parasite or predator control
Indirect Costs
• Facility modifications (more frequent animal handling)
• Safety devices (added protection/reduced liability, for animals and handlers)
• Enhanced/additional nutrition (minerals, vitamins, etc., for high-value genetics)
• Depreciation on equipment/facilities
• Consultation fees
• Interest on capital improvement expenditures

DIAGNOSIS

Reproductive decision costs: direct and indirect
Direct Costs
• Labor/specialized training
• Estrus synchronization techniques and drugs
• Semen, semen tanks, liquid nitrogen, artificial insemination gun, etc.
• Embryo transfer fees (drugs, professional fees, equipment, etc.)

DIFFERENTIAL DIAGNOSIS
A variety of unforeseen factors may be considered diagnostic factors associated with reproductive decisions.

CBC/BIOCHEMISTRY/URINALYSIS
N/A

OTHER LABORATORY TESTS
N/A

IMAGING
N/A

DIAGNOSTIC PROCEDURES
• Concerned record keeping efforts

ECONOMICS OF BEEF CATTLE REPRODUCTIVE DECISIONS

- Accessing available information and advice (university extension service, consultants, beef journals, etc.)
- Comparisons among beef operations
- Goals/accomplishments

 TREATMENT

Economic decisions should be:
- Based on best-available information
- Strictly adhered to
- Consistently reevaluated
- Compared based upon ROI

 MEDICATIONS

DRUGS OF CHOICE
N/A

CONTRAINDICATIONS
N/A

PRECAUTIONS
The aim and scope of all economic decisions should be based on:
- Farm income
- Financial return of "added value"
- Debt-to-income ratio
- Current (and future) agricultural markets and economics

POSSIBLE INTERACTIONS
N/A

 FOLLOW-UP

PATIENT MONITORING
N/A

POSSIBLE COMPLICATIONS
N/A

EXPECTED COURSE AND PROGNOSIS
The ROI for the economics of beef cattle reproductive decisions should be quantified and consistently evaluated to determine the quality (and the cost) of the individual decisions.

 MISCELLANEOUS

ASSOCIATED CONDITIONS
N/A

AGE-RELATED FACTORS
N/A

ZOONOTIC POTENTIAL
N/A

PREGNANCY
N/A

BIOSECURITY
N/A

PRODUCTION MANAGEMENT
Capacity and history of management schemes can be key indicators of ability to adequately understand economics of reproductive decisions.

RUMINANT SPECIES AFFECTED
Cattle

SEE ALSO
N/A

ABBREVIATIONS
AI = artificial insemination
ET = embryo transfer
IVP = in vitro embryo production
ROI = return on investment

Suggested Reading
Cunningham, M., Latour, M.A., Acker, D. 2005. *Animal science and industry*. 7th ed. Upper Saddle River, N.J. Pearson-Prentice Hall. Chapters 2, 10, 22, 26.
Dargatz, D. A., Dewell, G. A., Mortimer, R. G. 2003. Calving and calving management of beef cows and heifers on cow-calf operations in the United States. *Theriogenology* 61: 997–1007.
Fogleman, S. L., Jones, R. 2003. *Beef cow-calf enterprise*. Farm Management Guide, MF-266. Department of Agricultural Economics, Kansas State University, Manhattan, Kansas 66506-4011.
Johnson, S. K., Jones, R. 2003. Costs and comparisons of estrous synchronization systems. Kansas State Research and Extension Bulletin(s). Kansas State University, Manhattan, Kansas 66506-4011.

Author: John Gibbons

ECTROPION

 BASICS

OVERVIEW
• Ectropion is an eversion or rolling out of the eyelid. This condition can be congenital or acquired. Ectropion allows exposure of the globe and buildup of debris in the ventral conjunctival sac, which can predispose to chronic keratitis or conjunctivitis. Deformed or notched upper eyelid may also be present.
• Irritation of the eyeballs often results from this condition.
• It can be corrected by surgery, if necessary.

Types of Ectropion
• Developmental
• Cicatricial ectropion
• Traumatic
• Postoperative iatrogenic secondary to entropion surgery
• Neurological
• Senile ectropion—connective tissue loses elasticity as it ages.
• Anatomic ectropion—usually congenital, but may intensify as animal ages; can be heritable in some breeds.

PATHOPHYSIOLOGY
Hereditary, congenital, or secondary to trauma/postoperative

ORGAN SYSTEMS AFFECTED
Ophthalmic

GENETICS
• May be an inherited eye defect
• Congenitally rare: reported in piebald sheep

GEOGRAPHIC DISTRIBUTION
Worldwide

INCIDENCE/PREVALENCE
Rare

SIGNALMENT
Lambs are most commonly affected. But depending on the predisposing cause, all ruminant species may be affected.

SIGNS
Blepharospasm, ocular discharge, drooping eyelid, keratoconjunctivitis, eye irritation epiphora, secondary infections are common, exposure keratoconjunctivitis

CAUSES AND RISK FACTORS
Congenital in piebald sheep; the upper eyelid is notched and there is ectropion at the notch. Entropion generally occurs at either side of the notch.

 DIAGNOSIS

Clinically obvious, eyelid is abnormally rolled outward.

DIFFERENTIALS
Foreign body, neoplasia, ophthalmic debris, secondary epiphora

CBC/BIOCHEMISTRY/URINALYSIS
NA

OTHER LABORATORY TESTS
NA

IMAGING
NA

 TREATMENT

• Culling individuals (records)
• Surgical techniques to shorten lids and/or roll the lid inward
• Topical antibiotic/steroid combos to temporarily ease discomfort of secondary infections; surgical repair if conjunctivitis, keratitis, epiphora present

Surgical Technique
• There are numerous procedures available, but most of these are for minor cases of ectropion and include procedures such as V to Y, or trephine.
• Surgery is indicated in only those animals deemed valuable enough to warrant intervention. Surgery should not be attempted on breeding animals with a genetic predisposition.
• If the ectropion is moderately extensive, a full-thickness wedge resection may be indicated.

• If the ectropion is severe and is complicated by notching or other malformation of the eyelid, considerable reconstructive surgery may be necessary.

• The full-thickness wedge removal technique involves taking a full-thickness triangular wedge out of the lateral eyelid area. This procedure has a relatively high rate of dehiscence of the marginal portion of the incision. Close the conjunctiva first, using 6-0 absorbable suture and bury the knots under the conjunctiva, then close the skin with 4–0 or 5-0 silk. Use a "figure of 8" suture for the skin margin.

• May be wise to do a temporary tarsorrhaphy to minimize eyelid movement and stress on the incision site; sutures removed in 10-14 days

• Can use topical antibiotics and steroid afterward, but probably unnecessary

MEDICATIONS

DRUGS OF CHOICE
Topical antibiotics and steroids may be indicated.

CONTRAINDICATIONS
Appropriate milk and meat withdrawal times must be followed for all compounds administered to food-producing animals.

FOLLOW-UP

PATIENT MONITORING

PREVENTION/AVOIDANCE
Cull affected animals that appear as genetic carriers. Avoid ophthalmic trauma and, if at all possible, do not perform entropion surgery on immature animals.

POSSIBLE COMPLICATIONS
Keratoconjunctivitis, dehiscence after surgery, recurrence

EXPECTED COURSE AND PROGNOSIS
Fair to good with surgery

MISCELLANEOUS

ASSOCIATED CONDITIONS
This condition may predispose to keratoconjunctivitis.

AGE-RELATED FACTORS
Generally found in young animals or postsurgical patients

ZOONOTIC POTENTIAL
N/A

PREGNANCY
N/A

RUMINANT SPECIES AFFECTED
Sheep most commonly affected, but can occur in all ruminant species.

BIOSECURITY
N/A

PRODUCTION MANAGEMENT
Remove mothers and offspring from the breeding program as the condition may be hereditary.

SEE ALSO
Entropion
Keratoconjunctivitis

ABBREVIATIONS
N/A

Suggested Reading
Gelatt, K. N. 2000. *Essentials of veterinary ophthalmology.* Baltimore: Lippincott, Williams and Wilkins.
Lackner, P. A. 2001, Feb. Techniques for surgical correction of adnexal disease. *Clin Tech Small Anim Pract.* 16(1): 40–50.
Moore, C. P., Constantinescu, G. M. 1997, Sep. Surgery of the adnexa. *Vet Clin North Am Small Anim Pract.* 27(5): 1011–66.
Moore, C. P., Whitley, R. D. 1984, Nov. Ophthalmic diseases of small domestic ruminants. *Vet Clin North Am Large Anim Pract.* 6(3): 641–65.
Van Der Woerdt, A. 2004, Sep-Oct. Adnexal surgery in dogs and cats. *Vet Ophthalmol.* 7(5): 284–90.

Author: Melissa N. Carr

EDEMA, PERIPHERAL

 BASICS

OVERVIEW
• Edema is an abnormally increased accumulation of fluid in the interstitium.
• Edema in ruminants is most often caused by either increased intravascular hydrostatic pressure or decreased intravascular colloid osmotic (oncotic) pressure.

SYSTEMS AFFECTED
Multiple systems affected depending on underlying disease

GENETICS
N/A

INCIDENCE/PREVALENCE
Unknown

GEOGRAPHIC DISTRIBUTION
Worldwide

SIGNALMENT
Species
All ruminant species affected

Breed Predilections
N/A

Mean Age and Range
N/A

Predominant Sex
N/A

SIGNS
Edema can nearly always be distinguished from other causes of tissue swelling based upon whether or not a "pit" is left following firm, digital pressure applied to the tissue over several seconds. It is important to maintain the pressure over time to allow the excess fluid time to escape between the cells.

CAUSES AND RISK FACTORS
• Increased intravascular hydrostatic pressure:
  • Traumatic reticulopericarditis ("hardware disease") leading to cardiac tamponade
• Bacterial endocarditis
• Adult/enzootic/BLV associated lymphosarcoma affecting the right heart base
• Severe current or previous pneumonia or other primary lung disease leading to cor pulmonale
• High altitude disease/brisket disease
• Congenital heart defect
• Thymic/adolescent lymphosarcoma
• Decreased intravascular oncotic pressure:
  • Protein losing enteropathies:
    (a) Clinical parasitism.
    (b) Johne's disease/*Mycobacterium avium* subspecies *paratuberculosis*
    (c) Bovine viral diarrhea
    (d) Salmonellosis
  • Protein losing nephropathies:
    (a) Pyelonephritis
    (b) Renal amyloidosis
  • Failure of the liver to produce adequate albumin:
This is rare in ruminants but can occur (e.g., in cases of severe protein or caloric malnutrition).
• Other causes:
• Increased capillary permeability (e.g. insect or snake bite).
• Obstruction of lymphatic return (e.g. thymic/adolescent lymphosarcoma).
• Monensin or lasalocid toxicity.
• Copper deficiency.

 DIAGNOSIS

DIFFERENTIAL DIAGNOSES
• Cellulitis
• Urolithiasis
• Caval syndrome
• "Normal" edema in primiparous cows
• Neck chain or leg band applied too tightly restricting venous return
• Overzealous IV fluid administration

CBC/BIOCHEMISTRY/URINALYSIS
• Packed cell volume/total protein concentration
  • A PCV/TP is simple to run and can quickly help to distinguish between cardiac and oncotic causes of edema.
  • The TP must be interpreted with caution:
    (a) Oncotic causes of edema are typically due to low albumin. Total serum protein includes other proteins (primarily globulin) in addition to albumin and may be within normal limits despite hypoalbuminemia.
    (b) Dehydration can lead to the spurious conclusion that the total protein level is within normal limits in an animal with true hypoproteinemia. A PCV run on the same sample provides at least some reference for interpretation of the test vis-à-vis the animal's hydration status.
  • CBC/chemistry profile
• Hypoalbuminemia is suggestive of the low oncotic pressure causes of edema.
• Hyperglobulinemia is suggestive of a chronic inflammatory problem such as traumatic reticulopericarditis.
• Urinalysis
  • Proteinuria is highly suggestive of a protein losing nephropathy.
  • *Important note*: The pH of ruminant urine is often quite alkaline (high pH). At high pH, the protein indicator on urine test strips may be falsely positive.

OTHER LABORATORY TESTS
• Fecal flotation for parasite ova
• Johne's test

IMAGING
Ultrasound may help to distinguish between edema and cellulitis.

OTHER DIAGNOSTIC PROCEDURES
• Cardiac auscultation. Note rate, rhythm, and the presence of any murmur. If a cardiac cause of edema is suspected, then the heart rate will generally be at least mildly elevated.

• Observation and palpation of venous (primarily jugular) distension. Note that the head must be elevated above the scapulohumeral joint. The jugular vein is normally moderately distended ventral to the level of the scapulohumeral joint.
• Palpation of peripheral lymph nodes

PATHOLOGICAL FINDINGS
Findings will be dependent upon the underlying disease.

TREATMENT
• Edema is not a disease but rather a manifestation of disease. In general, the treatment for edema is to treat the underlying disease.
• Animals receiving intravenous fluid therapy (e.g., neonatal diarrhea) sometimes over time develop edema due to decreased intravascular oncotic pressure. In these cases, it is necessary to switch to plasma (preferred) or colloids for volume expansion.

MEDICATIONS
DRUGS OF CHOICE
• Furosemide: 0.05 to 1.0 mg/kg IV or IM
• Dexamethasone: Approximately 0.04 mg/kg IV or IM
• Naquasone (dexamethasone 5 mg and trichlormethiazide 200 mg) bolus: 1 to 2 boluses initially followed by 1/2 to 1 bolus daily for udder edema

CONTRAINDICATIONS/POSSIBLE INTERACTIONS
• Dexamethasone should be used cautiously when a concurrent infectious process is or may be present.

• Drug withdrawal time periods for meat and milk need to be followed.

FOLLOW-UP
N/A

MISCELLANEOUS
• Some degree of udder edema in primiparous dairy cows is normal. This is secondary to the changes that occur in the vascular system of the udder when the first calf is born.
• Severe edema can have deleterious effects (mastitis, increased susceptibility to herpes mamillitis, etc.).
• Investigations of herd problems with abnormally severe udder edema in first calf cows should initially focus upon the immediate prefresh diet of the heifers, specifically levels of minerals (sodium particularly), readily fermentable carbohydrate (starch), and protein.

ASSOCIATED CONDITIONS
N/A

AGE-RELATED FACTORS
N/A

ZOONOTIC POTENTIAL
N/A

PREGNANCY
N/A

RUMINANT SPECIES AFFECTED
Potentially all ruminant species may be affected.

BIOSECURITY
N/A

PRODUCTION MANAGEMENT
N/A

SYNONYMS
N/A

SEE ALSO
Urolithiasis
Specific disease sections

ABBREVIATIONS
BLV = bovine leukosis virus
CBC = complete blood count
IM = intramuscular
IV = intravenous
PCV = packed cell volume
pH = measure of acid/base concentration
TP = total protein

Suggested Reading
Angel, K. L., Tyler, J. W. 1992, Jul-Aug. Pulmonary hypertension and cardiac insufficiency in three cows with primary lung disease. *J Vet Intern Med*. 6(4): 214–19.
Guyton, A. C., Hall, J. E. 2000. The body fluid compartments: extracellular and intracellular fluids; interstitial fluid and edema. In: *Textbook of medical physiology*, 10th ed., pp. 264–78. Philadelphia. W. B. Saunders.
Kinsky, M. P., Milner, S. M., Button, B., Dubick, M. A., Kramer, G. C. 2000, Nov. Resuscitation of severe thermal injury with hypertonic saline dextran: effects on peripheral and visceral edema in sheep. *J Trauma* 49(5): 844–53.
Malven, P. V., Erb, R. E., D'Amico, M. F., Stewart, T. S., Chew, B. P. 1983, Feb. Factors associated with edema of the mammary gland in primigravid dairy heifers. *J Dairy Sci*. 66(2): 246–52.

Author: Lowell T. Midla

EMBRYO CRYOPRESERVATION

 BASICS

OVERVIEW
Embryo cryopreservation (or freezing) is a method of holding embryos in a suspended metabolic state for a number of reasons.
• Transfer into recipients at a more suitable time
• Transport embryos to a distant location
• Market high value genetics
• Schedule embryo transfer (ET) when recipients are available.
• Embryo cryopreservation is also a primary reason that bovine ET is a large industry in the United States (over half of the bovine embryos collected in 2003 in the United States were cryopreserved).

PATHOPHYSIOLOGY
Advantages of embryo cryopreservation compared to ET of fresh embryos:
• Allows calves to be born during a favorable season of the year
• Allows many embryos to be transferred at a single location
• Allows synchronized recipients to be utilized if few fresh embryos are collected on a given day

SYSTEMS AFFECTED
Endocrine/metabolic, reproductive

SIGNALMENT
Embryos from some breeds of cattle (i.e., *Bos indicus* and Jersey) may exhibit a low pregnancy rate following ET, perhaps due to lipid content in the cytoplasm of embryo cells.

SIGNS
N/A

CAUSES AND RISK FACTORS
The bovine uterus is highly immunocompetent; however, introduction of foreign material during ET (of fresh or frozen embryos) is possible.

 DIAGNOSIS

In order to recover embryos for cryopreservation, the uterus of the donor female is lavaged (usually 7 days after estrus) with a simple isotonic salt solution. Donor females are generally stimulated with FSH to produce multiple ovulations and are then inseminated (usually via AI) to allow for fertilization. Embryos are recovered and staged (according to the IETS) as the following (on day 7):
• Stage 3 = Degenerate
• Stage 4 = Morula
• Stage 5 = Early blastocyst
• Stage 6 = Full blastocyst
• Stage 7 = Expanding blastocyst
• Stage 8 = Hatched blastocyst
There may also be unfertilized ova. Within each stage classification embryos are graded (grade 1, 2, or 3 with 1 being the highest quality). Grade 3 embryos are usually not cryopreserved due to poor conception rates post thaw.

DIFFERENTIAL DIAGNOSIS
N/A

CBC/BIOCHEMISTRY/URINALYSIS
N/A

OTHER LABORATORY TESTS
N/A

IMAGING
Bovine embryos are approximately 150 μm in diameter and must be visualized with the aid of a microscope ($\geq$ 60x magnification).

DIAGNOSTIC PROCEDURES
Grading embryos is a subjective process.

 TREATMENT

Cryopreservation Technique
• Embryos can be equilibrated and cryopreserved in a variety of medias that contain different cryoprotectants usually involving a gradual cooling process:
  • Glycerol (1.0–1.5 M)
  • Ethylene glycol (1.0–2.0 M)
• Embryos can also be rapidly cryopreserved (vitrification) using a much higher concentration of cryoprotectants (Gly = 5.0–7.0 M, EG = 3.0–8.0 M). Regardless of technique, embryos are usually cryopreserved in 1/4 or 1/5 ml plastic straws and housed in properly identified goblets and canes.
• Gradual cooling protocols initiate freezing at -7.0°C and cool at a rate of about 0.5°C per minute to -35°C. Before the embryos begin the cooling ramp, they are "seeded" to initiate ice crystal formation and prevent negative effects of latent heat. Embryos are plunged into liquid nitrogen (-196°C) after reaching -35.0°C. Vitrification is a protocol in which the embryos in the highly concentrated cryoprotectant media are introduced into liquid nitrogen after a short time (1–10 minutes).

Thawing Technique
Most thawing protocols employ a 5–10 second air thaw, and then a 20–30 second submersion in a 30°C water bath. In order to slowly replace the Gly with water and prohibit embryo cells from rupturing, embryos cryopreserved in Gly require a stepwise removal of the Gly usually buffered with varying sucrose concentrations. Embryos cryopreserved with EG can be thawed and transferred directly (DT) to the waiting recipient. Depending upon concentration and type of cryoprotectants, vitrified embryos can be slowly rehydrated during the thawing process or transferred directly.

EMBRYO CRYOPRESERVATION

MEDICATIONS

DRUGS OF CHOICE
N/A

CONTRAINDICATIONS
N/A

PRECAUTIONS
Some cryoprotectants can be absorbed through the skin, and possibly the uterine endometrium following ET. Exposure effects of small amounts of cryoprotectants are not described.

POSSIBLE INTERACTIONS
N/A

FOLLOW-UP

PATIENT MONITORING
N/A

POSSIBLE COMPLICATIONS
N/A

EXPECTED COURSE AND PROGNOSIS
Pregnancy rates of embryos following cryopreservation, thawing, and ET are variable and related to many factors.
• Embryo/recipient synchrony
• Embryo quality
• Stage of embryo development
• Recipient quality

MISCELLANEOUS

ASSOCIATED CONDITIONS
• Advantages of DT embryos
  • No microscope needed
  • Limited assistance needed
  • Reduced thaw time
• Advantages of Gly embryos
  • Enables postthaw grading and evaluation of embryos
  • May be required by some breed registries
• Advantages of vitrified embryos
  • No intercellular ice crystals
  • Enables many embryos to be frozen in a short time

AGE-RELATED FACTORS
N/A

ZOONOTIC POTENTIAL
N/A

PREGNANCY
Pregnancy rates following ET of cryopreserved/thawed bovine embryos range (40%–60%).

RUMINANT SPECIES AFFECTED
Cattle

BIOSECURITY
Embryos should be frozen in sealed straws regardless of protocol to prevent viral/bacterial contamination.

PRODUCTION MANAGEMENT
DT embryos have distinct time and resource management advantages.

SEE ALSO
Embryo collection
Embryo quality
Embryo transfer
Pregnancy

ABBREVIATIONS
AETA = American Embryo Transfer Association
AI = artificial insemination
DT = direct transfer
EG = ethylene glycol
ET = embryo transfer
FSH = follicle stimulating hormone
Gly = glycerol
IETS = International Embryo Transfer Society

Suggested Reading
Beardon, H. J., Fuquay, J. W., Wilard, S. T. 2004. *Applied animal reproduction.* 6th ed. Upper Saddle River, NJ: Pearson-Prentice Hall.
Mitchell, J. R., Doak, G. A. 2004. *The AI and ET of dairy and beef cattle; a handbook and laboratory manual.* 7th ed. Upper Saddle River, NJ: Pearson-Prentice Hall.
Nedambale, T. L., Dinnyes, A., Groen, W., Dobrinsky, J. R., Tian, X. C., Yang, X. 2004. Comparison of in vitro fertilized bovine embryos cultured in KSOM or SOF and cryopreserved by slow freezing or vitrification. *Theriogenology* 62(3):437–449.
Saha, S., Otoi, M., Takagi, M., Boedino, A., Sumantri, C., Suzuki, T. 1996. Normal calves obtained after direct transfer of vitrified bovine embryos using ethylene glycol, trehalose, and polyvinlypyrrolidone. *Cryobiology* 33: 291–99.

Authors: John Gibbons and Paul E. Maunisk

EMESIS

 BASICS

OVERVIEW

- Emesis, or vomiting, is a centrally mediated event originating in the medulla.
- The medullary vomiting center can be stimulated by visceral afferent stimuli or by stimulation of the chemoreceptor trigger zone.
- In ruminant species, activation of the chemoreceptor trigger zone most often results from stimulation via toxins.
- Emesis is an unusual occurrence in ruminant species.

GENETICS

No genetic factors have been identified in animals that vomit, however management factors may play a significant role when vomiting is observed in calves.

SIGNALMENT

Species
- All ruminant species may be affected.
- Sheep and goats may be more affected than cattle due to their dietary indiscretions but signs may be observed in any adult ruminant.

Breed Predilection
N/A

Mean Age and Range
- Emesis can occur in any age animal.
- In young animals, emesis may result from congenital anomalies such as persistent right aortic arch or esophageal diverticula.
- Young animals are also more prone to diseases such as meningitis and may suffer trauma to the central nervous system.
- It is very rare to observe vomiting in animals less then 6 months of age due to lack of exposure to agents that cause vomiting.

Predominant Sex
N/A

SIGNS
- Signs of anorexia and hypersalivation typically precede emesis.
- Emesis involves coordinated contractions of the abdominal and diaphragm muscles with concurrent relaxation of the cardia.

CAUSES AND RISK FACTORS

- Workup of a case involving emesis (true vomiting) must include attainment of an appropriate history, physical examination, and examination of the environment in which the animal or animals reside.
- History most commonly associated with signs of emesis includes potential exposure to various toxins or poisonous plants. This is especially pertinent when multiple animals are showing signs.
- Toxins that can result in emesis include methanol or ethanol, copper, phosphorus, arsenic, nitrates, snakebite, and petroleum products.
- Numerous poisonous plants can cause emesis and exposure is clearly dependent on plant availability. A partial list of plants includes

> Castor bean
> Cocklebur
> Cyanogenic plants (Arrow grass, Johnson grass, Sudan grass, chokecherry, elderberry, etc.)
> *Delphinium* (larkspur)
> Laurel
> *Melia* (chinaberry)
> Nitrate accumulators (pigweed, lamb's quarter, Jimson weed, fireweed, dock, Johnson grass, oats, millet, rye, corn, sorghum, etc.)
> Oleander
> *Solanum* spp.
> *Veratrum* (hellebore)
> *Zigandenus* spp. (death camas)

- Other conditions that have been associated are difficult dental eruptions or tooth root abscesses, late-stage hypocalcemia, grain overload, traumatic reticuloperitonitis, diaphragmatic hernia, abomasal impactions, and vagal indigestion.
- Outbreaks of vomiting in a herd situation are likely due to ingestion of spoiled corn silage or ingestion of toxic plants such as azaleas, rhododendrons, lily of the valley, or sneezeweed. A report of a flock outbreak in sheep was attributed to gram-negative endotoxins that had contaminated a shipment of prepared feed.

 DIAGNOSIS

Based on history and clinical signs

DIFFERENTIAL DIAGNOSIS
- Most cases of feed returning to the mouth of ruminants is due to regurgitation (i.e., reflux of esophageal or rumen contents into the mouth or nose).
- Excessive regurgitation typically results from physical blockage of the esophagus, cardia, or rumenoreticular outflow.
- Common conditions resulting in regurgitation include foreign bodies, tumors, papillomas, granulomas, abscesses, diaphragmatic hernia, or esophageal irritation.
- Pharyngeal lesions (e.g., balling gun injury) may also cause gagging or retching, but this is not true emesis.
- Passage of a stomach tube may aid in determining if the normal passage of ingesta from mouth to cardia is impeded.

CBC/BIOCHEMISTRY/URINALYSIS
In chronic cases, a CBC may be of benefit to identify elevated fibrinogen levels if the cause is associated with an esophageal abscess. Clinical signs of hypocalcemia will be confirmed with a biochemistry profile. Electrolyte profiles can be helpful in correcting bicarbonate deficits and hydration status.

OTHER LABORATORY TESTS
N/A

IMAGING
- None directly applicable to emesis; however, ultrasound, radiology (plain or contrast), and endoscopy may be considered to assist in ruling out pharyngeal or esophageal disease.
- Contrast radiography of the cervical and thoracic regions is beneficial in defining obstructive lesions associated with the esophagus. Barium studies can be helpful in small ruminants.

PATHOLOGICAL FINDINGS
- Toxins or toxic plants present in forestomachs
- CNS lesions involving medulla

TREATMENT

• Removal of animals from offending toxin or toxic plants
• Specific antidotes or treatments for various toxins may be indicated.
• Rumenotomy may be indicated.
• The use of laxatives or ruminotorics to increase forestomach motility and passage of ingesta is unlikely to be of practical benefit in an animal that is actively vomiting.
• Transfer of fresh rumen fluid from a healthy donor is likely to restore rumen flora and function once the vomiting has ceased.

MEDICATIONS

DRUGS OF CHOICE
Magnesium oxide, activated charcoal and mineral oil are indicated as an aid in removing or limiting absorption of toxins. Antibiotics may be used to prevent bacterial sepsis associated with rumenitis.

CONTRAINDICATIONS
• The use of anti-emetics (e.g., phenothiazines, antihistamines, metaclopramide) in ruminant species is not well documented.
• It may be contraindicated to chemically block the elimination of toxicants from the forestomach of an animal actively vomiting
• Appropriate milk and meat withdrawal times must be followed for all compounds administered to food producing animals.

FOLLOW-UP

PATIENT MONITORING
Monitor patient for continued signs of emesis and possible complications.

PREVENTION/AVOIDANCE
Avoid exposure to poisonous plants or toxic compounds.

POSSIBLE COMPLICATIONS
• Complications associated with emesis (or regurgitation) include aspiration pneumonia, dehydration, electrolyte derangements, or acid-base abnormalities.
• The term "internal vomiting" has been used to describe a form of vagal indigestion whereby abomasal outflow is blocked and the abomasal contents are refluxed into the reticulorumen.
• Hypochloremic metabolic alkalosis often results from internal vomiting, conceivably could occur with emesis.

EXPECTED COURSE AND PROGNOSIS
• Depending on the dose and duration of a toxic insult, prognosis is guarded to good if animals are immediately removed from the source of the toxin.
• Complications including metabolic derangements and aspiration pneumonia worsen the prognosis.

MISCELLANEOUS

ASSOCIATED CONDITIONS
N/A

AGE-RELATED FACTORS
• In young animals, emesis may result from congenital anomalies such as persistent right aortic arch or esophageal diverticula.
• Young animals are also more prone to diseases such as meningitis and may suffer trauma to the central nervous system.

ZOONOTIC POTENTIAL
N/A

PREGNANCY
N/A

BIOSECURITY
N/A

PRODUCTION MANAGEMENT
• Pharyngeal lesions (e.g., balling gun injury) may cause gagging or retching, but this is not true emesis.

• Passage of a stomach tube may aid in determining if the normal passage of ingesta from mouth to cardia is impeded.

SEE ALSO
Arsenic
Copper
Methanol or ethanol
Nitrates
Petroleum products
Phosphorus
Snakebite
Specific toxic plant chapters
Transfaunation

ABBREVIATIONS
CNS = central nervous system

Suggested Reading
Bizimenyera, E. S. 2003, Aug. Acute poisoning of Friesian heifers by *Solanum macrocarpon* L. ssp dasyphyllum. *Vet Hum Toxicol.* 45(4):222–23.
Galey, F. D., Holstege, D. M., Plumlee, K. H., Tor, E., Johnson, B., Anderson, M. L., Blanchard, P. C., Brown, F. 1996, Jul. Diagnosis of oleander poisoning in livestock. *J Vet Diagn Invest.* 8(3):358–64.
Plumlee, K., ed. 2003. *Clinical veterinary toxicology.* St. Louis: Mosby.
Porter, M. B., MacKay, R. J., Uhl, E., Platt, S. R., de Lahunta, A. 2003, Aug 15. Neurologic disease putatively associated with ingestion of *Solanum viarum* in goats. *J Am Vet Med Assoc.* 223(4): 456, 501–504.
Smith, B. P., ed. 2002. *Large animal internal medicine.* 3rd ed. St. Louis: Mosby.

Authors: George Barrington and Dennis D. French

ENDOMETRITIS

BASICS

DEFINITION
• Endometritis is inflammation of the lining of the uterus (endometrium) without systemic illness. It is associated with chronic bacterial infection of the uterus beyond 3 weeks postpartum and is characterized by purulent uterine discharge and delayed involution of the reproductive tract.
• Endometritis has clinical importance to the extent that it causes impaired fertility in the breeding period.
• There are few clinical trials with validated diagnostic criteria, economically meaningful outcomes, and correct analyses, resulting in controversy over the optimum methods of diagnosis and treatment.

PATHOPHYSIOLOGY
• Contamination of the uterus with a wide variety of bacteria is nearly universal after calving.
• The key element in the pathophysiology of endometritis is the immune response of the uterus to effect uterine involution and to clear bacterial infection.
• The central mechanism of bacterial clearance is nonspecific immunity (phagocytosis by neutrophils). By 3 to 4 weeks postpartum, the number of bacteria and the variety of species have diminished substantially in healthy cows.
• In cows with clinical endometritis, the most common isolates are *Arcanobacterium pyogenes*, *Streptococcus* spp., and *E. coli*.
• The only bacterium that is consistently associated with uterine inflammation is *A. pyogenes*. This opportunistic, gram-positive facultative anaerobe is commonly present in mixed culture with a wide variety of organisms, but most often with the gram-negative anaerobes *Fusobacterium necrophorum* and *Prevotella melaninogenica* (formerly *Bacteroides melaninogenicus*).
• Toxins and enzymes from these bacteria cause inflammation of the endometrium, which may impair ovarian function and inhibit establishment of pregnancy.

SYSTEMS AFFECTED
Reproductive

GENETICS
No known association

INCIDENCE/PREVALENCE
• The reported prevalence of postpartum endometritis varies widely, depending on the case definition and method of diagnosis, and the interval postpartum at examination. Unfortunately, in many studies, the case definition was not explicit, and in most cases was not validated as being associated with reproductive performance.
• The incidence of endometritis in a review of 43 studies ranged from 2% to 37.3%, with a median of 10%.
• Using validated diagnostic criteria, between 3 and 5 weeks postpartum the prevalence was 17%, varying among herds from 5% to 26%.

GEOGRAPHIC DISTRIBUTION
Worldwide, in intensively managed dairy cattle

SIGNALMENT
Species
Cattle; predominantly dairy cattle; 3 to 8 weeks after calving

Breed Predilections
None known

Mean Age and Range
Lactating adults; all parities affected, but more common in older (≥ third parity) than younger cattle

Predominant Sex
Females only

SIGNS
Mucopurulent or purulent discharge from the vulva, but this sign is frequently not observed by chance alone. Internal examination is required.

HISTORICAL FINDINGS
Cows with endometritis will frequently have been affected with one or more risk factors early in the current lactation.

PHYSICAL EXAMINATION FINDINGS
• It is important to interpret physical exam findings in light of normal postpartum involution of the reproductive tract, and to allow time for involution to occur in healthy cattle before making a diagnosis of endometritis.
• Although data on normal involution are piecemeal, on average, healthy cows achieve a stable uterine horn diameter of 4–5 cm by 25–30 DIM, and cervical diameter <5 cm by 40 DIM.
• Lochia is normally passed until 14–23 DIM and, over the course of involution, lochia changes from thin red-brown fluid to more viscous sanguineous-purulent to yellow-white mucous liquid. Complete microscopic involution takes until approximately 40 DIM. Therefore, examination of cattle for endometritis should be done no sooner than 3 weeks postpartum. Practically, diagnosis and treatment should only be initiated 4 weeks after calving (i.e., >28 to 30 DIM).
• Examination should include visual inspection of the perineum for fresh mucopurulent or purulent discharge. Vaginoscopy is recommended to improve both the sensitivity and specificity of diagnosis. Insertion of a clean-gloved hand after wiping the vulva with a paper towel is an alternative to vaginoscopy. At 4 weeks postpartum, mucopurulent or purulent discharge (but not mucus with flecks of pus) from the cervix, and cervical diameter >7.5 cm are significantly associated with increased time to pregnancy.
• Transrectal palpation of the uterus has traditionally been the means of diagnosis of endometritis, but this method is subjective and has poor sensitivity and specificity for identifying cows with impaired fertility.
• Given knowledge about cervical discharge and size, palpation of uterine size, symmetry, and texture had no predictive value for reproductive performance.
• There is some evidence to suggest that blanket treatment of cows with RP, dystocia, or purulent vulvar discharge noticed by the herd manager after 13 DIM, without any examination to specifically diagnose endometritis, may be economically advantageous at the herd level. However, the value of the effort for individual diagnosis and treatment depends on the sensitivity and specificity of the diagnostic criteria, the prevalence of endometritis, and the cost and efficacy of treatment.
• Additionally, there are cows without these risk factors that have clinical endometritis (detectable by examination of vaginal discharge).

CAUSES
• Failure of uterine immune defenses resulting in chronic bacterial infection of the uterus that persists beyond 3 weeks postpartum
• The central etiologic agent is *Arcanobacterium pyogenes*, although there is commonly a mixed infection with anaerobes (*Fusobacterium necrophorum, Prevotella melaninogenica*).

RISK FACTORS
RP, dystocia, twins, metritis, and clinical ketosis are risk factors for endometritis, the greatest of which is RP. However, in one large field trial with a validated case definition, over half the cows with clinical endometritis did not have any of the significant risk factors (twins, RP, or metritis).

DIAGNOSIS
For reproductive examinations before the breeding period to have value, they must identify cows at increased risk of failure to become pregnant in a timely way and that may benefit from treatment.

DIFFERENTIAL DIAGNOSIS
Pyometra (uterus filled with pus, with a CL present); metritis (more severe uterine infection with systemic signs including fever; occurs in the first week postpartum)

CBC/BIOCHEMISTRY/URINALYSIS
N/A

OTHER LABORATORY TESTS
• Uterine bacteriologic culture (collected transcervically using a guarded swab) or uterine biopsy (using mare biopsy forceps) might be useful to investigate unusual cases or epidemics but are not useful for routine diagnosis.
• Subclinical endometritis can be diagnosed by uterine cytology, either by transcervical cytobrush, or flush and aspiration of 20–60 ml of saline, centrifugation, and staining of smears. This technique is novel in cattle, but cows with >5% or >18% neutrophils at 5 weeks postpartum, or >1% at 40–60 DIM in the absence of clinical signs (see below) had reduced reproductive performance.

IMAGING
Subclinical endometritis can be diagnosed by transrectal ultrasonography on the basis of fluid in the uterine lumen.

DIAGNOSTIC PROCEDURES
Inspection of uterine/vaginal discharge by vaginoscopy or manual examination with a clean glove, as well as transrectal palpation of the diameter of the cervix; palpation of the diameter of the uterine horns (>8 cm diameter) may be useful in the absence of inspection of vaginal discharge, but is an insensitive method.

PATHOLOGIC FINDINGS
Histologically, disruption of the endometrial epithelium, infiltration of inflammatory cells, and accumulations of lymphocytes, vascular congestion, and stromal edema

TREATMENT

APPROPRIATE HEALTH CARE
Outpatient medical

NURSING CARE
N/A

ACTIVITY
As usual

DIET
As usual

CLIENT EDUCATION
See Prevention/Avoidance below.

SURGICAL CONSIDERATIONS
N/A

MEDICATIONS
• The general principle of therapy for endometritis is to reverse inflammatory changes that impair fertility by reducing the load of pathogenic bacteria and enhancing the processes of uterine defense and repair.

• Well-designed, appropriately analyzed, large-scale field studies of the diagnosis and treatment of endometritis with both an objective case definition and economically meaningful outcomes are lacking. Many therapeutic trials suffer from a lack of negative controls, small numbers of animals resulting in little statistical power, or both. Most investigations have used diagnostic criteria that were not validated as to their effect on reproductive performance, making it difficult or impossible to discern a true treatment effect.

DRUGS OF CHOICE
• IU Antibiotic—the principle is to reduce the load of pathogens. There are two valid studies showing that one treatment of 0.5 g cephapirin benzathine IU at approximately 30 DIM reduced time to pregnancy relative to untreated cases.
• PGF—the principle is to induce luteolysis and in turn, estrus. Reducing or removing the influence of progesterone on the uterus and causing myometrial contractions should enhance resolution of endometritis. There is controversy over whether PGF causes myometrial contraction or other benefits for treatment of endometritis in the absence of a CL. On balance, PGF is most effective when a CL is present. Although clear-cut data are lacking, IM injection of PGF (0.5 mg cloprostenol or 25 mg dinoprost) after approximately 30 DIM is likely beneficial as treatment for endometritis. A second administration of PGF 14 days later may provide additional benefit, although clinical trial data are lacking.

CONTRAINDICATIONS
Use of PGF before approximately 26 DIM is controversial. Some studies suggest beneficial effects, many suggest no benefit, and a few report a deleterious effect on subsequent reproductive performance among cows with endometritis.

PRECAUTIONS
• Cephapirin benzathine is approved for use in lactating cows in Canada and the European Union, but not in the United States. IU tetracycline and other antibiotics may result in violative drug residues in milk.
• Drug withdrawal times need to be determined and maintained for all treated food animals.

ENDOMETRITIS

POSSIBLE INTERACTIONS

None known

ALTERNATIVE DRUGS

There are reports of treatment of endometritis by IU infusion of oxytetracycline, crystalline penicillin G, and numerous other antibiotics, as well as Lugol's iodine, povidone iodine, and other disinfectants, and systemically administered estradiol, tetracycline, penicillin, and ceftiofur. There is little evidence that any of these improve reproductive performance, and several of the IU substances may cause damage to the endometrium or to uterine defenses.

 FOLLOW-UP

PATIENT MONITORING

Follow-up examination and repeated treatment 2 weeks after initial diagnosis and treatment (i.e., at approximately 45 DIM) might be useful to identify refractory cases. However, in almost 80% of cases, clinical signs will be resolved by this time, even if untreated.

PREVENTION/AVOIDANCE

• The key element in establishment of chronic uterine infection appears to be the effectiveness of uterine defense mechanisms in clearing the inevitable infection. However, there is little information on preventive measures specific to endometritis.
• Management and nutritional practices that prevent dystocia, RP, and metritis by favoring peripartum immune function (e.g., transition diet to meet or exceed NRC 2001 for >3 weeks prepartum with average DMI >12 kg/cow/day, >60 cm manger space/cow, calving at BCS = 3.5 out of 5) will plausibly reduce the incidence of endometritis.

POSSIBLE COMPLICATIONS

• Given the case definition of a localized uterine condition, there is no mortality attributable to endometritis, and no direct loss of milk production. Reports have shown an increase in the mean calving to pregnancy interval from 7 to 48 days for cows with endometritis compared to unaffected herd mates, despite various treatments administered to affected animals.

• A meta-analysis of 23 studies found that endometritis increased mean days open by 15, decreased the relative risk of pregnancy by 150 DIM by 31%, and reduced the rate at which cows became pregnant by 16%.
• Cows with mucopurulent or purulent cervical discharge or cervical diameter >7.5 cm at approximately 4 weeks postpartum had an increase of 32 days in median time to pregnancy over unaffected cows.

EXPECTED COURSE AND PROGNOSIS

Affected cows take longer, and are at increased risk of failure to become pregnant. Clinical signs will be resolved by 60 DIM in >95% of cases after one (or in a minority of cases, two) treatment with cephapirin IU or PGF. The issue is how many of these are truly cured as opposed to cases of ongoing subclinical endometritis.

 MISCELLANEOUS

ASSOCIATED CONDITIONS

Cows with endometritis may be at greater risk of pyometra.

AGE-RELATED FACTORS

N/A

ZOONOTIC POTENTIAL

N/A

PREGNANCY

N/A

RUMINANT SPECIES AFFECTED

Bovine (common), caprine, ovine, camelid (uncommon)

BIOSECURITY

The bacteria that appear to be a necessary cause of endometritis are ubiquitous opportunists and there is no evidence that they are contagious; their presence on the farm or even in the reproductive tract is not by itself sufficient to cause disease. Therefore, prevention of new cases should be directed as nonspecific enhancement of immunity in peripartum animals.

PRODUCTION MANAGEMENT

N/A

SYNONYMS

Uterine infection (commonly but incorrectly referred to interchangeably with metritis)

SEE ALSO

Metritis
Pyometra

ABBREVIATIONS

BCS = body condition score
CL = corpus luteum
DIM = days in milk (days after calving)
DMI = dry matter intake
IM = intramuscular
IU = intrauterine
NRC = National Research Council
PGF = prostaglandin F2γ
RP = retained placenta

Suggested Reading
Gilbert, R. O. 1992. Bovine endometritis: the burden of proof. *Cornell Vet.* 82:11–14.
LeBlanc, S. J., Duffield, T., Leslie, K., Bateman, K., Keefe, G., Walton, J., Johnson, W. 2002. Defining and diagnosing postpartum clinical endometritis, and its impact on reproductive performance in dairy cows. *J Dairy Sci.* 85:2223–36.
LeBlanc, S. J., Duffield, T., Leslie, K., Bateman, K., Keefe, G., Walton, J., Johnson, W. 2002. The effect of treatment of clinical endometritis on reproductive performance in dairy cows. *J Dairy Sci.* 85:2237–49.
Lewis, G. S. 1997. Uterine health and disorders. *J Dairy Sci.* 80:984–94.
Youngquist, R. S., Shore, M. D. 1997. Postpartum uterine infections. In: *Current therapy in large animal theriogenology*, ed. R. S. Youngquist. Philadelphia: W. B. Saunders.

Author: Stephen LeBlanc

ENTROPION

BASICS

DEFINITION
Entropion is an inversion or rolling in of the eyelid, most commonly the lower lid. The condition can be congenital or acquired, and usually leads to trichiasis, which can cause severe corneal damage. This in turn causes blepharospasm, which aggravates the entropion.

PATHOPHYSIOLOGY
Hereditary, congenital, or secondary to trauma/irritation; causes pain and damage to the cornea when the eyelashes, skin, and hair rub on the cornea

SYSTEMS AFFECTED
Ophthalmic: may cause blindness if chronic

GENETICS
Hereditary; entropion can be either congenital or acquired. Congenital entropion may not manifest itself initially, and it may be inherited in certain breeds.

INCIDENCE/PREVALENCE
Can range from 1 to 80% in a given flock

GEOGRAPHIC DISTRIBUTION
Worldwide depending on species

SIGNALMENT

Species
• Common in lambs, uncommon in cattle, usually dehydrated neonates. Has been observed in camels.
• Potentially, all ruminant species

Breed Predilections
N/A

Mean Age and Range
Common in lambs, usually the lower eyelid; uncommon in cattle, usually dehydrated neonates.

Predominant Sex
N/A

SIGNS

HISTORICAL FINDINGS
Types
• *Spastic entropion*—Due to painful lesion of the globe (e.g., keratitis, corneal ulcer); almost always a complication of entropion due to other causes
• *Cicatricial entropion*—Following inflammation, trauma, or surgery of eyelids
• *Anatomic entropion*—Usually congenital but may become worse as postnatal development progresses and is often heritable; many of these animals have an abnormally long eyelid, particularly on the lower lid margin.

PHYSICAL EXAMINATION FINDINGS
• Blepharospasm, ocular discharge, corneal ulceration in chronic cases
• The eyelids are examined for abnormalities of position, function, and structure, such as lagophthalmos, ptosis, trichiasis, ectropion, entropion, blepharitis, lid neoplasms.
• Clinical signs seen with entropion include epiphora, blepharospasm, conjunctivitis, and keratitis. The amount and type of signs varies with the extent of involvement and duration.
• Medial entropion may occlude the lower lacrimal punctum.

CAUSES AND RISK FACTORS
May be secondary to keratoconjunctivitis; inflammation causes a predisposed eyelid to roll inward.

DIAGNOSIS

DIFFERENTIAL DIAGNOSIS
• Clinically obvious, rolling the thumb under the eye and seeing the lid unroll confirms presence of entropion
• *Chlamydia psittaci* is unilateral, becoming bilateral in 7 to 14 days. Early in the disease, the conjunctiva is chemotic, glistening, and grayish-pink, and the ocular discharge is serous. Sneezing is present early in the disease.

ENTROPION

Severe blepharospasm occurs and may cause a secondary spastic entropion.
• Differentiate between primary and secondary entropion, however, need to treat either way.
• Differential for persistent corneal ulcer: entropion, KCS, foreign bodies, ectopic cilia, and infection

CBC/BIOCHEMISTRY/URINALYSIS
N/A

OTHER LABORATORY TESTS
• Culture and cytology of ocular secretions if underlying cause suspected
• Cultures of the external ocular structures must be done before extensive cleaning is done and before drugs are instilled.
• Sterile swabs are used to collect material for culture. The swab should be moistened. The moistened swab is rubbed over the area to be cultured taking care to avoid skin, hair, and other nearby structures.
• Bacterial identification and disc sensitivity tests aid in the choice of antimicrobial therapy.

IMAGING
N/A

OTHER DIAGNOSTIC PROCEDURES
• Examination of the cornea is incomplete without utilization of topical ophthalmic stains.
• Fluorescein is used to demonstrate the presence or absence of corneal ulcers. For topical use, fluorescein-impregnated paper strips are preferred to fluorescein solution to insure sterility.
• The corneal epithelium is lipid selective and prevents any appreciable corneal penetration by fluorescein. In the presence of a corneal epithelial defect, the dye rapidly diffuses into the corneal stroma.

PATHOLOGIC FINDINGS
N/A

TREATMENT

• In lambs, the eyelid often needs to be everted long term, until maturity normalizes the conformation.
• Always evaluate the problem after topical anesthesia to decrease the spastic component. Surgical correction should only involve the anatomic or cicatricial component.
• Medical treatment of entropion involves ocular lubricant ointments, such as Lacrilube, Dura Tears, or Hypotears.
• There are many methods of correction, but the simplest and usually most effective is the skin and muscle resection.
• With large flocks of affected lambs, it may be impractical to do surgery. In this case, 0.5–1.5 ml of 70% ethanol injected subcutaneously in the affected eyelid in the area of the entropion (about 0.5–1.0 cm below eyelid margin) will usually cure the entropion. Penicillin can be substituted for the ethanol.

ACTIVITY
N/A

DIET
N/A

CLIENT EDUCATION
Due to the hereditary nature of this condition, the client should be discouraged from breeding the same lines of sheep to prevent the occurrence in the future.

SURGICAL CONSIDERATIONS
• If the cause of the entropion is excessive eyelid length, the treatment involves shortening the eyelid. You may choose to do a simple full-thickness wedge resection; the resection should be within the lateral one-third of the eyelid.
• Surgical Technique: under anesthesia, a modified Hotz-Celsus resection can be performed in which a section of skin is removed from under the eyelid and the resulting sutures pull the eyelid out. Towel clamps or forceps can be used to initially decide how much tissue needs to be removed, and then the incisions are made parallel to and 2 mm from the eyelid to remove a strip of tissue. Nonabsorbable interrupted sutures close the defect and hold the lid out. Slight undercorrection is advised due to wound contracture. Be sure loose ends of the stitches do not rub the cornea.

MEDICATIONS

DRUGS OF CHOICE
Broad-spectrum antibiotics are usually administered if corneal ulceration is present; culture and sensitivity tests can guide selection in recurring, nonhealing, or infected ulcers.

CONTRAINDICATIONS

• Appropriate milk and meat withdrawal times must be followed for all compounds administered to food-producing animals.
• Topical corticosteroids and anesthetics are contraindicated when the cornea retains fluorescein stain.

PRECAUTIONS

N/A

POSSIBLE INTERACTIONS

Concurrent corneal disease (e.g., ulcer from eyelid rubbing) also should be treated.

POSSIBLE COMPLICATIONS

Corneal ulcers, dehiscence of sutures/staples, recurrence

 FOLLOW-UP

EXPECTED COURSE AND PROGNOSIS

Immediate relief from pain and epiphora unless there is underlying infection. Prognosis is good as long as lid eversion is maintained.

 MISCELLANEOUS

ASSOCIATED CONDITIONS

Secondary to or predisposes to keratoconjunctivitis

AGE-RELATED FACTORS

Young most commonly affected (lambs by day 2 or 3 of age).

ZOONOTIC POTENTIAL

Chlamydia psittaci may cause disease in humans.

PREGNANCY

N/A

RUMINANT SPECIES AFFECTED

Sheep most commonly; potentially all ruminant species are affected.

BIOSECURITY

N/A

PRODUCTION MANAGEMENT

Remove mothers and offspring from the breeding program, as the condition is hereditary.

SYNONYMS

SEE ALSO

Blindness
Corneal ulceration
Enucleation
Keratoconjunctivitis
Microphthalmia
Ocular surgery

ABBREVIATIONS

KCS = keratoconjunctivitis sicca

Suggested Reading
Basrur, P. K., Yadav, B. R. 1990, Nov. Genetic diseases of sheep and goats. *Vet Clin North Am Food Anim Pract.* 6(3):779–802.
Green, L. 1991, Aug 10. Treatment of entropion in lambs. *Vet Rec.* 129(6):128.
Taylor, M., Catchpole, J. 1986, Mar 29. Incidence of entropion in lambs from two ewe flocks put to the same rams. *Vet Rec.* 118(13): 361.
Yeruh, I., van Straten, M., Elad, D. 2002, Oct. Entropion, corneal ulcer and corneal haemorrhages in a one-humped camel (*Camelus dromedarius*). *J Vet Med B Infect Dis Vet Public Health.* 49(8):409–10.

Author: Melissa N. Carr

ENZOOTIC ATAXIA

BASICS

OVERVIEW
Enzootic ataxia is a disease of newborn or young lambs. It is most frequently associated with lambs born of ewes with a deficiency of copper in the diet.

PATHOPHYSIOLOGY
• Abnormal bone growth and increased fragility of bones predisposing to fractures of long bones is apparently due to defects in development of connective tissue and growth plates.
• Hypomyelinogenesis occurs in utero or shortly after birth in affected kids and lambs resulting in a progressive ataxia, muscle atrophy, paresis, and paralysis.
• Affected animals have stiffness of the back and legs and are reluctant to rise. When individuals do stand, there is a characteristic swaying of the hindquarters.
• Other neurologic signs can include blindness, obtundation, and head tremor.
• There may be persistent diarrhea, unthriftiness, and poor fleece in lambs.
• The pathogenesis is not known.

SYSTEMS AFFECTED
Musculoskeletal, CNS, hair/wool, production management

GENETICS
There is a possible familial predisposition.

INCIDENCE/PREVALENCE
Unknown

GEOGRAPHIC DISTRIBUTION
Worldwide distribution

SIGNALMENT

Species
Sheep, goats, blesbok (*Damaliscus dorcas phillipsi*), black wildebeest (*Connochaetes gnou*), sika deer (*Cervus nippon Temminck*), bactrian camels, red deer, *Cervus elaphus*, beef cattle, and piglets may be affected.

SIGNS
• Affected animals may appear normal at birth.
• Clinical signs usually occur within the first 6 months of life.
• Ewes are often asymptomatic, but may have "stringy" appearance to the wool or osteoporosis.
• Depigmentation of hair coat is noticeable in darker colored animals. Commonly occurs around the eyes giving a "spectacled" appearance.

CAUSES AND RISK FACTORS
• Copper deficiency in the dam's diet is responsible for the clinical signs; however, the pathogenesis is not known. It is speculated that copper deficiency results in altered cellular respiration and reduced synthesis of myelin. It may also result in reduced synthesis of noradrenaline and increase dopamine in tissues.
• Animals raised on pasture with copper deficient soil are at greater risk of disease.
• There is a possible familial predisposition.

DIAGNOSIS

DIFFERENTIAL DIAGNOSIS
• Molybdenum toxicity causes improper copper metabolism and causes the same clinical signs as copper deficiency.
• Sulfur
• In young kids, signs resemble the neurologic form of caprine arthritis and encephalitis (CAE) virus infection.
• The diarrhea associated with enzootic ataxia is commonly mistaken for internal parasitism, although it is possible for both conditions to be present, especially in animals raised on pasture.

CBC/BIOCHEMISTRY/URINALYSIS
Ewes may be anemic.

OTHER LABORATORY TESTS
There may be decreased copper levels in blood and liver.

IMAGING
N/A

DIAGNOSTIC PROCEDURES
Generally diagnosed based on clinical signs with possible decreased blood or liver copper levels.

PATHOLOGIC FINDINGS

GROSS FINDINGS
• Possible symmetric cavitations in the subcortical white matter can lead to secondary hydrocephalus.
• In severe cases, little is left of the hemispheres except the cortical shell of gray matter.

HISTOPATHOLOGICAL FINDINGS
• White matter neuronal degeneration or necrosis can be found in the central portions of the cerebral hemispheres, brain stem, and spinal cord.
• Demyelination occurs in the brain stem and spinal cord. Myelinated tracts may have a spongy appearance with some collections of gitter cells.
• Chromatolysis of neurons in the red nucleus may occur.

TREATMENT
Evaluate copper status of the herd and soils where animals are pastured. Copper supplementation should be provided as needed.

MEDICATIONS
None

CONTRAINDICATIONS
N/A

FOLLOW-UP

PATIENT MONITORING
N/A

PREVENTION/AVOIDANCE
Provide appropriate copper/mineral supplements. Supplements can be administered in various forms such as a top dressing to pasture or feed, or a weekly drench given to individual animals.

POSSIBLE COMPLICATIONS
None

EXPECTED COURSE AND PROGNOSIS
• Prompt supplementation with copper may improve signs.
• Severely affected animals may have permanent neurologic deficits.

MISCELLANEOUS

ASSOCIATED CONDITIONS
Copper supplementation can be toxic to treated animals.

AGE-RELATED FACTORS
The onset of clinical signs usually occurs between 1 week and 6 months of age.

ZOONOTIC POTENTIAL
None

PREGNANCY
Maternal copper deficiency is cause of clinical disease in lambs and kids.

SYNONYMS
Swayback

SEE ALSO
Caprine arthritis-encephalitis (CAE) virus infection
Internal parasitism
Molybdenum toxicity
Sulfur

ABBREVIATIONS
CAE = caprine arthritis encephalitis
CNS = central nervous system

Suggested Reading
Bourke, C. A. 1995, Jun. The clinical differentiation of nervous and muscular locomotor disorders of sheep in Australia. *Aust Vet J.* 72(6): 228–34.
Jones, T. C., Hunt, R. D., King, N. W., ed. 1997. Congenital demyelinating disease of lambs (swayback, enzootic ataxia). In: *Veterinary pathology.* 6th ed. Baltimore, Maryland: Williams & Wilkins.
Lofstedt, J., Jakowski, R., Sharko, P. 1988, Nov 15. Enzootic ataxia and caprine arthritis/encephalitis virus infection in a New England goat herd [corrected]. *J Am Vet Med Assoc.* 193(10): 1295–98.
Millar, M., Barlow, A., Gunning, R., Cosser, J. 2003, Mar 29. Enzootic ataxia in farmed red deer. *Vet Rec.* 152(13): 408.
Penrith, M. L., Tustin, R. C., Thornton, D. J., Burdett, P. D. 1996, Jun. Swayback in a blesbok (*Damaliscus dorcas phillipsi*) and a black wildebeest (*Connochaetes gnou*). *J S Afr Vet Assoc.* 67(2): 93–96.
Suttle, N. F. 1988, Oct. The role of comparative pathology in the study of copper and cobalt deficiencies in ruminants. *J Comp Pathol.* 99(3): 241–58.

Author: Lisa Nashold

ENZOOTIC PNEUMONIA OF CALVES

BASICS

DEFINITION
Respiratory disease complex of young calves less than 6 months of age caused by multiple etiologic agents, a decreased host defense system, and environmental risk factors such as poor ventilation and overcrowding.

PATHOPHYSIOLOGY
• The bacterial pathogens involved with this disease are normal inhabitants of the nasal and pharyngeal mucosa.
• Host and environmental factors combine to weaken the normal pulmonary defense mechanisms.
• Viral infections cause damage to the mucosal lining of the upper respiratory tract and may reduce the production of secretory defenses.
• Viral infections may also have an effect on alveolar macrophages or neutrophils, which can enhance bacterial adherence.
• Factors such as failure of passive transfer, stressors such as overcrowding and mixing, poor ventilation, and high relative humidity also allow the proliferation of these opportunistic bacteria.

SYSTEMS AFFECTED
Respiratory

GENETICS
N/A

INCIDENCE/PREVALENCE
• Based on producer diagnosis, 7.4%–11% of dairy calves
• Based on veterinary diagnosis, 25.6%–29% of dairy calves

GEOGRAPHIC DISTRIBUTION
N/A

SIGNALMENT
Species
• Most common in housed dairy calves and veal calves
• Beef calves in crowded conditions

Breed Predilections
N/A

Mean Age and Range
• Calves less than 6 months of age
• Peak incidence at 5–6 weeks of age

Predominant Sex
N/A

SIGNS
N/A

HISTORICAL FINDINGS
• Multiple animals depressed and febrile
• Partial anorexia
• Increased respiratory rates
• Coughing
• Nasal discharge
• Lacrimation
• Decreased weight gains
• Rough hair coats
• High morbidity
• Low mortality

PHYSICAL EXAMINATION FINDINGS
• Fever (39.5°C–40.5°C)
• Polypnea
• Mild to severe dyspnea
• Abnormal cranioventral lung sounds such as loud harsh breath sounds, crackles, and wheezes
• Harsh, dry, cough response on tracheal compression
• Intensity of heart sounds is increased dorsal to heart base.

CAUSES
Multifactorial etiology

Primary Infectious Agents
• *Mycoplasma bovis*
• *Mycoplasma dispar*
• Other *Mycoplasma* spp.
• Bovine respiratory syncytial virus
• Parainfluenza-3 virus
• Bovine herpesvirus-1
• Bovine viral diarrhea virus
• Bovine adenovirus
• Bovine coronavirus

Secondary Agents
• *Mannheimia haemolytica*
• *Pasteurella multocida*
• *Histophilus somnus*
• *Arcanobacterium pyogenes*

RISK FACTORS
• Inadequate housing
• Poor ventilation
• Housing calves together in large groups
• Grouping calves together of various ages
• Direct contact with older animals
• Low colostral immunity
• Birth outside the maternity pen
• Overcrowding
• High relative humidity
• Large daily temperature range

DIAGNOSIS

DIFFERENTIAL DIAGNOSIS
• Pneumonia caused by *Mannheimia haemolytica*
• Aspiration pneumonia
• Congenital cardiac defects
• *Histophilus somnus* pneumonia

CBC/BIOCHEMISTRY/URINALYSIS
N/A

OTHER LABORATORY TESTS
Isolation and identification of organisms
• Nasopharyngeal swabs
• Transtracheal washes
• Lung lavage samples
• Serological tests for confirmation of BRSV infections
• Immunohistochemistry, virus isolation or antigen capture ELISA for identification of persistently infected BVDV calves

IMAGING
N/A

DIAGNOSTIC PROCEDURES
N/A

PATHOLOGIC FINDINGS
• Extensive anteroventral lung consolidation
• Fibrinous pleuritis
• Suppuration and abscessation of lungs
• Severe interstitial pneumonia associated with BRSV infections
• Inflammation of nasal mucosa

TREATMENT

APPROPRIATE HEALTH CARE
• Medical management: use and selection of appropriate antibiotics
• Appropriate selection and treatment of cases
• Consider mass medication of calves in outbreak situations.
• Sick calves should be isolated from healthy calves.

NURSING CARE
• Fluid therapy such as oral electrolyte solutions or intravenous fluids may be indicated in dehydrated animals.
• Well-ventilated, draft-free environment provided

ENZOOTIC PNEUMONIA OF CALVES

ACTIVITY
N/A

DIET
N/A

CLIENT EDUCATION
• Discuss probable causes and risk factors.
• Warn that viral or *Mycoplasma* pneumonias may not respond to antimicrobial therapy.

SURGICAL CONSIDERATIONS
N/A

 MEDICATIONS

DRUGS OF CHOICE
Any antimicrobials labeled for use in the bovine for undifferentiated respiratory disease would be suitable. These may include:
• Short-acting or long-acting oxytetracyclines
• Tilmicosin
• Trimethoprim-potentiated sulfonamides
• Ceftiofur
• Florfenicol
• Enrofloxacin (beef calves only)

CONTRAINDICATIONS
N/A

PRECAUTIONS
• Failure to respond to treatment may indicate predominantly viral infections, *Mycoplasma* infections, or late selection and treatment of cases.
• Drug withdrawal times must be determined and maintained for treated animals.

POSSIBLE INTERACTIONS
N/A

ALTERNATIVE DRUGS
Efficacy of NSAIDs in these cases is questionable.

 FOLLOW-UP

PATIENT MONITORING
Pyrexia may be utilized as a measure of response to therapy. Calves that are still febrile after 3 days of therapy could be categorized as a relapse and considered for an alternative antimicrobial.

PREVENTION/AVOIDANCE
• Improving air quality is an important criterion for control.
• Dairy calves should not share the same air space as adult animals.
• Rearing dairy calves in calf hutches is an excellent method for reducing the potential risk factors associated with enzootic calf pneumonia.
• Alternatively, use group housing in cold well-ventilated facilities.
• Humidity levels between 55% and 75% are optimal.
• Avoid mixing of various age groups of calves.
• Utilize all-in–all-out approach in group housing, if possible.
• Avoid overcrowding.
• Ensuring calves have high levels of passive immunity by ensuring adequate colostrum ingestion shortly after birth.
• There is lack of evidence to support that vaccines administered to young calves are beneficial in preventing enzootic pneumonia.

POSSIBLE COMPLICATIONS
N/A

EXPECTED COURSE AND PROGNOSIS
• Response to antimicrobial therapy should be evident within 48 hours if the primary pathogen is bacterial.
• *Mycoplasma* and viral infections may not respond to antimicrobial therapy.
• Calves that are selected early in the course of the disease for treatment will generally have a very low case fatality rate.
• Case fatality rates have been reported at 2.25%.

 MISCELLANEOUS

ASSOCIATED CONDITIONS
Neonatal diarrhea may be associated with enzootic pneumonia, as many of the same risk factors are shared.

AGE-RELATED FACTORS
N/A

ZOONOTIC POTENTIAL
N/A

PREGNANCY
N/A

RUMINANT SPECIES AFFECTED
Cattle

BIOSECURITY
• Keeping age groups of calves separate is a significant preventive measure.
• Avoid mixing of calves from various sources.
• Purchased calves may be persistently infected with bovine viral diarrhea virus, which may predispose infected animals to enzootic pneumonia.

PRODUCTION MANAGEMENT
• Heifers that do not experience enzootic pneumonia are twice as likely to calve and will calve 6 months earlier than heifers that did have enzootic pneumonia.
• Enzootic pneumonia cases are at an increased risk of culling.

SYNONYMS
N/A

SEE ALSO
Aspiration pneumonia
Congenital cardiac defects
Histophilus somnus pneumonia
Pneumonia caused by *Mannheimia haemolytica*

ABBREVIATIONS
BRSV = bovine respiratory syncytial virus
BVDV = bovine viral diarrhea virus
ELISA = enzyme-linked immunosorbent assay
NSAIDs = nonsteroidal anti-inflammatory drugs

Suggested Reading
Ames, T. R. 1997. Dairy calf pneumonia: the disease and its impact. *Vet Clin NA Food Anim* 13: 379–90.
Kiorpes, A. L., Butler, D. G., Dubielzig, R. R., Beck, K. A. 1988. Enzootic pneumonia in calves: clinical and morphologic features. *Comp Cont Educ Pract Vet.* 10:247–61.
Van Donkersgoed, J., Ribble, C. S., Boyer, L. G., Townsend, H. G. G. 1993. Epidemiological study of enzootic pneumonia in dairy calves in Saskatchewan. *Can J Vet Res.* 57: 247–54.

Author: John R. Campbell

EPERYTHROZOONOSIS

 BASICS

DEFINITION
• Eperythrozoonosis (Candidatus *Mycoplasma* spp.) is often considered to be a subclinical disease of cattle, small ruminants, and camelids. However, it can be a significant cause of hemolytic anemia in immunologically naïve, immunosuppressed, or debilitated individuals.
• Current nomenclature recommendations are as follows: *Mycoplasma (Eperythrozoon) wenyoni* in cattle, *Mycoplasma (Eperythrozoon) ovis* in sheep, and *Mycoplasma haemolamae* in camelids.

PATHOPHYSIOLOGY
• Eperythrozoonosis is contractible via inoculation of infected blood. Biting insects are considered vectors, though a specific insect has not been identified as the principal vector. Transmission may also occur vertically and via blood-contaminated needles or instruments.
• Parasitemia develops within days of inoculation, but the rapid onset of an effective immune response curtails proliferation, halting further progression. Thus, latent infection can be common in endemic herds and the organism often coexists symbiotically within the host without causing clinical signs of anemia.
• The recent development of highly sensitive PCR assays have detected the organism in the blood of otherwise apparently healthy individuals.
• Debilitated, immunosuppressed, or immunologically naïve individuals are susceptible to uncontrolled parasitemia and clinical signs of disease develop. The organism is found on the surface of erythrocytes, which are primarily removed from the circulation by the mononuclear phagocytes in the spleen and liver.
• Icterus without hemoglobinemia or hemoglobinuria is a cardinal clinical sign. In sheep, intravascular hemolysis may also occur. Anemia develops, and in severe cases, death from hypoxemia may ensue.

SYSTEMS AFFECTED
• Hemic/lymphatic: anemia, extravascular hemolysis, icterus; dependent edema in cattle
• Cardiovascular: hypoxemia
• Skin: poor wool quality in sheep
• Reproductive: scrotal edema and reduced fertility in bulls

GENETICS
N/A

INCIDENCE/PREVALENCE
The disease is often subclinical, and widely used diagnostic methods (examination of blood smears or serology) are not sensitive enough to detect latent infection. Thus, it is difficult to actually determine the prevalence of the disease. The use of a recently developed and highly sensitive PCR assay has thus far detected latent infection in approximately 20% of New World camelids in the United States, Canada, and Australia. Use of PCR assays in other species will be helpful in determining the true prevalence of the disease.

GEOGRAPHIC DISTRIBUTION
Cases have been reported worldwide.

SIGNALMENT
Species
Cattle, small ruminants, camelids, mule deer, elk

Breed Predilections
N/A

Mean Age and Range
Any age may be affected but younger immunosuppressed or immunologically naïve ruminants may be more susceptible.

Predominant Sex
N/A

SIGNS
GENERAL COMMENTS
• Eperythrozoonosis rarely causes clinical signs of disease and its presence may be a coincidental finding. Severely debilitated or immunosuppressed individuals are more susceptible to clinical eperythrozoonosis.
• The signs of the primary disease process that are responsible for immunosuppression often overshadow the clinical signs of eperythrozoonosis.

HISTORICAL FINDINGS
Concurrent illness, progressive depression, weakness and lethargy, poor growth or chronic weight loss, poor coat quality, anorexia, and icterus

PHYSICAL EXAMINATION FINDINGS
• Clinical signs of disease infrequently occur in cattle and the presence of *Eperythrozoon* species may be a coincidental finding in some individuals.
• Immunosuppression from concurrent systemic disease may predispose individuals to eperythrozoonosis; however, the primary disease process may conceal the signs of eperythrozoonosis.
• Sheep appear to be most susceptible.

• Fever, weakness, and recumbency are expected if the condition progresses. In severe cases, tachycardia, tachypnea, pallor of the mucous membranes, lack of episcleral vessels, and icterus develop.
• Although hemolysis is primarily extravascular, intravascular hemolysis can occur in sheep and thus hemoglobinuria may be present.
• In chronic infection, signs of anemia may be present without signs of active hemolysis (e.g., icterus). In cattle, dependent edema, reduced fertility, and lymphadenopathy may be the predominant signs.

CAUSES
• Eperythrozoonosis is caused by a small (0.5 μm) coccoid prokaryotic organism that lacks a cell wall and cannot be cultivated. Although historically classified as a rickettsial organism, recent studies suggest that it is more closely related to mycoplasma.
• Current nomenclature recommendations are as follows: *Mycoplasma (Eperythrozoon) wenyoni* in cattle, *Mycoplasma (Eperythrozoon) ovis* in sheep, and *Mycoplasma haemolamae* in camelids.

RISK FACTORS
Eperythrozoonosis is most commonly considered to be an opportunistic infection that infrequently results in clinical disease, unless an individual is severely immunosuppressed or systemically compromised.

 DIAGNOSIS

DIFFERENTIAL DIAGNOSIS
• Any cause of extravascular hemolysis in cattle would cause similar signs including anaplasmosis and autoimmune hemolytic anemia.
• The absence of hemoglobinemia and hemoglobinuria distinguishes eperythrozoonosis from causes of intravascular hemolysis in cattle.
• With the occasional occurrence of intravascular hemolysis, leptospirosis and copper toxicity should be considered as differential diagnoses in sheep.

CBC/BIOCHEMISTRY/URINALYSIS
• Anemia: regenerative anemia 5 to 7 days after onset (signs of regeneration include an increased MCV, anisocytosis, polychromasia, basophilic stippling, reticulocytes, Howell Jolly bodies, nucleated red blood cells); nonregenerative anemia may occur in chronic cases.

- Hemoglobinemia (pink plasma, MCH, and MCHC increased) and/or hemoglobinuria may occur in sheep.
- Hyperbilirubinemia (unconjugated)
- Hypoglycemia
- Acidosis

OTHER LABORATORY TESTS

- Eperythrozoon species may be seen in a peripheral blood smear on the surface of erythrocytes as a coccoid, rod, or ring-shaped organism.
- Giemsa, Romanowsky, and acridine orange stains are particularly helpful to highlight the organisms. Parasitemia is often low, or affected cells are removed from the circulation by the mononuclear phagocytic system, therefore absence of visible *Eperythrozoon* species does not preclude the diagnosis.
- Complement fixation and indirect fluorescent antibody tests are positive within a few days of onset of clinical disease but, in some cases, may remain positive for only a short period of time. Unless paired serology is used, a single positive titer cannot distinguish between recent infection and previous exposure.
- A PCR test has been developed to detect the organism in camelids and cattle and is more sensitive in detecting the organism than examination of blood smears.
- The evolution of an immune attack directed at the organism on the surface of red blood cells may lead to a positive Coomb's test.

IMAGING
N/A

DIAGNOSTIC PROCEDURES
N/A

PATHOLOGIC FINDINGS
Splenomegaly, edema, body cavity effusion, and widespread icterus

TREATMENT

APPROPRIATE HEALTH CARE
Inpatient or outpatient care

NURSING CARE
- If anemia is severe and clinical or laboratory evidence of hypoxemia is evident (intense lethargy or weakness, profound tachycardia or tachypnea, severe anemia, acidosis, increased anion gap), a whole blood transfusion is indicated.
- The normal total blood volume is approximately 8% of the body weight (i.e., 0.08 x body weight in kilograms equals the total blood volume in liters). Typically, transfusing one-fourth to one-third of the total blood volume is adequate.

ACTIVITY
Confined

DIET
N/A

CLIENT EDUCATION
N/A

SURGICAL CONSIDERATIONS
N/A

MEDICATIONS

DRUGS OF CHOICE
Tetracycline (10 mg/kg IV q 12–24 hours for 3 to 5 days) is effective in controlling acute parasitemia in sheep and camelids, but it may be less effective in eliminating latency.

CONTRAINDICATIONS
Appropriate milk and meat withdrawal times must be followed for all compounds administered to food-producing animals.

PRECAUTIONS
N/A

POSSIBLE INTERACTIONS
N/A

ALTERNATIVE DRUGS
N/A

FOLLOW-UP

PATIENT MONITORING
Heart rate, respiratory rate, attitude, appetite, PCV

PREVENTION/AVOIDANCE
Currently, there is no vaccine for eperythrozoonosis.

POSSIBLE COMPLICATIONS
Death from hypoxemia, poor wool quality, reduced fertility, chronic weight loss

EXPECTED COURSE AND PROGNOSIS
The prognosis is good with treatment.

MISCELLANEOUS

ASSOCIATED CONDITIONS
N/A

AGE-RELATED FACTORS
N/A

ZOONOTIC POTENTIAL
N/A

PREGNANCY
N/A

RUMINANT SPECIES AFFECTED
Cattle, small ruminants, camelids, mule deer, elk. Sheep and camelids appear to be most susceptible to clinical disease.

BIOSECURITY
N/A

PRODUCTION MANAGEMENT
N/A

SYNONYMS
N/A

SEE ALSO
Extravascular hemolysis in cattle: anaplasmosis and autoimmune hemolytic anemia
Intravascular hemolysis, leptospirosis, and copper toxicity in sheep

ABBREVIATIONS
MCV = mean corpuscular volume
MCH = mean corpuscular hemoglobin
MCHC = mean corpuscular hemoglobin concentration
PCR = polymerase chain reaction

Suggested Reading
Neimark, H., Hoff, B., Ganter, M. 2004. *Mycoplasma ovis* comb. nov., (formerly *Eperythrozoon ovis*), an eperythrocytic agent of hemolytic anemia in sheep and goats. *Intern. J Systemic Evol Micro.* 54:365–71.
Reagan, W. J., Garry, F., Thrall, M. A., Colgan, S., Hutchison, J., Weiser, M. G. 1990. The clinicopathologic, light and scanning electron microscopic features of eperythrozoonosis in four naturally infected llamas. *Vet Pathol.* 27(6): 426–31.
Smith, J. A., Thrall, M. A., Smith, J. L., Salman, M. D., Ching, S. V., Collins, J. K. 1990. *Eperythrozoon wenyonii* infection in dairy cattle. *J Am Vet Med Assoc.* 196(8): 1244–50.
Vandervoort, J. M., Bourne, C., Carson, R. L., Health, A. M., Boudreaux, M. K. 2001. Use of a PCR assay to detect infection with Eperythrozoon wenyoni in cattle. *J Am Vet Med Assoc.* 219(10): 1432–34.
Welles, E. G., Tyler, J. W., Wolfe, D. F., Moore, A. 1995. Eperythrozoon infection in young bulls with scrotal and hindlimb edema, a herd outbreak. *Theriogenology* 43(3): 557–67.

Author: Michelle Henry Barton

ESCHERICHIA COLI O157:H7, CHALLENGES IN FOOD SAFETY

BASICS

OVERVIEW
• Shiga-toxigenic *Escherichia coli* O157:H7 emerged as a significant enteric pathogen following a human outbreak in 1993 due to undercooked hamburgers.
• It may be transmitted by food, water, or direct contact.
• The infectious dose is considered to be very small; even one organism is believed to cause disease especially in children and the elderly or immunocompromised. These populations are more susceptible and may succumb to hemorrhagic colitis and hemolytic uremic syndrome.
• Humans have been reported to contract *Escherichia coli* O157:H7 from petting zoos, contaminated and undercooked ground meat, raw milk, water, as well as inadequately pasteurized apple cider and various fruits and vegetables.
• Cattle and most ruminants are considered a reservoir of *Escherichia coli* O157:H7.
• In 1997, this significant pathogen was declared an adulterant in ground beef by the U. S. Department of Agriculture because the infectious dose is very low and common cooking practices may not kill the organism.

SYSTEMS AFFECTED
Production management, gastrointestinal

GENETICS
N/A

INCIDENCE/PREVALENCE
N/A

GEOGRAPHIC DISTRIBUTION
Worldwide, depending on species and environment

SIGNALMENT
Species
Potentially, all ruminant species
Breed Predilections
N/A
Mean Age and Range
N/A
Predominant Sex
N/A

CAUSES AND RISK FACTORS
• *Escherichia coli* O157:H7 is a ubiquitous organism and is prevalent in ruminant feces.
• Beef and dairy cattle and other infected animals are asymptomatic.
• Fecal shedding is greater in summer months.
• The organism can be found in water and feed and can survive for extended periods (13 weeks in cold water such as lakes, wells, and rivers).
• Disabled, nonambulatory "downer" cattle have been reported to have a higher prevalence than healthy cattle.
• Seasonal variation in infectivity occurs in the summer months, with an increase in fecal shedding in cattle and corresponding increase in human illness.
• The CDC reported that risk factors for human illness from *Escherichia coli* O157:H7 are eating undercooked ground beef and contact with farms or farm animals.
• Cooking ground beef to 160°F internal temperature, hand washing, and separating food and animal areas are protective practices that reduce human exposure.

DIAGNOSIS

DIFFERENTIAL DIAGNOSIS
N/A

OTHER LABORATORY TESTS
N/A

IMAGING
N/A

DIAGNOSTIC PROCEDURES
Escherichia coli O157:H7 may be best isolated by selective enrichment and immunomagnetic separation (IMS) to enhance sensitivity due to the low prevalence of the organism.

PATHOLOGIC FINDINGS
N/A

TREATMENT

• Potential animal production practices that reduce *Escherichia coli* O157:H7 include cleaning and disinfecting water troughs, feeding probiotics or competitive exclusion products, administering bacteriophages, vaccines, genetically modified feeds, sodium chlorate in feed or water, manure treatment, and good management practices to reduce fecal contamination.
• Chlorination of water troughs does not seem to significantly decrease *Escherichia coli* O157:H7 due to the amount of organic material present and constant recontamination.
• Most experts believe there will be no single magic bullet, but that multiple interventions will need to be applied.

ESCHERICHIA COLI O157:H7, CHALLENGES IN FOOD SAFETY

MISCELLANEOUS

ASSOCIATED CONDITIONS
• Humans have been reported to contract *Escherichia coli* O157:H7 from petting zoos, contaminated and undercooked ground meat, raw milk, water, as well as inadequately pasteurized apple cider and various fruits and vegetables.
• Cattle and most ruminants are considered a reservoir of *Escherichia coli* O157:H7.
• Hemorrhagic colitis and hemolytic uremic syndrome in humans

AGE-RELATED FACTORS
• The infectious dose is considered to be very small; even one organism is believed to cause disease especially in children and the elderly or immunocompromised. These populations are more susceptible and may succumb to hemorrhagic colitis and hemolytic uremic syndrome.
• Prevalence of *Escherichia coli* O157:H7 varies with stages of production: unweaned dairy calves approximately 2%, weaned calves 5%, and adult cattle at slaughter 13–28%.
• Children, the elderly, and immunocompromised people are more susceptible and may succumb to hemorrhagic colitis and hemolytic uremic syndrome (HUS).

ZOONOTIC POTENTIAL
• Shiga-toxigenic *Escherichia coli* O157:H7 emerged as a significant enteric pathogen following a human outbreak in 1993 due to undercooked hamburgers.
• It may be transmitted by food, water, or direct contact.

• Humans have been reported to contract *Escherichia coli* O157:H7 from petting zoos, contaminated and undercooked ground meat, raw milk, water, as well as inadequately pasteurized apple cider and various fruits and vegetables.

PREGNANCY
N/A

RUMINANT SPECIES AFFECTED
Potentially, all ruminant species can be affected.

BIOSECURITY
The CDC reported that risk factors for human illness from *Escherichia coli* O157:H7 are eating undercooked ground beef and contact with farms or farm animals.

PRODUCTION MANAGEMENT
Research in potential animal production practices that reduce *Escherichia coli* O157:H7 include cleaning and disinfecting water troughs, feeding probiotics or competitive exclusion products, administering bacteriophages, vaccines, genetically modified foods, sodium chlorate in feed or water, manure treatment, and good management practices to reduce fecal contamination.

SYNONYMS
N/A

SEE ALSO
Animals as reservoirs for *E. coli*
Animals as reservoirs for *Salmonella*
E. coli
Manure management
Manure pathogens
Salmonella
Zoonotic bacterial diseases

ABBREVIATIONS
CDC = Centers for Disease Control
HUS = hemolytic uremic syndrome
IMS = immunomagnetic separation

Suggested Reading
Armstrong, G. I., Hollingsworth, J., Morris, J. G. 1996. Emerging food-borne pathogens: *Escherichia coli* O157:H7 as a model of entry of a new pathogen into the food supply of the developed world. *Epidemiol Rev.* 18:29–51.
Besser, T. E. 1999. The ecology of shigatoxic *E. coli* O157 and prospects of on the farm control. *Proceedings 32nd Annu Meet Am Assoc Bovine Pract.*, pp. 6–9.
Byrne, C. M., Erol, I., Call, J. E., Kasper, C. W., Buege, D. R., Miemke, C. J., Fedorka-Cray, P. J., Benson, A. K., Wallace, F. M. Luchansky, J. B. 2003. Characterization of *Escherichia coli* O157:H7 from downer and healthy dairy cattle in the upper Midwest region of the United States. *Applied and Environmental Microbiology* 69: 4683–88.
Centers for Disease Control and Prevention. 2001. Outbreaks of *Escherichia coli* O1576:H7 among children associated with farm visits—Pennsylvania and Washington, 2000. *MMWR Morb Mortal Wky Rep.* 50:293–97.
Dunn, J. R., Ken, J. E., Thompson, R. A. 2004. Prevalence of shiga-toxigenic *Escherichia coli* O157:H7 in adult dairy cattle. *JAVMA* 7:1151–58.
Gansheroff, L. J., O'Brien, A. D. 2000. *Escherichia coli* O157:H7 in beef cattle presented for slaughter in the US: higher prevalence rates than previously estimated. *Proc Natl Acad Sci U S A* 97:2959–61.
Laegried, W. W., Elder, R. O., Keen, J. E. 1999. Prevalence of *Escherichia coli* O157:H7 in range beef calves at weaning. *Epidemiol Infec.* 123:291–98.

Author: Bonnie Buntain

ESOPHAGEAL DISORDERS

 BASICS

DEFINITION
- Choke, megaesophagus, stricture, rupture
- Esophageal disorders refer to any disorders that disrupt the normal function of the esophagus.
- Most common is esophageal obstruction (*choke*), which is defined as the partial or complete obstruction of the esophageal lumen resulting in the inability to swallow effectively. The obstruction may be caused by an intraluminal obstruction such as feed material or foreign body, or by an extraluminal obstruction such as abscess or neoplasia. In addition to obstruction, the esophagus may be affected by stricture, rupture, or megaesophagus.

PATHOPHYSIOLOGY
- Intraluminal esophageal obstruction occurs most commonly in areas of decreased dilation such as the cranial cervical esophagus, thoracic inlet, or base of the heart.
- Ingested feed is the most common cause of obstruction, particularly large objects such as apples, corncobs and potatoes, or dry materials such as pelleted feed.
- Ruminants are notoriously indiscriminant eaters and esophageal obstruction can also be caused by ingestion of foreign bodies.
- Esophageal obstruction can be potentiated by the presence of an extraluminal space-occupying lesion such as an abscess or neoplasia or by underlying neurologic dysfunction.

SYSTEMS AFFECTED
Gastrointestinal
- Esophageal obstruction causes dysphagia and ptyalorrhea.
- Bloat results from complete obstruction of the esophagus, as gas produced by reticulorumen fermentation is unable to escape.
- Esophageal damage from obstruction may result in rupture, fibrosis, or stricture formation.

Endocrine/Metabolic
Esophageal obstruction may cause metabolic acidosis if unrelieved due to a persistent loss of sodium bicarbonate and sodium phosphate in the saliva.

Cardiovascular
Tachycardia may be present due to stress or dehydration. Ruminants frequently become dehydrated due to loss of saliva and the inability to drink.

Respiratory
Aspiration pneumonia may result secondary to esophageal obstruction.

Skin/Exocrine
Cellulitis may be present in the cervical region if the obstruction has resulted in esophageal rupture.

GENETICS
None

INCIDENCE/PREVALENCE
- Esophageal obstruction is rare in cattle, sheep, and goats. Of the ruminants, it is most common in cattle due to their indiscriminant eating habits.
- Megaesophagus is rare in ruminants.

GEOGRAPHIC DISTRIBUTION
None

SIGNALMENT
- May be seen in cattle as well as sheep and goats
- There does not appear to be any age, breed, or sex disposition.
- Any ruminant exposed to solid feedstuff, pelleted feed, or foreign objects is susceptible.

SIGNS
GENERAL COMMENTS
- The most consistent clinical signs of esophageal obstruction are ptyalism, rumen tympany, coughing, and repeated extension of the head and neck.
- The presence of clinical signs varies with the duration (acute to chronic) and severity of the obstructive lesion (partial to complete).

HISTORICAL FINDINGS
- Ptyalism
- Extension of the head and neck
- Anxiety and restlessness
- Frequent swallowing
- Nasal discharge containing feed material

PHYSICAL EXAMINATION FINDINGS
- Ptyalism
- Dysphagia
- Coughing
- Nasal discharge
- Anxiety
- Tachycardia/tachypnea
- Respiratory distress
- Bruxism
- Bloat
- Repeated attempts to swallow
- Staggering
- Dehydration

CAUSES
- Esophageal obstruction is usually caused by impaction of feed material in the esophagus or ingestion of foreign bodies.

- Eating large items such as corncobs, apples, and potatoes, whole or in large pieces, can be the sole cause of the obstruction without any underlying disease.
- Foreign material (e.g., glass or metallic objects) can also be consumed and lodge in the esophagus.
- Consuming dry or pelleted feeds can also cause esophageal obstruction if the bolus is not moist enough to allow passage through the esophagus. Of the ruminants, this is most common in sheep.
- Esophageal obstruction may be secondary to other disorders of the esophagus such as strictures, diverticula, neoplasia such as squamous cell carcinoma, or abscesses.

RISK FACTORS
- Gluttony
- Ingestion of dry or pelleted feed
- Incomplete mastication of feedstuffs
- History of esophageal obstruction or stricture
- Dehydration

 DIAGNOSIS

DIFFERENTIAL DIAGNOSIS
- Various infectious agents may cause dysphagia similar to that seen with esophageal obstruction.
- Botulism, tetanus, and rabies can all cause bloat, dysphagia, and ptyalism. Toxic plants—such as milkweed, larkspur, sneezeweed, and *Rhizoctonia leguminicola*–infected red clover—also cause ptyalism.
- Traumatic damage to the pharynx can also cause ptyalism and cellulitis.
- Bloat can be caused by vagal indigestion or trauma and inflammation associated with the vagal nerve.

CBC/BIOCHEMISTRY/URINALYSIS
- Packed cell volume and serum protein level may be elevated due to dehydration.
- Metabolic acidosis, hyponatremia, and hypokalemia may be present due to the loss of saliva.
- The leukogram and fibrinogen levels may be altered due to inflammatory changes associated with the primary disease process or secondary aspiration pneumonia.

IMAGING
Radiography
- Both survey and contrast radiography may be helpful to determine the etiology and severity of esophageal obstruction.

- Both the cervical and thoracic esophagus can be visualized by radiography.
- Diagnosis of stricture, perforation, and diverticula can also be made by contrast esophageal radiology.
- Contrast media can be easily administered via oroesophageal or nasoesophageal tube.
- Fluoroscopy may be helpful to diagnose motility disorders although restraint in the ruminant can be frustrating.

DIAGNOSTIC PROCEDURES
- In small ruminants, the object may be palpated in the cervical esophagus. This is often not possible in the bovine patient and passage of a nasogastric tube is necessary to establish the location of the obstruction. The tube should be passed through an oral speculum and should be advanced gently to avoid damage to affected mucosa.
- The overall condition of the patient should be evaluated.
- The thorax should be carefully auscultated for evidence of aspiration pneumonia.

Endoscopy
- Esophagoscopy will aid in localizing and characterizing the lesion as well as determining the severity of esophageal damage.
- Strictures and diverticula can also be visualized with esophagoscopy. A 2–3-m endoscope may be necessary to visualize the extent of the bovine esophagus, however a 1-m or pediatric endoscope is adequate for the small ruminant. The animal should be restrained in a head gate or stanchion and the head should be controlled. Use of an oral speculum is necessary to prevent damage to the endoscope. Insufflation with air will help to visualize the esophagus especially in cases where a large amount of saliva is present.

TREATMENT

MEDICAL MANAGEMENT
- Some cases of esophageal obstruction will resolve spontaneously but each should be treated as quickly as possible to decrease inflammation and reduce the incidence of complications.
- In cases where the obstruction is palpable within the cervical esophagus, it may be manually extracted by applying gentle and steady pressure in the jugular groove aboral to the obstruction and pushing it in an oral direction.

- Sedation is usually necessary, but once the object is in the proximal esophagus it may be propelled into the pharynx or grasped and removed. A speculum and manipulation of the tongue will be helpful with this technique.
- If the obstruction is in the thoracic esophagus, an attempt can be made to push the object into the rumen as the esophagus widens as it courses toward the cardia. Then, if it is a foreign body, it can be retrieved via rumenotomy. This should not be performed if the object has sharp edges as identified by endoscopy, as it could potentially lacerate the esophagus.
- Objects in the cervical esophagus should not be pushed aborally due to the narrowing of the esophagus at the thoracic inlet.
- Sedation should be given to reduce anxiety and promote esophageal relaxation around the object. A nasogastric tube can be passed to the level of the obstruction and the obstruction, if it is feed material, may be broken down with a gentle lavage of warm water.
- The use of lubricants such as mineral oil or surfactants (DSS) is controversial due to the risk of aspiration.
- The animal should be sedated (see Medication below) to allow the head to drop as low as possible, preventing aspiration of lavage material. Additionally, a large-bore endotracheal tube can be inserted into the esophagus, cuff inflated, and the smaller oroesophageal tube inserted through the larger tube. This allows lavage material and fluid to pass through the ET tube and reduce risk of aspiration. If available, progress can be evaluated with endoscopy. Several attempts may need to be made to break down the obstruction, and it may take several hours to do so. Breaks should be taken to allow the animal to rest and breathe without risk of aspiration.
- If the obstruction cannot be relieved with the animal standing, general anesthesia may be required. The patient is placed in lateral recumbency with the head lowered and the same lavage techniques are used. If this does not allow relief of the obstruction, esophagotomy may be required.
- If there is evidence of esophageal rupture based on clinical signs, endoscopy, or radiography, surgical management may be necessary. If the rupture is acute, survival with surgery is possible.
- If the rupture is long-standing, involves contamination of the thorax, or involves extensive soft tissue contamination, the prognosis is extremely guarded and slaughter is recommended.

SURGICAL MANAGEMENT
- If the obstruction cannot be alleviated with sedation, lavage, and manual extraction, or if the object is sharp or irregular, surgical correction by esophagotomy becomes necessary.
- Perforation or rupture of the esophagus requires surgical intervention. Due to the risk of contamination of the surgery site, general anesthesia is usually required. Alternatively, the procedure has been performed under sedation and local anesthesia. Preoperative antimicrobials should be given and continued after surgery. An esophageal tube should be placed at the level of the obstruction for easier identification of the esophagus.
- Cervical esophagotomy is considerably easier to perform than transthoracic esophagotomy, as rib resection and positive pressure ventilation are required for the latter.
- If damage to the esophagus is severe, resection and anastomosis may be required. Detailed description of each of these surgeries is beyond the scope of this text and can be found elsewhere.
- Esophageal surgery carries a high complication rate and includes contamination of soft tissues, dehiscence of the incision, stenosis or diverticulum formation, pleuritis, and aspiration pneumonia.

NURSING CARE
- The animal should be held off feed and water until the obstruction is resolved. In cases of dehydration, the patient may require intravenous fluid therapy.
- The type of intravenous fluid used should be based on electrolyte and acid-base imbalances.

DIET
- Diet associated with esophageal disorders is dependent on type and severity of the disease present.
- Ruminants with resolved esophageal obstruction and minimal mucosal damage with no decrease in motility can be fed frequent small amounts for the first 24–72 hours.
- More severe esophageal damage, decreased motility, or surgical correction will require alternative alimentation.
- Placement of an esophagostomy tube distal to the obstruction site is one option. This is best reserved for calves that are not yet functional ruminants, as the regurgitated food material and saliva will leak around the tube. Daily passage of an orogastric tube can be used for feeding if done cautiously to avoid damage to the already compromised esophagus.

ESOPHAGEAL DISORDERS

• Ideally, ruminants can be fed through a temporary rumenostomy cannula. This allows a complete bypass of the damaged esophagus while maintaining an acceptable level of nutrition.

CLIENT EDUCATION
• The practice of feeding poor-quality feed or whole food items should be discouraged.
• Due to the indiscriminant eating habits of ruminants, producers should be encouraged to keep pastures free of foreign objects that could pose a risk if consumed.

MEDICATIONS

DRUGS OF CHOICE
• Xylazine (.01–.02 mg/kg/IV) can be given for sedation and esophageal relaxation.
• Broad-spectrum antimicrobials should be given in cases of esophageal necrosis, aspiration pneumonia, or esophageal surgery.
• Flunixin meglumine can be given (1.1 mg/kg q 24h) for inflammation and pain but withdrawal times should be followed.
• Oxytocin is not effective for treatment of esophageal obstruction in ruminants (unlike its possible use in Equidae) due to the presence of striated muscle for the length of the esophagus.

CONTRAINDICATIONS
The use of lubricants, such as mineral oil or surfactants (DSS) to relieve an esophageal obstruction, is controversial due to the risk of aspiration.

PRECAUTIONS
• Antibiotic and nonsteroidal anti-inflammatory (NSAIDs) choices should be made with regard to meat and milk withdrawal times.

• NSAIDs should be given judiciously to the dehydrated patient due to the risk of nephrotoxicity.

FOLLOW-UP

PATIENT MONITORING

PREVENTION/AVOIDANCE

POSSIBLE COMPLICATIONS
• Esophageal perforation
• Esophageal stricture
• Recurrent obstructions
• Aspiration pneumonia
• Altered esophageal motility
• Esophageal diverticulum
• Pleuritis
• Incisional dehiscence (surgery cases)

EXPECTED COURSE AND PROGNOSIS
• Prognosis is dependent on duration and severity of the lesion as well as occurrence of complications.
• Prognosis is good if resolution of the obstruction occurs spontaneously or with minimal manipulation and mucosal damage.
• Prognosis is guarded with more aggressive manipulation or if surgical correction is required, and grave to poor with prolonged obstruction and rupture of the esophagus.

MISCELLANEOUS

ASSOCIATED CONDITIONS
Aspiration pneumonia; bloat; rabies; rumen fistula; squamous cell carcinoma

RUMINANT SPECIES AFFECTED
All ruminant species

PRODUCTION MANAGEMENT
See Client Education above.

SYNONYMS
Choke

SEE ALSO
Botulism
Rabies
Tetanus
Toxic plants, such as milkweed, larkspur, sneezeweed, and *Rhizoctonia leguminicola*–infected red clover.
Vagal indigestion

ABBREVIATIONS
DSS = dioctyl sodium sulfosuccinate
ET = endotracheal tube
IV = intravenous
NSAIDs = nonsteroidal anti-inflammatory drugs

Suggested Reading
Bargai, U., Pharr, J. W., *et al*. 1989. The esophagus. In: *Bovine radiology*, ed. J. P. Morgan. Ames: Iowa State University Press.
Fubini, S. L., Pease, A. P. 2004. Esophageal surgery. In: *Farm animal surgery*, ed. S. L. Fubini and N. G. Ducharme. Philadelphia: W. B. Saunders.
Haven, M. L. 1990. Bovine esophageal surgery. In: Surgery of the bovine digestive tract. *Vet Clin North Am Food Anim Pract.* 6:359–69.
Navarre, C. B., Lowder, M. Q., Pugh, D. G. 2002. Oro-esophageal diseases. In: *Sheep and goat medicine*, ed. D. G. Pugh. Philadelphia: W. B. Saunders.

Author: Laura M. Riggs

BASICS

OVERVIEW
• Facial eczema is a hepatogenous photosensitization.
• Hepatotoxic sporidesmins A to H are produced by the fungus *Pithomyces chartarum,* a saprophyte of pasture leaf litter.
• Sporidesmins are pyrrolidiones.
• All grazing ruminants can be affected.

PATHOPHYSIOLOGY

SYSTEMS AFFECTED
Liver and lightly pigmented skin are affected, typically: ears, eyelids, face, lips, and dorsum of the trunk, vulva, mammary gland, and coronets.

GENETICS
N/A

INCIDENCE/PREVALENCE
Unknown

GEOGRAPHIC DISTRIBUTION
Sporidesmin toxicosis occurs primarily in autumn, but only in warm humid coastal areas of northern New Zealand, and sometimes Australia, South Africa, and Europe.

SIGNALMENT
• Only ruminants and camelids grazing at pasture are affected.
• Fallow deer, New World camelids, and sheep are most susceptible. Cattle and red deer are moderately susceptible. Goats are least susceptible.
• Morbidity can approach 50%; mortality is typically <5%.
• Subclinical effects are of great economic importance.
• Merino sheep are less susceptible to liver damage than British breeds. In sheep, the heritability of susceptibility to facial eczema is 0.42.
• Pastures predominantly made up of ryegrass are more hazardous than pastures of other plant species.

SIGNS
• Exposed nonpigmented and lightly pigmented skin is affected, typically: ears, eyelids, face, lips, and dorsum of the trunk, vulva, mammary gland, and coronets.
• Direct sunlight elicits cutaneous hyperaesthesia. Signs include: restlessness, head shaking, rubbing or scratching the affected part, and seeking shade.
• Initially, there is cutaneous erythema and edema of the ears, face, udder, and escutcheon. The ears droop, and there is copious lacrimation.

• Affected patches of skin have superficial necrosis that exudes serous fluid, and scabs form.
• Rubbing often results in self-trauma and secondary suppurative dermatitis.
• When affected sheep with short wool or open fleeces are exposed to direct sunlight, they often assume a characteristic posture with exaggerated lordosis and run to seek shade. The abnormal behavior appears to be a pain response.
• The milk production of affected cows drops dramatically. Cattle are restless, seek shade, and lick at the peeling skin.
• Affected fallow and red deer have mild skin lesions, but are more restless and irritable than other species, and actively seek shade. Deer deteriorate rapidly; some become temporarily blind (keratosis), and compared with other species, a greater proportion die.
• Severely affected animals of all species develop jaundice.

CAUSES AND RISK FACTORS
• Sporidesmin toxicosis from grazing the spores of the leaf litter fungus *Pithomyces chartarum.*
• The amount of sporidesmins on pasture is directly proportional to spore numbers. Spore production peaks when humidity approaches 100%, at temperatures between 20 and 24 degrees C, with night minimum temperatures

FACIAL ECZEMA

>14 degrees C. Spore numbers increase within 48 hours after >4 mm of rain followed by grass minimum temperatures of >12 degrees C, typically 16 to 18 degrees C for two consecutive nights.
• Several such periods are necessary for spore numbers to exceed the "danger level" of >100 000 spores per gram of grass.
• Other risk factors include; stocking rate, closeness of grazing, class of livestock, time spent grazing, and previous recent exposure to sporidesmins.

 DIAGNOSIS

DIFFERENTIAL DIAGNOSES
All other causes of photosensitivity include rape scald (*Brassica napus*); musky storksbill toxicosis (*Erodium moschatum*); lupinosis from phomopsin mycotoxins produced by *Diaporthe toxica*; pyrrolizidine alkaloid poisoning; lantadene poisoning; ngaio poisoning (*Myoporum laetum*); hypericism (*Hypericium* sp.); trefoil dermatitis following ingestion of bur medic (*Medicago polymorpha*), hay made from flood-damaged alfalfa (*Medicago sativa*) or Alsike clover (*Trefolium hybridum*); fagopyrin toxicosis from seeds and dried plants of buckwheat (*Polygonum fagopyrum*); ergotism (*Claviceps*

purpurea); mycotoxicosis from *Periconia* sp. on Bermuda grass; blue-green algal poisoning (*Microcystis* sp.); heritable porphyra; postpartum photosensitivity; ovine white liver disease; and toxicosis from administration of synthetic chemicals such as carbon tetrachloride.

CBC/BIOCHEMISTRY/URINALYSIS
Liver damage is reflected by elevated serum gamma glutamyltransferase (GGT).

OTHER LABORATORY TESTS
N/A

IMAGING
N/A

DIAGNOSTIC PROCEDURES
N/A

PATHOLOGIC FINDINGS
• Sporidesmins are nonspecific toxins that in sufficient concentration cause permeability changes in many tissues.
• Grazing animals absorb ingested sporidesmins from the intestine.
• Unconjugated sporidesmins are excreted and concentrated in bile. Initially there is dose-dependent degeneration/necrosis of the biliary epithelium. Leakage of bile into mesenchymal tissue of portal triads initiates pericholangitis.

• Severe or repeated insults result in progressive obliterative cholangitis, with biliary and periportal fibrosis. The reparative phase is characterized by bridging periportal fibrosis and proliferation of many small-diameter bile ducts.
• The liver lesions are asymmetrically distributed.
• The left lobe is primarily affected due to portal streaming. After repeated or chronic poisoning, there is fibrosis and atrophy of the left liver lobe and compensatory hypertrophy of the right and caudate lobes, which gives the liver a typical "boxing glove" gross appearance.
• Consequent to cholestasis, phylloerythrin, which is a photoactive metabolite of chlorophyll, cannot be excreted via the biliary system and accumulates in tissues. Similarly, endogenous photoactive porphyrins accumulate in tissues, resulting in mild jaundice.
• Accumulated photoactive metabolites in superficial tissues undergo a photodynamic reaction with sunlight and adjacent tissue is damaged.

 TREATMENT

Remove from toxic pasture and provide shade. Allow animals to graze outside at night.

MEDICATIONS

DRUGS OF CHOICE
N/A

CONTRAINDICATIONS
N/A

FOLLOW-UP

PATIENT MONITORING
N/A

PREVENTION/AVOIDANCE
Spore count monitoring is actively pursued at regional level. Farmers can monitor individual paddocks.

POSSIBLE COMPLICATIONS
Death

EXPECTED COURSE AND PROGNOSIS
• Once removed from toxic pasture, if provided with adequate shade, food and water, both the skin and liver heal within 1 to 3 weeks.
• Recovery of lost weight takes longer. Chronic ill thrift is a sequel of severe outbreaks.

MISCELLANEOUS

ASSOCIATED CONDITIONS
The milk production of affected cows drops dramatically. Cattle are restless, seek shade, and lick at the peeling skin.

AGE-RELATED FACTORS
N/A

ZOONOTIC POTENTIAL
N/A

PREGNANCY
Ewe fertility and fecundity can be markedly reduced, because the facial eczema danger period coincides with the mating season of sheep.

RUMINANT SPECIES AFFECTED
• All ruminant species grazing at pasture.
• Merino sheep are less susceptible to liver damage than British breeds. In sheep, the heritability of susceptibility to facial eczema is 0.42.

BIOSECURITY
N/A

PRODUCTION MANAGEMENT
• Manage pasture to minimize the amount of leaf litter substrate in the sward.
• Plan grazing management so that warm, humid paddocks are grazed before the danger period, and exposed, cool paddocks are reserved for the danger period.
• Avoid grazing to the base of pastures by ensuring light grazing pressure.
• Zinc administration before exposure reduces liver damage. Intraruminal slow-release zinc capsules of various sizes are available for cattle and sheep.
• Oral dosing of sheep and cattle with zinc oxide slurry, at frequencies ranging from daily to weekly, is progressively less effective as the interval is increased.
• Zinc sulphate in the drinking water is effective only for dairy cattle with no alternate source of water.
• Pastures can be sprayed with fungicides before spore counts rise, to provide safe pastures for 4 to 6 weeks.

SEE ALSO
Blue-green algal poisoning (*Microcystis* sp.)
Ergotism (*Claviceps purpurea*)
Lantadene poisoning
Mycotoxicosis from *Periconia* sp. on Bermuda grass
Photosensitivity
Pyrrolizidine alkaloid poisoning
Rape scald (*Brassica napus*)
Zinc

ABBREVIATIONS
GGT = gamma glutamyltransferase

Suggested Reading
Bruere, A. N., West, D. M. 1993. *The sheep: health, disease and production*. Palmerston North: Foundation for Continuing Education of the N. Z. Veterinary Association.
Cheeke, P. R. 1995, Mar. Endogenous toxins and mycotoxins in forage grasses and their effects on livestock. *J Anim Sci*. 73(3): 909–18.
Greenwood, P. E., Williamson, G. N. 1985, Feb. An outbreak of facial eczema in sheep. *Aust Vet J*. 62(2): 65–66.
Le Bars, J., Le Bars, P. 1996. Recent acute and subacute mycotoxicoses recognized in France. *Vet Res*. 27(4–5): 383–94.
McKenzie, R. A. 2002. *Toxicology for Australian veterinarians* [CD-ROM]. University of Queensland School of Veterinary Science, Brisbane, Australia ABN 63 942 912 684.
Seawright, A. A. 1989. *Animal health in Australia*: Volume 2 (*2nd ed.*), *Chemical and plant poisons*. Canberra: Australian Government Publishing Service.
Towers, N. 1999. *AgFact* (Nos. 135, 136, 137, 138, 139). www.agresearch.cri.nz/agr/pubs/AgFact/Search.asp (accessed Mar 13, 2004).

Author: A. D. (Sandy) McLachlan

FAILURE OF PASSIVE TRANSFER

 BASICS

DEFINITION
• Newborn ruminants are born hypogammaglobulinemic due to the nature of their placentation.
• Although immunocompetent at birth, neonatal ruminants are immunonaïve and thus dependant on maternally derived immunoglobulin and other factors absorbed from colostrum.
• Neonates that fail to acquire adequate passive immunity are said to suffer failure of passive transfer.

SYSTEMS AFFECTED
Immune system, gastrointestinal system, musculoskeletal system, and respiratory system; also production management

GENETICS
N/A

INCIDENCE/PREVALENCE
• Unknown but in many instances of poor colostral management extremely high
• An association exists between higher IgG (or protein) levels and lower disease incidence.
• This association appears to have a greater influence in herds with high disease incidence compared to herds with low disease incidence.

GEOGRAPHIC DISTRIBUTION
Worldwide

SIGNS

HISTORICAL FINDINGS
These animals are at increased risk for the development of diseases such as septicemia, enteritis, diarrhea, omphalitis, arthritis, and respiratory disease.

CAUSES AND RISK FACTORS
Factors to consider in assessing disease risk include general hygiene, pathogen virulence, pathogen concentration, the physical environment (e.g., temperature, humidity, wind chill), nutritional status, and miscellaneous stresses (e.g., transportation, handling, surgery).

Composition and Formation of Colostrum
• Colostrum is a complex fluid that in addition to immunoglobulins contains various immune cells, immunoactive substances such as cytokines, and nutritional elements.
• The concept of failure of passive transfer has largely been used to describe situations in which neonates do not absorb adequate levels of colostral immunoglobulin.
• This narrowly focused concept is due to the fact that immunoglobulins are such a large constituent of colostrum and they have been the most thoroughly studied component.

• Immunoglobulin G1 (IgG_1) is the primary immunoglobulin in bovine colostrum, making up >85% of the total colostral immunoglobulin mass.
• Colostral IgG_1 originates from maternal serum and is transferred into colostrum during the last 4 to 6 weeks of gestation.
• Transfer involves active, IgG_1-specific, Fc receptors located on the basilateral membrane of mammary secretory epithelial cells.
• These receptors appear to be under the control of lactogenic hormones as well as local mechanisms within the mammary gland.

Colostral Cellular Makeup
• Colostrum contains greater than 1×10^6 cells per milliliter.
• Although the particular cell types present in colostrum vary between species, time of lactation, and other physiologic conditions, it is clear that neonates receive a significant number of immune cells via colostrums.
• In sheep and cattle, lymphocytes make up approximately 20%–30% of colostral cells.
• Studies in cattle suggest that these colostral lymphocytes differ from those in maternal circulation and that they function by modulating the neonatal immune system and the secretion of various cytokines, as well as the secretion of immunoglobulin A.
• Macrophages and neutrophils make up the remainder of colostral cells.
• Macrophages are thought to serve as cytokine-producing and antigen-presenting cells.
• The neutrophils are likely involved in the protection of the mammary gland rather than the neonate.
• While interleukin-2 (IL-2) and tumor necrosis factor (TNF) have been found in colostrum, their role as yet is unknown.
• Colostrum is rich in insulinlike growth factor-1 (IGF-1), which helps regulate newborn growth and may enhance the early neonatal immune response.
• Finally, transforming growth factor is present in high concentrations in bovine colostrum but decreases by 30 days postpartum.

Absorption of Colostrum
• Whereas the transfer of immunoglobulin from maternal circulation into colostrum involves an active, specific, receptor-mediated process, absorption across the gut wall of the neonate is nonselective and in fact does not appear to differentiate between macromolecules.
• Absorption and transfer across intestinal epithelial cells occur via nonselective pinocytosis initiated by the presence of macromolecules.
• The efficiency of immunoglobulin absorption effectively declines to zero over the first approximately 24 hours of life.

• The term "closure" is used to define the point at which absorption by the gut of immunoglobulins ceases.
• NOTE: the absorptive process across the gut epithelium appears to be saturable. That is, a finite capacity exists for the absorption of all macromolecules.
• The presence of high levels of nonimmunoglobulin molecules fed during the first 24 hours of life may adversely compete with the absorption of colostral immunoglobulins.

CBC/BIOCHEMISTRY/URINALYSIS
N/A

OTHER LABORATORY TESTS

Determination of Passive Transfer Status
• Many methods are available to measure immunoglobulin concentrations in calf serum after absorption from colostrum.
• In conjunction with specific guidelines, these techniques are used to define if a neonate has attained adequate passive transfer or suffers failure of passive transfer.
• By convention, serum IgG_1 concentration of 10 mg/ml at 48 hours of age is the objective value for defining the threshold between adequate passive transfer and failure of passive transfer.
• The various tests for immunoglobulin concentration vary in their speed, accuracy, and equipment required for operation. The first step of all tests involves the acquisition of serum from the calf.
• Single radial immunodiffusion (SRID) and the enzyme-linked immunosorbent assay (ELISA) are the only tests that directly measure serum IgG concentration. Other tests including zinc sulfate turbidity, sodium sulfite precipitation, whole blood glutaraldehyde coagulation, total serum solids by refractometry, and gamma-glutamyl transferase activity indirectly estimate serum IgG concentration based on colostral total proteins.
• The techniques for performing these tests and the values used for their interpretation can be found in numerous texts (e.g., Bovine neonatal immunology, see below).
• NOTE: results of the various testing methods on any particular operation must be kept in perspective and their use not overinterpreted.

Assessing Disease Risk
• An association exists between higher IgG (or protein) levels and lower disease incidence.
• This association appears to have a greater influence in herds with high disease incidence compared to herds with low disease incidence.
• The rate of disease occurrence is obviously a balance between a calf's ability to resist disease and the severity of disease challenging the calf.

• Serum immunoglobulin concentration is only one factor that contributes to disease resistance, yet it provides no information regarding the degree of disease challenge.

• Additional factors to consider in assessing disease risk include general hygiene, pathogen virulence, pathogen concentration, physical environment (e.g., temperature, humidity, wind chill), nutritional status, and miscellaneous stresses (e.g., transportation, handling, surgery).

• Furthermore, other factors that influence disease resistance might include the less-studied nonimmunoglobulin components of colostrum (cells, cytokines, etc.).

Test Accuracy

• Accurate measurement of serum immunoglobulin in a particular calf does not necessarily guarantee protection from disease for the following reasons:

  • First, the tests described only quantify a calf's serum immunoglobulin concentration. They do not determine specific protective capabilities of the absorbed immunoglobulins.

  • Second, these tests cannot determine if the absorbed immunoglobulins will reach the appropriate site of challenge in a calf in sufficient concentrations to neutralize a particular pathogen.

• These two points are not meant to conclude that there is no benefit in measuring serum immunoglobulin levels as an indicator of passive transfer of immunity. Rather, they illustrate the potential limitations of measuring immunoglobulin levels.

IMAGING
N/A

OTHER DIAGNOSTIC PROCEDURES
N/A

CLIENT EDUCATION

• The efficiency of immunoglobulin absorption effectively declines to zero over the first approximately 24 hours of life.

• The term "closure" is used to define the point at which absorption by the gut of immunoglobulins ceases.

TREATMENT

Transfusions may prove helpful.

MEDICATIONS

N/A

DRUGS OF CHOICE
N/A

CONTRAINDICATIONS
N/A

PRECAUTIONS
N/A

POSSIBLE INTERACTIONS
N/A

ALTERNATIVE DRUGS
N/A

FOLLOW-UP

PREVENTION/AVOIDANCE
Proper colostral management

POSSIBLE COMPLICATIONS
N/A

EXPECTED COURSE AND PROGNOSIS
Clinical course and prognosis vary and are associated with the underlying disease conditions. Without additional quality colostrum or transfusions, typically failure of passive transfer warrants a guarded to poor prognosis.

MISCELLANEOUS

ASSOCIATED CONDITIONS
Septicemia, enteritis, diarrhea, omphalitis, arthritis, and respiratory disease

AGE-RELATED FACTORS
First 24–48 hours of life

ZOONOTIC POTENTIAL
N/A

PREGNANCY
N/A

RUMINANT SPECIES AFFECTED
All domestic and wild ruminant species can be affected.

BIOSECURITY
Selection of donors:
• Identify on-farm disease problems that can be influenced by colostral management.
• Do not pool colostrum. Feed colostrum from an individual preselected dam to individual young stock.

• Minimize disease transfer via colostrum (e.g., Johne's disease, CAE, BLV) by preselecting negative dams.
• Only first milking colostrum should be fed to the newborn during the first 12 hours of life.

PRODUCTION MANAGEMENT
• Young stock whose dam produces inadequate colostrum, should be fed colostrum from a preselected donor.
• Frozen colostrum should be stored from individual donors, identified, and marked prior to freezing.
• Maintain a bank of frozen, high-quality colostrum for use in emergency situations.
• Feed young stock first within 2 hours of birth and again within 12 hours of birth.

SYNONYMS
Failure to thrive

ABBREVIATIONS
CAE = caprine arthritis encephalitis
ELISA = enzyme-linked immunosorbent assay
Fc = IgG_1 specific Fc receptors
IGF-1 = insulinlike growth factor-1
IgG_1 = immunoglobulin G1
IL-2 = interleukin-2 (IL-2)
SRID = single radial immunodiffusion
TNF = tumor necrosis factor

Suggested Reading
Barrington, G. M., Parish, S. M. 2001. Bovine neonatal immunology. *Vet Clin N Am, Food An Pract*. 17:463–76.
Better, T. E., Gay, C. C. 1985. Septicemic colibacillosis and failure of passive transfer of colostral immunoglobulins in calves. *Vet Clin N Am, Food An Pract*. 1:445–59.
Dudek, J. E. 1983. Bovine immunoglobulins: an augmented review. *Vet Immunol Immunopathol* 4:43–152
Hutchison, J. M, Garry, F. B., Belknap, E. B., Getzy, D. M., Johnson, L. W., Ellis, R. P., Quackenbush, S. L., Rovnak, J., Hoover, E. A., Cockerell, G. L. 1995, Dec. Prospective characterization of the clinicopathologic and immunologic features of an immunodeficiency syndrome affecting juvenile llamas. *Vet Immunol Immunopathol*. 49(3):209–27.
Le Jan, C. 1996. Cellular components of mammary secretions and neonatal immunity. *Vet Res*. 27:403–17.

Author: George Barrington

FASCIOLIASIS (LIVER FLUKE)

 BASICS

OVERVIEW
• Liver flukes are platyhelminths (flatworms) of the class Trematoda. They have a long, complex life cycle that requires a snail intermediate host. Stages in the snail are not infective to mammalian hosts.
• After the fluke completes a complex asexual development within the snail, the stage called cercaria penetrates out of the snail onto pasture and develops into metacercariae. Livestock can become infected only if they ingest the free-living metacercariae while grazing pasture.
• There are two species of liver fluke that infect livestock: *Fasciola hepatica* and *Fascioloides magna*.

Fasciola hepatica
• *Fasciola hepatica*, the common liver fluke, is the most important liver fluke species of ruminants, but also will infect horses, swine, rabbits, and humans.
• Distribution of *F. hepatica* is strictly limited by the distribution of its snail's intermediate hosts and is most common in the Gulf Coast and the Pacific northwest regions of the United States.
• Cattle infected with *F. hepatica* rarely demonstrate clinical disease, but subclinical impairment of feed efficiency, growth, and fertility can have an important impact on productivity
• Though bovine fascioliasis is most often a subclinical disease, where extremely high fluke burdens rapidly accumulate, outbreaks of acute disease can occur
• Ovine/caprine fascioliasis may present with severe clinical symptoms such as anemia, anorexia, weight loss, submandibular edema, ascites, and death.
• Life cycle of *F. hepatica* does not change, but seasonal transmission profiles differ for each geographic region and these differences mean that treatment programs also differ by region.
• Only two flukicidal drugs are labeled for use in the United States, and both are extremely limited in their ability to kill the immature migrating stages less than 8 weeks old.

Fascioloides magna
• *Fascioloides magna*, the large American fluke, is a normal parasite of deer, but also infects cattle, small ruminants, and swine.
• Distribution of *F. magna* parallels that of *F. hepatica* but also is present in many areas where *F. hepatica* is not found.
• *F. magna* is considered to have low pathogenicity in deer, cattle, and swine, but will cause severe disease in small ruminants.
• Infections with *F. magna* do not become patent in nondeer hosts, so definitive diagnosis is possible only at necropsy.
• Treatments effective against *F. hepatica*, are poorly effective against *F. magna*, making treatment and control in ruminants/swine difficult.

SIGNALMENT
Fasciola hepatica
• All ages of ruminants; disease rare in other hosts
• Young animals are more susceptible to infection and more likely to demonstrate clinical disease.
• Small ruminants are more likely than cattle to develop clinical disease.

Fascioloides magna
• Cattle and swine may become infected, but symptoms of disease are very unlikely.
• Small ruminants of any age may become infected and may demonstrate severe disease.

SIGNS
Fasciola hepatica
Cattle
• Usually no clinical symptoms
• Major impact is decreased animal productivity.
• May see poor growth, weight loss, unthriftiness
• Calves with heavy infections may demonstrate anemia, submandibular edema, ascites.

Sheep/Goats
• Clinical symptoms are more severe than in cattle.
• May be none in light infections
• Anemia, anorexia, weight loss, submandibular edema, ascites, and death in moderate to heavy infections
• May see acute disease caused by large numbers of juvenile flukes. Symptoms resemble acute haemonchosis; may see as outbreak.

Complications
May include:
• Infectious necrotic hepatitis (Black disease, *Clostridium novyi*)
• Bacillary hemoglobinuria (*C. haemolyticum*)

Fascioloides magna
• Cattle and swine—symptoms of disease are very uncommon.
• Sheep and goats—weight loss, lethargy, sudden death

CAUSES AND RISK FACTORS
• *Fasciola hepatica, Fasciola gigantica, Fascioloides magna* and *Dicrocoelium dendriticum*.
• *Fasciola hepatica* is present worldwide.
• *Fasciola gigantica* is restricted to warmer climates including Africa and Asia.
• *Fascioloides magna* is present only in parts of North America and Europe.
• *Dicrocoelium dendriticum* is common in Europe and Asia, but is infrequently diagnosed in North America and the United Kingdom.
• *Dicrocoelium dendriticum* is substantially less pathogenic than the other fluke species.

Fasciola hepatica
• Snails of the genus *Fossaria* serve as the primary intermediate host in the United States. Characteristics of *Fossaria*
  • Amphibious; lives in wet mud along edges of shallow water
  • Typically inhabits semipermanent ponds and temporary pools (e.g., tire ruts)
  • Found in areas with neutral soils (pH 6–8) and poor drainage
  • Has the ability to aestivate (burrow in mud and enter arrested state)
• Ruminants grazing low-lying wet pastures in enzootic regions. Major enzootic areas: Gulf Coast states, California/ Northwest/Pacific Northwest, Puerto Rico, Hawaii. Sporadic cases diagnosed elsewhere
• Ruminants in enzootic regions not on a liver fluke control program
• Years with above-normal rainfall provide increased risk of infection.

Fascioloides magna
• In addition to *Fossaria*, there are a number of other snail species that serve as intermediate hosts for *F. magna*.

FASCIOLIASIS (LIVER FLUKE)

• Ruminants/swine grazing low-lying wet pastures or pastures containing lakes/ponds in enzootic regions.
  • Major enzootic areas: everywhere in the United States where *F. hepatica* is enzootic, plus additional areas in southeast United States in moist lowland and swampy areas, Great Lakes states, especially Minnesota, Wisconsin, Michigan, Adirondack Mountains of New York, western United States
  • Enzootic regions where there are large populations of deer

Life Cycle (Fasciola hepatica, Fasciola gigantica, Fascioloides magna)

• Adult flukes reside in either the bile ducts (*Fasciola hepatica*, *Fasciola gigantica*) or thin-walled cysts of the definitive host, which communicate with the bile ducts (*Fascioloides magna*) producing operculated ova, which are passed in the feces.
• The most common definitive host of *Fasciola hepatica* and *Fasciola gigantica* are cattle and sheep; however, other species may be affected.
• The definitive hosts of *Fascioloides magna* are wild cervidae including deer and moose. Fluke eggs hatch releasing miracidia, which seek out, invade the tissues of *Lymnaea* spp. or *Galba* spp. snails, and undergo asexual replication.
• Flukes escape from snails as cercariae, attach to pasture forage, and mature to metacercariae. Metacercariae are ingested by the definitive or aberrant host and immature flukes are released in the intestine, migrate across the intestinal wall and peritoneal cavity reaching the liver. Flukes migrate through the liver parenchyma and finally take up residence in either the bile ducts or hepatic cysts.
• In sheep and goats, *Fascioloides magna* will tend to migrate continuously rather than becoming encysted; hence, small numbers of these flukes may cause sufficient hepatic damage to result in the patient's demise.

Life Cycle (Dicrocoelium dendriticum)

• The lifecycle of *Dicrocoelium dendriticum* exhibits substantial pattern differences from that of *Fasciola* or *Fascioloides*. The intermediate hosts are land snails with broad distribution. Additionally, cercariae that leave snails infect a second intermediate host (*Formica* spp. ants) where they mature to metacercariae. Ants are ingested by grazing herbivores.

• Flukes migrate up the common bile duct and there is no significant or destructive tissue migration phase.

Environmental and Host Factors Affecting the Life Cycle

• In general, fluke eggs hatch only at temperatures above 40°F. Intermediate hosts (snails) are able to replicate only at temperatures above 50°F.
• Immature fluke forms fail to mature at cool environmental temperatures; however, these forms will overwinter within snails and replicate and are released with the advent of more temperate conditions in the spring.
• Metacercariae present on pastures are readily destroyed by severe cold (harsh winters) or hot, dry conditions. Consequently, the risk of infection is impacted by both seasonal and geographic risks producing a distinct local pattern.

DIAGNOSIS

Fasciola hepatica

• Based on clinical signs (if present), time of year, grazing history, and knowledge of herd history and area
• Demonstration of eggs in feces; with acute disease, there may be no eggs in feces; caused by juvenile flukes
• Characteristic liver lesions and/or demonstration of liver flukes in bile ducts

Fascioloides magna

• Premortem diagnosis very difficult—eggs are rarely shed in the feces livestock hosts
• Cattle, pigs—no clinical signs, eggs not passed in feces, usually incidental finding at slaughter/necropsy
• Sheep, goats—tentative diagnosis by clinical signs (similar to acute fascioliasis) and history of area/geography. Definitive diagnosis at necropsy—no eggs in feces

DIFFERENTIAL DIAGNOSES

• Gastrointestinal nematodes, particularly *Haemonchus contortus*
• *Taenia hydatigena* larvae in hepatic parenchyma (when helminths found in liver at necropsy)

CBC/BIOCHEMISTRY/URINALYSIS

• Anemia
• Hypoproteinemia
• Elevated GGT and/or GLDH

OTHER LABORATORY TESTS

• Fecal sedimentation technique—eggs will not float. Eggs are large, golden brown, operculated ($140 \times 80\mu$).

• Flukefinder modified sedimentation method improves ease of fecal diagnosis and is recommended.
• ELISA for *F. hepatica* if available (few labs perform this test)
• A PCR-RFLP assay for the distinction between *Fasciola hepatica* and *Fasciola gigantica* has recently been developed.

IMAGING

Ultrasound findings can aid in the diagnosis after 9 weeks postinfection. Ductal dilatation is shown by ultrasound, and moving echogenic forms in the dilated bile ducts can be observed after 9 weeks postinfection in sheep.

DIAGNOSTIC PROCEDURES

N/A

PATHOLOGIC FINDINGS

Fasciola. hepatica

Most lesions due to chronic infections
• Hyperplastic cholangitis—bile duct dilation, thickening, and fibrosis. In cattle, get calcification of bile ducts so called pipestem lesion
• Hepatic fibrosis — Liver is pale and firm with irregular outline.
• In acute disease
  • Enlarged liver with hemorrhagic tracts
  • Surface of liver covered with a fibrinous exudate
  • Serosanguineous fluid in abdominal cavity
  • Flukes may be too small to see with naked eye.

Fasciola magna

• Cattle and pigs—young flukes migrate in liver parenchyma, but adult flukes become encapsulated in thick-walled cysts that do not communication with bile ducts. Necrotizing tracts in the liver containing black hematin pigmentation
• Sheep and goats—young flukes migrate extensively through liver causing severe damage to liver parenchyma (adults do not encyst). Necrotizing tracts in the liver containing black hematin pigmentation. Black pigmentation also may be present in other organs.

TREATMENT

Available flukicidal drugs (see below) do not kill juvenile and/or immature liver fluke stages. Therefore, timing of treatments is critical and is based on local patterns of transmission.

FASCIOLIASIS (LIVER FLUKE)

Table 1

	Curatrem (clorsulon)	Ivomec-Plus (clorsulon + ivermectin)	Valbazen (albendazole)
Drugs Available in the United States for Treatment of Liver Flukes			
Dose	7 mg/kg	2 mg/kg + 200 g/kg	10 mg/kg
Kills adult flukes	+ (> 99%)	+ (97–99%)	+ (76–92%)
Kills immature flukes (8–12 weeks)	+ (85–95%)	—	—
Kills juvenile flukes (0–8 weeks)	—	—	—
Route of administration	Oral drench	Subcutaneous injection	Oral drench
Spectrum	Narrow (flukes only)	Broad (flukes, nematodes, ectoparasites)	Broad (flukes, nematodes, tapeworms)
Meat withdrawal times	8 days	49 days	27 days
Other information	Treatment of choice if treating at a time of year when it is expected that juvenile and/or immature stages will be present		Withholding feed for 24 hr prior to treatment will improve efficacy.

Source: Table modified from Kaplan (2001).

Suggested treatment times:
• Gulf Coast region—Treat in late summer or early fall; supplemental treatment in the spring in unusually wet years and on properties with a history of problems with liver fluke.
• Northwest United States (where winters are cold, e.g., Idaho, Montana)—Treat in late winter or early spring.
• Pacific Northwest/California (mild winters)—Fluke transmission may occur year round; no strategic treatment plan has been developed.

MEDICATIONS

DRUGS OF CHOICE
Only two drugs are available to treat liver fluke infections in the United States. (See Table 1)
• Clorsulon: two products available (Curatrem, Ivomec-Plus)
• Albendazole (Valbazen)
No drugs have FDA label approval for treatment of *F. magna* and effectiveness of treatments has not been well established. It is suggested to use albendazole at twice the recommended label dose for 2 or 3 consecutive days.

CONTRAINDICATIONS
• Drug withdrawal times for meat must be monitored and followed.
• None of the drugs are approved for use in lactating dairy cattle.

FOLLOW-UP
N/A

PATIENT MONITORING
N/A

PREVENTION/AVOIDANCE
• Improve pasture drainage
• Fence off ponds
• Move cattle off of "fluky" pastures during high transmission periods

POSSIBLE COMPLICATIONS
N/A

EXPECTED COURSE AND PROGNOSIS
• Prognosis is very good in chronic infections.
• Prognosis is guarded in acute disease.

MISCELLANEOUS

ASSOCIATED CONDITIONS
• Infections with gastrointestinal nematodes will almost always be present in fluke-infected animals, which will exacerbate the impact on the host.
• Associated conditions include anorexia, lethargy, pale mucous membranes, peripheral edema, weight loss, ill thrift, poor performance, and sudden death.

AGE-RELATED FACTORS
All ages are susceptible, but young animals are more likely to suffer severe disease.

ZOONOTIC POTENTIAL
• Metacercariae of *F. hepatica* are infective to humans, but this parasitic stage is found only on pasture.
• There is no possible zoonotic transmission directly from animals to humans.

PREGNANCY
N/A

RUMINANT SPECIES AFFECTED
All ruminants are susceptible to infection.

BIOSECURITY
- *F. hepatica* can be spread between farms by infected rabbits and deer, making eradication almost impossible.
- Fencing of pastures (and ponds) with "deer-proof" fencing should prevent *F. magna* infections in livestock in enzootic areas.

PRODUCTION MANAGEMENT
- Fence off marshy areas from grazing ruminants.
- Strategic deworming of cattle and sheep in the spring or early summer may limit the degree to which snail populations become infected with immature stages of flukes and limit amplification of infection.
- Deworming prior to introduction of livestock into low-lying pastures will have a long-term beneficial effect.

SEE ALSO
Bacillary hemoglobinuria (*Clostridium haemolyticum*)
Gastrointestinal nematodes, particularly *Haemonchus contortus*
Infectious necrotic hepatitis (black disease, *Clostridium novyi*)
Taenia hydatigena larvae in hepatic parenchyma

ABBREVIATIONS
FDA = Food and Drug Administration
GGT = serum gamma glutamyltransferase
GLDH = glutamic dehydrogenase

Suggested Reading
Duff, J. P., Maxwell, A. J., Claxton, J. R. 1999, Sep 11. Chronic and fatal fascioliasis in llamas in the UK. *Vet Rec.* 145(11):315–16.
Fairweather, I., Boray, J. C. 1999. Fasciolicides: efficacy, actions, resistance and its management. *Veterinary Journal* 2:81–112.

Kaplan, R. M. 1994. Liver flukes in cattle—control based on seasonal transmission dynamics. *Compendium on Continuing Education for the Practicing Veterinarian* 5:687–94.
Kaplan, R. M. 2001. Liver flukes in cattle: a review of the economic impact and considerations for control. *Veterinary Therapeutics* 1:40–50.
Loyacano, A. F., Williams, J. C., Gurie, J., DeRosa, A. A. 2002. Effect of gastrointestinal nematode and liver fluke infections on weight gain and reproductive performance of beef heifers. *Veterinary Parasitology* 3:227–34.
Marcilla, A., Bargues, M. D., Mas-Coma, S. 2002, Oct. A PCR-RFLP assay for the distinction between *Fasciola hepatica* and *Fasciola gigantica*. *Mol Cell Probes*. 16(5):327–33.

Authors: Ray M. Kaplan and Jeff W. Tyler

FATTY LIVER

BASICS

OVERVIEW
• Hepatocellular accumulation of fat results from overfeeding of dry dairy cows in the preparturient period; by the postparturient period, a damaging amount of fat has accumulated in the liver. It may appear as an individual case or as a herd problem in dairy cows. It is uncommon in beef cattle where it appears as an individual case prepartum.
• Fatty liver often appears in association with other diseases of the postparturient cow such as ketosis, retained placenta, metritis, milk fever and displaced abomasum.
• The development of fatty liver is a slow, insidious process and may range from progressively decreased milk production to a full-blown liver injury.
• The fundamental metabolic-nutritional defect is in the livers of cows where triglycerides (TG) are synthesized in excess of the liver's ability to synthesize the proteins of very low density lipoprotein (VLDL).

PATHOPHYSIOLOGY
• Overfeeding during the dry period induces excessive body fat stores.
• In the postparturient period, development of a negative energy balance leads to an intense mobilization of lipid from these stores.
• In the process, stored lipids are hydrolyzed by lipolytic enzymes to their constituent fatty acids and glycerol, which are then transported to the liver via the circulation as nonesterified fatty acids (NEFA) and glycerol.
• NEFA are taken up by the liver and enter the lipid metabolic pathways and glycerol enters the carbohydrate metabolic pathways. NEFA is resynthesized into TG or further metabolized.
• Normally, TG are transported out of the liver as components of lipoproteins of which VLDL is the major TG transporter. When there is insufficient lipoprotein synthesis, the TG cannot be transported out of the liver and they accumulate in the hepatocyte.
• These stores of TG physically damage the hepatocytes and/or disturb their normal metabolic pathways to induce the clinical syndrome of fatty liver.

SYSTEMS AFFECTED
Hepatic, metabolic, production management, nutrition

GENETICS
N/A

INCIDENCE/PREVALENCE
Unknown

GEOGRAPHIC DISTRIBUTION
Worldwide

SIGNALMENT
• Fatty liver is seen primarily in the high-producing dairy cow that is in its second to fourth lactation and is recognizably overconditioned.
• The more severely affected cows with depression and anorexia may be poorly conditioned. It may appear in individual cows or as a herd problem.
• When fatty liver appears in beef cattle, it occurs prior to calving and as an individual case.

Species
Bovine

Breed Predilections
N/A

Mean Age and Range
N/A

Predominant Sex
N/A

SIGNS
• Clinical signs of fatty liver are related to the degree of liver damage and/or to the associated diseases of parturition that may be present.
• Affected cows have a history of overfeeding during the dry period, possibly with difficulties in calving or postparturient disorders such as metritis, retained placenta, parturient paresis, ketosis, or displaced abomasum.
• They are characterized by being overly fat, anorexic, depressed, and weak with decreased milk production. Clinical signs of liver injury such as icterus are not usually apparent.

DIAGNOSIS

DIFFERENTIAL DIAGNOSIS
• All diseases of the high-producing dairy cow in early lactation are included in the differential. The more important differentials are ketosis, parturient paresis, retained placenta, metritis, and displaced abomasum. These are often seen concurrently with fatty liver.
• Secondary differentials include toxic hepatitis, biliary cholangitis, cholestasis, hepatic encephalopathy, and hepatoma.

CBC/BIOCHEMISTRY/URINALYSIS
• The CBC often has a leukopenia, neutropenia, lymphopenia, and degenerative left shift. Fibrinogen and Hp may also be increased. These are nonspecific signs of general inflammation and do not point directly to fatty liver.
• The common biochemical profiles are variable regarding the standard indices for liver injury.
• These include serum bili and serum liver enzymes such as AST, GD, GGT, ID, and AlP. The bile acids, urea, proteins, albumin, or NH_3 are also variable so judicious interpretation of any positive results correlating with history and clinical signs are required to arrive at a diagnosis.
• BSP or ICG clearance T1/2 are generally increased but both tests are time consuming, BSP is not generally available, and ICG is expensive.
• Serum lipid analyses including NEFA, TG, Chol, and LP fractions are definitive, noninvasive tests but are time and equipment expensive. NEFA increase; TG, Chol, and VLDL decrease.
• Urine ketones will be present in concurrent ketosis and urobilinogen may be absent if there is advanced cholestasis.
• Liver biopsy with compatible serum lipid analyses is the definitive diagnostic test for fatty liver. The specimen is distinctly yellow, is extremely friable, and floats in water. Microscopically, excessive hepatocyte accumulation of fat is seen.
• At necropsy, there is excessive abdominal and omental fat with some degree of icterus throughout the abdominal cavity. The liver is enlarged with rounded edges, greasy to the touch, extremely friable, and yellow.

TREATMENT

• Concurrent diseases, which may be present, must be treated.
• Restore anorexia or decreased rumen motility by transfaunation and provide good-quality, highly palatable hay.
• Correct the nutritional energy imbalance, restore carbohydrate metabolism, and promote liver protein synthesis.
• The therapy of fatty liver is supportive with the goal of correcting the negative energy balance, reducing fat mobilization, promoting carbohydrate metabolism, and increasing transport of TG out of the liver by promoting LP synthesis. All therapeutic approaches are empirical and largely symptomatic.

MEDICATIONS

DRUGS OF CHOICE

• Give an initial bolus of 250–500 ml of 50% glucose followed by a continuous intravenous infusion of glucose at 50–60 g/h to restore energy balance.
• Glucose precursors such as propylene glycol may be given per os initially at 250 mg bid for 2 days followed by 125 mg per os bid for 2 more days.
• Glucose is monitored two to three times per day using a portable glucose meter. Urine ketone is monitored at the same time using dipsticks.
• Choline, a component of LP, may be given at 50 g/d S.C. with some success in promoting the movement of TG out of the liver.
• PZI may be given at 200 U bid for several days to promote glucose utilization and hepatic LP synthesis, which will aid the movement of TG out of the liver.
• Glucocorticoids as used for bovine ketosis may be used to promote gluconeogenesis.
• Glucagon at 10 mg/day has been used experimentally at a constant intravenous infusion for 14 days and shown to be effective in increasing plasma glucose, and decreasing NEFA and TG. When given S.C. at 2.5 or 5.0 mg/day every 8 hours for 14 days, similar results were obtained in older cows but not in younger cows.

CONTRAINDICATIONS

Appropriate milk and meat withdrawal times must be followed for all compounds administered to food-producing animals.

FOLLOW-UP

PREVENTION

• The most effective means of preventing fatty liver is to avoid overfeeding during the dry period. The goal is to prevent the positive energy balance, which results in an overly fat or overconditioned cow with excess fat stores. In these cows, shortly postpartum, the demands of lactation create a marked negative energy balance, which then calls upon the fat stores for energy.
• As a result of the lipolysis, NEFA and glycerol are delivered to the liver in excess of its ability to transport the reformed TG out of the liver. These TG accumulate in the hepatocyte to eventually cause liver injury.

EXPECTED COURSE AND PROGNOSIS

The prognosis is generally poor in the advanced and complicated cases of fatty liver. Early diagnosis and rapid corrective measures will markedly improve the outcome.

MISCELLANEOUS

ASSOCIATED CONDITIONS

• Clinical signs of fatty liver are related to the degree of liver damage and/or to the associated diseases of parturition that may be present.
• They are characterized by being overly fat, anorexic, depressed, and weak with decreased milk production. Clinical signs of liver injury such as icterus are not usually apparent.

AGE-RELATED FACTORS

Generally, animals in their second through fourth lactation.

ZOONOTIC POTENTIAL

N/A

PREGNANCY

Clinical signs of fatty liver are related to the degree of liver damage and/or to the associated diseases of parturition that may be present.

RUMINANT SPECIES AFFECTED

Cattle: dairy and beef breeds

BIOSECURITY

N/A

PRODUCTION MANAGEMENT

• Affected cows have a history of overfeeding during the dry period, and may have had difficulties in calving or postparturient disorders such as metritis, retained placenta, parturient paresis, ketosis, or displaced abomasum.

• The most effective means of preventing fatty liver is to avoid overfeeding during the dry period.

SYNONYMS

Hepatic lipidosis

SEE ALSO

Biliary cholangitis
Cholestasis
Hepatic encephalopathy
Hepatoma
Ketosis
Metritis and displaced abomasum
Parturient paresis
Retained placenta
Toxic hepatitis

ABBREVIATIONS

AlP = alkaline phosphatase
AST = aspartate aminotransferase
BSP = bromosulphonthalein
CBC = complete blood count
Chol = cholesterol
GD = glutamate dehydrogenase
GGT = γ-glutamyl transferase
HDL = high density lipoprotein
Hp = haptoglobin
ICG (CG) = indocyanine green (cardiogreen)
id (sdh) = iditol dehydrogenase (sorbitol dehydrogenase)
LP = lipoprotein
NEFA = nonesterified fatty acid
NH$_3$ = ammonia
PZI = protamine zinc insulin
T1/2 = half-time
TG = triglyceride
VLDL = very low density lipoprotein

Suggested Reading
Bobe, G., Ametaj, B. N., Young, J. W., Beitz, D. C. 2003. Potential treatment of fatty liver with 14-day subcutaneous injections of glucagon. *J Dairy Sci.* 86:3138–47.
Bruss, M. L. 1997. Lipids and ketones. In: *Clinical biochemistry of domestic animals*, ed. J. J. Kaneko, J. W. Harvey, M. L. Bruss. 5th ed. San Diego: Academic Press.
Hippen, A. R., She, P., Young, J. W., Lindberg, G. L., Richardson, L. F., Tucker, R. W. 1999. Alleviation of fatty liver in dairy cows with 14-day intravenous infusions of glucagon. *J Dairy Sci.* 82:1130–52.

Author: J. Jerry Kaneko

FESCUE TOXICITY

BASICS

OVERVIEW
• Fescue toxicosis is a disease affecting primarily the cardiovascular and endocrine systems.
• Tall fescue (*Festuca arundinacea Schreb.*) is a cool season perennial grass grown worldwide.
• Noninfected varieties of tall fescue are available but they do not withstand extreme environmental conditions (overgrazing, drought, heat, etc.) as well as the endophyte-infected varieties.
• The fungus has a symbiotic relationship with the fescue, which makes the plant hardier.
• *Neotyphodium coenophialum* is present within the seed and throughout the plant.
• *N. coenophialum* produces several ergot-type and pyrrolizidine-type alkaloids, which cause the clinical signs associated with fescue toxicity.
• Three syndromes are seen in ruminants: fescue foot, summer slump, and fat necrosis.
• Another syndrome causing severe reproductive abnormalities in pregnant mares is not generally seen in ruminants.

PATHOPHYSIOLOGY
• The grass itself is not believed to be the cause of toxicity, but rather an endophytic fungus that infects it, *Neotyphodium coenophialum* (endophyte-infected).
• These toxins primarily cause peripheral vasoconstriction.

SYSTEMS AFFECTED
Cardiovascular and endocrine systems.

GENETICS
N/A

INCIDENCE/PREVALENCE
Unknown

GEOGRAPHIC DISTRIBUTION
Tall fescue (*Festuca arundinacea Schreb.*) is a cool season perennial grass grown worldwide.

SIGNALMENT
• This toxicosis affects cattle, sheep, and goats, as well as horses.
• Any animal that is grazing or consuming fescue hay can be affected.

Species
• Summer slump (most common syndrome—seen in all ruminants)
• Fescue foot (only in cattle)
• Fat necrosis in cattle/lipomatosis/abdominal necrotic fat (only in cattle)

Breed Predilections
N/A

Mean Age and Range
N/A

Predominant Sex
N/A

SIGNS
• Fescue foot (only in cattle)
  • Early: mild lameness particularly in rear limbs, walking with back arched
  • Redness and swelling around coronary band
  • Limb edema may be present.
  • Cold extremities
  • Hair on pastern easily rubbed off
  • With progression, a sharp line of demarcation appears at the level of the pastern or fetlock.
  • Skin below line becomes dry and gangrenous.
  • Hoof wall and skin may necrose.
  • Tips of ears and switch of tail may also necrose.
  • Affected animals are generally underweight and have dull hair coat.
• Summer slump (most common syndrome—seen in all ruminants)
  • Hirsutism
  • Elevated temperature and respiratory rate
  • Poor weight gain
  • Heat intolerance
  • Diarrhea
  • Hypersalivation
  • Photosensitization
  • Delayed puberty in heifers
  • Decreased conception and pregnancy rates
  • Decreased milk production
• Fat necrosis in cattle/lipomatosis/abdominal necrotic fat (only in cattle). Signs are related to obstruction of abdominal organs: bloat, colic.

CAUSES AND RISK FACTORS
• Consumption of tall fescue that is infected with *N. coenophialum*
• Fescue foot is more commonly seen in cold ambient temperatures.
• Summer slump is seen in warm to hot ambient temperatures.

DIAGNOSIS

DIFFERENTIAL DIAGNOSES
• Fescue foot
  • Ergot toxicosis/ *Claviceps purpurea* toxicity (history of consuming nonfescue forages, examination of forage for fungus)
  • Trauma (examination of foot)
  • Foot rot (examination of foot)
  • Frostbite (history of ambient conditions)
  • Selenium toxicosis (elevated serum selenium, history of consuming nonfescue forages)
• Summer slump
  • Internal parasites (fecal examination)
  • Nutritional deficiencies (analysis of feeding practices—including trace mineral supplements)
  • Chronic organophosphate toxicity—particularly in sheep (history of exposure, clinical signs of neurologic disease/axonal degeneration)
  • Molybdenum toxicity (located in an area of high molybdenum soil; signs attributable to copper deficiency: hypotrichosis, diarrhea, joint swelling, low serum or liver copper, and high liver molybdenum)
• Fat Necrosis
  • Lymphosarcoma (necropsy)
  • Intestinal obstruction (exploratory laparotomy, inflammatory leukogram, abdomenocentesis)
  • Peritonitis (inflammatory leukogram, abdomenocentesis)
  • Intussusception (exploratory laparotomy, inflammatory leukogram, abdomenocentesis)
  • Intestinal torsion (exploratory laparotomy, inflammatory leukogram, abdomenocentesis)

CBC/BIOCHEMISTRY/URINALYSIS
N/A

IMAGING
N/A

FESCUE TOXICITY

DIAGNOSTIC PROCEDURES
• Clinical signs matching syndromes noted above
• History of consuming fescue (pasture or hay) for weeks or months
• Microscopic examination of fescue for fungus
  • Should examine many tillers or seeds of the grass
  • Clinical signs have been seen in animals consuming fescue with as little as 20% if the grass is infected with *N. coenophialum.*

PATHOLOGIC FINDINGS

GROSS FINDINGS
• All syndromes
  • Poor body condition
  • Rough hair coat
• Fescue foot: gangrenous tissue on extremities, particularly rear limbs, with a line of demarcation from normal tissue.
• Fat necrosis: presence of calcified fat in abdomen, particularly the omentum

HISTOPATHOLOGICAL FINDINGS
Fescue foot: vascular thrombosis, tissue necrosis in lower limbs

TREATMENT
• Fescue foot: if disease is recognized early (before tissues necrose), remove fescue from diet or dilute with forage source that is not infected.
• Summer slump: remove from fescue
• Fat necrosis—none

MEDICATIONS

DRUGS OF CHOICE
Fescue foot: broad-spectrum antibiotic therapy for secondary bacterial infections (observe appropriate withdrawal times).

CONTRAINDICATIONS
• Appropriate milk and meat withdrawal times must be followed for all compounds administered to food-producing animals.
• Steroids should not be used in pregnant animals.

POSSIBLE INTERACTIONS

FOLLOW-UP
N/A

MISCELLANEOUS
• Recent research suggests that treatment of fescue or direct feeding of seaweed extract (*Ascophyllum nodosum*) may decrease the toxic effects of endophyte-infected fescue.
• Nontoxic varieties of endophyte-infected fescue have been developed and appear to be hardier than noninfected fescue but with a much lower potential to cause the untoward effects seen with toxic endophyte infected varieties.

ASSOCIATED CONDITIONS
N/A

AGE-RELATED FACTORS
N/A

ZOONOTIC POTENTIAL
N/A

PREGNANCY
N/A

RUMINANT SPECIES AFFECTED
Potentially, all ruminant species are affected.

BIOSECURITY
N/A

PRODUCTION MANAGEMENT
N/A

SYNONYMS
N/A

SEE ALSO
Chronic organophosphate toxicity
Claviceps purpurea toxicity
Ergot toxicosis
Foot rot
Frostbite
Internal parasites
Intestinal obstruction
Intussusception
Lymphosarcoma
Molybdenum toxicity
Nutritional deficiencies
Peritonitis
Selenium toxicosis

ABBREVIATIONS
N/A

Suggested Reading
Baird, A. N. 1999. Fescue foot. In: *Current veterinary therapy 4: food animal practice*, ed. J, L, Howard, R. A. Smith. Philadelphia: W. B. Saunders.
Brendemuehl, J. P. 2002. Fescue toxicosis. In: *Large animal internal medicine*, ed. B. P. Smith. Philadelphia: Mosby.
Davis, E. W. 2002. Fescue foot. In: *Large animal internal medicine*, ed. B. P. Smith. Philadelphia: Mosby.
Fike, J. H., Allen, V. G., Schmidt, R. E., Zhang, X., Fontenot, J. P., Bagley, C. P., Ivy, R. L., Evans, R. R., Coelho, R. W., Wester, D. B. 2001. Tasco-forage: I. influence of seaweed extract on antioxidant activity in tall fescue and in ruminants. *J Anim Sci.* 79:1011–21.
Kerr, L. A., Kelch, W. J. 1999. Fescue toxicosis. In: *Current veterinary therapy 4: food animal practice*, ed. J. L. Howard, R. A. Smith. Philadelphia: W. B. Saunders.

Author: Dawn J. Capucille

FLOPPY KID SYNDROME

 BASICS

OVERVIEW
• A floppy kid syndrome (fading kid syndrome, FKS) case is defined as one that is normal at birth but develops a sudden onset of profound muscular weakness (flaccid paresis or paralysis) or ataxia at 3–10 days of age.
• Kids with this clinical syndrome were first reported in the spring of 1987, although there were anecdotal reports of herds with this syndrome several years earlier.
• First recognized in herds in Canada and the west coast of the United States, this syndrome has since been diagnosed throughout the United States and Canada.

SIGNALMENT
• Affected kids have been found in dam-reared, pasteurized milk hand-reared, and unpasteurized milk hand-reared herds.
• There does not seem to be a breed predilection.

SIGNS
• Profound muscular weakness (flaccid paresis or paralysis) or ataxia
• Affected kids cannot use their tongues to suckle but can swallow.
• Affected kids have no other signs of illness such as diarrhea or respiratory disease.

CAUSES AND RISK FACTORS
• *Clostridium botulinum, E. coli*, and caprine herpes virus have been incriminated as possible etiologic agents.
• Cases tend to occur most commonly late in the kidding season.
• Herd morbidity ranges from 10%–50%.
• No specific management or goat-related risk factors have been identified.

 DIAGNOSIS

DIFFERENTIAL DIAGNOSIS
• Diagnosis is made on the basis of clinical signs of paresis/paralysis in 3–10-day-old kids with metabolic acidosis.
• These cases may be confused with white muscle disease, abomasal bloat, colibacillosis, septicemia, or enterotoxemia.

CBC/BIOCHEMISTRY/URINALYSIS
• A marked metabolic acidosis with an increased anion gap and decreased bicarbonate is present.
• Chloride levels are normal.
• Some affected kids are hypokalemic.
• There are no other detectable, repeatable serum biochemical abnormalities.

OTHER LABORATORY TESTS
N/A

IMAGING
N/A

DIAGNOSTIC PROCEDURES
N/A

PATHOLOGIC FINDINGS
N/A

 TREATMENT

• Early recognition of the syndrome and immediate treatment of the base deficit as well as supportive care are critical.
• If clinical chemistries are available, the base deficit can be calculated and the kid can be given fluids spiked with bicarbonate.
• Less severely affected kids can be treated with sodium bicarbonate (baking soda) at the rate of teaspoons in a small amount of water given orally.
• In addition, kids may need supportive therapy such as tube feeding.

MEDICATIONS
DRUGS OF CHOICE
Oral or intravenous sodium bicarbonate
CONTRAINDICATIONS
N/A

FOLLOW-UP
N/A

MISCELLANEOUS
• Spontaneous recovery without treatment has been reported in a few cases; however, case fatality rates have been as high as 30%–50% in untreated animals.
• Because the cause is unknown, no preventative measures can be specifically recommended.
• Necropsy of dead kids is encouraged to rule out other causes of neonatal mortality.

ASSOCIATED CONDITIONS
N/A
AGE-RELATED FACTORS
First 2 weeks of life
ZOONOTIC POTENTIAL
N/A
PREGNANCY
N/A
RUMINANT SPECIES AFFECTED
Goat kids
BIOSECURITY
N/A
PRODUCTION MANAGEMENT
N/A
SYNONYMS
Fading kid syndrome
FKS
SEE ALSO
Abomasal bloat
Caprine herpes virus
Caprine arthritis encephalitis
Colibacillosis
E. coli
Enterotoxemia
Septicemia
White muscle disease

ABBREVIATIONS
FKS = fading kid syndrome

Suggested Reading
Bureau, M. A., Begin, R. 1982. Depression of respiration induced by metabolic acidosis in newborn lambs. *Biol Neonate.* 42(5–6):279–83.
Herdt, T. H., Emery, R. S. 1992, Mar. Therapy of diseases of ruminant intermediary metabolism. *Vet Clin North Am Food Anim Pract.* 8(1):91–106.
Jorquera, P., Wu, J., Bockenhauer, D. 1999, Apr. Nonanion gap metabolic acidosis in a newborn. *Curr Opin Pediatr.* 11(2):169–73.
Rowe, J. D., East, N. E. 1998. Floppy kid syndrome (metabolic acidosis without dehydration in kids). *Proceedings of the 1998 Symposium on the Health and Disease of Small Ruminants,* Western Veterinary Conference, Las Vegas, NV.

Author: M. S. Gill

FLUID THERAPY

BASICS

OVERVIEW
• Fluid therapy is indicated when patients are severely dehydrated or unable or unwilling to ingest oral fluids.
• General goals are to replace fluid and electrolyte deficits and meet ongoing needs and losses.

SYSTEMS AFFECTED
Hemolymphatic

GENETICS
N/A

INCIDENCE/PREVALENCE
N/A

GEOGRAPHIC DISTRIBUTION
Worldwide

SIGNALMENT
Species
All ruminant species

Breed Predilections
N/A

Mean Age and Range
N/A

Predominant Sex
N/A

DIAGNOSIS

CLINICAL EXAMINATION
• The degree of patient dehydration is typically determined by physical examination.

Assessing Hydration Status in Ruminants			
% Dehydration	Demeanor	Sunken Eye	Skin Tenting
<6%	Normal	−	−
6–8%	Depressed	+	+/−
8–10%	Depressed	++	2–5 sec
10–12%	Comatose	+++	5–10 sec
>12%	Dead	++++	>10 sec

• Skin turgor and elasticity, position of the eye within the orbit, tenacity of mucus within the oral cavity, capillary refill time, and patient demeanor are all indicators of patient hydration status.
• As a general rule of thumb, fluid deficits less than 6% of body weight cannot be detected on clinical examination and deficits greater than 12% of body weight are generally fatal. The following table provides attempts to summarize expected clinical signs of dehydration in cattle.
• Clinical demeanor also has been associated with acid/base status in neonatal calves with diarrhea.
• The following table summarizes expected base deficits in calves of varying ages. It should be emphasized that this information is relevant only in neonatal calves with primary uncomplicated gastrointestinal disease.
• Calves with septicemia will have highly variable acid/base status. Furthermore, these rules of thumb are not appropriate in adult ruminants.

• Under ideal circumstances fluid and electrolyte disorders are confirmed by inexpensive, minimally invasive laboratory procedures.

CBC/BIOCHEMISTRY/URINALYSIS
• Hematocrit and serum protein concentration are readily determined in most veterinary practices.
• These procedures are useful adjuncts to physical examination in confirming the presence of dehydration.
• Serum chemistry analyzers suitable for clinic and ambulatory practice are becoming more common.
• Although panel composition varies with instrument and test kit, patient side confirmation of azotemia, acid/base status, and serum calcium and potassium is now possible. It should be noted that many of these instruments have not been validated for use in ruminants; however, most practitioners find them useful adjuncts in the development of fluid therapy protocols.

OTHER LABORATORY TESTS
N/A

Estimating Base Deficit (mmol/L) in Calves of Various Ages with Diarrhea		
Calf Demeanor	=<8 days	>=8 days
Bright, alert, ambulatory	0	5
Depressed, stands only with assistance	5	10
Unable to stand, suckling reflex intact	10	15
Comatose, suckling reflex absent	10	20

IMAGING
N/A

DIAGNOSTIC PROCEDURES
N/A

TREATMENT

GENERAL PRINCIPLES OF FLUID THERAPY

1. Oral fluids are generally preferred unless medically contraindicated. Oral fluids are inexpensive and safe and can be administered rapidly in field conditions.
2. Hypoglycemia is rare in adult ruminants, but occurs occasionally in neonates. Diseases of adult ruminants, which result in hypoglycemia, include fatty liver, ketosis, and pregnancy disease.
3. Mild hypocalcemia is common in anorectic adult cattle.
4. Mild metabolic alkalosis is common and expected in anorectic adult cattle.

5. Metabolic alkalosis and increased serum concentrations of albumin may decrease serum-ionized calcium. Metabolic acidosis and hypoalbuminemia may increase serum-ionized calcium. Many laboratories measure total calcium; however, animals recognize and regulate serum-ionized calcium. Correction factors developed for companion animals are inaccurate in ruminants.
6. Sodium bicarbonate administration is appropriate only for correction of metabolic acidosis. Metabolic acidosis is common in neonates with diarrhea, grain engorgement, and salivary loss, but rare in most other conditions of ruminants.
7. Maximum short-term IV fluid administration rates should not exceed 80–90 ml/kg/hr (20 ml/kg/hr in llamas).
8. Maximum long-term IV fluid administration rates for cattle should not exceed 20 ml/kg/hr.
9. Hypokalemia is common in anorectic adult cattle.

10. Neonates with diarrhea often have hyperkalemia (increased serum potassium concentrations); however, body stores of potassium (intracellular potassium) are often very low.
11. Potassium administration rates should not exceed 0.5 mmol/kg/hr unless the patient is severely hypokalemic, or glucose and/or bicarbonate are administered concurrently. Glucose and bicarbonate administration will cause extracellular potassium to shift to the intracellular space.
12. Near isotonic (300 mOsm/L) fluids should be used under most conditions.
13. Fluid deficit is generally calculated as follows: Body weight (kg) × (% dehydration/100) = deficit (L).
14. Estimates of daily maintenance requirements vary from 60–120 ml/kg/day, depending on severity of ongoing losses (diarrhea, renal losses). The values above include ongoing losses. Maintenance requirements are calculated as follows: Body weight (kg) × [(60–120 ml/kg/day)/1000 ml/kg] = (L).
15. Total daily fluid needs are calculated by adding deficits and daily maintenance requirements.
16. Base deficit is typically calculated as follows: Body weight (kg) × [measured deficit (mmol/L)] × [bicarbonate space]. Bicarbonate space is typically estimated as 0.5 to 0.6 in cattle. Bicarbonate replacement is used to replace 50–100% of base deficit. Higher percentages of deficit replacement, approaching 100%, are appropriate in neonates with diarrhea.

FLUID THERAPY

17. The core electrolyte abnormalities in calves with diarrhea include dehydration, acidosis, low systemic potassium with serum hyperkalemia due to acidosis, and occasionally hypoglycemia.
18. Isotonic = 300 mOsm/L, Isotonic sodium bicarbonate = 1.3% = 1.3 g/100mL = 13 g/L, Isotonic sodium chloride = 0.9% = 0.9 g/100 mL = 9 g/L
19. Do not withhold milk from calves with diarrhea. Do not feed beef calves more than 1 L/feeding. Beef calves are acclimated to small, frequent meals.
20. Oral fluids are probably adequate in mildly dehydrated calves (≤8%). Severely dehydrated calves probably require at least short-term intravenous fluids.

TREATMENT

In general, fluid therapy can be reduced to the following set of questions:
1. What is the fluid deficit?
2. What is the daily maintenance requirement for fluids?
3. What will the total fluid needs be over the next 24 hrs?
4. What is the base deficit?
5. What volume of isotonic sodium bicarbonate will replace this deficit?
6. How would you prepare this volume of isotonic sodium bicarbonate solution?
7. What is the maximum rate of fluid administration in the first hour?
8. How much 50% dextrose will we add to the first hour's fluids to create a 1% solution?
9. What is the theoretical maximum concentration of potassium for fluids administered in the first hour of therapy?
10. Based on the above answers, design a fluid therapy protocol for the patient.

EXAMPLE

You are examining a 50-kg Holstein heifer calf with profuse diarrhea. The calf is 15 days old. On physical examination, the calf is severely dehydrated (estimate 10%) and is comatose.

1. **What is the calf's fluid deficit?**
   Body weight (kg) × (% dehydration)/100 = 50 kg × 10/100 = 5 L
2. **What is the calf's daily maintenance requirement for fluids?**
   Body weight (kg) × 100 ml/kg = 50 kg × 100 ml/kg = 5000 ml = 5 L
3. **What will the calf's total fluid needs be over the next 24 hrs?**
   Deficit + Maintenance = 5 L + 5 L = 10 L
4. **What is the calf's base deficit?**
   Body weight (kg) × (estimated base deficit) × bicarbonate space = Estimated deficit based on the calf's demeanor (comatose) and age (>8 days) is 20 mmol/L
   50 kg × 20 mmol/L × 0.6 = 600 mmol HCO_3^-
   Alternatively, base deficit can be calculated from measured blood bicarbonate. For purposes of this calculation, we will assume the calf has a pure metabolic acidosis and serum bicarbonate of 5 mmol/L, and that normal is 25 mmol/L.
   Body weight (kg) × (normal bicarbonate - measured bicarbonate) × 0.6 = 50 kg × (25 - 5) × 0.6 = 600 mmol/L HCO_3^-
5. **What volume of isotonic sodium bicarbonate (1.3%) will replace this deficit?**
   Each liter of an isotonic solution has 300 mOsm/L. In the case of isotonic sodium bicarbonate, half the particles in solution are Na^+ and half are HCO_3^-. Therefore,

each liter of isotonic sodium bicarbonate contains 150 mmol/L of HCO_3^-. [Calculated deficit (mmol)]/150 mmol/L = [600]/150 = 4 L 1.3% sodium bicarbonate ($NaHCO_3$)

6. **How would you prepare this volume of isotonic sodium bicarbonate solution?**
   1.3% = 1.3 g/100 ml = 13 g/L
   Volumes required × 13 g/L = 4 L × 13 g/L = 52 g $NaHCO_3$ in 4 L sterile water
   It is important that base deficit be corrected using isotonic solutions.
7. **What is the maximum rate of fluid administration in this calf for the first hour?**
   Calves may be administered as much as 40 to 80 ml/kg during the first hour of therapy without creating an inordinate risk of pulmonary edema. Thereafter, administration rates should not exceed 20 ml/hr. Maintenance fluid rates in calves are approximately 4 ml/kg/hr.
   Body weight (kg) × 80 ml/kg/hr = 50 kg × 80 ml/kg/hr = 4000 ml = 4 L
8. **How much 50% dextrose will we add to the first hour's fluids to create a 1% solution?**
   We desire a 1% dextrose solution. Standard solutions, which we carry in our truck, are 50% solutions. Consequently, we will need to make a 1:50 dilution to create a 1% solution.
   1 L = 1000 mL, 1000 mL/50 = 20 mL
   Therefore, we add 20 mL of 50% dextrose to each of the 4 L we administer in the first hour. Remember, not all calves with diarrhea are hypoglycemic and excessive glucose supplementation will cause serum glucose to exceed the renal threshold, causing an osmotic diuresis, an undesirable effect in a dehydrated patient.

9. **What is the theoretical maximum concentration of potassium for fluids administered in the first hour of therapy?**

Generally, we limit potassium administration to a maximum of 0.5 mmol/kg/hr.

(Body weight (kg) × 0.5 mmol/kg)/volume administered (50 × 0.5)/4 = 6.25 mEq/L

Having performed this calculation, we recognize that the concurrent administration of bicarbonate and glucose will cause potassium to move intracellular, resulting in a precipitous decline in serum potassium. Consequently, we will typically administer 8 to 12 mmol/L potassium in bicarbonate-containing fluids.

10. **Based on the above answers, we design a fluid therapy protocol for a calf.**

Obviously, these are not exact calculations. Here is a rough plan.

a. Hour 1: 4 L isotonic sodium bicarbonate, each liter supplemented with 10 mmol K/L. Each of the first 2 L is supplemented with 20 ml 50% dextrose.

b. Hour 2: 2 L of a commercially available oral electrolyte solution (total volume 6 liters)

c. Hour 8: 2 L whole milk (total volume 8 liters)

d. Hour 14: 2 L of a commercially available oral electrolyte solution (total volume 10 liters)

If the calf is readily nursing, alternate oral electrolytes and milk at 6-hour intervals. If hydration appears normal, one or both daily electrolyte feedings may be discontinued. Do not use stool characteristics as a criteria for administration of milk.

FOLLOW-UP

In animals receiving extensive fluid therapy, the need to reassess hydration and acid base at frequent intervals should be considered.

MISCELLANEOUS

• Many practitioners use hypertonic fluids. These solutions can be rapidly administered in an ambulatory setting.

• As general rule, 7–8% sodium chloride solution is administered at a rate of 5 ml/kg IV.

• When using such protocols, oral fluids should be provided or administered.

ASSOCIATED CONDITIONS
N/A

AGE-RELATED FACTORS
N/A

ZOONOTIC POTENTIAL
N/A

PREGNANCY
N/A

RUMINANT SPECIES AFFECTED
Potentially all ruminant species are affected.

BIOSECURITY
N/A

PRODUCTION MANAGEMENT
N/A

SYNONYMS
N/A

SEE ALSO
Colostrum and milk replacers
Laboratory tests
Oral fluid therapy

ABBREVIATIONS
IV = intravenous
Kg = kilogram
mg /kg= milligram per kilogram
NaHCO$_3$ = sodium bicarbonate
Sec = second

Suggested Reading
Naylor, J. M. 1996. Neonatal ruminant diarrhea. In: *Large animal internal medicine* ed. B. P. Smith., 2nd ed., pp. 396–417. St. Louis: Mosby.
Radostits, O. M., Gay, C. C., Blood, D. C., Hinchcliff, K. W. 2000. *Veterinary medicine*, 9th ed. New York: W. B. Saunders.
Roussel, A. J. 1999. Fluid therapy in mature cattle. *Vet Clinics NA: Food Animal Pract*. 15:545–57.
Roussel, A. J., Cohen, N. D., Holland, P. S., Taliaoferro, L., Green, R., Benson, P. Navarre, C. B., Hooper, R. N. 1998. Alterations in acid-base balance and serum electrolyte concentrations in cattle: 632 cases (1984–1994). *J Am Vet Med Assoc*. 212:1769–75.

Author: Jeffrey W. Tyler

FLUORIDE TOXICITY

BASICS

OVERVIEW
• Fluoride (F^-) is absorbed by the gastrointestinal tract and lungs.
• Clinical signs associated with chronic F^- exposure are manifest primarily in skeletal and dental abnormalities and may take months to years to become apparent depending on the solubility of the fluoride compound, amount of F^- absorbed, and duration of exposure.
• Chronic fluorosis is commonly due to ingestion of mineral supplements with high F^- content or consumption of contaminated forage and water by industrial emissions containing F^-.
• Acute toxicity is rare but may result from inhalation of gases containing fluoride or ingestion of highly toxic rodenticides containing fluoride. In acute cases, clinical signs are referable to the nervous system and death results from respiratory or cardiac failure.

SIGNALMENT
Dairy cattle are considered more at risk of chronic toxicity due to their longer lifetime in production. There is no breed, sex predilection, or genetic basis for fluorosis.

SIGNS
• Dental abnormalities occur only if animals are exposed during permanent tooth development prior to eruption and include dullness, mottling, pitting, and discoloration of tooth enamel, and abnormal tooth wear and loss, particularly in pairs of teeth that erupt at the same time.
• Dental problems may result in decreased feed and water intake, difficulty with mastication, weight loss, and general unthriftiness.

• Other clinical signs include decreased milk production and skeletal abnormalities; lameness, arthritis, fractures of the pedal bones; bilateral enlargement and roughening of metatarsals, metacarpals, ribs and mandible; and abnormal hoof wear resulting from altered gait with elongated toe, especially on hind feet.

CAUSES AND RISK FACTORS
• >40–100 mg F^-/kg feed cattle, >60 mg F^-/kg feed ewes, >150 mg F^-/kg feed lambs
• Rock phosphate deposits, nondefluorinated or inadequately defluorinated mineral supplements, monoammonium, diammonium, and gypsum phosphate fertilizers or other sources of phosphorus containing less than 100:1 parts phosphorus to fluoride, contaminated forage and water from industrial aerial emissions, deep well and thermal spring water, fluorinated municipal water, sewage effluent from municipalities using fluorinated water, forage and water contamination by volcanic gas and ash pose a risk.
• Forage usually has a low level of fluoride but levels are variable and should be considered.
• A calcium deficient diet may increase F^- accumulation. Animals in poor body condition may be more susceptible.
• Rodenticides containing sodium monofluoroacetate (1080) or fluoroacetamide are highly toxic and may account for acute toxicity. Due to the highly lethal nature of these compounds, their use is restricted in the United States.
• Fluoride absorption is related to solubility; sodium fluoride > rock phosphate >dicalcium phosphate > defluorinated phosphate

DIAGNOSIS

Clinical signs, history of exposure/mineral supplementation, radiography and feed/bone/urine F^- levels

DIFFERENTIAL DIAGNOSIS
Arthritis; osteoporosis; deficiencies in calcium, phosporus, or vitamin D; traumatic injury

CBC/BIOCHEMISTRY/URINALYSIS
Eosinophilia, anemia, hypoglycemia, increased ALP

OTHER LABORATORY TESTS
• F^-, Ca^{2+}, P concentrations in forage, mineral supplements, soil, and water
• F^- content in bone (normal content will vary with bone selected), antler, kidney, serum
• >10 ppm F^- in urine
• T_4, T_3 hypothroidism

IMAGING
Radiography: periosteal hyperostosis, exostosis, sclerosis in metacarpals, metatarsal, mandible, and ribs

DIAGNOSTIC PROCEDURES

PATHOLOGICAL FINDINGS
• Gross—teeth:pitting, discoloration,chalkiness of enamel, irregular wear, and tooth loss
• Skeletal—exostoses, sclerosis, arthritis, stunted growth
• Histopathological—abnormal remodeling of bone, atrophy of osteoblasts and bone marrow cells, retardation of cartilage cell differentiation

TREATMENT
Remove from source. Provide feeds that are easily masticated, symptomatic treatment for osteoarthritis/lameness

MEDICATIONS

DRUGS OF CHOICE
None

CONTRAINDICATIONS
.

POSSIBLE INTERACTIONS
N/A

FOLLOW-UP

PATIENT MONITORING

PREVENTION/AVOIDANCE
• Aluminum sulfate, aluminum chloride, calcium aluminate, and calcium carbonate reduce absorption of fluorides.
• Use only feed grade sources of phosphorus supplements.

POSSIBLE COMPLICATIONS
N/A

EXPECTED COURSE AND PROGNOSIS
In mild cases, improvement may be seen over weeks to months as fluoride body stores are depleted. In severe cases of lameness or inability to consume adequate forage, euthanasia may be required as some bony lesions are irreversible.

MISCELLANEOUS

ASSOCIATED CONDITIONS

AGE-RELATED FACTORS
Young animals with growing bones are most severely affected. Exposure of adult animals will result in normal dentition with skeletal lesions.

ZOONOTIC POTENTIAL
None

PREGNANCY
Congenital fluorosis has been reported in calves born to fluoride intoxicated cows.

RUMINANT SPECIES AFFECTED
All ruminants are susceptible.

BIOSECURITY
None

SEE ALSO
Arthritis
Deficiencies in calcium, phosporus, or vitamin D
Osteoporosis
Traumatic injury

ABBREVIATIONS
ALP = alkaline phosphatase
Ca^{2+} = calcium
F = fluoride
P = phosphorus
ppm = parts per million

Suggested Reading
Bourke, C. A., Ottaway, S. J. 1998. Chronic gypsum fertiliser ingestion as a significant contributor to a multifactorial cattle mortality. *Aust Vet J*. 76(8): 565–69.
Jubb, T. F., et al., 1993. Phosphorus supplements and fluorosis in cattle—a northern Australian experience. *Aust Vet J*. 70(10): 379–83.
Osheim, D. L., Rasmusson, M. C. 1998. Determination of fluoride in bovine urine. *J AOAC Int*. 81(4): 839–43.
Osweiler, G. 2004. In: *Clinical veterinary toxicology*, ed. K. Plumlee. St. Louis: Mosby.
Patra, R. C, et al. 2000. Industrial fluorosis in cattle and buffalo around Udaipur, India. *Sci Total Environ*. 253(1–3):145–50.
Schultheiss, W. A., Van Niekerk, J. C. 1994. Suspected chronic fluorosis in a sheep flock. *J S Afr Vet Assoc*. 65(4): 84.
Vikoren, T., et al. 1996. Fluoride exposure in cervids inhabiting areas adjacent to aluminum smelters in Norway. I. Residue levels. *J Wildl Dis*. 32(2):169–80.

Author: Lauren Palmer

FOOT-AND-MOUTH DISEASE

BASICS

OVERVIEW
• Foot-and-mouth disease (FMD) is a very contagious, viral disease of cloven-hoofed livestock and some wild animals, characterized by fever and vesicular lesions with subsequent erosions of the epithelium of the mouth, tongue, nostrils, feet, and teats.
• Sheep and goats are considered "maintenance" hosts. They can have very mild signs; therefore, diagnosis may be delayed allowing time for aerosol and contact spread as well as environmental contamination.
• Compared to other species, pigs produce extremely high concentrations of virus particle in aerosols. They are considered "amplifying" hosts.
• Cattle are considered "indicators" of this disease because they generally are the first species to show signs of infection. Their lesions are more severe and progress more rapidly.
• Recovered or vaccinated cattle exposed to diseased animals can be healthy carriers for 6–24 months. Sheep can be carriers for 4–6 months. Pigs are not carriers of FMDV.

PATHOPHYSIOLOGY
• FMDV is a single-stranded RNA virus and a member of the family Picornaviridae, genus *Aphthovirus*.
• There are seven immunologically and serologically distinct types of FMDV: O, A, C, Southern African Territories (SAT) -1, SAT-2, SAT-3, and Asia-1. Currently there are more than 60 subtypes.
• FMDV usually enters the host via the respiratory tract and can be transmitted by aerosols, ingestion, direct contact, artificial insemination, and meat products.
• Feeding of infected animal products such as meat, milk, bones, glands, and cheese can also spread the disease.
• Incubation of the virus is from 1 to 14 days and clinical signs usually develop in 3 to 5 days.
• The disease usually runs its clinical course in 1 to 3 weeks.

SYSTEMS AFFECTED
Skin, herd health, reproductive, cardiovascular, renal

GENETICS
There is no particular mode of inheritance for this disease.

INCIDENCE/PREVALENCE
• The morbidity rate may approach 100% in susceptible populations, particularly when the disease or serotype is not endemic to the population.
• Mortality is usually between 1% and 5%, although may be higher in young animals or in certain wildlife populations exposed to certain strains.

GEOGRAPHIC DISTRIBUTION
• Generally, endemic areas include Asia, Africa, and parts of South America. In South America, Chile and Guyana are free of the disease without vaccination.
• North and Central America, Australia, and New Zealand have been free of FMD for many years. Despite the 2001 outbreak in the United Kingdom, it and most European countries are recognized as free without vaccination.
• The OIE designates member countries as being in one of five categories: (1) free without vaccination, (2) free with vaccination, (3) having free zones without vaccination, (4) free zones with vaccination, and (5) having endemic FMD. This list is updated each May and can be accessed at www.oie.int.
• Serotypes are somewhat geographically represented. O and A occur in many parts of the world, serotypes SAT-1, 2, 3 are generally limited to Southern Africa, and Asia-1 is generally found in Asia.

SIGNALMENT
Species/Host Range
• Cloven-hoofed domestic livestock (e.g., cattle, pigs, sheep, goats, water buffalo) and cloven-hoofed wild animals (e.g., deer, elk, bison, antelopes, wildebeest) predominant. Other susceptible animals include elephants, nutrias, armadillos, and hedgehogs and may serve as sources of transmission to ruminants.

• South American camelids have low susceptibility to FMDV, whereas camels are resistant to natural infection.
• FMDV does not discriminate on the basis of breed, age, or sex, although mortality may be higher in younger animals.
• Immunity to one virus serotype is not protective against other serotypes.

SIGNS
• Initial clinical signs are fever, lethargy, salivation, lameness, blanching of the coronary bands, and inappetence.
• Foot-and-mouth disease is characterized by vesicles (blisters), which progress to erosions in the mouth, nares, muzzle, feet, or teats.
• Vesicles on the tongue, dental pad, gums, soft palate, nostrils, or muzzle characterize oral lesions. Severe oral lesions may lead to complete sloughing of the epithelial lining of the tongue.
• Hoof lesions are in the area of the coronary band and interdigital space. Severe lesions may lead to complete sloughing of the hoof.
• Infection with FMD is accompanied by a high fever in the range of 103–106°F.
• Depression, anorexia, excessive salivation, serous nasal discharge, decreased milk production, lameness, and reluctance to move are commonly observed.
• Abortion may occur in pregnant animals.
• Young animals may die acutely without clinical signs.

CAUSES AND RISK FACTORS
• Contact with infected animals; spread from aerosols; exposure to contaminated meat, milk, cheese, blood, etc.; contact with mechanical vectors (e.g., contaminated people's hands, footwear, etc.).
• It is important to note exposure to infected pigs can spread the disease very rapidly because they are efficient amplifiers of FMDV and that sheep can produce infectious aerosols while not displaying pronounced clinical signs.
• Risk factors include naïve population exposed to exotic FMD virus or serotype, unvaccinated population in endemic areas, poor biosecurity, and feeding contaminated feed to susceptible animals.

DIAGNOSIS

DIFFERENTIAL DIAGNOSIS
- Vesicular stomatitis
- Papular stomatitis
- Bovine viral diarrhea-mucosal disease
- Malignant catarrhal fever
- Foot rot
- Herpes mammillitis
- Pseudocowpox
- Rinderpest
- Bluetongue
- Contagious ecthyma (orf) in sheep
- Infectious bovine rhinotracheitis
- Chemical and thermal burns

CBC/BIOCHEMISTRY/URINALYSIS
N/A

OTHER LABORATORY TESTS
- Antigen detection: virus isolation (gold standard), complement fixation, ELISA
- Nucleic acid detection: PCR
- Antibody detection: virus neutralization, ELISA

IMAGING
N/A

DIAGNOSTIC PROCEDURES
- In the United States, contact the authorities immediately upon suspicions of a vesicular disease. Only under the direction of a foreign animal disease diagnostician (FADD) will samples be collected in the initial case. All samples must be sent to the Foreign Animal Disease Diagnostic Laboratory (FADDL) in Plum Island, New York.
- Vesicular fluid, the epithelium that covers vesicles, whole blood, serum (acute and convalescent), and esophageal-pharyngeal fluid from convalescent animals (probang test) in cell culture fluid are important samples for diagnosis.

GROSS FINDINGS
- The diagnostic lesions of foot-and-mouth disease are single or multiple vesicles from 2 mm to 10 cm in size.
- Lesions may be seen in any stage of development from a small white area to a fluid-filled blister, sometimes joining with adjacent lesions. The vesicles rupture, leaving a red, eroded area, which is then covered with a gray fibrinous coating. This coating becomes yellow, brown, or green, and is then replaced by new epithelium.
- "Tiger heart" lesions may also be seen; these lesions are characterized by a gray or yellow streaking in the myocardium caused by degeneration and necrosis. These are most commonly seen in young animals that die acutely.
- Denuded rumen papillae

TREATMENT

In endemic areas, generally supportive treatment of infected individuals is warranted. Milking time hygiene is of utmost importance. In areas where FMD is exotic, health care is usually swift and terminal.

MEDICATIONS
N/A

CONTRAINDICATIONS/POSSIBLE INTERACTIONS
N/A

FOLLOW-UP

PREVENTION/AVOIDANCE
- FMD is prevented thru the implementation of stringent biosecurity procedures.
- It is possible for humans to act as vectors of the disease with virus surviving for 24 to 48 hours on oral mucosa.
- At the farm level, basic animal husbandry practices that limit spread of endemic organisms (e.g., restriction of high-risk visitors, quarantine of high-risk animals and animal products, etc.) will aid in the exclusion of FMD.
- At the country level, control of importation of animals and products, decontamination of at-risk garbage, and a strong animal health infrastructure will mitigate the risk of FMD transmission.
- The virus is inactivated when exposed to pH below 6.5 or above 11; however, it can survive for extended periods (days to weeks) when protected in milk, meat, serum, or other organic material.
- Sodium hydroxide (2%), sodium carbonate (4%), and citric acid (0.2%) are effective disinfectants. FMDV is resistant to iodophors, quaternary ammonium compounds, hypochlorite, and phenol, especially in the presence of organic matter.

PRODUCTION MANAGEMENT
Vaccination
- Vaccines against FMD are available and are used primarily in endemic areas or as an aid in eradicating the disease.

FOOT-AND-MOUTH DISEASE

• Cross protection between different serotypes is limited. Therefore, it is important that the vaccine contain the same subtype of virus as is in the area. This necessitates frequent checking of the serotype and subtype during an outbreak as FMD virus frequently changes during natural passage through various species.
  • Protective immunity develops within 14 days (often by 4 days)
• Protection from aluminum hydroxide vaccines decreases rapidly in 4–6 months. A double-emulsion oil vaccine can protect for up to 1 year.
  • Vaccinated animals infected with live virus may shed FMDV without detectable clinical signs.
  • It is difficult to distinguish between animals that have been vaccinated and those that have been exposed to live FMDV by conventional serologic methods.
  • It is imperative that vaccinated animals have permanent identification and are marked as vaccinated.

Control and Prevention
• In countries free of FMD (see Geographic Distribution above), the OIE suggests controlling outbreaks by: (1) slaughter of all clinicals and in-contact susceptibles; (2) slaughter of all clinicals and in-contact susceptibles with vaccination and subsequent slaughter of at-risk animals; (3) slaughter of all clinicals and in-contact susceptibles with vaccination of at-risk animals without their slaughter; or (4) vaccination without slaughter of affected or vaccinated animals.
• Use of vaccine in an outbreak affects OIE FMD status and subsequent ability for international trade. For example, if an outbreak occurs in a country free of FMD where vaccination is not routinely employed and it is used during the outbreak, there is a 3-month waiting period if all animals are slaughtered, but a 6-month waiting period after the last case or vaccination before free status and free trade is regained. If no vaccine is used, it is a 3-month waiting period. More details are available in the Terrestrial Animal Health Code (http://www.oie.int/eng/normes/mcode/en_chapitre_2.2.10.htm).

• In Africa, the prevalence of six serotypes, maintenance in buffalo, and widespread intercontinental trade make eradication from the continent unlikely in the near future.
• Vaccination is used widely in some countries (e.g., the Middle East) to prevent economic losses associated with the disease not necessarily to eradicate the disease.

POSSIBLE COMPLICATIONS
Secondary bacterial infection of eroded foot-and-mouth lesions are common as is low milk production, failure to thrive, mastitis, and reproductive inefficiency.

EXPECTED COURSE AND PROGNOSIS
• The disease usually runs its course in 1 to 3 weeks.
• Some animals may become carriers. Cattle may carry the virus for a few years, while sheep and goats usually carry it for less than a year.
• The duration of immunity from naturally occurring disease is relatively short and is serotype, and often subtype, specific.

MISCELLANEOUS

ASSOCIATED CONDITIONS
N/A

AGE-RELATED FACTORS
All ages of animals are susceptible to infection with FMD. Neonates are more susceptible to fatal cardiac disease related to FMD infection.

ZOONOTIC POTENTIAL
FMD has been isolated from only about 40 human cases, despite widespread occurrence of the disease in animals. Vesicular lesions can be seen, but signs are mild. Because of this, FMD is not considered a public health concern.

PREGNANCY
Some pregnant animals may abort.

RUMINANT SPECIES AFFECTED
Domestic and wild, even-toed ungulates: cattle, goats, sheep, bison, South American camelids, water buffalo, deer, reindeer, elk, mouse, antelopes, chamois, gazelles, impala, giraffe, wildebeest

SEE ALSO
Bluetongue
Bovine viral diarrhea
Chemical and thermal burns
Contagious ecthyma (orf) in sheep
Foot rot
Infectious bovine rhinotracheitis
Malignant catarrhal fever
Papular stomatitis
Rinderpest
Vesicular stomatitis

ABBREVIATIONS
ELISA = enzyme-linked immunosorbent assay
FMD = foot-and-mouth disease
FMDV = foot-and-mouth disease virus
OIE = Office International des Epizooties
PCR = polymerase chain reaction

Suggested Reading
Bartleling, S. J. 2002. Development and performance of inactivated vaccines against foot and mouth disease. *Rev Sci Tech.* 21:577–88.
Grubman, M. J. 2003, Dec. New approaches to rapidly control foot-and-mouth disease outbreaks. *Expert Rev Anti Infect Ther.* 1(4):579–86.
Mebus, C. A., House, J. 1998. Foot and mouth disease. In: *Foreign Animal Diseases Book* ("The Gray Book"), 6th ed. Richmond: United States Animal Health Association.
Musser, J. M.. 2004, Apr 15. A practitioner's primer on foot-and-mouth disease. *J Am Vet Med Assoc.* 224(8): 1261–68.
Perez, A. M., Ward, M. P., Carpenter, T. E. 2004, Jun 19. Epidemiological investigations of the 2001 foot-and-mouth disease outbreak in Argentina. *Vet Rec.* 154(25):777–82.
Wernery, U., Kaaden, O. R. 2004, Sep. Foot-and-mouth disease in camelids: a review. *Vet J.* 168(2):134–42.

Authors: Daniel L. Grooms and Daryl V. Nydam

BASICS

DEFINITION
• Interdigital phlegmon (foot rot) is an acute or subacute necrotizing infection of the interdigital skin in cattle that extends into the underlying tissues and results in diffuse digital swelling and lameness.
• A second form of the disease has been reported in the UK and the United States, "superfoul," "super foot rot," or peracute foot rot, which is much less responsive to antimicrobial therapy than the normal form.
• Super foot rot will have a peracute onset (i.e., less than 12 hours after infection).

PATHOPHYSIOLOGY
• Trauma to the interdigital skin causes a local dermatitis and allows the infection from *Fusobacterium necrophorum* and *Prevotella levii* or other synergistic bacterium to get established.
• The early infection produces dermal and hypodermal necrosis with subsequent involvement of the whole interdigital skin. The necrotizing dermatitis spreads to the underlying tissues and causes an inflammatory response, which leads to generalized digital swelling and acute lameness due to pain. The foot becomes swollen from the fetlock to the coronary band.

SYSTEMS AFFECTED
Skin (primary), musculoskeletal (secondary)

GENETICS
Incidence may be higher in *Bos taurus* than *Bos indicus*.

INCIDENCE/PREVALENCE
Usually sporadic but can be epidemic under some conditions

GEOGRAPHIC DISTRIBUTION
Worldwide

SIGNALMENT
Species
Bovine

Breed Predilections
Jersey cattle are reported to have lower risk than other dairy breeds.

Mean Age and Range
More common in younger animals but found in all age groups

Predominant Sex
None

SIGNS
HISTORICAL FINDINGS
• Sporadic occurrence of lameness with swelling around the coronary band

PHYSICAL EXAMINATION FINDINGS
• Swollen, painful foot with necrotic, foul-smelling interdigital lesion; usually only one foot involved, more common in rear feet

CAUSES
• *Fusobacterium necrophorum* is always present and *Porphorymonas levii* is the most common secondary organism. Other *Porphorymonas* species are also found as secondary invaders as well as members of the genera *Prevotella*, *Peptostreptococcus*, and other *Fusobacterium*.
• Isolates of *Fusobacterium* have been found to have great differences in virulence, with isolates from "super foot rot" being at the higher end of the virulence scale.

• *Fusobacterium necrophorum* and *Prevotella levii* are considered to be part of the normal flora of bovine intestinal tracts. Spirochetes are occasionally isolated from lesions.

RISK FACTORS
Major risk factor is trauma to the interdigital skin, which can be due to mechanical trauma (e.g., stones, stubble, frozen ground, etc.) or hydropic maceration due to constant moisture (e.g., wet ground or manure slurry); may be more common during warmer weather.

DIAGNOSIS

DIFFERENTIAL DIAGNOSIS
Septic arthritis as a sequel to sole ulcer, white line abscess, or vertical fissure. Septic arthritis will usually have swelling of only one digit and will not have the necrotizing interdigital lesion unless the cellulitis has become more diffuse.

CBC/BIOCHEMISTRY/URINALYSIS
N/A

OTHER LABORATORY TESTS
N/A

IMAGING
N/A

DIAGNOSTIC PROCEDURES
• Acute to peracute onset of lameness, symmetrical swelling around the coronary band and in the interdigital space
• Usually only found on one foot and is more common on rear feet
• Pyrexia and decreased feed intake are commonly seen in both beef and dairy cattle and decreased milk production is common in dairy cattle.

FOOT ROT IN CATTLE

• Microbiological culture is seldom used due to the time and expense involved in culturing anaerobic organisms.
• In herd outbreaks, culture may be useful to confirm the presence of *F. necrophorum*.

PATHOLOGIC FINDINGS
• Necrotizing, usually caseous, necrosis of the interdigital skin with a characteristic foul odor and swelling of the foot around the coronary band
• Extensive inflammation of the skin and underlying tissues

TREATMENT

APPROPRIATE HEALTH CARE
• Currently, there are two vaccines licensed for prevention of interdigital phlegmon but this author is unaware of any peer-reviewed studies on vaccine efficacy.
• Hoof trimmers will commonly treat lesions with a topical antimicrobial and wrap the foot with a bandage.
• Sometimes it is necessary to remove the interdigital fat pad to facilitate healing of the interdigital skin.

NURSING CARE
• If bandages are applied, they should be removed after 3–4 days.
• Affected cattle should be given the full course of parenteral antimicrobials and be monitored for improvement and clinical cure.

ACTIVITY
Should be limited during recovery

DIET
Nutrition is sometimes blamed, but there is little or no evidence of any specific nutritional deficiency or excess that causes the skin to be invaded by bacteria more easily.

CLIENT EDUCATION
• If wet conditions are associated with an outbreak, cattle should be moved to drier areas, if possible.
• Good corral and freestall management and removal of any trauma inducing objects should attenuate the incidence.
• During an outbreak, it would be prudent to isolate affected animals from the remainder of the herd.

SURGICAL CONSIDERATIONS
Amputation of a claw may become necessary if septic arthritis occurs secondary to the interdigital phlegmon.

MEDICATIONS

DRUGS OF CHOICE
• The following drugs have labels specifically for foot rot and can be used on all dairy cattle as well as beef cattle:
  Amoxicillin (Amoxi-inject): 3–5 mg/lb IM or SC for ≤ 5 days (withdrawal: meat 25 days; milk 96 hours)

Ceftiofur HCl (Excenel): 1.1–2.2 mg/lb IM or SC once per day for 3–5 days (withdrawal: meat 2 days; milk 0 days)
Ceftiofur HCl (Naxcel): 1.1–2.2 mg/lb IM once per day for 3–5 days (withdrawal: meat 0 days; milk 0 days)
Sulfadimethoxine bolus (Albon bolus): 25 mg/lb PO once per day for first day, 12.5 mg/lb once per day, should not exceed 5 days (withdrawal: meat 7 days; milk 60 hours)
Sulfadimethoxine injectable, 40% solution (several manufacturers): 25 mg/lb IV once per day as initial dose, 12.5 mg/lb IV once per day; continue for 2 days after clinical signs are gone.
Penicillin or oxytetracycline can be used for treatment of susceptible bacterial infections in nonlactating dairy cattle and beef cattle. Check label for dosage and withdrawal times.
Nonsteroidal anti-inflammatory drugs (NSAIDs) may be helpful on a case-by-case basis.

CONTRAINDICATIONS
Appropriate milk and meat withdrawal times must be followed for all compounds administered to food-producing animals.

PRECAUTIONS
Do not treat for longer than period stated on label.

POSSIBLE INTERACTIONS
N/A

ALTERNATIVE DRUGS
Extralabel antimicrobials might be used but practitioners would have to show that labeled products were not efficacious.

FOLLOW-UP

PATIENT MONITORING
Monitor affected cattle during treatment for indications that pain and swelling are abating.

PREVENTION/AVOIDANCE
• Footbaths with antiseptic solutions are commonly used on dairies to prevent new cases of infectious foot diseases including interdigital phlegmon.
• Commonly used footbath compounds are $CuSO_4$ or $ZnSO_4$ (5%–10%) or formalin (3%–5%).
• Footbaths require good management to be effective since contamination of the footbath solution with fecal and urine will render the solution ineffective.
• It is commonly recommended that the footbath be drained, cleaned, and refilled after every 100–300 animals pass through.
• Footbath programs have to be carefully monitored and tend to be site specific.

POSSIBLE COMPLICATIONS
Suppurative arthritis, septic tenosynovitis, rupture of the flexor tendon, abscessation of the interdigital space, and phalangeal osteomyelitis

EXPECTED COURSE AND PROGNOSIS
Recovery is usually uneventful if the disease is diagnosed and treated promptly. "Super foot rot" is usually not responsive to antibiotics.

MISCELLANEOUS

ASSOCIATED CONDITIONS
Other infectious causes of lameness exacerbated by poor foot hygiene or wet or muddy conditions, such as interdigital dermatitis, digital dermatitis, and heel horn erosion

AGE-RELATED FACTORS
Found in all ages but more common in younger animals

ZOONOTIC POTENTIAL
No

PREGNANCY
N/A

RUMINANT SPECIES AFFECTED
Bovine, both dairy and beef

BIOSECURITY
Introduction of new cattle onto a facility may introduce new, highly virulent strains of the bacteria and cause outbreaks of interdigital phlegmon.

PRODUCTION MANAGEMENT

SYNONYMS
Acute foot rot
Acute necrotic pododermatitis
Foul in the foot
Infectious pododermatitis

Interdigital necrobacillosis
Interdigital pododermatitis
Phlegmona interdigitalis

SEE ALSO
Digital dermatitis
Heel horn erosion
Interdigital dermatitis
Interdigital fibroma
Septic arthritis

ABBREVIATIONS
NSAIDs = nonsteroidal anti-inflammatory drugs

Suggested Reading
Berg, J. N., Franklin, C. L. 2000. Interdigital phlegmon a.k.a. interdigital necrobacillosis a.k.a. acute foot rot of cattle: considerations in etiology, diagnosis and treatment. *Proc. XI Intl. Symp. on Disorders of the Ruminant Digit & III Intl. Conf. on Bovine Lameness.* Parma, Italy.
Berry, S. L. 2001. Diseases of the digital soft tissues. *Vet Clin N Amer Food Anim Pr.* 17:129–42.
Demirkan, I., Murray, R., Du Carter, S. D. 2000. Skin diseases of the bovine digit associated with lameness. *Vet Bull.* 70:149–71.
Guard, C. 2000. Environmental risk factors contributing to lameness in dairy cattle. *Proc Ontario Assoc Bov Pract.* 2000:10–16.
Stokka, G. L., Lechtenberg, K., Edwards, T., MacGregor, S., Voss, K., Griffin, D., Grotelueschen, D. M., Smith, R. A., Perino, L. J. 2001. Lameness in feedlot cattle. *Vet Clin N Amer Food Anim Pr.* 17:189–208.

Author: Steven L. Berry

FRACTURES AND LUXATIONS

 BASICS

DEFINITION
• Luxation: complete dislocation or displacement of a joint
• Subluxation: partial dislocation (displacement) of a joint
• Fractures are classified as *complete* or *incomplete*: *closed* (simple), when the overlying tissue is intact; *compound*, when the fracture site communicates with the skin surface; *comminuted*, when the bone is splintered; or *displaced*, when the ends of the bone are no longer aligned.

PATHOPHYSIOLOGY
Luxations and Subluxations
• Subluxations/luxations of the fetlock joint are rare.
• Generally, both fetlock joints of a foot are affected and displacement may occur dorsally or laterally, with dorsal subluxation being more common.
• Luxation of the patella may occur dorsally, laterally, or medially and may be intermittent or permanent.
• When luxated dorsally (intermittent upward fixation), the patella is hooked over the proximal aspect of the medial trochlear ridge of the femur during flexion.
• This has been associated with desmitis of the patellar ligament as well as ligamentous laxity.
• Dorsal luxation generally occurs unilaterally; it may however be bilateral.
• Lateral and medial luxations are rare.
• Lateral luxation is congenital or may be associated with trauma to the medial femeropatellar ligament.
• The llama has a single patellar ligament; all other ruminants have three distal patellar ligaments. Patellar luxation in goats and llamas is usually congenital in origin.
• Coxofemoral luxations occur when an animal slips or falls.
• Excessive traction during dystocia may cause coxofemoral luxation in calves.
• Craniodorsal luxations are most common.
• Luxation of the sacroiliac joint is rare and is usually associated with calving.

Fractures
• Fractures of the distal phalanx are usually closed and intra-articular and involve the palmar (plantar) third of the bone.

• The inside claws of the forelimbs and the outside claws of the hind limbs are affected most commonly.
• P2 fractures are rare and are generally compression fractures associated with jumping on hard ground.
• Transverse and oblique fractures of P1 may not involve the pastern or fetlock joint.
• Sagittal, comminuted, and avulsion P1 fractures are usually intra-articular.
• Trauma is the most common cause of long-bone fractures in both ruminants and llamas.
• Capital physeal fracture of the femur can occur during forced extraction, in particular in breeds of beef cattle with a large birth weight and muscle mass.
• In young bulls, the shear forces associated with their pushing against one another may cause physeal fractures of the head of the femur.
• Fractures of the pelvis are rare and are caused by severe traumatic insult with the wing of the ileum fracturing most commonly.
• Fractures of the mandible and maxilla are usually traumatic in origin and occur more commonly in younger animals.

SYSTEMS AFFECTED
Musculoskeletal, production management, nervous, skin

GENETICS
• The Brahman breed has been associated with an increased risk of upward fixation of the patella.
• Heritability of patellar luxation in llamas has not been established but owners should be advised against using a llama with congenital patellar luxation as breeding stock.

INCIDENCE/PREVELANCE
Unknown

GEOGRAPHIC DISTRIBUTION
Worldwide

SIGNALMENT
Species
All ruminant species are affected.

Breed Predilections
• Potential heritability of patellar luxation in llamas
• The Brahman breed has been associated with an increased risk of upward fixation of the patella.

Mean Age and Range
Animals of all age groups are affected.

Predominant Sex
There is no sex predilection.

SIGNS
• Fetlock subluxation/luxation is characterized by severe alteration of the axis of the distal limb, buckling of this joint, moderate to severe lameness, abnormal range of motion, and effusion of this joint as well as pain on rotation and flexion of the distal limb.
• Upward fixation of the patella is characterized by a sudden locking of the extremity in extension (the distal limb is flexed and dragged along).
• In lateral patellar luxation, the patella is palpable on the lateral aspect of the joint and the quadriceps muscle loses its extensor function so that the stifle and hock are permanently flexed.
• Congenital lateral patellar luxation can affect both legs, and a crouching stance with inward rotation of the stifles is characteristic.
• Clinical signs of patellar luxation in small ruminants and llamas are similar to those described in cattle and a click may be audible as the patella is disengaged from a locked position.
• Signs of ileosacral luxation/subluxation range from ataxia and knuckling of the hind limbs (due to fibular nerve paresis) to recumbency.
• With ileosacral luxation the sacral region appears dropped, the head of the tail elevated, and rectal palpation reveals a dorsoventral narrowing of the pelvic canal.
• Craniodorsal coxofemoral luxations cause lameness with minimal weight bearing.
• Caudoventral and cranioventral luxations are associated with a recumbent animal.
• In order to compensate for fracture of P1 of the inside claw of the forelimb, crossing of the legs may be seen. In the hind limb the outside claw is more commonly affected and a strong abduction of the limb is noted.
• Long-bone fractures present as sudden onset non–weight bearing lameness, the patient may be recumbent and an unphysiological angle to the limb may be evident.
• With a slipped capital physis, the animal will bear weight but is noticeably lame, crepitus may be palpable over the greater trochanter, and, in chronic cases, muscle atrophy and varus deformity of the contralateral limb are evident.
• Fractures of the tuber coxae are characterized by the "knock down hip" appearance associated with the bony displacement and a slow anterior phase to the stride.

• With pelvic wing fractures, a dragging of the toe as it is advanced and the anterior and ventral location of the fracture segment may also be appreciated.

DIAGNOSIS

DIFFERENTIAL DIAGNOSIS
Differential diagnoses for the presenting signs include:
• Subsolar abscess
• Laminitis
• Sprain (distorsion)
• DJD
• Septic arthritis
• Hip dysplasia (young bulls)
• Neurological deficits
• Spastic paresis (Differentiate from upward fixation of patella: with spastic paresis the limb is held in extension but passive flexion is possible.)
• Neurogenic atrophy of the quadriceps femoris muscle (due to femoral nerve damage at birth) resulting in lateral patellar luxation (Differentiate from congenital lateral luxation as surgery will not correct this lesion.)
• Soft-tissue trauma (joint capsule, ligament, muscle tears)
• Cranial cruciate ligament rupture
• Medial and lateral collateral ligament injury to the stifle
• OCD/subchondral bone cysts
• Angular limb deformities

CBC/BIOCHEMISTRY/URINALYSIS
N/A

OTHER LABORATORY TESTS
N/A

IMAGING
• High quality radiographs are often required in order to localize and confirm the presence of a luxation/subluxation or fracture and to determine the prognosis.
• Imaging of the upper limb and pelvis can be challenging and requires a high-output machine.
• The large udder in adult cows complicates radiography of the pelvis.
• If general anesthesia is not practical, sedation may be sufficient to obtain a ventral-to-dorsal image of the affected limb in lateral recumbency.

DIAGNOSTIC PROCEDURES
• External palpation of the pelvis and upper limb for crepitus (both standing and at a walk) provides valuable information in localizing a lesion

• Use of a stethoscope for audible crepitus in the upper limb may also prove helpful.
• Rectal palpation of the bony pelvis is necessary if a pelvic fracture is suspected.

PATHOLOGIC FINDINGS
• In fetlock luxation/subluxation, the medial or lateral collateral ligament is usually completely torn with the other being detached from the bone.
• Soft-tissue trauma at the site of fracture may cause pain, swelling, and a hematoma that palpates as a fluctuant mass.
• Crepitus may be evident
• In large animals with femoral and humeral fractures, crepitus may only be detectable on auscultation.

TREATMENT
See Surgical Considerations below.

APPROPRIATE HEALTH CARE
N/A

NURSING CARE
N/A

ACTIVITY
• With any of the conditions described isolated strict stall confinement of the affected animal, in order to minimize movement is desirable
• Upward fixation of the patella in small ruminants and calves is an exception where restricted exercise is advocated in order to strengthen the muscles that stabilize the stifle joint.

DIET
In general no change in diet is necessary.

CLIENT EDUCATION
• The client must be informed that activity should be kept to a minimum.
• In the case of cast application, it must be monitored for signs of strike-through (drainage) and foul odor, and the animal's degree of lameness must be followed closely.

SURGICAL CONSIDERATIONS
• Subluxations/luxations of the fetlock joint can be treated by repositioning the joint and applying a cast (usually for a period of 6–8 weeks).
• Arthrodesis of the fetlock joint may be considered in the case of compound luxations.
• Successful use of collateral ligament prosthesis has been described in the fetlock.
• Upward fixation can be corrected through standing desmotomy of the medial femoropatellar ligament.

• Desmotomy of the lateral and imbrication of the medial patellar ligament are appropriate for lateral luxation of the patella.
• Osteotomy and relocation of the tibial crest and trochleoplasty (deepening of the trochlear groove) have been described in ruminants.
• In adult cattle, simple, closed fractures of the digit can be managed with stall rest, application of a block on the other claw, and cast application.
• Comminuted or open fractures may require amputation of the digit.
• In small ruminants, young cattle, and llamas, phalangeal fractures and those of the long bones may be treated with cast application alone or transfixation pins in combination with a cast.
• Tibial and radial fractures may be stabilized using the Thomas splint.
• Internal fixation using dynamic compression plates, intramedullary pins, or interlocking nails may be successfully implemented for the repair of metacarpal/tarsal, tibial, radial, humeral, and femoral fractures.
• External support for transport to a referral center should involve the placement of two sections of PVC pipe (positioned at right angles to one another) secured firmly over a bandage.
• Internal fixation with pins or screws is advocated for the treatment of a slipped capital physis of the femur.
• Closed reduction of coxofemoral luxations may be attempted in acute injury (within 24 hours) whereby the affected limb of the sedated, recumbent animal is secured by a heavy rope running through the inguinal region, and traction is applied to a second rope attached to the distal metatarsal area.
• The aim of open reduction for coxofemoral luxation is to remove the debris, preventing relocation of the femoral head, from within the acetabulum.
• Sequestrum formation associated with fracture of the tuber coxae may require surgical removal of the bony fragment.
• Rostral fractures of the mandible and maxilla can often be treated conservatively or through circumdental wire placement.
• More caudal jaw fractures may require external or internal fixation.

MEDICATIONS

DRUGS OF CHOICE
• In the case of open luxation/subluxation or fracture or if surgery is performed, broad-spectrum antibiotic coverage is indicated.

FRACTURES AND LUXATIONS

• For all conditions described, nonsteroidal anti-inflammatory medication is indicated to provide pain relief and a reduction in inflammation.

CONTRAINDICATIONS
• Appropriate milk and meat withdrawal times must be followed for all compounds administered to food-producing animals.
• Steroids should not be used in pregnant animals.

POSSIBLE INTERACTIONS
N/A

ALTERNATIVE DRUGS
N/A

 FOLLOW-UP

PATIENT MONITORING
• Monitor for degree of lameness, joint effusion, soft-tissue swelling, problems in the contralateral limb, muscle atrophy, ability to feed and drink.
• In the case of cast placement, this should be monitored for strike-through and foul odor.
• Surgery sites should be closely monitored for incisional infections.

PREVENTION/AVOIDANCE
N/A

POSSIBLE COMPLICATIONS
Those commonly associated with surgical procedures especially fracture repair

EXPECTED COURSE AND PROGNOSIS
• In young animals with fetlock subluxation, the prognosis is good, with luxation it is guarded. In adult animals, the prognosis is guarded to poor.
• With upward fixation of the patella and the appropriate surgical treatment, the prognosis is fair.
• In the case of lateral and medial patellar luxation, the prognosis is guarded to poor.

• Mild subluxations of the sacroiliac joint are associated with a good prognosis however may pose problems during parturition in the future.
• Prognosis for fractures of the digit depends on fracture configuration and the degree of joint involvement.
• Mild residual lameness is to be expected following long-bone fracture repair.
• Prognosis for successful repair of a long-bone fracture deteriorates with increasing complexity of fracture and increasing age and weight of animal.
• Stall rest alone for slipped capital physis of the femur is associated with a poor prognosis.
• Fractures of the tuber coxae generally have a good prognosis.
• Fractures of the bony pelvis are associated with callus formation and a narrowing of the birth canal.
• The prognosis for animals with coxofemoral luxation depends on their ability to stand, the direction of the luxation, and the time that passes before correction.
• Mandibular/maxillary fractures are generally associated with a good prognosis.

 MISCELLANEOUS

ASSOCIATED CONDITIONS
See Differential Diagnosis above.

AGE-RELATED FACTORS
N/A

ZOONOTIC POTENTIAL
N/A

PREGNANCY
Steroids should not be used in pregnant animals.

RUMINANT SPECIES AFFECTED
All species are affected.

BIOSECURITY
N/A

PRODUCTION MANAGEMENT
N/A

SYNONYMS
N/A

SEE ALSO
Anesthesia and analgesia
Angular limb deformities
Cranial cruciate ligament rupture
DJD
Laminitis
Luxations
Medial and lateral collateral ligament injury to the stifle
Neurogenic atrophy
OCD
Septic arthritis
Spastic paresis

ABBREVIATIONS
DCP = dynamic compression plate
DJD = degenerative joint disease
OCD = osteochondrosis dissecans
PVC = polyvinyl chloride

Suggested Reading
Ducharm, N. G. 1996. Stifle injuries in cattle. *Vet Clin North Am Food Animal Pract*. 12:59–84.
Hull, B. L. 1996. Fractures and luxations of the pelvis and proximal femur. *Vet Clin North Am Food Animal Pract*. 12: 54–58.
Kaneps, A. J. 1996. Orthopedic conditions in small ruminants (llama, sheep, goat, and deer). *Vet Clin North Am Food Animal Pract*. 12:221–31.
Röthlisberger, J., Schwalder, P., Kircher, P., Steiner, A. 2000. Collateral ligament prosthesis for the repair of subluxation of the metatarsophalangeal joint in a Jersey cow. *Vet Rec*. 146:640–43.

Author: Stefan Witte

BASICS

OVERVIEW
• A freemartin is a XX/XY chimera that results from the fusion of the placental circulation of at least one male and one female fetus.
• Freemartinism most commonly occurs when a single female twin calf is born with a single bull calf twin, but in cattle, sheep, and goats, it can occur with triplets or quadruplets provided there are dual-sex fetuses present.
• Affected female twins most commonly appear phenotypically female at birth but may demonstrate masculinization of external genitalia peripubertally.

SYSTEMS AFFECTED
Reproductive

GENETICS
N/A

INCIDENCE/PREVALENCE
Unknown

GEOGRAPHIC DISTRIBUTION
Worldwide distribution

SIGNALMENT
Female calves, lambs, or goat kids that are born with at least one male sibling

Species
Cattle, sheep, and goats; more common in cattle

Breed Predilections
N/A

Mean Age and Range
Newborn

Predominant Sex
N/A

SIGNS
• The only clinical signs of relevance relate to androgenization of the gonadal and genital phenotype
• Elongation of the hair at the ventral vulva
• Exaggerated prominence to the clitoris
• Short blind ending vagina
• Absence of ovaries and uterine structures
• Inguinal, abdominal, or paranephric testes

DIAGNOSIS
• In postpubertal heifers: palpation of pelvis for absence of normal uterine anatomy and absent ovaries
• Physical appearance of vulva and clitoris
• Karyotyping of peripheral blood sample to demonstrate XX/XY intersex status and/or demonstration of male cells in blood or tissues of heifer by PCR
• Vaginal length less than 12 cm and the absence of an external os to the cervix on vaginoscopy can be used to assist in the diagnosis of suspect freemartinism at 3–6 weeks of age.

TREATMENT

MEDICATIONS
N/A

FOLLOW-UP
N/A

MISCELLANEOUS

ASSOCIATED CONDITIONS
N/A

AGE-RELATED FACTORS
Congenital condition

ZOONOTIC POTENTIAL
N/A

PREGNANCY
N/A

RUMINANT SPECIES AFFECTED
Freemartinism can occur in cattle, sheep, and goats; it is not documented in camelids.

BIOSECURITY
N/A

PRODUCTION MANAGEMENT
Cull affected breeding animals.

SEE ALSO
Arthrogryposis
Chondrodysplasia (spider lamb disease)
Ovine hereditary

ABBREVIATIONS
PCR = polymerase chain reaction

Suggested Reading
Ennis, S., Vaughan, L., Gallagher, T. F. 1999, Aug. The diagnosis of freemartinism in cattle using sex-specific DNA sequences. *Res Vet Sci.* 67(1): 111–12.
Khan, M. Z., Foley, G. L. 1994. Retrospective studies on the measurements, karyotyping and pathology of reproductive organs of bovine freemartins. *J Comp Pathol.* 110(1): 25–36.
Pessa-Morikawa, T., Niku, M., Iivanainen, A. 2004, Jan. Persistent differences in the level of chimerism in B versus T cells of Freemartin cattle. *Dev Comp Immunol.* 28(1): 77–87.
Smith, K. C., Parkinson, T. J., Long, S. E., Barr, F. J. 2000, May 13. Anatomical, cytogenetic and behavioural studies of freemartin ewes. *Vet Rec.* 146(20): 574–78.
Smith, K. C., Parkinson, T. J., Pearson, G. R., Sylvester, L., Long, S. E. 2003, Feb 8. Morphological, histological and histochemical studies of the gonads of ovine freemartins. *Vet Rec.* 152(6): 164–69.

Author: Simon F. Peek

FROSTBITE

BASICS

DEFINITION
Damage or injury to the skin and body tissues resulting from their freezing following exposure to excessive cold or windchill.

OVERVIEW
- Severe frostbite is a grave physiological condition with potentially life-threatening consequences.
- All species are susceptible.
- Uncommon injury in well-nourished animals when environmental temperatures are above 10°F (−12.22°C)
- Frostbite is not uncommon when temperatures are at or below 0°F (−17.78°C) or windchill lowers the temperature to those low temperatures.
- Neonates are at greatest risk due to wet, thin skin at birth, lack of substantial quantities of subcutaneous fat, high surface area: volume ratio.
- Frostbite may be primary or secondary to debilitating disease or malnutrition.
  - Sick calves may suffer frostbite despite adequate housing and nutrition.
  - Frostbite may occur at higher environmental temperatures in compromised animals.
- Cold injury most commonly affects ears, tail, teats, scrotum, and distal extremities (feet; hind limbs more than forelimbs).
- May be associated with systemic disease
- Tissue damage is substantially exaggerated if thawing is followed by refreezing (freeze-thaw-freeze-thaw syndrome).
- Tissue previously damaged by freezing is more prone to injury on subsequent exposure to cold temperatures.

PATHOPHYSIOLOGY
- Exact mechanism of tissue damage is difficult to define.
- Multiple pathologic mechanisms occurring concurrently
- Frostbite involves direct cellular injury from freezing, injury from progressive vasoconstriction and subsequent arterial thrombosis, and ischemic necrosis.
- Four phases describe mechanisms of cell damage during freezing:
  - Phase I (prefreeze phase): congestion and leakage of fluid from vascular compartment due to arterial constriction and venous dilation
  - Phase II (freeze-thaw phase): extracellular ice crystal formation causes cell membrane rupture or cellular dehydration.
  - Phase III (vascular stasis phase): more severe and persistent arterial spasm and venous dilation leading to arteriovenous shunting and tissue hypoxia
  - Phase IV (ischemia phase): neural tissue damage due to prolonged tissue hypoxia
- Additional injury occurs during rewarming:

- Return of blood flow and warming of affected tissue
- Interstitial edema due to capillary hyperpermeability following release of histamine and bradykinin from damaged mast cells; edema persists for about a week.
- Subcutaneous hemorrhage
- Skin develops vesicles or raised, red-purple lesions.
- Thromboxane and norepinephrine release cause severe vasoconstriction at line of demarcation between viable and damaged tissue; prostaglandin I_2 release has a membrane stabilizing effect.
- Specific enzymes (NADH-diaphorase, alkaline phosphatase, esterase) are found in dermal fibroblasts, sebaceous glands, and hair follicles and at high concentrations in viable tissue; may help to define line of demarcation of viable and nonviable tissue in dermis.
- During frostbite, inappropriate upregulation of neutrophil-endothelial cell adhesion results in sequestration of granulocytes in damaged tissue. Hypoxia and inflammation result in release of their cytoplasmic granules and additional cellular damage.
- Altered elasticity of granulocytes and vasoconstriction lead to trapping of cells in capillary beds and microthrombi formation.
- Direct cellular destruction, release of catecholamines, and tissue anoxia have potentially significant secondary effects in severe frostbite resulting in damage to other organs.
- Affected skin is usually anesthetic.
- Rapid rewarming is painful but results in less cellular and tissue damage than does slow rewarming.

SIGNALMENT
- Neonates
- Debilitated, sick, or dehydrated animals
- Animals with heavily pigmented skin
- Milking cattle and goats turned outside in cold weather with inadequately dried udders and teats
- Animals with preexisting vascular damage (e.g., ergotism, fescue toxicosis, vasculitis)
- Malnourished animals with reduced metabolic heat generation

SIGNS
- Signs of chilling including piloerection, shivering, peripheral vasoconstriction
- Mild frostbite causes blanching of tissue and reduced sensation followed by painful erythema, scaling, and alopecia.
- Severe frostbite results in necrosis, dry gangrene, sloughing of affected part(s); affected skin is usually anesthetic.
- Death from low core body temperature can result if not treated before vital organs are compromised.
- Frozen teats
  - Initially appear reddened or pale
  - If severe, progress to scab formation over distal half of teat.

- Scab loosens over days and exposes raw denuded teat end.
- As second scab develops, duct may become occluded and milking difficult.
- Milk-fed calves may show superficial muzzle sloughing.
- Pain with rewarming of affected area
- Line of demarcation between viable and nonviable tissue usually appears within 3 days of rewarming affected areas.
- Demarcation line is initially diffuse but becomes more distinct within 7 days, but may take weeks before clearly defined.
- Vesicles and blisters develop on affected areas.
- After sloughing, ears are rounded, alopecic, and have pinna of variable length.

CAUSES AND RISK FACTORS
- Exposure to subnormal temperatures and wetness
- Windchill accelerates evaporation and cooling of exposed areas.
- Wet neonates or adults with wet udders, teats, testicles
- Heifers with severe periparturient udder edema and reduced perfusion to teats
- Poor nutrition
- Hypoglycemic neonates
- Previous tissue damage due to cold injury

DIAGNOSIS
- Diagnosis is based upon history and clinical signs.
- Appearance of skin and tissue of affected area(s)

POSTMORTEM LESIONS
- Decreased subcutaneous and perirenal fat deposits
- Edema
- Subcutaneous hemorrhage of tarsal region
- Edema, vesicles, or bullae over affected tissue
- Skin and tissue necrosis
- Histology: adiposities filled with eosinophilic cytoplasm instead of lipid; tissue microthrombosis, vasculitis

DIFFERENTIAL DIAGNOSIS
- Inherited, small pinna of American La Mancha goat
- Traumatic injury
- Previous tissue damage from ergot toxicosis

CBC/BIOCHEMISTRY/URINALYSIS
- Metabolic acidosis
- Dehydration
- ±Hypoglycemia (primarily neonates)
- ±Reflect secondary infection or organ compromise

OTHER LABORATORY TESTS
N/A

IMAGING
N/A

DIAGNOSTIC PROCEDURES
N/A

TREATMENT

- Only amenable to treatment in early stages
- Treatment depends on severity of injury; mild cases may not require therapy.
- Rewarming should be initiated as soon as possible but not until it is known that refreezing can be prevented; thawing and refreezing increases tissue damage.
- Incomplete or partial rewarming decreases chances for successful recovery.
- Move animal to areas (warm housing) where refreezing is not possible.
- Handle frozen tissue gently.
- Rapid thawing reduces physical effects of frostbite without causing further cellular damage.
- Thaw rapidly in warm water (plain or with a dilute antiseptic solution).
  - Recommended water temperature range: 100.2–111.1°F, 38–44°C
  - Water should be 104–106°F.
- Rewarming process should be repeated twice daily for 2 to 3 days.
- Application of lanolin or bland, protective ointment or cream after rewarming completed
- Apply aloe vera topically for its antithromboxane, anti-inflammatory, and analgesic effects.
- Leave damaged area exposed during healing.
- Analgesia
  - Nonsteroidal anti-inflammatory drugs for analgesia and systemic anti-inflammatory effects
  - Flunixin meglumine; 1.1 mg/kg IV, IM every 12 to 24 hours
  - Ketoprofen: 2.2 mg/kg/day IV, IM
  - Hind limb pain: ± use of epidural during rewarming period for analgesia
- Broad-spectrum antimicrobials to prevent secondary infection
- Correction of dehydration and metabolic acidosis by administration of oral or intravenous fluids
- Fluid administration advised even if not dehydrated for vascular support and to help correct hyperviscosity, improve capillary circulation, and prevent hypovolemic shock that may occur after peripheral rewarming and subsequent fluid shifts
- Protect animal from subnormal temperature until healing has occurred.
- Inspect skin for blisters and bullae.
  - Blisters that are filled with clear or opaque fluid should be debrided to prevent further tissue contact with thromboxane and prostaglandin E_2, which may mediate progression of dermal ischemia.
  - Hemorrhagic blisters should be left intact to avoid further damage to microvasculature.
- Supportive care
  - High-protein, high-calorie diet
  - Vitamin supplement
- Tetanus immunization in animals with extensive frostbite
- Use of glucocorticoids is controversial.

- Short-term use may be beneficial in decreasing capillary permeability, maintaining microcirculation, stabilizing cell membrane, and reducing induced histamine.
  - Long-term use should be avoided.
- Restrain to avoid self-mutilation
- Edges of healthy and gangrenous tissue should be kept clean, protected, and allowed to slough naturally.
- Check daily under sloughing skin for infection.
- If necessary, debride necrotic tissue to facilitate healing and limit secondary infection.
- Postpone debridement or surgical excision of limbs until boundary between viable and nonviable tissue is clearly obvious, which may take 8 weeks (impractical for most large animals).
- Treatment of frostbitten teats:
  - Keep teat duct patent; may require surgery.
  - Prevent development of mastitis.
  - Topical aloe vera
  - Severely affected cows may need to be culled.

MEDICATIONS

N/A

DRUGS OF CHOICE
N/A

CONTRAINDICATIONS
Appropriate milk and meat withdrawal times must be followed for all compounds administered to food-producing animals.

PRECAUTIONS
- Avoid massaging or rubbing tissue during warming as this can prolong resolution of edema and recovery period.
- Do not use occlusive bandages over damaged areas.
- Avoid premature debridement of affected area; more tissue may be viable than initially apparent.

FOLLOW-UP

Full recovery is usually possible after mild to moderate frostbite provided appropriate and proper treatment is given.

MISCELLANEOUS

ASSOCIATED CONDITIONS
Secondary bacterial infection

ZOONOTIC POTENTIAL
N/A

RUMINANT SPECIES AFFECTED
Cattle, goats, sheep, other ruminants

BIOSECURITY
N/A

PRODUCTION MANAGEMENT
- Change management to avoid occurrence of frostbite.
- Give special attention to drying off calves, kids, and lambs born in cold environments.
- Ensure susceptible body parts remain dry during exposure to subnormal temperatures.
- Provide adequate, clean, dry bedding to neonates to minimize heat loss by convection and evaporation.
- Provide easily accessible shelter.
- Provide consistent feeding management.
- With ambient temperatures below 0° C management should include:
  - Dry udder and teats completely before animal leaves parlor.
  - Provide adequate windbreaks and shelter.
  - Dip just the teat end during very cold weather.
- Provide windbreaks and bedding for calving cow when windchill temperatures are below 10–20°F.
- House calving cows and calves less than 1 day old when windchills are below 10°F and calves cannot be kept dry because of rain or snow.
- Keep dairy animals clean, dry, and out of the wind with adequate dry bedding daily when temperatures are subnormal.

SYNONYMS
Cold-induced injury

SEE ALSO
Ergot toxicosis
Fescue toxicosis
Traumatic injury
Wound care

ABBREVIATIONS
IM = intramuscular
IV = intravenous
NADH = nicotinamide adenine dinucleotide reduced form

Suggested Reading
Pelton, J. A., Callan, R. J., Barrington, G. M., Parish, S. M. 2000. Frostbite in calves. *Comp Cont Edu.* 22(10): S136–41.
Pugh, D. 2002. Diseases of the integumentary system. In: *Sheep and goat medicine*. Philadelphia: W. B. Saunders.
Rebhun W. C. 1995. Skin diseases. In: *Diseases of dairy cattle*. Baltimore: Williams and Wilkins.
Scott, D. W. 1999. Environmental skin diseases. In: *Current veterinary therapy 4: food animal practice*, ed. J. L. Howard, R. A. Smith. Philadelphia: W. B. Saunders.
Smith, M. C., Sherman, D. M. 1994. Skin. In: *Goat medicine*. Philadelphia: Lea & Febiger.

Authors: Susan Semrad and Karen A. Moriello

FUNGAL TREMORGENS

 BASICS

OVERVIEW
• Tremorgens are mycotoxins that have been reported to cause tremoring conditions in cattle, goats, sheep, deer, horses, and camelids.
• Clinical signs associated with ingestion of these neurotoxins are collectively known as "staggers" and include ataxia, muscle tremors, rigid stance, recumbency, and paddling convulsions. The tremors are accentuated by exercise and can lead to tetany and collapse.
• The mycotoxins are produced by fungal genera such as *Aspergillus, Neotyphodium, Penicillium, Phalaris,* and *Claviceps,* and are often associated with specific grasses, such as dallis grass, bahia grass, canary grass, Bermuda grass, and perennial ryegrass.

PATHOPHYSIOLOGY
• The endophyte *Neotyphodium lolii* is associated with perennial ryegrass (*Lolium perenne*) and produces tremogenic toxins known as lolitrems A, B, C, and D. These toxins are indole compounds that are derivatives of lysergic acid that exert their effects in a similar fashion to paspalitrems in that they inhibit GABA and glycine.
• The seed heads of dallis and bahia grasses can be infected by *Claviceps paspali*. The fungus produces alkaloids including indole compounds derived from lysergic acid known as paspalitrems. These alkaloids include paspalinine, paspalitrem A, and paspalitrem B, which may exert their effects by inhibiting the inhibitory neurotransmitter, gamma-aminobutyric acid (GABA).
• Loss of inhibitory neurotransmitters leads to increased neurotransmission and prolonged depolarization, resulting in the neurologic signs of incoordinated movements, ataxia, and muscle tremors.

SIGNALMENT
Reports of tremogenic mycotoxin intoxication have occurred in cattle, horses, goats, sheep, deer and camelids. There are no age, species, or breed predilections.

SIGNS
As described above

CAUSES AND RISK FACTORS
• Risk factors and inciting conditions vary between tremorgenic compounds.
• Paspalitrems proliferate in warm, humid climates of the southeastern United States. Wet conditions following dallis grass seed head formation result in increased toxin formation.
• Factors that promote formation of *Phalaris* mycotoxin include decreased light intensity, humidity, and high nitrogen levels.
• Outbreaks of ryegrass staggers have been documented in New Zealand, Australia, and North America during the summer and early fall during drought conditions.
• Seventy-five percent of the fungal species associated with mycotoxin production are found in the lower 2 cm of the plant, therefore, outbreaks usually occur on overgrazed pastures. Toxin levels increase within days of heavy dew or light rainfall.

Fungal Varieties
• The seed heads of dallis and bahia grasses can be infected by *Claviceps paspali*. The fungus infects the pistil of the grass flower and produces a sticky fluid, "honeydew," which hardens into mature sclerotia containing a high concentration of toxin.
• The fungus produces alkaloids including indole compounds derived from lysergic acid known as paspalitrems. These alkaloids include paspalinine, paspalitrem A, and paspalitrem B, which may exert their effects by inhibiting the inhibitory neurotransmitter, gamma-aminobutyric acid (GABA).

• Loss of inhibitory neurotransmitters leads to increased neurotransmission and prolonged depolarization, resulting in neurologic signs of incoordinated movements, ataxia, and muscle tremors.
• The condition is known as dallis grass staggers or nervous ergotism.
• The fungal genera *Phalaris* can be found in canary grass and produce tryptamine alkaloids (dimethylated indolealkylamines).
• These mycotoxins produce their neurogenic effects by competitively inhibiting the initial step in the breakdown of serotonin by monoamine oxidase. There are two clinical forms of *Phalaris* grass staggers: acute death from cardiovascular collapse and the chronic nervous form. The cardiovascular form often results in sudden death within 12–72 hours of exposure to the toxin.
• Clinical signs prior to death reflect cardiovascular failure (e.g., cardiac arrhythmias, dyspnea, cyanosis, and extreme tachycardia). The nervous form may occur after repeated exposures over 2–3 weeks. Clinical signs include those listed above and a "rabbit hopping" gait seen in sheep, when both rear legs move in unison.
• Bermuda grass is also associated with staggers in cattle, sheep, goats, and horses. The toxic principle has yet to be identified but the clinical signs are similar to those seen in ryegrass staggers and can develop as soon as 36 hours following ingestion or after several days of exposure.
• The toxin endures through the drying process and may be found in hay several years after the initial cutting.
• The endophyte *Neotyphodium lolii* is associated with perennial ryegrass (*Lolium perenne*) and produces tremogenic toxins known as lolitrems A, B, C, and D. Lolitrem B is most commonly associated with clinical signs of ryegrass staggers in ruminants and horses.

FUNGAL TREMORGENS

• These toxins are indole compounds, which are derivatives of lysergic acid that exert their effects in a similar fashion to paspalitrems in that they inhibit GABA and glycine. Signs may be mild until the animal is stimulated or excited when the prominent clinical sign becomes muscle tremors of the head and neck.
• Signs may progress to ataxia, stiffness, hypermetria, generalized tremors, or seizures.
• Other mycotoxins that may contribute to ryegrass staggers include those produced by the genera *Penicillium* and *Aspergillus*. The mycotoxins produced by *Penicillium* spp. include penitrem A, verruculogen, and fumitremogen B. *Aspergillus* spp. produces verruculogen and penitrem A.
• These toxins are produced by fungus in the soil and are absorbed by plant roots and accumulate in vegetation. The toxic mechanism on the CNS is as described above.

DIAGNOSIS

• Diagnosis is based on clinical signs and history of exposure.
• Analysis of forage to identify specific mycotoxins can be performed by most state diagnostic laboratories; but it is not commonly performed, and obtaining a forage sample with adequate mycotoxin levels is difficult.
• Extracts of the fungus-infected feed material can be analyzed by thin-layer chromatography, high-performance liquid chromatography, or bioassay.

DIFFERENTIAL DIAGNOSES

• Other plants that may contain mycotoxins and cause tremorgenic conditions include white snakeroot, rayless goldenrod, jimmy fern, and mountain laurel.
• Other conditions that can cause similar neurologic signs include hypomagnesemia in ruminants, rabies, yew (*Taxus* spp.) poisoning, and selenium poisoning.

CBC/BIOCHEMISTRY/URINALYSIS

Tremorgens cause no changes in clinical pathology. An elevation in serum creatinine kinase or aspartate aminotransferase may be seen due to muscle cell damage from ataxia or incoordination.

PATHOLOGIC FINDINGS

TREATMENT

• There is no specific treatment or antidote for tremorgenic mycotoxin intoxication.
• Removal from affected pastures or contaminated forages and supportive care may allow for recovery in 3–14 days.

MEDICATIONS

FOLLOW-UP

MISCELLANEOUS

ASSOCIATED CONDITIONS
N/A

AGE-RELATED FACTORS
N/A

ZOONOTIC POTENTIAL
N/A

PREGNANCY
N/A

RUMINANT SPECIES AFFECTED
Cattle, goats, sheep, deer, horses, camelids.

BIOSECURITY
N/A

PRODUCTION MANAGEMENT
N/A

SYNONYMS
N/A

SEE ALSO

Hypomagnesemia
Jimmy fern
Mountain laurel.
Rabies
Rayless goldenrod
Selenium poisoning.
White snakeroot
Yew (*Taxus* spp.) poisoning

ABBREVIATIONS

CNS = central nervous system
GABA = gamma-aminobutyric acid

Suggested Reading

Cheeke, P. R. 1995. Endogenous toxins and mycotoxins in forage grasses and their effects on livestock. *Journal of Animal Science* 73: 909–18.

Fowler, M. E. 1998. Toxicology. In: *Medicine and surgery of South American camelids: llama, alpaca, vicuna, guanaco.* Ames: Iowa State University Press.

Osweiler, G. D. 2001. Mycotoxins. *Toxicology: the veterinary clinics of North America* (17) 3: 559–61.

Plumlee, K. H., Galey, F. D. 1994. Neuromycotoxins: a review of fungal toxins that cause neurological disease in large animals. *Journal of Veterinary Internal Medicine* 8 (1): 49–54.

Rebhun, W.C. 1995. Miscellaneous toxicities and deficiencies. In: *Diseases in dairy cattle.* Baltimore: Williams and Wilkins.

Author: Natalie Coffer

GASTROINTESTINAL MICROBIOLOGY

BASICS

OVERVIEW
• Diseases of the digestive tract of ruminants are common among farm animals.
• GI tract infections are primarily spread throughout the population by means of fecal to oral transmission.
• Many of the pathogens are zoonotic and pose both a herd safety issue as well as a food safety concern.
• The digestive tract of ruminants is a complex environment composed of normal microflora, which provide both a defense mechanism against colonization of pathogens and a major source of nutritional and metabolic components for the ruminant.
• Normal microflora of the ruminant digestive tract include but are not limited to:
  Bacteroides spp.
  Butyrivibrio spp.
  Candida spp.
  Clostridium spp.
  Eubacterium spp.
  Lactobacillus spp.
  Methanobacterium spp.
  Ruminococcus spp.
  Selenomonas spp.
  Streptococcus spp.
  Trichosporon spp.
  Vibrio spp.
• Some of the most common pathogens associated with ruminant digestive tract infections include but are not limited to:
  Campylobacter jejuni
  Cryptosporidium spp.
  E. coli O157:H7
  Listeria monocytogenes
  Mycobacterium avium paratuberculosis
  Salmonella spp.

SYSTEMS AFFECTED
Gastrointestinal

GENETICS
N/A

INCIDENCE/PREVALENCE
N/A

GEOGRAPHIC DISTRIBUTION
Potentially worldwide, depending on species and environment

SIGNALMENT
Neonates are most susceptible due to the lack of an established GI tract microflora and the lack of a fully established immune system.

Species
Potentially, all ruminant species

Breed Predilections
N/A

Mean Age and Range
N/A

Predominant Sex
N/A

SIGNS
Dehydration
Diarrhea
Fever
Weakness
Weight loss

CAUSES AND RISK FACTORS
• Transmission is primarily fecal to oral.
• Risk factors include anything contaminated with feces such as water, feed, equipment, or the environment.
• Newborn calves can be infected by coming in contact with the mother's udders that have been contaminated with feces, or in some instances through the mother's colostrum.
• Neonates are most susceptible due to lack of an established GI tract microflora.
• Neonates are most susceptible due to lack of a fully established immune system.
• Pathogenic strains of *Escherichia coli* recovered from the intestinal tract of animals fall into categories called enterotoxigenic, enteropathogenic, enterohemorrhagic, and necrotoxigenic. Two categories— enteroaggressive and enteroinvasive—have not been reported in domestic livestock.
• The pathogenicity of bacterial strains is determined by the genetic presence of adhesins and toxins.
• The genes encoding for these adhesions and toxins are generally organized in chromosomes, large plasmids, or phages, and are often transmitted horizontally between strains. Bacterial antibiotic resistance is passed on in this way.

Neonatal Diarrhea
• Numerous pathogens are implicated in the occurrence of neonatal diarrhea, but only a limited number is commonly involved in the infection process. Most bacteria are actually secondary opportunists and not primary pathogens. Most of these bacteria are present within the gastrointestinal tract of many healthy, mature adults.
• Infectious diarrhea is an important cause of neonatal calf morbidity and mortality that

results in significant economic losses in the sheep, dairy goat, beef, and dairy cattle industries.
• The immune status of the newborn (the level of passively acquired immunity through colostrum) is the major risk factor related to the occurrence of diarrhea.
• The environmental conditions in which neonates may reside vary tremendously between facilities.
• Numerous risk factors related to the occurrence of neonatal diarrhea have been identified. These factors can be categorized as: those that are related to the neonate, the pathogens involved in the infection, and the environment of the neonate.
• Risk factors related to bacterial pathogens associated with neonatal calf diarrhea include the occurrence of multiple infections and the size of the infective inoculum.

DIAGNOSIS

DIFFERENTIAL DIAGNOSIS
N/A

CBC/BIOCHEMISTRY/URINALYSIS
N/A

OTHER LABORATORY TESTS
Common techniques for identifying digestive tract pathogens:

Selective Growth
Depending on the type of pathogen suspected in the disease, one can use selective media and growth conditions specific to the pathogen in order to select for the growth of the pathogen over other organisms. This technique should help to reduce the presence of normal microflora.

Antibiotic Susceptibility
Various organisms can be identified based on their resistance or susceptibility to specific antibiotics.

Biochemical Assays
Once a pure culture is isolated from a fecal sample, there exist numerous biochemical assays that identify biochemical and metabolic properties that are unique to the organism or group of organisms in question.

Serology
Employs the use of antibodies in order to identify the presence of antigenic factors, which may be unique to a specific pathogen. Antibodies can cross react with other

organisms resulting in false-positive test results. Pathogens can also undergo mutations involving antigenic factors, which can lead to false negative results.

Verotoxin Assays

Gene-probe methods directed at toxin gene sequences

Polymerase Chain Reaction (PCR)

DNA extractions can either be performed after the organism has been cultured and selected for growth, or in some cases DNA extractions can be performed directly on the fecal samples without the need for culture. PCR utilizes primers and/or probes, which identify organisms by targeting specific genes, DNA sequences, or polymorphisms unique to the organism.

Enzyme-Linked Immunosorbent Assay (ELISA)

The use of ELISA and immunoblotting assays to examine the serum antibody response of cattle to bacteria is another diagnostic tool. Evidence of infection utilizing an LPS-based ELISA in association with an immunoblotting procedure, can be used to supplement existing bacteriological procedures. ELISA can also be employed to examine cell-free broth filtrates for enterotoxin production and cytotoxin production. Viable bacteria can be examined for invasive properties by an ELISA with the immunoglobulin fraction of antiserum to formalin-killed bacteria of an invasive strain.

IMAGING
N/A

DIAGNOSTIC PROCEDURES
N/A

TREATMENT

MEDICATIONS

DRUGS OF CHOICE
N/A

CONTRAINDICATIONS
N/A

FOLLOW-UP

PREVENTION

Farm management practices can reduce digestive tract related diseases:
• Waste management practices in order to reduce active pathogens
• Managing the calving season so that it overlaps as little as possible with the rainfall season
• Manipulating grazing so that fecal deposition occurs away from the water
• Setting up fencing to keep livestock away from the water
• Established milking, feeding, and calving practices that limit exposure to feces
• Proper storage of feed
• Keeping neonates and calves away from feces
• Keeping the housing clean and disinfected, and monitoring the housing
• Monitoring of the herd through diagnostics and clinical signs of illness
• Isolating infected ruminates once they have been identified
• Monitoring critical control points such as: carrier cows, replacement stocks, feces of sick cows, dirty environments, recycled flush water, feedstuffs, feed commodities, infected rodents and birds, and rendering trucks

MISCELLANEOUS

ASSOCIATED CONDITIONS
N/A

AGE-RELATED FACTORS
N/A

ZOONOTIC POTENTIAL

Depends on the specific pathogen. However, *Campylobacter jejuni, Cryptosporidium* sp., *Listeria monocytogenes, Salmonella* sp., *E. coli* O157:H7, *Mycobacterium avium paratuberculosis* are all potential zoonotic pathogens. Cattle are an important reservoir of Shiga-toxin-producing *Escherichia coli* O157:H7 and other enterohemorrhagic *E. coli* (EHEC) that cause diarrhea, hemorrhagic colitis, and hemorrhagic uremic syndrome in humans. One strategy for reducing human foodborne EHEC infections is to reduce the levels of EHEC in cattle.

PREGNANCY
N/A

RUMINANT SPECIES AFFECTED
Potentially, all ruminant species are affected.

BIOSECURITY
N/A

PRODUCTION MANAGEMENT
N/A

SYNONYMS

SEE ALSO
Campylobacter jejuni
Cryptosporidium spp.
E. coli O157:H7
Listeria monocytogenes
Mycobacterium avium paratuberculosis
Salmonella spp.

ABBREVIATIONS
ELISA = enzyme-linked immunosorbent assay
GI = gastrointestinal
PCR = polymerase chain reaction

Suggested Reading
Barrington, G. M., Gay, J. M., Evermann, J. F. 2002, Mar. Biosecurity for neonatal gastrointestinal diseases. *Vet Clin North Am Food Anim Pract*. 18(1): 7–34.
Dean-Nystrom, E. A., Bosworth, B. T., Moon, H. W. 1999. Pathogenesis of *Escherichia coli* O157:H7 in weaned calves. *Adv Exp Med Biol*. 473:173–77.
DebRoy, C., Maddox, C. W. 2001, Dec. Identification of virulence attributes of gastrointestinal *Escherichia coli* isolates of veterinary significance. *Anim Health Res Rev*. 2(2): 129–40.
Kang, S. J., Ryu, S. J., Chae, J. S., Eo, S. K., Woo, G. J., Lee, J. H. 2004, Mar. 5. Occurrence and characteristics of enterohemorrhagic *Escherichia coli* O157 in calves associated with diarrhea. *Vet Microbiol*. 98(3–4): 323–28.
Smith, D. G., Naylor, S. W., Gally, D. L. 2002, Sep. Consequences of EHEC colonization in humans and cattle. *Int J Med Microbiol*. 292(3–4): 169–83.

Author: Gabriel J. Rensen

GASTROINTESTINAL PHARMACOLOGY

 BASICS

OVERVIEW
• The importance of motility modifiers in ruminants is for the treatment of a myriad of gastrointestinal dysmotilities or malfunctions of the esophageal groove reflex, or as an aid in placement of reticular magnets.
• Diseases of ruminants that are caused by motility disorders and could potentially benefit from motility modification include paralytic ileus, cecal dilatation, and displacements of the abomasum.
• Paralytic ileus frequently occurs with the presence of severe hypocalcemia, but is rarely observed postoperatively.
• Well-documented data about modifiers of gastrointestinal (GI) motility in ruminants are sparse due to the complex nature of the control systems responsible for motility in the bovine.

PATHOPHYSIOLOGY
• Gastrointestinal motility is known to be regulated by myogenic, neural, and chemical systems, with a fourth regulatory system involving the interstitial cells of Cajal believed to have a function in establishing the pacemaker activity of the GI cells.
• It is important to recognize that the neural control of GI motility refers to the extrinsic system that includes the vagus nerve and the sympathetic pelvic, lumbar colonic, and hypogastric nerves and the intrinsic system. This system consists of ganglia with efferent axons to the smooth muscle cells, afferent sensory axons, and the interconnective nerve strands located in the myenteric and submucosal plexuses.
• Chemical control of GI motility is performed by various hormones and neurotransmitters. These compounds are released from nerve endings of both the extrinsic and intrinsic nervous systems that supply the GI tract.

SYSTEMS AFFECTED
Gastrointestinal

GENETICS
N/A

INCIDENCE/PREVALENCE
N/A

GEOGRAPHIC DISTRIBUTION
Worldwide

SIGNALMENT

Species
Potentially, all ruminant species

Breed Predilections
N/A

Mean Age and Range
N/A

Predominant Sex
N/A

Gastrointestinal Pharmacology
• Pharmacologic compounds capable of influencing GI motility either imitate or antagonize the effects of endogenous transmitters.
• Motility modifiers are categorized as cholinergics, adrenergics, antidopaminergics, serotoninergics, motilin agonists, opioid receptor-blockers, or lidocaine based upon their mechanism of action and their main target receptor. A key factor in the cascade of smooth muscle contractions is the serum calcium concentration of the affected animal.
• Correction of preexisting hypocalcemia and other electrolyte imbalances and rehydration is crucial to every protocol dealing with the treatment of GI motility disorder.

Cholinergics
• Acetylcholine (Ach) is the natural cholinergic neurotransmitter released from cholinergic axonic terminals.
• In the GI tract, Ach binds to the muscarinic receptors released from nerve terminals that originate from the intrinsic nervous system of the gut. All of the compounds that follow have an effect on either the release or breakdown of Ach and provide some ability to affect GI motility.

Bethanechol
• Bethanechol mimics the effect of Ach and is classified as a directly acting parasympathetic agonist. This compound has high affinity to muscarinic receptors of the GI tract with a much lower affinity for the smooth muscle cells of the vascular system.
• When dosed at 0.07 mg/kg subcutaneously (SC), this compound was found to increase overall myoelectric spiking activity in cows.

Neostigmine
• Neostigmine is classified as an indirectly acting parasympathetic agonist due to its ability to inhibit acetylcholinesterase, which hydrolyzes Ach. The effect of neostigmine is less restricted to the GI tract than that of bethanechol.

• This compound dosed at 0.02 mg/kg SC increased myoelectric activity but the effect was most pronounced upon uncoordinated spikes.

Metoclopramide
• Metoclopramide represents a first-generation prokinetic compound. Prokinetics have the ability to stimulate, coordinate, and restore gastric, pyloric, and small intestinal motility. Metoclopramide works by enhancing the release of Ach from postganglionic cholinergic nerve terminals, sensitizing muscarinic receptors and reducing hydrolysis of Ach by inhibiting acetylcholinesterase.
• Numerous studies at varied dosages have discovered that this compound alone does not affect GI motility and have identified that it does have the ability to cross the blood-brain barrier leading to restlessness and excitement. However, when metoclopramide (0.1 mg/kg SC) was used in combination with bethanechol (0.07 mg/kg SC), increased spike rates were reported.

Atropine and Scopolamine
• Atropine and scopolamine are naturally occurring alkaloids. They bind competitively to muscarinic receptors and are classified as parasympathetic antagonists.
• Atropine (0.04 mg/kg IV) completely eradicates abomasal myoelectric activity for up to 3 hours. Adverse effects are ruminal bloat and tachycardia.

Adrenergics
• Norepinephrine is the naturally occurring neurotransmitter of most sympathetic postganglionic nerve terminals, binding to both alpha and beta adrenergic receptors. These terminals are located postsynaptically on intestinal smooth muscle cells.
• Presynaptic stimulation by inhibition of Ach release is more important than postsynaptic stimulation because smooth muscle cells receive little postganglionic sympathetic innervation.

Xylaxine and Detomidine
• Xylazine and detomidine have potent alpha-2 agonistic properties; yohimbine represents an alpha-2 receptor blocker; tolazoline is an alpha-1 and -2 receptor blocker and D1-propanolol is a beta-receptor blocker. Stimulation of adrenergic receptors results in inhibition of GI motility.

• The stimulating effect of adrenoceptor blockers is restricted to disease processes accompanied by a hyperactive state of the sympathetic nervous system.
• D1-propanolol has been shown to have no significant effect on contractility in vitro on bovine colonic tissue or in vivo on the ileocecocolic area of healthy cows when dosed at 0.2 mg/kg IM.
• Xylazine induces widespread reduction in GI motility when dosed at 0.2 mg/kg IM, and adverse effects have included salivation, ruminal bloat, hypothermia, and bradycardia.
• Yohimbine (0.125 mg/kg IV) or tolazoline (0.25–0.5 mg/kg IV) may be used for xylazine reversal.

Antidopaminergics
Dopamine is the precursor of norepinephrine and epinephrine. Dopaminergic receptors have been demonstrated in the GI tract of laboratory animals and sheep but not cattle.

Domperidone
Domperidone is a potent and specific dopamine-receptor antagonist that binds to dopaminergic receptors and does not cross the blood-brain barrier. The effect of this compound on the rumen and forestomachs of goats is to block the stimulatory effects of dopamine.

Serotoninergics
Serotonin is stored in the GI tract mainly in the enterochromaffin cells and is involved in regulation of GI motility by either enhancing or inhibiting it by binding to the receptors.

Cisapride
Cisapride represents a prokinetic drug that has been studied as a potential excitatory agent that would exert its effects by increasing the release of Ach at postganglionic nerve terminals. However, cisapride did not affect myoelectric activity at the ileocecocolic area of healthy cows in vivo or produce any increased contractility of smooth muscle preparations in vitro at a dose of 0.08 mg/kg IV.

Other Compounds
• Motilin is a hormone that initiates contractile activity by binding to specific receptors situated on smooth muscle cells.
• Erythromycin lactobionate has been demonstrated to bind to motilin receptors situated on smooth muscle cells. This compound increases myoelectric activity in the abomasum and duodenum for up to 8 hours following either IV or IM injections in healthy cattle.

• Opioid peptides in the gut are represented by met-enkephalin and leu-enkephalin. Receptors for these peptides are present in the myenteric plexus and activation causes inhibitory effects by hyperpolarization of neurons, preventing neuronal excitation.
• Naloxone did not affect myoelectric activity of the ileocecocolic area of experimental cows when given at 0.05 mg/kg IV.
• Lidocaine blocks voltage-gated channels and this blockade is thought to contribute to a motility-promoting effect in postoperative ileus in other species. However, lidocaine does not have significant effects on in vitro abomasal or duodenal tissues of healthy cows.

 TREATMENT

• Most cases of paralytic ileus, cecal dilatation/dislocation, and displacement of the abomasum are multifactorial diseases.
• Treatment protocols should not be restricted to the administration of motility modifiers and should always include treatment of the concurrent metabolic disorders, infectious diseases, and supervision of management practices.
• Many of the compounds described in this chapter do not have veterinary-approved products available for use in cattle in the United States. In this area of study, well-documented results are rare and intensive research in this field is warranted in the future.

MEDICATIONS

DRUGS OF CHOICE

CONTRAINDICATIONS
Appropriate milk and meat withdrawal times must be followed for all compounds administered to food-producing animals.

PRECAUTIONS
N/A

POSSIBLE INTERACTIONS
N/A

 MISCELLANEOUS

ASSOCIATED CONDITIONS
N/A

AGE-RELATED FACTORS
N/A

ZOONOTIC POTENTIAL
N/A

PREGNANCY
Effect on pregnancy depends on specific pharmacologic agent utilized. Read package insert. Follow instructions as directed.

RUMINANT SPECIES AFFECTED
Potentially, all ruminant species are affected.

BIOSECURITY
N/A

PRODUCTION MANAGEMENT
N/A

SYNONYMS
N/A

SEE ALSO
Farad
Fluid therapy
Gastrointestinal disease

ABBREVIATIONS
Ach = acetylcholine
FARAD = Food Animal Residue Avoidance Databank
GI = gastrointestinal
IM = intramuscular
IV = intravenous
SC = subcutaneous

Suggested Reading
Braun, U., Gansohr, B., Haessig, M. 2002, Aug. Ultrasonographic evaluation of reticular motility in cows after administration of atropine, scopolamine and xylazine. *J Vet Med A Physiol Pathol Clin Med*. 49(6): 299–302.
Gerring, E. L. 1989, Aug. Effects of pharmacological agents on gastrointestinal motility. *Vet Clin North Am Equine Pract*. 5(2): 283–94.
Navarre, C. B., Roussel, A. J. 1996, Mar–Apr. Gastrointestinal motility and disease in large animals. *J Vet Intern Med*. 10(2): 51–59.
Sherman, D. M. 1983, Nov. Unexplained weight loss in sheep and goats. A guide to differential diagnosis, therapy, and management. *Vet Clin North Am Large Anim Pract*. 5(3): 571–90.
Steiner, A. 2003. Modifiers of gastrointestinal motility of cattle. *Vet Clinics Food Anim*. 19:647–60.
Steiner, A., Roussel, A. J. 1995, Dec. Drugs coordinating and restoring gastrointestinal motility and their effect on selected hypodynamic gastrointestinal disorders in horses and cattle. *Zentralbl Veterinarmed A*. 42(10): 613–31.
Van Metre, D. C., Tyler, J. W., Stehman, S. M. 2000, Mar. Diagnosis of enteric disease in small ruminants. *Vet Clin North Am Food Anim Pract*. 16(1): vi, 87–115.

Author: Dennis D. French

GOSSYPOL TOXICOSIS

BASICS

OVERVIEW
• Gossypol is a bi-napthyl-aldehyde that occurs naturally in the cotton plant (*Gossypium* spp.).
• Whole cottonseed (WCS) and cottonseed meal (CSM) are a good source of energy, fiber, and protein in diets of adult cattle, calves, and sheep.
• Because gossypol has been recognized since the turn of the century to be toxic to animals, a limiting factor of whole cottonseed and cottonseed meal as feed sources to ruminant livestock is their gossypol content.

SYSTEMS AFFECTED
Reproductive, musculoskeletal, respiratory, hepatic

GENETICS
N/A

INCIDENCE/PREVALENCE
Unknown

GEOGRAPHIC DISTRIBUTION
Worldwide in areas feeding cottonseed meal

SIGNALMENT
• Ruminants have been reported to detoxify gossypol in the rumen by binding to soluble proteins. However, the protein-binding detoxifying mechanism in adult cattle can be overwhelmed if the total gossypol content is excessive, or low protein content is present in the rumen.
• Preruminant cattle such as lambs and calves are commonly affected.

Species
Potentially all ruminants feeding on cottonseed meal

Breed Predilections
N/A

Mean Age and Range
N/A

Predominant Sex
N/A

SIGNS
• The clinical signs of gossypol toxicity seen in ruminants and preruminant cattle include sudden death as well as physiological and reproductive effects without death.
• Adult cattle reduced milk production and respiratory stress
• Preruminant calves show respiratory signs and congestive heart failure.
• Infertility in cows
• Reduced spermatogenesis and impaired sperm motility associated with morphological aberrations of the sperm midpiece. Damaged spermatogenic epithelium with an increase in sperm cell midpiece abnormality and erythrocyte fragility.

CAUSES AND RISK FACTORS
• Consumption of diets containing excessive amounts of gossypol from whole cottonseed and cottonseed hulls or meal is the route of exposure that causes toxicity.
• The level predisposing the animal to toxicity depends on the species, rumen function, level of protein in the diet, and duration of consumption.

DIAGNOSIS

History of Feeding Cottonseed Products
• Young calves—cottonseed meal or cottonseed hulls in starter or grower rations
• Ruminants—whole cottonseed fed above recommended levels

Clinical Picture
• Multiple animals involved
• Sudden death syndrome
• Chronic respiratory problems, unresponsive to antibiotics
• Animals not doing well, depressed
• History of infertility

DIFFERENTIAL DIAGNOSIS
• Monensin toxicity
• Vitamin E and selenium toxicity
• Toxic plants such as coffee, senna, bracken fern, white snakeroot, lantana, and milkweed

CBC/BIOCHEMISTRY/URINALYSIS
There are minimal changes in blood chemistry and erythrocyte parameters during toxicity. However, changes such as an increase in erythrocyte fragility, hemoglobinuria, anemia, and a decrease in hemoglobin content have been reported.

OTHER LABORATORY TESTS
Estimation of Gossypol Intake from Rations Containing Cotton Products
• Send representative samples of the cotton by-product (WCS or CSM) to a qualified laboratory for total and free gossypol analysis. Note that the standard analytical method will not give accurate results of gossypol levels in a total mixed ration (TMR) sample, therefore, the cotton by-products should be analyzed individually
• Laboratory results will be in percent (%). Convert to mg/kg, as shown in Table 1.
  For example, a typical result from a sample of WCS may be 1.1% total gossypol. According to Table 1, this would be equivalent to 11,000 ppm, or 11,000 mg/kg.
• To calculate the amount of gossypol in the seed kernel of the whole seed, the result must be multiplied by 0.55 to get an accurate gossypol level as fed. In the above example, this would lead to a value of (11,000 mg/kg) × (0.55) = 6050 mg/kg.

Table 1

Given	To obtain	Multiply by
Percent (%)	Parts per million (ppm)	10,000
Parts per million (ppm)	mg/kg	1.0

• Estimate the amount of each cotton by-product fed per cow on a daily basis. For example, a TMR might contain 15% WCS on a dry matter basis. If a cow consumes 22.5 kg/day of this TMR on average, then she consumes (22.5 kg) × (0.15) = 3.4 kg of WCS daily.
• Multiply the amount of cotton by-product consumed by the amount of gossypol in mg/kg. In the example, this would be (3.4 kg) × (6050 mg/kg) = 20,570 mg (20.5 g) of gossypol per cow from WCS on a daily basis.
• Add the gossypol from each source to calculate the animal's total daily gossypol intake.

PATHOLOGIC FINDINGS
Gross Necropsy Findings
• Lesions are compatible with failure of the cardiovascular and respiratory system similar to those reported for swine.
• Hepatomegaly
• Cardiomegaly
• Gelatinous, yellow-brown color fluid in the thoracic and peritoneal cavity

Histopathology
Centrilobular hepatic congestion and necrosis related to hepatic anoxia

TREATMENT
N/A

MEDICATIONS

FOLLOW-UP

PREVENTION/AVOIDANCE
• Stage of rumen development is critical in detoxifying gossypol. While the young ruminant is being fed milk, rumen development and function are minimal. During this time, the animal functions essentially as a preruminant and tolerable levels of free gossypol in the diet are similar to nonruminant species, which is 200 ppm.

• When considering toxicity levels of free gossypol in ruminants, the source—whole cottonseed vs. cottonseed meal—should be considered. Detoxification of free gossypol in the rumen appears to be more efficient with whole cottonseed.
• Guidelines for safe levels of gossypol intake should not exceed 20 g/day for lactating dairy cows, 8 g/day for breeding bulls.

MISCELLANEOUS

ASSOCIATED CONDITIONS
• The clinical signs of gossypol toxicity seen in ruminants and preruminant cattle include sudden death as well as physiological and reproductive effects without death.
• Adult cattle reduced milk production and respiratory stress.
• Infertility in cows
• Reduced spermatogenesis and impaired sperm motility associated with morphological aberrations of the sperm midpiece. Damaged spermatogenic epithelium with an increase in sperm cell midpiece abnormality and erythrocyte fragility.

AGE-RELATED FACTORS
• Preruminants such as lambs and calves are commonly affected.
• Preruminant calves show respiratory signs and congestive heart failure.

ZOONOTIC POTENTIAL
N/A

PREGNANCY
Infertility in cows

RUMINANT SPECIES AFFECTED
Potentially all ruminants feeding on cottonseed meal

BIOSECURITY
N/A

PRODUCTION MANAGEMENT
• Consumption of diets containing excessive amounts of gossypol from whole cottonseed and cottonseed hulls or meal is the route of exposure that causes toxicity.

• The level predisposing the animal to toxicity depends on the species, rumen function, level of protein in the diet, and duration of consumption.

SYNONYMS
N/A

SEE ALSO
Monensin toxicity
Vitamin E and selenium toxicity
Toxic plants such as coffee, senna, bracken fern, white snakeroot, lantana, and milkweed

ABBREVIATIONS
CSM = cottonseed meal
TMR = total mixed ration
WCS = whole cottonseed

Suggested Reading
Risco, C. A., Adams, A. L., Seebohm, S., Thatcher, M. J., Staples, C. R., Van Horn, H. H., McDowell, L. R., Calhoun, M. C., Thatcher, W. W. 2002. Effects of gossypol from cottonseed on hematological responses and plasma α-tocopherol concentration of dairy cows. *J Dairy Sci.* 85:3,3575–3402.
Risco, C. A., Chase, C.,Jr. Gossypol Toxicity. In: D'Mello F.E. (ed) *Handbook of plant and fungal toxicant*. CRC Press, Inc. 1997. pp 87–95.
Risco, C. A., Chenoweth, P. J., Larsen, R. E., Velez, J., Shaw, N., Tran, T., Chase, C. C. 1993. The effect of gossypol in cottonseed meal on performance, hematological and semen traits in post pubertal Brahman bulls. *Theriogenology* 40:3, 629–42.
Risco, C. A., Holmberg, C., Kutches, A. 1992. Effect of graded levels of gossypol on calf performance: toxicological and pathological considerations. *J Dairy Science* 75:10, 2787–98.

Author: Carlos A. Risco

GRASS TETANY/HYPOMAGNESEMIA

 BASICS

OVERVIEW
• Magnesium (Mg) deficiency affects the central nervous system of ruminants.
• Mg is absorbed from the rumen and excreted in urine.
• High dietary potassium decreases absorption of Mg.
• Rapidly growing grasses contain relatively high concentrations of potassium and low concentrations of Mg.

PATHOPHYSIOLOGY
• Mg is necessary for most major cellular metabolic pathways and is vital to maintenance of resting membrane potentials at synapses.
• Because adenosine triphosphate (ATP) requires Mg to form the high-energy bond between phosphates, Mg is required for all enzymatic reactions requiring ATP.
• Mg is also necessary for ATPase activity; therefore, myofibril contractions are sustained in hypomagnesemia, leading to tetanic spasms.
• Most Mg is present in teeth and bones, which is not readily mobilized.
• There is no direct hormonal control of Mg uptake, so daily intake is necessary.

SYSTEMS AFFECTED
CNS, musculoskeletal, production management

GENETICS
N/A

INCIDENCE/PREVALENCE
Unknown

GEOGRAPHIC DISTRIBUTION
Worldwide in distribution

SIGNALMENT
• Most commonly seen in lactating beef cattle within the first 2 months of calving, particularly if grazing cool season grasses.
• Lactating dairy cattle are affected less commonly because of differences in nutritional management. Grazing dairy cattle would be at greater risk.

• Ewes and dairy goats are also susceptible.
• Calves on all milk diets without added Mg may develop the disease as well.

Species
Potentially, all ruminant species

Breed Predilections
N/A

Mean Age and Range
N/A

Predominant Sex
N/A

SIGNS
• Affected animals are often found dead.
• Anorexia and separation from the herd
• Early in the course, ears will be erect and twitching and hyperesthesia will be noted.
• Alert, hyperexcitable, may charge
• Muscle fasciculations and head tremors may be noted.
• Nystagmus and fluttering of the eyelids
• Ataxia
• Recumbency
• Clonic convulsions, opisthotonus, or tetanic muscle spasms
• Elevated body temperature because of excess muscle activity
• Increased heart and respiratory rate

CAUSES AND RISK FACTORS
• Mature ruminants just prior to calving and during early lactation have the highest demand for Mg.
• Periods of rapid grass growth, particularly cool season grasses and cereal crops, are the most common time for clinical signs to occur (spring and/or fall).
• Heavy fertilization of pastures increases the risk of grass tetany. Use of recycled poultry bedding as a feed supplement or fertilizer has commonly been associated with an increased incidence of hypomagnesemia.

 DIAGNOSIS

DIFFERENTIAL DIAGNOSIS
• Hypocalcemia (serum Ca)
• Nervous ketosis (urine ketones)

• Nervous coccidiosis (fecal float)
• Heavy metal toxicities: for example, arsenic and lead (history of exposure to heavy metals, elevated blood, kidney or liver concentration of heavy metal)
• Salt poisoning (history, necropsy)
• Tetanus (response to therapy, necropsy)
• Rabies (necropsy)
• Viral encephalitides (history of herd and surrounding area, increasing antibody titers)

CBC/BIOCHEMISTRY/URINALYSIS
• Serum Mg less than 1.2 mg/dl
• Cerebrospinal fluid Mg less than 1.45 mg/dl
• Urine Mg less than 2.5 mg/dl
• Postmortem ocular Mg less than 1 mg/dl (within 24 hours of death)
• Affected animals are often hypocalcemic.
• After episodes of tetany, animals will often have elevated potassium, aspartate aminotransferase (AST), and creatinine phosphokinase (CK) due to muscle damage.

IMAGING
N/A

DIAGNOSTIC PROCEDURES
• Diagnosis is most often made on the basis of clinical signs or history because of the need for immediate treatment.
• Decreased serum, CSF, ocular or urine Mg concentrations are confirmatory.

PATHOLOGIC FINDINGS
.

GROSS FINDINGS
• May note evidence of thrashing on ground around where the animal died.
• No gross findings directly attributable to hypomagnesemia
• Trauma and bruising are common findings because of seizures.
• Rumen contents may be aspirated into lungs.
• Ecchymotic hemorrhages
• Agonal pulmonary emphysema

HISTOPATHOLOGICAL FINDINGS
Calves dying of hypomagnesemia may have microscopic calcium deposits in arterial walls of the heart, lungs, and spleen.

GRASS TETANY/HYPOMAGNESEMIA

TREATMENT

- Minimize handling to decrease the chance of initiating tetanic seizures.
- It may be necessary to administer intramuscular sedation prior to initiating Mg therapy to control seizure activity. Avoid intravenous sedative administration.
- Heart rate should be monitored closely while administering Mg solutions and treatment should be slowed or discontinued if heart rate drops substantially.
- Respiratory failure may occur if Mg solutions are given too quickly due to medullary depression.

MEDICATIONS

DRUGS OF CHOICE

- Animals with hypomagnesemia are often hypocalcemic as well and should receive therapy containing calcium.
- Administer intravenous calcium borogluconate solution containing 5% Mg (500 ml for adult cattle; 50–100 ml for calves and small ruminants).
- Many animals relapse several hours after treatment, so an additional source of Mg should be provided with initial treatment.
  - Oral Mg salts: (1) 50% Mg sulfate solution (125–150 ml for adult cattle). (2) Mg oxide (60 g in gelatin capsule for adult cattle).
  - Subcutaneous injection of 100–200 ml (for adult cattle) of a 20%–50% Mg sulfate solution. Limit to 50 ml per site to avoid tissue damage.
  - Mg enema —60 g of Mg in 250–500 ml of water. Solution should not be more concentrated than this to avoid mucosal sloughing.

CONTRAINDICATIONS

- Avoid potassium-containing solutions for therapy because they will interfere with Mg absorption.
- Appropriate milk and meat withdrawal times must be followed for all compounds administered to food-producing animals.

FOLLOW-UP

- Allowing animals access to only hay or mature grass for a portion of the day will increase Mg in the diet and may prevent further cases.
- Mg is unpalatable and will not be consumed in significant quantities unless mixed with some other dietary component.
- Mg can be added to feed or water to encourage intake
  - If feeding Mg in water, animals must be given access to only supplemented water to ensure intake of Mg.
  - Spraying or dusting pastures with Mg fertilizers in the spring will increase dietary Mg.
  - Mg will be readily consumed in concentrate mixtures or molasses licks.

MISCELLANEOUS

Therapy is often unrewarding, especially in cases where seizures have already occurred.

ASSOCIATED CONDITIONS
N/A

AGE-RELATED FACTORS

- Most commonly seen in lactating beef cattle within the first 2 months of calving, particularly if grazing cool season grasses.
- Lactating dairy cattle are affected less commonly because of differences in nutritional management. Grazing dairy cattle would be at greater risk.
- Calves on all-milk diets without added Mg may develop the disease as well.
- Calves dying of hypomagnesemia may have microscopic calcium deposits in arterial walls of the heart, lungs, and spleen.

ZOONOTIC POTENTIAL
Hypomagnesemia is neither contagious nor zoonotic.

PREGNANCY
N/A

RUMINANT SPECIES AFFECTED
Cattle, sheep, and goats

BIOSECURITY
N/A

PRODUCTION MANAGEMENT

- Periods of rapid grass growth, particularly cool season grasses and cereal crops, are the most common times for clinical signs to occur (spring and/or fall).
- Heavy fertilization of pastures increases the risk of grass tetany. Use of recycled poultry bedding as a feed supplement or fertilizer has commonly been associated with an increased incidence of hypomagnesemia.

SYNONYMS
Hypomagnesemia, tetany

SEE ALSO
Heavy metal toxicities
Hypocalcemia
Nervous coccidiosis
Nervous ketosis
Rabies
Salt poisoning
Tetanus
Viral encephalitides

ABBREVIATIONS
AST = aspartate aminotransferase
ATP = adenosine triphosphate
Ca = calcium
CK = creatinine phosphokinase
CNS = central nervous system
CSF = cerebral spinal fluid
Mg = magnesium

Suggested Reading
Blackwelder, J. T., Hunt, E. 2002. Disorders of magnesium metabolism. In: *Large animal internal medicine*, ed. B. P. Smith, Philadelphia: Mosby.
Goff, J. P. 1999. Ruminant hypomagnesemic tetanies. In: *Current veterinary therapy 4: food animal practice*, ed. J. L. Howard, R. A. Smith. Philadelphia: W. B. Saunders.
Wilson, G. F. 2002. Metabolic diseases of grazing cattle: from clinical event to production disease. *NZ Vet J* 50: S85–87.

Author: Dawn J. Capucille

HAEMONCHOSIS

 BASICS

OVERVIEW
• Haemonchus is a voracious blood-sucking parasite that causes anemia, hypoproteinemia, and death losses especially in small ruminants.
• Diarrhea and weight loss are seldom important in haemonchosis.
• In warm moist environments, *Haemonchus* is by far the dominant gastrointestinal nematode.
• *Haemonchus* species tend to be host specific but there is some host cross infection.
• Populations of *Haemonchus contortus* have become resistant to all currently available anthelmintics.

SIGNALMENT
• All ages of sheep, goats, camelids, deer, and cattle may become infected, but young and lactating adult small ruminants are at greater risk of disease.
• Until young animals have been exposed to *Haemonchus* and are older than 4 to 7 months of age, they do not develop resistance to the parasite.
• Hosts adversely affected may vary with environment and vegetation consumed. Where sheep and goats graze on short grass and legumes, the disease is seen most often in goats. When there is plentiful browse, goats are unlikely to be exposed to large numbers of infective larvae.
• Adult females are unable to mount a protective immune response against helminths during the periparturient period.
• Breeds and species that evolved in humid tropical areas are more likely to have the genetic traits that make them resistant to infection.

SIGNS
• The primary signs of disease are those of anemia and hypoproteinemia.
• The onset of disease can be sudden with apparently healthy animals becoming weak and lying down unable to rise.
• Diarrhea is seldom seen in haemonchosis although the stool may be soft.
• In chronic cases, there may be a loss of wool, decreased fiber diameter, and weight loss.
• Depending on the physiologic status of the host and the number of parasites with which it is infected, the disease may present differently.

Peracute Disease
Sudden death, very few clinical signs, the PCV falls to less than 10. Only a few individuals in the flock will be affected. The anemia is responsive and immature erythrocytes will be seen in the survivors. There may be a soft stool.

Acute Disease
• More individuals in the flock will be affected. Anemia, pale mucous membranes, and hypoproteinemia (bottle jaw) are the most common clinical signs. May be constipated.
• A common sequela to acute haemonchosis is wool break, in which wool breaks off weeks following the acute signs of disease.

Chronic Disease
Anemia becomes unresponsive—ill thrift with poor-quality wool, weight loss, or failure to gain

Host Immunity
• Immunity to *Haemonchus* infections is slow in development and fragile when exposed to large numbers of larvae.
• Disease is seen in all ages but more in young and during the periparturient relaxation of resistance.
• There is genetic resistance to haemonchosis, which is usually manifest as an acquired protective immunity, with fewer worms establishing and those worms producing fewer eggs.
• There maybe an allergic response to massive larval exposure known as self-cure. Adult worms are expelled and the larvae that triggered the response may eventually take their place or are lost.

Parasite Survival Strategies
• Adult females produce 5000–6000 eggs per day.
• Larvae feed on fecal bacteria, molts do not shed the cuticle. This sheath protects the L3 infective larva from desiccation.
• The L3 larvae are infective to the host. It takes 5 to 10 days from the eggs being passed for development to the infective stage.
• The larvae can only exit the fecal pellet then ascend vegetation in a film of moisture.
• The ruminant, while grazing, ingests larvae.
• The L3 exsheaths in rumen, moves to abomasum, enters gastric pits, and molts to L4.
• The L4 feeds on blood and molts to the adult, who mates and produces eggs approximately 3 weeks after being acquired.

• Adult worms live for months in susceptible hosts.
• The worms produce so many eggs that some offspring will survive unfavorable conditions within or outside the host.
• During prolonged periods of drought or winter weather conditions, ensheathed larvae survive in the fecal pellet. They are inactive and apparently do not utilize stored energy. When rains occur, they rapidly exit the fecal pellet.
• Following dry periods, the livestock graze closer to the fecal pat than normal and their chances of becoming infected are increased.
• Hypobiosis, or arrested development within the host's abomasum during the early fourth stage. These larvae are in a state of inactivity and are not affected by the host's immune system. They survive until conditions either within the host or in the environment are more favorable.
• *Haemonchus contortus* have such a rich genome that some individuals in populations have genes that enable them to resist the effects of anthelmintics.
• With the extreme fecundity of the worm, it has rapidly adapted to the use of anthelmintics and some populations have become resistant to every anthelmintic currently available.

CAUSES AND RISK FACTORS
• Haemonchus is a tropical parasite that does well in warm, humid, temperate climates during the warm season.
• Young or lactating animals
• Heavily stocked and grazed pastures
• Breeds that evolved in arid or cold climates are at greater risk.
• Grazing pastures a few days following rains increases the likelihood of acquiring infection.

 DIAGNOSIS

DIFFERENTIAL DIAGNOSIS
• Anemia due to other parasites and bacteria such as *Fasciola, Fascioloides, Bunostomum, Ostertagia, Teladorsaiga, Babesia, Anaplasma, Mycoplasma* (*Eperythrozoon*), fleas, lice, and biting flies.
• Chronic copper poisoning in sheep may be differentiated by time of the year, age of affected animals, icterus, and access to sources of copper.

• Poisoning caused by sweet clover, pokeweed, or plants that cause intestinal or other bleeding may resemble haemonchosis. Age of animals and time of year may help differentiate.

CBC/BIOCHEMISTRY/URINALYSIS
• Erythrocyte and hemoglobin levels will be depressed.
• At first strictly blood loss, low packed cell volume with normal erythrocytes. Surviving animals quickly mount a response as the body attempts to replace lost erythrocytes.
• A macrocytic normochromic anemia is the most common finding with acute haemonchosis.
• In chronic haemonchosis with iron, cobalt, copper levels depleted, a microcytic, hypochromic anemia will be seen.
• Serum protein levels are low.
• Protein loss occurs through the gastrointestinal tract so both albumen and globulin levels are lowered by a similar amount.

OTHER LABORATORY TESTS
• Fecal flotation using a saline or sugar flotation media with a specific gravity of 1.18 or greater will float the eggs of *Haemonchus* and other nematodes.
• Fecal examination will reveal strongylid thin-shelled segmented eggs.
• A quantitative test such as the modified McMaster method will aid the clinician in determining if there are sufficient numbers of worms to cause disease.
• There is a more or less linear relationship between the egg count and the number of adult worms. Fecal egg counts of more than 4000 eggs per gram of feces are associated with haemonchosis.
• Measuring before and after treatment egg counts can be vital in determining if anthelmintics used are actually effective in specific herds and flocks.
• Eggs are not diagnostic for *Haemonchus,* as other genera of strongylids produce identical eggs.
• In humid areas during the warm portion of the year, *Haemonchus* is usually the dominant parasite especially where it is resistant to anthelmintics.

PATHOLOGIC FINDINGS
GROSS FINDINGS
• Postmortem examination demonstrating the presence of adult worms in the abomasum is the most accurate diagnostic method.
• The body cavities may be fluid filled.
• Intermandibular edema, pallor of the mucous membranes are indicative of haemonchosis.
• The fecal material will be of normal consistency, dark, and dry, or an unformed stool may be seen.

HISTOPATHOLOGICAL FINDINGS
• The histological findings are those associated with anemia due to erythrocyte loss.
• Bone marrow changes will be a function of the duration of the disease.
• There will be no specific changes in the abomasum, however, in hosts undergoing an immunologic response, there may be increased cellularity with mast cells, eosinophils, or globular leukocytes.
• None of these findings are consistent or diagnostic.

 TREATMENT

• Broad-spectrum safe anthelmintics are the primary means of treatment and control.
• Early after the development of broad-spectrum anthelmintics, many *Haemonchus contortus* populations became resistant to anthelmintics. Resistance has become common in many geographic regions.
• Selection by treatment not mutation appears to be the driving force in the establishment of resistance.
• *Haemonchus* in cattle and in small ruminants in cooler climates is susceptible to some benzimidazoles, levamisole/morantel, or macrocyclic lactones if administered in an adequate dose to the specific host.
• In warmer climates with elevated precipitation, worm populations have been selected for resistance.

• Tolerant or resistant worms often accompany livestock being introduced into new areas. The worms accompanying their hosts are likely to be those with resistant features; clinical disease thus happens more rapidly than in areas where there may still be susceptible worms.
• Underdosing: Either by underestimating weight or by selecting a dose for the average size of animal in a flock, worms will be exposed to a less than lethal level of anthelmintic.
• Goats and cervids metabolize anthelmintics more quickly than do cattle or sheep. Therefore, a sheep dose is an underdose in a goat.
• Injecting anthelmintics may be a form of underdosing. When persistent anthelmintics are used, the injectable formulation will maintain a blood level over a prolonged period of time. As long as the blood level is sufficient to kill all incoming worms, this may be an advantage rendering the host largely free of parasitism for weeks. As the blood levels drop, only those worms with some level of tolerance of the drug will be able to establish in the host.
• Cattle pour-on formulations are not absorbed as well by many other species, and when used are a form of underdosing in other species.

Anthelmintic Resistance
• Treating to keep parasite levels at the minimum is selecting for resistance if every worm is not killed. Treating every 3 to 4 weeks year-round or during the transmission season insures that only those worms with tolerance to an anthelmintic have only similar worms to mate with.
• Strategic worming practices, such as treat and move if the new pasture has few if any parasitic larvae in them, insure that the survivor worms can mate only with survivors.
• Anthelmintic resistance by *Haemonchus* has few apparent drawbacks; the benzimidazole-resistant worms are larger, produce more eggs, and therefore suck more blood than the susceptible worms.

HAEMONCHOSIS

• Macrocyclic lactone resistant *Haemonchus* may not be as cold tolerant as larvae in the pasture and may die out over winter if exposed to sufficient chilling.
• At least some of the levamisole/morantel-resistant *Haemonchus* revert to susceptibility, as the resistance gene trait is linked to the sex gene.
• Almost without exception, the anthelmintics labeled for use in small ruminants in North America are not effective against *Haemonchus* in the southern states.
• The most important aspect of the use of anthelmintics is to determine if the product is actually effective on the farm on which a control program is contemplated.
• Fecal egg count reduction test: Animals are administered what is believed to be an adequate dose of anthelmintic after collection of feces to determine the quantity of eggs present. A reevaluation of egg counts 7 to 14 days later will determine if there has been an adequate reduction in egg counts.
• Because of the natural variation of the number of worms in individual hosts, the average difference must be determined in 12 to 20 individual animals within a herd or flock to be certain that the test is valid.
• From a practical aspect, 6 to 10 individuals who are identified and resampled may be sufficient especially if they are younger animals.
• Allowing some animals to remain as untreated controls increases the value of the test but is often impractical under field conditions.
• In some instances, an anthelmintic cannot be identified that is effective against the worm population on a farm.

Enhancement of Anthelmintics
• The effectiveness of benzimidazoles may be enhanced by dividing the dose over several days or by fasting the animals overnight in a dry lot.
• Combining anthelmintics by administration of two or more drugs each from a different family of anthelmintics simultaneously
• Which two or three drugs should be used on an individual farm? The answer is what works on that farm. Proprietary drugs using all three families of anthelmintics are being used in other countries with *Haemonchus*-resistance problems.

Rotation of Anthelmintics
• Fast rotation: use a drug in a different family each time an anthelmintic is utilized. This method selects for resistance to all the compounds in the rotation.
• Slow rotation: use a product for a year then switch to a compound in another family. May work for a while but resistance will occur.
• There may be nothing to rotate to.
• Some rotation systems are not rotation at all, just other compounds in the same family all of which affect the worm in the same fashion.
• Use a product until it fails, then switch to something in a different family.

Effective Use of Anthelmintics
• Once an anthelmintic is identified that is effective on the farm in question, then decide what is desired in a control program.
• In the early spring, reduced pasture contamination is the most important aspect. The ewe or doe in the periparturient relaxation of resistance phase, even if she has the genetic capacity for resistance, will be a source of eggs for the environment.
• Strategic deworming to remove arrested or recently emerged larvae before they contaminate the pasture may have the greatest impact on pasture contamination.
• A few individual animals will have a much greater number of worms and worm eggs than the remainder of the population.
• If the worm-wealthy individuals can be identified, treating them rather than the entire host population can have as much impact on lessening the number of larvae subsequently on pasture as treating the entire flock.
• Identification of wormy individuals can be made by determining egg counts or by measuring the color of the ocular mucous membranes.
• Treating these animals will reduce the worm population but will not ensure the survival of only resistant worms, as those in the untreated animals will not be selected.
• A corollary to individual treatment is the culling of those animals that are treated most often. They are not resistant to worms and their offspring will likely have similar traits.
• Another approach is treatment of hosts after they have been exposed to large numbers of worms. Treatment 2 weeks following rain should remove much of that acquired population of worms before they can begin passing eggs.

• Zero grazing for a period of time after a disease outbreak may enable the host to recover both in terms of reestablishment of a protective immune response and production of erythrocytes and serum protein levels.

Prevention Management
• Management systems that lower the exposure of hosts to parasites can be devised. These systems may not optimize the value of forages but they result in healthier livestock.
• Rapid pasture rotation systems where pastures are vacated for as few as 30 days before returning animals may be of value in warm, humid climates, during the hottest time of the year in high rainfall areas or on irrigated pastures.
• Rapid pasture rotation otherwise will insure that the worms are waiting for the hosts when they return to the pasture.
• Utilizing pastures that have been used for cropping, especially in the last half of the grazing season, is grazing parasite-free pastures and, by the following year, any larvae deposited on the cropland will not survive until the next grazing.
• Alternate or cograzing with other species or classes of livestock may harvest *Haemonchus* larvae from the pasture.
• In general, the *Haemonchus* in sheep and goats do not do well in cattle. Recent observation questions this assumption, as some populations of *Haemonchus contortus* may thrive in calves.
• Horses do not share *Haemonchus* and can be safely grazed in areas dangerous to ruminants.
• Older cattle may become infected but are highly resistant to effects of the worms and can be used to clear larvae from a pasture.

Nutrition
• In general, *Haemonchus* does not cause weight loss and animals may appear to be thrifty up to the time they become extremely anemic.
• Providing sufficient protein is vital with haemonchosis as that is what is being lost.
• During the periparturient period, increased protein, not energy levels will lessen egg production by gastrointestinal nematodes.
• To be sure, you cannot feed animals through the disease but it is vital in recovery, especially for those whose immune response is compromised.

Natural Biological Control
• Pastures containing plants high in condensed tannins are safer grazing for hosts as the incoming larvae are adversely affected.
• The physical structure of some plants is also a challenge for larvae to ascend the vegetation.
• If animals browse, their chances of acquiring larvae diminish as the distance from the ground increases. Most infective larvae are found with in 2 inches (50 mm) of the soil surface.
• Predaceous fungi have been evaluated as agents that kill larvae in pastures. One species, *Duddingtonia flagrans*, is able to traverse the digestive tract and is present in the fecal pat when the larvae hatch. Feeding spores or incorporating them in ruminal boluses has the capacity to lower pasture contamination.

Vaccination
• Vaccination is an approach deemed likely to be successful because animals naturally develop resistance to *Haemonchus*. However, the requirement for multiple exposure and maturation of the host immune system appears to be important in natural immunity and also appears to be the case with whole-worm antigens, selected antigens, or irradiated larval vaccines.
• A different approach—the production of vaccines directed against antigens the host normally never encounters (cryptic antigens)—has shown promise. Antigens derived form the intestinal lining of the worm were identified, and vaccinated sheep produce antibody against these antigens. When the worm begins to suck blood, the antigen-antibody reaction destroys the intestinal lining of the worm.
• As with anthelmintics, the ability of the worm to rapidly select populations with possible different antigenic determinants is a concern.
• Cryptic antigen–vaccinated animals are not boosted by natural infection, so vaccination will have to be repeated frequently.

Genetics
• The selection of individual animals with a level of resistance to the parasite or those that have the capacity to rebound from the effects of parasitism seems to be a logical approach. The offspring of resistant hosts are likely to also be resistant. Therefore, resistance to *Haemonchus* could be a selection criterion used in a flock.

• The genetic aspect of resistance to gastrointestinal parasites is not well understood. It appears that multiple genes are involved in aspects of the protective response and that different genes may be more important at different times in the course of infection.
• Some breeds have more individual animals with sufficient factors, and they are more likely to survive exposure levels that would kill other animals.
• Even in resistant breeds, all animals are not equal, and factors such as lactation, age, or nutritional status may influence the course of disease.
• When animals are producing at their genetic maximum, they are at greater risk of parasitic disease because they are immunologically and nutritionally challenged.
• Other phenotypic characteristics such as production of milk, fiber, multiple births, and resistance to other agents may be at odds with resistance to helminths. Research does not indicate that the traits, which lead to increased production, are linked to those of increased susceptibility.
• To determine if genetic resistance is the answer to the problem of haemonchosis, as currently appears to be the case, much more knowledge is needed.

Summary
• There is no overall approach that fits with the environment—and management practices—that will control haemonchosis.
• Schemes that recognize that some animals are much more at risk than others and that strive to assure that the at-risk population is exposed to fewer worms or, if exposed, is treated differently may have a chance of success.
• Programs based on chemical control alone will likely fail unless the season of transmission is very short or new anthelmintics with completely different modes of action are discovered.
• Effective vaccines may be produced but will not likely be practical in young animals at highest risk. However, they may lessen pasture contamination and subsequent exposure.

 MISCELLANEOUS

SEE ALSO
Anemia due to other parasites and bacteria such as *Fasciola, Fascioloides, Bunostomum, Ostertagia, Teladorsaiga, Babesia, Anaplasma, Mycoplasma* (*Eperythrozoon*), fleas, lice, and biting flies
Chronic copper poisoning in sheep
Plants that cause intestinal or other bleeding
Poisoning caused by sweet clover, pokeweed

ABBREVIATIONS
PCV = packed cell volume

Suggested Reading
Adams, D. B. 1984. Infection with *Haemonchus contortus* in sheep and the role of adaptive immunity in selection of the parasite. *International J Parasitol.* 18:1071–75.
Gray, G. D., Barger, I. A., LeJambre, L. F., et al. 1992. Parasitological and immunological responses of genetically resistant Merino sheep on pastures contaminated with parasitic nematodes. *International J Parasitol.* 22:417–25.
Knox, D. P., Smith, W. D. 2001. Vaccination against gastrointestinal nematode parasites of ruminants using gut-expressed antigens. *Vet Parasitol.* 100:21–32.
Larsen, M. 1999. Biological control of helminths. *International J Parasitol.* 29:139–46.
Urquhart, G. M., Armour, J., Duncan, J. L., et al. 1996. *Veterinary parasitology.* 2nd ed. Oxford: Blackwell Science.
VanWyk, J. A., Stenson, M. O., VanDerMerwe, J. S., et al. 1999. Anthelmintic resistance in South Africa; Surveys indicate an extremely serious situation in sheep and goat farming. *Onderstepoort J Vet Res.* 66:273–84.
Waller, P. J. 2003. Global perspectives on nematode parasite control in ruminant livestock: the need to adopt alternatives to chemotherapy, with emphasis on biological control. *Anim Hlth Res Rev.* 4:35–43.

Author: Thomas Craig

HAEMOPHILUS SOMNUS COMPLEX

 BASICS

DEFINITION
• *Haemophilus somnus* is a small, pleomorphic, gram-negative bacteria.
• It was first identified in 1960 as the cause of thrombotic meningoencephalitis (TME) in feedlot cattle. Since this time, it has been confirmed as contributing to or causing disease involving multiple organ systems.

PATHOPHYSIOLOGY
• *H. somnus* can be isolated from respiratory and reproductive tracts of healthy animals.
• Method of transmission is unclear, possibly spread via respiratory secretions, urine, or venereal contact.
• Organism can survive in biologic fluids for several weeks in the environment.
• *H. somnus* initially colonizes mucous membranes. It then invades the circulatory system leading to vasculitis and septicemia with localization in various tissues and organs.
• Entry via the respiratory tract is the probable route of respiratory infection.
• Reproductive disease is possibly spread through venereal contact or respiratory route.

SYSTEMS AFFECTED
• Respiratory—important bacterial pathogen in bronchopneumonia/pleuropneumonia (bovine respiratory disease complex, BRDC); also associated with pleuritis, laryngitis, otitis media
• Nervous—TME
• Reproductive—abortion, infertility (due to endometritis), vaginitis, orchitis, mastitis

• Cardiovascular—myocarditis, pericarditis, septicemia
• Musculoskeletal—infectious polyarthritis
• Ophthalmic—conjunctivitis, retinal hemorrhage

GENETICS
N/A

INCIDENCE/PREVALENCE
• Culture of normal animals and serologic evidence suggests infection is widespread. Clinical disease is less common.
• In Canada and the northern United States, *H. somnus* infection is considered to be a significant cause of morbidity and mortality in feedlot cattle.

GEOGRAPHIC DISTRIBUTION
• Commonly isolated in Canada, western and midwestern United States. Rarely isolated in northeastern and southeastern United States.
• Identified in South America, Europe, Australia, New Zealand, Russia, Israel, and Japan

SIGNALMENT

Species
Bovine—similar disease syndromes seen in sheep infected with *Haemophilus agni* and *Histophilus ovis*.

Breed Predilection
• Systemic disease is seen predominantly in beef cattle.
• Reproductive disease can be seen in both beef and dairy cattle.

Mean Age and Range
• Respiratory, neurologic, and cardiovascular disease are predominantly in feedlot cattle (6–24 months of age).
• Reproductive disease is seen in breeding-age animals.

Predominant Sex
• Systemic disease affects both sexes.
• Reproductive disease is seen predominantly in females.

SIGNS

GENERAL COMMENTS
• Signs will differ based on system(s) affected.
• Combinations of respiratory, nervous, cardiovascular, musculoskeletal, and/or ophthalmic disease can occur in an affected individual or in a group of animals.
• Reproductive involvement typically occurs without other system involvement.

HISTORICAL FINDINGS
• Onset of systemic disease can range from acute death with no premonitory signs to chronic disease.
• Sporadic abortion is the typical reproductive manifestation.

PHYSICAL EXAMINATION FINDINGS
• Systemic disease—fever, depression, possibly a high morbidity
  • Respiratory—dyspnea, nasal discharge, lacrimation; similar to other causes of bacterial pneumonia
  • Nervous—severe depression, partially closed eyes, muscle weakness, ataxia, recumbency
• Occasionally, opisthotonus, nystagmus, strabismus, unilateral or bilateral blindness, hyperasthesia, and/or convulsions can occur.
• Ophthalmic—retinal hemorrhage with accumulation of exudates. Typically seen with other system involvement.
• Musculoskeletal—swelling, heat, and pain in one or multiple joints
• Myocarditis—typically, cattle that have had prior case of respiratory disease. Often found acutely dead. May present as congestive heart failure.

• Reproductive disease—sporadic abortion with little to no clinical signs in the dam

CAUSES

Infectious disease: organism—*Haemophilus somnus*
• Pathogenic and commensal strains
• Pathogenic strains are resistant to complement and serum antibodies.
• Pathogenic strains can survive within macrophages and PMNs.

RISK FACTORS

• Disease typically seen during the first 3–4 weeks following feedlot arrival.
• Imunologically naïve cattle experience higher morbidity and mortality following feedlot entry.
• Possible seasonal effect (increased diagnostic lab submissions during November, December, and January)

DIAGNOSIS

DIFFERENTIAL DIAGNOSIS

Respiratory

• Clinically indistinguishable from other differentials; requires culture, virology, serology, and/or histopathology for differentiation
• Other bacterial pathogens in BRDC—*Manheimia haemolytica*, *Pasteurella multocida*
• Primary viral respiratory infection—IBR, BVDV, BRSV, etc.

Neurologic

• Polioencephalomalacia—high sulfate/sulfur level in feed and/or water, typically afebrile, cortical blindness, different pathologic lesions
• Listeria meningoencephalitis
• Hypovitaminosis-A—insufficient levels of vitamin A in feed, low plasma and liver vitamin A levels
• Salt toxicity—history of water deprivation, typically afebrile, cortical blindness, high serum and CSF sodium levels, different pathologic lesions
• Lead toxicity—opportunity for exposure to lead, typically afebrile, cortical blindness, high blood lead level, different pathologic lesions
• Viral encephalomyelitis—rabies, malignant catarrhal fever, etc.
• Cranial trauma

Reproductive

• Indistinguishable clinically from other causes of abortion. Requires culture, virology, and/or histopathology of abortus and placenta for differentiation.
• Other bacterial causes of abortion—*Leptospira* spp., *Listeria monocytogenes*, *Brucella abortus*, etc.
• Protozoal causes of abortion—*Neospora caninum*
• Viral causes of abortion—IBR, BVDV
• Other causes of abortion—Mycotic infection, idiopathic, toxicity (plant, nitrate, etc.), trauma

CBC/BIOCHEMISTRY/URINALYSIS

No unique or specific changes. Nonspecific changes associated with inflammation could be seen—increased fibrinogen, leukocytosis, increased neutrophil:lymphocyte ratio, increased serum globulin

OTHER LABORATORY TESTS

• Bacterial culture
 • Slow-growing nature can lead to overgrowth of contaminants
 • Requires blood-containing media for growth
 • Requires an atmosphere containing increased CO_2
 • Previous antibiotic treatment may decrease ability to isolate organism.
• Serology—requires acute and convalescent samples for accurate interpretation
• Other testing modalities—immunohistochemistry and PCR testing developed, but not commercially available at this time

IMAGING

N/A

DIAGNOSTIC PROCEDURES

CSF tap—Fluid typically contains increased total protein, increased globulin, and increased cell count (predominantly neutrophils).

PATHOLOGIC FINDINGS

• Gross lesions
 • Respiratory—fibrinopurulent bronchopneumonia with a cranioventral distribution. Fibrinous pleuritis may be present with or without pneumonia lesions.
 • Neurologic—multifocal areas of hemorrhage and necrosis throughout all areas of the brain. Meninges may appear cloudy and hyperemic. CSF is typically cloudy.
 • Musculoskeletal—serofibrinous polyarthritis

HAEMOPHILUS SOMNUS COMPLEX

• Cardiovascular—Myocarditis lesions are typically found in the papillary muscle of the left ventricle, range from a round area of hemorrhage and necrosis acutely to an exudative abscess.
• Reproductive—characterized by a necrotizing placentitis. Fetal septicemia may result in petechial hemorrhages.
• Histopathologic lesions: Septic thrombosis and vasculitis are seen in the affected organ(s).

TREATMENT

APPROPRIATE HEALTH CARE
• Clinically affected animals should have constant access to fresh, palatable feedstuffs and clean water.
• Animals should be cared for in a low-stress, low-competition environment.
• If affected individuals become laterally recumbent and are unable to rise, or if their condition has severely deteriorated, euthanasia is appropriate.

NURSING CARE
Normal

ACTIVITY
Physical activity should be minimized.

DIET
Normal

CLIENT EDUCATION
None

SURGICAL CONSIDERATIONS
N/A

MEDICATIONS

DRUGS OF CHOICE
Respiratory Disease
• Typically treated as undifferentiated BRDC
• Several antibiotics are specifically labeled for treatment of *H. somnus*:
  • Ceftiofur (1.1–2.2 mg/kg SQ for 3–5 days)
  • Enrofloxacin (7.5–12.5 mg/kg SQ)
  • Florfenicol (40 mg/kg SQ)
• Many other antibiotics labeled for treatment of BRDC may be effective as well.

Neurologic Disease
• No drugs are labeled for this use in the United States. Extralabel use requires that the practitioner provide an appropriate drug withdrawal time.
• Antibiotic must pass blood-brain barrier:
  • Florfenicol
  • Oxytetracycline

CONTRAINDICATIONS
None

PRECAUTIONS
Appropriate drug withdrawal time should be followed before slaughter.

POSSIBLE INTERACTIONS
None

ALTERNATIVE DRUGS
None

FOLLOW-UP

PATIENT MONITORING
Typically involves evaluation of improvement or deterioration of clinical signs (attitude, appetite, rectal temperature, system-associated signs).

PREVENTION/AVOIDANCE
• Many nonspecific control measures for BRDC (viral vaccination, stress reduction, etc.) would be effective in control of *H. somnus*.
• Commercial *H. somnus* bacterin is available.
  • Requires two doses at 2- to 3-week interval.
  • Results of trials to evaluate clinical efficacy have yielded conflicting results.
• Postarrival mass medication with antibiotics can be used when high BRDC morbidity is expected.

POSSIBLE COMPLICATIONS

Poor response to therapy may require euthanasia.

EXPECTED COURSE AND PROGNOSIS

• Generally, cattle treated in the early stages of disease have a better chance of recovery than those with more advanced disease regardless of the affected system.
• Cattle with advanced neurologic disease have a poor to grave prognosis even with aggressive treatment.
• Polyarthritis often has a poor response to therapy leading to chronic lameness.

MISCELLANEOUS

ASSOCIATED CONDITIONS

None

AGE-RELATED FACTORS

• Systemic disease typically is seen in feedlot cattle (age 6–24 months).
• Reproductive disease is seen in breeding age animals.

ZOONOTIC POTENTIAL

None

PREGNANCY

Organism can cause abortion.

RUMINANT SPECIES AFFECTED

• Bovine
• Ovine—affected by similar disease caused by *Haemophilus agni* and *Histophilus ovis*

BIOSECURITY

Biosecurity is difficult to attain in a feedlot setting due to movement of cattle from multiple sources onto the premises.

PRODUCTION MANAGEMENT

H. somnus plays a role in BRDC, which is the most economically significant disease in the beef industry.

SYNONYMS

Neurologic disease—"brainer," "sleeper"

SEE ALSO

• Bovine respiratory disease complex
  • BRDC—*Mannheimia haemolytica, Pasteurella multocida*
  • Primary viral respiratory infection—IBR, BVDV, BRSV
• Neurologic: polioencephalomalacia, *Listeria* meningoencephalitis, hypovitaminosis-A, salt toxicity, lead toxicity, viral encephalomyelitis, rabies, malignant catarrhal fever
• Reproductive
  • Bacterial causes of abortion—*Leptospira* spp., *Listeria monocytogenes, Brucella abortus*
  • Protozoal causes of abortion—*Neospora caninum*
  • Viral causes of abortion—IBR, BVDV
  • Other causes of abortion—mycotic infection, idiopathic, toxicity (plant, nitrate, etc.), trauma

ABBREVIATIONS

BRDC = bovine respiratory disease complex
BRSV = bovine respiratory syncitial virus
BVDV = bovine viral diarrhea virus
CSF = cerebrospinal fluid
IBR = infectious bovine rhinotracheitis (bovine herpesvirus-1)
PCR = polymerase chain reaction
PMNs = polymorphonuclear leukocytes

Suggested Reading
Apley, M. D., Fajt, V. R. 1998. Feedlot therapeutics. *Vet Clin North Am: Food Anim Pract*. 14:291–314.
Guichon, P. T., Jim, G. K., Booker, C. W., Schunicht, O. C. 1996. *Haemophilus somnus*: an important feedlot pathogen. In: *Bovine respiratory disease—sourcebook for the veterinary professional*. Trenton, NJ: Veterinary Learning Systems.
Inzana, T. J. 1999. The *Haemophilus somnus* complex. In: *Current veterinary therapy: food animal practice*, ed. J. L. Howard, R. A. Smith. 4th ed. Philadelphia: W. B. Saunders.
Kwiecien, J. M., Little, P. B. 1991. *Haemophilus somnus* and reproductive disease in the cow: a review. *Can Vet J*. 32:595–601.
Perino, L. J., Hunsaker, B. D. 1997. A review of bovine respiratory disease vaccine field efficacy. *Bovine Pract*. 31(1):59–66.

Author: William R. DuBois

HEARTWATER (COWDRIOSIS)

BASICS

DEFINITION
• A tick-borne rickettsial disease of domestic and wild ruminants is caused by *Erlichia* (formerly *Cowdria*) *ruminantium*. This rickettsial agent is transmitted by ticks of the genus *Amblyomma*, particularly the tropical bont tick (*A. variegatum*).
• The disease is enzootic throughout sub-Saharan Africa, Madagascar, and the Caribbean islands of Guadeloupe, Marie-Galante, and Antigua. The disease is exotic to the United States.
• At least two *Amblyomma* species found in North America are potential vectors and this poses the threat of the disease introduction. Introduction of the vector is also possible through importation of wildlife from endemic areas.
• It is colloquially called "heartwater" due to the common finding of hydropericardium in infected cattle.

SIGNALMENT
• Most domestic ruminants are susceptible.
• Sheep and goats are more susceptible. Among sheep breeds, Persian and Afrikaner are more tolerant than European breeds. Angora goats are highly susceptible.
• *Bos indicus* breeds are more tolerant than *Bos taurus* breeds.
• Among wild ruminants, water buffalo and bison are highly susceptible. Infection has been observed in eland, wildebeest, blesbuck, and Cape buffalo.
• Age resistance, or a reduction in severity of clinical signs after infection, occurs in very young animals (calves <4 weeks of age, lambs and goat kids <1 week), and results in immunity to reinfection with the same strain and a carrier state.

SIGNS
• Incubation period following bite from infected tick is 9–29 days in cattle, 5–35 days in sheep.
• Signs can be peracute, acute (most common), subacute, or subclinical.
• Peracute signs include rapid development of fever, hyperesthesia, lacrimation, convulsions, and sudden death. This form occurs in susceptible breeds introduced into endemic areas and is the rarest form.
• Acute signs include several days of high fever, anorexia, depression, exaggerated gait, excessive blinking, chewing movements, circling, aggression, and most animals die. This is the most common form.
• Subacute form is characterized by mild fever and mild nervous signs and occurs in animals with some natural resistance.
• The subclinical form has been reported in animals with natural resistance including neonates.
• Hydropericardium (hence the name heartwater) and hydrothorax are some of the pathological findings observed on necropsy.

CAUSES
• Cowdriosis is caused by *Ehrlichia* (formerly *Cowdria*) *ruminantium*, a rickettsial agent transmitted by ticks of the genus *Amblyomma*.
• Important tick species that transmit the organism are *A. variegatum, A. habraeum,* and *A. pomposum.*

RISK FACTORS
• Naïve animals introduced to endemic areas are highly susceptible. Introduction of vectors carrying *E. ruminantium* may also result in outbreaks.
• In endemic areas, reduced tick populations may lower herd immunity through less-frequent challenge and thereby put herds at greater risk for an epidemic of illness when tick populations rebound.

• In the United States, Gulf Coast states from Florida to Texas are at risk for introduction of the tropical bont tick, and possibly *E. ruminantium,* from the Caribbean.
• Zebu breeds of cattle appear more resistant to infection than European breeds.
• Animals 3–18 months are most susceptible, while young calves, lambs, and goat kids exhibit age resistance.

DIAGNOSIS

• Cowdriosis should be suspected when an animal is infested with *Amblyomma* ticks and develops fever and nervous signs and dies.
• In fatal cases, presence of characteristic gross lesions and demonstration of *E. ruminantium* colonies using Giemsa stain on endothelial cells of brain smears.

DIFFERENTIAL DIAGNOSIS
• Includes diseases that cause sudden death (peracute form) or cortical signs. These include anthrax, lightning strike, polioencephalomalacia, salt poisoning, lead poisoning, and rabies.
• The acute form may resemble babesiosis, theileriosis, and trypanosomiasis especially in endemic areas.
• Nervous system abnormalities may suggest other diseases such as rabies, hypomagnesemia, nervous ketosis, listeriosis, tetanus, meningitis or encephalitis, or poisoning by some toxins.

CBC/BIOCHEMISTRY/URINALYSIS
N/A

OTHER LABORATORY TESTS
Serologic assays (e.g., ELISA) are available but suffer from cross-reactions with other rickettsiae.

IMAGING
N/A

DIAGNOSTIC PROCEDURES
May be definitively diagnosed by observation of organisms in smears of affected tissue, usually brain.

PATHOLOGIC FINDINGS
• Pathogenesis is the result of damage to vascular endothelium and subsequent increased vascular permeability.
• Gross lesions include hydrothorax, hydropericardium, pulmonary edema, splenomegaly, petechiae, and ecchymoses of mucosa.

TREATMENT
• Tetracyclines are the treatment of choice but must be given early in the course of the disease.
• Chemoprophylaxis with tetracyclines has been suggested in animals introduced to endemic areas.
• Short-acting formulations of oxytetracycline, 10–20-mg/kg body weight, given two times at 24-hour intervals
• Various vaccines are available in endemic areas with varying successes.
• Tick control is essential.
• Exposure of young animals may permit development of resistance.

MEDICATIONS

CONTRAINDICATIONS
Appropriate milk and meat withdrawal times must be followed for all compounds administered to food-producing animals.

MISCELLANEOUS

ASSOCIATED CONDITIONS
N/A

AGE-RELATED FACTORS
Young animals are more resistant to infection.

ZOONOTIC POTENTIAL
N/A

PREGNANCY
N/A

RUMINANT SPECIES AFFECTED
• Sheep and goats are more susceptible. Among sheep breeds, Persian and Afrikaner are more tolerant than European breeds. Angora goats are highly susceptible.
• *Bos indicus* breeds are more tolerant than *Bos taurus* breeds. Among wild ruminants, water buffalo and bison are highly susceptible.

BIOSECURITY
Heartwater is a foreign animal disease in the United States. Contact appropriate animal health officials (e.g., USDA—APHIS Veterinary Services http://www.aphis.usda.gov/vs) for suspected cases.

PRODUCTION MANAGEMENT
N/A

SYNONYMS
Heartwater

SEE ALSO
Anthrax
Babesiosis
Hypomagnesemia
Lead poisoning
Lightning strike
Listeriosis
Nervous ketosis
Polioencephalomalacia
Rabies
Salt poisoning
Theileriosis
Trypanosomiasis

ABBREVIATIONS
APHIS = Animal and Plant Health Inspection Service
CSF = cerebrospinal fluid
ELISA = enzyme-linked immunosorbent assay
i.v. = intravenous
USDA = United States Department of Agriculture

Suggested Reading
Mebus, C. A., Logan, L. L. 1988. Heartwater disease of domestic and wild ruminants. *J Am Vet Med Assoc.* 192:395–98.
Peter, T. F., Burridge, M. J., Mahan, S. M. 2002. *Ehrlichia ruminantium* infection (heartwater) in wild animals. *Trends in Parasitology.* 18:(5) 214–18.
Radostits, O. M., Gay, C. C., Blood, D. C., Hinchcliff, K. W. 2000. *Veterinary medicine.* 9th ed. New York: W. B. Saunders.
Wagner, G. G., Holman, P., Waghela, S. 2002. Babesiosis and heartwater: threats without boundaries. *Vet Clin North Am Food Anim Pract.* 18:417–30.

Authors: Munashe Chigerwe, Curtis L. Fritz, and Anne M. Kjemtrup

HEAT STRESS IN SOUTH AMERICAN CAMELIDS

BASICS

OVERVIEW

DEFINITION
Disease syndrome in South American camelids secondary to exposure to conditions of excessively high ambient temperature or combinations of high ambient temperature and high humidity.

PATHOPHYSIOLOGY
• The preoptic area of the anterior hypothalamus receives and processes information from thermosensors throughout the body.
• Hyperthermia arises from thermoregulatory malfunction. In cases of heat stress, malfunction arises due to an elevated thermal burden that the body is incapable of handling.

SYSTEMS AFFECTED
• Cardiovascular, respiratory, digestive, hemic/lymphatic, hepatobiliary, renal/urologic, reproductive, nervous.
• The extent of body system damage is dependent upon the severity of the exposure.
• Animals that have undergone prolonged severe heat stress may have systemic complications that far outlast the inciting hyperthermic incident.

GENETICS
N/A

INCIDENCE/PREVALENCE
N/A

GEOGRAPHIC DISTRIBUTION
Heat stress can occur in any part of the world where ambient temperature rises above 80° F.

SIGNALMENT
Species
Potentially all camelid species

Breed Predilections
N/A

Mean Age and Range
N/A

Predominant Sex
N/A

SIGNS
Fever, widely fluctuating rectal temperature, tachycardia, tachypnea, anorexia, weakness, sweating, open mouth breathing, cyanosis, droopy lip with froth at commissures, ventral edema, scrotal edema in males, depression, marked weakness, colic, recumbency, DIC, hypovolemic shock, multiorgan failure (kidney, liver)

HISTORICAL FINDINGS
Exposure to high ambient temperature or a combination of high heat and high humidity is required for animals to become heat stressed.

PHYSICAL EXAMINATION FINDINGS
• Physical examination findings vary based on the severity of disease.
• Elevated rectal temperature is typically present. If animals are examined early in the course of disease or at a cooler time of day, rectal temperature may not be excessively high.
• Increased heart and respiratory rates are often present.
• Sweating and open mouth breathing are common as disease progresses. Weakness and incoordination become marked and can progress to recumbency.
• Ventral edema, particularly scrotal edema in males, is common in affected individuals.
• In severely affected animals, petechial and ecchymotic hemorrhages associated with the onset of DIC, uremic smell to the breath and ulcers in the mouth associated with renal failure may also be seen.

CAUSES
Breakdown of thermoregulatory function due to exposure to periods of high heat ± high humidity

RISK FACTORS
Environmental Factors
• Temperature
• Humidity
• Air movement

Animal Factors
• Dehydration
• Exercise
• Heavy, dark fleece
• Obesity
• Pregnancy
• Lactation
• Current or recent illness

Nutritional Factors
• High concentrate diet
• High protein hay
• Selenium deficient diets
• Vitamin and mineral deficient diets
• Salt-deficient diets

Management Factors
• Availability of fresh drinking water
• Availability of shade
• Availability of cooling water
• Presence of fans
• Timing of stressful activity

DIAGNOSIS

DIFFERENTIAL DIAGNOSIS
Differential diagnosis varies depending on observed clinical signs:
• Infectious diseases that generate fever
• Polioencephalomalacia
• Tick paralysis
• Parelaphostrongylosis
• GI causes of colic
• C3 ulcers

• Urethral rupture (animals with severe ventral edema)
• Testicular abscess (males with scrotal swelling)
• Testicular hydrocele (males with scrotal swelling)

CBC/BIOCHEMISTRY/URINALYSIS
• CBC often shows a mature neutrophilia with no left shift, platelet count may decrease with time.
• Biochemistry—abnormalities vary depending on organ systems involved. Increases can be seen in creatinine, urea nitrogen, AST, CK, bilirubin, and SDH. Hypoproteinemia may be present. Electrolytes (Na, and Cl) may be decreased. Whole body potassium is often decreased, but serum levels may be increased in the presence of academia. Metabolic and respiratory acidosis also may be present.
• Urinalysis—initially increased specific gravity that may become isosthenuric if renal failure ensues, tubular casts may be present in individuals with severe disease, positive blood and protein also may be present.

OTHER LABORATORY TESTS
Clotting profiles—clotting times may be increased.

IMAGING
N/A

OTHER DIAGNOSTIC PROCEDURES
CSF—used to rule out other causes of neurologic disease

PATHOLOGIC FINDINGS
Gross Postmortem
• Autolysis beyond what is expected for time of death
• Hemorrhages and other signs consistent with DIC
• Serous atrophy of fat

Histologic Changes
• Renal necrosis
• Hepatic necrosis
• Coagulation necrosis of neurons
• Vascular congestion in the lungs, liver, spleen, and myocardium

TREATMENT

SUPPORTIVE CARE
• Cooling to within a normal rectal temperature—care should be taken as these animals may lack the ability to warm themselves if overcooled. Focus of cooling efforts should be on the ventral body surface because evaporative cooling is best here. Intact fleece will help insulate the animal even when wet, so water must soak through to the skin.
• IV fluids—correction of dehydration, electrolyte disturbances and acidosis. Adult camelids require 30–40 ml/kg/day and crias

require 80–120 ml/kg/day. Camelids are prone to pulmonary edema at rapid infusion rates. Administration rate should not exceed 20 ml/kg/hr.
• Intranasal oxygen therapy if indicated.
• Shearing—if not already shorn will increase area for heat loss.

ACTIVITY
Limit activity as muscle activity increases heat production.

DIET
• High-quality forages should be fed during warmer times of the year. This will decrease the heat increment of digestion.
• It is important to ensure that overfeeding does not occur as it predisposes to obesity and the necessity to process the excess energy at a metabolic level.
• Mineral supplements that contain salt or an additional salt supplement should always be available.

CLIENT EDUCATION
• Clients should be educated on risk factors and prevention techniques as well as early recognition of affected animals.
• Use the comfort index (ambient temperature + % humidity) to anticipate problems.
CI <120—Problems are unlikely.
CI 120–180—Caution. Problems are possible.
CI >180—Danger. Problems are likely, observe animals closely.

MEDICATIONS
DRUGS OF CHOICE
Anti-inflammatory Agents
• Steroids—for shock
  • Dexamethasone—0.1 mg/kg IV
  • Prednisolone sodium succinate—0.5–1.0 mg/kg
• Nonsteroidal anti-inflammatory agents—flunixin meglumine 1.1 mg/kg. NSAIDs should be used cautiously as many heat-stressed animals may have severe renal compromise at presentation.

Antimicrobial Agents—for Prevention of Secondary Infection
• Ceftiofur hydrochloride—1.1–2.2 mg/kg IM or SC q 24 hours. Ceftiofur sodium can be used IV at the same dose.
• Ampicillin trihydrate—10 mg/kg IM q 24 hours. Sodium ampicillin can be used q 8 hours at the same dose.
• Penicillin—22,000 IU/kg IM or SC q 12 hours. Potassium penicillin can be used IV q 6 hours at the same dose.

Antioxidant Agents
• Vitamin E—immediate antioxidant activity: 1 ml/100 lbs SC or IM (300 IU/ml)

• Selenium—antioxidant activity will take 7–10 days for effect:
Bo-Se—1 ml/50 lb
Mu-Se—1 ml/200 lb

CONTRAINDICATIONS
• NSAIDs should be used with caution because severe renal compromise is often present at presentation.
• None of the drugs listed are approved for use in camelids and none have an established withdrawal time.
• Appropriate milk and meat withdrawal times must be followed for all compounds administered to food-producing animals.

PRECAUTIONS
N/A

POSSIBLE INTERACTIONS
N/A

ALTERNATIVE DRUGS

FOLLOW UP
PATIENT MONITORING
• Rectal temperature should be monitored regularly (every 0.5 hours) until stabilized, then several times daily.
• Serum biochemistry should initially be monitored every 1 to 2 days depending on severity of disease to assess progress and provide a basis for alteration in fluid therapy.

PREVENTION/AVOIDANCE
• Shear animals for hot humid months.
• Adequate access to clean drinking water.
• Adequate access to a mineral and salt supplement.
• Provide shade, fans, and other cooling mechanisms for animals during high heat and humidity.
• Observe animals and institute immediate treatment at signs of trouble.

POSSIBLE COMPLICATIONS
• Affected animals are more predisposed in the future.
• Infertility:
Male—excessive heat is spermicidal to primary spermatocytes.
Female—ovarian activity will decrease in times of high heat.
• Pregnancy loss
• Congenital abnormalities in the fetus

EXPECTED COURSE AND PROGNOSIS
• Prognosis varies from good to grave depending on condition at the time of admission.
• Early heat stress with no systemic complications will often resolve with cooling and several days in a cooler environment.
• Individuals with organ failure and other serious manifestations may not survive despite aggressive therapy.

MISCELLANEOUS
ASSOCIATED CONDITIONS
N/A

AGE-RELATED FACTORS
N/A

ZOONOTIC POTENTIAL
N/A

PREGNANCY
• Steroid use during pregnancy may induce abortion.
• Thermal damage to the developing fetus may result in congenital abnormalities, particularly of the CNS.

RUMINANT SPECIES AFFECTED
Potentially all camelid species are affected.

BIOSECURITY
N/A

PRODUCTION MANAGEMENT
N/A

SYNONYMS
N/A

SEE ALSO
Body condition scoring camelids

ABBREVIATIONS
AST = aspartate aminotransferase
CI = comfort index
CK = creatine kinase
CNS = central nervous system
CSF = cerebrospinal fluid
DIC = disseminated intravascular coagulation
GI = gastrointestinal
IM = intramuscular
IV = intravenous
NSAIDs = nonsteroidal anti-inflammatory drugs
SC = subcutaneous
SDH = sorbitol dehydrogenase

Suggested Reading
Evans, C. N. *Veterinary llama field manual.* 2nd ed. Madisonville, KT. Self published by author.
Fowler, M. E. 1994. Hyperthermia in llamas and alpacas. *Vet Clin Food Anim.* 10(2): 309–17.
Fowler, M. E. 1998. *Medicine and surgery of South American camelids.* 2nd ed. Ames: Iowa State University Press.
Middleton, J. R., and Parish, S.M. 1999. Heat stress in a llama (*Lama glama*): a case report and review of the syndrome. *J Camel Practice and Research* 6(2): 265–69.
Strain, M. G., and Strain, S. S. 1998. Handling heat stress syndrome in llamas. *Vet Med.* 83(5): 494–98.

Author: Dusty W. Nagy

HEAT STRESS IN DAIRY CATTLE

 BASICS

OVERVIEW
• The thermoneutral zone for dairy cattle is between 41°F and 77°F.
• When dairy cattle are exposed to ambient temperatures above 77°F or a temperature-humidity index (THI) greater than 72, physiological changes occur that affect milk production, reproduction, and general health.

PATHOPHYSIOLOGY
• Total body heat load is the sum of metabolic heat production and heat from solar radiation.
• Cattle are able to dissipate heat by nonevaporative mechanisms such as conduction, convection, or radiation, or evaporation of water from the skin and respiratory tract.
• If high temperature and humidity prevent the dissipation of heat through either evaporative or nonevaporative mechanisms, the cow's body temperature will rise resulting in:
1. Reduced DMI to lower endogenous heat production with subsequent reduction in milk production of 10%–20% or more.

2. The shift of blood flow from internal organs to the skin surface. Alterations in blood flow to the uterus and ovaries and changes in maternal-fetal hormone levels lead to reduced follicular activity, early embryonic death, and reduced milk yield in the following lactation.
3. Panting and respiratory alkalosis with compensatory output of bicarbonate in urine leading to acidosis and contributing to laminitis, sole ulcers, and white line disease.

SIGNALMENT
Cattle of any age or stage of production; however, high-producing dairy cows will experience heat stress before dry cows or youngstock due to the increase in metabolic heat production associated with high milk production and dry matter intake (DMI).

SIGNS
Individual Cows
• Standing in stall, decrease in activity including activity during estrus
• Will seek shade and wind
• Increased respiratory rate, open-mouth breathing
• Sweating, increased rectal temperature
• Increased saliva production
• Reduced DMI
• Increased water intake

Herd
• Decreased milk production
• Decreased conception rate

CAUSES AND RISK FACTORS
• Climate—air temperature greater than 77°F or high relative humidity combined with high ambient temperature resulting in THI greater than 72
• Inadequate shade structure

 TREATMENT

Modify the Environment
• Shade: Provide 60 sq ft of shade per cow. Provide feed and water in shaded areas.
• Ventilation: Avoid overcrowding. Raise the roof and open the sides of the shade structure. Install a ridge vent. Allow 50 ft between structures.
• Reduce air temperature: In arid environments, the use of evaporative cooling pads and fans, high-pressure foggers, and misters cool air by using energy from the air to evaporate water.
• Cool the cow: Forcing air over a wet hair coat cools the cow by evaporating water from the hair and skin. Sprinkler and fan systems may be used in holding areas and shade structures. Human-made cooling ponds and sprayers have been shown to reduce body temperature.

Modify the Ration
• Forage: Feed high-quality forage with an ADF no less than 18%.
• Protein: Feed a ration of 18% protein (or less) on a DM basis with RDP not to exceed 61% of dietary CP. Excess protein requires energy to excrete; do not feed excess N.
• Energy: Fat can be added to a ration up to 6%–7% on a DM basis.
• Buffer: Sodium bicarbonate may be fed at a rate of 0.75% of DMI.
• Minerals: Increase K to 1.5% DM, Na to 0.45%, and Mg to 0.35% DM for lactating cattle.
• Feeding smaller quantities of feed more frequently at cooler times of the day may help to maintain DMI. Provide a minimum of one watering station per 20 cows and maintain water temperature between 70°F–86°F.

 MISCELLANEOUS

ASSOCIATED CONDITIONS
Panting and respiratory alkalosis with compensatory output of bicarbonate in urine leading to acidosis and contributing to laminitis, sole ulcers and white line disease.

AGE-RELATED FACTORS
N/A

ZOONOTIC POTENTIAL
N/A

PREGNANCY
Alterations in blood flow to the uterus and ovaries and changes in maternal-fetal hormone levels lead to reduced follicular activity, early embryonic death, and reduced milk yield in the following lactation.

RUMINANT SPECIES AFFECTED
Lactating dairy cattle

BIOSECURITY
N/A

PRODUCTION MANAGEMENT
• Modify the environment
• Modify the ration

SYNONYMS
N/A

SEE ALSO
Dairy cattle nutrition
Dairy heifer management
Dairy heifer nutrition

ABBREVIATIONS
ADF = acid detergent fiber
DM = dry matter
DMI = dry matter intake
RDP = rumen degradable protein
THI = temperature-humidity index

Suggested Reading
Jones, G. M., Stallings, C. C. 1999. *Reducing heat stress for dairy cattle*. Dairy Publication 404–200, Virginia Cooperative Extension. Available at: http://www.ext.vt.edu/pubs/dairy/404-200/404-200.html. Accessed August 28, 2004.
Shearer, J. K. 2004. Heat stress in dairy cattle. In: *Bovine medicine*, ed. A. H. Andrews, R. W. Blowey, H. Boyd, R. G. Eddy. 2nd ed. Ames, IA: Blackwell Science.
West, J. W. 2003. Effects of heat-stress on production in dairy cattle. *J Dairy Science* 86:2131–44.

Author: Victoria Olson

HEATH FAMILY: GRAYANOTOXIN

BASICS

OVERVIEW
- Laurels (*Kalmia*), pieris (*Pieris*), and rhododendrons and azaleas (*Rhododendron*) are all members of the Ericaceae (Heath) family.
- Usually an evergreen shrub or small tree, but may be a climber
- Leaves are tough, leathery, glossy, smooth marginated, and alternate.
- Flowers are large and showy in terminal clusters and have five white or colored petals.
- Due to domestication for ornamentation, the geographical distribution is worldwide
- Grow in acidic habitats
- Toxicity occurs with ingestion of 0.15%–0.6% of body weight of the green plant.
- Dried plant is toxic

PATHOPHYSIOLOGY
- Grayanotoxins are principal toxins.
- Andromedotoxin, acetylandromedol, rhodotoxin, and asebotoxin are all names for grayanotoxin I.
- Deacetylanhydroandromedotoxin is grayanotoxin II.
- Deacetylandromedotoxin is grayanotoxin III.
- Grayanotoxin I and III are the most potent with grayanotoxin I being the most common.
- The grayanotoxins increase Na+ permeability resulting in increased resting membrane potentials of heart and nervous tissue although this may not be the mechanism of all clinical signs.
- Pyrethroid intoxication has a similar mechanism of action, but a different site of action on the sodium channels.

- Grayanotoxin has digitalislike cardiac effects, but is structurally different from digitalis.
- Grayanotoxin III prolongs ventricular depolarization.
- Intoxication causes upper GI abnormalities such as, colic, excessive salivation, odontoprisis, vocalization, and projectile vomiting.
- Onset of clinical signs is acute ~ 6 hours.
- First clinical sign is GI related.
- May cause irregular heart rate
- Cardiovascular deficits may cause weakness and depression.

SIGNALMENT
- Seen frequently in camelids and small ruminants
- Any animal ingesting the plant is at risk.

SIGNS
- Colic
- Depression
- Weakness
- Anorexia
- Rumen atony
- Frequent swallowing
- Excessive salivation
- Bloat
- Irregular heart rate; initially bradycardia, then tachycardia
- Dullness
- Dyspnea
- Vomiting, may be projectile
- Nasal discharge
- Frequent defecation
- Ataxia
- Recumbency
- Loss of PLR
- Coma
- Sudden death

CAUSES AND RISK FACTORS
Any ruminant ingesting a plant from the Ericaceae family is at risk.

DIAGNOSIS

DIFFERENTIAL DIAGNOSIS
- Other plant toxicities
- Pyrethroid toxicity

CBC/BIOCHEMISTRY/URINALYSIS
- Hemoconcentration
- Hyperkalemia
- Hyperchloremia
- Prerenal azotemia
- Elevations in glucose

OTHER LABORATORY TESTS
- Hypoxemia
- Acidemia

IMAGING
N/A

DIAGNOSTIC PROCEDURES
- Evidence of leaves in rumen
- Analysis for grayanotoxin in rumen, vomitus, urine, and fecal samples

PATHOLOGIC FINDINGS
- Nonspecific gastrointestinal irritation and hemorrhage
- Liver damage
- Kidney damage
- Evidence of regurgitated ruminal contents in mouth and pharynx
- Aspiration pneumonia
- Sheep may develop a secondary pasteurellosis.

HEATH FAMILY: GRAYANOTOXIN

TREATMENT

- Supportive care
- Rumenotomy to remove plant parts and prevent continuing toxicity

MEDICATIONS

DRUGS OF CHOICE

- Analgesics
- Activated charcoal (AC) (2–5 g/kg PO in a water slurry)
- Evidence in other species of recycling through gastrointestinal system; repeat doses of AC may be beneficial.
- Atropine 1 mg/kg given IV to effect
- Cathartics
- Antibiotics for treatment of aspiration pneumonia

CONTRAINDICATIONS

- Avoid fluids with calcium and potassium.
- Aspiration pneumonia is a possible complication that may be worsened by aspiration of oral administered drugs.
- Drug withdrawal times must be determined and maintained.

FOLLOW-UP

PATIENT MONITORING

- Monitor acid/base.
- Monitor potassium levels.

PREVENTION/AVOIDANCE

- Animals do not normally ingest plants, but will when there is little else to eat.
- Camelid poisoning commonly occurs from tying pack animals within reach of plant.
- Limit exposure to toxic plants.

POSSIBLE COMPLICATIONS

- Aspiration pneumonia
- Ischemia secondary to hypoperfusion
- Respiratory failure

EXPECTED COURSE AND PROGNOSIS

- With supportive care, mortality is low.
- Animals that survive recover completely.
- Aspiration pneumonia may occur and lead to respiratory failure.
- Neurologic abnormalities may lead to respiratory failure.
- Depending on amount ingested, may present as sudden death.

MISCELLANEOUS

ASSOCIATED CONDITIONS

Aspiration pneumonia

AGE-RELATED FACTORS

N/A

ZOONOTIC POTENTIAL

Honey made from bees pollinating plants of the Ericaceae family is the cause of "mad honey disease" in humans.

PREGNANCY

Not likely, although one reported case of fetal mummification after ingestion at 100 days of gestation in a goat.

RUMINANT SPECIES AFFECTED

All species affected

BIOSECURITY

Frequently poisoning is from neighbors/owners feeding hedge clippings.

PRODUCTION MANAGEMENT

N/A

SEE ALSO

Cardiotoxic agents
Colic
Other plant toxicities
Pyrethroid toxicity
Vomiting

ABBREVIATIONS

AC = activated charcoal
GI = gastrointestinal
PLR = consensual pupillary light response

Suggested Reading
Galey, F. D. 2002. Cardiac glycosides. In: *Large animal internal medicine*, ed. B. P. Smith. St. Louis: Mosby.
Puschner, B., Holstege, D. M., Lamberski, N. 2001. Grayanotoxin poisoning in three goats. *JAVMA* 218 (4): 573–75.

Author: Benjamin R. Buchanan

HEAVY METAL TOXICOSIS

 BASICS

OVERVIEW
• Toxicity arising from exposure (mostly by ingestion) to heavy metals.
• The term "heavy metals" has been given a wide range of inconsistent meanings and has not been defined by any authoritative body such as IUPAC.
• Here "heavy metals" describes a group of metals and metalloids (semimetals), specifically arsenic (As), copper (Cu), lead (Pb), molybdenum (Mo), and zinc (Zn), which have been associated with toxicity in ruminants under natural conditions.

PATHOPHYSIOLOGY
• Arsenic (As)—exists in trivalent and pentavalent forms. Trivalent arsenicals bind to sulfhydryl (–SH) groups leading to inactivation of enzymes and enzyme cofactors including those involved in cellular respiration (TCA cycle). They also impair capillary integrity resulting in plasma transudation into the GI tract. Pentavalent arsenicals uncouple oxidative phosphorylation leading to cellular energy deficits.
• Copper (Cu)—acute exposure causes irritation and coagulative necrosis of GI mucosa. Chronic toxicity occurs when the capacity of the liver to regulate Cu (by sequestration and excretion) is exceeded. Excess Cu undergoes redox cycling (Cu$^+$ ⇔ Cu^{++}) and generates reactive oxygen species that cause membrane lipid peroxidation and necrosis of hepatocytes. Cu is then released from necrotic hepatocytes to blood circulation and damages RBC causing intravascular hemolysis and release of hemoglobin. Damage to RBC causes anoxia, more centrilobular hepatic necrosis, and more release of Cu, which accumulates in and damages the kidney. Cu also inactivates proteins and enzymes by binding to –SH groups and may displace other essential trace metals (e.g., Zn) from their proteins.
• Lead (Pb)—binds to –SH groups and inactivates several enzymes including those involved in heme synthesis, impairs nerve and muscle transmission by competing with calcium (Ca), displaces Ca in bone and Ca-binding proteins (e.g., calmodulin), impairs membrane-bound enzymes (e.g., Na$^+$, K$^+$-ATPase) leading to RBC fragility and renal tubular injury, impairs vitamin D metabolism, and interferes with GABA production and activity in the CNS. Pb is also irritating (GI mucous membrane), gametotoxic, teratogenic, and immunosuppressive.

• Molybdenum (Mo)—interferes with Cu metabolism leading to Cu deficiency—Mo and sulfur (S) form insoluble thiomolybdates in the rumen, which bind and reduce absorption of Cu—and stimulate urinary loss of Cu. Some thiomolybdates increase hepatobiliary excretion of Cu, decrease blood Cu availability, and directly inhibit Cu-dependent enzymes. Mo may also alter Zn metabolism and impair myelin maintenance and function leading to enzootic ataxia in lambs.
• Zinc (Zn)—exact pathophysiology of Zn toxicity in ruminants is unknown. However, Zn irritates the GI tract; antagonizes Ca, Cu, and iron (Fe) metabolism; and injures the pancreas and pancreatic ducts.

SYSTEMS AFFECTED
• As—virtually all (GI, renal, hepatic, CNS, respiratory, cardiovascular, etc.)
• Cu—GI, hepatic, renal, hematic, cardiovascular
• Pb—CNS, GI, hematic, skeletal, renal
• Mo—GI, hematic, musculoskeletal, CNS, cardiovascular, dermal
• Zn—hepatic, hematic, renal, pancreas, GI

GENETICS
Compelling scientific evidence supports genetic predisposition of certain breeds of sheep to Cu toxicity (see Breed Predilections below).

INCIDENCE/PREVALENCE
• Incidence of heavy metal toxicosis is to some extent influenced by nutrition and other management factors, age, sex, and breed (see Species and Breed Predilections below for specifics).
• As toxicity is now less frequent because of reduced use of As-containing compounds as pesticides.
• Peak incidence of Cu toxicity occurs in the fall and winter while most cases of Pb toxicity are associated with seeding and harvesting activities.

GEOGRAPHIC DISTRIBUTION
• Heavy metal toxicoses can occur virtually anywhere.
• In the United States, Cu toxicosis is more common in western states.
• Mo is naturally high in soils in some U.S. states (Florida, Oregon, California, Utah, Hawaii, Montana, Colorado, and Nevada) and in several areas of other countries around the world.

SIGNALMENT

Species
• All ruminants are susceptible to heavy metal toxicosis.

• Sheep are very sensitive to Cu, while Pb most commonly poisons cattle.
• Ruminants are more sensitive than nonruminants to Mo.

Breed Predilections
• As, Pb and Zn toxicities have no breed predilections.
• Cu—British breeds of sheep (i.e., Suffolk, Oxford, and Shropshire), Texel sheep, and Jersey cattle are more susceptible.
• Mo—Scottish Blackface and Finnish Landrace sheep are apparently more prone to develop swayback.

Mean Age and Range
Young and old animals are more susceptible to heavy metal toxicosis.

Predominant Sex
N/A

SIGNS
• As—abdominal pain, weakness, staggering, ataxia, watery diarrhea, ruminal atony, weak rapid pulse and shock, oliguria, proteinuria, dehydration, uremia, and acidosis.
• Cu—*acute toxicity*: vomiting, anorexia, hypersalivation, abdominal pain, greenish diarrhea, dehydration, shock, collapse, and death. *Chronic:* sudden onset of hemolytic crisis with weakness, anorexia, thirst, depression, hyperventilation, trembling, anemia, hemoglobinemia, methemoglobinemia, hemoglobinuria (port wine urine), icterus, dyspnea, and death.
• Pb—depression, hyperesthesia, muscle tremors, convulsions, blindness, ataxia, seizures, incoordination, aggression, head pressing, spastic twitching of eyelids, bloat, tenesmus, diarrhea, teeth grinding, jaw champing, and death
• Mo—sudden death, anorexia, severe diarrhea with gas bubbles, emaciation, reduced growth, anemia, lameness, ataxia, swayback in lambs, recumbency, protrusion of nictitating membrane, blindness, achromotrichia (depigmentation of hair/wool), rough hair coat, alopecia, deformity of limbs, muscular degeneration, decreased milk production, and decreased reproductive performance
• Zn—green-colored diarrhea, dehydration, anemia, jaundice, weakness, paresis, anorexia, reduced weight gains, decreased milk yield, subcutaneous edema, polydipsia, polyuria, polyphagia, depression, listlessness, chemosis, exopthalmia, convulsions, and death

CAUSES AND RISK FACTORS
• As—grazing in areas around As mining and smelting sites, exposure to herbicides or old pesticides that have been improperly discarded or stored

- Cu—excessive administration of Cu formulations or ingestion of improperly formulated rations, feeding sheep feeds formulated for other animals, consumption of vegetation or water contaminated with Cu (e.g., near mining/smelting operations or pastures amended with poultry or swine manure), consumption of forage/feeds low in Mo and S and grazing animals in areas containing hepatotoxic plants (e.g., plants containing pyrrolizidine alkaloids). Chronic toxicity is precipitated by stress (e.g., shipping, bad weather, deteriorating plane of nutrition or lactation).
- Pb—consumption of forages contaminated by airborne emissions near Pb smelters or along roadsides, consumption of contaminated water or feed from Pb-lined pipes and drinking/feeding utensils, ingestion of Pb-containing products (automotive batteries, farm machinery grease or oil, paints, putties, and pesticides). In cattle, many cases are associated with seeding and harvesting activities when used oil and batteries are likely to be improperly disposed. Toxicity is exacerbated in animals deficient in Ca, Zn, iron (Fe), and vitamin D. The restricted use of leaded gasoline and oils has significantly reduced environmental contamination of Pb.
- Mo—consumption of contaminated pastures (near mining or metal production plants) or forage grown with heavy application molybdic or phosphate fertilizers and lime. Low dietary Cu and high dietary S exacerbate the toxicity. High soil pH increases Mo absorption and decreases Cu absorption.
- Zn—consumption of improperly formulated diets or zinc-contaminated forage (e.g., near galvanizing factories and mines), access to substances containing Zn, and careless use of Zn sulfate as a prophylactic and treatment of diseases (e.g., ovine foot rot, facial eczema, and lupinosis)

 DIAGNOSIS

DIFFERENTIAL DIAGNOSIS
- As—Pb toxicity, insecticide poisoning, selenium (Se) toxicity, Mo toxicity, Cu toxicity, bovine viral diarrhea
- Cu—infectious gastroenteritis, leptospirosis, arsenic or selenium toxicoses, phenothiazine and other anthelmintic poisonings, bacillary hemoglobinuria, nitrate/nitrite poisoning, postparturient hemoglobinuria, babesiosis, *Corynebacterium renale* infection

- Pb—other diseases with nervous signs including rabies, PEM, TEME, listeriosis, ammoniated feed toxicosis, hepatic encephalopathy, nervous coccidiosis, tetanus, hypovitaminosis A, thiamine deficiency, sodium (Na) ion toxicosis, hypomagnesemic tetany, nervous acetonemia, As poisoning, brain abscess or neoplasia, *Haemophilus* meningoencephalitis.
- Mo—primary Cu deficiency, enzootic ataxia, infectious gastroenteritis, internal parasitisms, leptospirosis, anthelmintic poisoning, As toxicosis, Se toxicosis
- Zn—other causes of diarrhea or anemia, such as acute autoimmune hemolytic anemia

CBC/BIOCHEMISTRY/URINALYSIS
- As—elevated hematocrit, BUN and urine specific gravity, and proteinuria
- Cu—hemoglobinemia, methemoglobinemia, reduced blood glutathione, reduced PCV, increased WBC, AST, LDH, AP, GGT, SDH, and bilirubin
- Pb—microcytic hypochromic to normocytic normochromic anemia, basophilic stippling, high nucleated RBC counts, mature leukocytosis, decreased myeloid/erythroid ratio, increased RBC fragility leading to anisocytosis, polychromasia, echinocytosis, poikilocytosis, and target cells. Also urinary ALA levels are elevated; RBC ALAD and porphyrin levels are reduced and elevated, respectively.
- Mo—microcytic hypochromic anemia, elevated AST, GGT, GDH, CK, SDH, bilirubin, creatinine, and Ca, and increased or decreased BUN (depending on the stage of the toxicosis)
- Zn—anemia, neutrophilia, immature RBCs, uremia, reduced erythrocyte ALAD, elevated blood Na, glucose, LDH, GGT, AP, and SDH

OTHER LABORATORY TESTS
- As—analyze for As concentration in liver, kidney, urine, GI contents, feces, and in suspected feeds.
- Cu—analyze for Cu concentration in serum, liver, kidneys, and in suspected feed.
- Pb—analyze for Pb concentration in whole blood (>0.6 ppm is diagnostic), kidney, and liver as well as urinary ALA.
- Mo—determine Mo concentration in blood, liver, and kidney. Blood levels that result in toxicity depend on dietary intake of Cu and S. Quantify Mo and Cu in feeds and forage.

- Zn—analyze for Zn concentration in serum and tissues (e.g., kidney, liver, pancreas) and urine. Special royal-blue top tubes are recommended for blood collection to avoid contamination.

PATHOLOGIC FINDINGS
- As—abomasum and intestines show redness and congestion of mucosa, submucosal edema, and epithelial necrosis.
- Cu—acute toxicity results in severe gastroenteritis with hemorrhage, edema, erosions, and ulcerations in the abomasum, faint-blue color of GI contents, generalized icterus, and swollen friable livers. In chronic toxicity, livers appear yellowish, swollen, and friable; kidneys are dark-red or bluish-black (gunmetal blue kidneys); and gall bladders are distended with greenish bile. Histopathology reveals centrilobular coagulative necrosis with fibrosis of portal areas and lymphocytic inflammation in liver, proliferation and apoptosis of bile ducts with bile stasis, necrosis of renal tubular and glomerular cells and hemoglobin in renal tubules, brown-black and enlarged spleen with numerous fragmented RBCs, and status spongiosus in the CNS white matter.
- Pb—emaciation, muscle wasting, and degenerative changes in the nervous system and kidney. Histopathology reveals laminar cortical cerebral necrosis, necrosis of renal tubules with high numbers of mitotic figures, and osteoporosis.
- Mo—emaciation, coarse and poorly pigmented hair/wool, osteoporosis and fractures, swollen friable livers, and swollen kidneys with perirenal edema. Histopathology shows hydropic hepatocellular degeneration and periacinar hemorrhagic necrosis, hydropic renal degeneration with tubular necrosis, lysis of cerebral white matter, and demyelination and degeneration of motor tracts in the spinal cord and neurons (in lambs with swayback).
- Zn—poor body condition, abomasitis and duodenitis with greenish mucosa, submucosal edema in the rumen and abomasum, catarrhal enteritis and congestion of small intestines, subcutaneous edema, hydrothorax, hydropericardium, and pancreatic atrophy. Cattle also show pulmonary emphysema, pale flabby myocardium, severe hepatic degeneration, and lesions in the pancreas. Histopathology reveals fibrosing pancreatitis, renal glomerular and tubular lesions, multifocal granulomas in the liver, and proliferation of neck cells of gastric glands.

HEAVY METAL TOXICOSIS

TREATMENT

General Principles
Stabilize the patient, eliminate source of heavy metal, decontaminate (e.g., by physical removal through rumenotomy, washing off topically or by administration of cathartics), administer antidote (chelation therapy), enhance elimination, and provide symptomatic and supportive care.

MEDICATIONS
• As—dimercaprol (BAL) 3 mg/kg IM q8h (before clinical signs) or 6 mg/kg IM q8h (after onset of clinical signs) for 3–5 days; sodium thiosulfate (30–60 g PO q6h for 3–4 days)
• Cu—ammonium molybdate (50–500 mg PO sid per head) and sodium thiosulfate (300–1000 mg PO sid per head) for 3 weeks (an aqueous mixture of the two salts can be sprayed on the feed to reduce labor); three treatments of ammonium tetrathiomolybdate (sheep, 1.7–3.4 mg/head IV or SC) on alternate days; D-penicillamine (52 mg/kg/day PO for 6 days), but it is expensive for treating on a flock basis.
• Pb—diazepam (0.55–1.5 mg/kg IM) for seizures; Ca-EDTA (73.3 mg/kg slow IV, divided sid or tid) for 3–5 days; BAL (3–6 mg/kg IM q8h for 3–5 days). Thiamine 250–1000 mg q12h is a useful adjunct to Ca-EDTA.
• Mo—copper glycinate (60 mg/calf and 120 mg/adult cattle SC); 1000 mg copper sulfate per adult cow; copper sulfate (1–5% depending on Mo levels in the feed) in salt-mineral mix
• Zn—chelation therapy with Ca-EDTA as for Pb and supplementation of ration with Cu.

CONTRAINDICATIONS
• Ca-EDTA and BAL—use with extreme caution and adjust dose in patients with impaired renal function.
• Ca-EDTA and BAL should not be used in patients with anuria and impaired liver function, respectively.
• Exercise extra caution when using Cu compounds in sheep (very sensitive to Cu).
• Appropriate milk and meat withdrawal times must be followed for all compounds administered to food-producing animals.

POSSIBLE INTERACTIONS
• Ca-EDTA—use with caution with nephrotoxic drugs (e.g., aminoglycosides) and glucocorticoids.

• BAL—do not administer with Fe and Se salts (forms toxic complexes).
• Chelation therapy can cause depletion of essential minerals (e.g., Zn and Fe).

FOLLOW-UP

PREVENTION/AVOIDANCE
Prevent access to sources of heavy metals and ensure correct mineral nutrition and proper pasture management.

EXPECTED COURSE AND PROGNOSIS
• Generally favorable in animals with mild to moderate signs provided that the source of the heavy metal can be identified and removed from the animal's environment.
• Guarded to poor in animals with severe signs (e.g., hemolytic crisis, severe CNS signs)

MISCELLANEOUS

ASSOCIATED CONDITIONS
As and Pb toxicities—none; Cu toxicity—Zn deficiency, possibly Mo deficiency; Mo and Zn toxicities—Cu deficiency

ZOONOTIC POTENTIAL
• None. However, organ meat may contain levels of heavy metals that pose a risk to humans (e.g., livers containing >500 mg/kg Cu are considered a risk to public health).
• Lead and Mo are secreted in milk and can present a risk to humans.

PREGNANCY
• Pb crosses placental barrier and is secreted in milk and thus can cause fetal and neonatal poisoning.
• Zn exposure in ewes can cause fetal and/or neonatal Cu deficiency.
• Pregnant ruminants are more susceptible to Zn toxicity.

BIOSECURITY
N/A

PRODUCTION MANAGEMENT
• Nutrition—Ca, Zn, S, Fe, and vitamin D supplementation can reduce incidence of heavy metal toxicity. For example, the maintenance of correct Cu-to-Mo-to-S ratio in feeds is imperative to reduce incidence of Mo toxicity.
• Pasture management—use of some fertilizers may induce mineral imbalances in forage, hepatotoxic plants increase toxicity of Cu, and some plants may reduce bioavailability of essential heavy metals such as Cu.

SYNONYMS
As toxicity—arsenic toxicosis. Other names for As-containing compounds include arsenicals, arsenites, arsenates, arsine. Cu toxicity—enzootic icterus of sheep, copper toxicosis, copper poisoning, copper sulfate poisoning
Pb toxicity—plumbism, saturnism, lead intoxication, lead poisoning, lead toxicosis
Mo toxicity—molybdenosis, molybdenum toxicosis, teart disease, peat scours
Zn toxicity—zinc poisoning, new wire disease (in birds), zincalism (in humans)

SEE ALSO
N/A

ABBREVIATIONS
ALA = δ-aminolevulinic acid
ALAD = δ-aminolevulinic acid dehydratase
AP = alkaline phosphatase
AST = aspartate aminotransferase
BAL = British anti-Lewisite
Bid = twice a day
CK = creatinine kinase
EDTA = ethylenediaminetetraacetic acid
GABA = gamma aminobutyric acid
GDH = glutamate dehydrogenase
GGT = gamma-glutamyl transferase
GI = gastrointestinal
IM = intramuscular
IUPAC = International Union of Pure and Applied Chemistry
LDH = lactate dehydrogenase
Na⁺, K⁺-ATPase = sodium, potassium adenosine triphosphatase (sodium pump)
PCV = packed cell volume
PEM = polioencephalomalacia
PO = per os (by mouth)
q = every
SDH = sorbitol dehydrogenase
Sid = once a day
RBC = red blood cell
TCA = tricarboxylic cycle (Krebs cycle)
TEME = thromboembolic meningoencephalitis
Tid = three times a day
WBC = white blood cell

Suggested Reading
Beasley, V. R., Dorman, D. C., Fikes, J. D., Diana, S. G., Woshner, V. 1999. *A systems affected approach to veterinary toxicology.* Urbana: University of Illinois.
Duffus, J. H. 2001. "Heavy metals"—a meaningless term. *Chemistry International* 23(6).
Plumlee, K. H. 2004. *Clinical veterinary toxicology.* St. Louis: Mosby.

Author: Collins N. Kamunde

HEMORRHAGIC BOWEL SYNDROME

 BASICS

DEFINITION
• Hemorrhagic bowel syndrome (HBS) is a severe, highly fatal disease that presents as acute intestinal dysfunction in dairy cattle characterized by submucosal hemorrhage of the jejunum and often intraluminal blood clots.
• The syndrome can be diagnosed by history, clinical signs, and consistent diagnostic findings, and definitively by exploratory laparotomy or necropsy. Efforts to treat the disease are supportive coupled with surgical intervention.

PATHOPHYSIOLOGY
• The complete etiology and pathogenesis of HBS have not been completely elucidated, however, the consistent identification of *Clostridium perfringens* type A, and its associated alpha and beta 2 toxins provides evidence for their role in the syndrome.
• Dietary factors are also thought to be a contributory factor in the development of HBS.

SYSTEMS AFFECTED
• Gastrointestinal: Findings most frequently include hemorrhagic enteritis, devitalized or ischemic portions of the small intestine, distended loops of bowel, dark red to purple discoloration of the serosa of the bowel, and intraluminal blood clots that are closely adherent to the mucosal surface.
• Cardiovascular: Inflammatory mediators released during necrosis of the small intestine secondarily affect the cardiovascular system. Tachycardia and cool extremities due to decreased peripheral perfusion are the most common findings.

GENETICS
N/A

INCIDENCE/PREVALENCE
Reports of HBS have increased in frequency in the United States. Fifty percent of respondents to a survey of Minnesota dairy farms had reported at least one case of HBS in the previous 12 months. Greater than half of these respondents reported multiple cases. Ninety-four percent of the affected herds contained greater than 50 cows, and 83% of these affected herds were being fed a total mix ration.

GEOGRAPHIC DISTRIBUTION
N/A

SIGNALMENT
Hemorrhagic bowel syndrome is most commonly diagnosed in high-producing, adult, female dairy cattle.

SIGNS

HISTORICAL FINDINGS
Reports suggest cattle consuming a total mixed ration are more likely to be affected. In addition, affected cattle tend to be approximately 3 months postpartum.

PHYSICAL EXAMINATION FINDINGS
Signs include acute anorexia, decreased milk production, scant feces, and abdominal pain. Abdominal distention, tachycardia, bloody stool, cool extremities, and pale mucous membranes are often observed as well.

CAUSES
The specific cause of HBS is undetermined. However, the beta 2 toxin liberated by *Clostridium perfringens* type A has been incriminated in the development of the syndrome.

RISK FACTORS
High-producing dairy cows fed total mix rations high in energy and low in fiber appear to be at greater risk. One study found that larger herds (>50 cows) were more likely to have cases of HBS than smaller herds.

 DIAGNOSIS

DIFFERENTIAL DIAGNOSIS

Intussusception
Intussusception is the most likely rule out in cases of HBS due to similarities in presentation. Cattle with intussusception often have a history of a more prolonged progression of illness and gradual abdominal distention than those with HBS. Cattle with HBS often present with more severe depression and higher heart and respiratory rates than those with intussusception.

Abomasal Lymphosarcoma/Pyloric Outflow Obstruction
Tumors, foreign bodies, or abscesses that obstruct the outflow of the pylorus could present with clinical signs similar to HBS. Occult blood tests may or may not be positive in this instance, depending on the nature of the obstruction. Serum biochemical findings, however, may mimic HBS. Clinicians should look for other signs of enzootic lymphosarcoma. Cattle with pyloric outflow obstruction do not present with acute onset of signs and are not as depressed as those with HBS. In addition, the characteristic "papple"-shaped abdominal contour observed from the rear in cases of pyloric obstruction is not a consistent finding in HBS.

Abomasal Ulcer
Occult blood tests may be positive and the animal may present with some degree of abdominal pain with abomasal ulceration. Ultrasonography is useful to differentiate between HBS and abomasal ulcers; however, exploratory laparotomy may be required to make a definitive diagnosis.

Salmonellosis
The depression, acute onset, anorexia, and passage of blood in the feces associated with salmonellosis can be suggestive of HBS. Leukopenia and the continued passage of stool, albeit abnormal, aids in the differentiation of salmonellosis from HBS.

Mesenteric Root Volvulus/Intestinal Incarceration
Exploratory laparotomy may be the only means to definitively differentiate between these conditions and HBS.

HEMORRHAGIC BOWEL SYNDROME

CBC/BIOCHEMISTRY/URINALYSIS

Complete Blood Count/Fibrinogen
Cattle with HBS frequently have a leukocytosis accompanied by a left shift. Packed cell volume and total protein vary depending on the hydration status of the animal.

Serum Chemistry
• Results of a serum chemical profile reflect the gastrointestinal stasis associated with the disease.
• Findings include a metabolic alkalosis, hypochloremia, hypokalemia, azotemia, hypo- or hypercalcemia, hypo- or hyperphosphatemia, and hyperglycemia. Hyperglycemia is thought to be a result of endogenous release of steroid and epinephrine due to the stress of disease.
• Serum enzymes including creatinine, AST, GGT, and SDH tend to be elevated.

Urinalysis
Ketonuria is a common finding in cows with HBS due to anorexia and potentially negative energy balance.

OTHER LABORATORY TESTS

Fecal Occult Blood
Fecal occult blood tests are positive in cases of HBS due to the submucosal hemorrhage associated with the disease.

Rumen Chloride
Elevation in rumen chloride (>30 mEq/dL) is a consistent finding in HBS due to the tendency for obstruction of the proximal jejunum with clotted blood. However, rumen chloride levels may be within the normal range if complete obstruction of the jejunum does not occur, or if the obstruction is more distal in the jejunum and the test is performed prior to backflow of gastrointestinal content into the rumen.

IMAGING
Ultrasound: Transabdominal ultrasonography in the ventral region of the right paralumbar fossa consistently reveals dilatation of small intestinal bowel loops. Often, homogenous echogenic material consistent with clotted blood is evident within the dilated loops of intestine.

DIAGNOSTIC PROCEDURES

Abdominocentesis
Cytologic examination of abdominal fluid is often unremarkable in cases of HBS; however, this diagnostic tool can be of benefit to rule out other causes of acute gastrointestinal stasis, hemorrhage, and obstruction.

Rectal Exam
Rectal findings may reveal distended bowel loops, however, inability to palpate these does not rule out the disease.

Exploratory Laparotomy
Exploratory right-sided laparotomy, in most cases, should serve as the definitive diagnostic tool.

PATHOLOGIC FINDINGS
• Necropsy findings include segmental necrosis with hemorrhage of the jejunum. Frequently, a large blood clot that may or may not be adhered to the mucosa occludes the lumen of the affected segment of bowel.
• Occasionally, fibrinous peritonitis is discovered in addition to the jejunum lesions.

TREATMENT

APPROPRIATE HEALTH CARE
Hemorrhagic bowel syndrome requires intensive inpatient management coupled with surgical exploration and intervention to identify and remove affected jejunum.

NURSING CARE
Nursing care of HBS cases requires intravenous fluids to correct the electrolyte derangements associated with the disease.

ACTIVITY
Due to the severity of the disease, the activity level of cattle with HBS will be depressed; therefore, altering activity is not a factor in the management of HBS.

DIET
Animals with HBS are anorexic, therefore, the goal of the clinician is to stimulate intake of its normal diet. Rumen transfaunation is often a helpful tool to restore active rumen bacteria and protozoa. The diet of the herd should be examined to ensure adequate fiber content and reduce excessive energy intake.

CLIENT EDUCATION
• Clients should be instructed to examine the ration of the herd to ensure adequate fiber length and content.
• Animals with HBS that recover from the disease should be monitored, and owners should expect continued passage of feces and increases in appetite and milk production as the animal convalesces.

SURGICAL CONSIDERATIONS
• In cases of HBS, a right-sided exploratory laparotomy is indicated not only to arrive at a definitive diagnosis, but also to remove the offending segment(s) of bowel. Intestinal resection of affected areas and anastomosis appear to provide the best postoperative prognosis.
• Enterotomy, with either manual removal of the blood clot or intraluminal lavage, is a reported means of relieving the intestinal obstruction. Manual dissolution of the clot without enterotomy has also been described, but is associated with a poor prognosis.

MEDICATIONS

DRUGS OF CHOICE
• Antibiotics are indicated in cases of HBS due to the assumption that *Clostridium*

perfringens plays a role in the syndrome. Specifically, procaine penicillin G at 40,000 IU/kg once a day IM is active against clostridial species and also serves as supportive therapy postoperatively to guard against the development of peritonitis.
• Currently, FARAD recommends a 45-day slaughter withdrawal on extralabel use of procaine penicillin G and a 96-hour milk withdrawal.

CONTRAINDICATIONS
N/A

PRECAUTIONS
Animals with a history of allergic reaction to penicillin should not be treated with procaine penicillin G.

POSSIBLE INTERACTIONS
N/A

ALTERNATIVE DRUGS
N/A

 FOLLOW-UP

PATIENT MONITORING
• The most important sign indicating successful surgical treatment is the passage of a normal amount of feces within 24 hours postoperatively. However, the consistency of the stool may be abnormal for some time and some blood may pass for an additional 48 hours or so.
• Rumen motility should also be monitored daily and should gradually return to normal function. The heart rate and respiratory rate should be observed every 4 hours until they are within normal limits.
• Rectal temperature should be recorded daily for at least 1 week following recovery in an attempt to detect postoperative peritonitis.

PREVENTION/AVOIDANCE
• Due to the fact that the pathogenesis of HBS is still under investigation, efforts to prevent or reduce the number of cases of HBS are primarily centered on providing immunity to *Clostridium perfringens* type A and carefully monitoring dietary factors.

• Currently, there are no commercially available vaccines that contain *Clostridium perfringens* type A or its beta-2-toxin gene, and vaccines containing *Clostridium perfringens* types C and D are not apparently protective against HBS. However, autogenous vaccines using farm-specific isolates are available from various laboratories and are being used in the herd of origin as a preventative measure.
• Preliminary results suggest these vaccines have some efficacy in the prevention of HBS.
• Diets high in energy and low in fiber have been incriminated as risk factors in the development of HBS. Therefore, dietary adjustments may also benefit herds experiencing cases of HBS.

POSSIBLE COMPLICATIONS
Peritonitis is a potential complication of cattle that recover from HBS. Peritonitis may develop due to rupture or leakage of necrotic bowel or following resection and anastomosis of compromised sections of jejunum. Postoperative ileus of the gastrointestinal tract is also a frequent complication.

EXPECTED COURSE AND PROGNOSIS
• The prognosis for HBS is poor to grave. The more quickly the condition is recognized and subjected to surgical treatment, the better the chances for survival. In addition, more aggressive surgical management (resection and anastomosis) is associated with a better survival rate.
• Often, the progression of the syndrome is so rapid that even the most astute managers fail to appreciate the severity of the disease, and damage to the jejunum is beyond repair or intervention.

 MISCELLANEOUS

ASSOCIATED CONDITIONS
N/A

AGE-RELATED FACTORS
Hemorrhagic bowel syndrome has been reported only in adult cattle.

ZOONOTIC POTENTIAL
N/A

PREGNANCY
Cows with HBS are postpartum.

RUMINANT SPECIES AFFECTED
Bovine

BIOSECURITY
N/A

PRODUCTION MANAGEMENT
If the animal has been on a total mix lactating cow ration, it should be examined to determine if fiber length is adequate.

SYNONYMS
Fatal jejunal hemorrhage syndrome
Hemorrhagic enteritis
Intraluminal-intramural hemorrhage of the small intestine

SEE ALSO
Abomasal ulcer
Intussusception
Lymphosarcoma
Ruminal transfaunation
Salmonella
Volvulus

ABBREVIATIONS
AST = aspartate aminotransferase
Cl = chloride
FARAD = Food Animal Residue Avoidance Databank
GGT = gamma glutamyl-transferase
HBS = hemorrhagic bowel syndrome
SDH = sorbitol dehydrogenase

Suggested Reading
Dennison, A. C., VanMetre, D. C., Callan, R. J., Dinsmore, P., Mason, G. L., Ellis, R. P. 2002. Hemorrhagic bowel syndrome in dairy cattle. *J Am Vet Med Assoc.* 221(5): 686–89.
Godden, S., Frank, R., Ames, T. 2001. Survey of Minnesota dairy veterinarians on the occurrence of and potential risk factors for jejunal hemorrhage syndrome in adult dairy cows. *The Bovine Practitioner* 35(2): 97–103.

Author: Kevin Washburn

HEPATITIS (FUNGAL, TOXIC, AND INFECTIOUS)

BASICS

OVERVIEW
• Many agents can cause diffuse degenerative and inflammatory diseases of the liver in ruminants, categorized under the general term "hepatitis."
• Fungal agents include *Aspergillus* and *Fusarium*. Toxic agents include inorganic and organic poisons and poisonous plants.
• Infectious agents include clostridia and liver flukes.

PATHOPHYSIOLOGY
• Fungal and toxic agents—typically cause centrilobular swelling, decreased hepatic blood flow, lysosomal damage, and decreased mitochondrial function, leading to liver cell death and necrosis. Necrosis leads to decreased gluconeogenesis and eventually to fibrosis.
• Infectious agents—*Clostridium* spp. are normally found in the ruminant gastrointestinal tract, including the liver. Anaerobic conditions (e.g., from migrating liver fluke larvae) can cause clostridia to multiply and release exotoxins, which cause coagulative necrosis in the liver.
• Large numbers of migrating liver flukes may cause enough liver damage to cause an acute hepatic insufficiency, with decreased production of serum proteins causing submandibular edema.

SYSTEMS AFFECTED
Hepatic system

GENETICS
N/A

INCIDENCE/PREVALENCE
N/A

GEOGRAPHIC DISTRIBUTION
Worldwide

SIGNALMENT
Species
All ruminant species

Breed Predilections
N/A

Mean Age and Range
N/A

Predominant Sex
N/A

SIGNS

HISTORICAL FINDINGS
Exposure to fertilizers or presence of poisonous plants on the farm

PHYSICAL EXAMINATION FINDINGS
Icterus (may not be visible even with hyperbilirubinemia in ruminants), hepatic encephalopathy signs (dullness or hyperexcitability, muscle tremors, convulsions, weakness, head pressing), emaciation, edema, diarrhea or constipation, photosensitization, liver enlargement (the liver is normally palpable in ruminants, on the right side behind the costal arch, only if it is enlarged).

CAUSES AND RISK FACTORS
• Causes—fungal causes include toxins from *Aspergillus* and *Fusarium*. Toxic causes include inorganic poisons (i.e., copper, arsenic, phosphorus) and organic poisons (i.e., gossypol, creosol, coal tar).
 • Toxic causes also include poisonous plants (i.e., the weeds senecio and crotalaria), pasture plants (i.e., Alsike clover [Trifolium hybridum], water-damaged alfalfa hay), and trees and shrubs (i.e., lantana).
 • Infectious causes include clostridia, chlamydia, liver flukes, and ascarid infections.
• Risk factors—include inadvertent exposure to toxic causes in the form of fertilizers, cottonseed oil, or industrial waste.

DIAGNOSIS

DIFFERENTIAL DIAGNOSIS
• Encephalomyelitis—liver enzymes normal
• Encephalomalacia—liver enzymes normal
• Cerebral edema—liver enzymes normal

CBC/BIOCHEMISTRY/URINALYSIS
Biochemistry
Liver enzymes, bilirubin, and bile acids. Liver enzymes (e.g., SDH, GGT, Alk phos, AST) are important measures of disease. SDH is liver specific, found in cytoplasm of hepatocytes; short half-life therefore elevated in acute liver disease but may be normal in chronic liver disease.
• GGT, Alk phos, and AST are not liver specific, are membrane bound, are found in liver but also in other tissues like muscle, bone, kidney. Long half-life therefore elevated in chronic liver disease but may be normal in acute liver disease.
• GGT is found mainly in the biliary tract, so it is a good indicator of biliary obstruction.
• Serum bilirubin is not a sensitive indicator of liver function in ruminants, since it is only slightly elevated in liver disease. However, in the absence of hemolytic anemia, a bilirubin level >2 mg/dl (mainly conjugated bilirubin in ruminants) indicates impaired liver function in ruminants.
• Bile acids are a specific liver function test in ruminants. A bile acid concentration >60 micromol/L indicates liver dysfunction in ruminants.

OTHER LABORATORY TESTS
Liver biopsy/histopathology

IMAGING
Ultrasound can visualize the gallbladder and a portion of the liver on the right side of the abdomen, high up and caudal to the last rib and between the ribs.

OTHER DIAGNOSTIC PROCEDURES
N/A

PATHOLOGIC FINDINGS
• Enlarged liver with swollen edges
• In toxic hepatitis, tend to see pronounced generalized lobulation due to engorged centrilobular vessels, icterus, edema, possibly photosensitization
• In infectious hepatitis, tend to see more focal lesions, with necrosis, lobulation, fatty infiltration. In parasitic hepatitis, tend to see focal hemorrhages under the liver capsule, and necrotic tracks.

HEPATITIS (FUNGAL, TOXIC, AND INFECTIOUS)

 TREATMENT

ACTIVITY
N/A

DIET
Ideal diet for animals with hepatitis is low in protein and fat, due to the diminished ability of the liver to detoxify ammonia and other nitrogenous substances, and high in carbohydrates and calcium, but affected animals are usually anorexic.

CLIENT EDUCATION
Applying fertilizers safely and correctly to avoid exposing animals to toxic levels, recognizing and eliminating poisonous plants on pasture, clostridial vaccination, liver fluke control

 MEDICATIONS

• Oral antibiotics to control protein digestion and putrefaction (works better in monogastric animals than in ruminants)
• Supplement feed or inject with multivitamins and minerals.
• Oral or intravenous glucose to maintain blood glucose levels
• Activated charcoal 500 g PO as a laxative if acute intoxication suspected

DRUGS OF CHOICE
Oral neomycin or chlortetracycline

CONTRAINDICATIONS
Appropriate milk and meat withdrawal times must be followed for all compounds administered to food-producing animals.

PRECAUTIONS
N/A

POSSIBLE INTERACTIONS
Oral antibiotics tend to alter rumen microflora, often resulting in indigestion and acidosis.

ALTERNATIVE DRUGS
N/A

 FOLLOW-UP
N/A

PATIENT MONITORING
N/A

PREVENTION/AVOIDANCE
See Client Education above.

POSSIBLE COMPLICATIONS
N/A

EXPECTED COURSE AND PROGNOSIS
Prognosis poor if hepatic fibrosis seen on liver biopsy/histopathology; otherwise prognosis guarded.

 MISCELLANEOUS

ASSOCIATED CONDITIONS
N/A

AGE-RELATED FACTORS
N/A

ZOONOTIC POTENTIAL
N/A

PREGNANCY
Fetus typically will be aborted in cases of severe hepatitis.

RUMINANT SPECIES AFFECTED
All

BIOSECURITY
N/A

PRODUCTION MANAGEMENT
Applying fertilizers safely and correctly to avoid exposing animals to toxic levels, recognizing and eliminating poisonous plants on pasture, clostridial vaccination, liver fluke control

SYNONYMS
N/A

SEE ALSO
Arsenic
Ascarid infection
Aspergillus and *Fusarium*
Cerebral edema
Chlamydia infection
Clostridium infection
Copper
Creosol and coal tar
Encephalomalacia
Encephalomyelitis
Fungal infections
Gossypol
Liver flukes
Phosphorus
Poisonous plants: senecio and crotalaria, Alsike clover (Trifolium hydridum), water-damaged alfalfa hay, lantana
Serology
Transfaunation

ABBREVIATIONS
Alk phos = alkaline phosphatase
AST = aspartate aminotransferase
GGT = gamma glutamyltransferase
PO = per os, by mouth
SDH = sorbitol dehydrogenase

Suggested Reading
Pugh, D.G., ed. 2002. *Sheep and goat medicine*. Philadelphia: W. B. Saunders.
Radostits, O. M., Gay, C. C., Blood, D. C., Hinchcliff, K. W., eds. 2000. *Veterinary medicine*. 9th ed. London: W. B. Saunders.
Smith, B. P., ed. 2002. *Large animal internal medicine*. 3rd ed. St. Louis: Mosby.

Author: David McKenzie

HEREDITARY CHONDRODYSPLASIA: OVINE

BASICS

Ovine hereditary chondrodysplasia (spider lamb syndrome)
• *Heritable* congenital defect that produces multiple, severe skeletal deformities in young lambs. "Spider" relates to severe valgus limb deformities that create a "spider legged" appearance.
• *Genetic defect* disrupts normal ossification processes involving transformation of cartilage to bone.
  • Semilethal— affected lambs seldom survive past 6 months of age.
  • Most common in black-faced breeds of sheep
  • First described in United States in 1980s in popular lines of Suffolk and Hampshire sheep
  • Documented in Suffolk, Hampshire, Shropshire, Oxford, Southdown, and associated crossbred sheep
  • Entered non-black-faced breeds (*ex: Southdown*) through crossbreeding programs
• Prior to availability of DNA testing, *white* and *gray* pedigrees used to define carriers. *Grey* individuals— pedigrees linked to suspected carriers. *White* individuals— pedigrees with no apparent incidence of carriers. Pedigrees often inaccurate— now DNA testing a better option.
• Inheritance pattern—simple autosomal recessive. NN = normal; NS = carrier; SS = clinically affected lamb.

PATHOPHYSIOLOGY

Genetic defect linked to fibroblast growth factor receptor 3 (FGFR3)
• FGFR3 normally down regulates chondrocyte growth in bone development process.
• Homozygous SS disrupts down regulation of process resulting in excessive and disorderly proliferation and transformation of chondrocytes to bone.

SYSTEMS AFFECTED

Musculoskeletal

INCIDENCE/PREVALENCE

United States and Canada (also other countries where carrier sheep have been imported)
• Regions where black-faced breeds are common (Midwest)
• Rare but not uncommon

RISK FACTORS

• Breeds commonly associated with the problem
• Mating carrier sheep—(NN X NN = 100% NN), (NS X NS = 25% SS + 50%NS + 25% NN)

DIAGNOSIS

• DNA isolated from blood or semen can identify NN, NS or SS status
• Clinical signs (suggestive), radiological and necropsy findings (supportive)

• Clinical presentation
  • Two distinct clinical entities can confuse practitioners.
  • *Affected lambs that appear grossly normal at birth.* While subtle deformities are present at birth, typical limb deformities and muscle atrophy associated with SLS may not be readily apparent until the lamb is 4 to 6 weeks old.
  • *Affected lambs with visible deformities at birth.* Severe skeletal deformities obvious at birth, may affect neonatal survival.
• Clinical description of skeletal deformities observed in both groups include
  • Abnormally long, thin-boned legs with a long fine neck (extreme type for breed)
  • Small rounded head (Roman nose) with occasional lateral deviation to the nose
  • Moderate to severe muscle atrophy—progresses with age
  • Scoliosis (usually) and/or kyphosis (less common) of the spine
  • Wide, flattened appearing sternum with small palpable "dimple"
  • Moderate to severe valgus deformities distal to the hock and/or carpus; severity increases with age and growth.

DIFFERENTIAL DIAGNOSIS

• AGH syndrome (arthrogryposis hydranencephaly syndrome) and/or limb deformities
• Cache Valley virus— joints feel "frozen," lack of articulation; die at birth
• Plant toxicities— *Veratrum californicum,* locoweed (*Astragalus or Oxytropis* sp.)

HEREDITARY CHONDRODYSPLASIA: OVINE

DIAGNOSTIC PROCEDURES

• Radiographic findings— abnormal areas of ossification observed throughout skeleton.
  • Live animal or postmortem: flexed lateral of the elbow reveals multiple irregular "islands" of ossification in the olecranon.
  • Postmortem: VD or DV view sternum (disarticulated from ribs) reveals multiple irregular islands of ossification instead of normal symmetrical bipartite pattern.
• Blood or semen can be submitted for DNA testing to confirm genotype.
• Laboratory findings— Nondiagnostic: slightly increased alkaline phosphatase activity associated with bone lesions

GROSS FINDINGS

• *Skull*: rounding of dorsal silhouette (Roman nose appearance) with elongation and erosion of cartilage on the occipital condyles
• *Sternum*: sternebrae irregular shape and size, failure to fuse, malalignment and dorsal deviation of second to sixth sternebrae
• *Vertebrae*: consistent scoliosis, misshapen, excessive amounts and abnormal configuration to vertebral body cartilage
• *Appendicular skeleton*: excessive cartilage in olecranon and scapula, lateral "bowing" of distal radius and ulna, hind limbs usually less severely affected, erosion of articular cartilage in most joints

TREATMENT

None. Euthanasia suggested once diagnosis confirmed

FOLLOW-UP

PREVENTION/AVOIDANCE

Where appropriate, DNA test and utilize only NN rams in the breeding program.

MISCELLANEOUS

ZOONOTIC POTENTIAL

N/A

SYNONYMS

Congenital chondrodysplasia in sheep
Ovine hereditary chondrodysplasia or hereditary chondrodysplasia
SLS
Spider lamb syndrome
Spider leg syndrome
Spider syndrome

SEE ALSO

Cache Valley virus
Euthanasia and disposal
Plant toxicities— *Veratrum californicum,* locoweed *(Astragalus or Oxytropis* sp.)

ABBREVIATIONS

DV = dorsoventral
FGFR3 = fibroblast growth factor receptor 3
SLS = spider lamb syndrome
VD = ventrodorsal

Suggested Reading

Doherty, M. L., Kelley, E. P., Healy, A. M., Callanan, J. J., Crosby, T. F., Skelly, C., Boland, M. P. 2000, Jun 24. Congenital arthrogryposis: an inherited limb deformity in pedigree Suffolk lambs. *Vet Rec.* 146(26): 748–53.
Rook, J. S., Trapp, A. L., Krehbiel, J., et al. 1988. Diagnosis of hereditary chondrodysplasia (spider lamb syndrome) in sheep. *J Am Vet Med Assoc.* 193(6): 713–18.
Whittington, R. J., Glastonbury, J. R., Plant, J. W., Barry, M. R. 1988, Apr. Congenital hydranencephaly and arthrogryposis of Corriedale sheep. *Aust Vet J.* 65(4): 124–27.

Author: Joseph S. Rook

HIGH MOUNTAIN DISEASE

 BASICS

DEFINITION
This disease is right-heart failure secondary to hypoxic pulmonary vasoconstriction associated with living at high altitudes where the oxygen content of the air is lower than at lower altitudes. This is a form of cor pulmonale, which is right-heart failure secondary to pulmonary hypertension due to disease of the pulmonary vasculature.

PATHOPHYSIOLOGY
• Chronic pulmonary hypertension is the primary cause of this condition. In cattle, a hypoxic (high altitude) environment leads to pulmonary vasoconstriction, the severity of which depends on the amount of smooth muscle in the arterial and arteriolar walls.
• Altered myocardial metabolism and chemoreceptor activity may be contributory factors. There also may be phenotypic changes in smooth muscle cells with hypoxic or pressure-induced injury causing the deposition of elastin and collagen in pulmonary vasculature. A pressure overload on the right ventricle results from chronic pulmonary arterial hypertension. Depending on the rapidity of the development of the hypertension, the right ventricle may respond with failure, dilation, or hypertrophy. If acute failure does not occur and the animal remains in a hypoxic environment, the disease is progressive and right-heart failure will result when the right ventricle dilates and is unable to compensate.
• Ingestion of locoweed (*Oxytropis* and *Astragalus* spp.) can worsen the disease due to myocardial damage caused by the plant toxins.
• Other chronic pulmonary diseases, such as lungworm infestation and bronchopneumonia, can lead to cor pulmonale in ruminants by causing pulmonary hypertension, and these conditions can exacerbate the effects of high mountain disease.

SYSTEMS AFFECTED
• Cardiovascular—Right-heart dilation or hypertrophy leads to right-heart failure, which causes increased venous blood pressure due to diminished return of blood through the right heart. The increased pressure causes vascular leakage, which leads to ventral subcutaneous edema, ascites, and pulmonary/pleural effusion.
• Gastrointestinal—Diarrhea is a common finding.
• Hepatobiliary—Hepatic congestion is common because of decreased return of blood to the right heart.
• Musculoskeletal—Affected animals are usually weak and exercise intolerant. This is secondary to heart failure.
• Respiratory—Pneumonia, emphysema, and atelectasis are commonly found in addition to pleural and pulmonary effusion.

GENETICS
The predisposition to this condition appears to be heritable, as calves from affected cows are more likely to have the disease. The mode of inheritance is unknown.

INCIDENCE/PREVALENCE
• The incidence is estimated at 0.5 to 2.0% in cattle pastured at elevations greater than 6000 feet in the western United States and South America.
• The incidence is increased in areas or conditions where locoweed ingestion is a problem. In addition, the incidence can be increased in certain herds if proper selection pressures are not applied because there is a heritable component of the disease.

GEOGRAPHIC DISTRIBUTION
• The disease is most common in the western United States and in South America, although it has been reported in other mountainous regions of the world. It most commonly occurs at altitudes greater than 6000 feet, although similar conditions have been reported at lower elevations.
• Areas where locoweed grows are more likely to have the condition reported.

SIGNALMENT
Species
Cattle are most commonly affected, although the disease has been reported in sheep and deer under extreme stress. Acquired heart failure in small ruminants is most commonly attributed to other sources.

Breed Predilections
None.

Mean Age and Range
The disease is more common in calves than adult cattle, but all ages are affected.

Predominant Sex
None

SIGNS
• The most common primary sign is subcutaneous edema of the brisket, ventral thorax, and sometimes limbs and submandibular region.
• Increased distension and/or pulsation of the jugular vein, dyspnea, tachypnea, cyanosis, weakness, and exercise intolerance are usually evident and usually precede the formation of edema.
• Ascites and diarrhea may be present also.
• Occasionally marked subcutaneous edema does not form and instead the animals become emaciated in conjunction with the presence of the other signs.

HISTORICAL FINDINGS
Affected animal are usually first noted to be depressed or lethargic, followed by the slow onset of the above-mentioned signs. Often a stressor such as movement or extremely cold weather precedes the onset of clinical signs.

PHYSICAL EXAMINATION FINDINGS
1. Ventral subcutaneous edema (thorax, limbs, brisket, and submandibular)
2. Jugular venous distension and/or pulsation
3. Lethargy, exercise intolerance, weakness
4. Tachypnea, dyspnea
5. Heart murmur
6. Diarrhea
7. Ascites
8. Cyanosis

CAUSES
• The cause of this condition is a hypoxic environment. The disease can be exacerbated by concurrent lung disease, severe stress, or locoweed ingestion.
• There is a genetic predilection.

RISK FACTORS
• Living at altitude greater than 6000 feet
• Pulmonary disease
• Stress
• Cold weather
• Availability of locoweed
• Genetic predisposition (the animal's sire or dam was affected)

 DIAGNOSIS

DIFFERENTIAL DIAGNOSIS
• Any other cause of right-heart failure, such as tricuspid insufficiency, cardiac lymphosarcoma, other thoracic neoplasia, bacterial endocarditis, pulmonic stenosis, and dilative cardiomyopathy can be difficult to differentiate.

• Pericarditis, traumatic pericarditis—Heart sounds may be muffled or a "washing machine murmur" may be heard with these conditions. Animals with traumatic reticulopericarditis are likely to be painful (positive grunt test, expiratory grunt, abducted elbows) febrile, and toxemic. Pericardiocentesis or ultrasound may differentiate these conditions.
• Chronic pneumonia—Thoracic auscultation may differentiate, as harsh lung sounds or areas of consolidation may be heard with pneumonia. Transtracheal wash cytology and culture can rule in or out, and a neutrophilia on a CBC rules in an infectious process.
• Parasitic bronchitis—A fecal exam (Baerman sedimentation technique) will rule in or out. Eosinophilia in transtracheal wash cytology is indicative of larval migrans.
• Left-heart failure—This causes weak peripheral pulses, pulmonary edema, and pleural effusion. Pulmonary edema is evidenced by crackles on thoracic auscultation.
• Pleuritis—This is almost always a secondary condition in ruminants. Thoracic auscultation reveals pleural friction rubs and a horizontal fluid line. Ultrasound can be helpful. Evaluation of pleural fluid is diagnostic (total protein greater than 2 g/dl or greater than 10,000 cells/ml is abnormal).

CBC/BIOCHEMISTRY/URINALYSIS
N/A

OTHER LABORATORY TESTS
• Transtracheal wash—Cytology and culture can rule in or out parasitic bronchitis or primary bronchopneumonia.

HIGH MOUNTAIN DISEASE

• Fecal sedimentation can diagnose parasitic bronchitis.
• Cardiac catheterization—With cor pulmonale there are increased pressures in the right ventricle, right atrium, and pulmonary artery. Right-heart failure is indicated by increased right ventricular end diastolic pressure.

IMAGING
Radiology and ultrasound are useful only to rule out other primary lung disease, pleuritis, and pericarditis. An echocardiogram can verify right-heart dysfunction.

OTHER DIAGNOSTIC PROCEDURES
None

PATHOLOGIC FINDINGS
• On necropsy, there are findings indicative of right-heart failure such as ventral subcutaneous edema, ascites, hepatic congestion (nutmeg liver), and myocardial damage (dilation and/or hypertrophy of the right ventricle).
• The lungs may have lesions of bronchitis, pneumonia, emphysema, or bronchiectasis. Lesions of locoweed toxicosis may be present in other organs.

TREATMENT

APPROPRIATE HEALTH CARE
• The disease is reversible if caught early on and the affected animals are treated appropriately.
• Moving affected animals to lower altitudes (less than 5000 feet) and treating any primary or secondary pulmonary disease are most important.

• Animals may be treated on an inpatient or outpatient basis but should be confined in a suitable low-stress environment to minimize the need for exercise.
• If locoweed ingestion is a problem for the herd, it should be moved, or supplemental feed should be provided to minimize ingestion of locoweed.

NURSING CARE
• Oxygen therapy is beneficial if economically feasible as reversal of hypoxia helps relieve the pulmonary hypertension.
• Diuretics are beneficial. Avoid overhydration, stress, and exercise. Large effusions can be removed via paracentesis.
• Digitalis and digoxin can be used if heart failure is present; however, the prognosis is poor once signs of heart failure are present, and there are economic considerations with the use of these drugs.

ACTIVITY
The patient's activity should be restricted as much as possible.

DIET
Avoid locoweed.

CLIENT EDUCATION
• Affected animals that recover should not return to high altitude or be used for breeding.
• Prognosis for recovery of individual animals is good unless heart failure is present.

SURGICAL CONSIDERATIONS
N/A

MEDICATIONS

DRUGS OF CHOICE
• Broad-spectrum antibiotics should be used if pneumonia is present. Examples are florfenicol at 40 mg/kg sub-Q once (slaughter withdrawal 38 days), oxytetracyline at 20 mg/kg IM q 48 hours (200 mg/ml product, cattle dose, or 10 mg/kg IM q 24 hours for sheep and goats).
• Nonsteroidal anti-inflammatory drugs may be beneficial (i.e., flunixin meglumine at 1.1–2.2 mg/kg IV q 24 hours for up to three days; 4-day slaughter withdrawal).
• Diuretics such as furosemide (500 mg once daily for 1–2 days in cattle) may help speed up the resolution of edema but should be avoided in patients with diarrhea or if aspirin is used.
• Digoxin may be used to treat heart failure if economically feasible (0.25 mg/100 lb, the titrate dose to achieve normal atrial rate; cattle dose, no withdrawal time available).
• Drug withdrawal times must be determined and maintained for all treated food-producing animals.

CONTRAINDICATIONS
• Avoid overhydration.
• Do not use diuretics in patients with possible electrolyte or acid/ base disturbances, such as diarrhea, or in patients on aspirin therapy.
• Appropriate milk and meat withdrawal times must be followed for all compounds administered to food-producing animals.

PRECAUTIONS
None

POSSIBLE INTERACTIONS
None

HIGH MOUNTAIN DISEASE

ALTERNATIVE DRUGS
• There are many broad-spectrum antibiotics for treatment of bacterial pneumonia in ruminants.
• Other NSAIDS, such as aspirin, may be used if necessary.

FOLLOW-UP

PATIENT MONITORING
Frequency of monitoring is dependent upon the severity of the patient's condition, but once-daily monitoring of clinical signs should give an indication of the animal's progress.

PREVENTION/AVOIDANCE
• Do not breed recovered animals, as there is a heritable component to this disease. Recovered animals should not be moved back to high altitude.
• Avoidance of primary lung disease such as pneumonia and lungworm infestation (via biosecurity, judicious vaccination, deworming protocols, etc.) can prevent secondary cor pulmonale and decrease the severity of clinical signs in animals that become affected with brisket disease.
• Avoid locoweed ingestion by avoiding locoweed or providing supplemental feed in pastures where locoweed exists. (Locoweed is not a first-choice forage, generally.) Cattle can become addicted to locoweed, however, so if locoweed ingestion becomes a problem, cattle may have to be moved.
• Avoid severe stress, especially during extremely cold weather.

POSSIBLE COMPLICATIONS
Complications that could occur with any serious disease or stressor are likely in affected animals (such as abortion).

EXPECTED COURSE AND PROGNOSIS
Onset of the disease takes 1 to 2 weeks. Prognosis for recovery is good unless heart failure is present. Full recovery may take several days to more than a week.

MISCELLANEOUS

ASSOCIATED CONDITIONS
None

AGE-RELATED FACTORS
The disease is most common in young animals but all ages may be affected.

ZOONOTIC POTENTIAL
None

PREGNANCY
Abortion is possible in pregnant animals due to fetal stress.

RUMINANT SPECIES AFFECTED
Cattle are by far the most susceptible, but the disease has been reported in sheep and deer under extreme stress.

BIOSECURITY
N/A

PRODUCTION MANAGEMENT
See "Avoidance" section above. In addition, measurement of pulmonary arterial pressures may be useful in selection of breeding stock (mean arterial pressure should be less than 35 mm Hg at elevations of 5000 feet or greater).

SYNONYMS
Brisket disease
Brisket edema
Dropsy
High altitude disease
Pulmonary hypertensive heart disease

SEE ALSO
Bacterial endocarditis
Cardiac lymphosarcoma, other thoracic neoplasia
Cor pulmonale
Locoweed toxicosis
Right-heart failure, such as tricuspid insufficiency

ABBREVIATIONS
NSAIDS = nonsteroidal anti-inflammatory drugs
CBC = complete blood count
IM = intramuscular
IV = intravenous

Suggested Reading
Aiello, S. E., ed. 1998. High mountain disease. In: *The Merck veterinary manual*, 8th ed. Whitehouse Station, NJ: Merck & Co., Inc.
Ishmael, W. 1999, Oct. 1. Faint of heart. *Beef,* available at http://beef.mag.com/mag/beef_faint_heart/
McGuirk, S. M., and Reef, V. B. 2002. Brisket disease: Cor pulmonale/pulmonary hypertension. In: *Large animal internal medicine*, B. P. Smith, ed., 3d ed. St. Louis: Mosby.
Pasquini, C., and Pasquini, S. 1996. High mountain disease. In: *Guide to bovine clinics*, 3d ed. Pilot Point, TX: Sudz.

Author: Robert C. Bamberg, IV

HORNER'S SYNDROME

 BASICS

OVERVIEW
Horner's syndrome is a group of clinical signs associated with interruption of ocular sympathetic nerve pathways.

SIGNALMENT
Can occur in any species

SIGNS
• Miosis
• Ptosis
• Enophthalmos
• Protrusion of the third eyelid
• Anisocoria
• Cattle manifest miosis, enophthalmos, and loss of sweat on the ipsilateral side of the muzzle, unlike horses where there is excessive sweating of the face and neck to the level of C2 on the affected side.
• Sheep and goats generally only exhibit mild ptosis.
• Visual deficits do not usually occur.

CAUSES AND RISK FACTORS
• Lesions anywhere along the preganglionic or postganglionic ocular sympathetic nerve fibers result in the characteristic clinical signs known as Horner's syndrome.
  • Preganglionic sympathetic nerve fibers:
    1. Originate from the mesencephalic tectum in the brain stem.
    2. Descend through cervical spinal cord.
    3. At the level of T1–T3 spinal cord segments, they enter the gray matter of the spinal cord.
    4. Exit the ventral spinal nerves and run through the brachial plexus.
    5. Ascend the neck in the vagosympathetic trunk.
    6. Continue to the cranial cervical ganglion under the tympanic bulla where they synapse with postganglionic sympathetic nerve fibers.

• Postganglionic sympathetic nerve fibers:
  1. Pass through the petrous temporal bone area.
  2. Follow the ciliary nerve and innervate the following:
    a. Periorbital smooth muscles that are responsible for pulling the globe toward the surface of the orbit
    b. Eyelid muscles and third eyelid muscles in some species
    c. Dilator muscle of the pupil
    d. Periarteriolar musculature
    e. Sweat glands of the head
    f. Ciliary muscles
• Specific injuries or disease that can result in Horner's syndrome include:
  • Trauma to the neck or avulsive injuries
  • Abscesses in the periorbital, mediastinal, or thoracic region
  • Compressive lesions in the T1 – T3 spinal segments
  • Neoplasms that have been associated with Horner's syndrome include lymphosarcoma, melanoma, squamous cell carcinoma, neurofibroma, and respiratory epithelial carcinoma
  • Esophageal perforation
  • Otitis interna and otitis media
  • Complications associated with surgical ligation of the carotid artery
  • Necrotizing perivascular drug injections
• Transient Horner's syndrome can occur after IV injection of drugs. It has been associated most frequently with xylazine, but can also occur after IV injection of vitamin E/selenium or phenylbutazone.

 DIAGNOSIS

DIFFERENTIAL DIAGNOSIS
• Anisocoria may be caused by ocular diseases such as abnormalities of the iris, cornea, lens, or retina.
• Miosis can be caused by ocular pain especially if uveitis is present.

• Paralysis of the eyelid(s) can be caused by trauma or injury to the palpebral branch of the facial nerve as it crosses the zygomatic arch. This can occur in cattle that struggle in stanchions.
• Facial paralysis can be caused by injury to the buccal branches of the facial nerve on the side of the jaw.

CBC/BIOCHEMISTRY/URINALYSIS
N/A

OTHER LABORATORY TESTS
N/A

IMAGING
• Cervical and/or thoracic radiographs may reveal abnormalities such as vertebral fracture or luxation, abscesses or other space occupying masses, esophageal perforation or other abnormalities that would result in injury to the sympathetic pathway.
• Ultrasound may be useful in identifying retrobulbar masses.

DIAGNOSTIC PROCEDURES
Localizing the site of injury can be attempted using the following methods:
• Evaluate associated clinical signs that may be present such as concurrent neurologic signs that can be localized to particular areas of the CNS.
• Application of epinephrine (0.1 ml of 1:1000 epinephrine) topically to the eye to cause mydriasis
  • Postganglionic lesions demonstrate onset of dilation in < 20 minutes.
  • Preganglionic lesions demonstrate onset of dilation in 30–50 minutes.
• Evaluate response to application of direct-acting vs. indirect-acting agents.
  • Indirect-acting agents (1% hydroxyamphetamine) cause good dilation of a normal eye or one with a preganglionic or a central pathway lesion.
  • Direct-acting agents (1% phenylephrine) cause good dilation of an eye with a postganglionic lesion.

PATHOLOGIC FINDINGS

GROSS FINDINGS
Depend on the underlying cause

HISTOPATHOLOGICAL FINDINGS
No findings are considered specific for Horner's syndrome.

TREATMENT
• Treat the underlying cause of denervation.
• Drain abscesses when possible.
• Lavage perivascular drug injection sites and administer systemic NSAIDs or dexamethasone to prevent tissue necrosis.

MEDICATIONS
Depend on the underlying cause of denervation

CONTRAINDICATIONS
• Appropriate milk and meat withdrawal times must be followed for all compounds administered to food-producing animals.
• Steroids should not be used in pregnant animals.

FOLLOW-UP

PATIENT MONITORING
N/A

PREVENTION/AVOIDANCE
N/A

POSSIBLE COMPLICATIONS
N/A

EXPECTED COURSE AND PROGNOSIS
• Signs are often irreversible even when the underlying cause is successfully treated.
• IV administration of xylazine causes Horner's syndrome but resolves spontaneously; however, necrotizing perivascular injections can result in permanent neurologic deficits if not treated immediately.

MISCELLANEOUS

ASSOCIATED CONDITIONS
Transient Horner's syndrome can occur after IV injection of drugs. It has been most frequently associated with xylazine but also can occur after IV injection of vitamin E/selenium or phenylbutazone.

AGE-RELATED FACTORS
N/A

ZOONOTIC POTENTIAL
N/A

PREGNANCY
N/A

SEE ALSO
Anisocoria
Culling decisions
Facial paralysis
Miosis
Ophthalmic surgery
Paralysis of the eyelid(s)

ABBREVIATIONS
CNS = central nervous system
NSAIDs = nonsteroidal anti-inflammatory drugs

Suggested Reading

Aiello, S. E., ed. 1998. Facial paralysis. In: *Merck veterinary manual*. 8th ed. Whitehouse Station, NJ: Merck & Co.
Guard, C. L., Rebhun, W. C., Perdrizet, J. A. 1984, Oct. Cranial tumors in aged cattle causing Horner's syndrome and exophthalmos. *Cornell Vet.* 74(4):361–65.
Oliver, J. E., Jr., Lorenz, M. D., Kornegay, J. N., ed. 1997. *Handbook of veterinary neurology*. 3rd ed. Philadelphia: W. B. Saunders.
Pace, L. W., Wallace, L., Rosenfeld, C. S., Sansone, J. 1997, Jan. Intracranial squamous cell carcinoma causing Horner's syndrome in a cow. *J Vet Diagn Invest.* 9(1):106–8.
Smith, B. P., ed. 2002. Horner's syndrome. In: *Large animal internal medicine*. 3rd ed. St. Louis: Mosby.

Author: Lisa Nashold

HYPOCALCEMIA: BOVINE

 BASICS

DEFINITION
Hypocalcemia, also known as milk fever and postparturient paresis, is an afebrile disease characterized by acute-to-peracute flaccid paralysis in lactating dairy cows. It occurs most commonly in high producing dairy cows within 72 hours after parturition.

PATHOPHYSIOLOGY
• Muscular contraction is impaired several ways by hypocalcemia: (1) loss of the membrane-stabilizing effect of calcium on peripheral nerves resulting in hyperesthesia and mild tetany, and (2) impaired role of calcium in the release of acetylcholine at the neuromuscular junction resulting in paralysis due to blockade of the transmission of nerve impulses to the muscle fibers.
• Increased disease susceptibility has been observed around the time of parturition. Low extracellular calcium in vitro decreases phagocytosis and intracellular killing by polymorphonuclear neutrophils.

SYSTEMS AFFECTED
Metabolic and musculoskeletal

GENETICS
N/A

INCIDENCE/PREVALENCE
• Postparturient paresis occurs commonly in older dairy cows. The condition is uncommon in second-calf cows and rare in first-calf heifers. The effect of age and parity is likely related to capacity for milk yield and mobilization of calcium.
• The incidence of parturient paresis is 3%–8% of cows, but may be as high as 25%–30% in individual herds. Jersey cattle appear to be the most susceptible breed.

Calcium and Phosphorus Homeostasis
• Circulating concentrations of calcium and phosphorus are precisely regulated by parathyroid hormone (PTH) secreted by the parathyroid glands, calcitonin secreted by the C cells of the thyroid gland, and 1, 25-dihydroxycholecalciferol (1,25-[OH]$_2$D; vitamin D) produced by the kidney. Phosphorus is less strictly controlled than is calcium. Both minerals are absorbed in the small intestine, with phosphorus being absorbed in the proximal small intestine.

• Hypocalcemia stimulates production of PTH, which in turn stimulates synthesis of vitamin D by the kidney. The efficiency of calcium absorption is increased by vitamin D.
• When excess calcium is present, calcitonin inhibits resorption of calcium by the kidney leading to urinary loss.
• Plasma concentrations of calcium and phosphate are maintained during periods of dietary deficiencies. The early lactation period in dairy cattle is characterized by hypocalcemia, which stimulates the synthesis of PTH. The increased concentrations of PTH enhance resorption of calcium from bones and from the renal tubules. Low plasma concentrations of phosphorus trigger production of vitamin D, which in turn increases the uptake of phosphorus.
• With adequate dietary concentrations of phosphorus, active absorption of the mineral becomes saturated, and passive absorption predominates.
• In contrast to most species, ruminants must secrete excess phosphate in the saliva, and to a lesser extent, in the urine. A fraction of phosphate excreted in saliva is resorbed in the small intestine, while the remainder is eliminated from the body in the feces.
• Cows with chronic hypomagnesemia also have profound alterations in calcium homeostasis. Hypomagnesemia prevents production or secretion of both PTH and 1,25-(OH)$_2$.

GEOGRAPHIC DISTRIBUTION
Worldwide, depending on species and environment

SIGNALMENT
Species
Potentially all ruminant species

Breed Predilections
Jersey cattle appear to be the most susceptible breed.

Mean Age and Range
• Postparturient paresis occurs commonly in older dairy cows. The condition is uncommon in second-calf cows and rare in first-calf heifers.
• The effect of age and parity is likely related to capacity for milk yield and mobilization of calcium.

Predominant Sex
Female

SIGNS
HISTORICAL FINDINGS
• Parturient paresis occurs in cows with the combination of hypophosphatemia (~2.1 mg/dl), hypermagnesemia (2.2–2.7 mg/dl), and hyperglycemia (95–130 mg/dl). In contrast to parturient paresis, nonparturient hypocalcemia is often associated with hypomagnesemia and hyperphosphatemia.
• Common clinical pathologic findings in cows with parturient paresis are neutrophilia, lymphopenia, and eosinopenia, along with moderately increased serum concentrations of creatinine phosphokinase.
• There are three discernible stages of milk fever:
  • Stage I is short in duration and animals exhibit hypersensitivity, excitability, and muscle tremors. Head bobbing, ear twitching, and fine tremors over flank will be seen. Affected animals have a reduced appetite and most resist walking. If affected animals are willing to move, they tend to be ataxic and fall easily. Animals will proceed into stage II, if treatment is not instituted.
  • Stage II milk fever is characterized by sternal recumbency and the inability to rise. Many cows appear drowsy with a characteristic kink (S-curve) in their neck. The muzzle is dry, and ears and other extremities are cold with a body temperature of 97°F to 101°F (36.1°C to 38.3°C). Most affected cows have a faint pulse and the heart rate is increased (80/min). Constipation and rumen stasis are common findings in stage two milk fever.
  • Stage III milk fever is characterized by lateral recumbency and progression to a comatose state. Bloat may result due to an inability to eructate gas. Cardiac output decreases, the heart rate may reach 120 beats/min, and the pulse is nearly undetectable. If treatment is not instituted quickly, affected cows will die from cardiac arrest or respiratory failure within a few hours.

CAUSES AND RISK FACTORS
• The increase in milk yield capacity and ability to mobilize calcium stores are likely the reasons why age and parity are associated with an increased incidence of milk fever in older high-producing cows.
• The most consistent abnormality of milk fever is the acute hypocalcemia in which the plasma calcium concentration decreases from approximately 10 mg/dl to 3–7 mg/dl (see Table 1).

Table 1

Blood Serum Analysis of Normal Dairy Cows and Dairy Cows with Milk Fever			
	Mineral (mg/ml)		
Condition	Calcium	Phosphorus	Magnesium
Normal	9.4	4.6	1.7*
Normal at parturition	7.3	3.9	
Milk fever			
Stage I	6.2+/−1.3	2.4+/−1.4	3.2+/−0.7
Stage II	5.5+/−1.3	1.8+/−1.2	3.1+/−0.8
Stage III	4.6+/−1.1	1.6+/−1.0	3.3+/−0.8

Note: Mean+/-standard deviation.

DIAGNOSIS

DIFFERENTIAL DIAGNOSIS
Metritis, mastitis, grass tetany, acute indigestion, traumatic gastritis, coxofemoral luxations, obturator paralysis, lymphosarcoma, spinal compression and fracture of the pelvis, aspiration pneumonia, degenerative myopathy

CBC/BIOCHEMISTRY/URINALYSIS
Common clinical pathologic findings in cows with parturient paresis are neutrophilia, lymphopenia, and eosinopenia, along with moderately increased serum concentrations of creatinine phosphokinase.

OTHER LABORATORY TESTS
Parturient paresis occurs in cows with the combination of hypophosphatemia (~2.1 mg/dl), hypermagnesemia (2.2–2.7 mg/dl), and hyperglycemia (95–130 mg/dl). In contrast to parturient paresis, nonparturient hypocalcemia is often associated with hypomagnesemia and hyperphosphatemia.

IMAGING
N/A

OTHER DIAGNOSTIC PROCEDURES
N/A

TREATMENT

• Treatment efforts are intended for returning serum calcium to within the normal range. The treatment should be administered as soon as possible to avoid muscular and nerve damage.
• Calcium borogluconate is commonly administered IV but can be administered via subcutaneous and IP routes. Subcutaneous administration allows for slow calcium absorption, which may reduce the risk of cardiac arrest. Animals that relapse or fail to respond should be reexamined and treated in 8 to 12 hr.
• Calcium is directly cardiotoxic; any calcium-containing solution should be administered slowly (over about 10 to 20 min) during cardiac auscultation. Administration of calcium should be discontinued if dysrhythmias develop. To eradicate cardiac dysrhythmias associated with administration of calcium, atropine can be given intravenously. The cardioexcitatory consequences of intravenous calcium can be reduced by rapid administration of MgSO₄.

• In the case of mild parturient paresis, oral calcium can be administered. Oral calcium administration will decrease the risk of cardiotoxicity. The best combination of calcium preparation is calcium propionate in a propylene glycol gel. Reaching a 4 g rise of calcium in the blood requires oral administration of about 50 g soluble calcium. Calcium propionate is a better alternative than calcium chloride.
• The administration of calcium chloride has a tendency to cause a slight metabolic acidosis.

Chronic Cases
• For the 15% of parturient paresis cows that do not react to calcium therapy, administer 1α- hydroxycholecalciferol, 1α- (OH)₃, a synthetic analog of vitamin D₃. It should be administered at 1 μg/kg of body weight, half IV and half IM.
• The advantages and disadvantages of vitamin D₃ in treating milk fever have been reported elsewhere.

ACTIVITY
N/A

DIET
• Dietary manipulation of the dry cow ration with the addition of anionic salts has been used routinely to prevent milk fever.
• The acid-base status of a cow dictates the sensitivity of the tissue to PTH stimulation, and metabolic alkalosis is responsible for the blunting of PTH responsiveness.
• Formulation of rations to reduce this metabolic alkalosis and/or induce a compensated metabolic acidosis in prepartum cows is widely used.

CLIENT EDUCATION
• Reduced feed intake before calving, due to palatability of anionic salts, may reduce caloric intake creating problems other than milk fever, such as displaced abomasums.
• Prophylactic use of calcium and vitamin D preparations demands a lot of labor and is costly. Use of vitamin D metabolites to prevent hypocalcemia, may result in postparturient paresis that is more clinically severe than normal postparturient paresis.

HYPOCALCEMIA: BOVINE

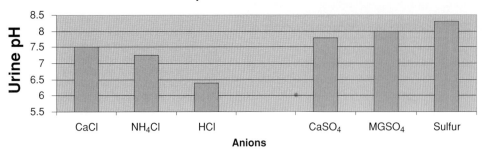

2 Eq of each anionic source fed

Figure 1.

Mean urine pH of Jersey cows fed 2 Eq of anion using hydrochloric acid, ammonium chloride, calcium chloride, calcium sulfate, magnesium sulfate, or elemental sulfur as a source of anions (n = 6). (Adapted from Goff and Horst, 2004).

Control/Prevention

• Dietary manipulation of the dry cow ration with the addition of anionic salts has been used routinely to prevent milk fever. The acid-base status of a cow dictates the sensitivity of the tissue to PTH stimulation, and metabolic alkalosis is responsible for the blunting of PTH responsiveness. Formulation of rations to reduce this metabolic alkalosis and/or induce a compensated metabolic acidosis in the prepartum cows is widely used.

• Feeding of anionic salts in the prepartum dairy ration results in a negative dietary cation-anion difference diet (DCAD), which causes a mild acidosis. This mild acidosis mobilizes calcium and may enhance absorption of Ca from gut.

• Anions are usually added as anionic salts, such as $CaCl_2$ or $MgSO_4$. Urine pH is routinely monitored to assess the degree of metabolic acidification. A urine pH of 8.25 has been proposed as the basis for the screening of milk fever within 48 hr of parturition.

• Prepartum diets supplemented with commercial preparations of HCl mixed into commercial feed appears to lower the urine pH over anionic salts (Figure 1).

DCAD Guidelines

• Dietary cation-anion differences (DCAD: mEq [(NA + K) – (Cl + S)]/100 g.

• Assess the prefresh ration for added cations, such as sodium from sodium bicarbonate.

• Urine pH is a practical indicator of metabolic pH status and reflects the effectiveness of anionic products. Urine pH should be 6.0–6.5 for Holsteins and 5.5–6.0 for Jerseys for optimal effect.

• An incremental introduction of anionic products may reduce palatability problems of supplemental rations.

• Low dietary calcium administration has been considered a method to reduce the incidence of milk fever. The method of low dietary calcium administration, however, has been almost abandoned. It has been difficult to keep calcium administration low with commercially available feeds. The addition of 1 kg/d of zeolite (sodium aluminum zeolite, Dedima 100, Degussa-Huls AG, D-60287, Frankfurt am Main, Germany) to the diet during the last month of pregnancy has been considered as a prevention of postparturient paresis. The zeolite prevented postparturient paresis as well as subclinical hypocalcemia in Jersey cows.

Precautions and Considerations

• The aim of feeding a diet with a DCAD of -10 to -15 mEq/100 g dry matter to dry cows may raise the levels higher than the optimal level required to control or prevent hypocalcemia. This DCAD range may be difficult to achieve when dietary potassium exceeds 1.2% of dietary dry matter.

• Reduced feed intake before calving due to palatability of anionic salts may reduce caloric intake creating problems other than milk fever, such as displaced abomasums.

• Prophylactic use of calcium and vitamin D preparations demands a lot of labor and is costly. Use of vitamin D metabolites to prevent hypocalcemia may result in postparturient paresis that is more clinically severe than normal postparturient paresis. These preparations are best used only in high-risk cases.

 MEDICATIONS

DRUGS OF CHOICE

See Treatment above

CONTRAINDICATIONS

Appropriate milk and meat withdrawal times must be followed for all compounds administered to food-producing animals.

PRECAUTIONS

N/A

POSSIBLE INTERACTIONS

N/A

ALTERNATIVE DRUGS

N/A

 MISCELLANEOUS

ASSOCIATED CONDITIONS

See Calcium and Phosphorus Homeostasis above

AGE-RELATED FACTORS

• Postparturient paresis occurs commonly in older dairy cows. The condition is uncommon in second-calf cows and rare in first calf-heifers.
• The effect of age and parity is likely related to capacity for milk yield and mobilization of calcium.

ZOONOTIC POTENTIAL

N/A

PREGNANCY

See Age-Related Factors and Historical Findings above

RUMINANT SPECIES AFFECTED

All ruminant species are affected.

BIOSECURITY

N/A

PRODUCTION MANAGEMENT

See Diet and Control/Prevention above

SYNONYMS

• Hypocalcemia
• Milk fever
• Postparturient paresis

SEE ALSO

Acute indigestion
Aspiration pneumonia
Coxofemoral luxations
Degenerative myopathy
Grass tetany
Lymphosarcoma
Mastitis
Metritis
Obturator paralysis
Spinal compression and fracture of the pelvis
Traumatic gastritis

ABBREVIATIONS

AP = alkaline phosphatase
BW = body weight
DCAD = dietary cation-anion difference
E2 = estradiol-beta
IM = intramuscular
IP = intraperitoneal
IV = intravenous
PO = per os, by mouth
PTH = parathyroid hormone

Suggested Reading
Ducusin, R. J. T., Uzuka, Y., Satoh, E., Otani, M., Nishimura, M., Tanabe, S., Sarashina, T. 2003. Effects of extracellular Ca^{2+} and intracellular Ca^{2+} concentrations in polymorphonuclear leukocytes of postpartum cows. *Res Vet Sci*. 75:27–32.

Goff, J.P., Horst, R.L. 1998. Use of hydrochloric acid as a source of anions for prevention of milk fever; *J Dairy Sci*. 81(11):2874–2880.
Goff, J. P., Ruiz, R., Horst, R. L. 2004. Relative acidifying activity of anionic salts commonly used to prevent milk fever. *J Dairy Sci*. 87:1245–55.
Horst, R. L., Goff, J. P., Reinhardt, T. A. 2003. Role of vitamin D in calcium homeostasis and its use in prevention of bovine periparturient paresis. *Acta Vet Scand Suppl*. 97:35–50.
Moore, S. J., VandeHaar, M.J., Sharma, B. K., Pilbeam, T. E., Beede, D. K., Bucholtz, H.F., Leisman, J. S., Horst, R. L., Goff, J. P. 2000. Effects of altering dietary cation-anion difference on calcium and energy metabolism in peripartum cow. *J Dairy Sci*. 83:2095–2104.
Seifi, H. A., Mohri, M., Kalamati Zadeh, J. 2004. Use of prepartum urine pH to predict the risk of milk fever in dairy cows. *Vet J*. 167:281–85
Shearer, J. K., Van Horn, H. H. 1992. Metabolic diseases of dairy cattle. In: *Large dairy herd management*, ed. H. H. Van Horn, C. J. Wilcox. Champaign, IL: American Dairy Science Association.

Author: Douglas C. Donovan

HYPOCALCEMIA: SMALL RUMINANT

 BASICS

DEFINITION
• Hypocalcemia in ewes is most common during the last 4 to 6 weeks of gestation. The developing ovine fetus has a relatively high demand for calcium compared to the bovine fetus. However, hypocalcemia may occur during the first 6 weeks of lactation even in the face of relatively low milk yield.
• In dairy goats during lactation, hypocalcemia may occur and can be diagnosed several weeks into lactation.
• Sheep and goats are affected less frequently by hypocalcemia than are dairy cows.
• Plasma calcium tends to be higher during pregnancy and peaks at 5 to 7 weeks prepartum in cervidae. Hypocalcemia can be observed 1–2 weeks postpartum.
• Nonparturient hypocalcemia makes up a higher proportion of cases in small ruminants.
• Clinical signs of hypocalcemia in sheep and goats include hyperesthesia and tetany rather than flaccid paralysis that occurs in dairy cattle.
• Prompt hypocalcemia therapy reduces the incidence of secondary complications (e.g., muscle damage and mastitis).

PATHOPHYSIOLOGY
• Muscular contraction is impaired several ways by hypocalcemia: (1) loss of the membrane-stabilizing effect of calcium on peripheral nerves resulting in hyperesthesia and mild tetany, and (2) impaired role of calcium in the release of acetylcholine at the neuromuscular junction resulting in paralysis due to blockade of the transmission of nerve impulses to the muscle fibers.
• Increased disease susceptibility has been observed around the time of parturition. Low extracellular calcium in vitro decreases phagocytosis and intracellular killing in polymorphonuclear neutrophils.
• In contrast to most species, ruminants must secrete excess phosphate in the saliva and, to a lesser extent, in the urine. A fraction of phosphate excreted in saliva is resorbed in the small intestine while the remainder is eliminated from the body in the feces.

• Sheep with chronic hypomagnesemia also have profound alterations in calcium homeostasis. Hypomagnesemia prevents production or secretion of both PTH and $1,25\text{-}(OH)_2$.
• Physiological hyperparathyroidism in pregnant deer has been observed during the last trimester of pregnancy.
• The hyperparathyroidism of pregnant deer is manifested by increased concentration of alkaline phosphatase (AP), parathyroid hormone (PTH), and estradiol-beta (E2).

SYSTEMS AFFECTED
Production management, metabolic, nutritional, and musculoskeletal

GENETICS
N/A

INCIDENCE/PREVALENCE
• During late gestation, 25% of the sheep flock may have hypocalcemia.
• The incidence of hypocalcemia is increased in does carrying multiple fetuses during late lactation.
• In one study of the hypocalcemic cases that recovered, approximately 25% required more than one treatment. Ewes that developed hypocalcemia before lambing and that recovered, lost 22% of their lambs, the main reason probably being premature birth.

GEOGRAPHIC DISTRIBUTION
Worldwide depending on species and environment

SIGNALMENT
Species
Small ruminant species

Breed Predilections

Mean Age and Range
• The effect of age and parity is likely related to capacity for milk yield and mobilization of calcium.
• In sheep, the tendency to develop hypocalcemia increases with increasing age.

Predominant Sex
Female

SIGNS
Ovine Hypocalcemia
Incidence/Prevalence
During late gestation, 25% of the flock may have hypocalcemia.

Clinical Signs
• Tetany is detected in sheep and goats more often than in cattle where flaccid paralysis is the primary sign of hypocalcemia.
• Hypocalcemia may be difficult to differentiate from pregnancy toxemia, so assessment of urine for ketones may be helpful.
• Transit tetany may occur in pregnant ewes and lambs following the stress of transportation. Lambs will present with muscle tremors and tetany rather than flaccid paralysis.

Treatment
The administration of intravenous calcium solutions (1 g Ca/45 kg of BW) will usually resolve hypocalcemia. However, ewes are more likely to relapse than cows after calcium treatment.

Dietary Prevention
A continuously increasing plane of nutrition during the last 6 weeks of gestation will increase calcium intake and prevent hypocalcemia and pregnancy toxemia in most cases.

Caprine Hypocalcemia
In dairy goats during lactation, hypocalcemia may occur and can be diagnosed several weeks into lactation.

Incidence
The incidence of hypocalcemia is increased in does carrying multiple fetuses during late lactation.

Clinical Signs
Hyperexcitability or mild depression and ataxia are the most common signs of hypocalcemia. Goats do not often exhibit signs of recumbency or coma.

Treatment
The administration of intravenous calcium solutions (1 g Ca/45 kg of BW) will usually resolve hypocalcemia.

Prevention
Limiting calcium intake for 30 days before parturition is helpful in prevention programs. The removal of alfalfa hay from the diet will lower the concentration of calcium in the diet, which may reduce hypocalcemia.

Cervidae Hypocalcemia
• Plasma calcium tends to be higher during pregnancy and peaks at 5 to 7 weeks prepartum in cervidae. Hypocalcemia can be observed 1–2 weeks postpartum.
• Elevated concentrations of plasma calcium and phosphorus are observed during lactation.
• Physiological hyperparathyroidism in pregnant deer has been observed during the last trimester of pregnancy.
• The hyperparathyroidism of pregnant deer is manifested by increased concentration of alkaline phosphatase (AP), parathyroid hormone (PTH), and estradiol-beta (E2).
• An increase in calcium absorption and mobilization during pregnancy may be facilitated by increased AP and PTH.
• Elevated plasma E2 may function to block excessive bone resorption. After parturition, lowered E2 and elevated calcitonin may protect the skeleton against excessive bone resorption.

MEDICATIONS

CONTRAINDICATIONS
• Appropriate milk and meat withdrawal times must be followed for all compounds administered to food-producing animals.
• Steroids should not be used in pregnant animals.

MISCELLANEOUS

ASSOCIATED CONDITIONS
• Subclinical hypocalcemia in ewes is probably a consequence of vaginal prolapse rather than a cause.

• Sheep with chronic hypomagnesemia also have profound alterations in calcium homeostasis. Hypomagnesemia prevents production or secretion of both PTH and 1,25-$(OH)_2$.
• Physiological hyperparathyroidism in pregnant deer has been observed during the last trimester of pregnancy.
• The hyperparathyroidism of pregnant deer is manifested by increased concentration of alkaline phosphatase (AP), parathyroid hormone (PTH), and estradiol-beta (E2).

AGE-RELATED FACTORS
• The effect of age and parity is likely related to capacity for milk yield and mobilization of calcium in heavily lactating dairy goats.
• In sheep, the tendency to develop hypocalcemia increases with increasing age.

ZOONOTIC POTENTIAL
N/A

PREGNANCY
Physiological hyperparathyroidism in pregnant deer has been observed during the last trimester of pregnancy.

RUMINANT SPECIES AFFECTED
All small ruminant species are affected.

BIOSECURITY
N/A

PRODUCTION MANAGEMENT
See Age-Related Factors and Incidence/Prevalence above

SYNONYMS
Hypocalcemia
Milk fever
Postparturient paresis

SEE ALSO
Body condition by species
Cervid reproduction
Ewe flock nutrition
Grass tetany
Mastitis
Sheep and goat nutrition

ABBREVIATIONS
AP = alkaline phosphatase
BW = body weight
E2 = estradiol-beta
PTH = parathyroid hormone

Suggested Reading
Chao, C. C., Brown, R. D., Deftos, L. J. 1985, Jun. Metabolism of calcium and phosphorus during pregnancy and lactation in white-tailed deer. *Acta Endocrinol (Copenh)*. 109(2):269–75.
Cockcroft, P. D., Whiteley, P. 1999, May 8. Hypocalcaemia in 23 ataxic/recumbent ewes: clinical signs and likelihood ratios. *Vet Rec*. 144(19):529–32.
Martens, H., Schweigel, M. 2000, Jul. Pathophysiology of grass tetany and other hypomagnesemias. Implications for clinical management. *Vet Clin North Am Food Anim Pract*. 16(2):339–68.
Nosdol, G., Waage, S. 1981, Jun–Aug. Hypocalcaemia in the ewe. *Nord Vet Med*. 33(6–8):310–26.
Oetzel, G.R. 1988, Jul. Parturient paresis and hypocalcemia in ruminant livestock. *Vet Clin North Am Food Anim Pract*. 4(2):351–64.
Sweeney, H. J., Cuddeford, D. 1987, Jan 31. An outbreak of hypocalcaemia in ewes associated with dietary mismanagement. *Vet Rec*. 120(5):114.

Author: Douglas C. Donovan

HYPODERMATOSIS

 BASICS

DEFINITION
Infestation with and lesions caused by the larvae of two *Hypoderma* species

OVERVIEW

Hypodermatosis in Cattle
• Common parasitic disease of economic importance in cattle; also reported in goats, sheep, horses, and humans
• *Hypoderma* spp. widely distributed in Northern Hemisphere (North America, Europe, Africa, and Asia). Southern limit is reached in Punjab India, Libya, northern Mexico, and Hawaii
• Not reported south of the equator
• *Hypoderma bovis* (northern cattle grub, bomb fly) and *Hypoderma lineatum* (common cattle grub, heel fly) parasitize cattle.
• *H. bovis* occurs in northern United States and Canada. *H. lineatum* occurs in southern, warmer areas of United States.
• Adult are hairy, beelike flies without functional mouth parts so they do not sting or bite host.
• Complete life cycle is about 1 year, but adult flies are short-lived (7–8 days), being active in spring to early summer.
• Female fly can lay as many as 100 eggs on a single host; total egg production is 500 to 800 eggs per female.
• First-stage larval migration through connective tissue initially leads to inflammation and edema; final migration to dorsum of animals results in formation of warbles (nodules with breathing pores containing larvae).
• Cattle may be infected with 1 to 300 warbles.
• Infections are most severe in younger animals.
• Larvae are most pathogenic during two phases of their development: (1) Late autumn and winter when larvae in epidural fat and esophagus: if large numbers present or if animal treated and larva killed in situ, the anaphylactic reaction may cause damage to spinal tissue or difficulty swallowing or eructating. (2) Preemergence phase when damage occurs in subdermal tissue, skin of back, and subsequently hide and carcass
• In species other than cattle, the life cycle of *Hypoderma* spp. is rarely completed; aberrant migration may result in neurologic disorders.

Hypoderma in Goats
Przhevalskiana silenus
• Synonyms: *Hypoderma silenus, H. crossi, P. crossi, P. aegagi*
• Parasitizes goats, sheep, and occasionally horses in Europe, Mediterranean countries, and Asia
• Goats frequently have numerous lesions, sheep often only minor infestation.
• *Przhevalskiana silenus* flies lay eggs on hairs of leg and chest in spring. Larvae migrate directly to dorsum of animal.
  • First-stage larvae reside under cutaneous trunci muscle causing muscle necrosis and neutrophilic infiltration.
  • Larvae migrate through overlying muscle, penetrate skin, and molt to second stage.
  • Wall of granulation tissue forms around larvae and creates nodule.
  • Third-stage larvae drop to ground and pupate.
  • Damages leg and back muscles and hides
• *Hypoderma aeratum* parasitize goats in Cyrus, Crete, and Turkey.
• *H. crossi* infest goats in India.
• *H. lineatum* is not documented to infest goats.
• Sheep also parasitized by *H. aeratum, H. crossi,* and occasionally *H. diana.*
• *H. diana* parasitizes deer.

PATHOPHYSIOLOGY
Life cycles of cattle *Hypoderma* are similar except stages of *H. lineatum* occur 3 to 8 weeks earlier than *H. bovis.*
• Geographic and climatic conditions cause the life cycle of these parasites to vary as to specific time of year for the appearance of various stages.
• In the United States in spring or early summer, adult *H. lineatum* appear 3–4 weeks before *H. bovis.*
• Female *H. lineatum* deposit eggs in linear rows on hairs associated with the heels of forelegs, dewlap, or lower body of cattle.
• Female *H. bovis* deposit eggs singly on hairs of the rump or upper parts of the hind limbs of cattle.
• Tiny first-stage larvae hatch from eggs within 3–7 days, crawl down the hair, penetrate the skin, and migrate through the connective tissue.
• Larvae release enzymes to break down tissue and facilitate movement as they migrate to the host's back. Tissue through which larvae travel becomes greenish-yellow.

• *H. bovis* larvae migrate directly toward the spinal canal.
• *H. lineatum* larvae migrate to the subcutaneous connective tissues along the esophageal wall.
• Larvae remain at these sites for the winter and molt to second stage of development.
• During later winter months (January and February), both species resume migration through the connective tissues to the subdermal tissue of the host's dorsum and cut a breathing hole through the hide.
• Larvae form warbles (swellings) between the layers of the hide and undergo two molts within a cystlike structure in nodules during a 4–6-week period.
• Third-stage larvae (grub) emerge from the breathing pore in the skin, causing a disease called cutaneous myiasis.
• Larvae fall to the ground and burrow into the soil to pupate; metamorphosis from grub to adult fly takes 2 to 8 weeks.
• Adult flies emerge from the pupae and mate soon after. Adults active from late May through August with peak activity during June and July.
• Life cycle takes about a year, 8 to 11 months of which are spent as grubs in the bodies of cattle.
• Healing occurs after emergence of grub but carcass and hide remain damaged.
• Allergic reactions may occur if larvae die naturally or are damaged during attempts to remove them manually.

SIGNALMENT
• Younger animals are most severely affected.
• Older animals develop a degree of immunity to the grub larvae.
• Infections become lighter with age.
• No sex or breed predilection

SIGNS
• Cattle bothered by adult flies during spring and summer demonstrate a behavior called "fly worry" or "gadding."
  • Stampeding behavior
  • Running back and forth with tails in air
  • Stamping feet
  • Decreased feeding and production
  • May inflict self-injury
• Larvae cause irritation, rashes, sores as they penetrate skin.
• Heavy infestations result in poor growth, condition, and production.

- Signs and lesions due to first-stage larvae migration
  - *H. bovis*: fat necrosis, inflammation, and edema of connective tissue around spinal canal, posterior paresis, and/or paralysis, secondary periostitis, osteomyelitis
  - *H. lineatum*: inflammation and edema around esophagus may interfere with swallowing and eructation, weight loss, bloat, and respiratory compromise.
- Signs and lesions due to third-stage larvae
  - Firm to fluctuant, ~ 3 cm, raised nodules (warbles) with breathing pore along dorsum of animal
  - Lesions are painful to touch.
  - Yellowish fluid may exude from breathing pore.
  - Surrounding tissue is necrotic.
  - Secondary infection of cysts and abscess formation
- *Przhevalskiana silenus* flies lay eggs on hairs of leg and chest in spring. Larvae migrate directly to dorsum of animal.
  - First-stage larvae reside under cutaneous trunci muscle causing muscle necrosis and neutrophilic infiltration.
  - Larvae migrate through overlying muscle, penetrate skin, and molt to second stage.
  - Wall of granulation tissue forms around larvae and creates nodule.
  - Third-stage larvae drop to ground and pupate.
  - Cause muscle and hide damage
- Anaphylactic reaction
  - Response to larvae killed in situ in treated animals or crushed during removal from cyst on back
  - Depression, salivation, lacrimation, defecation, edema of head and anus, dyspnea and death

CAUSES AND RISK FACTORS
- Warble flies present in Northern Hemisphere between 25 and 60 degrees latitude in North America, Europe, Africa, and Asia.
- Local climate and geographic factors affect life cycle of *Hypoderma*

DIAGNOSIS
- Season, location, and presence of characteristic lesion
- Cystlike bumps on cattle's backline with visible breathing hole
- Extraction of larvae after enlarging breathing hole
- ELISA test to detect antibody to migrating larvae

DIFFERENTIAL DIAGNOSIS
- Trauma
- Infectious granulomas
- Parafilariasis in cattle
- Epidermoid or dermoid cysts
- Neoplasia
- Other causes of spinal cord disease
- Other causes of esophageal dysfunction and bloat

CBC/BIOCHEMICAL/URINALYSIS
N/A

OTHER LABORATORY TESTING
N/A

IMAGING
N/A

DIAGNOSTIC PROCEDURES
Skin biopsy
- Larvae in a subcutaneous and dermal cyst
- Cyst walls contain dense connective tissue with neutrophilic and eosinophilic infiltrate.
- ±suppurative pyogranulomatous or granulomatous reactions containing eosinophils and larval segments

TREATMENT
- If small number of lesions are present, carefully remove entire grub and cyst manually by aseptically enlarging breathing hole.
- Breaking of cyst or larvae by trauma, squeezing nodule, or manual removal may result in severe systemic reaction.

- Protect ruptured nodular lesions from fly strike and secondary bacterial infections with topical ointments.
- Fly control measures to minimize environmental factors that favor propagation of fly numbers include fly repellents or tags and dust bags
- Systemic insecticides (pour-ons, spot-ons, injectable, drench, boluses, dipping vat, pressure spray, feed additives) for nonlactating cattle; proper timing is essential for safe, effective treatment and control.
  - Ideal time for treatment varies with geographical area, temperatures, and species of *Hypoderma* involved.
  - Treat after adult heel fly activity ceases but before migrating larvae reach the esophagus or spinal cord.
  - In the United States, administer drugs in early autumn (after eggs hatch) to eliminate first-stage larvae during early phase of migration.
  - In the northern United States and Canada, do not treat between November 1 and March 1.
  - Treatment after November 1 may cause severe allergic reactions in animals, resulting in bloat, paralysis, and death.
  - Third-stage larvae are less susceptible to treatment.
  - Further treatment in spring (after March 1)
- Organophosphates
  - Not approved for use in lactating cattle
  - Trichlorphon, crufomate, fenthion, phosmet, bromphos, coumaphos, fenchlorphos
  - Observe dosage recommendations and precautions.
  - Observe withdrawal periods for meat and milk.
- Ivermectin, moxidectin, doramectin (pour-ons, injectables, sustained release bolus); not approved for lactating cattle
- Treatment in goats
  - Ideal treatment time varies with geographical locations.
  - 2% trichorfon backwash
  - Ivermectin

• Topical application of rotenone directly on grub; repeat every 4 weeks as needed—will kill grub but not protect hide from damage
• Ear tags impregnated with organophosphorous compound or synthetic pyrethroid may help reduce egg disposition by adults.
• No approved cattle grub treatment for lactating animals
• Heifers and dry cows may be treated only if the days to freshening exceed that period listed on product label.
• Apply treatments only as recommended for given geographical area and latitude.

MEDICATIONS
N/A

DRUGS OF CHOICE
Ivermectin: cattle
• 200 ug/kg SQ
• Topical 5% solution poured along back at dosage of 500 ug/kg

CONTRAINDICATIONS
• Organophosphate toxicosis
  • Signs: lacrimation, pollakiuria, diarrhea, muscle fasciculations, ptyalism, bloat
  • Antidotal therapy: atropine if needed; caution—may exacerbate bloat
• Anaphylactic reaction if animals treated when grub are in situ or during removal from cyst
  • Anti-inflammatory drugs
  • Antimicrobials
• Death of *H. lineatum* in wall of esophagus or of *H. bovis* in spinal canal
  • Esophagitis, bloat
  • Meningitis, periostitis, osteomyelitis, posterior paresis or paralysis

PRECAUTIONS
• Do not treat cattle with systemic insecticides when larvae are in their overwintering sites as death in situ and subsequent lysis may result in anaphylaxis.
• Do not treat cattle after November 1.
• Before using any pesticide, read label and follow all precautions.
• Appropriate milk and meat withdrawal times must be followed for all compounds administered to food-producing animals.

FOLLOW-UP
• Lesions can persist for up to 12 weeks.
• Recovered cattle have immunity for months.

MISCELLANEOUS

ASSOCIATED CONDITIONS
• Secondary bacterial infections or abscess formation
• Spinal cord inflammation and neurologic signs
• Esophageal dysfunction

ZOONOTIC POTENTIAL
N/A

RUMINANT SPECIES AFFECTED
Cattle, goats, sheep, deer

BIOSECURITY
N/A

PRODUCTION MANAGEMENT
• Confine cattle to barns from May to August; heel flies are unlikely to enter barn to lay their eggs.
• Develop regional, community-based fly control program through treating all nonlactating cattle with systemically active insecticide
• Monitor for grub infection
  • Inspect backs of cattle in March and April for presence of warbles.
  • Most important to examine animals under 5 years of age
  • Calves born after fly season and those kept indoors during summer are unlikely to have cattle grubs.
  • Observe for gadding behavior in cattle during late spring and summer.
  • Examine pastured animals for eggs on hairs of animal's legs, udder, escutcheon, and rump.
• Economic losses due to decreased milk production, loss of body condition, and injury during "gadding" behavior
• Beef cattle infected with grubs do not finish well and sell at lower prices than grub-free cattle.

• Devaluation loss: devalued carcass due to damage to tissue from tunneling of grub larvae
• Trim loss: meat around warbles is discolored and must be discarded
• Hide loss: breathing holes damage valuable portion of hide
• Heavy infestation in replacement cattle can result in poor weight gain, delayed time to first lactation, and long-term production losses.

SYNONYMS
Bomb flies
Cutaneous myiasis
Gad fly
Grubs or cattle grubs
Heel flies
Hypoderma infestation
Warble flies
Warbles
Wolves

SEE ALSO
Epidermoid or dermoid cysts
Infectious granulomas
Neoplasia
Other causes of esophageal dysfunction and bloat
Other causes of spinal cord disease
Parafilariasis in cattle
Trauma

ABBREVIATIONS
ELISA = enzyme-linked immunosorbent assay
SQ = subcutaneous

Suggested Reading
Lloyd, J. E. 1999. Flies, lice and grubs. In: *Current veterinary therapy 4: food animal practice*, ed. J. L. Howard, R. A. Smith. Philadelphia: W. B. Saunders.
Rebhun, W. C. 1995. Skin diseases. In: *Diseases of dairy cattle*. Baltimore: Williams & Wilkins.
Smith, M. C., Sherman, D. M. 1994. *Goat medicine*. Philadelphia: Lea & Febiger.
Taylor, S. M., Andrews, A. H. 1996. Endoparasites and ectoparasites. In: *Bovine medicine; disease and husbandry of cattle*, ed. A. H. Andrews. Oxford: Blackwell Science.
White, S. D. 2002. Diseases of the skin. In: *Large animal internal medicine*, ed. B. P. Smith. 3rd ed. St. Louis: Mosby.

Authors: Susan Semrad and Karen A. Moriello

BASICS

OVERVIEW
• Naturally occurring hypothyroidism is rare in large animals.
• Etiologies in large animals include iodine deficiency and inherited abnormalities.
• Characterized by an array of clinical signs associated with a decrease in thyroid hormone activity
• Goiter is a subacute or chronic disease characterized by thyroid gland enlargement resulting from a deficiency of biologically active iodine
  • Inadequate iodine intake in feedstuffs or water
  • Excessive intake of goitrogenic plants interfering with iodine metabolism
• Deficiency may be an absolute iodine dietary deficiency or from a decrease in iodine absorption from the intestine due to high nitrates or other minerals in diet or water.
• Dietary deficiency results in low plasma iodine concentrates with a subsequent decrease in the normal accumulation and trapping of iodides in the thyroid gland causing suppression of thyroid hormone synthesis (induced-hypothyroidism).
• Low plasma thyroid hormone levels triggers the anterior pituitary to release thyroid-stimulating hormone (TSH), which stimulates thyroid gland activity resulting in follicular hyperplasia and glandular enlargement.
• Geographically, goiter occurs commonly in areas with iodine-deficient soil
  • Western Canada
  • Northeast or northwest (Pacific coast) United States
  • Great Lakes, Great Plains, Rocky Mountains
  • Western states of Latin America, Venezuela, Colombia
  • Himalayas
  • Highland regions of the continents

Hereditary Congenital Goiter
• Inherited congenital goiter with hypothyroidism reported in Merino and Polled Dorset sheep and in Dutch (mixed seaman and dwarf goats), pygmy, Boer, and Nubian goats, and Afrikaner cattle
• Afrikaner cattle
  • Abnormality of the basic RNA
  • May have concurrent inherited grey coat color
• Dutch goats and Merino sheep due to defect in thyroglobulin synthesis
  • Affected Merinos sheep may develop a lustrous, fine, straight, (silky) wool.
  • Lambs have impaired development of wool-producing follicles, thick, scaly skin, sparse wool, goiter, ± respiratory difficulty.

• Autosomal recessive trait in Dutch goats
  • Thyroid weights: affected 15–300 g, unaffected 1–4 g
  • Decreased plasma T_3 and T_4
  • On necropsy, thyroid was hypertrophic and hyperplastic, colloid was almost absent.
  • Signs in kids included sluggishness, poor growth, recurrent bloat, thick and scaly skin, sparse, rough haircoat. If not supplemented with iodine, haircoat disappeared and skin thickened and became scaly
  • Responded to iodide (1 mg per day orally)

Iodine Deficiency (Induced Hypothyroidism)
• Iodine deficiency results in hypothyroidism and goiter.
• Sheep are more susceptible to iodine deficiency than cattle.
• Referred to as "endemic goiter" in goats
• Primary iodine deficiency or goiter is caused by an inadequate dietary intake of iodine, which often reflects low iodine content in soil.
  • Especially affects unborn fetus and neonates
  • Associated with increased calf mortality rates
  • Clinical signs range from dry skin and sparse hair coat in mild cases to diffuse alopecia, myxedema, ± goiter in more severely affected animals.
• Secondary goiter due to decreased uptake of dietary iodine may be due to interference by high calcium, nitrates, goitrogens, or goitrogenic plants in the diet.
• Goitrogens are compounds that interfere with the intestinal uptake of dietary iodine or with its metabolism during thyroxine formation.
• Overall, goitrogens increase the iodine requirement.
• Iodine deficiency is most commonly seen in neonates of dams that consumed goitrogenic plants during gestation.
• Goitrogenic plants disrupt iodine metabolism.
  • Impaired uptake of iodine by thyroid gland by thiocyanates, nitrate type in *Brassicas* or legume crops
  • Impaired iodination of tyrosine residues within the gland by thiouracil in brassica seeds
• Iodine supplementation may overcome deficiency signs from thiocyanate-type goitrogens but can only partially suppress those caused by thiouracil-type goitrogens.

Neonatal Hypothyroidism (Cretinism, Iodine Deficiency)
• Hyperplastic goiter in neonates is the most common thyroid disorder in small ruminants and horses.
• Due to excess consumption of iodine (e.g., kelp-feed supplements) or goitrogenic plants by dam during gestation

• Few "idiopathic" cases reported in western Canada.
• Neonatal hypothyroidism in Angora goats
  • Signs included retarded growth, shortened heads, droopy eyelids, dullness, weight gain, prognathism, bilateral goiter.
  • Probable cause was ingestion of a thiocyanate goitrogen by dams during gestation.
  • Iodine responsive
• In neonatal hypothyroidism, the thyroid glands are abnormal and pituitary gland is normal.
• Inadequate circulating thyroid hormone concentrations result in release of thyroid stimulating hormone (TSH) from the pituitary gland and subsequent thyroid enlargement.
• Goiter is the most consistent, but not always present, clinical sign.
• In sheep, plasma thyroxine of < 20 nmol/l and pasture content of iodine of < 0.09 mg/kg are associated with high incidence of congenital goiter.
• High incidence of neonatal hypothyroid cases reported in western Canada.
• In affected herds or flocks, neonatal mortality rate is greatly increased.
• Animal surviving initial period after birth may recover except for partial persistence of the goiter.

SIGNALMENT
• May occur in all ages, sexes, and breeds
• Most commonly see hypothyroid signs in
  • Fetuses and neonates more than yearlings
  • Young and growing lambs and kids
  • Geriatric animals
  • Heavily producing goats and ewes
• Adult ewes affected more frequently than rams
• Polled Dorset, Dorset horn, and Merino sheep and Boer and Angora goats appear more susceptible to iodine deficiency (induced hypothyroidism).

SIGNS

Signs of Inherited Goiter
• Sheep: high mortality rate, goiter, "silky" appearance to wool, edema, floppiness of ears, enlarged and inwardly bowed carpi, dorsoventral flattening of the nose, dyspnea
• Goats: goiter, growth retardation, sluggishness, rough sparse hair coat that worsens with age, thick scaly skin, respiratory distress
• Afrikaner cattle: high incidence of stillbirths and neonatal deaths, tracheal compression from enlarged gland, ± coat color defect

Neonatal Hypothyroidism
• Thyroid enlargement or goiter
• Late abortion, stillborn, or weakness in newborns
• Dry skin

HYPOTHYROIDISM AND IODINE DEFICIENCY-INDUCED HYPOTHYROIDISM

- Poor quality and sparse wool and hair
- In one outbreak, affected Angora kids showed no hair or skin abnormalities.
- Tendon laxity or failure to form normal bone insertions
- Retarded central nervous system development (hypomyelinization)
- Behavioral abnormalities
- Incoordination
- Poor suckling and right reflexes
- Hypothermia
- Tendon contraction
- Skeletal defects
- Lambs have impaired development of wool-producing follicles, thick, scaly skin, sparse wool, goiter, ± respiratory difficulty.
- Death due to weakness, hypothermia, hypoglycemia

Signs of Iodine Deficiency
- Goiter
- Affected adult goats generally show no skin changes ± dry skin
- Poor wool growth
- Poor quality wool
- Rough and matted fleece
- Weight loss or obesity
- Subcutaneous edema
- Routine activities reduced
- Hypolactia
- Decreased weight gain
- Infertility in both sexes
- Poor libido in male
- Low semen quality
- Irregular estrus
- Abnormal conception rates
- Resorption of embryos; abortion; fetal hydrops
- Prolonged gestation

Goiter May Be Associated With
- Respiratory distress
- "Thyroid thrill" due to increased arterial supply to thyroid gland and heard or felt over jugular furrow
- Pulsation of gland concurrent with arterial pulse
- Edema of the neck

CAUSES AND RISK FACTORS
- Goitrogenic plants: Cruciferae family
  - Brassica spp. contain glucosinolates that are hydrolyzed to thiocyanates and include rape, kale, turnips, Chinese cabbage, cauliflower, broccoli, cole, rutabaga, swede
  - Legume family including white clover (cyanogenic glycosides), subterranean clover, soybeans, and peanuts (thiocyanates)
  - Plant goitrin (in kale), thiourea, and thiouracil interfere with iodination of tyrosine.

- Other goitrogenic plants
  - Prune family (cherries, apricots)
  - Some grains (sorghum, flaxseed, linseed meal, rapeseed meal)
  - Mimosine in Leucaena leucocephala is metabolically broken down into a goitrogen in ruminants.
  - Stargrass (Cynodon nlemfuensis) contains cyanides, act through effects of thiocyanate,
  - Turnipweed, radish
  - Rapeseed oil cake
- High dietary calcium or nitrates
- Selenium deficiency
  - Associated with susceptibility to goiter
  - Essential for deioinase activity during thyroxine metabolism
- Cereal grains and hay are low in iodine.
- Winter or heavy rainfall
- Heavily fertilized pastures
- Bacterial pollution of water or feedstuffs
- Feeding sewage sludge
- Interrelationships that affect iodine metabolism include high arsenic, fluorine, or calcium; deficient or high cobalt, and low manganese concentrations in diet.

DIAGNOSIS
- Diagnosis of iodine deficiency may be difficult.
- History of intake of excess iodine (e.g., kelp, seaweed supplement), low dietary iodine, or goitrogenic plants by dam during gestation
- Clinical signs of hypothyroidism/iodine deficiency
- Aborted fetus, stillborn or dead neonate with appropriate clinical signs/lesions
- Decreased plasma-bound iodine (PBI) concentrations in blood (normal 2.4–14 μg of PBI/dl of plasma)
- Decreased iodine concentration in blood, serum, plasma, milk, urine, and forage content
  - Blood iodine concentrations normally between 5 and 10 μg/dl
  - Serum iodine concentrations normally between 2.1 and 9.3 μg/dl
- Decreased plasma and serum thyroxine concentrations
  - Normal serum thyroxine: Ewes: >60 nmol/l, Lambs: >90 nmol/l
  - Normal serum thyroxine concentrations for goats: 5.0–7.0 μg/dl; 6.1–8.3 μg/dl
  - Normal serum thyroxine concentrations for 2-week to 6-year-old goats: mean 6.53 μg/dl, range 2.0–17.0 μg/dl 5.0–7.0 μg/dl; 6.1–8.3 μg/dl
  - Normal T_3 levels in goats 124–151 ng/dl

- Iodine levels in blood and milk are reliable indicators of thyroxine status of the animal
- In ewe, milk iodine concentration below 8 μg/L is indicative of dietary iodine deficiency.
- Blood thyroxine concentrations affected by level and stage of production. Level may drop as much as 30% in the first week after parturition.
- In ewes, premating and during pregnancy, thyroid hormone concentrations were not reliable indicators of iodine deficiency.
- Urinary iodine concentration is good marker of iodine intake.
- Pasture iodine content is not helpful if problem is due to intake of goitrogenic plants.
- Heterozygous Afrikaner cattle can be identified by blot hybridization analysis.
- Skin biopsy reveals orthokeratotic, hyperkeratosis, follicular keratosis and atrophy, telogenization of hair follicles, sebaceous gland atrophy, and diffuse dermal mucinous degeneration (myxedema)
- Necropsy lesions

Necropsy Lesions
- Gross lesions
  - Adult sheep: Bilateral enlargement of thyroid gland (most cases) with edema in and around thyroid gland
  - Lambs: Enlarged thyroid (up to 10 times or more of normal size) and edema
  - Transudates in body cavities
- Histologic lesions
  - Epidermal atrophy, sebaceous gland hypoplasia, diffuse mucinous degeneration (myxedema)
  - Scarce hair follicles that are hypoplastic,
  - Absence of colloid in follicles
  - Hyperplasia of follicular lining cells, which invaginate into lumen
- Sheep: Thyroid gland–to–body weight ratio of more than 0.46:1 or greater than 0.9 g/kg fresh weight indicates goiter (0.4–0.9 g/kg indicates marginal iodine deprivation)
- Total thyroid gland weight of >2.8 g for congenital goiter in lambs
- Characteristic histologic lesions in thyroid gland of normal or increased weight

DIFFERENTIAL DIAGNOSIS
- Thymic gland enlargement in newborn
- Abscesses
- Wattles cyst
- Cobalt and vitamin B_{12} deficiency
- Causes of infectious abortion
- Hypovitaminosis A

CBC/BIOCHEMISTRY/URINALYSIS
- ± increased plasma protein, serum triglyceride, cholesterol, phospholipid
- CBC and serum chemistry panels are nondiagnostic.

HYPOTHYROIDISM AND IODINE DEFICIENCY-INDUCED HYPOTHYROIDISM

OTHER LABORATORY TESTS
• TSH or TRH response test
• ± increased plasma protein, serum triglyceride, cholesterol, phospholipid
• CBC and serum chemistry panels are nondiagnostic.
• Basal serum levels of T_3 and T_4 are unrealiable for diagnosing hypothyroidism.

DIAGNOSTIC PROCEDURES
Skin biopsy

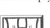

TREATMENT
• Developmental lesions cannot be reversed because thyroid hormone therapy is effective only during period of low plasma concentrations of thyroid hormone.
• Treatment of clinically affected neonates is seldom undertaken due to high case fatality rate.
• Clinical and subclinical effects of simple iodine deficiency may respond to iodine supplementation during pregnancy.
• Iodine supplements are effective against thiocyanate- and nitrate-type goitrogens but not effective against thiouracil-type goitrogens.
• Iodine supplementation
  • Iodized poppyseed oil IM (1 ml per ewe) 7–9 weeks before lambing: may provide iodine for up to 2 years
  • Mineral blocks or loose mineral with iodine
  • Iodized salt containing 0.007% to 0.01% iodine in iodate form (as only salt source)
  • Supplement with organoiodine or periodates
  • Drench in potassium iodine (200–300 mg orally) once in late gestation
  • Lugol's in the drinking water (one drop of Lugol's in 1 gallon of water)
  • 7% iodine applied sparingly one time along the topline (7% iodine may be irritating, avoid sunlight after application)
  • Weekly application of tincture of iodine (1 ml) along back of goats during gestation
  • Weekly application of tincture of iodine (4 ml for cattle, 1–2 ml for sheep) to inside of flank during gestation
  • Monitor for signs of iodine toxicity
• Iodine supplementation for beef cattle
  • Recommended level of supplementation of iodine is 0.5 ppm.
  • ppm iodine supplement is required for diets containing 25% goitrogenic feeds.
  • Sources of supplemental iodine that are highly available to the ruminant but are unstable because of oxidation include calcium iodide, sodium iodide, and potassium iodide.
  • More stable forms of iodine supplement include potassium iodate or pentacalcium orthoperiodate.

• Organic iodide, ethylenediamine dihydroiodine (EDDI) used as feed supplement.
• Current Food and Drug Administration (FDA) regulations set the maximum limit of iodine supplementation at 10 mg/head/day.
• Treatment for affected neonates or young stock
  • Lugol's iodine (3–5 drops) in milk
  • Potassium iodine (20 mg) orally

MEDICATIONS

CONTRAINDICATIONS
Appropriate milk and meat withdrawal times must be followed for all compounds administered to food-producing animals.

PRECAUTIONS
• Potassium iodide is potentially toxic and abortogenic.
• Oversupplementation with iodine may induce iodism.
• Signs of iodism include coughing, seromucoid nasal discharge, excessive lacrimation, and generalized scaling of the skin, partial alopecia, variable appetite, and joint pain.
• Iodine is rapidly metabolized and excreted by the body so removal of supplement generally results in rapid recovery from iodism.

MISCELLANEOUS

ASSOCIATED CONDITIONS
• May be relationship between inherited dwarfism and hypothyroidism
• May be relationship between stillbirth/perinatal weak calf syndrome and hypothyroidism

RUMINANT SPECIES AFFECTED
• Sheep
• Goats
• Cattle

PRODUCTION MANAGEMENT
• Economic losses due to
  • Abortion
  • Increased perinatal mortality
  • Infertility problems
  • Poor growth
  • Poor wool quality
• Maintain adequate amounts of iodine in the diet
  • Lactating cow and dry cow need 0.6 to 0.8–1.0 mg/kg dry weight feed.
  • Nonpregnant cows and calves require 0.1 to 0.3 mg/kg dry weight feed.
  • Sheep need from 0.1 to 0.4 mg iodine/kg dry matter.

• Lactating does require 0.8 mg/kg dry matter.
• Nonlactating goats require 0.2 mg/kg dry matter.
• Cruciferous plants increase ration iodine requirement up ~2 mg/kg.
• Amount of iodine required in diet is effected by many factors
  • Geographic region
  • Weather, rainfall
  • Season
  • Access to goitrogenic plants
  • Degree of pasture fertilization

ZOONOTIC POTENTIAL
N/A

PREGNANCY
N/A

BIOSECURITY
N/A

SYNONYMS

SEE ALSO
Abscesses
Causes of infectious abortion
Cobalt and vitamin B_{12} deficiency
Hypovitaminosis A
Thymic gland enlargement in newborn
Wattles cyst

ABBREVIATIONS
CBC = complete blood count
EDDI = ethylenediamine dihydroiodine
FDA = Food and Drug Administration
IM = intramuscular
PBI = plasma bound iodine
TRH = thyrotropin-releasing hormone
TSH= thyroid-stimulating hormone

Suggested Reading
Dybdal, N. O. 2002. Endocrine and metabolic diseases. In: *Large animal internal medicine*, ed. B. P. Smith. 3rd ed. St. Louis: Mosby.
Pugh, D. G. 2002. *Sheep and goat medicine*. Philadelphia: W. B. Saunders.
Radostits, O. M., et al. 1999. *Veterinary medicine: a textbook of the diseases of cattle, sheep, pigs, goats, and horses*. 9th ed. New York: W. B. Saunders.
Smith, M. C., Sherman, D. M. 1994. *Goat medicine*. Philadelphia: Lea & Febiger.
Suttle, N. F., Jones, D. G. 2000. Micronutrient imbalances. In: *Diseases of sheep*, ed. W. B. Martin, I. D. Aitken. Oxford: Blackwell Science.

Authors: Susan Semrad and Karen A. Moriello

INDIGESTION

BASICS

DEFINITION
• Simple indigestion is a form of gastrointestinal upset causing transient anorexia and minimal symptoms of systemic illness.
• Defined as being a less-severe illness than other forms of rumen indigestion
• Results from an abrupt change in feed

PATHOPHYSIOLOGY
• Animals are exposed to feedstuffs to which they are previously unaccustomed in either type or amount.
• This results in a change in the rumen environment by the presence of unusual substrates.
• The rumen microflora change in population as a result of change in feed substrate.
• Microflora then produce fermentation products that have deleterious effects on rumen motility, digestion, and nutrient absorption.

SYSTEMS AFFECTED
Gastrointestinal

GENETICS
There is not generally thought to be a genetic predilection for simple indigestion.

INCIDENCE/PREVALENCE
Simple indigestion is a common disease of nongrazing animals and is the most common sequela of an abrupt change in ration.

GEOGRAPHIC DISTRIBUTION
Distributed in areas in which conditions or production systems limit grazing

SIGNALMENT
Species
Any ruminant species is susceptible.

Breed Predilections
No breed predilection exists.

Mean Age and Range
• Any age animal is susceptible.
• Primary animals affected are young animals being intensively fed for growth and adult dairy cattle being fed for production.

Predominant Sex
No sex predilection exists

SIGNS

GENERAL COMMENTS
• Signs are generally less severe and more transient than other rumen indigestion disorders.
• May present as an individual animal or herd problem
• Due to adaptability of rumen flora, different animals may respond variably to management changes.

HISTORICAL FINDINGS
• Acute onset
• Anorexia of 1–2 days duration
• Decrease in milk production
• Malodorous diarrhea 12–24 hours after onset

PHYSICAL EXAMINATION FINDINGS
• General lack of evidence of significant systemic illness
• Rumen motility reduced, but often present
• Rumen fill is nearly normal, but contents are fluid.
• Bloat is mild, if present.
• Malodorous diarrhea may be noted.

CAUSES
• Abrupt change in feed type or amount
  • Rumen microflora are exposed to substrates to which they are not accustomed or in greater quantities than that to which they are acclimated.
  • Production of inhibitory substances directly from feed presence or as a result of fermentation and its products
• Implicated feeds
  • Moldy, overheated feed
  • Frosted forages
  • Incompletely fermented, spoiled, sour silage
  • High-quality feeds fed at a suddenly high rate or a change in one or more components

RISK FACTORS
• Lack or complete absence of grazing time
• Provision of large amounts or accidental exposure to novel feeds

DIAGNOSIS

DIFFERENTIAL DIAGNOSIS
• Traumatic reticuloperitonitis
• Left displaced abomasum
• Ketosis
• Lactic acidosis
• Rumen alkalosis
• Rumen putrefaction
• Vagal indigestion
• Peritonitis
• Any systemic illness early in development causing anorexia

CBC/BIOCHEMISTRY/URINALYSIS
May indicate mild dehydration: Elevations in total serum protein, hematocrit, BUN, and creatinine

OTHER LABORATORY TESTS
Rumen fluid analysis
• Microflora inactive under light microscopy
• Rumen fluid pH may be slightly acid or alkaline, depending on nature of offending feedstuff

IMAGING
Not required to diagnose simple indigestion, but survey radiography may be useful in diagnosing traumatic reticuloperitonitis

DIAGNOSTIC PROCEDURES
Diagnosis generally based on physical examination excluding more-severe sources of indigestion

GROSS FINDINGS
Uncomplicated cases of simple indigestion are transient and rarely result in death.

HISTOPATHOLOGICAL FINDINGS
N/A

TREATMENT

APPROPRIATE HEALTH CARE
• Patients with simple indigestion may be treated as outpatients.
• Valuable animals may warrant hospitalization for monitoring of their condition for timely improvement and intervention should their condition worsen.
• Remainder of herd should be closely monitored by producer for further incidence.
• Treatment of affected animals
  • Transfaunation of 8–16 L of healthy rumen fluid : may be obtained from healthy donor or from slaughter house
  • Provide good quality grass hay or straw
  • If rumen pH alterations confirmed:
    • Acidosis: magnesium hydroxide or magnesium oxide (450 g per adult cow) PO
    • Alkalosis: Acetic acid (4–10 L) PO

NURSING CARE
Oral or parenteral polyionic fluid therapy may be indicated depending on severity of dehydration or electrolyte imbalances.

ACTIVITY
Activity may be limited in order to allow close monitoring of the animal's condition.

DIET
• Offending feedstuffs should be removed from the affected animals and the herd.
• Animals should be provided unlimited access to good quality grass hay or straw.
• Unless the offending feedstuff is inherently damaged (i.e., moldy, spoiled, contaminated), it may be reintroduced in small, graduated amounts, along with good-quality hay or other forage source.

CLIENT EDUCATION

• Animals being fed for production should be introduced to concentrated feeds gradually and provided quality forage.
• When new feedstuffs are incorporated into a production system, they should be incorporated prior to full depletion of previous feedstuffs, in order to allow gradual introduction.
• Feed should be inspected immediately prior to feeding for signs of damage or contamination.
• Silages and other stored feeds should be properly protected from environmental damage (moisture, oxygen, feces).

SURGICAL CONSIDERATIONS

In cases of simple indigestion, surgery such as rumenotomy is rarely required.

MEDICATIONS

DRUGS OF CHOICE

• Medication outside of supportive care and dietary management rarely required in uncomplicated cases of simple indigestion
• Ruminatorics are of limited use in simple indigestion
  • Nux vomica
  • Ginger
  • Tartar
  • Parasympathomimetic agents:
  • Neostigmine—may be of value if motility is reduced but still present; requires vagal tone to produce action; atonic animals are unable to respond.
  • Carbamylcholine—induces forestomach contractions, which are not productive and uncoordinated

CONTRAINDICATIONS

• Appropriate milk and meat withdrawal times must be followed for all compounds administered to food-producing animals.
• Important to confirm rumen pH before administering corrective substances: Magnesium oxide contraindicated in absence of rumen acidosis

PRECAUTIONS

N/A

POSSIBLE INTERACTIONS

N/A

ALTERNATIVE DRUGS

N/A

FOLLOW-UP

PATIENT MONITORING

• Monitor closely for return to feed in 24–48 hours.
• May require additional transfaunations or additional diagnostics if not responding

PREVENTION

• Provide animals on feed with smaller meals more frequently, more closely mimicking grazing.
• Add buffers to feed ($NaHCO_3$).
• Avoid rapid changes in feeding practices.

POSSIBLE COMPLICATIONS

Rumen environment may further deteriorate and require more intensive therapy.

EXPECTED COURSE AND PROGNOSIS

• Typical course of anorexia is 1–2 days, with diarrhea occurring 12–24 hours after onset.
• If uncomplicated and managed by removal of offending feed, prognosis is good.
• Animals return to normal once rumen microflora and fermentation products achieve homeostasis and inhibitory products have been eliminated.
• Transfaunation encourages more rapid return of stable rumen environment.

MISCELLANEOUS

ASSOCIATED CONDITIONS

Lactic acidosis; rumen alkalosis

AGE-RELATED FACTORS

Young animals may be more inclined to overindulge in concentrated feeds.

ZOONOTIC POTENTIAL

None

PREGNANCY

If condition is mild and has a short course, it is unlikely to result in loss of pregnancy.

RUMINANT SPECIES AFFECTED

Any ruminant species may be affected.

BIOSECURITY

PRODUCTION MANAGEMENT

• Silage and other processed feeds should be properly prepared and stored to prevent spoilage.
• Animals should be gradually introduced to increasing amounts or different types of feeds.
• New feedstuffs should be ordered and introduced prior to depletion of previous feed to allow for mixing and gradual introduction.

SYNONYMS

N/A

SEE ALSO

Rumen acidosis
Rumen alkalosis

ABBREVIATIONS

BUN = blood urea nitrogen
$NaHCO_3$ = sodium bicarbonate
PO = per os

Suggested Reading

Constable, P. D. 1999. The ruminant forestomach: Simple indigestion. In: *Current veterinary therapy 4: food animal practice*, ed. J. L. Howard, R. A. Smith. Philadelphia: W. B Saunders.

Edwards, J. L., Tozer, P. R. 2004, Feb. Using activity and milk yield as predictors of fresh cow disorders. *J Dairy Sci.* 87(2): 524–31.

Garry, F. B. 2002. Indigestion in ruminants: Simple indigestion. In: *Large animal internal medicine*, ed. B. P. Smith. 3rd ed. Saint Louis: Mosby.

Stocker, H., Lutz, H., Kaufmann, C., Rusch, P. 1999, Sep 18. Acid-base disorders in milk-fed calves with chronic indigestion. *Vet Rec.* 145(12): 340–46.

Stocker, H., Lutz, H., Rusch, P. 1999, Sep 11. Clinical, haematological and biochemical findings in milk-fed calves with chronic indigestion. *Vet Rec.* 145(11): 307–11.

Van Metre, D. C., Fecteau, G., House, J. K., George, L. W. 1995, Mar 1. Indigestion of late pregnancy in a cow. *J Am Vet Med Assoc.* 206(5): 625–27; discussion 627–8.

Author: Meredyth Jones

INFECTIOUS BOVINE RHINOTRACHEITIS

 BASICS

DEFINITION

• Infectious bovine rhinotracheitis (IBR) is a mild to severe upper respiratory disease in cattle caused by bovine herpesvirus-1 (BHV-1). IBR viral infection is one of the viral factors in bovine respiratory disease complex (BRDC).
• BHV-1 can also cause conjunctivitis, reproductive disease, and abortion. A variant of BHV-1, bovine herpesvirus-5 (BHV-5) can cause viral encephalitis.
   • The virus may remain latent in tissues and be reactivated after stress. Genomes of several different viral strains may be latent in the same animal at the same time.
   • Infection with BHV-1 may occur simultaneously with other bacterial and viral infections (e.g., *Mannheimia* [*Pasteurella*] *haemolytica*, bovine viral diarrhea [BVD] virus, and parainfluenza virus type 3) leading to severe respiratory infection.
   • Infection with IBRV may also enhance bovine keratoconjunctivitis (IBK) caused by *Moraxella bovis*.

PATHOPHYSIOLOGY

• BHV-1 is spread through nasal exudate, droplets, genital secretions, semen, frozen embryos, and fetal fluids.
• Cattle are the only significant source of viral spread. Although other species may become infected, they probably do not contribute to the spread of BHV-1.
• BHV-1 multiplies in the nasal cavities and upper respiratory tract resulting in rhinitis, laryngitis, and tracheitis. The virus spreads from the nasal cavity to the ocular system by the lacrimal gland. BHV-1 induces damage to the upper respiratory tract (URT) epithelium and conjunctiva of the eye. The damage to URT epithelium coupled with inflammatory changes increases the susceptibility of the lung to secondary bacterial infection.

• Conjunctivitis results from inflammation and edema of the conjunctiva. BHV-1 can induce late-term abortions in pregnant cattle by causing a viremia that results in BHV-1 infection of the ovary, placenta, and corpus luteum.
• In Europe, BHV-1 is associated with genital tract infections of both the male (infectious pustular balanoposthitis, IPB) and female (infectious pustular vulvovaginitis, IPV). BHV-5 infections spread rapidly up the peripheral nervous system to the brain and cause encephalitis.
• Once animals are infected with BHV-1 or BHV-5 in the URT, the virus spreads to the nervous system becomes latently infected in the nervous and lymphoid system, and the animals are a life-long source of infectious virus.
• Airborne transmission of the virus is believed to be of minor importance.

SYSTEMS AFFECTED

Respiratory, reproductive, ocular, immune, gastrointestinal, central nervous system

GENETICS

N/A

INCIDENCE/PREVALANCE

• BHV-1 is endemic in cattle.
• IBR is seldom seen in calves less than 6 months of age and is most prevalent and severe in animals between 6 and 18 months of age.
• Nonvaccinated pregnant cattle are highly susceptible to BHV-1 infection and up to 25% can abort (so-called abortion storm).

GEOGRAPHIC DISTRIBUTION

Worldwide

SIGNALMENT

Species

Widely present in bovines and many wild species, American bison (*Bison bison*), African buffalo (*Syncerus caffer*), and sheep

SIGNS

• Symptoms in BHV-1 infected calves can vary from subclinical to severe disease with 100% morbidity and 10% mortality.
• Clinical signs of rhinotracheitis can occur within 1 or 2 days of infection with an increased rectal temperature of 104–108°F (40–42°C).
• Respiratory signs may consist of pink muzzle, nasal discharge (initially serous and later mucopurulent), inappetance, fever, depression, salivation, drop in milk production, red conjunctiva, and ocular discharge.
• In the presence of secondary bacterial infections (*Mannheimia haemolytica, Pasteurella multocida, Haemophilus somnus* or *Mycoplasma bovis*) respiration becomes labored followed by hyperpnea, open-mouth breathing, and death.
• Conjunctivitis can occur with respiratory disease or it may appear alone. Conjunctivitis originates from the cornenosceral line and is usually bilateral.
• Abortion occurs in the last trimester of gestation.
• In calves, both respiratory and digestive tracts are involved.
• IPV, also known as coital exanthema, is characterized by small pustules on vulva and vagina. These pustules may later enlarge and spread over the whole epithelium and cause edema and hyperemia. The loss of epithelium encourages secondary infections.
• Lesions in IPB are limited to the prepuce, penis, and urethra.
• In Europe, BHV-1 is mainly responsible for genital tract infections. The respiratory tract disease varies in intensity and prevalence. In Belgium, digestive disorders are common in calves.
• Virus strains causing abortion, encephalitis, and mastitis are present only in a few countries. Dermatitis and lesions in the interdigital space are also rare.
• Infection becomes latent and may recrudesce with stress. The virus may be shed intermittently or continuously after recrudescence.

INFECTIOUS BOVINE RHINOTRACHEITIS

CAUSES
• BHV-1 is an enveloped double-stranded DNA virus of the genus *Varicellovirus*, in the subfamily Alphaherpesvirinae, family Herpesviridae.
• The virus is easily inactivated by desiccation, heat, and disinfectants.

RISK FACTORS
Stress (e.g., weaning, shipping, etc.) will increase the risk. Maternal antibody will inhibit vaccine response.

DIAGNOSIS

DIFFERENTIAL DIAGNOSIS
Respiratory
• Pneumonia
  • Shipping fever
  • Enzootic calf pneumonia
  • *Haemophilus somnus* pneumonia
  • Atypical interstitial pneumonia
  • Early bacterial pneumonia
  • Verminous pneumonia
• Septicemia—neonates
• Virus
  • Bovine coronavirus (BCV) has also been associated with respiratory disease. In younger calves, it is also seen with enteritis and diarrhea. BCV in 5- to 13-month-old cattle causes symptoms of dyspnea, nasal discharge, and increased respiratory rate.
  • Infectious bovine rhinotracheitis (IBR)
  • Bovine respiratory syncytial virus (BRSV) is characterized by increased harshness in respiratory sounds to severe with dyspnea, forced expiration, and open-mouth breathing. Spontaneous cough can be easily induced and can vary from dry and nonproductive to moist.
  • Parainfluenza-3 virus (PI-3) infection is usually a mild, lower respiratory disease.
  • Bovine viral diarrhea virus (BVDV) is associated with oral ulcers, mucopurulent discharge, and upper respiratory disease.

Abortion—Infectious
• Anaplasmosis
• Bluetongue
• Bovine viral diarrhea virus (BVDV) mucosal disease
• Brucellosis
• Campylobacteriosis
• Epizootic bovine abortion
• Leptospirosis
• *Mycoplasma*
• Mycotic abortions
• Q fever
• Salmonellosis
• Trichomoniasis

BHV-5 Encephalitis
The differential diagnoses include listeriosis, pseudorabies, rabies, and *Haemophilus somnus*.

CBC/BIOCHEMSTRY/URINALYSIS
N/A

OTHER LABORATORY TESTS
• Other procedures that have proved useful in detection of BHV-1 are fluorescent antibody tests of fresh tissue and immunohistochemistry staining of cell cultures or formalin-fixed paraffin embedded tissues.
• Intranuclear inclusion bodies are often present in the liver of BHV-1–infected fetuses.
• A rise in serum neutralizing antibody titer also can be used to confirm BHV-1 infection. Paired serum samples collected 2 to 3 weeks apart are necessary; a single sample, even if it has a high titer, is of little value. It is not possible to detect a rising antibody titer in abortions, because infection generally occurs a considerable length of time before the abortion, and titers are already maximal.
• BHV-1 ELISA antibody detection tests are also available.

IMAGING
N/A

DIAGNOSTIC PROCEDURES
• BHV-1 is readily detected by virus isolation. Clinical specimens should be collected during the febrile, acute phase of infection. Respiratory and ocular specimens can be collected antemortem using swabs. Swabs can also be used for the detection of genital infections.
• On postmortem, virus isolation samples from IBR animals can be collected from the upper respiratory tract and trachea.
• From aborted fetuses, the liver, adrenal, kidney, and lung are the preferred tissues. In animals with encephalitis, several regions (olfactory lobes, midbrain, cortex, etc.) should be sampled. BHV-1 can also be detected using polymerase chain reaction (PCR).

PATHOLOGIC FINDINGS
Gross Lesions
• Gross lesions of uncomplicated IBR are restricted to the upper respiratory tract and trachea.
  • Petechial to ecchymotic hemorrhages with edema are found in the mucous membranes of the nasal cavity and the sinuses. There may be focal areas of necrosis in the nose, pharynx, larynx, and trachea that may coalesce to form plaques. The sinuses may be filled with a serous or serofibrinous exudate.
  • As the disease progresses, the pharynx becomes covered with a serofibrinous exudate, and blood-tinged fluid may be found in the trachea.
  • The pharyngeal and pulmonary lymph nodes may be acutely swollen and hemorrhagic. The tracheitis may extend into the bronchi and bronchioles; when this occurs, epithelium is sloughed in the airways.
  • In animals with bacterial bronchopneumonia, the viral lesions are often masked.
  • Aborted fetuses may have pale, focal, necrotic lesions in all tissues, which are especially visible in the liver.

INFECTIOUS BOVINE RHINOTRACHEITIS

• In digestive tract infection, one can see erosions and ulceration of buccal mucosa, lips, gums, hard palate, esophagus, and abomasums.
• In IPV and IPB, inflammatory lesions can be seen in vulva, vagina, cervical mucosa, prepuce, and penile mucosa.

Histologic Examination
• Histologic examination of IBR tissues reveals acute catarrhal inflammation of the mucosa with rare inclusion bodies as well as lymphocytic infiltration in the mucosa, edema in the lamina propria, and type A eosinophilic inclusion bodies can be seen.
• In BHV-5 encephalitic calves, histological changes consist of a widespread nonsuppurative meningoencephalitis, more severe in the anterior cerebrum, the dorsolateral cortex and, to a lesser extent, the posterior cerebrum and the midbrain.
• The lesions are characterized by gliosis, disruption of the neutrophil and perivascular cuffing, consisting of macrophages, histiocytes, and lymphocytes. In aborted fetuses, intranuclear inclusion bodies are often present in the liver.

TREATMENT

APPROPRIATE HEALTH CARE
The therapy for IBR is supportive. Severely diseased animals that are dehydrated may receive oral and/or intravenous fluids.

ACTIVITY
Handling of BHV-1-infected animals should be minimal to decrease the risk of secondary bacterial infections.

DIET
N/A

CLIENT EDUCATION
Minimize handling of animals and use preventative vaccines.

SURGICAL CONSIDERATIONS
N/A

MEDICATIONS

DRUGS OF CHOICE
Nonsteroidal anti-inflammatory drugs (NSAIDs) may have some benefit to lessen the severity of BHV-1 disease. Antimicrobial treatment is used to reduce secondary bacterial infections.

CONTRAINDICATIONS
N/A

PRECAUTIONS
N/A

POSSIBLE INTERACTIONS
N/A

ALTERNATIVE DRUGS
N/A

FOLLOW-UP

PATIENT MONITORING
Respiratory characteristics along with rectal body temperature should be frequently monitored to assess IBR clinical progression and also the development of secondary bacterial infections that would result in bovine respiratory disease complex (BRDC).

PREVENTION/AVOIDANCE

Immunity and Vaccination
• Infection leads to the development of humoral and cell-mediated immunity. The humoral immunity and not the cellular immunity can be transmitted to neonates via colostrum.
  • Both modified-live virus (MLV) and inactivated virus BHV-1 vaccines are on the market. The MLV vaccines are available as either a parenteral (intramuscular, IM or subcutaneous, SC) or intranasal (IN) vaccine.
  • Use of MLV vaccines is not without risk due to persistence of the virus and its potential for reactivation.

• Although conventional vaccines can prevent clinical signs of IBR, their use has not resulted in reduction of the prevalence of infection. Similarly, marker vaccines can prevent disease but not infection and/or subsequent latency. The continued excretion of virus from vaccinated animals results in environmental contamination making the control of the disease more difficult.
• No vaccine has been shown to overcome viral latency.
• BHV-1 vaccines are cross-reactive and should be efficacious against BHV-5.

Control and Eradication
• Marker vaccines can be used in conjunction with companion diagnostic tests to differentiate between infected and vaccinated cattle, a property that is useful in eradication and control programs.
• Eradication of herpesviruses is extremely difficult because of their ability to establish latent infections. In addition, these viruses have a wide range of genes and proteins (envelope glycoproteins and cytokine inhibitors, for example) that can counteract host immune response.
• Many European countries were forced to eradicate BHV-1 because of international trade restrictions on the import/export of seropositive cattle whereby importing countries consider only vaccinated animals for import and require that the animals be seronegative prior to vaccination.
• Eradication programs in Austria, Denmark, and Switzerland have removed most of the seropositive cattle from their bovine populations. The Swiss program consisted of four phases (e.g., prevention of virus transmission by restrictions on trade of bovines, slaughter of antibody-positive animals in breeding herds, detection and eradication of BHV-1 reservoirs, and enforcement of monitoring program by legal action). Currently, a similar program is being tried in Germany.

POSSIBLE COMPLICATIONS
• IM MLV BHV-1 vaccines may cause abortion in pregnant cattle.
• Maternal antibodies in calves interfere with development of an effective IBR immune response with parenteral MLV vaccines.
• Maternal antibodies have no effect on IN MLV vaccines.

EXPECTED COURSE AND PROGNOSIS
• Uncomplicated BHV-1 respiratory infections will resolve in 5–7 days.
• Animals that have secondary infections usually will develop bronchopneumonia with varying levels of morbidity and mortality.

 MISCELLANEOUS

ASSOCIATED CONDITIONS
• BRDC is a frequent sequela to IBR.
• Retained placenta and metritis are possible sequelae to BHV-1 abortion.
• Virus strains causing abortion, encephalitis, and mastitis are present only in a few countries. Dermatitis and lesions in the interdigital space are also rare.

AGE-RELATED FACTORS
A rare, generalized disease may occur in neonatal calves less than 2 weeks of age. Most IBR and BHV-5 disease is seen in animals > 6 months of age.

ZOONOTIC POTENTIAL
N/A

PREGNANCY
BHV-1 infections result in late-term abortions that occur as long as 100 days following infection.

RUMINANT SPECIES AFFECTED
Bovine

BIOSECURITY
• BHV-1 survives very poorly in the environment and is susceptible to UV light, desiccation, heat, and disinfectants. The virus will survive better in the winter.

• Animals exhibiting clinical signs of IBR or BHV-5 should be isolated from other cattle as transmission of these viruses occurs by the oronasal route.

PRODUCTION MANAGEMENT
• In herds with a history of IBR, BHV-1 abortion, or BHV-5 encephalitis, a BHV-1 vaccine program should be implemented.
• Although conventional vaccines can prevent clinical signs of IBR, their use has not resulted in reduction of the prevalence of infection. Similarly, marker vaccines can prevent disease but not infection and/or subsequent latency. The continued excretion of virus from vaccinated animals results in environmental contamination making the control of the disease more difficult.

SYNONYMS
IBR
Rednose

SEE ALSO
Bovine coronavirus (BCV)
Bovine parainfluenza 3 virus (PI-3)
Bovine respiratory syncytial virus (BRSV)
Bovine viral diarrhea virus (BVDV)
Haemophilus somnus
Listeriosis
Parainfluenza-3 virus (PI-3)
Pseudorabies
Rabies

ABBREVIATIONS
BCV = bovine coronavirus
BHV-1 = bovine herpesvirus-1
BHV-5 = bovine herpesvirus-5
BRSV = bovine respiratory syncytial virus
BVDV = bovine viral diarrhea virus
ELISA = enzyme-linked immunosorbent assay
IBK = infectious bovine keratoconjunctivitis
IBR = infectious bovine rhinotracheitis
IM = intramuscular

IN = intranasal
IPB = infectious pustular balanoposthitis
IPV = infectious pustular vulvovaginitis
MLV = modified-live virus
NSAIDs = nonsteroidal anti-inflammatory drugs
PCR = polymerase chain reaction
PI-3 = bovine parainfluenza-3 virus
SC = subcutaneous
SN = serum neutralization
URT = upper respiratory tract

Suggested Reading
Fulton, R. W., Briggs, R. E., Payton, M. E., Confer, A. W., Saliki, J. T., Ridpath, J. F., Burge, L. J., Duff, G. C. 2004. Maternally derived humoral immunity to bovine viral diarrhea virus (BVDV) 1a, BVDV1b, BVDV2, bovine herpesvirus-1, parainfluenza-3 virus, bovine respiratory syncytial virus, *Mannheimia haemolytica* and *Pasteurella multocida* in beef calves, antibody decline by half-life studies and effect on response to vaccination. *Vaccine* 22:643–49.
Jones, C. 2003. Herpes simplex virus type 1 and bovine herpesvirus 1 latency. *Clin Microbiol Rev*. 16: 79–95.
Meyer, G., Lemaire, M., Ros, C., Belak, K., Gabriel, A., Cassart, D., Coignoul, F., Belak, S., Thiry, E. 2001. Comparative pathogenesis of acute and latent infections of calves with bovine herpesvirus types 1 and 5. *Arch Virol*. 146:633–52.
Schwyzer, M., Ackermann, M. 1996, Nov. Molecular virology of ruminant herpesviruses. *Vet Microbiol*. 53(1–2):17–29.
Turin, L., Russo, S., Poli, G. 1999, May. BHV-1: new molecular approaches to control a common and widespread infection. *Mol Med*. 5(5):261–84.

Authors: Christopher C. L. Chase and Sagar Goyal

INFECTIOUS NECROTIC HEPATITIS

 BASICS

DEFINITION
Infectious necrotic hepatitis is a disease affecting mainly animals on pasture and causing sudden death.

PATHOPHYSIOLOGY
• *Clostridium novyi* type B is a gram-positive spore-forming anaerobic bacteria, and is a normal inhabitant of soil. Spores are ingested by animals in the process of grazing, and occasionally cross the intestinal mucosa and are carried through the lymphatic drainage by the mononuclear macrophage system to the Kupffer cells of the liver.
• Liver damage, typically from larval migration of the common liver fluke *Fasciola hepatica*, and occasionally from other liver parasites such as *Fascioloides magna*, *Dicrocoelium dendriticum*, and *Cysticercus tenuicollis*, can cause localized anaerobic conditions, allowing the clostridial spores to germinate and proliferate. This releases exotoxins (mainly lethal alpha toxin and necrotizing and hemolytic beta toxin), which cause coagulative necrosis in the liver. The exotoxins enter the general circulation, damaging vascular endothelium and neurons in multiple organs, causing sudden death.

SYSTEMS AFFECTED
Hepatic

GENETICS
N/A

INCIDENCE/PREVALENCE
• Tends to be a seasonal disease related to the liver fluke life cycle, occurring in the warmer months when fluke transmission is active.
• Incidence in affected sheep flocks 5%–10%; incidence in cattle difficult to determine.

GEOGRAPHIC DISTRIBUTION
• Worldwide, wherever liver flukes are present.
• Important problem in Australia and New Zealand, lesser importance in Europe, the United Kingdom, and the United States

SIGNALMENT

Species
Mainly sheep and cattle. Disease appears to progress more rapidly in sheep.

Breed Predilections
N/A

Mean Age and Range
Age: 2–4 years; adult animals in good body condition

Predominant Sex
N/A

SIGNS

HISTORICAL FINDINGS
• Sudden death in a liver-fluke-endemic area during the warmer months of the year in animals unvaccinated against clostridia
• History of liver fluke infestation in the past

PHYSICAL EXAMINATION FINDINGS
• Animals most often found dead, in lateral recumbency with no signs of struggle and in apparently advanced decomposition even if death was recent.
• Signs nonspecific before death occurs (e.g., depression, anorexia, dyspnea, fever initially but subnormal temperature before death)

CAUSES AND RISK FACTORS
• Causes—toxins produced by the gram-positive anaerobic bacteria *Clostridium novyi* type B proliferating in liver tissue damaged by migrating liver flukes
• Risk factors—failure to vaccinate against clostridia; exposure to liver flukes

 DIAGNOSIS

DIFFERENTIAL DIAGNOSIS
• Other clostridial diseases (e.g., bacillary hemoglobinuria)—see red urine, bleeding from nose or rectum
• Anthrax—see bleeding from orifices
• Acute fascioliasis in sheep

CBC/BIOCHEMISTRY/URINALYSIS
N/A

OTHER LABORATORY TESTS
• Anaerobic culture
• Fluorescent antibody
• Gram-stain and microscopic inspection of an impression smear of the liver shows numerous large gram-positive rods.
• Specific toxin identification

IMAGING
N/A

OTHER DIAGNOSTIC PROCEDURES
N/A

PATHOLOGIC FINDINGS
• Generalized autolysis of all body tissues, especially the liver and kidneys
• Foci of coagulative necrosis in the liver
• Migrating fluke channels in the liver
• Engorged and hemorrhagic subcutaneous blood vessels
• Blood-tinged fluid in all body cavities (urine appears normal in color)

 TREATMENT

Rarely treated since animals are usually found dead prior to diagnosis

INFECTIOUS NECROTIC HEPATITIS

ACTIVITY
Restrict movement of animals being treated, since stress of physical exertion can precipitate sudden death.

DIET
N/A

CLIENT EDUCATION
• Routine vaccination against clostridia
• Control of liver fluke infestation by pasture management, limiting access to streams and ponds, and strategic flukicide treatment.

MEDICATIONS
• Vaccinate herd
• Mass medicate herd with long-acting penicillin or tetracycline. Use flukicide (e.g., clorsulon).

DRUGS OF CHOICE
• Penicillin: 20,000–40,000 IU/kg IV q 6 hours
• Clorsulon: 7 mg/kg PO

CONTRAINDICATIONS
Appropriate milk and meat withdrawal times must be followed for all compounds administered to food-producing animals.

PRECAUTIONS
N/A

POSSIBLE INTERACTIONS
N/A

ALTERNATIVE DRUGS
N/A

FOLLOW-UP
N/A

PATIENT MONITORING
N/A

PREVENTION/AVOIDANCE
• Vaccination with clostridial toxoid with booster in 4–6 weeks and annual revaccination preferably in early summer at least 1 month before expected fluke exposure
• Use of molluscicides in streams, flukicides in animals, and drainage of marshy areas

POSSIBLE COMPLICATIONS
N/A

EXPECTED COURSE AND PROGNOSIS
• Prognosis is grave in animals showing clinical signs.
• Rapid clinical course in sheep usually found dead before clinical signs noted.
• Short clinical course in cattle, with nonspecific clinical signs (depression, anorexia) seen just before death

MISCELLANEOUS

ASSOCIATED CONDITIONS
Fascioliasis

AGE-RELATED FACTORS
Typically, adult animals 2–4 years of age

ZOONOTIC POTENTIAL
N/A

PREGNANCY
N/A

RUMINANT SPECIES AFFECTED
Sheep, cattle

BIOSECURITY
Carcasses should be buried deeply, burned, or removed from the premises to avoid spread of spores.

PRODUCTION MANAGEMENT
N/A

SYNONYMS
Black disease

SEE ALSO
Acute fascioliasis
Anthrax
Bacillary hemoglobinuria
Body condition scoring
Hepatitis
Liver flukes
Serology

ABBREVIATIONS
IV = intravenous
PO = per os, by mouth

Suggested Reading
Pugh, D. G., ed. 2002. *Sheep and goat medicine.* Philadelphia: W. B. Saunders.
Radostits, O. M., Gay, C. C., Blood, D. C., Hinchcliff, K. W., eds. 2000. *Veterinary medicine.* 9th ed. London: W. B. Saunders.
Smith, B. P., ed. 2002. *Large animal internal medicine.* 3rd ed. St. Louis: Mosby.

Author: David McKenzie

INFECTIOUS PUSTULAR VULVOVAGINITIS

BASICS

OVERVIEW
• Infectious pustular vulvovaginitis (IPV) is characterized by vulvitis and vaginitis and it is part of the granular venereal diseases.
• Infectious pustular vulvovaginitis is caused by alphaherpesvirus, bovine herpes virus (BHV) type 1, subtype 2, of the Herpesviridae family.
• Bovine herpesvirus-1 is divided in two subtypes (BHV-1.1 and BHV-1.2) according to genetic differences and the systems that it affects.
• BHV-1.1 affects the respiratory system causing infectious bovine rhinotracheitis (IBR), while BHV-1.2 affects the reproductive system causing IPV in females and infectious pustular balanoposthitis (IPB) in males. Bovine herpesvirus 5 is formerly known as BHV-1.3, which is responsible for the encephalitic form of the disease.
• Rarely IPV and IBR occur concurrently.
• Agent: bovine herpesvirus type-1 subtype-2 (BHV-1.2)

GENETICS
• Bovine herpesvirus 1 is the herpesvirus serologically related to IBR or IPV/IPB, and is divided in two main subtypes according to genetic differences (BHV-1.1 and BHV-1.2).
• The genetic differences may be responsible for the diverse epidemiological and pathological patterns of virus behavior. While BHV-1.1 is related to IBR, the respiratory form of the disease, BHV-1.2 is related to the genital form of the ailment (IPV/IPB).
• Bovine herpesvirus 1.2b is a different strain of the virus and it is usually related to the occurrence of IPV/IPB and outbreaks of low/medium virulence of IBR.
• Some specific genotypes of bovine animals are more resistant to challenges with BHV-1, developing less-severe disease. This is an indication that breeding programs that increase the occurrence of these specific genes may alter the sensitivity of populations to BHV-1 infection.

INCIDENCE/PREVALENCE
Infectious pustular vulvovaginitis was considered endemic in Europe during the 1960s and 1970s. However, due to control measures such as vaccination and elimination of serologically positive animals, its prevalence has been reduced greatly.
• Outbreaks of IPV were frequent in Europe and more specifically in Great Britain in the 1960s and 1970s. However, it has become less common in the past few years due to implemented control measures.
• Seroprevalence surveys have indicated that 10%–50% of cattle may be serologically positive for BHV, but the prevalence depends on vaccination practices.

GEOGRAPHIC DISTRIBUTION
Bovine herpesvirus has been isolated in Africa, Asia, North America, Australia, New Zealand, and Europe.

Transmission
• Infectious pustular vulvovaginitis is transmitted directly by coitus or artificial insemination.
• Mechanical means are also possibilities for the transmission of the causal agent.

Epidemiology
• The incubation period for BHV-1.2 is usually between 1 and 3 days.
• Transmission of BHV-1.2 is rapid and can affect 60% –90% of the herd.

SIGNALMENT
Species
Bovine, ovine, and wild ruminants

Breed Predilections
N/A

Mean Age and Range
• Animals in the breeding age are more likely to be infected.
• Unbred animals can also be affected.

Predominant Sex
Female
• Female: bovine females infected with BHV-1.2 usually develop IPV.
• Male: bovine herpesvirus 1.2 is responsible for IPB in males.

DIAGNOSIS
• Indirect: Serology—ELISA and virus neutralization test; Skin test—delayed-type hypersensitivity (DTH) reaction
• Direct: Fluorescent microscope; polymerase chain reaction (PCR)

DIFFERENTIAL DIAGNOSIS
• Granular venereal disease caused by mycoplasma, ureaplasma, *Haemophilus somnus*, and *A. pyogenes*
• Transmissible fibropapilloma
• Granular vulvitis
• Necrotic vulvitis

CBC/BIOCHEMISTRY/URINALYSIS
N/A

OTHER LABORATORY TESTS
N/A

IMAGING
N/A

PATHOLOGIC FINDINGS
• Females develop mucopurulent secretion from the vagina and inflammation of the vulva and vagina.
• Lymphoid follicles present pustules that develop from small-sized ulcers to coalescing erosions.
• Male bovines infected with BHV-1.2 that develop infectious pustular balanoposthitis (IPB) are reluctant to mate.
• The animals tend to recover within 10 to 30 days of the beginning of signs and remain transiently immune.

TREATMENT
Although, lavage of the vagina with antiseptic solutions and emollients has been recommended, treatment is usually not required. Animals usually recover within 30 days of the initial infection.

INFECTIOUS PUSTULAR VULVOVAGINITIS

MEDICATIONS

FOLLOW-UP

PATIENT MONITORING
N/A

PREVENTION/AVOIDANCE
• Vaccination can be of benefit. However, in the face of an outbreak, vaccination has little effect.
• Avoid mating among infected animals to decrease the risk of dissemination of the disease.
• BHV-1.2 can survive cryopreservation. Therefore, semen donors and semen should be tested and free of BHV-1.2.
• Eradication of the disease requires vaccination and often elimination of animals that are carriers of the genital form of BHV

POSSIBLE COMPLICATIONS
• Not uncommonly, female bovine infected with BHV-1.2 that develop IPV have an increased rate of return to estrus after insemination. This can have a major impact in the breeding programs and consequently to the profitability of dairy and beef operations.
• Rarely IPV is followed by abortion outbreaks.

EXPECTED COURSE AND PROGNOSIS
• Animals usually develop signs of infection within 1 to 3 days after exposure.
• Initial signs are mucopurulent vaginal secretion and vulvar/vaginal inflammation.

• Lymphoid tissue develops pustules that become small ulcers (< 3 mm) and may result in coalescing erosions. The vulvar mucosa in the latter stages of the disease presents small but numerous necrotic focal areas.
• Within 10 to 30 days of infection, animals recover spontaneously.
• Infectious pustular vulvovaginitis has a very good prognosis.

MISCELLANEOUS

ASSOCIATED CONDITIONS
• During the initial phases of the disease, animals may present less-specific signs such as pyrexia and milk drop.
• Animals in the breeding age infected with BHV-1.2 may present increased rate of return to estrus.
• Conjunctivitis with serous discharge and bilateral nasal discharge are signs of BHV-1.2 when the respiratory tract is affected.

AGE-RELATED FACTORS
Although, breeding-age animals are more likely to develop the condition, unbred heifers can also be infected.

ZOONOTIC POTENTIAL
N/A

PREGNANCY
Infectious pustular vulvovaginitis is rarely related to abortion outbreaks.

RUMINANT SPECIES AFFECTED
Bovine, ovine, wild ruminants

BIOSECURITY
• Vaccination
• Testing of bulls and frozen semen
• Avoid the use of shared hired bulls

SEE ALSO
A. pyogenes
Granular venereal disease caused by mycoplasma, ureaplasma
Granular vulvovaginitis
Haemophilus somnus vulvovaginitis
Infectious bovine rhinotracheitis
Necrotic vulvitis
Transmissible fibropapilloma

ABBREVIATIONS
BHV = bovine herpesvirus
DTH = delayed-type hypersensitivity
ELISA = enzyme-linked immunosorbent assay
IBR = infectious bovine rhinotracheitis
IPB = infectious pustular balanoposthitis
IPV = infectious pustular vulvovaginitis
PCR = polymerase chain reaction

Suggested Reading
Ackermann, M., Belak, S., Bitsch, V., Edwards, S., Moussa, A., Rockborn, G., Thiry, E. 1990, Jun. Round table on infectious bovine rhinotracheitis/infectious pustular vulvovaginitis virus infection diagnosis and control. *Vet Microbiol*. 23(1–4): 361–63.
Miller, J. M., Van Der Maaten, M. J., Whetstone, C. A. 1988, Oct. Effects of a bovine herpesvirus-1 isolate on reproductive function in heifers: classification as a type-2 (infectious pustular vulvovaginitis) virus by a restriction endonuclease analysis of viral DNA. *Am J Vet Res*. 49(10): 1653–56.
Pritchard, G., Cook, N., Banks, M. 1997, May 31. Infectious pustular vulvovaginitis/infectious pustular balanoposthitis in cattle. *Vet Rec*. 140(22): 587.
Whetstone, C. A., Miller, J. M., Bortner, D. M., Van Der Maaten, M. J. 1989, Oct. Changes in the bovine herpesvirus 1 genome during acute infection, after reactivation from latency, and after superinfection in the host animal. *Arch Virol*. 106(3–4): 261–79.

Author: Ricardo Carbonari Chebel

INHALATION PNEUMONIA

 BASICS

DEFINITION
Inhalation or aspiration pneumonia is caused by inhalation of large amounts of foreign material.

PATHOPHYSIOLOGY
• Inhalation of large amounts of foreign material into the lungs sets up an inflammatory reaction.
• Irritation of the lung tissues results in infection by a mixed population of organisms (e.g., *Corynebacterium* spp., *Fusobacterium* spp., *E. coli*, *Klebsiella* spp., etc.) leading to cell and tissue death and a gangrenous pneumonia.

SYSTEMS AFFECTED
Respiratory

GENETICS
N/A

INCIDENCE/PREVALENCE
N/A

GEOGRAPHIC DISTRIBUTION
Worldwide

SIGNALMENT
Species
All

Breed Predilections
N/A

Mean Age and Range
N/A

Predominant Sex
N/A

SIGNS
N/A

HISTORICAL FINDINGS
Typically, a neonate being bottle fed or tube fed milk or a milk substitute, or any age animal being administered liquid medication via a nasogastric tube or orogastric tube or dosing syringe

PHYSICAL EXAMINATION FINDINGS
Coughing, frothing at the nose and mouth, foul breath odor, depression, polypnea, dyspnea, coughing, fever, gurgling sounds over trachea, crackles and wheezes over lung fields, occasional pleural friction rubs

CAUSES AND RISK FACTORS
• Caused by inadvertent inhalation of foreign material, usually milk, a milk replacer, or liquid medication
• Risk factors include administration of milk, milk replacers, or liquid medication by untrained personnel, or administration of these substances to a struggling animal or a weak animal with an inadequate suckling or swallowing ability (e.g., pharyngeal paresis).
• Can occur also in pail-fed calves, calves that have aspirated meconium secondary to fetal distress/dystocia, animals put through dipping vats, lambs with nutritional myodegeneration, cattle ingesting crude oil, or subsequent to vomiting in downer cattle with parturient paresis

 DIAGNOSIS

DIFFERENTIAL DIAGNOSIS
• Acute bronchopneumonia
• Septicemia

CBC/BIOCHEMISTRY/URINALYSIS
Marked leukopenia due to neutropenia early in course of disease, with elevated fibrinogen.

OTHER LABORATORY TESTS
Transtracheal aspirate with culture and sensitivity

IMAGING
Radiography—cranioventral lung consolidation

OTHER DIAGNOSTIC PROCEDURES
N/A

PATHOLOGIC FINDINGS
• Cranioventral lung consolidation with hemorrhage in acute cases and necrosis in subacute cases
• Diffuse alveolitis

 TREATMENT

ACTIVITY
Restrict activity

DIET
N/A

CLIENT EDUCATION
Proper administration of liquid food and medication

 MEDICATIONS

• Prolonged treatment with broad-spectrum antibiotics
• NSAIDs and/or corticosteroids immediately following suspected aspiration.

DRUGS OF CHOICE
• Procaine penicillin G 22,000 U/kg IM bid
• Florfenicol 20 mg/kg IM repeat in 48 hours
• Flunixin meglumine 1.1 mg/kg IV or IM bid
• Dexamethasone 2 mg/kg IV

CONTRAINDICATIONS

Appropriate milk and meat withdrawal times must be followed for all compounds administered to food-producing animals.

PRECAUTIONS

• Florfenicol is not to be used in veal calves or female dairy cattle 20 months of age or older.
• Dexamethasone may induce parturition.

POSSIBLE INTERACTIONS

N/A

ALTERNATIVE DRUGS

N/A

 FOLLOW-UP

N/A

PATIENT MONITORING

Monitor for improvement in attitude, appetite, lung sounds.

PREVENTION/AVOIDANCE

• Ensure that liquid food and medications are administered by trained personnel.
• Ensure proper placement of tubes into stomach/rumen by blowing into tube and auscultating over left paralumbar fossa.

POSSIBLE COMPLICATIONS

N/A

EXPECTED COURSE AND PROGNOSIS

Prognosis is fair if small quantities of foreign material inhaled and/or immediate treatment instituted, otherwise prognosis is guarded to poor.

 MISCELLANEOUS

ASSOCIATED CONDITIONS

N/A

AGE-RELATED FACTORS

Typically, a neonatal animal

ZOONOTIC POTENTIAL

N/A

PREGNANCY

N/A

RUMINANT SPECIES AFFECTED

All ruminant species can be affected.

BIOSECURITY

N/A

PRODUCTION MANAGEMENT

• Ensure that trained personnel administer liquid food and medications.
• Caused by inadvertent inhalation of foreign material, usually milk, milk replacer, or liquid medication.
• Risk factors include administration of milk, milk replacers, or liquid medication by untrained personnel, or administration of these substances to a struggling animal or a weak animal with an inadequate suckling or swallowing ability.

SYNONYMS

Aspiration pneumonia
Foreign-body pneumonia
Gangrenous pneumonia
Lipid pneumonia
Medication pneumonia

SEE ALSO

NSAIDs
Pneumonia
Respiratory pharmacology

ABBREVIATIONS

bid = twice daily
IM = intramuscular
IV = intravenous
NSAIDs = nonsteroidal anti-inflammatory drugs

Suggested Reading

Pugh, D.G., ed. 2002. *Sheep and goat medicine*. Philadelphia: W. B. Saunders.
Radostits, O. M., Gay, C. C., Blood, D. C., Hinchcliff, K. W., eds. 2000. *Veterinary medicine*. 9th ed. London: W. B. Saunders.
Smith, B. P., ed. 2002. *Large animal internal medicine*. 3rd ed. St. Louis: Mosby.

Author: David McKenzie

IODINE DEFICIENCY AND TOXICITY

BASICS

OVERVIEW
• Iodine is essential for normal formation and function of the thyroid hormones thyroxine (T_4) and triiodothyronine (T_3). Inadequate intake of iodine results in the formation of inactive thyroid hormones. In a negative feedback system, the pituitary responds to decreased serum thyroid hormones by increasing secretion of thyroid stimulating hormone (TSH) resulting in a compensatory hypertrophy and hyperlasia of the thyroid gland (goiter) especially in neonates.
• Goiter is usually the first clinical sign of an iodine deficiency. The concentration of iodine in water, soil, and plants is highly variable but is readily absorbed from the gastrointestinal tract as iodide (I^-). The body stores iodide in the thyroid gland, salivary glands, gastric mucosa, and mammary glands.
• Short periods of decreased intake rarely results in clinical signs of deficiency in adult animals.
• Toxicity (iodinism), a result of prolonged ingestion of plants or supplements containing iodine (0.4 mg/kg–2.2. mg/kg), also produces clincial signs of goiter. Iodine is excreted in urine and to a lesser degree in milk, sweat, and feces.

SYSTEMS AFFECTED
• Cardiovascular—tachycardia
• Endocrine/metabolic—hyperthermia, hypothermia, goiter
• Gastrointestinal—anorexia, weight loss
• Musculoskeletal—enlarged neck
• Nervous system—depression
• Respiratory—persistent cough, naso-ocular discharge, bronchopneumonia
• Reproductive—decreased milk yield, reproductive disorders, abortion, increased mortality of neonates
• Skin/exocrine—dermatitis, alopecia, flabby edematous skin

GENETICS
Familial dyshormonogenetic goiter—an autosomal recessive trait affecting mRNA for thyroglobulin in goats, Afrikaner cattle, and Corriedale, Dorset horn, Merino, and Romney Marsh sheep

INCIDENCE/PREVALENCE
N/A

GEOGRAPHIC DISTRIBUTION
Geographic areas known to be deficient in soil iodine include the Great Lakes region, Pacific Northwest, Central Plains, Rocky Mountains, and northeastern United States; parts of eastern Europe, Swiss Alps, parts of the Andes, and Himalayas

SIGNALMENT
All ruminants and all ages are susceptible but newborns are at greater risk of deficiency as well as toxicity. Sheep may be more tolerant of higher doses of iodine than are cattle.

Species
Potentially all ruminant species

Breed Predilections
Afrikaner cattle and Corriedale, Dorset horn, Merino, and Romney Marsh sheep may be more affected by goiter

Mean Age and Range
N/A

Predominant Sex
N/A

SIGNS
Deficiency
Enlargement of the thyroid gland, skin of the neck may be thickened and edematous, calves and lambs may be born without hair or wool, may be born weak, or die shortly after birth; iodine deficiency in cows may result in reproductive disorders characterized by decreased conception rates, fetal resorption, abortions, and stillbirths. In bulls, decreased libido and semen quality are observed.

Toxicity
• Signs are highly variable depending on dose, nature of the compound ingested, and length of time of exposure.
• Clinical signs may take months to more than a year to develop in adults, and adults may not exhibit clinical signs unless stressed or have concurrent disease.
• Symptoms include enlarged thyroid gland; lacrimation; salivation; dry, flaky skin; cough; naso-ocular discharge; bronchopneumonia; decreased feed consumption; decreased weight gain; decreased milk production; tachycardia

CAUSES AND RISK FACTORS
Deficiency
• Geographic areas known to be deficient in soil iodine include the Great Lakes region, Pacific Northwest, Central Plains, Rocky Mountains, and northeastern United States; parts of eastern Europe, Swiss Alps, parts of the Andes, and Himalayas
• Consumption of goitrogenic plants increases the dietary need for iodine 2–4x. Goitrogenic substances alter the uptake of iodine by the thyroid gland or the incorporation of iodine into the thyroid hormone producing clinical signs of iodine deficiency.
• Known goitrogenic plants include soybean, soybean meal, cottonseed, cassava, millet, sweet potatoes, cabbage, rape, kale, turnips, white clover, onions, garlic (heating or processing usually destroys goitrogenic substances). An increase in dietary iodine will compensate in most cases.

Toxicity
• In newborns, goiter is usually a result of ingestion of excess iodine by the cow/ewe/doe.
• Sources include excess mineral supplements containing ethylenediamine dihydroiodide (EDDI), calcium iodate, kelp, potassium iodide, and sodium iodide. Iodine is widely used for its antibacterial properties. Treatment doses of EDDI for therapy or prevention of infectious pododermatitis are higher than recommended daily requirements and pose a risk.

IODINE DEFICIENCY AND TOXICITY

DIAGNOSIS

DIFFERENTIAL DIAGNOSIS
Consumption of goitrogenic plants, abscess, trauma, hematoma, foreign body, neoplasia of thyroid gland (especially in older bulls), familial dyshormonogenetic goiter—an autosomal recessive trait affecting mRNA for thyroglobulin in goats, Afrikaner cattle, and Corriedale, Dorset horn, Merino, and Romney Marsh sheep. Selenium deficiency aggravates iodine-deficient goiter, diets high in nitrates inhibit iodine uptake by the thyroid gland.

CBC/ BIOCHEMISTRY/URINALYSIS
Biochemical changes are inconclusive for iodine deficiency/toxicosis.

OTHER LABORATORY TESTS
• Iodine levels in serum, milk, and urine (Lactating animals will have lower serum iodine and higher milk iodine levels due to iodine excretion in milk.)
• Iodine levels in soil, forage, and water
• Serum T_3 and T_4 levels

IMAGING
Ultrasonography or radiography may rule out other causes of swelling in neck region.

DIAGNOSTIC PROCEDURES

PATHOLOGIC FINDINGS
Gross Pathology
• Uniformly enlarged thyroid gland may be twice normal size.
• Respiratory system: tracheitis, bronchopneumonia, inflammatory exudate
Histopathology
Histopathology of thyroid gland is variable.

TREATMENT
• In cases of deficiency, diet may be supplemented with stabilized iodized salt containing 0.007% iodine.
• In cases of toxicosis, removal from source of excess iodine is the only treatment.

MEDICATIONS

DRUGS OF CHOICE
None

CONTRAINDICATIONS

FOLLOW-UP

PATIENT MONITORING

PREVENTION/AVOIDANCE
• Forage analysis in iodine deficient areas and supplementation with a stable iodized salt
• Species requirements
  • Dairy cows 0.33 mg I/kg DM for nonlactating, 0.45 mg I/kg DM for lactating animals
  • Sheep 0.10–0.80 mg I/kg DM the higher range for pregnant and lactating animals
  • Goats 0.2–0.8 mg I/kg DM the higher range for lactating animals
  • Beef cattle 0.5 mg I/kg diet

POSSIBLE COMPLICATIONS

EXPECTED COURSE AND PROGNOSIS
In mild cases, goiter will resolve with supplementation/removal, but young animals affected in utero may not survive.

MISCELLANEOUS

ASSOCIATED CONDITIONS
Hypothyroidism

AGE-RELATED FACTORS
Newborns are at greatest risk.

ZOONOTIC POTENTIAL
None

PREGNANCY
• If dietary iodine levels are marginal or deficient during pregnancy, developmental abnormalities, neonatal weakness, signs of goiter at birth or shortly thereafter, and death of the neonate may result even though pregnant females may not show any clinical signs of iodine deficiency.
• Clinical signs in the neonate depend on the stage of development at the time of deficiency and are not usually reversible.

RUMINANT SPECIES AFFECTED
All species susceptible

BIOSECURITY
N/A

PRODUCTION MANAGEMENT
Prevention is more effecctive than treatment.

SEE ALSO
Abscess
Diets high in nitrates
Familial dyshormonogenetic goiter
Foreign body
Goitrogenic plants
Hematoma
Neoplasia of thyroid gland
Selenium deficiency
Trauma

ABBREVIATIONS
DM = dry matter
EDDI = ethylenediamine dihydroiodide
T_3 = triiodothyronine
T_4 = thyroxine
TSH = thyroid stimulating hormone

Suggested Reading
Merck veterinary manual, 8th ed. 1998. Whitehouse Station, NJ: Merck & Co.
Morgan, S. E. 2004. Iodine. In: *Clinical veterinary toxicology*, ed. K. Plumlee. St. Louis: Mosby.
Olson, W. G., et al. 1984. Iodine toxicosis in six herds of dairy cattle. *J Am Vet Med Assoc.* 184:179–81.
Smith, B. P. 2002. *Large animal internal medicine*. 3rd ed. St. Louis: Mosby.
Smith, M. C., Sherman, D. M. 1994. *Goat medicine*. Baltimore: Williams & Wilkins.

Author: Lauren Palmer

JIMSONWEED TOXICITY (*DATURA STRAMONIUM*)

 BASICS

OVERVIEW
• Caused by ingestion of jimsonweed (Jamestown weed or *Datura stramonium*) and its toxic tropane alkaloids.
• All parts of the green or dried plant are toxic including the seeds. Plants become more toxic as they mature. Seeds are considered to be the most toxic part of the plant.
• Contain two tropane alkaloids: (1) L-hyoscyamine (atropine) and (2) scopalamine (L-hyoscine)
• Tropane alkaloids act as a competitive antagonist of acetylcholine at muscarinic cholinergic receptors of the parasympathetic nervous system.
• Clinical signs are attributable to this receptor blockade and are manifest as (1) blockage of contraction of the muscles of the iris and mydriasis, (2) decreased smooth muscle contraction of the gastrointestinal system, (3) decreased salivary secretions, and (4) increased vagal tone.
• Jimsonweed is commonly found in fencerows, barnyards, and roadsides throughout much of the United States.
• The green plant is generally unpalatable due to its strong odor. Thus, lack of other forage, drying of the plant in hay, or contamination of cereal grains or feed with the seeds are the primary routes of ingestion and toxicity.

• Toxicity is often somewhat self-limiting as anorexia is induced early in the toxic process limiting ingestion of further toxins.
• Signs predominantly involve the neuromuscular, ophthalmic, and gastrointestinal systems.

SIGNALMENT
• All ruminant species and swine can be affected.
• Cattle appear to be more susceptible than other ruminants.
• No sex, age, or breed predilection among animals consuming the plant

SIGNS
• Mydriasis
• Depression
• Restlessness
• Anorexia
• Sinus tachycardia
• Weakness
• Photophobia
• Dry mucous membranes
• Constipation/ileus
• Rumen atony

CAUSES AND RISK FACTORS
Associated with ingestion of toxin-containing plant. Consumption of feed or cereal grains containing 1000 seeds/kg can be toxic in cattle.

 DIAGNOSIS

DIFFERENTIAL DIAGNOSIS
• Other toxic plants with tropane alkaloids including moonflower, angel's trumpet, deadly nightshade, belladonna, black henbane, horse or bull nettle, Texas thistle, tropical soda apple, and ground cherries.
• Parenteral or topical atropine therapy

CBC/BIOCHEMISTRY/URINALYSIS
No changes specific for jimsonweed toxicity

OTHER LABORATORY TESTS
• Urine and gastrointestinal contents can be tested for tropane alkaloids.
• Test administration of parasympathomimetic drugs *may not* cause appreciable improvement.

IMAGING
N/A

DIAGNOSTIC PROCEDURES
• If acute consumption is suspected, a rumenotomy with confirmation of plant material or seeds in the ingesta would be diagnostic and may be indicated.
• Urine from affected animal is said to induce mydriasis if applied topically to the eye of a test animal.

PATHOLOGIC FINDINGS
• Identification of seed or plant material in the rumen
• No distinct lesions
• May see hemorrhages of the liver or kidney or effusions of the pericardium

JIMSONWEED TOXICITY (*DATURA STRAMONIUM*)

TREATMENT

• Remove animals from source of toxin (plants or seed).
• If acute ingestion of large volumes of toxin are suspected, rumenotomy with evacuation of the ingesta may be beneficial.
• Often self-limiting due to anorexia, an early sign.

MEDICATIONS

DRUGS OF CHOICE

• Orogastric administration of mineral oil or activated charcoal may decrease absorption of the toxin.
• Rarely administration of a cholinergic drug (such as physostigmine, pilocarpine, or arecoline) is used, however, no clear benefit to the use of these drugs has been demonstrated.

CONTRAINDICATIONS

Atropine

POSSIBLE INTERACTIONS

FOLLOW-UP

PATIENT MONITORING

Monitor for signs of continued ileus or intestinal obstruction secondary to ileus.

PREVENTION/AVOIDANCE

Do not pasture animals on fields with jimsonweed or feed hay or grain containing the plant or seed.

POSSIBLE COMPLICATIONS

N/A

EXPECTED COURSE AND PROGNOSIS

• Often self-limiting due to decreased ingestion of the toxin after initial signs of toxicity.
• Most have a good prognosis with supportive care

MISCELLANEOUS

ASSOCIATED CONDITIONS

N/A

AGE-RELATED FACTORS

N/A

ZOONOTIC POTENTIAL

N/A

PREGNANCY

• Some studies have demonstrated teratogenic properties of tropane alkaloids, however more recent studies have not been able to clearly demonstrate a cause and effect relationship.
• Until further work is done, tropane alkaloids should be considered possible teratogens.

RUMINANT SPECIES AFFECTED

• All ruminant species and swine
• Cattle appear to be most susceptible.

BIOSECURITY

N/A

PRODUCTION MANAGEMENT

N/A

SEE ALSO

N/A

ABBREVIATIONS

N/A

Suggested Reading

Burrows, G. E., Tyrl, R. J., ed. 2001. *Toxic plants of North America*. Ames: Iowa State University Press.

Nelson, P. D., Mercer, H. D., Essig, H. W., Minyard, J. P. 1982, Oct. Jimson weed seed toxicity in cattle. *Vet Hum Toxicol*. 24(5):321–25.

Piva, G., Piva, A. 1995. Anti-nutritional factors of *Datura* in feedstuffs. *Nat Toxins*. 3(4):238–41; discussion 242.

Schulman, M. L., Bolton, L. A. 1998, Mar. *Datura* seed intoxication in two horses. *J S Afr Vet Assoc*. 69(1):27–29.

Author: Paul J. Plummer

JOHNE'S DISEASE

BASICS

OVERVIEW
• Johne's disease (pronounced Yo-nees) is a serious disease of most ruminants that can cause significant economic loss if not controlled.
• Species affected by Johne's disease include cattle, sheep, goats, and camelids.
• It is estimated that greater than 50% of the dairy and 20% of the beef cow-calf operations in the United States have at least one animal infected with Johne's disease.
• Johne's disease is caused by the bacteria *Mycobacterium avium* subsp. *paratuberculosis.*
• Animals less than 6 months of age are most susceptible to infection. Older animals are less susceptible to infection.
• The primary source of infection is feces that contain the causative bacteria. Infected animals can produce large amounts of the bacteria and shed this organism in their feces.
• Most infected animals do not begin shedding the Johne's organism until they are adults.
• Any method by which young stock become exposed to fecal material from adult animals may serve as a source of infection with the Johne's disease organism.
• This may include being born in a dirty maternity pen, nursing a dirty teat, being housed in direct contact with adult animals, using common feeding/manure handling equipment (skid-loader), or having manure run-off from mature cow areas going through the environments of young stock.
• Another important source of transmission is milk and colostrum. About one-third of cows infected with Johne's disease, whether they are showing clinical signs or not, will shed the bacteria in their colostrum or milk.
• Approximately 20% of cows with Johne's disease will pass the causative bacteria across their placenta to the developing fetus. The risk of this happening increases dramatically in cows with clinical signs of Johne's disease.

SIGNALMENT
• Newborn animals are most susceptible to infection with Johne's disease. As they get older, risk of infection decreases. In cattle, most infections likely occur in the first 6 months of life.
• Following a long incubation period of months to years, clinical disease typically occurs in an adult animal.
• All breeds of cattle, sheep, and goats are susceptible to Johne's disease.

SIGNS
• There is a long incubation period between infection and the appearance of clinical signs. In cattle, this period of time may range from 1 year to several years.
• Prior to the development of observable clinical signs, animals may be affected subclinically. Syndromes that have been associated with subclinical Johne's disease in cattle include reduced milk production, reduced reproductive performance, and increased disease susceptibility.
• The classical clinical sign of Johne's disease in cattle is chronic, watery diarrhea. This diarrhea may be intermittent at first, but eventually progresses to chronic and unrelenting. Diarrhea is not as evident in sheep and goats.
• The diarrhea has no distinguishing characteristics such as blood, mucus, or foul odor. It is often referred to as "pipe stream" in nature because of its watery and projectile appearance.
• Secondary to diarrhea, animals lose weight despite the maintenance of a good appetite. Weight loss is the primary clinical sign in sheep and goats.
• Depending on concurrent metabolic loads (milk production, pregnancy), weight loss may occur gradually over months or very rapidly over the course of a few weeks.
• In advanced cases, the development of submandibular edema may occur secondary to a decrease in total serum protein.

CAUSES AND RISK FACTORS
Johne's disease is caused by the bacteria *Mycobacterium avium* subsp. *paratuberculosis.*

DIAGNOSIS

DIFFERENTIAL DIAGNOSIS
• Parasitism
• Copper deficiency
• Bovine leukosis
• Salmonellosis
• Amyloidosis
• Chronic reticuloperitonitis/peritonitis

CBC/BIOCHEMISTRY/URINALYSIS
Hypoproteinemia, characterized by low serum albumin, may be present in advanced clinical cases of Johne's disease.

OTHER LABORATORY TESTS
N/A

IMAGING
N/A

DIAGNOSTIC PROCEDURES
• Fecal culture—standard culture methods require 10–16 weeks to complete. New rapid culture methods can shorten the culture time to 8–10 weeks.
• PCR/DNA probe—organism detection assay used on feces or tissue
• ELISA, immunodiffusion, complement fixation—antibody detection assays
• Acid-fast stain—direct visualization of organism in appropriate tissue samples such as ileum or ileal cecal lymph nodes

GROSS FINDINGS
• In cattle, lesions are primarily found in the distal jejunum, ileum, cecum, proximal colon, and associated lymph nodes.
• Thickening of the intestine three to four times normal thickness is characteristic.
• Affected mucosa takes on a corrugated appearance.
• The ileocecal valve is typically thickened and often reddened in color.
• In sheep, intestinal mucosal may be thickened, but it does not typically become corrugated.
• Mesenteric lymph nodes are enlarged and edematous in cattle. In sheep, they have areas of necrosis and calcification.

HISTOPATHOLOGICAL FINDINGS
• The earliest cellular changes are increased numbers of macrophages and lymphocytes.
• As the infection progresses, the mononuclear inflammatory infiltrate becomes pronounced and giant cells become more numerous. The inflammation is diffuse; the lesions are not walled off or circumscribed by fibrous connective tissue.
• Acid-fast bacteria will be present in areas of mononuclear inflammation.

TREATMENT

• There are no chemotherapeutic agents approved for use in food-producing animals for the treatment of *Mycobacterium paratuberculosis*.
• Use of antimycobacterial chemotherapeutic agents has largely been ineffective. Isoniazid, rifampin, Clofazimine, dapsone, aminoglycosides, and ethambutol may result in transient reduction in clinical signs and slowing of disease progression, but response is inconsistent and they have failed to cure the disease.
• Drug withdrawal times must be determined and maintained for food-producing animals.

MEDICATIONS

N/A

CONTRAINDICATIONS

N/A

FOLLOW-UP

PATIENT MONITORING

N/A

PREVENTION/AVOIDANCE

• Stopping the transmission from infected cattle that are shedding the bacteria (generally adult animals) to susceptible animals (generally young animals) is key to controlling the disease.
• Specific recommendations include making sure newborns are born into and housed in a clean environment, reducing the chance of spread through colostrum and milk by not sharing colostrum and milk between multiple young stock or feeding only pasteurized sources of milk or milk replacers, making sure that weaned young stock are separated from adult animals.
• Infected animals should be identified and either culled or managed so as to reduce the chance they are spreading the disease to susceptible animals.

POSSIBLE COMPLICATIONS

N/A

EXPECTED COURSE AND PROGNOSIS

• Johne's is a chronic progressive disease.
• Progression of Johne's disease typically occurs over a 2–3-year period.
• Johne's disease progression can be divided into four stages. Stage 1 is the period of inapparent infection that occurs early in the disease progression. Stage 2 is a subclinical phase where shedding of the organism is intermittent. Stage 3 is characterized by consistent heavy shedding. Stage 4 is the clinical stage of the disease.
• Johne's disease is inevitably a fatal disease if allowed to progress.

MISCELLANEOUS

ASSOCIATED CONDITIONS

N/A

AGE-RELATED FACTORS

• Calves are most at risk for becoming infected with Johne's disease. As cattle get older, infection becomes less likely.
• Because of the long incubation period, clinical signs of disease typically do not appear until adulthood.

ZOONOTIC POTENTIAL

There has been some association of *Mycobacterium paratuberculosis* with Crohn's disease in humans, but no definitive link has been made.

PREGNANCY

Mycobacterium paratuberculosis can cross the placenta and infect the fetus. This occurs about 20% of the time in Johne's-infected cows. The risk of fetal transmission in utero increases as the disease progresses in the dam.

SYNONYMS

Paratuberculosis

SEE ALSO

Amyloidosis
Bovine leukosis
Chronic reticuloperitonitis/peritonitis
Copper deficiency
Parasitism
Salmonellosis

ABBREVIATIONS

ELISA = enzyme-linked immunosorbent assay
PCR/DNA = polymerase chain reaction/deoxyribonucleic acid

Suggested Reading

Rossiter C.A., Burhans W.S. 1996, July Farm-specific approach to paratuberculosis (Johne's disease) control. *Vet Clin North Am Food Anim Pract.* 12(2):383–415.

Sweeney, R. W. Transmission of paratuberculosis. 1996. In: Sweeny, R.W. (ed), Paratuberculosis (Johne's disease), *Veterinary Clinics of North America – Food Anim Pract*, Philadelphia. W.B. Saunders Co., pp. 305–12.

Tavornpanich, S., Gardner, I. A., Anderson, R. J., Shin, S., Whitlock, R. H., Fyock, T., Adaska, J. M., Walker, R. L., Hietala, S. K. 2004, Aug. Evaluation of microbial culture of pooled fecal samples for detection of *Mycobacterium avium* subsp *paratuberculosis* in large dairy herds. *Am J Vet Res.* 65(8):1061–70.

Waters, W. R. 2001, Nov. Immunology of inflammatory diseases of the bowel. *Vet Clin North Am Food Anim Pract.* 17(3):517–34.

Wells, S. J., Dee, S., Godden, S. 2002, Mar. Biosecurity for gastrointestinal diseases of adult dairy cattle. *Vet Clin North Am Food Anim Pract.* 18(1):35–55, v–vi.

Author: Daniel L. Grooms

JOHNE'S DISEASE—SMALL RUMINANTS AND EXOTICS

 BASICS

OVERVIEW
• Johne's disease (paratuberculosis) is an insidious, chronic, diarrheal disease of domestic and wild ruminant species that occurs worldwide.
• Ruminant species infected include domesticated cattle, sheep, goats, and camelids, as well as several species of deer (white-tailed, sika, red, axis, roe, fallow), moose, Rocky Mountain bighorn sheep, Rocky Mountain bighorn goats, tule elk, American buffalo, antelope, aoudad, mouflon, water buffalo, yak, gnu, and wild rabbits.
• Monogastric animals infected include mules, horses, swine, chickens, monkeys, and mandrills.
• The causative agent is *Mycobacterium avium* subsp. *paratuberculosis (Map)*
• Based on culture characteristics and molecular typing, two strains of *Map* have been described. These include the cattle (C) strain, which predominantly affects cattle as well as goats, camelids, and wildlife; and the sheep (S) strain, which primarily affects sheep.
• Cross-species transmission of *Map* between cattle and sheep can occur.
• The role of wildlife in maintaining infection cycles in domesticated ruminants is unknown. Natural transmission of *Map* from wildlife to domesticated animals has not been documented, however, domesticated animals have been implicated in natural outbreaks of Johne's disease in wildlife populations.
• The majority of information available regarding the epidemiology, biology, pathology, and diagnosis of Johne's disease is based on studies performed on cattle. While many of the features of Johne's in small ruminants and exotics are likely similar to those found in cattle, differences do exist.
• Transmission studies in most species indicate the primary route to be fecal-oral. Transmission can also occur via colostrum and milk, as well as across the placenta (intrauterine).
• Though age-related resistance has been primarily studied in cattle, it is believed that young animals (<30 days) are most susceptible to infection.

SYSTEMS AFFECTED
Production management, nutrition, gastrointestinal, musculoskeletal

GENETICS
N/A

INCIDENCE/PREVALENCE
Unknown

GEOGRAPHIC DISTRIBUTION
Worldwide, depending on species and environment

SIGNALMENT
Species
Many domestic and wild ruminant species as well as monogastric species
Breed Predilection
N/A
Mean Age and Range
2–7 years
Predominant Sex
N/A

SIGNS
• Chronic weight loss is the most consistent finding in sheep, goats, camelids, and deer.
• Diarrhea or softening of stool is observed at the end stages of disease in the minority (10%–20%) of cases.
• Hypoproteinemia with intermandibular edema (bottle jaw) can be seen in sheep, camelids, and deer.
• Wool break and poor fleece condition can be observed in sheep.
• Patchy alopecia can be observed in deer.
• Clinical signs often appear with, or are exacerbated by, periods of stress (parturition, etc.).

CAUSES AND RISK FACTORS
• Manure management
• Water contamination
• Acid soils
• Colostrum feeding
• Milk feeding and pasteurization
• Note: Bacterial shedding in feces, milk, colostrum, as well as transplacental transmission is more common in animals displaying clinical signs of disease.

 DIAGNOSIS

DIFFERENTIAL DIAGNOSIS
• Parasitism
• Internal abscessation (*C. pseudotuberculosis*)
• Caprine arthritis and encephalitis (CAE)
• Ovine progressive pneumonia (OPP)
• Protein/energy malnutrition
• Copper deficiency
• Cobalt deficiency
• Other diseases causing chronic weight loss

CBC/BIOCHEMISTRY/URINALYSIS
Hypoproteinemia and hypoalbuminemia are typically manifest in the later stages of disease.

OTHER LABORATORY TESTS
N/A

DIAGNOSTIC PROCEDURES
• Fecal culture —Test sensitivity is dependant on the *Map* strain and stage of infection. The S strain of *Map* is difficult to grow in culture and can take up to 12 months. In all small and wild ruminants, test sensitivity is increased in the later stages of disease.
• Serologic testing (AGID, ELISA)—Test sensitivity is increased in the later stages of disease. Cross-reacting antibodies to *Corynebacterium pseudotuberculosis* can affect test specificity.
• Polymerase chain reaction (PCR)
• Histopathologic examination of ileocecal lymph nodes, mesenteric lymph nodes, and ileocecal junction

PATHOLOGIC FINDINGS
• Variable weight loss or cachexia
• Variable thickening (mild to severe corrugation of mucosa) of distal small intestine and cecum
• Enlargement and edema of associated lymph nodes
• Lymphangectasia
• Histology: epitheliod cell infiltration into mucosa and submucosa with presence of acid-fast organisms, caseous necrosis, sinus histiocytosis of intestinal lymph nodes.
• Note: severity of pathologic findings may not correlate with disease severity.

JOHNE'S DISEASE—SMALL RUMINANTS AND EXOTICS

TREATMENT

While supportive therapy may prolong life, no practical treatment is available.

MEDICATIONS

N/A

CONTRAINDICATIONS

N/A

FOLLOW-UP

N/A

PREVENTION/AVOIDANCE

- Control fecal/oral transmission (sanitation, hygiene, etc.).
- Prevent feeding of colostrum and milk from test-positive animals.
- Purchase replacement animals from Johne's-free herds or herds with no evidence of infection.
- Annual serologic testing of herd
- Segregation and culling of test-positive animals or clinical cases
- Culling of offspring from known Johne's-infected dams

POSSIBLE COMPLICATIONS

N/A

EXPECTED COURSE AND PROGNOSIS

- Animals exposed to *Map* can either clear the infection or proceed to develop chronic diarrheal disease.
- Animals diagnosed with and displaying signs of Johne's disease are expected to continue to suffer decreased production, ill thrift, and weight loss, and finally succumb to the disease.

MISCELLANEOUS

N/A

ASSOCIATED CONDITIONS

N/A

AGE-RELATED FACTORS

Young animals (<30 days of age) are believed to be most susceptible to infection. Infection of older animals is possible, however, definitive proof of susceptibility is hampered by limitations of current diagnostic techniques.

ZOONOTIC POTENTIAL

While humans can be infected with *Map*, currently insufficient evidence exists to determine if *Map* is a pathogen of real significance. Concern also exists whether or not *Map* is associated with Crohn's disease, a chronic granulomatous ileocolitis of humans. Again, there is currently insufficient evidence to determine if *Map* is a cause of Crohn's disease.

PREGNANCY

N/A

SEE ALSO

Caprine arthritis and encephalitis (CAE)
Cobalt deficiency
Copper deficiency
Internal abscessation (*C. pseudotuberculosis*)
Other diseases causing chronic weight loss
Ovine progressive pneumonia (OPP)
Parasitism
Protein/energy malnutrition

ABBREVIATIONS

AGID = agar gel immunodiffusion
ELISA = enzyme-linked immunosorbent assay
Map = *Mycobacterium avium* ssp. *paratuberculosis*
PCR = polymerase chain reaction

Suggested Reading
Benedictus, G., Kalis, C. J. 2003. Paratuberculosis: eradication, control and diagnostic methods. *Acta Vet Scand*. 44(3–4): 231–41.
National Research Council of the National Academies. 2003. *Diagnosis and control of Johne's disease, final report*. Washington, DC: National Academies Press.
Reddacliff, L. A., Whittington, R. J. 2003, Dec. Culture of pooled tissues for the detection of *Mycobacterium avium* subsp *paratuberculosis* infection in individual sheep. *Aust Vet J*. 81(12): 766–67.
Stehman, S. M. 1996. Paratuberculosis in small ruminants, deer and South American camelids. *Vet Clin North Am: Food An Pract*. 12(2): 441–55.
Whittington, R. J., Eamens, G. J., Cousins, D. V. 2003, Jan-Feb. Specificity of absorbed ELISA and agar gel immuno-diffusion tests for paratuberculosis in goats with observations about use of these tests in infected goats. *Aust Vet J*. 81(1–2): 71–75.
Whittington, R. J., Marsh, I. B., Taylor, P. J., Marshall, D. J., Taragel, C., Reddacliff, L. A. 2003, Sep. Isolation of *Mycobacterium avium* subsp *paratuberculosis* from environmental samples collected from farms before and after destocking sheep with paratuberculosis. *Aust Vet J*. 81(9): 559–63.

Author: George M. Barrington

JUVENILE LLAMA IMMUNODEFICIENCY SYNDROME (JLIDS)

BASICS

DEFINITION
• JLIDS is a syndrome in young llamas characterized by failure to grow/gain weight as expected and generalized ill thrift, which routinely progresses to multiple and/or chronic systemic infections and eventually to death.
• Recent research suggests an inherited impairment in B-cell development as a potential primary cause.

PATHOPHYSIOLOGY
• Poorly understood
• The specific immunodeficiency has not been determined, but an autosomal recessive defect in B-cell development has been proposed.
• Immunodeficiency leads to opportunistic or overwhelming systemic infections, and failure of the animal to respond to appropriate therapies, ultimately resulting in death.

SYSTEMS AFFECTED
Primarily the immune system is affected. Secondary infections can affect the respiratory, hematologic, gastrointestinal, musculoskeletal, urogenital, and/or ocular systems.

GENETICS
An autosomal recessive inherited basis is suspected but not proven for JLIDS.

INCIDENCE/PREVALENCE
Not well established. One report suggests immune dysfunction is responsible for 7% or greater of llama deaths.

SIGNALMENT
• Juvenile llamas, usually between the ages of 6 and 18 months, of either sex
• Not documented in alpacas

SIGNS
• There are no pathognomonic signs—signs vary with the organ system(s) involved and the stage of the disease, including respiratory signs, lameness, dermatitis, ocular signs, or CNS signs/ataxia.
• Common reported complaints include:
  • Poor body condition and/or poor growth as compared to herdmates
  • Recurring infections or infections that fail to respond to treatment
  • Anemia, with pale mucous membranes, tachycardia, and mild heart murmur
  • Lethargy, depression
  • Occasionally, peracute infection may lead to rapid weight loss and death without prior signs.

RISK FACTORS
• No specific risk factors have been identified.
• A hereditary component to the development of the clinical disease is likely, but a specific inheritance pattern has not been elucidated.

DIAGNOSIS

DIFFERENTIAL DIAGNOSES
Malnutrition, nutritional deficiency (copper, zinc, or selenium), iron deficiency, intestinal parasitism, and hypothyroidism

CBC/BIOCHEMISTRY/URINALYSIS
• Anemia— usually mild, normocytic, normochromic, and nonregenerative, though if the animal is infected with the erythrocyte parasite *Eperythrozoon* spp., the anemia can be severe and mildly regenerative.
• Hypoproteinemia with hypoalbuminemia and low to low-normal globulin levels, even in the face of infection
• Low serum iron concentration with low to low-normal total iron binding capacity

IMAGING
Radiography may be indicated if clinical signs of lower respiratory tract disease and/or septic arthritis is present.

OTHER DIAGNOSTIC PROCEDURES
• *Clostridium perfringens* C and D antibody ELISA: paired serum samples are collected prior to and 2 weeks after vaccination with *C. perfringens* C and D toxoid, and antibody levels are measured. Healthy llamas show at least a twofold increase in titers, while JLIDS llamas have a low initial titer and fail to show any significant rise in titer after vaccination.
• Lymph node biopsy: affected llamas show regions of paracortical lymphocyte depletion.
• Immunologic testing: lymphocyte blastogenesis assays, serum protein electrophoresis, and flow cytometry can be used to characterize the specific immunodeficiency in an affected llama. Although these tests are still in the process of being validated for camelids, initial reports suggest consistent findings in JLIDS llamas include low levels of serum IgG and low numbers of B-lymphocytes.

TREATMENT/PREVENTION

• In the early stages, rule out intestinal parasitism as a cause for ill thrift with appropriate anthelmintic therapy.
• Antimicrobial therapy is indicated to treat systemic infections, with the caveat that infections in llamas with JLIDS routinely fail to respond to therapy and ultimately are fatal.
• Appropriate milk and meat withdrawal times must be followed for all compounds administered to food-producing animals.

JUVENILE LLAMA IMMUNODEFICIENCY SYNDROME (JLIDS)

MISCELLANEOUS

ASSOCIATED CONDITIONS
• Eperythrozoonosis is a common incidental finding in camelids in North America, but is rarely associated with clinical anemia except in animals with underlying immune dysfunction. The detection of the organism in the blood smear in an animal with severe anemia with or without hemolysis is suggestive of immunodeficiency, such as JLIDS.
• Secondary infections with typically nonpathogenic organisms, such as *Pneumocystis carinii, Bordatella* sp*.,* or fungal organisms, are commonly associated with JLIDS.

AGE-RELATED FACTORS
Juvenile llamas (aged 6–18 months, typically)

ZOONOTIC POTENTIAL
N/A

PREGNANCY
N/A

BIOSECURITY
N/A

PRODUCTION MANAGEMENT
• The specific immunodeficiency has not been determined, but an autosomal recessive defect in B-cell development has been proposed.

• Recent research suggests an inherited impairment in B-cell development as a potential primary cause.
• Cull/euthanize affected animals; evaluate parental records for possible genetic correlation.

SYNONYMS
Failure to thrive

SEE ALSO
BCS camelids
Hypothyroidism
Intestinal parasitism
Iron deficiency
Malnutrition
Nutritional deficiency (copper, zinc, or selenium)

ABBREVIATIONS
BCS = body condition score
CNS = central nervous system
ELISA = enzyme-linked immunosorbent assay
JLIDS = juvenile llama immunodeficiency syndrome

Suggested Reading
Davis, W. C., Heirman, L. R., Hamilton, M. J., Parish, S. M., Barrington, G. M., Loftis, A., Rogers, M. 2000. Flow cytometric analysis of an immunodeficiency affecting juvenile llamas. *Vet Immunol Immunopathol.* 74: 103–20.

Hutchison, J. M., Garry, F. 1994. Ill thrift and juvenile llama immunodeficiency syndrome. *Update on Llama Medicine, Veterinary Clinics of North America: Food Animal Practice* 10(2): 331–43.
Hutchison, J. M., Garry, F. B., Belknap, E. B., Getzy, D. M., Johnson, L. W., Ellis, R. P., Quackenbush, S. L., Rovnak, J., Hoover, E. A., Cockerell, G. L. 1995, Dec. Prospective characterization of the clinicopathologic and immunologic features of an immunodeficiency syndrome affecting juvenile llamas. *Vet Immunol Immunopathol.* 49(3):209–27.
Hutchison, J. M., Garry, F. B., Johnson, L. W., Quackenbush, S. L., Getzy, D. M., Jensen, W. A., Hoover, E. A. 1992. Immunodeficiency syndrome associated with wasting and opportunistic infection in juvenile llamas: 12 cases (1988–1990). *J Amer Vet Med Assoc.* 201(7): 1070–76.

Author: Kelsey A. Hart

KERATOCONJUNCTIVITIS/CONJUNCTIVITIS

 BASICS

OVERVIEW
• Infectious bovine keratoconjunctivitis (IBK) is the inflammation/infection of the cornea and conjunctiva.
• Interactions between the animal, its environment, season, vector availability, physical abrasions, and concurrent infection influence the prevalence of IBK.
• IBK vaccination has in many cases been less than successful.
• Affected animals must be separated from the herd/flock. Vector transmission is important in the longevity of the disease state.
• Carrier animals are common and must be identified and removed from the flock/herd.
• Conjunctivitis: inflammation of the conjunctiva, the membrane that covers the eyelids, and the exposed surface of the eyeball

PATHOPHYSIOLOGY
• Primary: infectious, allergic, foreign body, irritation
• Secondary: underlying disease, deep eye disease, and systemic disease
• *Moraxella bovis* may utilize host iron sources for growth. Iron-repressible outer membrane proteins may accomplish this.
• *Mycoplasma* spp. or infectious bovine rhinotracheitis (IBR) virus may exacerbate the disease process.
• Virulent strains of *M. bovis* produce hemolysin
• *Moraxella bovis* pili antigen cross-reactivity, variable bacterial strains, and uncontrolled environmental factors influence vaccine efficacy.

SYSTEMS AFFECTED
Ophthalmic, musculoskeletal, reproductive, production management

GEOGRAPHIC DISTRIBUTION
Worldwide

SIGNALMENT
• All species, all ages
• Seen most often in young animals

SIGNS

HISTORICAL FINDINGS
• Blepharospasm, epiphora, conjunctival vessel injection, chemosis, lymphoid follicles, corneal opacity, neovascularization, and ulceration
• IBK symptoms may range from mild conjunctivitis to severe corneal ulceration. Chronic corneal perforation and blindness may occur.
• Intense redness of the conjunctival tissues occurs unilateral or bilateral often associated with discomfort and epiphora. Epiphora can be serous, sanguineous, purulent, mucoid, and/or a combination of these.
• Severe cases are often associated with photophobia, blepharospasm, and corneal ulcers, with or without partial or complete loss of vision.

CAUSES AND RISK FACTORS
• Seen most often in young animals. Dust and shipping exacerbate the condition. Flies irritate the eyes further and help spread disease. Tall grass and dusty feeds may physically irritate corneal surfaces.
• In most common outbreak situations where infectious agents are involved, ruminant species are predisposed to *Moraxella bovis* (in cattle), *Chlamydia psittaci*, and *Mycoplasma* spp. (in sheep and goats).

Bacteria
• *Chlamydia psittaci*—may cause abortions and polyarthritis in addition to ocular signs, most common during lambing
• *Branhamella ovis* (*Neisseria*)—aerobic bacteria found in one or both eyes, may be normal flora, found with concurrent mycoplasmal and chlamydial disease and in normal eyes. Can also be cultured from cattle.

Mycoplasma
• May show neovascularization, corneal ulceration, hypopion, and anterior uveitis; is usually unilateral.
• Goats generally do not develop hypopion and ulceration but can have corneal opacification and blindness.
• Camelids have not been reported to be infected by mycoplasmal conjunctivitis.
• *Moraxella* spp. infections in llamas, spread by flies from infected cattle, can occur.
• Neonatal septicemia of all species.

Virus
• Parainfluenza virus, adenovirus, and other respiratory viruses can cause ocular discharge.
• Equine herpesvirus type 1—in llamas, causes blindness and retinal degeneration.

Foreign Body
Foreign objects—seeds or awns of plants, grasses, windblown debris

Entropion
Infolding of eyelid causing abrasion to the corneal surface and tissue irritation; predisposing to ulceration and bacterial infections

Ectopic Cilia
Eyelashes grow inward toward the corneal surface causing irritation to the cornea predisposing to ulcers and infections.

Parasites
• *Oestrus ovis*—nasal bot of sheep can migrate from the nasal passages through the nasolacrimal duct into the eye.
• *Elaeophora schneideri* (sore head)—usually found in deer, spread by biting flies, is most common in the western United States and Canada. Can cause cataracts and blindness due to migration of the parasite.
• *Thelazia californiensis*—ophthalmic parasite seen in ruminants and camelids.

DIAGNOSIS

DIFFERENTIAL DIAGNOSIS
Distinguish primary eye lesions from secondary systemic and parasitic conditions.

Cattle
• Pink eye/infectious bovine keratoconjunctivitis caused by *Moraxella bovis* with acute herd outbreaks of up to 90% morbidity, especially in young.
• Foreign bodies—grass awns, thistle thorns, tall pasture grass
• Allergic, physical, chemical, or smoke irritation
• Cancer— squamous cell carcinoma with predisposition in white faced breeds and unpigmented conjunctiva/adnexa

• IBR—infectious bovine rhinotracheitis associated with respiratory signs, cough
• Phytotoxicity—ingestion of photosensitizing plants and materials such as lush clover, lupinosis, lantana, lucerne. Other toxic agents include: mycotoxins, phenothiazines, motor oil, lubricating oils, and timber preservatives.
• Entropion—congenital defect usually of the lower eyelid
• Eye worms—*Thelazia* sp., habronemiasis
• Vitamin A deficiency—lack of green, fresh, feedstuffs, drought, calves on skim milk
• Cobalt deficiency—unthrifty, poor coat, anemia
• Riboflavin deficiency
• Dermoid cysts
• Toxic ingestion—vitamin D, iodine, phenothiazines, polybrominated biphenyls, chlorinated napthalenes
• Listeriosis—neurological signs
• Other causes—East coast fever, besnoitosis, lumpy skin disease, bluetongue, actinomycosis, mucosal disease, cholangitis, ephemeral fever, moniliasis, transfusion reaction, respiratory syncytial virus, angioneurotic edema, theileriosis (caused by *Theileria parva* and *T. annulata*), ant bite, rinderpest, trypanosomiasis, malignant catarrhal fever, pneumonic pasturellosis.

Sheep and Goats
• Pink eye—outbreaks of conjunctivitis and corneal ulcers of one or both eyes most often associated in sheep with *Chlamydia psittaci* and in goats with *Mycoplasma* sp.; either agent can be the primary causative infecting organism in both species.
• Chlamydial outbreaks are highly infectious striking up to 90% in herd/flock; often associated with abortion outbreaks in does and lameness/arthritis of stifle, carpal, and tarsal joints. Chlamydiosis is also usually associated with severe eyelid edema and marked conjunctival lymphoid hyperplasia.
• Mycoplasma-related conjunctivitis often associated with less-severe conjunctivitis, but more severe nasal discharge, coughing, and pneumonia.
• *Mycoplasma* sp. also associated with mastitis and arthritis, but much less severe conjunctivitis
• *Neisseria ovis*
• Entropion/ectropion
• Foreign body/grass awn
• Cancer
• Cobalt deficiency
• Fly-strike
• Photosensitization—St. John's wort, heliotrope
• Vitamin A deficiency
• Listeriosis
• Sepsis

KERATOCONJUNCTIVITIS/CONJUNCTIVITIS

CBC/BIOCHEMISTRY/URINALYSIS
Changes consistent with possible underlying disease

OTHER LABORATORY TESTS
• Cornea staining with fluorescein (corneal ulcers exam)
• Topically applied anesthesia, evaluate orbit and adnexa for foreign bodies
• Microbial culture/sensitivity of eye fluids or conjunctival scrapes
• Conjunctival scrapings with cytologic evaluation—show inflammatory cells
• New methylene blue, Wright's, or Giemsa stains may show intracytoplasmic inclusions in epithelial cells. This occurs in one-third of chlamydial cases. Giemsa or Gram stain may show intracytoplasmic coccobacillary/ring-shaped bodies with mycoplasma.

Serology
• IFA for chlamydia, ELISA with mycoplasma to detect carrier animals
• Milk cultures in dairy goats for *M. mycoides* spp. *mycoides*

IMAGING
N/A

TREATMENT
• Isolation of affected animals and fly control.
• For parasitic external infections, mechanical removal and flushing may prove helpful; antibiotics topically or systemically for secondary infections; topical or systemic organophosphates (products approved for ophthalmic use only); steroid ointment may help with inflammation (cases without concomitant ulceration).

• Uncomplicated mycoplasmal and chlamydial eye infections are generally self-limiting without treatment; however, treatment may shorten course and decrease carrier state.
• Treatment of IBK is determined by economic considerations, drug efficacy, and withdrawal times, and feasibility of drug administration.

MEDICATIONS

DRUGS OF CHOICE
• Culture and sensitivity are indicated for appropriate therapeutic choice. Antibiotic therapy should be aimed at achieving drug concentrations in titers at a level high enough to meet or exceed the minimum inhibitory concentration (MIC) for an adequately sustained time period.
• Oxytetracycline ophthalmic ointment 3–4 times daily for 3–4 weeks
• Steroid ophthalmic ointment 2–3 times daily to decrease inflammation (cases without concomitant ulceration)
• Neomycin/polymyxin-B/bacitracin ophthalmic ointment 3–4 times daily for sensitive organisms
• Oxytetracycline systemically for mycoplasmal or chlamydial infections
• Tylosin systemically where culture and sensitivity indicate use for *Branhamella*.
• Atropine 1% ointment 1–2 times daily. If uveitis is present, provide shade from the sun. Llamas are very sensitive to atropine and may need atropine once every 3 days. Monitor pupil diameter to determine reapplication protocol.

• Treatment of isolated affected animals as early as possible with subcutaneous injections 48–72 hours apart with a long-acting tetracycline drug or florfenicol.
• Severe corneal ulceration cases may be given a subconjunctival injection of a long-acting penicillin or tetracycline. Possibly an eyelid flap procedure using absorbable suture material may be indicated. Similar treatment for sheep and goats may be indicated.

CONTRAINDICATIONS
• Do not use steroid preparations topically or systemically if a corneal ulcer is present.
• Appropriate milk and meat withdrawal times must be followed for all compounds administered to food-producing animals.
• Steroids should not be used in pregnant animals.

FOLLOW-UP

PATIENT MONITORING
Recheck corneal surface for ulceration weekly.

PREVENTION/AVOIDANCE
• Quarantine all new animals when entering the flock/herd, milk screening of dairy goats for mycoplasma, fly, and dust control.
• Mow fields to prevent physical abrasions.
• Decrease environmental stress (e.g., heat, particulate matter, bioaerosol level).
• Asymptomatic carriers can potentiate repeat outbreaks in following years.
• Resistance to repeat infection in the same animals is strong, but wanes after 2 to 3 years.

• Provision for uncrowded, shaded areas, fly control with insecticide bags hung near feeders and pyrethrum ear tags, keeping pastures mowed and free of thistle and grass awns and phytotoxic plants, possible vaccination program to be administered at least 30 days prior to sunny dry seasons.
• Do not vaccinate sheep and goat flocks that are unaffected, as this affects sera titer screens.
• Can vaccinate sheep and goats prior to breeding season, but carriers can maintain presence in flock.

POSSIBLE COMPLICATIONS
Blindness, abortions, lameness, and complications due to systemic disease

EXPECTED COURSE AND PROGNOSIS
• Mycoplasma generally resolves in 10 days, but may have recurring episodes for weeks; carriers possibly develop.
• Chlamydial infection generally resolves in 30 days with recurrence and carriers possible.

 MISCELLANEOUS

ASSOCIATED CONDITIONS
Ulceration, blindness, abortions, lameness

AGE-RELATED FACTORS
Generally in younger stock; however, all ages are susceptible.

ZOONOTIC POTENTIAL
• *Chlamydia* sp. can cause flulike symptoms in humans.
• Several of these diseases are zoonotic. Care must be taken in the collection of laboratory samples and the diagnosis/treatment of affected animals.

PREGNANCY
Some causes of keratoconjunctivitis can also cause abortion.

RUMINANT SPECIES AFFECTED
Cattle, sheep, and goats are most commonly affected. Llamas have not been reported with mycoplasmal conjunctivitis

BIOSECURITY
• Isolation and quarantine of new stock entering the herd/flock.
• Treat and or cull new animals for disease conditions prior to herd introduction.

PRODUCTION MANAGEMENT
Many eyelid disorders and ectopic cilia are hereditary problems. Avoid using these animals for breeding.

SEE ALSO
Blindness
Chlamydia spp.
Corneal ulcers
Entropion/ectropion
Mycoplasma spp.
Ophthalmic surgery

ABBREVIATIONS
ELISA = enzyme-linked immunoabsorbent assay
IBK = infectious bovine keratoconjunctivitis
IBR = infectious bovine rhinotracheitis
IFA = immunofluorescent antibody test
MIC = minimum inhibitory concentration

Suggested Reading
Brown, M. H., Brightman, A. H., Fenwick, B. W., Rider, M. A. 1998, Jul-Aug. Infectious bovine keratoconjunctivitis: a review. *J Vet Intern Med*. 12(4): 259–66.
Fowler, M. E. 1998. *Medicine and surgery of South American camelids*. 2nd ed. Ames: Iowa State University Press.
Gelatt, K. N. 2000. *Essentials of veterinary ophthalmology*. Baltimore: Lippincott, Williams and Wilkins.
Otter, A., Twomey, D. F., Rowe, N. S., Tipp, J. W., McElligott, W. S., Griffiths, P. C., O'Neill, P. 2003, Jun 21. Suspected chlamydial keratoconjunctivitis in British cattle. *Vet Rec*. 152(25): 787–88.
Shryock, T. R., White, D. W., Werner, C. S. 1998, Apr 15. Antimicrobial susceptibility of *Moraxella bovis*. *Vet Microbiol*. 61(4): 305–9.

Authors: Melissa N. Carr and Larry P. Occhipinti

KETOSIS (ACETONEMIA—DAIRY CATTLE)

BASICS

DEFINITION
• Ketosis is a metabolic disorder of lactating dairy cows resulting from an abnormal buildup of ketones in body tissues and fluids.
• The disorder is generally more common 4 to 6 weeks after calving, but can occur as early as a few days after parturition.
• Ketosis is characterized by hypoglycemia, ketonemia, ketonuria, acetone on breath, inappetance, either lethargy or high excitability, loss of weight, depressed milk production, and occasionally incoordination.

PATHOPHYSIOLOGY
• Contributory factors for ketosis have been attributed to two abnormalities in fatty acid oxidation and ketogenesis. The first abnormality is an insufficiency in carnitine palmitolyltransferase activity, which results in decreased entry of long chain fatty acids into the mitochondria.
• Bovine carnitine palmitolyltransferase is inhibited by lipogenic enzymes, such as malonyl-CoA carboxylase and fatty acid synthethase, which are induced by insulin and inhibited by glucagon.
• Lack of a continual insulin response and the resulting increase in the glucagon-to-insulin ratio in plasma of cows treated with glucagon may have been a factor in the increased rate of oxidation of fatty acids.
• The second contributory factor, oxaloacetate, is necessary for acetyl-CoA to enter the Krebs cycle and be oxidized to carbon dioxide.
• In addition, oxaloacetate is an intermediate in the synthesis of glucose from lactate, propionate, pyruvate and glucogenic amino acids. Oxaloacetate is formed during the conversion of pyruvate to phosphoenolpyruvate by pyruvate carboxylase.
• In dairy cows, glucagon increases expression of messenger RNA for pyruvate carboxylase.
• Administration of glucagon addresses the two factors that contribute to the development of ketosis, namely decreased activity of carnitine palmitoyltransferase and oxaloacetate insufficiency.

SYSTEMS AFFECTED
Hepatic, musculoskeletal

GENETICS
N/A

INCIDENCE/PREVALENCE
N/A

GEOGRAPHIC DISTRIBUTION
Worldwide, depending on production management

SIGNALMENT
Species
Bovine

Breed Predilections
N/A

Mean Age and Range
N/A

Predominant Sex
N/A

SIGNS

HISTORICAL FINDINGS
• The most commonly encountered clinical signs of ketosis include inappetance, constipation, mucus-covered feces, depression, a staring expression, loss of body weight, decreased milk production, and a humped back posture suggestive of mild abdominal pain. Acetone odor is also detected on the cow's breath. These signs are evident a few days to few weeks after calving in affected cows.
• Other common signs include circling, staggering, licking, chewing, bellowing, hyperesthesia, compulsive walking, and head pressing. These occur in episodes of approximately an hour in duration.

CAUSES AND RISK FACTORS
• Ketosis may occur as either primary or secondary ketosis.
• Primary ketosis is caused either by a negative energy balance due to a reduction in feed intake or absorption of dietary carbohydrate precursors.
• In contrast, secondary ketosis occurs due to a decrease in feed intake, commonly due to a preexisting condition such as metritis, mastitis, traumatic reticulitis, or abomasal displacement.

• The onset of ketosis is triggered by a drain on the cow's glucose reserve. As blood glucose concentrations decrease, body fat is mobilized to meet energy demands.
• A corresponding increase in the concentration of nonesterified fatty acids (NEFA) in blood is indicative of this fat mobilization (see Table 1). Although NEFA are metabolized in the liver, incomplete β-oxidation of NEFA leads to the formation of ketone bodies.

TREATMENT

Medicinal
• Cows with ketosis can be treated by intravenous infusion of 500 ml of dextrose. However, this treatment is only beneficial for a few hours, as most of the dextrose is excreted in the urine and thus can not be recommended as the sole treatment for ketosis.
• Glucocorticoids, such as dexamethasone (0.04 mg/kg) or betamethasone (0.04 mg/kg), reduce cellular uptake of glucose and are commonly used to extend the duration of the hyperglycemia caused by administration of dextrose.
• Overuse of glucocorticoids may result in a reduction of feed intake and exacerbate problems in cows with fatty liver.
• In addition, the treatment of ketosis is aimed at providing glucose precursors, such as glycerol, propylene glycol, and sodium propionate. Glycerol should be given 180 ml/day for 2 days then 90 ml/day for 2 days.
• Cattle with ketosis also can be drenched with propylene glycol (oral liquid, Crown) at 200 ml for the first day then 100 ml/day for 3 days.
• Sodium propionate should be administered orally at 100–250 g daily. Sodium propionate may be considered a more effective treatment of metabolic acidosis in diseases such as ketosis. The added propionate serves as a source for glucose for the cow.

Therapeutics
The concentration of glucose in the blood is regulated by insulin and glucagon, hormones produced by cells in the islets of Langerhans in the pancreas. The islets contain three major types of cells: alpha, beta, and delta.

KETOSIS (ACETONEMIA—DAIRY CATTLE)

Table 1

Blood Changes Associated with Ketosis		
Blood parameter	Normal	Ketosis
Blood glucose (mg/100 ml)	52	28
Blood ketones (mg/100 ml)	3	41
Plasma NEFA (mg/100 ml)[1]	3	33

Source: Adapted from Schultz (1978).
[1]NEFA = nonesterified fatty acids.

MEDICATIONS

CONTRAINDICATIONS
Appropriate milk and meat withdrawal times must be followed for all compounds administered to food-producing animals.

FOLLOW-UP

PREVENTION/AVOIDANCE
• The underlying mechanism responsible for clinical and subclinical ketosis is negative energy balance during the first 8 weeks of lactation.
• During late lactation and the dry period, feeding programs should be designed to promote good body condition scores at the time of calving. The model ration for early lactation cows should be highly palatable and energy dense, and introduced in a stepwise fashion.
• Prophylactic use of slow release insulin at a low dose (0.14 IU/kg of BW) has proven effective in preventing ketosis and hepatic lipidosis.

Energy Substrates
• Inclusion of specific precursors that increase the energy density of the diet during the last 3 weeks prepartum may be warranted.
• An increase in the amount of glucose precursors should promote hepatic gluconeogenesis and increase circulating concentrations of insulin. This should decrease hepatic triglyceride accumulation and NEFA mobilization.
• Supplementation of the diet with propylene glycol increases blood glucose and reduces NEFA mobilization and liver fat accumulation.
• Increasing the amount of starch in the diet may be the most effective strategy to increase energy density, and may increase plasma insulin concentration by as much as 300%.

Dietary Fat
• Altering the energy status of the dry cow by increasing dietary fat has not provided much improvement in the energy status of the dry cow.

Insulin
• Insulin, a peptide hormone composed of acidic and basic chains attached by disulphide bonds, is produced by beta cells. Insulin is an anabolic hormone and acts to preserve nutrients in their storage forms by stimulating glycogenesis, lipogenesis, and glycerol synthesis by inhibiting gluconeogenesis, glycogenolysis, and lipolysis.
• In ruminants, insulin can be a potent regulator of feed intake and nutrient partitioning. Therapeutic and physiological effects of coadministration of insulin and glucose have been evaluated for efficacy in treating cows with ketosis.
• The results of one study indicated that circulating concentrations of ketone bodies and nonesterified fatty acids were significantly lower in cows receiving glucose plus insulin (22.1 μU/ml and 0.79 mEq/L, respectively) than in cows receiving glucose alone (63.8 μU/ml and 0.98 mEq/L, respectively). Therefore, the concurrent use of glucose and insulin may be useful in the treatment of ketosis.

Glucagon
• Glucagon, a peptide hormone containing 29 amino acids, is a pancreatic hormone produced by the alpha cells of the islets of Langerhan. Glucagon stimulates hepatic gluconeogenesis, glycogenolysis, amino acid uptake, and ureagenesis.
• Continuous, intravenous infusion of glucagon in one study for 14 days beginning 21 days postpartum resulted in decreased liver triacylglycerol concentrations and the incidence of ketosis in dairy cows that were given 1,3-butanediol in the diet to induce fatty liver and ketosis.

• Intravenous infusion of glucagon also improves the carbohydrate status of lactating dairy cows without increasing plasma concentrations of NEFA. Because continuous intravenous infusion of glucagon is not practical for on-farm use, studies have been performed comparing single or multiple 5 mg injections of glucagon over a 14-day period. The results of these studies suggest that this treatment improves the carbohydrate status of dairy cows and decreases plasma concentrations of NEFA and β-hydroxybutyrate. Repeated daily, 15 mg injections of glucagon decreased hepatic concentrations of triacyclglycerol in cows older than 3.5 years, but failed to produce similar results in younger cows.
• Glucagon is not currently used in the treatment of ketosis, and it appears that its use would only be effective in animals older than 3.5 years.

DIET
• Because blood and liver concentrations of vitamin B_{12} decrease in cows after parturition, it has been recommended that niacin (6 g/day) be incorporated into the ration for up to 10 weeks after calving.
• Reduced concentrations of cobalt and vitamin B_{12} have been implicated as a cause of ketosis. Metabolism of propionate through the Krebs cycle requires vitamin B_{12}. Vitamin B_{12} can be added to the diet, but the efficacy of this vitamin in the treatment of ketosis has not been proven.

KETOSIS (ACETONEMIA—DAIRY CATTLE)

• Dietary fat does not decrease plasma concentrations of NEFA, liver triglycerides, or the development of metabolic diseases. In contrast, the results of one research trial indicated that inclusion of fat in the diet resulted in lower liver triglyceride concentrations, despite higher NEFA concentrations.

Pregnancy Toxemia of Beef Cattle: Protein Energy Malnutrition
Basics
Definition
• Pregnancy toxemia in beef cattle occurs as a result of a negative energy balance due to concurrent increases in energy demands and decreases in the quality and quantity of feed when caloric requirements are increased.
• The increased energy demand is due to fetal development and cold weather.

Signs

Historical Findings
Affected beef cows are usually thin with long hair coats, and their body temperature often is lower than normal. Affected cows that develop diarrhea die 7–14 days after becoming recumbent.

Diagnosis
Differential Diagnosis
• Hypocalcemia
• Listeriosis
• Polioencephalomalacia
• Hypomagnesemia
• Trauma
• Parasitism

CBC/Biochemistry/Urinalysis
• Serum calcium concentrations, packed cell volume, and insulin may be decreased. The liver is smaller than normal at necropsy, since fatty infiltration of hepatocytes occurs transitorily in protein-energy malnutrition.
• Ketonuria is not a common clinical manifestation of ketosis in beef cattle.

Pathologic Findings
Lesions from concurrent diseases may be observed if protein energy malnutrition is acute. A yellow fatty liver and decreased muscle mass often is present. Atrophy of fat has been observed in the coronary groove, bone marrow, and perirenal region.

Treatment
The administration of glucose precursors, such as propylene glycol (150–200 ml, orally), can be helpful to alleviate symptoms of pregnancy toxemia.

Prevention and Nutritional Control
The key to preventing pregnancy toxemia and hepatic lipidosis in pregnant beef cows is to ensure sufficient body condition (body condition score: 5 to 7) as the cow enters the last trimester of her pregnancy. An environmental temperature, at 0°C increases energy needs by 20%.

Contraindications
Appropriate milk and meat withdrawal times must be followed for all compounds administered to food-producing animals.

Miscellaneous
Associated Conditions
Overuse of glucocorticoids in treatment may result in a reduction of feed intake and exacerbate problems in cows with fatty liver.

Age-Related Factors
N/A

Zoonotic Potential
N/A

Pregnancy
N/A

Ruminant Species Affected
Bovine

Biosecurity
N/A

Production Management
• Because blood and liver concentrations of vitamin B$_{12}$ decrease in cows after parturition, it has been recommended that niacin (6 g/day) be incorporated into the ration for up to 10 weeks after calving.
• During late lactation and the dry period, feeding programs should be designed to promote good body condition scores at the time of calving. The model ration for early lactation cows should be highly palatable and energy dense, and introduced in a stepwise fashion.

 MISCELLANEOUS

SYNONYMS
N/A

SEE ALSO
Hypocalcemia
Hypomagnesemia
Listeriosis
Polioencephalomalacia
Pregnancy toxemia in small ruminants, body condition scoring by species

ABBREVIATIONS
BW = body weight
NEFA = nonesterified fatty acids

Suggested Reading
Aiello, R. J., Kenna, T. M., Herbein, J. H. 1984. Hepatic gluconeogenic and ketogenic interrelationships in the lactating cow. *J Dairy Sci.* 67:1707–15.
Bobe, G., Ametaj, B. N., Young, J. W., Beitz, D. C. 2003. Potential treatment of fatty liver with 14-day subcutaneous injections of glucagons. *J Dairy Sci.* 86:3138–47.
Bobe, G., Sonon, R. N., Ametaj, B. N., Young, J. W., Beitz, D. C. 2003. Metabolic response of lactating dairy cows to single and multiple subcutaneous injections of glucagons. *J Dairy Sci.* 86:2072–81.
Fleming, S. A. 1996. Metabolic disorders. In: *Large animal internal medicine: diseases of horses, cattle, sheep, and goats*, ed. B. P. Smith. 3rd ed. St. Louis: Mosby.
Grummer, R. R. 1993. Etiology of lipid-related metabolic disorders in preparturient dairy cows. *J Dairy Sci.* 76:3882–96.
Hayirli, A., Bertics, S. J., Grummer, R. R. 2002. Effects of slow–release insulin on production, liver triglyceride, and metabolic profiles of Holsteins in early lactation. *J Dairy Sci.* 85:2180–91.
Schultz, L.H. 1974. Ketosis. In: *Lactation, vol. 2.* New York: Academic Press.

Author: Douglas C. Donovan

LACTATION FAILURE (DYSGALACTIA, AGALACTIA, HYPOGALACTIA)

BASICS

OVERVIEW
• Agalactia is a clinical sign characterized by the absence of milk secretion, or the inability of a dam to lactate after parturition.
• Hypogalactia refers to an abrupt reduction in the normal amount of milk produced, and the term "dysgalactia" is sometimes used as a synonym.
• True agalactia can be present in situations of mammary gland aplasia or endocrinology problems that compromise milk synthesis.
• Secondary agalactia is much more common and is present as one of the clinical signs of infectious diseases, intoxications, or neoplasia.
• Contagious agalactia of small ruminants is a syndrome that principally affects the mammary glands, joints, and eyes. The main causal agents are *Mycoplasma agalactiae* in sheep, and *M. agalactiae*, *M. mycoides* subsp. *mycoides* large colony type, and *M. capricolum* subsp. *capricolum* in goats. In addition, *M. putrefaciens* can produce a similar clinical picture, particularly in goats.

SIGNALMENT
• Females just after parturition are most commonly affected.
• Contagious agalactia occurs on all five continents and is often enzootic.

SIGNS
In secondary agalactia or hypogalactia, some of the specific signs for the primary disease can be present, including:
• Depression
• Inappetence (feed refusal)
• Fever
• Swollen or inflamed quarter(s)
• Conjunctivitis and arthritis (infectious agalactia of small ruminants)

CAUSES
• Mammarian aplasia, dysplasia
• Peracute toxigenic mastitis (agalactia)
• Clinical mastitis (hypogalactia)
• Mycoplasma mastitis in small ruminants (agalactia)
• Leptospirosis (hypogalactia)
• Self-suckling or others suckling
• Water deprivation
• Intoxication (fungal toxins)
• Nutritional deficiency or imbalance (hypogalactia)
• Injury
• Neoplasia

RISK FACTORS
• Cows affected by peracute toxigenic mastitis caused by *Staphylococcus aureus*, *Escherichia coli*, or *Klebsiella* spp. show signs of severe toxemia, such as high fever (104°F–107°F), rumen stasis, and inappetence. Although not all quarters are usually affected, agalactia as a consequence of severe systemic illness can be present. The lactation curve is compromised and loss of the affected quarter is not uncommon. However, if treatment is successful, cows can reestablish milk production within 1 to 3 days.
• Contagious agalactia of sheep and goats is caused by *Mycoplasma agalactia* and can manifest in an acute, subacute, or chronic form. The udder shows signs of inflammation at the beginning of infection, milk secretion is watery and becomes purulent as the disease progresses, and agalactia is observed in the latter stages. Herd outbreaks may be accompanied by conjunctivitis and lameness (joint inflammation).
• Dysgalactia and agalactia caused by leptospirosis outbreaks have been described in cow and sheep herds.
• Grazing of tall fescue (*Festuca arundinacea*) that is contaminated with fungus (*Acremonium coenophialum*) has been shown to cause hypogalactia in cows. Feeding of grains contaminated with ergot (*Claviceps purpurea* in rye or *Clavicles africana* in sorghum) has produced clinical symptoms characterized by hypogalactia and eventual gangrene of extremities.

DIAGNOSIS

DIFFERENTIAL DIAGNOSIS
• Inability to secrete milk needs to be differentiated from inability to release milk from the alveolus or to pass it through the teat canal. Blockages need to be more fully examined.
• Primiparous females after parturition sometimes have trouble adapting to the new environment in the milking parlor and the administration of exogenous oxytocin (20 IU) may be necessary the first few days of lactation to accomplish milk release. This procedure may need to be repeated for some days until the animal has completely adapted.
• Proliferative granulation tissue or fibrosis (pencil obstruction) consequent to teat injury can cause partial or total obstruction of a teat canal, compromising milk flow. This is more common in one or two teats rather than hypogalactia or agalactia of the entire gland.

CBC/BIOCHEMISTRY/URINALYSIS
N/A

OTHER LABORATORY TESTS
N/A

IMAGING
N/A

DIAGNOSTIC PROCEDURES
Diagnostics should be based on case history, and specific laboratory analyses may be necessary depending on the primary disease.

TREATMENT
Treatment should be directed against the primary disease that is causing agalactia or hypogalactia.

LACTATION FAILURE (DYSGALACTIA, AGALACTIA, HYPOGALACTIA)

 MEDICATIONS

N/A

DRUGS OF CHOICE

N/A

CONTRAINDICATIONS

Appropriate milk and meat withdrawal times must be followed for all compounds administered to food-producing animals.

PRECAUTIONS

N/A

POSSIBLE INTERACTIONS

 FOLLOW-UP

N/A

POSSIBLE COMPLICATIONS

N/A

 MISCELLANEOUS

ASSOCIATED CONDITIONS

Contagious agalactia of small ruminants is a syndrome that principally affects the mammary glands, joints, and eyes.

AGE-RELATED FACTORS

N/A

ZOONOTIC POTENTIAL

Certain strains of *Leptospira*, *Chlamydiophila*, and *Mycoplasma* are considered zoonotic.

PREGNANCY

Mycoplasma spp. can cause abortions in ruminants.

RUMINANT SPECIES AFFECTED

Potentially, all ruminant species are affected.

BIOSECURITY

N/A

PRODUCTION MANAGEMENT

N/A

SYNONYMS

Hypogalactia, dysgalactia, and agalactia

SEE ALSO

Caprine and ovine mastitis
Mastitis microbial diagnosis
Mastitis microbiology
Milk quality
Mycoplasmal mastitis
Specific mastitis sections

ABBREVIATIONS

A = agalactia
H = hypogalactia
IU = international units

Suggested Reading

Bergonier, D., Berthelot, X., Poumarat, F. 1997, Dec. Contagious agalactia of small ruminants: current knowledge concerning epidemiology, diagnosis and control. *Rev Sci Tech.* 16(3):848–73.

Blaney, B. J., McKenzie, R. A., Walters, J. R., Taylor, L. F., Bewg, W. S., Ryley, M. J., Maryam, R. 2000, Feb. Sorghum ergot (*Claviceps africana*) associated with agalactia and feed refusal in pigs and dairy cattle. *Aust Vet J.* 78(2):102–107.

Kinde, H., DaMassa, A. J., Wakenell, P. S., Petty, R. 1994, Oct. Mycoplasma infection in a commercial goat dairy caused by Mycoplasma agalactiae and Mycoplasma mycoides subsp. mycoides (caprine biotype). *J Vet Diagn Invest.* 6(4):423–27.

Madanat, A., Zendulková, D., Pospisil, Z. 2001. Contagious agalactia of sheep and goats: a review. *ACTA Vet Brno.* 70:403–12.

McKeown, J. D., Ellis, W. A. 1986, Apr 26. *Leptospira hardjo* agalactia in sheep. *Vet Rec.* 118(17):482.

Quinlan, J. F., McNicholl, V. J. 1993. Agalactia and infertility due to *Leptospira interrogans* serovar *hardjo* infection in a vaccinated dairy herd. *Irish Vet J.* 46:97–98.

Author: Sérgio O. Juchem

LAMENESS IN SHEEP

BASICS

OVERVIEW
• Lameness is common in sheep.
• It is an important cause of economic loss due to decreased productivity, decreased fertility, and increased culling as well as the indirect costs associated with treating and managing the lame animals.
• The significant welfare implications of lameness cannot be over overestimated. Lameness in sheep should always be addressed and never ignored.
• Sheep may go lame for any number of reasons and generally it is possible to extrapolate from our knowledge of other species. There are, however, a number of conditions specific to sheep that require special consideration due to their infectious nature, the severity of the disease, and the economic and welfare costs associated with disease.
• Like all ruminants, the hooves of sheep grow continuously. Regular hoof care will decrease the chances of the animals developing severe lameness and will also allow the identification of more serious disease before it spreads throughout the flock.
• The three most important causes of lameness in sheep are: (1) infectious foot rot, (2) interdigital dermatitis, (3) contagious ovine digital dermatitis.

SIGNALMENT
• These conditions are most commonly seen in flock outbreaks of mature sheep, although they may affect all ages and breeds.
• Certain breeds of sheep (e.g., merino) appear to be more susceptible to foot rot.

SIGNS
• Lameness in one leg should be easily recognized by even inexperienced shepherds, however, in most cases, more than one limb are affected.
• Bilateral forelimb lameness often results in the animals flexing their carpi and "walking on their knees" with the development of severe calluses.
• In severe cases, the animal may become recumbent and be unable to reach feed and water resulting in severe loss of body condition.
• In some cases, fly-strike may complicate a foot rot lesion.
• Close examination of the feet is an absolute requirement of the examination of any lame sheep.

Interdigital Dermatitis (Scald)
• Lameness may be severe.
• The lesion is restricted to the interdigital skin especially in the heel region.
• The skin may be reddened or pale; there may be swelling and possible hair loss.
• Although the lesion appears mild, it causes significant discomfort.

Foot Rot
• Lameness is severe.
• There is severe underrunning of the hard horn. The lesion typically starts on the axial surface of the heel and in severe cases may result in complete separation of the axial wall and the sole from the underlying tissues.
• There is a characteristic malodorous exudate from the lesions.

Contagious Ovine Digital Dermatitis (CODD)—Hairy Heel Wart
• This unusual cause of lameness has been recently described in the United Kingdom.
• The lesion typically affects only one limb; there is severe undermining of the hoof wall and extreme pain.

CAUSES AND RISK FACTORS
• Interdigital dermatitis is caused by *Fusibacterium necrophorum* and nonvirulent strains of *Dichelobacter nodosus*.
• Contagious foot rot is caused by a number of virulent strains of *Dichelobacter nodosus* (previously *Bacteroides*).
• Prior infection of the foot with either *Fusobacterium necrophorum* or *Arcanobacterium pyogenes* may make it more susceptible to infection.
• The virulence of *D. nodosus* strains is associated with the production of heat-stable proteases and an increase in keratolytic activity.
• The cause of CODD is unknown. Analysis of samples from the lesions has demonstrated the presence of spirochetes, which appear to be similar to those associated with digital dermatitis in cattle.
• Severe lameness in sheep is generally associated with warm, wet conditions.
• The etiological agents of contagious foot rot and CODD do not survive for long periods in the environment (16 days maximum).
• The main mechanism of spreading the disease is by the purchase and introduction of clinically affected animals or subclinical carrier animals.

DIAGNOSIS

DIFFERENTIAL DIAGNOSIS
There are few conditions that can be confused with these causes of lameness:
• Foot and mouth disease virus
• Laminitis due to excessive carbohydrate consumption
• White line abscess formation
• Postdipping lameness—poorly maintained parasiticide dips resulting in infection with *Erysipelothrix rhusipathiae* (*E. rhusiopathiae*).

CBC/BIOCHEMISTRY/URINALYSIS
N/A

OTHER LABORATORY TESTS
N/A

IMAGING
N/A

DIAGNOSTIC PROCEDURES
• Not usually performed
• *Dichelobacter nodosus* may be cultured but requires special transport media.
• A biopsy of CODD lesions may be used to demonstrate the presence of spirochetes.

TREATMENT
• The mainstay of therapy for any form of lameness is proper hoof trimming.
• All animals should have their feet trimmed. The flock should be separated into clean and affected animals (trimming equipment should be disinfected between animals).
• Move animals through a 15% zinc sulfate footbath (150 g/L). If possible, affected animals should stand in the solution for at least 15 minutes.
• Animals should then be turned out to a clean (previous unused for a least 3 weeks) pasture.
• The process should be repeated at weekly intervals until the disease is controlled.
• Severely affected animals or those responding poorly to treatment should be culled.

MEDICATIONS

DRUGS OF CHOICE
• Animals with severe foot rot should be treated with a long-acting oxytetracycline product (20 mg/kg).
• Anecdotal evidence suggests that an oxytetracycline footbath (similar to that used for cattle) may be of benefit for the treatment of CODD.

CONTRAINDICATIONS
• Most drugs are not licensed for use in sheep, therefore these recommendations constitute an off-label use of the drugs.
• Appropriate milk and meat withdrawal times must be followed for all compounds administered to food-producing animals.
• Steroids should not be used in pregnant animals.

FOLLOW-UP

PATIENT MONITORING
• Dealing with these diseases is extremely costly and time consuming.
• Repeated treatments are necessary.

PREVENTION/AVOIDANCE
• Due to the high costs associated with the disease, prevention is the goal.
• Sheep that are new to the flock from an unknown source should always have their feet trimmed and treated.
• They should then be placed in isolation for 2 weeks prior to introduction to the rest of the flock.
• Multivalent vaccines are available in some parts of the world and are an effective means of control, however, immunity is short lived.

EXPECTED COURSE AND PROGNOSIS
• Foot rot: The majority of animals will recover without incident.
• CODD: The prognosis for this condition is guarded.

MISCELLANEOUS

ASSOCIATED CONDITIONS
Lameness, loss of productivity, and subsequent culling from the flock

AGE-RELATED FACTORS
N/A

ZOONOTIC POTENTIAL
N/A

PREGNANCY
N/A

RUMINANT SPECIES AFFECTED
Sheep

BIOSECURITY
• A good biosecurity program is the most effective way of preventing an outbreak of severe lameness in sheep.
• Sheep that are new to the flock from an unknown source should always have their feet trimmed and treated.
• They should then be placed in isolation for 2 weeks prior to introduction to the rest of the flock.

PRODUCTION MANAGEMENT
All animals should have their feet trimmed. The flock should be separated into clean and affected animals (trimming equipment should be disinfected between animals).

SYNONYMS
Hairy heel wart
Scald
Strawberry foot rot

SEE ALSO
Ewe flock nutrition
Foot rot in sheep
Laminitis
Sheep nutrition
Sheep selection and breeding

ABBREVIATIONS
CODD = contagious ovine digital dermatitis

Suggested Reading
Clements, A. C., Mellor, D. J., Fitzpatrick, J. L. 2002, Jun 29. Reporting of sheep lameness conditions to veterinarians in the Scottish borders. *Vet Rec.* 150(26): 815–17.
Hosie, B. 2004, Jan 10. Foot rot and lameness in sheep. *Vet Rec.* 154(2): 37–38.
Reilly, L.K., Baird, A.N. and Pugh, D.G. 2002. Diseases of the musculoskeletal system. In: *Sheep and goat medicine*, ed. D.G. Pugh. Philadelphia: W. B. Saunders Company.
Wassink, G. J., Grogono-Thomas, R., Moore, L. J., Green, L. E. 2004, May 1. Risk factors associated with the prevalence of interdigital dermatitis in sheep from 1999 to 2000. *Vet Rec.* 154(18). 551–55.

Author: Chris Clark

LAMINITIS IN CATTLE

 BASICS

OVERVIEW
• Laminitis is a common, multifactorial disease causing lameness in cattle.
• Laminitis is the most common lameness causing disease in dairy cattle and is often found in beef cattle on high-concentrate diets. Laminitis is a diffuse aseptic inflammation of the dermis (corium) of the claw that can be acute, subacute, or chronic.
• The lesions attributable to laminitis are the result of systemic disease associated with dysfunction of the digital vasculature and/or sinkage of the third phalanx with subsequent production of poor-quality horn in the sole, wall, heel, and white line of the hoof capsule.
• Laminitis rarely occurs as acute laminitis, but when it does it is a medical emergency (grain overload).
• Subacute, or chronic, laminitis is much more common in both dairy and beef cattle.
• Subclinical laminitis is sometimes referred to, and is characterized by soft yellow sole and heel horn with hemorrhages in the sole and white line but no concurrent lameness.

PATHOPHYSIOLOGY
• There is speculation that excess production of histamines from protein sources or endotoxins from gram-negative bacteria occur after feeding high-concentrate diets under acid conditions (subacute rumen acidosis, SARA).
• The histamines or endotoxins may then set up a metabolic cascade resulting in decreased oxygen and nutrient supply to the corium. Once the corium is damaged, poor-quality horn is produced, which leads to further damage from mechanical or environmental conditions (high moisture, manure slurry). If the vascular insult lasts long enough, the distal phalanx sinks within the hoof capsule causing further damage to the corium.
• Sinkage of the distal phalanx is thought to be irreversible. There has been speculation that the vascular insult results in separation of the laminae, which leads to sinking of the third phalanx; however, separation of the laminae has not been found to be a prominent feature in pathological samples examined.
• A more current theory is that laminitis is due to failure of the suspensory apparatus for the third phalanx, which occurs around the time of parturition and allows the distal phalanx to sink.
• It has also been noted that the digital cushion in animals with laminitis has more connective tissue and less fat and provides less protection of the corium from concussion.
• Other researchers have proposed a role of metaloproteinases in allowing the suspensory apparatus to relax with resultant sinking of the distal phalanx.

SYSTEMS AFFECTED
• Dermatologic
• Musculoskeletal (secondary to complicated laminitis lesions)

GENETICS
Laminitis has an estimated heritability of 0.14–0.22.

INCIDENCE/PREVALENCE
Variable, from 5%–50% or greater

GEOGRAPHIC DISTRIBUTION
Worldwide

SIGNALMENT
Species
Bovine, both dairy and beef
Breed Predilections
• Laminitis is seen most often in dairy breeds due to long periods of feeding high-concentrate rations to promote milk yield.
• In beef cattle, it is more often seen in feedlot cattle than cattle housed on pasture or range.
Mean Age and Range
First-calf cows are more likely to have subacute lesions (sole and white line hemorrhage) due to factors associated with first calving, such as large change in energy density of feed and change in housing, lactation, and growth, all occurring simultaneously.
Predominant Sex
Seen more in dairy cows

SIGNS
HISTORICAL FINDINGS
Increased lameness as a herd problem with laminitis-associated lesions (see Physical Examination Findings and Risk Factors).
PHYSICAL EXAMINATION FINDINGS
• In acute laminitis, animals are clinically lame and walk with arched backs.
• Affected cattle may shift weight from foot to foot and are reluctant to move.
• Hooves are tender to hoof testers.
• Pyrexia and anorexia are commonly seen.
• There are no visible alterations in the hoof; however, increased warmth and pulsation may be discernable.
• In subacute laminitis, the sole will have hemorrhage or yellow discoloration, which will be visible 6–8 weeks after the initial insult.
• In chronic or recurrent-chronic laminitis, the shape of the claw is altered, where the claw becomes broad with concavity of the dorsal wall ("slipper foot").
Lesions Related to Laminitis
• Red and/or yellowish discoloration and softness of sole horn
• Horizontal grooves and fissures on the wall (hardship grooves, thimbles)
• Abnormal shape of the claw—becomes broader and flatter, and dorsal wall becomes furrowed and concave (slipper foot)

• Sole and heel ulcers
• Toe ulcers and abscesses
• Double sole
• White line separation, hemorrhages, or abscesses
• Dropped sole

CAUSES
• A combination of predisposing factors leads to displacement of the third phalanx and/or disruption of digital-vascular system causing production of poor-quality horn.
• Manure slurry and constant moisture will soften the already damaged horn.
• Hard floors will cause increased pressure to the damaged corium, which can lead to full thickness ulcers or allow abscesses to form.

RISK FACTORS
Housing conditions (concrete flooring, wet floors, manure slurry, time standing on concrete, bedding, stall comfort), genetics, breeding, nutrition and feeding management (high-concentrate, low effective fiber, wet feeds, slug feeding, ruminal acidosis), periparturient period (calving, transition to lactating cow rations, hormonal changes)

 DIAGNOSIS

DIFFERENTIAL DIAGNOSIS
Other causes of lameness: digital dermatitis, interdigital phlegmon, hoof overgrowth due to imbalance of growth and wear, thin soles due to excessive wear

CBC/BIOCHEMISTRY/URINALYSIS
N/A

OTHER LABORATORY TESTS
N/A

IMAGING
N/A

DIAGNOSTIC PROCEDURES
History and clinical observation

PATHOLOGIC FINDINGS
Sinkage of the third phalanx, decreased fat content of the digital cushion, inflammation of the corium and epidermis, exostosis of third phalanx, decreased thickness of corium, abnormal claw shape, overgrowth of lateral, hind claws

 TREATMENT

APPROPRIATE HEALTH CARE
• Functional hoof trimming should be performed at least one to two times per year, which will help to redistribute weight bearing and allow normal horn formation to resume.
• Sole ulcers should have the surrounding horn thinned to allow growth of new horn.

• An orthopedic block should be applied to the sound claw to allow the diseased claw to rest and heal.
• White line abscesses will need to be opened and all necrotic tissue removed.
• Lesion borders should be thin so that corium is not pinched during the healing process.

NURSING CARE
Affected dairy cows should be placed in pens close to the milking parlor. If treated cattle are bandaged, the bandages will need to be removed after 3–5 days.

ACTIVITY
Walking should be limited as much as possible for lame cattle.

DIET
Normal

CLIENT EDUCATION
• Clients should understand the relationship between various risk factors and laminitis.
• Nutrition and feeding management as well as cow comfort should be monitored and changes made as necessary to keep laminitis (and lameness) at an acceptable level.

SURGICAL CONSIDERATIONS
Deeper infections (septic arthritis or tenosynovitis) seen as sequelae to sole ulcers or white line disease may require claw amputation as a salvage operation.

MEDICATIONS

DRUGS OF CHOICE
For treatment of acute laminitis (grain overload):
• Flunixin meglumine (1.1–2.2 mg/lb once per day for ≤ 3 days) is not labeled for lactating or dry dairy cows.
• Dexamethasone (see label for dose, withdrawal, and class of animals).

CONTRAINDICATIONS
• Dexamethazone can cause abortion in pregnant cows with possible dystocia, retained placenta, and metritis.
• Appropriate milk and meat withdrawal times must be followed for all compounds administered to food-producing animals.

PRECAUTIONS
See Causes and Risk Factors above.

POSSIBLE INTERACTIONS
N/A

ALTERNATIVE DRUGS
N/A

FOLLOW-UP

PATIENT MONITORING
• Animals with sole ulcers or white line disease should be rechecked after 1–2 weeks. Lesion

should be cleaned and the wall or sole thinned again at the edge of the lesion, if necessary.
• If granulation tissue is present, it must be removed.

PREVENTION/AVOIDANCE
• Periodic locomotion scoring of cows will alert management when lameness incidence is increasing and allow timely investigation and action to prevent laminitis (or other lameness-causing diseases).
• Animal comfort with good bedding, comfortable stalls, and yielding walking surfaces will help decrease incidence.
• Proper nutrition and feeding management are critical.
• Make sure that there is a gradual transition from dry cow to lactating rations in dairy cattle and that cows have adequate effective fiber.
• Zinc methionine and biotin have been shown to decrease lesions associated with laminitis.
• Research has shown that the digital cushions in heifers contain less fat and therefore provide less cushion than in cows.
• Heifers should have enough time (i.e., 2 months, if going from dirt to concrete) to adapt to new corrals or freestalls before calving.
• For beef cattle, a gradual transition from high roughage to concentrate feeding should attenuate the incidence of laminitis.

POSSIBLE COMPLICATIONS
Sole or toe ulcers or white line abscesses, if not treated early, can progress into deeper infections with involvement of the bones, joints, tendons, and ligaments of the foot.

EXPECTED COURSE AND PROGNOSIS
• Most cases of laminitis that cause lameness can be treated by functional hoof trimming and treating the lesion and will have a good prognosis for recovery.
• If animals have had chronic or recurrent-chronic laminitis and the pedal bone has dropped in the claw capsule, the prognosis for recovery is worse.
• Sole ulcers, toe ulcers, white line abscesses, and heel ulcers will require follow-up care and may require replacement of orthopedic blocks after several weeks.

MISCELLANEOUS

ASSOCIATED CONDITIONS
Subacute ruminal acidosis

AGE-RELATED FACTORS
First lactation dairy cows are especially prone to laminitis-related lesions (sole and white line hemorrhage).

ZOONOTIC POTENTIAL
N/A

PREGNANCY
Changes in hormonal balance, relaxing of the pedal bone suspensory apparatus, changes in

diet due to dry cow to lactating rations are predisposing factors for laminitis.

RUMINANT SPECIES AFFECTED
Bovine

BIOSECURITY
N/A

PRODUCTION MANAGEMENT
• Good cow comfort, especially for springing heifers, is critical to allow cows to spend an adequate amount of time lying.
• Time standing on concrete, whether due to overcrowding, poor stall design or bedding, or long times in the holding area and milking parlor, will increase laminitis.
• Slug-feeding, sorting feed, or overmixing total mixed rations will predispose to subacute rumen acidosis, which, in turn will predispose to laminitis.

SYNONYMS
Coriosis, diffuse pododermatitis aseptica, pododermatitis

SEE ALSO
• (Papillomatous) digital dermatitis
• Heel horn erosion
• Hoof overgrowth
• Hoof trimming
• Rumen dysfunction: acidosis

ABBREVIATIONS
SARA = subacute ruminal acidosis

Suggested Reading
Bergsten, C. 2003. Causes, risk factors, and prevention of laminitis and related claw lesions. *Acta Vet Scand Suppl*. 98:157–66.
Cook, N. B., Nordlund, K. V., Oetzel, G. R. 2004. Environmental influences on claw horn lesions associated with laminitis and subacute ruminal acidosis in dairy cows. *J Dairy Sci*. 87:E36–E46.
Donovan, G. A., Risco, C. A., DeChant Temple, G. M., Tran, T. Q., Van Horn, H. H. 2004. Influence of transition diets on occurrence of subclinical laminitis in Holstein dairy cows. *J Dairy Sci*. 87:73–84.
Lischer, Ch. J., Ossent, P., Raber, M., Geyer, H. 2002. Suspensory structures and supporting tissues of the third phalanx of cows and their relevance to the development of typical sole ulcers (Rusterholz ulcers). *Vet Rec*. 151:694–98.
Nordlund, K. V., Cook, N. B., Oetzel, G. R. 2004. Investigation strategies for laminitis problem herds. *J Dairy Sci*. 87:E27–E35.
Stokka, G. L., Lechtenberg, K., Edwards, T., MacGregor, S., Voss, K., Griffin, D., Grotelueschen, D. M., Smith, R. A., Perino, L. J. 2001. Lameness in feedlot cattle. *Vet Clin N Amer Food Anim Pr*. 17:189–208.
van Amstel, S. R., Shearer, J. K. 2001. Abnormalities of hoof growth and development. *Vet Clin N Amer Food Anim Pr*. 17:73–92.

Author: Steven L. Berry

LANTANA TOXICOSIS

 BASICS

OVERVIEW

• Lantana is thought to have originated in Central America, but today is widely spread throughout the tropics and subtropics of the world. Some 150–160 species and more than 75 named varieties exist.
• Resides in the Verbenaceae, commonly known as the verbena or vervain family.
• An uncommon cause of intoxication, lantana can be a significant cause of poisoning and death losses where it grows wild.
• Mortality is high in severe cases.
• Cattle are most frequently affected.
• It primarily affects the hepatobiliary system and skin. Renal and gastrointestinal systems are often involved as well.
• A squarestemmed perennial herb or shrub ranging between 0.5 and 1.2 m tall, lantana produces flowers in dense spikes from spring to fall.
• The plants are often used as ornamentals because of their showy flowers that come in a wide variety of colors—white, red, yellow, orange, blue, and purple. Different colors may exist on the same plant and colors change as the flowers mature.
• Fruits occur in clusters, initially green then becoming dark purple to black when ripe.
• Simple leaves with serrated margins are ovate to lanceolate in shape and are arranged in opposite or whorled patterns. They emit an aromatic odor when crushed.
• Stems are erect and prickly with yellow, orange, and red petals on *Lantana camara*. Common name—"ham and eggs."
• Stems on *Lantana montevidensis* are trailing and smooth, with red to purple petals.
• Poisonings are most common in summer and fall, often due to clippings being consumed.
• Frequently planted as an ornamental, lantana has often escaped and become wild.

SIGNALMENT

• Although ruminants tend to be more commonly poisoned, most animal species, including sheep, goats, horses, dogs, wildlife, and children, are susceptible.
• There are no known breed, species, or sex predilections.

SIGNS

• Intoxication and related clinical signs depend upon the amount consumed and the rate of ingestion.
• Signs of acute intoxication may be seen within 24 hours postconsumption.
• Initially depression, weakness, anorexia, depressed ruminal motility, and constipation (often severe) occur.
• Within 2 to 4 days, icterus, bloody diarrhea, skin changes associated with photosensitization, paralysis, and death can be seen.
• Death may be prolonged over several weeks and is due to hepatic disease and renal failure.
• Dehydration and electrolyte imbalances (metabolic acidosis) also play roles in the pathogenesis.
• Chronic poisoning develops over several weeks and primarily involves photosensitization.
• Icterus, oronasal ulcerations, keratitis, and increased sensitivity to light may also be found.

CAUSES AND RISK FACTORS

• Lantadenes are hepatotoxic triterpene acids. Lantadene A is considered the most toxic; lantadene B is less toxic.
• Numerous cultivars and hybrids exist, possessing varying amounts of lantadenes with differing levels of toxicity.
• Leaves are the primary source of lantadene.
• Green fruits may possess other toxins—children have been poisoned with the absence of liver disease after consumption of green fruit. Ripened fruit and seeds are not toxic and reportedly are sometimes sought after by sheep and goats.

• Five to 10 g of dried leaves/kg of body weight will produce severe, often fatal poisoning in sheep and cattle.
• Lantadenes are absorbed primarily from the small intestine, but also the rumen. They are transformed in the liver and excreted in the bile, resulting in an obstructive cholangitis. Conjugated bilirubin and phylloerythrin are retained. Phylloerythrin accumulates in hepatocytes and the skin. When activated by sunlight, it results in tissue damage—photosensitization.
• The effects of lantadenes are cumulative. Subacute poisoning over 1 to 2 days is more common than acute intoxication.
• Lantadenes also have a direct effect on the GI tract, causing severe mucosal irritation. Ruminal stasis, secondary to liver disease, decreases rumen microflora activity. This leads to an increase in pH and ammonia nitrogen.

 DIAGNOSIS

DIFFERENTIAL DIAGNOSIS

• The signs of lantana intoxication are nonspecific. A number of hepatotoxic plants are listed.
  • *Helenium* spp.—sneezeweed
  • *Hymenoxys* spp.—rubber weed, bitterweed
  • *Senecia* spp.
  • *Crotolaria* spp.
• Oak poisoning may also produce signs similar to acute lantana intoxication.
• Clinical signs, history of ingestion, finding plants in feed, hay, or rumen contents are supportive of a diagnosis.

CBC/BIOCHEMISTRY/URINALYSIS

• Serum bilirubin is elevated; the majority of which is conjugated.
• Serum hepatic enzymes, SDH and AST, are elevated.
• BSP clearance is decreased.

OTHER LABORATORY TESTS
N/A

IMAGING
N/A

DIAGNOSTIC PROCEDURES
N/A

PATHOLOGIC FINDINGS
- Icteric tissues
- Skin lesions due to photosensitization
- Keratitis
- Gastroenteritis
- Obstructive cholangitis
- Enlarged orange-tinted liver
- Enlarged gall bladder
- Enlarged kidneys with perirenal edema
- Periportal degeneration, portal fibrosis, bile duct hyperplasia, centrilobular necrosis
- Hepatocyte enlargement with multiple nuclei
- Renal tubular necrosis with casts
- Hyperemic and edematous GI mucosa

TREATMENT

- Remove affected animals from sunlight, provide shade.
- Prevent animal access to lantana.
- Removal/destruction of lantana—it is susceptible to 2, 4-D herbicides.
- Support patient, treat symptomatically, maintain hydration and electrolytes.
- Rumenotomy with evacuation of contents may be worthwhile if performed early.

MEDICATIONS

- Control absorption of toxins from the GI tract—activated charcoal—2–5 g/kg in a water slurry given orally (1 g charcoal per 5 ml water).
- Na thiosulfate—0.5 g/kg BW IV may be beneficial.
- Systemic and topical antibiotics

CONTRAINDICATIONS
Appropriate milk and meat withdrawal times must be followed for all compounds administered to food-producing animals.

POSSIBLE INTERACTIONS

FOLLOW-UP

PATIENT MONITORING
N/A

PREVENTION/AVOIDANCE
- Providing a proper diet and adequate nutrition to animals will minimize the intake of many toxic plants.
- Protective immunization has been studied and provided limited protection. Results were thought to be promising.

POSSIBLE COMPLICATIONS
None

EXPECTED COURSE AND PROGNOSIS
- Variable, dependent upon the amount and rate of consumption
- High mortality is expected with acute cases.
- Many animals will survive moderate cases of intoxication.

MISCELLANEOUS

ASSOCIATED CONDITIONS
None

AGE-RELATED FACTORS
None

ZOONOTIC POTENTIAL
None

PREGNANCY
None

RUMINANT SPECIES AFFECTED
All ruminant species can be affected.

BIOSECURITY
N/A

PRODUCTION MANAGEMENT
N/A

SEE ALSO
Specific toxicology agent chapter

ABBREVIATIONS
AST = aspartate aminotransferase or aspartate transaminase
BSP = bromosulfophthalein
BW = body weight
GI = gastrointestinal
IV = intravenous
SDH = sorbitol dehydrogenase

Suggested Reading
Burrows, G. E., Tyrl, R. J., ed. 2001. *Toxic plants of North America*. Ames: Iowa State University Press.
Hammond, A. C. 1995, May. Leucaena toxicosis and its control in ruminants. *J Anim Sci*. 73(5):1487–92.
Ide, A., Tutt, C. L. 1998, Mar. Acute *Lantana camara* poisoning in a Boer goat kid. *J S Afr Vet Assoc*. 69(1):30–32.
McLennan, M. W., Amos, M. L. 1989, Mar. Treatment of lantana poisoning in cattle. *Aust Vet J*. 66(3):93–94.
Pass, M. A. 1986, Jun. Current ideas on the pathophysiology and treatment of lantana poisoning of ruminants. *Aust Vet J*. 63(6):169–71.
Sharma, O. P., Singh, A., Sharma, S. 2000, Sep. Levels of lantadenes, bioactive pentacyclic triterpenoids, in young and mature leaves of *Lantana camara* var. *aculeata*. *Fitoterapia*. 71(5):487–91.

Author: Matt G. Welborn

LARYNGEAL OBSTRUCTION

 BASICS

DEFINITION
Laryngeal obstruction in ruminants has many causes, including abscesses, granulomas, papillomas, chondritis, trauma, edema, and foreign bodies.

SYSTEMS AFFECTED
Respiratory

GENETICS
N/A

INCIDENCE/PREVALENCE
N/A

GEOGRAPHIC DISTRIBUTION
Worldwide

SIGNALMENT
Species
• All ruminant species are susceptible.
• Abscesses of the arytenoid cartilages tend to occur in calves and sheep.
• Laryngeal granulomas and papillomas tend to occur in feedlot cattle.
• Laryngeal chondritis can occur in sheep.
• Foreign bodies tend to be ingested more readily by cattle.

Breed Predilections
• Laryngeal abscesses in sheep may occur more commonly in Texel and Southdown breeds.
• Laryngeal chondritis in sheep may occur more commonly in the Texel breed.

Mean Age and Range
N/A

Predominant Sex
Laryngeal abscesses in sheep may occur more commonly in rams than in ewes.

SIGNS

HISTORICAL FINDINGS
May be history of recent medication with a balling gun or dosing syringe, or exposure to a feedlot environment, or smoke inhalation, or participation in a roping event.

PHYSICAL EXAMINATION FINDINGS
Dyspnea and/or stertorous breathing exaggerated by palpation of the larynx, extended neck, palpable laryngeal swelling, hypersalivation, cyanosis in severe cases

CAUSES AND RISK FACTORS
• Laryngeal abscesses, chronic laryngitis, laryngeal granulomas and papillomas, edema, chondritis, and foreign bodies may all cause laryngeal obstruction.
• Laryngeal abscesses may be caused by bacterial infection—mainly *Arcanobacterium* (*Actinomyces*) *pyogenes*—of the arytenoid cartilages secondary to laryngeal trauma (e.g., from a balling gun or dosing syringe). Chronic laryngitis due to *A. pyogenes* infection in sheep may also cause laryngeal obstruction.
• Laryngeal granulomas may originate from chronic laryngeal contact ulcers (e.g., in feedlot cattle).
• Laryngeal papillomas are caused by a papovavirus, which enters chronic laryngeal contact ulcers.
• Edema of the larynx may be caused by smoke inhalation or anaphylactic reactions, or by laryngeal chondritis in sheep.
• Foreign bodies may lodge in the larynx, although they more commonly lodge in the pharynx.

 DIAGNOSIS

DIFFERENTIAL DIAGNOSIS
• Necrotic laryngitis
• Actinobacillosis
• Tumors
• Pharyngeal trauma and/or obstruction

CBC/BIOCHEMISTRY/URINALYSIS
Inflammatory profile or stress leukogram

OTHER LABORATORY TESTS
• Biopsy/histopathology of laryngeal mass
• Cytology and culture of aspirated material from a laryngeal abscess

IMAGING
• Endoscopy is useful for direct visualization of the obstruction, and may be used for transendoscopic removal of the obstruction.
• Radiology of upper respiratory system

OTHER DIAGNOSTIC PROCEDURES
N/A

PATHOLOGIC FINDINGS
• Laryngeal abscesses—encapsulated abscesses in the arytenoid cartilages near the vocal fold.
• Laryngeal papillomas—sessile to pedunculated yellow frondlike growths over the vocal processes of the arytenoid cartilages.

 TREATMENT

• Tracheostomy in severe cases of laryngeal obstruction
• Surgical or transendoscopic removal of obstructing mass or object

ACTIVITY
Restrict activity due to dyspnea

DIET
Softened feed may be less irritating to the laryngeal region following removal of the obstruction.

CLIENT EDUCATION
Proper use of a balling gun and/or dosing syringe so as to minimize trauma.

MEDICATIONS
• Broad-spectrum antibiotics, and NSAIDs
• Epinephrine if obstruction due to anaphylaxis (4–8 ml of 1:1000 solution per 500 kg IV for cattle, 1–3 ml of 1:1000 solution IM or SQ for average adult sheep or goat)

DRUGS OF CHOICE
N/A

CONTRAINDICATIONS
Appropriate milk and meat withdrawal times must be followed for all compounds administered to food-producing animals.

PRECAUTIONS
N/A

POSSIBLE INTERACTIONS
N/A

ALTERNATIVE DRUGS
N/A

FOLLOW-UP
Tracheostomy site may need to be surgically closed.

PATIENT MONITORING
Tracheostomy site needs to be regularly monitored and cleaned.

PREVENTION/AVOIDANCE
• See Client Education above.
• Decreasing laryngeal contact ulcers in feedlot cattle by dust control and routine vaccination for respiratory pathogens may reduce the incidence of laryngeal granulomas and papillomas.

POSSIBLE COMPLICATIONS
Tracheostomy can predispose animal to lower respiratory infections since the filtering and humidifying action of the upper respiratory passages is bypassed.

EXPECTED COURSE AND PROGNOSIS
Laryngeal abscesses have a guarded prognosis unless detected and treated early.

MISCELLANEOUS

ASSOCIATED CONDITIONS
N/A

AGE-RELATED FACTORS
N/A

ZOONOTIC POTENTIAL
N/A

PREGNANCY
N/A

RUMINANT SPECIES AFFECTED
All ruminant species

BIOSECURITY
N/A

PRODUCTION MANAGEMENT
Proper use of a balling gun and/or dosing syringe so as to minimize trauma

SYNONYMS
N/A

SEE ALSO
Actinobacillosis
Necrotic laryngitis
Necrotic stomatitis
Pharyngeal trauma and/or obstruction
Pneumonia
Respiratory pharmacology
Tumors

ABBREVIATIONS
NSAIDs = nonsteroidal anti-inflammatory drugs
IM = intramuscular
IV = intravenous
SQ = subcutaneous

Suggested Reading
Pugh, D. G., ed. 2002. *Sheep and goat medicine.* Philadelphia: W. B. Saunders.
Radostits, O. M., Gay, C. C., Blood, D. C., Hinchcliff, K. W., eds. 2000. *Veterinary medicine.* 9th ed. London: W. B. Saunders.
Smith, B. P., ed. 2002. *Large animal internal medicine.* 3rd ed. St. Louis: Mosby.

Author: David McKenzie

LEAD TOXICOSIS

 BASICS

OVERVIEW
- Most cases of lead poisoning occur in cattle.
- The vast majority of lead poisoning cases is the result of acute oral exposures; chronic exposures are rare in ruminants.
- Lead sources are many, but most poisonings result from ingesting battery plates.
- The onset of signs is abrupt, and typically includes signs associated with the gastrointestinal tract and central (and to a lesser extent, peripheral) nervous systems.
- Death with few to no premonitory signs may be observed in calves and young animals.
- Death or euthanasia is a common sequelae, due to the severity of neurological signs.
- Antemortem diagnosis relies on elevated blood lead levels and evidence of radiodense objects in the gastrointestinal tract (more common to find in the reticulum). Excessive liver and kidney lead levels; evidence of lead particles in the GIT (reticulum, rumen); and histologic evidence of laminar cortical necrosis provide postmortem evidence for a diagnosis of lead poisoning.
- Treatment, if possible and economically viable, includes administration of oral magnesium sulfate, thiamine, Ca-EDTA, along with supportive care targeted to those signs observed.
- Prognosis is generally poor, and care must be taken in considering home or custom slaughter due to tissue residues.

PATHOPHYSIOLOGY
- Lead salts are absorbed from the gastrointestinal tract.
- The majority of lead is bound to surface proteins of red blood cells.
- Lead has a wide tissue distribution and long half-life (approximately 9 days), and ultimately forms deposits in bone where it resides for years and is considered biologically inert.
- Any bone remodeling can lead to the release of stored lead.
- Lead can cross the placenta and be secreted into the milk.
- Lead affects multiple systems, and the effects are varied depending on whether the exposure is acute or chronic.
- Lead interferes with sulfhydryl and zinc containing enzymes, leading to erythrocyte fragility, bone marrow suppression, and interference with heme synthesis (more common to see these changes with chronic exposures), along with interfering with various neurotransmitters in the CNS.
- Neurological signs may be due to cerebral edema as a result of increased vascular permeability.
- Segmental demyelination of peripheral nerves (e.g., pharyngeal) may be seen.
- Pb will interfere with calcium absorption from the gut, along with displacing calcium in multiple sites.
- Lead, in people, is immunotoxic and carcinogenic.

SYSTEMS AFFECTED
Gastrointestinal and central (and possibly) peripheral nervous systems are the primary targets; other systems affected may include red blood cells, bone marrow, kidney, and liver.

Toxic Dose
- The toxic dose for cattle has been determined experimentally. The acute toxic dose may range from 400–800 mg/kg and the acute dose may range from 1–7 mg/kg/day. These are from experimental exposures and differ from clinical cases where the amount and form of lead ingested is generally not known.
- Cattle—intakes of greater than 6 mg/kg body weight can lead to chronic poisoning, and intakes greater than 10 mg/kg BW may cause acute lead poisoning.
- Sheep—generally occurs only in lambs; symptoms of poisoning appear at intakes greater than 4.5 mg/kg BW.
- Goats—more resistant than sheep or cows. Very minor signs of poisoning occur at intakes of 60 mg/kg BW. This is equal to blood concentrations of 130 micrograms per dl.

Sources
- Lead storage (car) batteries
- Lead shot
- Old lead arsenate
- Lead contamination of soils (smelters)
- Crop production enhancement agents: many crop yields are increased with the use of fertilizers, fungicides, and herbicides that contain lead (e.g., lead arsenate).
- Old lead-based paints
- Mining: strip mining can cause lead to leech into groundwater and soil and into the air as dust particles.

GENETICS
N/A

INCIDENCE/PREVALENCE
Unpredictable, but most cases occur in cattle in the spring, when they are turned out in pastures where they have access to broken batteries.

GEOGRAPHIC DISTRIBUTION
Worldwide

SIGNALMENT
Species
- All ruminant species are at risk.
- Young animals are perhaps more susceptible due to their curiosity and greater absorption of lead from the gastrointestinal tract.
- Cattle more likely than other ruminants due to less-discriminating grazing.

Breed Predilections
N/A

Mean Age and Range
- All ages are susceptible.
- Younger animals are at greater risk of intoxication due to increased capacity to absorb lead from the intestines.

Predominant Sex
N/A

SIGNS
- Signs appear to occur abruptly, though there may be a delay of several days (depending on the lead source) from the time of lead ingestion and the onset of signs.
- Blindness, circling, aimless wandering, head pressing
- Grinding of the teeth
- Rhythmic twitching of the muscles, often involving the face (e.g., eyelids)
- Tucked and painful abdomen; rumen atony, constipation, or diarrhea may be present.
- Salivation, due to pain or pharyngeal paralysis
- Excitement and/or seizures (depression may also be observed)
- Bradycardia and hypertension have both been observed in cattle.

CAUSES AND RISK FACTORS
- Discarded broken batteries are by far the most common source of lead poisoning in ruminants. The interior lead plates often contain > 90% lead.
- Other less common sources of lead include machinery grease, old used motor oil, paint, pesticides, caulk and putty, contamination from mines and smelters, water, and grazing pastures contaminated with lead shot.
- Burning batteries does not destroy lead; this practice only provides animals a more concentrated lead source in the remaining ash.
- Acute oral toxic dose for calves and cattle is approximately 400–800 mg/kg BW.
- Pb can be excreted in the feces, urine and bile. Chelation therapy enhances renal excretion.

DIAGNOSIS

• Based on clinical signs and history of possible exposure
• Definitive diagnosis requires detection of lead in appropriate clinical specimen
• Diagnostic samples:
  • Whole blood
  • Lead concentrations of greater than 0.35 ppm with appropriate clinical signs are diagnostic
  • Kidneys (> 10 ppm Pb wet weight are diagnostic)
  • Liver (> 10 ppm Pb wet weight are diagnostic)

DIFFERENTIAL DIAGNOSIS

• Polioencephalomalacia, salt poisoning, and/or water deprivation, vitamin A deficiency, rabies, listeriosis, abscess, thromboembolic meningoencephalitis, nervous coccidiosis, and hepatic encephalopathy
• There are many differentials for "sudden" death in calves or cows; these could include enterotoxemia, water hemlock (*Cicuta*), botulism, nonprotein nitrogen intoxication, cyanobacteria (blue-green algae), *Delphinium* (larkspur), *Zigadenus* (death camas), *Astragalus* (locoweed), nitrate poisoning

CBC/BIOCHEMISTRY/URINALYSIS

• Basophilic stippling is commonly mentioned as a potential alteration: inconsistent; may be mistaken for other disease processes
• Anemia (subchronic to chronic lead toxicosis)
• Increased RBC fragility

OTHER LABORATORY TESTS

• Whole blood lead, EDTA, or heparin. Levels greater than 0.3 ppm indicate excessive exposure, > 0.6 ppm is compatible with poisoning.
• Even though blood lead levels are diagnostic for confirming exposure, blood Pb levels sometimes do not correlate well with clinical signs. For instance, one might see a blood lead level of 0.30 ppm in a cow that is seizing; and one might see a blood lead level of 0.90 ppm in a cow that is not showing any clinical disease. Because of this, when you diagnose lead poisoning in an individual animal, remaining animals in the "exposed" group should be tested, regardless of whether they are showing signs or not.
• Liver *and* kidney concentrations greater than 5.0 ppm wet weight are consistent with excessive lead exposure.

IMAGING

Radiography done antemortem or postmortem may show radiographic densities in the GIT, most commonly in the reticulum.

DIAGNOSTIC PROCEDURES

One should find the source (through history, pasture examination, etc.) and remove it from the animal's environment; or remove the animals from the contaminated environment. Sometimes batteries can be so disintegrated and ground into the soil that little visible evidence remains.

PATHOLOGIC FINDINGS

• No findings are pathognomonic for lead poisoning.
• Cerebral edema and mild gastritis and enteritis are sometimes observed grossly.
• Histologically, laminar cortical necrosis, centrilobular degeneration, and proximal renal tubule degeneration and necrosis have been observed. These are uncommon lesions.
• Intranuclear inclusion bodies in the kidney and brain can be seen with chronic exposures or massive acute oral exposures.

Gross Necropsy Findings

• None that is pathognomonic
• CNS
• Flattened or yellow cerebral cortical gyri

HISTOPATHOLOGICAL FINDINGS

• CNS
  • Laminar cortical necrosis with swelling of the capillary endothelium within the brain
• Renal
  • Lead inclusion bodies are often found in the proximal renal tubules.
  • Inclusions are described as intranuclear inclusions in the proximal tubules with periglomerular nephritis.

TREATMENT

• Find and remove the suspect source or remove animals from the contaminated environment.
• Removal of the lead from the multicompartmental ruminant GIT has been shown to be next to impossible.
• Treatment of lead intoxication may not be rewarding and deaths may occur prior to the initiation of antidotal therapy.
• The prolonged retention of lead may be due to continued release and absorption of lead from metal particles in the reticulum or rumen.

• Chelation therapy
  • Ca-EDTA—55–90 mg/kg body weight slowly IV or IM, bid
  • Treat for 3–5 days.
  • Wait for several days and reevaluate neurologic status; another round of chelation may be indicated.
• Symptomatic therapy—thiamine HCL—administer 2 mg/kg IM, bid. Treat for up to 2 weeks.
• Supportive therapy—mineral supplementation may be required if there is prolonged chelation therapy.

MEDICATIONS

• Magnesium sulfate can be added to the diet to help bind lead within the gastrointestinal tract (one recommended dosage: 0.5 g/lb BW daily).
• Thiamine hydrochloride, 250–1000 mg twice daily, IM or SQ, for 5–10 days. This is not a chelator, but many affected animals will improve clinically and when combined with a chelator, it has been shown to enhance the renal excretion of lead.
• Ca-EDTA is an effective chelator, but may not be an economically viable option for many clients. One recommended dosage is 72 mg/kg, slow IV, divided twice to three times daily for 3 to 5 days. This may be repeated after a few days if clinical signs persist. Blood leads should be periodically monitored to evaluate the effectiveness of the chelation therapy.
• Depending on the severity and signs, symptomatic care may include diazepam or barbiturates for seizure control, IV fluid therapy to correct dehydration, monitoring for the development of electrolyte abnormalities, monitoring feed and caloric intake and addressing deficiencies accordingly, zinc supplementation (1.0 mg/kg/day).
• British anti-Lewisite (dimercaprol or BAL) penetrates into the brain, and can be a helpful chelator in animals showing severe neurological signs. One suggested dosage is 3.0 mg/kg IM as a 5% solution in a 10% solution of benzyl benzoate in peanut oil every 4 hours for 2 days, every 6 hours on day 3, then bid for the next 10 days. BAL is potentially nephrotoxic and is painful when injected. It can be difficult to obtain and expensive to use.

CONTRAINDICATIONS

• Ca-EDTA is potentially nephrotoxic, so monitoring renal parameters and maintaining adequate hydration status are recommended.
• Lead may interfere with copper, calcium, zinc, iron, and selenium metabolism.
• Appropriate milk and meat withdrawal times must be followed for all compounds administered to food-producing animals.

LEAD TOXICOSIS •

FOLLOW-UP

• Blood lead levels should be monitored periodically to determine the efficacy of chelation therapy, along with assisting with decision making in regard to slaughter withdrawal times. Normal blood levels should be < 0.10 ppm.
• Lead can be secreted into milk; milk should be tested and discarded if levels are too high.

PATIENT MONITORING

It is common for the neurological signs (e.g., blindness) to persist. Ill thrift may be present in "recovered" young.

PREVENTION/AVOIDANCE

• Knowledge of the common sources of lead should help producers avoid this potentially devastating disease.
• Keep at-risk animals away from junk or "resource" piles located on the property.

POSSIBLE COMPLICATIONS

N/A

EXPECTED COURSE AND PROGNOSIS

• The more severely affected animals have a poor prognosis. It is often impossible to remove the lead from the gastrointestinal tract, and patients showing severe neurological signs often do not respond well to treatment.
• Mild or moderately affected animals may improve if you can remove the lead from the gastrointestinal tract, and enhance renal excretion through chelation therapy.

MISCELLANEOUS

ASSOCIATED CONDITIONS

• The half-life of lead in an intoxicated animal depends on a number of factors including age and physiological status.
• In some references, the half-life of lead is reported to be several weeks to 2 months. This may underestimate the half-life of elimination of lead.
• A study from Michigan examined the half-life of lead in poisoned animals and reports that pregnant or lactating cattle tended to have a shortened half-life as compared to a castrated bull.
• If there is any question of toxicity, a whole blood sample can be collected and analyzed for lead.

AGE-RELATED FACTORS

Younger animals are at greater risk of intoxication due to increased capacity to absorb lead from the intestines.

ZOONOTIC POTENTIAL

• Lead is immunosuppressive and carcinogenic in people. The developing fetus and young children are very susceptible to lead's toxic effect on the nervous system. Care should be taken when using meat or milk from lead contaminated carcasses for human consumption.
• There is potential for lead exposure to animals from milk and meat of poisoned animals.
• In some states, there are restrictions on movement or marketing of cattle poisoned with lead.
• The veterinarian should consult the local diagnostic laboratory or department of public health for questions specific to their practice area.

PREGNANCY

• Lead has been shown to cross the placenta in humans; it is conceivable that lead may exert a deleterious effect on the developing ruminant fetus.
• Pregnant cattle that suffer from lead toxicosis may transfer significant amounts of lead to the developing fetus.
• The amount of lead transferred across the placenta or into the milk is highest when the blood concentrations of lead are greatest.

RUMINANT SPECIES AFFECTED

All ruminant species are susceptible.

BIOSECURITY

N/A

PRODUCTION MANAGEMENT

• Restrict animal access to lead sources (e.g., paint-cribbing, batteries, grease, etc.). Avoid access to junk piles in the pastures.
• Removing nonclinical, exposed animals from the source is very successful in preventing new cases.

SYNONYMS

Pb
Plumbism
Saturnism

SEE ALSO

Abscess
Astragalus (locoweed)
Botulism
Cyanobacteria (blue-green algae)
Delphinium (larkspur)

Enterotoxemia
Hepatic encephalopathy
Listeriosis
Nervous coccidiosis
Nitrate poisoning
Nonprotein nitrogen intoxication
Polioencephalomalacia
Rabies
Salt poisoning and/or water deprivation
Thromboembolic meningoencephalitis
Vitamin A deficiency
Water hemlock (*Cicuta*)
Zigadenus (death camas)

ABBREVIATIONS

BAL = British anti-Lewisite
Bid = twice daily
BW = body weight
Ca-EDTA = calcium disodium ethylenediaminetetraacetic acid
CNS = central nervous system
GIT = gastrointestinal tract
IM = intramuscular
IV = intravenous
Pb = lead
ppm = parts per million
RBC = red blood cell
SQ = subcutaneous

Suggested Reading
Galey, F. D., Slenning, B. D., Anderson, M. L., Breneman, P. C., Littlefield, E. S., Melton, L. A., Tracy, M. L. 1990, Jul. Lead concentrations in blood and milk from periparturient dairy heifers seven months after an episode of acute lead toxicosis. *J Vet Diagn Invest*. 2(3): 222–26.
Gwaltney-Brant, S. 2004. Lead. In: *Clinical veterinary toxicology*, ed. K. H. Plumlee. St. Louis: Mosby.
Rumbeiha, W. K., Braselton, W. E., Donch, D. 2001. A retrospective study on the disappearance of blood lead in cattle with accidental lead toxicosis. *J Vet Diagn Invest*. 13(5): 373–78.
Waldner, C., Checkley, S., Blakley, B., Pollock, C., Mitchell, B. 2002, Nov. Managing lead exposure and toxicity in cow-calf herds to minimize the potential for food residues. *J Vet Diagn Invest*. 14(6): 481–86.

Authors: Patricia Talcott and Joe Roder

BASICS

OVERVIEW
• Leptospirosis is a zoonotic, acute febrile disease with clinical manifestations depending on the animal species and the serovar (serological variant) involved of a spirochete in the genus *Leptospira*.
• Leptospirosis causes acute and chronic disease (septicemia, agalactia, hepatitis, nephritis, and abortion) in a wide range of domestic livestock and wildlife hosts.
• Vaccination is serovar specific.

PATHOPHYSIOLOGY
• Leptospires enter the body through cutaneous or mucosal abrasions or by direct penetration of moist skin. Rarely transmission can occur by venereal or transplacental routes.
• Septicemia follows for 4–7 days resulting in systemic dispersion of bacterial toxins causing fever, capillary damage (petechia), hepatic necrosis, renal tubular damage, and agalactia. In calves, hemolysin toxin may cause intravascular hemolysis, hemolytic anemia, and hemoglobinuria.
• Humoral response creates rising serum antibody levels resolving the septicemia and fever with the bacteria localizing in the liver and renal parenchyma causing hepatitis, interstitial nephritis, and persistent leptospiruria.
• Animals may succumb acutely to septicemia and hemolytic anemia or later due to interstitial nephritis.
• Animals in the second half of gestation (> 4 months) can have invasion of the placenta and fetus during the septicemic phase resulting in abortion several weeks later.
• Sheep and goats can develop encephalitis due to localization of the leptospires in the nervous system.

SYSTEMS AFFECTED
• Renal and urologic including interstitial nephritis, tubular damage, and chronic renal failure
• Hepatobiliary including hepatitis, necrosis
• Cardiovascular including endothelial cell damage
• Nervous system including meningitis
• Reproductive including abortion, stillbirth, and retention of fetal membranes
• Mammary including agalactia and abnormal milk

GENETICS
N/A

INCIDENCE/PREVALENCE
• A survey of cattle at slaughter in the United States reported 2% of mature cattle were renal carriers of leptospires with serovars *hardjo, pomona*, and *grippotyphosa* being isolated.
• *L. hardjo* is host adapted to cattle and has caused epidemiologic or endemic reproductive problems in cattle in the United States.
• *L. pomona* is most common in calves.

GEOGRAPHICAL DISTRIBUTION
• Worldwide distribution favoring warm, wet climates and surviving in standing water for prolonged periods.
• Leptospirosis has been reported in most parts of the globe with different serovars predominant in different regions.

SIGNALMENT
Species
• Cattle, sheep, goats, wild ruminants, water buffalo, deer, and other cervids
• A survey isolating leptospires from kidneys of cattle at slaughter in the United States reported higher isolation rates from beef cattle than dairy cattle.
• The host-adapted serovars generally cause a mild or unapparent disease developing into a carrier state. For example:
  • *Leptospira borgpetersenii* serovar *hardjo-bovis* is adapted to cattle.
  • *Leptospira interrogans* serovar *hardjo-prajitno* is adapted to sheep.
• Animals infected by a non-host-adapted serovar may develop acute, severe clinical disease, especially young animals; it also may cause abortion in pregnant dams. Examples are *Leptospira interrogans* serovars *pomona, grippotyphosa, canicola*, and *icterohaemorrhagiae* in cattle.

Breed Predilections
N/A

Mean Age and Range
Calves and lambs are more typically affected by the acute form, subacute form in adult cattle, and chronic form in sheep, goats, and occasionally adult cattle.

Predominant Sex
• A survey isolating leptospires from kidneys of cattle at slaughter in the United States reported higher isolation rates from bulls than cows.
• Males are often nonsymptomatic carriers that may excrete *Leptospira* in the urine and semen.

SIGNS
Cattle: Herd Level
• Sudden drop in milk production in 5%–50% of lactating cows
• Increased rate of abortion
• Increase in infertility (lower conception rates) may be seen.

Individual Cow
• Host-adapted serovars
  • Depression, anorexia, transient, slight pyrexia, recumbency ranging from 1 to 7 days
  • Agalactia—sudden sharp drop in milk yield, which lasts from 7 to 14 days. Characterized by a flabby, nonpainful udder, affecting all four quarters. Milk is thick, yellowy, and may contain clots.
  • Abortion, stillbirths, and infertility
• Non-host-adapted serovars: depression, anorexia, pyrexia (40.0°C–41.5°C or 104°F–107°F), hemoglobinuria, jaundice, mucosal surface hemorrhages, mastitis with blood tinged milk, anemia, lameness (due to synovitis), abortion, death

Sheep and Goats
• Rarely cases of clinical disease
• In young stock: pyrexia, dyspnea, depression, anorexia, may be hemoglobinuria, pale or yellowish mucous membranes; death due to septicemia may occur within 12 hours.

GENERAL COMMENTS
• Presentation will vary dependent on age, pathogenicity of the serovar, and environmental factors affecting the agent's survival.
• Primary reservoir hosts (*L. hardjo* in cattle) may shed leptospires in urine with insidious clinical signs and weak antibody responses.
• Incidental hosts (*L. pomona* in cattle) present with more acute signs and a stronger antibody response.

PHYSICAL EXAMINATION FINDINGS
• Calves present with fever, anorexia, depression, (with *L. hardjo*) hemolytic anemia, hemoglobinuria, icterus, and petechia (with *L. pomona*.)
• Hemoglobinuria typically resolves within 72 hours; anemia begins to resolve at 4–5 days and is typically resolved 7–10 days later.
• Mortality rate in calves is higher than in adult cattle.

LEPTOSPIROSIS

- Adult cattle present with abnormal milk (thick, yellow, blood tinged) without obvious inflammation of the mammary gland, or later with abortions.
- In endemically affected herds, younger animals may have an increased incidence of sporadic abortions.

CAUSES
- Pathogenic serovars of the *Leptospira* spirochete
- Pathogenic leptospires are classified as a single species, *Leptospira interrogans*, with more than 200 serovars in 23 serogroups. At least 7 serovars are identified in cattle in the United States including: *pomona, hardjo, canicola, grippotyphosa, ictohaemorrhagiae, swaijzak*, and *bratislava*.

RISK FACTORS
- Direct transmission through contact with urine, vaginal discharge, postabortion discharge, or the fetus of an infected host.
- Indirect transmission through contact with contaminated environment (water sources)

DIAGNOSIS

DIFFERENTIAL DIAGNOSIS
- Acute to subacute disease (hemoglobinuria and icterus)
- Water toxicosis (young calves)
- Postparturient hemoglobinuria
- Anaplasmosis
- Babesiosis
- Bacillary hemoglobinuria
- Enzootic hematuria
- Snakebite
- Acute hepatitis
- Cholangiohepatitis
- Poisonings: rape, kale, brassica, copper (chronic), acorn, cassia, senna, gossypol (cottonseed), dinitrophenol, mercury, monensin, ionophores, oxalate, ethylene glycol, vetch, pyrrolizidine alkaloids, phosphate fertilizer, solanum
- Copper toxicity

Reproductive Disease
- Anaplasmosis
- Bluetongue
- Bovine viral diarrhea mucosal disease
- Brucellosis
- Campylobacteriosis
- Trichomoniasis
- Infectious bovine rhinotracheitis (IBR)
- Malnutrition
- Mycoplasma
- Mycosis

CBC/BIOCHEMISTRY/URINALYSIS
- CBC may show a hemolytic anemia and leukocytosis; may be leukopenia.
- Urinalysis: may be increased bilirubin, hemoglobin, and albumin. *Note:* urine may be infectious!
- Biochemistry may show increased liver enzymes (AST and ALT), bilirubinemia, and azotemia.

OTHER LABORATORY TESTS
- Serology—microscopic agglutination test (MAT) on acute and convalescent (7–10 days later) sera is a commonly used test for leptospirosis.
- MAT titers are considered diagnostic when greater than 1:800 in an animal with coinciding clinical signs or by a fourfold rise in paired samples.
- In cases of abortion, MAT titers are declining so identification of titers of 300 or greater in several cows would be significant in an unvaccinated herd.
- Results of samples taken in early infection may show cross-reactivity to other serovars.
- As titers drop after several months to low or negative levels, chronic carriers and animals that abort may be seronegative.
- Individual animal serology may not be diagnostic; therefore, leptospirosis should be diagnosed on a herd level. It is important to sample several suspect animals.
- Serological titers due to vaccination cannot be distinguished from those due to infection, although they tend to be lower and more transient.
- Vaccination with a bacterin may produce a low titer on the MAT test; protective immunity can last up to 12 months.
- Chronic carriers or animals with infections isolated in the kidneys may not have diagnostic titers.
- Dark-field microscopic examination of urine, fluorescent antibody staining of urine or tissues, and PCR are other techniques that can be used to diagnose leptospirosis.
- Warthin-Starry silver staining can be attempted on formalin-fixed samples.
- Isolation is not usually performed due to the difficulty in culturing the organism.

Culture
Not generally performed for diagnostic purposes due to high risk of culture contamination and prolonged isolation period ranging from weeks to months

Dark-Field Microscopy
Tentative indication but not specific

Immunofluorescence
- Urine: fast and specific if urine arrives to lab quickly and chilled
- Can add formalin to a final concentration of 0.8% to preserve the bacteria in the sample
- As excretion in cattle is intermittent, a negative result does not preclude the disease.
- FA has also been reported to be used with variable success to detect *Leptospira* in aborted fetal tissues.

IMAGING
N/A

GROSS AND HISTOPATHOLOGICAL FINDINGS
- Anemia, icterus, and hemoglobinuria (young calves)
- Subcutaneous and subserosal hemorrhage
- Autolytic fetus
- Centrilobular hepatic necrosis
- Diffuse interstitial nephritis
- Fetal hepatitis and nephritis

TREATMENT

- Infected animals can be treated with antibiotics to prevent irreversible liver and kidney damage, abortion, establishment of a carrier state, and hemolytic anemia.
- Animals with acute disease may require blood transfusions, oral or intravenous fluid therapy, and other supportive nursing care.
- Treating lactating dairy cattle with agalactia may hasten return to near normal yields, but requires discarding the milk for the withdrawal period. Treatment at this time may also reduce the likelihood of abortion.
- Acute disease in calves should be treated aggressively both symptomatically and with antibiotics.
- No treatment has been proven 100% effective in eliminating the carrier state of a host-adapted serovar.

ACTIVITY
N/A

DIET
N/A

CLIENT EDUCATION
Leptospirosis has zoonotic potential through contact with contaminated urine and the environment.

MEDICATIONS

- Antimicrobial therapy
  - Single injection of oxytetracycline, 20 mg/kg of body weight IM
  - Tetracycline, 10–15 mg/kg bid for 3–5 days.
  - Long-acting oxytetracycline, 20 mg/kg twice at 10 day intervals
  - Long-acting amoxicillin, 15 mg/kg, two doses 48 hours apart
  - Tilmicosin, 10 mg/kg SQ
  - Ceftiofur sodium 2.2 or 5 mg/kg IM SID for 5 days or 20 mg/kg IM SID for 3 days
  - Streptomycin or dihydrostreptomycin, 12.5 mg/kg bid for 3 days. A single dose of 25 mg/kg will usually clear the carrier state from *L. pomona* or other non-host-adapted serovars.
- Appropriate meat and milk withdrawal times must be considered.

CONTRAINDICATIONS
N/A

PRECAUTIONS
Previously, streptomycin, dihydrostreptomycin, or dihydrostreptomycin-pencillin G was used for treatment but is no longer available in certain countries for use in food-producing animals.

POSSIBLE INTERACTIONS
N/A

FOLLOW-UP

- Minimizing access to wildlife, rodents, and contaminated water sources can reduce the exposure in domestic stock.
- Vaccination with bacterins containing multiple serovars generally confers protection to abortion and death and significantly reduces renal colonization.
- Selection of seronegative replacement stock will help prevent introduction into the herd.

MISCELLANEOUS

- Prompt vaccination and antimicrobial therapy for pregnant beef cows early in the epizoonosis can prevent further abortions.
- Leptospirosis is a zoonotic agent so appropriate hygiene and sanitary methods must be followed by practitioners and owners to prevent transmission.

ASSOCIATED CONDITIONS
N/A

AGE-RELATED FACTORS
The acute form more typically affects calves and lambs, subacute form in adult cattle, and chronic form in sheep, goats, and occasionally adult cattle.

ZOONOTIC POTENTIAL

- Leptospirosis has zoonotic potential through contact with contaminated urine and the environment. All pathogenic *Leptospira* serovars are zoonotic.
- People are generally infected by means of aerosol or direct contact with infected urine or urine-contaminated water, which penetrates through mucous membranes or wet or abraded skin.
- People working with infected cattle should take precautionary measures such as protective clothing, rubber boots, latex gloves, and protective eyeglasses or facemasks.
- All cases of unexplained fever or influenzalike syndromes in contact workers should be reported to the attending general practitioner to determine the possible implication of *Leptospira*.

PREGNANCY

- In endemically affected herds, younger animals may have an increased incidence of sporadic abortions.
- Animals in the second half of gestation (> 4 months) can have invasion of the placenta and fetus during the septicemic phase resulting in abortion several weeks later.

RUMINANT SPECIES AFFECTED
Potentially, all ruminant species are affected.

BIOSECURITY
N/A

PRODUCTION MANAGEMENT
N/A

SYNONYMS
Red water

SEE ALSO
Acute hepatitis
Anaplasmosis
Babesiosis
Bacillary hemoglobinuria
Bluetongue
Bovine viral diarrhea mucosal disease
Brucellosis
Campylobacteriosis
Cholangiohepatitis
Copper toxicity
Enzootic hematuria

Infectious bovine rhinotracheitis (IBR)
Malnutrition
Mycoplasma
Mycosis
Postparturient hemoglobinuria
Pyrrolizidine alkaloid toxicity
Snakebite
Trichomoniasis
Water toxicosis (young calves)

ABBREVIATIONS
ALT = alanine aminotransferase
AST = aspartate transaminase
BID = twice a day
FA = fluorescent antibody
IBR = infectious bovine rhinotracheitis
IM = intramuscular
MAT = microscopic agglutination test
PCR = polymerase chain reaction
SID = once daily
SQ = subcutaneous

Suggested Reading

Aiello, S. E., ed. 1998. Leptospirosis in cattle. In: *Merck veterinary manual*, 8th ed. Whitehouse Station, NJ: Merck and Co. [online] Available at: http://www.merckvetmanual.com/mvm/index.jsp?cfile=htm/bc/51202.htm&word=Leptospirosis%2ccattle. Accessed September 18, 2004.

Alt, D. P., Zuerner, R. L., Bolin, C. A. 2001, Sep 1. Evaluation of antibiotics for treatment of cattle infected with *Leptospira borgpetersenii* serovar *hardjo*. *J Am Vet Med Assoc.* 219(5):636–39.

Bolin, C. A., Alt, D. P. 2001, Jul. Use of a monovalent leptospiral vaccine to prevent renal colonization and urinary shedding in cattle exposed to *Leptospira borgpetersenii* serovar *hardjo*. *Am J Vet Res.* 62(7):995–1000.

Levett, P. N. 2001, Apr. Leptospirosis. *Clin Microbiol Rev.* 14(2):296–326.

Rebhun, W. C. 1995. *Diseases of dairy cattle.* Philadelphia: Lippincott, Williams & Wilkins.

Authors: Noah Barka and Michael D. Bernstein

LEUKOCYTE RESPONSES IN CATTLE

 BASICS

OVERVIEW
- Types of leukocytes in cattle:
  - Neutrophils
  - Lymphocytes
  - Monocytes
  - Eosinophils
  - Basophils
- Production of leukocytes:
  - Neutrophils, eosinophils, basophils, and monocytes are produced in the bone marrow.
  - Lymphocytes are produced in lymph nodes, bone marrow, spleen, thymus, and Peyer's patches.

DEFINITION
- Leukocytosis refers to an increase in the numbers of leukocytes in blood. Neutrophilia, lymphocytosis, monocytosis, eosinophilia, and basophilia refer to increased total numbers of the specific cell.
- Leukopenia refers to a decrease in the numbers of leukocytes in blood. Neutropenia, lymphopenia, and monocytopenia refer to decreased total numbers of the specific cell.
- Evaluation of the leukocyte portion of the hemogram is preformed on the basis of the absolute numbers of each cell type and not on the percentages of the cell types.
- Left shift indicates that immature neutrophils, which are usually bands but may also include less mature cells such as myelocytes and metamyelocytes, are increased. Regenerative left shift indicates that the total neutrophil count is increased and there is a concomitant left shift. Degenerative left shift indicates that the total neutrophil count is low (or at the low end of normal) and there is a concomitant left shift. Often with a degenerative left shift, the total number of immature neutrophils (band neutrophils, metamyelocytes, etc.) is greater than the total number of mature neutrophils.

PATHOPHYSIOLOGY
General
- Leukocyte counts are higher in calves than in adults. Young adults have higher leukocyte counts than older adults.
- Adult cattle are considered a "small storage pool" species. As such they have fewer neutrophils in reserve in their bone marrow (the storage pool) than do "large storage pool" species such as dogs. "Small storage pool" animals such as adult cattle deplete the storage pool more rapidly when they develop significant inflammation than do large storage pool species.
- Because cattle tend to deplete their storage pool rapidly, they frequently develop neutropenia with inflammation. Increased myelopoiesis occurs in an attempt to produce more neutrophils. Frequently, especially with severe inflammation, immature neutrophils (especially band neutrophils) are released from the marrow, which causes a left shift, which frequently is degenerative.
- With inflammation cattle tend to produce large amounts of fibrinogen. Thus, variable neutrophil counts (neutrophilia, normal neutrophil count, or neutropenia), which may be accompanied by a left shift with hyperfibrinogenemia are often found with inflammation.
- Leukocyte changes with stress are similar in cattle to those of other species. Excitement (epinephrine induced physiologic leukocytosis) results in leukocytosis, which is due to neutrophilia and lymphocytosis. Corticosteroid-induced changes consist of neutrophilia without a left shift and lymphopenia, monocytosis, and eosinopenia.
- Toxic changes in neutrophils indicate the presence of bacterial toxins and inflammatory cytokines. Usually toxic changes indicate bacterial disease. Features of toxicity include Döhle bodies (blue inclusion bodies in the cytoplasm), diffuse cytoplasmic basophilia, cytoplasmic vacuolation or foaminess, and granulation (these features are listed in order from least to most severe).

- Reactive lymphocytes in blood indicate immune response to antigens. The most obvious feature of reactive lymphocytes is very basophilic cytoplasm. Reactive lymphocytes are generally slightly larger and have a greater amount of cytoplasm than normal lymphocytes. Slight irregularity such as indentations and fissures of their nuclei may be recognized.

Neutrophilia
- Neutrophilia in cattle is usually modest and total neutrophil counts above $15,000/\mu l$ are rare.
- Neutrophilia accompanied by lymphocytosis occurs with physical exertion, excitement and acute stress.
- Neutrophilia accompanied by lymphopenia and occasionally by monocytosis occurs with stress that causes release of corticosteroids and glucocorticoid administration.
- Many infectious diseases of bacterial etiology cause neutrophilia provided that the inflammatory reaction is not of such severity that the bone marrow storage pool is depleted (see neutropenia). Left shift with toxic neutrophils may be found.
- Noninfectious causes of inflammation such as cholangiohepatitis result in moderate neutrophilia.
- Fungal infections, traumatic tissue injury, neoplasia and immune mediated disease may cause neutrophilia.

Lymphocytosis
- Calves have higher lymphocyte counts than adults. Younger adults also have higher lymphocyte counts than older animals.
- Lymphocytosis accompanied by neutrophilia occurs with physical exertion, excitement, and acute stress.
- Lymphocytosis occurs with immune responses. It may be found with infectious diseases, after vaccination, and in young animals reacting to environmental organisms and other antigens.
- Persistent lymphocytosis occurs with many cattle infected with bovine leukemia virus.

- Occasionally, lymphocytosis in which the lymphocytes are bizarre and anaplastic may be seen with lymphoma.

Monocytosis
- Monocytosis may occur with stress that causes release of corticosteroids and glucocorticoid administration.
- Chronic infectious disease may produce monocytosis, particularly if the agent causes granulomatous inflammation.
- Fungal infections may produce monocytosis.

Eosinophilia
- Eosinophilia is rare.
- Migration of multicellular parasites may cause eosinophilia.
- Eosinophilia may be found with emphysema.
- Eosinophilia may be found with allergy.

Neutropenia
- Severe inflammation often depletes the neutrophil storage pool resulting in neutropenia, which is often accompanied by a left shift that includes neutrophilic myelocytes and neutrophilic metamyelocytes as well as band neutrophils.
- Bacteria infections, especially with endotoxin-producing organisms or release of endotoxin through devitalized intestinal barriers, result in toxic cytoplasmic features of neutrophils.
- Bone marrow suppression from toxins such as bracken fern or from myelophthisis such as with rare cases of bone marrow involvement with lymphoma causes marked neutropenia. Nonregenerative anemia and thrombocytopenia are often found as well, which suggests generalized hematopoietic hypo- or aplasia.

Lymphopenia
- Lymphopenia accompanied by neutrophilia occurs with stress that causes release of corticosteroids and with administration of glucocorticoids.
- Viral infectious disease such as bovine virus diarrhea may cause lymphopenia.

Bovine Leukocyte Adhesion Deficiency (BLAD)
- BLAD is a fatal granulocytopathy of Holsteins that is inherited in an autosomal recessive manner.
- It is caused by a defect in CD18 unit of β_2-integrins, which are expressed primarily on leukocytes. The β_2-integrins are heterodimers consisting of the β subunit (CD18) and one of several α subunits (CD11a, CD11b, CD11c, and CD11d). Mac-1, the heterodimer of CD11b and C18, mediates tight adherence of neutrophils to postcapillary venule endothelial cells, which is an early activity of neutrophil migration into tissues. The inability of the neutrophils to adhere to endothelium prevents them from moving into infected tissue. Calves die soon because the neutrophils are unable to extravasate into infected tissues.
- BLAD calves have recurrent soft tissue infections. They do not develop significant inflammation at these sites. Calves may have a history of respiratory disease and diarrhea, periodontal gingivitis, and gingival recession.
- They have marked neutrophilia (> 40,000/μl to well over 100,000/μl) that persists and continues to increase. The marked and progressive neutrophilia is due to continued stimulation of myelopoiesis, which is a frustrated attempt to provide neutrophils to combat infections. Additionally, the inability of the neutrophils to leave the circulation causes them to remain in blood for a prolonged period of time.
- Presumptive diagnosis of BLAD may be made on the basis of the leukogram findings of persistent and progressive neutrophilia in a young calf. Flow cytometric analysis with fluorescent labeled antiCD18 antibody reveals markedly reduced amounts of CD18. A DNA-polymerase chain reaction (PCR)-restricted technique fragment length polymorphism (RTLP) technique, which unequivocally identifies the genotype of cattle at the CD18 locus, has been developed. It is available through Immgen Inc., College

Station, Texas, as well as the Bovine Blood Typing Laboratory of Canada, Saskatoon, Saskatchewan. In the United States, all testing is coordinated and recorded through the Holstein Association of America.

Chédiak-Higashi Syndrome
- Chédiak-Higashi syndrome (CHS) is a rare inherited disease that is transmitted as an autosomal recessive trait that is characterized by hypopigmentation, enlarged or giant granules in granule-containing cells, and a platelet storage pool disease.
- In addition to hypopigmentation (often described as partial albinism) and bleeding diathesis, cattle with CHS have increased susceptibility to bacterial infections. This susceptibility is due to multiple defects of neutrophils and other cells of defense.
- CHS has been described in Hereford, Brangus, and Japanese Black (Wagyu) cattle.
- Diagnosis is based on clinical features coupled with recognition of enlarged granules in phagocytes. In most species, the enlarged granules are best recognized in eosinophils.
- A PCR method for detection of the abnormal CHS gene has been described.

SYSTEMS AFFECTED
- The primary tissues affected are the bone marrow and lymphatic tissue, which are the location for production of the various leukocytes. There may be evidence of increased production such as increased M:E in the marrow or immune reactivity in lymph nodes.
- Any tissue or organ can be affected since leukocytes, especially neutrophils, migrate into them under the influence of a variety of stimuli.
- BLAD calves have numerous soft tissue infections. Very little pus is found in these sites because of the inability of neutrophils to adhere to endothelial cells during the initial stages of inflammation.

LEUKOCYTE RESPONSES IN CATTLE

GENETICS
• Bovine leukocyte adhesion deficiency (BLAD) occurs in Holstein calves. It is inherited as an autosomal recessive trait.
• Chédiak-Higashi syndrome has been described in Hereford, Brangus, and Japanese Black (Wagyu) cattle. It is inherited as an autosomal recessive trait.

INCIDENCE/PREVALENCE
BLV infection may be as high as 75% in some diary herds.

GEOGRAPHIC DISTRIBUTION
Since leukocytes are vital for combating infectious and noninfectious causes of diseases, cattle throughout the world may have hemogram features reflecting leukocyte reactions.

SIGNALMENT
• All cattle may have some abnormality in leukocyte parameters or morphology due to a wide variety of diseases and physiological conditions.
• BLAD is a disease of young Holstein calves.
• CHS is a disease of Herefords, Brangus, and Japanese Black (Wagyu) cattle.

Breed Predilections
• BLAD occurs in Holstein cattle.
• CHS has been described in Hereford, Brangus, and Japanese Black (Wagyu) cattle.

Mean Age and Range
• Animals of all ages are susceptible to conditions that cause inflammation and immune reactions.

• Severe, multiple infections are found in young, generally less than 1 month of age, Holstein calves with BLAD.

Predominant Sex
N/A

SIGNS

HISTORICAL FINDINGS

PHYSICAL EXAMINATION FINDINGS

CAUSES AND RISK FACTORS
Bacterial Diseases
• Bacterial infections usually cause suppurative inflammation, which develops through migration of blood neutrophils into tissues. Inflammation often causes neutrophilia if the insult is not markedly severe. Often hyperfibrinogenemia accompanies an inflammatory leukogram.
• However, severe infection with accompanying marked inflammation causes large numbers of neutrophils to migrate from the blood into the inflamed tissue and with subsequent depletion of the neutrophil storage pool resulting in neutropenia with a degenerative left shift. The neutrophils may be toxic, especially with gram-negative infections.
• When the infection and the accompanying inflammatory reaction do not resolve in a few days, myelopoiesis increases to satisfy the demand for neutrophils. Such established inflammation results in neutrophilia without a left shift. Additionally, there may be monocytosis, normal to mildly increased lymphocyte count, and reactive lymphocytes.

• Endotoxin released by bacteria also affects the leukogram. Severe endotoxemia results in marked leukopenia due to neutropenia and lymphopenia. There may also be a degenerative left shift.
• Mastitis, metritis, and other bacterial diseases of tissues and organs that may have multiple etiologies cause similar neutrophil responses as described above.

Viral Diseases
• There are many different viral diseases of cattle which require diagnostic evaluation (see Bovine Blood Chemistry, Diagnostic Techniques–Sampling for Microbiology, and Serologic Testing).
• Lymphopenia is found with many viral infections, particularly during the initial phases. If secondary bacterial infections develop, neutrophilia may occur as a response to inflammation.
• Persistent lymphocytosis occurs in cattle infected with BLV.

Parasitic Diseases
• Leukogram change may be found with many parasite infections. Such changes are nonspecific.
• Occasionally, eosinophilia develops during the migratory phase of multicellular parasites.

Neoplasia
• Neoplasia can cause a variety of leukogram changes. If a neoplasm itself becomes necrotic or if it damages invaded tissue or adjacent organs, neutrophilia and monocytosis may be found.
• Lymphocytosis with large, bizarre mononuclear lymphoblasts is occasionally found in cattle with lymphoma.

DIAGNOSIS

• Leukocyte parameters are evaluated as part of the information used to diagnose many diseases.
• A DNA-polymerase chain reaction (PCR)-restricted technique fragment length polymorphism (RTLP) technique for diagnosis of BLAD is available through Immgen Inc., College Station, Texas as well as the Bovine Blood Typing Laboratory of Canada, Saskatoon, Saskatchewan (see Diagnostic Techniques–PCR to Detect Microorganisms).

DIFFERENTIAL DIAGNOSIS

CBC/BIOCHEMISTRY/URINALYSIS
See Bovine Blood Chemistry, Bovine Leukemia, Diagnostic Techniques–Sampling for Microbiology, Serologic Testing, Lymphocytosis, and Lymphosarcoma.

OTHER LABORATORY TESTS
Evidence of an inflammatory reaction in the CBC that is suggestive of bacterial infection often suggests culture of the involved tissue or organ should be performed.

IMAGING

OTHER DIAGNOSTIC PROCEDURES

PATHOLOGIC FINDINGS
Inflammation may be detected in organs and tissues by histopathological evaluation.

TREATMENT

ACTIVITY

DIET

CLIENT EDUCATION

MEDICATIONS

DRUGS OF CHOICE
Bacterial infections may be treated with an appropriate antibiotic depending upon the organism's sensitivity and the legality of using a particular antibiotic in food-producing animals.

CONTRAINDICATIONS
Appropriate milk and meat withdrawal times must be followed for all compounds administered to food-producing animals.

MISCELLANEOUS

ASSOCIATED CONDITIONS
N/A

AGE-RELATED FACTORS
N/A

ZOONOTIC POTENTIAL
N/A

PREGNANCY
N/A

RUMINANT SPECIES AFFECTED
Bovine

BIOSECURITY
N/A

PRODUCTION MANAGEMENT
N/A

SYNONYMS
N/A

SEE ALSO
• Anemia, camelids
• Anemia, nonregenerative: bovine
• Anemia, regenerative: bovine

ABBREVIATIONS
• BLAD = bovine leukocyte adhesion deficiency
• BLV = bovine leukemia virus
• CHS = Chédiak-Higashi syndrome

Suggested Reading
Feldman, B. F., Zinkl, J. G., Jain, N. C. 2000. *Schalm's veterinary hematology*. 5th ed. Baltimore: Lippincott, Williams and Wilkins.
Jain, N. C. 1986. *Schalm's veterinary hematology*. 4th ed. Philadelphia: Lea and Febiger.
Zinkl, J. G. The leukocytes. 1981, May. *Vet Clin North Am Small Anim Pract*. 11(2):237–63.

Authors: Joseph G. Zinkl and Bernard F. Feldman

LIGHTNING STRIKE—SUDDEN DEATH

 BASICS

DEFINITION
• A discharge of electricity occurring in association with thunderstorms.
• Sudden death in groups of animals without signs of struggle is strongly suggestive of lightning strike.

OVERVIEW
Lightning may cause death after
• Direct strike—lightning strikes animals directly
• Contact—electrical charge passing through object such as tree or fence to animals
• Side flash—jumps one path to animals
• Step voltage—lightning strikes object that allows radiation of energy in all directions including where animals are standing thereby killing animals instantly
• Blunt trauma—lightning strike injures animal by knocking it to ground or via falling objects

PATHOPHYSIOLOGY
• The massive electrical current and voltage applied to animals by lightning most commonly results in subacute cardiac and respiratory arrest.
• Neurologic damage in animals can be observed in or around the 4th ventricle leading to cardiac and respiratory arrest.
• Survivors may develop multiple organ system dysfunction including severe burns, vascular injury (subcutaneous hemorrhages to DIC), traumatic injury to limbs (falling, blunt trauma), or nerve excitation resulting in massive muscle contraction and thermal injury to muscle. This may result in myonecrosis, rhabdomyolysis that may lead to renal compromise.
• Renal damage associated with rhabdomyolysis and myoglobinuria can also result in hyperkalemia, hypocalcemia, hyperglycemia, and acidosis.
• Gastrointestinal effects may be due to direct effect of electrical injury on abdominal organs leading to hemorrhage or the result of blunt trauma secondary to falling or objects striking the animal.

SYSTEMS AFFECTED
Any system can potentially be affected; skin lesions on animals struck directly by lightning, others may have minimal or no observable lesions.

GENETICS
N/A

INCIDENCE/PREVALENCE
Commonly observed in specific geographic locations during the spring, summer, and early fall months of the year. Thunderstorms are prevalent in the middle latitudes of the United States and some states have very high incidence of storms (Arizona, Colorado, and Florida).

GEOGRAPHIC DISTRIBUTION
Worldwide distribution

SIGNALMENT
Any animal; more commonly observed in pastured animals

Species
All ruminant species

Breed Predilections
N/A

Mean Age and Range
N/A

Predominant Sex
N/A

SIGNS
• Animal(s) found dead often after severe weather storms in areas where thunderstorms are frequent. Animals may be found dead where they were standing. Single or multiple animals may be found near large trees, against fences, or near watering holes, dead or unconscious.
• Feed (hay, grass) may be present within the oral cavity. Burn or singe marks on the animal and damage to the environment may be present; however, animals that are electrocuted secondary to charged water or earth or objects (step voltage) may not have visible signs of electrocution (burns).
• Death is usually instantaneous, and therefore little sign of struggle is evident.

• Singe or burn marks on animals are most commonly observed and are commonly present on medial surface of limbs, jaw, neck, and shoulders. Often, singe marks are located at one end of treelike scorch lines.
• Peripheral blood vessels are often distended with blood that clots poorly. There is capillary damage leading to subcutaneous hemorrhage and in some instances subcutaneous gas is noted.
• Ruminal distension may produce venous blood from abdomen to cranial aspect of animal.
• Nasal mucosal and frontal sinus congestion are observed in some cases, and linear mucosal hemorrhages of the larynx, trachea, and bronchi are present in most cases of lightning-induced death. This may lead to blood-tinged frothy fluid or ropes of clotted blood draining from mouth and nares.
• Infrequently, animals rendered unconscious by lightning strike followed by recovery may manifest neurologic signs and evidence of struggling may be present.
• A recent report of ocular disease in dairy cows following lightning strike indicates that electrical or blunt trauma to eyes may occur as is observed in human victims.
• Swine in outdoor pens struck by lightning manifested acute hind-limb paralysis.
• Lesions were limited to fractures of caudal lumbar and sacral vertebrae with dorsal displacement of sacral spine and transection of the spinal cord.
• Bilateral femur fractures were also observed in two calves associated with lightning strike.

 DIAGNOSIS

• Careful evaluation of animal(s) and immediate environment (up to 40 meters in diameter), for signs of burns, burnt or damaged trees, or other objects.
• Useful information may include number of animals affected, number in herd, specific management practices (feeding, watering, housing), recent medical history of animals, last observation of animal, and time of death (if known).

- History of recent severe weather, although this may confuse some cases.
- Necropsy of animal(s) is highly recommended. Transport to local state diagnostic laboratory, or a veterinarian should perform field necropsy.

DIFFERENTIAL DIAGNOSIS
- Any cause of acute death in livestock
- Anthrax (*Bacillus anthracis*), clostridial intoxications (*Clostridium hemolyticum, Clostridium chauvoei, Cl. perfringens, Clostridium botulinum*), *Mannheimia hemolytica, Haemophilus somnus, Listeria monocytogenes* septicemia, organophosphate, carbamate, lead, ionophore, gossypol, toxic gases, blue-green algae intoxication, Japanese yew, nitrates, cyanogenic plants, salt poisoning, and other toxicants

CBC/BIOCHEMISTRY/URINALYSIS
N/A

OTHER LABORATORY TESTS
- Samples to collect would include heart, lung, liver, spleen, kidneys, gut, lymph nodes, endocrine glands (thyroid, pancreas, adrenals), rumen content, skin and subcutaneous tissues, muscle (especially from limbs), paying particular attention to lesions or abnormalities observed.
- Samples should be saved for histopathology (10% buffered formalin), toxicology (frozen organs such as liver, kidney, rumen content, whole eyes, or ocular fluid aspirates), and microbiology (blood, brain, liver spleen, lymph-nodes, kidney and muscle, thoracic or abdominal fluids, CSF, urine).
- Samples for microbiology should be collected in sterile containers and stored on ice but not frozen. Feed or plants consumed may also be evaluated for pesticides, herbicides, and heavy metals.

IMAGING
N/A

TREATMENT
- Treatment of survivors should focus on clinical signs.
- Neurologic sequela are common, and nonsteroidal and steroidal anti-inflammatory agents, hyperosmolar agents (mannitol, 50% dextrose, hypertonic saline) to reduce inflammation and swelling in critical locations (CNS, muscle) are recommended.

- Local wound care for burns and systemic antimicrobial agents
- Appropriate milk and meat withdrawal times must be followed for all compounds administered to food-producing animals.
- Euthanasia for more severely affected animals may be appropriate.

MEDICATIONS

FOLLOW-UP

MISCELLANEOUS

ASSOCIATED CONDITIONS
N/A

AGE-RELATED FACTORS
N/A

ZOONOTIC POTENTIAL
N/A

PREGNANCY
N/A

RUMINANT SPECIES AFFECTED
Potentially all ruminant species

BIOSECURITY
N/A

PRODUCTION MANAGEMENT
Useful information may include number of animals affected, number in herd, specific management practices (feeding, watering, housing), recent medical history of animals, last observation of animal, and time of death (if known).

SYNONYMS
N/A

SEE ALSO
Anthrax (*Bacillus anthracis*)
Blue-green algae intoxication
Carbamate

Clostridial intoxications (*Clostridium hemolyticum, Clostridium chauvoei, Cl. perfringens, Clostridium botulinum*)
Cyanogenic plants
Euthanasia and disposal
Gossypol
Haemophilus somnus
Ionophore
Japanese yew
Lead
Listeria monocytogenes septicemia
Mannheimia hemolytica
Nitrates
Organophosphate
Salt poisoning and other toxicants
Toxic gases

ABBREVIATIONS
CNS = central nervous system
CSF = cerebral spinal fluid
DIC = disseminated intravascular coaggulopathy

Suggested Reading
Blackwell, J. G. 1976. Lightning incriminated in the sudden death of 18 steers. *Veterinary Medicine/Small Animal Clinician* 71: 1375–77.
Boeve, M. H., Huijben, R., Grinwis, G., Djajadiningrat-Laanen, S. C. 2004. Visual impairment after suspected lightning strike in a herd of Holstein-Friesian cattle. *Veterinary Record* 154: 402–4.
Casteel, S. W., Turk, J. R. 2002. Collapse/sudden death. In: *Large animal internal medicine*, ed. B. P. Smith. St. Louis: Mosby.
Ramsey, F. K., Howard, J. R. 1970. Diagnosis of lightning strike. *Journal of the American Veterinary Medical Association* 156: 1472–74.
Van Alstine, W. G., Widmer, W. R. 2003. Lightning injury in an outdoor swine herd. *Journal of Veterinary Diagnostic Investigation* 15: 289–91.

Author: Jeff Lakritz

LISTERIOSIS

 BASICS

OVERVIEW
• The most common clinical presentation of listeriosis in ruminants is a multifocal, assymetrical cranial nerve deficit with varying degrees of cortical involvement. Less common clinical presentations include septicemia, abortion, and mastitis.
• The primary cause of listeriosis is *Listeria monocytogenes*. *Listeria ivanovii* is less pathogenic and a less frequent cause of clinical disease. *Listeria monocytogenes* is common in the environment both as a free-living bacteria and as a contaminant shed by clinically or subclinically infected animals.

SIGNALMENT
The neurologic disease is observed in cattle, sheep, goats, and other ruminants. Septicemic disease may be observed in both ruminants and monogastrics.

SIGNS
• A detailed neurologic examination is the single most important step in determining a diagnosis of listeriosis.
• Affected animals typically have clinical signs suggestive of cortical and multifocal asymmetrical cranial nerve deficits. Referable to the cortical component of the disease, affected animals are usually somnolent and depressed.
• Propulsive walking also may be observed. Occasionally, a primary spinal cord disease is observed in ruminants.
• The most consistent, prominent, and helpful clinical signs are referable to multiple, asymmetrical cranial nerve deficits. Like cattle with otitis, these clinical signs often include drooped or immobile ears, inability to close palpebrae, loss of facial sensation, strabismus, and nystagmus.
• Cranial nerve VIII involvement is common, resulting in head tilt and circling toward the lesion. In contrast to otitis, involvement of additional cranial nerves and cortical involvement are common. Consequently, additional clinical signs including ptosis, inability to swallow, dropped or assymetrical jaw, difficulty ingesting food and water, asymmetry and deviation of the tongue may be observed. Right- and left-sided cranial nerve deficits in the same animal are common.

• Ataxia of varying degree is usually present.
• Dramatic dehydration is common due to loss of saliva and inability to prehend and swallow food and water. Prolonged skin tenting, sunken eyes, and very firm rumen contents confirm dehydration.

CAUSES
• The primary cause of listeriosis is *Listeria monocytogenes*. *Listeria ivanovii* is less pathogenic and a less-frequent cause of clinical disease. *Listeria monocytogenes* is common in the environment both as a free-living bacteria and as a contaminant shed by clinically or subclinically infected animals.
• The bacteria will persist for extended intervals following contamination.
• *Listeria* grows at temperatures ranging from 0°C to 45°C and at a pH as low as 4.5.

RISK FACTORS
• The most common and easily recognized risk factor for listeriosis is the feeding of poorly preserved ensiled forages. These forages will generally have a pH greater than 4.0. Visible spoilage may or may not be present.
• Factors that limit the efficacy of silage fermentation include long fiber length, drier than optimal silage, inadequate packing of forage, use of bunker rather than tower silos, absence of silo covers, and relatively slow feeding, which permits spoilage at the face of a bunker silo or top of a tower silo.
• Baled silage probably increases the risk of listeriosis because the quality of fermentation is generally less adequate.
• Contamination of silage with soil also is a potential risk factor.
• It should be noted that many outbreaks have no history of silage feeding, particularly in the case of small ruminants. In these instances, the presumption is that pasture contamination and persistence of the bacteria create an increased risk for clinical disease.
• Additional risk factors implicated in some outbreaks include abrupt changes in rainfall or temperature, calving, transportation, and poor body condition.

 DIAGNOSIS

DIFFERENTIAL DIAGNOSIS
• Common differential diagnoses include otitis, thromboembolic meningoencephalitis caused by *Hemophilus somnus*, and brain stem abscesses.

• Asymmetrical cortical diseases may be considered initially as differential diagnoses because affected animals often circle; however, these animals will not have the characteristic cranial nerve deficits usually seen in ruminants with listeriosis.
• Diseases that cause diffuse cortical disease like polioencephalomalacia and lead intoxication are sufficiently dissimilar in appearance that they may be discounted by the initial neurologic examination.

CBC/BIOCHEMISTRY/URINALYSIS
• Laboratory tests that may be helpful in the diagnosis and treatment of listeriosis include packed cell volume, serum protein, and serum chemistries.
• Increased hematocrit and serum protein concentrations are often dramatic. Serum chemistries often reveal very low serum bicarbonate or total CO_2, suggesting a metabolic acidosis, low serum urea concentrations, and hypokalemia; however, these results are not pathognomonic. These results will often prove useful during treatment.

IMAGING
N/A

OTHER DIAGNOSTIC PROCEDURES
• Cerebrospinal fluid (CSF) analysis may be helpful in differentiating causes of asymmetrical brain stem disease in feedlot cattle.
• Listeriosis will generally cause mild increases in CSF cell counts and protein concentrations with the predominant cells being mononuclear cells, lymphocytes, and monocytes. In contrast, thromboembolic meningoencephalitis will typically result in a CSF that has a high cell count, a high protein concentration, a visible yellow color, and a preponderance of neutrophils.
• Likewise, culture of the CSF may support specific differential diagnoses; however, negative CSF cultures are expected in most animals with listeriosis.
• Bacterial cultures of CSF or, in the cases of postmortem specimens, brain tissue may permit isolation of *Listeria monocytogenes*. It should be stressed that the sensitivity of this procedure is limited and negative cultures do not rule out listeriosis. Additionally, isolation of *Listeria* spp. typically requires cold enrichment procedures and extended incubation times, which limit the timely diagnosis and preventive intervention.

TREATMENT

• A number of antibiotics have been advocated for the treatment of listeriosis. The two antibiotics most commonly recommended are penicillin (20,000 to 40,000 IU/kg BID) and oxytetracycline (10 mg/kg SID). Various sources strongly advocate one or the other antibiotic; however, no controlled comparative efficacy data are available.
• Drug withdrawal times must be determined and maintained for all drugs utilized in food-producing animals.
• Fluid and electrolyte therapy is critical for optimal patient care. Affected animals are typically profoundly dehydrated with severe metabolic acidosis.
• Additional abnormalities often observed include hypokalemia and hypocalcemia. Efforts to replace fluid and base deficits, meet maintenance requirements, and correct hypokalemia and hypocalcemia should be directed by serum chemistry results because the severity of these abnormalities is highly variable. Fluid therapy is discussed in more detail in a separate chapter.
• Oral fluids are a reasonable, low-cost alternative in most affected animals. Mature cattle readily tolerate administration of 20–40 L of oral fluid several times per day.

DIET

CLIENT EDUCATION
• Parenteral nutrition is costly and probably contraindicated in most cases of listeriosis.
• In expensive animals or pet food animals, the practitioner may consider performing a rumenostomy to facilitate administration of food, water, and electrolytes.

MEDICATIONS

DRUGS OF CHOICE

CONTRAINDICATIONS
Appropriate milk and meat withdrawal times must be followed for all compounds administered to food-producing animals.

FOLLOW-UP

• Prognosis varies between cattle and small ruminants.
• The disease in sheep and goats progresses more rapidly, responds poorly to treatment, and usually is fatal. The prognosis in affected cattle is guarded.
• In cattle, early intervention and appropriate fluid, electrolyte, and nutritional support improve the prognosis.
• Cattle that recover from listeriosis will generally begin to eat and drink within 2 to 3 days after the start of treatment.
• In cattle with severe, progressive clinical signs and no improvement after 2 to 3 days of treatment, euthanasia should be considered.

MISCELLANEOUS

ASSOCIATED CONDITIONS
Affected animals typically have clinical signs suggestive of cortical and multifocal asymmetrical cranial nerve deficits.

AGE-RELATED FACTORS
N/A

ZOONOTIC POTENTIAL
• The disease in humans occurs primarily as a food-borne disease affecting the immunosuppressed, fetal, young or old host.
• Contaminated raw milk products pose a particular risk.
• Practitioners and livestock producers should take precautions when handling aborted fetuses or infected tissues because the organism can be spread by direct contact.

PREGNANCY
N/A

RUMINANT SPECIES AFFECTED
Potentially, all ruminant species are affected.

BIOSECURITY
N/A

PRODUCTION MANAGEMENT
• Factors that limit the efficacy of silage fermentation include long fiber length, drier than optimal silage, inadequate packing of forage, use of bunker rather than tower silos, absence of silo covers, and relatively slow feeding, which permits spoilage at the face of a bunker silo or top of a tower silo.
• Baled silage probably increases the risk of listeriosis because the quality of fermentation is generally less adequate.
• Contamination of silage with soil also is potential risk factor.

SYNONYMS
N/A

SEE ALSO
Asymmetrical cortical diseases
Brain stem abscesses
Lead intoxication
Otitis
Polioencephalomalacia
Thromboembolic meningoencephalitis caused by *Hemophilus somnus*

ABBREVIATIONS
BID = given twice daily
CSF = cerebral spinal fluid
SID = given once daily

Suggested Reading
Radostits, O. M., Gay, C. C., Blood, D. C., Hinchcliff, K. W. 2000. *Veterinary medicine.* 9th ed. New York: W. B. Saunders.
Rebhun, W. C., de Lahunta, A. 1982. Diagnosis and treatment of bovine listeriosis. *J Am Vet Med Assoc.* 180:395–98.

Author: Jeffrey W. Tyler

LIVER ABSCESSES

 BASICS

DEFINITION
• Hepatic abscesses are common as a sequela to rumen acidosis in cattle fed highly fermentable diets.
• Neonatal calves are susceptible to ascending navel infections, which can occasionally result in hepatic abscesses.
• Foreign bodies can cause abscessation by penetrating the liver parenchyma.
• The most common bacterial species cultured from hepatic abscesses, in cattle and sheep, are *Fusobacterium necrophorum* (predominantly found), *Streptococcus, Staphylococcus, Bacteroides*, and *Arcanobacterium pyogenes* (formerly known as *Corynebacterium pyogenes*).
• Liver abscesses represent a major economic loss to producers of feedlot cattle.
• Goats that have hepatic abscess are usually older than a year of age and in poor nutritional condition. The abscesses are usually secondary to a primary disorder. The most common bacterial species found in the abscesses are *Corynebacterium pseudotuberculosis, Escherichia coli*, and *Corynebacterium* spp.

PATHOPHYSIOLOGY
• Liver abscessation in ruminants is a result of compromise to the integrity of the ruminal wall. The compromise can be a sequela of rumen acidosis and/or objects penetrating the ruminal wall. The objects can range from coarse hay to foreign material.
• The primary organism involved in 85% of liver abscesses cultured is *Fusobacterium necrophorum*. This organism is a commensal microbe of the ruminal flora. Its primary energy substrate is lactate, allowing it to proliferate in an anaerobic environment that is using highly fermentable substrates to produce lactate.

• As bacteria colonize the ruminal wall, they shed bacterial emboli into the vascular drainage of the rumen and enter in the portal circulation. Bacteria and other foreign debris are phagocytized from the blood by Kupffer cells and leukocytes in the liver.
• The liver is a highly vascular and well-oxygenated organ. Since most of the bacteria and primarily *Fusobacterium necrophorum* are anaerobic bacteria, they have special virulence factors that allow them to establish an anaerobic microenvironment in which they can proliferate and produce an abscess.
• *Fusobacterium necrophorum* has leukotoxin and endotoxic lipopolysaccharides that help defend the bacteria from phagocytosis, and also promote intravascular coagulation, which results in infarcts in the parenchyma of the liver.
• As the abscess forms, it becomes encapsulated with connective tissue. In time, fluid reabsorption and connective tissue infiltration result in scar tissue formation in the liver with a net loss of parenchymal tissue.
• Occasionally, the abscess may rupture into the venous circulation resulting in anaphylaxis or showering the lungs with bacterial emboli. Ruptured abscesses can also cause formation of a thrombus in the caudal vena cava, which can result in portal hypertension and lead to ascites. If an abscess continues to increase in size, it may occlude the common bile duct and prevent bile secretion into the gastrointestinal tract.
• Liver abscesses do result from ascending umbilical vein infections in neonates. Neonates that have failure of passive transfer can also form liver abscesses independent of the nidus as they become bacteremic.
• Liver abscesses have also been reported in cattle infected with *Fasciola hepatica*.

SYSTEMS AFFECTED
• Hepatobiliary—loss of parenchymal tissue resulting in a decrease in metabolism of glucose and production of albumin. If the bile duct becomes obstructed, there is a decrease in bilirubin excretion and bile production.
• Musculoskeletal—decrease in weight gain and possible loss in muscle mass. If liver abscesses rupture into the venous circulation, it could result in laminitis.
• Skin—obstruction of the bile duct could prevent the excretion of phylloerythrin, which is a photodynamic agent to the dermis. The animal's dermis becomes photosensitized to UV light.
• Respiratory—occasionally, liver abscesses rupture into the caudal vena cava resulting in bacterial emboli being carried through the right heart chambers and into the lungs. Once in the lungs, the emboli can form abscesses that may erode through vessels in the lungs and cause hemorrhage into the bronchioles. Bilateral epistaxis and potentially exsanguination may result.
• Nervous—if enough of the liver is compromised, ammonia will not be converted to urea and neurological damage may result.
• Metabolic—destruction of liver parenchyma will prevent proper metabolism of glucose and glucose precursors in the blood. The animals will have poor weight gain and can have weight loss.
• Gastrointestinal—ruminal acidosis is the most consistent finding in animals with abscesses.

GENETICS
N/A

INCIDENCE/PREVALENCE
• In general, the incidence of liver abscesses is increased in ruminants fed diets high in carbohydrates and low in roughage.
• Holsteins are fed a consistently higher energy diet than beef cattle for longer periods; therefore, they have a higher incidence of liver abscesses.
• Feedlot steers have a somewhat higher incidence than heifers, which is believed to be related to higher amounts of feed intake.
• Cattle fed long-stem, dry, coarse hay are more prone to rumen wall penetration and abscess formation.
• Calves born in a dirty environment or that do not receive adequate colostrum are predisposed to ascending umbilical vein infections.
• Cattle in areas where liver flukes are endemic and not provided adequate prophylaxis can have abscesses form along the parasites' migratory tract.

GEOGRAPHIC DISTRIBUTION
None

SIGNALMENT
Species
Liver abscesses have been identified in bovine, ovine, and caprine species. In cattle and in sheep, the appearance of abscesses is primarily associated with animals that are being fed a highly fermentable diet with low roughage, leading to ruminal acidosis. In goats, the animals are usually older than a year and in poor body condition, with an accompanying pathologic disorder.

Breed Predilections
N/A

Mean Age and Range
Caprine, older than one year; beef and dairy cattle old enough to be fed a highly fermentable diet

Predominant Sex
N/A

SIGNS
GENERAL COMMENTS
Most cases of hepatic abscesses are subclinical and do not become recognized until the animals are slaughtered.

HISTORICAL FINDINGS
• Loss of weight
• Reduction in feed intake
• Decrease in feed efficiency
• Dairy cows or dairy goats may have a decrease in milk production.

PHYSICAL EXAMINATION FINDINGS
May have fevers, anorexia, exhibit pain when moving, diarrhea, ascites, peritonitis, and septic joints

CAUSES
• Rumen acidosis
• Septicemia and or bacteremia
• Ascending umbilical vein infection
• Liver flukes

RISK FACTORS
• Highly fermentable feeds
• Long-stem, dry coarse hay
• Dirty environment for neonates

DIAGNOSIS
Liver abscesses are usually detected only at the time of slaughter, since two-thirds of the liver must be affected before clinical signs manifest themselves.

DIFFERENTIAL DIAGNOSIS
• Parasitism
• Malnutrition
• Poor-quality feed
• Johne's disease
• Lymphosarcoma
• Traumatic reticuloperitonitis
• Hepatic lipidosis
• Polioencephalomalacia
• Septicemia

CBC/BIOCHEMISTRY/URINALYSIS
• In general, CBC and biochemistry tests are not reliable indicators of hepatic abscesses. If alterations are observed, they usually support the diagnosis but are not specific.
• CBC—can have a leukocytosis characterized by a neutrophilia and may or may not show an increase or decrease in total proteins. Anemia may be present due to chronic inflammation.
• Biochemistry—elevations in liver enzymes such as sorbitol dehydrogenase, gamma-glutamyltransferase, and aspartate aminotransferase may be present. Total bilirubin may not be elevated, but if there is a bile duct obstruction, there could be elevations in direct bilirubin.

OTHER LABORATORY TESTS
Liver function tests are not very informative and usually are cost and time prohibitive in ruminants.

IMAGING
Ultrasound of the liver can be rewarding if the abscess is in an area where it can be visualized.

DIAGNOSTIC PROCEDURES
An ultrasound guided liver aspirate may be useful if the abscess is in an area that can be visualized and aspirated.

PATHOLOGIC FINDINGS
• Abscesses in the liver can appear as large single abscesses or multiple irregular, granular yellow lesions randomly distributed (telangiectasis).

LIVER ABSCESSES

• There are two different types of gross pathologic lesions found in the liver. The first is an abscess with a thin capsule and a central area of necrosis and purulent material. The second is a thick, fibrous capsule with a central cavity and little to no purulent material.
• Some of the lesions with a thickened capsule may have central mineralization.
• Histologically, the abscesses that are a result of bacterial emboli appear as having a central area of coagulative necrosis with numerous phagocytic cells. Depending on the length of time the abscess has been forming, there may be bacteria present in the center, but more likely they are concentrated in the periphery of the necrotic core.
• Abscesses resulting from the migration of hepatic parasites include focal and multifocal coalescence of eosinophils forming granulomatous inflammation.

TREATMENT

• Treatment of animals identified with abscesses is often unrewarding due to the diffuse nature of the abscesses and limited blood supply to the heavy capsular lining. However, high doses of penicillin and oxytetracycline along with supportive therapy may be effective.
• If the abscess is in an area where it can be accessed surgically, it can be drained. This procedure is cost prohibitive in most food-animal cases.
• Anti-inflammatory agents can be administered to reduce damage from inflammatory factors and provide pain management.

APPROPRIATE HEALTH CARE

• There is very little that can be done that is cost effective in production animals. Most of these animals are culled due to poor performance.

• Supportive therapy and high levels of antibiotics can be administered to ruminants that are nonproduction animals.

NURSING CARE

Appropriate supportive care as warranted by the presenting clinical signs

ACTIVITY

• The animal's activity does not need to be restricted if it does not have pulmonary involvement.
• Pulmonary arterial thromboembolism will require that the animal be kept quiet. Activity should be limited to prevent the rupture of abscesses that could lead to hemorrhage.

DIET

• It is important to make sure that highly fermentable feeds are introduced slowly into the diet.
• If an animal is receiving a highly fermentable diet, adequate amounts of roughage need to be added to ensure proper buffering from saliva and ruminal motility.
• Feed additives that contain antibiotics help to decrease the numbers of bacteria responsible for producing acidic agents in the rumen.
• An adequate quantity of high-quality colostrum ingested by neonates will help to prevent septicemia and omphalophlebitis in calves.

CLIENT EDUCATION

• Educating clients on how to introduce highly fermentable feeds into the diet
• Feeding a balanced ration with enough fiber and roughage
• Proper neonatal management to prevent septicemia and failure of passive transfer
• Making sure the client has a proper parasite management program to eliminate the possibility of liver fluke infestation

SURGICAL CONSIDERATIONS

• Abscesses can be drained to the outside of the body if in an anatomic location that will allow for it.
• It is often cost prohibitive and impractical to do surgery on affected animals.

MEDICATIONS

DRUGS OF CHOICE

• Penicillins, ampicillin, and oxytetracycline are the drugs of choice to treat animals diagnosed with liver abscesses. The drugs are usually administered at very high doses for long periods of time, to try to facilitate penetration of the abscess capsular lining. Sometimes these drugs are combined with rifampin and metronidazole.
• Drugs used as feed additives for the prevention of abscess formation are bacitracin, lasalocid, monensin, oxytetracycline, tylosin, tilmicosin, and virginiamycin.

CONTRAINDICATIONS

Since most of the ruminants predisposed to liver abscess are production animals, which will have products that enter the human food chain, antibiotic residue avoidance needs to be taken into consideration.

PRECAUTIONS

• Any time antibiotics are introduced into a ruminant, they have the potential to alter normal ruminal microflora. Altered ruminal flora populations may either increase or decrease feed efficiency.
• Administering high levels of oxytetracyclines can cause hypocalcemia in cattle.

POSSIBLE INTERACTIONS

Any antibiotics or drugs that require metabolism by the liver should not be used if there is indication that the majority of the liver is affected.

ALTERNATIVE DRUGS

Alternative antibiotics may be used if the ruminant is not an animal that could end up in the food chain.

FOLLOW-UP

N/A

PATIENT MONITORING

There is very little patient monitoring that can be done for ruminants with liver abscesses. Depending on the extent of liver involvement, clinical signs associated with hepatic insufficiency may be evident. However, usually these animals will be "poor doers" and have a decrease in weight gain and increase in the amount of time it takes to achieve production goals.

PREVENTION/AVOIDANCE

• Prevention of ruminal acidosis by feeding adequate amounts of roughage is a key factor in reducing the incidence of liver abscesses in animals being fed highly fermentable feeds.
• The roughage will increase the amount of saliva produced to buffer VFA in the rumen. It will also help to maintain a healthy population distribution of lactobacillus organisms in the rumen.
• Introducing highly fermentable feeds slowly into the diets of ruminants will allow for adaptation of the microflora and absorptive capacity of the rumen to prevent a buildup of acidic agents.
• There are a number of feed additives that are used to decrease the incidence of ruminal acidosis and consequently liver abscesses. These additives can be ionophore antibiotics, which control the growth of gram-positive bacteria in the rumen and reduce the number of lactic acid–producing bacteria present.
• Tylosin is another antibiotic that is added to feeds. It directly decreases the number of *Fusobacterium necrophorum* and *Arcanobacterium pyogenes* bacteria in the rumen, and reduces the incidence of bacterial emboli formed in the ruminal wall that can travel to the liver.

• Regular preventive anthelmintics may reduce the risk of liver flukes producing migratory tracts in the liver that can become infected.
• Proper environmental management, along with navel dipping and assuring adequate colostrums, will help to prevent ascending umbilical vein infections.

POSSIBLE COMPLICATIONS

• The primary problem resulting from liver abscesses is a decrease in feed utilization by the animal. This in turn means a decrease in weight gain and possible weight loss as well as an increase in feed cost.
• Ruminants with liver abscesses also have an increased incidence of other medical complications, resulting in loss of income due to veterinary service and treatment cost.

EXPECTED COURSE AND PROGNOSIS

Since the vast majority of liver abscesses are undetected until slaughter, this is primarily a subclinical disease with major economic impact in the cattle industry.

MISCELLANEOUS

ASSOCIATED CONDITIONS

• Rumen acidosis
• Bloat
• Caudal vena cava thrombosis
• Pulmonary arterial thromboembolism
• Laminitis
• Polioencephalomalacia

AGE-RELATED FACTORS

N/A

ZOONOTIC POTENTIAL

N/A

PREGNANCY

N/A

RUMINANT SPECIES AFFECTED

Bovine, caprine, ovine, cervid

BIOSECURITY

N/A

PRODUCTION MANAGEMENT

See Prevention/Avoidance above.

SYNONYMS

Saw dust liver
Septic cholangiohepatitis
Telangiectasis

SEE ALSO

Caudal vena cava syndrome
Laminitis
Liver flukes
Omphalophlebitis
Polioencephalomalacia
Pulmonary arterial thromboembolism
Rumen acidosis
Rumenitis

ABBREVIATIONS

VFAs = volatile fatty acids

Suggested Reading

Brent, B. E. 1976. Relationship of acidosis to other feedlot ailments. *J Anim Sci.* 43:930–35.

Brink, D. R., Lowry, R. A., Parrott, J. C. 1990. Severity of liver abscesses and efficiency of feed utilization of feedlot cattle. *J Anim Sci.* 68:1201–7.

Johnson, B. 1991, Mar. Nutritional and dietary interrelationships with diseases of feedlot cattle. In: *The veterinary clinics of North America, food animal practice*, ed. J. Mass. Philadelphia: W. B. Saunders.

Nagaraja, T. G., Chengappa, M. M. 1998. Liver abscesses in feedlot cattle. *J Anim Sci.* 76:287–98.

O'Sullivan, E. N. 1999. Two-year study of bovine hepatic abscessation in 10 abattoirs in County Cork, Ireland. *Vet Rec.* 145:389–93.

Pearson, E. G., Mass, J. 2002. Liver abscesses. In: *Large animal internal medicine*, ed. B. P. Smith. 3rd ed. St. Louis: Mosby.

Author: Margo R. Machen

LOUPING ILL

 BASICS

OVERVIEW
• Louping ill is a term used to describe an acute tick-transmitted encephalomyelitis that affects mainly sheep, but is found in many other vertebrate animals. Louping ill virus is a single-stranded, neurotropic, RNA virus in the genus *Flavivirus* in the family Flaviviridae. The virus belongs to a subgroup of related viruses known as the tick-borne encephalitis complex.
• Small mammals and birds such as hares, red grouse, and ptarmigan are believed reservoirs that maintain the virus in the environment.

PATHOPHYSIOLOGY
• Louping ill is transmitted from animal to animal by a tick vector. *Ixodes ricinus* is thought to be the natural vector and other species including *Rhipicephalus appendiculatus*, *Ixodes persulcatus*, and *Haemaphysalis anatolicum* have been found carrying the virus. The larva, nymph, and adult may carry the virus by feeding on a viremic host. Transmission between life cycles of the tick appears to be only transstadially.
• Clinical signs of louping ill occur in two phases. The initial phase may be mild or unapparent with most animals suffering from a mild fever. Infected animals will either recover at this point or the virus will enter the central nervous system leading to associated clinical signs.
• Lactating goats can excrete high numbers of virus in milk, which can lead to a fatal infection in newborn kids. Louping ill virus can also be transmitted to various host species through exposure to aerosols and by parenteral routes.

SYSTEMS AFFECTED
• Nervous—primarily central nervous system
• Respiratory—primarily lungs
• Gastrointestinal

GENETICS
N/A

INCIDENCE/PREVALANCE
• All ages of sheep can be infected with Louping ill virus; however, lambs born to immune dams are passively protected for the first year. Yearlings are most susceptible and may have mortality rates as high as 60%. The prevalence of infection may be as high as 60% in adult sheep, but the incidence of disease is low unless the sheep have been moved from a nonendemic area to an endemic area.
• The disease is most prevalent during April through June and again in September due to the annual periodicity of tick activity.

GEOGRAPHIC DISTRIBUTION
Louping ill can be found strictly in the upland areas of the British Isles and Norway. A similar related disease of sheep has been reported in Bulgaria, Turkey, and the Basque region of Spain.

SIGNALMENT
Species
Sheep, cattle, goats, deer
Breed Predilections
None
Mean Age and Range
Mean—<2 years of age; Age range—all ages
Predominant Sex
None

SIGNS
HISTORICAL FINDINGS
• Depression
• Anorexia
• Muscle tremors
• Incoordination
• Salivation
• Protrusion of the tongue
• Chomping of the jaws
• Hopping "louping" gait
• Hypersensitivity to noise and touch

PHYSICAL EXAMINATION FINDINGS
• Fever—42°C, 107.6°F
• Depression
• Muscle tremors
• Incoordination
• Ataxia
• Hyperesthesia
• Louping gait
• Head-pressing
• Paraplegia
• Convulsions
• Opisthotonus
• Coma
• Constipation

CAUSES
A single-stranded, neurotropic RNA virus of the genus *Flavivirus*, family Flaviviridae, causes louping ill.

RISK FACTORS
• Grazing pastures infested with infected ticks is the most common way to acquire infection. The larva, nymph, and adult may carry the virus by feeding on a viremic host.
• Transmission between life cycles of the tick appears to be only transstadially.
• Concurrent infection with *Cytoecetes plagocytophila* or *Toxoplasma gondii* can exert a profound immunosuppressive effect on the immune system.

 DIAGNOSIS

DIFFERENTIAL DIAGNOSIS
Sheep
• Scrapie
• Maedi visna
• Pregnancy toxemia
• Hypocalcemia
• Tetanus
• Listeriosis
• Tick pyemia
• Hypocuprosis
• Rabies
• Hydatid disease
• Heavy metal toxicity
• Plant toxicosis
Cattle
• Malignant catarrhal fever
• Listeriosis
• Pseudorabies
• Bovine spongiform encephalopathy
• Rabies
• Hypomagnesemia
• Hypocalcemia
• Acute lead poisoning
• Plant toxicosis

CBC/BIOCHEMISTRY/URINALYSIS
None

OTHER LABORATORY TESTS
• Virus isolation from the blood during the febrile stage
• Hemagglutination inhibition test during febrile stage to detect IgM antibodies
• Fourfold or greater rise in antibody titer after central nervous system signs have developed
• ELISA for tick-borne encephalitis virus

IMAGING
N/A

DIAGNOSTIC PROCEDURES
Virus isolation from necropsy samples of the brain and spinal cord. Sterile unfixed samples should be placed in 50% glycerol and normal saline or frozen on dry ice.

PATHOLOGIC FINDINGS
• Gross lesions: congested meningeal vessels, secondary pneumonia
• Histopathology: nonsuppurative polio- and mengioencephalomyelitis with gliosis, perivascular infiltration, and neuronal degeneration. Lesions are primarily located in the brain stem.

TREATMENT

APPROPRIATE HEALTH CARE
• No specific treatment for individual animals
• Herd preventative care—vaccination with an inactivated, tissue-culture-propagated vaccine, pour-on acaricidal preparations

NURSING CARE
Infected animals should be provided with basic supportive care and sedation to prevent convulsions. Unlike sheep, cattle may fare well with basic nursing care.

ACTIVITY
Animals should be kept in a quiet location to prevent agitation, convulsions, and injury.

DIET
Animals showing clinical signs should be hand-fed to ensure adequate nutrition.

CLIENT EDUCATION
Clients need to be educated in the importance of tick control and vaccination protocols to prevent infection.

SURGICAL CONSIDERATIONS
N/A

MEDICATIONS

DRUGS OF CHOICE
None available

CONTRAINDICATIONS
N/A

PRECAUTIONS
N/A

POSSIBLE INTERACTIONS
N/A

ALTERNATIVE DRUGS
N/A

FOLLOW-UP

PATIENT MONITORING
Affected animals should be monitored frequently for convulsions due to noise or touch.

PREVENTION/AVOIDANCE
• An inactivated, tissue-culture-propagated vaccine is available for sheep, cattle, and goats. One injection will provide protection for >2 years. All animals kept for breeding should be vaccinated at 6–12 months of age.
• Pour-on insecticides should be used to reduce tick exposure.

POSSIBLE COMPLICATIONS
Animals that survive clinical disease have residual central nervous system deficits of variable severity.

EXPECTED COURSE AND PROGNOSIS
• In most cases, animals that show clinical signs will succumb after a clinical course of 1 to 12 days. Those that survive clinical disease never regain full health.
• Animals infected with louping ill virus are immune for life.

MISCELLANEOUS

ASSOCIATED CONDITIONS
CNS disorders

AGE-RELATED FACTORS
Where the disease is endemic, it is most often confined to animals <2 years of age because the adults are immune from previous infection and lambs are protected by colostral antibody.

ZOONOTIC POTENTIAL
Louping ill virus may infect humans through tick bites, contamination of skin wounds, and aerosol exposure. Ingestion of contaminated sheep or goat's milk may also result in infection. Infected humans may develop an illness that resembles influenza, polio, biphasic encephalitis, or a hemorrhagic fever.

PREGNANCY
Lambs born to nonimmune ewes that are exposed to the virus may develop a peracute illness with death occurring within 48 hours from the onset of clinical signs.

RUMINANT SPECIES AFFECTED
Sheep, goats, cattle, deer

SYNONYMS
Infectious encephalomyelitis of sheep
Ovine encephalomyelitis
Trembling ill

SEE ALSO
Brain lesions
CNS
Hypocalcemia
Listeriosis
Maedi visna
Pregnancy toxemia
Rabies
Scrapie
Tetanus

ABBREVIATIONS
CNS = central nervous system
IgM = immunoglobulin M
RNA = ribonucleic acid

Suggested Reading
Callan, R. J., Van Metre, D. C. 2004, Jul. Viral diseases of the ruminant nervous system. *Vet Clin North Am Food Anim Pract.* 20(2):327–62, vii.
Gritsun, T. S., Nuttall, P. A., Gould, E. A. 2003. Tick-borne flaviviruses. *Adv Virus Res.* 61:317–71.
Laurenson, M. K., Norman, R., Reid, H. W., Pow, I., Newborn, D., Hudson, P. J. 2000, Feb. The role of lambs in louping-ill virus amplification. *Parasitology* 120 (Pt 2):97–104.
Sheahan, B. J., Moore, M., Atkins, G. J. 2002, Feb-Apr. The pathogenicity of louping ill virus for mice and lambs. *J Comp Pathol.* 126(2–3):137–46.
Simpson, V. R. 2002, Mar. Wild animals as reservoirs of infectious diseases in the UK. *Vet J.* 163(2):128–46.
Timoney, P. J. 1998. Louping ill. In: *Foreign animal diseases.* Richmond, VA: United States Animal Health Association, http://www.vet.uga.edu/wpp/gray book/FAD.

Author: Stacy M. Holzbauer

LOW-FAT MILK SYNDROME

BASICS

OVERVIEW
• Low-fat milk syndrome is characterized by a decrease in milk fat content accompanied by a decrease in milk yield.
• Milk fat content and yield are highly responsive to nutrition; however, fatty acid composition of milk fat is affected to a lesser extent by the biohydrogenation of unsaturated fatty acids by rumen bacteria.
• Fat is the most variable constituent in ruminants' milk and also the major energy component. Triglycerides are the main form of fat secretion into milk, accounting for 97%–98% of the total milk lipids.
• The fatty acids can be either synthesized in the mammary gland from acetate and butyrate or taken up directly from the blood as preformed fatty acids. The mammary gland synthesizes short and medium carbon chain fatty acids (C4:0 to C14:0) and some palmitic acid (C16:0). The long carbon chain fatty acids (>C16:0) incorporated into milk fat arise from dietary lipids and from the mobilization of body fat stores available in the blood.
• Although different milk pricing systems are available worldwide, milk fat is still an important component in most countries and decreased milk fat percentage and yield can have a direct negative effect on dairy farm profitability.

PATHOPHYSIOLOGY
• Many theories exist as to pathophysiology.
• In one theory, biohydrogenation is compromised in animals that are fed diets that do not maintain a favorable rumen environment. Dietary factors that contribute to low rumen pH conditions reduce biohydrogenation of unsaturated fatty acids. Products from the incomplete biohydrogenation of unsaturated fatty acids in the rumen have a negative impact on lipid synthesis in the lactating mammary gland.
• In one study, cows fed low-forage diets (17.5% NDF) had lower milk fat content and yield. In addition, activity of key enzymes involved in de novo fatty acid synthesis in the mammary gland were dramatically reduced, by 62% and 44%, for acetyl-CoA-carboxylase and fatty acid synthase, respectively.
• *Trans*-octadecenoic acid (C18:1, *trans-10*) was shown to be negatively related to milk fat content; however, a direct cause-effect association has not been established.
• In another study, abomasal infusion of 10 g/d of conjugated linoleic acid (CLA; C18:2 *trans-10, cis-12*) resulted in 42% and 44% reduction in milk fat percentage and yield, respectively, mimicking the effect of a milk fat–depressing diet.

• Both fatty acids (C18:1, *trans-10*, and C18:2, *trans-10, cis-12*) originate in the rumen as intermediates in the biohydrogenation process of polyunsaturated fatty acids (Figure 1).
• Collectively, these data suggest that milk fat depression is caused by a direct effect of fatty acids originated from incomplete biohydrogenation in the rumen on mammary gland lipid synthesis. The precise role of specific fatty acids and possibly their interactions with mammary gland lipid metabolism is still unknown.

SIGNALMENT
• Holstein cows at or after peak lactation are more predisposed to the disease.
• Early lactating cows are under severe body fat mobilization and down regulation of mammary gland lipid synthesis during this period has little effect on milk fat content.
• Actually, early lactating cows have a higher milk fat content in the first weeks of lactation.

SIGNS
N/A

CAUSES AND RISK FACTORS
Milk fat depression is a consequence of incomplete biohydrogenation of polyunsaturated fatty acids in the rumen and exposure of the mammary gland to the detrimental effect of trans-fatty acids, intermediates in the process.

Risk Factors
• The feeding of polyunsaturated fatty acids. Milk fat depression has been shown in diets that contained at least 4%–4.5% crude fat.
• Dietary supplementation of oil is more likely to depress milk fat than oil seed incorporation.
• Low-forage diets (see Table 1 for fiber requirements).
• Excessively processed forages will result in poor particle size, decreased chewing time, and total buffer production.
• Feeding of marine oils
• Feeding corn silage as the only forage source in diets with a high level of NFC

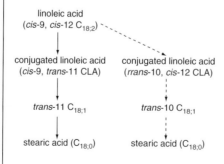

Figure 1.

Pathways of rumen biohydrogenation of linoleic acid (adapted from Bauman and Griinari, 2003).

DIAGNOSIS

DIFFERENTIAL DIAGNOSIS
N/A

CBC/BIOCHEMISTRY/URINALYSIS
N/A

OTHER LABORATORY TESTS
N/A

IMAGING
N/A

DIAGNOSTIC PROCEDURES
• Low-fat milk syndrome is diagnosed comparatively rather than by absolute milk fat percentage or yield. Therefore, knowledge of herd history, nutrition programs, and genetic background can be useful.
• Diagnosis is based on examination of milk production and composition records. In more chronic situations, symptoms related to subclinical ruminal acidosis may also be present. These symptoms include decreased feed intake, higher incidence of laminitis, and increased body condition loss.

TREATMENT
• Adjustment of the diet to maintain rumen health should be the main management goal.
• Low milk fat is frequently associated with dietary fiber (e.g., low forage content, high processed forages, or forages with lower effective fiber). The total NDF requirement in the NRC (2001) varies according to the amount of forage NDF and NFC in the diet. An increase in total diet NDF content for low-particle diets is recommended (Table 1).

Table 1

Minimal NDF Requirements for Diets of Lactating Cows Fed TMR with Adequate Particle Size and Ground Corn as the Predominant Starch		
Forage NDF (%)	Total dietary NDF (%)	Maximum dietary NFC (%)
19	25	44
18	27	42
17	29	40
16	31	38
15	33	36

Source: Adapted from NRC (2001).
Note: NDF = neutral detergent fiber; NFC = nonfiber carbohydrate; TMR = total mixed ration; NDF requirements should be increased when very processed forages are fed.

- Addition of buffers should be considered.
- Partial replacement of starch in the diet by fibrous by-products (e.g., almond hulls, whole cotton seed, soy hulls, beet or citrus pulp) is a useful tool to minimize decreased rumen pH.
- If marine oils are fed at more than 1% of diet DM, consider substitution of fat source.

MEDICATIONS
N/A

DRUGS OF CHOICE
- Addition of buffers to diet, including sodium bicarbonate and magnesium oxide, has improved rumen pH and diminished the negative effects of low-forage diets on milk fat.
- Sodium bicarbonate added at 0.7%–1.0% of diet DM has been effective in correcting milk fat depression. However, literature results can be inconsistent with respect to the effectiveness of buffers in controlling rumen pH (NRC, 2001).
- Buffer supplementation of high-forage diets or in pasture-based systems has produced poor results.

CONTRAINDICATIONS
N/A

POSSIBLE INTERACTIONS
N/A

PRECAUTIONS
Marine oils seem to directly affect biohydrogenation and cause milk fat depression even in situations of normal rumen pH. In one study, high levels of fish oil (2%–3% of DM) in diets with 50% forage (1:1, alfalfa/corn silage) had a linear negative effect on milk fat content and yield.

FOLLOW-UP
- Careful evaluation of diet composition is important and should account for:
  - NDF content
  - NDF from forage
  - Nonfiber carbohydrate
  - Source of starch in the diet
  - Processing characteristics of grains
  - Total lipid (ether extract) content
  - Type of fat supplement (vegetable oils, marine oils, oil seeds, protected fat, animal fat, etc.), which considers fatty acid composition of the lipid fraction

- Fiber content (NDF) of the diet is a critical issue in maintaining adequate rumen pH, but forage-particle size is also a contributing factor. Regular evaluation of diet particle size and processing characteristics of new forage feeds is recommended.
- Excessive mixing of TMR diets can reduce particle size and is a common mistake observed in the feeding routine.
- Adequate training of farm staff involved in feed activities is warranted in order to keep the feeding procedure as standardized as possible.

MISCELLANEOUS

ASSOCIATED CONDITIONS
Health problems associated with ruminal acidosis

AGE-RELATED FACTORS
N/A

ZOONOTIC POTENTIAL
N/A

PREGNANCY
N/A

RUMINANT SPECIES AFFECTED
Lactating dairy cattle

BIOSECURITY
N/A

PRODUCTION MANAGEMENT
- Adjustment of the diet to maintain rumen health should be the main management goal.
- Low milk fat is frequently associated with dietary fiber.
- Addition of buffers should be considered.
- Partial replacement of starch in the diet by fibrous by-products (e.g., almond hulls, whole cotton seed, soy hulls, beet or citrus pulp) is a useful tool to minimize decreased rumen pH.
- If marine oils are fed at more than 1% of diet DM, consider substitution of fat source.

SYNONYMS
N/A

SEE ALSO
Body condition scoring: dairy
Dairy heifer nutrient requirements
Dairy heifer nutrition
Dairy nutrition

ABBREVIATIONS
CLA = conjugated linoleic acid
DM = dry matter
NDF = neutral detergent fiber
NRC = National Research Council
TMR = total mixed ration
NFC = nonfiber carbohydrate

Suggested Reading
Bauman, D. E., Griinari, J. K. 2003. Nutritional regulation of milk fat synthesis. *Annu Rev Nutr*. 23:203–27.
Baumgard, L. H., Corl, B., Dwyer, D. A., Saebo, A., Bauman, D.E. 2000. Identification of the conjugated linoleic acid isomer that inhibits milk fat synthesis. *Am J Physiol Regulatory Integrative Comp Physiol*. 278: R179–R184.
Chilliard, Y., Ferlay, A., Mansbridge, R. M., Doreu, M. 2000. Ruminant milk fat plasticity: nutritional control of saturated, polyunsaturated, *trans* and conjugated fatty acids. *Ann Zootech*. 49:181–205.
Dovovan, D. C., Schingoethe, D. J., Baer, R. J., Ryalli, J., Hippen, A. R., Franklin, S.T. 2000. Influence of dietary fish oil on conjugated linoleic acid and other fatty acids in milk fat from dairy cows. *J Dairy Sci*. 83: 2620–28.
Griinari, J. M., Dwyer, D. A., Mcguire, M. A., Bauman, D. E., Palmquist, D. L., Nurmela, K. V. V. 1998. *Trans*-octadecenoic acids and milk fat depression in lactating dairy cows. *J Dairy Sci*. 81: 1251–61.
Kalscheur, K. F., Teter, B. B., Piperova, L. S., Erdman, R. A. 1997. Effect of dietary forage concentration and buffer addition on duodenal flow of *trans*-$C_{18:1}$ fatty acids and milk fat production in dairy cows. *J Dairy Sci*. 80: 2104–14.
National Research Council. 2001. *Nutrient requirements of dairy cattle*. 7th ed., Washington, DC: Natl. Acad. Sci.
Piperova, L. S., Teter, B. B., Bruckental, I., Sampugna, J., Mills, S. E., Yurawecz, M. P., Fritsche, J., Ku, K., Erdman, R. A. 2000. Mammary lipogenic enzyme activity, trans-fatty acids and conjugated linoleic acids are altered in lactating dairy cows fed a milk fat-depressing diet. *J Nutrition*, 2568–74.

Author: Sérgio O. Juchem

LUMPY SKIN DISEASE

 BASICS

OVERVIEW
• Lumpy skin disease (LSD) is a viral disease of cattle characterized by deep dermal skin nodules that eventually undergo central necrosis.
• Affected animals also usually have a high fever and a generalized lymphadenitis.
• LSD is caused by a capripoxvirus that is closely related to sheep and goat pox.
• The disease is endemic throughout most of Africa with occasional incursions into the Middle East. The virus primarily affects cattle but has experimentally infected giraffes and impalas.

SIGNALMENT
• Incubation period for the disease varies between 7 and 21 days with most cases being seen 10–12 days after exposure.
• Depending on the susceptibility of the cattle (Channel Island breeds are most susceptible), morbidity may range from 3% to 80% with mortality usually very low (1–3% in most cases).
• Animals with some other debilitating disease (parasitism, nutritional deficiency, or chronic disease) are more likely to die from infections.
• Calves tend to be more susceptible than adult cattle.

SIGNS
• Animals first develop a fever of 104–107°F (40–41.5°C). The fever may persist throughout the disease period and last up to 4 weeks.
• Large (1–5 cm) nodules develop under the skin usually within 2 days after the fever develops. Nodules develop primarily in the skin of the neck, muzzle, nares, eyelids, back, front and back legs, scrotum, perineum, mammary gland, teats, and tail. The oral mucosa may also become involved.
• Nodules become enlarged and involve the epidermis, dermis, and subcutaneous tissues and may involve the superficial muscles. Nodules are often painful to the touch.
• Edematous nodules eventually become necrotic and collapse centrally leaving an umbilicated lesion with a central necrotic core covered by a scab (sitfast). These heal slowly and are often complicated by secondary bacterial infections. Lesions that involve the mammary gland may become severely infected causing a severe mastitis and loss of the affected glands. Necrotic lesions may take up to 5 to 6 weeks to heal. Nodules may remain for some time in the skin until they resolve.
• In severe infections, the animal becomes lame due to the cutaneous nodules causing swelling and inflammation in the joints, tendon sheaths, and coronary band region.

• Large, swollen lymph nodes draining infected regions are often noted.
• Late-term abortions have been noted in infected animals; however, most abortions are believed due to the high fever and not infection of the fetus.
• Bulls may become sterile due to the high temperature or due to mechanical damage to the prepuce and penis from the virus.

CAUSES AND RISK FACTORS
• Transmission is believed to be by biting insect vectors. *Culex mirificus* and *Aedes natronius* are suspected.
• Disease outbreaks tend to occur most commonly during the rainy seasons.
• Contact with virally infected scabs and fomites can also spread the disease but to a lesser extent.
• The movement of contaminated raw hides has been implicated in some outbreaks.

 DIAGNOSIS

DIFFERENTIAL DIAGNOSIS
• Insect bites and associated urticaria: Lesions are often edematous and usually rise quickly after the animal is exposed. Lesions may itch but are not generally painful. Biopsies identify abundant edema and some eosinophils in the associated dermis.
• *Hypoderma bovis* infections: These are large nodules in the dermis that are usually seen in the skin of the dorsal back. Nodules have a central cavitary hole with fly larva present.
• Photosensitization: Nonpigmented regions are affected. The skin undergoes pronounced swelling and necrosis with flaking of the skin from the affected regions.
• Bovine papular stomatitis: Proliferative pox lesions are seen on the lips, muzzle, and oral and esophageal mucosa. Young animals are usually the only animals affected in the herd. Animals rarely have fever or pain associated with lesions.
• Allerton virus (Bovine herpes mammillitis, bovine herpesvirus type 2): Superficial epidermal lesions are identified primarily on the teats and muzzle but may be generalized. Lesions are small, raised nodules that scab over quickly and resolve leaving a hairless region with no damage to the hide.
• *Dermatophilus congolensis*: Lesions are usually generalized and characterized by some edema of the skin with scabs over affected areas. When the scabs are removed, normal epithelium is present. Characteristic bacteria consisting of numerous rows of coccoid organisms stacking up in the inflammation are present in the scab.

CBC/BIOCHEMISTRY/URINALYSIS
N/A

OTHER LABORATORY PROCEDURES
N/A

IMAGING
N/A

DIAGNOSTIC PROCEDURES
• Biopsies of early lesions that have not developed a scab can be used for virus isolation, histopathology, and electron microscopy.
• Aspirates of swollen lymph nodes should be placed in viral media and shipped on ice for virus isolation.
• Acute and convalescent sera should be obtained for serological testing.

PATHOLOGICAL FINDINGS

GROSS FINDINGS
• Animals develop generalized skin nodules 1–5 cm in diameter. Older nodules have a central area of necrosis with a central scab present (sitfast). Nodules are composed of edema, hemorrhage, and necrotic debris involving the epidermis, dermis, and subcuticular tissues and may extend into adjacent muscles.
• Individual or coalescing pox lesions can be present in the oral cavity, nares, pharynx, esophagus, and trachea. These lesions have coalescing thickening of the mucosa and submucosa with some edema, hemorrhage, and necrosis.
• Lymph nodes are swollen and enlarged.
• Lung lesions can occur with atelectasis and some edema present in affected lobules.
• Fibrin may be present in joints and tendon sheaths.

HISTOPATHOLOGIC FINDINGS
• Early skin lesions consist of swelling of the dermis with edema and some hemorrhage.
• Variable numbers of lymphocytes, neutrophils, and macrophages are present in the dermis with some fibroblastic proliferation present. Older lesions have vasculitis and thrombosis of vessels with necrosis of the associated tissues.
• The epidermis is acanthotic with orthokeratotic and parakeratotic hyperkeratosis, ballooning degeneration of the stratum spinosum, and necrosis of keratinocytes.
• Eosinophilic intracytoplasmic inclusions are present in swollen keratinocytes in the epidermis and in macrophages, fibroblasts, and endothelial cells in the affected dermis and subcutis. In old infarcted lesions, inclusion bodies are usually absent.

TREATMENT
• In most areas of the world, this is considered a reportable disease. Notification of state and/or federal veterinary authorities is important on suspicion of this disease.
• Treatment is supportive with antipyretic drugs (e.g., aspirin, flunixin meglumine) given to relieve the fever and improve the appetite of the affected animals.
• Antibiotics can be used for secondary bacterial infections that may occur in the skin, mammary gland, joints, or tendon sheaths.

MEDICATIONS
Appropriate antibiotics for treatment of bacterial complications should be made based on sensitivity of the bacterial agent.

CONTRAINDICATIONS/POSSIBLE INTERACTIONS
• Appropriate milk and meat withdrawal times must be followed for all compounds administered to food-producing animals.
• Steroids should not be used in pregnant animals.

FOLLOW-UP
PATIENT MONITORING
PREVENTION/AVOIDANCE
• In endemic areas of the world, vaccination has been successful in controlling outbreaks.
• Vaccinations with an attenuated LSD vaccine or with a sheep and goat pox vaccine have been successful.
• The control of insects has not proven effective at stopping the spread of the disease.

POSSIBLE COMPLICATIONS
• Secondary bacterial infections of the necrotic lesion are a common finding.
• Secondary bacterial infections of lesions of the mammary gland, joints, and penis can cause serious complications.

EXPECTED COURSE AND PROGNOSIS
• In naïve animals, mortality is usually low with most outbreaks having a mortality of less than 3%.
• Lesions may persist in severely affected animals for up to 6 months.
• Secondary bacterial infections can complicate the outcome of the disease.

MISCELLANEOUS
ASSOCIATED CONDITIONS
• Secondary bacterial infections of the necrotic lesion are a common finding.
• Secondary bacterial infections of lesions of the mammary gland, joints, and penis can cause serious complications.

AGE-RELATED FACTORS
N/A

ZOONOTIC POTENTIAL
N/A

PREGNANCY
Late-term abortions have been noted in infected animals; however, most abortions are believed to be due to the high fever and not infection of the fetus.

RUMINANT SPECIES AFFECTED
Channel Island breeds of cattle are most susceptible. Giraffes and impalas have been experimentally infected.

BIOSECURITY
• Quarantine all new stock entering the herd.
• Treat and/or cull animals with disease conditions prior to herd introduction.
• Contact with virus-infected scabs and fomites can also spread the disease but to a lesser extent.
• The movement of contaminated raw hides has been implicated in some outbreaks.

PRODUCTION MANAGEMENT
Bulls may become sterile due to the high temperature or due to mechanical damage to the prepuce and penis from the virus.

SYNONYMS
N/A

SEE ALSO
Allerton virus
Bovine herpes mammillitis
Bovine herpesvirus type 2
Bovine papular stomatitis
Dermatophilus congolensis
Hypoderma bovis
Insect bites and associated urticaria
Photosensitization

ABBREVIATIONS
LSD = lumpy skin disease

Suggested Reading
Hunter, P., Wallace, D. 2001. Lumpy skin disease in southern Africa: a review of the disease and aspects of control. *J S Afr Vet Assoc.* 72 (2):68 71.
Kitching, R. P. 2003. Vaccines for lumpy skin disease, sheep pox and goat pox. *Dev Biol (Basel).* 114:161–67.
Rweyemamu, M., Paskin, R., Benkirane, A., Martin, V., Roeder, P., Wojciechowski, K. 2000. Emerging diseases of Africa and the Middle East. *Ann N Y Acad Sci.* 916:61–70.
USAHA. 1998. Lumpy skin disease. In: *Foreign animal diseases.* Richmond, VA: United States Animal Health Association, http://www.vet.uga.edu/wpp/gray_book/FAD.

Author: Robert B. Moeller, Jr.

LUPINE TOXICITY

BASICS

OVERVIEW
• Lupines (*Lupinus* spp.) cause two distinct forms of poisoning in livestock: lupine poisoning and lupinosis. Alkaloid-containing lupines, *Lupinus formosus*, and *L. arbustus*.
• Lupine poisoning is a nervous syndrome caused by alkaloids present in bitter lupines.
• Lupinosis is a mycotic disease.
• The genus *Lupinus* contains a large number of species. In some parts of the world they form a useful fodder crop.
• Lupines are found in climax and grassy habits and are toxic even when dry.
• Many species of lupines contain quinolizidine or piperidine alkaloids known to be toxic or teratogenic to livestock.
• Defects caused by quinolizidine and piperidine teratogens include cleft palate and contracture-type skeletal defects such as arthrogryposis, scoliosis, torticollis, and kyphosis.
• Cleft palate and minor front limb contractures are induced in calves by maternal ingestion of the piperidine alkaloid-containing lupines, *Lupinus formosus* and *L. arbustus*. Crooked-calf disease, which includes an occasional cleft palate, is a congenital condition of widespread occurrence in cattle in the western United States and Canada. It is known to occur after maternal ingestion of certain species of *Lupinus* during specific gestational periods.

PATHOPHYSIOLOGY
• The toxic and teratogenic effects from these plant species have distinct similarities including maternal muscular weakness and ataxia and fetal contracture-type skeletal defects and cleft palate.
• It is believed that the mechanism of action of the piperidine and quinolizidine alkaloid-induced teratogenesis is the same; however, there are some differences in incidence, susceptible gestational periods, and severity between livestock species.

• Although many lupine species contain quinolizidine alkaloids including the teratogenic alkaloid anagyrine, *L. formosus* and *L. arbustus* produce piperidine alkaloids including the reported teratogen ammodendrine. In addition to ammodendrine, *L. formosus* contains both N-acetyl hystrine and N-methyl ammodendrine, whereas *L. arbustus* contains ammodendrine, trace amounts of N-methyl ammodendrine, and no N-acetyl hystrine.

SIGNALMENT
• Sheep, cattle, horses, pigs
• Most common in sheep and cattle

SIGNS
Lupine Poisoning
• Inappetence and dyspnea, usually followed by violent struggles, convulsions, and hyperexcitablility
• Death is due to respiratory paralysis.
• There is no icterus.
• Defects caused by quinolizidine and piperidine teratogens include cleft palate and contracture-type skeletal defects such as arthrogryposis, scoliosis, torticollis, and kyphosis.

Lupinosis
• Early signs in sheep and cattle are inappetence and listlessness, complete anorexia and jaundice follows, and ketosis is common.
• Cattle may show lacrimation and salivation.
• Sheep may become photosensitive.
• In acute outbreaks, death occurs in 2–14 days.

CAUSES AND RISK FACTORS
Lupine Poisoning
• Acute poisoning occurs when a considerable amount of the plant is eaten in a short time.
• Lupins contain a number of alkaloids, D-Lupanine is the most toxic and the most widely distributed.
• The concentration of alkaloid is greatest in the seeds, and the plants are most dangerous at the seeding stage.
• The alkaloids are not destroyed by drying.

• Lupine-induced "crooked calf disease": Crooked calf disease is characterized as skeletal contracture-type malformations and occasional cleft palate in calves after maternal ingestion of lupines containing the quinolizidine alkaloid anagyrine during gestation days 40–100.
• Toxic and teratogenic effects have been linked to structural aspects of these alkaloids, and the mechanism of action is believed to be associated with an alkaloid-induced inhibition of fetal movement during specific gestational periods.

Lupinosis
• The causal fungus is *Phomopsis leptostromiformis*, a phytopathogen causing phomosis stem blight, especially in white and yellow lupines; blue varieties are very resistant.
• The fungus is also a saprophyte and under favorable conditions grows well on dead lupine material.
• The fungus produces hepatotoxic secondary metabolites. The main one is phomopsin A.

DIAGNOSIS

DIFFERENTIAL DIAGNOSIS
Lupinosis
Acute aflatoxicosis

Photosensitization
• Chronic fluke damage
• Congenital porphyria
• Liver disease
• Phenothiazines
• St. John's wort
• Toxin absorption

Arthrogryposis
• BVD, IBR, bluetongue virus, akabane virus, and Cache Valley virus
• Arthrogryposis-hydranencephaly syndrome (AHS) in lambs may be confused with spider lamb syndrome (SLS), in which there is characteristic hyperflexion of forelimbs, cranial overextension of hind limbs, with a corkscrew deviation of the spine. In lambs with AHS, severe deformities result from primary abnormalities of the CNS and not of the skeleton. Hydranencephaly, micromyelia, hydrocephalus, and cerebellar hypoplasia are also seen with AHS.

CBC/BIOCHEMISTRY/URINALYSIS

Lupine Poisoning
Elevated serum GGT, AST, LDH, and GDH concentrations

OTHER LABORATORY TESTS
N/A

IMAGING
N/A

PATHOLOGIC FINDING

Lupine Poisoning
• No icterus
• No characteristic postmortem lesions

Lupinosis
• In acute disease, icterus is marked. Livers are enlarged, orange-yellow, and fatty.
• Chronic disease shows bronze- or tan-colored livers that are firm, contracted in size and fibrosed, and often likened to a boxing glove.
• Copious transudate may be found in the abdominal and the pericardial sac.

HISTOPATHOLOGICAL FINDINGS
N/A

TREATMENT

Lupine Poisoning
Remove animals from the source.

Lupinosis
• Frequent surveillance of sheep or cattle, and of lupine fodder material for characteristic black spot fungal infestation, especially after rain.
• The utilization of lupine cultivars, bred and developed for resistance to *P. leptostromiformis* is advocated.

MEDICATIONS

Lupinosis
Oral doses of zinc (0.5 g of zinc or more, per day) are useful in protection from phomopsin-induced liver injury in sheep.

CONTRAINDICATIONS
Appropriate milk and meat withdrawal times must be followed for all compounds administered to food-producing animals.

FOLLOW-UP

POSSIBLE COMPLICATIONS
Lupines have a marked teratogenic effect on cattle and give rise to crooked calf disease, characterized by arthrogryposis, scoliosis, torticollis, and cleft palate.

EXPECTED COURSE AND PROGNOSIS
With acute lupine poisoning, if the animal survives it will likely make a full recovery, because the lupine alkaloid is readily excreted in the urine.

MISCELLANEOUS

ASSOCIATED CONDITIONS
• Liver failure, respiratory failure, cleft palate and contracture-type skeletal defects such as arthrogryposis, scoliosis, torticollis, and kyphosis
• Cleft palate and minor front limb contractures are induced in calves by maternal ingestion (crooked calf disease).

AGE-RELATED FACTORS
N/A

ZOONOTIC POTENTIAL
N/A

PREGNANCY
Crooked calf disease is characterized as skeletal contracture-type malformations and occasional cleft palate in calves after maternal ingestion of lupines containing the quinolizidine alkaloid anagyrine during gestation days 40–100.

RUMINANT SPECIES AFFECTED
Potentially, all ruminant species are affected.

BIOSECURITY
N/A

PRODUCTION MANAGEMENT
• Producers should be aware of the association between certain toxic plants (e.g., lupines) and angular limb deformities such as CCD.

• To reduce the incidence of crooked calf syndrome, graze lupines during their least hazardous growth period and reduce exposure of pregnant cows. Lupines are most hazardous when either young or in the mature seed stage.
• Fence off heavily infested pasture areas and use intermittent, short-term grazing of lupine pastures.

SYNONYMS
Crooked calf syndrome

SEE ALSO
Acute aflatoxicosis
Arthrogryposis
Liver disease

ABBREVIATIONS
AHS = arthrogryposis-hydranencephaly syndrome
AST = aspartate aminotransferase
BVD = bovine viral diarrhea
CNS = central nervous system
GDH = glutamate dehydrogenase
GGT = gamma-glutamyl transferase
IBR = infectious bovine rhinotracheitis
LDH = lactate dehydrogenase
SLS = spider lamb syndrome

Suggested Reading
Panter, K. E., Gardner, D. R., Molyneux, R. J. 1998, Jun. Teratogenic and fetotoxic effects of two piperidine alkaloid-containing lupines (*L. formosus* and *L. arbustus*) in cows. *J Nat Toxins* 7(2):131–40.
Panter, K. E., James, L. F., Gardner, D. R. 1999, Feb. Lupines, poison-hemlock and *Nicotiana* spp. toxicity and teratogenicity in livestock. *J Nat Toxins* 8(1):117–34.
Panter, K. E., Keeler, R. F. 1993, Mar. Quinolizidine and piperidine alkaloid teratogens from poisonous plants and their mechanism of action in animals. *Vet Clin North Am Food Anim Pract.* 9(1):33–40.
Panter, K. E., Keeler, R. F., Bunch, T. D., Callan, R. J. 1990. Congenital skeletal malformations and cleft palate induced in goats by ingestion of *Lupinus, Conium* and *Nicotiana* species. *Toxicon* 28(12):1377–85.

Author: Troy Holder

LUXATIONS

 BASICS

OVERVIEW
• Luxation is a displacement of the bones in a joint, resulting in abnormal articulation (subluxation) or lack of articulation (complete luxation).
• Luxations seen in cattle include coxofemoral, patellar, tarsal, metacarpophalangeal/metatarsophalangeal, and scapulohumeral
• Coxofemoral luxations are usually craniodorsal, but cranioventral and caudoventral luxations are also seen.
• Patellar luxations are almost always lateral.
• Tarsal luxations usually involve plantarodistal movement of the calcaneus, but lateral and medial luxations in the small tarsal bones can occur secondary to trauma.
• Metacarpophalangeal/metatarsophalangeal luxations are usually lateral or medial.
• Scapulohumeral luxation is rare but usually occurs in a craniolateral direction.
• Luxations can involve any joint, but the most common in ruminants and South American camelids (SACs) are patellar and coxofemoral luxations. Other luxations, such as sacroiliac, metacarpophalangeal, metatarsophalangeal, carpal, tarsal, and scapulohumeral are less common.
• Luxations can occur concurrently with fractures and other musculoskeletal or neurologic injuries.

PATHOPHYSIOLOGY
• Most luxations are caused by falls or trauma
• Falls can be caused by systemic electrolyte disturbances, systemic weakness, poor footing, crowding.
• Luxations can be caused by cows riding each other during heat cycles.

SYSTEMS AFFECTED
Musculoskeletal

INCIDENCE/PREVALENCE
Unknown

SIGNALMENT
• Luxations are most common in bovines, but have been reported in all farm animal species.
• Adult cows are most commonly affected, but young calves can also be affected. Patellar luxations are commonly seen as a congenital condition in young animals. In newborn calves, they often occur in association with femoral neuropathy.

SIGNS
• Findings depend on the joint affected, but in general involve abnormal ambulation or stance.
• Historical findings may include a fall, especially on concrete, recumbency with struggling to stand, recent dystocia, recent estrus, trauma, abnormal stance, or abnormal angle of a limb.
• Physical exam findings
  • Abnormal limb position
  • Abnormal mobility or range of motion of limb distal to luxation
  • Lameness
  • Skeletal asymmetry when viewed from front or back of animal
  • Inability to bear weight on the limb
  • Lack of crepitus
  • Recumbency

Coxofemoral Luxation
• Pelvic asymmetry is present in all cases of coxofemoral luxation. The measured distances between the tuber coxae, greater trochanter, and ischium will be different on the affected and unaffected sides.
• Coxofemoral luxations are most often craniodorsal, with the femoral head and neck resting on the dorsal aspect of the ilium. Consequently, the affected limb appears shorter than the unaffected limb, the greater trochanter is more dorsal and the distance from the greater trochanter to the ischium is greater on the affected limb. The limb also tends to be externally rotated, which makes the stifle appear more prominent.
• Caudoventral luxations occur less commonly, and cranioventral luxations are rare. Ventral luxations in cattle are more often associated with other musculoskeletal injuries, and the animals are often unable to stand. In animals that can stand, pelvic asymmetry is present, the affected limb may appear longer, and the greater trochanter is more ventral than the opposite leg.

Patellar Luxation
• Patellar luxation results in the inability to maintain the stifle in extension, which causes the animal to have a crouched stance on the affected limb because of increased flexion of the femorotibial joint. When unilateral, they may appear to be resting the limb. In some animals, the luxation is intermittent; therefore, the abnormal joint angulation is also intermittent.
• Adult llamas with intermittent luxations may ambulate with the limb locked in extension. On palpation, the patella is palpable in a more lateral or medial location or it can be manually displaced from the trochlear groove in animals with intermittent patellar luxation.

Sacroiliac Luxation
Signs of a sacroiliac luxation include prominence of the wings of the ileum relative to the lumbar spine, and pain on palpation of the sacroiliac region. Animals with sacroiliac luxation may be unable to rise.

CAUSES AND RISK FACTORS
• Falls
• Trauma
• Hypocalcemia/hypophosphatemia/hypokalemia
• Riding during estrus
• Paralysis/paresis causing limb malfunction
• Forced extraction of calf during dystocia
• Dystocia
• Hypocalcemia/hypophosphatemia/hypokalemia
• Slippery floors
• Crowding
• Femoral nerve paralysis (for patellar luxation)

Coxofemoral Luxation
• Coxofemoral luxations in adult animals occur most commonly during falls on hard or slippery surfaces. In cows, these often occur in the postpartum period when ligamentous laxity, weakness, or metabolic derangements, such as hypocalcemia, may be present.
• Coxofemoral luxations also occur in cattle during estrus while being ridden, which is also a cause of sacroiliac luxations.
• Coxofemoral luxations can occur when the rear limb is caught in a gate, fence, or other structure. They occur in neonates, particularly calves, as a result of excessive traction during delivery.
• Excessive traction can also result in sacroiliac luxations or subluxations in cows.

Patellar Luxation
• Patellar luxations in adult cattle are typically traumatic luxations, and lateral luxations occur in calves due either to direct trauma or injury to the femoral nerve during delivery (hip lock).
• Lateral patellar luxations due to trauma have been reported most often in llamas, although congenital and traumatic medial patellar luxations have been reported.
• A genetic predisposition was a likely cause of patellar luxations (predominantly medial) reported in a flock of sheep.
• Congenital skeletal abnormalities involving the angle of the femoral neck and positioning of the tibial tuberosity may result in predisposition of patellar luxation (as described in dogs).
• Hypoplasia of the trochlear ridges, resulting in a shallow trochlear groove, may be present in animals with either lateral or medial patellar luxation. Severe osteochondrosis of the trochlear ridges can result in patellar luxation.

DIAGNOSIS

DIFFERENTIAL DIAGNOSES
• Fracture
• Paralysis/paresis
• Hypocalcemia/hypophosphatemia/hypokalemia
• Systemic disease causing weakness
• Muscle or tendon trauma or rupture

IMAGING
• Radiographs are often useful for differentiating luxation from fracture.
• The direction of luxation can be determined and coexisting articular fractures or fragments noted.
• Pelvic radiography for diagnosis of coxofemoral luxation may require general anesthesia.
• Ultrasonography is useful in evaluating the depth of the trochlear groove in animals with congenital patellar luxation if surgical repair is being considered. In young animals, the trochlear ridges are incompletely ossified resulting in the appearance of a shallow trochlear groove on radiographs even when the depth of the groove is normal.

OTHER DIAGNOSTIC PROCEDURES
• Clinical examination is generally important and reliable in making a diagnosis of luxation, but concurrent fractures may not be recognized.
• Electromyography (EMG) is useful in confirming the diagnosis of femoral neuropathy in calves with congenital patellar luxation. Since femoral neuropathy can develop because of hip lock during delivery and EMG changes take a week to develop, electromyography is not generally useful before that time.

PATHOLOGIC FINDINGS
• Necropsy will show luxation of the joint affected, associated muscle trauma, concomitant fractures, and bony debris.
• With patellar luxation secondary to femoral nerve paralysis, there may be lack of quadriceps muscle development or histologic degeneration of the femoral nerve.

TREATMENT

Coxofemoral Luxation
• Treatment can be by closed or open reduction.
• Reduction is best performed under general anesthesia, either injectable or inhalant, that provides good muscle relaxation. Sedation (e.g., xylazine) may be adequate if closed reduction is performed within a short time of the luxation; however, the animal will experience more pain and distress.
• Closed reduction should be attempted in calves and other young animals with acute luxations. If unsuccessful, open reduction should be performed if economically feasible.
• To correct a craniodorsal luxation, the animal is placed in lateral recumbency with the affected leg up, and traction is applied to the limb.
• In adult cattle, a calf jack, come-along, or winch is used to apply traction, while the animal is secured with ropes around the chest and abdomen, and the pelvis is held with a rope placed in the inguinal area, to oppose the traction applied to the limb. While traction is applied, the leg is externally rotated and the distal limb is adducted, which will allow the femoral head to externally rotate and "unhook" from the ileum. Once returned to the acetabulum, the limb is abducted and internally rotated. In a ventral luxation, the same manipulation is performed (traction, external rotation, and adduction of the distal limb). Once the femoral head is rotated out of the obturator foramen or other site ventral to the ilium, traction can be released and the femoral head should return to the acetabulum.

Surgical Approach
• Open reduction is performed under general anesthesia at a surgical facility, most often using a craniodorsal approach. While traction, external rotation, and adduction of the distal limb are performed, a hip skid can be used to facilitate reduction or a large Steinmann pin can be placed in the trochanteric fossa to help lever the proximal femur into position. Clotted blood, fibrin, tissue fragments, and any other material should be removed from the acetabulum. The joint capsule may need to be elevated from the joint space, which also helps reposition the normal fibrocartilaginous rim of the dorsal acetabulum, which is important in preventing reluxation.

• Correction of the luxation should be confirmed radiographically.
• Femoral head and neck excision has been used as a salvage procedure in calves, and extracapsular stabilization with sutures placed between the femoral neck and dorsal acetabulum has been successful in an alpaca.

Patellar Luxation
Correction of lateral patellar luxation requires surgical repair under general anesthesia, although mild intermittent luxations (grade I) can be managed conservatively.

Surgical Approach
• Several procedures are used to correct patellar luxations depending on the underlying cause and the anatomic abnormalities present. These include medial imbrication for lateral luxations (lateral imbrication for medial), with or without lateral release for lateral luxations (medial release for medial luxations), trochleoplasty, and/or transposition of the tibial tuberosity for lateral luxations. Placement of two large sutures between the cartilage on the medial aspect of the patella and the periosteum of the femur at the normal insertion of the medial femoropatellar ligament helps prevent recurrence of lateral luxations.
• Medial luxations more often require transposition of the tibial tuberosity to align the quadriceps, patella, and patellar ligament with the trochlear groove. Trochleoplasty is performed if the trochlear groove is too shallow to prevent reluxation.

Other Luxations
• Correction of other luxations, such as metacarpophalangeal, metatarsophalangeal, carpal, or tarsal luxations generally involves closed reduction under general anesthesia and stabilization in a cast for 4–12 weeks.
• Prolonged casting in young animals results in laxity of soft tissues and possible disuse osteopenia of bone, as well as loss of joint mobility. Surgical arthrodesis can be used in metacarpophalangeal, metatarsophalangeal, carpal, and distal tarsal joint luxations.
• Closed and open reduction with and without internal fixation or arthrodesis has been reported as a treatment for scapulohumeral luxation.

LUXATIONS

APPROPRIATE HEALTH CARE
• Luxations require emergency medical care.
• Closed reduction of a luxation should occur within 6 hours of the injury for best prognosis.
• Reduction should be performed under heavy sedation or anesthesia, and mechanical pulling devices may be required (e.g., calf jack, come-along, etc.)
• If closed reduction is unsuccessful, surgical reduction can be performed when the patient is stable.
• Following reduction, casts or splints may be used to stabilize the joints of the distal limbs until adequate scar tissue can form to replace disrupted ligaments.

NURSING CARE
• Good footing and bedding should be provided, especially if the animal is recumbent.
• If recumbent, the animal should be rolled from side to side and/or assisted to stand with slings or hip lifters to avoid dependent muscle necrosis and compartmental syndrome.
• Hobbles are useful for providing stability to cows with coxofemoral luxation.
• Feed and water should be easily available.
• Casts and splints must be carefully monitored and replaced if necessary.
• Animals should be confined for at least 4 to 6 weeks after reduction of luxation to reduce stress on the joint. Coxofemoral and scapulohumeral joint luxations should be stall rested for 2 to 3 months following reduction.

SURGICAL CONSIDERATIONS
• Surgical repair by open reduction is possible in most luxations, and can be particularly successful when closed reduction has failed due to debris present in the joint cavity.
• Recumbent animals are less likely to have a favorable outcome after coxofemoral surgery than are animals that were ambulatory prior to surgery.
• Surgical reduction is more expensive than closed reduction, and therefore may not be elected in many farm animals due to the economics of raising farm animals.
• Careful examination of the animal, consultation of radiographs, and knowledge of anatomy of the region should determine surgical approach. Consultation with or referral to a surgical facility is recommended.
• Surgical repair must be performed under general anesthesia to obtain complete relaxation of opposing muscles around the joint.
• Surgical repair should be performed as soon as possible after diagnosis to avoid contracture of the musculature around the joint with further displacement of the luxation.

MEDICATIONS

DRUGS OF CHOICE
• For closed reductions, NSAIDs/analgesics (flunixin meglumine 1.1–2.2 mg/kg IV q12 to 24 hours) should be administered for 1 to 3 days after reduction of luxation to reduce swelling and make the patient more comfortable.
• Antibiotics should not be required for closed reductions.
• Broad-spectrum antibiotics and analgesics are recommended for 7 to 10 days following open surgical reduction.

CONTRAINDICATIONS
• Appropriate milk and meat withdrawal times must be followed for all compounds administered to food-producing animals.
• Steroids can cause abortions in pregnant females.

PRECAUTIONS
None

POSSIBLE INTERACTIONS
Steroids should not be used for pain relief if the animal is pregnant.

ALTERNATIVE DRUGS
Any analgesics can be used for pain relief as long as they fall within the AMDUCA regulations.

FOLLOW-UP
• Stall confinement is necessary after correction of a luxation. Animals treated by cast fixation should be in a stall while the limb is cast to minimize the risk of pressure sores.
• Neonates and young animals should be kept in a stall for a minimum of 4 weeks after closed reduction of coxofemoral luxation, although some have done well with a shorter period of confinement.
• An Ehmer sling, to keep the limb abducted and internally rotated, can be used in calves in which reduction was difficult or instability remains, but otherwise is not recommended.
• Animals treated for luxations, particularly of the hip and patella, that lie with the affected limb down should be assisted to stand in the early postoperative period. Adult cattle that had ventral luxations may benefit from hobbles applied above the fetlock to prevent abduction of the affected limb.

• Use of a sling after surgery to correct patellar luxation in llamas has been recommended to allow gradual return to weight bearing and exercise.
• Adult cattle with coxofemoral or patellar luxations treated surgically require a minimum of 8 weeks of confinement to a stall with good footing followed by gradual increase in activity level.
• Skin sutures should be removed 10 days to 2 weeks after surgical correction of coxofemoral, patellar, or other luxations.

PATIENT MONITORING
• The animal should be confined after reduction and monitored for any signs of reluxation, for return to weight bearing, and for signs of secondary paresis caused by nerve compression during the luxation.
• Recovery is usually quick following closed reduction.

PREVENTION/AVOIDANCE
• Provision of excellent footing to cattle at all times will reduce the number of spontaneous falls and falls due to riding during estrus.
• Do not crowd or rush cows, especially if not on good footing.
• Avoid dystocia, as both cow and calf are at risk of coxofemoral luxation, and calves are at risk of femoral nerve damage, which could lead to patellar luxation.
• Treat weak cows as soon as possible to restore normal ambulation.

POSSIBLE COMPLICATIONS
• Failure of reduction
• Nerve paresis/paralysis
• Muscle damage
• Arthritis
• Compartmental syndrome (if recumbent)

EXPECTED COURSE AND PROGNOSIS
• Prognosis is good for early closed reduction.
• Prognosis is fair to good for open reduction of coxofemoral luxations.
• Prognosis is good for open reduction of other luxations.
• Prognosis is fair for patella luxation, as the underlying cause often cannot be corrected.

Coxofemoral Luxation
• Untreated coxofemoral luxation results in serious lameness and a very poor prognosis in cattle.

• The prognosis for coxofemoral luxations in young animals is favorable if treated soon after occurrence. The prognosis is fair to poor for correction of chronic luxations, and it is poor for luxations with concurrent fractures of the femoral head, neck, or diaphysis. The prognosis is fair for open reduction of acute coxofemoral luxations in adult animals, but it is poor if they are chronic.
• Some chronic luxations are not reducible even with the animal under general anesthesia. The prognosis is better for cattle with craniodorsal luxations than ventral luxations, most likely because the latter tend to be associated with other musculoskeletal injuries.
• Reluxation has been reported in 17% of calves and 40% of adult cattle after open reduction. In general, smaller species are less likely to develop recurrence of luxation and more likely to have a successful outcome.

Patellar Luxation
• The prognosis for surgical correction of congenital patellar luxation in calves is guarded if femoral neuropathy is also present, since the outcome of the neuropathy is uncertain; however, many do well after the imbrication procedure. Failure to stabilize a luxated patella in an animal with femoral neuropathy ensures a poor outcome.
• In the absence of femoral neuropathy, the prognosis for surgical correction of patellar luxation is fair to good, particularly if done at a young age, if severe anatomic abnormalities are not present, and if the trochlear groove is sufficiently deep to retain the patella without performing a trochleoplasty.
• Correction of medial patellar luxation by imbrication, release, wedge trochleoplasty, and tibial tuberosity transposition has resulted in a good outcome in sheep.
• Correction of patellar luxations in adult cattle has a guarded to poor prognosis because of the size and weight of the animal.

Sacroiliac Luxation
Cases of subluxations generally improve over several days, but generally have reduced pelvic diameter that could result in dystocia. Cows with sacroiliac luxations do not tend to recover.

Other Luxation
• The prognosis for other closed luxations that can be stabilized by cast fixation is favorable with appropriate stabilization, although chronic lameness due to degenerative joint disease is possible.
• Open luxations have a guarded prognosis because of the possibility of joint infection; however, the outcome can be favorable with appropriate treatment.
• The overall results reported for open reduction and stabilization of shoulder luxations are poor. The best success for correction of scapulohumeral luxation occurs in cases in which the luxation can be corrected by closed reduction.

MISCELLANEOUS

ASSOCIATED CONDITIONS
Hypocalcemia, hypophosphatemia, hypokalemia, laminitis/foot problems, dystocia, femoral nerve paralysis, paralysis/paresis, fractures, hip dysplasia, femoral neuropathy (with patellar luxation), osteochondrosis, congenital limb anomalies

AGE-RELATED FACTORS
• Luxations may be easier to reduce in young animals due to the lack of muscle mass and the pliability of the muscles and tendons.
• Coxofemoral luxations have better prognosis in small and young animals than in large or old animals.

ZOONOTIC POTENTIAL
None

PREGNANCY
• Do not use steroids for pain relief.
• Sedation and anesthesia can cause fetal distress and potentially fetal loss, though the incidence is rare.

RUMINANT SPECIES AFFECTED
Cattle, sheep, goats, llamas, alpacas, camels

BIOSECURITY
N/A

PRODUCTION MANAGEMENT
N/A

SYNONYMS
N/A

SEE ALSO
Anesthesia and analgesia
Angular limb deformity
Arthrogryposis
FARAD
Femoral nerve paralysis
Fractures
Hypocalcemia/milk fever
Lameness: joint
NSAIDs
Osteochondrosis

ABBREVIATIONS
AMDUCA = Animal Medicinal Drug Use Clarification Act
EMG = electromyography
FARAD = Food Animal Residue Avoidance Databank
IV = intravenous
NSAIDS = nonsteroidal anti-inflammatory drugs
SAC = South American camelids

Suggested Reading
Ducharme, N. G. 1996. Stifle injuries in cattle. *Vet Clin North Am Food Anim Pract.* 12(1): 59–85.
Ducharme, N. G., Trostle, S. S. 2004. Luxations/subluxations: coxofemoral, patellar, tarsal, and scapulohumeral. In: *Farm animal surgery*, ed. S. L. Fubini, N. G. Ducharme. St. Louis: Elsevier.
Hull, B. L. 1996. Fractures and luxations of the pelvis and proximal femur. *Vet Clin North Amer Food Anim Pract.* 12:47–58.
Shettko, D. L., Trostle, S. S. 2000. Diagnosis and surgical repair of patellar luxations in a flock of sheep. *J Am Vet Med Assoc.* 216(4):564–66.
Tulleners, E. P., Nunamaker, D. M., Richardson, D. W. 1987. Coxofemoral luxations in cattle: 22 cases. *J Am Vet Med Assoc.* 191:569–74.
Van Hoogmoed, L., Snyder, J. R., Vasseur, P. 1998. Surgical repair of patellar luxation in llamas: 7 cases. *J Am Vet Med Assoc.* 212(6):860–65.

Authors: Jill Parker and Jennifer M. Ivany Ewoldt

LYME BORRELIOSIS

BASICS

OVERVIEW
• Lyme borreliosis is a zoonotic disease caused by *Borrelia burgdorferi*, a bacterium in the order Spirochetae.
• *Borrelia burgdorferi* is transmitted to humans and other animals through the bite of ticks in the *Ixodes* genus. *Ixodes* ticks are most commonly found in moist wooded areas or naturally vegetated habitats with grasses and shrubs.
• Small mammals such as white-footed mice (*Peromyscus leucopus*) serve as the primary reservoir for *B. burgdorferi*.
• Domestic and nondomestic ruminants, except in rare ecologic circumstances, are not likely to serve as reservoirs for *B. burgdorferi*.

PATHOPHYSIOLOGY
• The Lyme borreliosis *Borrelia* complex is divided into *B. burgdorferi* sensu stricto (*B. burgdoreri* ss; those *Borrelia* genetically identical to the type-strain B31, recovered from an *Ixodes scapularis* tick from Long Island, New York) and *B. burgdorferi* sensu lato (*B. burgdorferi* sl; all other closely related *Borrelia*.).
• *Borrelia burgdorferi* ss, *B. afzelii*, and *B. garinii* cause Lyme borreliosis in humans and animals in Europe and Japan. Only *B. burgdorferi* ss is recognized as a cause of Lyme borreliosis in the United States.
• Serologic evidence of *B. burgdorferi* infection has been detected in large and small domestic ruminants, but significant clinical disease in these species is not common.
• Clinical Lyme borreliosis in ruminants manifests most commonly as large joint arthritis, but systemic, dermatologic, reproductive, and central nervous system signs can also rarely occur.

SIGNALMENT
• Where infected vector ticks exist and bite cattle.
• Clinical signs often occur as a herd problem with first-calf heifers most severely affected.
• One report of affected lambs

SYSTEMS AFFECTED
• Joint capsules
• Synovial membranes

GENETICS
No evidence of a genetic predisposition to infection has been shown in large animals.

GEOGRAPHIC DISTRIBUTION
Worldwide distribution is possible. Currently, cases in Europe, Japan, and the United States.

SIGNS
• Infection of ruminants with *B. burgdorferi* is most commonly subclinical.
• Joint swelling, usually distal to the carpus or tarsus. May be recurrent.
• Lameness, stiff gait
• Decreased milk production
• Occasionally reported: laminitis, fever, weight loss, abortion
• Rarely reported: erythematous skin rash on udder

CAUSES AND RISK FACTORS
• Exposure to pastures where infected ticks occur may predicate infection.
• *Borrelia burgdorferi* spirochetes commonly establish infection in joints. Some animal models have suggested that the resulting inflammation, which is often disproportionate to the spirochetal load, is possibly an immune-mediated response.
• *Borrelia burgdorferi* has been recovered from tissues in cattle such as synovial fluid, lung, liver, and rarely blood, colostrum, and aborted fetal tissue.
• Aside from the synovial fluid, disease manifestations do not appear to correlate with tissue location of *Borrelia* isolation.
• Cow-to-cow or cow-to-human transmission via infected blood, urine, or milk has not been shown.

DIAGNOSIS

DIFFERENTIAL DIAGNOSIS
• Other infectious and noninfectious causes of lameness and joint swelling include trauma, septic arthritis, and spirochete-associated digital dermatitis.
• Infection with *Borrelia theileri*, a tick-borne spirochete reported from Africa, Eastern Europe, Australia, South America, Mexico, and Texas, can cause fever, hemoglobinuria, and anemia.

CBC/BIOCHEMISTRY/ URINALYSIS
• Not specific
• Reported abnormalities: leukocytosis with left shift, anemia

OTHER LABORATORY TESTS
Anti-*Borrelia* antibodies may be detected in CSF and synovial fluid.

IMAGING
Radiography of affected joints may help to rule out other causes (e.g., fracture) of inflammation and swelling.

DIAGNOSTIC PROCEDURES
• Definitive diagnosis can be achieved only through detection of *B. burgdorferi* in synovial fluid from affected joints. Polymerase chain reaction (PCR) tests and culture for *B. burgdorferi* by experienced research laboratories are often unrewarding.
• Testing of serum or synovial fluids for antibodies to *B. burgdorferi* using immunofluorescent antibody tests and/or western blots has been used. High titers may be indicative of infection, but cross-reactivity with other ruminant spirochetes or nonclinical infection must also be considered.
• Serologic tests for *B. burgdorferi* must be interpreted carefully in ruminants as there is great potential for cross reactivity with other spirochetal agents that infect ruminants such as treponemes causing digital dermatitis and the tick-borne *Borrelia theileri*.

PATHOLOGIC FINDINGS

GROSS FINDINGS
• Marked thickening of affected joint capsules
• Affected joints may contain excessive amounts of synovial fluid, usually clear.

HISTOPATHOLOGIC FINDINGS
• Affected joint capsules may have layers of granulation tissue and necrotic debris.
• Villus proliferation of the synovial membranes

LYME BORRELIOSIS

TREATMENT

MEDICATIONS

• No standard treatment protocol is established for ruminants. Penicillin and tetracycline derivatives have proven effective in other species. Three weeks of antibiotics are recommended to clear the infection, but clinical improvement may be seen with shorter protocols.
• Anti-inflammatory agents may decrease the incidence of postinfectious laminitis.

CONTRAINDICATIONS
• Treatment for Lyme borreliosis with penicillin, oxytetracycline, and ceftiofur has been reported but is off-label usage.
• Appropriate milk and meat withdrawal times must be followed for all compounds administered to food-producing animals.

FOLLOW-UP

PATIENT MONITORING
N/A

PREVENTION/AVOIDANCE
• Implement a tick-control program, including regular inspection of resident and introduced animals and pastures for ticks.
• Eliminate the vector tick on cattle through the use of acaricides.
• Elimination of the vector tick from pasture requires an integrated approach targeting hosts (e.g., cattle and deer) and the environment. Contact local extension professionals for appropriate pasture vector control approaches.
• Vaccination against *Leptospira* appears to confer no cross-protection against *Borrelia* spirochetes.

POSSIBLE COMPLICATIONS
N/A

EXPECTED COURSE AND PROGNOSIS
Reports of treatment success range from complete remission in weeks to slow (months) response to treatment.

MISCELLANEOUS

ASSOCIATED CONDITIONS
• Joint swelling, usually distal to the carpus or tarsus; may be recurrent
• Lameness, stiff gait
• Decreased milk production
• Occasionally reported: laminitis, fever, weight loss, abortion

AGE-RELATED FACTORS
Heifers seem to be predominantly affected.

ZOONOTIC POTENTIAL
• While it had been postulated that *B. burgdorferi* recovered from milk and urine of cattle could be infective to humans, such transmission has not been conclusively demonstrated. A study in an endemic area demonstrated no significant difference in *B. burgdorferi* titers among dairy farmers and crop farmers.
• Farmers, ranchers, and others working in the same area where ruminants are infected with Lyme borreliosis may themselves be at risk of tick bite and infection with *B. burgdorferi*.

PREGNANCY
While *B. burgdorferi* spirochetes have been recovered from aborted fetal bovine tissues, abortion due to *B. burgdorferi* infection has not been conclusively shown.

SEE ALSO
Ehrlichiosis
Other infectious and noninfectious causes of lameness and joint swelling
Septic arthritis
Spirochete-associated digital dermatitis
Trauma

ABBREVIATIONS
CSF = cerebral spinal fluid
PCR = polymerase chain reaction

Suggested Reading
Bushmich, S. L. 1994. Lyme borreliosis in domestic animals. *J Spirochet and Tick-Borne Dis.* 1 (1): 24–28.
Fritz, C. L., Kjemtrup, A. M. 2003. Lyme borreliosis. *J Am Vet Med Assoc.* 223 (9): 1261–70.
Gray, J. S., Kahl, O., Lane, R. S., Stanek, G., eds. 2002. Lyme borreliosis biology, epidemiology, and control. Wallingford, Oxfordshire, United Kingdom: CABI Publishing.
Lischer, C. J., Leutenegger, C. M., Braun, U., Lutz, H. I. 2000. Diagnosis of Lyme disease in two cows by the detection of *Borrelia burgdorferi* DNA. *Vet Rec.* 146: 497–99.
Parker, J. L., White, K. K. 1992. Lyme borreliosis in cattle and horses: a review of the literature. *Cornell Vet.* 82:253–74.

Authors: Anne M. Kjemtrup and Curtis L. Fritz

LYMPHOCYTOSIS

 BASICS

DEFINITION
• Absolute number of lymphocytes greater than the reference range: Bovine >7500/μl; Ovine >9000/μl; Caprine >9000/μl; Camelids >7000/μl
• Absolute lymphocyte counts are greater in juvenile animals than adults.

PATHOPHYSIOLOGY
• Lymphocytes are produced in the bone marrow, lymph nodes, spleen, thymus, and Peyer's patches.
• Lymphocytes retain mitotic capability and can recirculate from the blood to lymphoid tissue. The number of lymphocytes in the blood represents a balance between cells leaving and entering circulation. Therefore, changes in peripheral lymphocyte counts may not necessarily indicate altered lymphopoiesis.
• Blood lymphocytes represent an assorted set of lymphocyte subpopulations including B and T lymphocytes. B cells are involved with humoral immunity and produce antibodies, while T lymphocytes are responsible for cell-mediated immunity and cytokine responses involved in immune system regulation.
• Approximately 95% of all lymphocytes are B and T lymphocytes with T cells predominating. The remaining lymphocytes make up a third group classified as "null" cells. Null cells consist of several subtypes including large granular lymphocytes and natural killer cells.
• In general, most lymphocyte subtypes cannot be identified on a blood film examination. However, large granular lymphocytes are occasionally observed in ruminant blood and can be recognized by the presence of small, red cytoplasmic granules.
• Infrequently, activated B lymphocytes (i.e., immunoblasts) are identified on blood film evaluation by their large size, deep blue cytoplasm, and perinuclear clear zone.
• Ruminant lymphocytes generally have diameters equal to those of neutrophils, but can be quite irregular in size.

SYSTEMS AFFECTED
• Hemic/lymphatic/immune—hepatosplenomegaly may occur as a result of hyperplasia or neoplasia; bone marrow may be hyperplastic; neoplastic populations of lymphocytes may rarely result in anemia and thrombocytopenia due to myelophthisis.
• Lymphosarcoma may affect all organ systems and cause specific problems such as cardiovascular, gastrointestinal, renal, and CNS.

GENETICS
N/A

INCIDENCE/PREVALENCE
• Pathologic lymphocytosis is uncommon in ruminants except cattle infected with BLV.
• Sporadic lymphosarcoma with concurrent lymphocytosis (also known as calf or juvenile form) is extremely rare and multiple cases within the same herd are even less common.

GEOGRAPHIC DISTRIBUTION
N/A

SIGNALMENT
• Reference values for absolute lymphocyte counts vary with ruminant species. Sheep and goats have higher mean absolute lymphocyte counts than cattle or camelids. However, alpacas and llamas generally have lower lymphocyte counts than camels.
• Sporadic lymphosarcoma (calf or juvenile form) generally affects calves 3–6 months of age, but may be observed in calves as young as 1 month or cattle as old as 3 years.
• Lymphocytic leukemia and BLV-associated lymphosarcoma affect adult ruminants >4 years of age.

SIGNS
• If cause is physiologic (rare cause in ruminants), excited or fearful
• If cause is pathologic (sporadic lymphosarcoma, lymphosarcoma, or lymphocytic leukemia), lymphadenopathy, anorexia, decreased milk production, poor body condition. Depending on the involvement of other organ systems, melena or diarrhea (intestinal tract), heart failure (myocardium), posterior paralysis (spinal canal), and exophthalmia (retrobulbar tissue) may be observed. Anemia may result in pale mucous membranes, tachypnea, and tachycardia.
• If cause is persistent lymphocytosis associated with subclinical stage of BLV infection, affected cattle rarely exhibit clinical signs.

CAUSES

Physiologic
Epinephrine release due to excitement, pain, fear, restraint. The change occurs within minutes and usually lasts less than 30 minutes. Effect is usually observed in young healthy animals. Physiologic lymphocytosis is uncommon in most ruminants.

Antigenic Stimulation
Uncommon cause, but may occur occasionally with chronic viral or bacterial infections (e.g., caprine arthritis encephalitis virus, bacterial pneumonia) and within 10–14 days of vaccination.

Autoimmune Disease
Rare

Persistent Lymphocytosis
Subclinical BLV infection in cattle results in decreased B cell turnover and an inverted B:T cell ratio. B cells in this condition are non-neoplastic.

Sporadic Lymphosarcoma
Cause is unknown.

Lymphosarcoma or Lymphocytic Leukemia
• Although reported in all ruminant species, lymphosarcoma with lymphocytosis and lymphocytic leukemia are rare except in cattle infected with BLV.
• Approximately 30% of BLV-infected cattle are leukemic. Lymphocytosis is primarily due to decreased cell death of B cells.

RISK FACTORS
N/A

 DIAGNOSIS

DIFFERENTIAL DIAGNOSIS
• Transient physiologic lymphocytosis typically occurs in young, healthy, and excitable animals.
• Persistent lymphocytosis (3-months duration) in cattle without clinical signs is associated with subclinical BLV infection.
• Ill cattle with absolute lymphocytosis—consider lymphosarcoma or lymphocytic leukemia; may be seropositive for BLV.

CBC/BIOCHEMISTRY/URINALYSIS

Physiologic Lymphocytosis
• CBC
• Mild lymphocytosis
• Rarely, mild increases in RBC, Hgb, and PCV due to epinephrine-mediated splenic contraction
• Mild neutrophilia
• Plasma proteins typically normal

Serum Biochemistry/Urinalysis
No characteristic changes

Persistent Lymphocytosis of Cattle
• CBC
• Mild to moderate lymphocytosis that persists over an interval of at least 3 months
• Morphologically atypical and large lymphocytes may be present on blood film examination, but similar lymphocytes may occasionally be observed in normal cattle or cattle with various non-BLV-associated conditions.

Serum Biochemistry/Urinalysis
No characteristic changes

Lymphocytic Leukemia
• CBC
• Marked to severe lymphocytosis with atypical lymphocytes observed in approximately 50% of the cases. (Approximately 5%–10% of BLV-infected cattle manifest with massive increases in circulating neoplastic lymphoblasts, but <2% develop lymphosarcoma.)
• Anemia (may be regenerative or nonregenerative depending on cause)
• Plasma proteins may be decreased if there is neoplastic involvement of gastrointestinal tract.

Serum Biochemistry/Urinalysis
No characteristic changes.

OTHER LABORATORY TESTS
• For cattle with persistent lymphocytosis: anti-BLV antibody test (anti-GP51 agar gel immunodiffusion (AGID) test is most common)
• Bone marrow evaluation in cases of lymphocytic leukemia often reveals a large population of infiltrating lymphoblasts.

IMAGING
Radiographic or ultrasonographic imaging may reveal evidence of hepatosplenomegaly or internal iliac lymph node enlargement associated with lymphosarcoma.

OTHER DIAGNOSTIC PROCEDURES
• Fine needle aspiration cytology and culture of enlarged lymph nodes is occasionally helpful in differentiating an abscess from lymphosarcoma.
• Histopathologic examination of tumor or lymph node biopsies may be more useful than cytology in confirming lymphosarcoma.

TREATMENT

Physiologic Lymphocytosis
Treatment is not warranted as lymphocyte counts typically return to normal within 30 minutes.

Lymphocytosis Due to Antigenic Stimulation
Treatment should be directed at the primary disease causing the lymphocytosis.

Lymphosarcoma and Lymphocytic Leukemia
No curative treatment for lymphosarcoma or lymphocytic leukemia exists in ruminants. Supportive or palliative therapy may be indicated to reduce discomfort.

ACTIVITY
Restrict

CLIENT EDUCATION
N/A

MEDICATIONS

DRUGS OF CHOICE
Chemotherapeutics
Case report data regarding chemotherapy are rare. A few reports summarizing unsuccessful attempts in treating lymphosarcoma and lymphocytic leukemia with dexamethasone and cylcophosphamide exist. Drug withdrawal periods must be determined and maintained.

Fluid Therapy
Rehydration with IV fluids appropriate for the primary cause (e.g., polyuric renal failure, diarrhea, etc.) and to correct any electrolyte and acid-base imbalances

CONTRAINDICATIONS
N/A

POSSIBLE INTERACTIONS
N/A

ALTERNATIVE DRUGS
N/A

FOLLOW-UP

PATIENT MONITORING
N/A

PREVENTION/AVOIDANCE
See Bovine Leukemia, Leukocyte Responses in Cattle and Lymphosarcoma for control suggestions.

POSSIBLE COMPLICATIONS
Chemotherapy-induced bone marrow suppression with subsequent anemia, leukopenia, and thrombocytopenia.

EXPECTED COURSE AND PROGNOSIS
Persistent Lymphocytosis of Cattle
Precedes the onset of lymphosarcoma in approximately 65% of the cases, but less than 5% of cows with persistent lymphocytosis develop lymphosarcoma.

Sporadic Lymphosarcoma
Rapidly progressive and usually fatal within 2 to 8 weeks of onset

Lymphosarcoma or Lymphocytic Leukemia
The prognosis for patients with lymphosarcoma or lymphocytic leukemia is poor with median survival times following diagnosis of <2–3 months.

MISCELLANEOUS

ASSOCIATED CONDITIONS
Persistent lymphocytosis of cattle is associated with BLV infection.

AGE-RELATED FACTORS
• Young animals—lymphocyte counts generally increase from birth to a maximum at approximately 11–12 months of age. Absolute lymphocyte counts begin to slowly decline in adult animals.
• Physiologic lymphocytosis occurs in young healthy animals.
• Sporadic lymphosarcoma occurs most commonly in 3–6–month–old calves.
• Lymphosarcoma and lymphocytic leukemia generally occur in adult animals >4 years.

ZOONOTIC POTENTIAL
N/A

PREGNANCY
N/A

RUMINANT SPECIES AFFECTED
Bovine, ovine, caprine, camelids

BIOSECURITY
N/A

PRODUCTION MANAGEMENT
N/A

SYNONYMS
Bovine leukosis
Bovine lymphoma
Chronic lymphocytic leukemia
Malignant lymphoma

SEE ALSO
Bovine leukemia virus

ABBREVIATIONS
AGID = agar gel immunodiffusion
BLV = bovine leukemia virus
CNS = central nervous system
Hct = hematocrit
Hgb = hemoglobin
IV= intravenous
PCV = packed cell volume
Plts = platelets
PP = plasma protein
RBC = red blood cells
WBC = white blood cells

Suggested Reading
Thurmond, M. 1996. Bovine lymphosarcoma. In: *Large animal internal medicine*, ed. B. P. Smith. 2nd ed. St. Louis: Mosby.
Valentine, B. A., McDonough, S. P. 2003. B-cell leukemia in a sheep. *Vet Path.* 40: 117–19.

Author: Frederic S. Almy

LYMPHOSARCOMA

 BASICS

DEFINITION
• Lymphosarcoma is a lymphoid cancer caused by a single stranded RNA retrovirus that integrates into the host cell genome.
• The cause of lymphosarcoma in cattle and sheep is believed to be bovine leukemia virus. Cattle are the natural host for BLV. However, only about 30% of BLV-positive cattle develop persistent lymphocytosis and only 5% of these develop lymphosarcoma.

OVERVIEW
• There are four forms of bovine leukemia: juvenile, thymic, cutaneous, and enzootic. The first three are considered sporadic because the animals are BLV negative for antibodies. The enzootic bovine leukemia animals are positive for BLV antibodies, have persistent lymphocytosis, and can develop lymphosarcoma.
• It can be hard to distinguish between the thymic form of BLV and lymphosarcoma.
• There are no indicators to predict which animals with persistent lymphocytosis will develop lymphosarcoma.
• BLV has not been associated with goats that develop lymphosarcoma.

PATHOPHYSIOLOGY
• In cattle and sheep, seroconversion occurs after exposure to the virus between 14 and 98 days. The wide temporal range of conversion is attributable to dose, route of infection, and immune status of the animal. Concurrent infection with a retro- or herpes virus may make the BLV infection more pathogenic.
• Currently it is believed that the virus is necessary only to initiate tumor development, but after initiation, the tumor self-replicates. The "tat" gene is the only gene identified that appears critical for tumor cell maintenance.
• Tumors can occur in every organ but primarily develop in lymph nodes.

SYSTEMS AFFECTED
Cardiac, musculoskeletal, gastrointestinal, lymphatic, ocular, reproductive, and metabolic

GENETICS
Cattle that have been identified with the BoLA-A allele w8.1 are more resistant to BLV infections and therefore have a lower incidence of lymphosarcoma.

INCIDENCE/PREVALENCE
• In the cattle industry, BLV-positive cattle are estimated to account for more than 44 million dollars in losses a year. These losses are in the form of genetics, carcass condemnation, trade restrictions, and veterinary costs.
• The dairy industry is believed to harbor more BLV-positive cattle because of the increased potential for transmission between cows.
• Male bull calves that have BLV-positive dams are believed to have a higher incidence of utero transmission.

GEOGRAPHIC DISTRIBUTION
Widespread throughout the United States

SIGNALMENT

Species
Cattle are the natural host for BLV. Sheep are highly susceptible to forming lymphosarcoma once exposed to BLV. Goats tend to form tumors but do not seroconvert.

Breed Predilections
None

Mean Age and Range
Cattle and sheep have the highest incidence of tumor formation between the ages of 2 and 4. Goats older than 2 years of age tend to be identified with tumors.

Predominant Sex
None

SIGNS

GENERAL COMMENTS
Depending on location of the developing tumor, animals will present with a wide variety of clinical signs.

PHYSICAL EXAMINATION FINDINGS
• Cattle and sheep: peripheral lymphadenopathy (prescapular, femoral, suprascapular, supramammary), weight loss, anorexia, decreased milk production, ketosis, diarrhea, ataxia, edema on ventral abdomen and udder due to blocked lymphatic drainage, exophthalmia, melena from gastrointestinal ulcers, dyspnea, cardiac dysrhythmia, pounding jugular pulse, masses in the reproductive tract, dog-sitting, and recumbent animals.
• Goats: pyrexia, emaciation, diarrhea, and dyspnea.

CAUSES
• Transmission of BLV occurs both horizontally and vertically.
• Horizontal transmission primarily occurs through fomites during normal cattle processing procedures. These include dehorning, rectal palpation, injections, tattoos, and surgeries. When instruments are not properly sterilized between procedures, contamination of naïve animals with the virus may occur. Body secretions from saliva, nasal discharge, broncho-alveolar fluids and urine have all been demonstrated to seroconvert exposed ruminants. Insects have been hypothesized to be a transmitting vector, but to date, experimental infection has not been demonstrated between animals.
• Experimental vertical transmission of virus can occur through semen, ova, and embryos. It is not believed that these reproductive products are a significant source of infection. None of these products may be sold internationally if the animals are identified as having BLV. In utero, cell-free transmission of virus to offspring occurs through the placenta in 3% to 25% of infected dams after the third month of gestation. Male calves born to an infected dam appear to have a higher incidence of infection than female calves. Colostrum and milk from BLV-positive cows are not believed capable of causing an infection in calves that ingest them if given after gut closure.

RISK FACTORS
• Fomites contaminated with whole blood from an infected cow that are not cleaned properly
• Sheep that are comingled with infected cattle
• Dairy cattle have more intense management and interaction than most beef cattle, which accounts for a higher incidence of transmission.

DIAGNOSIS

• Physical examination revealing peripheral lymphadenopathy
• Rectal palpation revealing large masses
• Virus isolation from the lymphocytes
• PCR testing for viral DNA, although specific and sensitive, is often cost-prohibitive. PCR testing distinguishes between calves that are positive for serology due to passive transfer of antibodies versus animals that have been administered vaccine. Positive results can occur when testing virus-infected lymphocytes within 3 days of exposure. Certain primers have been designed that specifically identify the 3′ end of the viral genome that is necessary for lymphosarcoma formation.
• Microscopic identification of viral particle in the lymphocyte. This will not tell you if the animals will develop lymphosarcoma.
• Testing blood samples for tumor specific antigen with monoclonal antibodies
• Serology—all of the serological tests depend on the host immune response to infection. Ruminants must seroconvert prior to detecting antibodies in the serum. The tests are designed to identify antibodies produced to either the gp51 or p24 viral antigen. Lymphosarcoma cattle are usually positive for p24 antibodies. This is not a common test done in labs. Cattle that are preparturient 2 to 3 weeks and postpartum up to 6 weeks may have a false negative test due to antibody compartmentalization in the udder. False positive results may occur in calves up to 6 months of age due to ingestion of antibodies from the dam in colostrum.
  • *Agar gel immunodiffusion (AGID)*—this is the primary test used to screen cattle and the official test for export of cattle. Most labs that run this test are identifying antibodies to gp51 viral antigen, which appears to be more sensitive than testing for p24. Antibodies to gp51 can occur as early as 3 weeks postexposure. A negative test indicates that the animal has not been exposed to BLV for 3 to 12 weeks prior to testing. A strong response to gp51 does not necessarily indicate that the animals will develop lymphosarcoma.
  • *Radioimmunoassay (RIA)*—this test is more sensitive than AGID and can detect smaller amounts of antibody within the first 2 weeks of infection. It has been developed for both the detection of p24 and gp51. Both serum and milk can be used for testing.
  • *Enzyme-linked immunosorbent assay (ELISA)*—sensitivity and specificity of this test are equal to RIA.

DIFFERENTIAL DIAGNOSIS
• Lymphadenopathy due to systemic infection
• Fat necrosis
• Melanomas
• Carcinomas
• Internal abscesses
• Caseous lymphadenitis in goats and sheep

CBC/BIOCHEMISTRY/URINALYSIS
• Cattle
  • CBC may be normal.
  • May see a lymphocytosis but rare
  • May be anemic, due to gastrointestinal bleeding (microcytic, hypochromic)
  • Can have an increase in liver enzymes if there is hepatic involvement
  • Hyperglobulinemia
  • Hypoalbuminemia
• Sheep and goats
  • Anemia that is nonregenerative
  • Hyperglobulinemia
  • Hypoalbuminemia

OTHER LABORATORY TESTS
A bone marrow aspirate and cytological examination may reveal clonal expansion of lymphoid precursors.

IMAGING
Can see masses on survey radiographs in the cranial thorax in ruminants that could be heart-based tumors

DIAGNOSTIC PROCEDURES
• Fine needle aspirate of the mass and cytological examination. Examination of the aspirate may reveal a large number of lymphoblasts, but it may be hard to distinguish between lymphadenopathy and systemic infections.
• Lymph node biopsy during a laparotomy

PATHOLOGIC FINDINGS
• Grossly, tumors appear to have a heavy fibrous capsular lining with cream-colored, friable inner contents and a necrotic, soft center.
• Tumor masses can occur in one or multiple organs and lymph nodes. The most common sites for development are:
  • Cardiac tumors primarily occur in the myocardium and right atrium. They are very rarely seen in the left side of the heart.
  • Gastrointestinal involvement of the pylorus is common and often will result in ulcers.
  • Ocular masses develop in the retrobulbar region.
  • Lymphatics in the area of the cranial udder
  • Uterine masses diffusely distributed throughout the tissues
  • Ventral spinal cord masses are readily palatable rectally.
  • Liver diffusely
  • Lungs diffusely but rare to find
  • Spleen diffusely
• Histologically, the masses have a large number of lymphoblast cells.

TREATMENT
None

APPROPRIATE HEALTH CARE
Some affected animals with high genetic value may need supportive care until they can have ova or semen harvested from them. Also, pregnant animals may need nursing care until they have their offspring.

NURSING CARE
Depending on what the animals are presenting as clinical signs, nursing care could range from soft bedding if the animal is recumbent or ataxic to slinging animals to prevent pressure necrosis.

ACTIVITY
Limit activity to prevent further injury if the animal is ataxic or recumbent and struggling.

DIET
Normal diet

CLIENT EDUCATION
It is important to educate your clients on the modes of horizontal transmission to prevent use of contaminated equipment on BLV-negative ruminants. It is important to discuss the economic impact of the disease on the production goals of the farm, to determine if testing and culling of infected animals are reasonable options. There are a number of international shipping restrictions that prevent the sale of breeding stock and their reproductive by-products if they are BLV positive.

SURGICAL CONSIDERATIONS
If the diagnosis is difficult to obtain through noninvasive techniques, an exploratory laparotomy and biopsy of lymph nodes may be warranted.

MEDICATIONS

DRUGS OF CHOICE
None

CONTRAINDICATIONS
None

PRECAUTIONS
None

POSSIBLE INTERACTIONS
None

ALTERNATIVE DRUGS
None

LYMPHOSARCOMA

FOLLOW-UP

Animals are usually culled from the herd once they present with clinical signs and are diagnosed as having lymphosarcoma.

PATIENT MONITORING
Monitor patients as their health degenerates to ensure they are humanely treated.

PREVENTION/AVOIDANCE
• Identify BLV-positive animals and keep them isolated from BLV-negative animals.
• Properly clean instruments that have whole blood contamination.
• Due not reuse needles.
• Test bulls that are used for natural service for BLV and do not use them if they are positive.
• Vector control—although to date experimental transmission of BLV by vectors has not been shown to be a primary infectious route
• Cull positive animals from the herd and maintain strict testing and biosecurity when introducing new animals to the herd.
• If the owners have BLV-positive cows, they can harvest the ova, rinse them, and implant them into a BLV-negative recipient.

POSSIBLE COMPLICATIONS
None

EXPECTED COURSE AND PROGNOSIS
Ruminants with lymphosarcoma generally deteriorate within a week to 2 months after presenting with clinical signs and eventually need to be humanely euthanized.

MISCELLANEOUS

ASSOCIATED CONDITIONS
Ataxia, anemia, ascites, ventral edema, bloat, choke

AGE-RELATED FACTORS
Lymphosarcoma occurs in mature ruminants, usually over the age of 4 years.

ZOONOTIC POTENTIAL
None

PREGNANCY
There is cell-free transmission of the virus after 3 months of gestation through the placenta to the fetus.

RUMINANT SPECIES AFFECTED
Cattle, sheep, and goats

BIOSECURITY
The optimal biosecurity measures would be to test and cull positive BLV ruminants from the herd. Culling positive animals is cost-prohibitive for most producers, so reducing the rates of transmission is a practical approach to eliminating the disease from the herd. Testing and adding only BLV-negative animals to the herd and eliminating positive animals through natural attrition and preferential selection can accomplish reducing the number of infected ruminants.

PRODUCTION MANAGEMENT
• There are several approaches to eradicating BLV from the herd. The producer is going to have to determine if the cost benefit of eradication is greater or less than having the disease present.
• There is a federally supported voluntary eradication program that has restrictions that vary by state.
• Eradicating or reducing BLV from the herd begins with testing all the animals in the herd. This primarily applies to cattle and sheep. All negative animals need to be retested in 12 weeks, and calves less than 6 months need to be retested at 6 months of age. Once producers have this information, they have three options:
 • Culling all positive animals identified can eliminate BLV from the herd in a few months. However, the economic hardship is extreme if the herd has a high rate of infection. There is also the loss of genetic material from the herd when culling.
 • Segregating infected animals from negative animals and slowly eliminating them from the herd and replacing with negative animals is another option. It takes longer to eliminate BLV from the herd this way, and requires more frequent serologic testing of the herd. Segregating positive from negative animals also requires essentially two separate facilities and equipment.
 • Managerial practices can be altered to prevent the transmission of the disease and allow for natural attrition of infected animals. This takes a long time to eliminate BLV from the herd, and requires frequent serological testing and a long-term commitment by the producer.

SYNONYMS
Enzootic bovine leucosis
Persistent lymphocytosis

SEE ALSO
Bovine leukemia virus
Cutaneous lymphosarcoma
Disposal
Euthanasia
Juvenile lymphosarcoma
Serology
Thymic lymphosarcoma

ABBREVIATIONS
AGID = agar gel immunodiffusion
BLV = bovine leukemia virus
ELISA = enzyme-linked immunosorbent assay
PCR = polymerase chain reaction
RIA = radioimmunoassay

Suggested Reading
Agresti, A., Ponti, W., Rocchi, M., et al. 1993. Use of polymerase chain reaction to diagnose bovine leukemia virus infection in calves at birth. *Am J Vet Res.* 54:373–78.
Digiacomo, R. F. 1992, March. Horizontal transmission of bovine leukemia virus. *Vet Med.* 263–70.
Digiacomo, R. F. 1992, March. Vertical transmission of bovine leukemia virus. *Vet Med.* 258–62.
Jacobs, R. M., Song, Z., Poon, H., et al. 1992. Proviral detection and serology in bovine leukemia virus-exposed normal cattle and cattle with lymphoma. *Can J Vet Res.* 56:339–48.
Johnson, R., Kaneene, J. B. 1991. Bovine leukemia virus. Part I. Descriptive epidemiology, clinical manifestations, and diagnostic tests. *Compendium Food Anim.* 13:315–24.
Johnson, R., Kaneene, J. B. 1991. Bovine leukemia virus. Part III. Zoonotic potential, molecular epidemiology, and an animal model. *Compendium Food Anim.* 13:1631–39.

Author: M. R. Machen

MAEDI-VISNA (VISNA-MAEDI)

BASICS

OVERVIEW
• Visna-maedi (VM), or maedi-visna (MV), is a chronic, multisystemic disease of sheep caused by visna-maedi virus (VMV).
• In the United States, the disease is known as ovine progressive pneumonia (OPP). Other names given to this disease include Graaff-Reinet disease in South Africa, la bouhite in France, and zwoegersiekte in Holland.
• VMV is the prototype species of the ovine/caprine lentivirus group of the genus *Lentivirus* in the family Retroviridae. VMV is closely related to other human and animal lentiviruses, particularly caprine arthritis encephalitis virus (CAEV).
• Like other lentiviruses, the genome of VMV is single-stranded RNA. After infection, the VMV genome is reverse transcribed into a double-stranded DNA copy that integrates into the host cellular DNA. As a result, VMV persists in cells of infected sheep for life, irrespective of the presence of neutralizing antibodies and cell-mediated immunity.
• MV has been reported in most sheep-producing countries of the world.
• In the United States, the average reported prevalence of VMV antibodies in sheep sera is 26%. However, there is a wide range of variation between states and among individual flocks.
• In west Texas, where the majority of U. S. sheep is raised, the VMV seroprevalence is 0.5%. The difference in VM seroprevalence between Texas and other U. S. states is probably due to differences in management between regions. In Texas, most sheep are raised on range conditions in a hot, dry climate and lambing occurs on pasture.
• Transmission of VMV occurs more often during periods when infected and noninfected sheep are housed close together, such as during lambing or in winter.

• During lambing and the postpartum period, transmission occurs by contact of newborns with either contaminated birth products or aerosols from the infected dam. Ingestion of infected colostrum or milk seems to play a less important role. Close contact between infected and noninfected sheep after weaning may also result in transmission.
• Coexistence of other chronic respiratory diseases in the flock, such as ovine pulmonary adenomatosis or lung parasites, seems to increase the risk of transmission.
• Vertical intrauterine transmission from infected ewes to the fetus occurs in 5%–10% of cases.
• Venereal transmission of VMV has not been shown to occur, but sheep experimentally infected with VMV and coinfected with *Brucella ovis* shed VMV in semen.
• Seroconversion usually occurs between 2 and 8 weeks postinfection (PI). Some sheep may remain seronegative for several months or longer in spite of being infected.

SIGNALMENT
• Sheep are the natural host of VMV infection. Goats can be infected experimentally with VMV. Phylogenetic analyses indicate that cross-species transmission of small ruminant lentiviruses (VMV and CAEV) occurs regularly under natural conditions. Feeding VMV-contaminated sheep colostrum or milk to goats can result in infection.
• The percentage of seropositive sheep in a flock increases with age.
• Although VMV transmission may occur at an early age, clinical signs of the disease are rarely shown before 2–3 years of age.
• Some breeds of sheep may be more susceptible to VMV infection than others. Finnish breeds seem to have a greater tendency to infection by VMV than the Ile de France, Rambouillet, or Columbia breeds. Some results may be difficult to interpret because of uncertainty in the exposure histories.

• Breed-related resistance to VMV-induced disease has been described in crosses between Icelandic and Border Leicester, pure Awassi, and Columbia breeds. Texel sheep are considered highly susceptible.
• Individual genetic susceptibility to VMV-induced pulmonary lesions has been demonstrated in artificially created isogenetic twin lambs.

SIGNS
• Several factors including virus strain, age, breed, and genetics of the animal, route of exposure, secondary infections, and management conditions may influence the clinical outcome of VMV-infection.
• The majority of sheep infected with VMV remains clinically healthy for life.
• In a proportion of infected sheep, VMV infection can lead to a disease complex characterized by cachexia and chronic inflammation in the lungs, lymph nodes, joints, mammary gland, and central nervous system (CNS).
• In North America, the most common manifestation of VM is chronic pneumonia with signs of afebrile, progressive respiratory failure in sheep 2–3 years or older. Affected sheep develop gradual emaciation and loss of body condition despite good appetite. They often remain behind the rest of the flock when driven to pasture and open-mouth breathing and dry cough are common.
• In the latter stages of disease, fever, purulent nasal discharge, cough, and depression are common as a result of secondary bacterial infection. Sheep usually die within 6 to 8 months after clinical signs become apparent.
• In some flocks, more than 60% of infected ewes may present evidence of mammary gland inflammation. In these cases, there is diffuse bilateral enlargement and hardening of the udder (hardbag). Milk may be normal in appearance but scant in quantity.

• Sheep with VMV-associated arthritis become lame and exhibit cachexia despite having a good appetite. There is weight loss and swelling of the carpal and tarsal joints. Clinical signs of arthritis normally appear 2–3 years after infection.

• Neurological manifestations of VM are seldom seen in the United States, but are common in Europe. In this form of the disease, there is aberration of gait affecting primarily the hindquarters. There is gradual weakening, leading first to paraplegia and then quadriplegia up to the point that animals are unable to rise. Affected animals lose weight, and jerking of the lips and facial muscles or blindness may be observed. Spinal taps reveal elevated numbers of mononuclear inflammatory cells in the cerebrospinal fluid.

DIAGNOSIS

DIFFERENTIAL DIAGNOSIS

• Other causes of chronic weight loss include caseous lymphadenitis, paratuberculosis (Johne's disease), chronic parasite infestations, and malnutrition.

• Other forms of chronic pulmonary disease include *Corynebacterium pseudotuberculosis*–induced mediastinal lymph node and lung abscesses, ovine pulmonary adenomatosis (jaagsiekte), chronic suppurative pneumonia, and parasitic pneumonia.

• Bacterial mastitis (bluebag)

• Arthritis by bacteria (*Chlamydia* and *Mycoplasma*)

• The neurologic form of VM can be confused with other CNS diseases such as scrapie, rabies, brain abscesses, and trauma of the spinal cord or parasitic lesions.

DIAGNOSTIC PROCEDURES

• In the United States, the agar gel immunodiffusion (AGID) test is the most commonly used serological technique to identify infected animals because of its low cost, simplicity, and high specificity. However, the sensitivity of the AGID test generally is considered low.

• Indirect ELISA tests utilizing either whole virus or recombinant OvLV proteins are used widely in Europe.

• The sensitivity of ELISA tests is considered to be better than the AGID test. Some studies have found the effectiveness of indirect ELISA and AGID test to be similar. A major problem is that none of the tests are standardized across laboratories, making comparative evaluations difficult.

• Virus isolation from "buffy coats" is the most definite way to confirm VM. However, this technique is expensive, cumbersome, often unsuccessful, and not recommended as a routine diagnostic test.

• Although PCR is a highly sensitive technique, its usefulness for the detection of VMV in clinical samples from naturally infected goats still requires validation.

PATHOLOGIC FINDINGS

Gross Findings

• The lungs of sheep with VMV-induced chronic interstitial pneumonia do not collapse fully after the thoracic cavity is opened, and they have a white or gray color. Impression lines as a result of rib compression on the costal surface of the lungs can be observed. The lungs are heavier than normal and firm on palpation. Multifocal, discrete, 1 to 2 mm or larger, gray foci may be observed throughout the lung parenchyma. Well-demarcated areas of consolidation without exudate in the airways are sometimes found in the cranioventral lobes. Mediastinal and peribronchial lymph nodes may be five to ten times larger than normal.

• The mammary gland in ewes affected with mastitis is symmetrically enlarged and firm on palpation.

• In sheep with arthritis, there is swelling of the carpal and tarsal joints and bursa. Other joints are less frequently affected. In these sheep, there is increased synovial fluid, discoloration and thickening of the synovial membrane, as well as erosion of the articular cartilage.

• Gross lesions are not observed in the CNS of sheep affected with the neurological form of VM.

Microscopic Findings

• Lymphoid interstitial pneumonia is the characteristic lesion in the lungs of sheep affected by the pulmonary form of VM. There is thickening of the interalveolar septa due to infiltration of mononuclear cells, hyperplasia of smooth muscle, and fibrosis. Numerous lymph follicles with active germinal centers are found adjacent to bronchioles and small vessels. Discrete nodules of lymphocytes are found unrelated to airways and blood vessels. In more severe infections, the alveoli are obliterated due to exudation of macrophages into the lumen.

• Lymphoid hyperplasia of associated lymph nodes is present.

• The mammary gland of ewes with VMV-induced mastitis shows follicular lymphoid hyperplasia around lactiferous ducts, interstitial infiltration of mononuclear cells, and fibrosis.

• Joint swelling is characterized by severe infiltration of lymphocytes, plasma cells, and macrophages as well as villi proliferation of the synovium. Degeneration of the articular cartilage, mineralization of the joint capsule, and periosteal replacement growth can be seen in more advanced cases.

• In the brain of sheep affected by the neurological form of the disease, there is periventricular encephalitis characterized by ependymal necrosis, widespread demyelination, and prominent perivascular lymphocytic cuffing.

TREATMENT

There are no commercial treatments available to control VM.

MEDICATIONS
N/A

CONTRAINDICATIONS
N/A

POSSIBLE INTERACTIONS
N/A

FOLLOW-UP
N/A

PATIENT MONITORING
N/A

PREVENTION/AVOIDANCE
• There are no commercial vaccines available to prevent VMV infection.
• Serological testing and segregation of positive reactors can achieve eradication of VM from a flock.
• Some VMV-infected sheep may remain seronegative for weeks or months after infection. These sheep may shed virus at irregular intervals, thus representing a major roadblock in VM control.
• Retesting every 3 to 6 months and elimination of new positive reactors is necessary until 3 to 5 consecutive tests result in 100% of the sheep being seronegative. Then, yearly testing and acquisition of replacements from VMV-free flocks are recommended.

• Separation of offspring from their mothers prior to the ingestion of colostrum and the use of heat-inactivated colostrum (56°C for 60 min) and milk substitutes have been used and found ineffective in the past. This method is labor intensive and not always effective.

MISCELLANEOUS

ASSOCIATED CONDITIONS
N/A

AGE-RELATED FACTORS
Clinical signs of VM are seen in animals 2–3 years old and older due to the long incubation period.

ZOONOTIC POTENTIAL
There is no evidence to indicate that VMV is infectious to humans.

PREGNANCY
Vertical transmission from mother to fetus occurs in a small proportion of cases, but there are no clinicopathological changes in infected fetuses.

SYNONYMS
Graaff-Reinet disease
La bouhite
Ovine progressive pneumonia (OPP)
Zwoegerziekte

SEE ALSO
Ovine progressive pneumonia

ABBREVIATIONS
AGID = agar gel immunodiffusion
CAEV = caprine arthritis encephalitis virus
ELISA = enzyme-linked immunosorbent assay
OPP = ovine progressive pneumonia
PCR = polymerase chain reaction
VMV = visna-maedi virus

Suggested Reading
Brodie, S. J., de la Concha-Bermejillo, A., Snowder, G. D., DeMartini, J. C. 1998. Current concepts in the epizootiology, diagnosis, and economic importance of ovine progressive pneumonia in North America: a review. *Small Ruminant Res.* 27:1–17.
de la Concha-Bermejillo A. 1997. Maedi-visna and ovine progressive pneumonia. *Vet Clin North Amer Food Anim Pract.* 13:13–33.
DeMartini, J. C., de la Concha-Bermejillo, A., Carlson, J. O., Bowen, R. A. 1999. Diseases caused by maedi-visna and other ovine lentiviruses. In: *Breeding for disease resistance in farm animals*, ed. R. F. E. Axford, S. C. Bishop, F. W. Nicholas, J. B. Owen. 2nd ed. Wallingford: CABI Publishing.
Juste, R. A., Kwang, J., de la Concha-Bermejillo, A. 1998. Dynamics of cell-associated viremia and antibody responses during the early phase of lentivirus infection in sheep. *Am J Vet Res.* 59:563–68.
Ritchie, C., Synge, B. 2004, Feb 14. Testing for maedi-visna. *Vet Rec.* 154(7):214–15.
Straub, O. C. 2004, Jan. Maedi-visna virus infection in sheep. History and present knowledge. *Comp Immunol Microbiol Infect Dis.* 27(1):1–5.

Author: Andrés de la Concha-Bermejillo

MAGNESIUM DEFICIENCY/EXCESS

 BASICS

DEFINITION
• Hypomagnesemia: measured serum magnesium concentration below established laboratory reference intervals for the species and breed; generally serum concentrations <1.4 mg/dL considered clinically significant in ruminants.
• Hypermagnesemia: measured serum magnesium concentration above established laboratory reference intervals for the species and breed; generally, serum concentrations > 3.0 mg/dL in ruminants.

PATHOPHYSIOLOGY
• Magnesium (Mg) represents 0.05% of total body weight and is the fourth most prevalent cation in the body following Ca, Na, and K.
• Mg is distributed in bones (60%), soft tissue (38%—mostly muscle), and extracellular fluids (2%—blood, CSF).
• Serum Mg concentration is composed of three fractions: free ionized portion (55%—regulated by hormones), protein-bound portion (30%—albumin, globulins), anion-bound portion (15%—PO_4, citrate).
• Several hormones influence concentration of free ionized Mg fraction.
  • Parathyroid hormone (PTH) increases reabsorption of Mg from the renal tubules, bone, and absorption from the gastrointestinal (GI) tract.
  • Thyroxine increases renal loss of Mg.
  • Aldosterone favors decreased GI absorption of Mg.
  • Activated vitamin D (1,25-DHCC) favors decreased serum Mg concentration via reduced PTH concentrations.
• Total daily body loss of Mg through feces, urine, and lactation can represent total amount of extracellular Mg.
• Limited reserves of mobile Mg in bone and extracellular sources for maintenance of homeostasis of extracellular Mg concentrations (capacity decreases with age).

• Ruminants are dependent upon daily oral intake of Mg (~20 g/day) and its absorption (adults—rumen; neonates—jejunum) to maintain adequate extracellular (CSF, blood) concentrations.
• Mg is an essential element and serves as a catalyst with over 300 different enzymes with particular importance to ATP reactions, bone formation, maintenance of cell membrane potentials, methyl group transfers, protein and fat catabolism, and regulation of RNA and DNA structure.
• Mg regulates CNS excitability by inhibiting Ca-dependant presynaptic excitation-secretion of neurotransmitters.
• Decreased CSF Mg concentrations lead to increased excitation.
• Increased CSF Mg concentrations lead to sedation.
• Mg is important in the production and decomposition of acetylcholine at neuromuscular junctions.
• Decreased Mg concentrations lead to increased acetylcholine at neuromuscular junctions predisposing to tetany.
• Increased Mg concentrations lead to muscle weakness and paralysis.

SYSTEMS AFFECTED
• Skeletal muscle—tetany (Mg decreased)/paralysis (Mg increased)
• CNS—excitement (Mg decreased)/sedation (Mg increased)
• Respiration—increased rate (Mg decreased)/decreased rate (Mg increased)
• Heart —increased rate (Mg decreased)/decreased rate (Mg increased)
• Reproduction —reduced fertility, retained placenta (Mg decreased)
• Renal —urolith formation (Mg increased)

GENETICS
N/A

INCIDENCE/PREVALENCE
• Hypomagnesemia-associated disorders seen in 10% of cattle herds.
• Hypomagnesemia-associated disorders responsible for 1%–3% of cattle, sheep, and goat deaths per year.

GEOGRAPHIC DISTRIBUTION
Worldwide

Species
All ruminants; cattle > sheep > goats.

Breed Predilection
• Adult cattle: beef cattle (Angus > Brahman) > dairy cattle (shorthorn > Holstein)
• Calf: dairy cattle

Mean Age and Range
• Adult cattle—3rd–5th lactation
• Calf—2–4 months
• Sheep—older ewes

Predominate Sex
N/A

SIGNS

Hypomagnesemia, Acute (Adult—Grass Tetany; Juvenile—Milk Tetany)
• Unusual vocalization (bellowing)
• Frenzied running
• Muscle fasiculations
• Erect ears
• Hyperesthesia and hyperexcitability
• Recumbent with seizure activity/nystagmus/limb paddling
• Increased body temperature
• Forceful respiration with tachycardia and loud heart sounds

Hypomagnesemia, Chronic (Adult—Winter Tetany)
• Unthriftiness
• Anorexia
• Frequent urination
• Mild ataxia
• Decreased milk production
• Reduced reproductive rate/retained placenta

Hypermagnesemia (rare)
• Possible hypotension
• Mental sedation
• Cardiac bradycardia, arrest
• Respiration depression, paralysis
• Skeletal muscle weakness

CAUSES

Hypomagnesemia
• Inadequate GI absorption of Mg
  • Anorexia
  • Starvation

- Type of diet: (1) Lush spring pastures (orchard grass, small grain, fescue) that contain high concentrations of potassium (K), PO_4, and nitrogen and low concentrations of Mg and sodium (Na). K interferes with GI absorption of Mg. (2) Whole milk diet for calves is low in Mg concentration and absorptive ability decreases with age.
- Infiltrative rumen disease
- Increased serum aldosterone concentrations—increased GI secretion of K, which interferes with Mg absorption
- Forages with increased concentrations of Ca or aluminum may interfere with Mg absorption.
- Excess urinary loss of Mg—impaired/reduced tubular reabsorption
  - Osmotic, loop diuresis
  - Hypercalciuria
  - Tubular acidosis
  - Aminoglycoside toxicities
  - Ketonuria

Hypermagnesemia
- Decreased urinary excretion
  - Reduced glomerular filtration due to dehydration or glomerular renal disease
  - Reduced renal tubular reabsorption due to renal failure
- Increased intestinal absorption of Mg without including PTH—excess oral administration of Mg
- Other
  - Milk fever/parturient hypocalcemia/paresis—possible mechanism: hypocalcemia -> ↑PTH -> ↑Mg bone, renal, and GI absorption
  - Excess intravenous Mg
  - Possibly hypoaldosteronism and hypothyroidism (both reported only in humans)

RISK FACTORS
All
- Environmental stress
- Poor body condition
- Overbody condition
- Abrupt change of diet

Adult Cattle
- Feeding forage with a ratio defined by $K/(Mg + Ca) > 2.2$
- Grazing forage with a Mg concentration <0.2%
- Grazing lush nonlegume pastures (*Phalaris Tuerosa*, orchard grass, fescue-bluegrass, small grains) low in Mg and Na—in order of decreasing risk: wheat > oats > barely > rye
- Soils high in K
- Treatment of pastures with fertilizers with high concentrations of nitrogen, potash, and poultry litter
- Beef cattle last 60 days of pregnancy
- Spring calving
- Poor-quality wintering diet
  - Winter diet deficient in Mg and Ca leads to ↑PTH -> depletion of bone Mg
  - Spring grass has ↑ Ca -> ↓PTH -> ↓ Mg bone, renal and GI absorption -> hypomagnesemia
- Pregnancy
- Lactation
- Third to fifth lactation cycle

Calf
- Diarrhea
- Fast growth rate

Ewe
- Pregnancy with twins
- Older animal
- Dental problems

DIAGNOSIS

DIFFERENTIAL DIAGNOSIS
Hypomagnesemia

Infectious
- Rabies
- Other viral encephalitites
- Enterotoxemia
- Tetanus

Toxicity
- Lead poisoning
- Strychnine poisoning
- Salt poisoning
- *Claviceps paspali* ingestion (ryegrass staggers)

Degenerative
Polioencephalomalacia (thiamin deficiency and other causes)

Metabolic
- Nervous ketosis
- Parturient hypocalcemia/paresis (milk fever)—urine Mg concentration > 10 mg/dL in milk fever, <1.0–3.0 mg/dL in grass tetany

CBC/BIOCHEMISTRY/URINALYSIS
Hypomagnesemia
CBC—no typical alteration

Blood Chemistry
- Serum preferred over plasma
  - Avoid use of EDTA and citrate collection tubes (chelate Mg)
  - Hemolysis will not elevate Mg concentration in sample (ruminants only)
- Mg <1.2–1.5 mg/dL
- Often moderate concurrent hypocalcemia (<8 mg/dL)
- Elevation in muscle enzyme activity (Ck, AST) if downer-animal or convulsive activity

Urine
- Mg <2 mg/dL indicator of danger for hypomagnesemia, 2–10 mg/dL marginal, and > 10 Mg/dL adequate
- Fractional excretion % of Mg decreased (normally 6.5–8.3% ± 3.7%)—[Mg_{Urine}/Mg_{Serum}] × [Cr_{Serum}/Cr_{Urine}] × 100

Hypermagnesemia
CBC—no typical alteration

Blood Chemistry
- Elevated serum Mg concentration
- Reduced serum Ca concentration

Urine
Fractional excretion % of Mg increased (normally 6.5–8.3% ± 3.7%)—[Mg_{Urine}/Mg_{Serum}] × [Cr_{Serum}/Cr_{Urine}] × 100

OTHER LABORATORY TESTS
Hypomagnesemia
- Cerebrospinal fluid Mg concentration (<1 mg/dL, can be used up to 12 hours postmortem)
- Measurement of Mg concentration in switch hair sample (correlates with serum concentration)

MAGNESIUM DEFICIENCY/EXCESS

IMAGING
N/A

DIAGNOSTIC PROCEDURES
Hypomagnesemia
- Forage Mg analysis (<0.2% increased risk)
- Calculate forage ratio of K \ (Mg + Ca). Values <2.2 indicate increased risk.
- Monogram for calculating risk factor using serum and forage Mg concentration
- In calves, bone analysis to evaluating the ratio of Ca:Mg, which is 70:1 normally but > 90:1 in hypomagnesemia conditions
- Vitreous fluid (up to 48 hours postmortem) <1.4 mg/dL (controversial)

PATHOLOGIC FINDINGS
Hypomagnesemia
Gross Pathology
- Muscle and head trauma due to seizure activity
- Petechiation in white matter of the midbrain and brain stem
- Agonal emphysema
- Aspiration of rumen contents

Histopathology
- Tissue mineralization in heart, spleen, and lung arteries
- Diapedesis of red blood cell in periventricular nuclei of the brain

Hypermagnesemia
Gross Pathology
Urinary calculi

TREATMENT

APPROPRIATE HEALTH CARE
Hypomagnesemia
- Cattle: remove from lush pasture, increase dry forage and legume consumption. Reduce stressor elements and environmental stimuli.
- Calf: reduce stressor elements and environmental stimuli.

Hypermagnesemia
Discontinue any dietary Mg supplementation.

ACTIVITY
N/A

CLIENT EDUCATION
- Risk of fatal cardiac arrythmias or arrest with IV Mg therapy
- Relapse following therapy likely if further prevention steps not taken

SURGICAL CONSIDERATION
N/A

MEDICATIONS

DRUGS OF CHOICE
Hypomagnesemia (Acute)
- Intravenous (IV) Ca borogluconate solution with 5% Mg hypophosphate (preferred medication)
- Sedation with chloral hydrate 50 mg/kg IV (cases of seizure activity)
- 10% magnesium sulfate (100 ml) subcutaneously (supplemental medication)
- Mg-rich enema (optional supplemental medication)
- 2 oz oral Mg oxide/day to prevent relapse

Hypomagnesemia (Chronic)
- 1–2 oz oral Mg oxide/day
- Acute Rx in cases with more severe symptoms

Hypermagnesemia
N/A

CONTRAINDICATIONS
Appropriate milk and meat withdrawal times must be followed for all compounds administered to food-producing animals.

PRECAUTIONS
Monitor heart during IV Mg therapy for arrythmias or bradycardia.

POSSIBLE INTERACTIONS
N/A

ALTERNATIVE DRUGS
N/A

FOLLOW-UP

PATIENT MONITORING
Hypomagnesemia
Herd urine concentration of Mg between 3.7 and 9.8 mg/dL indicates adequate herd status.

PREVENTION/AVOIDANCE
Hypomagnesemia
Calf
Offer oral starter ration (beginning at 2 weeks of age)

Cattle
- Forage analysis (see diagnostic procedures)
- Supplement with 1–2 oz Mg oxide/head/day
  - Mix Mg with molasses and water and spray on hay
  - Free choice 1:1:1 ratio of Mg oxide:dicalcium phosphate:ground barley
  - Free choice Mg mineral blocks
  - Apply 2% Mg sulfate dust every 2 weeks to pastures during spring danger period.
- Pasture management
  - Oversow grass with legume.
  - Avoid use of heavy potash and nitrogen fertilizers.
- Transition to a fall calving program
- Maintain adequate nutritional levels in winter months to avoid loss of body condition.

Hypermagnesemia
Avoid rations with Mg concentrations > 1.65%.

POSSIBLE COMPLICATIONS
- Mortality
- Unthriftiness
- Reduced reproduction rates
- Reduced milk production rates

EXPECTED COURSE AND PROGNOSIS

Hypomagnesemia

• Poor prognosis in cases that are comatose or have severe seizure activity
• Fair-good prognosis with IV therapy in less-severe cases
  • Improvement expected in 3–5 hours
  • Additional supplemental therapy and preventive steps vital to prevent relapse

Hypermagnesemia

Poor prognosis with serum Mg concentration > 3.5 mg/dL in association of renal disease

 MISCELLANEOUS

ASSOCIATED CONDITIONS
N/A

AGE-RELATED FACTORS
Hypomagnesemia
• Calves between 2 to 4 months of age
• Older adults

ZOONOTIC POTENTIAL
N/A

PREGNANCY
Increased risk for hypomagnesemia

RUMINANT SPECIES AFFECTED
All ruminants

BIOSECURITY
N/A

PRODUCTION MANAGEMENT
See also Prevention/Avoidance and Risk Factors above

SYNONYMS
Hypomagnesemia conditions: grass tetany, winter tetany, milk tetany, wheat pasture poisoning, green oat poisoning, and transport tetany

SEE ALSO
Degenerative—polioencephalomalacia (thiamin deficiency and other causes)
Infectious—rabies, other viral encephalitides, enterotoxemia, tetanus
Metabolic—nervous ketosis, parturient hypocalcemia/paresis (milk fever)
Nutritional diseases, body condition scores by species
Toxicity—lead poisoning, strychnine poisoning, salt poisoning, *Claviceps paspali* ingestion (ryegrass staggers)

ABBREVIATIONS
AST = aspartate transferase
Ca = calcium
CBC = complete blood count
Ck = creatine kinase
Cr = creatinine
CSF = cerebrospinal fluid
dL = deciliter
DNA = deoxyribonucleic acid
GI = gastrointestinal
IV = intravenous
K = potassium
mg = milligram
Mg = magnesium
Na = sodium
RNA = ribonucleic acid

Suggested Reading
Caple, I. W. 1998. Hypomagnesemic tetany in cattle and sheep. In: *Merck veterinary manual*, ed. S. E. Aiello. 8th ed. Whitehouse Station, NJ: Merck & Co.
Goff, J. P. 1999. Treatment of calcium, phosphorus, and magnesium balance disorders. *Vet Clin North Am Food Anim Pract*. 15:619–39, viii.
Hunt, E. 1996. Disorders of magnesium metabolism. In: *Large animal internal medicine*, ed. B. P. Smith. 2nd ed. St. Louis: Mosby.
McCaughan, C. J. 1992. Treatment of mineral disorders in cattle. *Vet Clin North Am Food Anim Pract*. 8:107–45.
Rosol, T. J., Capen, C. C. 1997. Calcium-regulating hormones and diseases of abnormal mineral metabolism. In: *Clinical biochemistry of domestic animals*, ed. J. J. Kaneko, J. W. Harvey, M. Bruss. 5th ed. San Diego, CA: Academic Press.
Stockham, S. L., Scott, M. A. 2002. Calcium, phosphorus, magnesium, and their regulatory hormones. *Fundamentals of veterinary clinical pathology*. Ames: Iowa State University Press.

Authors: Kurt L. Zimmerman and Daniel C. Rule

MALIGNANT CATARRHAL FEVER

BASICS

DEFINITION
• Peracute, acute, subacute, or chronic generalized infectious herpes viral disease characterized by sudden death, severe diarrhea, dyspnea, CNS symptoms, and oral lesions.
• Found in bovidae and cervidae with an extremely high mortality but generally a low morbidity.

PATHOPHYSIOLOGY
• Vasculitis of the endothelium and epithelium disruption characterizes this disease.
• Two or more distinct agents are thought to cause the disease.
• Ovine herpes virus 2 (OHV-2) and alcelaphine herpes virus 1 (AHV-1): OHV-2 is found in sheep and goats while AHV-1 is found in wildebeest.
• Alcelaphine herpes virus 2 (AHV-2) virus, which is similar to AHV-1, has been found in topi, hartebeest, and antelope. Infection of immunoregulatory granular lymphocytes with natural-killer (NK) activity is thought to occur.
• Polyclonal response through T-lymphocyte hyperplasia mediates tissue destruction.
• The disease appears to be an autoimmune phenomenon.

SYSTEMS AFFECTED
Gastrointestinal, CNS, respiratory, musculoskeletal, skin, generalized

GENETICS
N/A

INCIDENCE/PREVALENCE
• Very low morbidity, extremely high mortality in bovidae; high morbidity and extremely high mortality in cervidae
• There is some species variation within cervidae.

GEOGRAPHIC DISTRIBUTION
• Worldwide
• AHV-1 is found in Africa and in zoological and wildlife parks worldwide.
• OHV-2 is found in both wild and domestic sheep and goats worldwide.

Epidemiology
• Fomites are a common method of infection, especially postparturient.
• Nasal, ocular, and fecal contamination is common and the virus is cell associated.
• Serologic evidence supports the theory that deer and cattle may become subclinically infected and precipitate the disease following severe stress or concurrent infection.
• Transmission is primarily vertical; however, in wildebeest, transmission is vertical and horizontal.

SIGNALMENT

Species
• Bovine, caprine, ovine, bison, and wild ruminants
• Wildebeest, sheep, and goats act as asymptomatic carriers.
• Cattle usually experience the acute disease while deer generally exhibit the peracute form of the disease.

Breed Predilections
• Pere David's deer, Bali cattle, wapiti deer, red deer, Sitka deer, and white-tailed deer are all affected.
• Fallow deer may be resistant.

Mean Age and Range
• MCF usually affects adults (greater than 1 year of age) in the wild and in intensive production systems.
• Juvenile animals also may be affected in zoological and wildlife parks.
• Wildebeest are generally infected by 6 months of age.

Predominant Sex
N/A

SIGNS
• After an incubation period of 3–10 weeks (can be up to 6 months); serous nasal and ocular discharge are common.
• Erosions of the buccal papillae as well as erosive lesions of the mucosa of the upper respiratory tract are evident.
• The acute form is generally considered the "head and eye" form.
• Deer generally exhibit the peracute disease.
• Disseminated intravascular coagulation is usually followed by sudden death in cervidae.
• In all species, ulceration of the coronet, interdigital skin, teats, vulva, and the perineum may occur.
• Behavioral changes, nystagmus, weakness, tremors, paralysis, lameness, vasculitis, thickened skin, profuse mucopurulent nasal and conjunctival discharge, dyspnea, severe dysentery and diarrhea, oral and upper respiratory system ulcers, hypopion, muzzle encrustation, sudden death, generalized lymphadenopathy, fever, epithelial bleeding, and ulcers have all been reported.
• Some animals will progress to CNS signs of hyperesthesia, muscle fasciculation, and aggressive behavior.

GENERAL COMMENTS
Commonly spread from sheep, goats, and wildebeest to cattle, bison, deer, and other wild ruminants though shared grazing contact.

HISTORICAL FINDINGS
Generally found in grazing ruminants associated with sheep, goats, and wildebeest.

PHYSICAL EXAMINATION FINDINGS
• Disseminated intravascular coagulopathy is generally evident in deer.
• Nystagmus, weakness, tremors, paralysis, lameness, vasculitis, thickened skin, profuse mucopurulent nasal and conjunctival discharge, dyspnea, severe dysentery and diarrhea, oral and upper respiratory system ulcers, hypopion, muzzle encrustation, sudden death, generalized lymphadenopathy, fever, epithelial bleeding, and ulcers.
• Mucosal, GI, and respiratory necrosis are associated with lymphoid infiltration.

CAUSES
Generalized infectious herpes viral disease associated with the grazing of sheep, goats, and wildebeest.

RISK FACTORS
• Transmitted horizontally and vertically in wildebeest, vertical transmission in other species
• Nasal, ocular, and fecal contamination is common and is thought to be spread by fomites.

DIAGNOSIS

DIFFERENTIAL DIAGNOSIS
Foot-and-mouth disease, rinderpest, BVD/MD, vesicular stomatitis, IBR, bluetongue, East Coast tick fever (*Theileria parva*) encephalitis, shipping fever, arsenic toxicity, C naphthalene toxicity, rabies, yersiniosis, tick-borne diseases, and any vesicular disease.

CBC/BIOCHEMISTRY/URINALYSIS
• CBC initially will show a lymphocytosis with subsequent lymphopenia.
• When severe tissue damage is evident, neutrophilia occurs.

OTHER LABORATORY TESTS
Buffy coat analysis for virus isolation of AHV-1, AHV-2, and OHV-2.

IMAGING
N/A

OTHER DIAGNOSTIC PROCEDURES
• Virus neutralization and a CIE titer of 1:4 or higher are the most diagnostic tests.
• Polymerase chain reaction (PCR) is highly specific and is the best test for the determination of carriers within a clinically normal population.
• Other tests include immunoperoxidase and indirect immunofluorescence.

GROSS AND HISTOPATHOLOGICAL FINDINGS
• Confirmation is generally through histopathological findings including disseminated vasculitis, multifocal degenerative epithelial lesions, and multisystemic lymphoid tissue infiltration.
• Vascular lesions can vary from mild to fibrinoid necrosis.
• The kidney will generally show gross white raised capsular foci.
• Most lymph nodes are hyperplastic with a prominent paracortex. Multifocal ecchymotic hemorrhage in the colonic serosa occurs.
• In deer, luminal hemorrhage occurs in the colon, ileum, and cecum.
• The carotid rete is the most demonstrative tissue for the evaluation of vascular lesions.
• Other affected organs include: adrenal gland, kidney, liver, heart, meninges, and CNS perivascular spaces.

TREATMENT
• Usually ineffective
• Surviving animals may become disease carriers.

CLIENT EDUCATION
• Physically separate susceptible species from sheep, goats, and wildebeest in known infective areas.
• Wildlife populations may also spread the disease, so ensuring separation is essential to prevent disease introduction.
• Recovery is rare and may lead to a persistent carrier state.

MEDICATIONS

DRUGS OF CHOICE
• Antibiotics can be used as an adjunctive therapy to control secondary infections.
• Fluids and parenteral nutrition may be helpful as supportive measures.

CONTRAINDICATIONS
Survivors may become carriers.

PRECAUTIONS
N/A

POSSIBLE INTERACTIONS
N/A

ALTERNATE DRUGS
None

FOLLOW-UP

PATIENT MONITORING
N/A

PREVENTION/AVOIDANCE
• In areas infected with MCF, do not graze sheep, goats, and wildebeest with cattle or deer.
• Elimination of fomites, especially those contaminated with postparturient fluids, is essential. Insect control is also indicated.

POSSIBLE COMPLICATIONS
N/A

EXPECTED COURSE AND PROGNOSIS
• Disease course is generally 3–7 days.
• Prognosis is grave.
• Very low morbidity, extremely high mortality in bovine; high morbidity and extremely high mortality in cervidae.
• There is some species variation in cervidae.

MISCELLANEOUS

PREVENTION
• Separate grazing species.
• No vaccine is currently available.

ASSOCIATED CONDITIONS
None

AGE-RELATED FACTORS
None

ZOONOTIC POTENTIAL
None

PREGNANCY
N/A

SYNONYMS
• Catarrhal fever
• Gangrenous coryza
• Malignant head catarrh
• Snotsiekte

SEE ALSO
Arsenic toxicity
Bluetongue
BVD/MD
C naphthalene toxicity
East Coast tick fever (*Theileria parva*)
Encephalitis
Foot-and-mouth disease
IBR
Rabies

Rinderpest
Shipping fever
Tick-borne diseases
Vesicular stomatitis
Yersiniosis

ABBREVIATIONS
AHV-1 = alcelaphine herpes virus 1
BVD/MD = bovine viral diarrhea/mucosal disease
CIE = competitive inhibition ELISA test
CNS = central nervous system
ELISA = enzyme-linked immunosorbent assay
MCF = malignant catarrhal fever
OHV-2 = ovine herpes virus 2

Suggested Reading
Brenner, J., Perl, S., Lahav, D., Garazi, S., Oved, Z., Shlosberg, A., David, D. 2002, Aug. An unusual outbreak of malignant catarrhal fever in a beef herd in Israel. *J Vet Med B Infect Dis Vet Public Health* 49(6): 304–7.
Frolich, K., Thiede, S., Kozikowski, T., Jakob, W. 2002, Oct. A review of mutual transmission of malignant catarrhal fever between livestock and wildlife in Europe. *Ann N Y Acad Sci.* 969:4–13.
Hew, Y., Li, H., Crawford, T.B. 1999, Mar. Quantitation of sheep-associated malignant catarrhal fever viral DNA by competitive polymerase chain reaction. *J Vet Diagn Invest.* 11(2): 117–21.
Li, H., Keller, J., Knowles, D. P., Crawford, T. B. 2001, Jan. Recognition of another member of the malignant catarrhal fever virus group: an endemic gamma herpesvirus in domestic goats. *J Gen Virol.* 82(Pt 1): 227–32.
Schultheiss, P. C., Collins, J. K., Spraker, T. R., DeMartini, J. C. 2000, Nov. Epizootic malignant catarrhal fever in three bison herds: differences from cattle and association with ovine herpesvirus-2. *J Vet Diagn Invest.* 12(6): 497–502.

Author: Dan Grooms

MAMMARY GLAND SURGERIES: TEAT AMPUTATION, MASTECTOMY

BASICS

DEFINITION
Mastectomy is defined as excision of the udder with or without removal of the regional lymph nodes. Teat amputation involves removal of a portion of or the whole teat to allow drainage of the udder in severe cases of mastitis. Supranumery teats are usually removed in dairy heifers at a young age as a management practice.

SYSTEMS AFFECTED
Mammary gland

GENETICS
N/A

INCIDENCE/PREVALENCE
N/A

GEOGRAPHIC DISTRIBUTION
Potentially worldwide

SIGNALMENT

Species
Potentially, all lactating ruminant species

Breed Predilections
N/A

Mean Age and Range
Adult lactating animals

Predominant Sex
Female

History
• Adult female cattle, sheep, and goats. It appears that goats may require mastectomy more often than cattle.
• A recent retrospective study showed that 17 of 20 patients presented for mastectomy were goats. Many of the patients (70%) in this study were kept as pets and had never lactated, but had chronic bilateral or unilateral mammary gland enlargement.

SIGNS
With the exception of supranumery teat removal, teat amputation and mastectomy are regarded as salvage procedures when the conditions listed below cannot be resolved with medical therapy.

Teat Amputation
• Removal of supranumery teats
• Drainage of toxins and inflammatory products
  • Peracute coliform mastitis
  • Peracute/acute gangrenous mastitis
• Drainage of a chronic suppurative mastitis
• Prevent milking of a chronically infected mammary quarter

Mastectomy
• Chronic suppurative mastitis
• Mammary gland neoplasia
  • Adenoma
  • Adenocarcinoma
  • Lymphoma
  • Squamous cell carcinoma
• Mammary gland hyperplasia
• Peracute/acute gangrenous mastitis

DIAGNOSIS

• Chronic suppurative mastitis and acute gangrenous mastitis are usually diagnosed based on physical examination.
• Gangrenous mastitis is characterized by avascular necrosis of the udder tissue rendering the udder cool to the touch with blue or dark discoloration of the udder tissue. Crepitation may be present also with gas-forming organisms.
• Systemic clinical signs such as toxemia, acid/base and electrolyte imbalances, and dehydration may be seen in cases of peracute gangrenous mastitis.
• Chronic suppurative mastitis is characterized by purulent material draining from the teat orifice or abscessation of the udder.
• Ancillary testing such as milk culture and ultrasound of the udder may be included in the diagnostic workup.

TREATMENT

The decision of whether to perform a teat amputation or mastectomy will be based on the extent and severity of the mastitis, the degree of pain the animal is suffering, and the desired aesthetic outcome of surgery.

Teat Amputation: Surgical Procedure
• The teat is anesthetized using a 2% lidocaine ring block at the base of the teat.
• In cases of gangrenous mastitis, regional anesthesia is not necessary. The surgery can be performed in a cattle chute or milking parlor.
• The teat can be amputated at the base or midway between the base and tip. The tip of the teat is amputated with scissors by cutting horizontally across the base or middle of the teat. Hemostasis is not needed in cases of gangrenous mastitis.

• In cases of nongangrenous mastitis, hemostasis can be afforded by placing a plastic stent made from a 3 ml disposable syringe in the bore of the teat followed by a circumferential ligature placed over the teat and exerting pressure on the stent. The plunger of the syringe is removed and discarded. Two small holes are made in the fingerholds of the syringe case using an 18-gauge needle and the syringe case is circumferentially cut approximately 1 inch (2.5 cm) distal to the fingerholds to remove the tip. The syringe case is inverted and inserted into the bore of the remaining portion of the teat. The holes in the fingerhold portion of the syringe case are used to suture the cases to the end of the teat. A circumferential suture is then placed around the teat applying pressure against the syringe case stent inside the bore of the teat thus facilitating hemostasis. The syringe case stent can be removed in 48–72 hours.

Mastectomy: Surgical Procedure
• There are two techniques for performing a mastectomy.
• Surgical mastectomy involves the removal of the whole or part of the udder.
• An alternative approach is to ligate the external pudendal artery and vein either through a laparotomy incision (the vessels are ligated blindly through a paralumbar fossa incision just proximal to the internal inguinal ring using a sterile cable tie) or inguinal incision.
• The latter methods cause ischemia and gradual sloughing of the mammary tissue on the ligated side. One or both sides can be ligated depending on the distribution of the udder lesions. While the latter methods are less aesthetically pleasing, they may be the best option in cases where the patient is toxemic or severely debilitated, because general anesthesia is not required.
• It may be advantageous to amputate the teats on the ligated side to facilitate drainage and sloughing of the mammary gland parenchyma following ligation.
• Surgical mastectomies are usually performed under general anesthesia with the animal in dorsal recumbency. The udder is clipped and aseptically prepared. An elliptical skin incision is made one-third of the way up the side of the udder from its base. The subcutaneous tissues are bluntly dissected starting laterally and moving cranial and caudal. In cattle, assistance retracting the excised tissue is usually needed. The external pudendal artery and vein, smaller branch of the ventral perineal artery, and subcutaneous abdominal vein are the major vessels that should be ligated.

MAMMARY GLAND SURGERIES: TEAT AMPUTATION, MASTECTOMY

Note: Investigators recommend ligating the external pudendal artery prior to the external pudendal vein to minimize blood loss. The lateral and medial suspensory apparatus is dissected and the mammary gland removed from the body wall. Small bleeders can be ligated or cauterized using electrocautery. The skin edges are apposed using tension-relieving sutures such as vertical mattress sutures. The skin is then closed with a continuous Ford-interlocking suture pattern using a monofilament nonabsorbable suture material.
• Penrose drains can be placed to reduce seroma formation. Drains should be removed 48 to 72 hours after surgery.
• Skin sutures are usually removed in 10 to 14 days.

MEDICATIONS

• Perioperative antibiotics are warranted given the size and location of the surgery site. Postoperative pain management can be achieved with nonsteroidal anti-inflammatory drugs (NSAIDs) such as flunixin meglumine.
• Epidural administration of opioids via an in-dwelling epidural catheter has been described in goats for postoperative pain management.
• If excessive hemorrhage occurs, blood transfusion may be indicated to normalize the animal's packed cell volume.
• Intravenous fluid therapy during and after surgery will help maintain circulating volume.

CONTRAINDICATIONS

• Appropriate milk and meat withdrawal times must be followed for all compounds administered to food-producing animals.
• Goats are highly sensitive to the effects of lidocaine. Care needs to be implemented in its use.

FOLLOW-UP

POSSIBLE COMPLICATIONS

• The most common postoperative complication is hemorrhage.
• Hemorrhage is reported to be a greater problem in cattle than goats.
• If excessive tension is placed on the skin during closure, wound dehiscence may occur, and given the ventral location of the surgery site, wound infection is always a potential complication.
• Abscesses at the surgery site should be drained.

EXPECTED COURSE AND PROGNOSIS

In a recent study evaluating 20 cases of radical mastectomy in ruminants, 90% of cases were discharged from the hospital and of the animals for which follow-up data were available, the 1-year survival rate was 80%.

MISCELLANEOUS

ASSOCIATED CONDITIONS

Seroma/hematoma/abscess formation secondary to surgery; mastitis in surviving quarters/halves.

AGE-RELATED FACTORS

N/A

ZOONOTIC POTENTIAL

N/A

PREGNANCY

N/A

RUMINANT SPECIES AFFECTED

Potentially, all lactating ruminant species are affected.

BIOSECURITY

N/A

PRODUCTION MANAGEMENT

N/A

SYNONYMS

N/A

SEE ALSO

Anesthesia and analgesia
Animal welfare
FARAD
Mastitis section
Wound management

ABBREVIATIONS

FARAD = Food Animal Residue Avoidance Databank
NSAIDs = nonsteroidal anti-inflammatory drugs

Suggested Reading
Cable, C. S., Peery, K., Fubini, S. L. 2004, May–Jun. Radical mastectomy in 20 ruminants. *Vet Surg*. 33(3): 263–66.
Stevenson, J. S., Knoppel, E. L., Minton, J. E., Salfen, B. E., Garverick, H. A. 1994, Mar. Estrus, ovulation, luteinizing hormone, and suckling-induced hormones in mastectomized cows with and without unrestricted presence of the calf. *J Anim Sci*. 72(3): 690–99.
Viker, S. D., Larson, R. L., Kiracofe, G. H., Stewart, R. E., Stevenson, J. S. 1993, Apr. Prolonged postpartum anovulation in mastectomized cows requires tactile stimulation by the calf. *J Anim Sci*. 71(4): 999–1003.

Author: John R. Middleton

MAMMARY GLAND: ULTRASOUND

BASICS

OVERVIEW
• Many bovine practices are now equipped with ultrasound for reproductive cases, and there is a desire to use the machine for other applications.
• Ultrasound is an excellent tool for diagnostic imaging in large animals because it is portable, easy to use in the field, produces results at the time of the examination, and can be used for most soft tissue and some orthopedic problems.
• Ultrasounding is totally noninvasive. Palpation of a gland can detect only certain levels of disease. Ultrasound, in contrast, can give an "insider's" perception of mammary health, a picture of the inside anatomy and pathology.
• Tumors, growths, scarring, stones, trauma, hematoma formation, and level of mastitic damage can all be evaluated using ultrasound.
• Though culturing or other diagnostic tools are still primary, ultrasounding gives yet another dimension to the hard-to-diagnose case. It will also allow a better estimate of treatment prognosis to aid in deciding whether to cull or treat a cow.

• Ultrasound examination of the mammary gland can confirm diagnoses of tissue destruction, scarring, nonpalpable stones, or tumors. However, it should be emphasized that in many cases ultrasounding is not indicated and other forms of diagnosis are superior. Particularly for cows of low value, an ultrasound diagnosis would not be indicated.
• A limitation of the use of ultrasound in bovine practice is the knowledge and comfort of the practitioner with the technology and the transducer available. Ultrasound transducers intended for rectal examination of the reproductive system are ideal for examination of the mammary gland and teats.

SYSTEMS AFFECTED
Lactational and musculoskeletal

GENETICS
N/A

INCIDENCE/PREVALENCE
N/A

GEOGRAPHIC DISTRIBUTION
Worldwide

SIGNALMENT
Species
Lactating dairy species of cattle, sheep, and goats

Breed Predilections
Lactating dairy breeds
Mean Age and Range
Lactating dairy animals
Predominant Sex
Female

MISCELLANEOUS

Image Production
• Piezoelectric (pressure electric) crystals within the ultrasound transducer are deformed when a pulsed electrical current is applied to them. The deformations produce a sound beam.
• Ultrasound frequencies range from 20 to 1 MHz. These frequencies are above that which can be detected by the human ear.
• A transducer can produce a single frequency or a range of frequencies. A higher frequency transducer produces an image with better resolution than a lower frequency transducer but the sound beam cannot penetrate as far.
• In selecting a transducer, the transducer with the highest frequency that can provide an adequate depth of penetration for the structure imaged is chosen.

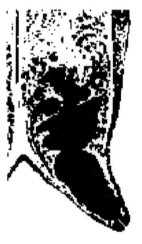

Figure 1.

Teat cistern.

• Once emitted from the transducer, the sound wave passes through the tissues and is eventually reflected back to the transducer. The transducer then acts as a receiver for the sound waves. The returning sound wave deforms the piezoelectric crystal producing an electrical signal. The electrical signal is converted into a series of dots on the monitor that form the image. The transducer acts as a receiver 99% of the time and as a transmitter 1% of the time.

Acoustic Impedance

• The number, strength, and time delay of sound waves returning from the tissues determine the ultrasound image.
• The location of the dot corresponds to the anatomic location of the imaged structure. The brightness of the dot is dependent on the difference in acoustic impedance (density and stiffness) of the tissue interfaces.
• Dense tissues such as bone or fibrous tissue produce high intensity (hyperechoic) images, which appear bright white.
• Low-density tissues such as fluid reflect very little sound wave and produce very low intensity (anechoic) images that appear black. See Figures 2 and 3.

• Because air has very low acoustic impedance and tissue has relatively high acoustic impedance, the marked difference in acoustic impedance between air and soft tissue causes near complete reflection of the ultrasound beam from the air-filled tissue back to the transducer forming a bright hyperechoic image.
• Because air is a near perfect reflector of the ultrasound beam, no ultrasound waves can penetrate air and any tissues deep to the air cannot be imaged.

Transducer Selection and Patient Preparation

• Appropriate preparation of the site to be imaged will enhance the quality of the image. Clean off any loose hair and dirt. Wet the skin and hair with alcohol. An image can be obtained, in some cases, with just alcohol applied to the skin. Be sure that the probe will not be damaged by the use of alcohol.
• Ultrasound gel can be applied and rubbed in if there is no significant hair growth (i.e., teat) or if the hair has been clipped. Ultrasound gel acts as a coupling agent to prevent air from trapping between the transducer and skin.
• A 7.5 MHz transducer with a stand off pad is ideal for imaging the teats. A 5.0 MHz transducer provides an adequate image. A stand off pad can be purchased separately or can be made from a glove filled with ultrasound gel.

• Many transducers are sold with stand off pads that fit the head of the transducer and these are the easiest to use.
• The mammary gland should be scanned with a 5.0–3.5 MHz transducer to give adequate penetration. All structures should be scanned in cross section and longitudinal planes.

ANATOMY

• The gland is made up of alveoli and alveolar ducts. The alveoli are grouped into lobes and lobules. The collecting ducts open into the gland cistern or lactiferous sinus.
• The gland cistern is separated from the teat cistern by a fibrous annular ring.
• The wall of the teat cistern is composed of 5 layers: the outer stratified squamous epithelium, muscular layer with longitudinal and circular layers, connective tissue which contains the major blood supply, the submucosa, and the inner mucosa.
• The streak canal is closed by a sphincter of smooth muscle and elastic tissue. The junction of the mucosa of the teat cistern and the stratified squamous epithelium of the streak canal is the rosette of Furstenburg.

Ultrasonographic Appearance of the Normal Bovine Mammary Gland

• The glandular parenchyma appears as a mixed trabecular pattern of anechoic (black) areas compartmentalized by hyperechoic (white) partitions. The anechoic areas represent milk within the gland.

MAMMARY GLAND: ULTRASOUND

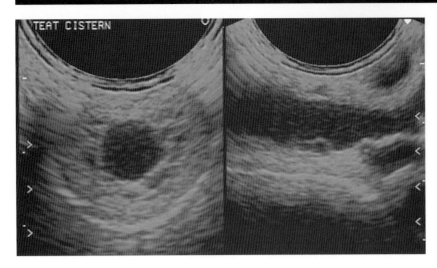

Figure 2.

Ultrasonographic image of a teat in cross sectional (left) and longitudinal (right) planes. The lumen of the teat is anechoic (black). Note the blood vessels surrounding the lumen.

• Small ducts in the matrix of the gland lead into larger lactiferous ducts that lead into the gland cistern. Blood vessels are seen within the mammary gland, but are difficult to differentiate from lactiferous ducts.

• The pattern formed by the lactiferous ducts and glandular parenchyma may vary among individuals. Nonlactating mammary glands appear as dense hyperechoic tissue with few visible blood vessels and lactiferous ducts.

• Periparturient cows will exhibit subcutaneous edema of the udder several days before and after freshening.

• The gland cistern appears as a large anechoic area. The lining of the gland cistern appears hyperechoic. See Figure 1.

• The annular ring can be detected as a hyperechoic band of tissue separating the gland cistern from the teat cistern.

• The teat cistern has an anechoic lumen surrounded by four layers visible on ultrasonographic examination.

• The outermost layer represents the skin air interface. The next inner layer is intermediate in echogenicity and represents the muscular layer.

• The two layers of longitudinal and circular muscle are difficult to differentiate on ultrasonography. The next inner layer is thin and hypoechoic to anechoic and represents the blood vessels known as the plexus venosus papillaris and the circulus venosus papillae. See Figures 2 and 3.

• The innermost layer is hyperechoic and represents the submucosa and the mucosa. The muscular layer of the streak canal appears hyperechoic.

Mastitis

• Acute purulent mastitis is denoted by marked udder enlargement with engorgement of the lactiferous ducts with fluid.

• If the cell content of the milk is high, the fluid in the ducts may appear hypoechoic as a result of the increased particulate matter. The demarcation between fluid within the lactiferous ducts and the glandular parenchyma may be diminished due to edema within the gland.

• A discrete abscess may be visualized anywhere within the glandular parenchyma. A thick hyperechoic fibrous wall may be present surrounding the abscess. Occasionally, draining tracts can be followed to the abscess. Chronic diffuse mastitis results in an increase in fibrous tissue within the glandular parenchyma and a decrease in the lactiferous ducts, giving the gland an overall hyperechoic appearance.

Obstruction of the Teat

• Obstruction of the teat may occur as a congenital anomaly (membranous shelf) or secondary to a traumatic occurrence. The obstruction may occur anywhere from the teat orifice to the gland cistern.

• Ultrasound can be used to determine the location of the obstruction and its extent. If the teat is completely obstructed, the teat will be filled with milk proximal to the obstruction.

• Distal to the obstruction, the teat will appear collapsed and does not contain milk. To further delineate the thickness, structure, and extent of the obstruction, saline can be infused retrograde into the teat canal. This technique will outline the obstruction and provide information to obtain a treatment plan and prognosis. In the case of a membranous shelf, once filled with saline the teat cistern may have normal anatomy and the proximal obstruction can be defined.

• Obstruction of the teat cistern may also be due to complete fibrosis. No anechoic milk will be visualized within the teat cistern, and instead it will be replaced with hypo- to hyperechoic dense tissue. A teat cannula cannot be passed in this case.

• Trauma or chronic mastitis may form a web within the teat cistern causing teat obstruction. The teat cistern will be filled with anechoic milk but thin hypoechoic strands can be visualized emanating from the walls of the teat cistern. See Figure 1.

• If the streak canal is obstructed, the teat cistern will be filled with anechoic milk. Fibrous clots may form in the lumen of the teat at the streak canal subsequent to trauma preventing milk flow.

Conclusions

• For the veterinary practitioner currently doing reproductive ultrasounding, it is very

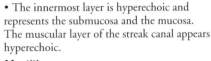

Figure 3.

Ultrasonographic image of a teat in longitudinal (left) and cross to sectional (right) planes. The lumen of the teat is anechoic (black). Note the obstruction at the streak canal (arrows).

simple to make mammary diagnoses with their ultrasound unit.

• Most schools and colleges of veterinary medicine offer ultrasounding short courses if the practitioner needs more specialized training.

• In many cases, ultrasounding is invaluable in determining the prognosis of a case and whether it is economically feasible to treat further.

• Ultrasound diagnosis can provide a more definitive diagnosis on those cases where the veterinarian is just not 100% sure. By no means is it indicated in cows of poor value or lactation performance.

ASSOCIATED CONDITIONS

Hematomas, mastitis, abscesses, tears, and ruptures

AGE-RELATED FACTORS

N/A

ZOONOTIC POTENTIAL

N/A

PREGNANCY

N/A

RUMINANT SPECIES AFFECTED

Lactating dairy animals

BIOSECURITY

N/A

PRODUCTION MANAGEMENT

N/A

SYNONYMS

N/A

SEE ALSO

Mastitis chapters
Ultrasounding by species

ABBREVIATIONS

MHz = megahertz

Suggested Reading

Cartee, R. E., Ibrahim, A. K., McLeary, D. 1986. B-mode ultrasonography of the bovine udder and teat. *J Am Vet Med Assoc.* 188:1284–87.

Dreyfuss, D. J., Madison, J. B., Reef, V. B. 1990. Surgical treatment of a mural teat abscess in a cow. *J Am Vet Med Assoc.* 197:1629–30.

Metcalf, J. A., Roberts, S. J., Sutton, J. D. 1992. Variations in blood flow to and from the bovine mammary gland measured using transit time ultrasound and dye dilution. *Res Vet Sci.* 53:59–63.

Takeda, T. 1989. Diagnostic ultrasonography of the bovine udder. *Jpn J Vet Res.* 37:133.

Trostle, S. S., O'Brien, R. T. 1998. Ultrasonography of the bovine mammary gland. *Compen Cont Edu Pract Vet.* 20:S64–S71.

Author: Abbey M. Sage

MANAGEMENT OF GUNSHOT WOUNDS

BASICS

OVERVIEW
• The pathology associated with gunshot wounds (GSWs) can vary dramatically with the part of the body affected and the ballistics (shape, weight, stability in flight, and velocity) associated with the bullet.
• Radiographs are indicated to assist in evaluating damage. GSWs may be minor and heal with little or no intervention, may require significant intervention in order to heal, or may be fatal with or without intervention.
• The degree of tissue injury depends on bullet weight, velocity, and the affected tissues' expansile ability.
• Contamination must always be suspected in gunshot injuries.

SYSTEMS AFFECTED
Musculoskeletal, CNS, gastrointestinal, cardiovascular, respiratory, either alone or in combination

GENETICS
N/A

INCIDENCE/PREVALENCE
Sporadic

GEOGRAPHIC DISTRIBUTION
Worldwide

SIGNALMENT
Species
All ruminant species

Breed Predilections
N/A

Mean Age and Range
N/A

Predominant Sex
N/A

SIGNS
Variable with anatomical location of GSW
• GSWs may be inapparent during physical examination. Hemorrhage may or may not be visible.
• Hemodynamic instability
• Animal may be asymptomatic.
• Dyspnea
• Hemoptysis
• Epistaxis

• Abdominal tenderness
• Hematuria
• Rectal bleeding
• Infection
• Lameness
• Bony fracture
• Neurologic abnormality

CAUSES AND RISK FACTORS
Wound severity is a function of bullet size, shape, velocity, and tissue characteristics.
• Larger bullets cause more damage simply as a function of size.
• Bullets that fragment or deform (e.g., hollow points) create larger holes.
• Higher velocity bullets cause more damage via shock waves through tissue along bullet path.
• More expansile tissues (e.g., bladder, bowel) struck by a bullet might be perforated only, while less-expansile tissues (e.g., encapsulated organs, kidney) might be severely disrupted.
• Bone can fragment, producing bone shards that act as additional missiles.

DIAGNOSIS

DIFFERENTIAL DIAGNOSIS
Varies with affected system(s)

CBC/BIOCHEMISTRY/URINALYSIS
PCV may be helpful to determine the extent of blood loss and potential anemia/transfusion requirements of valuable animals.

OTHER LABORATORY TESTS
As needed

IMAGING
Radiographs recommended for all GSWs. Anatomical placement of projectile fragments is important in formulating the final prognosis.

DIAGNOSTIC PROCEDURES
History, physical examination (entrance/exit wounds), plus radiographs provide information about bullet path and location.

SEVERITY OF INJURY: DETERMINANT FACTORS
Action of bullet (physical properties):
1. Bullet velocity
   • Velocity is the most important single factor responsible for wound damage.

   • Impact velocity is the speed at which the bullet meets target tissue and is important to the wound characteristics.
   • When impact velocities are low (nonmilitary-civilian bullets) wounds have less tissue damage and do not exhibit explosive effect. High-velocity injuries can exhibit explosive effects.
   • High-impact velocity wounds reflect maximum tissue destruction with remote injury.
2. Bullet mass: Projectile kinetic energy varies directly with the mass of the bullet.
3. Ballistic shape: Bullets of different weights, shapes, and calibers do not pass through the air in similar patterns.
4. Bullet composition
   • Soft-point bullets will mushroom or expand upon impact.
   • Hollow-point bullets behave similar to soft-point jacketed bullets and will mushroom or expand upon impact.
5. Bullet yaw
   • Yaw results from inherent asymmetry of the bullet.
   • Yaw in part explains the aberrant bullet wounds seen in veterinary practice. Because animal tissues are much less dense than air, yaw is magnified.
6. Tissue reaction
   • Tissue retentiveness to the passing bullet contributes to its severity. Wound extent is determined by the projectile's energy upon impact and tissue energy transfer. An entering bullet's kinetic energy is transferred to the surrounding tissue when producing the wound.
   • Tissue elasticity, cohesiveness, and density properties tend to oppose the bullet's inertia and slow it down.
7. Tissue elasticity
   • Tissues of different densities variably alter the kinetic energy transfer.
   • Tissue absorption of the kinetic energy is the determinant of wound severity.
8. Tissue cohesiveness
   • Penetrating wounds reflect sufficient tissue resistance to cause dissipation of the bullet's kinetic energy.
   • Perforating wounds reflect the difference between energy at wound entry and that remaining at exit.

9. Tissue density
- Damage to bone may result from the bullet striking the long bone directly. Effects depend on the type of bone structure, the physical characteristics of the bullet, and the periosteal supporting structures.
- "Indirect fracture" occurs when a high-velocity bullet passes near a bone but does not strike it directly.

TREATMENT

- Varies with injury; proper management of bullet wounds requires a working knowledge of physical factors involved in the creation of such injuries and the way in which they interact.
- Antibiotics may be indicated as GSWs are contaminated with dirt, hair, and skin fragments.
- Conservative treatment is usually sufficient in limb wounds not associated with fractures. Wounds should be allowed to heal as open wounds, or repaired surgically after infection is controlled.
- Extremity wounds rarely require tissue debridement. Thorough but mild irrigation with physiologic saline to remove surface debris and contaminants is indicated. Excision of devitalized exposed skin, muscle, and fascia may be indicated. Foreign bodies such as shotgun wads must be removed, but probing of the wound is generally avoided if at all possible.
- Fracture treatment varies. Casts or splints may be sufficient in some cases. More serious fractures require bone plating or external fixation. Severe fractures may require amputation or even animal euthanasia.
- GSWs to the abdomen usually require exploratory laparotomy to thoroughly evaluate viscera and repair any damage found.

- Thoracic GSWs are frequently fatal (blood loss). Surgery and blood transfusions can be attempted but may be unsuccessful. Ruminants with thoracic GSWs that are stable, not in shock, and eupneic generally should not undergo a thoracotomy.
- Euthanasia may be indicated for less-valuable animals.

MEDICATIONS

- Antibiotic choice varies with location of GSW.
- Analgesia as needed
- Fly repellent

CONTRAINDICATIONS

Appropriate milk and meat withdrawal times must be followed for all compounds administered to food-producing animals.

MISCELLANEOUS

ASSOCIATED CONDITIONS

- Lead poisoning symptoms may develop if one or more lead slugs are left in the body. Risk depends on body size, size of bullet, and location in body.
- Shotgun pellets decelerate rapidly, resulting in severe damage over a wide area. Devitalization secondary to vascular disruption occurs. Widespread skin and muscular avulsion is noted.
- Contamination must always be suspected in gunshot injuries.

AGE-RELATED FACTORS
N/A

ZOONOTIC POTENTIAL
N/A

PREGNANCY
N/A

RUMINANT SPECIES AFFECTED
Potentially all ruminant species

BIOSECURITY
N/A

PRODUCTION MANAGEMENT
N/A

SYNONYMS
N/A

SEE ALSO
Anesthesia and analgesia
Euthanasia and disposal
Wound management

ABBREVIATIONS
GSW = gunshot wound

Suggested Reading
Bebchuk, T. N., Harari, J. 1995, Sep. Gunshot injuries: pathophysiology and treatments. *Vet Clin North Am Small Anim Pract*. 25(5):1111–26.
Dicpinigaitis, P. A., Fay, R., Egol, K. A., Wolinsky, P., Tejwani, N., Koval, K. J. 2002, May. Gunshot wounds to the lower extremities. *Am J Orthop*. 31(5):282–93.
Doherty, M. A., Smith, M. M. 1995, Jan 15. Contamination and infection of fractures resulting from gunshot trauma in dogs: 20 cases (1987–1992). *J Am Vet Med Assoc*. 206(2):203–5.
Fullington, R. J., Otto, C. M. 1997, Mar 1. Characteristics and management of gunshot wounds in dogs and cats: 84 cases (1986–1995). *J Am Vet Med Assoc*. 210(5):658–62.
Velmahos, G. C., Demetriades, D., Cornwell, E. E., III. 1998, Oct. Transpelvic gunshot wounds: routine laparotomy or selective management? *World J Surg*. 22(10):1034–38.
Vincent, J., DiMaia, M. 1999. *Gunshot wounds, practical aspects of firearms, ballistics and forensic techniques*. CRC Press. Boca Raton, FL 33487, USA.

Author: Kent M. Jackson

MAST CELL TUMORS

BASICS

OVERVIEW
• Mast cell tumors are a round cell tumor (mesenchymal neoplasm) that may be benign or malignant.
• Tumors arise from cutaneous mast cells.
• Disease may be familial in cattle.
• Mast cell tumors account for approximately 3% of cutaneous and subcutaneous tumors of cattle.

SYSTEMS AFFECTED

GENETICS
May be congenital in calves

INCIDENCE/PREVALENCE
Unknown

GEOGRAPHIC DISTRIBUTION
Unknown

SIGNALMENT
Species
Mast cell tumors are uncommon in cattle and unreported in sheep or goats.

Breed Predilections
None reported

Mean Age and Range
• In cattle, tumors occur in animals 6 months to 7 years of age with no breed or sex predilection.
• May occur in calves

Predominant Sex
There does not appear to be a sexual predisposition.

SIGNS
• Lesions are commonly multiple.
• Size varies from 1 to 40 cm in diameter.
• Masses may be firm to fluctuant, dermal or subcutaneous, alopecic or ulcerated.
• Pruritus is common.
• Most commonly seen on the neck and trunk.
• Tumors are usually malignant and metastatic to local lymph nodes, kidney, and other organs.
• Congenital mast cell tumors in calves appear as small, raised skin nodules fixed to the overlying skin with no predilection for pigmented or nonpigmented skin. Lesions have a dry grey-crusted surface and are pruritic.

CAUSES
Unknown

DIAGNOSIS

DIFFERENTIAL DIAGNOSIS
Mast cell tumors may mimic other tumors, abscesses, or granulomatous lesions.

CBC/BIOCHEMISTRY/URINALYSIS
N/A

OTHER LABORATORY TESTS
N/A

IMAGING
N/A

OTHER DIAGNOSTIC PROCEDURES
• Skin biopsy reveals diffuse to multi-nodular proliferations of mast cells. Tissue eosinophilia and focal areas of collagen necrosis may be seen.
• Biopsy specimens should be stained with toluidine blue to aid in diagnosis.
• Fine needle aspiration may be helpful in diagnosis; many large round mast cells with an eosinophilic infiltrate may be seen; not all mast cells stain with in-house fast Giemsa stains.

PATHOLOGIC FINDINGS
Tumors have been found in skin and dermis and also spleen, skeletal muscle, omentum, abomasums, tongue, uterus, and in a disseminated form.

MAST CELL TUMORS

TREATMENT
• Culling affected animals
• Wide surgical excision, if practical
• Radiation and cryosurgery are other treatment options.

MEDICATIONS
N/A

FOLLOW-UP
• Most tumors in cattle are malignant and metastatic.
• Removal of a cutaneous lesion may give rise to metastasis.

MISCELLANEOUS

RUMINANT SPECIES AFFECTED
Cattle, rare in other species

BIOSECURITY
N/A

SYNONYMS
Mast cell tumor, mastocytoma

SEE ALSO
CLA
Dermatology chapters
SCC
Wound management

ABBREVIATIONS
CLA = caseous lymphadenitis
SCC = squamous cell carcinoma

Suggested Reading
Mullowney, P. C. 1984. Non-infectious skin diseases of cattle. In: *Symposium on large animal dermatology, veterinary clinics of North America* 6:185.
Scott, D. W. 1984. Neoplastic diseases. In: *Large animal dermatology*. Philadelphia: W. B. Saunders.
Scott, D. W. 1999. Neoplastic skin diseases. In: *Current veterinary therapy 4: food animal practice*, ed. J. L. Howard, R. A. Smith. Philadelphia: W. B. Saunders.
Yeruham, I., Perl, S., Orgad, U. 1999. Congenital skin neoplasia in cattle. *Veterinary Dermatology* 10:149–56.

Authors: Karen A. Moriello and Susan D. Semrad

MASTITIS: COLIFORM

BASICS

OVERVIEW
• Acute coliform mastitis (ACM) is the most prevalent cause of mastitis in dairy herds that effectively control contagious mastitis pathogens and has become the most economically important form of mastitis.
• The source of infecting organisms (e.g., *E. coli, Klebsiella pneumoniae, Enterobacter aerogenes, Pasteurella multocida, Serratia marcescens,* etc.) is the environment.
• Infections occur primarily at the time of milking, between milking times, or during the dry period.
• Cow-to-cow transmission has minimal impact on disease transmission.
• The severity of disease caused by coliform mastitis can vary from mild to peracute. The majority (60%–80%) of coliform intramammary infections results in clinical disease, whereas only 15%–23% result in acute systemic signs
• The disparate nature of clinical coliform mastitis suggests that a wide range of pathologic events and physiologic responses can occur.
• Bacteremia develops in a substantial proportion of cows with ACM concurrently showing systemic signs.
• Severity classification of cows with ACM based on systemic disease signs is simple and rapid, and may prove useful in determining therapy and outcome of an ACM episode.
• Despite decades of research, no universally accepted control measures or approaches to treatment have been definitively established.

SIGNALMENT
Species
• Coliform mastitis can occur in any species of domestic or wild ruminant.
• Coliform mastitis is most prevalent and clinically relevant in dairy cattle.

Breed Predilection
N/A

Mean Age and Range
Primarily in lactating cows or cows in a dry period

Predominant Sex
Female

SIGNS
• Signs vary in severity from those involving only localized changes of the mammary gland and secretion, to those involving systemic signs of peracute septicemia and even death.
• Varying levels of heat, pain, swelling, and discoloration of the infected gland(s)
• The appearance of the secretion is variable and can range from that which appears to be grossly normal milk to secretions that more closely resemble serum. Additional manifestations can include the presence of flakes, clots, or even blood.
• General systemic signs can include fever, anorexia, rumen stasis, diarrhea, dehydration, and recumbency.
• Signs of septicemia can include petechiation or scleral injection, injected mucous membranes with toxic ring at gingival margins, prolonged capillary refill time, hypothermia, tachycardia, and altered mentation (depression, coma).

CAUSES AND RISK FACTORS
• Poor environmental hygiene
• Poor premilking hygiene (milking wet udders, use of communal towels to dry teats, etc.)
• Poor milking hygiene
• Failure to manage cows properly after milking

DIAGNOSIS

DIFFERENTIAL DIAGNOSIS
• Acute mastitis characterized by swelling and pain can be caused by numerous organisms in addition to coliforms. A partial list includes *S. agalactiae, S. aureus, S. dysgalactiae, S. uberis, Clostridium* spp*., and Bacillus* spp.
• Common conditions that may be manifest by signs of septicemia (in addition to coliform mastitis) include endometritis, peritonitis, and pneumonia.

CBC/BIOCHEMISTRY/URINALYSIS
• CBC is variable and may include hemoconcentration, leukocytosis with neutrophilia, left shift, and leukopenia with neutropenia. Toxic changes to neutrophils may also be observed (Doehle bodies, toxic granulation, cytoplasmic vacuolization, and basophilia)
• Hyperfibrinogenemia
• Nonspecific changes in serum biochemical parameters may include hypocalcemia, hypokalemia, hypergammaglobulinemia, hyperglycemia, or hypoglycemia

OTHER LABORATORY TESTS
• Positive milk bacterial culture
• Positive blood bacterial culture. *Note:* in cows suffering severe ACM, positive blood cultures may isolate coliform organisms originating from the mammary gland or noncoliform organisms (e.g., *Bacillus* spp., *Pasteurella* spp.), which presumably originate from other organ systems (e.g., respiratory, gastrointestinal).

IMAGING
N/A

PATHOLOGIC FINDINGS
Gross and histologic postmortem findings either can be confined to local mammary changes associated with inflammation or may include signs of sepsis.

TREATMENT
• The majority of cases of ACM (>70%) are localized to the udder and exhibit only mild, if any, systemic signs of disease. Affected glands may be warm, firm, and swollen, often with an abnormal secretion. These cases are likely to respond to conservative therapy including frequent stripping of the affected gland, administration of anti-inflammatory agents, and oral fluid therapy (e.g., 16–24 liters of water containing 8 oz NaCl, 2 oz KCl, and 12 oz calcium propionate). Antimicrobial administration, either by systemic or intramammary routes, is unlikely to be warranted.

MASTITIS: COLIFORM

• Approximately 10%–15% of ACM-affected cows show severe systemic signs of disease. Signs may include significant dehydration, weakness, hypothermia, injected mucous membranes, marked gastrointestinal stasis, and diarrhea. Studies suggest these cows have a high likelihood of bacteremia. The use of systemic antimicrobials should be strongly considered.

• In severely affected cows exhibiting marked systemic signs, fluid therapy is an important consideration. Because oral administration is generally ineffective in cows with marked gastrointestinal stasis, intravenous administration is preferred. The type and volume of fluid for intravenous administration should be based on abnormalities in blood parameters and clinical interpretation. Most cows with ACM are hypoglycemic, hypocalcemic, hypokalemic, and alkalotic.

• Administration of hypertonic saline (7.5% NaCl, 5 ml/kg) is a reasonable alternative to administration of large volume intravenous fluids.

MEDICATIONS

DRUGS OF CHOICE
• Ceftiofur (1.1–2.2 mg/kg, IM, SC, IV, q 24 h)
• Flunixin meglumine (0.5–1.1 mg/kg, IV, q 12 h)

CONTRAINDICATIONS
Appropriate milk and meat withdrawal times must be followed for all compounds administered.

FOLLOW-UP

PATIENT MONITORING
• Monitor local changes to mammary gland and secretion.
• Physical examination
• CBC and biochemistry as clinically indicated

PREVENTION/AVOIDANCE
• Ensure proper environmental hygiene.
• Ensure proper premilking and milking hygiene.
• Provide fresh, palatable feeds and management conditions to help ensure cows remain standing for approximately 30 minutes after milking to allow formation of the keratin plug.

POSSIBLE COMPLICATIONS
Possibility of persistent (chronic) infections

EXPECTED COURSE AND PROGNOSIS
• The majority of cows diagnosed with ACM resolves within 5 days and returns to production.
• Cows with marked systemic signs and prolonged disease have a guarded to poor prognosis.
• Cows with marked systemic signs and concurrent bacteremia have a poor to grave prognosis.

MISCELLANEOUS

ASSOCIATED CONDITIONS
N/A

AGE-RELATED FACTORS
N/A

ZOONOTIC POTENTIAL
Coliform agents can be zoonotic.

PREGNANCY
Bacteremia develops in a substantial proportion of cows with ACM concurrently showing systemic signs and possible abortion.

ABBREVIATIONS
ACM = acute coliform mastitis
CBC = complete blood count
KCl = potassium chloride
NaCl = sodium chloride

SEE ALSO
Specific mastitis chapters

Suggested Reading
Cebra, C. K., Garry, F. B., Dinsmore, R. P. 1996. Naturally occurring acute coliform mastitis in Holstein cattle. *J Vet Int Med*. 10:252–57.
Tyler, J. W., Cullor, J. S. 2002. In: *Large animal internal medicine*, ed. B. P. Smith. 3rd ed. St. Louis: Mosby.
Wenz, J. R., Barrington, G. M., Garry, F. B., Dinsmore, R. P. 2001. Use of systemic disease signs to assess disease severity in dairy cows with acute coliform mastitis. *JAVMA* 218(4): 567–72.
Wenz, J. R., Barrington, G. M., Garry, F. B., McSweeney, K. D., Dinsmore, R. P., Goodell, G., Callan, R. J. 2001. Bacteremia associated with naturally occurring acute coliform mastitis in dairy cattle. *JAVMA* 219(7): 976–81.

Author: George Barrington

MASTITIS: FUNGAL

BASICS

OVERVIEW
• A variety of yeast and fungi has been found to cause bovine mastitis.
• Yeast and fungi compose part of the normal makeup of the soil and environmental microflora and, if given the opportunity, will colonize the udder resulting in intramammary infection.
• Fungal mastitis is a problem of machine-milked, high-producing dairy animals.
• Etiologic agents are ubiquitous environmental pathogens found worldwide in soil, organic matter, and water.
• Infections are usually sporadic, opportunistic, and limited to affected glands.
• Antimicrobials are suspected to depress host defense mechanisms and stimulate fungal growth.
• The most common etiological agents of fungal mastitis are *Cryptococcus neoformans* and *Candida albicans.*
• Most cases of fungal mastitis are mild and self-limiting; however, cases involving *Cryptococcus neoformans* can result in severe mastitis and permanent damage to the mammary gland.
• Yeast and fungi associated with bovine intramammary infections include:
  • *Candida* spp.
  • *Trichosporon beigelii*
  • *Trichosporon cutaneum*
  • *Rhodotorula* spp.
  • *Hansenula fabianii*
  • *Hansenula holisti*
  • *Hansenula polymorpha*
  • *Hansenula anomala*

PATHOPHYSIOLOGY
Etiologic agents include *Candida* spp. (77% of cases), *Cryptococcus* spp., and *Prototheca* spp. Rare genera include *Trichosporon, Aspergillus, Torulopsis, Saccharomyces, Rhodotorula, Pichia,* and *Hansenula.*

SYSTEMS AFFECTED
Infections are localized and rarely extend beyond the infected udder with limited spread to supramammary lymph nodes.

GENETICS
There is no evidence of genetic predisposition.

INCIDENCE/PREVALENCE
Unknown

GEOGRAPHIC DISTRIBUTION
Worldwide distribution in milking animals

SIGNALMENT
• Fungal mastitis is seen in ruminants but with low frequencies of occurrence. There is no mean age or age range associated with fungal mastitis, and there is no genetic basis associated with fungal mastitis.

• Infections often associated with unsanitary use of intramammary therapeutics.
• Poor milking technique and the buildup of contaminated environmental organic matter are often seen with this disease.
• Infections are more frequent in warm, wet weather.

Species
Potentially, all species used for milk production

Breed Predilections
N/A

Mean Age And Range
Lactating animals

Predominant Sex
Female

SIGNS

HISTORICAL FINDINGS
• Initial localized udder swelling, heat, and hardness are prominent.
• Sharp drop in milk yield with watery secretions containing clots and flakes.
• A 104°F–106°F spiking fever is often seen.
• Affected quarters are positive using the California Mastitis Test (CMT).
• Subclinical cases in herd mates are common.
• The likelihood of infection increases with parity and is most often seen in the second month of lactation.

PHYSICAL EXAMINATION FINDINGS
• Swelling of the affected gland
• Fever
• Reduction in milk production
• Lack of positive response to antibiotic therapy
• Abnormal mammary secretions
• Anorexia

CAUSES AND RISK FACTORS
• Yeast and fungi often gain entrance into the mammary gland through contaminated antibiotics and needles following antibiotic treatment for bacterial mastitis
• Injured or damaged regions of the mammary gland can provide the opportunity for the colonization of environmental yeast and fungi.
• Previous bacterial mastitis increases host susceptibility to fungal mastitis.
• Fungal mastitis is seen with milking machine malfunction and is associated with teat end damage.
• Inadequately sterilized milking units may act as fomites and result in epidemic infections.
• There is increased incidence and severity during warm, wet environmental conditions conducive to pathogen growth.

DIAGNOSIS
Diagnosis of fungal mastitis should be made based upon milk culture.

DIFFERENTIAL DIAGNOSIS
Confusion and misidentification between prototbecal mastitis and fungal mastitis is common based on colony morphology. Prototheca is an algae, which produce colonies similar to *Cryptococcus neoformans.*

CBC/BIOCHEMISTRY/URINALYSIS
• Leukocytosis and neutrophilia were found in experimental infections.
• Elevated urine ketones are possible.

OTHER LABORATORY TESTS
Positive California Mastitis Test (CMT)

Microbiologic Laboratory Tests
• *Candida albicans:* fermentation of various sugars
• *Cryptococcus neoformans:* production of the enzyme urease and the assimilation of carbon substrates

Candida albicans
• *Germ tube test:* rapid and reliable. This test utilizes media in which blastospores of *C. albicans* are suspended in serum and incubated at 37°C for 2–3 hours. The suspension must be examined between 2–3 hours for the presence of hyphal outgrowths.
• *Culture on cornmeal agar at 25°C:* Upon microscopic analysis, *C. albicans* will form chlamydospores, which are morphologically unique.

Cryptococcus neoformans
• *Direct culture:* *C. neoformans* is inhibited by cyclohexamide, but grows well on standard nonselective mycologic media. Identification is made on the presence of a capsule. Direct culture is the definitive test for identifying *C. neoformans.*
• *India ink preparation:* Upon microscopic examination, *C. neoformans* appears as a budding yeast or single cell with a clear halo surrounding it due to the presence of a polysaccharide capsule.

IMAGING
Direct microscopic examination of colonies or mammary secretions reveals yeast and fungi to be morphologically different from bacterial bacilli or cocci.

DIAGNOSTIC PROCEDURES
• The presence of hyphae or spores on direct microscopic examination of defatted milk smears renders a positive diagnosis.
• Predominant cultures on blood and/or Sabouraud's agar at room temperature or 37°F is suggestive of a positive diagnosis.
• Both yeast and *Prototheca* are larger than bacteria with yeast having buds and *Prototheca* being multinucleate.

- In the event of available histologic sections, Gomori methenamine silver (GMS) and periodic acid-Schiff (PAS) stains highlight morphology.
- Fluorescent antibody staining can be used with sections and cultures.

TREATMENT

- Antibiotic therapy should be discontinued upon recognizing fungal mastitis.
- Separate milking of infected animals, sterilization of milking units between animals, and CMT screening may reduce spread to herd mates.
- Frequent milking of affected teats increases the chances of a favorable prognosis.
- Hydrotherapy reduces localized inflammation.
- The cow should be culled from the herd.

MEDICATIONS

DRUGS OF CHOICE

- Antimycotic drugs have been used; however, there exists no substantial evidence in regards to the efficacy of antimycotic drug therapy. There are no USDA/FDA approved antimycotic treatments for fungal mastitis in milking animals. Prudent withdrawal times should be utilized.
- Fungal mastitis is usually self limiting; however, clinically recovered cows may shed yeast/fungi for up to 8 months.
- Fungal mastitis is refractory to most drug treatments and there is little evidence to support such therapy modifies the course of disease.
- Antipyretics (flunixin meglumine 1 mg/kg IM/IV q 24 h, aspirin 960 gr p.o. q 12 h) are useful to help reduce high fevers and inflammation. Follow directions and abide by meat and milk withdrawal periods.
- Intravenous sodium iodide (66 mg/kg body weight IV 1x / week) and oil-based intramammary iodine solutions have been reported to be of some value.
- While resistant to most antibiotics, experimental *Prototheca* infections have been treated with limited success using tertamisole hydrochloride or levamisole hydrochloride.

CONTRAINDICATIONS

Appropriate milk and meat withdrawal times must be followed for all compounds administered to food-producing animals.

FOLLOW-UP

PATIENT MONITORING

Monitoring temperature and milk secretions in addition to follow-up milk cultures are useful to gauge therapy effectiveness.

PREVENTION/AVOIDANCE

- During the administration of antibiotics, one should use a single-dose sterile treatment tube and use clean or sterile applicators during antibiotic treatments.
- Teat end hygiene is extremely important in preventing fungal contamination.
- Cull persistently infected animals.
- Use aseptic udder infusion techniques.
- Reduce environmental organic matter buildup.
- Practice aseptic milking hygiene.

POSSIBLE COMPLICATIONS

There are rare incidences of systemic mycosis.

EXPECTED COURSE AND PROGNOSIS

- Due to loss of production and persistent shedding, culling is a consideration.
- There is often irreversible tissue damage with near complete agalactia.
- Fungal mastitis does not respond well to antimicrobials.
- Tissue damage and infection are usually confined to the affected udder with rare systemic infections.

MISCELLANEOUS

ASSOCIATED CONDITIONS

Bacterial and mycoplasmal mastitis

AGE-RELATED FACTORS

Incidence of fungal mastitis increases with parity.

ZOONOTIC POTENTIAL

N/A

PREGNANCY

Sodium iodide may lead to abortion.

RUMINANT SPECIES AFFECTED

All lactating females

BIOSECURITY

N/A

PRODUCTION MANAGEMENT

- Yeast and fungi compose part of the normal makeup of the soil and environmental microflora and, if given the opportunity, will colonize the udder resulting in intramammary infection.
- Injured or damaged regions of the mammary gland can provide the opportunity for the colonization of environmental yeast and fungi.
- Affected cows should be culled from the herd.

SYNONYMS

N/A

SEE ALSO

Epidemiology of mastitis
FARAD
Monitoring mastitis
Specific mastitis organisms

ABBREVIATIONS

CMT = California Mastitis Test
FARAD = Food Animal Residue Avoidance Databank
GMS = Gomori methenamine silver
Gr p.o. q = grains per os (by mouth) every
IM = intramammary
IV = intravenous
PAS = periodic acid-Schiff
USDA/FDA = United States Department of Agriculture/Food and Drug Administration

Suggested Reading
Corbellini, L. G., Driemeier, D., Cruz, C., Dias, M. M., Ferreiro, L. 2001. Bovine mastitis due to *Prototheca zopfii*: clinical epidemiological and pathological aspects in a Brazilian dairy herd. *Trop Anim Health Prod*. 33(6): 463–70.
Erksine, R. J., Kirk, J. H., Tyler, J. W., DeGraves, F. J. Advances in the therapy for mastitis. *Veterinary Clinics of North America: Food Animal Practice* 9(3):499–517.
Gonzalez, R. N. *Prototheca*, yeast, and *Bacillus* as a cause of mastitis. National Mastitis Council, www.nmconline.org/articles/prototheca.htm
Perez, V., Corpa, J. M., Garcia Marin, J. F., Aduriz, J. J., Jensen, H. E. 1998. Mammary and systemic aspergillosis in dairy sheep. *Vet Pathol*. 35(4): 235–40.
Watts, J. L. 1988. Etiological agents of bovine mastitis. *Veterinary Microbiology* 16:41–66.

Authors: Gabriel J. Rensen and Michael Goedken

MASTITIS: MINOR BACTERIA

BASICS

DEFINITION
• Most cases of mastitis are caused by the major mastitis bacterial pathogens: *Staphylococcus aureus, Streptococcus agalactia, Mycoplasma* spp. (contagious mastitis pathogens), the coliform group, and *Streptococcus* spp. (environmental pathogens). Mastitis can be caused by many other bacterial and fungal pathogens as well.
• The National Mastitis Council considers the primary minor bacterial mastitis pathogens to be *Corynebacterium bovis, Arcanobacterium pyogenes* (formerly *Actinomyces*), and *Nocardia* spp.
• Other uncommon bacterial causes of mastitis to be considered here are coagulase-negative *Staphylococcus* spp., *Pseudomonas aeruginosa*, and *Serratia* spp.
• The classification of mastitis pathogens as common or uncommon causes of mastitis is relative due to the variation of environment, housing, nutrition, management, and diagnostic capability between regions.

PATHOPHYSIOLOGY
• Mastitis is inflammation of the mammary gland, usually as a result of bacterial infection. Pathogens gain entry into the gland either through ascending colonization of the streak canal (*Streptococcus* spp. and *Staphylococcus* spp.), by reverse-impaction during machine milking, or by contaminated intramammary treatments.
• Infection in the gland results in tissue damage either as the direct effect of infection in cells (e.g., *Staphylococcus* spp.) or from the immune response to the pathogen (e.g., gram-negative bacteria).
• Inflammatory responses range from mild to severe, depending on the bacteria, the infectious dose, and the host immune function. Within the gland, the response can range from coagulation of milk or serum proteins (gargut), damage or destruction of secretory tissue, blockage of ductules with necrotic debris and purulent material, endothelial leakage of serum and blood, fibrosis, abscess formation, granulomatous lesions, to gangrene.
• Diapodesis of white blood cells, primarily neutrophils, into the gland results from chemotactic signals by macrophages (the primary leukocyte in healthy glands).
• The leukocyte response, or somatic cell count (SCC), is a useful measure of inflammation in the mammary gland.
• Infections from coagulase-negative *Staphylococcus* and *Corynebacterium* usually result in mild to moderate inflammation, and the gland returns to normal after the infection is cleared.
• Infections from *Nocardia* spp., *Arcanobacterium pyogenes, Pseudomonas aeruginosa*, and *Serratia* spp. often cause serious tissue damage and can become chronic with abscesses or granuloma formation (*Nocardia*).

SYSTEMS AFFECTED
Mammary

GENETICS
N/A

INCIDENCE/PREVALENCE
Usually sporadic cases

GEOGRAPHIC DISTRIBUTION
Varies due to regional differences in housing, milking sanitation, intramammary treatments, teat dips, and use of pasture. "Summer mastitis" is seen with *Arcanobacter* infections of cows on pasture in England and Europe.

Epidemiology
• These organisms generally cause sporadic cases of mastitis. They are associated with poor teat hygiene premilking or postmilking, contaminated udder infusions, and teat end damage.
• *Pseudomonas* spp. are found in organic bedding and water and can contaminate water sources, milking equipment, and rubber parts in hoses and the milking system.
• Sources of *Nocardia* spp. are soil, water, and udder skin.
• The reservoir for *Corynebacterium bovis* is normal teat skin and infected udders. Cases of *Corynebacterium bovis* mastitis are often associated with inadequate teat dipping or sanitizing.
• Purulent discharge from wounds, teat injuries, and abscesses are the major sources for *Arcanobacterium pyogenes* infections.
• *Serratia* spp. are saprophytes found in soil and plants. Most of the mastitis-causing coagulase-negative *Staphylococcus* spp. are associated with teat skin.

SIGNALMENT

Species Affected
Cattle; occasionally sheep and goats

Breed Predilections
N/A

Mean Age and Range
Adults; *Corynebacterium bovis* can affect heifers prepartum.

Predominant Sex
Females

SIGNS

GENERAL COMMENTS
The primary clinical signs of mastitis are the hallmarks of inflammation: swelling, heat, pain, redness, and firmness. These early palpable signs precede visible changes to the milk.

HISTORICAL FINDINGS
• Postmilking dipping of teats with noniodine products is commonly associated with *Corynebacterium* and *Serratia* mastitis.
• Intramammary infusions with nonsterile products (i.e., other than commercial intramammary treatments).

PHYSICAL EXAMINATION FINDINGS
• Palpation of the mammary gland reveals swelling, heat, firmness, or pain. The milk secretion may have small flakes or large pieces of gargut (coagulations of protein and purulent material) and actual pus (in the case of *Arcanobacter*), or may be watery from serum leakage into the gland (with *Serratia*).
• Abscesses or granulomas may be palpable (especially with *Nocardia*). Milk production may be decreased due to damage to secretory cells or fibrosis.
• Fever and tachycardia are usually present in acute infections but not in chronic mastitis.

CAUSES
• Contaminated intramammary infusions, bedding, or water used to sanitize teats or milking machines.
• Not employing postmilking teat dipping, improper teat dipping, or the use of ineffective teat dip preparations are associated with *Corynebacterium* and *Serratia* mastitis.
• Hyperkeratosis or damaged teat ends predispose for coagulase-negative *Staphylococcus* mastitis. Maintaining cows with *Arcanobacter* mastitis or draining abscesses in the herd may also lead to infection.

RISK FACTORS
• Using common medications for intramammary infusion (e.g., bottles of medication rather than individual treatment tubes); warm, moist organic bedding (*Pseudomonas* and *Serratia*); not employing postmilking teat dipping or use of ineffective products (*Corynebacterium, Serratia*, and coagulase-negative *Staphylococcus*)
• Maintaining animals with *Arcanobacter* or *Nocardia* abscesses or nodules in the herd.

DIAGNOSIS

DIFFERENTIAL DIAGNOSIS
• Subclinical cases must be differentiated from mastitis caused by *Streptococcus agalactia, Corynebacterium bovis,* and minor udder pathogens.
• Clinical cases must be differentiated from mastitis caused by coliform bacteria, mycoplasma, and environmental streptococci.
• Gangrenous mastitis with bloody secretion must be differentiated from trauma to the gland.
• Acute mastitis, characterized by swelling, pain, and numerous organisms in addition to coliforms, can cause heat and increased firmness of the gland. A partial list includes *S. agalactiae, S. aureus, S. dysgalactiae, S. uberis, Clostridium* spp., *and Bacillus* spp.
• Common conditions that may be manifest by signs of septicemia (in addition to coliform

mastitis) include endometritis, peritonitis, and pneumonia.

CBC/BIOCHEMISTRY/URINALYSIS
N/A

OTHER LABORATORY TESTS
• Indirect tests are available to detect subclinical mastitis.
• Somatic cell count (SCC) or California Mastitis Test (CMT) of milk from quarter or composite samples will indicate if excessive inflammation is present. SCC over 200,000 or CMT score of 2 or 3 indicates mastitis is present. SCC is often reported as the log-linear score, in which case a score over 4 is considered mastitis.
• Other indirect tests include the NAGase test (N-acetyl-β-D-glucosamidase) and electrical conductivity. NAGase increases with somatic cell count and can be used instead of SCC.
• Sodium and chloride in the milk secretion tends to increase with mastitis, thus increasing the electrical conductivity of the secretion. Normal variation of ions in milk makes conductivity less sensitive in detecting subclinical mastitis than other methods.
• Microbiological testing of an aseptically collected milk sample from the affected gland is the only way to determine the causative organism.
• The National Mastitis Council *Laboratory Handbook on Bovine Mastitis* describes acceptable laboratory techniques for differentiating mastitis pathogens.

IMAGING
Ultrasounding the teat canal may be a helpful adjunct to diagnosis.

OTHER DIAGNOSTIC PROCEDURES
• Finding inflammation in the mammary gland during physical exam or seeing abnormal milk secretion (flakes, gargut, discoloration, pus, watery milk, or serum) are usual ways of initially diagnosing mammary gland infection.
• The specific bacteria causing mastitis can be determined only by aseptically collecting a milk sample from the affected quarter and performing appropriate microbiological tests.

GROSS AND HISTOPATHOLOGIC FINDINGS
Gross pathology will show inflamed tissue in the affected glands, ranging from discoloration to fibrosis to severe tissue damage.

TREATMENT
• *Corynebacterium* and coagulase-negative *Staphylococcus* spp. may self-cure but treatment with commercial intramammary antibiotics is advised.
• *Serratia* spp. and *Pseudomonas* mastitis usually respond poorly to antibiotic treatment.

• *Nocardia* and *Arcanobacter* mastitis are often refractory to treatment due to abscessation and purulent material.

Inpatient Versus Outpatient
N/A

CLIENT EDUCATION
Primary concerns are milking hygiene and cattle housing sanitation. Insist on proper postmilking teat dipping with an effective product. Never use medications from common bottles for intramammary infusions; always use separate commercial mastitis tubes.

MEDICATIONS

DRUGS OF CHOICE
Commercial mastitis preparations are advised for cases of *Corynebacterium* and coagulase-negative mastitis.

CONTRAINDICATIONS
Appropriate milk and meat withdrawal times must be followed for all compounds administered to food-producing animals.

PRECAUTIONS
N/A

POSSIBLE INTERACTIONS
N/A

ALTERNATIVE DRUGS
N/A

FOLLOW-UP

PATIENT MONITORING
Monitor for eating, drinking, reduction of inflammation in the gland, and return of normal milk secretion.

PREVENTION/AVOIDANCE
• Use only separate commercial preparations to treat mastitis; house animals in clean and dry conditions; disinfect teats prior to milking; use effective postmilking teat dip.
• Cull animals affected with chronic *Arcanobacter* or *Nocardia* infections.
• Vaccination with rough mutant gram-negative vaccines (e.g., J-5) may reduce the severity and incidence of *Serratia* mastitis.

POSSIBLE COMPLICATIONS
N/A

EXPECTED COURSE AND PROGNOSIS
• Complete recovery of normal mammary tissue after treatment for cases of *Corynebacterium* and coagulase-negative *Staphylococcus* spp. mastitis.
• *Serratia* often becomes chronic and continues through many subsequent lactation cycles.
• *Nocardia* and *Arcanobacter* mastitis usually becomes chronic.

MISCELLANEOUS

PREVENTION
Milking hygiene, sanitary housing, vaccination with J-5 type vaccines for *Serratia*

ASSOCIATED CONDITIONS
N/A

AGE-RELATED FACTORS
Postpuberty

ZOONOTIC POTENTIAL
Nocardia spp. infections are zoonotic and cultures should be considered dangerous. Colonies should be killed with formalin before opening the plates for examination.

PREGNANCY
N/A

SYNONYMS
Environmental staphylococcus or "other Staphylococcus" = coagulase-negative *Staphylococcus* spp.
Summer mastitis = *Arcanobacterium pyogenes* mastitis

SEE ALSO
Other bacterial and fungal causes of mastitis

ABBREVIATIONS
CMT = California Mastitis Test
NAGase = N-acetyl-β-D-glucosamidase
SCC = somatic cell count

Suggested Reading
Barkema, H. W., Schukken, Y. H., Lam, T. J., Beiboer, M. L., Benedictus, G., Brand, A. 1999, Aug. Management practices associated with the incidence rate of clinical mastitis. *J Dairy Sci.* 82(8): 1643–54.
Laboratory handbook on bovine mastitis. 1999. Madison, WI: National Mastitis Council.
Radostits, O. M., Gay, C. C., Blood, D. C., Hinchcliff, K. W., eds. 2000. *Veterinary medicine: a textbook of diseases of cattle, sheep, pigs, goats and horses.* 9th ed. London: W. B. Saunders.
Sargeant, J. M., Scott, H. M., Leslie, K. E., Ireland, M. J., Bashiri, A. 1998, Jan. Clinical mastitis in dairy cattle in Ontario: frequency of occurrence and bacteriological isolates. *Can Vet J.* 39(1): 33–38.
Wilson, D. J., Herer, P. S., Sears, P. M. 1991, May. N-acetyl-beta-D-glucosaminidase, etiologic agent, and duration of clinical signs for sequential episodes of chronic clinical mastitis in dairy cows. *J Dairy Sci.* 74(5): 1539–43.

Author: James P. Reynolds

MASTITIS: MYCOPLASMAL

BASICS

DEFINITION
• Mycoplasmal mastitis is an inflammation of the mammary gland in association with infection by various *Mycoplasma* spp.
• It is a contagious form of mastitis, capable of causing outbreaks of clinical mastitis not responsive to treatment.
• Mycoplasmal mastitis is spread primarily cow to cow at milking.

OVERVIEW
• Mycoplasmas are contagious mastitis pathogens that can cause clinical, subclinical, and chronic intramammary infections (IMI).
• Although *Mycoplasma bovis* is the most important agent of outbreaks of mycoplasmal mastitis in dairy herds, *M. alkalescens*, *M. arginini*, *M. bovigenitalium*, *M. bovirhinis*, *M. californicum*, and *M. canadense* have also been isolated from mastitic milk in the United States.
• Mastitis produced by different *Mycoplasma* is similar but may vary in severity, is unresponsive to antibiotic therapy, and has the potential to cause severe losses in a herd's milk production.

PATHOPHYSIOLOGY
• Mycoplasmas are extremely small self-replicating organisms, with a very small amount of genetic material. The organisms lack a cell wall and, therefore, are not affected by antimicrobials, which act via an effect on the cell wall.
• Because of the organism's limitations, mycoplasmas live in close association with host cells. They tend to produce chronic infections.
• Important in the pathogenesis of mycoplasmal mastitis are the variable surface lipoproteins (Vsps) from the plasma membrane, also referred to as membrane surface proteins. It has been proposed that the Vsps may be involved in attachment to host epithelium, stimulation of the host immune response, and/or in protecting mycoplasmas from destruction by host defenses.
• Changes in Vsps and membrane proteins are important in the pathophysiology of mycoplasmal mastitis.
• Most damage in mycoplasmal mastitis is reportedly from the cow's immune response. However, metabolic by-products and toxins from mycoplasmas also contribute to tissue damage and reduction of milk production.
• Inflammatory cells accumulate in alveoli and ducts, and ductular cells divide and reduce duct lumen space. Cells in alveoli regress and fluid accumulates, with an attendant drop in milk production. In the most severe reactions, fibrous tissue replaces alveoli and ducts, being a permanent loss. In less severe reactions, the cow may regain production, but at a lower level.

• Multiple abscesses, variable in size, can be found in cases of mastitis caused by *M. bovis*. These abscesses may contain *M. bovis*, which can cause long-term shedding.

SYSTEMS AFFECTED
Mammary gland—the primary effect is mastitis, with associated inflammatory changes, increased SCC, abnormal secretions, and loss of milk production.

GENETICS
N/A

INCIDENCE/PREVALENCE
• The disease is reportedly found worldwide.
• The incidence/prevalence is variable among geographic regions and among herds in a region. There is a wide variation in quarter infection rates in herds. The condition is endemic in some areas.
• Based upon culture of a single bulk tank sample, 7.9% of dairies tested positive in a 2002 USDA survey. There was a higher isolation rate (9.4%) in the West, as compared to the Midwest (2.2%), Northeast (2.8%), or Southeast (6.6%). Larger herds (>500 cows) had higher isolation rates (21.9%) than smaller herds.

SIGNALMENT

Species
Bovine

Breed Predilection
None

Mean Age and Range
All ages of cows are susceptible and at any time during lactation and in the dry period. Cows in early lactation may show more pronounced changes.

Predominant Sex
Female

SIGNS
In lactating cows, signs can include the following:
• Can be cause of subclinical, clinical, and/or chronic mastitis
• Sudden onset swelling of udder
• Swollen, meaty quarters that don't soften normally during milking
• Decrease in milk production, sometimes dramatic
• Lack of systemic signs; maintenance of appetite and thirst (Experimentally infected cows show fever briefly 3–4 days after inoculation; spontaneous cases may also show brief fever, which is usually not detected.)
• Lack of response to therapy
• Agalactia/atrophy
• Increased SCC
• Purulent mastitis (sometimes severe) without systemic signs
• Supramammary lymph nodes may be enlarged.
• Acute arthritis with swollen joints and lameness
• Multiple quarter involvement; sometimes all quarters are involved.
• Variable changes in secretions:

• Cows can, in some instances, be infected and show no changes in the appearance of secretions.
• In other cases, secretions in early infections may be normal at first appearance, but with settling may form a sediment and a whey-looking supernatant. With other cases, the secretion may be watery with clots, serous, or thick.
• The secretion may also appear tan to brown with flakes, or as a colostrum-like secretion, or purulent.
• It is reported that the majority of milk samples positive for mycoplasmas have normal secretions.
• A given quarter can be infected with multiple organisms, leading to variable signs.

HISTORICAL FINDINGS
Usually mastitis in multiple quarters without systemic signs; nonresponsive to therapy

PHYSICAL EXAMINATION FINDINGS
See above under Signs.

CAUSES
• Infection of the mammary gland with various species of mycoplasma. As few as 70 colony-forming units of *M. bovis* introduced via the teat canal can initiate mastitis.
• Characteristics of mastitis produced by various *Mycoplasma* spp. are generally similar, but may vary in degree.
• At least 11 species have been reported in milk in natural or experimental cases:
  1. *Mycoplasma bovis* is the most significant and, usually, the most common mycoplasmal agent of bovine mastitis. The NAHMS Dairy Survey 2002 found that *M. bovis* was isolated from 86% of operations that were positive for a mycoplasma.
  2. *M. alkalescens*, *M. arginini*, *M. bovigenitalium*, *M. bovirhinis*, *M. californicum*, *M. canadense*, *M. dispar*, *M.* spp. Group 7, *M. F-38*, *M. capricolum*
  3. *Acholeplasma laidlawii* (generally considered nonpathogen), *A. axanthum*

Sources of Infection
• The most common source of IMI due to mycoplasmas is the udder of infected cows.
• The purchase of replacement heifers and cows is frequently the origin of mycoplasmal mastitis outbreaks in previously *Mycoplasma*-free herds.
• *Mycoplasma* spp. are commonly spread from infected cows to uninfected cows at milking via milking machines or milkers' hands.
• Mycoplasmal udder infections usually persist through the current lactation and into subsequent lactations.
• Cattle of all ages and at any stage of lactation as well as nonlactating cattle are susceptible to mycoplasmal infections.
• Mycoplasmas present in the respiratory and urogenital tracts of healthy cattle may possibly serve as a source of IMI.

• Herds with and without mycoplasmal mastitis may contain both young and mature asymptomatic carriers.
• Mycoplasmas are sensitive to heat, sunlight, and environmental pressures but can survive on teat skin and in cool, moist, and protein-rich environments for variable periods.
• Contaminated intramammary treatments or improper teat sanitation during or at the end of lactation and airborne transmission in poorly ventilated facilities are also means of new infections.

RISK FACTORS
• Risk factors vary with the particular herd and situation. In California, large herd size is recognized as a risk factor, but this has not been found in New York.
• Herds purchasing outside replacements and expansion herds are at increased risk of infection.
• Four groups of animals at high risk of getting infection or spreading it: (1) first calf heifers, (2) new additions to herds, (3) fresh cows, (4) sick cows leaving/entering treatment herd.

DIAGNOSIS
DIFFERENTIAL DIAGNOSIS
• Other causes of chronic mastitis unresponsive to therapy
• *Acholeplasma laidlawii*, a nonpathogenic saprophytic contaminant resembling mycoplasmas, may be occasionally found in milk arising from the environment during wet weather or from teat skin.
• Bacterial L-forms, which can be induced by antibiotics used in dairy cows for the treatment of mastitis, also have a fried-egg appearance but have a coarser structure.

CBC/BIOCHEMISTRY/URINALYSIS
• One text reports that a marked leukopenia may be seen early in the disease course.
• Leukocyte numbers markedly increase in the milk. Often, secretions contain over 20 million cells/ml.

OTHER LABORATORY TESTS
N/A

IMAGING
N/A.

DIAGNOSTIC PROCEDURES
• Diagnosis is most commonly made using microbiological procedures on aseptically collected quarter or composite milk samples or on culture of bulk tank milk samples.
• Isolation is most commonly attempted using direct inoculation onto plates containing modified Hayflick medium. Plates are incubated in moist 10% CO_2 at 35–37°C. They are observed for growth with a microscope at intervals after plating. Plates are not called negative for growth until incubated for 7–10 days. Intermittent

shedding by carriers not demonstrating symptoms may make diagnosis difficult.
• Results are most favorable when fresh samples of milk kept on ice are plated right after collection. It is also acceptable to refrigerate samples for up to 2–3 days and to freeze samples.
• A variety of methods is used to detect the organisms or their antigens. A variety of serologic/immunologic tests is used. Polymerase chain reaction (PCR) assays are being developed for mycoplasmal diagnostics.
• Serologic methods, most commonly immunofluorescence, are used for species identification. DNA probes have also been used to identify mycoplasmas to species level.

Other Diagnostic Tests
• Diagnosis of infection at the herd level is usually made by isolation of mycoplasmas from either bulk tank milk (BTM) or samples from cows with clinical and subclinical IMI.
• In large herds, culture of partial BTM samples collected after milking each production group or the use of string sampling or milk-line sampling may be used as a method to locate groups in which cows infected with mycoplasmas exist.
• It is critical that no cows be moved to a different pen until culture results are back from the laboratory.
• Bulk tank milk samples are valuable for screening and surveillance on a herd basis.
• Large numbers of mycoplasmas are usually present in milk samples from cows with clinical disease.
• False-negative diagnosis may occur in BTM because dilution could mask several low-level *Mycoplasma* shedders in the herd.
• Culture of milk samples may be less effective in detecting convalescent carrier cattle that may only shed mycoplasmas intermittently.
• A low level of *Mycoplasma* excretion in milk from latent infections or carrier cattle may also impair diagnosis of IMI.
• Milk samples for culture of *Mycoplasma* must be collected aseptically, kept cool during transportation to the diagnostic laboratory or storage, and plated promptly to maximize isolation.
• If delay of more than 1 day is anticipated from collection to culturing, milk samples should be frozen at −30°C or below to assure viability, or stored in liquid nitrogen.
• Mycoplasmas that cause IMI in cows need a special agar medium for growth in the laboratory, usually modified Hayflick, and plates should be incubated for up to 7–10 days at 35°C to 37°C in a moist 10% carbon dioxide incubator.
• Mycoplasmal colonies have a fried-egg appearance on solid medium because colonies have a dense, central core that grows down into the medium.
• The polymerase chain reaction (PCR) is a highly sensitive, specific, and rapid procedure for laboratory diagnosis, but several practical

problems must be solved before full-scale adoption of this diagnostic procedure.
• Mycoplasmal shedding in milk will not impact the standard plate count (SPC), preliminary incubation count (PIC), or the laboratory pasteurized count (LPC).

PATHOLOGIC FINDINGS
• The pathology in mycoplasmal mastitis is most commonly described as a purulent interstitial mastitis. Widespread, scattered fibrosis and granulomatous changes with pus are found in the gland. Teat sinus and ductular linings are seen as thick and rough.
• Evidence of granulomatous mastitis is seen on histopathology.

TREATMENT
APPROPRIATE HEALTH CARE
• In general, the opinion is that there is no known effective treatment.
• Short-term improvement has been reported with parenteral oxytetracycline treatment. Intramammary tylosin and tetracycline have been reported to cure infections.

NURSING CARE
No specific recommendations; provide supportive care similar to that for other cases of mastitis.

ACTIVITY
N/A

DIET
N/A

CLIENT EDUCATION
• Even though a dairy is not currently experiencing mycoplasmal mastitis, the organisms are very likely present within the herd and the possibility of a mastitis outbreak exists.
• Mycoplasmal organisms capable of causing mastitis may be present in young and mature animals without disease. Young animals may acquire mycoplasmal organisms via contact with the urogenital tract and nasal discharges of mothers or in milk.
• At calving, heifers infected earlier in life may produce mycoplasmas in nasal secretions and in the vagina. Infected cows may be brought into a herd.
• The organism can persist long term in animals without showing serious clinical mastitis. Exposure may also occur when animals are brought to livestock shows.
• Transmission has also been proposed to occur between farms, transported by individuals such as veterinarians, milkers, owners, or livestock dealers.

SURGICAL CONSIDERATIONS
N/A

MEDICATIONS

DRUGS OF CHOICE
It is generally held that there is no known effective treatment (see Appropriate Health Care above).

CONTRAINDICATIONS
Appropriate milk and meat withdrawal times must be followed for all compounds administered to food-producing animals.

PRECAUTIONS
N/A

POSSIBLE INTERACTIONS
N/A

ALTERNATE DRUGS
N/A

FOLLOW-UP

PATIENT MONITORING
N/A

PREVENTION/AVOIDANCE
• Mycoplasmas survive for variable, but sometimes extensive, periods of time on teat skin and multiple environmental sites.
• The ability of mycoplasmas to survive is influenced by the site, the ambient temperature, and the presence of light and moisture. In manure at 23–28°C, survival was 236 days in the dark and 145 days in the light, but only 108 days at 37°C. In drinking water, mycoplasmas survived 23 days at 23–28°C in the dark and 1 day in the light, but less than a day at 37°C. *M. bovis* survived at 4°C in sponges for 57 days and 54 days in milk.

PREVENTION/CONTROL
Prevention
Mycoplasmal mastitis may be prevented by the following steps intended to help to keep mycoplasmal mastitis out of a herd:
• Isolate or quarantine new additions
• Culture new additions using procedures described under Diagnostic Procedures above.
• Investigate herd of origin of any animals brought into the herd
• If milk from animals was not cultured at purchase, milks from these animals should be cultured as they calve
• Culture all clinical cases of mastitis and all fresh cows for mycoplasma and screen bulk tank samples for mycoplasmas.
• Workers should practice strict hygienic milking and intramammary treatment procedures.
• Avoid any use of bulk intramammary treatment.
• Practice effective biosecurity.

Control
• There are widely divergent opinions and practices with respect to management and control of mycoplasmal mastitis.

• The epidemiology of the disease is incompletely understood and new knowledge is constantly being acquired. Consult current sources of information and current experts when dealing with cases of mycoplasmal mastitis.
• Provisional identification of a mycoplasmal species from milk sample(s) from a herd should be followed by confirmation of the isolate as a pathogenic mycoplasmal species.
• Depending upon factors such as the experience and capability of the laboratory, this procedure may involve sending the organism to a reference laboratory for species typing. It can take several days to complete this procedure.
• Some factors to consider in the management of the herd in the interim:
  1. Advise the owner that an organism appearing to be a mycoplasma has been isolated from a sample or samples of milk from the herd and is being tested for confirmation. Advise the owner of the potential seriousness of the disease.
  2. Educate the owner about the disease in general, emphasizing epidemiological aspects, focusing on specifics of treatment, control, and prevention. Advise the owner of the specific groups at particular risk.
  3. Advise the owner not to move cows among groups in the herd until results of testing are available.
  4. Assure that intramammary treatment from a bulk source is not being used and that all treatment of mastitis by the intramammary route is done with the strictest hygiene.
  5. Emphasize application of all measures focused on hygiene in milking and at calving.
• Mode of handling will vary from dairy to dairy based on the owner's attitude, facilities, number of infected animals, level of milk production, and reproductive status of carrier animals, and the availability of replacements.
• Control of the disease, when present, is often based upon finding infected cows via culture of all lactating and dry cows in the herd, as well as all clinical cases and all animals at calving.
• An alternative approach is to use culture of bulk tank milk or string/group samples to identify infected groups. Alternative strategies have been proposed to deal with mycoplasmal mastitis.

Types of Approaches to Consider
If mycoplasma is diagnosed in a herd, there are two general types of approaches to be considered:
1. Attempt to eliminate the organism from the herd:
  • Culture all cows, identify infected animals and cull those infected, (particularly if the number is limited)
  • Culture milks from cows at dry-off, freshening and from all clinical cases

• Culture bulk tank milks at appropriate intervals to monitor new infections
• Don't move cows between production groups until all cows cultured and classified as infected or not (realizing limitations of a single culture)
2. Limit spread and live animals with the disease:
  • Separate mycoplasma-positive cows, and milk them last or with separate equipment.
  • Cull cows with clinical mastitis or decreased production.
  • Strict milking time hygiene—passed by fomites, such as the milking machine, hands, wash cloths.
  • Culture milk for mycoplasmas—fresh cows, clinical cases, dry cows, bulk tanks.
  • Either don't feed mastitic milk to calves or feed only after pasteurization following current recommendations.
  • Back flushing—variable effects, some question of cost-effectiveness
  • Strict teat dipping, iodine products preferred by some
3. The following apply in all situations:
  • Practice strict milking time hygiene (passed by fomites, such as milking machines, hands, wash cloths).
  • Practice thorough teat dipping, iodine products preferred by some for mycoplasmal herds.
  • Assure milking machine is functioning to standards.
  • Use single-service towels for drying cows.
  • Use gloves, disinfect between cows.
  • Use single-service intramammary treatments.
  • Vaccines to date are generally considered of questionable effectiveness; trials are under way evaluating some products. It is suggested that the practitioner ask manufacturer for evidence of effectiveness of the vaccine prior to consideration of use.
  • Either don't feed mastitic milk to calves or feed only after pasteurizing using current recommendations.
  • Monitor appropriate milk samples for mycoplasmas: bulk tanks, clinical cases, fresh cows, introduced cows, etc.
4. Further recommendations
  • Infected cows should be identified by culture of composite or quarter milk samples from all milking and dry cows in the herd.
  • Cows diagnosed with *Mycoplasma* IMI should be considered positive for life.
  • Any management plan for mycoplasmal mastitis following a whole herd culture should include segregation and/or removal of infected animals from the herd.
  • Removal of infected animals from the herd to slaughter is advised when prevalence of infection is low and segregation is not practical.
  • Segregation can be used when prevalence of mycoplasmal mastitis is high in the herd and culling is not economically feasible, but needs adequate facilities and

management, and monitoring of the herd by repeated culturing of animals and BTM.

• Segregated cows should be milked last or with a separate milking unit from those used on uninfected cows to minimize the risk of infection for other cows.

• Mycoplasmal mastitis can be controlled with testing and discipline in the management of the disease, including the understanding by dairy personnel of the seriousness of the disease and their role to minimize its spread.

• Culture all replacements entering the herd, cows and heifers at calving, all mammary quarters with signs of clinical mastitis, cows with persistent high somatic cell counts and BTM frequently.

• Use strict milking hygiene, including the wearing of nitrile or latex gloves by milkers, foremilking, pre- and postmilking teat disinfection with a high-quality product that covers almost the entire teat, and single use of paper or cloth towels.

• Clearly identify each infected animal by using a double identification system like leg bands and ear tags.

• Cows with blind quarters harboring mycoplasmas can spread the disease in the herd with uninformed or careless milkers and make isolation inconsistent from BTM.

• Avoid stresses, like the pressure effects of transportation, overcrowding, calving, and milking, particularly for the first calvers because they can be important contributors to the disease.

• A dairy's hospital pen or treatment group is usually a key area for spreading the disease when treatments are administered without following aseptic procedures, including disinfection of gloved hands between treated cows.

POSSIBLE COMPLICATIONS
N/A

EXPECTED COURSE AND PROGNOSIS
• The effect of mycoplasmas on a particular herd is highly variable, depending upon bacterial, host, and management factors. Outcome is also variable, depending upon cow and bacterial factors.

• Some cows may become agalactic and/or develop complications (e.g., arthritis, etc.), may continue in production and produce normal-appearing milk with a high SCC, may be chronically infected with abnormal milk, or may return to production, go through a dry period, and calve again, still shedding mycoplasmas.

• Spontaneous cures may occur, usually after going through a dry period. A "spontaneous and complete recovery" from *M. bovis* has been reported.

• It is generally recommended that cows diagnosed as positively infected be considered positive for life.

 MISCELLANEOUS

ASSOCIATED CONDITIONS
See Systems Affected above.

AGE-RELATED FACTORS
Cows susceptible at all ages

ZOONOTIC POTENTIAL
Very limited reports of human infections. *M. bovis* reportedly isolated from two human cases with respiratory disease.

PREGNANCY
N/A

RUMINANT SPECIES AFFECTED
M. bovis is highly adapted to the bovine species, with uncommon isolations reported from buffaloes and small ruminants.

BIOSECURITY
Since many infections are introduced into a herd by bringing replacements on a farm, quarantine of newly introduced animals and milk culturing, as well as careful investigation into the status of the herd of origin of any introduced animals, will help limit this possibility.

PRODUCTION MANAGEMENT
• Many, if not most, new mycoplasmal mastitis infections are introduced when animals are brought into a herd.

• Mastitis has been proposed to occur following hematogenous spread of a respiratory infection to the mammary gland.

• Transmission is primarily at milking by fomites such as milking machines, milkers' hands.

• The organism can also be spread when bulk mastitis treatments are administered from a contaminated vial or via a contaminated syringe or with unsanitary treatment practices.

SYNONYMS
N/A

SEE ALSO
Cleaning and disinfection
Dairy heifer management
Fungal mastitis
Mastitis section
Unresponsive mastitis

ABBREVIATIONS
BTM = bulk tank milk
IMI = intramammary infections
LPS = laboratory pasteurized count
NAHMS = National Animal Health Monitoring System
PCR = polymerase chain reaction
PIC = preliminary incubation count
SCC = somatic cell concentration
SPC = standard plate count
USDA = United States Department of Agriculture
Vsps = variable surface lipoproteins

Suggested Reading

Animal Disease Exclusion Practices on U.S. Dairy Operations, 2002. USDA:APHIS:VS:CEAH, NRRC Building B, M.S. 2E7 2150 Centre Avenue Fort Collins, CO 80526–8117

Boddie, R. L., Owens, W. E., Ray, C. H., Nickerson, S. C., Boddie, N. T. 2002. Germicidal activities of representatives of five different teat dip classes against three bovine mycoplasma species using a modified excised teat model. *J Dairy Sci.* 85:1909–12.

Brandes, T., Kersting, K. W. 1999. Mycoplasma mastitis in dairy cattle. *Iowa State Veterinarian* 61(2): 76–81.

Butler, J. A., Sickles, S. A., Johanns, C. J., Rosenbusch, R. F. 2000. Pasteurization of discard mycoplasma mastitic milk used to feed calves: Thermal effect on various mycoplasmas. *J Dairy Sci.* 83:2285–88.

González, R. N., Wilson, D. J. 2003. Mycoplasmal mastitis in dairy herds. *Vet Clin NA, Food Animal Practice* 19:199–221.

Kirk, J. H., Lauerman, L. H. 1994. Mycoplasma mastitis in dairy cows. *Compend Contin Ed Pract Vet.* 16(4): 541–58.

Nicholas, R. A. J., Ayling, R. D. 2003. Mycoplasma bovis: disease, diagnosis and control. *Res in Vet Sci.* 74:105–12.

Oliver, S. P., González, R. N., Hogan, J. S., Jayarao, B. M., Owens, W. E. 2004. *Microbiological procedures for the diagnosis of bovine udder infection and determination of milk quality.* 4th ed. Verona, WI: National Mastitis Council, Inc.

United States Department of Agriculture. 2002 National Animal Health Monitoring System: Dairy 2002.

Authors: Kevin L. Anderson and Rubén N. González

MASTITIS: NO GROWTH

 BASICS

DEFINTION
Mastitis caused by noninfectious reasons or no growth on culture.

PATHOPHYSIOLOGY
Because most cases of no growth clinical mastitis are thought to be caused by bacteria, the pathophysiology would be the same as infectious mastitis.

SYSTEMS AFFECTED
Mammary gland

GENETICS
N/A

INCIDENCE/PREVALENCE
Noninfectious causes of clinical mastitis are relatively rare. Ten percent to 40% of clinical cases of mastitis yield no growth on culture.

GEOGRAPHIC DISTRIBUTION
Worldwide

SIGNALMENT
Typically seen in lactating ruminants but also can occur during the dry period and in prepartum heifers

SIGNS
• Signs are almost always restricted to changes in the milk, such as clots or flakes.
• Systemic signs in the animal are quite rare in true no growth cases of clinical mastitis.

CAUSES
• Trauma such as bruises or contusions may result in noninfectious clinical mastitis.
• Trauma from environmental hazards that result in perforations into the gland or teat can be expected to eventually result in bacterial mastitis. However, the vast majority of cases of clinical mastitis that result in no growth is largely thought to be due to bacteria.
• Antigen-based studies indicate that gram-negative bacteria may be a more likely cause than gram-positive bacteria; yet there is good evidence for both occurring. There are several other reasons for lack of growth on culture.

• Other reasons: the offending organism has already been eliminated by the cow's immune system, antibiotic inhibition, phagocytized bacteria (within white blood cells but alive), L-forms of *Staphylococcus aureus*, inappropriate culture medium (e.g., *Mycoplasma* does not grow on blood agar), numbers of bacteria are too low to be detected by the quantity of milk cultured, freezer kill (*Escherichia coli* tends to be more susceptible than gram-positive organisms), and in some cases an inaccurate assessment of the significance of culture growth reported as no growth.

RISK FACTORS
Risk factors would be the same as other forms of mastitis. The major risk factor for trauma with subsequent clinical mastitis is a pendulous udder.

 DIAGNOSIS

DIFFERENTIAL DIAGNOSIS
• Bacteria cleared by immune system
• Bacteria alive but phagocytized
• Bacteria numbers too low to detect by standard culture methods
• L-forms (*S. aureus*)
• Viral (sheep and goats)
• Organism does not grow on standard media (*Mycoplasma,* anaerobes)
• Trauma (noninfectious)
• Antibiotic or milk product inhibition
• Storage kill
• Inaccurate interpretation of culture result

CBC/BIOCHEMISTRY/URINALYSIS
N/A

OTHER LABORATORY TESTS
• No additional tests need to be performed routinely on the initial or sporadic case of clinical mastitis that yields no growth, especially in herds with no history of *Mycoplasma* mastitis. However, specialized media should be utilized when multiple cases of clinical mastitis in a single cow or in a group of cows yield no growth.
• Specifically, samples should be cultured for *Mycoplasma.*

IMAGING
N/A

DIAGNOSTIC PROCEDURES
As above

PATHOLOGIC FINDINGS
N/A

 TREATMENT

APPROPRIATE HEALTH CARE
• No specific therapy is warranted for cows with clinical mastitis with no growth as the culture result.
• Cases are almost always mild with clots or flakes in the milk with no swelling of the affected quarter(s) and no systemic affects on the cow.

NURSING CARE

ACTIVITY
Normal

DIET
Normal

CLIENT EDUCATION
Clients trained to obtain culture results prior to treatment should be able to reduce drug usage, thereby decreasing the chance of antibiotic residues in bulk tank milk.

SURGICAL CONSIDERATIONS
N/A

 MEDICATIONS

DRUGS OF CHOICE
• It would be difficult to justify the use of antimicrobial drugs for cases of no growth clinical mastitis.
• If treatment must be given, oxytocin at 1–2 ml to aid milk-out of the affected quarter should do no harm. There are no studies that document the beneficial effects of oxytocin in the treatment of clinical mastitis.
• Intramammary antibiotic therapy (by label) of clinical mastitis will usually occur prior to knowledge of culture results. This treatment does not appear to affect time to cure.

CONTRAINDICATIONS

Appropriate milk and meat withdrawal times must be followed for all compounds administered to food-producing animals.

PRECAUTIONS

Long-term use of oxytocin may result in cows becoming dependent on oxytocin for milk letdown.

POSSIBLE INTERACTIONS

None

ALTERNATIVE DRUGS

None

 FOLLOW-UP

PATIENT MONITORING

• Any cow with clinical mastitis, especially those that are not being treated, should be evaluated on a daily basis to assess disease progression. Cows that have truly cleared the infection but are still showing clinical signs (abnormal milk) will show improvement.

• Any cow with repeated episodes of no growth clinical mastitis should be cultured for *Mycoplasma*. Cultures of cows with severe clinical mastitis that are reported as no growth should be held in suspicion.

• In a Virginia Tech study in which cows with clinical mastitis were cultured daily for 8 days, all cases of no growth were mild and did not progress to a more severe condition, whereas all cases of severe clinical mastitis yielded ample growth.

PREVENTION/AVOIDANCE

Standard mastitis control measures should always be utilized.

POSSIBLE COMPLICATIONS

N/A

EXPECTED COURSE AND PROGNOSIS

• In a Virginia Tech study, cows with clinical mastitis were cultured and evaluated once a day for 8 days, then once a week for 1 month, then monthly until completely cured.

• The geometric mean time to clinical cure of 21 no growth cases of clinical mastitis that were not treated with anything was 4.8 days (range 1–26 days) and time until the quarter somatic cell count (SCC) was < 500,000 cells/ml was 10.5 days (range 1–66 days).

• In comparison, the geometric mean time to clinical cure of 19 no growth cases of clinical mastitis that were treated with intramammary cephapirin (by label) was 5.2 days (range 2–26 days) and time until the quarter SCC was < 500,000 cells/ml was 10.7 days (range 1–111). Providing culture results remain negative and no *Mycoplasma* is cultured, the prognosis is good.

 MISCELLANEOUS

ASSOCIATED CONDITIONS

Vast majority of cases of clinical mastitis that result in no growth largely thought to be due to bacteria.

AGE-RELATED FACTORS

N/A

ZOONOTIC POTENTIAL

N/A

PREGNANCY

N/A

RUMINANT SPECIES AFFECTED

Bovine, ovine, caprine

BIOSECURITY

Closed herds decrease the chance of *Mycoplasma* spp. introduction.

PRODUCTION MANAGEMENT

• Any cow with clinical mastitis, especially those that are not being treated, should be evaluated on a daily basis to assess disease progression.

• Any cow with repeated episodes of no growth clinical mastitis should be cultured for *Mycoplasma* spp.

SYNONYMS

N/A

SEE ALSO

Bacterial culture methods
Fungal mastitis
Mammary ultrasound
Mycoplasma spp.
PCR
Traumatic (noninfectious) lesions of the udder

ABBREVIATIONS

PCR = polymerase chain reaction
SCC = somatic cell count

Suggested Reading
Beaudeau, F., Fourichon, C., Seegers, H., Barelle, N. 2002, Feb 14. Risk of clinical mastitis in dairy herds with a high proportion of low individual milk somatic-cell counts. *Prev Vet Med*. 53(1–2): 43–54.
Sargeant, J. M., Scott, H. M., Leslie, K. E., Ireland, M. J., Bashiri, A. 1998, Jan. Clinical mastitis in dairy cattle in Ontario: frequency of occurrence and bacteriological isolates. *Can Vet J*. 39(1): 33–38.
Schreiner, D. A., Ruegg, P. L. 2003, Nov. Relationship between udder and leg hygiene scores and subclinical mastitis. *J Dairy Sci*. 86(11): 3460–5.
Suriyasathaporn, W., Schukken, Y. H., Nielen, M., Brand, A. 2000, Jun. Low somatic cell count: a risk factor for subsequent clinical mastitis in a dairy herd. *J Dairy Sci*. 83(6): 1248–55.

Author: Jerry Roberson

MASTITIS: SHEEP AND GOATS

 BASICS

DEFINITION
Inflammation of the mammary gland due to either infection or trauma, and typified by one or all of the following: loss of milk production, increase in inflammatory cells, abnormal milk, changes in gland size and/or consistency, and occasionally systemic illness or death of the animal.

PATHOPHYSIOLOGY
• Infection is most commonly ascending from the teat sphincter to teat cistern and potentially to the glandular tissue.
• The pathogenicity of the bacteria dictates the potential for severe disease: from subclinical mastitis to peracute toxic mastitis.
• The infectious agent may produce a toxin that is absorbed by the blood stream or the agent may invade the alveoli and interstitial tissues causing inflammation. Some infections may be hematogenous (e.g., retroviruses, some *Mycoplasma*).

SYSTEMS AFFECTED
Mammary gland and, occasionally, systemic illness.

GENETICS
There is a genetic association with logarithmic somatic cell counts (SCC) in some breeds of dairy sheep (e.g., Lacaune). There is also some evidence that selecting for longevity without incidence of mastitis may select against mastitis.

INCIDENCE / PREVALENCE
• Subclinical mastitis is considered to be very common in sheep and goats, dairy and meat.
• The annual flock-level incidence of severe clinical mastitis in which an animal becomes ill or loses a gland, is 3%–15%.
• The prevalence of mastitis in culled sheep is often greater than 30%, indicating that it is an important reason for culling.

GEOGRAPHIC DISTRIBUTION
Found in all sheep- and goat-raising countries, regardless of management

SIGNALMENT
Species
Sheep and goats, both as dairy and meat animals

Breed Predilections
None known

Mean Age and Range
Any lactating animal but prevalence of mastitis increases with age.

Predominant Sex
Female

GENERAL COMMENTS
N/A

HISTORICAL FINDINGS
Peracute Systemic Mastitis
• Highest risk is 2–4 weeks postlambing/kidding (first one-third of lactation) or just after weaning.

• Animal may be found dead or down from effects of toxemia/septicemia.
• If animal is not down, then severely depressed, gaunt/off feed, and may also appear lame.
• Gland or entire udder may appear bluish to black and cold.

Clinical Mastitis
• Animal may go off feed for a day or two. May appear mildly lame from the swollen udder.
• Owner may notice abnormal gland (hard, fibrotic, swollen). In meat animals, abnormal milk/udder may not be noticed until weaning or the subsequent lambing/kidding.

Subclinical Mastitis
• May not be detected in meat animals.
• If routinely screening dairy animals:
  • Dairy sheep: elevated somatic cell count (SCC) or California Mastitis Test (CMT) result.
  • Dairy goats: may only be detected with milk culture unless markedly elevated SCC.

PHYSICAL EXAMINATION FINDINGS
Peracute Systemic Mastitis
• High fever initially (> 40.5°C), severe dehydration and depression but temperature may become subnormal terminally. Systemic signs are compatible with toxemia or septicemia.
• The affected gland is swollen, hard, purple in color, and cold to the touch if gangrene is present.
• Serum, occasionally with gas, is expressed from the teat; no milk is present.
• Often the gangrene extends into the groin area and beyond.
• If the animal survives, the gangrenous gland is sloughed.

Clinical Mastitis
• Affected gland is swollen and hard or if more chronic, fibrotic. May contain abscesses.
• Milk is discolored (yellow or tan) and may contain clots. Milk may also appear serum-colored to watery or thickened.

Subclinical Mastitis
• Milk appears normal but gland may be slightly swollen or slightly hypoplastic, depending on severity and chronicity of mastitis, or may appear normal.
• Scarring and occlusion of the teat canal may occur secondarily to infection with *Staphylococcus chromogenes.*

CAUSES
Peracute Systemic Mastitis
• Most cases are due to *Staphylococcus aureus* and *Mannheimia haemolytica,* and less commonly *Pseudomonas aeroginosa* (from water sources) and coliforms such as *E. coli, Salmonella* spp., and *Klebsiella pneumonia.*
• May be secondarily infected with *Clostridium septicum* (gas gangrene).

Clinical and Subclinical Mastitis
• Bacteria
• See Table 1.
  • Coagulase negative staphylococcus (CNS) are by far the most common isolates. There are many species that have variable pathogenicity (70%–80%). Next in importance is *Staphylococcus aureus* (3%–8%), *Streptococcus uberis* (goats mostly), *Arcanobacterium pyogenes, Corynebacterium bovis, Listeria monocytogenes,* rarely *Streptococcus agalactia* (goats).
  • Species of CNS that are considered more pathogenic include *S. epidermidis, S. simulans, S. chromogenes, S. xylosus* (sheep), *S. caprae* (goats). Many of CNS isolates from small ruminants are hemolytic, indicating higher pathogenicity than strains found in cattle.
• Mycoplasma
  • *Mycoplasma agalactia* (contagious agalactia) is a common cause of severe mastitis in sheep and goats in the Mediterranean areas but is considered exotic to North America.
  • *Mycoplasma mycoides* ssp. *mycoides,* large colony type, occurs in North American goats and causes mastitis and septicemia in adult goats and septicemia, septic arthritis, and pneumonia in kids.
  • *Mycoplasma capricolum* and *M. putrifasciens* also cause caprine mastitis.

Table 1

Common Bacterial Etiologies for Mastitis in Sheep and Goats	
Acute/Clinical Mastitis	**Subclinical Mastitis**
Escherichia coli	*Arcanobacterium pyogenes*
Klebsiella spp.	*Bacillus* spp.
Mannheimia haemolytica	Coliforms
Pseudomonas spp.	*Corynebacterium pseudotuberculosis*
Staphylococcus aureus	*Pseudomonas* spp.
	Staphylococcus spp.
	Streptococcus spp.

- Viruses
  - Maedi visna virus (ovine progressive pneumonia virus) causes an interstitial mastitis in sheep.
  - Caprine arthritis encephalitis virus causes an interstitial mastitis in goats.
- Other: occasionally a variety of fungi is isolated from sheep or goat mastitis, most commonly *Aspergillus*. Yeast and *Prototheca* infections may also occur.

RISK FACTORS

- Compromised teat sphincter by one the following:
  - Contagious ecthyma infection (orf, soremouth) of the teat end
  - Over-milking or high teat-end vacuum pressure in dairy sheep and goats
  - Insufficient vacuum reserve so that back-splashing occurs when a milking unit is removed.
  - Possibly trauma from biting or aggressive nursing
- Presence of contagious bacteria, in particular *S. aureus* and CNS or rarely *Streptococcus agalactia* may infect by its presence on the teat end. Occasionally, sheep and goats may have a marked dermatitis from *S. aureus* infection on the udder, which may increase the risk of mastitis.
- Humans may be carriers of *S aureus* and transmit through poor hygiene.
- *M. mycoides* ssp *mycoides* is highly contagious and can be spread through poor milking hygiene. Does that consume infected milk as kids, may become shedders when they start to lactate.
- A dirty environment (e.g., manure, mud, dirty water) will contaminate the teat end. Water is the most important source of infection due to *P. aeruginosa*. Milking equipment with cracked liners or poorly cleaned after use, may also serve as an important reservoir for environmental bacteria.
- Mastitis due to *M. haemolytica* may be due to the presence of the bacteria in the nasopharynx of the nursing lambs or kids.
- Increased housing density is associated with a higher prevalence of mastitis in dairy and meat sheep.

 DIAGNOSIS

DIFFERENTIAL DIAGNOSIS

- Gangrene may occur secondary to a wound.
- Swelling of the udder may occur secondary to trauma.

CBC / BIOCHEMISTRY / URINALYSIS

A complete blood count (CBC) may provide evidence of sepsis and/or toxemia. A clinical chemistry profile may be useful in characterizing acid/base and electrolyte abnormalities and organ dysfunction in peracute disease. Serology and viral isolation can be used to diagnose retroviral mastitis.

OTHER LABORATORY TESTS

Detecting Inflammatory Cells

- CMT —there is a good correlation between CMT results and SCC. It has been suggested that all glands with a CMT reaction of 1+ or greater (a reaction associated with SCC $\geq 0.8 \times 10^6$ cells/mL) on a five-point scale (neg, trace, 1+, 2+, 3+) should be cultured, although up to 30% of infected glands may be missed using this screening test.
- SCC—a more useful screening test for mastitis in sheep than in goats. Sheep have a similar response to infection as cattle and a threshold of 0.5×10^6 cells/mL is a reasonable point above which the gland should be cultured. The SCC in goats is very high at the end of lactation, and is often greater than 1.0×10^6 cells/mL, making it difficult to differentiate between infection and effect of stage of lactation. While it is useful to culture goats with SCC greater than 1.0×10^6 cells/mL, using this cut-point may miss infections due to CNS or even *S. aureus*.
- NAGase—not commonly used but shows good correlation in midlactation with infection.

Detecting Infectious Agents

- A milk sample taken using aseptic technique should reveal a minimum of 5 cfu/mL milk in pure culture, for the organism to be considered significant. Freezing may increase the chances of isolation of some bacteria (e.g., *S. aureus*) but may lower the isolation rate of other bacteria. A high SCC may interfere with isolation of some bacteria, notably *S. aureus*, in which case repeated sampling (e.g., every other day for three samples, frozen and submitted for culture) may increase the rate of diagnosis in cases where infection is strongly suspected but single culture is unrewarding.
- In North America, it is prudent to request culture for *Mycoplasma* when investigating goat mastitis associated with disease in kids.
- Serology for MV-v/CAE-v is alone not diagnostic for interstitial mastitis due to these retroviruses. However, a positive test (ELISA or AGID) would suggest flock infection indicating that control measures are warranted.

IMAGING

Ultrasonography may be useful in the identification of fibrosis and abscesses within the mammary gland parenchyma.

DIAGNOSTIC PROCEDURES

N/A

PATHOLOGIC FINDINGS

- Necropsy of animals dying of peracute systemic mastitis reveals changes associated with severe toxemia or septicemia.
- Histology of glandular tissue affected with MV-v or CAE-v will reveal lymphoid follicles throughout the udder tissue and secondary scarring.

 TREATMENT

APPROPRIATE HEALTH CARE

- Peracute systemic mastitis
  - Most cases are noted after gangrene has set in, which can occur within a few hours after becoming ill. Care should focus on supportive therapy (intravenous fluids, nonsteroidal anti-inflammatory drugs), stripping of milk if possible, and administration of broad-spectrum antibiotics.
  - Antibiotics should be selected based on spectrum of activity, ability to be used in dairy animals (if applicable), and the drug's ability to cross into the mammary gland. For meat sheep, tilmicosin (Micotil, Provel) has been shown to be efficacious against *S. aureus* and *M. haemolytica* udder infections, but cannot be used in dairy sheep because of milk withdrawals. Tilmicosin should not be used in goats because of potential toxic effects.
- Treatment of clinical and subclinical mastitis during lactation
  - Cases in which damage has already occurred (e.g., severe fibrosis or abscessation) will not respond to treatment and culling should be considered.
  - Very little work is published on the efficacy of intramammary infusions of antibiotics during lactation in either sheep or goats. Care must be taken not to damage the teat sphincter, and to investigate appropriate withdrawals for milk and meat through FARAD or gFARAD. Parenteral treatment with tilmicosin (Micotil, Provel) has been shown to clear up *S. aureus* dermatitis and mastitis in dairy sheep.
  - Most work has been done on dry period treatment. Cure rates and new infection rates vary between studies, but it appears useful only if a flock or herd has a significant level of mastitis. Again, extreme care must be taken when infusing teats not to cause damage or contaminate the gland. A single injection of tilmicosin (Micotil, Provel) 1 month prior to lambing has been shown to increase lamb weight gains in multiparous ewes at weaning and to reduce the prevalence of abnormal udders regardless of culture results. Routine dry period therapy may be more useful in goats with a shorter dry period although little is published on this. Again, care must be taken to avoid residues with extralabel drug use.
  - CNS infections in particular experience a level of self-cure.
- Mycoplasma infections are not considered to be amenable to treatment, and infected animals, once identified, should be culled to slaughter.

MASTITIS: SHEEP AND GOATS

• Treatment of fungal mastitis is rarely successful and there are no specific treatments for viral mastitis. Hence, culling the affected animals from the herd is usually recommended.

NURSING CARE
See Appropriate Health Care section above.

ACTIVITY
N/A

DIET
N/A

CLIENT EDUCATION
• Cases of *S. aureus* that do not respond to treatment should be culled.
• Milking equipment and technique should be checked semiannually.

SURGICAL CONSIDERATIONS
Chronic suppurative mastitis or severe gangrenous mastitis may require partial (udder half) or total mastectomy to eliminate the source of infection and/or toxemia. Surgery of the mammary gland is covered in a separate chapter (Mammary Gland Surgeries: Teat Amputation, Mastectomy).

MEDICATIONS

DRUGS OF CHOICE
See Appropriate Health Care section above.

CONTRAINDICATIONS

PRECAUTIONS
• Withdrawal periods for milk cannot be extrapolated from those published for dairy cattle.
• Splitting a tube of mastitis ointment is contraindicated because of the risk of contamination.

POSSIBLE INTERACTIONS

ALTERNATIVE DRUGS
N/A

FOLLOW-UP

PATIENT MONITORING
Response to treatment can be monitored most easily by CMT, although SCC is preferable in dairy animals.

PREVENTION / AVOIDANCE
• Cull ewes at weaning that have severe udder damage or that are infected with *S. aureus*.
• Environment should be clean and dry. Use straw and avoid softwood shavings for bedding.
• Dairy sheep and goats:
  • Semiannual check of milking equipment to make sure it is clean, calibrated, and functioning appropriately.
  • Milk primiparous animals first and *S. aureus* carriers last (or cull).
  • Wash water should contain an appropriate sanitizer and udder should be thoroughly dried with a single-use towel before putting on machine. Predipping is optional but udder prep time should be kept to a minimum.
  • Do not overmilk (milk-out time ~ 2–3 minutes). Use an appropriate registered teat dip.
  • Dry period therapy should be used if infection rates warrant.
  • Dairy sheep SCC values should be monitored several times during their lactation in order to select infected animals for culture.

POSSIBLE COMPLICATIONS
N/A

EXPECTED COURSE AND PROGNOSIS
• Course of disease and prognosis will depend on the infectious agent and chronicity and severity of infection. Gangrenous mastitis generally is associated with a poor to grave prognosis. Subclinical disease, while having a good prognosis for life, may have a poor prognosis for the herd or flock if the inciting agent is a contagious pathogen.
• Chronic infections tend to cause depressed milk production, which ultimately decreases profits from dairy animals and reduces growth rates in lambs and kids.

 MISCELLANEOUS

ASSOCIATED CONDITIONS
Decreased milk production and herd/flock profitability.

AGE-RELATED FACTORS
N/A

ZOONOTIC POTENTIAL
• Many infectious agents found commonly in milk have the capacity to cause illness in humans, which underlines the need to pasteurize all milk prior to consumption.
• The following agents are potentially zoonotic and can either be shed in the milk or contaminate raw milk of sheep and goats: *S. aureus, Salmonella* spp., verocytotoxin producing *E. coli* (e.g., H7:O157), *Listeria monocytogenes, Brucella* spp.*, Yersinia enterocolitica, Klebsiella* spp., *Streptococcus faecalis,* and the rickettsia *Coxiella burnetii,* the causative agent of Q fever. Many of these organisms do not cause clinical mastitis but have the capacity to cause illness in humans.

PREGNANCY
N/A

RUMINANT SPECIES AFFECTED
Sheep and goats

BIOSECURITY
• Dairy sheep—limit the number of animals purchased after lactation has begun to reduce risk of purchasing *S. aureus* infected animals.
• Dairy goats—make sure that purchases are from a herd free of *M. mycoides.*

PRODUCTION MANAGEMENT
See in Prevention/Avoidance section above.

SYNONYMS

SEE ALSO
Dairy goat milk quality
Dairy sheep
Diagnostic microbiology
Farad
Mycoplasma mastitis
Orf

ABBREVIATIONS
AGID = agar gel immunodiffusion
cfu = colony forming units
CMT = California Mastitis Test
CNS = coagulase negative *Staphylococcus* species
ELISA = enzyme-linked immunosorbent assay
FARAD = Food Animal Residue Avoidance Databank
gFARAD = global FARAD (for countries other than the United States)
NAGase = N-acetyl-β-D-glucosaminidase
SCC = somatic cell count

Suggested Reading
Bergoneir, D., De Crémoux, R., Rupp, R., Lagriffoul, G., et al. 2003. Mastitis of dairy small ruminants. *Vet Res.* 34:689–716.
Billon, P., Fernandez Martinez, N., Ronningen, O., Sangiorgi, R., et al. 2002. Quantitative recommendations for milking machine installations for small ruminants. *Bull Int Dairy Fed.* 370: 4–19.
Menzies, P. I., Ramanoon, S. Z. 2001. Mastitis of sheep and goats. *Vet Clin North Am Food Anim Pract.* 17:333–58.

Authors: Paula I. Menzies and John R. Middleton

MASTITIS: STAPHYLOCOCCAL

 BASICS

OVERVIEW

• Mastitis is inflammation of the mammary gland caused by microorganisms, usually bacterial, that invade the mammary gland, multiply, and produce toxins harmful to the gland.
• Mastitis compromises the well-being of the patient.
• Mastitis compromises the nutrition available to the offspring.
• All livestock species are affected by mastitis.
• Mastitis in dairy cattle and milk goats produces serious economic losses.
• Mastitis is the single most common disease in adult dairy cows.
• In milk producing animals, losses are due to:
  • Decreased milk production
  • Discarded milk
  • Increased treatment costs
  • Increased replacement costs due to deaths or involuntary culling
• Losses in sheep are associated with acute clinical disease of the ewe or subclinical forms that decrease milk production with resulting poor lamb growth or increased lamb mortality.
• Staphylococci are gram-positive bacteria.
• Staphylococci organisms that cause mastitis are usually identified as *Staphylococcus aureus* and coagulase-negative staphylococci (CNS) or *Staphylococcus* species.

SIGNALMENT

• Mastitis in cattle can occur any time during lactation.
  • No signs are typically noted with subclinical infections.
  • Brood ewes and does usually develop mastitis between parturition and weaning.
• History of acute cases may include anorexia, depression, and loss of milk production.

SIGNS

Signs vary from subclinical to clinical to gangrenous.

Subclinical Mastitis
• Characterized by lack of visible changes to the gland or the milk
• Causes elevation of somatic cell count of the infected gland

Clinical Mastitis
Associated with changes in the gland and the milk. The infected quarter may have signs of swelling, pain, and heat.

Peracute
• Gland has swelling, heat, and pain.
• Secretion is abnormal and may contain clots, flakes, or discolored serum and sometimes blood.
• Signs of systemic illness are present. These include anorexia, depression, increased pulse rate, sunken eyes, and weakness.
• Onset is rapid and mortality may be high.

Acute, Gangrenous
• Gangrenous form is due to staph alpha toxin.
• Acute systemic and local signs are due to toxemia.
• Starts with inflammation of the gland, then development of cold teats and bloody secretions
• The gland has sharply delineated, blue discolorations.
• Mortality may be high.

Acute
• Changes to the gland and secretion are similar to peracute infections.
• Systemic signs are present but less severe than peracute infections.

Subacute
• Mild to moderate alterations to the secretion and mammary gland
• No systemic signs

Clinical Signs in Small Ruminants
• Referred to as "blue bag"
• Fever of 41–42°C (105–107°F)
• Anorexia
• Refusal to lie down or lameness
• Skin of mammary gland is initially red and hot, then becomes cyanotic and cold.
• Milk decreases in volume, becomes watery or bloody, and contains debris.
• Mortality may approach 80% if not treated.

CAUSES AND RISK FACTORS

• Infection of the mammary gland follows introduction of staphylococci bacteria through the teat sphincter
• *Staphylococcus aureus* (*Staph aureus*)
  • In dairy cows, it is usually associated with transfer of infected milk from infected to noninfected quarters during the milking process.
  • Transfer has also been associated with flies and milkers' hands.
  • Primary source: infected udders
  • Secondary sites include teat skin, udder skin, nose, lips, vagina, and other body sites.
  • Method of spread: via transfer of bacteria-laden milk from infected to noninfected glands. The milking process is a primary means of transfer, but nursing calves, flies, and milkers' hands can also transfer the organisms.
  • Often introduced into a herd by infected, purchased additions
  • Flies have been associated with infection in prepartum heifers.
• Coagulase-negative staphylococci (CNS)
  • Also referred to as staph species bacteria
  • Are normal inhabitants of bovine teat skin and can be free living in the environment
  • Infections are more common in first lactation cows.
  • Prevalence is high at parturition, then declines through the first month of lactation.
  • Primary source: commonly found on teat skin and in the streak canal
  • Cow-to-cow spread is probably rare.
  • Most infections are transient.
  • May be associated with teat injuries or alteration of teat skin condition

 DIAGNOSIS

DIFFERENTIAL DIAGNOSIS
• Subclinical cases must be differentiated from mastitis caused by *Streptococcus agalactia*, *Corynebacterium bovis*, and minor udder pathogens.
• Clinical cases must be differentiated from mastitis caused by coliform bacteria, *Mycoplasma*, environmental streptococci.
• Gangrenous mastitis with bloody secretion must be differentiated from trauma to the gland.

CBC/BIOCHEMISTRY/URINALYSIS
Usually not performed

OTHER LABORATORY TESTS
Microbiological identification of the causative agent is essential in diagnosis.
• Requires plating organisms to evaluate the colonial characteristics and hemolytic patterns on blood agar
• The catalase test is used to differentiate staphylococci from streptococci by mixing the colony with hydrogen peroxide.
  • Staphylococci are catalase positive (produce bubbles).
  • Streptococci are catalase negative (do not produce bubbles).
• Colonies should be gram stained. Staphylococci are gram-positive cocci that appear in clumps.

Staph aureus
• Large colonies that are creamy, grayish-white, or yellowish in color
• Generally produce hemolysis, typically a double zone, around the colony
• Most are coagulase positive.

Coagulase-Negative Staphylococci (Staph Species)
• Large, creamy, grayish-white, or yellowish in color
• Generally have no hemolysis
• Most are coagulase negative.

Coagulase Test
To perform the coagulase test, a *Staphylococcus* colony is mixed with rabbit plasma and incubated. Clotting indicates a positive reaction.

IMAGING
N/A

DIAGNOSTIC PROCEDURES
• A strip cup or strip plate is used to identify changes in milk.
• The udder should be palpated for heat, swelling, and induration.
• Perform a physical exam of the animal to assess systemic signs including fever, appetite, and hydration.
• California Mastitis Test: Used to identify infected quarters, especially those with subclinical infections; will not identify the pathogen.
• Culture is the only method to identify the specific pathogen.

TREATMENT
• Both intramammary and systemic therapy have been used.
• Treatment of early cases of *Staph aureus* is often successful; the success of treatment for chronic infections is poor.
• Response to therapy of *Staph aureus* is poorer due to formation of L-forms, penicillinase production, and the formation of microabscesses within the udder parenchyma.
• When possible, treatment should be based on culture and angiobiograms (susceptibility information).
• Goal is to return the gland to production.
• Consider the economics of the treatment.
• Use only products approved for use in food-producing animals.
• Withholding times for milk and meat must be observed.
• Better response to treatment is attained during the dry period.

MEDICATIONS
• Base on culture and sensitivity test results, if possible
• Several commercial products for intramammary administration are available.
  • B-lactam antibiotics such as penicillin, hetacillin, and amoxicillin
  • Cephapirin
  • Novobiocin
  • Pirlimycin

• No products are labeled for systemic therapy but injectable ampicillin (3–5 mg/lb) and oxytetracycline (5 mg/lb) have been used in conjunction with intramammary therapy.
• Nonsteroidal anti-inflammatory drugs (NSAIDs) are used to control pain and fever.
• Treatment of small ruminants is the same as for cattle.
• Withholding times for milk and slaughter must be followed.

FOLLOW-UP
Infected quarters should be cultured 21–28 days after treatment to determine cure.

PREVENTION/AVOIDANCE
Control of Staph aureus
• Identify infected cows and isolate or milk last
• Cull chronically infected cows.
• Treat all cows with appropriate dry cow infusion products.
• Apply an effective teat disinfectant to each teat following milking.
• Backflushing systems have been used to reduce the bacterial load in the milking inflations.
• Promote good milking hygiene and proper milking techniques to minimize teat end trauma.
• Vaccines are available but of limited usefulness.

Control of CNS
• Treat all cows with appropriate dry cow infusion products.
• Apply an effective teat disinfectant to each teat following milking.

MISCELLANEOUS
ASSOCIATED CONDITIONS
• Mastitis in dairy cattle and milk goats produces serious economic losses.
• In milk-producing animals, losses are due to:
  • Decreased milk production
  • Discarded milk
  • Increased treatment costs
  • Increased replacement costs due to deaths or involuntary culling

• Losses in sheep are associated with acute clinical disease of the ewe or subclinical forms that decrease milk production with resulting poor lamb growth or increased lamb mortality.

AGE-RELATED FACTORS
Coagulase-negative staphylococci infections are more common in first lactation cows.

ZOONOTIC POTENTIAL
N/A

PREGNANCY
N/A

RUMINANT SPECIES AFFECTED
Bovine

BIOSECURITY
N/A

PRODUCTION MANAGEMENT
• Cull chronically infected cows.
• Treat all cows with appropriate dry cow infusion products.
• Apply an effective teat disinfectant to each teat following milking.
• Backflushing systems have been used to reduce the bacterial load in the milking inflations.
• Promote good milking hygiene and proper milking techniques to minimize teat-end trauma.

SYNONYMS
Blue bag in small ruminants
Gangrenous mastitis

SEE ALSO
Mastitis in sheep and goats
Specific mastitis chapters

ABBREVIATIONS
CNS = coagulase-negative staphylococci
NSAIDs = nonsteroidal anti-inflammatory drugs
Staph = *Staphylococcus*

Suggested Reading
Current concepts of bovine mastitis. 1996, 4th ed. National Mastitis Council, 421 S. Nine Mound Rd., Verona, WI 53593.
Laboratory handbook on bovine mastitis. Rev. ed. 1999. National Mastitis Council, 421 S. Nine Mound Rd., Verona, WI 53593.

Author: Richard W. Meiring

MASTITIS: STREPTOCOCCAL

 BASICS

OVERVIEW
In many dairy herds with different management approaches, at least one type of streptococcal mastitis is among the most prevalent intramammary infections (IMI), often financially important. These include contagious as well as environmental pathogens.

SYSTEMS AFFECTED
Mammary and production management

GENETICS
N/A

INCIDENCE/PREVALENCE
• Fifteen percent of dairy herds in the northeast United States have *Streptococcus agalactiae* infections present in the herd at any given time, while 85% are free of this eradicable organism.
• Researchers currently suggest prevalence between 11%–47% of herds in various states/regions of North America.
• Within infected herds, prevalence of *Streptococcus agalactia* varies considerably, ranging from 1%–77% of the herd in 2003.
• *Strep ag* is reported as a pathogen in many dairy ruminant species. *Strep ag* in goat milk occurs rarely.
• Of dairy herds in the United States, 96% have *Strep dysgalactiae* or *Strep uberis* infecting at least one cow at any given time.
• Many laboratories and commercial dairy herd mastitis control programs do not speciate between these two types of nonagalactiae streptococci, identifying them as *Strep sp.*
• Among cows, the prevalence of *Strep sp.* is 14%–16% in reports from the United States and other developed countries.

GEOGRAPHIC DISTRIBUTION
Worldwide depending on bacterial species and environment

SIGNALMENT

Species
Dairy cattle

Breed Predilections
Dairy breeds of cattle

Mean Age and Range
N/A

Predominant Sex
Female

Major Pathogens
• *Streptococcus agalactiae* (contagious, usually aggressively spreading pathogen)
• *Streptococcus dysgalactiae* (predominant source is the environment)
• *Streptococcus uberis* (predominant source is the environment)
• The latter two are often diagnosed as a group in mastitis and udder health programs as *Strep sp.*

SIGNS
In herd:
• There is no one classical presentation of these pathogens within dairy herds; however, in most cases, *Strep ag* first becomes evident within months to 1 year following purchase of infected animals.
• Three percent of heifers have infections with *Strep ag* at first calving, and should not be assumed to be risk free as herd additions.
• Ninety-six percent of *Strep ag* cases are subclinical.
• *Strep ag* results in bulk tank SCC usually > 400,000/ml, often > 750,000/ml at least intermittently. SCC often rises steadily once the increase begins.
• Sometimes associated with high bacteria counts in milk, can be > 200,000/ml SPC.
• Often high (> 10%/mo) new infection rate on DHIA (or other test service) monthly reports.
• May be high level (> 10%/mo) of chronic infections as well.
• *Strep sp.* can be major mastitis in any herd, including herd as described above.

• However, *Strep sp.* more likely to be at high level when tank SCC < 400,000/ml, especially when < 200,000/ml.
• *Strep sp.* often are subclinical but many cases can have severe clinical signs, or SCC LS > 5.0.
• Often notice many new infections on DHIA among fresh cows < 60 DIM.
• *Strep sp.* mastitis increases from June through September in many herds in North America.

RISK FACTORS
• Failure to employ standard milking time hygiene measures are risk factors for the spread of *S. agalactiae* IMI. Herds that do not utilize dry cow antibiotic therapy and herds that do not cull chronically high SCC cows would be at increased risk for *S. agalactiae*. There is also a suggestion that teat end hyperkeratosis increases the risk of *S. agalactiae*.
• Historically, the Environmental Streptococci (ES) are considered to be opportunist mastitis pathogens; however, the ES, especially *S. dysgalactiae*, may have some characteristics of contagious pathogens. A few studies have demonstrated a greater risk of ES IMI to cows with advancing age.
• Several studies have documented that straw bedding increases the risk of cows to ES IMI. Likewise, cows bedded on deep bedded straw packs that tend to be urine and feces contaminated are at increased risk. In an Ohio study, increased prevalence of ES was associated with poor sanitation, increased number of days dry, use of tie stalls, and lack of drying teats prior to milking. There is also a suggestion that the increased time associated with correcting liner squawks increases the risk of ES IMI.

 DIAGNOSIS

• Bulk tank milk culture is a useful way to screen a herd or group for *Strep ag*.

• Sensitivity for a single bulk tank culture is 77% (across all ranges of prevalence). Three bulk tank milk culture samples collected approximately 3 days apart should be collected and cultured separately; if all 3 samples are negative, the probability the herd is uninfected is 99%.

• Bulk tank milk cultures are frequently positive for *Strep* sp., and have no practical value in monitoring for these infections.

• Culture of aseptic milk samples is the only definitive way to diagnose either type of mastitis in individual cows at present.

 • Culture should be carried out on blood agar. Incubation overnight at 37°C. Streptococci appear as small, somewhat transparent colonies with or without hemolysis at 18–24 hours.

 • All mastitis associated streptococci are catalase negative (place a small amount of the colonies on a glass slide and add a drop of hydrogen peroxide); there will be no bubbling, which indicates a negative catalase. Gram's stain will typically reveal gram-positive cocci in chains.

 • The three primary mastitis-associated streptococci can then be effectively differentiated from each other by a few simple tests (Table 1).

TREATMENT

• Culture of entire lactating herd is usually necessary to eradicate *Strep ag*, with resampling of the herd 3 weeks after treatment is complete, repeated until eradication is accomplished.

Table 1

Streptococcus	Esculin	Camp
agalactiae	–	+
dysgalactiae	–	–
uberis	+	+/–

• Intramammary therapy (IMM) cure rates have declined in recent years to approximately 90% of *Strep ag* cases curing following any single course of treatment.

• Individual cows usually warrant two regimens of therapy before being considered nonresponsive; many animals will cure the second time. Cows that are positive on third culture after two rounds of therapy should be strongly considered for culling.

• IMM infusion of beta-lactam antibiotic in all four quarters for three milkings in a row should be done for all infected cows as soon as culture results are available, treating all *Strep ag*–infected cows at the same time.

• Teat dipping and other classical mastitis control measures are weakly associated with control of *Strep* sp.

• The definitive control program for *Strep* sp. has not been developed.

• Environmental sanitation is critical, including dry cow and replacement heifer housing.

• Bedding cultures are often useful. Counts < 100,000 cfu/g are good; some are much lower.

• *Strep* sp. > 1,000,000 cfu/g in bedding (some are billions/g) strongly associated with higher prevalence of the infection in cows.

• Bedding cultures often convince farm management that various types of housing and bedding really are in need of increased cleanliness efforts.

• *Strep* sp. control programs including bedding, housing repair, and milking clean, dry teats must be developed with managers and employees of each farm.

MEDICATIONS

DRUGS OF CHOICE

• Because the spontaneous cure rate for streptococcal mastitis is usually less than 20% and often results in chronically high SCC, timely treatment with an appropriate antibiotic is essential and usually economical.

• Penicillin-based products are the intramammary drugs of choice. Several studies have found that the streptococci are still quite susceptible to the penicillin products.

• The initial therapeutic protocol should be an approved intramammary antibiotic used according to label directions. If this therapy is not successful, there are other alternatives.

• Anecdotal evidence suggests that simply switching to a different class of approved intramammary antibiotic used according to label is often sufficient in obtaining a bacterial cure. Another option is to extend the intramammary antibiotic therapy two to three times the labeled dosage. Studies with pirlimycin and ceftiofur have demonstrated increasing bacterial cures with increasing dosage lengths. However, a study with extended amoxicillin did not demonstrate any benefit over the normal labeled dosage.

• One other option is to treat both intramammary and systemically. In a recent study, increased bacterial cures were obtained by using intramuscular ampicillin with intramammary amoxicillin.

• For herds with a high prevalence of *S. agalactiae*, blitz treatment during lactation should be considered as it is often effective (> 80%) and often proves to be economical. *Enterococcus* species tend to be considerably more resistant to successful treatment than the other streptococci.

CONTRAINDICATIONS

Appropriate milk and meat withdrawal times must be followed for all compounds administered to food-producing animals.

FOLLOW-UP

PATIENT MONITORING

• Follow-up cultures are recommended on any treated streptococci cases.

• Recommended times to culture are 1–4 days after the milk antibiotic withdrawal (a negative culture at this time is most suggestive of the efficacy of the antibiotic) and at 28–30 days (helps to document that an actual bacterial cure did occur).

MASTITIS: STREPTOCOCCAL

• Alternatively, a decrease in individual cow SCC to normal levels would be suggestive of a cure.

PREVENTION/AVOIDANCE

• Although the significance of standard mastitis control procedures varies in importance among the streptococci, a complete mastitis control program is essential in control of the streptococci.
• Milking time hygiene will have the most effect on controlling *S. agalactiae* but will also help with control of the ES.
• Complete teat predipping with an effective germicide, which should be left in place for 15–30 seconds. Avoid water usage in the parlor. Teats should be dried completely with individual udder cloths or paper towels. Milking machines should be properly maintained. Avoid over- or undermilking. Quickly adjust milking units once squawking is heard. One study found increased *S. uberis* IMI associated with delay in correctly liner squawking. In the limited studies performed on backflushing, no benefit was found for the ES. At the end of milking, teats should be dipped up to the base of the udder with an effective germicide. Cows that have been treated and did not cure should be retreated or culled to help remove the intramammary reservoir.

• All quarters of all cows should be treated with an approved intramammary antibiotic at the time of dry off. Studies have shown that around 50% of new streptococci infections occur during the dry period. Proper nutrition, especially in regards to appropriate levels of vitamin E and selenium, is important for mammary immune function.
• Avoid the use of straw bedding when possible, and when not possible, proper maintenance of bedding areas is essential. Inorganic bedding is preferred, however one study found ten times more ES on the teats of cows bedded on sand than on teats of cows bedded on sawdust. Even pasture areas may be heavily contaminated with ES (e.g., common shade area). These prevention measures are less effective against *S. uberis* possibly because of its ubiquitous nature on the dairy farm (shed in the feces). Vaccines are being studied and may be available in the future. However, several studies have found that *S. uberis* strains vary considerably among dairy herds and even within dairy herds, which becomes problematic in regards to an effective vaccine.

POSSIBLE COMPLICATIONS
N/A

EXPECTED COURSE AND PROGNOSIS
• Spontaneous cure rate is around 20% for ES. The spontaneous cure rate for *S. agalactiae* is < 10%. Even though the organisms are susceptible, bacterial cures occur only 50–70% of the time.
• Extended intramammary therapy has been shown to increase the bacterial cures up to 100% in some experimental studies.

 MISCELLANEOUS

ASSOCIATED CONDITIONS
Loss of milk production and increased culling rates

AGE-RELATED FACTORS
Three percent of heifers have infections with *Strep ag* at first calving, and should not be assumed to be risk free as herd additions.

ZOONOTIC POTENTIAL
Although relatively rare, some streptococci of bovine origin have been identified in human infections. In particular, *S. agalactiae* is one of the leading causes of human neonatal infection. However, most studies have found that the *S. agalactiae* cultured from human infants is of a different type than that found in bovine mastitis.

MASTITIS: STREPTOCOCCAL

PREGNANCY
N/A

RUMINANT SPECIES AFFECTED
Dairy cattle

BIOSECURITY
Among cows, the prevalence of *Strep* sp. is 14%–16% in reports from the United States and other developed countries.

PRODUCTION MANAGEMENT
• Intramammary therapy (IMM) cure rates have declined in recent years, to approximately 90% of *Strep ag* cases curing following any single course of treatment.
• Individual cows usually warrant two regimens of therapy before being considered nonresponsive; many animals will cure the second time. Cows that are positive on third culture after two rounds of therapy should be strongly considered for culling.
• Environmental sanitation is critical, including dry cow and replacement heifer housing.

SYNONYMS
N/A

SEE ALSO
Environmental factors affecting mastitis
Manure management
Mastitis of sheep and goats
Microbiologic techniques
Specific mastitis chapters

ABBREVIATIONS
DHIA = Dairy Herd Improvement Association
DIM = days in milk
IMM = intramammary infusion
SCC = somatic cell count
SPC = standard plate count
Strep ag = *Streptococcus agalactiae*
Strep sp. = *Streptococcus dysgalactiae* and *Streptococcus uberis*

Suggested Reading
Keefe, G. P. 1997. *Streptococcus agalactiae* mastitis: a review. *Can Vet J.* 38(7):429–37.
Leigh, J. A. 1999. *Streptococcus uberis*: a permanent barrier to the control of bovine mastitis? *Vet J.* 157(3):225–38.
Wilson, D. J., Gonzalez, R. N., Das, H. H. 1997. Bovine mastitis pathogens in New York and Pennsylvania: prevalence and effects on somatic cell count and milk production. *J Dairy Sci.* 80(10):2592–98.
Zdanowicz, M., Shelford, J. A., Tucker, C. B., Weary, D. M., von Keyserlingk, M. A. 2004. Bacterial populations on teat ends of dairy cows housed in free stalls and bedded with either sand or sawdust. *J Dairy Sci.* 87(6):1694–1701.

Authors: David J. Wilson and Jerry R. Roberson

MASTITIS: VIRAL

BASICS

DEFINITION
• Inflammation of the mammary gland due to viral agents
• In cattle, bovine herpes virus (BHV) 1 and 4, foot-and-mouth disease virus (FMDV), and parainfluenza-3 (PI3) have been associated with mastitis but their overall significance is minimal.
• Caprine arthritis-encephalitis (CAE) virus is an agent of caprine mastitis.
• Maedi visna (ovine progressive pneumonia) causes mastitis in sheep.

PATHOPHYSIOLOGY
• The pathophysiology of BHV in bovine mastitis is little understood.
• Bovine herpes virus 4 may influence bacterial intramammary infections but the exact role is not understood. Bovine herpes virus 4 does not appear to be a significant agent of bovine mastitis as experimental inoculation into the mammary gland did not result in clinical mastitis although it did cause an increase in SCC.
• Subclinical mastitis occurred in 50% of inoculated cattle (n = 4).
• Secretory cell necrosis is associated with FMDV.
• In both CAE and MV, the infection is typically spread via virus-infected macrophages, which then enter the reticuloendothelial system where the virus-infected cells spread to target tissues.
• Once the target tissues are reached, the virus replicates and induces a lymphoproliferative response, which eventually leads to scarring and fibrosis of the mammary parenchyma.

SYSTEMS AFFECTED
• Bovine herpes virus 4 may affect the mammary gland and skin, and the reproductive tract.
• Caprine arthritis-encephalitis primarily affects joints in older goats and the central nervous system of young goats but is also commonly associated with the mammary gland and occasionally the lungs.
• Maedi visna (MV) typically affects the lungs and mammary gland of sheep and more rarely the neurologic system and joints.

GENETICS
There appears to be no genetic predisposition to any of the viral mastitis agents.

INCIDENCE/PREVALENCE
• Studies of prevalence and incidence of viral mastitis agents have not been conducted.
• A study conducted in 24 U. S. states in the early 1980s indicated that the ~80% of tested goats were seropositive for CAE. This study was conducted relatively early in the recognition of the disease (1974).
• A recent prevalence study could not be found. Studies among individual herds typically find a within-herd seroprevalence of > 60%. Studies specifically directed toward CAE mastitis could not be found.
• A study conducted in the late 1970s in Idaho found a 58% seroprevalence for MV in three flocks. A more recent study in the United States found a 26% prevalence. Within-flock seroprevalence may reach 100%. Again, prevalence of MV mastitis could not be found.

GEOGRAPHIC DISTRIBUTION
• BHV4 and PI3 likely have a worldwide distribution. The geographic distribution of FMDV is limited.
• Both CAE and MV are found worldwide.

SIGNALMENT
• There is insufficient knowledge regarding a standard signalment for bovine viral mastitis diseases in cattle.
• For both CAE and MV, the typical presentation is an older adult female with a hard udder with scant normal appearing milk.

SIGNS
• There are no distinguishing signs for the mastitis caused by viral mastitis agents in cattle.
• For both CAE and MV, mastitis typically presents as a hard udder with hypogalactia or agalactiae even at parturition.
• Other clinical signs associated with the mastitis are rare in that there is rarely any pain, swelling, redness, edema, or abnormal milk noted. In fact, the udder looks full and normal and only by palpation is the problem of the extremely firm udder noted. The condition is often bilateral.
• Regional lymph nodes are usually enlarged.
• Given time, the other systems affected by the virus will predispose the ewe or doe to progressive weight loss and eventual death.

CAUSES
• There is only limited and weak evidence to suggest that BHV4 may directly result in mastitis in cattle. Foot-and-mouth disease virus has been shown to result in a clinical mastitis that is often a sequela to a systemic infection. Parainfluenza virus 3 has been isolated from the mammary gland of cattle but its significance is not known.
• Both CAE and MV are retroviruses (slow viruses) that have many similarities but are distinct.

RISK FACTORS
• Too little is known about the epidemiology of bovine viral mastitis agents to elaborate on potential risk factors.
• Major risk factors for both CAE and MV are positive animals in the herd, consumption of milk or colostrum from a positive dam, and close contact with positive individuals.
• Aerosol transmission appears to be especially important in sheep due to MV's predilection for the lungs. The lamb and also herd mates in close proximity to the infected animal are at increased risk. The virus may also be transmitted via milk in the milking parlor.

DIAGNOSIS

DIFFERENTIAL DIAGNOSIS
• For bovine viral mastitis, differentials include any of the more common agents (mostly bacterial) of mastitis.
• For both CAE and MV, there are only a few other viral agents that might be responsible and these are only rarely reported. It is possible that bacterial, fungal, or algal agents could be responsible, but these do not typically result in a completely hard quarter.

CBC/BIOCHEMISTRY/URINALYSIS
These tests are not considered very useful in diagnosing viral mastitis. However, mammary somatic cells may present with more lymphocytes than neutrophils, which may help differentiate bacterial agents from viral agents.

OTHER LABORATORY TESTS
N/A

IMAGING
Imaging is not useful for bovine viral mastitis. Studies have not been conducted for small ruminant viral mastitis.

DIAGNOSTIC PROCEDURES
• Viral isolation and acute/convalescent titers may be used to diagnose bovine viral mastitis.
• For both CAE and MV, definitive diagnosis occurs by histological examination.
• Serology can be conducted and, if negative, suggests that the mastitis is not due to CAE; this is also true for MV. The two most commonly used tests are AGID and ELISA with reported sensitivities of 90% and 98%. A positive serologic test is an excellent indication that the animal is persistently infected.

PATHOLOGIC FINDINGS
• Thorough investigation of bovine viral mastitis pathologic findings has not been conducted.
• For CAE and MV, histopathology reveals foci of inflammatory cells within the interstitium with nodular lymphoid proliferation around the alveolar ducts. In chronic cases, there is increased deposition of connective tissue replacing the parenchyma, which likely results in the firmness of the udder.

TREATMENT

APPROPRIATE HEALTH CARE
• Because bovine viral mastitis is not considered to be very significant and prevalence is low, cattle with clinical mastitis should be treated as if the infection were bacterial in origin. Treatment should be symptomatic.
• There is no known efficacious treatment for CAE or MV mastitis and in production systems affected stock should be culled.

NURSING CARE
N/A

ACTIVITY
Unrestricted

DIET
No special dietary management is known to be helpful.

CLIENT EDUCATION
• The client should be aware that the overall importance of bovine viral mastitis is not known.
• Eradication programs should be discussed with clients when either CAE or MV is diagnosed because antibody-positive stock are considered infected for life.
• Kids and lambs should be fed only colostrum and milk from negative dams or pasteurized colostrum and milk. Kids of dams with "hard bag" may succumb to starvation and should receive supplemental milk and colostrum.

SURGICAL CONSIDERATIONS
N/A

MEDICATIONS

DRUGS OF CHOICE
There is no effective treatment for viral mastitis.

CONTRAINDICATIONS
N/A

PRECAUTIONS
N/A

POSSIBLE INTERACTIONS
N/A

ALTERNATIVE DRUGS
N/A

FOLLOW-UP

PATIENT MONITORING
The patient should be monitored and treated symptomatically.

PREVENTION/AVOIDANCE
• In general, bovine viral mastitis is not common enough nor deemed significant enough to warrant measures of prevention.
• Prevention and eradication programs are essential if small ruminant viral mastitis is to be controlled/eliminated. There are no vaccines.
• Transmission is primarily via milk and colostrum ingestion in neonates but other methods of transmission may occur (transplacental and sexual).
• Cross infection between sheep and goats is also thought to occur. See Mastitis: Sheep and Goats for detailed eradication programs.

POSSIBLE COMPLICATIONS
N/A

EXPECTED COURSE AND PROGNOSIS
• The duration of naturally occurring IMI is not known, but with the exception of FMDV IMI, mastitis appears to be relatively mild.
• Once the mammary gland is affected with CAE or MV, most cases will not improve.

MISCELLANEOUS

ASSOCIATED CONDITIONS
N/A

AGE-RELATED FACTORS
N/A

ZOONOTIC POTENTIAL
None

PREGNANCY
N/A

RUMINANT SPECIES AFFECTED
BHV4 = bovine; CAE = caprine; OPP = ovine

BIOSECURITY
• Milk is not considered an important means of transferring bovine viral mastitis.
• In CAE- or MV-negative herds or flocks, additions should come only from negative herds or flocks. When the disease status of a herd or flock is unknown, the new addition should be quarantined until negative test results are received.

PRODUCTION MANAGEMENT
N/A

SYNONYMS
CAE, hard udder or hard bag, OPP

SEE ALSO
Bovine herpes virus
Caprine arthritis-encephalitis
Foot-and-mouth disease virus
Maedi visna
Mastitis chapters
Parainfluenza-3

ABBREVIATIONS
BHV = bovine herpes virus
CAE = caprine arthritis-encephalitis
FMDV = foot-and-mouth disease virus
IMI = intramammary infection
MV = maedi visna
PI3 = parainfluenza-3
SCC = somatic cell count

Suggested Reading
Kalman, D., Janosi, S., Egyed, L. 2004, Sep. Role of bovine herpesvirus 4 in bacterial bovine mastitis. *Microb Pathog.* 37(3):125–29.
Miyano, H., Haritani, M., et al. 2004, Apr. Mammary lesions associated with bovine herpesvirus type 4 in a cow with clinical mastitis. *J Vet Med Sci.* 66(4):457–60.
Peterhans, E., Greenland, T., et al. 2004. Routes of transmission and consequences of small ruminant lentiviruses (SRLVs) infection and eradication schemes. *Vet Res.* 35:257–74.
Wellenberg, G. J., Van Der Poel, W. H., Van Oirschot, J. T. 2002, Aug 2. Viral infections and bovine mastitis: a review. *Vet Microbiol.* 88(1):27–45.

Author: Jerry R. Roberson

MELANOMA

BASICS

OVERVIEW
• Melanoma is a neoplastic proliferation of melanocytes that occurs most commonly in the skin and subcutaneous tissues, but can also involve the ophthalmic system.
• Melanomas account for 5–6% of all bovine tumors, and approximately 25% of skin tumors.
• The majority of melanomas in cattle appear benign histopathologically, but local invasion can be seen.
• Metastasis to lymph nodes and distant organs has been reported but appears to be rare.
• Melanomas are rare in sheep and goats.

SIGNALMENT
• Melanomas are most common in cattle less than 2 years of age, but may occur congenitally and have been reported in animals as old as 15 years.
• There is no sex predilection.
• Angus, Angus-crosses, and other dark-skinned cattle appear to be more likely to develop melanomas.

SIGNS
• Most melanomas in cattle are dark in color, and may or may not have hair on the overlying skin.
• Symptoms related to the location of the tumor, for example, intraocular melanoma resulted in a painful eye with buphthalmos, corneal ulceration, and edema.
• Cattle with melanomas may have no clinical signs associated with the tumor (painless soft tissue mass).

CAUSES AND RISK FACTORS
Unknown

DIAGNOSIS

DIFFERENTIAL DIAGNOSIS
• Other skin/subcutaneous tumors (fibroma, papilloma, lipoma, sebaceous tumors)
  • Requires histopathology for differentiation of tumor type
• Abscess
  • Abscess may be inflamed/painful, where melanomas are not.
  • Melanomas continue to grow over time.
  • Aspiration/cytology will differentiate between an abscess and a melanoma.

CBC/BIOCHEMISTRY/URINALYSIS
N/A

OTHER LABORATORY TESTS
N/A

IMAGING
Chest radiographs can help determine if there is pulmonary metastasis present prior to attempting surgical excision of the primary mass in a young animal.

DIAGNOSTIC PROCEDURES
• Biopsy of a mass for histopathologic evaluation and culture/sensitivity testing
• Aspiration and cytology of draining lymph nodes to evaluate for the presence of metastasis

PATHOLOGIC FINDINGS
• Often pigmented on cut surface, may exude pigmented fluid.
• Can occur in the dermis or subcutis, may have junctional activity (extension between the epidermis and dermis).
• Melanocyte may be epithelioid or spindloid in appearance and are often highly pigmented.
• Mitotic figures are typically low in number.
• May be positive for vimentin intermediate filaments and S100 protein on immunohistochemistry
• Even though melanomas may appear malignant histologically, recurrence and metastasis is rare.

TREATMENT

• Surgical excision, even when histologically incomplete, often results in long-term local control.
• There are no effective treatments for metastatic melanoma.

MEDICATIONS

DRUGS OF CHOICE
N/A

CONTRAINDICATIONS
N/A

FOLLOW-UP

PATIENT MONITORING
Routine postoperative monitoring of the surgical site is recommended.

PREVENTION/AVOIDANCE
N/A

POSSIBLE COMPLICATIONS
Scarring or hair loss at surgical site may impact the show quality of an animal.

EXPECTED COURSE AND PROGNOSIS
• Most (> 90%) melanomas have a benign course after excision and do not recur or metastasize.
• If truly malignant, recurrence and metastasis have been reported to occur within a few months.

MISCELLANEOUS

ASSOCIATED CONDITIONS
N/A

AGE-RELATED FACTORS
• Can be present at birth, and most commonly first noted in young animals
• Animals may present after mass has existed for years.

ZOONOTIC POTENTIAL
N/A

PREGNANCY
N/A

RUMINANT SPECIES AFFECTED
• Cattle
• Rare in sheep and goats.

PRODUCTION MANAGEMENT
N/A

ABBREVIATIONS
N/A

Suggested Reading
Bush, D. J., Lillich, J., Anderson, D. E., Desrochers, A., St. Jean, G. 1998, July/Aug. Surgical excision of melanoma in seven cattle. *Large Animal Practice*, pp. 36–39.

Authors: Marlene L. Hauck

BASICS

DEFINITION
• Melioidosis is a disease that affects a wide variety of animal species. However, severe disease is most commonly seen in sheep and goats.
• It is caused by the bacterium *Burkholderia pseudomallei*, an opportunistic, aerobic, gram-negative motile bacillus.
• The disease causes caseous abscesses of the lungs and respiratory disease. In disseminated forms, lameness, arthritis or encephalitis may also be seen.
• Goats are also prone to mastitis from this organism.

PATHOPHYSIOLOGY
• Melioidosis is caused by *B. pseudomallei*, an aerobic, gram-negative motile bacterium. It is an opportunistic pathogen that produces exotoxin.
• Disease can develop from the exotoxin produced by the organism (acute disease) or from the survival of the organism within phagocytic cells (latent or chronic form of disease).

SYSTEMS AFFECTED
• Respiratory—caseous lung abscesses, pneumonia, dyspnea
• Musculoskeletal—lameness, arthritis
• Nervous—encephalitis
• Mammary—mastitis (in goats)

GENETICS
N/A

INCIDENCE/PREVALENCE
• Outbreaks and cases typically occur in endemic areas during the wet season or after periods of heavy rainfall in areas with high humidity or temperature.
• The organism is typically ingested or inhaled from contaminated soil or water by animals.
• Limited cases of transuterine transmission have been reported.

GEOGRAPHIC DISTRIBUTION
Melioidosis is endemic in tropical and subtropical regions, particularly southeast Asia, northern and central Australia, the Middle East, India, China, and the Caribbean.

SIGNALMENT
Species
Although melioidosis affects many species of animals, sheep and goats are the most severely affected species. Cattle are rarely affected.

Breed Predilections
N/A

Mean Age and Range
N/A

Predominant Sex
N/A

SIGNS

GENERAL COMMENTS
Incubation is variable ranging from a few days to many years.

HISTORICAL FINDINGS
N/A

PHYSICAL EXAMINATION FINDINGS
• *Sheep:* Fever, generalized weakness; respiratory distress or dyspnea, severe coughing, mucopurulent nasal discharge; possibly lameness with swollen joints or partial paralysis. Neurological signs may include circling, incoordination, nystagmus, spasms.
• *Goats:* More commonly develop chronic disease and lameness, lymphadenopathy, mastitis, possibly respiratory signs (less severe than in sheep).
• *Cattle:* Rarely affected

MELIOIDOSIS

CAUSES
Transmission of *Burkholderia pseudomallei* is most commonly through contact with infected soil or water, either by contamination of open wounds or cuts or by inhalation or ingestion. Person-to-person and animal-to-person transmission can occur but is very rare.

RISK FACTORS
The primary risk factor for melioidosis is exposure to the contaminated soil or water in endemic areas during the wet season or after periods of heavy rainfall in areas with high humidity or temperature.

 DIAGNOSIS

DIFFERENTIAL DIAGNOSIS
• Tuberculosis
• Caseous lymphadenitis
• Actinobacillosis

CBC/BIOCHEMISTRY/URINALYSIS
N/A

OTHER LABORATORY TESTS
N/A

IMAGING
N/A

DIAGNOSTIC PROCEDURES
• Diagnosis of melioidosis is difficult but may be suspected at necropsy (see below).
• Although there are no pathognomonic lesions for the disease, isolation and identification of the organism should be attempted from swabs of nasal discharge and/or abscesses.
• Organisms may also be found in the feces or milk of infected animals.
• Additionally, serological tests (e.g., ELISA, indirect hemagglutination tests, and immunofluorescent tests) may also be used for diagnosis; however, cross-reactions can occur with *B. mallei* (causative agent for glanders).

PATHOLOGIC FINDINGS
• On necropsy, multiple abscesses may be found in any organ, but particularly the lungs, liver, spleen, and lymph nodes.
• Purulent material from the abscesses is thick or caseous and green tinged.
• Polyarthritis may also be seen.

 TREATMENT

Treatment is often expensive, prolonged, and unsuccessful. Prevention of the disease is the best method of approach.

APPROPRIATE HEALTH CARE
N/A

NURSING CARE
N/A

ACTIVITY
N/A

DIET
N/A

CLIENT EDUCATION
There is a potential zoonotic risk to humans with this disease, so precautions should be taken.

SURGICAL CONSIDERATIONS
N/A

 MEDICATIONS

DRUGS OF CHOICE
Tetracycline may be tried, but antibiotic therapy is usually unsuccessful.

CONTRAINDICATIONS

Appropriate milk and meat withdrawal times must be followed for all compounds administered to food-producing animals.

PRECAUTIONS

N/A

POSSIBLE INTERACTIONS

N/A

ALTERNATIVE DRUGS

N/A

 FOLLOW-UP

PATIENT MONITORING

N/A

PREVENTION/AVOIDANCE

• Remove animals from any contaminated source.
• Raise animals from ground/soil via wooden slats, concrete, or paved floors.
• Use chlorinated water supply.
• The microorganism *Burkholderia pseudomallei* is killed by heat.

POSSIBLE COMPLICATIONS

N/A

EXPECTED COURSE AND PROGNOSIS

N/A

 MISCELLANEOUS

ASSOCIATED CONDITIONS

N/A

AGE-RELATED FACTORS

N/A

ZOONOTIC POTENTIAL

• Melioidosis is considered a zoonotic disease, however, transmission of the organism to humans from animals is considered very rare.
• Most cases acquired by humans are from environmental (contaminated soil or water) infection (i.e., aerosolization or direct contact with open wounds).

PREGNANCY

N/A

RUMINANT SPECIES AFFECTED

Sheep, goats

BIOSECURITY

• See Prevention /Avoidance above.
• Isolation and quarantine of new stock entering the herd/flock
• Cull new animals for disease conditions prior to herd introduction.

PRODUCTION MANAGEMENT

SYNONYMS

Pseudoglanders
Whitmore disease

SEE ALSO

Actinobacillosis
Caseous lymphadenitis
Tuberculosis

ABBREVIATIONS

ELISA = enzyme-linked immunosorbent assay

Suggested Reading
Aiello, S. E., ed. 1998. *Merck veterinary manual*. 8th ed. Whitehouse Station, NJ: Merck and Co.
Choy, J. L., Mayo, M., Janmaat, A., Currie, B. J. 2000. Animal melioidosis in Australia. *Acta Tropica* 74:153–158.
Dance, D. A. 2000, Feb 5. Ecology of *Burkholderia pseudomallei* and the interactions between environmental *Burkholderia* spp. and human-animal hosts. *Acta Trop.* 74(2–3):159–68.
Inglis, T. J., Foster, N. F., Gal, D., Powell, K., Mayo, M., Norton, R., Currie, B. J. 2004, Oct. Preliminary report on the northern Australian melioidosis environmental surveillance project. *Epidemiol Infect.* 132(5):813–20.

Author: Glenda Dvorak

METABOLIC PROFILING

BASICS

OVERVIEW
• A "metabolic profile" is defined as a series of specific analytical tests run in combination and used as a diagnostic aid. Use of a metabolic profile is the result of technologic improvements in analytical instrumentation, which can complete multiple analyses in a short time period.
• Application of this diagnostic procedure on a herd basis has been questioned relative to its validity and sensitivity in defining a problem as well as its cost.
  • Although diet and metabolic status influence fertility, many other factors confound interpretation.
  • Diet influences nutritional status, but interpretation of metabolic parameters relative to diet must be undertaken under controlled sampling procedures and with an understanding of underlying physiology and metabolism.
• In-spite-of past concerns about validity of metabolic profiling, recent advances in our understanding of physiologic and metabolic changes associated with the transition from pregnancy to lactation and improved metabolic tests have increased the diagnostic potential of metabolic profiling.

SYSTEMS AFFECTED
All systems can be potentially affected

GENETICS
N/A

INCIDENCE/PREVALENCE
N/A

GEOGRAPHIC DISTRIBUTION
Worldwide

SIGNALMENT
Species
Potentially all ruminant species are affected by metabolic diseases

Breed Predilections
N/A

Mean Age and Range
N/A

Predominant Sex
N/A

DIAGNOSIS

CBC/BIOCHEMISTRY/URINALYSIS

OTHER LABORATORY TESTS

Rationale for Test Use
• Blood analytes are influenced by nutritional and metabolic state of the animal. Relationship between dietary intake and blood nutrient concentrations have been well documented in experimental research under controlled conditions.
• Metabolic profiling can potentially provide a more direct confirmatory evaluation of metabolic health in relation to nutrition.
• *Assess nutritional status of feeding group or herd.* Ration evaluation is the cornerstone of herd nutritional assessment, but can be fraught with uncertainty. Metabolic profiling can be used to complement dietary evaluation procedure.
  • Evaluate current feeding program adequacy.
  • Evaluate response to a change in feeding program.
• *Identify potential risk for disease problems.* Specific blood analytes that are either high or low relative to reference values prior to calving or immediately postpartum can predict potential for increased risk of having periparturient disease problems.
• *Identify disease conditions early.* Metabolic profiling can be used to assess prevalence of subclinical metabolic disease in the absence of obvious clinical disease problems.
• *Survey for potential causes of disease problems.* Metabolic profiling can be used as a screening tool to direct the focus of a herd investigation. Results do not necessarily suggest diet is the problem source, but can help to focus more intensive investigation of potential causes of a current problem.

Application
• Metabolic profiling should not be a stand-alone diagnostic test, but part of an integrated diagnostic system including the following:
  • *Records analysis*—provides a historical and present perspective on the herd including animal inventories, clinical disease prevalence, production, milk composition, dry matter intake, and youngstock.
  • *Animal evaluation*—General appearance and attitude, cud chewing activity, body condition scoring, manure characteristics, and lameness scoring.
  • *Facilities evaluation*—Ventilation, cow comfort assessment (overcrowding, stall usage), stall design (size and bedding type), feed bunk design (space per animal, management), and water (sources, availability and quality).
• *Dietary evaluation*—for diets on the farm
  1. Formulated diet is the one generated as the goal for feeding. To evaluate, compare nutrient composition to NRC recommendations adjusted to environment.
  2. Mixed and delivered diet is the one placed into the feed bunk for consumption. To evaluate, compare nutrient density to formulated diet and particle size to individual ingredients. Also evaluate consistency of mix within feed bunk.
  3. Consumed diet is that portion of the delivered diet consumed by the cows. To evaluate, compare nutrient content and particle size between delivered and refused feed in bunk.
  4. Digested and absorbed diet is the proportion of the consumed diet that is available to the cow to support metabolic functions. To evaluate, compare production response to predictions of dynamic rumen models or use metabolic profiling.

Species Orientation

• Herd-based use of metabolic profiling has predominately been applied to dairy farms
• Larger dairy farms (>150 milking cows) are generally more willing to utilize metabolic profiling as a diagnostic tool as they can distribute the cost over more animals and can gain more opportunity dollars in preventing disease.
• Concepts and principles of metabolic profiling can be applied to other agricultural production systems including beef cattle, sheep flocks and goatherds.

Limitations

• *Costs*—Total costs associated with metabolic profiling may limit the use of this diagnostic testing strategy. Costs will range from $17 to $50 per sample depending upon the number of blood analytes measured. One can either reduce the number of tests or number of sampled animals to reduce costs, but this will compromise the quality of information to be derived. Diagnostic laboratories at a subsidized cost of $200–$400 offer traditional Compton Metabolic Profiles or some variation thereof.
• *Herd size*—Smaller herds, especially those of less than 100 cows will not have a large enough population of animals to be sampled within a defined physiologic state.
• *Availability*—A limited number of laboratories provide metabolic profiling and interpretation, especially in the United States.
• *Interpretation of results*—Blood analyte concentrations for metabolic profiling must be interpreted differently than for individual animal disease diagnosis. Different reference ranges must be developed.

• *Analyte variability*—A variety of factors can introduce variability into blood analyte concentrations and reduce ability to interpret differences relative to nutritional status. A number of important variability factors can be controlled by careful grouping strategies and sample collection and handling, thus maximizing the observed differences primarily due to environment, namely nutrition.
  • Random biologic variation
  • Genetic variation
  • Physiologic state (i.e., growth, lactation stage, gestation stage)
  • Circadian or seasonal variation
  • Health status
  • Sampling error or mishandling—especially hemolysis
  • Analytical technique—variation in laboratory methods
  • Environment—herd-specific nutrition and management

DIAGNOSTIC EVALUATION

Approach

Although inherently similar relative to the use of automated determinations of blood analytes, metabolic profiling is a different approach compared to diagnostic clinical chemistry analyses ("serum profiles").
• Blood chemistry profiles are commonly used in all veterinary hospitals as an aid in diagnosis of individual animal health problems.
  • Population selected for blood sampling is sick animals.
  • Results are compared to standard laboratory reference ranges (healthy population mean two standard deviations) to determine those outside the reference range.
  • Identified abnormal blood analytes are used to diagnose disease conditions (i.e., hypocalcemia, ketosis, hypoglycemia).

• Metabolic profiling uses these same blood analytes to assess potential for metabolic disease and nutritional status.
  • Population selected for blood sampling is a large number of healthy animals within specified age and physiologic groups within the herd.
  • Controlled research has shown specific blood analytes to reflect dietary intake
  • Metabolic profiling can be used to assess group/herd nutritional status and potential risk for disease problems.

Methods Used

• Metabolic profiling should not be a random sample collection process followed by measurements of various blood analytes. One should have a plan in mind in approaching a problem.
  • Define a problem by asking a specific question relative to a problem. This is akin to defining a scientific hypothesis and then setting up an experimental design to test the hypothesis.
  • Consider pertinent comparisons of interest relative to the defined problem and identify which populations of animals are of concern.
• Survey evaluation—Use of metabolic profiling as a broad-based diagnostic tool to identify potential problem areas or assess overall nutritional status.
  • Individual sampling
    1. Randomly select an appropriate number (7–10) of "healthy" cows within defined parity and physiologic stage-based groups for evaluation.
    2. Measured analytes can be interpreted relative to calculated mean value compared to reference value or percentage of individuals above or below a defined threshold value.
    3. Due to cost constraints, either number of groups tested or analyte numbers are reduced, thus limiting the scope of the metabolic profile.

METABOLIC PROFILING

- Pooled sample technique
  1. Individual samples can be pooled by defined groupings and a "mean" value determined by analysis.
  2. By pooling samples, you are obtaining information from a greater number of animals for much less cost.
  3. Limitations to this methodology are loss of statistical evaluation (i.e., population variance) and issues of interpretation.
- Targeted diagnostics—Use of specific individual tests to identify potential disease problems.
  - Threshold criteria—measured analyte has a defined value in which samples either above or below this value suggest increased risk for a disease process. Collect 12 samples and if 3 or more samples are beyond the threshold value, then the sampled population is at risk for a given disease process.
    1. NEFA—values greater than 0.4 mEq/L in prefresh cows are suggestive of potential risk for a variety of postpartum metabolic diseases.
    2. BHB—values greater than 14.4 mg/dl (1.4 mmol/L) in fresh cows are suggestive of subclinical ketosis problems in the herd.
    3. Rumen pH—values less than 5.5 pH units in any cow are suggestive of subacute ruminal acidosis problems.

- Mean analysis—measured analyte can be interpreted as a mean for a defined group of animals relative to a predefined reference range. Group means can both be above or below the reference range and be associated with problems.
  1. Urea nitrogen—mean values below 10 mg/dl and above 16 mg/dl are of concern.
  2. Urine pH—mean values should be between 6.5 and 7.0 or 6.0 and 6.5 pH units for prefresh Holstein or Jersey cows, respectively.

Animal Selection
- For metabolic profiling, the selected population of cows to be sampled should be apparently "healthy" cows. Cows without clinical disease signs may have metabolic measures consistent with subclinical disease, which may be masked when combined with results from clinical disease cows.
- To address a fresh cow problem, samples are collected from:
  - Early dry cows: defined as > 10 days following dry-off and < 30 days prior to expected calving
  - Close-up dry cows: defined as 3 to 21 days prior to expected calving
  - Fresh cows: defined as 3 to 30 days in milk
- To address a specific disease problem: clinically affected cows can be sampled and compared to normal cows that are matched according to parity and stage of lactation.

Sample Collection Procedures
- Blood samples should be taken from either jugular or coccygeal veins with a minimal amount of stress. Lower concentrations of P and K have been documented in jugular compared to coccygeal blood samples as a result of salivary gland uptake. Blood samples from the mammary veins are not appropriate given the loss of nutrients into the mammary gland.
- Time of sampling relative to feeding and feeding management may also influence metabolite concentrations and should be considered in the decision process of when to sample.
  - NEFA, glucose are best sampled prior to first feeding.
  - BHB, UN are best sampled 3 to 5 hours following a feeding.
- If herds are being repeatedly sampled as a monitoring tool, samples should be taken at approximately the same time of day to minimize diurnal and prandial variation.
- Vacuum tubes are colored coded for specific diagnostic test procedures based on the specific anticoagulant or additive present in the tube (Table 1). Plasma from green-top tubes is generally preferred, but red-top (serum) tubes can be used. It is best to ask the laboratory which sample is preferred.

Table 1

Stopper Color	Additive	Sample Obtained	Intended Use/Disadvantages
		Description of Blood Collection Tubes Used for Metabolic Profiles	
Red	None	Serum	Routine use for all tests. Prolonged clot exposure results in increased glucose, Ca and decreased phosphorus. Hemolysis problems in poorly handled samples.
Gray	Na fluoride or K oxalate	Serum	Glycolytic Inhibitor for sensitive glucose analysis
Royal blue	Plastic stopper Na heparin	Serum, plasma or whole blood	Trace mineral analysis, especially Zn
Lavender	EDTA	Whole blood, plasma	Routine use for Complete Blood Count/EDTA chelates Ca, Mg, and increased enzyme activities.
Green	Na heparin	Plasma, whole blood	Routine analyses for either plasma or whole blood / no effect on metabolites

• Extreme efforts should be taken to prevent hemolysis of the sample. All samples should be iced, but not frozen, immediately after collection and kept refrigerated until processed. For serum samples, the clot should be removed as quickly as possible (within hours of collection).

• All samples should be properly identified with animal and group identification and date of collection.

• Other pertinent information for interpretation of the metabolic profile would include animal age, lactation number, milk production level, milk composition, days in milk, pregnancy status, and body condition score.

 MISCELLANEOUS

ASSOCIATED CONDITIONS
N/A

AGE-RELATED FACTORS
N/A

ZOONOTIC POTENTIAL
N/A

PREGNANCY
N/A

RUMINANT SPECIES AFFECTED
Potentially, all ruminant species are affected.

BIOSECURITY
N/A

PRODUCTION MANAGEMENT
See above

SEE ALSO
Bovine blood chemistry
Differential diagnosis: philosophy of test usage
Rumen dysfunction: acidosis

ABBREVIATIONS
AST = aspartate aminotransferase
BHB = β-hydroxybutyrate
Ck = creatine kinase
Cr = creatinine
GGT = γ-glutamyltransferase
NEFA = nonesterified fatty acids
SDH = sorbitol dehydrogenase
UN = urea nitrogen

Suggested Reading
Herdt, T. H. 2000. Variability characteristics and test selection in herd-level nutritional and metabolic profile testing. *Vet Clinics NA: Food Anim Pract.* 16(2): 387–403.
Herdt, T. H., Dart, B., Neuder, L. 2001. Will large dairy herds lead to the revival of metabolic profile testing? *AABP Proceedings* 34:27–34.
Herdt, T. H., Rumbeiha, W., Braselton, W. E. 2000. The use of blood analyses to evaluate mineral status in livestock. *Vet Clinics NA: Food Anim Pract.* 16(3): 423–44.
Ingraham, R. H., Kappel, L. C. 1988. Metabolic profile testing. *Vet Clinics NA: Food Animal Pract.* 4(2): 391–411.
Oetzel, G. R. 2003. Herd-based biologic testing for metabolic disorders. Available at: http://www.vetmed.wisc.edu/dms/fapm/fapmtools/2nutr/herdtest.pdf, Accessed August 16, 2004.
Van Saun, R. J. 1997. Nutritional profiles: a new approach for dairy herds. *Bov Pract.* 31(2): 43–50.
Van Saun, R. J., Wustenberg, M. 1997. Metabolic profiling to evaluate nutritional and disease status. *Bov Pract.* 31(2): 37–42.

Author: Robert J. Van Saun

METALDEHYDE TOXICOSIS

BASICS

OVERVIEW
• Metaldehyde poisoning is characterized by the abrupt onset of severe neurologic signs.
• Metaldehyde is widely used for the control of slugs and snails. In some countries (outside the United States), metaldehyde is also used as a solid fuel in camping stoves and lamps.
• Available formulations include pellets, granules, liquids, or wettable powder. Baits may also contain other pesticides such as insecticides. The concentration of metaldehyde in baits sold in the United States is generally between 1.5% and 5%.
• Metaldehyde poisoning in ruminants is reported infrequently but has occurred in cattle, sheep, and goats.
• The onset of clinical effects may occur as soon as 30 to 60 minutes after ingestion and death may be seen as soon as 1 hour.
• The poisoning is commonly referred to as the "shake and bake syndrome" because of the development of tremors and hyperthermia in affected animals.
• Metaldehyde toxicosis results in the disruption of the GABA-ergic system and may also involve other neurotransmitters.
• The oral lethal dose of metaldehyde in sheep is estimated to be 300 mg/kg body weight and 200 mg/kg body weight in cattle.

SIGNALMENT
• All ruminant species are susceptible to metaldehyde.
• Cases in cattle, sheep, and goats are reported infrequently. Most reported cases involve dogs.

SIGNS
• Signs of poisoning generally begin within 30 to 60 minutes of exposure.
• Initial clinical signs include salivation, tremors of the fore and hind legs, staggering, and respiratory distress.

• This is quickly followed by weakness, ataxia, hyperventilation, hyperthermia, and convulsions. In severe cases, the animals become recumbent, unconscious, and show continuous convulsions with leg paddling.
• Disseminated intravascular coagulation may occur as a result of severe hyperthermia (body temperature may reach 110°F).
• Death may occur within 60 minutes of exposure as a result of respiratory failure.

CAUSES AND RISK FACTORS
• Geographic areas with a high slug and snail population present a greater risk due to the increased use of metaldehyde baits.
• Bran or molasses is commonly added to the bait to increase its palatability. However, some baits have chemicals added to make them less likely to be ingested by species other than slugs and snails.
• Wild ruminants with access to metaldehyde baits are at risk.

DIAGNOSIS

DIFFERENTIAL DIAGNOSIS
• Cyanide toxicosis—initially bright cherry-red blood, history of exposure to cyanide-containing plants
• Nitrate toxicosis—chocolate-brown discoloration of blood, history of exposure to nitrate-containing plants
• Lead poisoning—determination of blood lead concentration
• Organophosphorus or carbamate insecticide exposure—commonly associated with gastrointestinal upset and neurological signs, evaluation of cholinesterase activity, detection of pesticides in gastrointestinal contents
• Exposure to neurotoxic plants, such as poison hemlock, water hemlock, tree tobacco, lupine—history of presence of plants in the environment and identification of plant parts in gastrointestinal contents, chemical analysis for plant toxins in gastrointestinal contents

• Exposure to cardiotoxic plants, such as oleander, milkweed, and azalea—chemical analysis for plant toxins in gastrointestinal contents, history of presence of plants in the environment
• Nonprotein nitrogen toxicosis—history of NPN supplements in the feed ration, detection of toxic levels of ammonia in rumen content and blood
• Strychnine toxicosis—history of exposure to strychnine-containing bait, detection of strychnine in gastrointestinal contents or liver
• 4-Aminopyridine—history of exposure to the avicide, detection of 4-aminopyridine in gastrointestinal contents
• Neurotoxic blue-green algae toxins—peracute onset, access to pond water, detection of anatoxin-A in gastrointestinal contents
• Seizures—nontoxic etiologies (e.g., trauma, neoplasia, infection, metabolic disorder)

CBC/BIOCHEMISTRY/URINALYSIS
• No specific clinical pathologic changes occur.
• Metabolic acidosis may be present.

OTHER LABORATORY TESTS
Detection of metaldehyde in serum, urine, rumen content, or liver. Confirmation of metaldehyde in suspect material.

IMAGING
N/A

DIAGNOSTIC PROCEDURES
N/A

PATHOLOGIC FINDINGS
• There are no clearly distinctive changes due to the rapidity of death.
• Generalized renal, hepatic, and pulmonary congestion.
• Petechial and ecchymotic hemorrhages in the heart, lung, and gastrointestinal tract.
• Metaldehyde has a characteristic odor of formaldehyde that may be present in the rumen contents along with bait material.

TREATMENT

- Metaldehyde poisoning progresses so rapidly that immediate treatment is necessary.
- Control of CNS signs and hyperthermia is essential. Decontamination with activated charcoal should be considered after initial stabilization of the poisoned animal.
- Fluid therapy should be instituted to control acidosis and dehydration.
- Any possible stress should be avoided.

MEDICATIONS

DRUGS OF CHOICE
- No antidote available
- Pentobarbital at 20–30 mg/kg IV or diazepam at 0.5–1.5 mg/kg IV for control of seizures
- Lactated Ringer's or sodium bicarbonate solutions IV
- Activated charcoal at 2 g/kg orally

CONTRAINDICATIONS
- Pentobarbital can cause respiratory depression.
- Appropriate milk and meat withdrawal times must be followed for all compounds administered to food-producing animals.

POSSIBLE INTERACTIONS

FOLLOW-UP

PATIENT MONITORING
Monitor progression of clinical signs

PREVENTION/AVOIDANCE
- Avoid metaldehyde-containing baits in areas accessible to livestock.
- Use bait according to label instructions.
- Consider the use of less-toxic alternatives to control slugs and snails.

POSSIBLE COMPLICATIONS
Renal and hepatic disease may develop if poisoned animal survives the initial convulsive phase.

EXPECTED COURSE AND PROGNOSIS
- Animals poisoned with metaldehyde may be found dead.
- Metaldehyde poisoning progresses so rapidly that treatment is often too late. In most cases, the affected animals have a poor-to-grave prognosis.
- If treatment is initiated promptly after the onset of clinical signs, the prognosis is fair.

MISCELLANEOUS

ASSOCIATED CONDITIONS
Concurrent toxicosis from other herbicides or pesticides that are sometimes mixed in (most commonly carbamate insecticides)

AGE-RELATED FACTORS
N/A

ZOONOTIC POTENTIAL
N/A

PREGNANCY
N/A

RUMINANT SPECIES AFFECTED
Cattle, sheep, goats, deer, camelids

BIOSECURITY
N/A

PRODUCTION MANAGEMENT
Avoid metaldehyde-containing baits in areas accessible to livestock.

SEE ALSO
4-Aminopyridine
Cyanide toxicosis
Exposure to cardiotoxic plants such as oleander, milkweed, and azalea
Exposure to neurotoxic plants such as poison hemlock, water hemlock, tree tobacco, lupine
Lead poisoning
Neurotoxic blue-green algae
Nitrate
Nonprotein nitrogen toxicosis
Organophosphorus or carbamate insecticide exposure
Seizures—nontoxic etiologies (e.g., trauma, neoplasia, infection, metabolic disorder)
Strychnine toxicosis

ABBREVIATIONS
CNS = central nervous system
GABA = gamma aminobutyric acid
IV = intravenous
NPN = nonprotein nitrogen

Suggested Reading
Booze, T. F., Oehme, F. W. 1985. Metaldehyde toxicity: a review. *Vet Hum Toxicol.* 27:11–19.
Puschner, B. Metaldehyde. In: *Small animal toxicology*, ed. M. E. Peterson, P. A. Talcott. Philadelphia: W.B. Saunders.
Talcott, P. A. 2004. Metaldehyde. In: *Clinical veterinary toxicology*, ed. K. H. Plumlee. St. Louis: Mosby.

Author: Birgit Puschner

METRITIS

 BASICS

OVERVIEW
- Metritis is an inflammation of all layers (endometrium, myometrium, and serosa) of the uterus during the postpartum period.
- This condition is more commonly seen in dairy cattle.
- Economic losses from metritis are associated with systemic diseases that occur during the first few weeks postpartum.
- Affected cows become pyretic, have a fetid purulent discharge from the uterus, and in some cases the condition can become septic and life threatening. In addition, cows with metritis are more likely to develop other postpartum disorders such as ketosis, displacement of the abomasum, endometritis, and pyometra.
- Cows with metritis usually go off feed, produce less milk, and experience a delay in days to first service, lower conception rates, and increased days open.

PATHOPHYSIOLOGY
- The vulva, vulvar sphincter, and cervix are mechanical barriers that protect the uterus from bacterial contamination. However, during parturition and shortly thereafter, these barriers break down and allow pathogenic and nonpathogenic bacteria to contaminate the uterus. Most of these bacteria are transient residents and are eliminated by the defense mechanisms of the uterus.
- The bacterial population is mixed and consists of both aerobic and anaerobic gram-negative and gram-positive organisms.
- The most common organisms associated with metritis are *Arcanobacterium* (*Actinomyces*) *pyogenes, Fusobacterium necrophorum, Bacteroides melaninogenicus, Escherichia coli,* and *Staphylococcus aureus.* Bacteroides decreases chemotaxis-inhibiting phagocytosis by neutrophils allowing *A. pyogenes* to persist. Occasionally, *Clostridium* spp. infects the uterus and causes a gangrenous metritis.
- In cows with a normal parturition, the uterus resolves the bacterial infection by 4 weeks postpartum. However, in cows affected with dystocia, retained fetal membranes, and delivery of twins, the bacterial contamination may become more severe and persistent.
- Unsanitary calving conditions and traumatic obstetrical manipulation can also predispose the cow to uterine infections.
- Because of differences in husbandry practices and stress from lactation, postpartum metritis is more commonly seen in dairy cows than beef cows.

SYSTEMS AFFECTED
- Endocrine/metabolic
- Herd health
- Reproductive

GENETICS
Due to differences in calving environment and stress from lactation, metritis is more commonly seen in dairy than in beef cattle or other ruminant species.

INCIDENCE/PREVALENCE
- The postpartum incidence of metritis varies among reports and with the definition criteria used for diagnosis.
- A mean of 17% with a range of 8.8% to 24% has been reported. About one-half of the cows with an abnormal parturition (dystocia, retained fetal membranes, twins) can be expected to develop metritis.

GEOGRAPHIC DISTRIBUTION
Worldwide; in hot, warmer climates the incidence of metritis may be higher due to the effect of heat stress.

SIGNALMENT

Species
More commonly seen in bovine than in caprine or ovine species.

Breed Predilection
Dairy cattle

Mean Age and Range
Reports are conflicting as to the effect of parity on incidence. However, most agree that the incidence is higher in primiparous than multiparous animals.

SIGNS

GENERAL COMMENTS
- Clinical signs of metritis are influenced by the virulence of the bacteria and predisposing risk factors.
- During the first few weeks postpartum, lochia is normally expelled from the reproductive tract. Lochia is red to brown in color and should not be considered abnormal.
- Discharges from the reproductive tract should only be considered abnormal when they are fetid, serous, or purulent with accompanying systemic signs.

HISTORICAL FINDINGS
Metritis occurs more commonly in those cows that experienced an abnormal parturition and they should be monitored carefully during the first 2 weeks postpartum. Affected cows are usually off feed, have low milk production, and appear depressed.

PHYSICAL EXAMINATION FINDINGS
- Fever (> 103.0°F or 39.4°C)
- Partial or complete anorexia
- Low milk production
- Lethargy or depression
- Fetid serosanguineous discharge from the reproductive tract
- Ketosis
- Displaced abomasum
- Mastitis

RISK FACTORS
- Fat or overconditioned animals
- Retained fetal membranes
- Dystocia
- Twins
- Abortion
- Weather

 DIAGNOSIS

DIFFERENTIAL DIAGNOSIS
- Normal discharge from the uterus or lochia
- Endometritis

CBC/BIOCHEMISTRY/URINALYSIS
- In cows with a septic metritis, a degenerative left shift accompanied with a neutropenia
- Hypocalcemia
- Hypoglycemia
- Ketonemia

OTHER LABORATORY TESTS
Bacterial culture and sensitivity

IMAGING
Real-time ultrasonography can be used to illustrate postpartum uterine changes related to infection.
- Uterine lumen fluid associated with infection contains echogenic particles.
- Uterine wall appears more thickened.

DIAGNOSTIC PROCEDURES
A vaginal examination with a speculum can be used to characterize the type of exudates from the uterus.

PATHOLOGIC FINDINGS
Necropsy findings in cows that die from toxic or septic metritis: peritonitis; friable, gangrenous uterus

TREATMENT

APPROPRIATE HEALTH CARE
• Because of the differences in diagnostic criteria and the lack of controlled studies, treatment of this condition remains controversial among clinicians.
• Most cases of metritis do not require inpatient medical management and can be successfully treated and managed medically on the farm.
• Therapy generally includes antibiotics (systemic and or intrauterine) and hormonal and supportive treatment for hypocalcemia or ketosis.

NURSING CARE
Fluid and electrolyte replacement therapy may be indicated in cows with septic or toxic metritis.

ACTIVITY
N/A

DIET
N/A

CLIENT EDUCATION
Clients should be educated on management strategies to help reduce risk factors in parturient animals.

SURGICAL CONSIDERATION
N/A

MEDICATIONS

DRUGS OF CHOICE
• A variety of broad-spectrum antibiotics is recommended for systemic administration in cows with metritis, particularly those that are pyretic. Label recommendations to avoid antibiotic residues in salable milk should be followed when systemic antibiotics are used.
  • Penicillin or a synthetic analog: 20,000 to 30,000 IU/kg bid
  • Ceftiofur: 1–2.2 mg/kg bid
• Intrauterine antibiotic administrations with penicillin or oxytetracycline are used by some clinicians with questionable efficacy. The author is not aware of any antibiotic that is approved for intrauterine use in the United States.

CONTRAINDICATIONS
• Systemic oxytetracycline is not recommended because of difficulty in reaching the minimal inhibitory concentration required for *A. pyogenes* in the uterine lumen.
• Appropriate milk and meat withdrawal times must be followed for all compounds administered to food-producing animals.

PRECAUTIONS
Sanitary conditions and prevention of genital tract trauma must be carefully considered when intrauterine antibiotics are used.

POSSIBLE INTERACTIONS
N/A

ALTERNATIVE DRUGS
Hormones such as estrogens and oxytocin have been used to increase uterine contractions and help evacuate uterine contents.
• Research is lacking that supports the use of these hormones for the treatment of metritis.
• Estrogenic compounds have been used to improve uterine contractions. Contractions induced by estrogen have been associated with flushing septic uterine contents into the uterine tubes.
• Oxytocin causes contraction of the postpartum uterus if it is used within 48 hours after calving. Doses of 20–40 IU repeated every 3 to 6 hours are generally used.

FOLLOW-UP

PATIENT MONITORING
Metritis patients should be monitored for development of ketosis, displaced abomasum, and mastitis. In addition, if the condition does not improve by 3 days of antibiotic treatment, an alternative antibiotic should be considered.

PREVENTION/ AVOIDANCE
• To prevent the incidence of risk factors, producers should follow routine monitoring of prepartum cow management strategies.
• Postpartum health monitoring during the first 2 weeks postpartum should include rectal temperature, milk production monitoring, and attitude to help diagnose and treat the condition early.

POSSIBLE COMPLICATIONS
• Septicemia
• Ketosis
• Displaced abomasum
• Mastitis

EXPECTED COURSE AND PROGNOSIS
Cows treated promptly can be expected to recover fully from metritis. However, milk production and reproductive performance are affected in the current lactation. In some cases, cows can develop uterine abscesses and pyometra.

MISCELLANEOUS

ASSOCIATED CONDITIONS
Ketosis, displaced abomasum

AGE-RELATED FACTORS
In general, incidence of metritis is greater in primiparous than multiparous animals.

ZOONOTIC POTENTIAL
N/A

PREGNANCY
Metritis occurs in postpartum animals.

RUMINANT SPECIES AFFECTED
Cattle, ovine, caprine

BIOSECURITY
N/A

PRODUCTION MANAGEMENT
Clients should be educated and instructed on appropriate management strategies affecting the transition animal to help prevent metritis.

SYNONYMS
Metritis should be differentiated from endometritis and pyometra.

SEE ALSO
Cesarean operation
Displaced abomasum
Endometritis
Ketosis
Mastitis
Pyometra
Septicemia

ABBREVIATIONS
IU = international units

Suggested Reading
Bondurant, R. H. 1999. Inflammation in the bovine female reproductive tract. *J Anim Sci*. 77: suppl. 2, 101–10.
Markusfeld, O. 1987. Periparturient traits in seven high dairy herds. Incidence rates, association with parity, and interrelationships among traits. *J Dairy Sci*. 70:158.
Markusfeld, O. 1984. Factors responsible for post parturient metritis in dairy cattle. *Vet Rec*. 114:539.
Olson, J. D., Bretzlaff, K., Mortimer, R. G., Ball, L. 1986. The metritis-pyometra complex. In: *Current therapy in theriogenology*, ed. D. A. Morrow. Philadelphia: W. B. Saunders.
Younquist, R. S., Shore, M. D. 1997. Postpartum uterine infections. In: *Current therapy in large animal theriogenology*, ed. R. S. Youngquist. Philadelphia: W. B. Saunders.

Author: Carlos A. Risco

MICROPHTHALMIA

 BASICS

OVERVIEW
- The term "microphthalmia" encompasses all conditions where the globe, palpebral fissure, eyelids, and intraocular structures are abnormally small.
- This condition occurs occasionally and can be unilateral or bilateral.
- In severe cases, the microphthalmic eye may be represented only by a tiny, melanotic cyst, which is embedded in the orbit with a permanently closed eyelid. In less-severe forms, there may be a small, but well developed eye with normal vision; this is called nanophthalmia.
- Varying degrees of severity and functional deficits exist, and may be associated with one or multiple ocular structures affected.
- It may be associated with other body system anomalies, such as with posterior vertebral column disease in dairy and beef cattle.

PATHOPHYSIOLOGY
- Microphthalmia in Texel sheep has its lesional morphogenesis during embryonal development.
- In one study, the microphthalmic eyes showed an anteriorly located conus-shaped mass composed of connective tissue with cartilage, smooth muscle, and fat tissue, particularly in the posterior part of the conus, and often islets of lacrimal glands and cystic structures lined with squamous epithelium in the anterior part.
- The iris, ciliary body, and ciliary processes were incorporated in the periphery of the broad base of the conus. The study showed an abnormal development of the lens vesicle. In a later stage (45 days), a conus-shaped mass was seen in the anterior part of the eyes, which at 56 days consisted of mesenchymal tissue with focal differentiation to cartilage and epithelial structures in the anterior part of the conus. The primary event proved to be abnormal development of the lens vesicle, with disintegration of the lens and subsequent overgrowth of mesenchymal tissue. The mesenchymal tissue later differentiated in various directions, whereas the epithelial structures found in the microphthalmic eyes at days 56 and 132 and in the newborn lambs seemed to be remnants of the epithelial lens vesicle.

SYSTEMS AFFECTED
Ophthalmic

GENETICS
- Congenital microphthalmia has occurred in Texel sheep in New Zealand, and is likely inherited as an autosomal recessive trait.
- May be heritable in shorthorn cattle
- Often associated in Hereford cattle with congenital hydrocephalus and appears to be a simple autosomal recessive trait

INCIDENCE/PREVALENCE
- In one study, 10% of Texel sheep were found to carry the recessive gene defect.
- One or both eyes may be affected.

GEOGRAPHIC DISTRIBUTION
Microphthalmia occurs in all ruminants and has a worldwide distribution. It is one of the most frequently encountered ocular anomalies of ruminants.

SIGNALMENT
Species
Has been reported in sheep, goats, cattle, and white-tailed deer.

Breed Predilections
- Texel sheep and shorthorn cattle
- Often associated in Hereford cattle with congenital hydrocephalus and appears to be a simple autosomal recessive trait.

Mean Age and Range
N/A

Predominant Sex
N/A

CAUSES AND RISK FACTORS
- Multiple etiologies are suspected, including a genetic inherited defect in white shorthorn cattle and as a possible sequelae to teratogenic agent exposure.
- Often associated in Hereford cattle with congenital hydrocephalus and appears to be a simple autosomal recessive trait.
- May be a sequelae of calves born from cows with in utero infections of bovine viral diarrhea.
- *Veratrum californicum*, skunk cabbage, western hellebore, false hellebore, and wild corn may also predispose to microphthalmia. Alkaloids in the plant roots seem to affect globe development. Sheep are considered more susceptible than goats and goats more than cattle.

 DIAGNOSIS

DIFFERENTIAL DIAGNOSIS
- *Veratrum californicum*—skunk cabbage, western hellebore, false hellebore, wild corn
  - Sheep > goats > cattle
  - Alkaloids found in plant and concentrated in root (jervine, pseudojervine, veratrosine)
  - Globe abnormalities include anophthalmia, cyclopia, and synophthalmos
  - Highly susceptible on gestational day 14
  - On days 11,12,13,15, and 16, normally developed fetuses or embryos that die between 18th and 23rd day of development
- Selenium "blind staggers" in sheep
  - Microphthalmia, multiple cysts, colobomas, cornea, lens, iris defects; felt to be sulfur-related polioencephalomalacia (PEM)
- Maternal vitamin A deficiency: found in pigs; primarily microphthalmia; anophthalmos, macrophthalmia, retinal dysplasia may also occur.
- Other conditions
  - Bluetongue virus—sheep; ocular lesions induced by modified- live vaccine use in pregnant sheep
  - Bovine viral diarrhea—cataracts, retinal degeneration and dysplasia, optic nerve gliosis and neuritis, microphthalmia
  - Congenital cataracts reported in cattle, sheep, rare in goats. Autosomal recessive in several breeds: Jersey, Hereford, Holstein-Friesian. Can be associated with microphthalmia and retinal lesions from in utero exposure to BVD, 76–150 days of gestation
  - May be secondary to inflammation, toxins, metabolic disease
  - Cattle—secondary to IBK, malignant catarrhal fever, IBR

CBC/BIOCHEMISTRY/URINALYSIS
N/A

OTHER LABORATORY TESTS
N/A

IMAGING
N/A

OTHER DIAGNOSTIC PROCEDURES
N/A

PATHOLOGIC FINDINGS

• The microphthalmic eyes showed an anteriorly located conus-shaped mass composed of connective tissue with cartilage, smooth muscle, and fat tissue, particularly in the posterior part of the conus, and often islets of lacrimal glands and cystic structures lined with squamous epithelium in the anterior part.

• The iris, ciliary body, and ciliary processes were incorporated in the periphery of the broad base of the conus. The conus was covered by a detached and folded but normally developed retina. The morphogenetic study showed an abnormal development of the lens vesicle.

 TREATMENT

No treatment is available. Cull affected animals from the breeding herd/flock.

 FOLLOW-UP

EXPECTED COURSE AND PROGNOSIS

Grave, cull affected animals from the breeding herd/flock

 MISCELLANEOUS

ASSOCIATED CONDITIONS

• Varying degrees of severity and functional deficits exist, and may be associated with one or multiple ocular structures.

• May be associated with other body system anomalies, such as with posterior vertebral column disease in dairy and beef cattle.

AGE-RELATED FACTORS
N/A

ZOONOTIC POTENTIAL
N/A

PREGNANCY
N/A

RUMINANT SPECIES AFFECTED
Potentially, all ruminant species are affected.

BIOSECURITY
N/A

PRODUCTION MANAGEMENT
Possible genetic predisposition. Implement culling program.

SYNONYMS
Selenium "blind staggers" in sheep

SEE ALSO
Blindness
Bluetongue
Ectropion
Entropion
Selenium
Veratrum californicum

ABBREVIATIONS
BVD = bovine viral diarrhea
IBK = infectious bovine keratoconjunctivitis
IBR = infectious bovine rhinotracheitis
PEM = polioencephalomalacia

Suggested Reading
Cook, C. S. 1995. Emryogenesis of congenital eye malformations. *Vet Comp Opthalmol*. 5(2):109–23.
Fulton, A. B., Albert, D. M., Buyukmihci, N., Wyand, D. S., Stone, W. B. 1977, Oct. Spontaneous anophthalmia and microphthalmia in white-tailed deer. *J Comp Pathol*. 87(4):557–68.
Gelatt, K. N. 1976, Feb. Congenital ophthalmic anomalies in cattle. *Mod Vet Pract*. 57(2):105–9.
Jackson, E. K. 1990, Jun 30. Microphthalmia in sheep. *Vet Rec*. 126(26):650.
Leipold, H. W., Huston, K. 1968. Congenital syndrome of anophthalmia-microphthalmia with associated defects in cattle. *Pathol Vet*. 5(5):407–18.
van Der Linde-Sipman, J. S., van den Ingh, T. S., Vellema, P. 2003, May. Morphology and morphogenesis of hereditary microphthalmia in Texel sheep. *J Comp Pathol*. 128(4):269–75.

Author: Larry P. Occhipinti

MIDDLE UTERINE ARTERY RUPTURE

BASICS

OVERVIEW
• Middle uterine artery rupture is a rare, acute, life-threatening hemorrhagic event encountered in ruminants associated with parturition.
• Rupture is more commonly seen in association with forced fetal extraction or fetotomy compared to simple uncomplicated delivery.
• Rarely, it may accompany correction of uterine torsion using the "plank in the flank" technique.

SYSTEMS AFFECTED
Hemolymphatic

GENETICS
N/A

INCIDENCE/PREVALENCE
Unknown

GEOGRAPHIC DISTRIBUTION
N/A

SIGNALMENT
Species
Dairy cattle; potentially all ruminant species
Breed Predilections
N/A
Mean Age and Range
N/A
Predominant Sex
Female

SIGNS
• Sudden death during or soon after parturition may be the only signs noted.
• Severe blood loss anemia may give rise to tachycardia, tachypnea, and signs of anxiety immediately preceding death.
• Occasional cases may occur subsequent to uterine prolapse, particularly in multiparous cows; in these animals death may occur soon after, or during, repositioning of the everted uterus.

DIAGNOSIS

• Usually a postmortem diagnosis, demonstrating the location of the rupture within the uterine artery
• Antemortem it may be presumptive based upon severe pallor of mucous membranes and corroborative clinical evidence of anemia (elevated heart and respiratory rates) immediately following dystocia.
• Rectal palpation may reveal large soft tissue swelling (hematoma) within the broad ligament on the affected side.

• In cases of arterial rupture coincident with uterine rupture, hemorrhage may be evident at the vulva, but otherwise external evidence of hemorrhage is absent.
• Some less-severe cases are diagnosed days to weeks after parturition by incidental rectal findings of a soft tissue mass within the broad ligament and/or a corresponding defect or aneurysm in the miduterine artery.

DIFFERENTIAL DIAGNOSIS
• Acute blood loss anemia from other internal site (large abdominal, pelvic, or thoracic vessel hemorrhage)
• Acute septic peritonitis due to uterine rupture.

CBC/BIOCHEMISTRY/URINALYSIS
• Affected cattle may die so peracutely that diagnostic procedures are redundant.
• If the animal survives the first few hours, routine blood work may show evidence of blood loss anemia.

OTHER LABORATORY TESTS
N/A

IMAGING
Rectal ultrasound will show a variably sized heterogeneous soft tissue mass within the broad ligament on the affected side. Ultrasound may also demonstrate a defect in the affected miduterine artery.

DIAGNOSTIC PROCEDURES
N/A

PATHOLOGIC FINDINGS
• Grossly, the miduterine artery will be ruptured on the affected side with accompanying massive hemorrhage into the broad ligament.
• Hemoabdomen may also be noted grossly.
• Extreme pallor of mucous membranes

TREATMENT

• Whole blood transfusion (6–12 liters)
• Hypertonic saline given intravenously (2–4 ml/kg of 7% sodium chloride) may be of acute resuscitative value.
• Intravenous oxytocin (20–100 IU) to promote uterine contraction and involution—may be given repeatedly.
• Intravenous formalin—500 ml of normal saline to which 10 ml of formalin has been added; questionable value; contamination of meat and milk issues, no determined withhold time.
• Aminocarproic acid (10–20 mg/kg, diluted in 1 liter of normal saline and given slowly intravenously)
• Vessel ligation may be tried but will be possible only if a full thickness uterine tear accompanies miduterine artery rupture.
• Keep affected individuals in close confinement with box stall rest to promote clot formation and stabilization.

MEDICATIONS
N/A

CONTRAINDICATIONS
Appropriate milk and meat withdrawal times must be followed for all compounds administered to food-producing animals.

FOLLOW-UP
N/A

MISCELLANEOUS

ASSOCIATED CONDITIONS
Anemia and death

AGE-RELATED FACTORS
More common in multiparous dams

ZOONOTIC POTENTIAL
N/A

PREGNANCY
N/A

RUMINANT SPECIES AFFECTED
Only documented in cattle

BIOSECURITY
N/A

PRODUCTION MANAGEMENT
N/A

SEE ALSO
Acute blood loss anemia from other internal site (large abdominal, pelvic, or thoracic vessel hemorrhage)
Acute septic peritonitis due to uterine rupture

ABBREVIATIONS
IU = international units

Suggested Reading
Angelos, J. A., Anderson, B. H., Waurzyniak, B. J., Ames, T. R., Turner, T. A. 1995, Sep 1. Aneurysm of the cranial mesenteric artery in a cow. *J Am Vet Med Assoc.* 207(5): 623–25.
Roberts, S. J. 1986. Injuries and diseases of the puerperal period. In: *Veterinary obstetrics and genital diseases (theriogenology),* ed. S. J. Roberts. 3rd ed. Woodstock, VT: Published by the author.
Steverink, P. J., Kuiper, R., Gruys, E. 1995, Jan 21. Aneurysm of the cranial mesenteric artery in a cow. *Vet Rec.* 136(3): 69–72.

Author: Simon F. Peek.

MILK VEIN RUPTURE

BASICS

DEFINITION
Hemorrhage from the caudal superficial epigastric vein (milk vein).

PATHOPHYSIOLOGY
• The milk vein is a common site for veinapuncture by laypeople because it is very superficial cranial to the mammary gland on the ventral abdomen. It is an especially convenient vein for farmers and workers treating down cattle for conditions such as milk fever (hypocalcemia). The vessel is only thinly covered by skin and subcutaneous tissue.
• Perivascular hemorrhage or leakage of irritating products such as calcium, dextrose, or antimicrobials can cause small abscesses or fibrous tissues that weaken the covering over the milk vein, sometimes resulting in rupture.

SYSTEMS AFFECTED
Cardiovascular

SIGNALMENT
Species Affected
Bovine

Breed Predilections
N/A

Mean Age and Range
Usually adults after IV treatment

Predominant Sex
Females secondary to the propensity for hypocalcemia treatment

SIGNS
Bleeding from either of the caudal superficial epigastric veins

GENERAL COMMENTS
N/A

HISTORICAL FINDINGS
IV treatment in the milk vein some time prior to hemorrhage. May see an increased incidence during times of biting flies and other insect activity due to bunching of cattle and increased leg kicking for fly avoidance.

PHYSICAL EXAMINATION FINDINGS
Hemorrhage from milk vein

CAUSES
Weakened tissue superficial to the milk vein

RISK FACTORS
Conditions requiring IV treatments, such as hypocalcemia, ketosis, or some mastitis treatments. Farmers treating cattle IV in milking parlors without adequate restraint tend to favor the milk vein.

DIAGNOSIS

DIFFERENTIAL DIAGNOSIS
N/A

CBC/BIOCHEMISTRY/URINALYSIS
N/A

OTHER LABORATORY TESTS
N/A

IMAGING
N/A

OTHER DIAGNOSTIC PROCEDURES
N/A

GROSS AND HISTOPATHOLOGIC FINDINGS
Rupture in thin-walled area of milk vein

TREATMENT
Suture ruptured area. Suturing may be complicated by friable tissue. Fluid therapy or blood transfusion may be required.

INPATIENT VERSUS OUTPATIENT
N/A

CLIENT EDUCATION
Advise client not to utilize the milk vein for IV treatments.

MEDICATIONS

DRUGS OF CHOICE AND FLUIDS
Balanced electrolytes or whole blood transfusion if pale mucous membranes or low PCV.

CONTRAINDICATIONS
N/A

PRECAUTIONS
The rupture is often difficult to suture because of the friable tissue that resulted in the rupture. Purse-string sutures surrounding the friable area are often required. This is a medical emergency.

POSSIBLE INTERACTIONS
N/A

ALTERNATIVE DRUGS
N/A

FOLLOW-UP

PATIENT MONITORING
Recurrence of hemorrhage

PREVENTION/AVOIDANCE
Do not use milk vein for IV treatments. Control flies and insects.

POSSIBLE COMPLICATIONS
Hypovolemic shock and death

EXPECTED COURSE AND PROGNOSIS
Recovery, if vein is successfully sutured and hypovolemia is corrected.

MISCELLANEOUS

PREVENTION
N/A

ASSOCIATED CONDITIONS
N/A

AGE-RELATED FACTORS
Usually adult dairy cows

ZOONOTIC POTENTIAL
N/A

PREGNANCY
N/A

SYNONYMS
N/A

SEE ALSO
Fluid therapy
Lymphosarcoma
Mammary nodular hyperplasia

ABBREVIATIONS
IV = intravenous
PCV = packed cell volume

Suggested Reading
Davies, R. C. 1968, Nov. 16. Rupture of the mammary vein in the cow. *Vet Rec.* 83(20):528.
Giles, M. B. 1968, Sep 28. Hematomas over the mammary veins in cows. *Vet Rec.* 83(13):333.
Hong, C. B. 1994, Jan. Mammary nodular hyperplasia in a cow. *J Vet Diagn Invest.* 6(1): 116–8.
Swarbrick, O. 1968, Sep. 21. Hematoma over the mammary veins in cows. *Vet Rec.* 83(12): 305–6.

Author: James P. Reynolds

MILKWEED (*ASCLEPIAS* SPP.) TOXICOSIS

BASICS

OVERVIEW
• Toxicity associated with ingestion of one of many *Asclepias* spp. (milkweed)
• There are over 100 species of *Asclepias* spp. growing naturally in North America and all are potentially toxic.
• Two mechanisms of toxicity (1) cardiovascular and gastrointestinal toxicity associated with cardenolides (cardiac glycosides) and (2) neuromuscular toxicity associated with neurotoxic pregnane glycosides.
• Milkweed is considered to be one of the most toxic plants in North America and has been associated with mortality rates of greater then 50% in sheep grazing milkweed for 24 hours or less.
• Distribution of plants varies by species, however there is at least one species present over most of the continent.
• Two leaf types are present and vary in their expression of the relative amounts of toxins:
  • Wide leaf varieties (i.e., *A. speciosa* and *A. syriaca*) are more commonly associated with cardiac and gastrointestinal toxicity. Toxicity is less common as they are only eaten when no other feed choices are available.
  • Thin leaf (< 1 cm wide) varieties (i.e., *A. fascicularis* and *A. subverticillata*), which contain higher levels of the neurotoxin and are consumed more commonly due to their more palatable nature and the animal's difficulty in selectively not consuming them in hay.
• Plants are most toxic during rapid growth but retain their toxicity even when dried in hay. Toxicity tends to decrease with maturity.
• Clinical signs develop with consumption of 0.05%–2% of body weight depending on the species and toxin concentration of the plant
• The cardenolides produced by the wide leaf varieties inhibit the function of the Na^+/K^+-ATPase pump and allow accumulation of Na and Ca inside the cell and depletion of intracellular K. This leads to abnormal membrane potentials and irregular action potential initiation.
• The mechanism of action of the neurotoxin is not known.

SIGNALMENT
• Sheep are most commonly affected.
• Can occur in any ruminant species
• Cattle require ingestion of twice as much toxin as sheep.
• Animals are consuming toxin-producing forages either in the field green or in hay.

SIGNS
• Vary with the species of plant consumed (i.e., neurotoxin-producing thin leaf or cardiotoxin-producing wide leaf), amount consumed, and duration of toxicity.
• Acute death may be the only clinical sign.
• Signs generally develop within 12 to 18 hours of ingestion of cardiac glycosides and may be immediate or delayed (i.e., 12 hours) with ingestion of neurotoxic compounds.
• Cardiac glycoside (cardiac and gastrointestinal toxin) symptoms include depression, weakness, reluctance to stand, enteritis, bloat, labored respiration with grunt, and possibly cardiac arrhythmias.
• Neurotoxic symptoms include depression, mydriasis, ataxia, weakness, pelvic limb paresis, humped-up appearance, rabbitlike gait, seizures, opisthotonus, and death due to respiratory failure.

CAUSES AND RISK FACTORS
• Ingestion of toxin-containing *Asclepias* spp. in pastures or hay
• Ingestion of neurotoxic compounds may be cumulative.
• Cattle on ionophore-containing diets may have an increased risk.

DIAGNOSIS

DIFFERENTIAL DIAGNOSIS
• Other sources of cardiac glycosides, including dogbane, Indian hemp, lily of the valley, foxglove, and oleander
• Other cardiotoxic plants including yew, rhododendron, and laurels
• Other neurologic diseases including heavy metal toxicosis, buckeye toxicity, dallis grass toxicity, traumatic nerve damage (calving paralysis), spinal column lymphosarcoma, and rabies

• Other causes of recumbency including fractures, hypocalcemia, hypomagnesemia, hypophosphatemia, and hypokalemia.
• Other causes of cardiac arrhythmias including traumatic reticulopericarditis, electrolyte disorder associated atrial fibrillation, cardiac neoplasia

CBC/BIOCHEMISTRY/URINALYSIS
There may be an increase in serum creatinine kinase activity. However, this is not a specific indicator for milkweed toxicity.

OTHER LABORATORY TESTS
• Evaluation of the pasture or hay for evidence of milkweed contamination. Careful examination for the narrow leaf varieties must be done, as they are often hard to identify due to their similarity to grasses even when contained in large quantities in hay.
• Analysis of urine, serum, tissue, and stomach contents for cardiac glycosides is available using high-performance liquid chromatography.

IMAGING
Echocardiography would be helpful in excluding other differential diagnosis. However, it is technically challenging and requires expensive equipment and thus is not routinely done.

DIAGNOSTIC PROCEDURES
N/A

PATHOLOGIC FINDINGS
• Depends on the toxin consumed
• Cardiac glycoside toxicity is associated with a hyperemia with or without hemorrhage of the abomasum and small intestine, pulmonary congestion, acute ischemia associated glomerulopathy and tubular necrosis, and in some cases mild nonsuppurative myocardial cellular degeneration. Hemorrhage may be present on the surface of the lung, kidney, and heart.
• Ingestion of the neurotoxic compound is more difficult to determine on necropsy, but there may be evidence of external trauma; hemorrhages in the trachea, heart, and lungs; and often an empty urinary bladder.

MILKWEED (*ASCLEPIAS* SPP.) TOXICOSIS

TREATMENT

• If acute ingestion of large amounts of toxin are suspected, a rumenotomy to evacuate the ingesta may be beneficial.
• Other herd mates should be isolated from the source of the toxin (i.e., pasture or hay).

MEDICATIONS

DRUGS

• Orogastric intubation with activated charcoal, cathartics, or mineral oil may decrease intestinal absorption of the toxins and increase rate of excretion in feces.
• Administering balanced polyionic fluids as needed to maintain hydration and for renal diuresis may minimize effects of ischemic-induced kidney damage.
• Sedative and or anesthesia may be helpful in patients with severe convulsions associated with neurotoxin ingestion.
• Antiarrhythmic drugs such as procainamide, lidocaine, or atropine sulfate may be used in rare cases exhibiting arrhythmias. (Appropriate records for extralabel drug use must be maintained.)
• Appropriate drug withdrawal periods must be determined and maintained.

CONTRAINDICATIONS

Use of calcium-containing fluids is contraindicated as it may potentiate the affects of cardiac glycosides.

FOLLOW-UP

PATIENT MONITORING

• Evaluation of neurologic status and monitoring for seizure activity should be done frequently.

• Frequent auscultation of the heart should be performed to access for development of cardiac arrhythmias.
• Monitoring of urinalysis and serum chemistry for azotemia is indicated in patients that survive the acute toxicosis.

PREVENTION/AVOIDANCE

Prevent animals from grazing on pasture or eating hay containing milkweed.

POSSIBLE COMPLICATIONS

If the animals survive, they may develop acute to chronic renal failure.

EXPECTED COURSE AND PROGNOSIS

• Varies with amount of toxin ingested, duration of exposure, and response to treatment
• Most animals will start developing signs within 12 to 18 hours of ingesting toxin.
• If symptoms are severe, animals will often die within 24 hours.
• If animal develops seizures and convulsions, the prognosis is grave.
• If animals survive the first 24–36 hours, they often will remain weak for a period of time before improving

MISCELLANEOUS

ASSOCIATED CONDITIONS
N/A

AGE-RELATED FACTORS
N/A

ZOONOTIC POTENTIAL
N/A

PREGNANCY
N/A

RUMINANT SPECIES AFFECTED

• Sheep seem to be the most susceptible.
• All species of ruminants can become affected.

BIOSECURITY
N/A

PRODUCTION MANAGEMENT
N/A

SEE ALSO

Other cardiotoxic plants including yew, rhododendron, and laurel
Other causes of cardiac arrhythmias including traumatic reticulopericarditis, electrolyte disorder associated atrial fibrillation, cardiac neoplasia
Other causes of recumbency including fractures, hypocalcemia, hypomagnesemia, hypophosphatemia, and hypokalemia
Other neurologic diseases including heavy metal toxicosis, buckeye toxicity, dallis grass toxicity, traumatic nerve damage (calving paralysis), spinal column lymphosarcoma, and rabies
Other sources of cardiac glycosides including dogbane, Indian hemp, lily of the valley, foxglove, and oleander

ABBREVIATIONS
N/A

Suggested Reading

Benson, J. M., Seiber, J. N., Bagley, C. V., Keeler, R. F., Johnson, A. E., Young, S. 1979. Effects on sheep of the milkweeds *Asclepias eriocarpa* and *A. labriformis* and of cardiac glycoside-containing derivative material. *Toxicon.* 17(2):155–65.
Burrows, G. E., Tyrl, R. J., ed. 2001. *Toxic plants of North America*. Ames: Iowa State University Press.
Smith, R. A., Scharko, P., Bolin, D., Hong, C. B. 2000, Dec. Intoxication of sheep exposed to ozark milkweed (*Asclepias viridis* Walter). *Vet Hum Toxicol*. 42(6):349–50.

Author: Paul J. Plummer

MISCELLANEOUS CONDITIONS OF THE HOOF WALL

 BASICS

OVERVIEW
• There are some conditions that may affect the hoof wall of cattle that may result in severe lameness; however, most of the lesions are cosmetic with little significance for the animal, but because the lesions are so obvious to the producer they may be regarded as a serious problem.
• There are essentially three conditions of importance: (1) vertical fissures (sandcracks), (2) horizontal grooves (hardship lines), and (3) axial cracks.

SYSTEMS AFFECTED
Skin and musculoskeletal systems

GENETICS
N/A

INCIDENCE/PREVALENCE
Unknown

GEOGRAPHIC DISTRIBUTION
Potentially worldwide distribution

SIGNALMENT
Species
Dairy and beef cattle
Breed Predilections
N/A
Mean Age and Range
The prevalence of the lesions appears to be related to increasing age of the animal and increased weight.
Predominant Sex
N/A

SIGNS
Vertical Fissures
• Vertical fissures are a vertically orientated defect in the hoof wall of variable length. They are generally found on the cranio-abaxial aspect of the hoof and are most common on that lateral foreclaw.
• A classification of vertical fissures has been proposed:
1. Fissure starts at the coronary band and extends a short way down the hoof wall.
2. Fissure starts at the coronary band and extends more than half way down the hoof wall.
3. Fissure starts at the coronary band and extends the entire length of the hoof wall.
4. Fissure may start at any point on the hoof wall and extends all the way down to the toe.
5. Fissure is found in the center of the hoof wall and extends neither to the coronary band or the toe.

• Vertical fissures are extremely common affecting more than 20% of adult beef cattle in some areas; however, they rarely result in lameness. The fissure in the hoof wall typically results in a marked thickening of the hoof capsule that prevents debris from reaching the sensitive corium.
• The thickening of the hoof wall may be so marked that dorsal surface of the pedal bone becomes remodeled. On occasion, debris may reach the corium and an abscess may develop resulting in severe lameness.
• The presence of an abscess may be confirmed based upon the fact that the hoof feels warm and there is a marked response to focal pressure in the region of the sandcrack when "hoof testers" are applied.

Horizontal Grooves
• A horizontal groove is a groove found running around the circumference of the hoof capsule parallel to the coronary band. It may be found at any point on the hoof wall and be of variable depth. In extreme cases, the hoof capsule may fracture along the horizontal groove.
• In those affected, the distal portion of the hoof becomes a "thimble."
• The distal portion typically remains attached to the underlying corium in the region of the toe and any movement of the "thimble" causes great pain.
• This condition is also occasionally referred to as a "hangnail."

Axial Cracks
An axial crack is a full thickness vertical crack in the hoof wall found on the axial aspect of the hoof. The fact that the crack extends through the full thickness of the hoof wall is apparent, as there is typically a small amount of granulation tissue protruding from the fissure. Animals typically exhibit signs of great pain when the lesion is handled.

HISTORICAL FINDINGS
• Vertical fissures are seen almost exclusively in beef cattle, especially those on the western prairies of Canada. The prevalence of the lesions appears to be related to increasing age of the animal and increased weight.
• Horizontal grooves may be seen in cattle of almost any age and production type.
• Axial cracks are only seen in mature dairy cattle.

CAUSES AND RISK FACTORS
Vertical Fissures
• The cause of vertical fissures has been hotly debated for hundreds of years. The high incidence of this lesion has been explained by theories about nutritional deficiencies and horizontal grooves as a risk factor. Recent research has demonstrated that vertical fissure formation may be due simply to environmental effects. During long dry winters the hoof horn dehydrates.

• Biomechanical studies of equine hoof horn have shown that the fracture toughness of the horn decreases when the horn is dehydrated resulting in easier cracking. Consequently, vertical fissures may simply be a result of the environment in which we keep beef cattle.

Horizontal Grooves
• The wall horn of the hoof grows from the coronary band toward the toe at a rate of approximately 3 mm/month in beef cattle and 5 mm/ month in dairy cows.
• Any metabolic insult (change in diet, illness, etc.) may result in a change in horn formation. As the wall horn grows out toward the toe, the changes in horn formation appear as grooves. The depth of the groove is dependent on the severity of the insult.
• In beef cattle, a common cause of horizontal grooves is spring turn out, when the diet changes from old hay and grain to lush spring pasture. It is thought that the ingestion of large amounts of freely fermentable carbohydrate may result in ruminal acidosis and the release of compounds from the rumen that results in alterations in horn formation.
• In dairy cows, horizontal grooves are typically related to calving when there is again a sudden change in diet and there may also be concurrent problems such as a mastitis or metritis. If a horizontal groove is deep enough, it may act as an area of weakness in the hoof wall and eventually crack all the way around allowing debris to impact between the hoof wall and the underlying corium. The corium responds by forming a thin layer of horn tissue to protect it itself. However, the attachment between the corium and the hoof wall typically remains vascular and intact in the region of the toe, where the movement of the distal portion of the hoof wall results in great pain.

Axial Cracks
• The cause of axial cracks is not known. However, since axial cracks are commonly seen in dairy herds that also have a high incidence of digital dermatitis, a theory has developed to explain their formation. It is assumed that atypical cases of digital dermatitis may develop on the coronary band at the cranial extremity of the interdigital cleft and that as a result of this lesion there is irreversible damage to the tissue resulting in a failure of normal horn formation.
• New horn is laid down on either side of the lesion. A full thickness defect occurs in the hoof wall exposing the underlying corium resulting in great pain.

MISCELLANEOUS CONDITIONS OF THE HOOF WALL

DIAGNOSIS

DIFFERENTIAL DIAGNOSIS
Other than a traumatic injury to the hoof, there are no real differentials for these lesions.

CBC/BIOCHEMISTRY/URINALYSIS
N/A

OTHER LABORATORY TESTS
N/A

IMAGING
Radiographs may be helpful in diagnosing the specific condition and prognosis.

DIAGNOSTIC PROCEDURES
• All the above-described lesions are diagnosed on the basis of the characteristic clinical signs.
• Diagnosis is based on a necessary close examination of the foot.

TREATMENT

Vertical Fissures
• The majority of vertical fissures does not require treatment.
• If the lesion is associated with abscess formation, the fissure should be debrided using either the end of a hoof knife or a small rotary grinding tool (Dremel). This allows lesion identity while draining the abscess is indicated.
• Experience has shown that many abscesses are found at the tip of the pedal bone and commonly extend caudally below the sole. These require resection of a large portion of the sole.
• The application of an orthopedic block (Technovit or similar) to the opposite claw may be necessary to provide pain relief to the animal.

Horizontal Grooves
• Simple horizontal grooves do not require treatment. If the groove fissures result in a thimble, the distal portion of the hoof should be removed. This is best done with the distal limb anesthetized with an intravenous regional anesthetic. The horn should be slowly resected with hoof cutters and a hoof knife.
• A light bandage may need to be applied to the extremity of the pedal bone for control of hemorrhage.
• An orthopedic block should be applied to the opposite claw.

Axial Cracks
• Axial cracks are extremely painful and an intravenous regional anesthetic should be performed before attempting any examination of the area. The horn on either side of the lesion may be resected and granulation tissue trimmed back to the corium. A bandage will be necessary to control hemorrhage.
• It is the author's experience that it is not possible to permanently resolve such lesions due to the damage to the coronary band. An alternative is to amputate the affected digit.

MEDICATIONS

• Antibiotics are not indicated in the treatment of any of the above conditions.
• Depending on the severity of the lesion, some clinicians may elect to use a short course of NSAIDs for pain relief.
• Proper drug withdrawal periods for meat and milk must be maintained.

FOLLOW-UP

PATIENT MONITORING
Orthopedic blocks should always be removed within 7 weeks of application.

PREVENTION/AVOIDANCE
• There is some evidence to suggest that supplementing diets with biotin may help to reduce the incidence of vertical fissures.
• Biotin supplementation may not be cost effective when one considers the low likelihood of vertical fissures resulting in lameness.
• Avoiding sudden diet changes should help reduce the incidence of severe horizontal grooves.
• Maintaining an effective control program for digital dermatitis may also help reduce the incidence of axial cracks.

EXPECTED COURSE AND PROGNOSIS
• Vertical fissure: after adequate drainage of the abscess, the prognosis is extremely good. Complications such as spread of infection to the distal interphalangeal joint are extremely rare. It is not clear whether suitably debriding the vertical fissure will allow the formation of new horn at the coronary band that will in time grow without the formation of a new fissure. After removal of a thimble, the prognosis for such animals is excellent. The animal should be completely pain free in approximately 2–4 weeks. Complete resolution of the lesion requires that new horn grow down and cover the lesion. This may take several months depending on the rate of horn wall growth and the position of the lesion.
• The prognosis for axial cracks is poor.
• Debriding the lesion can typically make the animal pain free for several months; however, the lesion typically becomes extremely painful soon after.

MISCELLANEOUS

ASSOCIATED CONDITIONS
Lameness, loss of production

AGE-RELATED FACTORS
The prevalence of the lesions appears to be related to increasing age of the animal and increased weight.

ZOONOTIC POTENTIAL
N/A

PREGNANCY
N/A

RUMINANT SPECIES AFFECTED
Bovine; potentially, all ruminant species can be affected.

BIOSECURITY
N/A

PRODUCTION MANAGEMENT
N/A

SYNONYMS
Hangnail
Hardship lines
Sandcracks

SEE ALSO
Specific chapters on lameness, foot rot, heifer management, culling decisions, bull management

ABBREVIATIONS
NSAIDs = nonsteroidal anti-inflammatory drugs

Suggested Reading
Campbell, J. R., Greenough, P. R., Petrie, L. 2000. The effects of dietary biotin supplementation on vertical fissures of the claw wall in beef cattle. *Can Vet J*. 41:690–94.
Clark, C. R., Petrie, L., Waldner, C., Wendell, A. In press. Characteristics of the bovine claw associated with the presence of vertical fissures (sandcracks). *Canadian Veterinary Journal*.

Author: Chris Clark

MITES OF SHEEP AND GOATS

BASICS

OVERVIEW
• Mange is caused by parasitic arthropods of the subclass Acari in the class Arachnida.
• The mites affecting sheep and goats are obligate parasites.
• The entire life cycle is completed on the host.
• Mite species are either burrowing or nonburrowing.
• Heavy mite infestations cause dermatitis.
• Transmission is by direct skin-to-skin contact.

SYSTEMS AFFECTED
Production management, skin, reproductive, and hemopoietic

GENETICS
N/A

INCIDENCE/PREVALENCE
N/A

GEOGRAPHIC DISTRIBUTION
Worldwide, depending on species and environment

SIGNALMENT
• Sheep and goats are affected by species-specific or species-adapted strains of mites.
• Different mite species have predilections for different body regions.

Species
Sheep and goats

Breed Predilections
N/A

Mean Age and Range
N/A

Predominant Sex
N/A

CAUSES AND RISK FACTORS

Psoroptidae
Sheep
• *Psoroptes ovis* (sheep scab/psoroptic mange)
• Infestation is biphasic: a quiescent phase in the axillae, groin, and face during warmer months, alternating with an active multiplying phase affecting the whole body in winter
• The mites are nonburrowing but bite through the skin resulting in an exudative, scabby lesion that is severely pruritic.
• Psoroptic mange is highly contagious and occurs worldwide, except in Australia and New Zealand, which eradicated sheep scab in the 1890s.

Sheep and Goats
• *Chorioptes bovis* (scrotal mange/chorioptic mange)
• Haired skin, particularly of the lower body, is colonized. Most infestations are light and clinical signs are easily overlooked.
• The mites are nonburrowing and feed on the skin surface. Lesions range from mild epidermal hyperplasia, to severe exudative dermatitis with marked epidermal hyperplasia, and hyperkeratosis with encrusted dried serous exudate.
• Affected rams have impaired fertility secondary to increased intrascrotal temperature.
• Although infection is common, lesions are rarely seen on goats. Chorioptic mange has worldwide distribution.

Goats
• *Psoroptes cuniculi* (ear mange).
• Mites inhabit the external ear, feed on whole blood, and cause epidermitis with scab formation.

Cheyletidae
Sheep
• *Psorergates ovis* (itch mite) mostly affects fine-wooled sheep.
• The preferred site of infestation is the fleece-covered areas along the sides of the body.
• The mites live on the skin surface. Infestation spreads through flocks slowly; the population increases on host animals slowly and peaks in winter.
• Affected sheep are irritated by the mites; they rub and bite at their sides, and the fleece contains excessive debris.
• Itch mite occurs sporadically in the fine wool growing areas of Australia, South Africa, New Zealand, and North and South America.

Sarcoptidae
Sheep
• *Sarcoptes scabiei* (ovine-adapted strains)
• Haired areas of the skin are affected. The female mites burrow into the skin.
• There is intense pruritis and an exudative dermatitis consequent to both the direct action of the mites and to self-trauma.
• Sarcoptic mange of sheep is rare and no longer occurs in nations with advanced sheep industries.

Goats
• *Sarcoptes scabiei* (caprine-adapted strains)
• Female mites burrow into the skin.
• Initially, there is traumatic alopecia, excoriations, and encrustations.
• Chronic cases have marked epidermal hyperplasia.
• Caprine sarcoptic mange is of greatest importance in areas where goats are the primary domestic ruminant.

Demodicidae
Sheep and Goats
• *Demodex* species ordinarily live in the hair follicles and sebaceous glands as commensal organisms.
• Demodectic mange, with heavy infestation and seborrheic dermatitis, is rare and of little economic importance.

DIAGNOSIS
• Behavior and lesions of self-trauma consistent with pruritis

• Locally extensive exudative dermatitis and epidermal hyperplasia with crusting
• Demonstrate the mite in skin scrapings.

DIFFERENTIAL DIAGNOSIS
Louse infestation

CBC/BIOCHEMISTRY/URINALYSIS
N/A

OTHER LABORATORY TESTS
N/A

IMAGING
N/A

DIAGNOSTIC PROCEDURES
N/A

PATHOLOGIC FINDINGS
N/A

TREATMENT
N/A

MEDICATIONS

DRUGS OF CHOICE
• Topical organophosphates
• Ivermectin is universally effective, if given parenterally twice at an interval of 7 to 14 days (covers two life cycles of most mite species).

CONTRAINDICATIONS
• *Psorergates ovis* is not susceptible to synthetic pyrethroids.
• Appropriate milk and meat withdrawal times must be followed for all compounds administered to food-producing animals.

• Steroids should not be used in pregnant animals.

FOLLOW-UP
N/A

PATIENT MONITORING
N/A

PREVENTION/AVOIDANCE
Strict biosecurity

POSSIBLE COMPLICATIONS
N/A

EXPECTED COURSE AND PROGNOSIS
N/A

MISCELLANEOUS

ASSOCIATED CONDITIONS
Heavy mite infestations cause dermatitis

AGE-RELATED FACTORS
N/A

ZOONOTIC POTENTIAL
N/A

PREGNANCY
N/A

RUMINANT SPECIES AFFECTED
Sheep and goats

BIOSECURITY
• Sheep scab (*Psorergates ovis* infestation) is a notifiable disease in some countries, and control is effected under statutory direction in others.
• Transmission is by direct skin-to-skin contact.

• Isolation and quarantine of new stock entering the herd/flock
• Treat and or cull new animals for disease conditions prior to herd introduction.

PRODUCTION MANAGEMENT
N/A

SYNONYMS
Ear mite
Itch mite
Scab
Sheep scab

SEE ALSO
Differential diagnosis of pruritis
Lice of sheep and goats

ABBREVIATIONS
N/A

Suggested Reading
Coop, R. L., Taylor, M. A., Jacobs, D. E., Jackson, F. 2002, Feb. Ectoparasites: recent advances in control. *Trends Parasitol*. 18(2):55–56.
Kaufmann, J. 1996, *Parasitic infections of domestic animals, a diagnostic manual*. Basel; Boston; Berlin: Birkhäuser Verlag.
Pettit, D., Smith, W. D., Richardson, J., Munn, E. A. 2000, Apr 28. Localisation and characterisation of ovine immunglobulin within the sheep scab mite, *Psoroptes ovis*. *Vet Parasitol*. 89(3):231–39.
Taylor, M. A. 2001, May. Recent developments in ectoparasiticides. *Vet J*. 161(3):253–68.
Van Den Broek, A. H., Huntley, J. F., MacHell, J., Taylor, M., Bates, P., Groves, B., Miller, H. R. 2000, Aug. Cutaneous and systemic responses during primary and challenge infestations of sheep with the sheep scab mite, *Psoroptes ovis*. *Parasite Immunol*. 22(8):407–14.

Author: A. D. (Sandy) McLachlan

MOLYBDENUM TOXICITY

 BASICS

OVERVIEW
• Molybdenum (Mb) is an essential micronutrient, which forms molybdenoenzymes. Dietary intake of excess Mb causes, in part, secondary hypocuprosis.
• The metabolism of copper, molybdenum, and inorganic sulfate is a complex interrelationship. Mb toxicity is directly associated with copper deficiency and has similar signs.
• Ruminants are especially susceptible to dietary molybdenum excess, leading to depressed growth, diarrhea, neurologic defects, and eventually death, if untreated.
• The ruminal interaction of molybdates and sulfides gives rise to thiomolybdates. At high levels, these compounds decrease the availability of dietary copper and, when absorbed, slow the metabolism of tissue copper and inhibit copper enzymes. This leads to signs of copper deficiency.
• Increased levels in the east and west coasts, increased in acidic, wet soil (peat bogs)
• Forage plants can accumulate Mb. Concentration is lowest in winter, increased in summer and fall.
• Seen in contamination of soils, industrial contamination, fertilizers, feeding of forages and grain. When Cu levels of feed or forages in the normal range of 8–11 ppm, cattle can be poisoned with Mb levels above 5–6 ppm and sheep on levels above 10–12 ppm.
• If Cu level is below 8–11 ppm, or sulfate level is high, even 1–2 ppm Mb may be toxic in cattle.
• High level of Cu in diet to 13–16 ppm can protect Mb poisoning up to 150 ppm dietary Mb.

Species Affected
Ruminants tend to be more susceptible than nonruminants; cattle are more susceptible than sheep.

PATHOPHYSIOLOGY
Causes cytochrome oxidase deficiency and limits heme synthesis.

SIGNALMENT
• Young animals have increased susceptibility.
• Calves can be poisoned by milk from cows on increased Mb.
• Lambs under 1 month of age, severely uncoordinated, ataxic, and usually blind

SIGNS
• Defects in pigmentation, keratinization, bone formation, myelination of the spinal cord, connective tissue formation, and pica
• With chronic ingestion, get osteoporosis, bone fractures, beaded ribs, and overgrowth of long bone ends
• Emaciation, depressed growth
• Liquid diarrhea full of gas bubbles, called peat scours, or teart
• Swollen genitalia impaired reproductive performance
• Anemia from decreased hematopoiesis
• Achromotrichia (depigmentation) of the hair coat especially around the eyes, giving a "spectacled" appearance
• In sheep, depigmentation of dark wool, loss of crimp and quality of the fine wool
• In Australia, enzootic ataxia, in the UK "sway back" seen in the lysis of CNS white matter
• Death is the result of starvation, exposure, or pneumonia.

CAUSES AND RISK FACTORS
The susceptibility of ruminants to a high intake of molybdenum depends on a number of factors:

• The copper contents and intake of the animal: the tolerance to molybdenum decreases as the content and intake of copper fall.
• The inorganic sulfate content of the diet: high dietary sulfate with low copper levels exacerbates the condition; low dietary sulfate causes high blood molybdenum levels due to decreased excretion.
• The chemical form of the molybdenum: water soluble in growing herbage is the most toxic, and curing decreases toxicity.
• The presence of certain sulfur-containing amino acids
• The species of the animal: cattle are less tolerant then sheep.
• The age: young animals are more susceptible.
• The season of the year: plants concentrate molybdenum beginning in the spring with the maximum level in the fall.
• The botanic composition of the pasture: legumes take up more of the element than other plant species.
• In cattle forage as safe ratio of Cu:Mb > 2:1; when the ratio is less than 2:1, Mb poisoning occurs.

 DIAGNOSIS

Made by clinical appearance, response to Cu treatment

DIFFERENTIAL DIAGNOSIS
• Ca/phos/vit D metabolic imbalance
• Massive parasitism, GI parasites
• Johne's disease
• Demyelinating diseases of brain and spinal cord

CBC/BIOCHEMISTRY/URINALYSIS
• Decreased PCV, microcytic, hypochromic anemia
• Cu and Mb levels in forage and tissues
• Liver levels of Cu < 10–30 ppm, Mb > 5 ppm significant
• Whole blood Cu < 0.6 ppm, Mb > 0.1 ppm, significant
• Milk Mb up to 300 ppm significant

OTHER LABORATORY TESTS
N/A

IMAGING
N/A

DIAGNOSTIC PROCEDURES
N/A

PATHOLOGIC FINDINGS

GROSS FINDINGS
Cardiovascular hemorrhage

HISTOPATHOLOGICAL FINDINGS
• Lysis of white matter and degeneration of motor tracts of spinal cord
   Microscopic to massive subcortical destruction
• Neuronal degeneration and demyelination

TREATMENT
• Remove animal from feed source.
• Where Mb content of forage is < 5 ppm, Cu sulfate in salt mineral mixture 1%. With higher Mb, use 2%.

• Repository Cu glycinate SQ and 60 mg for calves, 120 mg for mature cattle. May need to be repeated for a good response.
• Can use as top dressing in pasture, trace mineral mix free choice in feed.

MEDICATIONS

DRUGS OF CHOICE
Copper sulfate oral drench

CONTRAINDICATIONS
• Sheep are highly susceptible to copper drench.
• Appropriate milk and meat withdrawal times must be followed for all compounds administered to food-producing animals.

MISCELLANEOUS

ASSOCIATED CONDITIONS

AGE-RELATED FACTORS
• Young animals have increased susceptibility.
• Calves can be poisoned by milk from cows on increased Mb.
• Lambs under 1 month of age, severely uncoordinated, ataxic, and usually blind.

ZOONOTIC POTENTIAL
N/A

PREGNANCY
Impaired reproductive performance

SYNONYMS
• Peat scours
• Teart

SEE ALSO
Ca/phos/vit D metabolic imbalance
Demyelinating diseases of brain and spinal cord
GI parasites
Johne's disease
Massive parasitism

ABBREVIATIONS
CNS = central nervous system
Cu = copper
GI = gastrointestinal
Mb = molybdenum
PCV = packed cell volume
ppm = parts per million
SQ = subcutaneous

Suggested Reading
Buck, W.B., Osweiler, G.D., and Van Gelder, G.A. 1976. *Clinical and diagnostic veterinary toxicology.* 2nd ed. Dubuque, IA: Kendall-Hunt Publishing Co.
Molybdenum Poisoning. 2005. In: *Merck veterinary manual.* Whitehouse Station, NJ: Merck and Co.
Roder, J. D. 2001. Veterinary toxicology. In: *The practical veterinarian.* Woburn, MA: Butterworth-Heinemann.

Author: Greg Stoner

MONENSIN TOXICITY

BASICS

DEFINITION
- Monensin is a carboxylic ionophore antibiotic produced by the fungus *Streptomyces cinnamonensis*.
- Monensin is commercially available as Rumensin and Coban. It is commonly added in feed to treat ruminant coccidiosis and to improve feed efficiency and growth by increasing the propionic acid in the rumen, therefore providing more energy for metabolism. It also spares dietary proteins in the rumen and prevents bloating and acidosis.
- Poisonings have been reported in cattle, sheep, and goats. Ingestion of toxic amounts of ionophores in these animals affects the cardiovascular, musculoskeletal, neuromuscular, hepatic, and renal systems.
- Toxicosis can result from overdosage and misuse. Mixing errors and ingestion of premix concentrates are the leading causes of such presentations.
- Clinical signs in affected animals may be evident within a day, or take several weeks, depending on the concentration of monensin in the diet. Some effects may persist for months and lead to permanent damages. In one incidence, signs persisted in sheep for months after removal of the high-monensin (160–550 ppm) feed.
- The following lethal doses have been reported for various ruminants on a body weight basis:
  - Cattle $LD_1 = 5.5$ mg/kg; $LD_{10} = 11$ mg/kg; $LD_{50} = 21.9$–80 mg/kg
  - Sheep $LD_0 = 4$ mg/kg; $LD_{50} = 10.7$–13.1 mg/kg
  - Goat $LD_{50} = 22.4$–30.4 mg/kg

- The FDA recommends 5.5–33 ppm monensin in the total diet of cattle and 22 ppm for goats.
  - 100 ppm, for about 1 year, had no effect on circulatory or reproductive functions of cattle.
  - 200–400 ppm monensin in feed for some days may lead to chronic toxicosis in cattle.
  - Goats consuming feed with 55 ppm monensin for 3 weeks may manifest hepatotoxicity. However, no such effect is seen in goats at 11 ppm for 3 weeks, or at 8 mg/kg BW × 5 days.
- Although not approved for sheep, monensin has been purposefully added to ovine feed at levels similar to that of cattle. In lambs < 1 month of age, diffuse gastrointestinal hemorrhage has been reported. Single dose of monensin at 12 mg/kg resulted in no muscular abnormality. At 2–4 mg/kg × 4 days, listlessness and feed refusal were observed; and at concentrations $> = 8$ mg/kg × 2 days, toxicity was observed.

PATHOPHYSIOLOGY
- Monensin is well absorbed from GIT, and undergoes hepatic metabolism by P-450s and glutathione. O-demethylation and hydroxylation are the primary pathways. Urinary excretion is very low, < 1%.
- Ionophores form dynamically reversible $Ca^{2+}/Mg^{2+}/Na^+/K^+$-lipid soluble complexes that are easily transported across membranes, following the gradient. This causes increased intracellular sodium, and loss of potassium from the cells, discharges the potential gradient, and hence leads to reduction in ATP. An increased ATP utilization is required to maintain the cation concentrations across the membranes. These responses lead to reduction in cellular function and cell death. Increased intracellular sodium also results in mitochondrial swelling and changes in osmotic pressure and thus causes cellular swelling, in addition to the defects in oxidative phosphorylation.

- Increased intracellular sodium also triggers the Ca^{2+}-Na^+ exchange cycle, resulting in an increased intracellular calcium concentration in order to maintain the osmotic balance. This increase in intracellular calcium increases catecholamine production and leads to a positive inotropic effect. This is then followed by a negative inotropic effect.

SYSTEMS AFFECTED

Cardiovascular
- The loss of potential gradient across the myocardial cells results in abnormal impulse transmission and therefore cardiac arrhythmias and congestive heart failure in some cases.
- In more chronic cases, the lack of ATP availability causes cell death or necrosis, and such areas are then replaced by nonfunctional connective tissues such as fibroblasts. Thus, monensin toxicosis results in permanent myocardial damage that appears as pale areas/streaks.

Musculoskeletal
- Effects on skeletal muscles are similar to those seen in the cardiac muscles. Cattle have about equal predilection to develop heart and skeletal muscle lesions.
- In animals surviving the acute exposure, scarring and pallor of certain muscle groups may be noted.

Neuromuscular
The alteration in the normal conduction of impulse can result in altered reflexes and muscular incoordination.

Renal/Urologic
Myoglobinurea and urinary bladder distension have been reported in some ruminants.

Hepatobiliary
Mottling of liver along with hepatocellular necrosis have been reported also.

Respiratory
Pulmonary edema and congestion have been reported in acute cases.

GENETICS
N/A

INCIDENCE/PREVALENCE
The incidences are sporadic, but not very prevalent because of the awareness of monensin toxicity among farmers.

GEOGRAPHIC DISTRIBUTION
N/A

SIGNALMENT
• Based on the LD_{50} values, among ruminants, sheep are more susceptible to monesin toxicosis than cattle or goats.
• No differentiation of toxicity on the basis of age, sex, or breed has been reported.

SIGNS
Acute Effects
• Death
• Recumbency
• Arrhythmias
• Dyspnea
• Stiffness
• Ataxia
• Tremors
• Anorexia
• Edema of abdomen and legs
• Weakness
• Myoglobinurea
• Diarrhea

Chronic Effects
• Anorexia
• Diarrhea
• Depression
• Dyspnea
• Arrhythmias
• Unthriftiness
• Poor exercise tolerance
• Death

CAUSES
Monensin toxicosis is generally a result of feeding of premix ration or other mixing errors.

RISK FACTORS
Presence of other natural cardiotoxins and absence of adequate amounts of selenium and vitamin E can result in aggravation of the ionophore toxicosis.

DIAGNOSIS

DIFFERENTIAL DIAGNOSIS
• Selenium deficiency—evaluated by measuring selenium concentrations in blood, serum, or liver.
• Vitamin E deficiency—evaluated by measuring vitamin E in serum or liver.
• Cardiotoxic plants—identification of plant in feed, testing of rumen content for plant alkaloids.

CBC/BIOCHEMISTRY/URINALYSIS
Goats
• Increased phenobarbital-induced sleeping time
• Increased SDH

Cattle
• Muscle damage causing—increased AST, increased CPK.
• Diarrhea/rumenitis causing—hypokalemia, hyponatremia, and hypocalcemia.
• Also seen is leukocytosis with increased PMN cells and decrease in lymphocytes.
• Myoglobinurea in severely affected animals

OTHER LABORATORY TESTS
• Analyze feed, GI contents, and molasses for identification and quantification of monensin. The analysis can be done using TLC, colorimetric, or the LC-MS method.

• Tissue samples are not diagnostic because of the rapid elimination and low concentrations in tissues.

IMAGING
Echocardiography may be used to determine the myocardial damage in live, chronic cases. However, animals with acute exposure cannot be diagnosed with this method, as the fibrosis is not present.

DIAGNOSTIC PROCEDURES
• Prolongation of Q-T interval and the QRS complex. Absence of P wave and increased amplitude of S and T waves have been observed.
• Atrial/ventricular fibrillation, ventricular tachycardia, and intermittent and premature ventricular contractions may be evident.
• ECG abnormalities are not consistent with severity of exposure or the amount of myocardial damage.

PATHOLOGICAL FINDINGS
Findings similar to congestive heart failure

GROSS FINDINGS
• Enlarged heart with hydropericardium, epicardial hemorrhages, and a tigroid appearance
• Diffusely pale and yellow myocardium with pale and ventricular dilatation
• Pulmonary congestion and edema.
• Hepatic congestion
• Abomassal and SI mucosal congestion
• Ecchymotic hemorrhages around subcutaneous layer and facia of the neck and forelimbs
• Yellow-to-grey necrotic streaks in skeletal muscles

HISTOPATHOLOGICAL FINDINGS
• Cattle—mitochondrial swelling and vacuolar degeneration of cardiac myositis. Pallor/pale streaking in ventricular walls and the septum was also seen, in addition to the centrilobular hepatic necrosis with vacuolar degeneration. Focal degeneration of active skeletal muscles may be evident.

MONENSIN TOXICITY

• Sheep—fibrosis and hyalinization with sarcoplasmic mineralization were reported in ewes consuming 160-ppm monensin over a period of 70 days. Mononuclear infiltration was also observed. Unlike in cattle, the skeletal-muscle lesions in sheep were more severe than cardiac lesions.

 TREATMENT

APPROPRIATE HEALTH CARE

• Intense medical management is generally not required, however it is recommended to monitor and correct the blood electrolyte imbalances, if any. There is no effective medical management procedure.
• Apart from isolation, GIT decontamination, and general supportive care, consider surgical evacuation of rumen contents in case of substantial exposure.
• Fluids can be administered to maintain hydration and enhance elimination or prevent renal casting by myoglobin.

NURSING CARE

• A couple of months of stall rest and a quiet environment are essential to reduce stress and limit the cardiac damage.
• A good management and plane of nutrition

ACTIVITY

Restricted exercise and excitement

DIET

N/A

CLIENT EDUCATION

Animals surviving a toxic exposure can have permanent cardiac damage that may make the animal susceptible to sudden death following stress.

SURGICAL CONSIDERATIONS

Rumenotomy may be considered in acute cases to evacuate the rumen, followed by activated charcoal or mineral oil.

 MEDICATIONS

DRUGS OF CHOICE

• No antidote
• AC/mineral oil/saline cathartics
• Vitamin E/Se to minimize secondary oxidative tissue damage

CONTRAINDICATIONS

IV fluids should not be administered in animals with cardiovascular problems.

PRECAUTIONS

N/A

POSSIBLE INTERACTIONS

Monensin toxicity may be potentiated by the concurrent use of tiamulin, oleandomycin, chloramphenicol, erythromycin, sulfonamides, furazolidone, and other cardiac glycosides.

ALTERNATIVE DRUGS

N/A

 FOLLOW-UP

PATIENT MONITORING

Serum chemistry, ECGs, and echocardiography are helpful to monitor progress, however, they cannot predict the prognosis.

PREVENTION/AVOIDANCE

• Proper storage of the premixes and concentrates
• Maintain a proper feed-management protocol to avoid mixing errors and possible miscalculations.
• Test feed to ensure monensin concentrations within the FDA recommended ranges (see Definition above).
• Keep animals at a good nutritional level, especially selenium and vitamin E.

POSSIBLE COMPLICATIONS

The myocardial damage may persist for a long period of time without clinically affecting the animal. This may predispose the animal to succumb to factors resulting in an elevated heart rate or requiring an increase in cardiac output.

EXPECTED COURSE AND PROGNOSIS

• Suspected animals may exhibit clinical signs within a few hours of exposure or, in some cases, may take months for the precipitation. Depending on the amount of exposure, the animals may manifest the acute or chronic effects (please see Signs listed above).
• The prognosis is guarded to poor for any animal with suspected myocardial damage. The animals can be maintained, but their performance may be decreased.

 MISCELLANEOUS

ASSOCIATED CONDITIONS
N/A

AGE-RELATED FACTORS
N/A

ZOONOTIC POTENTIAL
N/A

PREGNANCY

Ionophores have not been directly associated with reproductive problems. However, the compromised cardiovascular function may result in abortion.

RUMINANT SPECIES AFFECTED

Cattle, sheep, and goat have reportedly been affected. However, all ruminant species should be considered susceptible.

BIOSECURITY

The tolerance level of monensin in edible tissues of cattle is 0.05 ppm.

PRODUCTION MANAGEMENT

• Do not feed to lactating dairy cows.
• Ensure proper mixing and final concentration within the FDA-recommended range of 5.5–33 ppm.

SYNONYMS
N/A

SEE ALSO
Cardiotoxic plants
Selenium deficiency
Vitamin E deficiency

ABBREVIATIONS
AC = activated charcoal
AST = aspartate aminotransferase
BW = body weight
CPK = creatine phosphokinase
ECG = electrocardiogram
FDA = Food and Drug Administration
GIT = gastrointestinal tract
LC/MS = liquid chromatography/mass spectrometry.
LD_0 = highest estimated dose at which none of the population is expected to die
LD_{10} = estimated dose at which 10% of the population is expected to die
LD_{50} = estimated dose at which 50% of the population is expected to die
PMN = polymorphonuclear cells
SDH = sorbitol dehydrogenase
TLC = thin layer chromatography

Suggested Reading
Anderson, T. D., Van Alstine, W. G., Ficken, M. D., Miskimins, D. W., Carson, T. L., Osweiler, G. D. 1984. Acute monensin toxicosis in sheep: Light and electron microscopic changes. *Am J Vet Res.* 45(6): 1142–47.
Hall, J. O. 2000, Nov. Ionophore use and toxicosis in cattle. *Vet Clin North Am Food Anim Pract.* 16(3): 497–509.
Langston, V. C., Galey, F., Lovell, R., Buck, W. B. 1985, Oct. Toxicity and therapeutics of monensin: a review. *Vet Med.* 75–84.
Novilla, M. N. 1992. The veterinary importance of the toxic syndrome induced by ionophores. *Vet Hum Toxicol.* 34(1): 66–70.

Author: Asheesh K. Tiwary

MUCOSAL DISEASE

 BASICS

OVERVIEW
• Mucosal disease in nature is rare because of the special circumstances that are required for it to occur.
• Mucosal disease is invariably fatal.
• Mucosal disease occurs only in cattle immunotolerant to and persistently infected with bovine viral diarrhea virus (BVDV).
• This persistent infection occurs when a fetus becomes infected in utero between 1 and 4 months of gestation with noncytopathic bovine viral diarrhea virus.
• Mucosal disease occurs when cattle persistently infected with BVDV become superinfected with an antigenically homologous cytopathic BVDV virus.
• The most common source of the cytopathic BVDV is for a mutation to occur at specific sites in the noncytopathic virus genome of the persistent virus, converting it from a noncytopathic to cytopathic virus.
• The mutation does not change the antigenic makeup of the virus, therefore the cytopathic virus is not recognized by the host's immune system and is allowed to replicate without challenge.
• Other sources of cytopathic viruses would include modified live vaccines or other cattle with mucosal disease. Antigenic homology between the cytopathic and noncytopathic virus must be maintained for mucosal disease to occur.
• A form of mucosal disease, called chronic mucosal disease, has been described. However, instead of being antigenically identical to the original virus, slight differences exist in the antigenic makeup of the new cytopathic virus. This allows the persistently infected cow to mount an immune response against the cytopathic virus. However, the immune response is often incomplete and pathology slowly evolves leading to the eventual death of the animal.

SIGNALMENT
• Mucosal disease occurs only in cattle persistently infected with BVDV.
• Mucosal disease can occur in any age animal. However, the vast majority of cases occurs in younger animals, generally less than 2 years of age.

SIGNS
• Mucosal disease is inevitably fatal.
• The clinical course of mucosal disease ranges from days to weeks.
• Onset of mucosal disease is characterized by fever (103–105°F), depression, weakness, and anorexia.
• Erosive lesions of the lips, gingival margins, dental pad, tongue, and hard palate are generally present. Erosive lesions may also be present on the external nares, teats, and vulva.
• Profuse foul smelling watery diarrhea is common and may include clotted blood and intestinal casts.
• Similar signs may be observed in cattle with chronic mucosal disease, but less severe in nature.

CAUSES AND RISK FACTORS
Mucosal disease occurs only in cattle that are persistently infected with BVDV.

 DIAGNOSIS

DIFFERENTIAL DIAGNOSIS
• Any vesicular disease needs to be considered including vesicular stomatitis, papular stomatitis, foot-and-mouth disease, and malignant catarrhal fever.
• Diseases that may induce hemorrhagic diarrhea include salmonellosis and hemorrhagic enteritis.

CBC/BIOCHEMISTRY/URINALYSIS
A severe leukopenia is common with total leukocyte counts ranging from 1000 to 4000 cells/μl.

OTHER LABORATORY TESTS
Isolation of both a cytopathic and noncytopathic BVDV from serum, whole blood, nasal swabs, or lymphoid tissue in clinically affected cattle.

IMAGING
N/A

DIAGNOSTIC PROCEDURES
NA

GROSS FINDINGS
• Erosive lesions of the lips, gingival margins, dental pad, tongue, and hard palate are generally present. Lesions may coalesce leading to large areas of mucosal sloughing.
• Linear erosions in the esophagus are common.
• Erosions of the rumen papillae and omasal leaves may be present.
• The abomasum is usually severely congested and erosions may be present.
• Erosions of the mucosal surface covering the Peyer's patch area located in the small intestine are very common.
• Erosions in the cecum and colon may also be present.

HISTOPATHOLOGICAL FINDINGS
• Severe lymphoid depletion of the Peyer's patch areas is common.
• A lack of inflammatory cells around erosive lesions is often appreciated.

 TREATMENT

• Mucosal disease is invariably fatal.
• Animals suspected or confirmed with having mucosal disease antemortem should be humanely euthanized.

 MEDICATIONS

N/A

CONTRAINDICATIONS
N/A

MUCOSAL DISEASE

 FOLLOW-UP

PATIENT MONITORING
N/A

PREVENTION/AVOIDANCE
• Prevention of mucosal disease revolves around a comprehensive BVDV control program with the goal of preventing the birth of cattle persistently infected with BVDV.
• Preventing persistent infections requires reducing exposure to BVDV, especially during the first trimester of gestation, and developing solid immunity through a BVDV immunization program.
• If cattle persistently infected with BVDV are identified, they should be removed from the herd immediately to reduce the risk of their serving as a source of virus spread to naïve cohorts.

POSSIBLE COMPLICATIONS
N/A

EXPECTED COURSE AND PROGNOSIS
• Mucosal disease is invariably fatal.
• Cattle affected with classic mucosal disease usually die within 5–10 days.
• Cattle affected with chronic mucosal disease may live for months.

 MISCELLANEOUS

ASSOCIATED CONDITIONS
N/A

AGE-RELATED FACTORS
Most cases of mucosal disease occur in cattle less than 2 years of age.

ZOONOTIC POTENTIAL
BVDV is not considered a zoonotic agent.

PREGNANCY
N/A

SEE ALSO
Bovine viral diarrhea virus
Foot-and-mouth disease
Hemorrhagic diarrhea/enteritis
Malignant catarrhal fever
Papular stomatitis
Salmonellosis
Vesicular stomatitis

ABBREVIATIONS
BVDV = bovine viral diarrhea virus

Suggested Reading

Baker, J. C., Houe, H., eds. 1995, Nov. Bovine viral diarrhea virus. *Vet Clin North Am Food Anim Pract*. 11(3).
Barrington, G. M., Gay, J. M., Evermann, J. F. 2002, Mar. Biosecurity for neonatal gastrointestinal diseases. *Vet Clin North Am Food Anim Pract*. 18(1):7–34.
Grooms, D. L. 2004, Mar. Reproductive consequences of infection with bovine viral diarrhea virus. *Vet Clin North Am Food Anim Pract*. 20(1):5–19.
Viet, A. F., Fourichon, C., Seegers, H., Jacob, C., Guihenneuc-Jouyaux, C. 2004, May 14. A model of the spread of the bovine viral-diarrhoea virus within a dairy herd. *Prev Vet Med*. 63(3–4):211–36.

Author: Daniel L. Grooms

MYCOPLASMA INFECTIONS IN CATTLE

 BASICS

DEFINITION
- The genus *Mycoplasma* has been associated with a wide range of clinical presentations in cattle.
- In North America, common clinical presentations include pneumonia, polyarthritis, otitis media/interna, mastitis, and ocular disease.
- Outside of North America, contagious pleuropneumonia is a critically important production-limiting disease of cattle.

SIGNALMENT VARIES WITH MYCOPLASMA SPP. AND SPECIFIC SYNDROME
Clinical Syndromes
- Clinical syndromes commonly associated with *Mycoplasma* spp. include pneumonia, polyarthritis, mastitis, otitis, reproductive disease, and ocular disease.
- Recently weaned beef calves and stockers often have respiratory and/or ocular disease.
- Dairy calves, particularly group housed, raw milk fed dairy calves with inadequate passive transfer, will often have pneumonia and otitis.
- Mastitis affects primarily adult dairy cattle.
- Although the disease may shift its clinical presentation and jump between age groups of cattle housed on the same farm, this is not a common or consistent observation.
- *Mycoplasma* spp. infections rarely cause acute death losses. Rather, these infections tend to cause chronic persistent infections, which are refractory to treatment.
- The reader is referred to those chapters discussing specific clinical syndromes for more detailed descriptions.

Pneumonia
- *Mycoplasma bovis* and *M. disbar* have been isolated from cattle with pneumonia. In general, *Mycoplasma* spp. appears to require several predisposing factors before the bacteria can cause clinical pneumonic disease.
- Predisposing management and host factors include weaning and shipping stresses, mixing cattle from multiple sources, and inadequate preconditioning programs.

- Preceding infections with respiratory viruses and *Mannheimia haemolytica* are commonly recognized as predisposing factors and may be obligatory stressors for the onset of pneumonic mycoplasmosis.
- In contrast to clinical signs observed with other pneumonia syndromes, the onset of clinical signs occurs longer after exposure (feedlot arrival or mixing of groups), has less dramatic clinical signs, has a more persistent clinical course, and often resists therapeutic intervention.

Polyarthritis
- *Mycoplasma* polyarthritis is observed most commonly in young dairy calves. In dairy herds, the syndrome may be associated with previous pneumonia and polyarthritis outbreaks.
- Feeding raw milk from cows with mycoplasma mastitis has been implicated as an important risk factor. In beef cattle, the syndrome is most often seen in recently weaned calves mixed and assembled from multiple sources.
- Preexisting pneumonic disease is a common part of the history.
- Affected calves are moderately lame. The joints most commonly affected include the carpus, hock, and stifle.

Otitis Media/Interna
- Otitis caused by *Mycoplasma* spp. is observed most commonly in dairy calves fed raw milk.
- Clinical signs usually include head tilt, loss of facial sensation, and loss of motor activity in the muscles of facial expression.
- Purulent drainage from the ear also is common. Preexisting or concurrent respiratory disease is common.

Mastitis
- *Mycoplasma bovis*, *M. californicum*, *M. bovigenitalium*, and others have been associated with clinical and subclinical mastitis in dairy cattle. *Mycoplasma* spp. tend to behave as contagious intramammary pathogens.
- Both acute clinical mastitis and chronic subclinical mastitis are common with *Mycoplasma* spp.

- Introduction of the pathogen into a dairy herd may result in fulminate outbreaks of clinical mastitis if poor milking and intramammary treatment hygiene potentiates the spread of the organism.
- The presence of clinical mastitis in multiple quarters is a common observation in cattle infected with *Mycoplasma* spp.
- Death losses caused by mycoplasma mastitis are rare. The most common clinical presentation is one of persistent high milk somatic cell counts and decreased milk production.
- Mycoplasma mastitis resists intramammary or systemic antibiotic therapy during either the lactating or dry-cow period.

Keratitis
- The predominant clinical sign is that of keratitis and conjunctivitis. This disease is not readily distinguished from infectious bovine keratoconjunctivitis (IBK). *Mycoplasma* spp. have been isolated from outbreaks of infectious bovine keratoconjunctivitis.
- A mycoplasma component should be suspected when outbreaks occur outside the accepted vector seasons or in the face of rigorous implementation of accepted control measures for *Moraxella bovis*.
- Herds in which cattle are frequently added to existing groups appear to be at greatly increased for *Mycoplasma* spp. ocular disease.

 DIAGNOSIS

DIFFERENTIAL DIAGNOSIS
Varies with *Mycoplasma* sp. and specific syndrome.

DIAGNOSTIC PROCEDURES
- Definitive diagnostic testing is based upon identification of the organism. Culture of *Mycoplasma* spp. is often problematic. The organisms have strict and complex growth requirements, generally require a high CO_2 atmosphere and are very slow growing. Furthermore, species and isolates often vary with regard to their growth requirements.

• The advent of polymerase chain reaction (PCR) assays has greatly expedited the diagnosis of mycoplasmosis. Both species- and genus-specific assay systems have been described for use on host tissues and samples.
• Most *Mycoplasma* spp. infections produce an inflammatory response in which the predominant cellular infiltrate is mononuclear. The relatively paucity of neutrophils in an inflammatory response strongly supports the potential for *Mycoplasma* spp.

TREATMENT

• Varies with *Mycoplasma* sp. and specific syndrome
• *Mycoplasma* spp. have been reported to be sensitive to a broad range of antibiotics including tetracyclines, florfenicol, enrofloxacin, tylosin, and tilmicosin. It should be emphasized that methods to determine in vitro sensitivity are currently under development and have not been standardized. Furthermore, in vitro sensitivity has not been demonstrated to accurately predict response to treatment.
• Vaccines have been approved and marketed for *M. bovis* respiratory disease in the United States. However, at this time the efficacy and performance of these vaccines has yet not been demonstrated in controlled clinical trials.
• No data are available to demonstrate the efficacy of prophylactic antibiotics.
• In general, preventive management strategies including optimal passive transfer, maintaining closed herds, or all-in all-out processing and standard preconditioning programs will decrease the prevalence and severity of clinical signs attributable to mycoplasmosis.

MEDICATIONS

CONTRAINDICATIONS
Appropriate milk and meat withdrawal times must be followed for all compounds administered to food-producing animals.

FOLLOW-UP

MISCELLANEOUS

ASSOCIATED CONDITIONS
Otitis media/interna, pneumonia, polyarthritis, mastitis, keratitis

AGE-RELATED FACTORS
N/A

ZOONOTIC POTENTIAL
N/A

PREGNANCY
N/A

RUMINANT SPECIES AFFECTED
Bovine

BIOSECURITY
• Introduction of the pathogen into a dairy herd may result in fulminant outbreaks of clinical mastitis if poor milking and intramammary treatment hygiene potentiates the spread of the organism.
• Herds in which cattle are frequently added to existing groups appear to be at greater risk for *Mycoplasma* spp. ocular disease.

PRODUCTION MANAGEMENT
• Vaccines have been approved and marketed for *M. bovis* respiratory disease in the United States. However, at this time the efficacy and performance of these vaccines has yet not been demonstrated in controlled clinical trials.
• Mycoplasma mastitis resists intramammary or systemic antibiotic therapy during either the lactating or dry-cow period.
• Predisposing management and host factors include weaning and shipping stresses, mixing cattle from multiple sources, and inadequate preconditioning programs.
• Feeding raw milk from cows with mycoplasma mastitis has been implicated as an important risk factor. In beef cattle, the syndrome is most often seen in recently weaned calves mixed and assembled from multiple sources.

SYNONYMS
N/A

SEE ALSO
Cleaning and disinfection
Mycoplasma mastitis
Pneumonia
Respiratory pharmacology

ABBREVIATIONS
IBK = infectious bovine keratoconjunctivitis
PCR = polymerase chain reaction

Suggested Reading
Giacometti, M., Nicolet, J., Johansson, K. E., Naglic, T., Degiorgis, M. P., Frey, J. 1999, Apr. Detection and identification of mycoplasma conjunctivae in infectious keratoconjunctivitis by PCR based on the 16S rRNA gene. *Zentralbl Veterinarmed B*. 46(3):173–80.
Hirose, K., Kobayashi, H., Ito, N., Kawasaki, Y., Zako, M., Kotani, K., Ogawa, H., Sato, H. 2003, Sep. Isolation of mycoplasmas from nasal swabs of calves affected with respiratory diseases and antimicrobial susceptibility of their isolates. *J Vet Med B Infect Dis Vet Public Health* 50(7):347–51.
Kirk, J. H., Glenn, K., Ruiz, L., Smith, E. 1997, Oct 15. Epidemiologic analysis of *Mycoplasma* spp. isolated from bulk-tank milk samples obtained from dairy herds that were members of a milk cooperative. *J Am Vet Med Assoc*. 211(8):1036–38.
Nagatomo, H., Takegahara, Y., Sonoda, T., Yamaguchi, A., Uemura, R., Hagiwara, S., Sueyoshi, M. 2001, Sep 28. Comparative studies of the persistence of animal mycoplasmas under different environmental conditions. *Vet Microbiol*. 82(3):223–32.
Radostitis, O. M., Gay, C. C., Blood, D. C., Hinchcliff, K. W., eds. 2000. *Veterinary medicine*. 9th ed. New York: W. B. Saunders.

Author: Jeff W. Tyler

MYCOTOXINS

 BASICS

DEFINITION
• Mycotoxins are secondary metabolites that have no biochemical significance in fungal growth and development.
• They are produced mainly by the mycelial structure of filamentous fungi (molds).
• Toxigenic molds are known to produce one or more of these secondary metabolites. It is well established that not all molds are toxigenic and not all secondary metabolites from molds are toxic.
• Some molds are capable of producing more than one mycotoxin and some mycotoxins are produced by more than one fungal species. For example, aflatoxins (AF) are produced by several fungal species, have numerous structural variations, and have different modes of action depending on the target animal. Additionally it is common to find more than one mycotoxin in a contaminated feed.
• Despite isolation and chemical characterization of more than 300 mycotoxins, research has focused on those toxins that are known to cause significant damage to humans, livestock, and companion animals.
• Examples of mycotoxins of greatest public health and agroeconomic significance include AF, ochratoxins (OT), trichothecenes, zearalenone (ZEN), fumonisins, tremorgenic toxins, and ergot alkaloids.

• Mycotoxicosis are characterized as feed related, noncontagious, nontransferable, noninfectious, and nontraceable to microorganisms other than fungi. Clinical symptoms usually subside upon removal of contaminated feed.
• Mycotoxins that adversely affect ruminant health or production are found mainly in postharvest crops such as cereal grains or forages. These toxins are produced by saprophytic fungi during storage or by endophytic fungi during plant growth.
• Except for fumonisins, mycotoxins are lipophilic and therefore tend to accumulate in the lipid fraction of plants and animals.

OVERVIEW
• Worldwide contamination of foods and feeds with mycotoxins is increasingly becoming a significant problem.
• In general, mycotoxins have various acute and chronic effects on humans and nonruminant animals.
• Depending on the target species, mycotoxins are known for their immunosuppressive, mutagenic, and carcinogenic effects. Additionally, they are well known for causing life-threatening injuries to critical organs such as the liver and kidney.
• The economic impact of mycotoxins includes loss of human and animal life, increased health and veterinary care costs, reduced livestock production, disposal of contaminated foods and feeds, economic investment in research and applications to reduce severity of the mycotoxin problem.

SYSTEMS AFFECTED
Hepatic, respiratory, and renal

GENETICS
N/A

INCIDENCE/PREVALENCE
N/A

GEOGRAPHIC DISTRIBUTION
Worldwide, depending on species and environment

SIGNALMENT
Species
All ruminant species

Breed Predilections
N/A

Mean Age and Range
N/A

Predominant Sex
N/A

 MISCELLANEOUS

Types and Fungal Origin of Mycotoxins
Aflatoxins
• Over 20 AF are produced by different *Aspergillus* species (e.g., *A. flavus* produces AFB_1 and AFB_2; *A. parasiticus* produces AFB_1, AFB_2, AFG_1, and AFG_2).
• Variations in the magnitude of toxicity exist among AF (e.g., AFB_1 is the most toxic in both acute and chronic aflatoxicoses, whereas AFM_1 is as hepatotoxic as AFB_1 but not as carcinogenic).

Ochratoxins
• OT are produced by both *Aspergillus* and *Fusarium* species.
• They are nephrotoxic in poultry, acutely toxic in rats and mice; they can promote tumors in humans.
• The most toxic OT is OTA, produced by *A. ochraceus* and selected *Penicillium* species such as *P. cyclopium* and *P. viridicatum*.

Trichothecenes
• Trichothecenes are mainly produced by several *Fusarium* species such as *F. sporotrichioides, F. graminearum, F. poae,* and *F. culmorum*. They are also produced by members of other genera such as *Myrothecium* and *Trichothecium*.
• Trichothecenes include T-2 toxin, diacetoxyscirpenol (DAS), and deoxynivalenol (DON—also known as vomitoxin and nivalenol).
• Both T-2 toxin and DAS are considered the most toxic.

Zearalenone
• Zearalenone is a phytoestrogenic compound that is a metabolite primarily associated with several *Fusarium* species such as *F. culmorum, F. graminearum,* and *F. sporotrichioides*.
• *F. graminearum* is considered the fungal species most responsible for the estrogenic effects commonly found in farm animals.

Fumonisins
• Fumonisins (B_1 and B_2) are cancer-promoting metabolites of *F. proliferatum* and *F. verticillioides*.
• Fumonisin B_1 is the most toxic and has been shown to promote tumors in rats and to cause equine leukoencephalomalacia and porcine pulmonary edema.

Moniliformin
• Moniliformin is produced by several *Fusarium* species (mainly *F. proliferatum*) and is usually found on the corn kernel. It can be transferred to next generation crops and survives for years in the soil.
• Although both fumonisin B_1 and moniliformin are produced by the same fungal species (*F. proliferatum*), no structural resemblance is found between the two toxins. Both toxins are shown in several FDA studies to be ubiquitous in U.S. corn.

Endophytic Tremorgens and Ergot Alkaloids
• Several colonizing toxigenic fungal species (e.g., *Acremonium lolii, A. coenophialum, Claviceps purpurea,* and *Penicillium* spp.) may thrive exclusively on live forages, especially grasses such as tall fescue.
• *A. lolii* is an endophytic fungus that thrives on perennial ryegrass and produces indole-terpene neurotoxins called tremorgens such as lolitrem B toxin.
• Perennial ryegrass staggers in livestock have been linked to lolitrem B toxin from *A. lolii* and to other tremorgens (e.g., penetrem B and verruculogen) produced by several *Penicillium* species (e.g., *P. crustosum* and *P. verruculosum*, respectively).
• Fescue foot, summer fescue toxicosis, and fat necrosis in cattle have been linked to tall fescue with growth of *A. coenophialum*.

• Other *Acremonium* species and *C. purpurea* are also responsible for sleepygrass toxicosis in livestock. This is a result of the ergot alkaloids (e.g., ergotamine, ergostine, and ergocristine) produced by these fungal species.
• Ergotamine and other lysergic acid amide derivatives in the perennial grass *Stipa robusta* are commonly associated with toxicoses in sheep.
• The two types of ergotism known in humans and animals are convulsive and gangrenous.

Mycotoxins in Ruminant Feed
• There are physical, chemical, and biological factors that operate interdependently and affect fungal colonization and/or mycotoxin production in ruminant feeds.
• The physical factors include the environmental conditions (e.g., temperature, relative humidity, and insect infestation) conducive to fungal colonization and mycotoxin production.
• The chemical factors include the use of fungicides and/or fertilizers.
• The biological factors include fungal strain specificity, strain variation, and instability of toxigenic properties.
• In general, the environmental conditions related to storage can be controlled, whereas those extrinsic factors (e.g., climate) or intrinsic factors (e.g., fungus-related factors) are more difficult to control.
• Unseasonable conditions have been suggested to render crops and forages susceptible to mycotoxin production (e.g., cool and damp springtime weather favors germination of the sclerotia and thus ergot alkaloid formation in fescue and ryegrass).

MYCOTOXINS

Negative Effects of Mycotoxins on Ruminants

• Ruminants are less known to exhibit the life-threatening effects that mycotoxins usually demonstrate in humans and other animals.

• Growth, production (milk, meat, or wool), and reproduction can be altered when ruminants consume mycotoxin-contaminated feed for extended periods of time (e.g., decreased productivity in cattle by AF and ZEN in sheep).

Cattle

• The role of AFB_1 in inducing bovine immunosuppression has been attributed to suppressing mitogen-induced stimulation peripheral lymphocytes and inhibiting bovine lymphocyte blastogenesis. Rumen motility can be reduced in a dose-dependent manner by feeding graded levels of AF (200–800 μg/kg of feed). Increasing AFB_1 level (up to 108.5 μg/kg of feed) decreases feed intake and a higher level (600 μg/kg of feed) also may decrease feed efficiency and body weight gain. These effects can be attributed to compromised rumen function (i.e., decreased cellulose digestion, volatile fatty acid production, and rumen motility). Milk yield and quality decreases with the feeding of AFB_1 (13 mg per cow/day) and the carryover rate of AFM_1 in milk is higher in early lactation than late lactation.

• Ochratoxins have not been shown to cause toxicity when fed alone or in combination with AFB_1 in naturally occurring doses (up to 540 and 13 μg/kg of feed, respectively).

• Except for T-2 toxin, trichothecenes have not been shown to affect cattle. T-2 toxin can induce immunosuppression by lowering serum concentrations of IgM, IgG, and IgA; by decreasing neutrophil functions, lymphocyte blastogenesis, and lymphocyte response to phytohemagglutinin; and finally by inducing necrosis of lymphoid tissues. Infertility and abortion in the final trimester of gestation have been also caused by T-2 toxin. Other effects of T-2 toxin included hemorrhagic syndrome in dairy cattle and abomasal ulcers and the sloughing of rumen papillae in calves.

• Zearalenone has been suggested to cause infertility and to decrease milk production.

• Consumption of tall fescue infected with *A. coenophialum* may cause fescue foot, hyperthermia, and fat necrosis. Fescue foot (vasoconstriction and gangrene in the hooves and tail) is attributed to the relaxation of smooth muscles caused by ergot alkaloids. Hyperthermia (summer fescue toxicosis) is characterized by weight loss, salivation, and heat stress, whereas fat necrosis is characterized by hardening of body fat and constricting internal organs, reducing serum cholesterol levels, and elevating serum amylase levels. Consumption of tall fescue infected with *A. lolii* also causes staggers, excitability, increased rectal temperature, increased respiration rate, and loss of body weight.

Sheep

• Feeding diets contaminated with AF (2.5 or 5.0 mg/kg of feed) caused hepatotoxicity in ewes. Symptoms such as hepatic and nephritic lesions, altered mineral metabolism, and increased size and weight of the liver and kidney were reported for lambs consuming AF at 2.5 mg/kg of feed. This AF dose also lowered plasma concentrations of several minerals (Ca, P, Mg, K, and Zn) in response to decreased feed intake and to malfunctions of the liver and kidney in lambs. The same AF dose also decreased lamb weight gain, suppressed cellular immunity, and induced changes in extrinsic coagulation factors as illustrated in increased fibrinogen concentration.

• Effects of trichothecenes on sheep appear to vary greatly even when high levels are consumed. For example, exposing lambs to DON (15.6 mg/kg of feed) had no effect on body weight gain, hemacytology parameters, or liver function. Exposing lambs to DAS (5 mg/kg of feed), however, induced weight loss. Further weight loss was also reported when lambs were fed the same level of DAS in combination with AF (2.5 mg/kg of feed) suggesting a synergistic effect of these toxins.

• Zearalenone has been shown to affect reproductive performance of sheep negatively by reducing fertility and ovulation rates when the dietary levels approached 12 mg/kg of feed.

• Fumonisins at high doses (11.1–45.5 mg/kg of body weight) have been demonstrated as acutely and fatally nephrotoxic and hepatotoxic in lambs. These high levels, however, have not been found in fumonisins-contaminated feeds.

• Sheep have been affected by ryegrass toxicosis as shown in the resulting tremors, decreased productivity, and occasional death. Perennial ryegrass staggers have been observed in sheep consuming ryegrass contaminated with *A. lolii* and the symptoms included shaking with loss of coordination and inability to walk. Staggers have been demonstrated when *A. lolii*-contaminated ryegrass had lolitrem B toxin at levels ranging from 2.0 to 2.5 mg/kg.

Other Ruminants

• Ruminants other than cattle and sheep have shown variable resistance to mycotoxins.

• Exposing white-tailed deer to AF (800 mg/kg of feed) caused acute injuries in the liver as illustrated in the increased serum bile acid concentrations and hepatic lesions.

• Offering weaned goats fumonisins-containing feed (95 mg/kg) had no effect on body weight gain and did not show any toxicity-related symptoms.

Ruminal Degradation of Mycotoxins

• The great resistance of ruminants to the negative effects of several mycotoxins is due to degradation and detoxification of these compounds in the rumen environment.

• Ruminal microbial degradation of mycotoxins has been demonstrated in isolated cultures of rumen contents.

• The rumen function, however, is negatively affected by the presence of mycotoxins. The negative effects include decreased cellulose fermentation, volatile fatty acid production, ammonia production, and proteolysis.

• Degradation of AF, OT, ZEN, T-2 toxin, DON, and DAS was demonstrated by using rumen protozoa and (or) rumen bacteria. Contribution of protozoa to ruminal degradation of mycotoxins, however, appears to be more significant than that of bacteria.

ASSOCIATED CONDITIONS
N/A

AGE-RELATED FACTORS
N/A

ZOONOTIC POTENTIAL

Examples of mycotoxins of greatest public health and agroeconomic significance include AF, ochratoxins (OT), trichothecenes, zearalenone (ZEN), fumonisins, tremorgenic toxins, and ergot alkaloids.

PREGNANCY
N/A

RUMINANT SPECIES AFFECTED

All ruminant species are affected.

BIOSECURITY
N/A

PRODUCTION MANAGEMENT
N/A

SYNONYMS
N/A

SEE ALSO
N/A

ABBREVIATIONS

AF = aflatoxins
DAS = diacetoxyscirpenol
DON = deoxynivalenol
OT = ochratoxins
ZEN = zearalenone

Suggested Reading

Black, R. D., McVet, D. S., Oehme, F. W. 1992. Immunotoxicity in the bovine animal. *Vet Human Toxicol*. 34:438–42.

Cheeke, P. R. 1998. Mycotoxins in cereal grains and supplements. In: *Natural toxicants in feeds, forages, and poisonous plants*, ed. P. R. Cheeke. Danville, IL: Interstate Publishers, Inc.

Cheeke, P. R. 1998. Mycotoxins associated with forages. In: *Natural toxicants in feeds, forages, and poisonous plants*, ed. P. R. Cheeke. Danville, IL: Interstate Publishers, Inc.

D'Mello, J. P. F., Macdonald, A. M. C. 1997. Mycotoxins. *Anim Feed Sci Technol*. 69:155–66.

Hussein, H. S., Brasel, J. M. 2001. Toxicity, metabolism, and impact of mycotoxins on humans and animals. *Toxicology* 167:101–34.

Author: Hussein S. Hussein

MYIASIS

BASICS

DEFINITION
Invasion of living or dead tissue by larvae of dipteran flies causes myiasis in livestock. Myiasis can be facultative or obligatory. The condition is of economic importance especially in Africa, Asia, and Australia.

OVERVIEW
• Myiasis, also known as fly-strike, is the infestation of the body by fly larvae.
  • Obligator myiasis: fly larvae are completely parasitic and will die without a host.
  • Facultative myiasis: fly larvae are free-living but can adapt themselves to a parasitic dependence on a host under the right circumstances.
• There are eight major flies affecting cattle: face flies (*Musca autumnalis*), houseflies (*Musca domestica*), horn flies (*Haematobia irritans*), horseflies (*Hybontia* spp. and *Tabanus* spp.), deerflies (*Chrysops* spp.), heel flies (*Hypoderma lineatum* and *H. bovis*), screwworms or blowflies (*Cochliomyia hominivorax*).
• Blackflies (family Simuliidae) produce a salivary toxin.
• Can be vectors for other diseases

SYSTEMS AFFECTED
Dermatologic, ophthalmic, musculoskeletal

GENETICS
N/A

INCIDENCE/PREVALENCE
N/A

GEOGRAPHIC DISTRIBUTION
Worldwide, depending on dipteran species and environment; Africa, Asia, North America, and Australia

SIGNALMENT
Species
Potentially all ruminant species

Breed Predilections
N/A

Mean Age and Range
N/A

Predominant Sex
N/A

SIGNS
• Animals show signs of restlessness and may bite at affected areas. Affected areas produce a foul-smelling odor with exudates, and the mature larvae are usually observed on the lesions.
• Signs can be broken into general categories based on action of the flies.

• Annoyance/irritation (all flies)
  • Weight loss
  • Reduced performance (decreased feed intake due to constant avoidance behavior)
  • Decreased milk production
  • "Gadding"—stampeding, wild running
• Blood-sucking flies (horn flies, stable flies, horseflies, deerflies, black blackflies)
  • Dermal lesions, wounds
  • Anemia
  • Transmission of infectious diseases (anaplasmosis, bovine leukemia virus, anthrax, tularemia)
• Hide damage (heel flies, screwworms)
  • Warbles (cysts)—heel flies
  • Ventral midline lesions —horn flies
  • Liquefactive necrosis and cavernous lesions filled with larvae—screwworms
• Toxin production (blackflies): secrete a salivary toxin that increases capillary permeability and allows fluid to escape into extravascular tissues.

Other
Heel flies, if killed in the fall before migrating: anaphylaxis, weakness, ataxia, dyspnea, bloat

CAUSES
• Larvae of the flies *Cochliomyia hominivorax* (North America) and *Chrysomia bezziana* (Africa, Asia, and Persian Gulf) cause screwworm myiasis. They are obligatory myiasis-producing flies, and they depend on the host to complete their life cycles. They invade living tissues.
• Larvae from other dipteran flies including *Musca domestica* (the housefly) and flies from the genera *Phornia, Lucilia,* and *Calliphora* (blowflies) are facultative myiasis-producing flies. They invade cutaneous dead tissues and cause cutaneous myiasis.
• Understanding the life cycle of the flies allows a better opportunity to break the cycle and control the flies.
  • Face flies: overwinter in buildings. Females feed on facial secretions (tears, saliva, nasal secretions, milk on calves' faces.
  • Horn flies: reproduce only in bovine feces, but feed on horses, sheep, and goats as well as cattle. Flies can travel 7–10 miles in search of a host.
  • Horseflies: intermittent blood feeders. Females must have a blood meal to lay eggs. Larvae are aquatic or semiaquatic.
  • Stable flies: require a blood meal one to two times daily. Larvae develop in decaying organic matter, such as grass clippings.
  • Houseflies: breed in manure
  • Screwworms: blowfly lays eggs on a preexisting wound. Obligate myiasis requires live tissue. Disease is self-perpetuating and more common in hot, humid weather.

• Heel flies: 9–12-month life cycle. Eggs are attached to hairs on the lower limbs. Eggs hatch, enter skin, and migrate. *H. bovis* migrates to the epidural fat in the spinal cord region. *H. lineatum* migrates to the esophagus. Larvae migrate a second time to the back in January and February. Third-stage larvae emerge from warbles and drop to ground. In 1–3 months, flies emerge and live < 1 week.

RISK FACTORS
• Obligatory myiasis-causing flies lay their eggs only on fresh wounds. These include wounds created by procedures such as castration, dehorning, and docking. Sites such as the navel of newborns, perineum, vagina, and wounds from tick bites also are susceptible to invasion.
• The exudates and odor from these flies attract more flies including flies causing cutaneous myiasis.
• Cutaneous myiasis is of major economic importance in sheep. Flies are attracted to wet fleece, areas affected by fleece rot, foot rot, and perineum soiled by feces or urine staining. The most common area affected in sheep is the breech.
• Lush pastures and parasitic gastroenteritis predispose to cutaneous myiasis because of perineal soiling. In addition, dense thick pastures with wet plants keep the fleece wet.
• Fly numbers with screwworm myiasis or cutaneous myiasis are affected by ambient temperatures. Hot, humid weather favors development of the flies.

Life Cycles
Screwworm Myiasis
• Adult females lay eggs on fresh wounds. Larvae hatch in 12–24 hours, feed on tissue, and complete growth in 5–7 days. Larvae exit the wound, fall to the ground, and pupate in the soil.
• Pupal period depends on environmental conditions and varies from a few days to 2 months. Emerging adults mate and females can lay eggs as early 6 days of age.
• Adult flies can breed only once in life.

Cutaneous Myiasis
• Larvae hatch from eggs deposited by adult females that are attracted to sites with excessive moisture or exudates within 12–24 hours. After feeding on tissues, the larvae fall to the ground and pupate in the soil.
• Life cycle is shorter in hot, humid conditions.

DIAGNOSIS

• Larvae from dipteran flies can be differentiated based on morphology. Formalin-fixed samples must be submitted for identification.
• Predisposing factors such as foot rot, fleece rot, tick bites, and diarrhea can be easily differentiated from cutaneous myiasis.

GROSS FINDINGS
• Heel flies: summer months; yellow exudate on the distal limbs
• Spring: warbles (cysts) on back with breathing hole
• Screwworms: cavernous lesions filled with larvae that look like wood screws. Lesions are commonly found around the head (i.e., dehorning lesions)
• Horn flies: ventral midline lesions

TREATMENT

• *Cochliomyia hominivorax* has been eradicated in the United States by an ongoing sterile male release eradication program and this condition is considered a reportable disease.
• Ivermectin is effective in killing *Chrysomia bezziana* larvae. Ivermectin and organophosphates can be used in cutaneous myiasis. Ivermectin also kills adult flies.
• Appropriate milk and meat withdrawal times must be followed for all compounds administered to food-producing animals.
• Sanitation: Remove decaying vegetation and bedding, rotting silage. Remove manure at least twice weekly
• Topical: ear tags, back rubbers and dust bags, pour-ons
• Feed additives (to kill eggs and larvae in feces): diflubenzuron (chitin inhibitor), tetrachlorvinphos
• Surgical: surgical removal of warbles

MEDICATIONS

CONTRAINDICATIONS
• Steroids should not be used in pregnant animals.

• Pour-ons and ivermectin/moxidectin must be given before October 15 (Northern Hemisphere) if used for treating heel flies. If treated after migration to epidural fat or esophagus, an inflammatory response can occur and a granuloma can form around the dead parasite.
• Always follow label recommendations for meat and milk withdrawal times, as well as mixing directions.

FOLLOW-UP

PREVENTION/AVOIDANCE
Treatment of wounds, ear tags with larvicide can be used. Sterile male release eradication has been successful.

EXPECTED COURSE AND PROGNOSIS
• Prognosis depends on the number and type of flies, as well as success of preventive measures. In general, animals should make a full recovery. However, severe screwworm infestations can cause death.
• Large numbers of blood-sucking flies can cause death from anemia. Massive infestations of blackflies can cause death due to capillary permeability.

MISCELLANEOUS

ASSOCIATED CONDITIONS
• Secondary wound infections and subsequent septicemia
• Face flies transmit *Moraxella bovis* (pink eye). They are vectors for *Thelazia* spp. and *Parafilaria bovicola*.
• Horn flies are the intermediate host for *Stephanofilaria stilesi* (filarial dermatosis of cattle)
• Horseflies can transmit anthrax, anaplasmosis, and tularemia.
• Stable flies are vectors of anthrax and surra
• Screwworms can cause secondary bacterial infections and toxemia.

AGE-RELATED FACTORS
N/A

ZOONOTIC POTENTIAL
N/A

PREGNANCY
N/A

RUMINANT SPECIES AFFECTED
• Cutaneous myiasis is of major economic importance in sheep. Flies are attracted to wet fleece, areas affected by fleece rot, foot rot, and perineum soiled by feces or urine staining. The most common area affected in sheep is the breech.
• All ruminant species may be affected.

BIOSECURITY
Screwworms are a reportable disease. Contact state or federal veterinarians if screwworm infestation is suspected.

PRODUCTION MANAGEMENT
• Wound-control measures
• Fly-control measures
• Shearing sheep
• Docking sheep
• Prevention of fleece rot, foot rot, and diarrhea

SYNONYMS
Fly blown

SEE ALSO
Anthelmintic: small ruminant, pediculosis

ABBREVIATIONS
N/A

Suggested Reading
Catts, E. P. and G. R. Mullen. 2002. Myiasis (Muscoidea, Oestroidea). In: *Medical and veterinary entomology* (G. R. Mullen and L.A. Durden, Eds.), pp. 318–348. San Diego, CA: Elsevier Science.
Radostits, O. M., Gay, C. C., Blood, D. C., et al. 2000. *Veterinary medicine*. 9th ed. New York: W. B. Saunders.
Spradbery, J. P., Tozer, R. S., Pound, A. A. 1991. The efficacy of insecticides against screw-worm fly (*Chrysomyia bezziana*). *Aust Vet J.* 68:338–42.
Thompson, D. R., Eagleson, J. S., Rugg, D., et al. 1994. The efficacy of ivermectin jetting fluid for control of blow fly strike on sheep under field conditions. *Aust Vet J.* 71:44–46.

Authors: Tina Wismer and Charlotte Means

MYOCARDITIS

BASICS

DEFINITION
Myocarditis is an inflammation of the myocardium due to various organisms (bacterial, viral, parasitic) or due to a thromboembolism from a vegetative endocarditis caused by these organisms.

PATHOPHYSIOLOGY
Damage to the endocardium due to unknown causes (possibly secondary to monensin toxicity) may lead to penetration of various organisms (bacterial, viral, parasitic) into the myocardium causing inflammation of the myocardium.

SYSTEMS AFFECTED
Cardiovascular system

GENETICS
N/A

INCIDENCE/PREVALENCE
Difficult to assess due to the disease often being subclinical

GEOGRAPHIC DISTRIBUTION
N/A

SIGNALMENT
Species
Mainly cattle

Breed Predilections
N/A

Mean Age and Range
N/A

Predominant Sex
N/A

SIGNS

HISTORICAL FINDINGS
May be history of sudden death following stress, or failure to thrive, or recurrent fevers, or monensin toxicosis

PHYSICAL EXAMINATION FINDINGS
• Tachycardia, cardiac arrhythmias, dyspnea, fever
• May have pronounced gallop rhythm or cardiac murmur over mitral valve or tricuspid valve in acute myocarditis

CAUSES AND RISK FACTORS
• Bacterial causes include *Staphylococcus, Streptococcus, Clostridium, Hemophilus,* and *Mycobacterium.*
• Viral causes include foot-and-mouth disease virus, bovine lymphosarcoma virus or BLV, bluetongue virus in sheep.
• Parasitic causes include toxoplasmosis, cysticercosis, sarcocystis, and *Neospora caninum* in neonatal calves.
• May also be associated with monensin or gossypol ingestion, nutritional myodegeneration (vitamin E/selenium deficiency or white muscle disease), and copper and cobalt deficiency in lambs

DIAGNOSIS

DIFFERENTIAL DIAGNOSIS
• Endocarditis
• Cardiomyopathy
• Cardiac neoplasia
• Congestive heart failure
• Monensin or gossypol intoxication
• Nutritional myodegeneration

CBC/BIOCHEMISTRY/URINALYSIS
• Leukocytosis due to neutrophilia, decreased serum albumin. If congestive heart failure occurs, may have liver damage with serum albumin and increased SDH, GGT, and bilirubin.
• Hemoglobinuria may suggest monensin or gossypol intoxication or nutritional myodegeneration as a cause of the myocarditis.

OTHER LABORATORY TESTS
• Blood culture
• Elevated myocardial enzymes of creatine kinase (myocardial bound) and lactic dehydrogenase, or LDH (LDH_1), may be present, interpretation uncertain in large animals.
• Whole blood selenium to rule out nutritional myodegeneration

IMAGING
Ultrasound/echocardiography to check for increased ventricular size, decreased interventricular septum size, and decreased myocardial function

OTHER DIAGNOSTIC PROCEDURES
• Pericardiocentesis with culture and sensitivity to check for bacterial agents
• Electrocardiogram, or ECG, to assess tachycardia and arrhythmia

PATHOLOGIC FINDINGS
• May be coronary thrombi and infarctions, and pale streaking of cardiac muscle, or may be no gross lesions
• Microscopically, may see increased interstitial fibrous tissue, foci of inflammatory mononuclear cells, and degeneration, necrosis, and fibrosis of myocardial cells

TREATMENT

ACTIVITY
Animal must be rested.

DIET
More forage and additional protein sources and limited cottonseed meal feeding to reduce gossypol ingestion to less than 1–2 g/kg for adult cattle and less than 0.5–1 g/kg for immature cattle.

CLIENT EDUCATION

• Good general husbandry (nutrition, vaccination, deworming) to boost immunity and limit exposure to disease agents
• Proper mixing of feed containing monensin; limited feeding of cottonseed meal to control gossypol toxicity
• Adequate supplementation of selenium and vitamin E to prevent nutritional myodegeneration

MEDICATIONS

• Control cardiac arrhythmias using quinidine
• Broad-spectrum antibiotics

DRUGS OF CHOICE

Quinidine 48 mg/kg IV over a 4-hour period

CONTRAINDICATIONS

Appropriate milk and meat withdrawal times must be followed for all compounds administered to food-producing animals

PRECAUTIONS

Concurrent IV administration of a balanced electrolyte at 3–4 ml/kg/h along with quinidine can help maintain adequate electrolyte and acid-base balance and blood pressure.

POSSIBLE INTERACTIONS

N/A

ALTERNATIVE DRUGS

N/A

FOLLOW-UP

N/A

PATIENT MONITORING

Monitor carefully during quinidine administration for adverse side effects (e.g., sweating, weakness, restlessness, cardiac arrhythmias).

PREVENTION/AVOIDANCE

See Client Education above.

POSSIBLE COMPLICATIONS

May develop idiopathic dilated cardiomyopathy

EXPECTED COURSE AND PROGNOSIS

Prognosis is fair to good if no signs of congestive heart failure, guarded to poor if signs of congestive heart failure are present.

MISCELLANEOUS

ASSOCIATED CONDITIONS

• *Hemophilus somnus* disease complex
• Monensin and gossypol toxicity
• Nutritional myodegeneration

AGE-RELATED FACTORS

N/A

ZOONOTIC POTENTIAL

N/A

PREGNANCY

N/A

RUMINANT SPECIES AFFECTED

Mainly cattle but all ruminants can be affected.

BIOSECURITY

N/A

PRODUCTION MANAGEMENT

N/A

SYNONYMS

N/A

SEE ALSO

Cardiac neoplasia
Cardiomyopathy
Congestive heart failure
Endocarditis
Monensin or gossypol intoxication
Nutritional myodegeneration

ABBREVIATIONS

BLV = bovine leukemia virus
ECG = electrocardiogram
GGT = gamma glutamyltransferase
IV = intravenous
LDH = lactate dehydrogenase
SDH = sorbitol dehydrogenase

Suggested Reading

Radostits, O. M., Gay, C. C., Blood, D. C., Hinchcliff, K. W., eds. 2000. *Veterinary medicine.* 9th ed. London: W. B. Saunders.
Smith, B. P., ed. 2002. *Large animal internal medicine.* 3rd ed. St. Louis: Mosby.

Author: David McKenzie

NAIROBI SHEEP DISEASE

BASICS

DEFINITION
Nairobi sheep disease (NSD) is a highly pathogenic, tick-borne, viral disease of sheep and goats. It is a reportable disease in the United States and on List B of the International Office of Epizootics.

PATHOPHYSIOLOGY
• NSD is transmitted by the bite of the brown tick, *Rhipicephalus appendiculatus*.
• The tick maintains the virus through transovarial and transstadial transmission. Unfed adult ticks can remain infectious for up to 2 years.
• The African bont tick (*Amblyomma variegatum*) in Kenya and a population of *R. pulchellus* in Somalia also transmit the NSD virus.
• Under normal field conditions, the virus is not transmitted by contact with infected animals. Experimentally, animals have been infected through inoculations of infectious blood, serum, and organ suspension and through large oral doses (50 ml) of infected blood or serum.
• Sheep tend to be more susceptible to NSD than goats.

SYSTEMS AFFECTED
• Gastrointestinal—abomasum, cecum, rectum, and ileocecal valve
• Hemic/Lymphatic/Immune—spleen, lymph nodes
• Respiratory
• Reproductive
• All organs and tissues will be affected with nonspecific changes.

GENETICS
N/A

INCIDENCE/PREVALANCE
• Sheep and goats in endemic regions are generally immune to NSD as are most lambs exposed while still protected by colostral antibodies.
• Naïve animals entering endemic regions often develop severe infections with mortality rates ranging from 40% to 90%.

GEOGRAPHIC DISTRIBUTION
• NSD is found primarily in east Africa. Infected animals have been found in Kenya, Uganda, Tanzania, Somalia, Ethiopia, and Zaire.
• One report has suggested the presence of the virus in India and Sri Lanka.

SIGNALMENT
Species
Sheep, goats

Breed Predilections
Masai sheep are more susceptible to NSD than other breeds.

Mean Age and Range
All ages

Predominant Sex
None

SIGNS

HISTORICAL FINDINGS
• Depression
• Diarrhea
• Straining
• Anorexia
• Nasal discharge
• Recumbency
• Abortions

PHYSICAL EXAMINATION FINDINGS
• Depression
• Fever—104–106°F (40–41°C)
• Diarrhea—initially thin and watery then progressing to contain frank blood and mucus
• Straining
• Mucopurulent nasal discharge
• Dyspnea
• Conjunctivitis

CAUSES
NSD is caused by virus in the genus *Nairovirus* of the family Bunyaviridae.

RISK FACTORS
• Outbreaks occur when naïve animals are moved into endemic regions.
• Sporadic outbreaks in nonendemic regions may occur after excessive amounts of rainfall and subsequent expansion of the tick vector's range.

DIAGNOSIS

DIFFERENTIAL DIAGNOSIS
• Heartwater
• Rift Valley fever
• Anthrax
• Peste des petits ruminants
• Coccidiosis
• Plant and heavy metal poisonings

CBC/BIOCHEMISTRY/URINALYSIS
Leukopenia during febrile stage

OTHER LABORATORY TESTS
• Virus isolation from the noncoagulated blood during febrile stage
• Paired sera samples showing a fourfold or greater rise in antibody titer
• ELISA of serum for neutralizing antibodies
• AGID of serum for neutralizing antibodies
• ID of serum
• HA of serum

IMAGING
N/A

DIAGNOSTIC PROCEDURES
• Virus isolation from mesenteric lymph nodes and spleen using cell cultures or by inoculating laboratory animals
• Virus identification from mesenteric lymph nodes and spleen using AGID
• IFA of cell cultures or from inoculated laboratory animal brain material
• CF of cell cultures or from inoculated laboratory animal brain material

PATHOLOGIC FINDINGS

GROSS FINDINGS
• Generalized lymphadenitis; ecchymotic and petechial hemorrhages on serosa on thoracic and abdominal organs; bloodstained intestinal contents; hyperemia and petechial hemorrhages on mucosa of abomasums, cecum, rectum and ileocecal valve; "zebra striping" of rectum; hyperemia of genital tract; congested spleen
• Aborted fetuses will have hemorrhages throughout internal organs, fetal membranes may be swollen, edematous, and hemorrhagic

HISTOPATHOLOGY FINDINGS
Nonspecific congestion and petechial and ecchymotic hemorrhages in most organs and tissues, mucosal hemorrhages from the abomasum to the rectum, severe glomerulotubular nephritis, lymphoid hyperplasia, myocardial necrosis

NAIROBI SHEEP DISEASE

TREATMENT

APPROPRIATE HEALTH CARE
• No specific individual treatment
• Herd preventative care—vaccination of susceptible animals moving to an endemic area with an attenuated, tissue-culture-propagated vaccine, pour-on acaricidal preparations

NURSING CARE
Infected animals should be provided with basic supportive care by replacement of lost fluids and restoration of electrolytes.

ACTIVITY
Animals should be protected from climatic conditions and stress.

DIET
Infected animals should be fed good-quality feed, avoiding rough feeds with low nutrient values.

CLIENT EDUCATION
• Clients need to be educated in the importance of tick control and vaccination protocols to prevent infection.
• Strict quarantine is not necessary because NSDV is not transmitted through direct contact.
• Dead animals should be disposed of by incineration or burial.

SURGICAL CONSIDERATIONS
N/A

MEDICATIONS

DRUGS OF CHOICE
N/A

CONTRAINDICATIONS
N/A

PRECAUTIONS
N/A

POSSIBLE INTERACTIONS
N/A

ALTERNATIVE DRUGS
N/A

FOLLOW-UP

PATIENT MONITORING
Patients should be monitored frequently for signs of dehydration.

PREVENTION/AVOIDANCE
• Owners should avoid taking naïve animals into endemic areas. If this is impossible, animals should be vaccinated with an attenuated, tissue-culture-propagated vaccine.
• Susceptible sheep and goats may also be protected from the vector by weekly application of acaricides, but this is often not feasible.

POSSIBLE COMPLICATIONS
Exposure of naïve herds of sheep or goats to NSD may result in 90% mortality.

EXPECTED COURSE AND PROGNOSIS
• Prognosis is poor unless animals were exposed when young while still protected by colostral antibody.
• Goats have a better prognosis than sheep.
• All animals who recover are immune for life.

MISCELLANEOUS

ASSOCIATED CONDITIONS
N/A

AGE-RELATED FACTORS
Colostral antibodies protect young in endemic areas.

ZOONOTIC POTENTIAL
• NSD appears to cause rare, mild, influenza-like symptoms in humans. One naturally acquired infection has been reported in Uganda.
• Precaution should be taken against aerosol exposure when working with this virus.

PREGNANCY
Pregnant animals will abort when infected with NSD.

RUMINANT SPECIES AFFECTED
Sheep and goats

SYNONYMS
N/A

SEE ALSO
Anthrax
Coccidiosis
Heartwater
Peste des petits ruminants
Plant and heavy metal poisonings
Rift Valley fever

ABBREVIATIONS
AGID = agar gel immunodiffusion test
CF = complement fixation test
ELISA = enzyme-linked immunosorbent assay
HA = hemagglutination test
ID = immunodiffusion test
IFA = indirect fluorescent antibody test
NSD = Nairobi sheep disease
NSDV = Nairobi sheep disease virus

Suggested Reading
Aiello, S. E., ed. 1998. *Merck veterinary manual*. 8th ed. Whitehouse Station, NJ: Merck and Co.
Howard, J. L., Smith, R. A. 1999. *Current veterinary therapy- food animal practice*. 4th ed. Philadelphia: W. B. Saunders Co.
Martin, W. B., Aitken, I. D. 2000. *Diseases of sheep*. 3rd ed. Oxford: Blackwell Science.
Timoney, P. J. 1998. Louping ill. In: *Foreign animal diseases*. Richmond, VA: United States Animal Health Association, http://www.vet.uga.edu/wpp/gray_book/FAD.

Author: Stacy M. Holzbauer

NASAL ANOMALIES

 BASICS

OVERVIEW
• Several nasal anomalies can affect the ruminant respiratory system.
• These include rhinitis (inflammation of the nasal passages), mycotic nasal granuloma (fungal infection of the nasal passages leading to granuloma formation), nasal tumors, allergic rhinitis (allergic reactions due to exposure to plant or fungal allergens), foreign body, trauma, and paranasal sinusitis (bacterial inflammation of the paranasal sinuses, mainly the frontal sinus and maxillary sinus).

PATHOPHYSIOLOGY
Rhinitis
Viruses, bacteria, fungi, and exposure to allergens can all lead to inflammation of the nasal passages. *Oestrus ovis* larvae or bots can also cause inflammation. The female fly deposits eggs around nostrils during summer and fall. Eggs hatch, and larvae crawl up nasal passage to dorsal turbinates and frontal sinuses, remain for weeks to months, and eventually migrate back to nostrils. They are sneezed out, and pupate on the ground.

Mycotic Nasal Granuloma
Eroded nasal mucosa becomes inoculated with fungal spores, causing a delayed (type IV) hypersensitivity and eventual granuloma formation.

Nasal Tumor
Growth of tumors leads to progressive airway obstruction.

Allergic Rhinitis
Exposure to allergens results in development of antibodies (e.g., IgE). Subsequent exposure results in an immediate (type I) hypersensitivity reaction. Chronic exposure may lead to chronic tissue damage from mast cell enzymes, causing hyperplasia and granulomatous inflammation (enzootic nasal granuloma).

Foreign Body
The presence of the foreign object leads to irritation and decreased airflow.

Trauma
Trauma and fractures of the facial bones, sinuses, and turbinates can lead to swelling, airflow obstruction, and epistaxis.

Paranasal Sinusitis
Bacterial inflammation of the sinuses may lead to anorexia, fever, and nasal discharge, and cause a head tilt probably due to inflammation of the peripheral portion of the vestibulocochlear nerve (cranial nerve or CN VIII).

SYSTEMS AFFECTED
Respiratory

GENETICS
Allergic rhinitis may be a familial predisposition.

INCIDENCE/PREVALENCE
N/A

GEOGRAPHIC DISTRIBUTION
Worldwide

SIGNALMENT
Species
• Rhinitis—all ruminant species
• Mycotic nasal granuloma—all ruminant species, mainly cattle
• Nasal tumor—all ruminant species, but rare
• Allergic rhinitis—mainly cattle
• Foreign body—all ruminant species, mainly cattle probably due to more aggressive eating habits
• Trauma—all ruminant species
• Paranasal sinusitis—most common in cattle, infrequent in sheep and goats

Breed Predilections
• Rhinitis, mycotic nasal granuloma, nasal tumor, foreign body, trauma, paranasal sinusitis—N/A
• Allergic rhinitis—Jersey, Guernsey, Holstein cattle

Mean Age and Range
• Rhinitis, foreign body, paranasal sinusitis—any age
• Mycotic nasal granuloma, nasal tumor, trauma—mainly adult animals
• Allergic rhinitis—usually 6 months to 2 years old

Predominant Sex
N/A

SIGNS
N/A

HISTORICAL FINDINGS
• Rhinitis—history of previous *Oestrus ovis* infection
• Mycotic nasal granuloma—previous signs of nasal irritation
• Nasal tumor—progressive signs of airway obstruction
• Allergic rhinitis—usually seasonal (warm, moist conditions) onset of signs
• Foreign body—signs of allergic rhinitis, with frequent attempts to scratch nose by rubbing against objects
• Trauma—fighting, roping, improper restraint, and passage of excessively large nasogastric tubes
• Paranasal sinusitis—dehorning or injury to the horns, or infected cheek teeth

PHYSICAL EXAMINATION FINDINGS
• Rhinitis—mucoid to purulent nasal discharge, stertorous breathing, sneezing, and inspiratory dyspnea if due to *Oestrus ovis* in sheep with milder signs in goats
• Mycotic nasal granuloma—stridor, dyspnea, mucopurulent nasal discharge, epistaxis, granulomas appear as yellow to red nodules or polyps up to 5 cm in diameter
• Nasal tumor—dyspnea, stridor, head shaking, nasal discharge, sneezing, epistaxis, foul breath odor, distorted facial bones
• Allergic rhinitis—sneezing, intense nasal pruritus, profuse bilateral mucoid nasal discharge, may develop enzootic nasal granulomas seen as multiple firm white nodules or flat pink plaques scattered throughout nasal cavity
• Foreign body—head shaking, sneezing, snorting, frequent nose licking, unilateral nasal discharge, foul breath odor, decreased airflow
• Trauma—facial swelling, subcutaneous emphysema, airflow obstruction, stertorous breathing, epistaxis. Secondary bacterial infection may cause foul breath odor and mucopurulent nasal discharge.
• Paranasal sinusitis—anorexia and fever initially, then nasal discharge, stridor, foul breath odor, purulent discharge from dehorning site, head tilt

CAUSES AND RISK FACTORS
• Rhinitis—bacteria, viruses (e.g., IBR, fungi, allergens). In sheep and goats, mainly caused by parasites (e.g., *Oestrus ovis* larvae or bots)
• Mycotic nasal granuloma—*Rhinosporidium, Aspergillus, Phycomyces*, other fungal species, more common in warm, wet climates
• Nasal tumor—squamous cell carcinoma, osteosarcoma, adenocarcinoma in cattle (e.g., ethmoid adenocarcinoma, which tends to be unilateral in cattle and metastasize to lymph nodes and lungs in cattle 6–9 years old); adenocarcinoma in sheep and occasionally goats (e.g., nasal adenocarcinoma in yearling to adult sheep)
• Allergic rhinitis—plant pollen or fungal spores
• Foreign body—aggressive eating habits (mainly cattle) or attempts to scratch nose in animals with allergic rhinitis
• Trauma—fighting, improper restraint, and passage of excessively large nasogastric tubes
• Paranasal sinusitis—dehorning or injury to the horns can cause frontal sinusitis, infected cheek teeth (molars, premolars) can cause maxillary sinusitis. *Actinomyces pyogenes* and *Pasteurella multocida* are the most common bacterial causes. Respiratory viruses (e.g., IBR/BHV-1 and PI-3, and *Oestrus ovis* larvae or bots in sheep) can also cause sinusitis.

DIAGNOSIS

DIFFERENTIAL DIAGNOSIS
• Rhinitis—allergic rhinitis, *Oestrus ovis* infection in sheep
• Mycotic nasal granuloma—allergic rhinitis, foreign body, tumor, nasal actinobacillosis or actinomycosis
• Nasal tumor—fungal granuloma, foreign body, sinusitis, fracture, nasal actinobacillosis or actinomycosis, Oestrus ovis bots in sheep
• Allergic rhinitis—fungal granuloma, tumor, foreign body, respiratory virus, nasal actinobacillosis or actinomycosis
• Foreign body—allergic rhinitis, tumors, fungal granuloma, nasal actinobacillosis or actinomycosis, *Oestrus ovis* bots in sheep

• Trauma—snakebite, actinobacillosis, actinomycosis, cellulitis from *Clostridium* or *Fusobacterium*
• Paranasal sinusitis—facial fracture, nasal tumors, actinobacillosis, actinomycosis

CBC/BIOCHEMISTRY/URINALYSIS
• Rhinitis, trauma, paranasal sinusitis—nonspecific inflammatory profile
• Mycotic nasal granuloma, nasal tumors, foreign body—N/A
• Allergic rhinitis—nonspecific inflammatory profile, eosinophilia

OTHER LABORATORY TESTS
• Rhinitis—nasal swabs for cytology and culture (numerous eosinophils and mast cells if *Oestrus ovis* infection is present)
• Mycotic nasal granuloma—biopsy/histopathology
• Nasal tumor—biopsy/histopathology
• Allergic rhinitis—biopsy/histopathology, cultures (bacterial, viral, fungal)
• Foreign body, trauma, paranasal sinusitis—N/A

IMAGING
• Rhinitis, mycotic nasal granuloma, allergic rhinitis, foreign body—endoscopy
• Nasal tumors—endoscopy, radiography
• Trauma, paranasal sinusitis—radiography

OTHER DIAGNOSTIC PROCEDURES
• Rhinitis, mycotic nasal granuloma, nasal tumor, allergic rhinitis, foreign body, trauma—N/A
• Paranasal sinusitis—oral/dental examination, percussion, sinus centesis, and cytology and culture

PATHOLOGIC FINDINGS
• Rhinitis—inflamed mucous membranes
• Mycotic nasal granuloma—granulation tissue containing eosinophils, mononuclear cells, sporangia, occasional hyphae
• Nasal tumors are commonly noted on necropsy
• Allergic rhinitis—inflamed mucous membranes, granulation tissue if enzootic nasal granulomas present
• Foreign body—inflamed mucous membranes
• Trauma—inflamed mucous membranes, traumatized soft tissue
• Paranasal sinusitis—purulent debris in frontal or maxillary sinuses

TREATMENT
• Rhinitis—see Medications below.
• Mycotic nasal granuloma—difficult to treat; salvage is often the most practical option. Can try surgical removal with long-term sodium iodide 66 mg/kg IV as 20% solution repeated at 14-day intervals until remission or iodism occurs
• Nasal tumor—surgical removal
• Allergic rhinitis—remove allergen (i.e., remove animal from pasture, anti-inflammatory drugs) and treat with anti-inflammatory drugs (e.g., dexamethasone 0.04–0.22 mg/kg IM or IV sid, or an antihistamine — tripelennamine hydrochloride 1.1 mg/kg IV or IM bid to qid as needed).
• Foreign body—manual or transendoscopic removal
• Trauma—surgery not usually needed unless injury very severe or breathing compromised
• Paranasal sinusitis—sinusotomy by trephining, flush daily with dilute antiseptic solution (e.g., 0.1% povidone iodine or 0.1% chlorhexidine); however, the frontal sinus of sheep and goats is very compartmentalized making flushing difficult. Antibiotics may be indicated (e.g., procaine penicillin G) and NSAIDs (e.g., flunixin meglumine) if systemic signs present.

ACTIVITY
N/A

DIET
N/A

CLIENT EDUCATION
See Prevention/Avoidance below.

MEDICATIONS
• Rhinitis—anti-inflammatory drugs (e.g., flunixin meglumine); ivermectin 0.2 mg/kg PO if due to *Oestrus ovis*. Treat in late summer to prevent heavy infestation and treat again in winter to kill overwintering larvae.
• Mycotic nasal granuloma—sodium iodide 66 mg/kg IV as 20% solution

NASAL ANOMALIES

• Allergic rhinitis—dexamethasone 0.04–0.22 mg/kg IM or IV sid, prednisolone 1–2.2 mg/kg IM or IV sid, topical corticosteroids in severe cases
• Trauma—prophylactic antibiotics (e.g., procaine penicillin G 22,000 U/kg IM or SQ bid) to prevent infection or sinusitis, NSAIDs (e.g., flunixin meglumine)
• Paranasal sinusitis—procaine penicillin G

DRUGS OF CHOICE
• Flunixin meglumine 0.5–1.1 mg/kg IV or IM sid to tid
• Procaine penicillin G 22,000 U/kg IM or SQ bid

CONTRAINDICATIONS
• Appropriate milk and meat withdrawal times must be followed for all compounds administered to food-producing animals.
• Steroidal agents are contraindicated in pregnant animals.

PRECAUTIONS
Allergic rhinitis—corticosteroid treatment may decrease milk production.

POSSIBLE INTERACTIONS
N/A

ALTERNATIVE DRUGS
N/A

 FOLLOW-UP

N/A

PATIENT MONITORING
N/A

PREVENTION/AVOIDANCE
• Rhinitis—if due to *Oestrus ovis*, ivermectin 0.2 mg/kg PO in late summer to prevent heavy infestation, and treat again in winter to kill overwintering larvae

• Paranasal sinusitis—dehorn at early age, avoid dehorning during rainy or dusty conditions; fly control; bandage if necessary

POSSIBLE COMPLICATIONS
Nasal tumor—surgical removal may be accompanied by significant blood loss; should have blood donor animal available for blood transfusion.

EXPECTED COURSE AND PROGNOSIS
• Rhinitis—usually good prognosis
• Mycotic nasal granuloma—guarded to poor prognosis
• Nasal tumor—poor prognosis
• Allergic rhinitis—fair to guarded prognosis
• Foreign body—usually good prognosis
• Trauma—usually good prognosis
• Paranasal sinusitis—guarded to fair prognosis

 MISCELLANEOUS

ASSOCIATED CONDITIONS
N/A

AGE-RELATED FACTORS
N/A

ZOONOTIC POTENTIAL
N/A

PREGNANCY
Allergic rhinitis—corticosteroid treatment may induce abortion or parturition.

RUMINANT SPECIES AFFECTED
• Rhinitis—all ruminant species; *Oestrus ovis* mainly in sheep
• Mycotic nasal granuloma—all ruminant species, mainly cattle
• Nasal tumors—all ruminant species, but rare

• Allergic rhinitis—all ruminant species, mainly Jersey, Guernsey, and Holstein cattle
• Foreign body—all ruminant species, mainly cattle
• Trauma—all ruminant species
• Paranasal sinusitis—all ruminant species, mainly cattle

BIOSECURITY
N/A

PRODUCTION MANAGEMENT
N/A

SYNONYMS
Allergic rhinitis = atopic rhinitis

SEE ALSO
Oestrus ovis
Pneumonia
Respiratory pharmacology

ABBREVIATIONS
BHV = bovine herpesvirus
Bid = twice daily
IBR = infectious bovine rhinotracheitis
IM = intramuscular
IV = intravenous
NSAIDs = nonsteroidal anti-inflammatory drugs
PI = parainfluenza
PO = per os, by mouth
Qid = four times daily
Sid = once daily
SQ = subcutaneous
Tid = three times daily

Suggested Reading
Pugh, D. G., ed. 2002. *Sheep and goat medicine*. Philadelphia: W. B. Saunders.
Radostits, O. M., Gay, C. C., Blood, D. C., Hinchcliff, K. W., eds. 2000. *Veterinary medicine*. 9th ed. London: W. B. Saunders.
Smith, B. P., ed. 2002. *Large animal internal medicine*. 3rd ed. St. Louis: Mosby.

Author: David McKenzie

BASICS

DEFINITION
• Necrobacillosis is a term used to describe any lesion associated with the gram-negative, strictly anaerobic bacterium *Fusobacterium necrophorum*.
• Oral necrobacillosis is a term used to describe infections of the mouth and larynx with *F. necrophorum*.
• This syndrome includes "necrotic stomatitis" in which the lesions are restricted to the oral cavity and "calf diphtheria" in which the lesions are largely confined to the larynx, buccal, and pharyngeal mucosa.
• *F. necrophorum* is a ubiquitous bacterial organism commonly found in the environment (soil) and is considered part of the normal flora of the oral cavity, respiratory tract, gastrointestinal tract, and urogenital tract of many omnivores and herbivores. The organism is commonly isolated from the soil of feedlots.

PATHOPHYSIOLOGY
• The organisms gain access to the body through traumatic injuries to mucous membranes and are considered to be infectious but noncontagious.
• It is generally thought that *F. necrophorum* is unable to penetrate and invade intact mucous membranes. Underlying mucosal defects (such as mucositis and laryngeal contact ulcers caused by repeated closure of the larynx associated with reflex coughing and swallowing) and laryngeal ulcers associated with mixed upper respiratory tract infections likely serve as portals of entry for bacterial organisms.
• *F. necrophorum* is thought to be a secondary bacterial invader and is often found in mixed infections. The ability of *F. necrophorum* to cause disease is enhanced by concurrent bacterial infections (e.g., *Arcanobacterium pyogenes*) and this synergy may play an important role in mixed infections.
• The organism produces a number of toxins associated with virulence, including necrotizing exotoxin, leukotoxin, hemolysins, hemagglutinin, adhesins, platelet-aggregating factor, extracellular enzymes, and endotoxins. The leukotoxin is known to be cytotoxic and causes vascular thrombosis.
• Infection leads to localized inflammation and edema of the laryngeal mucosa and cartilage; however, bacteremia and dissemination of organisms to the liver and other organs can occur in some cases.

SYSTEMS AFFECTED
• Gastrointestinal—primary (oral cavity, tongue, pharynx) and secondary (liver)
• Respiratory—primary (larynx/lungs)

GENETICS
N/A

INCIDENCE/PREVALENCE
The incidence of necrotic stomatitis is considered to be sporadic, with only a few calves in a herd becoming infected (low group morbidity rate). Outbreaks can occur in areas with poor hygiene or in areas with high concentrations of animals. Clusters of cases may occur when predisposing factors are present in large groups of animals over a short period of time. The disease occurs year-round, but there tends to be a higher incidence in the fall and winter.

GEOGRAPHIC DISTRIBUTION
• Worldwide distribution
• More common in countries where animals are housed indoors in the winter (confined quarters), maintained in feedlots, or housed in unsanitary environments

SIGNALMENT

Species
Cattle (bovine), sheep (ovine), goats (caprine), pronghorn antelope (*Antilocapra americana*), white tailed deer (*Odocoileus virginianus*), mule deer (*Odocoileus hemionus*), elk (*Cervus elaphus*), caribou (*Rangifer tarandus*), and wild/exotic ruminant species (e.g., gazelles, impalas).

Breed Predilections
There are no breed predilections.

Mean Age and Range
• The oral infection (necrotic stomatitis) tends to occur in calves <3 months of age, most commonly between 2 weeks and 3 months of age.
• Involvement of the larynx (necrotic laryngitis) is more common in older calves (yearlings up to 18 months of age).

Predominant Sex
There is no sex predilection.

SIGNS

HISTORICAL FINDINGS
Swollen, distended cheeks, tongue, and throat region; acute onset of a moist painful cough; lethargy, anorexia, and depression; inspiratory stridor, tachypnea, loud wheezing respiratory sounds; ptyalism, frequent and painful swallowing, dysphagia; fetid/rancid odor to the breath/halitosis; acute cases may remain active and bright without a fever initially; purulent nasal discharge (often bilateral); difficulty and reluctance to nurse; affected animals often stand and sip water continually.

PHYSICAL EXAMINATION FINDINGS
• Fever: temperature tends to be higher for calf diphtheria: 106° F (41°C); body temperature is moderately elevated for necrotic stomatitis: 103–104°F (39.5–40°C).
• Swollen (edematous) and hyperemic oral, pharyngeal, or laryngeal mucous membranes.
• The pharyngeal region may be painful on external palpation.
• Laryngeal opening is often reduced by edema and inflammation.

• Inspiratory dyspnea progressing to open-mouth breathing with extended head and neck.
• Necrotic erosions and ulcers (with diphtheritic membranes) are usually visible in the larynx/pharynx.

CAUSES
• The etiologic agent is thought to be *Fusobacterium necrophorum*, a gram-negative, strictly anaerobic bacterium, although many of these cases involve mixed infections.
• *F. necrophorum* is an opportunistic pathogen that gains entry either through lesions of viral infections (IBR or papular stomatitis) or after traumatic injury to mucous membranes.
• Many predisposing factors to infection have been suggested, including:
  • Contact ulcers of the laryngeal mucosa
  • Debilitating diseases
  • Erupting teeth
  • Generalized mucositis
  • Inhaled irritants/allergens
  • Nutritional deficiencies (e.g., vitamin A)
  • Other upper respiratory infections (IBR, PI3, bacterial, mycoplasmas, etc.)
  • Poor hygiene
  • Teeth grinding (bruxism)
  • Traumatic injuries to the oral mucosa

RISK FACTORS
• The incidence of disease tends to be highest in groups of animals that are kept in confined quarters under unsanitary conditions.
• Coarse, abrasive feeds may increase the risk of disease.
• General debilitating diseases may also predispose animals to developing disease.

 DIAGNOSIS

DIFFERENTIAL DIAGNOSIS
• Infectious bovine rhinotracheitis (IBR)
• Bovine viral diarrhea virus (BVD)
• Pharyngeal trauma (including iatrogenic)
• Dental abscess; maxillary or mandibular fracture
• Nasal granuloma
• Severe viral laryngitis/tracheitis
• Actinobacillosis
• Laryngeal edema; laryngeal abscess
• Foreign body
• Mycotic stomatitis
• Tumor (neoplasm)

CBC/BIOCHEMISTRY/URINALYSIS
Acute cases show changes in the CBC consistent with acute septic conditions:
• Leukopenia
• Neutropenia with a left shift
• Nonregenerative anemia
• Absolute neutropenia
• Granulocytopenia
• Hypoproteinemia
• Increased fibrinogen levels

NECROTIC STOMATITIS

OTHER LABORATORY TESTS
Anaerobic bacterial cultures can be obtained from deep within the oral and laryngeal lesions.

IMAGING
• Direct examination can be aided with use of an oral speculum with a good light source.
• Laryngoscopy to examine the lesions and the extent of laryngeal immobility
• Endoscopy (via nasal passage)
• Radiographs of larynx and oral cavity

DIAGNOSTIC PROCEDURES
• Clinical signs are often sufficient in establishing a diagnosis.
• Thorough visual examination of the oral cavity and larynx with an oral speculum or the above-mentioned imaging techniques are recommended to confirm the diagnosis.
• Bacteriology may be useful in identifying bacterial organism(s); however, *F. necrophorum* is strictly anaerobic and is relatively difficult to cultivate. Smears taken from the margins of the lesions may assist in confirming the diagnosis.
• Postmortem examination of affected animals is recommended to confirm diagnosis and to rule out other diseases.

PATHOLOGIC FINDINGS
• The gross lesions are most commonly located in the vocal processes and/or the medial angles of the arytenoid cartilages.
• Acute lesions include edema and hyperemia surrounding large, central, well-demarcated, yellowish-gray necrotic ulcers in the mucosa of the mouth, pharynx, and/or larynx.
• The lesions may extend along the vocal folds and processes and can involve the cricoarytenoideus dorsalis muscle. The tongue, buccal mucosa, pharynx, cheeks, gums, palate, and trachea may also be involved.
• The necrotic tissue projects slightly above the normal surface and is friable and adherent. In time, this tissue may slough, leaving erosions and ulcers.
• Chronic cases contain necrotic cartilage often associated with draining tracts and granulation tissue. In severe cases, you may see occlusion of the airway.
• The regional lymph nodes may be swollen and/or hyperemic; may see necrosis of the palatine and pharyngeal tonsils.
• On histopathology, areas of coagulation necrosis are surrounded by a zone of vascular reaction, leukocytes, and granulation tissue.
• The bacteria are typically arranged in long filaments (sometimes as rods or cocci), but are relatively difficult to demonstrate in tissue sections.

TREATMENT

APPROPRIATE HEALTH CARE
• Mild cases can be treated with outpatient medical management.
• Severe cases with respiratory dyspnea may require immediate attention and possibly surgical intervention to maintain a patent airway.

NURSING CARE
• Good nursing and supportive care are critical in treatment of necrotic stomatitis and calf diphtheria.
• Easy access to food and fresh water, adequate ventilation, shelter, and oral electrolytes or intravenous fluids, if necessary.

ACTIVITY
• The activity level of these animals may likely be reduced due to respiratory dyspnea.
• High activity levels may exacerbate the condition and compromise the animal's respiration.
• Attempts should be made to keep affected animals calm and quiet to minimize stress.

DIET
• Avoidance of rough feed may minimize oral/pharyngeal abrasions.
• Affected animals may be reluctant to feed due to pain and swelling of the oral cavity and pharyngeal region.

CLIENT EDUCATION
• Care must be taken in examining affected animals not to compromise the respiratory tract. Visual examination and laryngeal imaging can be stressful and may result in additional insult to the animal's respiration.
• This condition is commonly associated with dry and dirty environmental conditions. Steps to minimize stressors and to clean up the environment may reduce the occurrence of this condition.

SURGICAL CONSIDERATIONS
• In severe cases, a tracheotomy can be performed if necessary to obtain a patent airway.
• Severe, chronic cases may require surgical debridement to remove necrotic and/or granulation tissue and to drain laryngeal abscesses.
• Subtotal arytenoidectomy may be indicated in severe cases involving chronic chondritis (inflammation of the cartilage).

MEDICATIONS

DRUGS OF CHOICE
Antibiotics:
• Sulfonamides such as sulfamethazine (initial/loading dose of 140 mg/kg IV, followed by 70 mg/kg IV SID/daily OR 150 mg/kg PO daily for 3–5 days). Treatment not to exceed 5 days.
• Initial parenteral administration of antibiotics followed by oral administration is recommended.
• Procaine penicillin (22,000 units/kg IM or SQ BID).
• Penicillin G procaine—15,000 units per pound IM or SQ SID for a minimum of 1 week. Withdrawal time = 10 days for cattle.
• Recommendations for antibiotic therapy should take into consideration that there may be multiple bacterial agents involved.

CONTRAINDICATIONS
• Oral medications should be avoided initially if possible to prevent additional damage to the irritated oropharynx and larynx and because affected animals have reduced ability to swallow.
• Crystalluria and renal disease have been reported in association with long-term administration of certain sulfonamides.
• Do not give oxytetracycline and penicillin at the same time.
• Drug withdrawal times must be determined and maintained for food-producing animals.

POSSIBLE INTERACTIONS
Please refer to the manufacturer's recommendations for specific drug dosages, timing, routes of administration, and withdrawal times.

ALTERNATIVE DRUGS
• Streptomycin, oxytetracycline, and tylosin are also effective antibiotics and have been used to treat calves with this syndrome.
• Nonsteroidal anti-inflammatory agents (NSAIDs) such as aspirin, phenylbutazone, or flunixin (0.5 mg/pound IM SID) can be used as adjunct therapy to reduce fever, swelling, inflammation, and edema.
• Corticosteroids and/or antihistamines may be used as supportive treatment to reduce laryngeal swelling and to prevent asphyxia.
• The use of mild topical disinfectants and antiseptics (e.g. Lugol's or povidone iodine) has been described.

NECROTIC STOMATITIS

FOLLOW-UP

PATIENT MONITORING

Affected animals should be monitored frequently, including body temperature, respiratory rate, oral and laryngeal examination. Identify infected animals early to prevent the spread of calf diphtheria.

PREVENTION/AVOIDANCE

• There are no specific control measures to prevent necrotic stomatitis.
• Minimizing predisposing factors, instituting good hygiene practices, avoiding rough feed, and minimizing exposure to dust and inhaled irritants may reduce the incidence of disease.
• In high incidence areas, prophylactic antibiotic feeding may minimize the impact of the disease.

POSSIBLE COMPLICATIONS

• Pneumonia, either from aspiration or hematogenous spread, is the most common complication.
• Septicemia/Fusobacteremia, toxemia. If the bacterial organisms gain access to the portal circulation, sequelae such as liver abscesses and ulcerative rumenitis may be seen.
• Necrosis of laryngeal cartilage can lead to laryngeal chondritis, resulting in a "chronic roarer." Permanent distortion of the larynx can lead to a harsh dry cough and inspiratory stridor.
• Extensive necrosis may lead to laryngeal paralysis (involvement of the cricoarytenoideus dorsalis muscle) and restriction of the laryngeal orifice. This results in increased efforts to breathe and this forced inhalation may lead to pneumonia.
• Venous drainage from the face into vascular sinuses of the meninges may lead to abscessation of the brain and pituitary gland.
• Severely affected animals that survive are often chronic "poor-doers."

EXPECTED COURSE AND PROGNOSIS

• If the condition is detected early and treated aggressively, the prognosis is guarded to good. Case mortality has been reported as approximately 15–20%.
• The disease course for acute cases ranges from 7–10 days, but may be as long as 2–3 months for chronic cases.
• Severe complications as listed above can occur, especially if the diagnosis is delayed. Several reports suggest that approximately 20% of affected animals progress to chronic cases. The prognosis for chronic cases (especially cases with bilateral involvement) is guarded to poor.

• Untreated calves tend to die from toxemia, upper airway obstruction/asphyxia, and pneumonia, usually within 2 to 7 days.
• A 60% success rate for surgical intervention in severe and chronic cases has been reported.
• Involvement of the laryngeal cartilage (ulcers and necrosis) often leads to a delay in healing or a failure to recover.
• It is recommended that chronic, unresponsive cases be culled.

MISCELLANEOUS

ASSOCIATED CONDITIONS

• Aspiration pneumonia
• Laryngeal chondritis

AGE-RELATED FACTORS

• Most calves affected are between 3 and 18 months of age; however, calves as young as 5 weeks and as old as 24 months have been affected.
• The oral form (necrotic stomatitis) is more common in younger calves less than 3 months of age.
• The laryngeal form (necrotic laryngitis/calf diphtheria) is most common in older calves up to 18 months of age.

ZOONOTIC POTENTIAL

• There have been case reports of *F. necrophorum* septicemia in humans; however, this syndrome is not commonly considered to be zoonotic. General precautions (e.g., wearing gloves) should be taken when working with infected animals.
• Oropharyngeal infection with anaerobic bacteria and subsequent thrombophlebitis and septic embolization in human patients is termed Lemierre's syndrome.

PREGNANCY

N/A

RUMINANT SPECIES AFFECTED

• Bovine, ovine, caprine, cervids, wild/exotic ruminant species
• There is a similar syndrome observed in housed lambs as a complication of contagious ecthyma (parapox infection).

BIOSECURITY

• Although the organism is fairly ubiquitous, measures taken to control other respiratory diseases may reduce the incidence of necrotic laryngitis.
• Proper hygiene precautions and disinfection of potential fomites in calf pens and feeding/drinking places

PRODUCTION MANAGEMENT

• Observation and early diagnosis of cases are critical to minimize the impact on a feedlot.

• Preventive measures and early treatment can reduce the total number of animals affected.
• This disease is usually sporadic in nature and the economic losses are primarily due to reduced live weights, inefficient feed conversion, expensive treatments, and deaths.

SYNONYMS

• Necrotic/necrotizing stomatitis, necrobacillary stomatitis, oral necrobacillosis
• Calf diphtheria, necrotic/necrotizing laryngitis, laryngeal necrobacillosis
• The organism *Fusobacterium necrophorum* was previously named: *Sphaerophorus necrophorus, Actinomyces necrophorus, Corynebacterium necrophorum,* and *Fusiformis necrophorus.*

SEE ALSO

Calf diphtheria
Foot rot/pododermatitis (contagious)
Hepatic necrobacillosis
Interdigital necrobacillosis
Liver abscess syndrome
Pneumonia (aspiration)
Rumen acidosis

ABBREVIATIONS

BID = twice daily
BVD = bovine viral diarrhea virus
IBR = infectious bovine rhinotracheitis virus
IM = intramuscular
IV = intravenous
NSAIDs = nonsteroidal anti-inflammatory agents
PI3 = parainfluenza virus 3
SID = once daily
SQ = subcutaneous

Suggested Reading

Aiello, S. E., ed. 1998. *Merck veterinary manual.* 8th ed. Whitehouse Station, NJ: Merck and Co.

Howard, J. L, Smith, R. A. 1999. *Current veterinary therapy: food animal practice.* 4th ed. Philadelphia: W. B. Saunders.

Jubb, K. V. F., Kennedy, P. C., Palmer, N. 1993. *Pathology of domestic animals,* vol. 2. 4th ed. San Diego: Academic Press.

Radostits, O. M., Gay, C. C., Blood, D. C., Hinchcliff, K. W. 2000. *Veterinary medicine: a textbook of the diseases of cattle, sheep, pigs, goats, and horses.* 9th ed. New York: W. B. Saunders.

Tan, Z. L., Nagaraja, T. G., Chengappa, M. M. 1996. *Fusobacterium necrophorum* infections: virulence factors, pathogenic mechanism and control measures. *Veterinary Research Communications* 20:113–40.

Author: Erik J. Olson

NEMATODIRUS

 BASICS

DEFINITION
Infestation with the intestinal roundworm *Nematodirus* spp.

PATHOPHYSIOLOGY
• Adult *Nematodirus* spp. reside in the anterior third of the small intestine of ruminants. Eggs are shed in the feces and, in the case of *N. spathiger* and *N. helvetianus*, development into the third stage larvae happens within the egg in 2 to 4 weeks. *N. battus* and *N. filicollis* have a delayed development and require conditioning by cold over winter. These infectious larvae remain within the egg until they are stimulated to hatch with rain and they can remain viable in the soil or on vegetation for many months. They are then ingested by the host during grazing and develop into mature adults in about 3 weeks.
• If the animal survives the effects of the parasite infestation, resistance to reinfection can develop.

SYSTEMS AFFECTED
Production management, gastrointestinal

GENETICS
N/A

INCIDENCE/PREVALENCE
N/A

GEOGRAPHIC DISTRIBUTION
• Worldwide depending on species and environment
• Varies with geographic location.
• UK, Europe, New Zealand, Australia, South Africa, North America

SIGNALMENT
Species
Potentially all ruminant species

Breed Predilections
N/A

Mean Age and Range
N/A

Predominant Sex
N/A

SIGNS

HISTORICAL FINDINGS
• Pasturing in an enzootic area
• Previous year's lambs, calves, or kids were infected and were on the premises.
• Asymptomatic in resistant animals to acute illness within 3 weeks of exposure in susceptible animals
• Most severe in young animals but older nonresistant animals can also be affected.
• Lack of adequate anthelmintic program

PHYSICAL EXAMINATION FINDINGS
• Diarrhea, anorexia, dehydration
• Poor body condition
• In severe cases, sudden onset and death

CAUSES AND RISK FACTORS
• *Nematodirus* spp.
• Cattle—*N. helvetianus* primarily, also *N. spathiger*, *N. filicollis*, and *N. battus*
• Sheep and goats—*N. battus*, *N. spathiger*, *N. helvetianus*, *N. abnormalis*, *N. davitiani*, *N. filicollis*, and *N. lanceolatus*
• Bighorn sheep, deer, gemsbok—*N. spathiger*
• Moufflon—*N. filicollis*
• Bison—*Nematodirus* spp.
• Feeding on infested pasture, usually early in the grazing period
• Inadequate use of anthelmintics and preventive pasturing practices

 DIAGNOSIS

DIFFERENTIAL DIAGNOSIS
The epidemiology of *N. spathiger* and *N. helvetianus* can resemble that of *Trichostrongylus* spp.

CBC/BIOCHEMISTRY/URINALYSIS
CBC and biochemistry are indicated in severely affected animals.

OTHER LABORATORY TESTS

IMAGING
N/A

OTHER DIAGNOSTIC PROCEDURES
• Identification of eggs in feces during the patent period; however, clinical signs start during the late prepatent period making diagnosis more difficult early in the outbreak.
• Eggs are distinctive and easily identified. They are large (180–230 microns by 90–170 microns), smooth and elongate, tapering at both ends. They are segmented (8 cells inside) when initially passed in the feces.

PATHOLOGIC FINDINGS
• Severe dark green diarrhea staining the escutcheon or breech
• Dehydration and possibly cachexia.
• Fluid mucoid content of upper small intestine and soft or fluid feces in the colon. Duodenal mucosa might show hyperemia with excess mucus, but is usually normal in appearance. Third-stage larvae reside in the deeper layers of the mucosa and crypts. Fourth- or fifth-stage larvae reside coiled among the villi, and if in high enough numbers, result in villous atrophy.
• Worm counts reveal tangled cottony masses of elongate, lightly coiled nematodes in heavy infestations.

 TREATMENT

• With clinical disease, adequate high-quality nutrition and water are essential.
• All animals in the group should be treated with anthelmintics to reduce exposure level.
• If possible, prevent reinfestation by moving to premises free of the parasite.

 MEDICATIONS

• Anthelmintics should be given initially when first animals are put to pasture in spring, then again in 3–5 weeks.
• Repeated treatments may be needed depending on environmental conditions and the species of *Nematodirus* in the area. Single treatments can be used with a delayed spring turnout or if transfer to noninfested premises is done.

- Protocols will vary with location making the experience of local veterinarians essential.
- Ivermectin or doramectin at 200 micrograms per kilogram body weight given subcutaneously
- Do not treat animals that produce milk for human consumption with ivermectin or doramectin.
- U.S. meat withdrawal times are: ivermectin and doramectin, 35 days.
- Other anthelmintics that may be effective include (use as directed and observe withdrawal times): levamisole—5 mg per kg body weight; morantel—numerous preparations available; benzimidazoles (fenbendazole, oxfendazole, and albendazole)—numerous preparations available.

POSSIBLE INTERACTIONS
N/A

CONTRAINDICATIONS
Appropriate milk and meat withdrawal times must be followed for all compounds administered to food-producing animals.

FOLLOW-UP

PREVENTION/AVOIDANCE
- Anthelmintics as above
- Avoid infested premises/pastures
- Without reinfestation, premises should be relatively free of infective larvae or eggs after two seasons, so pasture rotation at that interval will decrease potential of exposure.
- Potential pasturing of different, not susceptible livestock species in the off years.
- If calves, lambs, or kids are put on the pasture, follow them with adults who are likely resistant.

POSSIBLE COMPLICATIONS
In UK, New Zealand, and Australia, high mortality rates have been experienced.

EXPECTED COURSE AND PROGNOSIS
Full recovery with resistance to reinfestation if clinical disease is mild and treated early

MISCELLANEOUS

ASSOCIATED CONDITIONS
- Other intestinal parasites
- Diarrhea, anorexia, dehydration

AGE-RELATED FACTORS
- Clinical disease seen primarily in calves, lambs, and kids
- Most severe in young animals, but older nonresistant animals can be affected also.
- If calves, lambs, or kids are put on the pasture, follow them with adults who are likely resistant.

ZOONOTIC POTENTIAL
None

PREGNANCY
N/A

RUMINANT SPECIES AFFECTED
Potentially, all ruminant species can be affected.

BIOSECURITY
- Isolation and quarantine of new stock entering the herd/flock
- Treat and or cull new animals for disease conditions prior to herd introduction.
- If possible, prevent reinfestation by moving to premises free of the parasite.

PRODUCTION MANAGEMENT
- Avoid infested premises/pastures.
- Without reinfestation, premises should be relatively free of infective larvae or eggs after two seasons, so pasture rotation at that interval will decrease potential of exposure.
- Potential pasturing of different, not susceptible livestock species in the off years.

SYNONYMS

SEE ALSO
Anthelmintic drugs
Body condition scoring
Deworming programs for specific species
Diarrheal diseases
FARAD
Trichostrongylus spp.

ABBREVIATION
FARAD = Food Animal Residue Avoidance Databank

Suggested Reading
Darchies, P., et al. 2001. Efficacy of doramectin against *Oestrus ovis* and GI nematodes in sheep in the southwest of France. *Vet Parasitol*. 96(2):147–54.
Ivens, V. R., Mark, D. L., Levine, N. D. 2000. *Principal parasites of domestic animals in the United States*. Special Publication 52. Urbana-Champaign: Colleges of Agriculture and Veterinary Medicine, University of Illinois.
Jubb, K. V. F., Kennedy, P. C., Palmer, N., eds. 1993. *Pathology of domestic animals*, vol. 3. 4th ed. San Diego: Academic Press.
Ranjan S., et al. 1997. Nematode reinfection following treatment of cattle with doramectin and ivermectin. *Vet Parasitol*. 72(1):25–31.
Rehbein, S., et al. 2000. Efficacy of ivermectin controlled release capsule against some rarer nematode parasites of sheep. *Vet Parasitol*. 88(3–4):293–98.

Author: Edward L. Powers

NEONATAL DIARRHEA

 BASICS

OVERVIEW
- Neonatal diarrhea is the most prevalent illness in ruminants during the first 28 days of life.
- The development of diarrhea in neonates occurs because of a lack of adequate immunoglobulin transfer, an overwhelming exposure to enteric pathogens, or a combination of the two.
- Although diarrheas are discussed as being caused by a single disease entity, most cases of diarrhea are a result of mixed infections.
- Treatment centers on the correction of electrolyte imbalances and hydration status.
- Death occurs due to dehydration, metabolic derangements, and electrolyte imbalances.
- Prevention focuses on vaccination of the dams with appropriate antigens prepartum, ensuring adequate colostral intakes, and providing a clean birthing and housing environment.

PATHOPHYSIOLOGY
Secretory Diarrhea
- Results from the stimulation of intestinal cells to secrete fluid into the lumen of the intestine. Although the absorptive capacity of the intestine remains intact, the amount of fluid secreted overcomes the absorptive capacity resulting in diarrhea.
- *E. coli* and *Salmonella* secrete entero- or exotoxins, which stimulate intestinal epithelium to secrete sodium, chloride, and potassium along with fluid.
- The production of prostaglandins, as a result of inflammatory processes, will stimulate cellular secretions as well as cytokines which are commonly seen in salmonellosis infections.

Malabsorptive Diarrhea
Results from injury to the absorptive epithelium of the intestinal tract. Viral agents—coronavirus and rotavirus—and parasitic agents—cryptosporidia and coccidia—are the main agents involved in this type of diarrhea.

Injury to the Intestinal Epithelium
- Results not only in the loss of absorptive capacity but also the loss of the enzyme systems needed for the digestion of nutrients such as lactose.
- Osmotically active solutes result from improper digestion and subsequent bacterial fermentation of nondigested nutrients. These osmotically active solutes draw fluid into the intestine, overcoming the absorptive capacity of the gut.
- Because diarrhea is usually the result of the interaction of multiple disease agents, various mechanisms are involved in the development of diarrhea.

SYSTEMS AFFECTED
Gastrointestinal, cardiovascular, musculoskeletal

GENETICS
NA

INCIDENCE/PREVALENCE
Incidence is higher in neonates born to primiparous dams due to ingestion of poor-quality colostrum and limited volume. Incidence is variable depending on the neonate's colostral intake and the environment in which it is born and housed.

SIGNALMENT
Species
Bovine, caprine and ovine

Breed Predilections
NA

Mean Age and Range
- Enterotoxigenic *E. coli* — usually within the first 4 days of life, may extend to 2 weeks if the animal is infected with viral or parasitic agents
- Enteroinvasive *E. coli* —first week of life for septicemia, joint infections may develop during the first two weeks of life.
- Enteropathogenic and Enterohemorrhagic *E. coli* —usually in the second and third weeks of life, range 4–28 days
- Salmonella —14 days to 2 months
- Coronavirus —7–14 days of age
- Rotavirus —4 days to 2 weeks of age
- Cryptosporidiosis —7 days to 3 weeks of age
- Coccidiosis —16 days of age and older

Predominant Sex
NA

SIGNS

GENERAL COMMENTS
- The severity of the diarrhea is dependent on agent virulence factors as well as host factors. Some animals may remain bright and alert and only exhibit mild signs of diarrhea, while others may have a profuse watery diarrhea and exhibit systemic involvement resulting in death.
- Most of the clinical signs observed are related to hypovolemia as a result of dehydration.
- The characteristics of the diarrhea are not diagnostic, although the presence of blood and mucus indicates large-intestine involvement.
- The presence of milk curds in the feces indicates a malabsorptive and or maldigestive type condition often associated with viral agents.
- Clinical signs of septicemia are associated with animals that are agammaglobulinemic or infected with enteroinvasive *E. coli* or *Salmonella*.

HISTORICAL FINDINGS
In a herd or flock situation, the number of cases increases with the duration of calving, lambing, or kidding season as the pathogen load builds over time.

PHYSICAL EXAMINATION FINDINGS
• Animals will have soiled perineums and tails. Animals will have varying degrees of dehydration exhibited by increased skin tent, sunken eyes, and tacky mucous membranes.
• Animals may or may not be febrile. Heart rate is increased due to dehydration but some animals may be bradycardic due to hyperkalemia. Respiratory rate will be elevated depending on the animal's acid-base status.
• The abdomen may appear slab sided if the animal is not eating or may appear bloated, especially on the right side, due to ileus and collection of fluid in the intestines.
• The umbilicus may be enlarged indicating omphalitis often associated with failure of passive transfer.
• Scleral injection as well as hypopion may be observed in calves that are septicemic.
• Animals may be recumbent and unable to rise indicating severe dehydration and acidosis.

CAUSES
• Rotavirus
• Enterotoxigenic *E. coli*
• *Cryptosporidium parvum* and *muris*
• Coronavirus
• Enteropathogenic and enterohemorrhagic *E. coli*
• Enteroinvasive *E. coli*
• *Salmonella* spp.
• *Clostridium perfringens* type C
• *Eimeria* spp.
• Bovine viral diarrhea virus
• Breda virus
• Calici virus
• Astro virus
• Parvovirus
• *Campylobacter coli* and *jejuni*

RISK FACTORS
• Inadequate colostral transfer of immunoglobulins resulting in agammaglobulinemia or hypogammaglobulinemia
• Birthing areas contaminated with fecal material containing pathogenic agents
• Inadequate or improper nutrition
• Neonatal housing in which the buildup of fecal material occurs. Environments that are cold, wet, and drafty.

DIAGNOSIS

DIFFERENTIAL DIAGNOSIS
• If diarrhea contains blood, *Salmonella*, coronavirus, enterohemorrhagic *E. coli*, BVDV, and coccidia should be considered.
• If diarrhea contains mucus, *Salmonella*, coronavirus, enteropathogenic *E. coli*, enterohemorrhagic *E. coli*, and coccidia should be considered.
• If the animal is febrile, *Salmonella*, enteropathogenic and enterohemorrhagic *E. coli*, and coccidia should be considered.
• Although infectious agents are often associated with neonatal diarrhea, poor-quality milk replacers may cause diarrhea in neonates as well as sudden changes in the diet.

CBC/BIOCHEMISTRY/URINALYSIS
CBC
• Hemoconcentration, increased plasma proteins
• A left shift may be observed in animals in which the infectious agent invades the mucosa, produces endotoxins, or causes mucosal damage to an extent that allows invasion of intestinal bacteria.

Serum Chemistry
• Hypoglycemia, metabolic acidosis, and prerenal azotemia are commonly observed.
• Serum Na and Cl may appear normal due to hemoconcentration but are low.
• Hyperkalemia may be present due to acidosis but a whole body potassium deficit exists.

OTHER LABORATORY TESTS
Determination of immunoglobulin status during the first week of life:
• Plasma protein, determined by refractometer, <5 mg/dL indicates failure of passive transfer.
• Zinc sulfate or sodium sulfite turbidity tests can be performed to estimate immunoglobulin status.
• Fecal floatation for observation of coccidia and cryptosporidia oocysts.

PATHOLOGIC FINDINGS
Gross Findings
• The intestines are filled with fluid. The mucosa may be congested. Gross lesions are not observed with most of the common causes of neonatal diarrhea.
• Hemorrhagic enteritis is associated with *Clostridium perfringens* type C infections.
• Mucosal ulceration is associated with BVDV infections.
• Disruption of the mucosa and petechial hemorrhages may be observed in animals infected with *Salmonella* or coccidia.
• Congestion of the lungs, liver, and spleen along with petechial hemorrhages of the epicardium and serosal surfaces of organs are often observed in animals with septicemia due to *Salmonella* or enteroinvasive *E. coli*.

NEONATAL DIARRHEA

HISTOPATHOLOGY
• Colonization of intestinal epithelium by enterotoxigenic *E. coli*.
• Adherence and effacement of epithelial cells by enteropathogenic and enterohemorrhagic *E. coli*. Stages of cryptosporidia and coccidia development are observed.
• A desquamation of epithelial cells, shortening and possible fusion of villi are observed with viral infections.

 TREATMENT

APPROPRIATE HEALTH CARE
N/A

NURSING CARE
• Fluid therapy is needed to correct dehydration, circulatory impairment and electrolyte and metabolic imbalances. Fluid may be administered orally or intravenously. Commercial oral electrolyte solutions containing glucose and an alkalinizing agent are recommended if the neonate is still nursing. Neonates without a suckle response need IV fluids. IV administration of lactated Ringer solution is adequate.
• With severe acidosis, isotonic sodium bicarbonate solution (1.3%, 13 of sodium bicarbonate to 1 l of distilled water) may be used. Dextrose solutions (2.5–5%) are indicated in cases of hypoglycemia.
• With hypoglycemia and an unknown electrolyte and acid-base status, a 2.5% dextrose and 0.45% saline solution has been recommended.

ACTIVITY
N/A

DIET
• Neonates with a suckle response should be left with the dam and allowed to nurse. Animals being reared artificially should remain on their diet or switch to whole milk or colostrum. If the diarrhea becomes worse or the calf becomes depressed, removal from the dam or milk is warranted. In case of hand-fed neonates that are depressed and not interested in sucking, or neonates not nursing the dam, neonates should receive a high-energy electrolyte solution at a rate of 10% of body weight divided into a minimum of four feedings. Once neonates are suckling, feed milk 5% of body weight in four feedings a day increasing amount per feeding gradually so calf is back on full feed within 2 to 3 days.
• Oral electrolytes containing an alkalinizing agent, other than acetate, should not be fed when calves are receiving milk as milk digestion maybe disrupted.

CLIENT EDUCATION
• Neonates should be kept dry and in a draft-free environment.
• Equipment used to treat neonates should be cleaned between animals.
• Diarrheic animals should be isolated from healthy animals as they are sources for large numbers of pathogens.
• Caregivers should wash hands between animals and keep clothing free of fecal material.

 MEDICATIONS

Many causes of diarrhea in neonates are self-limiting and antibiotics are not indicated. However, approximately 30% of neonates with diarrhea will have a bacteremia in which antimicrobial therapy may be beneficial.

DRUGS OF CHOICE
Broad-Spectrum Antibiotics
• Oral amoxicillin trihydrate 10 mg/kg PO q 12 h for nonruminating calves, 20-day slaughter withdraw (extralabel in small ruminants); amoxicillin trihydrate-clavulanate potassium 12.5 mg combined drug/kg PO q 12 h for 3 days (extralabel usage)
• Parenteral ceftiofur 2.2 mg/kg IM/SC q 24 h for 3 days (extralabel usage)

NSAIDs
Flunixin meglumine (1.1 mg/kg IV or 2.2 mg/kg IM) has been shown to decrease secretion induced by *E. coli* enterotoxins and reduce morbid days in calves with fecal blood (extralabel usage).

Plasma Transfusion
In cases of failure of passive transfer and depending on value of the animal, plasma transfusion may be warranted.

CONTRAINDICATIONS
• Do not use kaolin and pectin as they may increase electrolyte loss.
• Drug withdrawal times must be determined and maintained for food-producing animals.

FOLLOW-UP

PATIENT MONITORING
• Monitor attitude, suckling response and appetite, fecal color and consistency, and hydration status.
• Monitor age cohorts for signs of diarrhea.

POSSIBLE COMPLICATIONS
• Sepsis
• Hypovolemic shock
• Septic arthritis

PREVENTION/AVOIDANCE
• Ensure adequate colostral quality and intake.
• Birthing area should be clean.
• Remove dam and neonate after birth from birthing area and place in a clean environment.
• Dip navels in an antiseptic.
• Eliminate areas of fecal buildup.
• Vaccines containing enterotoxigenic *E. coli*, rotavirus, and coronavirus antigens and autogenous *Salmonella* vaccines given to dams prepartum may be beneficial.

EXPECTED COURSE AND PROGNOSIS
• Most cases of neonatal diarrhea resolve over a 2- to 3-day period. Recovery is dependent on the cause of the diarrhea.
• Diarrhea is more severe in animals in which multiple disease agents are present, for example, a virus-induced diarrhea with secondary bacterial infection.
• The length of time to recover is proportional to the amount of mucosal damage the animal experiences.

• Prognosis is directly related to the ability of the animal to maintain hydration and its immunoglobulin status.
• Animals that are hypogammaglobulinemic or are septicemic are at increased risk of dying.

MISCELLANEOUS

ASSOCIATED CONDITIONS
• Septic arthritis
• Omphalitis
• Meningitis

AGE-RELATED FACTORS
Neonatal disease

ZOONOTIC POTENTIAL
• All diarrheic animals should be handled as having a zoonotic potential.
• *Salmonella*, cryptosporidia, *Campylobacter*, and some *E. coli* are potentially pathogenic to humans.

RUMINANT SPECIES AFFECTED
Bovine, caprine, ovine

SYNONYMS
N/A

SEE ALSO
• Astro virus
• Bovine viral diarrhea virus
• Breda virus
• Calici virus
• *Campylobacter coli* and *jejuni*
• *Clostridium perfringens* type C
• Coronavirus
• *Cryptosporidium parvum* and *muris*
• *Eimeria* spp.
• Enteroinvasive *E. coli*
• Enteropathogenic and enterohemorrhagic *E. coli*

• Enterotoxigenic *E. coli*
• Parvovirus
• Rotavirus
• *Salmonella* spp.

ABBREVIATIONS
BVDV = Bovine viral diarrhea virus
IM = intramuscular
IV = intravenously
NSAIDs = nonsteroidal anti-inflammatory drugs
PO = per os, by mouth
SC = subcutaneous

Suggested Reading
Barrington, G. M., Gay, J. M., Evermann, J. F. 2002, Mar. Biosecurity for neonatal gastrointestinal diseases. *Vet Clin North Am Food Anim Pract*. 18(1):7–34.
Bendali, F., Sanaa, M., Bichet, H., Schelcher, F. 1999, Sep–Oct. Risk factors associated with diarrhoea in newborn calves. *Vet Res*. 30(5):509–22.
Muccio, J. L., Grooms, D. L., Mansfield, L. S., Wise, A. G., Maes, R. K. 2004, Oct 1. Evaluation of two rapid assays for detecting Cryptosporidium parvum in calf feces. *J Am Vet Med Assoc*. 225(7):1090–92.
Naylor, J. M. 2002. Neonatal ruminant diarrhea. In: *Large animal internal medicine*, ed. B. P. Smith. 3rd ed. St Louis: Mosby.
Sanders, D. E. 1985, Nov. Field management of neonatal diarrhea. *Vet Clin North Am Food Anim Pract*. 1(3):621–37.
Townsend, H. G. 1994, Mar. Environmental factors and calving management practices that affect neonatal mortality in the beef calf. *Vet Clin North Am Food Anim Pract*. 10(1):119–26.

Author: Kevin D. Pelzer

NEONATAL SEPTIC ARTHRITIS

BASICS

DEFINITION
• An inflammatory disease confined to the synovial membrane and articular surfaces as a result of sequestered bacteria.
• Route of infection is hematogenous as a result of bacteremia, which often originates from umbilical infection.
• Often occurs in multiple joints

PATHOPHYSIOLOGY
• Bacterial infections of newborn ruminants occur largely as a result of hypogammaglo-bulinemia.
• Neonates become bacteremic or septicemic from an infection that often originates from the umbilical cord or via oral ingestion.
• Bacteria then sequester in the joint and cause inflammation of the synovial membrane.
• Multiple joints are often affected
• Synovitis causes distension of joint capsule with fluid.
• Arthritis may be suppurative or serofibrinous.
• Erosion of articular cartilage, infection of subchondral bone, and osteomyelitis can be sequelae.

SYSTEMS AFFECTED
Musculoskeletal

GENETICS
N/A

INCIDENCE/PREVALENCE
• Incidence is not well described.
• Usually sporadic
• Can cluster in herds where calving occurs in unhygienic conditions

GEOGRAPHIC DISTRIBUTION
N/A

SIGNALMENT

Species
Cattle, sheep, goats, camelids

Breed Predilections
More common in dairy calves than beef calves

Mean Age and Range
• Neonatal ruminants < 4 weeks of age
• Usually evident within 2–3 days after birth

Predominant Sex
N/A

SIGNS

HISTORICAL FINDINGS
• Unhygienic calving environment
• History of inadequate colostral intake in the first few hours of life
• Small weak calves that remain recumbent for some hours
• Beef cows that reject their calves

PHYSICAL EXAMINATION FINDINGS
• Lameness is sudden and severe
• Multiple joints may be involved
• Joint effusion
• Pain
• Fever
• Inappetence
• Recumbency
• Palpation and flexion of joints reveal heat and pain.
• Tachycardia and dehydration may be evident.
• Umbilical abscessation may be evident on palpation.
• Nervous symptoms associated with meningitis may be present.

CAUSES
• *Arcanobacterium pyogenes*
• *Escherichia coli*
• *Streptococcus* spp.
• *Salmonella* spp.
• *Mycoplasma bovis*
• *Histophilus somnus*
• *Chlamydia psittaci* (lambs)
• *Erysipelothrix rhusiopathiae* (lambs)

RISK FACTORS
• Hypogammaglobulinemia as a result of inadequate colostral intake
• Dystocia
• Mismothering or abandonment
• Hypothermia
• Poor-quality colostrum
• Unhygienic calving area
• Overcrowded calving area

DIAGNOSIS

DIFFERENTIAL DIAGNOSIS
• Infectious arthritis can occur from primary causes such as penetration of joint by foreign body.
• Infectious arthritis can also occur from extension from surrounding tissues such as decubital lesions.
• Myositis
• Degenerative myopathy
• Trauma
• Diseases of the nervous system that may cause recumbency or lameness
• Osteomyelitis

CBC/BIOCHEMISTRY/URINALYSIS
Elevated white blood cell counts

OTHER LABORATORY TESTS
• Assessment of passive transfer can be evaluated at 8–12 hours after birth.
• Serum total protein less than 4.2 g/L is indicative of failure of passive transfer (FPT).
• Sodium sulfite precipitation test: rapid and accurate field test to assess FPT
• Serum GGT correlates moderately well with serum IgG concentrations.
• Radial immunodiffusion is the gold standard test for FPT but is expensive and takes longer to perform.

IMAGING
• Radiology may only reveal soft tissue swelling in early stages.
• Destruction of articular cartilage and bone may be evident in advanced cases.
• Occasionally, new bone may be deposited at periphery of joint.

DIAGNOSTIC PROCEDURES
• Joint aspiration may reveal purulent synovial fluid.
• Total leukocyte counts range from 50,000–100,000 cells/uL.
• Leukocytes are usually >90% neutrophils.
• Synovial fluid has elevated protein content (> 4 g/dL).
• Joint culture is often unrewarding.

PATHOLOGIC FINDINGS
N/A

TREATMENT

APPROPRIATE HEALTH CARE
• Systemic antibiotic therapy should be initiated and maintained for 5 to 10 days.
• Treatment of failure of passive transfer should be considered if possible.
• Short-term analgesic therapy (24–48 hours) in the form of nonsteroidal anti-inflammatories (flunixin meglumine or ketoprofen) may be used to reduce pain.
• Drug withdrawal times must be determined and maintained in treated animals

NURSING CARE
• Calf may need to be assisted to stand and nurse if appropriate (beef cattle).
• Physiotherapy by gentle flexion and extension or regular exercise may improve return to function.

ACTIVITY
Restricted until resolution of symptoms

DIET
N/A

CLIENT EDUCATION
• Predisposing causes should be discussed and eliminated if possible.
• Colostral management should be evaluated.
• Calving area hygiene should be evaluated.
• Warn client of need for long-term antibiotics and guarded prognosis.

SURGICAL CONSIDERATIONS
• Joint lavage using a "through and through" technique with two 14-gauge needles placed on either side of the joint.
• Warmed lactated Ringer's should be flushed through joint to remove debris.
• A light dressing should be applied to joint for 24–48 hours after joint lavage.
• Arthroscopy may be considered if joint lavage is unsuccessful in valuable animals. Allows high-volume lavage and is quite effective.
• Arthrotomy can be attempted in advanced cases.

MEDICATIONS

DRUGS OF CHOICE
• Selection of antibiotic may be determined by results of joint culture and sensitivity.
• Procaine penicillin G
• Ampicillin
• Ceftiofur
• Oxytetracycline
• Potentiated sulphonamides

CONTRAINDICATIONS
Appropriate milk and meat withdrawal times must be followed for all compounds administered to food-producing animals.

PRECAUTIONS

POSSIBLE INTERACTIONS
N/A

ALTERNATIVE DRUGS
Ketoprofen or flunixin meglumine may be used for short-term pain relief (24–48 hours).

FOLLOW-UP

PATIENT MONITORING
Duration of antibiotic therapy should continue despite resolution of symptoms for up to 10 days.

PREVENTION/AVOIDANCE
• Ensure adequate colostral intake.
• Utilize tincture of iodine.

POSSIBLE COMPLICATIONS
• Chronic arthritis may result in severe degenerative joint disease.
• Recurrence of infection may occur if source of infection is not eliminated.
• Osteomyelitis
• Meningitis may occur in neonates with septicemia.

EXPECTED COURSE AND PROGNOSIS
• Prognosis is dependent on level of failure of passive transfer.
• Prognosis is poor if multiple joints or meningitis is evident.
• Delay in initial treatment will also cause prognosis to be poor.
• Cases involving a single joint that are treated early have a reasonably good prognosis (up to 80% of calves may recover).

MISCELLANEOUS

ASSOCIATED CONDITIONS
• Omphalophlebitis
• Failure of passive transfer
• Septicemia
• Meningitis

AGE-RELATED FACTORS
N/A

ZOONOTIC POTENTIAL
N/A

PREGNANCY
N/A

RUMINANT SPECIES AFFECTED
Cattle, sheep, goats, camelids

BIOSECURITY
Hygiene of calving area will aid in prevention.

PRODUCTION MANAGEMENT
N/A

SYNONYMS
Joint-ill

SEE ALSO
Degenerative myopathy
Diseases of the nervous system that may cause recumbency or lameness
Myositis
Omphalophlebitis
Osteomyelitis
Trauma

ABBREVIATIONS
• FPT = failure of passive transfer
• GGT = gammaglutamyl transpeptidase

Suggested Reading
Jackson, P. 1999. Treatment of septic arthritis in calves. *Practice*, 21:596–601.
Weaver, A. D. 1997. Joint conditions. In: *Lameness in cattle*, ed. P. R. Greenough. 3rd ed. Philadelphia: W. B. Saunders.

Author: John R. Campbell

NEONATOLOGY: BEEF

 BASICS

DEFINITION
• Common diseases found in beef calves within the first few weeks of life
• Neonatal mortality in beef calves ranges from 4%–10%, with approximately 50%–70% of neonatal mortality occurring during the first 3 days after birth.

PATHOPHYSIOLOGY
Various, depending on disease condition

SYSTEMS AFFECTED
• Hemo/immune—Failure of passive transfer of immunity is the most common predetermining factor for disease development in neonates. In cases of septicemia, the umbilicus is frequently the site of bacterial entrance to the body.
• Gastrointestinal—Diarrhea is the most common disease manifestation in neonates.
• Respiratory—Aspiration of meconium may occur during dystocia. Premature calves may have immature lungs and lack sufficient pulmonary surfactant production. Pneumonia usually affects older calves; however, neonates can be affected during disease outbreaks and due to septicemic spread of bacteria.
• Endocrine/metabolic—Hypovolemia leading to reduced perfusion and hypoxia can result in hypoglycemia, hyponatremia, and acidosis (respiratory or metabolic).
• Cardiovascular—Congenital cardiac defects such as PDA, ventricular septal defects, and Tetralogy of Fallot; hypovolemia leading to circulatory shock
• Musculoskeletal—Many musculoskeletal defects are due to congenital abnormalities. Dystocia may result in trauma to the calf. Lameness may result from septic arthritis.
• Renal/urologic—Umbilical abscess or infection; reduced renal perfusion due to hypovolemia

GENETICS
Some neonatal conditions are genetic (e.g., epitheliogenesis imperfecta in shorthorn and Angus; cerebellar hypoplasia in Hereford, Angus, and shorthorn).

INCIDENCE/PREVALANCE
Unknown

GEOGRAPHIC DISTRIBUTION
Worldwide

SIGNALMENT
Beef breed calves < 2 weeks of age

SIGNS

HISTORICAL FINDINGS
• Dystocia
• Premature delivery
• Weakness
• Anorexia
• Failure of passive transfer
• Diarrhea

PHYSICAL EXAMINATION FINDINGS
• Weakness/depression
• Dehydration
• Hypothermia
• Fever (may or may not be present)
• Congenital abnormalities (e.g., cleft palate, contracted tendons)

CAUSES

Congenital
Although rare in occurrence, there are numerous congenital defects that may affect calves.

Metabolic
• Hypoglycemia
• Hypoxia
• Acidosis
• Dehydration
• Hyponatremia

Nutritional
• Maternal malnutrition can greatly affect neonatal calf livability.
• Starvation due to weak calf, inability to stand, poor mothering ability, etc.

Immune
Failure of passive transfer is a leading cause of neonatal morbidity and mortality.

Infectious
• Bacterial, viral, and fungal agents can all cause infections in the neonate.
• Rotavirus, cryptosporidia, coronavirus, *Escherichia coli*, and *Salmonella* spp. are the most common causes of infectious diarrhea.

Traumatic
Fractured ribs or other bones due to dystocia

RISK FACTORS
• Failure of passive transfer
• Dystocia
• Pathogen buildup due to crowded calving area
• Maternal malnutrition

 DIAGNOSIS

DIFFERENTIAL DIAGNOSIS
• Diarrhea: *E. coli*, *Salmonella* spp., rotavirus, cryptosporidia, coronavirus, *Clostridium perfringens* type C
• Septicemia: *E. coli*, *Actinomyces pyogenes*, *Staphylococcus aureus*, *Streptococcus* spp.
• Umbilical infection: *Actinomyces pyogenes*, *E. coli*, *Proteus*, *Enterococcus* spp.
• Pneumonia (usually seen in older animals but can occur in neonates)
  • Aspiration pneumonia
  • Septicemic spread of bacteria
  • Bovine respiratory syncytial virus
  • Infectious bovine rhinotracheitis
  • Bovine viral diarrhea virus
• Congenital defects
• Lameness: Septic arthritis, trauma
• Hypothermia
• Abomasal bloat
• Cardiac abnormality (PDA, VSD, etc.)

CBC/BIOCHEMISTRY/URINALYSIS
• Hypoglycemia
• Acidosis (metabolic or respiratory)
• Hyponatremia
• Hyperkalemia
• Leukocytosis with left shift

OTHER LABORATORY TESTS
• Failure of passive transfer —IgG < 10 g/L or TP < 5.5 g/dL
• Positive blood culture for bacteria
• Positive fecal culture

IMAGING
• Thoracic radiographs
• Ultrasonography of umbilical structures

DIAGNOSTIC PROCEDURES
N/A

PATHOLOGIC FINDINGS
Varies based on disease condition

 TREATMENT

APPROPRIATE HEALTH CARE
Varies based on disease diagnosis.

NURSING CARE
• Fluid therapy to correct dehydration and acidosis
  • Oral solutions should contain 50–80 mmol/L of alkalinizing agent (acetate, lactate, citrate, gluconate, and bicarbonate are most common). Acetate solutions provide best results for calves still drinking milk.
  • IV fluids can be provided to recumbent calves that are unable to suckle.
• Provide heat source to correct hypothermia
• Supplemental oxygen
• Meet nutritional needs
• Keep recumbent neonates in sternal recumbency, if possible

ACTIVITY
• Restrict contact with other animals
• Minimize physical activity
• Minimize stress

DIET
• Maintain proper nutrition of pregnant cows
• Ensure adequate colostrum intake in calves
• Weak, recumbent calves with severe diarrhea may benefit from being held off milk. Malabsorption of milk can increase osmotic diarrhea and promote bacterial overgrowth.
  • Provide fluid therapy.
  • Withholding milk for extended periods will result in weight loss and can lead to severe cachexia. Most calves will respond to fluid therapy within 2 days.
  • Calves that are alert and interested in nursing should be allowed to do so.

CLIENT EDUCATION
• Discuss importance of colostrum.
• Discuss calving and environmental management protocols to minimize disease transmission.

SURGICAL CONSIDERATIONS
• Congenital defects and/or traumatic injuries may require surgery.
• Stabilize calf before anesthesia.

MEDICATIONS

DRUGS OF CHOICE
Varies based on disease condition and antimicrobial susceptibility

CONTRAINDICATIONS
• Drugs prohibited for use in food animals.
• Appropriate milk and meat withdrawal times must be followed for all compounds administered to food-producing animals.

PRECAUTIONS
• Prolonged use of some drugs may result in cartilage damage.
• Prolonged use of oral antibiotics can lead to diarrhea.

POSSIBLE INTERACTIONS
N/A

ALTERNATIVE DRUGS
• Oral IgG supplements
• Probiotics

FOLLOW-UP

PATIENT MONITORING
Watch neonates closely; they can go downhill very quickly.

PREVENTION/AVOIDANCE
• Calving area hygiene and colostrum management are important aspects of preventing neonatal disease.
• Monitor newborn calves closely for signs of disease and begin proper treatment as soon as a problem is recognized.
• Ensure proper vaccination of cows.
• Avoid genetic lines known to produce defects.

POSSIBLE COMPLICATIONS
N/A

EXPECTED COURSE AND PROGNOSIS
Varies depending on disease condition

MISCELLANEOUS

ASSOCIATED CONDITIONS
N/A

AGE-RELATED FACTORS
N/A

ZOONOTIC POTENTIAL
Some neonatal diseases have zoonotic potential: *Salmonella*, cryptosporidia, *E. coli*.

PREGNANCY
N/A

RUMINANT SPECIES AFFECTED
N/A

BIOSECURITY
• Isolate sick animals to prevent disease spread.
• Biosecurity protocols may help minimize disease introduction.

PRODUCTION MANAGEMENT
• Proper vaccination of cows will minimize disease transmission and help to maximize colostrum quality.
• Clean, hygienic calving areas are essential.
• Adult animals excrete disease agents in low numbers; minimizing stocking density can reduce pathogen buildup.

SYNONYMS
N/A

SEE ALSO
Colostrum management
Congenital anomalies
Neonatal diarrhea
Neonatology: dairy

ABBREVIATIONS
IgG = immunoglobulin G
PDA = patent ductus arteriosis
TP = total protein
VSD = ventricular septal defect

Suggested Reading
Koterba, A. M., House, J. K., Madigan, J. E. 1996. Manifestation of disease in the neonate. In: *Large animal internal medicine*, ed. B. P. Smith. 2nd ed. St. Louis: Mosby.
Larson, R. L., Tyler, J. W., Schultz, L. G., Tessman, R. K., Hostetler, D. E. 2004. Management strategies to decrease calf death losses in beef herds. *JAVMA* 224: 42–48.
Townsend, H. G. G. 1994. Environmental factors and calving management practices that affect neonatal mortality in the beef calf. *Vet Clin North Am Food Anim Pract.* 10:119–26.

Author: Carolyn Hammer

NEONATOLOGY: DAIRY

 BASICS

OVERVIEW

At birth, a calf is transferred from a nearly sterile environment to an environment containing a multitude of pathogenic and nonpathogenic organisms. The calf is born with a naïve immune system. Therefore, any alterations in the animal's physiological state may depress the already delicate protective responses. This means an increase in disease susceptibility in the newborn, often with a negative impact on growth and development. The health of the neonate depends on many factors occurring before, during, and after parturition.

GEOGRAPHIC DISTRIBUTION

Worldwide, depending on breed and environment

SIGNALMENT

Species
Dairy cattle

Breed Predilections
N/A

Mean Age and Range
Neonate

Predominant Sex
N/A

 MISCELLANEOUS

Prenatal Care (Conception to Parturition)
Proper care of the cow during gestation is essential to producing a healthy calf.
Two areas of most importance are
(1) providing protection for the dam and calf through appropriate maternal vaccination and (2) ensuring optimal maternal body condition and sufficient nutrition.

Table 1

Vaccines That May Be Used During the Dry Period
Leptospirosis, multivalent
Bovine respiratory syncytial virus, BRSV (modified live or killed virus)
Infectious bovine rhinotracheitis, IBR (altered or killed virus only)
Clostridium, multivalent bacterin/toxoid
Parainfluenza type 3, PI3 (modified live or killed virus)
E. coli (K99) vaccine
Bovine virus diarrhea, BVD (killed virus only)
E. coli J5 vaccine
Rotavirus
Coronavirus

Source: Adapted from LDHM, American Dairy Science Association, 1999, p. 399.

Maternal Vaccination
• Maternal vaccination strategies to protect the neonate should be targeted at enhancing disease-specific colostral immunity and early protection against organisms causing diarrhea and respiratory diseases in the neonate (see Table 1).
• Calves should not be vaccinated (actively immunized) during the period immediately after birth, as colostrum-derived antibodies passively immunize them. The priority for vaccinating against infectious agents will vary from herd to herd, and should be based on the incidence of disease in the herd.
• When after birth a calf can be successfully vaccinated depends on (1) the ecology of the host-parasite interaction for the agent, (2) quantity of antibody transferred from the dam at birth, (3) the quality and timing of colostrum ingested, and (4) absorption efficiency of colostral antibodies.

Table 2

Suggested Body Condition Score (BCS) for Various Stages of Lactation	
Stage of lactation	BCS Range[1]
Calving	3.00–3.75
Peak milk production	2.25–2.75
150–200 days in milk	3.00–3.50
Dry off	3.00–3.75

Source: Adapted from Gearhart et al., 1990.
[1] Range: 1(emaciated) to 5 (fat).

Maternal Body Condition Score
• It is essential that the cow be maintained in good condition throughout the dry period and the lactation cycle to provide energy and building blocks for calf development and growth (see Table 2).
• Dry cows should be managed to allow for transition from a period of relatively low metabolic demands during the dry period to extremely high metabolic demands during parturition and the onset of lactation.
• Dietary manipulations for sustaining the cow's body condition require appropriate planning. Late lactation cows are more efficient at utilizing metabolizable energy than cows in the dry period.
• Body condition is based on scale of 1 (emaciated) to 5 (fat).

Perinatal Care
Initial Management of the Neonate
• Initiation of respiration is critical in the neonatal calf. An extended period without gas exchange leads to acidosis and accumulation of mucus in respiratory passages.
• Fluid in the lungs may be removed by lifting the calf by the hind legs until the muzzle is off the ground.

• A prolonged period of calving may result in fetal hypoxia. Consequently, cows should receive assistance during calving, when necessary. Mild to moderate hypoxemia in calves will produce metabolic acidosis.

• Normal calves have a venous pH of 7.34, bicarbonate of 30 mmol/L, and base excess of 5 mmol/L. Acidotic calves have been observed with a pH as low as 7.03 and a base deficit of 18 mmol/L. This is crucial, since a significant negative correlation exists between the severity of metabolic acidosis and efficiency of colostrum ingestion.

• The most frequent causes of mortality in the neonatal calf are dehydration and acidosis. Consequently, the highest priority in treating a diarrheic calf is to return the calf to metabolic homeostasis (venous pH 7.25–7.45).

• A variety of alkalinizing agents have been used (lactate, acetate, gluconate), but bicarbonate is consistently effective in severely acidotic calves. Bicarbonate requirements can be calculated from base deficit values (based on blood gas measurements or estimated from physical examination findings):

$$\text{mmol bicarbonate} = \text{body weight (kg)} \times \text{base deficit (mmol/L)} \times 0.5$$

• An estimate of the severity of acidosis in the neonatal calves before 8 days of age can be ascertained by physical examination using indicators of body position, strength of suck reflex, and age. A standing calf with a strong suck reflex will not likely have any base deficit. In contrast, a calf that is in sternal or lateral recumbency will likely have a base deficit of 10 mmol/L or greater.

• Severely depressed calves are best treated with intravenous fluids. Moderately depressed calves should be treated with intravenous fluids, if the condition is progressing in severity rapidly. A no. 15 scalpel blade can be used to make catheterization easier. A calf can be suspended upside down to allow blood to pool and distend the jugular vein. Before inversion, the calf's neck should be clipped and prepared. The calf should be placed flat after catheter is placed.

Navel Dipping

Disinfecting the calf's navel can minimize the threat of navel infection and subsequent development of septicemia. The navel must be thoroughly saturated with 7% iodine solution. The navel cord should be filled and an area approximately 2 inches around the base of the navel saturated with iodine. This should be conducted within 2 hours of birth, when the calf is put in the hutch, and 12–18 hours later.

Neonatal Period (0–14 d)

• Adequate colostrum ingestion and neonatal nutrition will help the calf combat infection, such as septicemia and neonatal diarrhea, during the early neonatal period.

• Colostrum performs a crucial role in protecting the newborn against gastrointestinal and respiratory infections. A brief description of the components in colostrum (see below) will aid in an understanding of how colostrum provides protection for the neonate.

Immune Function

A brief explanation of the neonatal immune system is warranted here. However, this explanation should not be considered to be all inclusive. The author strongly suggests other reviews of bovine neonatal immunology.

General Parameters

Immunoglobulins

• Susceptibility of the neonate to contagious and opportunistic infections is a consequence of the immaturity of the immune system. Bovine colostrum contains a high concentration of IgG (45 mg/dL).

• Passively acquired immunoglobulins are essential to the neonatal calf, as most calves are born agammaglobulinemic. The function of colostral immunoglobulins in the protection of neonatal calves has been extensively studied.

Colostral Leukocytes

• Bovine colostrum contains about 106 leukocytes/mL. Colostral leukocytes appear to contribute to regulation of the cellular aspect of the neonate's immune responses.

• Newborn calves are able to absorb colostral leukocytes through the intestinal barrier, and the preferential route is through the follicle-associated epithelium of the Peyer's patches.

• The common practice of freezing colostrum may destroy essential colostral leukocytes and diminish the protection delivered to the neonate.

• Mammary secretions contain four types of cells: epithelial cells, macrophages (50% of leukocytes), lymphocytes (20% of leukocytes), and neutrophils (30% of leukocytes) at 1 to 2 days after parturition.

Colostral Components

Several components of colostrum, other than immunoglobulin, may help to protect the neonatal calf from infection. These components include lactoferrin, CD14, and cytokines that enhance both innate and adaptive immune responses.

Lactoferrin

• Lactoferrin is an iron-binding protein product of the transferrin gene family.

• Lactoferrin is a major constituent of the secondary granules of polymorphonuclear neutrophils (PMN) and is found in high concentrations in colostrum and milk during mastitis.

• Higher concentrations of this protein are found in bovine colostrums than milk (1–5 mg/dL). Oral lactoferrin is absorbed in calves, but does not alter PMN superoxide production or IgG absorption. Lactoferrin has direct activity against at least two pathogens, *Escherichia coli* and rotavirus.

CD14

• CD14 enhances and regulates the inflammatory response to the bacterial cell wall. CD14 is a glycosyl-phosphatidyl-inositol anchored membrane protein expressed on mature monocytes and macrophages. Lipopolysaccharide binding proteins help mediate lipopolysaccharide complexation with soluble CD14.

• A soluble form of CD14 is found in colostrum. In addition, postsuckling calves show evidence of transfer of maternal CD14 to the circulation. Soluble CD14 induces B cell development, and increases antibody secretions by the neonate.

Cytokine

• Limited data are available concerning the activity of cytokines present in bovine mammary secretions. The activity of IL-2 is detected in the mammary gland 2 weeks before parturition, but diminishes by the last week of gestation.
• Antiviral activity demonstrated in mammary secretions is assumed to result from tumor necrosis factor-α present in the secretion. Insulinlike growth factor is found in colostrum at high concentrations and may promote both growth and immune system development of the neonate.
• The level of transforming growth factor decreases rapidly in the milk. It is almost undetectable by 30 days postpartum.

Neonatal Diseases

Septicemia
Septicemia often affects multiple organ systems, especially respiratory and gastrointestinal. Calves may be lethargic with poor suckle reflex, weakness, tachycardia, tachypnea, and recumbency.

Neonatal Diarrhea
• *Escherichia coli* is an important pathogen in the domestic livestock industry. This organism causes enteric colibacillosis, characterized by severe diarrhea, and septicemia, an acutely fatal systemic infection.
• Neonatal diarrhea may be caused by viral, bacterial, parasitic, or dietary insult. The diarrhea caused by specific organisms is usually observed at specific ages of the neonate, but does not always occur at these ages.

• The viruses most commonly associated with neonatal calf diarrhea are rotavirus (4–14 days of age), coronavirus (4–30 days of age), and bovine viral diarrhea virus (any age). Bacterial infections are common in the neonate: *Clostridium perfringens* (less than 10 days of age), enterotoxigenic *Escherichia coli* (1–4 days of age), and *Salmonella typhimurium* (any age).
• Parasitic infections in calves are common caused by *Cryptosporidium parvum* (7–28 days, possibly older), *Eimeria bovis* (clinical signs, older than 3–4 weeks) and *Giardia* spp. (are thought not be major pathogens in calves).
• Neonatal diarrhea may be caused by a combination of dietary and infectious agents. Calves with diarrhea usually have a partially compensated metabolic acidosis with decreased pCO2, negative base excess, a decreased buffer base, and a lowered blood pH.
• Nutritional aspects include overfeeding, inadequate sanitation of equipment, feeding of waste milk, or poor-quality milk replacers. Restricting intake of milk replacers may be beneficial in calves with diarrhea, but the deliberate underfeeding of healthy calves predisposes them to diarrhea.

Neonatal Nutrition Requirements

• Proper nutrition in the neonatal period may help the neonate survive disease challenges.
• Neonatal calves must have a good source of energy; milk replacers should contain a minimum of 15% fat on a dry matter basis, but may contain more than 20% (see Table 3). High levels of fat often are included in milk replacers to provide extra energy for growth, and inclusion of fat may tend to reduce severity of diarrhea.

Table 3

Recommended Nutrient Content of Milk Replacers	
Nutrient	Amount
Metabolizable energy (Mcal/lb)	1.71
Crude protein (%)	22
Ether extract, fat (%, minimum)	15[a]
Vitamin A, K (IU/lb)	3.682[b]
Vitamin D (IU/lb)	245[b]
Vitamin E (IU/lb)	20.4[b,c]

[a]National Research Council, 1989.
[b]National Research Council, 2001
[c]Reddy. 1987.

• Milk replacers should contain 22% protein, all derived from animal sources, since plant proteins are less digestible. However, the use of animal proteins in milk replacers may not be feasible with the outlawing of feeding animal proteins to animals due to bovine spongiform encephalopathy (BSE).

• Although vitamins A, D, and E are necessary components of the calf's diet, some milk replacers supply excessive amounts of these fat-soluble vitamins. In addition, vitamin E appears be immunostimulatory at levels of 125 IU/day.

Additional Considerations

• Proper rearing of replacement heifers for today's dairy herds is filled with pitfalls for the producer and the veterinarian alike. When raising calves, producers should consider the threats of disease occurrence including general hygiene, pathogen density in the local environment of calves, pathogen virulence, physical environment (temperature, humidity, and wind chill), and nutritional status of calves.

• Knowing the level of antibody transferred may not be enough. Total circulating immunoglobulin is not necessarily indicative of the specific trafficking antibody.

• A high level of serum immunoglobulin does not guarantee that the immunoglobulins will reach the site of infection and neutralize the organism. A better understanding of the herd and maternal vaccination limitation will make quantitative immunoglobulin measurement more useful.

ASSOCIATED CONDITIONS
N/A

AGE-RELATED FACTORS
N/A

ZOONOTIC POTENTIAL
N/A

PREGNANCY
N/A

RUMINANT SPECIES AFFECTED
Potentially all dairy cattle

BIOSECURITY
N/A

PRODUCTION MANAGEMENT
See Neonatal Nutrition Requirements above

SYNONYMS

SEE ALSO
Body condition scoring dairy cattle
BVD
IBR
PI3

ABBREVIATIONS
BCS = body condition score
BSE = bovine spongiform encephalitis
BVD = bovine diarrhea
CD14 = cluster of differentiation 14; cell-fill surface molecule
IBR = infectious bovine rhinotracheitis
IgG = immunoglobulin G
IL-2 = interleukin-2
PI3 = parainfluenza 3
PMN = polymorphonuclear neutrophils

Suggested Reading
Aldridge, B. M., Garry, F. B., Adams, R. 1993. Neonatal septicemia in calves: 25 cases (1985–1990). *J Am Vet Med Assoc.* 230:1324–29.
Barrington, G. M., Parish, S. M. 2001. Bovine neonatal immunology. *Vet Clin North Am: Food Animal Practice* 17:463–476.
Besser, T. E., Gay, C. C., Pritchett, L. 1991. Comparison of three methods of feeding colostrum to dairy calves. *J Am Vet Med Assoc.* 198:419–22.
Donovan, G. A. 1992. Management of cow and newborn calf at calving. In: *Dairy herd management*, ed. H. H. VanHorn, C. J. Wilcox. Champaign, IL: American Dairy Science Association.
Flipp, D., Alizadeh-Khiavi, K., Richardson, C., Palma, A., Paredes, N., Takeuchi, O., Akira, S., Julius, M. 2001. Soluble CD14 enriched colostrum and milk induces B cell growth and differentiation. *PNAS* 98:603–8.
Gearhart, M. A., Curtis, C. R., Erb, H. N., Smith, R. D., Sniffen, C. J., Chase, L. E., Cooper, M. D. 1990. Relationship of changes in condition scores to cows health in Holsteins. *J Dairy Sci.* 73:3132.
National Research Council. 1989. *Nutritional requirements of dairy cattle.* 6th rev. ed. Washington, DC: National Academy of Sciences.
National Research Council. 2001. *Nutritional requirements of dairy cattle.* 7th rev. ed. Washington, DC: National Academy of Sciences.
Wilcox, C. J. *Large dairy herd management.* 1999. American Dairy Science Association. Champaign, Ill. 825 pages.

Author: Douglas C. Donovan

NEONATOLOGY: DAIRY GOATS

 BASICS

DEFINITION
Common diseases found in dairy goats from birth to 1 week of age
Management factors and environmental conditions play a very large part in the disease process of the neonate.

PATHOPHYSIOLOGY
Varies based on disease condition

SYSTEMS AFFECTED
- Hemolymphatic/Immune
- Gastrointestinal
- Respiratory
- Endocrine/Metabolic
- Musculoskeletal
- Renal/urologic
- Cardiac

GENETICS
Some conditions in neonates have a genetic predisposition.

INCIDENCE/PREVALENCE
Unknown

SIGNALMENT
N/A

SIGNS

GENERAL COMMENTS
Management and husbandry are important in the prevention of neonatal diseases.

HISTORICAL FINDINGS
- Premature delivery
- Failure of passive transfer
- Diarrhea
- Anorexia

PHYSICAL EXAMINATION FINDINGS
- Congenital defects (e.g., cleft palate, contracted tendons, VSD)
- Dehydration
- Hypothermia
- Depression
- Weakness

CAUSES
- Congenital defects
- Failure of passive transfer
- Dehydration
- Hypothermia
- Hypoxia
- Hypoglycemia
- Nutritional deficiency in doe or kid
- Trauma

RISK FACTORS
- Poor body condition or underlying disease in doe
- Failure of passive transfer
- Premature delivery
- Poor environmental conditions

 DIAGNOSIS

DIFFERENTIAL DIAGNOSIS
- Septicemia
- Floppy kid syndrome
- Hypothermia
- Starvation
- Meconium impaction
- Neuromusculoskeletal diseases: tetanus, white muscle disease, trauma
- Congenital defects
  - Cleft palate
  - Contracted tendons
  - Umbilical hernia
  - Patent urachus
  - Cardiac (i.e., VSD)
- Diarrhea
  - *E. coli*
  - *Salmonella* spp.
  - Adenovirus
  - Corona virus
  - Rotavirus
  - *Cryptosporidium* spp.
  - *Giardia* spp.
  - Clostridial enterotoxemia type B
- Respiratory disease: Aspiration pneumonia, *Mannheimia haemolytica*

CBC/BIOCHEMISTRY/URINALYSIS
- Hypoglycemia
- Hypoproteinemia
- Hyperfibrinogenemia
- Left shift in leukogram with neutropenia (toxic bands)
- Metabolic acidosis

OTHER LABORATORY TESTS
- IgG < 400 mg/dL or TP < 5.0 g/dL
- Positive on fecal culture
- Electron microscopy for viruses
- Bacteremia on blood culture
- Hypoxemia on blood gas
- Decreased serum vitamin E
- Decreased EDTA or heparin whole blood selenium

IMAGING
Radiography if suspect fractures or aspiration pneumonia

DIAGNOSTIC PROCEDURES
N/A

PATHOLOGIC FINDINGS
N/A

 TREATMENT

APPROPRIATE HEALTH CARE
Varies based on disease condition and the environment

NURSING CARE
- Warming neonate
- Oxygen supplementation
- Oral or intravenous fluids (correct electrolyte and acid-base disturbances)
- Meet caloric needs via PO or IV nutrition (i.e., oral sugar/syrup or IV dextrose for hypoglycemia)
- Enema for meconium impaction

ACTIVITY
- Passive range of motion
- Rolling from side to side
- Maintain sternal recumbency

DIET
- Proper nutrition of the prepartum doe
- Important to feed the kids a balanced diet that meets their caloric and nutritional requirements. This may help prevent starvation, hypoglycemia, and nutrient deficiencies.

CLIENT EDUCATION
Correct any deficiencies in husbandry or breeding selection.

SURGICAL CONSIDERATIONS
- Stabilize patient before beginning any surgical procedures.
- Congenital defects and/or traumatic injuries may need surgical correction.
- Neonates in many instances are not good surgical candidates.

MEDICATIONS

DRUGS OF CHOICE
• Antibiotics based on suspected problem and/or culture and sensitivity
• NSAIDS may be indicated. Care should be used in selection and hydration status of the neonate. Some NSAIDs are contraindicated in the neonate.
• Intravenous plasma, oral plasma, or oral colostrum
• Antidiarrhea medications

CONTRAINDICATIONS
Avoid using drugs prohibited or not labeled for use in food-producing animals (e.g., aminoglycosides, metronidazole). Follow drug withdrawal periods for meat and milk.

PRECAUTIONS
Beware of drugs that may affect growing tissues.

POSSIBLE INTERACTIONS
N/A

ALTERNATIVE DRUGS
Probiotics may be indicated.

FOLLOW-UP

PATIENT MONITORING
• Keep in contact with farm owner/manager.
• May recheck blood work results for changes in values

PREVENTION/AVOIDANCE
• Correct management deficiencies.
• Avoid poor husbandry and/or breeding selection.
• Ensure colostral quality.
• Ensure adequate amount of colostrum is administered within the first 24 hours after birth.
• Adequate nutrition and vaccination of prepartum does.

POSSIBLE COMPLICATIONS
N/A

EXPECTED COURSE AND PROGNOSIS
Varies based on disease(s) encountered

MISCELLANEOUS

ASSOCIATED CONDITIONS
N/A

AGE-RELATED FACTORS
N/A

ZOONOTIC POTENTIAL
Some diseases of small ruminants may have zoonotic potential (e.g., *Salmonella* spp., *E. coli*, *Campylobacter* spp., *Cryptosporidium* spp., *Giardia* spp.)

PREGNANCY
N/A

RUMINANT SPECIES AFFECTED
N/A

BIOSECURITY
• Biosecurity measures may help to decrease the severity and course of neonatal diseases and may improve the prognosis.
• Can decrease transmission among other neonates, adult goats, and humans
• Isolation and quarantine of new stock entering the herd/flock
• Treat and or cull new animals for disease conditions prior to herd introduction.

PRODUCTION MANAGEMENT
• A good environment is vital to neonatal health.
• Management of pregnant does is important to neonatal health and viability.
• Proper husbandry and breeding practices are crucial in selecting for healthy neonates.

SYNONYMS
N/A

SEE ALSO
Congenital defects
Diarrhea
Floppy kid syndrome
Hypothermia
Meconium impaction
Neuro/musculoskeletal diseases
Respiratory disease
Septicemia
Starvation

ABBREVIATIONS
BID = twice daily
IgG = immunoglobulin G
IM = intramuscular
IV = intravenous
NSAIDs = nonsteroidal anti-inflammatory drugs
PO = per os, by mouth
SID = one time daily
TP = total protein
VSD = ventricular septal defect

Suggested Reading
Bulgin, M. S., Anderson, B. C. 1981, Apr 1. Salmonellosis in goats. *J Am Vet Med Assoc.* 178(7): 720–23.
Foreyt, W. J. 1990, Nov. Coccidiosis and cryptosporidiosis in sheep and goats. *Vet Clin North Am Food Anim Pract.* 6(3): 655–70.
Van Der Lugt, J. J., Randles, J. L. 1993, Dec. Systemic herpesvirus infection in neonatal goats. *J S Afr Vet Assoc.* 64(4): 169–71.
Van Metre, D. C., Tyler, J. W., Stehman, S. M. 2000, Mar. Diagnosis of enteric disease in small ruminants. *Vet Clin North Am Food Anim Pract.* 16(1): 87–115, vi.
Weese, J. S., Kenney, D. G., O'Connor, A. 2000, Aug 1. Secondary lactose intolerance in a neonatal goat. *J Am Vet Med Assoc.* 217(3):340, 372–75.

Authors: Jessica M. Dinham and Amanda S. Denisen

NEONATOLOGY: LAMBS

BASICS

OVERVIEW
• Preweaning lamb mortality typically consumes 10%–35% of the lamb crop each year. The majority of loss occurs shortly after parturition and often goes unrecognized by producers.
• As is the case with neonates of other species, disease involving newborn lambs occurs with little warning. Consequences to the newborn lamb are usually severe and treatment is often unrewarding. Thus, from an economic perspective, prevention is more important than individual animal treatment.

PATHOPHYSIOLOGY
• In most flocks, the causes of lamb mortality can be divided into several basic categories that can be used to catalog 75%–85% of all preweaning mortality (See chapter on abortion in sheep and goats).

• Typically these basic categories include (1) starvation/hypothermia, (2) stillbirth/dystocia, (3) pneumonia, and (4) abortion (see Table 1). However, the relative importance of each category is generally defined by production system and management decisions. While these basic categories are useful for defining mortality patterns within a given flock, it is important to remember that the significance of each category will vary between flocks and from year to year (see Figure 3).
• Furthermore, it should also be obvious that production system design (producer decisions) often impacts lamb mortality to a greater extend than do infectious diseases (see Figures 1 and 2).
• Prevention programs need to address environment, weather, forage resources, available markets, disease prevention, nutrition, genetic selection, maternal behavior, labor, and facility resources.
• Due to the complex intertwined character of management factors affecting prevention programs, it is often difficult to affect a change in mortality patterns during the same lambing season.

SYSTEMS AFFECTED
Potentially all, depending on condition

GENETICS
N/A

INCIDENCE/PREVALENCE
N/A

GEOGRAPHIC DISTRIBUTION
Potentially worldwide depending on environment

SIGNALMENT
Species
Ovine

Breed Predilections
Commercial sheep breeds

Mean Age and Range
Neonates

Predominant Sex
N/A

Table 1

Common Lamb Mortality Issues, Flock and Individual Assessment and Treatment

Hypothermia/Starvation Complex

Individual Assessment and Treatment
1. Simple Hypothermia
• Age: 6–8 hr following birth
• Clinical signs
  • Weak, lethargic, often comatose
  • Cold mouth, weak to no suckle reflex
  • Gaunt, empty abdomen
  • Mild hypothermia: 99°–102°F
  • Severe hypothermia: below 99°F
  • Normal temp: 101°–102°F
• Adequate tan fat and blood sugar
  • Tan fat not depleted
• Problem: Excessive heat loss
  • Cold environmental temperature
  • Wet birth coat, evaporation
  • Wind chill
  • Small body mass (low birth weight)
    1. Large surface area to weight ratio increases susceptibility to heat loss when adverse conditions
    2. Poor mothering ability
    3. Lack of movement (no heat generated)
  • Hypoxia during delivery (due to dystocia): Can't regulate body temperature for several days.
• Treatment: Provide warmth!!
  • Producers fail to recognize the importance of thermal management
  • Remove from ewe and dry
  • Supplement with warm dry heat @ 100°–103°F maximum temp.
  • Tube feed with 120–200 ml of colostrum (dose at 20 ml/lb body weight)
  • Return to ewe when rectal temp. normal (1–3 hours)
  • Assure future nutrition (i.e., check ewe)

2. Hypothermia 2° to Starvation
• Age: over 6–8 hr old
• Clinical signs same as Simple Hypothermia above
• Problem: Inadequate heat production due to starvation
  • Depleted tan fat
  • Low blood sugar
• Compounded by limited intake of colostrum
• Treatment: Aimed at elevating blood sugar and providing warmth
  • If able to stand or in sternal recumbency and can support head: treat as for Simple Hypothermia above.
  • If comatose: also inject 40 cc of 20% warm dextrose solution intraperitoneally.

Table 1

Continued

Flock Prevention Issues (and Contributing Factors)
Simple Hypothermia and Hypothermia 2° to Starvation
- Gestational nutrition: Smaller lambs chill more rapidly.
- Less tan fat—less resistant to H/S
  - Energy levels during early and late gestation influence birth weight.
  - Failure to address increased energy demands associated with late gestation and/or increased fetal numbers (twins/triplets)
  - Available shelter and fleece status impact nutritional requirements (more energy needed).
  - Poor quality/quantity of colostrum
  - Weigh first lambs—document size, then correct nutrition: commercial lambs should weigh 9–11 lb at birth.
  - Underfeeding the ewe may also affect maternal bond.
- Replacement selection pressure
  - Breed variations in wool cover and tan fat deposition at term
  - Prolificacy: how much is too much?
  - Mothering instinct and lamb vigor
- Lactational nutrition: an issue if starvation occurring in older lambs
- Vitamin E–selenium: routinely add to feeds/salt in deficient areas.
- Protection from environmental conditions
  - Important in winter-lambing systems if housing suspect: *Weather issues* (temperature, wind chill, rain, snow and ice storms), especially if pasture lambing
  - schedule lambing for weather conducive to lamb survival
  - Utilize: Historical weather data; ground temperature data (start lambing when > 50°F); natural protection—rough areas, clump grasses, pine and artificial wind breaks
- Quantity and quality of help
- Lambing pen and group pen availability and use: need one lambing pen per 5–10 ewes
- Dam/lamb identification
- Unshorn ewes: prone to expose lambs to poor weather
- Lack of milk: due to secondary diseases
- On pasture: forced movement of lambs contributes to mismothering

Pneumonia

Individual Assessment and Treatment
- Confinement related—common in barn-reared lambs especially when lambing occurs during periods of transitional weather
- Uncommon in pasture operations
- Clinical signs typical of acute bacterial (*Pasteurella* spp.) pneumonia in other species
  - Elevated temp.—above 103.5°F
  - Moist, harsh lung sounds
  - Elevated respiratory rate
  - Depressed, lethargic; (+/−) nasal discharge or cough
- In problem flocks, sudden death may be only sign (*Pasteurella septicemia*)
- Severe lesions develop shortly after birth (first week)—difficult to treat
- Treated lambs that survive may relapse when stressed (weaning, weather, and transport)
- Common antibiotics used in treatment
  - SQ procaine penicillin or procaine penicillin/benzathine penicillin combination @ 10,000 to 20,000 IU/lb body weight SID (dose NA)
  - SQ long-acting tetracycline injectable products @ 5 mg/lb SID or 9 mg/lb every 48 hours (NA)
  - SQ ceftiofur @ 0.5–1.0 mg/lb SID (A)
  - SQ florfenicol @ 9 mg/lb every 48 hrs (NA)
  - SQ tilmicosin @ 4.5 mg/lb given once (NA). CAUTION: FATAL TO HUMANS, HORSES, AND PIGS
  - Oral and injectable sulfonamide or trimethoprim/sulfa combination products common
- Anti-inflammatory: SQ flunixin meglumine @ 0.5 mg–1.0 mg/lb

Flock Prevention Issues (and Contributing Factors)
- Inadequate ventilation is a primary issue
  - Facility overcrowding @ 12 sq ft/ewe common in problem flocks
  - Difficult for nonmechanical ventilation @ less than 20 sq ft/ewe
- Transitional weather compounds ventilation problems
  - Temperature fluctuations and increased humidity
  - Facilities—difficult to exchange enough air
- Addressing inadequate ventilation
- Remove solid sidewalls
  - Replace sidewalls with (1) side-wall curtains; (2) greenhouse shade cloth (80/20 fabric); (3) hinged/sliding panels.
  - Open ridge vent and square for "chimney" drafting effect.
  - Place shade cloth over sliding doors.
  - Cover open-sided barns with shade cloth to prevent draft and weather stress, yet allow ventilation.
  - Ventilate "dead spaces" with fans.

NEONATOLOGY: LAMBS

Table 1

Continued

- Prolonged lambing season—increases crowding, contamination, and stress and extends into transitional weather.
- Pneumonia secondary to starvation or selenium/tocopherol deficiency
- Excessive moisture in bedding at lamb level
  - Bedding quantity insufficient
  - Unshorn ewes "drag" moisture into barn.
- Drop-lot or "flow through/no mix" lambing systems helpful
  - Advantages
    1. Decreases crowding—fed outside
    2. Decreases pregnant ewe/newborn lamb contact (scours, pneumonia)
    3. Facilitates proper group feeding
    4. Facilitates observation
    5. Facilitates bulk feeding of round bales and silage
    6. Maximizes facilities
    7. Encourages routine procedures in lambing/group pens
  - Disadvantages
    1. Occasional ewe lambs outside.
    2. Producer comfort
    3. Wool frosting
    4. Feeder cost and mobility
- Pneumonia issues reduced by drop-lot lambing system (lambs and ewes go directly to grass by 5–7 days old) or with pasture lambing system (unless poor weather)
- Problem pneumonia flocks
  - Routine SQ long-acting antibiotics on days 1 and 3 after birth
    1. Benzathine/procaine penicillin-G combination (NA) *or*
    2. Slow release tetracycline (NA)

Stillbirth/Dystocia

Individual Assessment and Treatment
- Stillbirth—treatment not applicable
- Common presentations associated with dystocia
  - 26.4% anterior presentation with head back
  - 25.0% anterior presentation with one leg back
  - 16.7% anterior presentation with elbow lock
  - 11.1% anterior presentation with both legs back
  - 12.5% posterior presentation with true breech
  - 8.3% others (multiple tangles and deformities)
  - Posterior presentation normal in lamb

Flock Prevention Issues (and Contributing Factors)
- Stillbirth/dystocia mortality rate—constant in most flocks at 2%–3% of lambs born each year
- Difficult to reduce further
- Stillbirth/dystocia—Problem Flock Issues
  - Nutrition
    1. Overfeeding— increased birth weight with dystocia
    2. Underfeeding—weak and stillborn lambs
    3. Triplet/twins/single size related to nutrition
  - Lambing supervision—delayed assistance
  - Breed differences—especially in bred ewe lambs
  - Skeletal deformities
  - Secondary to abortion outbreaks
  - Typical 4%–5% dystocia rate

Abortion

Individual Assessment and Treatment
Individual lamb treatment not applicable

Abortion Outbreak (Practical Response Until Diagnosis)
- 400 mg oral tetracycline/hd/day immediately (first 2–3 days)
- Then reduce to 200 mg/hd/day after 2 or 3 days
- Small flocks: SQ long-acting tetracycline @ 5 mg/lb as switched to oral
- Continue oral tetracycline through lambing—unless diagnosis or response dictates otherwise
- When possible, feed in bunks— not on ground.
- Clean up abortions and placentas
- Isolate aborted ewes until discharge ceases (3 wk).
- Vaccinate late-lambing groups.
- Treat retained placentas as needed.

Table 1

Continued

Flock Prevention Issues (and Contributing Factors)
- Fairly constant at about 1%–2% of the ewe flock
- Greater than 2% in one flock is action level.
- Sheep abortions—transmission via ingesting contaminated material
  - Infected fetal fluid
  - Infected manure or urine from carrier ewes
  - Licking aborted fetuses
  - Infected hay or grain—especially if fed on ground
- *Campylobacter* and *Chlamydia* often follow new ewe additions to the flock.
  - Carrier ewes (in gallbladder to manure)
  - Bird vectors
  - Closed flock important for prevention
- Toxoplasmosis—cat feces contamination of hay and grain
  - No vaccine in United States
  - No treatment
  - Monensin added to gestation feed may help prevent (NA)
- Vaccination *Campylobacter* and/or *Chlamydia*
  - Effectiveness variable
  - Often unavailable
  - Use only ovine strain vaccines
  - If open flock or problem flock
    1. Two doses, to new arrivals or replacements, before breeding and midpregnancy
    2. Booster yearly before breeding
- Closed flock with no problems: no vaccine

Scours

Individual Assessment and Treatment
1. *E. coli* Scours
- Difficult to treat once signs appear; work at prevention in remaining lambs
- Predisposing factors
  - Insufficient colostrum
  - Hypo motile intestine—not eating
  - Contaminated environment
- Signs related to
  - Rapid multiplication of *E. coli* in intestine
  - Endotoxin release
  - Scours, dehydration, and death in 12–36 hours
- Treatment suggestions
  - Standing/depressed
    1. 5%–10% dehydrated
    2. Oral fluids and antibiotics
  - Sternal/depressed
    1. 10%–15% dehydrated
    2. SQ and IV fluids and antibiotics
  - Comatose
    1. 15%–20% dehydrated
    2. Death
- Antibiotics for treatment
  - Spectinomycin: common piglet scour medication in oral pump formulation—dose @ 5 mg/lb SID or BID (NA)
  - Trimethoprim/sulfa oral syrup or tablets @ 15–20 mg/lb SID or BID (NA)

2. Coccidia Scours
- Common cause of scours in 3–8-week-old lambs born in confinement
- Clinical scours may occur 4–5 days before oocysts appear in fecal material—often treat by history
- Nursing lambs require individual treatment with oral sulfa or amprolium drench for five consecutive days
  - Labor intensive/impractical with larger groups of lambs
  - Prevention better option

Flock Prevention Issues (and Contributing Factors)
1. *E. coli* Scours (Contributing Factors)
- Prolonged lambing season: Environmental *E. coli* conc. increased
- Environmental conditions conducive to *E. coli* survival and transmission
  - Humidity and warmth associated with transitional weather
  - Unshorn ewes increase moisture in facility.

Table 1

Continued

- Facilities concentrate organism: lambing pen and common entry areas
- Poor sanitation
- Lack of colostrum
- Flock outbreak
  - Change location of lambing pens
  - Increase bedding
  - Prophylactic antibiotic at birth
    1. Spectinomycin oral syrup or trimethoprim/sulfa oral syrup or tablet (NA)
    2. Time antibiotic before clinical signs occur; usually dose on days 1, 2, and 3 following birth.
    3. If annual problem, vaccinate ewes prior to lambing.

2. Coccidia Scours (Contributing Factors)
- Environmental and sanitation factors similar to those listed for *E. coli*
- Ewes are asymptomatic carriers—oocysts in manure
  - Prevention aimed at decreasing oocysts shed into lambing barn environment from the ewe flock
  - Ewes treated 30 days prior to entering lambing area with:
    1. Lasalocid in feed @ 30 grams/ton of feed *or*
    2. Monensin in feed @ 15 grams/ton of feed (NA) *or*
    3. Decoquinate in feed or free-choice salt mix (NA) *or*
    4. Amprolium or sulfonamide compounds in drinking water or feed (NA)
- Weaned lambs: treat as a group in drinking water with oral sulfa or amprolium medications.
- Unweaned lambs: treat as individuals or decide to not treat and let immunity develop (3–6 weeks).

Omphalophlebitis

Individual Assessment and Treatment
- Difficult to treat as infection localized in liver and joints
- Aim at prevention
- Clinical signs
  - 10-day to 3-week-old lamb
  - Lame, gaunt, depressed, weak
  - Elevated temperature 103.5°–106°F
  - Swollen, hot, fluid-filled joints
- Systemic treatment with antibiotics similar to those presented above in Pneumonia section

Flock Prevention Issues (and Contributing Factors)
- Commonly a flock problem when transitional weather, crowding, and lack of bedding cause poor environmental conditions in lambing area
- Same contributing factors and management suggestions as with Pneumonia and *E. coli* Scours above
- Often associated with failure/improper iodine application to navel
  - Use 7% strong tincture of iodine as a dip.
  - Use fresh solution to prevent contamination.
- In problem flocks, prevention using SQ long-acting penicillin or tetracycline in newborn lambs; see Pneumonia Prevention above

Enterotoxmia

Individual Assessment and Treatment
- Commonly referred to as "overeating disease"
- Difficult to treat as signs are acute
- May exhibit convulsions shortly before death
- Prevention is key issue.
- Oral antibiotics and antitoxin can be given, but are usually unsuccessful.

Flock Prevention Issues (and Contributing Factors)
- Commonly associated with feed changes to high-concentrate rations
- Also common in "orphan lambs" fed milk replacer
- Exercise caution when introducing lambs to grain rations
  - Vaccinate ewes 4–6 weeks prior to lambing to encourage passive protection in the colostrums
  - Vaccinate their lambs at 3–4 weeks and again at 6–8 weeks of age.
  - If ewes are not vaccinated prior to lambing, vaccinate lambs during first few days of life and again at about 4 weeks of age.

Example Of Basic Causes Of Mortality In A
Winter Lambing Production System

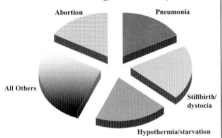

Figure 1.

Example Of Basic Causes Of Mortality In A
Spring Pasture Lambing Production System

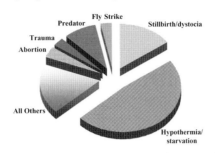

Note the basic unimportance of infectious causes!

Figure 2.

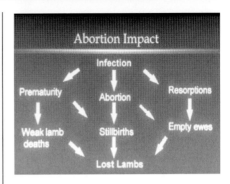

Figure 3.

Results of infection on conceptus.

MEDICATIONS

PRECAUTIONS
When treating food producing animals, drug withdrawal times must be determined and maintained.

MISCELLANEOUS

ASSOCIATED CONDITIONS
N/A

AGE-RELATED FACTORS
N/A

ZOONOTIC POTENTIAL
Caution: Use caution (especially women of childbearing age) when handling dead lambs and placentas, - especially if investigating an abortion problem.

PREGNANCY
N/A

RUMINANT SPECIES AFFECTED
Potentially, all ruminant species are affected.

BIOSECURITY
N/A

PRODUCTION MANAGEMENT
See chapters on replacement and culling strategies and abortion in sheep and goats, also see appendix on cleaning and disinfecting.

SYNONYMS
Neonatology

SEE ALSO
Lamb mortality

ABBREVIATIONS
(A) = approved
H/S = heat stress
(+/−) = may or may not be present
(NA) = unapproved use
SQ = subcutaneous

Suggested Reading
Rook, J. S., Schoolman, G., et al. 1990, Nov. Diagnosis and control of neonatal losses in sheep. *Advances in Sheep and Goat Medicine—The Veterinary Clinics of North America* 6(4):531–63.

Author: Joseph S. Rook

NEOSPORA

 BASICS

DEFINITION
Neospora caninum is a protozoa that is associated with abortion as well as the birth of congenitally infected, weak, and unthrifty calves in cattle. It is a very rare cause of reproductive failure in sheep and goats.

PATHOPHYSIOLOGY
• *Neospora caninum* is a protozoan; the dog is the definitive host.
• Cattle are dead-end hosts.
• Vertical transmission (transplacental) during pregnancy is the most common means of spread, but cattle may also become infected from consuming feed contaminated with dog feces.
• Most abortions occur at 5–6 months of gestation.
• Infected mature cattle usually develop an asymptomatic persistent infection that can undergo recrudescence during pregnancy with subsequent parasitemia to the fetus and placenta.
• Neospora may also be found in the semen of infected bulls.
• Transplacental infection and subsequent abortion are documented in sheep and goats due to *Neospora caninum* but appear to be less common than in cattle.

SYSTEMS AFFECTED
• Infection of the reproductive organs during pregnancy, specifically the fetus and placenta are the most pathologically significant targets for *Neospora* infection.
• Within the fetus, nervous, neuromuscular, and musculoskeletal systems can be affected.

GENETICS
There is no known genetic basis to the disease in cattle.

INCIDENCE/PREVALENCE
• Neosporosis in cattle has a widely variable prevalence on both a regional and individual herd basis.
• It can be associated with both endemic and epidemic abortion outbreaks.
• In some dairies in the United States, up to 90% of cows are seropositive.
• Abortion storms of up to one-third of all pregnant cows over a 2–3-month period have been documented.
• Quantitative studies have documented that between 12% and 42% of aborted fetuses from dairy cattle in the United States, Europe, and New Zealand are infected with *Neospora caninum.*

GEOGRAPHIC DISTRIBUTION
• Neosporosis can be found across the United States and has been documented in other countries, which include Australia, New Zealand, Argentina, United Kingdom, Italy, Portugal, Japan, and Korea.

• It is more commonly identified in higher density dairy areas of the United States.

SIGNALMENT
• Both dairy and beef cattle can be affected, but *Neospora* abortion is more common in dairy cattle.
• Clinical disease is not documented in males but infected bulls can shed the organism in semen.
• Abortions can occur year-round.
• No breed predilection is evident.
• Both multiparous and first-calf heifers can be affected by abortions.
• Both endemic and epidemic disease is reported.

SIGNS
• Abortion, usually between 5 and 6 months of gestation
• A small proportion (<5%) of cows will abort repeatedly in subsequent pregnancies.
• Fetuses may die in utero and be resorbed or become mummified.
• Following in utero exposure, calves may be born congenitally infected.
• Up to 95% of congenitally infected calves appear clinically normal at birth.
• Clinical signs due to *Neospora* infection are documented only in neonates (<2 months old).
• Neurologic signs include ataxia, weakness, and varying degrees of tetraparesis predominate in neonates, but congenitally infected calves may also be clinically normal.
• Congenital birth defects such as exophthalmia, hydrocephalus, torticollis, and arthrogryposis are reported but are rare.

CAUSES
Neospora caninum

RISK FACTORS
Self-rearing of heifer replacements, high stocking density, limited pasture access, and the presence of farm dogs have been documented to be risk factors for higher herd seropositivity rates.

 DIAGNOSIS

DIFFERENTIAL DIAGNOSIS
• Other protozoal causes of abortion—*Toxoplasma gondii* and *Sarcocystis cruzi* infection in cattle
• Viral causes of abortion—bovine viral diarrhea virus, infectious bovine rhinotracheitis, and bluetongue virus.
• Bacterial causes of abortion—*Salmonella* spp., *Leptospira interrogans*, *Haemophilus somnus*, *Arcanobacterium pyogenes*
• Miscellaneous causes of abortion—foothills abortion (Western United States), mycotic abortion

• Causes of weak and unthrifty neonatal calves—selenium deficiency (white muscle disease), iodine deficiency, persistent infection with BVDV, congenital infection with bluetongue virus, neonatal septicemia/failure of passive transfer

CBC/BIOCHEMISTRY/URINALYSIS
• Clinicopathologic data from cows that have aborted or congenitally affected calves is generally unremarkable and nondiagnostic.
• Congenitally infected calves may demonstrate elevations in muscle enzymes CK and AST due to recumbency.

OTHER LABORATORY TESTS
• CSF obtained from neurologically abnormal, congenitally infected calves may demonstrate a mild pleocytosis.
• Congenitally infected calves are at high risk for failure of passive transfer with hypogammaglobulinemia and septicemia if they demonstrate a weak suckle response.

IMAGING
N/A

DIAGNOSTIC PROCEDURES
• Serologic tests—ELISAs, IFAT, and NAT are all available and offer serologic confirmation of the presence of antibodies to *Neospora caninum* in blood obtained from a suspect animal.
• Due to widespread seropositivity in cattle populations, a positive antibody test does not incriminate *Neospora caninum* as the cause of an abortion.
• Refer to testing laboratory for arbitrary cutoffs in titer values that are considered more suggestive of disease.
• Consider serologic testing of comparably sized groups of cows with reproductive failure and those with normal reproductive histories when investigating putative problem herd, so as to gain data on background seropositivity in herd.
• Positive serologic tests on blood samples obtained from an aborted fetus or a presuckle blood sample from a newborn calf is diagnostic for congenital infection.
• Peritoneal fluid from an aborted fetus is a useful sample to submit for serology if heart blood is not available.
• Fetal tissues/placenta can also be examined by immunohistochemistry and/or PCR.

PATHOLOGIC FINDINGS
• Fetal brain, heart, liver, and placenta are best submitted for routine histopathology and immunohistochemistry.
• Fetal brain is the most consistently affected organ and shows signs of nonsuppurative focal encephalitis.
• Hepatitis, myocarditis, and myositis may also be present histologically in an aborted fetus.

- Placental lesions are also those of focal, nonsuppurative encephalitis.
- Protozoa are very rarely identified in histosections from aborted feti or placenta.
- Congenitally infected calves may be normal or may be born weak, unable to stand, and demonstrating a weak suckle reflex and diminished spinal reflexes.
- Some calves may appear comparatively normal at birth but develop progressive neurologic deterioration over the subsequent days to weeks.

TREATMENT

APPROPRIATE HEALTH CARE
- Health care of dams that have aborted can be managed on farm.
- Health issues of importance relate to complications of abortion—retained fetal membranes, metritis, delayed involution, and protracted return to service and conception.

NURSING CARE
N/A

ACTIVITY
Normal

DIET
Normal

CLIENT EDUCATION
Education of clients with respect to mode of transmission and preventative measures is highly relevant to the control of neosporosis.

SURGICAL CONSIDERATIONS
None

MEDICATIONS

DRUGS OF CHOICE
- There is no treatment for clearance of the infection in serologically positive individuals.
- Treatment of congenitally infected calves with weakness or neurologic signs is unrewarding.

CONTRAINDICATIONS
N/A

PRECAUTIONS
N/A

POSSIBLE INTERACTIONS
N/A

ALTERNATIVE DRUGS
N/A

FOLLOW-UP

PATIENT MONITORING
N/A

PREVENTION/AVOIDANCE
A commercial vaccine is available in the United States—vaccines may inspire a serologic response but the strength and duration of protection are uncertain.

POSSIBLE COMPLICATIONS
- Poor individual animal and herd reproductive performance can be a feature of both epidemic and endemic neosporosis.
- Milk production losses as the result of midpregnancy abortion

EXPECTED COURSE AND PROGNOSIS
Infected cows will often have a return to normal health and conceive again, but there is an increased chance of repeated abortion in subsequent pregnancies.

MISCELLANEOUS

ASSOCIATED CONDITIONS
N/A

AGE-RELATED FACTORS
The age of the dam, lactation number, and history of prior abortion do not appear to influence the rate of congenital infection.

ZOONOTIC POTENTIAL
None

PREGNANCY
Neosporosis is a prominent cause of abortion and fetal loss.

RUMINANT SPECIES AFFECTED
- Cattle, sheep, and goats
- Not reported in camelids

BIOSECURITY
- Embryo transfer appears to prevent vertical transmission of Neospora from seropositive donors to offspring provided the recipient is seronegative.
- Seropositive cows are more likely than seronegative cows to abort in subsequent pregnancies.
- Direct cow-to-cow transmission does not occur.
- Avoid contamination of cattle feedstuffs with dog feces.

PRODUCTION MANAGEMENT
- Serologic screening of new purchases may be considered, particularly for known negative herds.
- Consider presuckle serology of calves born to seropositive dams when attempting to reduce prevalence rate.
- Colostrum from seropositive dams does not appear to be a clinically significant means of vertical transmission

SYNONYMS
None

SEE ALSO
Bacterial causes of abortion—*Salmonella* spp., *Leptospira interrogans*, *Hemophilus somnus*, *Arcanobacterium pyogenes*
Causes of weak and unthrifty neonatal calves—selenium deficiency (white muscle disease), iodine deficiency, persistent infection with BVDV, congenital infection with bluetongue virus, neonatal septicemia/failure of passive transfer
Miscellaneous causes of abortion—foothills abortion (western United States), mycotic abortion
Protozoal causes of abortion—*Toxoplasma gondii* and *Sarcocystis cruzi* infection in cattle
Viral causes of abortion—bovine viral diarrhea virus, infectious bovine rhinotracheitis, and bluetongue virus.

ABBREVIATIONS
AST = aspartate aminotransferase
BVDV = bovine viral diarrhea virus
CK = creatine kinase
CSF = cerebrospinal fluid
ELISA = enzyme-linked immunosorbent assay
IFAT = indirect fluorescent antibody test
NAT = neospora agglutination test
PCR = polymerase chain reaction

Suggested Reading
Baillargeon, P., Fecteau, G., Pare, J., et al. 2001. Evaluation of the embryo transfer procedure proposed by the International Embryo Transfer Society as a method of controlling vertical transmission of *Neospora caninum* in cattle. *J Am Vet Med Assoc*. 218:1803–806.
Buxton, D., Maley, S. W., Wrught, S., et al. 1998. The pathogenesis of experimental neosporosis in pregnant sheep. *J Comp Pathol*. 118:267–70.
Buxton, D., McAllister, M. M., Dubey, J. P. 2002. The comparative pathogenesis of neosporosis. *Trends Parasitol*. 18(12): 546–52.
Dubey, J. P. 2003. Review of *Neospora caninum* and neosporosis in animals. *Korean J Parasitol*. 1:1–16.
Lindsay, D. S., Rippey, N. S., Powe, T. A., et al. 1995. Abortions, fetal death and stillbirths in pregnant pygmy goats inoculated with tachyzoites of *Neospora caninum*. *Am J Vet Res*. 56:1176–80.

Author: Simon F. Peek

NIGHTSHADE (SOLANUM SPP.) TOXICOSIS

BASICS

OVERVIEW
• Solanaceae family consists of many genera of which *Solanum* spp. (nightshade) has the largest number of species: > 1500 species worldwide
• Plants exist as herbs, shrubs, even small trees, annuals or perennials, some with thorns; fruits are fleshy berries.
• Plants may live in a wide range of habitats—pastures, gardens, waste areas, and in cultivated crops.
• Common species of *Solanum* in North America include *S. nigrum* (black nightshade), *S. carolinense* (horse nettle), *S. elaeagnifolium* (silverleaf nightshade), *S. rostratum* (buffalo bur), *S. tuberosum* (Irish potato), *S. ptychanthum* (eastern black nightshade).
• Gastrointestinal irritation, nervous system dysfunction, and terata are possible.

SIGNALMENT
All species affected (ruminants, swine, equine, humans, etc.)

SIGNS
• Salivation, vomiting, abdominal pain, diarrhea, or constipation may result from GI irritation.
• Decreased salivation, pupillary dilatation, decreased GI motility, and increased heart rate may result from anticholinergic effects.
• Neurologic signs reported in cattle, sheep, and goats: depression, incoordination, tremors, weakness, paralysis, seizures
• Rarely teratogenic effects

CAUSES AND RISK FACTORS
• Toxins primarily consist of steroidal alkaloids including solanidine and solanine. Numerous others exist.
• Toxins are found throughout the plant but are concentrated in the green (unripe) fruits and leaves.
• Activity of anticholinesterase is blocked, allowing accumulation of acetylcholine with resultant decreases in GI motility and salivation.
• Seasonality—most likely consumed in summer/fall. Could be fed throughout the year in hay or silage.
• Lack of available food sources increase likelihood of consumption.

DIAGNOSIS

DIFFERENTIAL DIAGNOSIS
• Numerous other plants and chemicals may produce similar signs of gastroenteritis or nervous dysfunction.
• Clinical signs, history of ingestion, finding plants in feed/hay, identifying plants in stomach/rumen contents are keys to diagnosis.

CBC/BIOCHEMISTRY/URINALYSIS
N/A

OTHER LABORATORY TESTS
N/A

IMAGING
N/A

DIAGNOSTIC PROCEDURES
N/A

PATHOLOGIC FINDINGS
• Gastroenteritis, possibly severe with hemorrhage and necrosis
• Hyperemia of intestinal mucosa
• Increased peritoneal fluid, especially in calves
• Purkinje cell swelling and/or loss
• Evidence of plant material/berries in rumen contents

TREATMENT
• Support patient, treat symptomatically.
• Rumenotomy and evacuation of contents may be useful early in the course of intoxication.
• Prevent further access to toxins.
• Maintain good source of nutrition.

MEDICATIONS

DRUGS OF CHOICE
• Dependent on clinical signs
• Atropine sulfate—if cholinergic signs predominate (salivation, diarrhea)—0.1–1.0 mg/kg IV, IM, or SQ. Give 1/4 IV and remainder SQ or IM. May repeat every 3–4 hours for 1–2 days.
• Physostigmine—if anticholinergic signs predominate (dilated pupils, GI stasis)—30–45 mg SQ cattle
• Activated charcoal—2–5g/kg in a water slurry given orally (1 g charcoal per 5 ml water)

CONTRAINDICATIONS
Appropriate milk and meat withdrawal times must be followed for all compounds administered to food-producing animals.

POSSIBLE INTERACTIONS

FOLLOW-UP

PATIENT MONITORING
N/A

PREVENTION/AVOIDANCE
• Providing a proper diet/adequate nutrition to animals will minimize intake of many poisonous plants.
• Do not allow access to areas or feeds that contain nightshades.

POSSIBLE COMPLICATIONS
None

EXPECTED COURSE AND PROGNOSIS
• Variable, dependent on amount consumed and time period of consumption.
• Prognosis often good with symptomatic treatment.

MISCELLANEOUS

ASSOCIATED CONDITIONS
None

AGE-RELATED FACTORS
None

ZOONOTIC POTENTIAL
None

PREGNANCY
Teratogenic effects such as craniofacial malformations have been reported in lab animals.

RUMINANT SPECIES AFFECTED
All ruminant species can be affected.

BIOSECURITY
N/A

PRODUCTION MANAGEMENT
N/A

SEE ALSO
Serology
Specific toxicosis by chapter
Toxicologic herd outbreaks

ABBREVIATIONS
GI = gastrointestinal
IM = intramuscular
IV = intravenous
SQ = subcutaneous

Suggested Reading
Burrows, G. E., Tyrl, R. J., ed. 2001. *Toxic plants of North America*. Ames: Iowa State University Press.
Keeler, R. F., Baker, D. C., Gaffield, W. 1990. Spirosolane-containing *Solanum* spp. and induction of congenital craniofacial malformations. *Toxicon* 28:873–84.
Menzies, J. S., Bridges, C. H., Bailey, E. M., Jr. 1979. A neurological disease associated with *Solanum dimidiatum*. *Southwest Vet* 32:45–49.
Porter, M. B., MacKay, R. J., Uhl, E., Platt, S. R., de Lahunta, A. 2003. Neurologic disease putatively associated with ingestion of *Solanum viarum* in goats. *J Am Vet Med Assoc*. 223(4):501–504.

Author: Matt G. Welborn

BASICS

OVERVIEW
• Most cases of nitrate (NO_3)/nitrite (NO_2) poisoning in ruminants occur as the result of consumption of nitrate-contaminated hay.
• Forages capable of accumulating toxic concentrations of nitrate include oat hay, *Sorghum* spp. and alfalfa. Pigweed (*Amaranthus* spp.), lambs quarter (*Chenopodium* spp.), Canada thistle (*Cirsium arvense*), and fireweed (*Kochia scoparia*) are several of many well-recognized nitrate-accumulating weeds, and can easily invade hay fields.
• Toxicities are acute, and animals suffer from hypoxia/anoxia secondary to methemoglobin formation.
• The onset of signs is rapid, and death can occur within a few hours of ingestion.
• Slow IV 1% methylene blue, 5–15 mg/kg, is the current drug of choice for treatment of clinically affected animals.
• Abortions due to fetal hypoxia may follow the initial outbreak.
• Many factors affect nitrate uptake by plants, and it is impossible to predict when problems may arise.
• Careful examination of pasture and hay for weed infestation and multiple random nitrate tests of the feed can be used to prevent losses.
• Nitrate/nitrite analysis of feed, water, and biological samples is readily available at many laboratories.

PATHOPHYSIOLOGY
• Nitrite is ten times more toxic than nitrate.
• Nitrate is converted to nitrite by rumen microorganisms.
• Nitrite, once absorbed systemically, oxidizes the ferrous iron to ferric in hemoglobin, converting it to methemoglobin.
• Lack of oxygen to the tissues is the ultimate cause of the signs observed.

SYSTEMS AFFECTED
Cardiovascular, leading to multiple organ failure

GENETICS
N/A

INCIDENCE/PREVALENCE
Generally unpredictable, but more likely to occur in times of drought and during the winter months.

GEOGRAPHIC DISTRIBUTION
Worldwide

SIGNALMENT
Potentially all ruminant species; adults appear to be more susceptible.

Species
All ruminant species at risk

Breed Predilections
N/A

Mean Age and Range
N/A

Predominant Sex
N/A

SIGNS
• Abrupt onset of dyspnea and weakness
• Recumbency
• Salivation
• Pale, cyanotic, or muddy mucous membranes
• Muscle tremors and seizures terminally
• Methemoglobin formation imparts a chocolate brown color to the blood. This color will disappear postmortem.
• Animals may appear to drop dead in their tracks, some with no signs of significant struggling.

CAUSES AND RISK FACTORS
• Animals that are more glutinous and higher on the pecking order, in an energy deficit or debilitated with a preexisting disease, may be more susceptible.
• Developing fetus in pregnant animal is susceptible to nitrate's anoxic effect.
• Clinical signs in animals and death can occur abruptly, despite history of feeding the same diet for days or weeks. This is not a cumulative or chronic problem. The sporadic nature of illness is directly related to the nonhomogenous distribution of nitrate in the feed and lack of rumen adaptation.
• An acute oral lethal dose is approximately 0.5 g nitrate/kg BW.
• Nitrate levels in the diet > 0.6% (equivalent to 6000 ppm nitrate [NO_3] or 1363 ppm nitrate-nitrogen [NO_3-N] are potentially toxic to animals. Divide ppm by 10,000 to convert to% (move decimal four to the left). To convert nitrate-nitrogen (NO_3-N) to nitrate (NO_3), multiply by 4.40.
• Many plants have been associated with nitrate accumulation: sorghums, alfalfa, oat hay, corn stalks, barley straw, *Amaranthus*, *Chenopodium*, *Kochia scoparia*, *Cirsium arvense*.

• Water can be the source of poisoning, but this is uncommon. Gross contamination of the water source and/or environment with nitrogen-containing fertilizers or use of tanks that once transported nitrogen-containing fertilizers as water troughs can be a risk. Nitrate levels < 200 ppm are generally considered safe, and most animals can tolerate much higher levels (1000–1500 ppm).
• Once the animal's rumen has become "acclimated" to nitrate, the animal can tolerate much higher dietary levels.
• Clinical signs generally occur within a few hours of ingesting a toxic dose, so often animals, particularly ones out on pasture or range, are showing signs of illness, or death occurs in large numbers of animals, when no one is around.
• Chronic exposures have been reported in clinical case reports, but this has been hard to experimentally reproduce and verify. Reported problems associated with chronic exposures include abortion, infertility, and hypovitaminosis A.
• Frost can stunt the growth of the plant in the field, but allows the plant to continue to accumulate nitrogen and nitrate from the soil.

DIAGNOSIS

Antemortem
• Muddy-colored mucous membranes, "chocolate brown" blood, and clinical signs suggestive of oxygen deprivation are consistent with nitrate/nitrite toxicosis.
• Nitrite is either converted to nitrate or excreted within 2 hours in cattle.
• Nitrate concentrations can be measured in refrigerated blood, serum or plasma, or urine using ion chromatography, for up to 24 hours after exposure.
• In blood, serum, or plasma, nitrate concentrations > 15 ppm are suggestive, and nitrate concentrations > 30 ppm are diagnostic of excessive exposure to nitrates.
• Suspect forages can be tested using diphenylamine to semiquantitatively estimate the nitrate concentration.
• Ion chromatography can be used to quantitatively analyze for nitrate and nitrite in suspect forages and water.
• Due to the instability of MHb and the need for phosphate buffers for storage of blood samples, determination of MHb concentrations is rarely performed.

NITRATE AND NITRITE TOXICOSIS

Postmortem
• Muddy-colored mucous membranes, "chocolate brown" blood, and postmortem changes suggestive of oxygen deprivation are consistent with nitrate/nitrite toxicosis.
• Ocular fluid (aqueous humor) nitrate concentrations can be determined, using diphenylamine (semiquantitative) or ion chromatography (quantitative) for up to a week after death in refrigerated samples.
• Ocular fluid nitrate concentrations > 10 ppm nitrate are suggestive, and ocular fluid nitrate concentrations > 20 ppm are diagnostic of exposure of nonneonates to excessive nitrates.
• Since neonatal calves normally have ocular fluid nitrate concentrations approximating 20 ppm during the first day of life, nitrate concentrations > 30 ppm are generally more consistent with nitrate/nitrite toxicosis in these animals.
• Nitrate concentrations can also be determined in urine, peritoneal, and pericardial fluids.
• Suspect forages can be tested using diphenylamine to semiquantitatively estimate the nitrate concentration, and ion chromatography can be used to quantitatively analyze for nitrate and nitrite in suspect forages and water.
• Rumen contents are not useful diagnostically because of postmortem instability associated with the activity of microorganisms.

DIFFERENTIAL DIAGNOSIS
• Chlorate, found in some fertilizers, is capable of causing methemoglobinemia.
• Other causes of "abrupt" onset of similar signs and death include *Cicuta* (water hemlock), cyanobacteria (blue-green algae), botulism, *Taxus* (yew), *Zigadenus* (death camas), *Delphinium* (larkspur), lightning strike, anthrax, organophosphate and carbamate insecticides, ionophores, and nonprotein nitrogen.

CBC/BIOCHEMISTRY/URINALYSIS
No remarkable abnormalities are observed, other than the blood appearing "chocolate" brown.

OTHER LABORATORY TESTS
• Methemoglobin levels can be run at select laboratories. Special sample preservation may be required.
• Diphenylamine kits or nitrate/nitrite qualitative or semiquantitative strip tests can be used on feed and water to confirm high nitrate levels.

• Nitrate/nitrite levels can be quantitatively assessed in serum, plasma, whole blood, feed, water, and ocular fluid. Eyes should be removed intact and sent to the laboratory for analysis. Levels in serum, plasma, whole blood, and ocular fluid > 20 ppm nitrate are generally indicative of excessive exposure and possible poisoning if accompanied by compatible history and signs; levels > 50 ppm nitrate are consistent with nitrate poisoning. Nitrate levels in ocular fluid may remain stable for up to 72 hours postmortem.
• Caution should be used when interpreting nitrate/nitrite levels of ocular fluid or gastrointestinal contents collected from aborted fetuses. This does not appear to be a very sensitive or specific diagnostic tool.

IMAGING
N/A

DIAGNOSTIC PROCEDURES
N/A

PATHOLOGIC FINDINGS
Nonspecific—congestion of major organs. Signs of a terminal struggle or seizure may be apparent.

TREATMENT
• Stress associated with handling must be minimized in severely hypoxic animals.
• Exposure to the identified source of the excessive nitrates should be discontinued.
• Rumen lavage with cold water and oral penicillin may slow the continuous reduction of nitrate to nitrite in the rumen.
• Methylene blue is a specific antidote for nitrate/nitrite toxicosis, but its commercial availability has become somewhat limited in the last several years.
• Methylene blue can be administered intravenously (5–15 mg/kg body weight) in a 1% solution in physiological saline.
• Since methylene blue is rapidly cleared from the circulation (serum half-life of 1.5 hours) and has a relatively wide margin of safety, additional, lower doses of the antidote can be administered to animals still exhibiting signs.
• Mild to moderately affected animals, if left untreated, can recover because of erythrocytic NADPH-dependent reduction of Fe^{3+} in MHb to functional Fe^{2+} in hemoglobin.

MEDICATIONS
• 1% Methylene blue, 5–15 mg/kg IV, slow. Response should be immediate.
• Ascorbic acid is thought to be less effective at reversing the methemoglobinemia.

CONTRAINDICATIONS
• The use of methylene blue is off-label. A recommended withdrawal period is 6 months.
• Methylene blue may not be available for much longer.

FOLLOW-UP
Pregnant animals may abort several days to a few weeks after the toxic insult, due to fetal anoxia.

PATIENT MONITORING
No long-term problems have been documented other than abortions. Animals can completely recover, with or without treatment (depending on exposure dose), within a few hours.

PREVENTION/AVOIDANCE
• Knowledge of the high-risk nitrate-accumulating plants and ability to recognize in the field or hay will hopefully minimize the risk.
• Knowledge of the risk factors predisposing high nitrates in the feed (e.g., fertilization, irrigation, soil conditions, environmental conditions) can lead one to be proactive in testing forages during the growing season and pre- and postharvest.
• Suspect forages or crops known to accumulate nitrate should be tested for nitrate concentrations prior to inclusion in the diet of ruminants, especially cattle.
• Forages containing < 5000 ppm nitrate are generally safe for consumption by ruminants.
• High nitrate-containing forages can be diluted with low-nitrate-containing forages prior to feeding to ruminants, or suspect forages can be divided into two feedings to prevent rapid intake.
• High nitrate-containing forages can be ensiled for at least 30 days to reduce the nitrate content prior to feeding to ruminants.
• Sorghums may contain toxic concentrations of cyanide. Lathrogenic compounds present has been associated with neuroaxonal degeneration in sheep. Chlorate, found in some fertilizers can also be toxic.

• The harvest of forages or crops grown under conditions conducive to nitrate accumulation should be delayed until conditions improve to allow nitrate levels in stalks to drop.
• If the harvest of forages or crops grown under conditions conducive to nitrate accumulation cannot be delayed, then the harvesting cutter-bar should be raised to 18 inches to leave the lower portions of the stems or stalks in the field.
• Gradual adaptation of ruminants to high-nitrate-containing forages can be performed over a period of 7 to 10 days.
• Feeding readily fermentable carbohydrate sources in conjunction with high-nitrate-containing forages will promote a denitrifying environment within the rumen.
• Feeding a supplement containing *Propionibacterium* spp. (Bova-Pro, Pro Brands LLC, Columbia, IL) for 10 days prior to anticipated exposure to high-nitrate-containing diets or administering a ruminal inoculum of the same product 10 days prior to nitrate exposure can reduce concentrations of nitrite in the rumen by enhancing denitrification.

POSSIBLE COMPLICATIONS
N/A

EXPECTED COURSE AND PROGNOSIS
• Nitrate poisoning can have a high morbidity and mortality rate; or only individuals may be affected.
• The course of the disease is relatively short, generally lasting within one feeding period.
• The prognosis is heavily dependent on the exposure dose within a short time frame, and levels of methemoglobinemia (blood levels > 80% are typically fatal).

 MISCELLANEOUS

ASSOCIATED CONDITIONS
N/A

AGE-RELATED FACTORS
• Younger animals with nonfunctional, nondenitrifying rumens are resistant to nitrate/nitrite toxicosis.

• The fetus has higher oxygen demands and is reported to be more susceptible to the adverse effects of methemoglobinemia.
• The influence of age-related factors in nitrate-nitrite toxicosis is somewhat dependent on the quality of the forage. If hay is primarily nitrate-containing stems, older, more dominant ruminants, especially cattle, will consume greater quantities of nitrate. If hay contains some leafy portions, which are consumed primarily by older, dominant animals, younger, less-dominant ruminants, especially cattle, will be forced to consume less-palatable portions of the hay dominated by nitrate-containing stems.

ZOONOTIC POTENTIAL
N/A

PREGNANCY
• Abortions may occur several days to a few weeks after the initial toxic insult in those animals that survive.
• Abortion is a common sequela in pregnant cattle consuming forages containing excessive nitrates (> 0.5% or 5000 ppm).

RUMINANT SPECIES AFFECTED
All ruminant species are susceptible.

BIOSECURITY
N/A

PRODUCTION MANAGEMENT
• Avoid feeding exceptionally weedy feeds, particularly avoiding those weeds that are well-recognized nitrate accumulators.
• Oral products (Bova-Pro) are sold as rumen adaptors; these products are marketed as altering the microflora population, allowing the animal the ability to tolerate high dietary nitrate levels.

SYNONYMS
N/A

SEE ALSO
Amaranthus spp. Anthrax
Botulism, *Taxus* (yew)
Cicuta (water hemlock)
Cyanobacteria (blue-green algae)
Delphinium (larkspur)

Ionophores
Lightning strike
Nonprotein nitrogen
Organophosphate and carbamate insecticides
Zigadenus (death camas)

ABBREVIATIONS
MHb = methemoglobin
NO_3 = nitrate
NO_3-N = nitrate-nitrogen
NO_2 = nitrite
NO_2-N = nitrite-nitrogen

Suggested Reading
Boermans, H. J. 1990, Mar. Diagnosis of nitrate toxicosis in cattle, using biological fluids and a rapid ion chromatographic method. *Am J Vet Res.* 51(3): 491–95.
Carson, T. L. 2000, Nov. Current knowledge of water quality and safety for livestock. *Vet Clin North Am Food Anim Pract.* 16(3): 455–64.
East, N. E. 1993, Oct 15. Accidental superphosphate fertilizer poisoning in a llama herd. *J Am Vet Med Assoc.* 203(8): 1176–77.
Galey, F. D. 2000, Nov. Diagnostic toxicology for the food animal practitioner. *Vet Clin North Am Food Anim Pract.* 16(3): 409–21.
Montgomery, J. F., Hum, S. 1995, Dec 2. Field diagnosis of nitrite poisoning in cattle by testing aqueous humour samples with urine test strips. *Vet Rec.* 137(23): 593–94.
Villar, D., Schwartz, K. J., Carson, T. L., Kinker, J. A., Barker, J. 2003, Mar. Acute poisoning of cattle by fertilizer-contaminated water. *Vet Hum Toxicol.* 45(2): 88–90.

Authors: Patricia Talcott and Tim J. Evans

OAK (*QUERCUS* SPP.) POISONING

BASICS

OVERVIEW
• Oak or acorn poisoning has been reported worldwide in different animal species for more than 300 years.
• Poisoning is associated with ingestion of oak buds, stems, leaves, or acorns. More than 60 species of oak are found in North America and many are reported to be toxic.
• Oak poisoning is most commonly seen in cattle and sheep, while the phenomenon is infrequently reported in horses. Pigs and deer are resistant, while goats are less susceptible than other ruminants.
• The toxic principles, tannins, are hydrolyzed in the rumen to gallic acid, pyrogallol, and other phenolic metabolites that induce gastrointestinal and renal dysfunction.
• Hydrolyzed tannins are absorbed and become bound to plasma proteins and endothelial proteins, which leads to GI ulceration, and hemorrhage and fluid loss from blood vessels resulting in edema.
• The main lesion associated with oak poisoning is renal tubular necrosis.
• Gallic acid and pyrogallols are extremely toxic to renal tubules causing acute renal tubular necrosis (ATN). ATN often leads to anuria, electrolyte imbalances, and uremia. Chronic poisoning results in chronic renal failure.
• Animals that survive acute renal insults often develop chronic renal disease and demonstrate poor weight gains compared with their cohorts.

SYSTEMS AFFECTED
Renal, gastrointestinal

SIGNALMENT
• Oak poisoning has been reported in cattle, sheep, goats, rabbits, and horses. Young buds and leaves are palatable to cattle, especially weaned calves.
• A history of ingestion for 2–14 days (average of 1 week) usually precedes clinical signs.

SIGNS
• Clinical signs include anorexia, depression, ruminal stasis, and constipation, which are often followed by hemorrhagic diarrhea. Polyuria and hematuria are often seen. A mucoid nasal discharge and/or epistaxis may also be seen in addition to dehydration, weakness, recumbency, ascites, hydrothorax, and ventral edema. In peracute poisoning, cattle may be found dead.
• Secondary complications such as bronchopneumonia, GI ulceration, perforation, and abscessation may also occur.

RISK FACTORS
• Immature leaves, stems, acorns, and buds are the most toxic and the most palatable.
• Oak poisoning associated with ingestion of leaves and buds is seen in the spring. Oak poisoning occurs in the autumn with ingestion of acorns.
• An increase in oak poisoning is often seen during droughts or other circumstances that lead to poor grazing.
• Cases may also be seen following wind or rain storms that drop leaves, acorns, or branches into pastures where cattle are grazing.
• Affected animals often develop a craving for acorns, occasionally to the exclusion of other available forage.

DIAGNOSIS

DIFFERENTIAL DIAGNOSIS
• Diagnosis of oak poisoning is made on history of exposure and characteristic clinical signs or necropsy findings.
• Primary differentials include diseases that cause acute or chronic renal failure in ruminants.
• Pigweed (*Amaranthus retroflexus*) poisoning, obstructive urolithiasis, clostridial diseases, heavy metal poisoning, leptospirosis, and renal injury due to nephrotoxic antibacterial drugs should be considered.

• Other differentials include diseases that cause gastrointestinal ulceration: infectious bovine rhinotracheitis, bovine viral diarrhea, foot-and-mouth disease, and bluetongue.

CBC/BIOCHEMISTRY/URINALYSIS
• Chemistry profiles of animals in peracute and acute disease states indicate elevated serum urea nitrogen and creatinine, hyponatremia, hyperkalemia, hypochloremia, hyperphosphatemia, and/or hypocalcemia.
• Mild metabolic acidosis with a high anion gap may also be seen. The animal may be anuric or urine may be isosthenuric with proteinuria, hematuria, and/or glucosuria.
• Granular or proteinaceous casts are often found on urinalysis.
• In chronic cases, elevated serum urea nitrogen, creatinine, and anion gap in addition to variable electrolyte imbalances may be seen.
• Some animals show chronic oral, esophageal, or gastrointestinal ulceration or perforation with abscessation.
• Elevated white blood cell counts usually indicate chronic GI ulceration or abscessation.
• Chronic inflammation may lead to a normocytic normochromic anemia. Serum protein levels may be abnormally low due to gastrointestinal and renal losses.

OTHER LABORATORY TESTS
Urinary phenolic content can be used to confirm diagnosis.

PATHOLOGIC FINDINGS
• Tubular necrosis and perirenal edema are prominent in ruminants. Grossly, the kidneys are pale and enlarged.
• Multifocal ulcerative lesions are found in the mouth and esophagus, and throughout the gastrointestinal tract. Ascites and hydrothorax are often present.
• Histopathologic examination reveals coagulation necrosis of the cortical tubular epithelium. Tubules are dilated and devoid of epithelium but with intact basement membranes. Many tubules contain granular, hyaline or cellular casts. Necropsy findings after 3–6 weeks of disease may show GI abscessation associated with perforated ulcers, and secondary bacterial pneumonia. Some tubular regeneration may also be seen.

OAK (*QUERCUS* SPP.) POISONING

TREATMENT
• There is no specific antidote for oak poisoning.
• The goal of therapy is to restore adequate renal perfusion and urine production. Intravenous fluid therapy is recommended to promote diuresis and correct acid-base and electrolyte abnormalities. Oral fluid therapy can be used in some cases, but is less effective.
• Antibiotic therapy should be initiated to treat secondary pneumonia and GI abscessation. Nephrotoxic antibiotics should be avoided.
• Transfaunation may be necessary to restore rumen motility. Remove affected animals from oak trees and provide fresh hay and water.
• Adding calcium hydroxide into feed as a 10% concentration has been shown to be effective in decreasing the incidence of intoxication and mortality rates.
• The mechanism of action is currently unknown.

MEDICATIONS
CONTRAINDICATIONS
Appropriate milk and meat withdrawal times must be followed for all compounds administered to food-producing animals.

FOLLOW-UP
N/A

MISCELLANEOUS
ASSOCIATED CONDITIONS
N/A
AGE-RELATED FACTORS
N/A
ZOONOTIC POTENTIAL
N/A
PREGNANCY
Ingestion of large numbers of acorns in the second trimester of pregnancy can result in congenitally malformed calves. "Acorn calves" seem to be a result of poor nutrition and ingestion of acorns.
RUMINANT SPECIES AFFECTED
Potentially, all ruminant species are affected.
BIOSECURITY
N/A
PRODUCTION MANAGEMENT
N/A
SYNONYMS
Acorn calves
Acorn toxicity
SEE ALSO
Clostridial diseases
Diseases that cause gastrointestinal ulceration: infectious bovine rhinotracheitis, bovine viral diarrhea, foot-and-mouth disease, and bluetongue
Heavy metal poisoning
Leptospirosis and renal injury due to nephrotoxic antibacterial drugs
Obstructive urolithiasis
Pigweed (*Amaranthus retroflexus*) poisoning

ABBREVIATIONS
ATN = acute (renal) tubular necrosis
GI = gastrointestinal

Suggested Reading
Anderson, G. A., Mount, M. E., Vrins, A. A., Ziemer, E. L. 1983. Fatal acorn poisoning in a horse: pathologic findings and diagnostic considerations. *Journal of American Veterinary Medical Association* 82(10): 1105–10.
Fletcher, A. 1985. Renal disease in cattle, part 1. Causative agents. *Compendium on Continuing Education.* 7(12):S702–7.
Howard, J. L., Smith, R. A. 1999. Physical and chemical diseases. In: *Current veterinary therapy 4: food animal practice*. Philadelphia: W.B. Saunders.
Pugh, G. D. 2002. Diseases of the urinary system. In: *Sheep and goat medicine*. Philadelphia: W.B. Saunders.
Rebhun, W. C. 1995. Miscellaneous toxicities and deficiencies. In: *Diseases in dairy cattle*. Baltimore: Williams & Wilkins.
Spier, S.J., Smith, B.P., Seawright, A. A., Norman, B. B., Ostrowski, S. R., Oliver, M. N. 1987. Oak toxicosis in cattle in northern California: clinical and pathologic findings. *Journal of American Veterinary Medical Association* 191(8): 958–64.

Author: Natalie Coffer

OBSTRUCTIVE UROLITHIASIS

BASICS

DEFINITION
Obstructive urolithiasis is the formation of calculi in the urinary system with obstruction and is almost exclusively a male-dominated condition.

PATHOPHYSIOLOGY
• Obstructive urolithiasis occurs when uroliths lodge in the excretory tract, most commonly in the urethra, traumatize the surrounding tissue, and either partially or completely obstruct urine outflow. Uroliths may form in both males and females (see Causes/Risk Factors below for urolith formation); however, the female outflow tract is short and distensible compared to the long, tortuous, and inelastic outflow tract of the male. This anatomic difference allows females to more easily excrete calculi.
• Although calculi may become lodged at any point along the urinary tract including the kidneys, ureters, and trigone area of the bladder, the locations along the urethra that have the smallest diameter are the most common sites for the obstructions to occur.
• In small ruminants, calculi most often are found in the urethral process and tip of the penis. In cattle, the most common site is the sigmoid flexure. In camelids, stones will lodge in the urethra at the level of the ischial arch to the glans penis.

SYSTEMS AFFECTED
Renal/urologic

GENETICS
There may be a genetic predisposition, which has not yet been proved.

GEOGRAPHICAL DISTRIBUTION
None

SIGNALMENT
Species
Cattle, camelids, goats, sheep

Breed Predilection
Texel sheep are predisposed to excreting increased amounts of phosphorus than other breeds of sheep. This may put them at greater risk to develop phosphatic calculi.

Mean Age and Range
Affected animals are 6 months of age or greater.

Predominant Sex
• The condition occurs almost exclusively in males.
• In small ruminants and cattle, the condition is more frequent in animals that have been castrated. In particular, those animals that were castrated before the onset of sexual maturity are more commonly affected.
• In camelids, obstructive urolithiasis occurs more often in intact males.

SIGNS
Clinical signs vary depending upon whether the condition is acute or chronic, with partial or complete obstruction, and whether or not the urinary tract is intact.

Acute or Partial Obstruction
• Dysuria, stranguria, dribbling urine
• Vocalization during episodes of straining
• Flagging of the tail
• Forceful contractions of the abdominal muscles while straining, accompanied by arching of the back and elevation of the head
• Abdominal discomfort may be demonstrated by stretching, kicking at the abdomen, and bruxism.
• Mild distension of the abdomen may be noted.
• Animal may appear normal between episodes.
• +/− Anorexia

Chronic or Complete Obstruction
• More pronounced clinical signs as outlined above
• Anorexia and depression
• No dribbling of urine and the preputial area is dry when obstruction is complete

If a rupture of the urethra or bladder occurs, the animal may temporarily appear comfortable since the pressure on the tract has been relieved. This comfort will be short-lived as urine accumulates in the abdomen (uroperitoneum) or in the subcutaneous tissues surrounding the penis and prepuce at the ventral abdomen.

Ruptured Bladder
• Bilaterally symmetrical distention of the abdomen; may not be noted in camelids
• A fluid wave may be noted in the opposite paralumbar fossa when the abdomen is balloted.
• Dribbling of urine may still be observed with a ruptured bladder.

Ruptured Urethra
• Plaquelike swelling surrounding the prepuce and penis on the ventral abdomen
• Swollen tissue gradually becomes cool and moist, and epilation may occur.
• Dribbling of urine may still be observed with a ruptured urethra.

CAUSES/RISK FACTORS
• There are multiple causes/risk factors for urolithiasis. Dietary factors play a major role.
• Chemical analysis of the stones (see urolith analysis laboratories below) and review of the ration to identify imbalances are crucial steps to the control and prevention of urolithiasis.

DIAGNOSIS

DIFFERENTIAL DIAGNOSIS
• With early or partial obstruction, animals with obstructive urolithiasis will display forceful abdominal contractions during their bouts of stranguria. Otherwise they will appear bright and alert. These signs are suggestive for urinary tract obstruction especially if accompanied by tail flagging, vocalization, dribbling of urine, or having a dry prepuce. It is common for owners to describe these signs and indicate that the animal may be constipated; however, constipation in male ruminants is much less common that obstructive urolithiasis.
• Chronic or complete obstruction accompanied by anorexia, depression, and/or colic, abdominal distension, and tachycardia are signs that are also associated with gastrointestinal disorders, such as rumen acidosis, abomasal emptying defect, abomasal impaction intestinal obstruction. However, with abdominal disorders, the animal's ability to urinate should be intact. Placing an animal in a stall with no bedding so that the presence or absence of pools of urine may be observed is useful to assess urination function.
• Rupture of the urinary bladder will create uroperitoneum, which will show as a progressive, bilaterally symmetrical distention of the abdomen. Many abdominal disorders that result in abdominal distension do not produce symmetrical distension. For example, the abdominal distension associated with rumen acidosis/atony is usually confined to the left abdomen, whereas abomasal emptying defect and abomasal impaction usually cause distension on the lower right side, with some involvement of the dorsal left paralumbar fossa.
• Rupture of the urethra is associated with ventral abdominal swelling surrounding the preputial area. Differentials for swelling in this area include umbilical hernia, abscess, or hematoma.

CBC/BIOCHEMISTRY/URINALYSIS
Early/Partial Obstruction
• CBC: usually within normal limits
• Serum biochemistry: possible increase in BUN, creatinine

Chronic/Complete Obstruction
• CBC: hemoconcentration, stress leukogram
• Serum biochemistry: increased BUN and creatinine, hypochloremia, normal or low potassium and sodium; potassium and phosphorus may be elevated in animals with uroperitoneum, and to a lesser extent in animals with rupture of the urethra

Commercial Laboratories That Perform Analysis on Uroliths
• Urinary Stone Analysis Laboratory, Department of Medicine and Epidemiology, School of Veterinary Medicine, University of California at Davis, Davis, CA 95616; 1–530-752-3228
• Dr. Carl Osborne, Department of Small Animal Clinical Medicine, 1352 Boyd Ave., St. Paul, MN 55108; 1-616-625-7744
• Urolithiasis Laboratory, P.O. Box 25375, Houston, TX 77265-5375; 1-800-235-4846

IMAGING
• History and physical examination findings in cases of obstructive urolithiasis are usually straightforward; however, abdominal ultrasonography of the bladder and kidneys may be useful for further diagnostic

confirmation and prognostic/therapeutic approach purposes.

• In small ruminants and camelids, a 3.5–5.0 MHz probe placed in the right inguinal area and directed toward the pelvic inlet should provide good visualization of the bladder. If this structure is not ruptured, its distended outline will be readily apparent.

• If rupture has occurred, free fluid in the abdomen will be seen. In cattle, transrectal ultrasonography using a 7.5 MHz probe can be used to visualize the pelvic urethra, bladder, and left kidney.

• If obstruction has been present for 48 hours or longer, it is likely that hydronephrosis has developed, which also can be seen using ultrasound imaging of the kidneys. Observation of this abnormality is associated with a poor prognosis.

• Abdominal radiography for survey and /or contrast studies of the urinary tract in cattle to ascertain the location of uroliths and abnormalities (bladder rupture, hydronephrosis) probably has limited availability in large cattle for most private practices. The equipment that is required is prohibitive.

• In small ruminants (including calves), lateral abdominal views may be useful in detecting radiodense uroliths on survey films, or radiolucent stones using contrast material. However, in animals where the penis cannot be extended (prepubertal males, males castrated before puberty) and the urethral process removed (sheep and goats), catheterization of the urethra to introduce contrast material is generally precluded.

DIAGNOSTIC PROCEDURES

• Abdominocentesis and chemical analysis of the retrieved sample for creatinine is useful to document uroperitoneum. Peritoneal fluid is most easily obtained from the right side of the abdomen, right of midline in the inguinal area.

• Abdominocentesis performed in an animal with a bladder rupture will yield a moderate to large amount of free flowing, clear, colorless to yellow-tinged, usually nonodiferous fluid. Comparison of peritoneal fluid creatinine to serum creatinine usually shows a 2:1 ratio.

PATHOLOGIC FINDINGS

• At the site(s) of the obstruction and proximal to this, the urethral mucosa will appear discolored from hemorrhage and necrosis. Discrete calculi may be found, or in the case of struvite crystals, sandlike granules may be compressed along the obstructed area. If the urethra has ruptured, subcutaneous accumulation of urine will be found surrounding the site of rupture.

• The bladder may be distended and thin or it may be thickened. The mucosa may appear hemorrhagic and/or necrotic.

• If the bladder has ruptured, uroperitoeum will be present and there may be blood clots in the abdomen. Hydroureters and hydronephrosis may also be noted.

 TREATMENT

• Once a diagnosis of obstructive urolithiasis is made, decisions concerning the affected animal should be made without delay and with consideration for the animal's utility and health status.

• The prognosis for recovery for an animal that is found early in the disease process with an intact bladder and urethra is considered good if supportive therapy (fluids, antibiotics, and frequent monitoring) and surgical intervention are provided.

• The prognosis declines somewhat if the urinary tract has ruptured. In cases where the obstruction is either partial or complete and chronic with or without rupture within the urinary tract, the prognosis is very poor to guarded even with supportive care and surgical intervention. Oftentimes these cases have sufficient urinary tract trauma including hydronephrosis that is irreversible.

APPROPRIATE HEALTH CARE

• Medical management consists of extension of the penis for examination and/or removal of the urethral process in those animals whose penis can be extended (sexually mature males and males castrated after the onset of puberty).

• A urinary catheter is placed in the urethra. The author prefers a semirigid type, 22-inch catheter for small ruminants and camelids. The 5–8 French size works well for animals that are less than 45 kg, whereas the 10–20+ French is used in larger animals. Use of epidural anesthesia and setting the small ruminant on its hindquarters aids in performing this procedure.

• Surgical management consists of performing a perineal urethrostomy (PU) or abdominal exploratory surgery combined with tube cystotomy.

• Perineal urethrostomy is an economical option as a salvage procedure since its prognosis as a long-term solution is fair to poor. It is an excellent option for an animal destined for slaughter. Abdominal exploratory surgery allows for repair of the bladder if a rupture has occurred and for placement of a urinary bladder catheter that exits through the body wall to provide a temporary outflow of urine directly from the bladder. This allows time for the traumatized urethra to heal. It is the recommended procedure for breeding animals and pets.

NURSING CARE

This consists of providing fluid therapy (usually intravenous) to correct electrolyte abnormalities. Assessing and addressing azotemia, maintaining good hydration and glomerular filtration rate are important components to adequate nursing care. Abdominal bandaging and urinary bladder catheter maintenance may also be required for those animals that have had abdominal surgery.

ACTIVITY

Animals that have intravenous and/or bladder catheters should be restricted to a small pen and housed alone so that other animals do not interfere with catheter lines.

DIET

Please see Table 1.

CLIENT EDUCATION

Clients should be informed of the possibility of condition recurrence. Even with surgical intervention and dietary management, the urethra may heal with a stricture/adhesion that may predispose an animal to future obstruction.

SURGICAL CONSIDERATIONS

See Appropriate Health Care above.

 MEDICATIONS

DRUGS OF CHOICE

Antimicrobial Therapy

Considerations should include drugs that achieve a high concentration in the urine, have a low potential for nephrotoxicity, have a broad spectrum of activity, and, if possible, are approved for use in the target species. Examples include ampicillin, sulfonamides, and third-generation cephalosporins such as ceftiofur. Additional considerations may include withdrawal times for food-producing animals, urine culture, and sensitivity. In general, tube cystotomy patients will require a more prolonged course of antimicrobial treatment (at least for several days past the removal of the indwelling bladder catheter) than those animals that undergo a perineal urethrostomy.

Anti-inflammatory Therapy

Nonsteroidal anti-inflammatory drugs such as flunixin meglumine (1–2 mg/kg, IV or SQ, q 12 hours for 1–3 days) and aspirin (100 mg/kg, PO, q 8 to 12 hours for 1–3 days) may be useful to decrease tissue irritation and inflammation. These drugs should be used with caution because of their nephrotoxic potential.

Sedatives/Analgesics

Sedation or epidural anesthesia is useful to aid in extension and examination of the penis. Diazepam (0.1 mg/kg IV) or acepromazine (0.05–0.1 mg/kg IV or IM) are recommended sedatives. Because xylazine has a diuretic effect, it may contribute to bladder distension and is not recommended unless immediate resolution of the obstruction is anticipated. Caudal epidural anesthesia (1 ml of 2% lidocaine/100 kg not to exceed 10 ml /450 kg in cattle or 3 ml in a 60 kg small ruminant for standing anesthesia) provides excellent relaxation of the retractor penis muscles, relief from urethral pain, and minimal side effects, and greatly facilitates examination of the penis and distal urethra.

OBSTRUCTIVE UROLITHIASIS

Table 1

Urolithiasis Analysis and Associated Risk Factors.			
Type of calculi	Risk factors	Radiodense	Prevention
Phosphatic: Magnesium ammonium phosphate (struvite) Calcium phosphate	High concentrate ($\uparrow$ P+):low roughage ($\downarrow$ Ca++) ration High magnesium (> 6%) Pelleted rations Alkaline urine (pH > 7.0)	No	Balance ration for calcium, magnesium, and phosphorus Adjust Ca:P ratio to 2:1 Add sodium chloride[1] or ammonium chloride[2] to ration Maximize water intake
Silicates	Western U.S. plants grown in sandy soils accumulate silicates. Hi silica-containing water Hi Ca: Low P ration	No	Adjust Ca:P ratio to 1:1 rather than 2:1 Maximize water intake
Oxalates: Calcium oxalate	Oxalate-containing plants	Yes	Maximize water intake
Calcium carbonate	Alfalfa diets (High in cations Ca++ and K+) Alkaline urine	Yes	Feed grass hay (better cation to anion balance) Add sodium chloride[1] or ammonium chloride[2] to ration Maximize water intake
Any of the above types	Castration, especially before the onset of puberty Inaccessible (distant location, frozen) or unpalatable water	See above	*Water management:* Fresh, clean, palatable, and accessible source Encourage water intake with addition of salts (sodium chloride[1] or ammonium chloride[2]) to the ration

[1] The addition of sodium chloride to a ration at a level of 2%–5%, or an individual dose of 1 tsp/45 kg, will encourage water intake, thus producing a greater volume of dilute urine (flushing action).

[2] The addition of ammonium chloride at 1%–2% (2–4 pounds/ton) of the ration, or an individual dose of 0.05–0.1 g/kg (1 tsp/45 kg), will encourage water intake with the same results as described for sodium chloride. Additionally, ammonium chloride may aid in decreasing urine pH, which is useful since some calculi, such as struvite, more readily precipitate in alkaline urine, which is the normal pH for ruminants.

CONTRAINDICATIONS
• Avoid drugs that are nephrotoxic. Stabilizing a patient with fluids and establishing urine flow may be necessary to accomplish first or concurrent with usage of drugs that have nephrotoxic potential, such as nonsteroidal anti-inflammatory agents.
• Appropriate milk and meat withdrawal times must be followed for all compounds administered to food-producing animals.

FOLLOW-UP

PATIENT MONITORING
Following medical or surgical treatment, an animal should be housed in an area that allows for observation of urination, either directly, or indirectly (removal of bedding and noting wet areas on the floor).

PREVENTION/AVOIDANCE
See Table 1.

POSSIBLE COMPLICATIONS
A range of complications may occur in an individual animal or group of animals in the case of a herd or flock outbreak. These may include: death, renal failure, reobstruction, peritonitis (postoperative and/or secondary to bladder rupture), and cellulitis (secondary to urethral rupture).

EXPECTED COURSE AND PROGNOSIS
See Treatment above.

MISCELLANEOUS

ASSOCIATED CONDITIONS
• Hydronephrosis/hydroureter
• Urethral rupture
• Bladder rupture

AGE-RELATED FACTORS
N/A

ZOONOTIC POTENTIAL
N/A

PREGNANCY
N/A

RUMINANT SPECIES AFFECTED
Cattle, sheep, goats, camelids

BIOSECURITY
N/A

PRODUCTION MANAGEMENT
See Cause and Risk Factors above, especially considering managing animals in a feedlot, and the influence that rations have on minimizing the occurrence of uroliths.

SYNONYMS
Water belly.

SEE ALSO
Abomasal emptying defect
Abomasal impaction intestinal obstruction
Chronic or complete obstruction
Constipation in male ruminants
Rumen acidosis
Rupture of the urethra
Rupture of the urinary bladder
Umbilical hernia, abscess, and hematoma

ABBREVIATIONS
BUN = blood urea nitrogen
IM = intramuscular
IV = intravenous
PU = perineal urethrostomy
SQ = subcutaneous

Suggested Reading
Pugh, D. G. 2002. *Sheep and goat medicine.* Philadelphia: W. B. Saunders.
Radostitis, O. M., Gay, C. C., Blood, D. C., Hinchcliff, K. W. 2000. *Veterinary medicine.* 9th ed. Philadelphia: W. B. Saunders.
Smith, B. D. 2002. *Large animal internal medicine.* 3rd ed. Philadelphia: Mosby.

Author: Michelle Kopcha

BASICS

OVERVIEW
• Ectropion is uncommon in farm animals, except when secondary to scar tissue formation.
• Entropion is seen as a congenital form, a traumatic form, which results from scarring, and secondary to other ocular disease, which causes squinting.
• Numerous other masses, growths, or lacerations can occur on the cornea, conjunctiva, eyelids, or nictitating membrane, which require surgery.
• The presence of ocular tumors on or around the eye may indicate the presence of tumors elsewhere in the body.

SIGNALMENT
• Entropion, ectropion, and other ocular lesions can occur in all ages and species of food animals.
• Entropion is more common in young animals, especially lambs, as a congenital defect.
• Cattle with nonpigmented periocular skin are more predisposed to squamous cell carcinoma (SCC).

SIGNS
• Anatomical abnormality can be directly observed.
• Epiphora
• Squinting
• Corneal edema
• Periocular masses
• Lacerations with associated hemorrhage
• Corneal defects

CAUSES
• Congenital
• Trauma
• Corneal ulcer/laceration
• Palpebral laceration
• Infectious conjunctivitis/keratitis
• Neoplastic

DIAGNOSIS

DIFFERENTIAL DIAGNOSIS
• Corneal ulcer
• Corneal laceration
• Conjunctivitis
• Keratitis
• Periorbital tumor
• Dermoid
• Ocular tumor
• Orbital fracture

TREATMENT

CONDITION

Congenital Entropion
• Repeated manual eversion of the lids
• Subconjunctival injection of saline or antibiotic
• Superglue can be used to plicate the lid to evert the margin.
• Skin staples or mattress sutures can be placed to plicate and evert the lid.
• Holtz-Celsus procedure to resect a wedge of skin in severe or recalcitrant cases

Traumatic Entropion
Surgical correction of laceration is required. Consultation with an ophthalmologist may be necessary to determine the best method of reconstructing the lid margins.

Secondary Entropion
• Diagnosis and treatment of the primary disease is essential.
• Pain relief usually results in resolution of the entropion.

Third Eyelid Masses
• Very small masses can be resected with scissors and topical or local anesthesia while leaving the rest of the nictitans intact.
• Larger masses or traumatized third eyelids can be resected entirely. Following topical and/or local anesthesia, hemostats are placed across the base of the nictitating membrane, and it is resected with scissors or scalpel. No suturing is required. Topical antibiotics are recommended to prevent infection.

Corneal Dermoids and Small SCC Lesions
• Superficial keratectomy can remove small lesions from the corneal surface with local and/or topical anesthesia.
• Hyperthermy can be used to remove small lesions or spreading thin lesions (< 10 mm thick). Repeated treatment and debulking may be required.
• Laser ablation can be used to remove some superficial lesions.

Corneal Lacerations and Ulcers
• Most ulcers and lacerations will heal with medical treatment.
• Severe lesions and lesions that could cause corneal rupture may benefit from protection.
• Conjunctival flaps can be performed, but may require consultation with an ophthalmologist.
• Tarsorrhaphy can be performed by suturing the outer eyelid margins closed. Absorbable suture can be used so that the sutures do not have to be removed, or nonabsorbable sutures can be used, but must be removed.
• A third eyelid flap can be performed to cover and protect the eye, and can be performed so that it can be raised and lowered for medicating the eye. A suture is placed through the lateral aspect of the upper eyelid, passed through the third eyelid around the cartilage to provide strength, and passed again through the upper eyelid. The suture is then drawn tight, pulling the third eyelid over the cornea to protect it. Avoid dragging or rubbing the suture on the cornea.

Eyelid Masses
• Wedge resection
• H-blepharoplasty
• Hyperthermy
• Cryotherapy
• Radiotherapy

Eyelid Lacerations
Careful surgical reconstruction in multiple layers

DRUGS OF CHOICE

CONTRAINDICATIONS
Appropriate milk and meat withdrawal times must be followed for all compounds administered to food-producing animals.

FOLLOW-UP

PATIENT MONITORING
• Careful monitoring of corneal damage is essential to avoid further damage or corneal rupture.
• Concurrent infections must be treated.
• Animals with ocular or periocular tumors should be monitored for new growths or recurrence of treated growths.

POSSIBLE COMPLICATIONS
• Corneal damage or rupture
• Ectropion, if entropion is overcorrected
• Recurrence of tumors

MISCELLANEOUS

ASSOCIATED CONDITIONS
• Squamous cell carcinoma (SCC)
• Infectious bovine keratoconjunctivitis

SEE ALSO
Anesthesia and analgesia
Enucleation/exenteration
Infectious bovine keratoconjunctivitis
Squamous cell carcinoma (SCC)

ABBREVIATIONS
SCC = squamous cell carcinoma

Suggested Reading
Irby, N. L. 2004. Surgical diseases of the eye in farm animals. In: *Farm animal surgery*, ed. S. L. Fubini, N. G. Ducharme. St. Louis, MO: Saunders.
Welker, B. 1995. Ocular surgery. *Vet Clin North Amer Food Anim Pract*. 11:149–57.

Author: Jennifer M. Ivany Ewoldt

OESTRUS OVIS INFESTATION

 BASICS

DEFINITION
• Infestation of the nasal cavity and/or sinuses with larval stages (bots or maggots) of *Oestrus ovis*.
• Infestation can produce a chronic rhinitis and sinusitis, most commonly associated with a mucopurulent nasal discharge.

PATHOPHYSIOLOGY
• *Oestrus ovis* is a dipteran fly in the same family as the warble fly of cattle.
• The adult fly is dark gray and is approximately 1 cm long.
• The adult fly has rudimentary or vestigial mouthparts and cannot feed.
• After mating, female flies deposit larvae (larviposit or oviposit) in and around the nostrils of the ruminant host. The fly does not land on the host in the process.
• Adult *Oestrus ovis* live 2–28 days and each female produces up to several hundred larvae.
• The parasite can "overwinter" as first-stage larvae in the nasal cavities of hosts and/or as pupae in the ground.
• The first-stage larvae, or instars, initially less than 2 mm long, enter the nasal cavity and feed upon mucus and exfoliated epithelial cells.
• The first-stage instars migrate in the nasal passages and undergo maturation to second-stage larvae or instars, which reside in the frontal and maxillary sinuses. Further maturation leads to third-stage instars. After a total larval period of weeks to several months, the fully developed third-stage larvae migrate back to the nostrils, are sneezed out, and pupate in the ground.
• The pupal period is 3–9 weeks.
• Adult flies arise after a period of approximately 4 weeks in summer but require much longer in cooler weather climates.
• Mechanical damage and trauma occur to the nasal mucosa due in part to attachment by the oral hooks and cuticular spines of the larvae.
• Hypersensitivity has been proposed to play a role in the pathophysiology; an increase in numbers of eosinophils and mast cells has been found in the mucosa. In the sinuses, dead larvae may produce an allergic and inflammatory response.
• Larvae and/or their products may produce inflammatory reactions in the lung.

SYSTEMS AFFECTED

Respiratory
• Rhinitis with nasal discharge, sneezing, and difficult, snoring respiration. The rhinitis is associated with a chronic catarrhal discharge, which may become purulent and which can contain many eosinophils.
• Chronic sinusitis and secondary pneumonia may be observed.

Nervous
• Rarely, the brain may be involved. Larvae enter the brain from the sinuses, or there is extension of purulent inflammation from the sinusoids.
• In "false gid," signs of incoordination and a high-stepping gait may simulate signs of gid, a parasitic invasion of the CNS due to larval stages of a canine tapeworm (*Coenurus cerebralis*) and related species (*Taenia multiceps*).

General
Heavy adult fly activity and/or larval burdens may cause sufficient annoyance to hosts to interfere with feeding and lead to loss of condition and/or reduced weight gains.

GENETICS
N/A

INCIDENCE/PREVALENCE
• The incidence/prevalence is variable among geographic regions and within flocks in a given region. The condition is endemic in some areas.
• The parasite is found worldwide. Various sources report it as widely distributed in Africa, Australia, Europe, countries of the Mediterranean basin, South Africa, some countries in South America, countries of the former USSR and the United States.

SIGNALMENT

Species
• Most common in sheep, reported less commonly in goats
• Has been reported in bighorn sheep (*Ovis canadensis*) and the European ibex (*Capra ibex*), some deer, elk, camels and camelids, dogs, and people

Breed Predilections
• Affects all breeds of sheep
• Larval burdens have been reported as lighter in goats than in sheep.

Mean Age and Range
• All ages are apparently affected.
• Larval burdens have been reported by some sources as being higher in younger animals.

Predominant Sex
Occurs in sheep of all sexes, breeds, and ages

SIGNS

GENERAL COMMENTS
Production effects may occur from larger parasite burdens when feeding is interfered with. Both the adult fly and larvae can affect the host. The effects include interference with feeding, complications of nasal infestations, and the results of aberrant larval migration.

HISTORICAL FINDINGS
The female adult flies bother sheep, causing one or more of the following signs: head shaking, sneezing, rubbing the nose on the ground or on other sheep, foot stamping, circling with nose to the ground, stamping feet and shaking heads, blowing, and interference with grazing.

PHYSICAL EXAMINATION FINDINGS
• Major findings include: rhinitis with nasal discharge (initially clear and mucoid; later mucopurulent and often with blood), sneezing, and difficult, snoring respiration.

• Chronic sinusitis, secondary bacterial pneumonia is possible in some cases.
• Very uncommonly, larvae may enter the brain from the sinuses or there can be the spread of purulent inflammation from the sinuses to the brain.

CAUSES
Infestation of the nasal cavity/sinuses with larvae or bots of *O. ovis*.

RISK FACTORS
• Environmental factors may play a major role in influencing the frequency of infestation.
• In North America, the adult fly is seen from spring to summer or autumn.
• The fly is particularly active in warm weather. In warm climates, the fly can be active over a greater portion of the year.

 DIAGNOSIS

DIFFERENTIAL DIAGNOSIS
Foreign bodies (visualization of foreign body in nasal cavity), nasal adenocarcinoma (visualization of tissue and/or biopsy), pneumonia (characteristic clinical signs, evidence of pulmonary pathology), sinusitis (clinical signs, lack of evidence of oestrosis), trauma (history), and others depending upon specific symptoms.

CBC/BIOCHEMISTRY/URINALYSIS
N/A.

OTHER LABORATORY TESTS
Serologic techniques such as an enzyme-linked immunosorbent assay (ELISA) test have been developed.

IMAGING
Techniques such as endoscopy may be used to visualize the parasite in the nasal cavity.

DIAGNOSTIC PROCEDURES
• Diagnosis is usually based upon clinical signs; it can be confirmed by necropsy postmortem or visualization of the larvae in the sinuses (e.g., endoscopy) antemortem.
• Diagnosis can also be based upon clinical signs and inferred from response to appropriate treatment.
• Diagnosis of problems associated with adult flies is based upon behavior of sheep. Larval identification may facilitate diagnosis also.

PATHOLOGIC FINDINGS
• Up to 20 or more larvae at different developmental stages may be found in the sinuses.
• Sinuses with live larvae may be seen as normal; sinuses with dead larvae may demonstrate edematous and thickened membranes and cavities with exudates.

TREATMENT

APPROPRIATE HEALTH CARE
• Treatment may be administered at various times during the year, based upon climatic factors and occurrence of infestations.
• In temperate climates, treatment in autumn has been recommended. The majority of larvae are small during this time period.

NURSING CARE
No specific recommendations

ACTIVITY
N/A.

DIET
N/A.

CLIENT EDUCATION
Strategic treatment may interrupt life cycle before the parasite becomes widely established.

SURGICAL CONSIDERATIONS
N/A

MEDICATIONS

DRUGS OF CHOICE
• These recommendations refer to treatment of the disease in the United States in sheep, the most commonly affected species.
• Obtain specific information for drug approvals by country and for other species.
• Some anthelmintics used in control/treatment programs for GI parasites may be effective in maintaining control of *O. ovis*.
• Ivermectin at 0.2 mg/kg (200 ug/kg) PO kills all instars and is reported as highly effective. A controlled-release form of ivermectin is available in some countries and has been shown to be effective over an extended period of time.
• Obtain country-specific meat and milk withdrawal times following drug use.
• It has been recommended in temperate zones to treat in autumn when the majority of larvae are small.

CONTRAINDICATIONS
• Ivermectin is not recommended for use in lactating animals due to its extended milk withdrawal time.
• Obtain current and complete information on any drugs used.
• Appropriate milk and meat withdrawal times must be followed for all compounds administered to food-producing animals.

PRECAUTIONS
N/A.

POSSIBLE INTERACTIONS
Check drug label and follow all regulations within individual country.

ALTERNATIVE DRUGS
• A variety of drugs has been used for treatment.

• Closantel, moxidectin, ruelene, rafoxanide, trichlorfon, and other systemic products have been reported in the literature.
• Some authors have recommended various treatments applied directly into the nostrils.

FOLLOW-UP

PATIENT MONITORING
N/A

PREVENTION/AVOIDANCE
• Treating at appropriate cycle stages can reduce the incidence of infection.
• Prevention is difficult. Attempts to minimize the effects of adult flies have been made by utilizing insecticides and by providing shelter or access to cool areas.
• Shelter or cool areas may decrease exposure to the adult flies, which are active in sunlight and warmth.
• The fly has a fairly narrow preferred temperature range.

POSSIBLE COMPLICATIONS
• Larvae may be unable to exit the sinuses and may die; calcified or septic sinusitis may result.
• Purulent inflammation in the sinuses may spread to the brain with the presence of dead larvae.
• Interstitial pneumonia and lung abscesses have been reported.
• Killing mature larvae may result in marked reactions in the membranes of the sinuses.

EXPECTED COURSE AND PROGNOSIS
Treatment at the appropriate life cycle with an effective drug should produce high cure rates.

MISCELLANEOUS

ASSOCIATED CONDITIONS
Chronic sinusitis, secondary bacterial pneumonia are possible in some cases.

AGE-RELATED FACTORS
Young animals may experience greater larval burdens.

ZOONOTIC POTENTIAL
• *Oestrus ovis* is a zoonosis.
• It most commonly causes ocular myiasis or ophthalmomyiasis, primarily among individuals with close contact to sheep or infested animals (e.g., shepherds).
• Affected individuals most commonly report the sensation of being struck in the eye by an insect or foreign body, followed by pain and inflammation in the ocular conjunctiva.
• Cases of conjunctival ophthalmomyiasis have been reported as caused by *O. ovis* larvae in locations such as Africa, the Middle East, countries of the former USSR, Europe, and the United States. The larvae are usually visualized and removed.

PREGNANCY
N/A.

RUMINANT SPECIES AFFECTED
Sheep (most commonly affected), goats, bighorn sheep (*Ovis canadensis*), blesbock (*Damaliscus albifrons*), camels and camelids, European ibex (*Capra ibex*), elk, and some species of deer.

BIOSECURITY
Spread of the parasite may be promoted by importation of infested animals.

PRODUCTION MANAGEMENT
• Moderate numbers of larvae cause little harm; heavy infestations may produce effects such as decreased grazing and feeding times.
• Infestations may cause a significant decline in production of milk or a decrease in weight gains.

SYNONYMS
Head bot
Head grub
Nasal bots
Nose bots
Nostril fly
Oestrosis
Oestrus ovis infestation
Sheep nasal bot fly infestation
Sheep nasal fly

SEE ALSO
Foreign bodies
Gun shot wound
Nasal adenocarcinoma
Pneumonia
Sinusitis
Trauma

ABBREVIATIONS
CNS = central nervous system
GI = gastrointestinal
N/A = not applicable
USSR = Union of Soviet Socialist Republics
PO = per os, by mouth

Suggested Reading
Acha, P. N., Szyfres, B. 2003. *Zoonoses and communicable diseases common to man and animals.* 3rd ed. Vol. III, *Parasitoses.* Scientific and Technical Publication No. 580. Washington, DC: Pan American Health Organization.
Dorchies, P., Duranton, C., Jacquiet, P. 1998. Pathophysiology of *Oestrus ovis* infection in sheep and goats: a review. *Vet Rec.* 142:487–89.
Georgi, J. R., Georgi, M. E., Theodorides, V. J. 1990. *Parasitology for veterinarians.* 5th ed. Philadelphia: W. B. Saunders.
Horak, I. G., Snijders, A. J. 1974. The effect of *Oestrus ovis* infestation on Merino lambs. *Vet Rec.* 94:12–16.
Kimberling, C. V. 1988. *Jensen and Swift's diseases of sheep.* 3rd ed. Philadelphia: Lea & Febiger.
Soulsby, E. J. L. 1968. Helminths, arthropods and protozoa of domesticated animals. In: *Monnig's veterinary helminthology and entomology.* 6th ed. Baltimore: Williams and Wilkins.

Author: Kevin L. Anderson

OLEANDER AND FOXGLOVE

 BASICS

OVERVIEW
• A member of the dogbane (Apocynum) family, oleander (*Nerium oleander*) is an evergreen ornamental shrub 15–25 feet tall.
• It has smooth, green bark and dark green leathery leaves, which are opposite at bottom, but appear whorled at the top.
• Multiple colors of flowers may bloom year round.
• The fruit is a hanging long slender pod and the seeds have tufts of hair.
• Foxglove (*Digitalis purpurea*) is tall with lanceolate dark green, hairy leaves that are low on the flowering stalk.
• Flowers are trumpet shaped, multiple colored, and profuse on the upper stalk.
• Additional plants include dogbane (*Apocynum cannabinum*), lily of the valley (*Convallaria majalis*), yellow oleander (*Thevetia peruviana*), squill (*Scillia maritime*), Ouabain (*Strophanthus* spp.), silkvine (*Periploca graeca*), and milkweed (*Asclepias*).
• Worldwide distribution due to cultivation as ornamentals
• Oleander is generally nonpalatable as a green plant, but most poisonings are associated with dried leaves from trimming.
• All parts of the oleander plant are toxic and only a small amount (0.005%–0.015% BW) must be ingested for toxicity

PATHOPHYSIOLOGY
• Foxglove is the natural source for digitalis.
• All parts of the plant are toxic.

• Toxicity due to oleander and foxglove ingestion is the same as digitalis toxicity.
• Na/K/ATP pump is affected leading to bradycardia, heart block, and asystole.
• Inhibition of pump leads to elevated intracellular Na and Ca and extracellular K.
• Cardiovascular compromise is predominant sign.
• Gastrointestinal and neurologic signs may also occur.
• Death usually occurs within 36 hours, but may take up to 14 days.
• Toxin is widely distributed in body, including milk, fetal fluids.
• Urinary excretion is primary route.

SIGNALMENT
All animals of all ages ingesting plants are at risk.

SIGNS
• Sudden death
• Neurologic
• Hyperexcitable nervous function
• Seizures
• Gastrointestinal
• Present following acute exposure
  • Vomiting and abdominal pain leading to severe diarrhea
  • Rumen atony
  • Increased salivation
  • Cardiovascular
• Present later in the course of intoxication
  • Bradycardia progressing to arrhythmia, paradoxic tachycardia, heart block, and then asystole
  • Weakness, depression, and coma occur secondary to cardiac insufficiency.

CAUSES AND RISK FACTORS
Any animal ingesting the plant is at risk of developing toxicity

 DIAGNOSIS

DIFFERENTIAL DIAGNOSIS
• Any cause of severe diarrhea
• Other plant toxicities

CBC/BIOCHEMISTRY/URINALYSIS
Hyperkalemia

OTHER LABORATORY TESTS
N/A

IMAGING
N/A

DIAGNOSTIC PROCEDURES
• Serum digitalis assay may cross-react with toxin.
• Presence of plant in intestinal content
• Evidence of plant consumption
• Laboratory assays have been developed for detection of oleander in ingesta.
• ECG alteration includes widening of the QRS complex, ST segment depression, enlarged P waves, and ventricular arrhythmias.

PATHOLOGIC FINDINGS
• Nonspecific
• Gastrointestinal irritation
• Pale mottling of heart with congestion
• Histological evidence of myocardial degeneration and necrosis

OLEANDER AND FOXGLOVE

TREATMENT

- Treatment is supportive and symptomatic.
- Rumenotomy to prevent further intoxication
- Prevent additional exposure.

MEDICATIONS

DRUGS OF CHOICE

- Activated charcoal (AC) (2–5 g/kg PO in a water slurry)
- Evidence in other species of recycling through gastrointestinal system; repeat doses of AC may be beneficial.
- Atropine for heart block (1 mg/kg to effect)
- Anti-arrhythmics
- Treatment for hyperkalemia
- Cathartics

CONTRAINDICATIONS

- Calcium-containing solutions are contraindicated.
- Potassium-containing solutions may be contraindicated with severe hyperkalemia and must be titrated.
- Drug withdrawal time must be determined and maintained.

POSSIBLE INTERACTIONS

FOLLOW-UP

PATIENT MONITORING

- Monitoring of serum potassium
- Monitoring of ECG

PREVENTION/AVOIDANCE

- Remove toxic plants from property
- Discard clippings appropriately

POSSIBLE COMPLICATIONS

EXPECTED COURSE AND PROGNOSIS

- Death is likely in severely affected animals.
- Treatment is often not cost effective.

MISCELLANEOUS

ASSOCIATED CONDITIONS

- Ischemia secondary to hypoperfusion
- Respiratory failure

AGE-RELATED FACTORS

N/A

ZOONOTIC POTENTIAL

Cardiac glycosides are toxic to humans.

PREGNANCY

N/A

RUMINANT SPECIES AFFECTED

All species are affected.

BIOSECURITY

Frequently, poisonings are from neighbors/owners feeding hedge clippings.

PRODUCTION MANAGEMENT

N/A

SEE ALSO

Arrhythmia
Diarrhea
Hyperkalemia
Other plant toxicities
Severe diarrhea, any cause

ABBREVIATIONS

AC = activated charcoal
ECG = electrocardiogram
PO = per os, by mouth

Suggested Reading

Dasgupta, A., Datta, P. 2004, Dec. Rapid detection of oleander poisoning using digoxin immunoassays: comparison of five assays. *Ther Drug Monit*. 26(6);658–63.
Downer, J., Craigmill, A., Holstege, D. 2003, Aug. Toxic potential of oleander derived compost and vegetables grown with oleander soil amendments. *Vet Hum Toxicol*. 45(4):219–21.
Galey, F. D. 2002. Cardiac glycosides. In: *Large animal internal medicine*, ed. B. P. Smith. St. Louis: Mosby.

Author: Benjamin R Buchanan

ONCHOCERCIASIS

 BASICS

OVERVIEW
• Filaroid of genus *Onchocerca*, superfamily Filarioidea
• Filamentous, threadlike nematode parasite
• May parasitize horse, cattle, sheep, goats, buffalo, pigs, humans, and others
• Filarial infection is an important cause of skin diseases of horses and cattle throughout the world.
• Three *Onchocerca* spp. associated with cutaneous lesions in cattle
   • *Onchocerca gibsoni* infests cattle in Africa, Asia, and Australia.
   • *Onchocerca gutturosa* infests cattle and horses in North America, Africa, Australia, and Europe.
   • *Onchocerca ochengi* infests African cattle.
• Other *Onchocerca* species in cattle
   • *Onchocerca lienalis* (synonym *O. bovis*) found in North America and worldwide in cattle; relatively nonpathogenic
   • There is debate about the speciation of these organisms that will most likely be decided via PCR testing. Some consider *O. lienalis* and *O. gutturosa* separate species but others consider them to be the same species.
   • *Onchocerca armillata* live in the aorta of cattle, buffalo, and goats of India and Iran.
• Prevalence of infection is very high (20%–100%) in a given population of animals.

PATHOPHYSIOLOGY
Life Cycle
• Indirect life cycle with arthropod intermediate host that serves as vector.
• Transmitted by intermediate hosts (bloodsucking insects, biting fly)
   • Each *Onchocerca* species has a particular intermediate host.
   • Intermediate hosts are primarily species of *Culicoides* (midge), *Simulium* (blackfly), or sandflies.
• Adults worms are tightly coiled and woven into deep connective tissues in "nodules" or "subcutaneous cysts."
   • *O. gibsoni* adult in nodules in fibrous tissue
   • *O. gutturosa* adults in connective tissue around nuchal ligament
   • *O. lienalis* found in gastrosplenic ligament, other ligaments, ligamentum nuchae, stifle, omentum, splenic capsule
   • *O. armillata* in the aorta
• Fertilized females produces vermiform embryos (microfilariae) into subcutaneous tissues and lymph spaces.
   • Microfilariae found in the skin and subcutaneous tissues at the feeding site of their intermediate host
   • Microfilaria of *O. gutturosa*, *O. lienalis*, and *O. ochengi* are found in the dermis.
   • *O. ochengi* hosts an endosymbiotic bacterium (genus *Wolbachia*) that is transovarially passed from female to offspring.

• Intermediate host, midge (*Culicoides* spp), sandfly, or blackfly (*Simulium* spp.), ingests microfilaria from lymph spaces and subcutaneous tissue when it feeds.
   • *Culicoides* spp. gnats are intermediate host for *O. gibsoni*.
   • Numerous *Simulium* spp. and *Culicoides* spp. gnats serve as intermediate hosts for *O. gutturosa*.
   • *Simulium* spp. gnats serve as intermediate hosts for *O. ochengi*, *O. lienalis*.
• Ingested microfilariae develop to the infective larval (juvenile) stage in the vector.
• Transmission takes place when infective larvae that develop in the vector are deposited on the skin of their definitive host at a subsequent feed.
• The larvae develop to adult at site of vector bite or after migrating to predilection site depending on species.
• Adults become surrounded by fibrotic tissue ("nodule") or encapsulated in connective tissue cyst as result of host's response to parasite.
• In bovine, cutaneous onchocerciasis
   • Necrosis, abscess formation, mineralization, and granulomatous to pyogranulomatous inflammation occur around adult worms.
   • Adult worms of some species may also affect muscle.
   • Microfilariae reside in the surrounding connective tissue and lymphatics.

• In some other species, cutaneous onchocerciasis is thought to represent a hypersensitivity reaction to microfilarial antigen(s) but the pathophysiology of the condition is not fully defined in cattle.
  • In humans, cutaneous reaction to *O. volvulus* microfilariae is thought to represent type I and type III hypersensitivity reactions.
  • In horses and humans, microfilarial therapy may provoke an intense inflammatory reaction. Exacerbation of cutaneous signs associated with dead and dying microfilariae (Mazzotti reaction).

SIGNALMENT
• No sex, or breed predilection
• Infestation prevalence tends to increase with age
• Onchocerciasis is seen worldwide but is more common in the tropics and subtropics.
• Putatively immune adult cattle exist in endemically exposed populations.

SIGNS
• Adult worm infestation is often symptomless but response varies with species.
• Several species, most notably *O. gibsoni*, cause subcutaneous nodules or "worm nests."
• *O. gutturosa, O. lienalis* are relatively nonpathogenic.
• *O. gutturosa*
  • Adult worms inhabit the ligamentum nuchae and connective tissue of scapula, stifle, and hip areas.
  • Few clinical signs
  • Firm, subcutaneous nodules or fibrous cyst under the (up to 3 cm diameter) skin over hip, stifle, and shoulder regions
  • Microfilariae are most numerous in the dermis of the face, neck, back, and ventral midline.

• *O. lienalis*
  • Few signs when found in ligamentum nuchae or gastrosplenic ligament
  • Occasional swelling over stifle joint
  • ± Disability if supporting ligaments are affected
• *O. gibsoni*
  • Causes unsightly firm subcutaneous nodules most notably over the brisket but also over hip, lateral stifle area, and lower limbs
  • Nodules are freely moveable.
  • Consist of worms encased in fibrous tissue
  • May cause rejection of beef carcasses
• *O. ochengi*
  • Adults produce asymptomatic, firm subcutaneous and dermal papules and nodules in scrotum and udder primarily, also on flanks, sides, and head.
  • Microfilariae are numerous in dermis of scrotum, udder, and ventral midline; cause mild to severe dermatitis resembling demodectic mange and pox.
• *O. armillata*—induces corrugation and swelling of inner aortic wall
• *Onchocerca* spp.
  • Sheep and goat may be parasitized.
  • Adults cause nodules in connective tissues.
  • Microfilariae migrate into dermis of ventral abdomen and thorax.
  • Host's response to dying larvae results in alopecia, erythema, and thickening of skin in area ± depigmentation.

CAUSES AND RISK FACTORS
• Three *Onchocerca* associated with cutaneous lesions in cattle are
  • *Onchocerca gibsoni* in Africa, Asia, and Australia

  • *Onchocerca gutturosa* in North America, Africa, Australia, and Europe.
  • *Onchocerca ochengi* infests African cattle
• Other *Onchocerca* species that infect cattle are
  • *Onchocerca linealis* (synonym *O. bovis*) found in North America and worldwide; relatively nonpathogenic
  • *Onchocerca armillata* affect cattle, water buffalo, and goats of India and Iran.
• Diseases are most common when seasonal insect populations are highest.
• Although all intermediate hosts are not fully defined, transmission is primarily by arthropod (*Culicoides* spp., *Simulium* spp.) vectors.
• It is not known how long the adults and microfilariae of the various *Onchocerca* spp. survive in the host. In humans, *O. volvulus* adults may live up to 16 years and the microfilariae up to 5 years.

 DIAGNOSIS
• Diagnosis is based upon history, clinical signs, presence of vectors, and skin biopsy.
• Identification of microfilariae from excised piece of skin or skin punch biopsy near nodules
• Skin biopsy—minced preparation to identify microfilariae
  • Punch biopsy (≥ 6 mm)
  • Mince specimen with a razor or scalpel blade
  • Place minced skin sample on a glass slide or in a Petri dish and cover it with room temperature physiologic saline.

ONCHOCERCIASIS

• Allow preparation to incubate at room temperature for 30 minutes.
• Examine specimen under a microscope for the rapid motion of the microfilariae in the saline.
• Do not use saline-containing preservatives (e.g., alcohol); they may kill microfilariae and not allow their migration from the minced skin.
• Technique only confirms the presence of *Onchocerca* spp, microfilariae but alone does not confirm diagnosis of cutaneous onchocerciasis.
• Must differentiate *Onchocerca* spp. microfilaria from those of other species (e.g., *Setaria* spp., *Stephanofilaria* spp., *Pelodera*, *Strongyloides*): *Setaria* are sheathed. *Onchocerca* spp. are nonsheathed; have short sharply pointed tails
• Skin biopsy: histologic section—distinguishing structural traits of adult female *Onchocerca* organisms
  • Thin and very long, threadlike worms
  • Found coiled in dense connective tissue, or some species form distinctive fibrous nodules
  • Cuticle has distinctive external circular ridges and striae in inner layer. Number of striae per ridge helps distinguish various species of *Onchocerca*.
  • Poorly developed muscle cells
  • Prominent hypodermal tissue
  • ± Hoeppli-Splendore material seen on the worm cuticle.
• Species: Size of adult worms and microfilaria
  • *O. gibsoni*: adult up to 20 cm long; microfilariae 240–280 μm long
  • *O. gutturosa*: adult up to 60 cm long; microfilariae 200–230 μm long

• *O. ochengi*: adult up to 25 cm; microfilariae 256–207 μm long
• Skin scrapings and direct smears are unreliable for the demonstration of microfilariae.
• Microfilariae are rarely found in the peripheral blood.

Postmortem Findings (Gross Findings)
• Single or clusters of firm fibrous nodules (0.5–5 cm in diameter)
• Nodules contain tightly coiled worms.
• Parasite tunnels
• Worms may be dead or calcified.
• Affected ligaments (e.g., nuchal, rumenosplenic, etc.) may appear gelatinous and brown with nodules.
• ±Roughening or calcification of aortic walls

Postmortem (or Biopsy) (Histolologic Findings)
• Edema
• Cellular infiltrations predominantly eosinophilic
• Hemorrhage
• Necrosis
• Chronic granulomatous to pyogranulomatous inflammation with macrophages, lymphocytes, plasma cells, giant cells, calcification, and fibrosis around degenerate or dead parasites
• Some have parasites with no tissue reaction.

DIFFERENTIAL DIAGNOSIS
• Skin tuberculosis
• Demodectic manage
• Bacterial and fungal granulomas
• Abscesses
• Parafilariasis, cysticercosis
• Eosinophilic myositis
• Viral nodules
• Neoplasia, neurofibromatosis

CBC/BIOCHEMISTRY/URINALYSIS
N/A

OTHER LABORATORY TESTING
N/A

IMAGING
N/A

DIAGNOSTIC PROCEDURES
• Skin biopsy
• Minced skin preparation to identify microfilariae

 TREATMENT

• Success of treatment of bovine onchocerciasis is doubtful.
• No currently available drug effectively kills adults or all developmental stages of *Onchocerca* spp. in cattle.
• Long-term oxytetracycline is macrofilaricidal in cattle with adult *O. ochengi* infection; possibly due to its action on the endobacteria *Wolbachia*.
• Avermectins/milbemycins have little effect on adults but induce sustained abrogation of embryogenesis. Repeated dosing may enhance the adulticide effect of drugs.
• In humans, ivermectin (Mectizan) is the only drug currently recommended for the treatment and control of onchocerciasis.

- All agents used for treatment of microfilariae/adults in ruminants must be evaluated for
  - Approval in species in which they are to be used
  - Appropriate dosage for species and age group in question
  - Particular side effects noted in species and age group in question.
  - Withdrawal times for lactating animals and for slaughter time
- Diethylcarbamazine citrate 4 mg/kg in feed may be helpful.
- Experimentally, prophylactic treatments with ivermectin or moxidectin prevented adult worm infection following field exposure of naïve calves.
- Ivermectin treatment at times of maximal transmission may help prevent infection and may have some therapeutic value against *O. ochengi* in cattle.
- Combinations of ivermectin with suramin, mebendazole, melfoquine, flubendazole, albendazole, levamisole on adult *O. gutturosa* and *O. volvulus*, in vitro, only showed a marginally increased effect on motility compared to ivermectin alone.

MEDICATIONS

N/A

DRUGS OF CHOICE
N/A

CONTRAINDICATIONS
Appropriate milk and meat withdrawal times must be followed for all compounds administered to food-producing animals.

FOLLOW-UP

PREVENTION/AVOIDANCE
- Control of arthropod intermediate host(s) is difficult to impossible.
- Avoid grazing areas with high insect population.
- Housing of animals during prime activity time of intermediate host
- Insect repellents, dusting bags

MISCELLANEOUS

ASSOCIATED CONDITIONS
Secondary bacterial or mycotic infections

ZOONOTIC POTENTIAL
Onchocerca volvulus causes human onchocerciasis and "river blindness."

RUMINANT SPECIES AFFECTED
Cattle, goats, sheep, buffalo

BIOSECURITY
N/A

PRODUCTION MANAGEMENT
- High morbidity (20%–100%), low mortality in a given group of animals
- Some species cause rejection of meat for human consumption
- Economic losses as a result of hide damage and carcass trimming

SYNONYMS
Skin nodular worm
Worm nodule disease

SEE ALSO
Abscesses
Bacterial and fungal granulomas
Demodectic mange
Eosinophilic myositis
Neoplasia, neurofibromatosis
Parafilariasis, cysticercosis
Skin tuberculosis
Viral nodules

ABBREVIATIONS
N/A

Suggested Reading

Awadzi, K. I. 2003. Clinical picture and outcome of serious adverse events in the treatment of onchocerciasis (review). *Filaria Journal* 2(suppl 1): S6.

Bowman, D. D., Lynn, R. C., Eberhard, M. L. 2003. *Georgis' parasitology for veterinarians*. 8th ed. St. Louis: Saunders (Elsevier Science).

Townsend, S., et al. 1990. The effects of ivermectin used in combination with other known antiparasitic drugs on adult *Onchocerca gutturosa* and *O. volvulus* in vitro. *Trans R Soc Trop Med Hyg*. 84(3): 411–16.

Trees, A. J., et al. 2000. *Onchocerca ochengi* infections in cattle as a model for human onchocerciasis: recent developments. *Parasitology* 120:S133–42.

Tschatoute, V. L., et al. 1999. Chemoprophylaxis of *Onchocerca* infections: in a controlled prospective study ivermectin prevents calves becoming infected with *O. ochengi*. *Parasitology* 118 (pt 2): 195–99.

Authors: Susan Semrad and Karen A. Moriello

ON-FARM PASTEURIZATION OF WASTE MILK

BASICS

OVERVIEW
• The use of waste or hospital milk to feed young stock is a very common practice among dairy farms. Although cost-effective, increased calf morbidity and mortality due to ingestion of pathogenic agents can be seen. Dairy producers are implementing on-farm pasteurization of their waste milk as a disease control procedure before feeding the milk to calves.
• Diarrhea, respiratory problems, pneumonia, arthritis, otitis media, and mastitis are diseases that have being associated with feeding nonpasteurized waste milk to calves.
• Proper pasteurization can reduce most pathogens in milk, providing a safe and nutritious feed.
• Calves fed pasteurized waste milk have higher mean body weight gain, lower mortality rates, and fewer days with diarrhea and pneumonia than calves fed with nonpasteurized waste milk.
• Pasteurization of waste milk decreases illnesses in calves compared with no pasteurization. If handled properly, waste milk is an economical and nutritious source of liquid feed for young dairy calves.
• Shedding of viable *M. paratuberculosis* has been documented in the colostrum and milk of infected dams.

SYSTEMS AFFECTED
Gastrointestinal, respiratory, central nervous system, mammary

GENETICS
N/A

INCIDENCE/PREVALENCE
• The 2002 NAHMS Dairy Survey indicated that 87.2% of dairy farms in the United States fed waste milk to their neonatal calves.

• National Animal Health Monitoring System (NAHMS) suggests between 20% and 40% of dairy herds in the United States have some level of Johne's disease.
• In one study, pasteurization of colostrum was found effective in the destruction of *M. paratuberculosis* but resulted in an average 25% reduction in colostral immunoglobulin.
• Discarded milk losses range from 48 to 136 pounds of milk per cow per year.

GEOGRAPHIC DISTRIBUTION
Worldwide depending on species and environment

SIGNALMENT

Species
Lactating bovine, ovine, and caprine species

Breed Predilections
Dairy breeds

Mean Age and Range
Calves, lambs, and kids

Predominant Sex
N/A

TREATMENT

• Two types of on-farm pasteurization are commonly utilized: (1) batch, where milk is heated to 63°C/145°F for 30 minutes and (2) HTST (high-temperature short-time) or flash pasteurization, where temperature reaches 72°C/162°F for 15 seconds.
• Waste milk has a much higher bacteria count than regular milk and therefore requires more than a 90% reduction in bacterial load.
• Farms that have problems with *Mycoplasma* spp. are especially problematic. *Mycoplasma canadense* is more heat resistant than other bacteria; it requires 5 min at 67.5°C or 2 min at 70°C to be eliminated.
• *M. paratuberculosis* may not be controlled by pasteurization and therefore on-farm pasteurization should not be considered as a way to control Johne's disease.

• There is no effect of pasteurization on antibiotics present in milk.
• Flash pasteurization of milk at 162°F (72°C) for 15 seconds kills most *Mycoplasma* spp. To effectively destroy *Mycoplasma* spp. in waste milk, a continuous-flow pasteurizer is necessary and must be monitored closely.
• Bacterial organisms in milk may bind together and not be effectively pasteurized with a batch-type pasteurization system.
• The need to handle large quantities of waste milk requires dairy operators to have the proper equipment. A small, used, bulk tank can store the daily production of waste milk.

CLIENT EDUCATION
• On-farm pasteurization has to be closely monitored to be efficient. Management and workers involved in the process must receive specific training in maintaining and operating the equipment, recording the data, cleaning the equipment, and general hygiene procedures.
• Maintain standard operating procedures (SOPs) for all the steps in the operation.
• Although it is recommended that waste milk be pasteurized, pasteurization of colostrum is not recommended. The elevated temperatures associated with pasteurization can destroy immunoglobulins.

PRECAUTIONS
• Refrigerate waste milk until pasteurization. Storage at room temperature will increase the microbial load and lower quality.
• Use milk immediately after pasteurization, but assure that the temperature is adequate to feed calves (around 38°C, 100.4°F).
• Do not pasteurize any milk that is acidic, bloody, or abnormal.
• Heat treatment can decrease the level of immunoglobulin (IgG).

ON-FARM PASTEURIZATION OF WASTE MILK

• If high-quality colostrum (>60 mg/ml) is pasteurized, there is a higher chance the postpasteurized product will exceed 50 mg/ml.
• Several bacterial organisms, including *E. coli*, bovine viral diarrhea (BVD), *Salmonella* spp., *Streptococcus* spp., and *Staphylococcus* spp., have been identified in waste milk.
• Pasteurization destroys bovine leukemia virus (BLV), so the pasteurized milk from BLV-positive cows can be fed to calves when BLV-free milk is not available.
• Pasteurization is not sterilization. A heavy bacterial load in waste milk will not be completely eliminated by pasteurization.
• Pasteurization does not remove antibiotics from waste milk.

 FOLLOW-UP

• Randomly check records, time, and temperature during pasteurization procedure.
• Regularly culture samples of pasteurized milk for pathogen load.

POSSIBLE COMPLICATIONS

• Complications originate from a failure in training and cleaning or equipment maintenance.
• If colostrum is pasteurized, the fluid characteristic of the liquid may become altered. This can cause problems in calf feeding and subsequent equipment cleaning.
• Do not feed waste milk to newborn calves on the first day of life. Bacteria can potentially penetrate the intestinal wall and cause illness.

 MISCELLANEOUS

ASSOCIATED CONDITIONS

Diarrhea, respiratory problems, pneumonia, arthritis, otitis media, and mastitis are diseases that have been associated with feeding nonpasteurized waste milk to calves.

AGE-RELATED FACTORS

• Calves fed pasteurized waste milk have higher mean body weight gain, lower mortality rates, and fewer days with diarrhea and pneumonia than calves fed with nonpasteurized waste milk.
• House calves and feed waste milk individually to prevent them from suckling one another. This should reduce possible transmission of infectious microorganisms that cause mastitis.

ZOONOTIC POTENTIAL

Brucellosis, Q-fever, and tuberculosis are zoonotic diseases that can be transmitted in waste milk if it is not pasteurized properly.

PREGNANCY

N/A

RUMINANT SPECIES AFFECTED

Lactating bovine, ovine, and caprine species

BIOSECURITY

• Maintain standard operating procedures (SOPs) for all the steps in the operation.
• HACCP (hazard analysis critical control points) and quality control programs can help manage the process and assure standardization.
• Do not feed waste milk from antibiotic-treated cows to calves intended for meat production. Antibiotic residues from the milk could be deposited in the tissues of the calves.

PRODUCTION MANAGEMENT

• On-farm pasteurization is indicated for calf ranches that receive waste milk from different sources.
• Before using as a calf feed, pasteurize waste milk to reduce microbial load.
• Do not feed waste milk to newborn calves.
• Use caution when feeding waste milk that may contain antibiotics to calves that are potentially to be used for beef production.
• House heifer calves individually (i.e., hutches) when feeding waste milk.
• Know the health status of the cows from which waste milk is obtained. Unless milk is pasteurized, do not feed milk from cows with BVD or Johne's, or from cows infected with *E. coli*, *Mannheimia*, or BLV.
• Refrigerate milk at all times until use.
• Discard waste milk that is excessively bloody, watery, or unusual in appearance.

SYNONYMS

N/A

SEE ALSO

Dairy heifer management
Heifer nutrition
Milk quality
Milk replacers

ABBREVIATIONS

BLV = bovine leukemia virus
BVDV = bovine viral diarrhea virus
CFU = colony forming unit
HACCP = hazard analysis critical control points
HTST = high-temperature short-time
IgG = immunoglobulin G
NAHMS = National Animal Health Monitoring System
SOP = standard operating procedure

Suggested Reading

Butler, J. A., Sickles, S. A., Johanns, C. J., Rosenbusch, R. F. 2000. Pasteurization of discard mycoplasma milk used to feed calves: thermal effects on various mycoplasmas. *J Dairy Sci.* 83:2285–88.

Godden, S. M., Smith, S., Feirtag, J. M., Green, L. R., Wells, S. J., Fetrow, J. P. 2003. Effect of on-farm commercial batch pasteurization of colostrum on colostrum and serum immunoglobulin concentration in dairy calves. *J Dairy Sci.* 86:1503–12.

Jamaluddin, A. A., Carpenter, T. E., Hird, D.W., Thurmond, M. C. 1996. Economics of feeding pasteurized colostrum and pasteurized waste milk to dairy calves. *J Am Vet Med Assoc.* 209:751–56.

Stabel, J. R. 2001, Feb. On-farm batch pasteurization destroys *Mycobacterium paratuberculosis* in waste milk. *J Dairy Sci.* 84(2):524–27.

Stabel, J. R., Hurd, S., Calvente, L., Rosenbusch, R. F. 2004, Jul. Destruction of *Mycobacterium paratuberculosis*, *Salmonella* spp., and *Mycoplasma* spp. in raw milk by a commercial on-farm high-temperature, short-time pasteurizer. *J Dairy Sci.* 87(7):2177–83.

Authors: Juliana M. Ruzante and James S. Cullor

ORCHITIS AND EPIDIDYMITIS

 BASICS

OVERVIEW
• Inflammation of the testicle and epididymis may occur separately but often occur concurrently and frequently have the same etiology. The inflammation may be the result of infection or trauma.
• Hematogenous spread from systemic infections is the most common route of infection. Retrograde extension from other parts of the urinary tract or secondary sex organs, particularly the epididymis, is also an important route of infection.
• Periorchitis of the tunica vaginalis testis within scrotum may be directly related to orchitis or an extension of severe peritonitis.

SIGNALMENT
• These conditions can occur in males of any breed and age but are most commonly seen in adults. The exceptions to this are several ram lamb diseases indicated below.
• Orchitis/epididymitis usually occurs unilaterally but both testicles/epididymi may be involved simultaneously.

SIGNS
• Warm, painful swelling of the entire testicle or one or more segments of the epididymis is the most common sign of acute disease.
• Epididymitis most frequently involves the tail segment.
• Some cases of *Brucella ovis* epididymitis in rams are subclinical and cannot be detected by palpation alone.
• Painful animals may refuse to mate or may be reluctant to move. Frequently they walk with a stilted gate.
• Chronic disease of these organs may not be accompanied by either heat or pain. Swelling of the head, body, or tail of the epididymis may be the only clinical sign of chronic epididymitis.
• Transient testicular degeneration usually occurs subsequent to inflammation of either the testicle or epididymitis. Severe inflammation of one or both testicles may lead to permanent testicular atrophy.

• Blood and/or pus in the semen may be seen in the ejaculate. In some cases, abscessation and liquefaction of the testicular parenchyma may occur with subsequent eruption and drainage through the scrotum. This is especially evident with cases of brucellosis in bulls and caseous lymphadenitis in goats.

CAUSES AND RISK FACTORS
Infectious
• *Brucella abortus* (bulls)—endemic areas
• *Brucella abortus* vaccine (bulls)
• *Brucella melitensis* (bucks) rare
• *Brucella ovis* epididymitis (mature rams)
• Epi-Vag virus (bulls) Africa
• Caseous lymphadenitis (CLA) (*Corynebacterium pseudotuberculosis*) (bucks, rams)
• Tuberculosis (*Mycobacterium tuberculosis*) (bulls) rare

Microbial
• *Actinomyces pyogenes* (*Corynebacterium*) (bulls and rams)
• *Actinomyces bovis* (bulls)
• *E. coli*
• *Hemophilus* spp. (bulls, young rams)
• *Salmonella*
• *Chlamydia psittaci*
• *Corynebacterium ovis* (young rams)
• *Actinobacillus seminis* (bulls, bucks, young rams)
• *Actinobacillus* spp. (young rams)
• *Histophilus ovis* (young rams)
• *Nocardia farcinica*
• *Pseudomonas* (bucks)
• *Salmonella abortus ovis* in Germany
• *Streptococcus* spp.
• *Staphylococcus* spp.
• *Yersinia* (*Pasteurella*) *pseudotuberculosis* in the United Kingdom

Nonspecific Bacteria
• *Mycoplasma* spp. (ram)
• Herpesvirus III (IBR-IPV) (bulls)

Parasitic
• Trypanosomiasis (bucks) Africa
• Besnoitosis (bucks) Africa

Traumatic
• Kick
• Butting
• Fighting

• Stepped on
• Barbed wire entanglement
• Penetrating wounds

Risk Factirs for Trauma
• Overcrowding of males
• Mixing young males with older males
• Introducing new males into the herd with an established dominance order
• Poor pasture/range management

Sadistic Behavior
• Shotgun pellets
• "BB" shot

 DIAGNOSIS

DIFFERENTIAL DIAGNOSIS
• Inguinal hernia
• Hydrocele
• Hematocele
• Spermatocele
• Varicocele
• Metastatic mesothelioma

CBC/BIOCHEMISTRY/URINALYSIS
Blood, pus, or increased WBCs in urine

OTHER LABORATORY TESTS
Blood, pus, or large numbers of WBCs in ejaculate

IMAGING
• Radiographs may reveal radiodense foreign bodies (BBs, buckshot, etc.)
• Ultrasonography may help differentiate hernia, hydrocele, varicocele, etc.
• Thermography may localize inflammation.

DIAGNOSTIC PROCEDURES
• Scrotal palpation
• Semen evaluation
• Semen culture
• Aseptic aspiration of peritesticular fluid for culture/cytology
• Testicular aspiration for culture—last resort, may lead to adhesions or abscessation and atrophy
• *Brucellosis ovis* serological test—complement fixation test

PATHOLOGIC FINDINGS

• Transient testicular degeneration
• Permanent testicular degeneration (atrophy)
• Occluded seminiferous tubules, rete testes, vas deferens, or epididymi

TREATMENT

• Unilateral castration if acute and the disease is limited to one testes
• Systemic antibiotic therapy for 7–14 days after the acute inflammatory stage subsides. Culture and sensitivity of the organism is indicated.
• Cool water hydrotherapy 30 minutes twice daily for 7–10 days
• Sexual rest

MEDICATIONS

DRUGS OF CHOICE

• Antibiotic selection based on culture and sensitivity results
• Systemic doses of procaine penicillin G or oxytetracycline
• Oxytetracycline 10 mg/kg plus dihydrostreptomycin 25 mg/kg twice daily for 7 days stopped shedding of *Brucella ovis* but is not recommended except for valuable rams that won't enter the food chain.

CONTRAINDICATIONS

Appropriate milk and meat withdrawal times must be followed for all compounds administered to food-producing animals.

FOLLOW-UP

PATIENT MONITORING

• Reevaluate scrotum and testes for adhesions or atrophy 1 month after the end of therapy.

• Reevaluate semen quality a minimum of 60 days after the end of the insult to the testicle(s) or removal of the affected testicle.

PREVENTION/AVOIDANCE

• *Brucella ovis* vaccination (rams)
• *Corynebacterium pseudotuberculosis* vaccination (caseous lymphadenitis)

POSSIBLE COMPLICATIONS

Reduced fertility and or sterility

EXPECTED COURSE AND PROGNOSIS

• Poor fertility prognosis for affected testicle/epididymis
• Guarded prognosis for normal fertility in adjacent testicle in cases of severe inflammation

MISCELLANEOUS

ASSOCIATED CONDITIONS

N/A

AGE RELATED FACTORS

N/A

ZOONOTIC POTENTIAL

Brucellosis abortus dangerous to people

PREGNANCY

N/A

RUMINANT SPECIES AFFECTED

Potentially all ruminant species

BIOSECURITY

• Report and cull *Brucellosis* spp. affected bulls—test herd.
• Cull epididymitis affected rams

PRODUCTION MANAGEMENT

N/A

SEE ALSO

Breeding soundness examination by species
Brucella abortus
Hematocele
Hydrocele
Inguinal hernia
Metastatic mesothelioma

Specific infectious diseases
Spermatocele
Varicocele

ABBREVIATIONS

CLA = caseous lymphadenitis
IBR-IPV = bovine rhinotracheitis/infectious pustular vulvovaginitis
WBCs = white blood cells

Suggested Reading
Ball, L., Young, S., Carroll, E. J. 1968, Jun. Seminal vesiculitis syndrome: lesions in genital organs of young bulls. *Am J Vet Res.* 29(6): 1173–84.
Johnson, W. H. 1997, Jul. The significance to bull fertility of morphologically abnormal sperm. *Vet Clin North Am Food Anim Pract.* 13(2): 255–70.
Memon, M. A. 1983, Nov. Male infertility. *Vet Clin North Am Large Anim Pract.* 5(3): 619–35.
Steffen, D. 1997, Jul. Genetic causes of bull infertility. *Vet Clin North Am Food Anim Pract.* 13(2): 243–53.
Van Camp, S. D. 1997, Jul. Common causes of infertility in the bull. *Vet Clin North Am Food Anim Pract.* 13(2): 203–31.

Author: Steven D. Van Camp

ORF/CONTAGIOUS ECTHYMA

 BASICS

OVERVIEW

• Orf, often referred to as contagious ecthyma, cutaneous pustular dermatitis, sore mouth, or scabby mouth, is a communicable disease characterized by the development of ulcero-pustulo-proliferative lesions in the skin of sheep, goats, wild ruminants, and humans.

• Orf is caused by orf virus (ORFV), the prototype species of the *Parapoxvirus* genus in the subfamily Chordopoxvirinae of the Poxviridae family.

• The precise geographic distribution of orf is not known, but it is thought to be present in most parts of the world where sheep and goats are raised.

• ORFV can be transmitted by close contact between infected and susceptible animals. Indirect transmission through contact with contaminated objects has been suspected, but it is difficult to demonstrate.

• ORFV does not cause latent infections in animals that recover from clinical disease, but clinically healthy animals that are moved from infected to noninfected premises or transported in contaminated vehicles can act as mechanical carriers.

• Before the eradication of screwworm flies (*Cochliomyia hominivorax*) from North America, orf was a major problem for the livestock industry. The fly larvae invade skin lesions, leading to secondary infections and high mortality among sheep and goats.

• Since the eradication of the screwworm fly from this region, mortality due to orf has decreased significantly. Still, outbreaks of orf continue to occur on a yearly basis. Although rarely fatal, orf is considered an economically important disease, particularly on premises where sanitary conditions are poor.

• Orf can lead to growth retardation, loss of body condition in young lambs and kids, and predisposition to secondary infections. The disease can also result in economic losses as a result of international trade barriers imposed on animal shipments.

SIGNALMENT

• Sheep, goats, and humans are the species most commonly affected by orf. The infection also has been reported in musk ox, takin, mule deer, camels, bighorn sheep, mountain goat, and the dog.

• With the exception of musk ox and takin, reports of orf in wild ruminants and other species have been limited to descriptions of the clinical and pathologic findings and to the identification of the virus by electron microscopy (EM). Therefore, the possibility of the etiological agent being a closely related parapoxvirus cannot be ruled out in those cases.

• Clinical orf is more common among lambs or goat kids after weaning. Animals that have recovered from orf, or that have been vaccinated, are potentially susceptible to reinfection. In reinfected animals, lesions usually are of less severity and the clinical course is shorter.

• Adult animals less often present clinically with orf with exception of does and ewes that may develop orf lesions in the teats while nursing affected kids/lambs.

SIGNS

• Orf is recognized by the appearance of macules in the skin that rapidly progress to form papules, vesicles, and pustules.

• Within a few days, the pustules rupture leaving an ulcerated area where a thick overlying crust is deposited giving rise to rapidly growing scabs. Papillomatous growths, resulting from continued epidermal proliferation, do occur.

• The lesions usually start at the commissures of the lips and spread around the lip margins to the muzzle. In more severe cases, the skin of other areas, such as the eyes, feet, vulva, or udder, may be affected.

• Occasionally, lesions may develop in the gingiva, dental pad, palate, tongue, and in the skin of the interdigital space. These lesions are painful, and affected animals may be reluctant to suckle, eat, or walk depending on the location of the lesions.

• In the majority of cases, the lesions are self-contained and heal spontaneously within 3 to 4 weeks after they first appear.

• A generalized, persistent form of orf, characterized by severe, multifocal, proliferative dermatitis, occurs in sheep and goats. Some individuals of the Boer goat breed seem to be more susceptible to this form of the disease. In these cases, secondary bacterial infections or maggot infestation of affected areas may occur.

• Morbidity often reaches 60 to 80% in susceptible animals. Occasionally, mortalities as high as 10% have been reported.

 DIAGNOSIS

DIFFERENTIAL DIAGNOSIS

Orf lesions may be confused with other ulcerative, vesicular or proliferative dermatitis, such as the ones caused by capri or sheep poxviruses, bluetongue virus, foot-and-mouth disease, or pearmouth, the latter a dermatitis of lips and muzzle caused by ingestion of prickly pear cactus.

DIAGNOSTIC PROCEDURES

• In the majority of cases, the diagnosis of orf is made by observation of clinical signs and lesions.

• The most common laboratory confirmatory test is the identification of parapoxvirus virons by negative staining EM in scab material. Several pieces of scab from various animals that are in the early phases of the infection should be submitted for diagnosis. Dry, late-stage scabs tend to contain smaller numbers of virus particles and larger numbers of bacteria reducing the possibilities of getting an accurate diagnosis.

• Gloves should be worn during the clinical exam and collection of samples from affected animals. Samples for diagnosis can be submitted at room temperature or refrigerated in a double-container to prevent infection of people handling the samples.

• The EM technique relies on the identification of typical ovoid-shaped parapoxvirus virons. A limitation of this technique is that all parapoxviruses, including bovine papular stomatitis virus (BPSV) and pseudocowpox virus (PCPV), are morphologically identical; and therefore, indistinguishable by EM.

• PCR has been used successfully to corroborate the clinical diagnosis. Most likely, this method will replace EM as the method of choice for confirmation of orf.

• Virus isolation is often unsuccessful. However, it can be attempted using a variety of primary cell cultures, including ovine and bovine kidney cells, ovine and bovine testis cells, and others. Typical cytopathic effect consists of cell rounding, clumping, and detachment. Intracytoplasmic eosinophilic inclusion bodies can be observed in stained cell culture.

• Serological tests such as serum neutralization, agar gel immunodiffusion (AGID) test, complement fixation, or agglutination, for the detection of anti-ORFV antibodies, are occasionally used, but have limited diagnostic value.

PATHOLOGIC FINDINGS

Gross Findings

• The predominant macroscopic lesions consist of ulcers, crusting, and papillomatous growths in the skin of lips and muzzle. These lesions range in size from a few millimeters to several centimeters. Macules, papules, vesicles, and pustules also can be observed, but in the majority of cases, these changes are transitory and rapidly progress to crusting lesions.

• Lymph nodes draining the affected areas of the skin are often enlarged.

• Secondary bacterial pneumonia and suppurative arthritis are common in animals with disseminated persistent orf.

Microscopic Findings

- Histologically, orf lesions in the skin are characterized by papillated, hyperplastic dermatitis with a mixture of epidermal and dermal proliferation.
- Hyperkeratosis, parakeratosis, and elongation of the rete pegs are evident, the latter particularly at the borders of the epidermis between areas of papillomatous proliferation and normal skin.
- Clusters of epidermal cells with vacuolated cytoplasm or cells with eosinophilic intracytoplasmic viral inclusions may be found in the stratum spongiosum. Subcorneal vesicles and pustules may be present throughout the epidermis. Ulcers covered by serocellular crust containing bacterial colonies or vegetable debris may be observed in the epidermis.
- The dermal component consists of proliferating connective tissue with various degrees of lymphocyte and plasma cell infiltration. Infiltration by neutrophils is more common in ulcerated areas. Capillary proliferation and edema of the dermis are also common.

TREATMENT

- There are no specific treatments for ORFV.
- Affected animals should be placed in shaded pens protected from the environment and provided with clean water and good quality hay or feed.
- Wide-spectrum antibiotics and topical insecticide should be used in animals with secondary bacterial infections or maggot infestations, respectively.
- Meat and milk withdrawal periods must be maintained for drug use.

MEDICATIONS

N/A

CONTRAINDICATIONS

Appropriate milk and meat withdrawal times must be followed for all compounds administered to food-producing animals.

FOLLOW-UP

PATIENT MONITORING

N/A

PREVENTION AND CONTROL

- The use of live ORFV vaccines, prepared by sheep skin passage or in cell culture, is a common practice.
- The vaccine should not be used in locations where the disease has never been diagnosed, but when used for the first time, all susceptible animals in the premises should be vaccinated.
- On premises where orf is endemic, all lambs and goat kids should be vaccinated at 6 to 8 weeks of age.
- In subsequent years, only the new lamb/kid crop and newly acquired animals should be vaccinated.
- Vaccines contain nonattenuated live virus and can induce disease in orf-naïve animals that share pens with vaccinated animals. Vaccine orf virus also can cause disease in humans and should be used with caution.
- First, scarify an area of the skin of animals at risk, most commonly in the medial aspect of the thigh, and then rub the vaccine in to apply the vaccine. The appearance of a localized lesion 2 to 3 days later indicates a successful vaccination.
- Although vaccinated animals or those that recover from natural infection are susceptible to reinfection, subsequent orf infections tend to be milder and of shorter duration. In practice, most vaccinated animals remain protected for several years after a primary infection.

MISCELLANEOUS

ASSOCIATED CONDITIONS

N/A

AGE-RELATED FACTORS

Most cases of orf occur in lambs and kid goats after weaning.

ZOONOTIC POTENTIAL

- In humans, orf is considered primarily an occupational hazard. The disease is common among farmers, sheep shearers, veterinarians, and producers that handle small ruminants. Slaughterhouse workers, butchers, and meat handlers are sometimes infected from carcasses.
- Orf in humans is manifested by the appearance of one or several localized pustules and scabby lesions on the hands and sometimes face or ears. The lesions progress to form large painful nodules that eventually regress and disappear in 4 to 6 weeks.
- Multifocal, widespread skin lesions in humans have been reported in immunocompromised people.
- Erythema multiforme may be a sequella in human orf.

PREGNANCY

- In ruminants, there are no indications that ORFV affects the fetus.
- In two cases of orf in pregnant women, the deliveries were uncomplicated, and the patients gave birth at term to normal babies.

SYNONYMS

Contagious ecthyma
Cutaneous pustular dermatitis
Scabby mouth
Sore mouth

SEE ALSO

Bluetongue virus
Capri or sheep poxviruses
Dermatologic chapters
Foot-and-mouth disease
Photosensitivity
Vaccinology

ABBREVIATIONS

AGID = agar gel immunodiffusion
EM = electron microscopy
ORFV = orf virus
PCR = polymerase chain reaction

Suggested Reading
de la Concha-Bermejillo, A. 1995. Poxviral diseases. In: *Health hazards in veterinary medicine*, ed. R. Farris, J. Mahlow, E. Newman, B. Nix. 3d ed., pp. 55–56. Schaumburg, IL: American Veterinary Medical Association.
de la Concha-Bermejillo, A., Guo, J., Zhang, Z., Waldron, D. 2003. Severe persistent orf in young goats. *J Vet Dig Invest*. 15:423–31.
Guo, J., Rasmussen, J., Wünschmann, A., de la Concha-Bermejillo, A. 2004. Genetic characterization of orf viruses isolated from various ruminant species of a zoo. *Vet Microbiol*. 99(2):81–92.
Guo, J., Zhang, Z., Edwards, J. F., Ermel, R. W., Taylor, Jr., C., de la Concha-Bermejillo A. 2003. Characterization of a North American orf virus isolated from a goat with persistent, proliferative dermatitis. *Virus Res*. 93:169–79.
Inoshima, Y., Morooka, A., Sentsui, H. 2000. Detection and diagnosis of parapoxvirus by the polymerase chain reaction. *J Virol Meth*. 84:201–8.

Author: Andrés de la Concha-Bermejillo

OSTEOCHONDROSIS

 BASICS

DEFINITION
• Osteochondrosis (OCD) is a disease that results from defective endochondral ossification. This defect may cause dissection cartilage flaps (osteochondrosis dessicans), subchondral bone cysts, or physitis.
• "Dyschondroplasia" and "chondrodysplasia" are other terms used for osteochondrosis.
• These conditions often progress to degenerative joint disease and chronic arthritis.

PATHOPHYSIOLOGY
• In osteochondrosis, cartilage cells fail to differentiate normally and calcification fails to occur; however, the cartilage cells continue to grow resulting in a zone of hypertrophied cartilage cells.
• Synovial fluid provides nutrition to the immature joint cartilage. A thicker zone of cartilage results in decreased nutrition to the basal layer of the cartilage cells. This results in degeneration and necrosis of the cartilage cells. The necrotic area can form the basis of a fissure that can lead to dissecting flaps, which present as osteochondrosis dessicans.
• Direct trauma has also been cited as a source of necrosis and eventual fragmentation.
• Subchondral bone cysts may result from thickened cartilage that infolds into subchondral bone of weight-bearing surfaces. Other studies suggest that subchondral bone cysts may develop from defective connective tissue or cartilage rather than endochondral ossification. This theory suggests that the cartilage cracks following mechanical trauma creates an opening and synovial fluid pumps through the defect into subchondral bone during weight bearing.
• Physitis is associated with thickening and weakening of the growth plate cartilage.

SYSTEMS AFFECTED
Musculoskeletal

GENETICS
May reflect the effects of genetic selection for rapid growth

INCIDENCE/PREVALENCE
N/A

GEOGRAPHIC DISTRIBUTION
Worldwide, depending on species and environment

SIGNALMENT

Species
Potentially all ruminant species

Breed Predilections
• There is no specific breed predilection in cattle, pigs, and goats.
• Hereditary dyschondroplasia, known as "spider lamb syndrome" in Suffolk and Suffolk crossbred lambs, has been recognized.

Mean Age and Range
Osteochondrosis has been reported in animals as young as 5 to 7 months, but overt clinical signs usually are observed in cattle between 12 and 24 months of age.

Predominant Sex
Osteochondrosis is more common in males than females. Among males, the disease is more common in bulls than steers.

SIGNS

HISTORICAL FINDINGS
• The primary clinical sign in cattle with osteochondrosis is lameness and joint effusion. Joint effusion is believed to be associated with joint capsule proliferation and synovial fluid production due to inflammation.
• The most commonly affected joints are the stifle, tarsus, carpus, and shoulder and multiple joint involvement is common and expected.
• Affected cattle are usually reluctant to move and typically walk with a short strided gait that entails minimal flexion of the stifle and hock. Animals often have a postlegged conformation with abnormally straight stifle and tarsus joints.
• Localization of lameness to a specific limb may be difficult.

CAUSES AND RISK FACTORS
The exact cause of osteochondrosis is unknown, but predisposing factors have been implicated.

Risk Factors
• The most important risk factor for OCD appears to be rapid weight gain during a young animal's period of cartilage maturation (prior to 2 years of age). More cases are reported in males than females, and among males the disease is more common in bulls than steers.
• High-energy and protein diets producing rapid growth have been implicated.
• The disease is more common among registered or valuable animals; however, this apparent predisposition probably reflects superimposed effects of genetic selection for rapid growth, diets composed to support maximum growth, and the increased likelihood of more definitive diagnostics in valuable animals.
• Among commercial beef and dairy replacements, the condition is rare because these animals are fed to support relatively slow growth.
• Although lesions are common in feedlot cattle, these animals rarely show clinical disease because they attain market weight before clinical signs become severe.
• This condition appears most common among registered beef bulls and male and female show cattle of both beef and, to a lesser extent, dairy breeds because these animals are fed diets supporting maximum growth for extended periods of time.
• Mineral imbalances including calcium, phosphorus, copper, and zinc are believed to

contribute to the development of osteochondrosis.
• Cattle raised on concrete floors with limited exercise are thought to be more predisposed to the development of osteochondrosis. These surfaces are thought to increase loading of the joints leading to mechanical trauma to the articular surface, increasing incidence of osteochondrosis.

 DIAGNOSIS

DIFFERENTIAL DIAGNOSIS
• Differential diagnoses include those diseases and conditions causing either polyarthritis or multiple limb lameness. Consequently, diseases such as mycoplasmosis, *Hemophilus somnus* infections, and bacterial endocarditis should be considered as differentials. Mycoplasmosis and *Hemophilus* infection are usually associated with respiratory signs. Mycoplasmosis can occur in neonates and may also be associated with otitis and feeding of dump milk. *Hemophilus* can also result in brain stem and cortical signs. Joint fluid analysis with both mycoplasmosis and *Hemophilus somnus* infections are associated with marked increase in white cell count and protein. PCR on joint fluid can be used to identify *Mycoplasma*. Signs of right-sided heart failure (distended jugular veins, increased jugular pulses, tachycardia, and submandibular edema) and presence of a systolic murmur are characteristic in endocarditis.
• Septic physitis, a common sequela to salmonellosis, may appear as a lameness involving multiple limbs and multiple swollen joints; however, joint distention is usually absent in this condition and close physical examination will generally reveal that swelling is localized to the physis, rather than joints.
• Both acute and chronic laminitis should be considered as likely differentials. The signalment, dietary composition, and management factors predisposing the two conditions are very similar and the two conditions often are present concurrently. Cattle with chronic laminitis will have altered hoof growth. Both acute and chronic laminitis will be confirmed by close examination and trimming of the hooves. Joint distention will be absent in cattle with laminitis.

CBC/BIOCHEMISTRY/URINALYSIS
N/A

OTHER LABORATORY TESTS
Joint fluid analysis reveals a nonseptic inflammation with mild to moderate increase in leukocyte count and protein.

IMAGING

Radiology
• Definitive diagnosis of osteochondrosis is confirmed by radiographic findings.

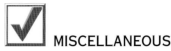

• Lesions are either the appearance of subchondral bone irregularity with bone fragmentation referred to as osteochondrosis dessicans or subchondral bone cysts characterized by periarticular focal areas of subchondral bone lucency.
• The stifle joint is the most commonly affected joint followed by the tarsal joint.
• Other joints reported as sites for osteochondrosis include the shoulder joint, distal radius, and phalanges.
• Osteochondrosis is radiographically apparent bilateral. Consequently, bilateral radiographs should be considered although clinical signs of bilateral disease might not occur.
• Radiographs of the shoulder and stifle are difficult (if not impossible) in most awake standing cattle.
• Osteochondrosis can lead to degenerative joint disease.

Arthroscopy
• Arthroscopy can be an effective technique for the diagnosis and treatment of osteochondrosis in cattle.
• Equipment costs and subsequent surgery may be prohibitive for most individuals.
• Arthroscopic techniques are also useful in the evaluation and treatment of osteochondrosis in sheep, goats, and camelids.

OTHER DIAGNOSTIC PROCEDURES
N/A

TREATMENT
• Conservative therapy includes stall rest for 1 to 3 months.
• Deep bedding and dirt-floored or pasture housing are recommended.
• Rations should be balanced with respect to mineral micronutrients. Energy content of the diet should be dramatically decreased and the patient's rate of gain limited.
• Nonsteroidal anti-inflammatory drugs may be considered for short-term palliative therapy.
• Surgical treatment involving removal of the osteochondral fragment and debridement of the fragment bed or debridement of the cyst in cases of subchondral bone cyst may be considered in valuable animals; however, no controlled clinical trials have examined the efficacy of these procedures in cattle.
• In feedlots, therapy should not be attempted and affected cattle should be marketed immediately.

ACTIVITY
Decrease activity

DIET
Rations should be balanced with respect to mineral micronutrients. Energy content of the diet should be dramatically decreased and the patient's rate of gain limited.

CLIENT EDUCATION
• Conservative therapy includes stall rest for 1 to 3 months. Deep bedding and dirt-floored or pasture housing are recommended. Rations should be balanced with respect to mineral micronutrients. Energy content of the diet should be dramatically decreased and the patient's rate of gain limited.
• Breeding stock with clinical disease will likely have a shortened productive lifespan due to the anticipated development of degenerative joint disease and culling should be considered.

MEDICATIONS
CONTRAINDICATIONS
Appropriate milk and meat withdrawal times must be followed for all compounds administered to food-producing animals.

PRECAUTIONS
N/A

POSSIBLE INTERACTIONS
N/A

ALTERNATIVE DRUGS
N/A

FOLLOW-UP
Monitor animal for appetite and pain response.

PATIENT MONITORING
N/A

PREVENTION/AVOIDANCE
• The diet and housing of herd mates in the same group as the affected animal should be examined.
• Rations should be balanced with respect to mineral micronutrients. Energy content of the diet should be decreased to the level needed to support economically relevant rates of gain.
• In feedlot animals, the energy density of the diet is not decreased.

POSSIBLE COMPLICATIONS
N/A

EXPECTED COURSE AND PROGNOSIS
• Most cases with signs of lameness and secondary degenerative joint disease have poor prognosis.
• Refractory lameness has been associated with medical management.
• Breeding stock with clinical disease will likely have a shortened productive lifespan due to the anticipated development of degenerative joint disease; culling should be considered.

MISCELLANEOUS
ASSOCIATED CONDITIONS
N/A

AGE-RELATED FACTORS
Osteochondrosis has been reported in animals as young as 5 to 7 months, but overt clinical signs usually are observed in cattle between 12 and 24 months of age.

ZOONOTIC POTENTIAL
N/A

PREGNANCY
N/A

RUMINANT SPECIES AFFECTED
Potentially, all ruminant species are affected.

BIOSECURITY
N/A

PRODUCTION MANAGEMENT
See Common Hoof Lameness of Cattle and Polyarthritis above.

SYNONYMS
Chondrodysplasia
Dyschondroplasia
Spider lamb syndrome

SEE ALSO
Acute and chronic laminitis
Analgesia
Bacterial endocarditis
Hemophilus somnus
Mycoplasmosis
Salmonellosis
Septic physitis

ABBREVIATIONS
OCD = osteochondrosis
PCR = polymerase chain reaction

Suggested Reading
Davies, I. H., Munro, R. 1999, Aug 21. Osteochondrosis in bull beef cattle following lack of dietary mineral and vitamin supplementation. *Vet Rec.* 145(8): 232–33.
Gaughan, E. M. 1996, Mar. Arthroscopy in food animal practice. *Vet Clin North Am Food Anim Pract.* 12(1): 233–47.
Hill, B. D., Sutton, R. H., Thompson, H. 1998, Mar. Investigation of osteochondrosis in grazing beef cattle. *Aust Vet J.* 76(3): 171–75.
Trostle, S. S., Nicoll, R. G., Forrest, L. J., et al. 1998. Bovine osteochondrosis. *Compendium on Continuing Education for the Practicing Veterinarian* 20: 856–63.
Trostle, S. S., Nicoll, R. G., Forrest, L. J., Markel, M. D. 1997, Dec 15. Clinical and radiographic findings, treatment, and outcome in cattle with osteochondrosis: 29 cases (1986–1996). *J Am Vet Med Assoc.* 211(12): 1566–70.
Tryon, K. A., Farrow, C. S. 1999. Osteochondrosis in cattle. *Vet Clin North Am Food Anim Pract.* 15:265–74.

Author: Munashe Chigerwe

OSTERTAGIOSIS

BASICS

OVERVIEW
• *Ostertagia* are nematode parasites of the gastric glands and lumen of the abomasum of ruminants.
• The subfamily ostertaginae has been divided into several morphologically distinguishable but biologically similar genera that are usually host specific but may be found in other ruminants.
• *Teladorsagia* of sheep and goats, *Mazamastrongylus* of American cervids, and *Spiculopteragia* of old world cervids plus other genera in cameloids and antelope appear to be able to cause similar syndromes in their respective hosts.
• The disease is associated with the emergence of larvae from the gastric glands causing increased abomasal pH, lowered serum protein, and anorexia.
• *Ostertagia ostertagi* is the most economically important nematode parasite of cattle in temperate regions and *Teladorsagia (Ostertagia) circumcincta* one of the most important parasites of sheep and goats in cool moist climates.

SIGNALMENT
• All ages may become infected but the young of the year are more at risk for disease.
• Stressed animals and those that have not been repeatedly exposed to the parasite are more likely to have signs of disease.
• Breeds that evolved in cool, moist environments are more likely to have genetic traits making them resistant to infection.

SIGNS
• Weight loss and diarrhea are the most common clinical signs.
• Hypoalbuminemia and dehydration may be seen in individual animals.
• The disease is seasonal and manifests in different ways depending on the epidemiology in a geographic region.

Type I Ostertagiosis
• Occurs in young animals during the early phases of exposure to larvae on pasture.

• Larvae enter the gastric glands a few days postinfection then emerge 2 to 3 weeks later.
• Most of the animals in a population will have some disease from anorexia to diarrhea and weight loss.

Pretype II Infection
• Occurs later in the grazing season as larvae acquired on pasture are programmed to enter hypobiosis.
• These larvae enter the gastric glands and cease development at the early fourth stage.
• They do not feed or develop and no disease is seen.

Type II Ostertagiosis
• Occurs when the previously arrested (hypobiotic) larvae resume development.
• The larvae tend to emerge from the gastric glands more or less en mass; those acquired over several months may emerge in weeks.
• The number of animals showing signs may be less but the disease is usually more serious from the numbers of gastric glands being destroyed.
• Watery diarrhea with type I—the forage is rapidly growing and a greenish diarrhea is seen. Type II varies with the forage—a brownish diarrhea if hay or silage is consumed or green if lush grass from autumn rains.
• Submandibular edema (bottle jaw), anemia, and dehydration with a dull hair coat are often seen.

Host Immunity
• Livestock develop resistance to infection following repeated exposure to larvae. However, the resistance is not complete and parasites can occur in any age animal.
• Cattle that have been treated with anthelmintics aimed at the transmission patterns of *Ostertagia* have increased milk production even though they are not showing signs of disease.
• A high-protein diet may mask some signs of disease but also may aid in the immune response of the host against the parasite.
• Apparently multiple exposures to the parasite are required to stimulate a protective response.

• Zebu cattle and zebu crosses are more likely to exhibit signs of disease than European breeds of cattle.
• *Ostertagia* cause a nonspecific suppression of immunity.
• Hypersensitivity reactions occur with infections, which may be deleterious to both host and parasite.

Parasite Survival Strategies
• Heat and desiccation are deleterious to larvae in pastures but survival under snow is common.
• Larvae can survive in pastures for up to a year during periods of drought if entrapped in dung pats.
• Arrested development of early fourth-stage larvae in the gastric glands enables the parasite to evade unfavorable conditions in the environment (extremes of hot, dry or cold) or immune response by host.
• Emergence from the arrested state often coincides with reproduction and the periparturient relaxation of resistance by the host allows the survival of worms for a sufficient period to ensure the next generation of worms is present in the pastures for acquisition by the offspring.

HISTORICAL FINDINGS
• Grazing history
• Age of animals with clinical signs
• History of anthelmintic use and evaluation of anthelmintics on the premises
• Weight loss, diarrhea, and no fever
• Season

CAUSES AND RISK FACTORS
• Ostertagids do well in most cool climates or during that portion of the year when those conditions are present.
• Young animals and those in early lactation are at greatest risk.
• Heavily stocked and overgrazed pastures
• Animals on low-protein diets
• Breeds that evolved in arid or tropical conditions are at greater risk.

DIAGNOSIS

DIFFERENTIAL DIAGNOSIS
• Diarrhea due to intestinal parasitism
• Hypoproteinemia due to haemonchosis or fascioliasis
• Enteric viral or bacterial diseases
• Malnutrition

CBC/BIOCHEMISTRY/URINALYSIS
• Anemia low packed cell volume but not clinically apparent
• Hypoproteinemia, especially low serum albumen levels
• Elevated serum pepsinogen levels >3.0 IU tyrosine, cattle or >2.0 sheep

OTHER LABORATORY TESTS
• Fecal flotation egg counts are usually elevated but the level may not be high, as individual ostertagids do not produce as many eggs as some other nematodes and there may be dilution due to diarrhea.
• Eggs are not diagnostic, as other genera of gastrointestinal nematodes produce identical eggs.
• Culturing larval nematodes to the infective L3 stage will enable a differential identification of worms at the generic level.

PATHOLOGICAL FINDINGS

GROSS FINDINGS
• Edematous roughened (Morocco leather) abomasal folds
• Enlarged regional lymph nodes
• Raised umbilicated nodules on surface of abomasum
• May be sloughing of mucosa
• Elevated abomasal pH
• Adult worms (ca. 1 cm) may be seen on surface of abomasum, easily overlooked if not fresh and moving.

HISTOPATHOLOGICAL FINDINGS
• Distended gastric glands may contain developing worms.
• Cells lining glands are undifferentiated with a scarcity of acid-producing cells.
• Reactive regional lymph nodes
• Edema and inflammatory cells in submucosa

TREATMENT

• Broad-spectrum safe anthelmintics are the primary means of treatment and control.
• Anthelmintic resistance by *Teladorsagia* is commonly seen in some geographic regions.
• Virtually all of the available anthelmintics are effective against adult and metabolically active larvae.
• Some benzimidazoles and all macrolides are effective against arrested larvae.
• Macrolides have a residual effect against incoming larvae that will kill them before they can establish. This residual period (several weeks) varies with the chemical and may be a powerful selection mechanism for resistance.
• Dose and move young, susceptible animals to a pasture with few parasite larvae in the summer in cool climates; summer dosing with a product effective against arrested larvae in the warm climates when the pasture larvae die out.
• Ruminal boluses containing anthelmintics may be used to clear pastures of infective larvae over periods of several months.
• Drug withdrawal times must be maintained.

Anthelmintic Resistance
• Treating to kill every worm will, if not 100% successful, select resistant worms. Those survivors will only have other survivors to mate with.
• Strategic deworming will select for anthelmintic-resistant worms but will also have a greater impact on total worm populations lowering numbers below the economic threshold for a longer time than will other approaches.
• Levamisole may appear to have resistant worms because it is only effective against adult worms. When the adults are removed, arrested larvae will rapidly mature, thereby causing clinical signs, and begin producing eggs. The drug may be effective but against the wrong stage of the life cycle.
• Resistance is usually seen in the geographic region where the ostertagids are the predominant worm and control programs have targeted them.
• Resistance must be evaluated at the farm level.

• Rotation of anthelmintics does not seem to slow the onset of resistance and may in fact result in resistance to all of the drugs in the rotation faster than if a product is used until it fails and another product in a different drug family is utilized.

Preventive Management
• Management systems that lower the exposure of hosts to parasites can be devised. These systems may not optimize the value of forages but they result in healthier livestock.
• Rapid pasture rotation systems, where pastures are vacated for as few as 30 days before returning animals, may be of value in warm humid climates during the hottest time of the year in high rainfall areas or on irrigated pastures.
• Rapid pasture rotation otherwise will insure that the worms are waiting for the hosts when they return to the pasture.
• Utilizing pastures that have been used for cropping, especially in the last half of the grazing season, is grazing parasite-free pastures and, by the following year, any larvae deposited on the cropland will not survive until the next grazing.
• Alternate or cograzing with other species or classes of livestock may harvest larvae from the pasture. In general, the *Ostertagia* species in sheep and goats do not do well in cattle. Horses do not share *Ostertagia* and can be safely grazed in areas dangerous to ruminants.
• Older cattle may become infected but are highly resistant to effects of the worms and can be used to clear larvae from a pasture.
• Providing sufficient protein is vital with ostertagiosis as that is what is being lost.
• During the periparturient period, increased protein, not energy, levels will lessen egg production by gastrointestinal nematodes.
• To be sure, you cannot feed animals through the disease, but it is vital in recovery especially for those whose immune response is compromised.
• Summer treat and move young animals to pastures with low numbers of parasitic larvae.

Natural Biological Control
• Pastures containing plants high in condensed tannins are safer grazing for hosts as the incoming larvae are adversely affected.
• The physical structure of some plants is also a challenge for larvae to ascend the vegetation.

OSTERTAGIOSIS

• If animals browse, their chances of acquiring larvae diminish as the distance from the ground increases. Most infective larvae are found within 2 inches (50 mm) of the soil surface.

• Predaceous fungi have been evaluated as agents that kill larvae in pastures. One species, *Duddingtonia flagrans*, is able to traverse the digestive tract and is present in the fecal pat when the larvae hatch. Feeding spores or incorporating them in ruminal boluses has the capacity to lower pasture contamination.

Vaccination

• Vaccination is an approach deemed likely to be successful because animals naturally develop resistance to gastrointestinal nematodes.

• The requirement for multiple exposure and maturation of the host immune system appears to be important in natural immunity and also appears to be the case with whole-worm antigens, selected antigens, or irradiated larval vaccines.

Genetics

• The selection of individual animals with a level of resistance to the parasite or those that have the capacity to rebound from the effects of parasitism seems to be a logical approach. The offspring of resistant hosts are likely to be resistant also. Therefore, resistance to *Ostertagia* could be a selection criterion used in a flock or herd.

• The genetic aspect of resistance to gastrointestinal parasites is not well understood. It appears that multiple genes are involved in aspects of the protective response and that different genes may be more important at different times in the course of infection.

• Some breeds have more individual animals with sufficient factors, and they are more likely to survive exposure levels that would kill other animals.

• Even in resistant breeds, all animals are not equal, and factors such as lactation, age, or nutritional status may influence the course of disease.

• When animals are producing at their genetic maximum, they are at greater risk of parasitic disease because they are immunologically and nutritionally challenged.

• Other phenotypic characteristics such as production of milk, fiber, multiple births, and resistance to other agents may be at odds with resistance to helminths. Research does not indicate that the traits, which lead to increased production, are linked to those of increased susceptibility.

• To determine if genetic resistance is the answer to the problem of ostertagiosis, as currently appears to be the case, much more knowledge is needed.

Summary

• There is no overall approach that fits with the environment—and management practices—that will control ostertagiosis.

• Schemes that recognize that some animals are much more at risk than others and that strive to assure that the at-risk population is exposed to fewer worms or, if exposed, is treated differently may have a chance of success.

• Programs based on chemical control alone will likely fail unless the season of transmission is very short or new anthelmintics with completely different modes of action are discovered.

• Effective vaccines may be produced, but will not likely be practical in young animals at highest risk. However, they may lessen pasture contamination and subsequent exposure.

MISCELLANEOUS

ASSOCIATED CONDITIONS
N/A

AGE-RELATED FACTORS
N/A

ZOONOTIC POTENTIAL
N/A

PREGNANCY
N/A

RUMINANT SPECIES AFFECTED
Potentially, all ruminant species are affected.

BIOSECURITY
N/A

PRODUCTION MANAGEMENT
N/A

SYNONYMS
N/A

SEE ALSO
Anemia
Diarrhea due to intestinal parasitism
Enteric viral or bacterial diseases
Haemonchosis or fascioliasis
Hypoproteinemia
Malnutrition

ABBREVIATIONS
IU = international units
L3 = larval stage 3

Suggested Reading
Lichtenfels, J. R., Hoberg, E. P. 1993. The systematics of nematodes that cause ostertagiosis in domestic and wild ruminants in North America: an update and key to species. *Vet Parasitol*. 46:33–53.
Ploeger, H. W., Kloosterman, A., Rietveld, F. W. 1995. Acquired immunity against *Cooperia* spp. and *Ostertagia* spp. in calves: effect of level of exposure and timing of the midsummer increase. *Vet Parasitol*. 58:61–74.
Steer, M. J., Strain, S., Bishop, S. C. 1999. Mechanisms underlying resistance to nematode infection. *Int J Parasitol*. 29:51–56.
Suarez, V. H., Busetti, M. R., Lorenzo, R. M. 1995. Comparative effects of nematode infection on *Bos taurus* and *Bos indicus* crossbred calves grazing on Argentina's western pampas. *Vet Parasitol*. 58:263–71.
Williams, J. C., Knox, J. W., Marbury, K. S., et al. 1987. The epidemiology of *Ostertagia ostertagi* and other gastrointestinal nematodes of cattle in Louisiana. *Parasitol*. 95:135–53.
Yang, C., Gibbs, H. C., Xiao, L. 1993. Immunologic changes in *Ostertagia ostertagi*-infected calves treated strategically with an anthelmintic. *Am J Vet Res*. 54:1074–83.

Author: Thomas Craig

BASICS

DEFINITION
Otitis is an infection of the middle and inner ear usually associated with respiratory infections caused by bacteria or *Mycoplasma* sp. These infections enter the ear either by ascending the eustachian tube or by hematogenous seeding.

PATHOPHYSIOLOGY

SYSTEMS AFFECTED
CNS

GENETICS
N/A

INCIDENCE/PREVALENCE
N/A

GEOGRAPHIC DISTRIBUTION
Worldwide

SIGNALMENT
• There is no apparent breed or sex predisposition. Incidence appears to be biphasic.
• Calves and lambs less than 1 month of age have a higher incidence, as do calves 6–9 months of age. The higher incidence in both age groups probably relates to an increased risk of respiratory disease caused by common management strategies.

SIGNS
• Affected calves typically have clinical signs suggestive of sepsis, scleral injection, and fever. Ataxia of varying degree is usually present. Severely affected animals, particularly neonates, may be moribund, complicating the diagnosis. In these animals, specific neurologic signs may be difficult to recognize.
• The most consistent and prominent clinical signs are neurologic and are usually referable to cranial nerve VII dysfunction. These include drooped or immobile ear, inability to close palpebrae, and a loss of facial sensation on the same side as the lesion.
• Cranial nerve VIII dysfunction also is common, resulting in head tilt and circling toward the lesion. Involvement of additional cranial nerves and cortical involvement are uncommon. Strabismus and nystagmus are often observed.
• Otoscopic examination is difficult in calves and probably of less value than in companion animals. In some cases, purulent discharge from the ear canal is present.
• Affected calves often have concomitant bacterial or mycoplasmal respiratory disease, and thoracic auscultation may reveal crackles. Dyspnea and hyperpnea also may be present.
• In outbreaks associated with *Mycoplasma* sp. pneumonia, polyarthritis and conjunctivitis may be present in affected calves or their herdmates.

CAUSES
• Respiratory pathogens *Mannheimia hemolytica* and *Mycoplasma* sp. are the most common isolates from animals with acute disease.
• *Arcanobacter pyogenes* is frequently isolated from chronic lesions, but these isolates probably do not reflect etiology. Rather, they can reflect the normal progression of a chronic inflammatory process in a ruminant.
• A variety of ubiquitous environmental bacteria has been isolated from affected animals.

RISK FACTORS
• Preexisting respiratory disease is likely the most important risk factor. Among older calves, 6–9 months, strategies that increase the incidence of shipping fever will likely increase disease incidence.
• Inadequate vaccination against respiratory disease, mixing animals from multiple sources, and inadequate preconditioning programs should all be considered risk factors.
• In neonatal calves, group housing, inadequate passive transfer of colostral immunoglobulins and feeding raw milk, particularly waste milk on dairies with endemic *Mycoplasma* mastitis, are important additional risk factors.

OTITIS MEDIA/INTERNA

DIAGNOSIS

DIFFERENTIAL DIAGNOSIS
• In older calves, common differential diagnoses include listeriosis, thromboembolic meningoencephalitis caused by *Haemophilus somnus* and brainstem abscesses.
• Otitis is usually differentiated from other differentials of asymmetrical brainstem disease because portions of the central nervous system exclusive of CN VII and VIII are rarely affected.
• In younger calves, the primary differential is bacteremia caused by coliform bacteria.

CBC/BIOCHEMISTRY/URINALYSIS
N/A

IMAGING
Radiography may be used to identify lesions in the bulla; however, this procedure is not recommended. Most food-animal practitioners lack the resources to produce quality skull films and experience interpreting films. Furthermore, this procedure is probably not justifiable based on cost and benefits.

OTHER DIAGNOSTIC PROCEDURES

Ancillary Diagnostic Procedures
• Ancillary diagnostic procedures are rarely needed to establish a diagnosis in individual animals. Specific etiologic diagnosis occasionally may be warranted to permit specific targeted diagnostic procedures and herd intervention strategies.
• Diagnostic necropsy should be performed on dead or moribund animals, particularly when multiple animals are affected.
• Cultures of brain and lung tissue should be performed. When necropsy specimens are not available, specific efforts should be made to characterize the source and etiology of ongoing herd respiratory disease.

• Transtracheal wash or bronchoalveolar lavage cytology and culture may permit identification of the offending pathogens.
• *Mycoplasma* sp. are laborious and difficult to culture, and some laboratories will use PCR to identify *Mycoplasma* sp.
• Cerebrospinal fluid analysis may be helpful in differentiating causes of asymmetrical brainstem disease in feedlot cattle. Otitis will cause either a normal CSF composition or, alternatively, a CSF with increased concentrations of protein and neutrophils.
• Thromboembolic meningoencephalitis will typically result in a CSF that has a high cell count, a high protein concentration, a visible yellow color, and a preponderance of neutrophils.
• Listeriosis will generally cause milder increases in CSF cell counts and protein concentrations with the predominant cell type being mononuclear cells. Likewise, culture of the CSF may support specific differential diagnoses; however, negative CSF cultures are common.
• In those animals with polyarthritis in concert with middle ear infections, arthrocentesis with culture and cytology may be useful in determination of the specific etiology.
• Septicemia and TEME tend to cause more dramatic changes in joint fluid composition and the predominant cell type is the neutrophil with both agents.

Herd Diagnostic Procedures
• In dairy herds with no previous history of *Mycoplasma* mastitis, the recognition of otitis should encourage practitioners to reevaluate the herd status with regard to *Mycoplasma* sp. mastitis, particularly if the herd has practiced feeding waste milk to calves.
• Bulk tank cultures performed on three sequential days are reasonable, low-cost strategies to screen herds for *Mycoplasma* sp. mastitis.

• When multiple cases of otitis are recognized in calves less than 1 month of age on a dairy, practitioners should establish the effectiveness of colostrum administration practices. Serum protein concentration should be determined on all calves less than 10 days of age. Calves with serum protein concentrations less than 5.2 g/dL should be classified as having inadequate passive transfer.
• If more than 20% of calves have less than adequate passive transfer status, immediately targeted intervention should be undertaken to correct deficiencies.

TREATMENT

• Antimicrobial treatment is generally used in affected calves. If *M. hemolytica* or *P. multocida* has recently been isolated from clinically ill calves on the premises, the sensitivity pattern of these isolates may be used to guide therapeutic decisions. Pending return of laboratory results, the practitioner may assume that antibiotics deemed effective in the treatment of bovine pneumonia are appropriate for treatment of otitis.
• If the practitioner suspects or has demonstrated the involvement of *Mycoplasma* sp., antibiotic selection should be based upon potential efficacy against *Mycoplasma* sp.
• Reasonable choices would include tylosin, tilmicosin, and florfenicol. Antibiotic sensitivity testing of *Mycoplasma* sp. isolates is problematic and most laboratories lack the ability to provide these results. Furthermore, in vitro susceptibility may have little relationship with in vivo efficacy.

MEDICATIONS

CONTRAINDICATIONS
Appropriate milk and meat withdrawal times must be followed for all compounds administered to food-producing animals.

FOLLOW-UP
• Correction of underlying conditions that predispose calves to respiratory disease should be a primary goal.
• In a feedlot setting adequate preconditioning programs including single sourcing of pen lots and immunization programs for respiratory viruses and *M. hemolytica* and bunk adjustment are important prevention factors.
• On dairy farms, efforts should focus on adequacy of passive transfer in calves, elimination of group housing for young calves, and avoiding the feeding of waste milk.

MISCELLANEOUS

ASSOCIATED CONDITIONS
N/A

AGE-RELATED FACTORS
• Among older calves, 6–9 months, strategies that increased the incidence of shipping fever will likely increase incidence. In neonatal calves, group housing, inadequate passive transfer of colostral immunoglobulins, and feeding raw milk, particularly waste milk on dairies with endemic *Mycoplasma* sp. mastitis, are important additional risk factors.
• When multiple cases of otitis are recognized in calves less than 1 month of age on a dairy, practitioners should establish the effectiveness of colostrum administration practices.

ZOONOTIC POTENTIAL
N/A

PREGNANCY
N/A

RUMINANT SPECIES AFFECTED
All ruminant species are affected.

BIOSECURITY
Avoid buying stock from comingled groupings (i.e., sale barns). Quarantine of newly arriving stock can be helpful in the diagnosis and prevention of the disease.

PRODUCTION MANAGEMENT
• Inadequate vaccination against respiratory disease, mixing animals from multiple sources, and inadequate preconditioning programs should all be considered risk factors.
• In a feedlot setting adequate preconditioning programs including single sourcing of pen lots and immunization programs for respiratory viruses and *M. hemolytica* and bunk adjustment are important prevention factors.
• On dairy farms, efforts should focus on adequacy of passive transfer in calves, elimination of group housing for young calves, and avoiding feeding of waste milk.

SYNONYMS
N/A

SEE ALSO
Brainstem abscesses
Listeriosis
Thromboembolic meningoencephalitis caused by *Haemophilus somnus*

ABBREVIATIONS
CN = cranial nerve
CSF = cerebral spinal fluid
PCR = polymerase chain reaction
TEME = thromboembolic meningoencephalitis

Suggested Reading
Jensen, R., Maki, L. R., Lauerman, L. H., Raths, W. R., Swift, B. L., Flack, D. E., Hoff, R. L., Hancock, H. A., Tucker, J. O., Horton, D. P., Weibel, J. L. 1983. Cause and pathogenesis of middle ear infection in young feedlot cattle. *J Am Vet Med Assoc.* 182:967–72.
Jensen, R., Pierson, R. E., Weibel, J. L., Tucker, J. O., Swift, B. L. 1982. Middle ear infection in feedlot lambs. *J Am Vet Med Assoc.* 181:805–7.
Walz, P. H., Mullaney, T. P., Render, J. A., Walker, R. D., Mosser, T., Baker, J. C. 1997. Otitis media in preweaned Holstein dairy calves in Michigan due to *Mycoplasma bovis*. *J Vet Diagn Invest.* 9:250–54.

Author: Jeff W. Tyler

OVARIAN CYSTIC DEGENERATION

 BASICS

DEFINITION
Ovarian cystic degeneration is a condition seen in dairy cattle that impairs reproductive performance. Although, the exact etiology is not known, the condition results from failure of dominant follicles to ovulate.

PATHOPHYSIOLOGY
• Disruption of the hypothalamic—pituitary—ovarian axis.
• Failure of a pulsatile or surge release of GnRH from the hypothalamus.

SYSTEMS AFFECTED
• Endocrine/metabolic
• Reproductive

GENETICS
A genetic predisposition has been suggested related to high milk production.

INCIDENCE/PREVALENCE
15%–20% in lactating dairy cows

GEOGRAPHIC DISTRIBUTION
N/A

SIGNALMENT
Species
Bovine

Breed Predilection
Reported more commonly in Holstein cattle, related to the predominance of this breed throughout the world and affinity for high milk production.

Mean Age and Range
There is no specific age distribution.

SIGNS
GENERAL COMMENTS
The majority of cases are found during diagnosis of pregnancy or in cows presented because of anestrus.

HISTORICAL FINDINGS
Cows may have a history of anestrus.

PHYSICAL EXAMINATION FINDINGS
• Examination of the genital tract to asses ovarian status
• Diagnosis of ovarian cystic degeneration is based on the finding of a follicle > 15 mm in diameter, the absence of uterine tone, and a corpus luteum.

RISK FACTORS
Any stressful condition including:
• Calving difficulty
• High milk production
• Mastitis
• Uterine infection (metritis)
• Lameness
• Poor body condition
• Excessive use of estrogenic hormones

 DIAGNOSIS

DIFFERENTIAL DIAGNOSIS
• Preovulatory follicle
• Cystic corpus luteum

CBC/BIOCHEMISTRY/URINALYSIS
N/A

OTHER LABORATORY TESTS
Milk or blood progesterone concentration may help distinguish a luteal from a follicular cyst.

IMAGING
Use of ultrasonography to evaluate ovarian structures

DIAGNOSTIC PROCEDURES
• Palpation of the uterus for tone
• Ultrasonography or palpation of the ovaries for presence of a folliclelike structure.
• History of anestrus

PATHOLOGIC FINDINGS
N/A

 TREATMENT

APPROPRIATE HEALTH CARE
N/A

NURSING CARE
N/A

ACTIVITY
N/A

DIET
N/A

CLIENT EDUCATION
Appropriate nutrition and health management strategies in dairy cattle

SURGICAL CONSIDERATION
N/A

 MEDICATIONS

DRUGS OF CHOICE
• Gonadotropin releasing hormone (GnRH)
• Prostaglandins F2α
• Progesterone

CONTRAINDICATIONS
• Estrogenic compounds
• Appropriate milk and meat withdrawal times must be followed for all compounds administered to food-producing animals.

PRECAUTIONS
It is imperative that the clinician differentiate the proestrus and estrus condition from a cystic ovary condition during examination of the genital tract.

POSSIBLE INTERACTIONS
N/A

ALTERNATIVE DRUGS
Progesterone

 FOLLOW-UP

PATIENT MONITORING
After hormonal treatment, careful observation for estrus is imperative in order to inseminate the cow on a timely basis.

PREVENTION/AVOIDANCE
Reduce stressful condition on dairy farms.

POSSIBLE COMPLICATIONS
N/A

EXPECTED COURSE AND PROGNOSIS
• Most cows affected with ovarian cystic degeneration respond favorably to treatment in terms of resumption of cyclicity.
• However, fertility is compromised in cows with this condition, who experience prolonged days open and calving interval.

 MISCELLANEOUS

ASSOCIATED CONDITIONS
N/A

AGE-RELATED FACTORS
A higher incidence has been observed in multiparous cows.

ZOONOTIC POTENTIAL
N/A

PREGNANCY
Affected cows experience lower pregnancy rates.

RUMINANT SPECIES AFFECTED
Bovine

BIOSECURITY
N/A

PRODUCTION MANAGEMENT
• Sound reproductive herd health management practices
• Nutrition and health management
• Cow comfort
• Early diagnosis and treatment
• Judicious use of estrus synchronization protocols that include GnRH, prostaglandins, and progesterone.

SYNONYMS
Anovular follicles
Follicular cysts

SEE ALSO
Cystic corpus luteum
Reproductive pharmacology
Ultrasound examination

ABBREVIATIONS
OCD = ovarian cystic degeneration
FC = follicular cysts
GnRH = gonadotropin releasing hormone

Suggested Reading
Borromeo, V., Berrini, A., Bramani, S., Sironi, G., Finazzi, M., Secchi, C. 1998, May. Plasma levels of GH and PRL and concentrations in the fluids of bovine ovarian cysts and follicles. *Theriogenology* 49(7): 1377–87.
Kubar, H., Jalakas, M. 2002, Sep. Pathological changes in the reproductive organs of cows and heifers culled because of infertility. *J Vet Med A Physiol Pathol Clin Med*. 49(7): 365–72.
Peter, A. T. 2004, Feb. An update on cystic ovarian degeneration in cattle. *Reprod Domest Anim*. 39(1): 1–7.
Younquist, R. S., Shore, M. D. 1997. Infertility due to abnormalities of the ovaries. In: *Current therapy in large animal theriogenology*, ed. R. S. Youngquist. Philadelphia: W. B. Saunders.

Author: Carlos A. Risco

OVARIAN HYPOPLASIA, BURSAL DISEASE, SALPINGITIS

 BASICS

DEFINITION
• Ovarian hypoplasia: hypoplastic degeneration of the ovary
• Bursal disease: diseases associated with the ovarian bursa
• Salpingitis: inflammation of uterine tube or oviduct
• Factors that interfere with ova transport in the bursa (i.e., bursitis) and uterine tube (i.e., salpingitis; occlusions) or impair semen viability and transport (uterine adhesion, endometritis, obstruction of the uterotubal junction) may be the cause of repeat breeding animals.

PATHOPHYSIOLOGY
Ovarian Hypoplasia
Occurs as an autosomal recessive trait. The condition can be partial or complete and unilateral or bilateral. The ovary undergoes incomplete development and a part or the whole affected ovary lacks a normal number of primordial follicles.

Bursal Disease
Causes include trauma; aggressive per-rectal palpation of the reproductive tract; developmental defects such as paraovarian cysts; and shallow, narrow, or closed bursa.

Salpingitis
Causes include ascending infection from the uterus, descending infection, anomalies such as segmental aplasia, and aggressive irrigation of infected uterus with inappropriate agents (including estrogen).

SYSTEMS AFFECTED
Reproductive

GENETICS
Ovarian hypoplasia: single recessive autosomal gene with incomplete penetration

INCIDENCE/PREVALENCE
• Slaughtered bovine reproductive tract examinations revealed the following incidence rates:
  • Ovarian hypoplasia—1.9% of slaughtered cattle of which 87.1% affected the left ovary, 4.3% affected the right ovary, and 9.6% affected both ovaries
  • Bursal disease—4.9% incidence rate in slaughter study
  • Salpingitis—10.5% incidence rate in study animals, of which only 4.8% were noted as detected by per-rectum palpation.
• In some instances, bursal disease and salpingitis occur together

GEOGRAPHIC DISTRIBUTION
N/A

Species
Bovine, ovine, caprine, camelids; potentially all ruminant species

Breed Predilections
• Ovarian hypoplasia: Swedish highland cattle, shorthorn cattle
• Salpingitis has been reported with a much higher incidence in water buffalo than in domestic cattle.

Mean Range and Range
None

Predominant Sex
Female

SIGNS

GENERAL COMMENTS

HISTORICAL FINDINGS
Infertility

PHYSICAL EXAMINATION FINDINGS
Ovarian Hypoplasia
The affected hypoplastic ovary is small, thin, narrow, and firm. It may be so small that it can difficult to locate by palpation alone. In severe cases, only a cordlike thickening can be found in the cranial border of the ovarian ligament. It may palpate as a pea or kidney-bean-like structure in partial hypoplasia or as a shrunken structure in total ovarian hypoplasia.

Bursal Disease
In cases of adhesion, the ovary is difficult to move. *Bursal cysts* develop from adhesions of the fimbria to the ovary and contain fluid from the tube that flows into the bursa causing distension.

Salpingitis
Tubo-ovarian cysts—in cases of salpingitis, clear fluid accumulates in the proximal portion to reflux into the bursa. The cranial portions of the uterine tube distend in a cystic manner.

CAUSES
Infectious
• Salpingitis and bursal disease: ascending infection from the uterus following abortion, retained placenta, septic metritis, and pyometra. A variety of infectious organisms including *Arcanobacterium pyogenes, Streptococci* spp., *Staphylococci* spp., *Campylobacter* spp., *Hemophilus somnus, Mycobacterium tuberculosis*

• *C. fetus* subsp. *venerealis*—is an obligate parasite of bovine genitalia. The organism localizes in the anterior vagina and cervix during the ovulatory phase but does not invade the uterus and oviducts until progesterone release. It then causes endometritis and salpingitis for several weeks to a few months during which the animal is infertile. Animals usually regain fertility within 5 months and the subsequent immunity lasts about a year.

Traumatic
Aggressive per-rectal palpation of reproductive tract

Degenerative and Anatomic
• Ovarian hypoplasia
• Partial hypoplasia and degenerative changes after BVD vaccination is reported.
• Salpingitis and bursal disease: anomalies such as segmental aplasia of the paramesonephric duct and paraovarian cyst

RISK FACTORS
• Ovarian hypoplasia: genetic and breed predisposition possible
• Salpingitis and bursal disease: genetic predisposition for segmental aplasia and paraovarian cyst, aggressive palpation, and intrauterine infusion of inappropriate agents

 DIAGNOSIS

DIFFERENTIAL DIAGNOSIS
Repeat Breeding
• Anaplasmosis
• Bad artificial insemination technique
• Bluetongue
• Brucellosis
• Campylobacteriosis
• Endometritis
• Erroneous artificial insemination timing
• Erroneous heat detection
• Fescue toxicity
• Follicular cysts
• Heat stress
• Inadequate number of bulls
• Inadequate uterine involution
• Leptospirosis
• Malnutrition
• Oviduct bursal adhesions
• Pneumovagina
• Poor semen quality
• Selenium deficiency
• Trichomoniasis
• Urine pooling
• Uterine tumors
• Zearalenone toxicity

Anestrus
- Erroneous heat detection
- Freemartinism
- Heat stress
- Luteal cysts
- Malnutrition
- Nursing beef cows
- Poor footing
- Postpartum period
- Pregnancy
- Pyometra

Cyclic Irregularities
- Bovine viral diarrhea virus (BVDV)
- Campylobacteriosis
- Cystic ovaries
- Endometritis
- Heat stress
- Infectious bovine rhinotracheitis (IBR)
- Intrauterine therapy
- Leptospirosis
- Poor heat detection
- Trichomoniasis

CBC/BIOCHEMISTRY/URINALYSIS
N/A

OTHER LABORATORY TESTS
Culture and sensitivity may be helpful to rule out bacterial causes.

IMAGING
Ultrasonographic imaging of the reproductive tract may help to increase the diagnostic accuracy.

DIAGNOSTIC PROCEDURES
Per-rectal palpation and ultrasonographic imaging of the reproductive tract is mandatory. The use of a dye-test or embryo-flush technique to diagnose the distended tube or oviductal blockage can be helpful. It allows differentiation of a unilateral or bilateral condition.

PATHOLOGIC FINDINGS
Ovarian Hypoplasia
- Hypoplastic ovaries are small, thin, narrow, and firm; the ovary may be so small that it is difficult to locate.
- In severe cases, only a cordlike thickening of the cranial border of the ovarian ligament may be evident. It may palpate as a pea or kidney-bean-like structure in partial hypoplasia or as a shrunken structure in total ovarian hypoplasia.

Bursal Disease
Pathologic lesions may range from mild adhesions of a few fibrous threads between the bursa and the ovary to extensive ovariobursal lesions. The lesions include narrow, shallow, or closed bursa, roughness of the internal wall of the bursa, and cysts of the bursa.

Salpingitis
- Hydrosalpinx—secondary to segmental aplasia or uterine/oviductal blockage due to adhesions distally, proximally, or at both ends of oviduct

- Pyosalpinx—accumulation of pus in the oviduct following extensive uterine infection
- The oviduct usually distends to a diameter of 0.5–2.0 cm (depending on species) containing clear mucus or pus; it is elongated, coiled, and thin walled on palpation.

TREATMENT
In general, treatment of these conditions is not satisfactory. However, correct diagnosis, chronicity, and specific disease agent may determine treatment success and failure.

APPROPRIATE HEALTH CARE
N/A

NURSING CARE
N/A

ACTIVITY
N/A

DIET
N/A

CLIENT EDUCATION
Ovarian Hypoplasia
Culling of affected animal

Salpingitis and Bursal Disease
Hygienic and clean procedures should be employed during abortion, dystocia, fetotomy, retained placenta, and prolapse of vagina to avoid ascending infections.

SURGICAL CONSIDERATIONS
N/A

MEDICATIONS

FOLLOW-UP

PATIENT MONITORING
N/A

PREVENTION/AVOIDANCE
In genetic conditions, culling of the affected animal may help reduce the incidence; hygienic and clean procedures should be employed in the treatment of abortion, dystocia, fetotomy, retained placenta, and prolapse of the uterus/vagina to avoid ascending infections.

POSSIBLE COMPLICATIONS
Infertility

EXPECTED COURSE AND PROGNOSIS
- Prognosis—guarded to poor
- Severe bilateral salpingitis carries a poor fertility prognosis for pregnancy by normal means.

MISCELLANEOUS

ASSOCIATED CONDITIONS
Infertility

AGE-RELATED FACTORS
N/A

ZOONOTIC POTENTIAL
Depends upon the causative organism

PREGNANCY
See Differential Diagnosis and Pathophysiology above

RUMINANT SPECIES AFFECTED
Bovine, ovine, camelid, and caprine; potentially all ruminant species

BIOSECURITY
N/A

PRODUCTION MANAGEMENT
N/A

SYNONYMS
N/A

SEE ALSO
Breeding soundness examination by species
Cervicitis and metritis
Reproductive ultrasound by species
Specific disease descriptions

ABBREVIATIONS
BVD = bovine viral diarrhea
IBR = infectious bovine rhinotracheitis

Suggested Reading
Farin, P.W., Estill, C.T. 1993, Jul. Infertility due to abnormalities of the ovaries in cattle. *Vet Clin North Am Food Anim Pract*. 9(2): 291–308.
Long, S. E. 1980, Feb 23. Some pathological conditions of the reproductive tract of the ewe. *Vet Rec*. 106(8): 175–77.
Rajamahendran, R., Ambrose, D. J., Burton, B. 1994, Sep. Clinical and research applications of real-time ultrasonography in bovine reproduction: a review. *Can Vet J* 35(9): 563–72.
Smith, K. C., Long, S. E., Parkinson, T. J. 1998, Dec 19–26. Abattoir survey of congenital reproductive abnormalities in ewes. *Vet Rec*. 143(25): 679–85.

Author: Ramanathan Kasimanickam

OVINE PROGRESSIVE PNEUMONIA

 BASICS

DEFINITION
• Ovine progressive pneumonia (OPP) is a chronic disease of adult sheep and goats. The etiological agent is ovine lentivirus (OvLV) (also known as visna-maedi virus, ovine progressive pneumonia virus) and the clinical signs include progressive emaciation, dyspnea, and the development of opportunistic infections.
• Chronic active inflammation can occur as well in the lymph nodes, joints, mammary glands, and central nervous system.

PATHOPHYSIOLOGY
• OvLV is transmitted in utero and also by aerosol, contact, and ingestion of infected milk. Infection is then established in monocytes and macrophages and spreads to the lungs, lymph nodes, choroids plexus, bone marrow, mammary glands and kidneys. OvLV causes a persistent infection in the face of humoral and cellular immunity and results in the development of immune-mediated lesions in multiple organ systems.
• Sheep infected tend to be afebrile and maintain a normal appetite.

SYSTEMS AFFECTED
Respiratory
• The lungs are the most common target organ. Infection of the lungs causes a diffuse lymphoproliferative interstitial pneumonia with infiltration of lymphocytes, plasma cells, and macrophages into the interalveolar septae.
• Hyperplasia of the alveolar epithelium and terminal bronchial smooth muscle may also occur. On necropsy, the lungs are grossly enlarged and very heavy.
• Vertical rib impressions may be seen on the exterior lung surface.

Mammary
• *Mastitis*: Indurative mastitis ("hardbag") is characterized by a large, hard udder with no abnormal secretions. The infection may be symmetrical or asymmetrical.
• In advanced cases, the udder is enlarged, teats are limp, and there is little milk in the teat cistern. The milk is normal in appearance.

Musculoskeletal
• *Arthritis:* The carpal joints are the most common joints infected and are obviously swollen. The swelling is bilateral.
• Lameness and emaciation are common sequelae.

Central Nervous System
• *Meningoencephalitis:* The initial signs of neurological involvement are ataxia, circling, stumbling, and unilateral proprioceptive deficits.
• Neurological signs can progress to rear limb paralysis and quadriplegia.

GENETICS
• Susceptibility to infection may vary due to breed.
• Rambouillet seem to be more resistant to infection, whereas Finnish Landrace and Texel are highly susceptible.

INCIDENCE/PREVALENCE
• Prevalence of infection varies between farms, breeds, and countries.
• Seroprevalence of OPP in ewes in the United States ranges from 1% to 70% and increases with age. Some flocks can approach 100% infectivity.
• Texas has an exceptionally low prevalence of infection (1%). Ewes culled in other states have seroprevalence rates of 30%–67%.
• The overall prevalence of the disease in the United States is not known.

GEOGRAPHIC DISTRIBUTION
• OPP occurs in all major sheep-producing countries with the exception of Australia, New Zealand, Iceland, and Finland.
• In the United States, the infection appears to be most common in the western states.

SIGNALMENT
Species
Ovine, rare in goats

Breed Predilection
• Texel and Finnish Landrace are the breeds that are most commonly affected.
• Rambouillet sheep appear to be most resistant to the infection.
• Highly susceptible breeds include Border Leicester, Finnsheep, Finn-crosses, Corriedales, Dorsets, and North Country Cheviots.
• The Ile de France has been shown to be resistant to infection.

Mean Age and Range
• OPP is rarely seen in animals less than 2 years of age and natural disease is usually observed in 2- to 3-year-old animals.
• Adults of any age, however, can be infected.

Predominant Sex
Both male and female animals can be infected.

SIGNS
• Emaciation and increasing respiratory distress are the most common signs.
• Animals maintain a normal appetite, are afebrile, rarely cough, and are not depressed.
• Indurative mastitis, arthritis, and meningioencephalitis may occur also.

 DIAGNOSIS

• Diagnosis is difficult, as many sheep show no clinical signs of infection. Symptoms, when evident, may reflect many different diseases.
• Clinical signs are compared to necropsy findings as well as serologic tests.
• Characteristic lung lesions include oversized, heavy, grayish-blue discolored lungs. There often are lesions of active secondary bacterial pneumonia in the anteroventral areas of the lung.

DIFFERENTIAL DIAGNOSIS
• Adenovirus/adenomatosis
• Caseous lymphadenitis
• Chlamydia
• Chronic pulmonary adenomatosis
• Mycoplasma
• Nasal bot
• Nasal myosis
• Neoplasia
• Parainfluenza type 3
• Parasitic bronchitis
• Pasteurellosis
• Selenium toxicity
• Tuberculosis

CBC/BIOCHEMISTRY/URINALYSIS
Not diagnostic

OTHER LABORATORY TESTS
• The two most commonly used laboratory serologic methods are agar gel immunodiffusion test (AGID), and enzyme-linked immunosorbent assay (ELISA) test.

• AGID is less sensitive than the ELISA, and is prone to false negative results. However, due to its ease of performance, it is generally the test of choice with most laboratories.
• The ELISA test is more sensitive than the AGID test because it can detect an infected animal 2 weeks postinfection.
• Detection of OPP virus can also be done through culture. This may require up to 12 weeks before results are available.

IMAGING
Not diagnostic

TREATMENT

• Treatment of OPP is not effective.
• Most sheep die due to secondary bacterial pneumonia. Antibiotics may be indicated to prolong the sheep's life a few weeks or months. However, humane euthanasia should be considered upon laboratory confirmation. Infected animals remaining in the flock can continue to infect.
• Control of the disease may include periodic flock testing, culling of positive animals, removing lambs from ewes at birth, feeding pasteurized colostrum/milk replacer, purchasing seronegative replacement stock and improved biosecurity measures.
• Two methods of control: test and remove infected individuals and isolate and artificially rear progeny.
• Using these methods, some producers have been successful in the eradication of OPP.
• The most important aspect of control is to ensure the purchase of replacement animals from flocks that test negative for OPP.
• Rams should also be tested and found negative prior to incorporation into the breeding flock.

MEDICATIONS
N/A

FOLLOW-UP

MISCELLANEOUS

ASSOCIATED CONDITIONS
N/A

AGE-RELATED FACTORS
N/A

ZOONOTIC POTENTIAL
N/A

PREGNANCY
• Since OPP is not treatable and is difficult to eradicate from flocks, lambs that are born to seropositve ewes should be removed from their dams before they nurse, raised in isolation, and fed bovine colostrum and milk replacer.
• An alternative to artificial rearing may be fostering lambs to seronegative ewes.

RUMINANT SPECIES AFFECTED
Sheep, goats

BIOSECURITY
• Control of infection requires testing of animals on an annual basis. This is a minimum time period with more frequent testing in known infected flocks.
• Seropositive animals and their progeny less then 1 year of age are culled.
• An alternative to culling is artificial rearing of lambs or fostering of lambs to seronegative ewes.
• Seronegative animals must remain isolated from infected sheep and any equipment that has been in contact with seropositive animals.
• Visitations to seronegative herds should be limited to personnel who have no contact with infected animals.
• New additions to the herd must be seronegative.

PRODUCTION MANAGEMENT
N/A

SYNONYMS
Maedi-visna
OPP
Progressive pneumonia

SEE ALSO
Adenovirus/adenomatosis
Chronic pulmonary adenomatosis
Mycoplasma
Parainfluenza type 3
Parasitic bronchitis
Tuberculosis

ABBREVIATIONS
OPP = ovine progressive pneumonia
OvLV = ovine lentivirus
AGID = agar gel immunodiffusion test
ELISA = enzyme-linked immunosorbent assay (ELISA) test

Suggested Reading
Aiello, S. E., et al., eds. 1998. *Merck veterinary manual*. 8th ed. Whitehouse, NJ: Merck and Co.
Bulgin, M. S. 1990, Nov. Ovine progressive pneumonia, caprine arthritis encephalitis, and the related lentivirus diseases of sheep and goats. *Vet Clin North Am Food Am Pract*. 6(3): 691–704.
De la Concha-Bermejillo, A., Juste, R. A., Kretschmer, R., Aguiliar, S. 1995, Winter. Ovine lentivirus infection: an animal model for pediatric HIV infection? *Arch Med Res*. 26(4): 345–54.
Demartini, J. C., Brodie, S. J., de la Concha-Bermejillo, A., Ellis, J. A., Lairmore, M. D. 1993, Aug. Pathogenesis of lymphoid interstitial pneumonia in natural and experimental ovine lentivirus infection. *Clin Infect Dis*. 17 (Suppl 1): S236–42.
Martin, W. B. 1996, Jun. Respiratory infections of sheep. *Comp Immunol Microbial Infect Dis*. 19(3): 171–79.
Pugh, D. G. 2002. *Sheep and goat medicine*. Philadelphia: W. B. Saunders Co.

Author: Penelope Collins

OVINE PULMONARY ADENOCARCINOMA

 BASICS

OVERVIEW
• A type D retrovirus called ovine pulmonary adenomatosis retrovirus (OPARV) causes a contagious disease characterized by the formation of pulmonary tumors in sheep.
• The disease is known as ovine pulmonary adenomatosis (OPA); however, it is also referred to as ovine pulmonary carcinoma, jaagsiekte, and sheep pulmonary adenocarcinoma.

SYSTEMS AFFECTED
Pulmonary and lymphoid tissues

GENETICS
• There appears to be some breed predilection.
• There is some evidence that the presence of endogenous viral sequences in ovine genomes may increase the OPA susceptibility in sheep.

INCIDENCE/PREVALENCE
Unknown

GEOGRAPHIC DISTRIBUTION
• OPA is found in sheep populations throughout the world; however, Australia and New Zealand are free from the disease.
• OPA is a significant problem in sheep-raising countries where it is enzootic. OPA is an economically important disease in Scotland, South Africa, and Peru; it is a minor disease in Canada and the United States.

SIGNALMENT
Species
• Sheep
• Goats: the disease has been experimentally transmitted from sheep to goats. Goats have a low susceptibility to infection. The disease appears to occur naturally at a low prevalence in goats.

Breed Predilections
Some breeds appear to be more susceptible to OPA.

Mean Age and Range
• The normal course of overt disease occurs in adult sheep between 3–4 years of age; lambs are more susceptible to infection if exposed prior to 10 weeks of age.
• The incubation period ranges from 3 weeks in lambs to several years in older animals.
• Average duration of clinical signs is 2 months (range of a few days to 6 months).
• Tumors were detected within 10–20 days following experimental inoculation of newborn lambs.
• The peak incidence of OPA after natural infection is thought to be 3 to 4 years.

Predominant Sex
N/A

SIGNS

HISTORICAL FINDINGS
• Marked dyspnea, sporadic coughing, and copious watery nasal exudate
• Weight loss and increased secretion from the lungs.

CAUSES AND RISK FACTORS
Lateral Transmission
Transmission occurs by aerosol and, experimentally, by contact. OPA is highly contagious and susceptibility is age dependent.

Vertical Transmission Via Embryos and Semen
OPA has not been detected in embryos or uterine fluids. However, during the later stages of disease, exposure of embryos, ova, and semen to virus may be possible.

 DIAGNOSIS

DIFFERENTIAL DIAGNOSIS
• Epithelial hyperplasia, a sequela to chronic infections of sheep
• Maedi-visna
• Verminous pneumonia

CBC/BIOCHEMISTRY/URINALYSIS
N/A

OTHER LABORATORY TESTS
• Detection of infected sheep prior to development of clinical disease may be extremely difficult.
• An ELISA using a recombinant protein component of the putative virus as the antigen has been utilized.
• Using PCR, major differences between endogenous and exogenous sequences have been identified in the env TM and 3′ unique sequence (U3) regions. Using primers in the U3 region, OPARV DNA can be detected in tumors in lung tissue, lung secretions of infected sheep, lymphoid tissues, and peripheral blood mononuclear cells.
• Blocking enzyme-linked immunosorbent assay (B-ELISA) and an immunohistochemical technique, which specifically detects OPARV in transformed epithelial cells of the alveoli of OPA-affected sheep, have been developed.
• A competition radioimmunoassay (RIA) has also been used to detect OPARV antigen in tumor cell homogenates, lung fluid, and cell culture supernatant fluids in sheep.

IMAGING
N/A

OTHER DIAGNOSTIC PROCEDURES
• Detection of subclinical infection is difficult. Field diagnosis relies on identifying overt animals within a flock with typical clinical and postmortem symptoms.
• The presence of the disease may not be recognized in flocks containing a predominance of animals less than 4 years of age.
• When purchasing new stock, the infection status of individual animals depends on the disease status of the originating flock.

OVINE PULMONARY ADENOCARCINOMA

PATHOLOGIC FINDINGS

Histopathology

• Pulmonary tissue pathological changes occur as multiple, well-circumscribed nodules of transformed secretory epithelial cells, multifocal nodules of neoplastic cuboidal epithelial cells in acinar or papillary patterns, peribronchiolar and interstitial lymphoid hyperplasia, type II pneumocytes and nonciliated bronchiolar (Clara) cells, and fibromuscular proliferation.

• Metastases are found most commonly in the bronchial or mediastinal lymph nodes in 10% to 50% of cases.

• Virus replicates actively in the transformed epithelial cells of the lung, and viral DNA and RNA have been detected in lymphoid tissues.

• Electron microscopically, cells have microvilli, tight junctions, and cytoplasmic lamellar bodies reflecting alveolar type II cells. Serum precipitating antibodies to ovine lentivirus are seen.

• Lung fluids have been shown to contain a 26 kd peptide that cross reacts with a primate-derived type D retrovirus as detected by immunoblotting or interspecies competition radioimmunoassay.

• Recent studies document the presence of type D-related retrovirus antigen in ovine pulmonary carcinoma (OPC) in the United States.

TREATMENT

Not effective. Humane euthanasia is indicated where infection is suspected.

MEDICATIONS

FOLLOW-UP

PREVENTION/AVOIDANCE

Due to the long preclinical incubation period, OPA may disseminate widely in a flock prior to disease recognition.

POSSIBLE COMPLICATIONS

N/A

EXPECTED COURSE AND PROGNOSIS

Grave; 95% of all clinical cases die. Surviving animals spread the disease.

MISCELLANEOUS

ASSOCIATED CONDITIONS

N/A

AGE-RELATED FACTORS

Adult sheep between 1 and 4 years of age with 4 years of age being the norm; lambs are more susceptible to infection if exposed prior to 10 weeks of age

ZOONOTIC POTENTIAL

N/A

PREGNANCY

N/A

RUMINANT SPECIES AFFECTED

Sheep, possibly goats

BIOSECURITY

• Restrict movement of sheep from known infected flocks.

• Purchase replacement stock from known disease-free farms and ranches.

PRODUCTION MANAGEMENT

Economic losses can arise from mortalities, the cost of eradication programs, and control measures.

SYNONYMS

Jaagsiekte
Jaagsiekte sheep retrovirus (jsrv)
Ovine pulmonary carcinoma
Sheep pulmonary adenocarcinoma

SEE ALSO

Caprine arthritis-encephalitis virus
Lentivirus
Maedi-visna
Verminous pneumonia

ABBREVIATIONS

DNA = deoxyribonucleic acid
ELISA = enzyme-linked immunosorbent assay
JSRV = jaagsiekte sheep retrovirus
OPA = ovine pulmonary adenomatosis
OPARV = adenomatosis retrovirus
PCR = polymerase chain reaction
RIA = radioimmunoassay

Suggested Reading

Demartini, J. C., Rosadio, R. H., Lairmore, M. D.1988. The etiology and pathogenesis of ovine pulmonary carcinoma (sheep pulmonary adenomatosis). *VetMicrobiol.* 17: 219–36.

Hecht, S. J., Sharp, J. M., De martini, J. C.1996. Retroviral aetiopathogenesis of ovine pulmonary carcinoma: a critical appraisal. *Br Vet J.* 152:395–409.

Palmarini, M., Sharp, J. M., de las Heras, M., Fan, H.1999. OPA sheep retrovirus is necessary and sufficient to induce a contagious lung cancer in sheep. *J Virol*, 73; 6964–72.

Parker, B. N. J., Wrathall, A. E., Saunders, R. W., Dawson, M., Done, S. H., Francis, P. G., Dexter, I., Bradley, R.1998. Prevention of transmission of sheep pulmonary adenomatosis by embryo transfer. *Vet Rec.* 142: 687–89.

Peterhans, E., Greenland, T., et al. 2004. Routes of transmission and consequences of small ruminant lentiviruses (SRLVs) infection and eradication schemes. *Vet Res.* 35:257–74.

Rosadio, R. H., Sharp, J. M., Lairmore, M. D., Dahlberg, J. E., De Martini, J. C. 1988. Lesions and retroviruses associated with naturally occurring ovine pulmonary carcinoma (sheep pulmonary adenomatosis). *Vet Pathol.* 25: 58–66.

Author: Scott R. R. Haskell

OXALATE TOXICITY

 BASICS

OVERVIEW
• Due to ingestion of plants containing large amounts of soluble potassium and sodium oxalate salts that when absorbed form insoluble calcium and magnesium oxalate salts
• Associated with ingestion of a number of different plant species: the most commonly seen include *Halogeton glomeratus* (halogeton), *Sarcobatus vermiculatus* (greaseweed, black greaseweed), and *Oxalis* (shamrock, soursob, sorrel).
• Many other plants contain oxalates but are less commonly associated with toxicity including, but not limited to, *Amaranthus* (red-pig root), *Chenopodium* (lamb's quarters), *Rheum rhaponticum* (rhubarb), *Panicum* spp. (elephant grass), and *Alocasia* (elephant's ear).
• Concentration of the oxalates depends on season, stage of plant growth, weather, soil, geographic area, and variation between plant species.
• Ruminants are able to detoxify oxalates in the rumen by bacterial degradation and this accounts for decreased toxicity in ruminants compared to some other species.
• Factors affecting the toxicity following ingestion include the amount and rate of ingestion, previous adaptation to the plant in allowing increased bacterial degradation (can occur over 2–3 days), and volume of other nontoxic plants in rumen.
• Rapid absorption of oxalates and formation of insoluble calcium and magnesium salts yields a rapid decline in serum calcium and magnesium levels. Acutely, these animals may present with signs commonly seen with hypocalcemia due to impaired cellular membrane function.
• More chronic ingestion will yield formation of oxalate-containing urinary stones and oxalate nephrosis (due to precipitation of these salts in the tubules).
• These plants grow throughout continental North America, however, the ones most commonly associated with toxicity (halogeton and greaseweed) are found mainly in the western portions of the country.

• Toxicity most commonly occurs when unadapted sheep or cattle are placed in or move through areas containing large stands of these plants.
• Local oxalate crystal formation in the rumen wall may induce a rumenitis or more severe gastroenteritis.

SIGNALMENT
• All ruminant species and swine can be affected, but the disease is seen more commonly in sheep.
• Acute exposure to the plant in unadapted animals is important in toxicity.

SIGNS
• Acute toxicity present with signs of hypocalcemia.
• Signs occur within several hours and death can occur within 12 hours.
• First signs may include dullness, anorexia, belligerence (mainly cattle), stiffness, weakness, muscle tremors, tetany, and recumbency. As disease progresses without treatment, coma and death may occur.
• Rumenitis, rumen stasis, and gastroenteritis
• If animal lives through acute stages, then azotemia and kidney failure ensue.
• Azotemia may be associated with increased depression, anorexia, and death.

CAUSES AND RISK FACTORS
• Ingestion of plants containing high levels of soluble oxalate salts
• Most commonly halogeton or greaseweed
• Ingestion of large amounts rapidly is a risk factor.
• Increased rumen fill by nontoxic forage is protective.
• Slow adaptation to oxalate plants over a period of 4 days can increase the rumen's ability to degrade the oxalates by up to 30%.
• Diets high in calcium may be protective due to formation of insoluble calcium oxalate salts in the GI tract.

 DIAGNOSIS

DIFFERENTIAL DIAGNOSIS
• Hypocalcemia of other causes, including lactational hypocalcemia (cattle) and gestational hypocalcemia (sheep and goats)
• Hypomagnesemia of other causes including grass tetany, lactation tetany, wheat pasture tetany, transport tetany, and grass staggers
• Other causes of acute renal failure—ischemia, heavy metal toxicosis (arsenic, mercury, lead), drug-related nephropathies, *Quercus* (oak toxicity), pigment nephropathies (hemoglobin, myoglobin), and monensin toxicity
• Other urinary tract disease—pyelonephritis, urolithiasis (struvite and silicates, calcium carbonate), and amyloidosis
• History of exposure to oxalate-containing plants is helpful in differentiating oxalate toxicity from other processes.

CBC/BIOCHEMISTRY/URINALYSIS
• Oxalate crystals in urine (may not be present in acute cases)
• With chronic toxicity, an azotemia would be consistent with but not diagnostic of oxalate toxicity.

OTHER LABORATORY TESTS
Quantification of oxalate levels in suspect forage

IMAGING
Transabdominal or transrectal ultrasound of the kidneys may demonstrate perirenal edema (especially if pigweed is the plant involved) or cortical hyperechogenicity due to deposition of crystals in tissue.

DIAGNOSTIC PROCEDURES
N/A

PATHOLOGIC FINDINGS
• Depends on the severity, chronicity, and plant of oxalate origin
• *Amaranthus* spp. (pigweed) often have perirenal edema in pig and cattle.

• Acute cases may have enlarged edematous, red kidneys, while more chronic cases may have smaller kidneys with histopathologic evidence of renal tubular nephrosis and oxalate crystal formation.
• Rumen wall may be hemorrhagic due to oxalates in the wall.
• Histopathology may demonstrate oxalate crystals in rumen wall.

TREATMENT

• Evaluate rest of the herd for early evidence of disease.
• Consider relocating rest of herd to a new area without plants or try to slowly introduce oxalate-containing forage and maintain intake with additional nontoxic forage to dilute the oxalates.
• Adaptation to oxalate forage should be done by cautiously allowing animals to graze for increasing periods of time over a minimum of 4 days.
• Add supplemental dicalcium phosphate to the diet to bind oxalates in the GI in the form of dicalcium phosphate–containing salts of alfalfa pellets.
• Hospitalization and fluid therapy to actively diurese the patient may slow down renal crystaluria and subsequent nephrosis.

MEDICATIONS

DRUGS OF CHOICE
• Hypocalcemic or hypomagnesimic patients should receive a slow IV infusion of 23% calcium gluconate or a commercially available mixture of calcium, magnesium, and glucose.
• IV fluids for diuresis is indicated.

CONTRAINDICATIONS
• Infusion of IV calcium should be done slowly and the heart rate and rhythm monitored. Calcium infusion should be discontinued if any abnormalities are observed.

• Appropriate milk and meat withdrawal times must be followed for all compounds administered to food-producing animals.

POSSIBLE INTERACTIONS

FOLLOW-UP

PATIENT MONITORING
• Cases with renal involvement should have repeated serum chemistries and urinalysis to monitor renal function, evaluate efficacy of diuresis, and determine when fluids can be safely discontinued.
• Electrolytes, PCV, acid-base status, and albumin should be monitored in cases that survive severe renal compromise, as alterations in these values may continue after treatment.

PREVENTION/AVOIDANCE
• If possible, avoid grazing oxalate-containing forages.
• Cautiously and slowly introduce oxalate forages over a period of 4 or more days.
• Increase calcium diphosphate in the diet (this may have an effect on DCAD balance and induce other metabolic syndromes if done long term).

POSSIBLE COMPLICATIONS
Chronic renal failure

EXPECTED COURSE AND PROGNOSIS
• Severely affected animals often succumb to renal failure if they survive the acute disease process.
• Early treatment of less-severely affected cases may be successful.
• Aggressive fluid therapy and diuresis may improve the prognosis in animals with renal involvement.

MISCELLANEOUS

ASSOCIATED CONDITIONS
N/A

AGE-RELATED FACTORS
N/A

ZOONOTIC POTENTIAL
N/A

PREGNANCY
N/A

RUMINANT SPECIES AFFECTED
• Sheep most common
• All ruminant species can be affected.
• Swine can be affected.

BIOSECURITY
N/A

PRODUCTION MANAGEMENT
N/A

SEE ALSO
Hypocalcemia of other causes, including lactational hypocalcemia (cattle) and gestational hypocalcemia (sheep and goats)
Hypomagnesemia of other causes, including grass tetany, lactation tetany, wheat pasture tetany, transport tetany, and grass staggers
Other causes of acute renal failure—ischemia, heavy metal toxicosis (arsenic, mercury, lead), drug-related nephropathion, Quercus (oak toxicity), pigment nephropathies (hemoglobin, myoglobin), and monensin toxicity
Other urinary tract disease—pyelonephritis, urolithiasis (struvite and silicates, calcium carbonate), and amyloidosis

ABBREVIATIONS
DCAD = dietary cation anion difference
GI = gastrointestinal
IV = intravenous
PCV = packed cell volume

Suggested Reading
Knight, A. P., Walter, R. G. 2001. *A guide to plant poisoning of animals in North America.* Jackson, WY: Teton New Media.

Author: Paul J. Plummer

PAPILLOMATOSIS

 ## BASICS

DEFINITION
• Papillomatosis occurs when ruminants are infected with one of several distinct papillomaviruses.
• Infection with a bovine papilloma virus can result in the formation of fibropapillomas or epithelial papillomas.

PATHOPHYSIOLOGY
• Six bovine papillomaviruses have been identified, with distinct tissue tropisms.
• Subgroup A contains BPV-1, -2, and -5 and causes fibropapillomas of the skin.
• Subgroup B contains BPV-3, -4, and -6, viruses that induce epithelial papillomas.
• Most papillomas spontaneously regress.
• With appropriate cofactors, progression to SCC or malignant bladder cancer may occur.

SYSTEMS AFFECTED
• Skin
• Gastrointestinal
• Urologic
• Reproductive

GENETICS
N/A

INCIDENCE/PREVALENCE
• PPD is more common in dairy cattle than beef cattle.
• At culling, 26% of dairy cattle demonstrated PPD compared with 4% of beef cattle.
• Cutaneous papillomatosis is a common disease in cattle.

GEOGRAPHIC DISTRIBUTION
Worldwide

SIGNALMENT
• Most cattle are infected under 18 months of age except for cattle infected with BPV-3.
• BPV-3 can infect cattle of any age.
• There is no reported gender or breed predilection in cattle.
• Saanen goats are more commonly infected than other goats.
• PPD is more common among dairy cattle than beef cattle.

SIGNS
• Lesions typically appear 1–4 months after infection.
• Typically, these are hairless tumors of the skin (head, neck, dewlap) and udder.
 • Often gray in color, firm with a dry, horny surface
 • Vary widely in size from 1 mm to several cms in diameter
 • May be wide based, cauliflowerlike in appearance, or pedunculated with a narrow base.
 • The number of lesions can vary from one to hundreds.

• Atypical warts are nonpedunculated, flat, circular masses, with delicate, frondlike protuberances. They may have hair growing through them.
• Can also involve the genital mucosa, alimentary tract, or bladder.
• Papillomas involving the cornea and interdigital space may also be viral in origin.
• Interdigital papillomatosis causes marked lameness with accompanying weight loss and decreased milk production.
• Papillomatosis of the alimentary tract can cause problems with breathing, eating, bloating, rumen atony, and weight loss.
• Many papillomas regress spontaneously.
• Teat papillomas may regress during the nonlactating period, and then recur at the next lactation.

CAUSES
• BPV-1 causes teat frond and penile fibropapillomas.
• BPV-2 infects the skin of the head and neck most commonly, but may involve contiguous skin as well.
• BPV-3 infects epithelial cells and is the cause of "atypical warts."
• BPV-4 typically causes papillomas in the alimentary tract and bladder.
• BPV-5 is the causative agent of the "rice-grain papillomas" of the teat and udder.
• BPV-6 has been isolated from teat frond papillomas.
• Immunity to one BPV does not protect against other types.
• PPD is thought to have a bacterial component to the development of this lesion.

RISK FACTORS
• Diffuse alimentary papillomatosis typically occurs in immunosuppressed animals, such as those ingesting bracken fern.
• Animals with inherent deficiencies in cell-mediated immunity may also be susceptible to widespread alimentary papillomatosis.
• Infection from one animal to another can occur through the presence of sharp or abrasive elements on the farm, or through the use of shared halters, brushes, etc.
• Exposure to cofactors, such as significant skin trauma (branding), ingestion of carcinogens/mutagens (such as bracken fern), or exposure to sunlight may result in malignant transformation to SCC and bladder cancer.
• Papillomatous digital dermatitis (or interdigital papillomatosis) is more commonly seen in first parity cows, in cows loose-housed, and in single-use cows (e.g., dairy).
• In herd situations, vaccination of uninfected cattle with an autogenous vaccine derived from the premises may be protective against infection.

 ## DIAGNOSIS

DIFFERENTIAL DIAGNOSIS
• Squamous cell carcinoma
• Dermatophilosis

CBC/CHEMISTRY/URINALYSIS
N/A

OTHER LABORATORY TESTS
N/A

IMAGING
N/A

DIAGNOSTIC PROCEDURES
• Diagnosis is typically based on examination of the lesion.
• Histopathology can be used to differentiate between papillomas and SCC.

PATHOLOGIC FINDINGS
• Fibropapillomas have a distinct fibromatous portion as well as a hyperplastic epithelial component.
• Purely epithelial papillomas demonstrate hyperplastic epidermis with extensive keratinization.
• In regressing lesions, the fibroblasts may appear to have shrunken nuclei and an indistinct cytoplasm, as well as fewer mitotic figures in both the fibromatous and epithelial components.

 ## TREATMENT

APPROPRIATE HEALTH CARE
• Many papillomas will regress spontaneously within 12 months.
• Vaccination with an autogenous or commercial vaccine may help prevent infection in other animals in the herd.
• Minor surgical procedures (such as dehorning) have been implicated in the spread of the virus.
• Although used in practice, there is little evidence that vaccination with an autogenous vaccine speeds regression of pre-existing papillomas, and may increase the duration of the disease.
• Partial excision combined with autogenous vaccine may be beneficial in calves with small papillomas.
• PPD is best treated with complete surgical removal of the involved tissue.
• Some cattle with PPD will respond to treatment with antibiotics.

ACTIVITY
N/A

DIET
No changes needed

CLIENT EDUCATION
• Depending upon site, lesions may regress and recur (teat papillomas) or regress and never recur.
• Avoidance of sharp or abrasive elements on farms with ongoing infections, as well as avoidance of shared halters, brushes, etc., will help prevent cow-to-cow transmission.

SURGICAL CONSIDERATIONS
None

MEDICATIONS

DRUGS OF CHOICE
• Topical oxytetracycline has shown some benefit in the treatment of PPD of the dewclaw or on the heels, but is less effective on lesions involving the interdigital cleft.
• Drug withdrawal periods must be maintained.

CONTRAINDICATIONS
N/A

PRECAUTIONS
N/A

POSSIBLE INTERACTIONS
N/A

ALTERNATIVE DRUGS
N/A

FOLLOW-UP

PATIENT MONITORING
N/A

PREVENTION/AVOIDANCE
Vaccination of uninfected cattle with an autogenous or commercial vaccination may prevent infection with BPV-1 or BPV-2.

POSSIBLE COMPLICATIONS
Infection with BPV can act as a cofactor in the neoplastic transformation of epithelial cells and the development of SCC and bladder tumors.

EXPECTED COURSE AND PROGNOSIS
• Most papillomas will regress spontaneously within 12 months.
• Animals with severe, generalized fibropapillomatosis have a poor prognosis (> 20% of the body affected).
• Atypical warts do not regress.
• PPD typically requires complete surgical excision for long-term control.

MISCELLANEOUS

ASSOCIATED CONDITIONS
Immunosuppression or defects in T-cell-mediated immunity play a role in the development of diffuse alimentary papillomatosis and generalized cutaneous fibropapillomatosis.

AGE-RELATED FACTORS
Most cattle are infected under 2 years of age.

ZOONOTIC POTENTIAL
None known

PREGNANCY
Lactation cycle can influence regression and recurrence of teat papillomas.

RUMINANT SPECIES AFFECTED
• Cattle are frequently affected.
• Sheep develop lesions similar to bovine papillomas in lightly haired regions such as the ear, muzzle, eye, and vulva.
• There has been successful transmission of papillomas from affected sheep to unaffected sheep using cell- and bacteria-free inocula.
• These lesions in sheep may undergo malignant transformation to SCC.

BIOSECURITY
N/A

PRODUCTION MANAGEMENT
• Vaccination of uninfected cattle with an autogenous or commercial vaccination against the L1 and L2 viral capsid proteins from BPV-2 and BPV-4 may prevent infection.
• Avoidance of sharp or abrasive elements on farms with ongoing infections, as well as avoidance of shared halters, brushes, etc., will help prevent cow-to-cow transmission.

SYNONYMS
Digital dermatitis,
Foot wart
Hairy heel warts
Interdigital papillomatosis
PPD
Strawberry foot rot

SEE ALSO
Dermatophilosis
Squamous cell carcinoma

ABBREVIATIONS
BPV = bovine papilloma virus
Cms = centimeters
Mm = millimeter
PPD = papillomatous digital dermatitis
SCC = squamous cell carcinoma

Suggested Reading
Goldschmidt, M. H. 2002. Tumors of the epidermis. In: *Tumors in domestic animals*, ed. D. J. Meuten. 4th ed. Ames: Iowa State University Press.
Hunt, E. 1984. Infectious skin diseases of cattle. In: *Large Animal Dermatology*. Veterinary Clinics North America, Vol. 6 (1) pp. 155–59
Jarrett, W. F. H., O'Neil, B. W., Gaukroger, J. M., et al. 1990. Studies on vaccination against papillomaviruses: the immunity after infection and vaccination with bovine papillomaviruses of different types. *Vet Rec.* 126:473–75.
Tsirimonaki, E., O'Neil, B. W., Williams, R., Campo, M. S. 2003. Extensive papillomatosis of the bovine upper gastrointestinal tract. *J Comp Path.* 129:93–99.
Vanselow, B. A., Spradbrow, P. B. 1982. Papillomaviruses, papillomas and squamous cell carcinomas in sheep. *Vet Rec.* 110:561–62.
Yeruham, I., Perl, S., Nyska, A. 1996. Skin tumors in cattle and sheep after freeze- or heat-branding. *J Comp Path.* 114:101–6.

Author: Marlene L. Hauck

PARAINFLUENZA-3 (PI-3)

 BASICS

OVERVIEW
• Parainfluenza-3 (PI-3) is an RNA virus in the paramyxovirus family.
• Worldwide distribution
• Infection is very common.

SIGNALMENT
Infection seen most commonly in young animals (2 months to 12 months of age)

SIGNS
• Most infections are subclinical with no detectable signs.
• Coughing, nasal discharge, slight fever, followed by recovery in a few days

CAUSES AND RISK FACTORS
• Aerosol and direct contact are the means of viral spread.
• Close contact, inadequate ventilation, and stress increase likelihood of spread.

 DIAGNOSIS

DIFFERENTIAL DIAGNOSIS
Other mild, uncomplicated viral respiratory infections:
• IBR
• BRSV
• BVDV
• Other viruses (bovine respiratory coronavirus, bovine adenovirus, etc.)

CBC/BIOCHEMISTRY/URINALYSIS
No specific changes

OTHER LABORATORY TESTS
• Virus isolation—lung tissue, transtracheal wash, nasal or laryngeal swab
• Serology
• Positive results on either test may not indicate the primary cause of disease since infection with PI-3 is very widespread.

IMAGING
N/A

DIAGNOSTIC PROCEDURES
N/A

PATHOLOGIC FINDINGS
• Gross lesions—PI-3 lesions are rarely seen on postmortem examination due to the high rate of recovery in uncomplicated cases. Mild inflammation and hyperemia of the mucosa of nasal passages and upper airways, enlargement of the respiratory lymph nodes, and mild pneumonitis may be seen.
• Histopathologic lesions—acute necrotizing bronchitis and bronchiolitis may be seen. Alveoli contain leukocytes, fibrin, and fluid. Cytoplasmic viral inclusion bodies may be seen.

 TREATMENT

• Clinically affected animals should have constant access to fresh, palatable feedstuffs and clean water.
• Animals should be cared for in a low-stress, low-competition environment.

 MEDICATIONS

DRUGS OF CHOICE
• No specific treatment
• Treat as undifferentiated bovine respiratory disease.

CONTRAINDICATIONS
None

POSSIBLE INTERACTIONS
None

 FOLLOW-UP

PATIENT MONITORING
Worsening of clinical signs may indicate secondary bacterial pneumonia (BRDC).

PREVENTION/AVOIDANCE
• Vaccination
• Both killed and modified-live parenteral vaccines are commercially available. Typically, PI-3 is included with other viral antigens in a multivalent vaccine.
• A vaccine for intranasal administration containing temperature-sensitive, modified-live strains of PI-3 and IBR is commercially available.
• Currently, there are no data from field trials supporting an advantage for PI-3 vaccination.
• Nonspecific BRDC prevention measures

POSSIBLE COMPLICATIONS

PI-3 infection can predispose to secondary bacterial pneumonia (BRDC).

EXPECTED COURSE AND PROGNOSIS

Spontaneous recovery following mild course of illness is likely in uncomplicated viral infection.

 MISCELLANEOUS

ASSOCIATED CONDITIONS

BRDC may follow PI-3 infection.

AGE-RELATED FACTORS

Infection is more common in young (2–12 months) animals.

ZOONOTIC POTENTIAL

None

PREGNANCY

Not associated with abortion or teratogenesis

RUMINANT SPECIES AFFECTED

Bovine, ovine, caprine

BIOSECURITY

None. Virus is ubiquitous in most cattle populations.

PRODUCTION MANAGEMENT

Uncomplicated PI-3 infection has minimal to no production importance. However, BRDC is the most economically significant disease in the beef industry.

SEE ALSO

Bovine respiratory disease complex
Bovine respiratory syncytial virus
Infectious bovine rhinotracheitis (bovine herpesvirus-1)

ABBREVIATIONS

BRDC = bovine respiratory disease complex
BRSV = bovine respiratory syncytial virus
BVDV = bovine viral diarrhea virus
IBR = infectious bovine rhinotracheitis (bovine herpesvirus-1)
PI-3 = parainfluenza-3

Suggested Reading

Alkan, F., Ozkul, A., Bilge-Dagalp, S., Yesilbag, K., Oguzoglu, T. C., Akca, Y., Burgu, I. 2000, May. Virological and serological studies on the role of PI-3 virus, BRSV, BVDV and BHV-1 on respiratory infections of cattle. I. The detection of etiological agents by direct immunofluorescence technique. *Dtsch Tierarztl Wochenschr*. 107(5): 193–95.

Kapil, S., Basaraba, R. J. 1997. Infectious bovine rhinotracheitis, parainfluenza-3, and respiratory coronavirus. *Vet Clin North Am: Food Anim Pract*. 13:455–69.

Loneragan, G. H., Gould, D. H., Mason, G. L., Garry, F. B., Yost, G. S., Miles, D. G., Hoffman, B. W., Mills, L. J. 2001, Oct. Involvement of microbial respiratory pathogens in acute interstitial pneumonia in feedlot cattle. *Am J Vet Res*. 62(10): 1519–24.

Morein, B., Hoglund, S., Bergman, R. 1973, Oct. Immunity against parainfluenza-3 virus in cattle: anti-neuraminidase activity in serum and nasal secretion. *Infect Immun*. 8(4): 650–56.

Stott, E. J., Thomas, L. H., Collins, A. P., Crouch, S., Jebbett, J., Smith, G. S., Luther, P. D., Caswell, R. 1980, Oct. A survey of virus infections of the respiratory tract of cattle and their association with disease. *J Hyg (Lond)*. 85(2): 257–70.

Author: William R. DuBois

PARASITE CONTROL ON DAIRIES

 BASICS

DEFINITION
Parasite control programs on dairies are aimed at decreasing clinical and subclinical disease. This is achieved by decreasing the exposure to parasites and by strategic treatment of exposed or infested animals.

OVERVIEW
• Because most internal parasites of cattle require pasture or grasslands in their life cycles, cattle in dry-lot or confinement dairies are at small or no risk for disease from the nematode parasites.
• Dairy cattle or replacements that are pastured are at risk, and parasite control programs should be considered.
• Young cattle are at risk of coccidiosis from oral-fecal contamination when they are raised in groups. Young cattle and cattle in their first year on pasture require parasite control.
• Adult cattle tend to develop immunity to nematodes and coccidia with exposure and may not benefit from anthelmintic treatment. Cattle on highly infected pastures will benefit from treatment.

SYSTEMS AFFECTED
Gastrointestinal, immune, and respiratory

GENETICS
N/A

INCIDENCE/PREVALENCE
• Nematode parasitism is common whenever cattle are pastured. Confined cattle are not at risk of nematode parasitism owing to the life cycle of the parasites.
• The reservoirs for coccidiosis and cryptosporidiosis are primarily the calves in a population, although older cattle can be a source of Coccidia and *Cryptosporidium parvum* on a farm.
• *Neospora* is very common in dairy cattle in North America.

GEOGRAPHIC DISTRIBUTION
Worldwide

Epidemiology
• Cattle exposed to the infectious portion of nematode and liver fluke (pasture) of parasites are at risk.
• Young cattle are at risk for coccidiosis and cryptosporidiosis. Cattle develop immunity to both with exposure history.
• Neosporosis has been associated with canine species interactions (the definitive host) but actual initial infection in a cow or herd has not been documented. Once infected, cattle remain infected and tachyzoites cross the placenta and infect the fetus (vertical transmission).
• Coccidia and cryptosporidia require fecal-oral contamination for transmission, and sanitation is the primary management factor associated with disease from either organism. The reservoir for all of the parasites is older cattle.

SIGNALMENT

Species Affected
Bovine

Breed Predilections
N/A

Mean Age and Range
• Because cattle develop immunity to most parasites with exposure, younger cattle are most susceptible. Exceptions are liver flukes and *Neospora*.
• Mean age and range of clinical disease and infection for cryptosporidia is from 5 days to 3 months and from 21 days to 12 months for coccidiosis.

Predominant Sex
N/A

 DIAGNOSIS

DIFFERENTIAL DIAGNOSIS
N/A

CBC/BIOCHEMISTRY/URINALYSIS
Parasitized cattle may have eosinophilia.

OTHER LABORATORY TESTS
• Fecal egg counts can be used to detect nematode parasitism, but the technique is not specific or sensitive for disease.
• Fecal sedimentation can diagnose liver flukes.
• Coccidia can be visualized on fecal flotation.
• Cryptosporidia can be diagnosed by using acid-fast stains on fecal smears.
• Serology can be used to diagnose cows infected with *Neospora*, but confirmation of abortion requires either necropsy of the fetus with detection of *Neospora* lesions associated with mortality or case-control studies using serology.

IMAGING
N/A

OTHER DIAGNOSTIC PROCEDURES
Necropsy exam with histochemistry is the most sensitive and specific way to diagnose parasitism in cattle.

 TREATMENT

CLIENT EDUCATION
Clients should be advised that they must adhere to the parasite control program in order to achieve decreased parasite loads in the pastures.

 MEDICATIONS

PRECAUTIONS
Anthelmintic drugs should be used only as labeled and the labeled withholding periods must be followed for each drug.

 FOLLOW-UP

PATIENT MONITORING
Fecal egg counts can be used to monitor parasitism in cattle and the effectiveness of the program.

PARASITE CONTROL ON DAIRIES

PREVENTION/AVOIDANCE
Maintain contagious disease control procedures in calves; do not overcrowd pastures.

POSSIBLE COMPLICATIONS
Animals should not be treated with avermectin drugs when the larval migration of *Hypoderma* is near CNS tissue.

 MISCELLANEOUS

Parasites of Dairy Cattle
• The nematode that causes the greatest pathology and economic loss in cattle is *Ostertagia*.
• Other nematodes that infect cattle include: *Cooperia, Haemonchus, Trichostrongylus,* and *Nematodirus*. Lungworms, *Dictyocaulus*, also parasitize cattle.
• Protozoal parasitism in dairy cattle includes coccidiosis from *Isospora* and *Eimeria*, cryptosporidiosis from *C. parvum* and sometimes *C. muris*, and neosporosis from *Neospora caninum*.
• Nematode and lungworm parasite control programs based on avermectins or moxidectin should be used when dairy cattle are grazing.
• A common program is to treat cattle twice early in the grazing season, approximately 6 to 8 weeks apart. Another approach is to treat at the beginning of the pasture season and again at the end. Heavily infested pastures may require treating every 3 weeks with nonivermectin drugs or every 5 weeks with ivermectin. Fecal egg counts can be used to monitor the program and estimate the level of infestation of the pasture.

• Coccidiosis is mainly a disease of young confined animals. The primary prevention measure is sanitation in the calf housing, especially the feed area, because the route of transmission is fecal-oral. Calves raised in individual hutches should not be exposed to coccidia and therefore do not need prophylaxis. The coccidiostats lasalocid or monensin (1 mg/kg bwt continuously) in the feed in group housing prevents clinical disease. Calves develop immunity as they age, and adult cattle do not require coccidiostats. Calves with clinical coccidiosis should be treated with sulfamethazine (110 mg/kg bwt for 5 days).
• Cryptosporidia have a short prepatent period (5 days) and a low infectious dose and often infect young calves. There are no documented effective drugs available for prevention or treatment of cryptosporidia in cattle in the United States. Contagious disease control procedures such as improved sanitation and strict adherence to working only from young to old animals during feeding and treatment should be employed in the calf housing system.
• *Neospora* infection in dairy cattle is common and the main route of transmission is vertical from dam to calf. Cattle are a secondary host for the parasite and are infected for life. *Neospora* can be a cause of second trimester abortions. A vaccine is licensed in the United States to control abortions from *Neospora*.

PREVENTION
N/A

ASSOCIATED CONDITIONS
Anemia, weakness, decreased growth, diarrhea, decreased immune response

AGE-RELATED FACTORS
N/A

ZOONOTIC POTENTIAL
Cryptosporidium parvum is a serious zoonotic pathogen.

PREGNANCY
N/A

SYNONYMS
Bottle jaw

SEE ALSO
Bovine anthelmintics
Bovine parasitology
FARAD
Ostertagia
Serology

ABBREVIATIONS
CNS = central nervous system
FARAD = Food Animal Residue Avoidance Databank

Suggested Reading
Barger, I. 1997, Nov. Control by management. *Vet Parasitol.* 72(3–4):493–500; discussion 500–506.
Coles, G. C. 2002, Aug 10. Sustainable use of anthelmintics in grazing animals. *Vet Rec.* 151(6):165–69.
Gasbarre, L. C., Stout, W. L., Leighton, E. A. 2001, Oct 31. Gastrointestinal nematodes of cattle in the northeastern US: results of a producer survey. *Vet Parasitol.* 101(1): 29–44.
Smith, B. P., ed. 2002. *Large animal internal medicine.* 3rd ed. St. Louis: Mosby.
Stromberg, B. E., Averbeck, G. A. 1999, Jan. The role of parasite epidemiology in the management of grazing cattle. *Int J Parasitol.* 29(1):33–39; discussion 49–50.
Williams, J. C. 1997, Nov. Anthelmintic treatment strategies: current status and future. *Vet Parasitol.* 72(3–4):461–70; discussion 470–77.

Author: Jim Reynolds

PARASITE CONTROL PROGRAMS—SMALL RUMINANTS

BASICS

OVERVIEW
• In most of North America, *Haemonchus contortus* is the most important nematode pathogen of small ruminants and *Trichostrongylus colubriformis* is the next most common and important. *Teladorsagia* (*Ostertagia*) *circumcincta* is an important pathogen in cool climates but is rarely seen in the southern United States. Other species such as *Trichostrongylus axei, Cooperia* spp., *Oesophagostomum, Trichuris ovis, Strongyloides papillosus*, and *Bunostomum* are less common and by themselves usually do not cause important levels of disease.
• The number of FDA-approved drugs available for use in the treatment of parasites in small ruminants is severely limited.
• Extralabel anthelmintic drug use is a standard practice in small ruminants, but this is an exclusive privilege of the veterinary profession and is only permitted when a bona fide veterinarian-client-patient relationship exists and an appropriate medical diagnosis has been made.
• Anthelmintic resistance is extremely prevalent in gastrointestinal nematodes (GIN) of small ruminants and camelids and must be calculated into all treatment decisions.
• Because multiple-drug-resistant parasites are becoming quite prevalent, now and in the future, anthelmintics must be thought of as extremely valuable and limited resources that must be preserved.

• Recipe-based anthelmintic treatment programs can no longer be recommended. An integrated scheme using "smart drenching" principles and a medically based selective approach to treatment should be implemented wherever possible.
• Goats metabolize drugs more rapidly than do other ruminants and therefore should receive a dose one and a half to two times greater than is required for sheep and cattle.

SYSTEMS AFFECTED
Predominantly gastrointestinal

SIGNALMENT
• Ruminants and pseudoruminants of all ages
• Young recently weaned and periparturient animals are at the greatest risk for severe disease.

SIGNS

Haemonchus contortus
Anemia, hypoproteinemia, weakness, weight loss, poor hair coat, death

Other GI Nematodes
Diarrhea, weight loss, anorexia, poor hair coat, and to a much lesser extent than in *H. contortus*, anemia and hypoproteinemia

CAUSES AND RISK FACTORS
• Poor nutrition
• Overstocking of pastures
• Young, recently weaned animals are highly susceptible to infection.
• Periparturient ewes/does from approximately 2 weeks before to 8 weeks after parturition have a clinically significant suppression in immunity of GI nematodes.
• Drug-resistant parasites

DIAGNOSIS

DIFFERENTIAL DIAGNOSES
See Parasitology section of this volume.

CBC/BIOCHEMISTRY/URINALYSIS
N/A

OTHER LABORATORY TESTS
See Parasitology section of this volume.

IMAGING
N/A

DIAGNOSTIC PROCEDURES
N/A

PATHOLOGIC FINDINGS
N/A

TREATMENT
N/A

MEDICATIONS

DRUGS OF CHOICE

CONTRAINDICATIONS
• Appropriate meat and milk withdrawal times must be followed for all anthelmintics administered to food-producing animals.

PARASITE CONTROL PROGRAMS—SMALL RUMINANTS

• Because most anthelmintics used in small ruminants are administered in an extralabel fashion, appropriate withdrawal times will not be listed on the product label, and it is the responsibility of the veterinarian to ensure that appropriate meat and milk withdrawal times are known by the farmer and followed. When in doubt, contact the Food Animal Residue Avoidance Databank (FARAD).

 FOLLOW-UP

N/A

 MISCELLANEOUS

ASSOCIATED CONDITIONS

Haemonchus contortus
Anemia, hypoproteinemia, weakness, weight loss, poor hair coat, death

Other GI Nematodes
Diarrhea, weight loss, anorexia, poor hair coat, and, to a much lesser extent than in *H. contortus*, anemia and hypoproteinemia

AGE-RELATED FACTORS
Young, recently weaned and periparturient animals are at the greatest risk for severe disease.

ZOONOTIC POTENTIAL
N/A

PREGNANCY
Periparturient ewes/does from approximately 2 weeks before to 8 weeks after parturition have a clinically significant suppression in immunity of GI nematodes.

RUMINANT SPECIES AFFECTED
Sheep, goats, and camelids

BIOSECURITY
N/A

PRODUCTION MANAGEMENT

Smart Drenching
Smart drenching is an approach whereby we use the current state of knowledge regarding host physiology, anthelmintic pharmacokinetics, parasite biology, dynamics of the genetic selection process for resistance, and the resistance status of worms on the farm to develop strategies that maximize the effectiveness of treatments while also decreasing the selection of drug resistance. A smart drenching approach requires that a medically-based program be used for parasite control, rather than adherence to some calendar-based recipe. The following are the components to a smart drenching program:

FAMACHA—Selective Rather Than Whole-Herd Treatment
• This is the newest approach to smart drenching and is probably the most important component of a program designed to delay the development of resistance.

• In this method, the ocular mucous membranes of sheep and goats are classified into five categories through color comparison of sheep conjunctivae. Using a laminated color chart illustrating the different classifications, FAMACHA enables identification of individual animals in need of anthelmintic treatment and provides a means to implement a selective treatment program.
• FAMACHA can be used only where *H. contortus* is the primary parasite.

Know the Resistance Status of the Worms Infecting the Herd
• With the prevalence of resistance so high, it is critical that anthelmintic efficacy be determined on each farm and be monitored every 2 to 3 years.
• There are two methods for determining resistance on a farm: (1) perform an on-farm fecal egg count (FEC) reduction test; (2) send in a fecal sample to a lab offering the DrenchRite larval development assay.

Keep Resistant Worms Off the Farm
• Anthelmintic-resistant worms can come from only two sources: either they are home-grown by selection with drug treatment or they are purchased.
• All new additions to the herd or flock should be quarantined in a dry lot (without any grass) or on concrete and aggressively dewormed upon arrival.

PARASITE CONTROL PROGRAMS—SMALL RUMINANTS

• Recommended protocol: withhold feed for 24 hours (free choice water), and then deworm sequentially with moxidectin, levamisole, and albendazole at recommended individual-drug dosage. After 14 days, a FEC should be performed and the animal should be allowed to enter the herd only if the fecal test is negative.

Administer the Proper Dose
• Underdosing exposes worms to sublethal concentrations of drug, which increases the selection for resistance, and several studies have demonstrated that sheep/goat producers often underestimate the weight of their animals.
• Animals should be weighed individually or dosed according to the heaviest animals in the group (except when treating with levamisole in goats where overdosing can be risky).
• Check accuracy of dosing equipment on a regular basis.

Utilize Host Physiology to Maximize Drug Availability and Efficacy
• All oral anthelmintics should be delivered into the rumen. This is accomplished by delivering drugs over the back of the tongue using a properly designed drenching apparatus. Presenting a drench to the buccal cavity, rather than into the pharynx/esophagus, can stimulate closure of the esophageal groove with significant drench bypassing the rumen.
• Once in the rumen, the duration of drug availability as it is absorbed from the rumen and flows to more distal sites of absorption is largely dependent on the flow-rate of the digesta. Restricting feed intake for 24 hours prior to treatment decreases digesta transit flow rate, thereby increasing drug availability and efficacy. This recommendation is most useful for BZ and AM drugs. It is not useful for levamisole.
• Similar increases in efficacy can be achieved by repeating the dose in 12 hours. For levamisole, treatment should be repeated after 24 hours.
• Pour-on formulations designed for cattle are poorly absorbed in small ruminants. If used, these products should be administered only orally.

Drug Selection and Rotation
• Two different anthelmintics (from different drug classes) given together will produce a synergistic effect, which may significantly increase the efficacy of treatment compared to the individual drugs. This synergistic effect is most pronounced when the level of resistance is low, but once high-level resistance to both drugs is present, the synergistic effect will be lost.
• Rotation of anthelmintics is an overblown concept that gives farmers and veterinarians a false sense that they are actually doing something worthwhile in terms of resistance prevention. Rotation actually does very little to prevent the development of anthelmintic resistance, and is not a replacement for proper resistance-prevention measures.
• Instead of a calendar-based rotation, drug choice should be made after considering many factors, the most important of which are the number of drugs that remain effective on that farm (and level of effectiveness) and the degree of parasite-induced illness in the animals being treated.

Reduce the Frequency of Treatment Through the Use of Sound Pasture Management
• Good pasture management can significantly reduce the impact of parasitism and the dependence on dewormers.
• History has taught us that anthelmintics alone will not successfully control parasites and a more sustainable approach to small ruminant parasite control and husbandry is required.
• Managing pastures so that safe grazing areas (low larval contamination) are available will permit movement of animals to a safe area, reducing the number of treatments that are needed.
• To prevent the rapid development of drug resistance, it is important that animals not be treated immediately before a move to safe pasture unless a significant proportion of the animals is left untreated.

• Few parasites are acquired when animals browse forage high off of the ground, therefore browse areas should be utilized as much as possible.
• Reducing stocking rates will greatly decrease the number of parasites that sheep and goats are exposed to and also will improve the quality and quantity of forage available to the animals. Overstocking can often make control of *H. contortus* nearly impossible.

SEE ALSO
FARAD
Ostertagiasis
Parasitic pneumonia
Parasitology chapters
Parelaphostrongylosis
Pediculosis: ovine and caprine

ABBREVIATIONS
AM = avermectin/milbemycins
BZ = benzimidazoles
FARAD = Food Animal Residue Avoidance Databank
FEC = fecal egg count
GIN = gastrointestinal nematodes
I/T = imidazothiazoles/tetrahydropyrimidines

Suggested Reading
Hennessy, D. R. 1997. Physiology, pharmacology and parasitology. *International Journal for Parasitology* 2:145–52.
Kaplan, R. M. 2004. Responding to the emergence of multiple-drug resistant *Haemonchus contortus*: smart drenching and FAMACHA. In: *Proceedings 93rd Annual Meeting of the Kentucky Veterinary Medical Association/31st Annual Mid-America Veterinary Conference*. Lousiville, KY: MAVC.
Mortensen, L. L., Williamson, L. H., Terrill, T. H., Kircher, R., Larsen, M., Kaplan, R. M. 2003. Evaluation of prevalence and clinical implications of anthelmintic resistance in gastrointestinal nematodes of goats. *Journal of the American Veterinary Medical Association* 4:495–500.
Small ruminant parasite control and FAMACHA: www.scsrpc.org
Van Wyk, J. A., Bath, G. F. 2002. The FAMACHA(c) system for managing haemonchosis in sheep and goats by clinically identifying individual animals for treatment. *Veterinary Research* 5:509–29.

Author: Ray M. Kaplan

PARASITE CONTROL PROGRAMS—SMALL RUMINANTS

Table 1

		Approved						
		Commonly Used Anthelmintics in Sheep and Goats						
Drug	Class	Sheep	Goats	Dosage (mg/kg)	How Supplied	Prevalence of Resistance[a]	Meat WDT	Milk WDT for Goats
Ivermectin	AM	Yes	No	Sheep: 0.2 Goats: 0.4	Sheep: oral drench	High	Sheep: 11 days Goats: 14 days	Not approved 8 days
Remarks: Injectable formulation not recommended								
Doramectin	AM	No	No	Sheep: 0.2 Goats: 0.4	Injectable	High	ND	NE
Remarks: Not recommended because residual activity promotes resistance								
Moxidectin	AM	No	No	Sheep: 0.2 Goats: 0.4	Cattle Pour-on	Moderate	Sheep: 14 days Goats: 23 days	NE
Remarks: Only use pour-on product orally. Use sparingly to preserve efficacy. Kills avermectin-resistant *Haemonchus*, but when used in this fashion, resistance to moxidectin may develop rapidly.								
Levamisole	I/T	Yes	No	Sheep: 8.0 Goats: 12.0	Soluble drench powder	Low	Sheep: 3 days Goats: ND	NE
Remarks: Toxic side effects = salivation, restlessness, muscle fasciculations. Recommend weighing goats before treatment.								
Morantel	I/T	No	Yes	10	Feed premix	Moderate to high	30 days	0 days
Remarks: Approved for use in lactating goats								
Fenbendazole	BZ	No[b]	Yes	Sheep: 5.0 Goats: 5.0[c]	Paste Suspension feed block, mineral pellets	High	Goats: 6 days[d] (suspension only)	Not approved 0 days[d]
Albendazole	BZ	Yes	No	Sheep: 7.5 Goats: 15–20	Paste Suspension	High	Sheep: 7 days Goats: ND	NE
Remarks: Do not use within 30 days of conception.								

Note: AM = avermectin/milbemycin; BZ = benzimidazole; I/T = imidazothiazole/tetrahydropyrimidine; WDT = withdrawal time, consult with FARAD for WDTs in small ruminants; NE = milk WDT has not been established in goats; product should not be used in lactating dairy goats; ND = meat withdrawal time has not been established in goats. To be safe, it is probably best to double sheep WDT.

[a]In the southern United States. Prevalence of resistance has not been established elsewhere.

[b]Approved in big-horned sheep and wildlife.

[c]Label dose is 5.0 mg/kg but 10 mg/kg is recommended.

[d]Listed WDTs are for the 5 mg/kg dose. If used at the 10 mg/kg level, these WDTs should be extended.

PARASITIC PNEUMONIA

 BASICS

DEFINITION
Alveolar and interstitial pneumonia in ruminants can be caused by the lungworm *Dictyocaulus viviparus* and aberrant migration of *Ascaris suum* larvae in cattle, and the lungworms *Dictyocaulus filaria*, *Protostrongylus rufescens*, and *Muellerius capillaris* in sheep and goats.

PATHOPHYSIOLOGY
• Generally, lungworms have a prepatent phase when larvae are migrating and adults are not present in large airways, and a patent phase when adults are present in large airways. *D. viviparus* and *D. filaria* have direct life cycles.
• Adults live in the trachea and bronchi, lay eggs, hatch quickly. First larval stage L1 are coughed up, swallowed, passed in feces, then develop in environment. Third larval stage L3 migrate onto grass and are ingested, penetrate intestine, and are taken by lymphatic drainage to mesenteric lymph nodes. Fourth larval stage L4 travel through blood and lymphatics to lungs, lodge in pulmonary capillaries of caudoventral lung lobes, enter alveoli, and molt to adults in bronchioles.
• *P. rufescens* and *M. capillaris* have indirect life cycles.
• Adults live in trachea and bronchi, lay eggs, hatch quickly. L1 are coughed up, swallowed, passed in feces. They enter snail or slug intermediate host, develop to L3. Intermediate host and L3 migrate onto grass and are ingested, penetrate intestine, and are taken by lymphatic drainage to mesenteric lymph nodes. L4 travel through blood and lymphatics to lungs, lodge in pulmonary capillaries of caudoventral lung lobes, enter alveoli, and molt to adults in bronchioles.
• *A. suum* can infect cattle exposed to large amounts of eggs in pens heavily contaminated by swine. Cattle are typically affected about 10 days after exposure, with signs due to allergic reaction to the larvae migrating through the lungs. Larvae in the alveoli initiate allergic reaction, with eosinophilic exudate being produced, causing coughing and tachypnea. More larvae tend to be aspirated into the caudoventral lung lobes, with consolidation developing there and in the interstitium as larvae migrate.

• Adult worms in the trachea and bronchi cause inflammation. Generally, larvae in the alveoli cause inflammatory reaction with eosinophilic exudate blocking bronchioles and causing coughing and tachypnea.
• Adult worms in larger airways cause marked inflammatory response with consolidation of caudoventral lung lobes.

SYSTEMS AFFECTED
Respiratory

GENETICS
N/A

INCIDENCE/PREVALENCE
• Mainly areas with mild climate, high rainfall, intense irrigation, in late summer through fall.
• In southern United States, maximum *D. viviparus* infection in calves may be from December to March.
• Typically occurs in groups of animals on pasture

GEOGRAPHIC DISTRIBUTION
Worldwide, mainly northern temperate climates

SIGNALMENT
Species
All ruminant species
Breed Predilections
• Beef cattle tend to be less affected by *D. viviparus* since management is more extensive, therefore infective larvae are not as concentrated.
• Mainly a disease of dairy calves
Mean Age and Range
• *D. viviparus* infection tends to occur in cattle less than 1 year old, or previously unexposed adults, turned out onto infected pasture.
• Infection also occurs in older cattle, previously infected and considered immune, reinfected when they are moved from nonendemic to endemic areas.
Predominant Sex
N/A

SIGNS
HISTORICAL FINDINGS
Areas of high rainfall or intense irrigation, young animals turned out onto infected pasture, older animals moved from nonendemic to endemic areas

PHYSICAL EXAMINATION FINDINGS
Marked coughing (inconsistent finding in sheep and goats), tachypnea, dyspnea, fever (high fever in *A. suum* larval migration), anorexia, weight loss, harsh breath sounds, and widespread crackles and wheezes on lung auscultation (crackles over dorsal half of lungs in *D. viviparus* infection in cattle)

CAUSES
• Cattle—*D. viviparus*, aberrant migration of *A. suum*
• Sheep and goats—*D. filaria*, adults in trachea and bronchi, most pathogenic. *P. rufescens*, adults in bronchioles, lesions smaller, less pathogenic. *M. capillaris*, adults in lung parenchyma, which become encysted so relatively benign; most common but least pathogenic lungworm of sheep and goats; more pathogenic in goats than in sheep; causes a more diffuse inflammation and interstitial pneumonia in goats.

RISK FACTORS
Exposure to vector (snail or slug) habitat (i.e., marshy land, wet muddy areas around waterholes, areas of high rainfall, intense irrigation)

 DIAGNOSIS

DIFFERENTIAL DIAGNOSIS
• Acute bovine pulmonary emphysema and edema or ABPEE (atypical interstitial pneumonia, fog fever) —cattle over 2 years old suddenly switched from sparse dry forage to lush green pasture.
• Bacterial/viral bronchopneumonia

CBC/BIOCHEMISTRY/URINALYSIS
May see increase in eosinophils from 2 to 6 weeks after infection

OTHER LABORATORY TESTS
Baermann sedimentation technique on feces or fluid from transtracheal aspirate to look for lungworm larvae; need to check several animals in herd

IMAGING
• Radiography—may see consolidation of caudoventral lung lobes
• Endoscopy—may see adult lungworms in large airways

OTHER DIAGNOSTIC PROCEDURES
N/A

PATHOLOGIC FINDINGS

• Prepatent phase—lungs grossly normal, few atelectic lobules in caudoventral lung lobes. May see larvae in microscopic smears of bronchial exudate, and eosinophilic infiltration
• Patent phase—bilaterally symmetrical caudoventral lung consolidation. See adult worms in trachea and bronchi, with hemorrhage and fluid exudate.
• *D. filaria*—adult worms mainly in caudodorsal diaphragmatic lung lobes
• *M. capillaris*—adult worms mainly in lung parenchyma, form grayish nodules 2–3 mm in diameter in subpleural tissue of sheep.

 TREATMENT

ACTIVITY
Restricted movement

DIET
N/A

CLIENT EDUCATION
• Avoid infected pastures
• Vector control (e.g., molluscicides)

 MEDICATIONS

• Ivermectin 0.2 mg/kg SQ
• Fenbendazole 5 mg/kg PO

DRUGS OF CHOICE
See Medications above.

CONTRAINDICATIONS
Appropriate milk and meat withdrawal times must be followed for all compounds administered to food-producing animals.

PRECAUTIONS
Move animals to fresh pasture after treatment to avoid reinfection.

POSSIBLE INTERACTIONS
N/A

ALTERNATIVE DRUGS
N/A

 FOLLOW-UP

N/A

PATIENT MONITORING
N/A

PREVENTION/AVOIDANCE
• Avoid infected pastures
• Vector control (e.g., molluscicides)
• Strategic deworming (e.g., ivermectin at 3, 8, and 13 weeks after turning out on new pasture).

POSSIBLE COMPLICATIONS
N/A

EXPECTED COURSE AND PROGNOSIS
• Good prognosis if animal only has cough and tachypnea
• Guarded prognosis if animal also has dyspnea, fever, or anorexia

 MISCELLANEOUS

ASSOCIATED CONDITIONS
N/A

AGE-RELATED FACTORS
Acute infection in young animals or previously unexposed adults turned out onto infected pasture, or re-infection in older animals previously infected and considered immune and moved from nonendemic to endemic areas.

ZOONOTIC POTENTIAL
N/A

PREGNANCY
Benzimidazoles (e.g., fenbendazole) may be teratogenic in first trimester of pregnancy; use with caution.

RUMINANT SPECIES AFFECTED
All

BIOSECURITY
N/A

PRODUCTION MANAGEMENT
N/A

SYNONYMS
Husk
Parasitic bronchitis
Parasitic pneumonitis
Verminous bronchitis
Verminous pneumonia

SEE ALSO
Acute bovine pulmonary emphysema and edema or ABPEE (atypical interstitial pneumonia, fog fever)
Bacterial/viral bronchopneumonia
FARAD
Specific parasite chapters

ABBREVIATIONS
FARAD = Food Animal Residue Avoidance Databank
ABPEE = acute bovine pulmonary emphysema and edema
PO = per os, by mouth
SQ = subcutaneous

Suggested Reading
Pugh, D. G., ed. 2002. *Sheep and goat medicine*. Philadelphia: W. B. Saunders.
Radostits, O. M., Gay, C. C., Blood, D. C., Hinchcliff, K. W., eds. 2000. *Veterinary medicine*. 9th ed. London: W. B. Saunders.
Smith, B. P., ed. 2002. *Large animal internal medicine*. 3rd ed. St. Louis: Mosby.

Author: David McKenzie

PARASITIC SKIN DISEASES

 BASICS

OVERVIEW
• Mange: parasitic skin disease of ruminants
• Infectious causes include *Chorioptes bovis, Sarcoptes scabiei- var ovis, Psoroptes ovis, Psoroptes cuniculi, Psororegates ovis.*
• In cattle, infestations with *P. ovis* are responsible for a severe dermatitis. The disease is very common in some breeds of beef cattle, whereas dairy cattle such as Friesian-Holstein are considered resistant. Immunological as well as nonimmunological factors may be responsible for the breed-related susceptibility or resistance to *P. ovis.*

SYSTEMS AFFECTED
Skin/exocrine, production management

GENETICS
Unknown

INCIDENCE/PREVALENCE
Unknown

GEOGRAPHIC DISTRIBUTION
• *Chorioptes bovis*—Eradicated and REPORTABLE; seen most often in Europe, New Zealand, and Australia
• *Sarcoptes scabiei-var ovis*—rare, REPORTABLE
• *Psoroptes ovis*—eradicated and REPORTABLE
• *Psoroptes cuniculi*—REPORTABLE in Texas only
• *Psororegates ovis*—REPORTABLE; common in many parts of the world

SIGNALMENT
• Any age or breed; the lesions of psoroptic mange are particularly severe in angora goats.
• Llamas are susceptible to sarcoptic, psoroptic, and chorioptic mange, and symptoms are similar to sheep and goats.

Species/Breed Predilections
Any age or breed may be affected. The lesions of psoroptic mange are particularly severe in angora goats.
Llamas are susceptible to sarcoptic, psoroptic, and chorioptic mange, and symptoms are similar to sheep and goats.
P. ovis is very common in some breeds of beef cattle, whereas dairy cattle such as Friesian-Holstein are considered resistant.

Mean Age and Range
Any age may be affected.

Predominant Sex
N/A

SIGNS
Sarcoptic Mange
• Very pruritic, crusts, scabs, and self-trauma/mutilation
• Goats—lesions may be generalized, lymphadenopathy may be seen.
• Sheep—affects nonwooly skin, usually seen on head and ears initially
• Llamas—thickened skin and lesions similar to sheep and goats

Chorioptic Mange
Pruritic papules, crusts, and ulcers usually start on feet and legs and spread to the hindquarters, scrotum. Can be generalized

Psoroptes Ovis
Pruritic scaly crusts mostly on the wooly parts of the body

Psoroptes Cuniculi
• Ears, causing excess wax production initially, but can spread to head, neck, and body
• Causes significant mohair damage in angora goats

Demodectic Mange
• Nonpruritic
• Goats—nodules and papules on face, neck, shoulders, and sides; nodules contain a thick grayish exudate full of mites.
• Sheep—nodular periocular lesions

Psororegates Ovis
• Pruritic and scaly, lesions on thorax, flanks, and thighs
• May cause weight loss and wool damage

CAUSES AND RISK FACTORS
• Chorioptic and psoroptic mange are seen most often in the winter.
• *Psoroptes cuniculi* is a common mite in rabbits.
• Demodex is a normal skin mite transmitted from the mother to neonate. Underlying diseases may predispose to demodex overgrowth.

 DIAGNOSIS

DIFFERENTIAL DIAGNOSIS
Dermatophilosis, lice, lymphosarcoma, dermatophytosis, photosensitization, *Staphylococcus* sp. dermatitis, tuberculosis, contagious ecthyma (ORF), foot-and-mouth disease, scrapie, poxvirus, pemphigus, herpes, contact dermatitis, trombiculidiasis, nutrient deficiency (selenium, zinc, vitamins A, D, or E), pseudorabies

CBC/BIOCHEMISTRY/UA
CBC may show an inflammatory leukogram.

OTHER LABORATORY TESTS
N/A

DIAGNOSTIC PROCEDURES
• Skin scrapings, biopsy, ear swabs, bacterial culture, and sensitivity
• The practitioner needs to differentiate demodex nodules from the nodules of tuberculosis. Mites may not always be found; a treatment trial may be warranted.

IMAGING
N/A

 TREATMENT

Nonpharmacologic: ensure feeding, management, nutrition, and hygiene procedures are adequate.
All in-contact animals need to be treated.
For reportable conditions, call the state/provincial/governmental veterinarian for specific quarantine and treatments.

 MEDICATIONS

DRUGS OF CHOICE
• Although not always approved for treatment of certain conditions in target species, ivermectin at 0.2 mg/kg SQ (may need to be repeated in 2 weeks) treats most external parasites. The determination of meat and milk drug withdrawal time needs to be determined prior to treatment.
• Various dips are approved for treatment: 2% lime sulfur for use in lactating goats once weekly for 4–12 dips.
• Antibiotics may be indicated for secondary skin infections.
• There are no effective treatments reported for *Demodex,* which may resolve spontaneously. Localized lesions may be incised, expressed, and infused with Lugol's iodine.

CONTRAINDICATIONS
• Steroid use will allow mites to proliferate and is contraindicated.
• Appropriate milk and meat withdrawal times must be followed for all compounds administered to food-producing animals.
• Steroids should not be used in pregnant animals.

 FOLLOW-UP

PATIENT MONITORING
Monitor clinical signs and/or repeat skin scrapings.

PREVENTION/AVOIDANCE
• Quarantine new animals before introducing into the herd/flock.
• *Psoroptes*—2-week life cycle on the host, can live off host for 3 weeks
• *Chorioptes*—2–3-week life cycle, live off host 3 days
• *Sarcoptes*—10–17-day life cycle, life cycle off host is variable
• *Psorergates*—35-day life cycle on host, can live 3–4 days off host

POSSIBLE COMPLICATIONS
Repeat infections are possible.

EXPECTED COURSE AND PROGNOSIS
Prognosis for *Demodex* sp. is guarded, for other mites is fair to good with adequate diagnosis and subsequent treatment.

 MISCELLANEOUS

ASSOCIATED CONDITIONS
• Pruritic, crusts, scabs, and self trauma/mutilation
• Goats—lesions may be generalized, lymphadenopathy may be seen.
• Sheep—affects nonwooly skin, usually seen on head and ears initially
• Llamas—thickened skin and lesions similar to sheep and goats

AGE-RELATED FACTORS

ZOONOTIC POTENTIAL
• *Sarcoptes scabiei* is zoonotic and can cross between species.
• The practitioner needs to differentiate demodex nodules from the nodules of tuberculosis.

PREGNANCY
N/A

BIOSECURITY
• Quarantine new animals before introducing into the herd/flock.
• Isolate affected herd members or whole herds/flocks.
• For reportable conditions, call the state/provincial/governmental veterinarian for specific quarantine and treatments.

RUMINANT SPECIES AFFECTED
All ruminant species

PRODUCTION MANAGEMENT
N/A

SEE ALSO
Contact dermatitis
Contagious ecthyma (ORF)
Dermatitis
Dermatophilosis
Dermatophytosis
FARAD
Foot-and-mouth disease
Herpes
Lice
Lymphosarcoma
Nutrient deficiency (selenium, zinc, vitamins A, D, or E)
Pemphigus
Photosensitization
Poxvirus
Pseudorabies
Scrapie
Staphylococcus sp.
Trombiculidiasis
Tuberculosis

ABBREVIATIONS
SQ = subcutaneous
FARAD = Food Animal Residue Avoidance Databank
ORF = contagious ecthyma
CBC = complete blood count
SQ = subcutaneous

Suggested Reading
Aiello, S. E., ed. 1998. *Merck veterinary manual*. 8th ed. Whitehouse Station, NJ: Merck & Co.
Losson, B. J., Lonneux, J. F., Lekimme, M. 1999, Jun 30. The pathology of *Psoroptes ovis* infestation in cattle with a special emphasis on breed difference. *Vet Parasitol*. 83(3–4):219–29.
Rehbein, S., Visser, M., Winter, R., Maciel, A. E. 2002, Dec. Efficacy of a new long-acting formulation of ivermectin and other injectable avermectins against induced *Psoroptes ovis* infestations in cattle. *Parasitol Res*. 88(12):1061–65. Epub 2002, Aug 13.
Rehbein, S., Visser, M., Winter, R., Trommer, B., Matthes, H. F., Maciel, A. E., Marley, S. E. 2003, Jun 25. Productivity effects of bovine mange and control with ivermectin. *Vet Parasitol*. 114(4):267–84.
Rooney, K.A., Illyes, E.F., Sunderland, S.J., Sarasola, P., Hendrickx, M.O. Keller, D.S., Meinert, T.R., Logan, N.B., Weatherley, A.J., Conder, G.A. 1999, Apr. Efficacy of a pour-on formulation of doramectin against lice, mites, and grubs of cattle. *Am J Vet Res*. 60(4):402–4.
Warnick, L. D., Nydam, D., Maciel, A., Guard, C. L., Wade, S. E. 2002, Jul 15. Udder cleft dermatitis and sarcoptic mange in a dairy herd. *J Am Vet Med Assoc*. 221(2):273–76.

Author: Melissa N. Carr

PARELAPHOSTRONGYLUS TENUIS: CEREBROSPINAL NEMATODIASIS

BASICS

DEFINITION
Aberrant migration of the larvae of *Parelaphostrongylus tenuis* into the central nervous system of small ruminants, camelids, and certain cervidae species.

PATHOPHYSIOLOGY
• The natural host for *P. tenuis* is the white-tailed deer (*Odocoileus virginianus*). Clinical signs or pathological findings associated with *P. tenuis* infestation in this species are rare. In white-tailed deer, adult meningeal worms reside in the subdural space and the cranial venous sinuses.
• Eggs laid in the meninges develop, hatch, penetrate blood vessels, and are carried to the lungs, whereas eggs deposited in the venous circulation are carried to the lungs where they embryonate and hatch. The first stage larvae move up the bronchi and trachea, are ingested, pass in the feces, and penetrate certain terrestrial slugs and snails.
• Development of infective larvae within the intermediate host requires three to four weeks. Ingesting infested slugs and snails infects white-tailed deer.
• Ingested larvae penetrate the abomasal wall, migrate through the peritoneal cavity via nerves to the dorsal gray columns of the spinal cord, and become adults in 20 to 30 days. They then migrate to the subarachnoid space, probably by the dorsal nerve rootlets.
• The prepatent period is approximately 90 days, and the life cycle is complete in 4 months.
• When aberrant hosts such as sheep, goats, camelids, and certain cervidae ingest infected snails and slugs, the larvae are released in the gut and migrate to the spinal cord and/or brain where they may cause inflammation and neural tissue damage. Generally, they do not reach maturity.

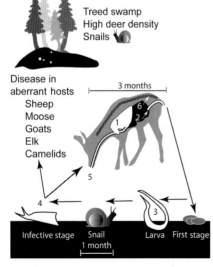

Treed swamp
High deer density
Snails

Disease in aberrant hosts
Sheep
Moose
Goats
Elk
Camelids

3 months

6
1 2
4 5
3

Infective stage   Snail   Larva   First stage
                   1 month

Figure 1.

SYSTEMS AFFECTED
Nervous

GENETICS
There is no known genetic basis for this condition.

INCIDENCE/PREVALANCE
There are no published reports regarding the incidence/prevalence of this condition.

GEOGRAPHIC DISTRIBUTION
The distribution of this problem reflects the range of the white-tailed deer, which is southern Canada, conterminous United States with the exception of parts of the Southwest, Mexico to Bolivia, and northeast Brazil. Additionally, the intermediate hosts (snails and slugs) prefer low-lying to swampy areas that have trees.

SIGNALMENT
Species
Sheep, goats, camelids, and certain species of cervidae including moose, elk, antelope, reindeer

Breed Predilection
There is no reported breed predilection. However, this problem is more likely to occur in animals that graze low-lying, treed areas with a high density of white-tailed deer. Therefore, it is more frequently observed in goats managed for meat and/or fiber rather than dairy goats based on housing differences. Meat and fiber animals are more likely to have access to pasture, whereas dairy goats more frequently are housed with limited access to pasture.

Mean Age and Range
Most clinically affected animals are at least 6 months of age, which may reflect the time required from ingestion of infective larvae to their arrival in the nervous system.

Predominant Sex
There is no sex predilection associated with this condition.

SIGNS
• The clinical signs vary and depend upon the number of migrating parasites present and the portion or portions of the nervous system affected. Both upper and lower motor neuron and brain signs have been reported including:
  • Blindness
  • Circling
  • Lameness
  • Paralysis and/or ataxia in one or more limbs (may see a dog sitting posture if both hind limbs are affected)
  • Paresis
  • Spastic gait
• The observed signs may change as the migratory pattern of the parasites change, they may remain static, spontaneous recovery may occur, especially if the neurologic damage is minor, or the animal may die. If only the spinal cord is involved, an affected animal will appear bright and alert, and usually display a normal appetite.

• Brain involvement can produce a variety of clinical signs that may mimic other central nervous system diseases.

CAUSES AND RISK FACTORS
• The major cause for cerebrospinal nematodiasis in North America is *Parelaphostrongylus tenuis*; however, other parasites such as *Oestrus ovis* and *Coenurus cerebralis* have also been reported.
• The major risk factor for infestation is grazing low-lying, treed pastures in the late summer and into the fall that are cohabited by the natural host for *P. tenuis* the white-tailed deer. After a killing frost, the risk for infestation to occur when susceptible animals utilize these types of pastures is greatly decreased.

DIFFERENTIAL DIAGNOSIS
The following list of rule-outs should be considered when brain-related neurologic signs are observed:
• Caprine arthritis-encephalitis (goats less than 6 months of age)
• Encephalitic listeriosis
• Heat stress (camelids)
• Metabolic disease
• Polioencephalomalacia
• Rabies
• Scrapie (rare in goats)
• Space occupying lesion in the brain, especially abscess
• Toxicity (lead, salt, plants)
• Trauma
The following list of rule-outs should be considered when spinal cord and/or peripheral nerve-related signs are observed:
• Heat stress (camelids)
• Metabolic disease
• Myositis
• Nutritional deficiencies, especially copper and vitamin E and selenium
• Rabies
• Space occupying lesion in or around the spinal cord, especially abscess
• Trauma

CBC/BIOCHEMISTRY/URINALYSIS/OTHER LABORATORY TESTS
There are no specific tests for diagnosis of *P. tenuis,* however, a complete blood count, serum chemistry analysis, and urinalysis may be useful to rule in or rule out other conditions.

IMAGING
There are no specific imaging examinations for detecting this condition, although these tests are useful for detecting spinal cord or brain trauma, and space-occupying lesions, which are differential diagnoses for the condition.

CEREBROSPINAL FLUID (CSF) ANALYSIS
The most useful ancillary diagnostic aid is CSF cytology and detection of an eosinophilic pleocytosis. Although this is not pathognomonic for *P. tenuis,* it is highly suggestive for cerebrospinal nematodiasis. A mononuclear pleocytosis may also be observed and is less specific for parasite migration.

PARELAPHOSTRONGYLUS TENUIS: CEREBROSPINAL NEMATODIASIS

PATHOLOGIC FINDINGS
There are no detectable gross postmortem findings. A definitive diagnosis requires histopathologic identification of the parasite within the brain or spinal cord.

TREATMENT
Nursing Care
• The amount of supportive care needed will be determined by the extent and location of the neurological damage in an affected animal. For example, an animal with mild impairment at the level of the spinal cord, associated with paresis in one or two limbs and no loss of appetite would require minimal assistance. In such cases, an animal should be penned by itself or with a few nonaggressive companions, in an area that is well bedded with a nonskid floor.
• Food and water should be readily accessible. Encouraging mild to moderate exercise is important to promoting muscle strength and function.
• Animals showing more severe signs, such as paralysis of the forelimbs, hind limbs (dog sitting posture), or both, will require intensive nursing care. This may include using a sling or a water floatation tank to support the animal and provide physical therapy. Food and water need to be immediately accessible.
• Animals that have signs associated with brain level lesions present the greatest challenge since these animals are often recumbent and inappetant. Besides physical therapy, enteral feeding via stomach tube or temporary rumen fistula may be required. Parenteral nutrition via intravenous feeding may also be a consideration.

CLIENT EDUCATION
Damaged nervous tissue may take 6 months or longer to heal, or for an animal to develop compensatory skills. It is useful to discuss with a client the fact that the more severe the neurologic damage, the poorer the prognosis, and, if recovery is to occur, it may take a long time and require intensive nursing care.

SURGICAL CONSIDERATIONS
NA

MEDICATIONS

DRUG(S) OF CHOICE
• Anthelmintic
• Fenbendazole—20 to 50 mg/kg, PO q24 for 5 days
• Anti-inflammatory
Flunixin meglumine—1 mg/kg IV (the preferred route since this product results in tissue irritation when used IM or SQ), q12, for 2 to 3 days
Dexamethazone— 0.1 mg/kg, IV, IM or SQ (Avoidance of the IM is recommended in food-producing animals to avoid injection-site lesions.) CAUTION: Do not use in pregnant animals since it may induce abortion.

• Vitamins and mineral supplements
• E/Se, B-complex, A, D—use as directed on an individual product label

CONTRAINDICATIONS
Appropriate milk and meat withdrawal times must be followed for all compounds administered to food-producing animals.

PRECAUTIONS
• An animal's pregnancy status is an important consideration if steroid-type anti-inflammatory drugs are being considered in the treatment protocol. Drugs such as dexamethazone may induce abortion.
• Use of anthelmintic products in the avermectin family (ivermectin) are not recommended for treatment. These products do not cross an intact blood brain barrier. With inflammation, as may be present with this disease, these products may cross and result in a toxic reaction (lethargy, ataxia, recumbency, death). Because the signs of toxicity resemble clinical signs of meningeal worm infestation, it may be difficult to identify a toxic reaction.

POSSIBLE INTERACTIONS
None

ALTERNATIVE DRUGS
NA

FOLLOW-UP

PATIENT MONITORING
See nursing care.

PREVENTION/AVOIDANCE
Prevention is directed toward the following:
1. Minimize exposure of susceptible animals to infected snails. In locations that have four distinct seasons, the potential for animals to ingest snails infested with the infective third-stage larvae of *P. tenuis* is greatest in late summer until the first killing frost. Therefore, restricting access to low-lying, snail and deer infested pastures during this time is recommended. During hot, dry summers, snail population growth will be inhibited; therefore, pasture access may be continued longer into the summer. Cool, moist summers will favor snail population growth, which will prompt limiting pasture access earlier in the season. In milder climates, access to these pastures should be restricted year round.
2. Strategic anthelmintic treatments. Before *P. tenuis* migrates into the CNS, it is susceptible to several commercially available products including ivermectin and fenbendazole using dosages recommended for treatment of gastrointestinal parasites in the species. The recommended interval of therapy varies from every 4 to 6 weeks to every 3 to 4 weeks since there may be some species and individual animal differences in how rapidly infective larvae reach the CNS. For some management

situations, using a continuous treatment approach with the addition of a product to the feed or providing it in combination with a supplement block may be effective and less labor intensive.

POSSIBLE COMPLICATIONS
NA

EXPECTED COURSE AND PROGNOSIS
See nursing care and client education.

MISCELLANEOUS

ASSOCIATED CONDITIONS
N/A

AGE-RELATED FACTORS
Because of the life cycle of the parasite, snail, and animal, it would be rare to see this problem in an animal that is less than 4 to 6 months of age.

ZOONOTIC POTENTIAL
None

PREGNANCY
See medications/contraindications.

RUMINANT SPECIES AFFECTED
Sheep, goats, camelids, and certain species of cervidae including moose, elk, antelope, reindeer

BIOSECURITY
N/A

PRODUCTION MANAGEMENT
See prevention/avoidance.

SYNONYMS
Deer worm, brain worm, meningeal worm

SEE ALSO
Caprine arthritis-encephalitis (goats less than 6 months of age)
Encephalitic listeriosis
Heat stress (camelids)
Metabolic disease
Polioencephalomalacia
Rabies
Scrapie (rare in goats)
Space occupying lesion in the brain, especially abscess
Toxicity (lead, salt, plants)
Trauma

ABBREVIATIONS
CNS= central nervous system
CSF= cerebral spinal fluid
IM= intramuscular
IV= intravenous
PO= per os, by mouth
SQ= subcutaneous

Suggested Reading
Fowler, M. E. 1989. *Medicine and surgery of South American camelids*, 2d ed. Ames: Iowa State University Press.
Smith, M. C., Sherman, D. M. 1994. *Goat medicine*. Philadelphia: Lea and Febiger.

Author: Michelle Kopcha

PATENT URACHUS

 BASICS

OVERVIEW
• The urachus connects the fetal bladder and the allantoic sac during gestation.
• The urachus normally shrinks and closes after birth and becomes the vestigial round ligament of the bladder.
• Patent urachus is the result of a persistent urachal stalk that remains open and dribbles urine in the neonate.
• This condition is much less common in calves than in foals.
• Patent urachus may predispose the neonate to septicemia.

SYSTEMS AFFECTED
Production management, musculoskeletal, hemolymphatic, urinary

GENETICS
N/A

INCIDENCE/PREVALENCE
N/A

GEOGRAPHIC DISTRIBUTION
Worldwide, depending on species

SIGNALMENT
Sporadic postnatal condition of calves, lambs, and kids; has been diagnosed in the white rhinoceros calf (*Ceratotherium simum simum*).

Species
Potentially all ruminant species

Breed Predilections
N/A

Mean Age and Range
N/A

Predominant Sex
N/A

SIGNS
The cardinal clinical sign of patent urachus is dribbling of urine from the umbilicus.

CAUSES AND RISK FACTORS
Umbilical infection may contribute to the development of patent urachus.

 DIAGNOSIS

DIFFERENTIAL DIAGNOSIS
Other umbilical masses, such as persistent urachus, urachal cyst, umbilical abscess, umbilical hernia, infected umbilical arteries, vein, and/or urachus

CBC/BIOCHEMISTRY/URINALYSIS
• A neutrophilic leukocytosis and hyperfibrinogenemia may be present in cases of septicemia.
• Neonates with concurrent failure of passive transfer usually have a low plasma protein level.

OTHER LABORATORY TESTS
BUN and creatinine analysis of the fluid should be identical to urine.

IMAGING
Ultrasonography may confirm that the structure attaches to the urinary bladder.

DIAGNOSTIC PROCEDURES
N/A

PATHOLOGIC FINDINGS
N/A

TREATMENT

• If the urachus does not close by 24 hours after birth, surgical resection is suggested to decrease the chances of development of septicemia.
• Surgical intervention also allows removal of other umbilical structures that may be affected.
• Surgery involves a ventral midline laparotomy with resection of the urachus and the tip of the bladder.
• If surgical resection can not be performed, broad-spectrum antimicrobial therapy should be initiated and the urachus chemically cauterized with silver nitrate or 7% iodine to promote closure.

MEDICATIONS

DRUGS OF CHOICE

Broad-spectrum parenteral antibiotics to prevent septicemia should be administered whether surgical or medical therapy is chosen.

CONTRAINDICATIONS

Appropriate milk and meat withdrawal times must be followed for all compounds administered to food-producing animals.

FOLLOW-UP

N/A

MISCELLANEOUS

ASSOCIATED CONDITIONS

Patent urachus may predispose the neonate to septicemia.

AGE-RELATED FACTORS

Sporadic postnatal condition

ZOONOTIC POTENTIAL

N/A

PREGNANCY

N/A

RUMINANT SPECIES AFFECTED

Potentially, all ruminant species can be affected.

BIOSECURITY

N/A

PRODUCTION MANAGEMENT

N/A

SYNONYMS

N/A

SEE ALSO

Failure of passive transfer
Neutrophilic leukocytosis
Septicemia
Umbilical abscess
Umbilical hernia

ABBREVIATIONS

BUN = blood urea nitrogen

Suggested Reading
Hunt, R. J., Allen, D., Jr. 1989, Apr. Treatment of patent urachus associated with a congenital imperforate urethra in a calf. *Cornell Vet.* 79(2): 157–60.
Langan, J., Ramsay, E., Schumacher, J., Chism, T., Adair, S. 2001, Mar. Diagnosis and management of a patent urachus in a white rhinoceros calf (*Ceratotherium simum simum*). *J Zoo Wildl Med.* 32(1): 118–22.
Stone, W. C., Bjorling, D. E., Trostle, S. S., Hanson, P. D., Markel, M. D. 1997, Apr 1. Prepubic urethrostomy for relief of urethral obstruction in a sheep and a goat. *J Am Vet Med Assoc.* 210(7): 939–41.
Wolfe, D. F., Moll, H. D. 1998. *Large animal urogenital surgery.* 2nd ed. Philadelphia. Williams and Wilkins.

Author: M. S. Gill

PEDICULOSIS OF SHEEP AND GOATS

BASICS

OVERVIEW
• Lice are small wingless insects 1 to 2 mm long belonging to the order Phthiraptera.
• Two suborders of lice are ectoparasites of veterinary importance: Mallophaga (biting/chewing lice), and Anoplura (sucking lice).
• Lice are highly specific with respect to host species.
• Sheep lice are specific with respect to the part of the body that is colonized.
• Lice are permanently ectoparasitic, spending the entire life cycle on the host.
• Transmission is by direct close contact.
• The most economically important species is the sheep body louse *Bovicola ovis.*

SYSTEMS AFFECTED
Skin, production management

GENETICS
N/A

INCIDENCE/PREVALENCE
Unknown

GEOGRAPHIC DISTRIBUTION
• Lice of sheep and goats have worldwide distribution, except *Linognathus africanus*, which is restricted to the subtropics.
• The ked, a wingless blood-sucking fly of the family Hippoboscidae, is an obligate ectoparasite with worldwide distribution.

SIGNALMENT
Species
Sheep and goats

Breed Predilections
N/A

Mean Age and Range
All age groups can be affected, but heavy infestation of preweaning animals is rare.

Predominant Sex
N/A

SIGNS
• Sheep infested with *Bovicola ovis* are irritated by the lice. Lousy sheep bite at their fleece and rub against fences, posts, and trees.

• The greatest numbers of lice are in the fleece along the dorsal midline near the withers, on the sides of the body between the elbow and flank, and along the throat.
• The fleece is damaged and wool lost from the fleece accumulates on structures within the sheep's environment.
• The fleece becomes felted (cotted), contains increased amounts of wool grease and suint, and is discolored yellow/brown.
• *Bovicola ovis* infestation has been linked to the pelt fault "cockle."
• Sheep keds cause signs of annoyance resembling heavy louse infestation. The wool is stained brown and has a musty odor.
• Local induration of the skin around ked bites results in "ked-cockle" of pelts.

HISTORICAL FINDINGS
Sheep
• Biting: *Bovicola ovis* (body louse)
• Sucking: *Linognathus pedalis* (foot louse), *Linognathus ovillus* (face louse), and *Lignonathus africanus* (African sheep louse/blue louse)
• Ked: *Melophagus ovinus*

Goats
• Biting: *Bovicola caprae* (common/milch goats), *Bovicola limbatus* and *Bovicola crassipes* (Angora goats)
• Sucking: *Linognathus stenopsis*
• Ked: *Melophagus ovinus* (rare).

Ecology
• Lice are sensitive to temperature and humidity.
• In temperate regions, louse populations on pastured sheep are greatest during the cooler months.
• *Bovicola ovis* infestation is absent from permanently very hot, dry areas.

CAUSES AND RISK FACTORS
Heavy lice infestation often reflects debilitation.

DIAGNOSIS

DIFFERENTIAL DIAGNOSES
Mite infestation, pruritic diseases, photosensitivity, topical allergies

CBC/BIOCHEMISTRY/URINALYSIS
N/A

OTHER LABORATORY TESTS
N/A

IMAGING
N/A

DIAGNOSTIC PROCEDURES
• Part the fleece to examine the staple for lice.
• Body lice cluster within the fleece, therefore multiple sites must be examined.
• Adult keds, pupae, and ked feces are readily apparent in the fleece. The wool is stained by ked feces and has a characteristic musty odor.

PATHOLOGIC FINDINGS
N/A

TREATMENT
Flocks can be kept free of lice and keds if strict quarantine is employed to prevent infestation.

MEDICATIONS

DRUGS OF CHOICE
• Saturation dipping with either synthetic pyrethroid or organophosphate insecticides eliminates louse infestation, if animals are thoroughly wetted to the skin.
• Saturation dipping is most effective if performed 6 to 8 weeks after shearing.
• Pour-on synthetic pyrethroid formulations can eliminate lice or reduce louse numbers, depending on wool length and type.
• Formulations of available insecticides vary widely. Recommendations for treatment must match the formulation, the treatment type (saturation/pour-on), the wool length, and the wool type, while taking into account seasonal factors and withholding periods.
• To achieve satisfactory results, the manufacturer's instructions must be followed precisely.
• Strict attention must be paid to worker health and safety, and environmental waste management.
• Eradication requires simultaneous treatment of the entire flock.

CONTRAINDICATIONS
• Diarrhea and fecal soiling: the dip-wash used for saturation dipping rapidly becomes polluted. Some formulations of chemical become adsorbed to organic particulates, then settle out and are degraded.
• Foot rot and foot abscesses: the dip-wash becomes contaminated with bacteria.
• Dirty/dusty sheep: the dip-wash becomes contaminated with dirt.
• Saturation dipping of sheep with long wool is ineffective because the dip-wash fails to penetrate the fleece to the skin.
• Appropriate milk and meat withdrawal times must be followed for all compounds administered to food-producing animals.
• Steroids should not be used in pregnant animals.

 FOLLOW-UP

PATIENT MONITORING
N/A

PREVENTION/AVOIDANCE
Maintain strict herd/flock quarantine.

POSSIBLE COMPLICATIONS
• Treatment failure due to inadequate insecticide application
• Immersion plunge or saturation shower dipping with heavily contaminated dip-wash can result in "post-dipping lameness"; a septic arthritis caused by *Erysipelothrix rhusiopathiae*.
• Saturation dipping late in the day, with insufficient time for sheep to dry before nightfall, can precipitate pneumonia, dermatophilosis ("mycotic" dermatitis) caused by *Dermatophilus congolensis*, fleece rot caused by *Pseudomonas aeruginosa*, or wool discoloration from chromogenic bacteria.

• Plunge or shower dipping sheep with unhealed shearing cuts can result in pyogenic infections, clostridial malignant edema, tetanus, other necrotizing anaerobic infections, and caseous lymphadenitis.
• Unrested sheep that are saturation dipped while hot are prone to pneumonia.

EXPECTED COURSE AND PROGNOSIS
Persistent without treatment

 MISCELLANEOUS

ASSOCIATED CONDITIONS
Melophagus ovinus transmits the nonpathogenic *Trypanosoma melophagium*.

AGE-RELATED FACTORS
All age groups can be affected, but heavy infestation of preweaning animals is rare.

ZOONOTIC POTENTIAL
N/A

PREGNANCY
N/A

RUMINANT SPECIES AFFECTED
Sheep and goats

BIOSECURITY
• Flocks can be kept free of lice and keds if strict quarantine is employed to prevent infestation.
• Isolation and quarantine of new stock entering the herd/flock
• Treat and or cull new animals for disease conditions prior to herd introduction.

PRODUCTION MANAGEMENT
Some countries have statutory provisions with respect to livestock movement and insecticide dipping in order to prevent lice spreading to noninfested properties.

SYNONYMS
Body louse
Face louse
Foot louse

SEE ALSO
Alopecia
Differential diagnosis of skin disease
Keds
Mites
Pruritus

ABBREVIATIONS
N/A

Suggested Reading
Bates, P. 1999, Aug 7. Control of sheep ectoparasites using shower dips, spray races, and jetting wands. *Vet Rec.* 145(6):175.
Coop, R. L., Taylor, M. A., Jacobs, D. E., Jackson, F. 2002, Feb. Ectoparasites: recent advances in control. *Trends Parasitol.* 18(2):55–56.
James, P. J., Riley, M. J. 2004, Sep. The prevalence of lice on sheep and control practices in South Australia. *Aust Vet J.* 82(9):563–68.
Kaufmann, J. 1996. *Parasitic infections of domestic animals, a diagnostic manual*. Basel; Boston; Berlin: Birkhäuser Verlag.
Taylor, M. A. 2001, May. Recent developments in ectoparasiticides. *Vet J.* 161(3):253–68.
Willadsen, P. 1997, Jul 31. Novel vaccines for ectoparasites. *Vet Parasitol.* 71(2–3):209–22.

Author: A. D. (Sandy) McLachlan

PENILE DEVIATIONS

 BASICS

OVERVIEW
• Penile deviation is a common cause of copulation failure in bulls.
• The heritability of penile deviation is low.
• The spiral or corkscrew penile deviation is the most common deviation observed in bulls.
• Spiral deviation of the penis occurs at the peak of erection.
• Up to 50% of normal bulls have been shown to develop spiral deviation during copulation.
• Spiral deviation is often noticed in normal bulls during masturbation, following intromission, and when erection is produced by an electroejaculator; it is not considered pathologic until its occurrence is observed on repeated natural breeding trials in which it occurs prior to intromission.
• Ventral or rainbow deviation is less common than spiral and also prevents intromission.
• S-shaped penile deviation is relatively rare.
• Lateral deviations may occur secondary to trauma of the penis or prepuce when resultant scars or adhesions of the elastic tissue pull the penis to one side or the other.

SIGNALMENT
The majority of penile deviations occur in the polled beef breeds such as polled Hereford and Angus.

SIGNS
• The spiral configuration, caused by the dorsal apical ligament slipping off to the left, results in a counterclockwise spiral of the penis as viewed from the rear.
• Ventral penile deviation occurs when the dorsal apical ligament is thin and stretched to the point that it is incapable of holding up the distal portion of the penis during erection.
• S-shaped deviation occurs when the dorsal apical ligament is sufficient in strength but insufficient in length resulting in the characteristic S-shape during erection

CAUSES AND RISK FACTORS
• Spiral deviation occurs in bulls between 2 1/2 and 5 years of age.
• The S-shaped deviation usually occurs in older bulls with an excessively long penis.

 DIAGNOSIS

DIFFERENTIAL DIAGNOSIS
Ventral penile deviation may be confused with persistent frenulum, which can also result in ventral position of the penis during erection.

CBC/BIOCHEMISTRY/URINALYSIS
N/A

OTHER LABORATORY TESTS
N/A

IMAGING
N/A

DIAGNOSTIC PROCEDURES
• Corkscrew deviation can only be definitively diagnosed by observation of its occurrence during natural breeding attempts.
• Ventral deviation can be diagnosed with the use of an electroejaculator.

PATHOLOGIC FINDINGS
Abnormalities of the dorsal apical ligament may result in corkscrew, ventral, or S-shaped deviations.

 TREATMENT

• The fascia lata or mesh implant techniques are used for repair of both spiral and ventral penile deviations.
• The objective of these techniques is to surgically create a firm union of the dorsal apical ligament to the tunica albuginea to prevent slippage or stretching of the dorsal apical ligament.
• There is no surgical treatment for S-shaped deviations.
• Lateral deviations may be corrected by careful removal of scar tissue.

 MEDICATIONS

DRUGS OF CHOICE
Postoperative antibiotics are administered for 7 days after surgical treatment.

CONTRAINDICATIONS
Appropriate milk and meat withdrawal times must be followed for all compounds administered to food-producing animals.

 FOLLOW-UP

The prognosis for return to breeding soundness after surgery is considered more favorable with spiral than ventral deviations.

 MISCELLANEOUS

Bulls undergoing surgical correction of penile deviations can be used for breeding at 60 days postop.

ASSOCIATED CONDITIONS
N/A

AGE-RELATED FACTORS
• Spiral deviation occurs in bulls between 2 1/2 and 5 years of age.
• The S-shaped deviation usually occurs in older bulls with an excessively long penis.

ZOONOTIC POTENTIAL
N/A

PREGNANCY
Repeat breeders, decreased conception rate

RUMINANT SPECIES AFFECTED
Primarily beef bulls

BIOSECURITY
N/A

PRODUCTION MANAGEMENT
• Breeding soundness examination of all breeding bulls
• Genetic selection

SYNONYMS
N/A

SEE ALSO
Beef bull management
Penile hematoma
Penile prolapse

ABBREVIATIONS
N/A

Suggested Reading
St. Jean, G. 1995, March. Male reproductive surgery. In: *Veterinary clinics of North America: food animal practice, soft tissue surgery*, ed. B. L. Hull, D. M. Rings. Philadelphia: W. B. Saunders.

Author: M. S. Gill

BASICS

OVERVIEW
• Hematoma of the penis, also referred to as "ruptured penis," "broken penis," or "fractured penis," is common in bovine species and rare in others
• Penile hematoma occurs during coitus when the cow slips or goes down under the weight of the bull or when the penis is thrust against the perineum of the cow during breeding attempts.
• The corpus cavernosum penis (CCP) is a closed system, and during erection, blood pressure within the CCP may exceed 14,000 mm of Hg.
• Sudden angulation of the penis may increase the blood pressure and result in a hematoma.
• Penile hematoma results from a tear of the tunica albuginea into the CCP; the tear usually occurs on the dorsum of the penis at the distal sigmoid flexure opposite the insertion of the retractor penis muscles where the tunica albuginea is thinner.
• Tears in the tunica albuginea are between 2–7.5 cm long, transverse, and usually do not extend over 180° circumferentially.
• The swelling due to hematoma is a result of blood from the CCP being forced into the peripenile tissues.
• The size of the hematoma is not related to the length of the tear in the tunica albuginea but to the number of coital attempts the bull makes following rupture.

SIGNALMENT
• Aggressive young bulls used in range breeding are prone to penile hematomas.
• Heavy beef bulls, commonly 2- to 4-year-old Herefords, have been reported to be predisposed to penile hematoma.
• Recurrence of penile hematoma is common, but surgical repair lessens the risk; 50% recur with medical treatment but only 25% recur with surgical treatment.

SIGNS
• Diagnosis is based on physical exam and the presence of a large swelling immediately cranial to the scrotum.
• Owners often first notice the presence of a prolapsed prepuce, which may result secondary to the swelling of the hematoma.
• The swelling is soft until the clot begins to form by about the fourth day; by 10 days the clot begins to organize and the swelling becomes quite firm.
• Bruising of the skin over the hematoma may be apparent in light-skinned bulls.

CAUSES AND RISK FACTORS
• Sudden angulation of the penis during erection may result in rupture of the tunica albuginea and hematoma formation.

• Factors contributing to penile hematoma might include excessive body weight causing awkwardness, partial desensitization, or deviations of the penis.

DIAGNOSIS

DIFFERENTIAL DIAGNOSIS
Preputial abscess and rupture of the urethra can be confused with the swelling created by a penile hematoma.

CBC/BIOCHEMISTRY/URINALYSIS
N/A

OTHER LABORATORY TESTS
N/A

IMAGING
N/A

DIAGNOSTIC PROCEDURES
Physical examination; ultrasonography

PATHOLOGIC FINDINGS
N/A

TREATMENT

• Medical treatment consists of parenteral antibiotics, warm local hydrotherapy for 2–3 weeks, and sexual rest for 60–90 days; spontaneous recovery occurs in > 50% of the cases given 90 days sexual rest.
• Surgical treatment involves removal of the blood clots and repair of the rent in the tunica albuginea.
• Surgery should be performed between 5 and 10 days posttrauma; a second chance for surgical repair is after 21 days when fibrosis dissipates.
• Surgical repair probably reduces the incidence of complications.
• Sexual rest should be provided for 60 days after surgery.

MEDICATIONS

DRUGS OF CHOICE
Parenteral antibiotics may be administered for 10 days during medical therapy or for 10 days postoperatively if surgery is performed.

CONTRAINDICATIONS
Appropriate milk and meat withdrawal times must be followed for all compounds administered to food-producing animals.

FOLLOW-UP

Undesirable sequelae that may occur secondary to penile hematoma and/or its treatment include recurrence of the hematoma, adhesions of elastic layers to the tunica albuginea or to the skin preventing complete extension of the penis, analgesia of the penis due to damage of the dorsal penile nerve, abscessation, or vascular shunts.

MISCELLANEOUS

ASSOCIATED CONDITIONS
Recurrence of penile hematoma is common, but surgical repair lessens the risk; 50% recur with medical treatment but only 25% recur with surgical treatment.

AGE-RELATED FACTORS
• Aggressive young bulls used in range breeding are prone to penile hematoma.
• Heavy beef bulls, commonly 2- to 4-year-old Herefords, have been reported to be predisposed to penile hematoma.

ZOONOTIC POTENTIAL
N/A

PREGNANCY
Reduced breeding rate may occur if the condition is not detected early.

RUMINANT SPECIES AFFECTED
Primarily beef bulls

BIOSECURITY
N/A

PRODUCTION MANAGEMENT
• Body condition scoring bulls to reduce excessive body weight
• Bull selection programs based on conformation

SYNONYMS
Broken penis
Fractured penis
Ruptured penis

SEE ALSO
Beef bull behavior
Beef bull management
Body condition scoring: beef
Penile deviation
Penile prolapse

ABBREVIATION
CCP = corpus cavernosum penis

Suggested Reading
St. Jean, G. 1995, March. Male reproductive surgery. In: *Veterinary clinics of North America: food animal practice, soft tissue surgery*, ed. B. L. Hull, D. M. Rings. Philadelphia: W. B. Saunders.

Author: M. S. Gill

PERICARDITIS

BASICS

DEFINITION
Inflammation of the pericardium that results in accumulation of fluid or exudate within the pericardial sac

OVERVIEW
• Uncommon disease
• In cattle, most commonly seen as traumatic pericarditis following perforation of pericardial sac by an infected, metallic, foreign body originating from the reticulum
• Less frequently occurs as result of blood-borne infection (septicemia) or direct extension of infection (pleuropneumonia, pleuritis, myocarditis)
• Three forms described: (1) effusive pericarditis with nonseptic fluid accumulation in pericardial sac, (2) fibrinous pericarditis with accumulation of fibrin ± fluid in pericardial sac, and (3) constrictive pericarditis with fibrosis and thickening of the pericardial sac
• Most cases are fibrinous and septic in ruminants but occasionally are idiopathic and nonseptic.

PATHOPHYSIOLOGY
• Results from trauma, hematogenous or direct spread of infection, or idiopathic
• Initially, inflammation of pericardium with hyperemia, fibrin deposition, and little exudate results in pain and "rubbing" sound when pericardium and epicardium move together during heart movement.
• As fluid accumulates in the pericardial sac, friction sounds decrease, heart sounds become muffled, and tachycardia progresses.
• Heart chambers become compressed due to presence of fluid and fibrin leading to incomplete filling and congestive heart failure.
• Gas will also be present in sac if infection is due to a gas-producing organism.

• Suppurative pericarditis results in toxemia following systemic absorption of bacterial toxins.
• Nonsuppurative pericarditis: fluid is resorbed and adhesion(s) formed between pericardium and epicardium during recovery stage.
• Suppurative pericarditis may result in organization of adhesion(s) and restriction of cardiac movement, and heart failure.
• Necropsy lesions
  • Fluid accumulation in pericardial sac
  • Fibrin tags on pericardial and epicardial surfaces
  • Thickening of epicardium and pericardium
  • ±Pericardium adhered to epicardium
  • Lesions of congestive heart failure
  • Embolic lesions to other organs

SIGNALMENT
• Seen worldwide
• Mature cattle
• Goats may be slightly more prone to disease than sheep because of eating habits.
• No sex or breed predilection

SIGNS
Septic Pericarditis
• *Early stages*
  • Pain, hypophagia, tachypnea, intermittent fever, elbow abduction, arched back
  • Tachycardia, pain on palpation of thoracic wall over cardiac region, "friction rub" on auscultation of heart
  • ±Signs of pnemonia, pleural effusion, peritonitis
• *As fluid accumulates in pericardial sac*
  • Muffling of heart sounds
  • Bilateral jugular distention ± abnormal pulsation
  • "Splashing or washing machine murmur" with heart beat if gas is present in pericardium
  • Decreased palpability of apex beat
  • Expanded area of cardiac dullness
  • Progressive tachycardia

• Weakened peripheral pulses
• Dyspnea
• Lung sound over ventral thorax may be decreased.
• Signs of toxemia
• Signs of congestive heart failure
• Death or survival
• Survivors experience stage of chronic pericarditis with additional signs
  • Myocarditis
  • ±Arrhythmias
  • Return of more normal heart sounds and heart rate as effusion resolves
• Complete recovery is uncommon

CAUSES AND RISK FACTORS
• In cattle, most commonly traumatic in origin secondary to "Hardware Disease"
• Extension from other focus of infection (i.e., pleuropneumonia)
• Secondary to lymphoma or other neoplasm
• Component of diseases causing polyserositis
• Idiopathic
• Penetrating foreign body
• Hypoproteinemia
• In goats: pericardial effusion or pericarditis seen with mycoplasmosis, viral goat dermatitis, false blackleg, enterotoxemia due to *Clostridium perfringens* type D, and caprine tuberculosis

DIAGNOSIS

• Suspected based on findings of pericardial rub or "sloushing" sound with heart beat, muffling of heart sound, venous congestion, and decreased pulse pressure
• Confirmed based on echocardiography and pericardiocentesis
• History and physical examination
  • Tachycardia
  • Pleural friction rub

- Muffling of heart sounds
- Decreased pulse pressure
- Venous congestion
- ±Fever
- ±Obvious sites of infection
- Complete blood cell count and fibrinogen concentration
- Echocardiography
  - Most valuable diagnostic procedure
  - Differential effusive from fibrinous pericarditis
- Pericardiocentesis
  - Fluid analysis (cell counts, protein concentration) and cytology
  - Bacterial and mycoplasma culture and sensitivity
  - Isolation of viral agent
  - Fluid not useful for diagnosis of heartwater (cowdriosis)
  - With systemic mycoplasmosis, organism is better isolated from other sites.
- Thoracic radiography
  - May be of limited value if pleural effusion present
  - Difficult to accurately evaluate size and shape of heart in mature cattle.
  - Serum chemistry panel often reflects accompanying changes in other organ(s).

DIFFERENTIAL DIAGNOSIS

- Pasteurellosis or mycoplasmosis in cattle, sheep, and goats
- Cattle: Black disease, infection with *Haemophilus* spp., *Pseudomonas aeruginosa*, *Actinobacillus suis*, sporadic bovine encephalomyelitis, tuberculosis
- Sheep and goats: *Staphylococcus aureus* infection

- Infectious endocarditis
- Right- or congestive heart failure
- Pleuropneumonia/pleuritis
- Mediastinal or pleural abscess or mass
- Hydropericardium
  - Gossypol toxicity
  - Clostridial intoxication in sheep
  - Lymphomatosis
- Toxic myocardial necrosis
- Heartwater (cowdriosis) in Africa and Caribbean

CBC/BIOCHEMICAL/URINALYSIS

- Complete blood cell count
  - ±Anemia of chronic disease
  - Primarily leukocytosis ± left shift; monocytosis
  - May have leukopenia with left shift
  - Hyperfibrinogenemia
  - Cattle have less consistent leukocyte response compared to other species.
- Serum chemistry panel often reflects accompanying changes in other organ systems, hydration status, or hypophagia.
  - Azotemia
  - Elevated GGT
  - Elevated creatine kinase if recumbent
  - Electrolyte or acid-base abnormalities from anorexia

OTHER LABORATORY TESTS

IMAGING

- Echocardiography
  - Determine presence, amount, and character of pericardial effusion

- Determine presence of chamber collapse; usually right atrium first and then right ventricle, followed by left side as fluid accumulation increases.
- Interventricular septal motion is increased or paradoxical.
- Pericardial effusion is imaged between the pericardium and epicardium, around both ventricles with less between the descending aorta and left ventricular free wall.
- Clear anechoic effusion is most consistent with a transudate.
- More echogenic fluid with fibrin is typical of septic or traumatic pericarditis.
- Thoracic radiography
  - Evaluate size and shape of heart—difficult in mature cattle.
  - Cardiomegaly, obscured cardiac silhouette, vena cava, and diaphragm, dorsal displacement of trachea
  - Enlarged pericardium, fluid line with gas cap above it
  - Determine presence and character of pleural fluid, evaluate lung parenchyma.
  - ±Identify metallic foreign body.

DIAGNOSTIC PROCEDURES

- Echocardiography
- Pericardiocentesis
  - Cattle: 18-gauge spinal needle (4–8 inches) or small chest tube
  - Clip and surgically prepare site on left thorax
  - Inject local anesthetic over dorsal aspect of 6th rib and around front of it blocking skin and subcutaneous tissue down to parietal pleura.

- Skin puncture with scalpel in left 5th intercostal space just dorsal to elbow
- Needle or trocar is advanced through skin incision, at the anterior aspect of the 6th rib.
- Normal pericardial fluid has protein content of < 2.5 g/dl; cell count < 5000/μl; mononuclear cell is predominant cell type.
- Goats: One source recommends using the right 4th intercostal space low on the chest wall as the procedure site to avoid lung and coronary arteries. Animal maybe standing or in lateral recumbency. Chemical restraint is advisable, diazepam.
- Risks: pneumothorax, cardiac puncture, hemorrhage due to laceration of coronary artery or myocardium, death from fatal arrhythmia or cardiac tamponade, contamination of pleural space with pericardial fluid
- Electrocardiogram
  - Diminished amplitude of QRS complexes
  - Arrhythmia present
  - Electrical alternans in cattle
- Thoracic radiographs

 TREATMENT

Septic Pericarditis
- Treatment is long term, costly, and often unsuccessful.
- Rumenotomy to remove penetrating foreign body, if present
- Ideally, choice of antimicrobial agents is based on culture and sensitivity results on pericardial fluid.
- Broad-spectrum, parenteral, bactericidal, antimicrobial therapy administered when causative agent not is identified
- Analgesic and anti-inflammatory drugs as needed
- Pericardiocentesis to drain fluid and lavage of pericardial space with isotonic, nonirritating fluid followed by installation of antimicrobial drug
- If unresponsive, thorocotomy and pericardectomy or pericardiostomy to provide drainage or to perform marsupialization of pericardium to body wall
- Diuretics and restriction of dietary salt if congestive heart failure is present
- Supportive care to maintain hydration and nutritional status and electrolyte and acid-base balance
- Appropriate treatment of secondary organ disease or dysfunction
- Early withdrawal of therapy may result in relapse.
- Often, extralabel use of antimicrobial is required because few are labeled for long-term therapy.

Idiopathic Effusive Pericarditis
- Drain fluid from pericardial sac.
- Corticosteroid therapy or nonsteroidal anti-inflammatory drugs; caution in pregnant animals (abortifactant)

- Supportive care to maintain hydration and nutritional status and electrolyte and acid-base balance
- Diuretics and restriction of dietary salt if congestive heart failure is present

 MEDICATIONS

DRUGS OF CHOICE
- Penicillin: 22,000 IU/kg: Aqueous potassium penicillin IV QID or procaine penicillin IM BID
- Amoxillin: 10 mg/kg IM BID
- ±Rifampin: 5 mg/kg PO BID, as supplemental therapy to enhance antibiotic penetration into lesion
- Anti-inflammatories
  - Flunixin meglumine (Banamine) 1.1 mg/kg SID or 0.5 mg/kg BID (caution: may induce abomasal ulcers)
  - Aspirin: 30–100 mg/kg PO every 12 to 24 hours
- Furosemide: 0.5 to 1.0 mg/kg IV every 12 to 24 hours
- Potassium supplement (50– 200 g/day PO) if on potassium-wasting diuretics
- Appropriate milk and meat withdrawal times must be followed for all compounds administered to food-producing animals.

FOLLOW-UP

EXPECTED COURSE AND PROGNOSIS
• Complete recovery is uncommon with septic pericarditis.
• Prognosis for septic pericarditis is not better than guarded (30%).
• Chronicity of condition is a major factor in outcome.

MISCELLANEOUS

ASSOCIATED CONDITIONS
• Reticuloperitonitis
• Cardiac arrhythmias including sinus tachycardia, premature ventricular contractions, and atrial fibrillation
• Toxemia
• Septic embolism to other organs
• Congestive heart failure
• Myocardial disease.

ZOONOTIC POTENTIAL
N/A

RUMINANT SPECIES AFFECTED
• Cattle
• Goats
• Sheep: kid with traumatic pericarditis

BIOSECURITY
N/A

PRODUCTION MANAGEMENT
• Prevention of traumatic reticulopericarditis and hardware disease is best management.
• Management to prevent exposure to metal objects; prophylactic magnet administration

SEE ALSO
Cattle: Black disease, infection with *Haemophilus* spp., *Pseudomonas aeruginosa*, *Actinobacillus suis*, sporadic bovine encephalomyelitis, tuberculosis
Heartwater (cowdriosis) in Africa and Caribbean
Hydropericardium
Gossypol toxicity
Clostridial intoxication in sheep
Lymphomatosis
Infectious endocarditis
Mediastinal or pleural abscess or mass
Pasteurellosis or mycoplasmosis in cattle, sheep, and goats
Pleuropneumonia/pleuritis
Right- or congestive heart failure
Sections on traumatic reticuloperitonitis (Hardware disease)
Sheep and goats: *Staphylococcus aureus* infection
Toxic myocardial necrosis

ABBREVIATIONS
BID = twice daily
GGT = gamma glutamyl transpeptidase
IM = intramuscular
IV= intravenous
PO = per os, by mouth
QID = four times daily
SID = once daily

Suggested Reading
Pugh, D. G. 2002. Diseases of the integumentary system. In: *Sheep and goat medicine*. Philadelphia: W. B. Saunders.
Radostits, O. M., Gay, C. C., Blood, D. C., Hinchcliff, K. W. 1999. Diseases of the heart. In: *Veterinary medicine: a textbook of diseases of cattle, sheep, pigs, goats and horses*, 9th ed., pp. 389–91. New York: W. B. Saunders.
Reef, V. B. 1998. Cardiovascular ultrasound. In: *Equine diagnostic ultrasound*, pp. 254–55. Philadelphia: W. B. Saunders.
Reef, V. B., McGuirk, S. 2002. Diseases of the cardiovascular system. In: *Large animal internal medicine*, ed. B. Smith, 3rd ed. St. Louis: Mosby.
Smith, M. C., Sherman, D. M. 1994. *Goat medicine*, pp. 233, 236. Philadelphia: Lea & Febiger.
Sojka, J. E., et al. 1990. An unusual case of traumatic pericarditis in a cow. *J Vet Diagn Invest* 2:139–42.

Authors: Susan Semrad and Sheila McGuirk

PERINATAL LAMB MORTALITY

BASICS

OVERVIEW
• Lamb mortality data suggest a regional lamb loss pattern influenced by weather, management practices, nutrition, housing, and genetic factors.
• Preweaning loss typically consumes 10%–35% of the annual lamb crop and is often viewed by producers as a "normal" event.
• Diseases involving neonates usually occur with little warning, consequences to the newborn are severe, and treatment is unrewarding. Consequently, prevention is more important than individual animal treatment.
• Prevention program strategy requires basic knowledge of when, where, and how lamb losses occur and the association involving management decisions and mortality.

Categorizing Lamb Losses
• Timing— most losses occur during first week of life (see Figure 1).
   • Especially first through third day following birth

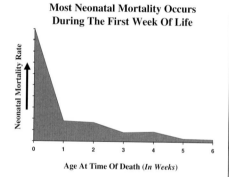

Most Neonatal Mortality Occurs During The First Week Of Life

Figure 1.

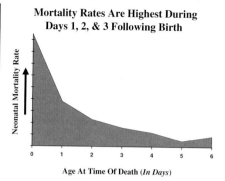

Mortality Rates Are Highest During Days 1, 2, & 3 Following Birth

Figure 2.

• Losses occurring during last 3 weeks of gestation and first 3 weeks following birth: prepartum (15% of mortality); partum (20% of mortality); postpartum (65% of mortality) (see Figure 2)
• Causes—management practices can both prevent and contribute to mortality.
   • Most due to management, not infectious processes
   • Intensive management systems increase importance of infectious diseases.
   • On-the-farm gross postmortem examination is useful in grouping losses into very basic categories.
   • Categorization focuses control measures
   • Four broad loss categories define 70%– 80% of mortality: (1) starvation, hypothermia, and exposure; (2) stillbirth or stillbirth/dystocia; (3) pneumonia; and (4) abortion (see Table 1).

Postmortem Examination of the Lamb
Gross postmortem by practitioner
• Economical means of confirming cause
• Diagnostic lab—for persistent or undiagnosed problems
• Educational tool for producers
• Examine all to document flock trends
• Focus control programs by classifying into four to six basic categories
• Caution: Use caution (especially women of childbearing age) when handling dead lambs and placentas, especially if abortion is a problem.

Production Management Summary
• Major losses occur early in life
   • Four major areas of loss with individual flock patterns
   • Often unable to affect change during the same lambing season
• Individual flock mortality information is a useful tool for directing disease control measures toward the appropriate management problem.
• Production goals for lamb loss
   • Less than 5% loss, difficult to achieve
   • 5%–10% range, a good goal
   • 15%–20% and up is typical
• Prevention programs should encompass environment, weather, forage resources, available markets, disease prevention, nutrition, genetic selection, maternal behavior, and labor and facility resources.

Table 1

Gross Postmortem Guide for Categorizing Ten Common Flock Loss Patterns			

Suggestive Lesions/Common Observations			
External	Thorax	Abdomen	Comments

1. Stillbirth (SB)

Term lamb by weight and wool	Adequate SQ fat cover over ribs	No excess fluid or blood	Stillborn lambs are a good
Commercial lambs 9–11 lb	Absence of rib fractures and bruising	Abomasum contains serum-colored	"normal" for comparing and
No evidence of fetal death	to chest wall	fluid and no milk	contrasting findings during
Wool tight to skin	Absence of SQ serosanguinous fluid	Kidney fat normal amount and	other postmortem exams
Lack of fetid odor	No excess fluid or blood in chest	color (tan fat)	SB typically involves 3%–5% of
No deformities	Nonaerated purple-colored lung	No adhesions, abscesses, or	the annual lamb crop
Covered w/ mucus	with liverlike consistency	discolored bowel	Difficult to reduce below the
Feet rounded and soft w/clean	Normal amount of fat in coronary	Liver firm, intact, and not swollen	3%–5% level
soles	groove		
Umbilical cord fresh, not dry			

2. Stillbirth Related to Dystocia (Same as SB above except. . .)

Meconium staining:	Rib fractures	Ruptured liver with blood in	Owner history may be helpful
mustard-colored mucus	• Bruising	abdomen common	Some lambs may exhibit small
Swollen tongue, head, limb, or	• Obvious fractures	Umbilical or abdominal herniation	areas of partially inflated lung
tail	• Blood in chest from lacerated	due to maternal straining	tissue resulting from attempts
Found in a position suggesting	veins or arteries, usually not		to breathe
dystocia	clotted		
	Agonal hemorrhage on pleural		
	surface common		

3. Hypothermia/Starvation Complex (H/S)[1]

Simple Hypothermia	Simple Hypothermia	Simple Hypothermia	50% of all lambs that die during
Less than 6 hr old	Lungs: pink, spongy, and inflated	Abomasum: may/may not contain	the first week of life die from
Often still wet	Small amount of serum-colored fluid	milk	H/S Complex
Weather and exposure +/– able	in thorax	Perirenal tan fat present, not	Presence and amount of milk in
to rise	Coronary groove fat present	depleted	abomasum can be variable.
If recumbent, rounded, soft, clean	External rib fat not depleted: same	Hypothermia 2⁰ to starvation	If weather severe, H/S can occur
soles	as SB lamb	Abomasum usually empty, thick,	in lambs with a full stomach!
If stood and walked, soles worn,	Evidence of rib trauma may/may not	muscular, and contracted	Milk may also be given by owner
hard w/ manure and dirt	be 2⁰ to H/S	Perirenal fat depleted	just prior to death
Umbilical cord fresh	Hypothermia 2⁰ to Starvation	Kidney easily visualized	In older lambs, often presence of
Hypothermia 2⁰ to Starvation	Lungs: pink, spongy, and inflated	Depleted fat a "watery"/ dark	odd feed and no milk.
Over 6 hr old	Coronary groove fat depleted	purple color	Brown/tan fat depletion and
Usually dry	External rib fat depleted	Adrenal gland enlarged and easily	adrenal gland changes most
Severe weather exposure	Evidence of rib trauma may/may	visualized	obvious if weather more
may/may not be present	not be 2⁰ to H/S		conducive to lamb survival (i.e.,
Evidence of standing and			lambs survives long enough for
walking: Soles worn, hard, and			changes to occur)
coated with manure/dirt			

4. Pneumonia

Usually > 4 hr old	Sharp line of demarcation between	Often concurrent lesions due to H/S	In farm flock management
Usually dry	normal pink/spongy and	or other causes: 1⁰ or 2⁰	systems losses occur very early
Evidence of standing and	consolidated red/purple affected	cause/effect relationship	in life.
walking: soles worn, hard, and	lung tissue	Abomasal ulcers common (stress)	
coated with manure/dirt	Cranioventral orientation to lesions:		
Weather often transitional	Abscesses +/–		
	Adhesions+/–Septicemia		
	• Entire lung purple and edematous		
	• Pericardial fluid +/– fibrin clots		
	• Petechial hemorrhage on heart		
	surface		

(Continued)

PERINATAL LAMB MORTALITY

Table 1

(Continued)			

Suggestive Lesions/Common Observations			
External	Thorax	Abdomen	Comments

5. Abortion

Campylobacteriosis Previously vibriosis Abortion, stillbirths, and weak lambs that die shortly after birth Abortions @ 132 days of gestation Fetus +/− "potbellied" appearance Ewes not sick Placenta unremarkable History: outside ewes added to flock *Toxoplasmosis* Abortion, stillbirth, mummified fetuses, weak lambs, open ewes Mummified fetuses common White focal 1–2 mm lesions on cotyledons No intercotyledonary lesions *Chlamydia (EAE)* Abortion, stillbirth, weak lambs Sick ewes Placenta Necrotic cotyledon Thickened intercotyledonary areas May occur in successive years	*Campylobacteriosis* Similar to SB lambs Often areas of partial inflation due to immature lung function (respiratory distress syndrome) *Toxoplasmosis* Lungs vary from stillbirth, normal to mummified Thoracic fluid: Toxoplasma titer good field diagnostic tool *Chlamydia (EAE)* Lungs vary from stillbirth to normal	*Campylobacteriosis* Serosanguinous fluid SQ Liver swollen (+/−) Gray/tan doughnut-shaped necrotic foci in liver *Toxoplasmosis* Variable: normal, mummified to stillbirth appearance *Chlamydia (EAE)* Variable: normal to stillbirth	Independent of cause, most occur during last month of gestation Individual farm problem usually 5%–25% rate 1%–2% rate considered "normal" Transmission oral via ingestion

6. Trauma

Fractured limbs Owner history Often 2⁰ to H/S, dystocia, and processing procedures	Fractured ribs Hemothorax Punctured lung	Ruptured liver Hemoperitoneum • Liver rupture • Postcastration • Postdocking	Suspect blood loss when generalized pallor to tissues

7. Scours

E. coli • First week of life • Mostly day 2 to 4 • Affected lambs down and dead within 24 to 48 hr Tail and rump area wet from scours Watery, white, feces *Coccidiosis* Common in 4–6-week-old lambs Rectal straining Blood in feces rare	*E. coli* Normal inflated lungs Septicemia: Petechial hemorrhage on heart surface *Coccidiosis* Normal inflated lungs	*E. coli* Bowel: thin, distended, fluid-filled, and discolored Perforation w/ adhesions and peritonitis often secondary *Coccidiosis* Bowel: thin, distended, fluid-filled	Secondary lesions consistent with H/S common Individual flock problem Often related to transitional weather

8. Navel-ill (Joint-ill)

Common in lambs 10–30 days old Thin/weight loss Lameness/swollen, infected joints	Normal inflated lungs 2⁰ pneumonia common	Liver abscesses Peritonitis Thick, infected umbilical vessels	Common following transitional weather Common in 2–3-week old lambs

(Continued)

Table 1

		(Continued)	
	Suggestive Lesions/Common Observations		
External	Thorax	Abdomen	Comments

9. Intestinal Blockages

Bloated, distended tight abdomen History of abdominal pain	Normal inflated lungs	Purple bowel discoloration localized to area of blockage: misdiagnosis as overeating disease Volvulus, torsion intussusception Strangulation of abdominal hernia	Common in lambs raised on milk replacer

10. Enterotoxemia (*Clostridium perfringens* type C & D)

Sudden death Type C: 1–3-day-old lambs Similar to *E. coli* except diarrhea rare Type D: lambs older than 4 weeks of age • Common in creep fed and feedlot lambs • Exception: common in orphan lambs on replacer	Normal inflated lungs Pericardial fluid +/− fibrin clots +/− petechial hemorrhage on heart surface	Type C— bowel • Milk engorged abomasum • Hemorrhagic abomasitis Type D—bowel • Change often minimal • Petechial hemorrhage • Purple bowel	

Note: 2^0 = secondary.

[1]Answer these three basic postmortem questions: (1) Did it breathe? (2) Did it nurse? (3) Fat cover?

MISCELLANEOUS

ZOONOTIC POTENTIAL
Caution: Use caution (especially women of childbearing age) when handling dead lambs and placentas, especially if investigating an abortion problem.

PRODUCTION MANAGEMENT
See Categorizing Lamb Losses above.

SYNONYMS
Lamb mortality
Neonatal mortality
Postmortem examination
Preweaning losses

SEE ALSO
See Categorizing Lamb Losses above.

ABBREVIATIONS
@ = at
EAE = enzootic abortion in ewes
H/S = hypothermia and starvation complex
(+/−) = may or may not be present
1^0 & 2^0 = primary and secondary
SB = stillbirth
SQ = subcutaneous
w/ = with

Suggested Reading
Daniel, J. A., Held, J. E., Brake, D. G., Wulf, D. M., Epperson, W. B. 2006. Evaluation of the prevalence and onset of lung lesions and their impact on growth of lambs. *Am J Vet Res.* 67: 890–94.

Kahn, C. M. (ed) 2006. Health-management interaction: sheep: introduction. In: *Merck veterinary manual.* Whitehouse State, New Jersey:Merck & Co., Inc.
Goodwin, K. A., Jackson, R., Brown, C., Davies, P. R., Morris, R. S., Perkins, N. R. 2005. Pneumonic lesions in lambs in New Zealand: patterns of prevalence and effects on production. *NZ Vet J.* 53:91–2.
Rook, J. S., Scholman, G., et al. 1990, Nov. Diagnosis and control of neonatal losses in sheep. *Advances in Sheep and Goat Medicine—The Veterinary Clinics of North America* 6(4):531–63.

Author: Joseph S. Rook

PERIORBITAL STAPHYLOCOCCAL DERMATITIS

BASICS

DEFINITION
• Periorbital facial dermatitis is a contagious bacterial infection of sheep caused by *Staphylococcus aureus*.
• This is of major economic impact as more than 50% of a flock can be affected and affected ewes may not suckle lambs.

PATHOPHYSIOLOGY
• Caused by combination of microtrauma to the skin and rapid replication of resident *S. aureus* organisms found in the nostrils and on the skin.
• Microtrauma to the skin of the face and legs may occur from trauma that occurs during feeding at troughs or while feeding on rough pastures (i..e., thistles).
• Large numbers of bacteria are found in the exudate and readily transmitted by direct contact to other sheep.
• Death is uncommon, but the infection may invade the deep dermal and subcutaneous tissues causing sepsis and ulcers.
• Immunity is short-lived as reinfection can occur within 40 days of resolution.

SYSTEMS AFFECTED
Skin

GENETICS
N/A

INCIDENCE/PREVALENCE
• Highly contagious and up to 50% of a flock may be affected
• Most common in later winter and early spring

GEOGRAPHIC DISTRIBUTION
Worldwide

SIGNALMENT
Most commonly affects adult sheep, no sex or breed predisposition

SIGNS
• Blood smears on face are often first signs; lesions bleed easily and large amounts of blood may be found on the face and wool.
• Small ulcers at site are found upon closer inspection especially on the nasal and maxillary bones, orbital rim, ears, and base of horns.
• Lesions involve both the pigmented and unpigmented skin of the face, and are present over the nasal and maxillary bones and around the eyes, ears, and base of horns.
• Swollen, painful necrotic ulcers exuding blood and pus are found at affected sites.
• Affected sites ulcerate and may be 4–5 cm in diameter and with time will form scabs that bleed readily if removed.
• Ulcerated areas heal by granulation tissue.
• Lesions take up to 1 month to heal, and it can take several months before disease resolves in a flock.
• Staphylococcal lesions may develop on the legs, udders, and teats of affected sheep.
• Mastitis may occur in sheep if teat/udder is involved.
• Affected sheep are afebrile and have normal appetites.

CAUSES AND RISK FACTORS
• Disease is caused by various strains of *S. aureus* that produce coagulase positive alpha, beta, and gamma hemolysins.
• Organism enters skin through small penetrating wounds around the face.
• The disease is highly contagious among sheep and is spread by close head-to-head contact among sheep.
• Overcrowding, inadequate space at feed troughs, and cold, wet weather may predispose sheep to disease.
• Disease is most common in sheep housed outdoors in winter and spring.

DIAGNOSIS

DIFFERENTIAL DIAGNOSIS
• Culture is needed to confirm diagnosis because ulcers on teats and udders can also be caused by *Pasturella haemolytica*.
• Lesions on the legs must be differentiated from dermatophilosis.
• Photosensitization caused by pithomycotoxicosis (facial eczema) occurs in the summer and autumn and is associated with liver toxicity; death is common.

CBC/BIOCHEMICAL/URINALYSIS
N/A

OTHER LABORATORY TESTS
N/A

IMAGING
N/A

DIAGNOSTIC PROCEDURES
Bacterial culture and sensitivity and isolation of *S. aureus*

PATHOLOGICAL FINDINGS
Skin biopsy shows suppurative intraepidermal pustular dermatitis and superficial folliculitis.

PERIORBITAL STAPHYLOCOCCAL DERMATITIS

TREATMENT

- Affected sheep should be separated from flock.
- Lesions will usually self-heal within several weeks.
- Individual sheep may benefit from parenteral antibiotic and hydrotherapy to remove exudate.
- Topical antibiotics and/or drying agents (iodine, chlorhexidine) applied to open ulcers may prevent secondary colonization of the lesions by other bacteria and speed healing.
- Trough space should be increased to limit contact of heads.
- Clinically affected sheep should be removed from flock to avoid spread of this contagious disease.

MEDICATIONS

Parenteral antibiotics selected through culture and susceptibility testing with sensitivity to the strain of *Staphylococcus aureus*

CONTRAINDICATIONS

- Appropriate milk and meat withdrawal times must be followed for all compounds administered to food-producing animals.
- Steroids should not be used in pregnant animals.

FOLLOW-UP

PATIENT MONITORING
N/A

PREVENTION/AVOIDANCE
Increase space at feed troughs to minimize head to head contact.

POSSIBLE COMPLICATIONS
- Mastitis in ewes
- Reluctance of ewes to suckle lambs

EXPECTED COURSE AND PROGROSIS
Outbreaks in a herd/flock may take several months to run their course.

MISCELLANEOUS

ASSOCIATED CONDITIONS
Mastitis

AGE-RELATED FACTORS
N/A

ZOONOTIC POTENTIAL
S. aureus is a primary bacterial pathogen of humans, and although there are no known reports of transmission from sheep to people, gloves should be worn when handling affected sheep.

PREGNANCY
N/A

RUMINANT SPECIES AFFECTED
Sheep

BIOSECURITY
N/A

PRODUCTION MANAGEMENT
This is of major economic impact as more than 50% of a flock can be affected and affected ewes may not suckle lambs.

SYNONYMS
Dermatologic differential diagnosis
Eye scab
Necrotic ulcerative dermatitis
Periorbital/facial eczema or dermatitis

SEE ALSO
Dermatophilosis
Facial eczema
Photosensitization caused by pithomycotoxicosis

ABBREVIATIONS
N/A

Suggested Reading
Lofstedt, J. 1983. Dermatologic diseases of sheep. In *Vet Clinic of N. America.* 5(3): 437–38.
Mullowney, P. C. 1984, Mar. Skin diseases of sheep. *Vet Clin North Am Large Anim Pract.* 6(1): 131–42.
Plant, J. Bacterial and fungal infections of the skin and wool. In: *Diseases of sheep*, ed. W. B. Martin, I. D. Aitken, 3rd ed. Edinburgh: Blackwell Science.
Scott, D. W. 1984. Environmental diseases. In *Large animal dermatology*. Philadelphia: W. B. Saunders.
Smith, M. C., Sherman, D. M. 1994. Staphylococcal dermatitis in goats. In: *Goat medicine*. Philadelphia: Lea & Febiger.

Authors: Karen A. Moriello and Susan D. Semrad

PESTE DES PETITS RUMINANTS

 BASICS

DEFINITION
Peste des petits ruminants (PPR) is an acute viral disease of small ruminants, especially goats. The course of the disease is similar to rinderpest in cattle and the two viruses are closely related.

PATHOPHYSIOLOGY
• PPR virus is transmitted by close contact and is present in ocular, nasal, oral, and fecal secretions.
• Most infections occur through inhalation of aerosols, and the virus invades the body through the upper respiratory tract epithelium. Fomites may play a role in infection.
• Once in the body, the virus has an affinity for lymphoid and epithelial tissue.
• Animals may be infectious during the incubation period, which lasts from 3 to 10 days, but no known carrier state exists.
• Sheep are less susceptible to PPR than goats.
• A peracute form with higher mortality occurs frequently in goats.

SYSTEMS AFFECTED
• Gastrointestinal—oral cavity, esophagus, abomasums, small intestine, large intestine
• Respiratory—nasal cavity, larynx, trachea, lungs
• Ophthalmic—conjunctiva
• Hemic/lymphatic/immune—spleen

GENETICS
N/A

INCIDENCE/PREVALANCE
• The prevalence of PPR in enzootic areas is low with new infections existing continuously.
• Epizootics may occur when a susceptible population moves into the area and are often characterized by ~100% mortality among sheep and goats.

GEOGRAPHIC DISTRIBUTION
PPR is found in west and central Africa, the Middle East, and India.

SIGNALMENT
Species
Goats, sheep, cattle, gazelle, gemsbok, deer
Breed Predilections
None
Mean Age and Range
4–8 months; all ages
Predominant Sex
None

SIGNS
HISTORICAL FINDINGS
• Decreased appetite
• Serous nasal discharge that becomes mucopurulent—may be profuse and block nasal passages
• Matted eyelids
• Diarrhea—profuse but nonhemorrhagic
• Coughing
• Dull coat
• Dry muzzle
• Abortions

PHYSICAL EXAMINATION FINDINGS
• Serous nasal discharge that becomes mucopurulent—may be profuse and block nasal passages
• Fever—104–106°F (40–41°C)
• Necrosis of nasal mucous membranes
• Necrotic foci on the gingiva, dental pad, hard palate, cheeks and associated papillae, and tongue
• Putrid odor of the mouth
• Diarrhea—profuse but nonhemorrhagic
• Congested conjunctiva
• Dyspnea
• Coughing
• Dehydration
• Emaciation

CAUSES
PPR is caused by PPRV, which is a paramyxovirus of the genus *Morbillivirus*. It is antigenically very similar to the rinderpest virus.

RISK FACTORS
Poor nutritional status, stress from movement, and concurrent parasitic and bacterial infections may enhance the severity of disease.

 DIAGNOSIS

DIFFERENTIAL DIAGNOSIS
• Rinderpest
• Pasteurellosis
• Foot-and-mouth disease
• Nairobi sheep disease
• Contagious caprine pleuropneumonia
• Contagious ecthyma
• Bluetongue
• Heartwater
• Coccidiosis
• Plant or mineral poisoning

CBC/BIOCHEMISTRY/URINALYSIS
None

OTHER LABORATORY TESTS
• Virus isolation from clear tears, noncoagulated blood, or antibiotic-treated erosion debris
• Hemagglutination inhibition test using tears and nasal fluids
• Virus neutralization of neutralizing antibodies
• ELISA of serum for neutralizing antibodies
• AGID of serum for neutralizing antibodies
• PCR
• Paired sera samples showing a fourfold or greater rise in antibody titer

IMAGING
N/A

DIAGNOSTIC PROCEDURES
• Virus isolation—unclotted blood, lymph nodes, tonsils, spleen, and lungs
• Immunohistochemistry—mesenteric lymph nodes, spleen, lung, tonsils, ileum, and large intestine
• Samples should be placed on frozen cold packs and delivered to the laboratory within 12 hours of necropsy.

PATHOLOGIC FINDINGS
Gross Lesions
Emaciation; conjunctivitis; erosive stomatitis of the lower lip, gingiva, tongue; commissures of the mouth, hard palate, pharynx, and upper third of the esophagus; erosions of the abomasum; mild erosions in the small intestine; severe ulceration of Peyer's patches; congestion around the ileocecal valve, ceco-colic junction, and in the rectum; congestion of the mucosal folds in the colon and rectum ("zebra stripes"); small erosions and petechiae of the nasal mucosa, turbinates, larynx, and trachea; lung infiltration; enlarged and congested spleen

Histopathology
Multinucleated giant cells with inclusions in the lungs; empty germinal centers in lymph nodes; eroded mucosa in oral and nasal cavities, gastrointestinal tract, and lungs; bronchopneumonia with consolidation and atelectasis

TREATMENT

APPROPRIATE HEALTH CARE
• No specific treatment for individual animals
• Control of secondary bacterial and parasitic infections
• Herd preventative care—vaccination with attenuated Nigerian 75/1 isolate of PPR in some parts of the world; not available in the United States

NURSING CARE
Infected animals should be provided with basic supportive care by replacement of lost fluids and restoration of electrolytes.

ACTIVITY
Restrict movement to prevent respiratory distress

DIET
Avoid feeding rough/coarse feeds to reduce irritation to mucosal erosions

CLIENT EDUCATION
Clients need to be educated in the importance of vaccination to prevent infection in countries where it is approved for use.

SURGICAL CONSIDERATIONS
None

 ## MEDICATIONS

DRUGS OF CHOICE
N/A

CONTRAINDICATIONS
N/A

PRECAUTIONS
N/A

POSSIBLE INTERACTIONS
N/A

ALTERNATIVE DRUGS
N/A

 ## FOLLOW-UP

PATIENT MONITORING
Animals should be monitored for respiratory distress due to blocked nasal passages.

PREVENTION/AVOIDANCE
Animals in endemic areas should be vaccinated with the attenuated Nigerian 75/1 isolate of PPR. The vaccine is protective for approximately 1 year.

POSSIBLE COMPLICATIONS
Exposure of naïve flocks/herds of sheep or goats to wild-type PPR may result in 100% mortality.

EXPECTED COURSE AND PROGNOSIS
• Animals suffering from acute PPR usually have a poor prognosis. The severity and outcome of the disease is correlated with the extent of the lesions in the mouth.
• Lesions that resolve in 2–3 days have a good prognosis.
• Respiratory symptoms and foul mouth odor are indicative of a poor prognosis.
• Recovered animals are immune for life.

 ## MISCELLANEOUS

ASSOCIATED CONDITIONS
Secondary bacterial and parasitic infections

AGE-RELATED FACTORS
Young animals, 4–8 months of age, often have worse clinical disease than adult animals.

ZOONOTIC POTENTIAL
N/A

PREGNANCY
Abortions may occur in pregnant animals.

RUMINANT SPECIES AFFECTED
Goats, sheep, cattle, gazelle, gemsbok, deer

SYNONYMS
Contagious pustular stomatitis
Goat plague
Kata
Pest of sheep and goats
Pest of small ruminants
Pneumoenteritis complex
Pneumoenteritis syndrome
Pseudorinderpest of small ruminants
Stomatitis

SEE ALSO
Bluetongue
Coccidiosis
Contagious caprine pleuropneumonia
Contagious ecthyma
Foot-and-mouth disease
Heartwater
Nairobi sheep disease
Pasteurellosis
Rinderpest

ABBREVIATIONS
AGID = agar gel immunodiffusion test
ELISA = enzyme-linked immunosorbent assay
PCR = polymerase chain reaction
PPR = peste des petits ruminants
PPRV = peste des petits ruminants virus

Suggested Reading
Anderson, J., McKay, J. A. 1994, Feb. The detection of antibodies against peste des petits ruminants virus in cattle, sheep and goats and the possible implications to rinderpest control programmes. *Epidemiol Infect.* 112(1):225–31.
Diallo, A., Libeau, G., Couacy-Hymann, E., Barbron, M. 1995, May. Recent developments in the diagnosis of rinderpest and peste des petits ruminants. *Vet Microbiol.* 44(2–4):307–17.
Haas, L., Barrett, T. 1996, Sep. Rinderpest and other animal morbillivirus infections: comparative aspects and recent developments. *Zentralbl Veterinarmed B.* 43(7):411–20.
Taylor, W. P., al Busaidy, S., Barrett, T. 1990, May. The epidemiology of peste des petits ruminants in the Sultanate of Oman. *Vet Microbiol.* 22(4):341–52.
Timoncy, P. J. 1998. Louping ill. In: *Foreign animal diseases.* Richmond, VA: United States Animal Health Association, http://www.vet.uga.edu/wpp/gray book/FAD.

Author: Stacy M. Holzbauer

PETROLEUM PRODUCT POISONING

 BASICS

DEFINITION
Ingestion, inhalation, or topical administration of petroluem products resulting in morbidity and mortality

PATHOPHYSIOLOGY
• Naturally occuring and refined petroleum products exist in complex mixtures often containing hundreds of compounds contributing to variability in clinical signs, pathology, and outcome.
• Products with highly volatile hydrocarbon fractions (e.g., gasoline, kerosene) are more likely to result in aspiration after ingestion compared to compounds of low volatility or high viscosity.
• Exposed or weathered products are less toxic if the volatile fractions have had time to evaporate.
• Ingestion of unweathered, highly volatile, petroleum products target the lung either by eructation and inhalation, aspiration during emesis, or hematogenous exposure.
• Hypoxia, chemical pnuemonia, and aspiration pneumonia are the most common sequelae.
• The gastrointestinal tract, liver, kidney, and brain are also targeted. Expansion of hydrocarbon in the rumen results in bloat and rumen stasis.
• Petroleum products and associated chemical additives are caustic to gastrointestinal mucosal resulting in gastroenteritis, colitis, mucosal edema, and hemorrhage.
• Dermal lesions occur when petroleum products are applied topically or used as a vehicle for insecticide sprays or dips resulting in contact dermatitis.

SYSTEMS AFFECTED
• Cardiovascular—dehydration, increased or decreased heart rate, arrhythmia, cardiac arrest
• Endocrine/metabolic—pyrexia
• Gastrointestinal—anorexia, salivation, vomiting, decreased rumen motility, bloat, oil in feces and rumen contents, diarrhea or constipation
• Hemic/lymphatic/immune
• Hepatobiliary
• Herd health—milk tainted with fuel odor, decreased milk production
• Musculoskeletal—reluctance to move, recumbency, weight loss, lameness
• Nervous—depression, excitability, shivering, head tremors, ataxia, decreased menace response and palpebral reflex, opisthotonos, coma, death
• Ophthalmic—blindness
• Renal/urologic
• Reproductive—abortion

• Respiratory—tachypnea, dyspnea, aspiration pneumonia, fuel/oil odor to breath, coughing
• Skin—blistering, drying, cracking, unthrifty

GENETICS
None

INCIDENCE/PREVALANCE
N/A

GEOGRAPHIC DISTRIBUTION
Common in areas where animals and oil production or petroleum waste exist within close proximity

SIGNALMENT

Breed Predilections
None

Mean Age and Range
None

Predominant Sex
None

SIGNS

GENERAL COMMENTS
Clinical signs or death commonly seen within 24 hours after ingestion

HISTORICAL FINDINGS
• Animals may be found dead; multiple animals are usually affected; younger animals may be more at risk due to curiosity and inquisitive nature.
• Animals that survive may do poorly for weeks after exposure.

PHYSICAL EXAMINATION FINDINGS
Oily, nasal discharge, dyspnea, tachypnea, petroleum odor on breath and feces, decreased rumen motility, bloat, recumbency, displaced abomasum, CNS signs, sudden death

CAUSES
• Ingestion or inhalation of petroleum products
• In cattle, reported toxic doses of unweathered oil and weathered oil are 2.5–5.0 ml/kg BW and 8.0 ml/kg BW, respectively.
• Experimental exposure of goats to kerosene resulted in morbidity at 10 and 20 ml/kg BW and mortality at 40 ml/kg BW.

RISK FACTORS

Environmental Factors
• Contamination of feed or water supply by petroleum product as a result of broken pipes; leaky valves; heating, fuel, or lubricating oil spills; contact with drilling muds and fluids; or leaking fuel storage tanks.
• Direct access to petroleum drilling slush or mud pits, used motor oil, or road-oil used for dust control are risk factors.
• Rainfall may bring petroleum products to water or soil surface long after a spill occurs.

• Poor-quality pasture may contribute to ingestion; however, animals willingly consume large volumes of petroleum even if uncontaminated, good-quality feed and water are available.

Animal Factors
• Age, preexisting health, hydration, and nutritional status, duration of exposure, duration of time to treatment
• Direct application of petroleum product either topically or by drench may result in toxicosis.

Petroleum Factors
Amount of petroleum product consumed, viscosity, volatility (higher volatility and lower viscosity increases the likelihood of aspiration), chemical composition of product, toxicity of chemical additives, weathered (less toxic) vs. unweathered product (more toxic)

 DIAGNOSIS

• History of exposure and petroleum odor on breath and in feces is supportive.
• Gas chromatography of GI contents and suspected source is diagnostic.

DIFFERENTIAL DIAGNOSIS
Lead or other heavy metal exposure, chemicals used in petroluem extraction, organophosphate ester poisoning

CBC/BIOCHEMISTRY/URINALYSIS
Results vary with exposure
• Increased PCV, HGB, Fib, TPP, leukopenia initially followed by leukocytosis
• Elevated AST, GGT, BUN, creatinine, LDH, CPK, cholesterol
• Decreased potassium, calcium, glucose

OTHER LABORATORY TESTS
• Gas chromatography "fingerprinting" of rumen contents or liver, lung, or kidney tissue, and the suspected source of poisoning
• Heavy metal analysis of liver, GI contents, kidney, and brain to rule out other causes
• Acetylcholinesterase level in blood and brain tissue to rule out organophosphate toxicity

IMAGING
Thoracic radiography in smaller ruminants has prognostic value.

DIAGNOSTIC PROCEDURES
Tracheal wash and culture

PATHOLOGICAL FINDINGS

GROSS PATHOLOGY

Respiratory Tract
Cranial and middle lung lobe most often affected; consolidation, dark red to purple, mottled, abscesses, lesions are usually bilateral, serofibrinous exudate, pleural adhesions, tracheitis.

Gastrointestinal

Esophagitis, bloat, enteritis, colitis, fuel odor to GI tract, petechial hemorrhages of GI tract, bloody intestinal contents.

Histopathogical Lesions

- Lung—necrotizing bronchopneumonia
- GI tract—mucosal and submucosal congestion and mucosal and serosal hemorrhage
- Heart—myocardial degeneration and necrosis, mineralization, congested myocardial and epicardial blood vessels, infiltrations of lymphocytes, macrophages, and neutrophils
- Kidney—renal tubular degeneration, interstitial nephritis, granular eosinophilic casts mixed with inflammatory cell infiltrates, renal vessel thrombi
- Liver—periacinar fatty degeneration and periportal infiltration of lymphocytes and plasma cells, bile duct hyperplasia
- Brain—meningeal hyperemia, meningeal/choroid edema, parenchymal hemorrhage

TREATMENT

Remove from source; use esophageal tube to relieve bloat (use of a trocar increases risk of peritonitis); administer saline laxative.

APPROPRIATE HEALTH CARE

NURSING CARE

IV fluids may be helpful, supportive care by system.

ACTIVITY

Restrict activity.

DIET

Modifications to diet will depend on rumen motility. Some animals continue to eat but are depressed, while others will be anorectic for days to weeks.

CLIENT EDUCATION

SURGICAL CONSIDERATIONS

Rumenotomy and transfaunation may be indicated.

MEDICATIONS

DRUGS OF CHOICE

Broad-spectrum antibiotics, IV or IM for more than 7 days may be indicated.

CONTRAINDICATIONS

- Rumen lavage via orogastric or nasogastric tube increases risk of aspiration.

- Appropriate milk and meat withdrawal times must be followed for all compounds administered to food-producing animals.

POSSIBLE INTERACTIONS

ALTERNATIVE DRUGS

Sheep who received artificial surfactant administered intratrachially after experimental exposure to kerosene via direct application to lungs have improved outcome over control animals.

FOLLOW-UP

PATIENT MONITORING

Physical examination and routine bloodwork as warranted by clinical findings.

PREVENTION/AVOIDANCE

- Fence off areas to keep animals away from potential sources.
- Locate petroleum storage tanks more than 500 feet and downhill from well or surface water.
- Inspect all tanks, pipes, and valves associated with petroleum storage and extraction facilities regularly for corrosion and leakage.
- Place used oil in secure containers prior to disposal.
- Do not reuse petroleum storage containers for feed or water.

POSSIBLE COMPLICATIONS

EXPECTED COURSE AND PROGNOSIS

- Highly variable depending on type of compound and severity of exposure
- Some animals that survive the initial exposure will have few clinical signs while others will do poorly for weeks to months requiring culling or euthansia.
- Animals with aspiration pneumonia have a guarded to poor prognosis.

MISCELLANEOUS

RELATED CONDITIONS

AGE-RELATED FACTORS

ZOONOTIC POTENTIAL

- Inhalation of petroleum vapors is potentially toxic.
- Many compounds associated with petroleum products are known carcinogens.

PREGNANCY

Abortions have been attributed to petroleum exposure.

RUMINANT SPECIES AFFECTED

All ruminant species are susceptible.

BIOSECURITY

N/A

PRODUCTION MANAGEMENT

- Poor-quality pasture may contribute to ingestion; however, animals willingly consume large volumes of petroleum even if uncontaminated, good-quality feed and water are available.
- Fence off areas to keep animals away from potential sources.

SYNONYMS

N/A

SEE ALSO

Agricultural chemical toxicity
Other toxicology chapters
Toxic gas toxicity
Toxicologic herd outbreak investigation

ABBREVIATIONS

AST = aspartate aminotranferase
BUN = blood urea nitrogen
BW = body weight
CNS = central nervous system
CPK = creatine phosphokinase
FIB = fibrinogen
GGT = gamma-glutamyl transferase
GI = gastrointestinal
HGB = hemoglobin
IM = intramuscular
IV = intravenous
LDH = lactate dehydrogenase
PCV = packed cell volume
TPP = total plasma protein

Suggested Reading

Adler, R., et al. 1992. Toxicosis in sheep following ingestion of natural gas condensate. *Vet Path*. 29:11–20.

Aiello, S. E., ed. 1998. *Merck veterinary manual*. 8th ed. Whitehouse Station, NJ: Merck and Co.

Coppock, R. W., et al. 1995. Toxicology of oil field pollutants in cattle: a review. *Vet Human Tox*. 37(6):569–75.

Edwards, W. C. 1991. Livestock poisoning from oil field drilling fluids, muds and additives. *Vet Human Tox*. 33(5):502–4.

Edwards, W. C., Coppock, R.W., Zinn, L. L. 1979. Toxicosis related to the petroleum industry. *Vet Human Tox*. 21:328–37.

Author: Lauren Palmer

PHARMACOLOGY OF MASTITIS: BOVINE

BASICS

OVERVIEW
• Mastitis is inflammation of the mammary gland caused by a pathogenic organism.
• Clinical mastitis is characterized by abnormal milk composition, gland swelling and/or pain, and/or illness of the cow. Bacteria are generally present in this milk. Decreased milk production is observed.
• Subclinical mastitis is characterized by seamingly normal milk with an increase in somatic cell count (SCC), and can also be determined by culturing high SCC milk. Bacteria are present in this milk. Decreased milk production is observed.
• Chronic mastitis is characterized as an infection that has a long duration and may show periodic clinical symptoms.
• Mastitis-control programs that are effective and cost efficient rely heavily on prevention rather than on treatment.
• Therapeutic intervention may be a necessary part of most control programs and may include antibacterial treatment as well as anti-inflammatory therapy.
• Homeopathy and other alternative therapies may offer improved and complementary mastitis treatment options.

SYSTEMS AFFECTED
Mammary

GENETICS
N/A

INCIDENCE/PREVALENCE
N/A

GEOGRAPHIC DISTRIBUTION
Potentially worldwide depending on species and environment

SIGNALMENT
Species
Bovine

Breed Predilections
N/A

Mean Age and Range
N/A

Predominant Sex
N/A

SIGNS
N/A

CAUSES AND RISK FACTORS
Contagious Mastitis
The major causes are *Streptococcus agalactiae* and *Staphylococcus aureus*. The major reservoir for these pathogens is infected udders.
• *Corynebacterium bovis* is a minor contagious mastitis pathogen that spreads rapidly in cases where proper teat dipping programs are not in place.
• *Mycoplasma* species are also contagious pathogens—of greatest concern is *M. bovis*.

• *Streptococcus dysgalactiae* is usually considered an environmental pathogen but is spread from cow to cow like other contagious pathogens.

Environmental Mastitis
Pathogens of an environmental origin can cause environmental mastitis.
• These pathogens include gram-negative rods (*Serratia* sp., *Pseudomonas* sp., and *Proteus* sp.), coliforms (*Escherichia coli*, *Klebsiella* sp., and *Enterobacter* sp.), and streptococci other than *agalactiae* (these organisms are usually referred to as environmental streptococci).
• Of these environmental streptococcal species, the most commonly isolated is *Strep. uberis*.

DIAGNOSIS

DIFFERENTIAL DIAGNOSIS
N/A

CBC/BIOCHEMISTRY/URINALYSIS
N/A

OTHER LABORATORY TESTS
N/A

IMAGING
N/A

DIAGNOSTIC PROCEDURES
N/A

TREATMENT

• Preventative measures for the control of mastitis caused by contagious bacteria (*Streptococcus agalactiae* and *Staphylococcus* aureus) should include the development of a program to prevent spread at milking time and culling or isolating chronic cows.
• Preventative measures for the control of mastitis caused by environmental bacteria center around controlling the number of bacteria to which the teat is exposed. A cow's environment should be clean and dry and free of manure, mud, or pools of standing water. Free stalls should be designed and maintained properly. Bedding materials should be selected to limit the amount of nutrients available to environmental bacteria—sand or crushed limestone will be lower in nutrients and moisture and therefore lower in bacteria.
• Germicidal teat dip, both premilking and postmilking, should be routinely used to prevent contagious and environmental mastitis.
• Proper milking procedures should be followed and all equipment needs to be adequately cleaned and maintained.
• Culling is a necessary part of any mastitis control program. It will help by eliminating the source (the infected cow) of contagious

bacteria—mainly *Mycoplasma* spp. and *Staph. aureus*. Hopeless cases of mastitis should not be treated. Cases of mastitis caused by *Nocardia* spp., *Prototheca* spp., *Serratia* spp., *Pseudomonas* spp., *Actinomyces* spp., *Mycobacterium* spp., yeasts, fungi, and other unusual pathogens are usually not responsive to antibiotic therapy and culling is the next logical choice in preventing the spread of infection to the rest of the herd.
• Segregation may be useful in herds that have significant *Mycoplasma* or *Staph. aureus* problems. However, this can be expensive because infected cows need to be identified. Culturing milk samples routinely does this. In order for this to be effective, infected cows must be identified early and accurate maintenance records must be kept.

MEDICATIONS

DRUGS OF CHOICE
• Therapeutic management of clinical mastitis should address the efficacy of the drug, the economics of the treatment, and the possible residues left in the milk after treatment. *Culture and sensitivity results should be evaluated for mastitic organisms prior to implementing a treatment program.*

• *Dry cow therapy*: treatment of all quarters is recommended after the last lactation with commercial intramammary (IMM) antibiotics to reduce the number of new infections during the dry period. This is more effective than treatment during lactation because higher doses of antibiotics can be used without risk of residues ending up in milk.
• *Treatment during lactation*: mastitis control based solely on therapy during lactation can be very expensive and is not very effective. Preventative measures should be the most important part of a mastitis control program. This method of mastitis treatment has been successful in herds with *Strep. agalactiae*. Antibiotic treatment of cows during lactation infected with *Staph. aureus* is of limited value. Cure rates are usually less than 50%. *Mycoplasma* infections are not responsive to antibiotic therapy.
• Aminoglycosides and cephalosporins may have a high proportion of susceptible isolates in vitro, and because of this, they are often selected for use in treating coliform mastitis.
• Ceftiofur sodium may be useful against gram-negative pathogens to help prevent or treat systemic infections. Because it does not diffuse into the mammary gland, it is approved for use in lactating cows if the labeled dose of 1–2.2 mg/kg q 24 hours is administered intramuscularly, and no milk withholding time is required. Ceftiofur is not recommended for intramammary infusion.

PHARMACOLOGY OF MASTITIS: BOVINE

• Dietary vitamin E and selenium may help in reducing the incidence of environmental mastitis, especially in dry cows. It is recommended that dry cows receive 1000 IU supplemental vitamin E per cow per day and that lactating cows receive 400 to 600 IU per cow per day. The selenium content of the diet should be 0.3 ppm for lactating cows and dry cows.

• Endotoxin-induced shock is a primary problem in cases of coliform mastitis and the infected cow may benefit most from fluid therapy and not antibiotic treatment.

• Anti-inflammatory drugs may be helpful when used to treat acute environmental mastitis. These are cyclooxygenase inhibitors (nonsteroidal anti-inflammatory drugs) and corticosteroids. There is no evidence that the treatment with anti-inflammatory drugs positively affects the survival or production of the cow.

• Nonsteroidal anti-inflammatory drugs (NSAIDs) have been advocated for the relief of symptoms of endotoxic shock and in therapy of coliform mastitis. Aspirin, flunixin meglumine, phenylbutazone, ibuprofen, carprofen, and flurbiprofen have all been used in experimental coliform mastitis and in experimental endotoxin-induced mastitis.

• Dexamethasone, fluoroprednisolone, betamethasone, and flumethasone have also been utilized in treating animals experimentally challenged with coliform mastitis.

• Vaccines: J-5 (R mutant) *E. coli* antigen vaccines are used to enhance resistance to intramammary coliform infections. Administration of the vaccine during the dry period has been reported to reduce the severity of coliform infections in intramammary challenge studies with *E. coli*.

• There is no vaccine that has proven successful in controlling mastitis caused by environmental streptococcus.

Antibiotic Treatment for Gram-Negative Bacteria

The following are antibiotic treatment options for acute mastitis caused by gram-negative bacteria. In some cases they have proven affective against some gram-positives as well. Culture and sensitivity results should be evaluated for mastitic organisms prior to implementing a treatment program.

• Sulfadiazine/trimethoprim or sulfadoxine/trimethoprim: 25 mg/kg IV or IM once daily for 2–4 days and polymyxin B sulfate 100 mg (cir. 8000 IU) or colistin sulfate 100 mg (cir. 20,000 IU) in 10–20 mL water for intramammary injection once daily for 2 or 3 days.

• Gentamicin sulfate 5 mg/kg IV or IM once daily for 3–5 days and gentamicin sulfate 100–150 mg intramammary once daily for 2 or 3 days.

• Ampicillin trihydrate 10 mg/kg IM twice daily for 2 or 3 days and cephapirin sodium 200 mg intramammary after each milking for three consecutive milkings.

• Polymyxin B sulfate or colistin sulfate 5 mg/kg IM twice daily for 2 days and cephapirin sodium 200 mg intramammary after each milking for three consecutive milkings.

Antibiotic Treatment for Gram-Positive Bacteria

The following are antibiotic treatment options for acute mastitis caused by gram-positive bacteria. Culture and sensitivity results should be evaluated for mastitic organisms prior to implementing a treatment program.

• Sulfadiazine/trimethoprim or sulfadoxine/trimethoprim 25 mg//kg IV or IM once daily for 3–5 days and hetacillin potassium 62.5 mg or amoxicillin sodium 62.5 mg intramammary after each milking for six consecutive milkings.

• Ampicillin trihydrate 10 mg/kg IM twice daily for 3–5 days and cloxacillin sodium 200 mg intramammary after each milking for six consecutive milkings.

• Erythromycin lactobionate or tylosin tartrate 10 mg/kg loading dose IV followed by erythromycin base or tylosin base 5 mg/kg IM twice daily for 3–5 days and erythromycin 300 mg intramammary after each milking for six consecutive milkings.

• Sulfamethazine sodium 100 mg/kg loading dose IV, followed by 50 mg/kg IV once daily for 3–5 days and amoxicillin sodium 62.5 mg intramammary after each milking for six consecutive milkings or cloxacillin sodium 200 mg intramammary after each milking for six consecutive milkings or procaine penicillin 100,000 IU intramammary after each milking for four to six consecutive milkings.

Homeopathy and Other Alternative Therapies

• Antibiotics are widely used in the treatment and prophylaxis of mastitis, but their antibacterial and therapeutic efficacy continues to decrease. New methods of mastitis prophylaxis including the use of vaccines and biological response modifiers have been reviewed.

• Different methods of immunomodulation for the prevention of mastitis have shown promise in experimental trials. Improving nutrition, housing, and the environment of dairy cattle are still crucial in the prevention of mastitis, especially during the most susceptible postparturient period.

• Other alternative immunomodulators that have shown promise in mastitis treatment during the lactating period include herbal gels, herbal extracts, ginseng, saponin, propolis, and antibacterial proteins.

• In a Swedish study on the effect of subcutaneous injections of ginseng on cows with subclinical *Staphylococcus aureus* mastitis, the results indicate that ginseng treatment can activate the innate immunity of cows and may contribute to the cow's recovery from mastitis. Ginseng may have potential to stimulate immune function in dairy cows.
• Anecdotally, combinations of silica, phytolacca, belladonna, *Calcarea fluorica*, bryonia, ipecacuanha, arnica, and conium have been found effective in the medical management of mastitis.
• Increasing the ongoing desire to decrease the use of antibiotic drugs, to cut down on treatment expense, and to find alternative treatment solutions when regular conventional therapies are not successful are factors that have increased interest in alternative therapies.
• Scientific research is needed to evaluate alternative therapeutic efficacy of currently used treatments.
• Qualified, well-trained homeopaths or herbalists are needed to assure quality treatment results.
• Complementary therapies such as homeopathy and alternative therapies are becoming increasingly needed in veterinary medicine today.

CONTRAINDICATIONS

Appropriate milk and meat withdrawal times must be followed for all compounds administered.

 FOLLOW-UP

N/A

POSSIBLE COMPLICATIONS

• Untested combinations of products should not be used.

• Compounding of intramammary products is illegal and may result in violative antibiotic residues in both meat and milk.
• Multiple dose containers should never be used between mammaries due to the risk of contamination with organisms such as *Mycoplasma* spp. or *Staph. aureus* that can be spread to other quarters or other cows in the herd. These bacteria are not susceptible to antibiotic therapy.
• Great care should be used when infusing dry cow products through the streak canal because environmental contaminants may be inadvertently forced through the canal and cause additional infections. Environmental contaminants are not susceptible to dry cow treatment products.
• Products approved by the FDA for use during lactation are uniformly ineffective against coliform bacteria.

 MISCELLANEOUS

ASSOCIATED CONDITIONS
N/A

AGE-RELATED FACTORS
N/A

ZOONOTIC POTENTIAL
N/A

PREGNANCY
N/A

RUMINANT SPECIES AFFECTED
Potentially, all ruminant species are affected.

BIOSECURITY
N/A

PRODUCTION MANAGEMENT
N/A

SYNONYMS
N/A

SEE ALSO
Drug storage requirements
Extralabel drug use
FARAD
Mastitis specific chapters

ABBREVIATIONS
FDA = Food and Drug Administration
IM = intramuscular
IMM = intramammary
IU = intrauterine
IV = intravenous
NSAIDs = nonsteroidal anti-inflammatory drugs
SCC = somatic cell count

Suggested Reading
Anderson, K. L. 1993, Nov. Update on bovine mastitis. *Veterinary Clinics of North America Food Animal Practice* 9 (3).
Hektoen, L. 2005, Aug 20. Review of the current involvement of homeopathy in veterinary practice and research. *Vet Rec.* 157(8):224–29.
Karreman, H. J. 2004. *Treating dairy cows naturally: thoughts and strategies.* Paradise, PA: Paradise Publications
National Mastitis Council. http://www.nmconline.org/articles.
Sears, P. M., Wilson, D. J. 2003, March. Mastitis. *Veterinary Clinics of North America Food Animal Practice* 19 (1).
Ziv, G. 1992, March. Treatment of preacute and acute mastitis. *The Veterinary Clinics of North America Food Animal Practice: Applied Pharmacology and Therapeutics* II8 (1).

Authors: Heather A. Johnson,
Brenda Kennedy-Wade,
Carmela Jaravata

PHENOXYL TOXICITY

 BASICS

OVERVIEW
• These are chlorophenoxylic herbicide compounds, such as 2,4-D and MCPA. They are used to control weeds and aquatic plants, to increase fruit durability in storage, and to prevent premature fruit dropping. Exposure is from accidental ingestion of concentrates or sprays, occasionally from chronic ingestion of treated forages. These herbicides are relatively nontoxic unless ingested in a concentrated form.
• Repeated and massive doses are needed to cause poisoning in ruminants.
• These agents can cause liver and kidney failure, hypotension, and increased cancer risk; also can see hemolysis.
• Types—2,4-D, 2,4-DB, dalapon, MCPA, Sivex, 2,4,5-T
• The advent of commercial farming prompted the development of selective weed control chemicals. These organic herbicides are plant growth regulators altering the metabolism of plants and are associated with potential teratogenicity.
• A side effect of the compound's use is the increased levels of nitrates or cyanide in plants that can cause secondary poisoning to ruminants prior to the plants death.
• Some toxic weeds become more palatable after treatment such as jimsonweed and nightshade.
• Essentially, usage has been stopped because of the toxic contaminants of dioxins (TCDD, HCDD).

SIGNALMENT
• Ten days exposure is required to produce poisoning.
• Calves have been poisoned by a single oral dose of 200 mg/kg BW.

SIGNS
• See clinical signs from massive and repeated exposures.
• Anorexia, depression, rumen atony, muscle weakness, especially hind limbs
• Diarrhea, ulceration of oral mucosa, bloating
• Animals progressively become emaciated and moribund.

CAUSES AND RISK FACTORS
• Feeding up to 2000 ppm herbicide in the diet amounted to 1 ppm in liver and kidneys and < 0.05 ppm in the muscle and fat.
• Herbicide residues are not likely to be at >300 ppm in or on forage immediately after treatment at recommended rates for brush and weed control. Residues decline rapidly. The forage t 1/2 is 1–2 weeks.
• Meat residues occur only with extremely high exposure during continuous ingestion of freshly treated vegetation.
• Withdrawal of animals from treated forages for 1–2 weeks prior to slaughter should decrease any residues.
• Herbicide-treated forages don't seem to affect rumen microbial functions or development in the rumen; they are not readily degraded by ruminal microorganisms.

 DIAGNOSIS

DIFFERENTIAL DIAGNOSIS
• Mb toxicity/Cu deficiency
• Severe parasitism
• Diseases causing anorexia, depression, rumen atony, muscle weakness, especially hind limbs
• Diseases causing diarrhea, ulceration of oral mucosa, bloating
  • Abomasal torsion
  • Acidosis/grain overload
  • Bovine viral diarrhea virus (BVD)
• Cathartic/laxatives
• Coccidiosis
• Colitis/typhilitis
• Displaced abomasum
• Enteritis
• Heart failure
• Indigestion
• Intussusception
• Jejunal hemorrhage syndrome
• Johne's disease
• Liver failure
• Malignant catarrhal fever
• Molybdenosis/copper deficiency
• Parasitism
• Parasympathomimetic drugs
• Peritonitis
• Poisonous plants: acorn (oak), *Brassica* spp., fungal toxicity, mushroom, oleander, pokeweed, pyrrolizidine alkaloids, rattlebox, selenium accumulators, *Solanum* spp., St. John's wort
• Salmonellosis
• Sepsis/toxemia/enterotoxemia
• Toxins: aflatoxin, arsenic, chlorpyrifos (Dursban), copper, herbicides, levamisole, lincomycin, monensin, nicotine, phosphorus fertilizers, propylene glycol, sodium bicarbonate, sulfur, trichothecene, zinc
• Uremia/renal failure
• Winter dysentery
• Xylazine, large doses
• Diseases causing weight loss and emaciation

CBC/BIOCHEMISTRY/URINALYSIS
• Major elimination by the kidneys
• CBC/biochemistry/urinalysis is indicated to monitor parameters for treatment.
• No parent compounds or metabolites found in milk from orally dosed cattle.

OTHER LABORATORY TESTS
High levels of compound in kidney and liver, decreased levels in fat and muscle

IMAGING
N/A

DIAGNOSTIC PROCEDURES
Feed analysis, chemical analysis

PATHOLOGICAL FINDINGS
• Epicardial hemorrhage
• Hydropericardium
• Bright green, undigested feed from ruminal stasis
• Liver swollen, friable
• Kidneys congested
• Hyperemia, enlargement of lymph nodes and mesenteric vessels
• High levels in liver and kidney, decreased levels in fat and muscle

TREATMENT
• Activated charcoal, alkaline diuresis
• Control seizures; diazepam, phenobarbital

MEDICATIONS

DRUGS OF CHOICE
Control seizures: diazepam, phenobarbital

CONTRAINDICATIONS
Appropriate milk and meat withdrawal times must be followed for all compounds administered to food-producing animals.

PRECAUTIONS
• Keep toxic chemicals away from livestock. Do not apply toxic chemicals to fields or crops on which animals may feed.
• Consult manufacturer and FARAD if accidental exposure occurs.

POSSIBLE INTERACTIONS
N/A

FOLLOW-UP

PREVENTION/AVOIDANCE
• Withdrawal of animals from treated forages for 1–2 weeks prior to slaughter would decrease any residues.
• Keep toxic chemicals away from livestock. Do not apply toxic chemicals to fields or crops on which animals may feed.
• Meat residues occur only with extremely high exposure during continuous ingestion of freshly treated vegetation.

POSSIBLE COMPLICATIONS
N/A

EXPECTED COURSE AND PROGNOSIS
Depends on quantity ingested; fair to poor depending on treatment and amount of agent consumed.

MISCELLANEOUS

ASSOCIATED CONDITIONS
• A side effect is the increased levels of nitrates or cyanide in plants that can cause secondary poisoning before the plant dies.
• Some toxic weeds become more palatable after treatment, such as jimsonweed and nightshade.

AGE-RELATED FACTORS
N/A

ZOONOTIC POTENTIAL
N/A

PREGNANCY
N/A

RUMINANT SPECIES AFFECTED
Potentially, all ruminant species are affected.

BIOSECURITY
N/A

PRODUCTION MANAGEMENT
Keep all chemicals and sprays away from feeding ruminants.

SYNONYMS
N/A

SEE ALSO
Diseases causing anorexia, depression, rumen atony, muscle weakness, especially hind limbs
Diseases causing diarrhea, ulceration of oral mucosa, bloating
Mb toxicity/Cu deficiency
Severe parasitism

ABBREVIATIONS
BVD = bovine viral diarrhea
BW = body weight
FARAD = Food Animal Residue Avoidance Databank
HCDD = dioxone; 1,2,3,4,5,6,7,8-HCDD
TCDD = the most toxic member of the dioxin and furan family—2,3,7,8-TCDD; 2,3,7,8-tetrachlorodibenzo-p-dioxin

Suggested Reading
Clark, D. E., Palmer, J. S. 1971, Jul-Aug. Residual aspects of 2,4,5-T and an ester in sheep and cattle with observations on concomitant toxicological effects. *J Agric Food Chem.* 19(4): 761–64.
Paulino, C. A., Oliveira, G. H., Palermo-Neto, J. 1994, Oct. Acute 2,4-dichlorophenoxyacetic acid intoxication in cattle. *Vet Hum Toxicol.* 36(5): 433–36.
Paulino, C. A., Palermo-Neto, J. 1995, Aug. Effects of acute 2,4-dichlorophenoxyacetic acid on cattle serum components and enzyme activities. *Vet Hum Toxicol.* 37(4): 329–32.
Rowe, V. K., Hymas, T. A. 1954, Oct. Summary of toxicological information on 2,4-D and 2,4,5-T type herbicides and an evaluation of the hazards to livestock associated with their use. *Am J Vet Res.* 15(57): 622–29.

Author: Greg Stoner

PHOSPHORUS DEFICIENCY/EXCESS

 BASICS

DEFINITION
- Phosphorus (P) deficiency = a disorder (hypophosphotosis) caused by decreased total body P, which can manifest with reduced serum P concentrations (hypophosphatemia ~ <2.0 mg/dL) below the established reference interval for a particular species and breed.
- Phosphorus excess = a condition reflected by elevated serum P concentrations (hyperphosphatemia ~ > 6.0 mg/dL) above the established reference interval for a particular species and breed due to endogenous or exogenous etiologies.

PATHOPHYSIOLOGY
- Altered bone growth and mineralization disorders are the primary manifestation related to P deficiency and excess with a few key exceptions.
  - Liver toxicosis with white/yellow P ingestion
  - Postparturient hemoglobinuria (PPH) with dietary P deficiency
- 80% of the P in the body is stored in bones and teeth of which 90% is stored in the form of hydroxyapatite used to form the mineralized matrix of bone.
- Remaining 20% of body P is in intracellular soft tissues (minor extracellular-serum portion) where it is involved in critical roles.
  - Maintenance of cellular structural proteins (phospholipids, nucleic acids, phosphoproteins)
  - Cellular energy transfer and storage and muscle contraction (ATP, ADP, AMP)
- Ruminant's absorption of dietary P primarily in the forestomachs and loss of excess body P via saliva (predominant) and urine with hormonal influence on both absorption and excretion. Grains generally lower in P concentration than forage and plant concentration correlates with soil concentration.
- Typical serum P assays measure only inorganic fraction (P_i), which exists in several forms (predominately HPO_4^{2-} and $H_2PO_4^-$ in a 4:1 ratio).
- There is rapid translocation between the intracellular and serum P pools. Serum P_i measurement is an unreliable indicator of total body P stores.
  - Hypophosphatemic animals likely have reduced body stores of P
  - Animals with reduced body stores of P may not be hypophosphatemic
- Serum P_i concentrations influenced by the following variables:

- Rate of renal clearance—decreased glomerular filtration rate (GFR) leads to elevation of serum P_i
- Rate of renal tubular reabsorption
  (1) Parathyroid hormone (PTH) decreases tubular reabsorption, decreasing serum P_i
  (2) Calcitonin hormone decreases tubular reabsorption, decreasing serum P_i
  (3) Growth hormone (GH) increases tubular reabsorption, increasing serum P_i
- Rate of gastrointestinal (GI) absorption
  (1) 1,25-dihydroxycholecalciferol (1,25-DHCC, calcitriol, active vitamin D) increases GI absorption, increasing serum P_i
  (2) Reduced dietary P results in decreased GI absorption, decreasing serum P_i
- Shift from serum pool to intracellular pool—insulin, carbohydrate loads, respiratory alkalosis shifts serum P_i to the intracellular pool, decreasing serum P_i
- Resorption rate of bone—PTH increases osteocyte and osteoclast release of P from bone
- Age of animal—younger animals have increased GH levels, which increases tubular reabsorption, increasing serum P_i
- Regulation of P absorption/secretion
- Decreased serum P_i >
- Increased active vitamin D from the kidney > increased GI P and Ca absorption > increases serum P_i and Ca
- Increased serum Ca >
  (a) Decreased PTH from parathyroid gland >
  (1) Increased renal tubule reabsorption of P > increases serum P_i
  (2) Decreased P secretion in saliva > decreased GI loss of P > increases serum P_i
  (b) Increased calcitonin from thyroid C cells > decreases renal tubule reabsorption of P and Ca > decreases serum P_i and Ca
- Increased serum P_i >
  (1) Decreased active vitamin D from the kidney > decreased GI P and Ca absorption > decreases serum P_i and Ca
  (2) Decreased serum Ca >
  (a) Increased PTH from the parathyroid gland >
  (1) Decreased renal tubule reabsorption of P > decreases serum P_i
  (2) Increased P secretion in saliva > increased GI loss of P > decreases serum P_i
  (b) Decreased calcitonin from thyroid C cells > increased renal tubule reabsorption of P and Ca > increases serum P_i and Ca

SYSTEMS AFFECTED
- Bone
  - P deficiency: osteopenia (reduced bone mass), osteomalacia (demineralized matrix), rickets (defective endochondral ossification, accumulation of unmineralized matrix)
  - P excess: osteodystrophia fibrosa (fibrous connective tissue replaces cortical bone)
- Red blood cells—hemolysis (P deficiency)
- White blood cells—reduced chemotaxis and phagocytosis (P deficiency)
- Muscle—weakness (P deficiency)
- Liver—periportal necrosis (white/yellow P toxicity) /central lobular necrosis (PPH)
- Reproduction—reduced reproductive rates (P deficiency)

GENETICS
N/A

INCIDENCE/PREVALENCE
- P deficiency: hypophosphotosis and hypophosphatemia: sporadic, 1–2 in herd
- P excess: P toxicosis and hyperphosphatemia: sporadic

GEOGRAPHIC DISTRIBUTION
P Deficiency: Hypophosphotosis and Hypophosphatemia
- Osteomalacia/rickets: worldwide but most cases South Africa, Australia, New Zealand, and dry tropical regions (regional soils deficient in P); southern and northern latitudes (reduced levels of sunlight with reduced amounts of active vitamin D)
- PPH: worldwide; North America, New Zealand

P Excess: P Toxicosis and Hyperphosphatemia
Osteodystrophia fibrosa/P toxicosis: worldwide

SIGNALMENT
Species
- P deficiency: hypophosphotosis and hypophosphatemia
  - Osteomalacia/rickets: all ruminants; cattle > sheep and goats
  - PPH: cattle
- P excess: P toxicosis and hyperphosphatemia—osteodystrophia fibrosa: all ruminants; goats > cattle and sheep

Breed Predilection
- P deficiency: hypophosphotosis and hypophosphatemia
  - Osteomalacia/rickets: N/A
  - PPH: dairy cattle
- P excess: P toxicosis and hyperphosphatemia—osteodystrophia fibrosa: N/A

PHOSPHORUS DEFICIENCY/EXCESS

Mean Age and Range
- P deficiency: hypophosphotosis and hypophosphatemia
  - Osteomalacia: older adult
  - Rickets: growing young <1 year
  - PPH: North America—older adult (3–10 years, within 6 weeks of calving), New Zealand —any age adult
- P excess: P toxicosis and hyperphosphatemia—osteodystrophia fibrosa: N/A

Predominant Sex
- P deficiency: hypophosphotosis and hypophosphatemia
  - Osteomalacia/rickets: N/A
  - PPH: cow
- P excess: P toxicosis and hyperphosphatemia—osteodystrophia fibrosa/P toxicosis: N/A

SIGNS

P Deficiency: Hypophosphotosis and Hypophosphatemia
- Osteomalacia: shifting lameness, poor growth rate, dull hair coat, decreased feed consumption, weight loss, reduced milk production, reduced reproductive performance, pica, kyphosis, lordosis, spontaneous nonhealing fractures, and a long and lean appearance
- Rickets: stiffness, lameness, joint enlargement, enlarged costochondral junction, arched back, bow-legged, and decreased growth rate.
- PPH: weakness, marked decrease in milk production, red-brown urine, pallor of mucous membranes, pounding jugular pulse, tachycardia, tachypnea, and jaundice. See signs of osteomalacia.

P Excess: P Toxicosis and Hyperphosphatemia
- Osteodystrophia fibrosa: stiffness, shifting laxness, loss of appetite, progressive cachexia, and anemia, swelling of jaw and mandible, and fractures
- P toxicosis: diarrhea, abdominal pain, garliclike breath odor, jaundice, and convulsions

CAUSES

P Deficiency: Hypophosphotosis and Hypophosphatemia
- Decreased GI absorption
  - Diet deficient in P (green grains, P poor soil)
  - P binding agents (diet high in Ca, Al, Mg, and fat)
  - Hypovitaminosis D (lack of sunshine; bile duct aplasia)
  - Intestinal malabsorption disease
  - Starvation, wasting disease

- Increased urinary excretion of P
  - Diuresis
  - Increased PTH due to primary hyperparathyroidism (functional tumor of parathyroid gland)
- Movement of extracellular P into the intracellular pool
  - Hyperinsulinism (glucose infusion; insulinoma)
  - Respiratory alkalosis
- Inadequate mobilization of P from bone stores (postparturient paresis)

P Excess: P Toxicosis and Hyperphosphatemia
- Spurious—hemolysis of sample or delay in removal of serum from clot (release of P from RBC)
- Decreased urinary excretion
  - Decreased GFR —dehydration; renal failure (renal hyperparathyroidism); obstruction of urinary tract
  - Rupture of urinary bladder
  - Decreased PTH concentration (primary hypoparathyroidism)
  - Acromegaly
- Increased P absorption from GI
  - Diet high in P content (nutritional hyperparathyroidism)
  - Hypervitaminosis D
  - Intestinal necrosis—shift of P from intracellular pool to serum and increased absorption of GI P
  - Ingestion of fertilizer
  - Ingestion of fireworks
  - Ingestion of rodenticides with P
- Shift of P from intracellular pool to extracellular pool (serum)
  - Myopathy, muscle necrosis
  - Tumor lysis syndrome
- Other
  - Osteolytic bone lesion (neoplasia)
  - Young animal

RISK FACTORS

P Deficiency: Hypophosphotosis and Hypophosphatemia
- All
  - P deficient soil (regional, heavy rains, continuous removal of crops)
  - Concurrent vitamin D, manganese, zinc, or vitamin A deficiency
  - Anorexia/starvation
  - Environmental stress
  - Winter (reduced sunlight)
  - Grazing green cereal crops
- Osteomalacia—older adult animal
- Rickets—weaned, young growing animal
- PPH
  - High production, early postpartum period, lactation

- Concurrent Cu deficiency
- Diet of lush rye, Egyptian clover, green alfalfa, turnips, beet pulp, rape, and kale
- New Zealand: late summer, first to second lactation cycle

P Excess: P Toxicosis and Hyperphosphatemia
Osteodystrophia fibrosa: diets high in P and deficient in Ca (high grain-to-forage ratio)

 DIAGNOSIS

DIFFERENTIAL DIAGNOSIS

P Deficiency: Hypophosphotosis and Hypophosphatemia
- Osteomalacia/rickets
  - Fluorosis arthritis
  - Cu or Mg dietary deficiency
  - Physitis due to any cause
  - Hyperparathyroidism
  - Vitamin D deficiency
- PPH
  - Babesiosis
  - Theileriosis
  - Bacillary hemoglobinuria

P Excess: P Toxicosis and Hyperphosphatemia
- Dehydration
- Renal failure or obstruction of urinary tract
- Myopathy
- Liver failure due to a variety of metabolic, toxic, and infectious causes

CBC/BIOCHEMISTRY/URINALYSIS

P Deficiency: Hypophosphotosis and Hypophosphatemia
CBC
- Osteomalacia/rickets—N/A
- PPH—moderate to marked anemia, polychromasia and basophilic stippling of RBC, nucleated red blood cells, anisocytosis of RBC

Blood Chemistry
- Osteomalacia/rickets
  - +/− Hypophosphatemia (1.5–3.5 mg/dL)
  - +/− Hypocalcemia
- PPH
  - Hypophosphatemia common (<1.5 mg/dL)
  - Increased AST activity (ischemic liver necrosis)
  - Increased total bilirubin concentration (intravascular hemolysis—primary indirect bilirubin)

PHOSPHORUS DEFICIENCY/EXCESS

Urine
- Osteomalacia/rickets
  - +/− Hypophosphatemia (1.5–3.5 mg/dL)
  - Decreased fractional excretion of P ($[P_{Urine}/P_{Serum}] \times [Cr_{Serum}/Cr_{Urine}] \times 100$), normally 0.0–0.53% in sheep
- PPH
  - Hemoglobinuria (without RBC)
  - Bilirubinuria
  - Proteinuria

P Excess: P Toxicosis and Hyperphosphatemia
CBC
Osteodystrophia fibrosa/P toxicosis—N/A

Blood Chemistry
- Osteodystrophia fibrosa
  - Hyperphosphatemia
  - +/− Hypocalcemia
  - Hyperphosphatasemia (increased ALP)
- P Toxicosis
  - +/− Hyperphosphatemia
  - +/− Hypocalcemia
  - Increased AST (liver necrosis)
  - Increased total bilirubin (liver necrosis)

Urine
Osteodystrophia fibrosa/P toxicosis— increased fractional excretion of P

OTHER LABORATORY TESTS
P toxicosis: calculate ingested dose of P—approximate lethal dose is 1–4 mg/kg

IMAGING
Radiographic

P Deficiency: Hypophosphotosis and Hypophosphatemia
- Osteomalacia: thin cortices of long bones, reduced bone density (30% loss of mineral matrix required for visualization), noncalloused bone fractures
- Rickets: diaphyses of bones are shorter and broader than normal, cortices are increased in width, clublike thickening in metaphysis, irregular persistence of cartilage at physis, bowed long bones, domed cranium, prominent costochondral junctions

P Excess: P Toxicosis and Hyperphosphatemia
Osteodystrophia fibrosa: reduced bone density, subperiosteal bone resorption, loss of dura dentes

DIAGNOSTIC PROCEDURES
- Measure bone ash:organic ratio with bone biopsy
  - Normal bone: ash:organic ratio of 3:2
  - Rickets/osteomalacia/osteodystrophia fibrosa: ash:organic ratio of 1:2–1:3
- Analysis of dietary P and Ca concentration

PATHOLOGIC FINDINGS
Osteomalacia
- Gross pathology—soft and brittle bones, thin cortices with large marrow cavities, noncalloused fractures
- Histopathology—accumulation of excess unmineralized osteoid on trabecular bone surfaces

Rickets
- *Gross pathology*—bowed long bones, domed cranium, prominent costochondral junctions, clublike thickening in metaphyseal region (rachitic metaphysis), retarded mandibular growth
- *Histopathology*—failure of osteoid and cartilaginous matrix to mineralize, overgrowth of fibrous tissue in metaphysis, persistent cartilage, and irregular physis

PPH
- *Gross pathology*—thin watery blood, jaundice of soft tissue, distended gall bladder, red-brown colored urine, liver with a nutmeg pattern
- *Histopathology*—central lobular coagulative hepatic necrosis, bile and hemosiderin pigment in renal tubular epithelial cells, and hemoglobin in tubules

Osteodystrophia Fibrosa
- *Gross pathology*—thickening of flat bones particularly of the jaw and skull, soft bones, noncalloused fractures
- *Histopathology*—extensive erosion of periosteal and cortical bone by numerous osteoclasts, compact bone replaced by fibrocellular tissue, herniatieblon of articular cartilage into the epiphysis

P Toxicosis
Severe icterus and fatty liver with periportal necrosis

TREATMENT

APPROPRIATE HEALTH CARE
Osteomalacia/Rickets/PPH
- Correct any dietary deficiency in P, Ca, or vitamin D. Ideal dietary ratio of Ca:P is 2:1
  - Cattle: 150–300 kg body weight require 9–18 g/day of P
  - Sheep: 10–100 kg body weight require 1.9–4.8 g/day of P
- Adequate sunlight (osteomalacia/rickets)

Osteodystrophia Fibrosa
- Nutritional cause: correct excess dietary P
- Renal cause

P Toxicosis
Remove source of exposure

ACTIVITY
N/A

CLIENT EDUCATION
Osteomalacia/Rickets/Osteodystrophia Fibrosa
Gross bone deformities unlikely to resolve following correction of dietary P concentration.

PPH
Animals that survive initial hemolytic crisis will likely succumb later due to hemoglobin-induced renal failure.

P Toxicosis
Recovery from acute abdominal pain often followed in 3–5 days by liver failure and death.

SURGICAL CONSIDERATION
N/A

MEDICATIONS

DRUGS OF CHOICE
Osteomalacia/Rickets
- Injectable vitamin D: 10,000–30,000 IU/kg
- Supplement ration with dicalcium phosphate or bone meal

PHOSPHORUS DEFICIENCY/EXCESS

PPH
• Adult cattle: whole blood transfusion (10–20 L)
• 60 g sodium acid phosphate in 300 ml of sterile distilled water IV and repeated every 12 hours for three treatments
• 120 g of bone meal oral daily for 5 days
• Fluid therapy to minimize renal damage from free hemoglobin

Osteodystrophia Fibrosa (Nutritional Cause)
N/A

P Toxicosis
• Oral activated charcoal
• Oral mineral oil

CONTRAINDICATIONS
Appropriate milk and meat withdrawal times must be followed for all compounds administered to food-producing animals.

PRECAUTIONS
N/A

POSSIBLE INTERACTIONS
N/A

ALTERNATIVE DRUGS
N/A

 FOLLOW-UP

PATIENT MONITORING
PPH
Degree of anemia, renal function

P Toxicosis
Liver function

PREVENTION/AVOIDANCE
Osteomalacia/Rickets/Osteodystrophia Fibrosa
See Causes section above.

POSSIBLE COMPLICATIONS
N/A

EXPECTED COURSE AND PROGRESS
Osteomalacia/Rickets/Osteodystrophia Fibrosa
Good with appropriate correction of dietary Ca and P intake

PPH
Grave prognosis with death in 2–5 days

P Toxicosis
Grave prognosis with initial improvement followed in 3–5 days with liver failure and hepatoencephalopathy-associated seizures and death

 MISCELLANEOUS

ASSOCIATED CONDITIONS
PPH
Renal failure

P Toxicosis
Liver failure

AGE-RELATED FACTORS
Rickets: unusual in newborn and nursing calves

ZOONOTIC POTENTIAL
N/A

PREGNANCY
PPH
Increases risk of disorder

RUMINANT SPECIES AFFECTED
All ruminants

BIOSECURITY
N/A

PRODUCTION MANAGEMENT
N/A

SYNONYMS
Osteodystrophia fibrosa = big head disease
Osteomalacia = adult rickets

SEE ALSO
Nutritional diseases
Osteomalacia/rickets—fluorosis arthritis; Cu or Mg dietary deficiency; physitis due to any cause; hyperparathyroidism; vitamin D deficiency
PPH—babesiosis; theileriosis; bacillary hemoglobinuria
P excess: P toxicosis and hyperphosphatemia—dehydration; renal failure or obstruction of urinary tract; myopathy; liver failure due to a variety of metabolic, toxic, and infectious causes

ABBREVIATIONS
1,25-DHCC = 1,25-dihydroxycholecalciferol
ADP = adenosine diphosphate
Al = aluminum
ALP = alkaline phosphatase
AMP = adenosine monophosphate
AST = aspartate transferase
ATP = adenosine triphosphate
Ca = calcium
CBC = complete blood count
Ck = creatine kinase
Cr = creatinine
dL = deciliter
GFR = glomerular filtration rate
GH = growth hormone
GI = gastrointestinal
g = gram
IV = intravenous
K = potassium
mg = milligram
Mg = magnesium
P = phosphorus
P_i = inorganic phosphorus
PPH = postparturient hemoglobinuria
PTH = parathyroid hormone
USPG = urine specific gravity

Suggested Reading
Fleming, S. A., Yates, D. J. 1996. Disorders of phosphorus metabolism. In: *Large animal internal medicine*, ed. B. P. Smith. 2nd ed. St. Louis, MO: Mosby.
Goff, J. P. 1999. Treatment of calcium, phosphorus, and magnesium balance disorders. *Vet Clin North Am Food Anim Pract*. 15:619–39, viii.
Hesters, N. L., Fleming, S. A., Yates, D. J. 1996. Calcium and phosphorus homeostasis. In: *Large animal internal medicine*, ed. B. P. Smith. 2nd ed. St. Louis, MO: Mosby.
McCaughan, C. J. 1992. Treatment of mineral disorders in cattle. *Vet Clin North Am Food Anim Pract*. 8:107–45.
Padgett, S. L. 1998. Dystrophies associated with calcium, phosphorus, and vitamin D. In: *Merck veterinary manual*, ed. S. E. Aiello. 8th ed. Whitehouse Station, NJ: Merck & Co.
Stockham, S. L., Scott, M. A. 2002. Calcium, phosphorus, magnesium, and their regulatory hormones. In: *Fundamentals of veterinary clinical pathology*. Ames: Iowa State University Press.

Authors: Kurt L. Zimmerman and Daniel C. Rule

PHOTODERMATITIS

 BASICS

DEFINITION
• Dermatitis caused by photodynamic agents present in the skin.
• The source of these photodynamic agents in livestock are endogenous substances or plant material.
• Stimulation of photodynamic agents by ultraviolet light results in generation of free radicals resulting in tissue damage.

SIGNALMENT
• Ruminants especially cattle and sheep and monogastrics are all affected.
• Congenital defective hepatic function leading to secondary photosensitization occurs in lambs of the Corriedale and Southdown breeds.

SIGNS
• Signs include erythema, edema, and sloughing off of skin around unpigmented areas or areas exposed to ultraviolet rays.
• Common sites include eyelids, conjunctiva, ears, muzzle, dorsum of the body, perineum, and teats.
• Icterus is associated with secondary photodermatitis due to hepatic insufficiency.

CAUSES
• The principal photodynamic agents are endogenous porphyrins and phylloerythrin from plant material.
• Primary photodermatitis is due to ingestion of exogenous photodynamic agents. Plants containing photodynamic agents include *Hypericum* spp. (St John's wort), *Lolium perenne* (perennial ryegrass), *Cymopterus* (wild carrot). Chemicals including phenothiazine and rose Bengal and acaridine dyes have been reported to cause photosensitization.
• Secondary photodermatitis results from accumulation of phylloerythrin in plasma due to insufficient hepatobiliary excretion. Plants that contain hepatotoxins include lantana, cyanobacteria, lupins, ragwort, *Crotalaria* spp., and *Tribulus* spp.
• Mycotoxins in stored feeds also can cause hepatotoxicity.
• Inherited aberrant defective functions of enzymes involved in porphyrin-heme synthesis may result in excessive production of porphyrins, which are photodynamic.
• Congenital photodermatitis occurs in Corriedale and Southdown breed of sheep and results from defective bile excretion.

RISK FACTORS
Exposure of animal to plants containing primary photodynamic agents or plant containing hepatotoxins predisposes animal to photodermatitis.

 DIAGNOSIS

DIFFERENTIAL DIAGNOSIS
• These include dermatophytosis and infectious bovine keratoconjunctivitis. Keratoconjunctivitis is not accompanied with dermatitis.
• Dermatophytosis will affect both pigmented and nonpigmented areas and the organisms can be isolated from the lesions.

CBC/BIOCHEMISTRY/URINALYSIS
There are no specific laboratory findings with photodermatitis. Elevated levels of plasma bilirubin may be observed with secondary photodermatitis. Liver enzymes may be elevated.

OTHER LABORATORY TESTS
Liver biopsies may be useful in secondary photodermatitis.

IMAGING
N/A

OTHER DIAGNOSTIC PROCEDURES
Submission of potential toxic plants to diagnostic laboratory for species confirmation

TREATMENT
• Animals should be removed from the source of dynamic agent or exposure to sunlight.
• Supportive therapy may be required for severe cases.

MISCELLANEOUS

ASSOCIATED CONDITIONS
Icterus is associated with secondary photodermatitis due to hepatic insufficiency.

AGE-RELATED FACTORS
N/A

ZOONOTIC POTENTIAL
N/A

PREGNANCY
N/A

RUMINANT SPECIES AFFECTED
Potentially, all ruminant species are affected.

BIOSECURITY
N/A

PRODUCTION MANAGEMENT
• Fence off pastures containing toxic plant species.
• Herbicide treatment of toxic plants
• Genetic selection in Corriedale and Southdown breeds of sheep

SYNONYMS
N/A

SEE ALSO
Crotalaria spp.
Cyanobacteria
Cymopterus (wild carrot)
Hypericum spp. (St John's wort)
Lantana
Lolium perenne (perennial ryegrass)
Lupines
Mycotoxins
Phenothiazines and rose Bengal
Ragwort
Tribulus spp.

ABBREVIATIONS
N/A

Suggested Reading
House, J. K, George, L. W., Karen, L., et al. 1996. Primary photosensitization related to ingestion of alfalfa silage by cattle. *J Am Vet Med Assoc*. 209:1604–7.
Radostits, O. M, Gay, C. C., Blood, D.C., et al. 2000. *Veterinary medicine*. 9th ed. New York: W. B. Saunders.
Rowe, L. D. 1989. Photosensitization problems in livestock. *Vet Clin North Am Food Anim Pract*. 5:301–23.
Scruggs, D.W, Blue, G. K. 1994. Toxic hepatopathy and photosensitization in cattle fed moldy alfalfa hay. *J Am Vet Med Assoc*. 204:264–66.

Author: Tina Wismer

PHOTOSENSITIZATION

 BASICS

OVERVIEW
• Photosensitization is an abnormal reaction of the skin to sunlight due to the presence of a photodynamic agent in the dermis. Photodynamic agents absorb certain wavelengths of ultraviolet (UV) light, producing free radicals, which react with proteins in the dermal tissue, causing damage.
• Photosensitization can be divided into three categories: Type I (primary photosensitization), Type II (photosensitization due to aberrant pigment synthesis), and Type III (secondary or hepatogenous photosensitization).

PATHOPHYSIOLOGY
• In Type I photosensitization, the photodynamic agents are absorbed into the blood from the gastrointestinal tract (GI) and react with UV light at the skin surface. Type I reactions may also occur with direct contact to the photodynamic agent (plant, chemical). Once in the dermis, the photodynamic agent absorbs the energy of a light photon and forms free radicals. The oxygen free radical reacts with amino acids, nucleic acids, and membrane lipids in the capillary endothelium and surrounding tissues, causing tissue destruction.
• Type II photosensitization is due to a genetic defect in the individual. The photodynamic agent is a pigment that is produced endogenously by an aberrant metabolic process.
• Type III photosensitization is secondary to liver damage. Chlorophyll is metabolized by microbes in the GI tract, forming phylloerythrin. Phylloerythrin, a photodynamic metabolite of chlorophyll, is absorbed into the blood stream. Normally phylloerythrin is removed from the blood by the liver, and excreted in bile. With liver damage or biliary obstruction, phylloerythrin cannot be excreted, and thus enters the general circulation. Liver damage can occur from toxins, bacteria, viruses, or neoplasia. Secondary photosensitization is intensified when the consumption of chlorophyll from green plants is high.

SYSTEMS AFFECTED
• Skin/exocrine
• Hepatobiliary

GENETICS
• White- or light-skinned breeds are at higher risk for Type I or Type III photosensitivity. Black-skinned animals are rarely affected with photosensitization of any type.
• Type II photosensitization has been reported to occur as an inherited autosomal recessive congenital disease in Holstein, Ayrshire, and Shorthorn cattle and Southdown and Corriedale sheep.

• In bovine erythropoietic porphyria ("pink tooth"), affected cattle are deficient in uroporphyrin III cosynthetase, an enzyme needed for proper formation of hemoglobin. Uroporphyrin and coproporphyrin accumulate in the bones, teeth, skin, and urine, as well as other tissues and secretions. Accumulations of porphyrin metabolites in the skin predispose the animals to photosensitization.
• Southdown lambs may have a congenital defect that can cause hyperbilirubinemia and results in hepatogenous photosensitization. Corriedale lambs can have a similar condition, which is characterized by a failure to excrete phylloerythrin and conjugated bilirubin that also results in hepatogenous photosensitization.

INCIDENCE/PREVALENCE
Late spring, summer, and early fall are most common, but if photosensitizing plants are baled into hay, signs may be seen year round.

GEOGRAPHIC DISTRIBUTION
Worldwide

SIGNALMENT
Species
All ruminant species
Breed Predilections
White- or light-colored breeds
Mean Age and Range
Affects all ages, but young may be more susceptible
Predominant Sex
Affects both sexes equally

SIGNS
• Photosensitization occurs most frequently in hairless and white-skinned areas of the body. Eyelids, lips, ears, nose, white blazes, coronary bands, and other white areas are most commonly involved.
• Signs may be more severe in areas of the body that receive more sunlight (head, neck, back).
• In contact photosensitization, only areas of contact with the photodynamic agent are affected. The affected area first becomes erythematous, edematous, and painful. Honey-colored serum begins to seep from the thickened skin, and extensive scabs can form

after 1–2 days. Secondary bacterial infections of the skin can occur.
• Animals tend to be very pruritic in the early stages. As signs progress, they resist handling and may not want to eat due to the discomfort. Occasionally, the eyes will be affected and these animals may become blind. Death is due to starvation or misadventure.
• Signs consistent with hepatic encephalopathy (e.g., ceaseless walking, head pressing, behavior changes, etc.) are seen with secondary photosensitization.

HISTORICAL FINDINGS
• With plant ingestion, signs may appear from 24 hours to several months after the first ingestion.
• With drug eruptions, cutaneous lesions are noted 24–48 hours after drug administration, although there may occasionally be a longer interval.

PHYSICAL EXAMINATION FINDINGS
Animals may be restless and pruritic with reddened and swollen eyelids, muzzle, and lips. Affected animals may also exhibit tachypnea, tachycardia, hyperthermia, diarrhea, salivation, and jaundice (if Type III).

CAUSES
Plants: see Tables 1 and 2
Pharmaceuticals
• Antibiotics (penicillin, sulfas, tetracycline)
• Anticonvulsants
• Local anesthetics
• Nonsteroidal anti-inflammatory agents (NSAIDs), antipyretics (aspirin, phenylbutazone)
• Phenothiazines
• Thiazides
Chemicals
• Carbon tetrachloride
• Copper
• Methylene blue
• Phenanthridium
• Phosphorus
Fungal
Pithomyces chartarum, *Aspergillus* spp., and *Fusarium* spp. can all produce hepatotoxic mycotoxins and cause secondary photosensitization.

Table 1

Plants That Cause Type I (Primary) Photosensitization		
Latin Name	Common Name	Toxin
Hypericum spp.	St. Johns wort	Conjugated quinone (hypericin)
Fagopyrum esculentum	Buckwheat	Conjugated quinone (fagopyrin)
Heracleum mantegazzianum	Giant hogweed	Furocoumarins
Ammi majus	St. Anne's lace	
Cymopterus spp.	Spring parsley	
Thamnosma texana	Dutchman's breeches	

PHOTOSENSITIZATION

Table 2

Plants That Cause Type III (Secondary) Photosensitization			
Latin Name	Common Name	Toxin	Mechanism of Action
Senecio spp. *Crotalaria* spp. *Amsinckia intermedia* *Echium* spp. *Heliotropium* spp. *Symphytum* spp. *Cynoglossum officinale*	Ragwort, groundsel, senecio Crotalaria, rattlebox Fiddleneck Blueweed, viper's bugloss Heliotrope Comfrey Hound's tongue	Pyrrolizidine Alkaloids (PA)	PAs are metabolized by the liver and the activated pyrrole form alkylates DNA in the hepatocyte, which impairs cell division. This prevents the hepatocyte from undergoing binary fission to regenerate hepatocytes, resulting in hepatocytomegaly and karyomegaly. When large numbers of hepatocytes die, the necrosis triggers a regenerative response accompanied by bile duct proliferation.
Microcystis *Anabaena* *Oscillatoria* *Nodularia spumigena*	Blue green algae	Microcystins	Microcystins cause disruption of the actin filaments of the hepatic cytoskeleton, leading to cellular collapse.
Lantana spp. *Lippia* spp.	Lantana, shrub verbena, yellow sage White brush	Triterpenoid compounds	Triterpenoids affect hepatocytes by inhibiting secretory function and decreasing bile canaliculi ATPase activity resulting in cholestasis and jaundice.
Helenium spp. *Hymenoxys* spp.	Sneezeweed Rubberweed, bitterweed	Sesquiterpene lactones	Sesquiterpene lactones bind to sulfhydryl groups and other nucleophilic components, inhibiting numerous aerobin and anaerobin enzymes.
Tetradymia and *Artemisia* spp.	Horsebrush Black sagebrush	Furanosesquiterpenens Sesquiterpene lactones	Tetradymol metabolites uncouple oxidative phosphorylation in electron transport. Phylloerythrin from other plants must be eaten to result in the development of photosensitization.
Panicum spp. *Tribulus terrestris* *Nolina* spp. *Agave lecheguilla*	Panicum, Kleingrass Puncture vine, goathead Sacahuiste, bunchgrass Agave, lecheguilla	Disogenin	Lithogenic steroidal saponins (disogenins) are responsible for formation of crystals in the bile ducts resulting in hepatogenous photosensitization.
Kochia scoparia	Kochia	Unknown, possibly saponins	Secondary photosensitization
Trifolium hybridum	Alsike clover	Unknown	Primary photosensitization has been seen with ingestion and possibly contact. Secondary photosensitization has been seen with long-term ingestions.
Phyllanthus abnormis *Descurainia pinnata* *D. sophia*	Abnormal-leaf Flower Tansymustard Flixweed	Unknown	Secondary photosensitization
Brassica rapa *B. napus* *B. oleracea*	Turnip Rape Kale	Nitriles?	Unknown photosensitization
Lotus corniculatus *Trifolium incarnatum* *T. subterraneum* *T. pratense* *Medicago denticulate* (polymorpha) *M. sativa* *M. lupulina* *M. minima* *Avena sativa* *Sorghum* *Triticum* *Chamaesyce (Euphorbia) maculata*	Bird's-foot trefoil Crimson clover Subterranean clover Red clover Burclover Alfalfa Black medic Small burclover Oats Sorghum Wheat Spotted spurge	Unknown	Unknown photosensitization

PHOTOSENSITIZATION

Neoplasia
Any neoplasia that affects hepatic function can cause secondary photosensitization.

RISK FACTORS
Any underlying liver disorder or genetic defect that decreases excretion of phylloerythrin

 DIAGNOSIS

DIFFERENTIAL DIAGNOSIS
• Pemphigus foliaceus
• Irritant dermatitis
• Allergic dermatitis
• Folliculitis/furunculosis
• Dermatophytosis
• Chemical burns
• Thermal burns
• Malignant catarrhal fever
• Pediculosis
• Demodectic mange

CBC/BIOCHEMISTRY/URINALYSIS
• Elevations in GGT, AST, and ALP (most common)
• Elevations in SDH, GLDH, LDH (early in syndrome)
• Hyperbilirubinemia
• Inflammatory leukogram may be present.

OTHER LABORATORY TESTS
• Elevated bile acids
• Prolonged BSP clearance time
• Plasma phylloerythrin ($> 10\ \mu g/dl$ is diagnostic)

IMAGING
N/A

DIAGNOSTIC PROCEDURES
Skin or liver biopsies can be performed on valuable animals.

PATHOLOGIC FINDINGS
• Dermal lesions vary from minimal reddening to urticarial lesions with erythema and swelling, to skin necrosis. The skin may have a gelatinous appearance extending down into the deeper corium. Microscopically, edema will be accompanied by necrosis and a polymorphonuclear infiltrate in the deeper corium. Both the epidermis and the superficial dermal vasculature may be damaged.
• Animals with secondary photosensitization will have hepatic and other systemic lesions. Bright yellow fat, hepatomegaly, liver cirrhosis, hepatic necrosis, and ascites are common. Depending on the extent of the liver damage, bruising and hemorrhage may be seen.
• If toxicosis is due to PAs, then hepatocytomegaly (always present), fibrosis, and bile duct proliferation may be seen.
• With disogens, birefringent crystals may be evident in the bile ducts (small ducts may be obstructed), skin, kidney, adrenal gland, and heart.

 TREATMENT

APPROPRIATE HEALTH CARE
Therapy involves removing the animal from sunlight and preventing reexposure to the photodynamic agent. All drugs being administered when photosensitization occurred should be stopped. If the liver is involved, appropriate therapy for liver disease must be given.

NURSING CARE
As many affected animals stop eating and drinking, supplemental feeding and fluid therapy are important. Mortality primarily occurs in lambs because the ewe's udders are so painful that lambs are not permitted to nurse. Cows also refuse to let calves nurse, but calf losses are usually low. Soothing skin medication or other pain relief can hasten healing.

ACTIVITY
Prevent animal exposure to UV light. Let out on dry pasture only at night.

DIET
Avoid any additional photosensitizing plants.

CLIENT EDUCATION
Clients need to inspect hay and pastures for any phototoxic plants.

SURGICAL CONSIDERATIONS
N/A

 MEDICATIONS

DRUGS OF CHOICE
• Pain relief with NSAIDs (e.g., flunixin 1.1–2.2 mg/kg PO or IV q 6–12 h; 72-hour milk withdrawal, 10–day meat withdrawal) if hepatopathy is not involved.
• Antibiotics if pyoderma is present (e.g., ceftiofur 1.1–2.2 mg/kg IM q 24 h; no milk or meat withdrawal)

CONTRAINDICATIONS
• If signs are due to a drug reaction, avoid using any related medications in the treatment of clinical signs.
• Appropriate milk and meat withdrawal times must be followed for all compounds administered to food-producing animals.

PRECAUTIONS

If secondary photosensitization, use caution when using drugs that must be metabolized by the liver.

POSSIBLE INTERACTIONS

ALTERNATIVE DRUGS

Liver protectants and blood transfusions may be attempted to prolong life in valuable animals.

FOLLOW-UP

PATIENT MONITORING

Monitor until dermal lesions have resolved or until liver values return to normal.

PREVENTION/AVOIDANCE

• Avoid future exposures to any implicated compounds and related substances.
• Avoid grain and hay contaminated by species of plants known to cause photosensitization.
• Control photosensitizing plants by spraying pastures and crop land with herbicides. Plants along trails and in shipping areas should be removed.
• Supplementation of phosphorus and cobalt may lessen PA effects.
• Less-valuable animals or more resistant species may be used to "pregraze" pastures (e.g., sheep/goats may be used to graze groundsel before cattle).
• Provide supplemental feeding with more nutritious and palatable forage with contaminated pastures and follow a range management program that prevents overgrazing.
• Avoid exposure to blue-green algae by fencing off contaminated ponds.
• Facial eczema can be prevented by breeding animals for resistance, oral dosing with zinc, and spraying pastures with fungicides.

POSSIBLE COMPLICATIONS

Prolonged grazing of *Echium* and *Heliotropium* may result in chronic copper poisoning of sheep.

EXPECTED COURSE AND PROGNOSIS

• Type I has a good prognosis. Type III has a poor prognosis due to liver involvement.
• The skin eruptions usually subside within 24 to 48 hours after exposure ceases, although lesions may persist up to 6 months.

MISCELLANEOUS

ASSOCIATED CONDITIONS

Pyoderma

AGE-RELATED FACTORS

Affects animals of all ages, but increased mortality in young animals

ZOONOTIC POTENTIAL

PA metabolites are secreted in milk.

PREGNANCY

PAs cross the placenta and can affect the fetus, leading to increased calf losses, even with clinically normal dams.

RUMINANT SPECIES AFFECTED

All ruminant species may be affected.

BIOSECURITY

N/A

SYNONYMS

Bighead = *Tribulus terrestris, Chamaesyce maculata*
Facial eczema = *Pithymyces chartarum*
Fagopyrism = *Fagopyrum esculentum*
Geeldikkop = *Tribulus terrestris*
Hard liver disease = chronic *Amsinkia intermedia* toxicosis
Seneciosis, Pictou disease, sleepy staggers = chronic *Senecio* spp. intoxication
Trifoliosis, dew poisoning, big liver disease = *Trifolium hybridum* intoxication

SEE ALSO

Demodectic mange
Dermatophytosis
Hepatitis
Malignant catarrhal fever
Pediculosis
Photodermatitis

ABBREVIATIONS

ALP = alkaline phosphatase
AST = aspartate aminotransferase
BSP = bromosulfophthalein
GGT = gamma-glutamyltransferase
GI = gastrointestinal
GLDH = glutamate dehydrogenase
LDH = lactate dehydrogenase
NSAIDs = nonsteroidal anti-inflammatory drugs
PA = pyrrolizidine alkaloids
SDH = sorbitol dehydrogenase
UV = ultraviolet

Suggested Reading
Burrows, G. E., Tyrl, R. J. 2001. *Toxic plants of North America*. Ames: Iowa State University Press.
Cheeke, P. R., Shull, L. R. 1985. *Natural toxicants in feeds and poisonous plants*. Westport, CT: AVI Publishing Company, Inc.
Flaoyen, A. 1996. Do steroidal saponins have a role in hepatogenous photosensitization diseases of sheep? *Adv Exp Med Biol.* 405:395–403.
Scruggs, D. W., Blue, G. K. 1994, Jan 15. Toxic hepatopathy and photosensitization in cattle fed moldy alfalfa hay. *J Am Vet Med Assoc.* 204(2):264–66.

Author: Tina Wismer

PINE NEEDLE TOXICITY

 BASICS

OVERVIEW
Ingestion of pine needles, bark, or new growth tips of several species of pine causes abortions in cattle and, less frequently, systemic toxicity in cattle and sheep.

PATHOPHYSIOLOGY
• Amount of toxic principle varies considerably with geographic location and season.
• Abortifacient effects most often occur with ingestion of 1 kg needles/day for several days or higher amounts for 2–3 days.
• Clinical signs: 24 hours to several weeks postexposure.
• Mechanism: It is thought that the diterpene acids, of which isocuppressic acid is the most common, are metabolized in the rumen or liver to abortifacient metabolites. The toxins appear to modify hormonal effects responsible for the normal increase in uterine blood flow that occurs with increasing pregnancy. Results are an increase in caruncular arterial tone and decrease in uterine blood flow, which causes premature parturition. There may also be an effect on progesterone-producing cells in the corpus luteum, causing a direct decrease in progesterone levels and termination of pregnancy.
• No effect on overall fertility
• Other abietane diterpenes present are thought to be responsible for systemic toxicity (higher concentration in new growth tips and bark than in needles).

SYSTEMS AFFECTED
Reproductive, respiratory, renal, systemic

GENETICS
N/A

INCIDENCE/PREVALENCE
Unknown

GEOGRAPHIC DISTRIBUTION
• *P. ponderosa* (ponderosa or western yellow pine) is the most widespread found across much of western North America.
• *P. contorta* (lodgepole or limber pine) is found in the Sierra-Cascade range and the Rockies.
• *P. radiata* (Monterey pine) found around Monterey, California and cultivated in New Zealand.
• Other plants containing toxic principle that also cause abortion in livestock: *Communis juniperus* (common juniper) in North America and New Zealand. *Cupressus macrocarpa* (Monterey cypress) is native to Monterey, California, and is a widespread ornamental.

SIGNALMENT
• Abortion: cattle and bison (though bison rarely eat pine needles) susceptible from midgestation to parturition. Risk increases with length of pregnancy.
• Toxicity: cattle, bison, sheep
• Goats, deer, and elk unaffected

SIGNS
Reproductive
• Early parturition with depression, mucoid vulvular discharge (often bloody), weak uterine contractions, incomplete cervical dilation, uterine hemorrhage, dystocia, birth of dead or small weak calf
• Maternal complications include retained placenta, septic metritis, agalactia, anorexia, rumen stasis, and death (if untreated).
• While significant exposure does not cause abortion in sheep, the number of dead lambs born at term may increase.

Systemic
• Toxicosis in cows from a diet of 10%–15% new growth tips or very high doses of pine needles: depression, anorexia, rumen stasis, dyspnea, peripheral neuropathy, nephrosis, and death.
• In cattle and sheep, when 15%–40% of their diet consisted of pine needles, there were altered rumen fluid dynamics including fluid rate of passage, decreased volatile fatty acids, and decreased nitrogen intake and digestibility (supplemental protein has no effect on symptoms).

CAUSES AND RISK FACTORS
• Ingestion of pine needles of any age or state, although green needles more likely to be ingested
• Pregnant cows at increasing risk from midgestation to term, with greatest risk in last trimester
• Decreased temperatures and/or increased snow cover in winter
• Harsh weather that forces cows to seek shelter under pine trees
• Crowded feeding areas

 DIAGNOSIS

DIFFERENTIAL DIAGNOSIS
Abortion caused by BVD or IBR viruses, neosporosis, leptospirosis, brucellosis, selenium deficiency, or foothill abortion (EBA).

CBC/BIOCHEMISTRY/URINALYSIS
Systemic toxicity: azotemia, hypercreatinemia, proteinuria, and elevation of AST and SDH

OTHER LABORATORY TESTS
N/A

IMAGING
N/A

DIAGNOSTIC PROCEDURES
Combination of access to pine needles, presence of risk factors, and clinical signs

PATHOLOGIC FINDINGS
• Reproductive—dams that die exhibit heavy uterine exudate with necrotic placental tissue, edema, and focal ulceration of endometrium and necrosis in the caruncles. Stillborn calves may show malacia of white brain (cerebral leukomalacia) matter or may appear normal.
• Systemic—nephrosis, vacuolation of basal ganglia neuropil, perivascular and myelinic edema

TREATMENT

• Supportive care for calf
• Removal of placenta and treatment for uterine infection in the cow
• Systemic treatment of bacterial infection, dehydration, and malnutrition in any affected animal

MEDICATIONS

DRUGS OF CHOICE
Broad-spectrum antibiotics to treat uterine and/or systemic bacterial infection

CONTRAINDICATIONS
Appropriate milk and meat withdrawal times must be followed for all compounds administered to food-producing animals.

POSSIBLE INTERACTIONS

FOLLOW-UP

PATIENT MONITORING
N/A

PREVENTION/AVOIDANCE
• Fence pregnant cows in the last trimester away from pines and provide supplemental feed.
• For all cattle, when feeding supplemental feed, do so over a larger area to ensure all animals access.
• Remove young stands of pines where appropriate

POSSIBLE COMPLICATIONS
Dams: retained placenta, septic metritis, agalactia, anorexia, rumen stasis, and death (if untreated)

EXPECTED COURSE AND PROGNOSIS
• Dams usually recover with treatment but death has been reported.
• Calf prognosis is dependent on stage of development at birth and supportive treatment for premature birth.
• Incidence of abortion 0%–100%

MISCELLANEOUS

ASSOCIATED CONDITIONS
Nutritional deficiency

AGE-RELATED FACTORS
N/A

ZOONOTIC POTENTIAL
N/A

PREGNANCY
Reproductive toxicity in last trimester of pregnancy

RUMINANT SPECIES AFFECTED
Cattle, bison, sheep

BIOSECURITY
N/A

PRODUCTION MANAGEMENT
• Fence pregnant cows in the last trimester away from pines and provide supplemental feed.

• For all cattle, when feeding supplemental feed, do so over a larger area to ensure all animals access.
• Remove young stands of pines where appropriate.

SEE ALSO
Abortion caused by BVD or IBR viruses, neosporosis, leptospirosis, brucellosis, selenium deficiency or foothill abortion (EBA).
EBA
Rumen stasis
Selenium deficiency

ABBREVIATIONS
AST = aspartate aminotransferase
BVD = bovine viral diarrhea
EBA = epizootic bovine abortion
IBR = infectious bovine rhinotracheitis
SDH = sorbitol dehydrogenase

Suggested Reading
Burrows, G. E., Tyrl, R. J., ed. 2001. *Toxic plants of North America*. Ames: Iowa State University Press.
Gardner, D. R., James, L. F., Panter, K. E., Pfister, J. A., Ralphs, M. H., Stegelmeier, B. L. 1999. Ponderosa pine and broom snakeweed: poisonous plants that affect livestock. *J Nat Toxins* 8(1): 27–34.
Stegelmeier, B. L., Gardner, D. R., James, L. F., Panter, K. E., Molyneux, R. J. 1996. The toxic and abortifacient effects of Ponderosa pine. *Veterinary Pathology* 33:22–28.

Author: Kristy A. Cortright

PLANTS PRODUCING ACUTE RESPIRATORY DISTRESS SYNDROME

 BASICS

OVERVIEW
• An afebrile pneumonia like disease of cattle but occasionally observed in other ruminants.
• Rapid death may result.
• Several etiologies exist for the disease including rapidly changing animals from poor to lush pasture, and the plant *Perilla frutescens* (purple mint, perilla mint). Moldy sweet potatoes, rape, kale, turnips, and moldy pink half-runner beans are also associated with the disease.
• Many lush grasses are associated with ARDS including Bermuda, fescue, alfalfa, and Kleingrass. In the southeastern United States, *Perilla frutescens*, or purple mint, is often associated with ARDS. *Perilla* is an annual weed that grows to a height of 1–2 meters. *Perilla* is readily identified by its square stem and is common along wood lines and waste areas. The plant has small terminal white flowers and a characteristic minty fragrance.
• Lush pasture of many grasses contains high quantities of L-tryptophan. Dry, nonsucculent pastures contain lower quantities of L-tryptophan.
• Perilla mint contains 3-substituted furans (perilla ketone, egomaketone, and isoegomaketone).
• L-tryptophan in high quantities can lead to pneumotoxicosis.
• Three-substituted furans can be pneumotoxic by their direct affects on the lung.
• The condition is often referred to as bovine asthma, or AIP, in the United States and fog fever in the United Kingdom.

SIGNALMENT
• All ruminants, but cattle primarily
• Horses have been affected by perilla mint.

SIGNS
• The clinical course is rapid and cattle may be found dead in 12–24 hours, especially if stressed.
• Animals are observed breathing very rapidly and shallow with their mouths open. Foam is evident around their mouth. An expiratory grunt is very audible from 100 feet or more. Animals may be extremely cyanotic and die quickly if stressed.

CAUSES AND RISK FACTORS
Animals are susceptible whenever moved from dry nonsucculent pasture to lush pasture. Signs may appear within 1 week following the transfer.
• L-tryptophan is metabolized by rumen microorganisms to indoleacetic acid, which is subsequently decarboxylated by *Lactobacillus* spp. to 3-methylindole (3-MI). The 3-methylindole is absorbed and metabolized by the lung mixed-function oxidase system to produce pneumotoxicosis.
• Usually observed in the fall when cattle are moved from summer pasture to lush fall growth, it has been observed in spring when cattle are turned out on lush pasture after being fed hay over the winter.
• If caused by *Perilla frutescens*, usually observed from August through October when this plant reaches maturity. The seed heads are the most toxic. Has been observed in cattle eating hay containing purple mint.

 DIAGNOSIS

DIFFERENTIAL DIAGNOSIS
• Other causes of pneumonia
• Hardware disease in cattle due to the pronounced expiratory grunt
• Organophosphate toxicosis

CBC/BIOCHEMISTRY/URINALYSIS
N/A

IMAGING
• Thoracic radiography
• Pulmonary emphysema and edema are common.
• Emphysematous bullae may be observed on the lung surface.

DIAGNOSTIC PROCEDURES
N/A

PATHOLOGIC FINDINGS
• Lungs are enlarged and heavy due to edema, cellular proliferation, and congestion. Foam fills many airways.
• Interlobular edema and emphysema are commonly observed. Emphysematous bullae are often observed on the lung surface.
• Emphysema may extend into the mediastinum and subcutaneous cervical and thoracic areas.
• Microscopically, alveolar epithelial hyperplasia of type 2 pneumocytes is common along with interstitial emphysema, edema, and hyaline membranes.

 TREATMENT

• No specific treatment
• Keeping animals as calm as possible is important.
• If stressed, animals often become anoxic and die.
• Remove animals from etiology (i.e., purple mint or lush pasture). Place on dry feed.

 MEDICATIONS

DRUGS OF CHOICE
• No specific drugs are effective.
• Symptomatic treatment such as corticosteroids, atropine, diuretics, antihistamines, and antibiotics.

PLANTS PRODUCING ACUTE RESPIRATORY DISTRESS SYNDROME

• Avoid stress (if possible) when treating.
• Weigh the value of therapeutic pharmacology versus the stress involved with handling and treatment.

CONTRAINDICATIONS
• Appropriate milk and meat withdrawal times must be followed for all compounds administered to food-producing animals.
• Steroids should not be used in pregnant animals.

FOLLOW-UP

PATIENT MONITORING
N/A

PREVENTION/AVOIDANCE
• Gradually introduce cattle to lush pasture after feeding on nonsucculent, if possible.
• Inhibit certain ruminal microflora that reduce L-tryptophan to 3-MI with monensin or lasalocid.
• Avoid exposure to perilla mint.
• Supply ample good pasture as perilla is usually consumed only when other better forage is lacking.

POSSIBLE COMPLICATIONS
N/A

EXPECTED COURSE AND PROGNOSIS
• Very guarded early prognosis as death may occur within 12–24 hours.
• Clinical course may last 2–3 weeks.

• If animals survive 2 or 3 days and are not stressed, prognosis improves.
• Even severely affected animals may return to normal in 2–3 weeks when the type 2 pneumocytes resolves to type 1.

MISCELLANEOUS

ASSOCIATED CONDITIONS
Animals are observed breathing very rapidly and shallow with mouths open. Foam is evident around mouth. An expiratory grunt is very audible from 100 feet or more. Animals may be extremely cyanotic and die quickly if stressed.

AGE-RELATED FACTORS
Calves fed the flowering perilla plant develop the toxic syndrome, while those fed earlier plants (collected before seed stage) and late plants (collected after frost) remain asymptomatic.

ZOONOTIC POTENTIAL
N/A

PREGNANCY
N/A

PRODUCTION MANAGEMENT
The time of year when perilla reaches the seed stage often corresponds to periods when pasture grass is scarce forcing cattle to consume plants not normally eaten when ample desirable forage is available.

SYNONYMS
AIP
Bovine asthma
Fog fever

SEE ALSO
Hardware disease in cattle
Moldy sweet potatoes, rape, kale, turnips
Organophosphate toxicosis
Other causes of pneumonia
Toxicosis herd outbreaks

ABBREVIATIONS
AIP = atypical interstitial pneumonia
ARDS = acute respiratory distress syndrome
3-MI = 3-methylindole

Suggested Reading
Apley, M. D., Fajt, V. R. 1998, Jul. Feedlot therapeutics. *Vet Clin North Am Food Anim Pract.* 14(2):291–313.
Burrows, G. E., Tyrl, R. J. *Toxic plants of North America.* Ames: Iowa State University Press.
Kerr, L. A., Johnson, B. J., Burrows, G. E. 1986, Oct. Intoxication of cattle by *Perilla frutescens* (purple mint). *Vet Hum Toxicol.* 28(5):412–16.
Kerr, L. A., Linnabary, R. D. 1989, Jun. Review of interstitial pneumonia in cattle. *Vet Hum Toxicol.* 31 (3):247–254.
Pearson, E. G., Andreasen, C. B., Blythe, L. L., Craig, A. M. 1996, Sep 15. Atypical pneumonia associated with ryegrass staggers in calves. *J Am Vet Med Assoc.* 209(6): 1137–42.

Author: Larry A. Kerr

PNEUMOTHORAX

 BASICS

OVERVIEW
• A pneumothorax is a collection of air or gas in the pleural space (the space surrounding the lungs).
• Pleural pressure is normally negative with respect to alveolar and atmospheric pressures throughout the respiratory cycle.
• A negative pleural pressure is maintained by two forces applied to the pleural space simultaneously and in opposition: (a) elastic forces that tend to collapse the lung and (b) recoil forces that tend to expand the chest wall.
• Normal end-expiratory pleural pressure is approximately –5 cm H_2O.
• Pleural pressure becomes more negative (–7.5 cm H_2O) during inspiration when the chest wall expands through the effort of the inspiratory muscles (diaphragm and external intercostal muscles).
• The onset of a pneumothorax disconnects the lung/chest wall unit and the chest wall expands controlled only by recoil forces, while the lung collapses under the influence of its own elastic properties.
• During pneumothorax, pleural and atmospheric pressures progressively equilibrate causing the lung to reach its minimal volume.

PATHOPHYSIOLOGY
• In cattle, there is evidence to support an association between rupture of emphysematous bullae during straining, coughing, and effort of parturition and the development of closed pneumothorax.

• Most commonly, the problem is confined to one hemithorax because cattle have a complete mediastinum. Occasionally, rupture of pulmonary bullae can occur bilaterally leading to severe dyspnea and acute death.
• Penetrating thoracic trauma, although rare in ruminants, can lead to pneumothorax by disruption of the integrity of the chest wall. Wounds that cause pneumothorax are most commonly located on the lateral chest wall and may be associated with rib fractures. Pectoral wounds are very rarely associated with pneumothorax.

SYSTEMS AFFECTED
Respiratory

GENETICS
N/A

INCIDENCE/PREVALENCE
• There is no specific incidence rate reported for pneumothorax.
• In feedlot cattle, however, mortality rates of up to 0.5% have been associated with atypical interstitial pneumonia, emphysema, and pneumothorax.

SIGNALMENT
• Not common in ruminants. When encountered, it is most common in dairy calves and adult dairy cattle. Case reports describe pneumothorax in bulls.
• In the beef feedlot industry, atypical interstitial pneumonia poses a substantial risk of pneumothorax.
• Chest trauma may result in a pneumothorax in other ruminant species, although the incidence of penetrating chest trauma is unknown in small ruminants and llamas.

SIGNS
• Inspiratory dyspnea
• Tachycardia
• Open-mouth breathing
• Cattle are alert and anxious.
• Pronounced abdominal effort during respiration
• Cyanosis in severe cases
• Auscultation: the affected side of the thorax (hemithorax) is almost silent while normal or slightly increased respiratory sounds are audible on the unaffected side.
• Percussion performed during auscultation may produce a "ping" on the affected hemithorax.
• Subcutaneous emphysema is not uncommon.

RISK FACTORS
• Pneumothorax in cattle is associated with bovine respiratory syncytial virus (BRSV) infection (acute interstitial pneumonia) and, less commonly, with acute pneumotoxicosis.
• Atypical interstitial pneumonia and acute respiratory distress may be predisposing factors in beef cattle.
• Trauma

 DIAGNOSIS

• Assessing the clinical presentation in conjunction with the predisposing factors mentioned above makes the diagnosis. Clinical signs are often sufficiently straightforward to allow a diagnosis.
• Presence of a thoracic wound should always warrant a thorough evaluation of chest wall integrity.
• The diagnosis is confirmed by obtaining thoracic radiographs.

TREATMENT

• In case of thoracic trauma, the wound should be explored to verify the presence of and remove any rib fragments. The wound should be closed primarily, if possible, or covered with a dressing that allows an airtight seal to occur.
• The hemithorax should be suctioned in order to aspirate the air contained in the pneumothorax. This can be accomplished by using standard suction/vacuum equipment attached via tubing to a sterile teat cannula placed in the dorsal-and caudal-most aspect of the thorax.
• Alternatively, air can be aspirated by using a large syringe connected to a teat cannula via a three-way stopcock.
• Placement of a chest tube connected to a commercially available continuous flow evacuation device has been reported as a successful and simple method for pneumothorax evacuation in bulls.
• These measures may fail in case of ruptured bullae because air continuously leaks through the disrupted lung parenchyma. In these cases, however, it is worth continuing the evacuation process chronically because the ruptured lung parenchyma will eventually heal.

• In mild cases, air will gradually reabsorb following healing of the lesion without evacuation.
• Broad-spectrum antibiotic administration is indicated in case of thoracic trauma or when concurrent bacterial pleuritis and pneumonia are suspected or in case of a chest wound.

MEDICATIONS

FOLLOW-UP

MISCELLANEOUS

ASSOCIATED CONDITIONS
• Bovine respiratory syncytial virus (BRSV)
• Acute pneumotoxicosis
• Atypical interstitial pneumonia
• Penetrating thoracic trauma
• Pleuritis and pneumonia

AGE-RELATED FACTORS
N/A

ZOONOTIC POTENTIAL
N/A

PREGNANCY
N/A

BIOSECURITY
N/A

PRODUCTION MANAGEMENT
N/A

SYNONYMS
N/A

SEE ALSO
Acute pneumotoxicosis
Atypical interstitial pneumonia
Bovine respiratory syncytial virus (BRSV)
Penetrating thoracic trauma
Pleuritis and pneumonia

ABBREVIATION
BRSV = bovine respiratory syncytial virus

Suggested Reading
Peek, S. E., Slack, J. A., McGuirk, S. M. 2003, Jan-Feb. Management of pneumothorax in cattle by continuous-flow evacuation. *J Vet Intern Med*. 17(1): 119–22.
Slack, J. A., Thomas, C. B., Peek, S. E. 2004. Pneumothorax in dairy cattle. *JAVMA* 225:5, 732.
Smith, J. A. 2002. Pneumothorax. In: *Large animal internal medicine*, ed. B. P. Smith. 3rd ed. St. Louis: Mosby.

Authors: S. John Peroni and Laura Riggs

POLIOENCEPHALOMALACIA

 BASICS

OVERVIEW
• Polioencephalomalacia is a syndrome/lesion that can have several underlying causes in ruminants but typically results from a disturbance in thiamine metabolism.
• Traditionally described as the result of thiamine deficiency but elevated dietary sulfur is also a cause of this syndrome. Within the rumen, the elevated dietary sulfur is transformed to hydrogen sulfide.
• High-concentrate diets that lower rumen pH have been implicated as a cause of polioencephalomalacia due to the increase in thiaminase-producing bacteria.
• The treatment of the syndrome, regardless of the cause, is similar.
• Prevention and management of the syndrome benefits from an understanding of causative factors.

SYSTEMS AFFECTED
CNS primarily

Sources
Sulfur toxicosis causing polioencephalomalacia; sources of sulfur:
• High sulfate water (gyp water)
• Molasses
• Elemental sulfur
• Gypsum or ammonium sulfate added to concentrate diets
• Cruciferous forages
• Some grain processing by-products
• Thiamine deficiency
  • Ingestion of thiaminase-containing plants (bracken fern)
  • Amprolium treatment for coccidiosis
• Acute lead intoxication can have similar lesions.
• Water deprivation/sodium ion toxicosis may have similar lesions.

Toxic Dose: Sulfur
• The NRC recommendation for sulfur intake is less than 0.3% of diet.
• The maximum tolerated dose is 0.4% of diet.

GENETICS
N/A

INCIDENCE/PREVALENCE
N/A

GEOGRAPHIC DISTRIBUTION
Some areas may have elevated sulfur concentration in the groundwater. These levels can increase the risk of toxicosis.

SIGNALMENT
Species
All ruminants are susceptible.

Breed Predilections
N/A

Mean Age and Range
Young animals are more susceptible to polioencephalomalacia.

Predominant Sex
N/A

SIGNS
• Alteration of vision
• Head pressing
• Ear twitching
• Muscle tremors
• Depression
• Lethargy
• Opisthotonus
• Ataxia
• Recumbency
• Coma
• Death

CAUSES AND RISK FACTORS
• High-sulfate-containing water: If the animal's only source of water contains high concentrations of sulfur, there is an increased risk of toxicosis.
• Young animals on a high-grain diet
• Treatment of coccidiosis with amprolium
• Young animals are more susceptible than older.

 DIAGNOSIS

• Presence of clinical signs
• Elevated sulfur content of feedstuff and/or water
• Possible odor of hydrogen sulfide (rotten eggs) of cattle

DIFFERENTIAL DIAGNOSIS
• Rabies
• Acute lead intoxication
• Water deprivation/sodium ion toxicosis
• Selenium "blind staggers"
• Vitamin A deficiency
• Ethylene glycol toxicity

CBC/BIOCHEMISTRY/URINALYSIS
Not specific for this syndrome

OTHER LABORATORY TESTS
Hydrogen sulfide gas from the gas cap of the rumen
• Draw off gas and test for hydrogen sulfide using a precision gas sampler
• Gastec sampler with sulfide analyzer tube (Sensidyne, Clearwater, Florida)

PATHOLOGIC FINDINGS
Gross Necropsy Findings
• Swelling and flattening of cerebral gyri
• Pale yellow discoloration of the cerebral cortical grey matter
• Necrotic lesions may autofluoresce under ultraviolet light.

HISTOPATHOLOGICAL FINDINGS
• Neurons are shrunken and necrotic.
• Nuclei are small and faded or absent.
• Evidence of phagocytic cells in the brain

TREATMENT

- Identification and removal of source
- Symptomatic and supportive therapy
  - Provide roughages for animals on high-concentrate diets
  - Thiamine (vitamin B_1) 10–20 mg/kg up to TID intramuscularly or subcutaneously depending on severity of clinical signs and suspected cause; often mixed results
  - Possibly corticosteroids to reduce swelling and edema
  - Appropriate milk and meat withdrawal times must be followed for all compounds administered to food-producing animals.

FOLLOW-UP

PREVENTION/AVOIDANCE

- Provide alternative sources of water
- Dilution of high-sulfate sources of water
- Careful attention to the addition of any type of sulfur to the diet (prevent a mixing error)
- Provide adequate dietary thiamine when being treated for coccidiosis as amprolium acts as a thiamine antagonist for coccidia.

MISCELLANEOUS

- The exact mechanism of action of sulfur in causing polioencephalomalacia is not fully elucidated; possible mechanisms:

- Sulfide has been shown to inhibit cellular respiration similar to cyanide by inhibiting cytochrome c oxidase
- The production of free radicals from sulfides has been proposed.
- When estimating the total intake of sulfur, both feed and water sources must be estimated.
  - Sulfur in water can be a significant source.
  - The sulfur in water is generally in the sulfate form.
  - The sulfate form needs to be converted to elemental sulfur.

ASSOCIATED CONDITIONS
N/A

AGE-RELATED FACTORS
Younger animals are more susceptible to polio than mature animals.

ZOONOTIC POTENTIAL
N/A

PREGNANCY
N/A

RUMINANT SPECIES AFFECTED
All ruminant species

BIOSECURITY
N/A

PRODUCTION MANAGEMENT

- High-sulfate-containing water must be monitored. If the animal's only source of water contains high concentrations of sulfur, there is an increased risk of toxicosis.
- Young animals on a high-grain diet need to be monitored for overconsumption.

SYNONYMS
Sulfur toxicosis
Thiamine or vitamin B deficiency

SEE ALSO
Specific CNS chapters: rabies, acute lead intoxication, water deprivation/sodium ion toxicosis, selenium "blind staggers"
Specific toxicology chapters

ABBREVIATIONS
CNS = central nervous system
NRC = National Research Council

Suggested Reading
Cebra, C. K., Cebra, M. L. 2004. Altered mentation caused by polioencephalomalacia, hypernatremia, and lead poisoning. *Vet Clin N A: Food Anim Pract*. 20:287–302.
Gould, D. H. 1998. Polioencephalomalacia. *J Anim Sci*. 76:309–14.
Gould, D. H. 2000. Update on sulfur-related polioencephalomalacia. *Vet Clin North Am Food Anim Pract*. 16:481–95.
Niles, G. A., Morgan, S. E., Edwards, W. C. 2000. Sulfur-induced polioencephalomalacia in stocker calves. *Vet Human Toxicol*. 42:290–91.
Niles, G. A., Morgan, S. E., Edwards, W. C. 2002. The relationship between sulfur, thiamine and polioencephalomalacia—a review. *Bov Pract*. 36:93–99.

Authors: Joe Roder and Danelle Bickett-Weddle

POLYARTHRITIS

 BASICS

DEFINITION
Inflammation of multiple joints resulting in persistent lameness

SIGNALMENT
Varies with the specific syndrome and etiology. All ruminant species can become affected.

SIGNS
• The clinical signs typically observed in cattle with polyarthritis include shifting leg lameness, stilted gait, and unwillingness to move. Close examination usually reveals multiple visibly swollen and distended joints.
• Joint capsules are palpably distended and pressure on the joint will cause increased distention of the joint at an alternate site. Warmth and pain upon palpation of joints may be observed.
• Clinical syndromes presenting with multiple distended and/or painful joints
  • *Mycoplasma* spp. arthritis
  • *Hemophilus somnus* arthritis
  • Chlamydial arthritis
  • Polyarthritis secondary to septicemia
  • Polyarthritis secondary to bacterial endocarditis
  • Osteochondrosis
  • Septic physitis secondary to salmonellosis

• The reader is referred to chapters discussing these syndromes and diseases for additional detail.

RISK FACTORS
Varies with the specific syndrome and etiology

 DIAGNOSIS

DIFFERENTIAL DIAGNOSIS
• *Mycoplasma* spp. arthritis
• *Hemophilus somnus* arthritis
• Chlamydial arthritis
• Polyarthritis secondary to septicemia
• Polyarthritis secondary to bacterial endocarditis
• Osteochondrosis
• Septic physitis secondary to salmonellosis

Diagnosis Critera
• Herd histories of preceding or concurrent outbreaks of respiratory disease will greatly increase the likelihood of mycoplasmal, *Hemophilus somnus,* or chlamydial disease.
• Polyarthritis secondary to septicemia is seen almost exclusively in calves less than 1 month of age. Most affected calves will have additional diagnoses of clinical signs strongly supportive of septicemia including omphalophlebitis, hypopion, fever, and scleral injection.

• Age of onset will vary among the common causes of polyarthritis. Polyarthritis secondary to calf septicemia is diagnosed in very young calves. Chlamydial arthritis is most common preweaning. *Mycoplasma* and *Hemophilus* polyarthritis are most common in recently weaned calves. Osteochondrosis is most common in cattle between 1 and 2 years of age. Polyarthritis secondary to endocarditis is typically seen in adult cattle.

CBC/BIOCHEMISTRY/URINALYSIS
N/A

OTHER LABORATORY TESTS

IMAGING
Radiography is a useful adjunct to the diagnosis of polyarthritis. Osteochondrosis with or without degenerative joint disease and septic physitis can readily be confirmed or ruled out by radiographic examination.

OTHER DIAGNOSTIC PROCEDURES
Ancillary diagnostic procedures:
• Arthrocentesis and analysis of joint fluid is the single most useful test in most animals with polyarthritis. Cattle with polyarthritis caused by *H. somnus* or endocarditis will generally have joint fluid with a profound increase in leukocytes and the predominant cell type being the neutrophil.
• Joint fluid in cattle with *Mycoplasma* spp. infection has a less dramatic increase in cell numbers and the predominant cell type is mononuclear cells.

• Cattle with either osteochondrosis or septic physitis secondary to salmonellosis will generally have near normal joint fluid composition.
• Microbiologic culture procedures or polymerase chain reaction (PCR) assays may be useful in the identification of the offending pathogens. However, it should be noted that negative results are common and should not exclude the possibility of a diagnosis.
• Serologic tests are available for chlamydia.

TREATMENT

Varies with the specific syndrome and etiology (see Weightloss: Bovine, Ligamentous Injuries of the Stifle, Common Hoof Lameness of Cattle, Septic Arthritis, Osetochondrosis, Cattle Lameness and Angular Limb Deformity).

MISCELLANEOUS

ASSOCIATED CONDITIONS

See Septic Arthritis, Osetochondrosis, Angular Limb Deformity, Common Hoof Lameness of Cattle, and Bovine Footrot above.

AGE-RELATED FACTORS

• Polyarthritis secondary to calf septicemia is diagnosed in very young calves. Chlamydial arthritis is most common preweaning.
• *Mycoplasma* and *Hemophilus* polyarthritis are most common in recently weaned calves.
• Osteochondrosis is most common in cattle between 1 and 2 years of age.
• Polyarthritis secondary to endocarditis is typically seen in adult cattle.
• Polyarthritis secondary to septicemia is seen almost exclusively in calves less than 1 month of age.

ZOONOTIC POTENTIAL

Chlamydia spp. and *Salmonella* spp. should be considered zoonotic agents and care should be used in sample collection.

PREGNANCY

Chlamydia spp. and *Salmonella* spp. can cause abortion in herds/flocks.

RUMINANT SPECIES AFFECTED

Potentially, all ruminant species are affected.

BIOSECURITY

See specific chapters, such as Bovine Footrot, Common Hoof Lameness of Cattle.

PRODUCTION MANAGEMENT

See specific chapters, such as Common Hoof Lameness of Cattle.

SYNONYMS

N/A

SEE ALSO

Anesthesia and analgesia
Chlamydial arthritis
Hemophilus somnus arthritis
Mycoplasma spp. arthritis
NSAIDs
Osteochondrosis
Polyarthritis secondary to bacterial endocarditis
Polyarthritis secondary to septicemia
Septic physitis secondary to salmonellosis

ABBREVIATIONS

NSAIDs = nonsteroidal anti-inflammatory drugs
PCR = polymerase chain reaction

Suggested Reading

Hughes, K. L., Edwards, M. J., Hartley, W. J., Murphy, S. 1966. Polyarthritis in calves caused by *Mycoplasma* spp. *Veterinary Record* 78:276–81.

Smith, B. P., Biberstein, E. L.. 1977. Septicemia and meningoencephalitis in pastured cattle caused by a Haemophilus-like organism (*Haemophilus somnus*). *Cornell Veterinarian* 67:300–305.

Storz, J., Shupe, J. L., Smart, R. A., Thornley, R.W. 1966. Polyarthritis in calves: isolation of psittacosis agents from affected joints. *American Journal of Veterinary Research* 27:633–41.

Van Pelt, R. W., Langham, R. F. 1966. Nonspecific polyarthritis secondary to primary systemic infection in calves. *Journal of the American Veterinary Medical Association* 149:505–11.

Author: Jeff W. Tyler

POLYCYTHEMIA

 BASICS

DEFINITION
• An increase in the RBC count, Hgb concentration, and PCV (or Hct) due to either a relative or absolute increase in the number of circulating RBCs
• The term "polycythemia" is used commonly, but because RBCs are primarily affected, a better term is "erythrocytosis."

PATHOPHYSIOLOGY
• RBC numbers are affected by changes in plasma volume, splenic contraction, erythrocyte attrition or destruction, erythropoietin secretion, and rate of bone marrow production (erythropoiesis). Erythropoiesis is also influenced by production of hormones from the adrenal cortex, ovaries, testes, anterior pituitary, and thyroid glands.
• A normal PCV is maintained by an endocrine feedback loop. Decreased arterial PO_2 results in renal hypoxia. The kidney responds by increasing EPO secretion. EPO acts on the bone marrow to increase the rate of erythropoiesis. Increased erythropoiesis results in an increase in the circulating RBC mass.
• Polycythemia, or erythrocytosis, can be classified as either "relative" or "absolute." Relative polycythemia may be transient or persistent. Transient relative polycythemia is caused by splenic contraction, which introduces high hematocrit blood into the circulation. Splenic contraction is mediated by epinephrine and primarily occurs in excitable animals. Transient relative polycythemia is a rare occurrence in ruminants.

• *Relative polycythemia* occurs when there is a decrease in plasma volume. Dehydration and fluid shifts are the most common cause and result in a relative increase in circulating RBC.
• *Absolute polycythemia* is caused by a true increase in the RBC mass as a result of increased erythropoiesis. Absolute polycythemia may be classified as either primary or secondary.
  • *Primary absolute polycythemia* (polycythemia vera) is considered a well-differentiated myeloproliferative disorder independent of EPO control.
  • *Secondary absolute polycythemia* is caused by overproduction of RBCs due to increased EPO concentration. Increased EPO secretion may be an appropriate response to chronic hypoxia (e.g., cardiac insufficiency), or an inappropriate and excessive production of EPO in an animal with normal PO_2 (e.g., erythropoietin-secreting renal tumor).

SYSTEMS AFFECTED
• Hemic/lymphatic/immune— moderate to marked erythrocyte hyperplasia in the bone marrow, hyperviscosity
• Cardiovascular— hyperviscosity results in sluggish blood flow and poor tissue perfusion/oxygenation.
• Respiratory— dyspnea, tachypnea, cyanosis result from poor tissue oxygenation.
• Nervous—lethargy, ataxia, blindness, and seizures due to decreased oxygen delivery to CNS tissue.
• Renal/urologic—chronic hypoxia and thrombosis may lead to renal tubular necrosis.

GENETICS
Familial erythrocytosis has been described in cattle.

INCIDENCE/PREVALENCE
Absolute polycythemia is rare in ruminants. Relative polycythemia is much more common.

GEOGRAPHIC DISTRIBUTION
• Animals at altitudes of > 6000 ft have higher RBC counts than animals at sea level.
• Among ruminants, cattle are the most susceptible to developing polycythemia due to high altitudes.

SIGNALMENT
Reference values for RBC, Hgb, and PCV vary with ruminant species. South American camelids have higher RBC counts and Hgb concentration than cattle, sheep, or goats, but PCVs are similar.

SIGNS

HISTORICAL FINDINGS
• *Transient relative polycythemia:* excitement or extreme pain
• *Relative polycythemia:* lethargy, anorexia
• *Absolute polycythemia:* weakness, lethargy, anorexia, dyspnea, tachypnea

PHYSICAL EXAMINATION FINDINGS
• *Relative polycythemia:* Dehydration (sunken eyes, decreased skin turgor, etc.) due to vomiting, diarrhea, or decreased water intake
• *Absolute polycythemia:* Depressed mental status, prominent sublingual and episcleral vessels, brick-red and/or cyanotic mucous membranes, retinal hemorrhage, ± epistaxis, increased bronchovesicular lung sounds (due to pulmonary congestion)
• *Primary absolute polycythemia:* possible splenomegaly and hepatomegaly as reported in people with polycythemia, but these signs as well as primary polycythemia are rarely observed in domestic animals. Polyuria and polydipsia due to impaired vasopressin release.

Table 1

Mechanism	Relative Polycythemia Dehydration	1° Absolute Polycythemia Myeloproliferative Disorder	2° Absolute Polycythemia Hypoxia	2° Absolute Polycythemia Increased EPO
PCV	↑ - ↑↑	↑↑ - ↑↑↑	↑↑ - ↑↑↑	↑↑ - ↑↑↑
Plasma protein	↑	N	N	N
EPO	N	N - ↓	↑↑	↑↑ - ↑↑↑
PO$_2$	N	N	↓	N
WBC	N	N - ↑	N	N
Plts	N - ↑	N - ↑	N - ↑	N

N = normal, ↑ = slight increase, ↑↑ = moderate increase, ↑↑↑ = extensive increase, and ↓ = slight decrease in the listed hematologic parameters

• *Secondary absolute polycythemia caused by hypoxia*: heart murmur, weak pulses, prominent jugular veins, cyanosis, dyspnea, and abnormal lung sounds
• *Secondary absolute polycythemia due to inappropriate EPO secretion*: clinical signs include those listed above in addition to signs of neoplasia, space-occupying renal or hepatic lesions, or an endocrine disorder.

CAUSES
• *Transient relative polycythemia*: excitement, pain, seizures, restraint
• *Relative polycythemia (common)*: vomiting, diarrhea, decreased water intake, diuresis, polyuric renal disease, internal H$_2$O shift from plasma to interstitial space (edema) or gastrointestinal tract lumen.
• *Primary absolute polycythemia*: *rare myeloproliferative disorder in ruminants and camelids*
• *Secondary absolute polycythemia due to hypoxia*: chronic primary pulmonary disease, cardiac disease, congenital heart defects that result in left to right shunting (e.g., Tetralogy of Fallot), high altitude

• *Secondary absolute polycythemia due to inappropriate EPO secretion (rare)*: renal cysts; hydronephrosis; renal, hepatic, or intestinal tumors secreting EPO or an EPO-like substance; endocrine disorders; androgenic steroids (endogenous or exogenous)

RISK FACTORS
N/A

DIAGNOSIS

DIFFERENTIAL DIAGNOSIS
• *Transient relative polycythemia* typically occurs in young, healthy, and excitable animals.
• A mildly to moderately increased PCV and total plasma protein with concurrent clinical findings of dehydration support a diagnosis of relative polycythemia.
• *Primary absolute polycythemia* (polycythemia vera) is diagnosed by eliminating causes of relative and secondary absolute polycythemia.
• *Secondary absolute polycythemia* is a physiologically appropriate response to conditions that cause tissue hypoxia.

CBC/BIOCHEMISTRY/URINALYSIS
Transient Relative Polycythemia
• CBC: (1) Mild to moderate increases in RBC, Hgb, and PCV; (2) leukocytosis, mild neutrophilia, and lymphocytosis; (3) plasma proteins typically normal.
• Serum biochemistry/Urinalysis: no characteristic changes

Relative Polycythemia and Absolute Polycythemia
Differentiation among the causes of relative and absolute polycythemia initially require assessment of a CBC and plasma protein (see Table 1). Additional tests confirm the diagnosis.

OTHER LABORATORY TESTS
• PO$_2$
• Renal, adrenal, and hepatic function tests
• EPO assay (low availability for ruminants)
• Bone marrow cytologic evaluation reveals erythroid hyperplasia in cases of any cause of absolute polycythemia.

POLYCYTHEMIA

IMAGING

Absolute Polycythemia
Radiographic or ultrasonographic imaging may reveal evidence of renal or hepatic neoplasms, renal cysts, hydronephrosis, or cardiopulmonary disease.

OTHER DIAGNOSTIC PROCEDURES
N/A

 ## TREATMENT

Transient Relative Polycythemia
Treatment is not warranted as RBC counts typically return to normal within a few hours.

Relative Polycythemia
Rehydration and correction of underlying condition leading to dehydration

Primary Absolute Polycythemia
Removal of excess RBCs by repeated phlebotomy

Secondary Absolute Polycythemia
• Removal of excess RBCs by phlebotomy is typically recommended when PCV > 60% to decrease blood viscosity, but may be offset by the need to maintain tissue oxygenation. Supplemental O_2 therapy may improve tissue oxygenation initially.

• Specific therapy for decreasing RBC mass: Phlebotomy to keep PCV less than 50% (or in the high normal range) to control hypervolemia and hyperviscosity. A guideline of 20 ml/kg of blood removed every 2 to 3 days is advised. Iron deficiency may ensue requiring decreased frequency of therapeutic phlebotomy or iron supplementation.

ACTIVITY
Restriction of activity may be indicated.

CLIENT EDUCATION
N/A

 ## MEDICATIONS

DRUGS OF CHOICE

Relative Polycythemia
Rehydration with IV fluids appropriate for the primary cause (e.g., polyuric renal failure, diarrhea, etc.) and to correct any electrolyte and acid-base imbalances.

Absolute Polycythemia
Hydroxyurea (30 mg/kg, PO q 24h) is used in people and occasionally in dogs with primary absolute polycythemia with some benefit.

CONTRAINDICATIONS
• Phlebotomy may be contraindicated in patients with hypoxia.
• Appropriate milk and meat withdrawal times must be followed for all compounds administered to food-producing animals.

PRECAUTIONS
Rapid removal of blood during phlebotomy can result in severe hypotension and cardiovascular collapse.

POSSIBLE INTERACTIONS
N/A

ALTERNATIVE DRUGS
For polycythemia vera: chlorambucil and bisulfan have been used with limited success in dogs and cats. A safe and effective dose in ruminants or camelids is unknown. Consultation with a veterinary oncologist is advised for current treatment options. Withdrawal periods have not been determined for these medications.

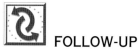 FOLLOW-UP

PATIENT MONITORING
• PCV, PP, and body weight 2–3 times per day in markedly dehydrated animals or until normovolemia has been reestablished

- Respiration and heart rate, mucous membrane color
- Initially, in patients with primary absolute polycythemia receiving myelosuppressive drugs, a CBC is advised at least weekly. Monthly CBCs (monitor RBC, WBC, and Plts) following stabilization of PCV for adjustment of chemotherapy dosage and as phlebotomies are required.

PREVENTION/AVOIDANCE
N/A

POSSIBLE COMPLICATIONS
- Chemotherapy-induced bone marrow suppression with subsequent leukopenia and thrombocytopenia
- Hyperviscosity associated with PCV > 60% may lead to thrombosis and/or hemorrhage (epistaxis most common).

EXPECTED COURSE AND PROGNOSIS
- The long-term prognosis for patients with absolute polycythemia is dependent upon the severity and cause for the disorder. Congenital cardiac defects and neoplastic diseases generally carry a guarded to poor prognosis.
- Familial erythrocytosis in cattle and primary polycythemia may be managed by phlebotomy, but long-term studies evaluating effectiveness of treatment in affected ruminants are lacking.

 MISCELLANEOUS

ASSOCIATED CONDITIONS
N/A

AGE-RELATED FACTORS
N/A

ZOONOTIC POTENTIAL
N/A

PREGNANCY
N/A

RUMINANT SPECIES AFFECTED
Bovine, ovine, caprine, camelids

BIOSECURITY
N/A

PRODUCTION MANAGEMENT
N/A

SYNONYMS
Erythrocytosis

SEE ALSO
Anemia
Fluid therapy
Hyperviscosity syndrome
Nonregenerative anemia

ABBREVIATIONS
EPO = erythropoietin
Hct = hematocrit
Hgb = hemoglobin
PCV = packed cell volume
Plts = platelets
RBC = red blood cells
WBC = white blood cells

Suggested Reading
Gentz, E. J., Pearson, E. G., Lassen, D., et al. 1994. Polycythemia in a llama. *J Am Vet Med Assoc.* 204:1490–92.
McKenna, S. L. B., Barkema, H. W., McClure, J. T., et al. 2003. Tetralogy of Fallot in a 2-year old Holstein heifer. *Can Vet J.* 44:312–13.
Morris, D. D. 1996. Erythrocytosis (polycythemia). In: *Large animal internal medicine*, ed. B. P. Smith. 2nd ed. St. Louis: Mosby.

Author: Frederic S. Almy

POSTERIOR VENA CAVA THROMBOSIS SYNDROME

 BASICS

DEFINITION
• An embolic pneumonia characterized by multifocal abscessation, which is caused by septic emboli that originate from a septic thrombus in the caudal vena cava.
• The septic thrombi in the vena cava are most often sequelae from liver abscesses caused by ruminal acidosis.

PATHOPHYSIOLOGY
• Feedlot cattle and dairy cattle that are fed rapidly fermentable high-carbohydrate grain diets commonly experience ruminal acidosis.
• Acidosis of rumen results in rumenitis and damage to rumen epithelium.
• Bacteria such as *Fusophorum necrophorum* and *Actinomyces pyogenes (Arcanobacterium pyogenes)* enter the portal blood stream and are transported to the liver.
• Liver abscessation occurs.
• If liver abscesses infiltrate the caudal vena cava, a septic thrombus can form.
• Septic emboli from thrombus then enter the pulmonary arterial system and cause an embolic pneumonia.
• Abscessation in the lung may erode pulmonary arterial vasculature in the lung and cause sudden death due to hemorrhage from the respiratory tract.

SYSTEMS AFFECTED
Gastrointestinal, hepatobiliary, respiratory

GENETICS
N/A

INCIDENCE/PREVALENCE
• 1.3% of feedlot deaths
• 1.6–7.3 cases per 100,000 head on feed

GEOGRAPHIC DISTRIBUTION
N/A

SIGNALMENT

Species
Cattle

Breed Predilections
• Feedlot cattle
• Dairy cows on high-grain diets

Mean Age and Range
• More common in yearling feedlot cattle and adult dairy cattle
• Uncommon in cattle less than 1 year of age
• 68% of cases in feedlot yearlings occur in first 90 days on feed

Predominant Sex
N/A

SIGNS

HISTORICAL FINDINGS
• Chronic history of weight loss
• Coughing
• History of episodes of epistaxis
• May exhibit acute respiratory distress
• May be found suddenly dead

PHYSICAL EXAMINATION FINDINGS
• Tachypnea
• Tachycardia
• May be febrile
• Respirations appear painful
• Mild expiratory grunt
• Epistaxis
• Hemoptysis
• Pale mucous membranes due to anemia
• Hemic murmurs
• Coughing
• Melena caused by coughing up and swallowing blood
• Subcutaneous emphysema
• Widespread rhonchi on auscultation of advanced cases
• Up to 50% of cases may die suddenly because of acute hemorrhage from the respiratory tract.

CAUSES

Primary Agents
• *Fusobacterium necrophorum*
• *Arcanobacterium pyogenes (Actinomyces pyogenes)*
• *Staphylococcus*
• *Streptococcus*
• *Escherichia coli*

Secondary Agents
N/A

RISK FACTORS
• Highly fermentable carbohydrate-based diets
• Sudden increase in the proportion of grain in the diet
• Thrombi may also originate from other sources of infection, such as jugular phlebitis, mastitis, metritis, foot rot

 DIAGNOSIS

DIFFERENTIAL DIAGNOSIS
• Anaphylaxis
• Atypical interstitial pneumonia
• Hypersensitivity pneumonitis
• Lungworm

CBC/BIOCHEMISTRY/URINALYSIS
• Anemia
• Neutrophilic leukocytosis with a left shift
• Hypergammaglobulinemia due to chronic infection

OTHER LABORATORY TESTS

IMAGING
• Increase in lung density
• Distinct opacities related to embolic infarcts may be evident.

DIAGNOSTIC PROCEDURES
N/A

POSTERIOR VENA CAVA THROMBOSIS SYNDROME

PATHOLOGIC FINDINGS
- Hepatic abscessation
- Thrombus in posterior vena cava
- Hepatomegaly
- Ascites
- Multiple pulmonary abscesses
- Intrapulmonary hemorrhage
- Swallowed blood evident in rumen

TREATMENT

APPROPRIATE HEALTH CARE
- Case fatality rate is close to 100%.
- Salvage is the only realistic option although condemnation of carcass is highly likely.
- Euthanasia should be considered.
- Antibiotic therapy may be attempted but is largely unsuccessful.

NURSING CARE
N/A

ACTIVITY
N/A

DIET
Evaluate reasons for occurrence of ruminal acidosis.

CLIENT EDUCATION
- Discuss potential risk factors
- Communicate grave prognosis for cases

SURGICAL CONSIDERATIONS
N/A

MEDICATIONS

DRUGS OF CHOICE
N/A

PRECAUTIONS
N/A

POSSIBLE INTERACTIONS
N/A

ALTERNATIVE DRUGS
N/A

FOLLOW-UP

PATIENT MONITORING
N/A

PREVENTION/AVOIDANCE
- Slowly adapt ruminants to high-carbohydrate rations.
- Utilize ionophores in ration to modulate feed intake and control acidosis.
- Antimicrobial feed additives such as tylosin, virginiamycin, chlortetracycline, or oxytetracycline can be used to prevent liver abscessation.
- Drug withdrawal times must be determined and maintained with antibiotic usage.
- Vaccines for *Fusobacterium necrophorum* may lower the incidence of liver abscesses.

POSSIBLE COMPLICATIONS
Many animals die because of blood loss from pulmonary arterial bleeds.

EXPECTED COURSE AND PROGNOSIS
- Most cases are fatal.
- Prognosis is very grave.

MISCELLANEOUS

ASSOCIATED CONDITIONS
- Rumenitis or grain overload
- Liver abscessation
- Embolic pneumonia
- Foot rot

AGE-RELATED FACTORS
N/A

ZOONOTIC POTENTIAL
N/A

PREGNANCY
N/A

RUMINANT SPECIES AFFECTED
Cattle

BIOSECURITY
N/A

PRODUCTION MANAGEMENT
N/A

SYNONYMS
Embolic pneumonia
Embolic pulmonary aneurysm
Metastatic pneumonia
Pulmonary thromboembolism

SEE ALSO
Anaphylaxis
Atypical interstitial pneumonia
Grain overload
Hypersensitivity pneumonitis
Lungworm

ABBREVIATIONS
N/A

Suggested Reading
Radostits, O. M., Gay, C. C., Blood, D. C., Hinchcliff, K. W., eds. 2000. *Veterinary medicine*. 9th ed. London: W. B. Saunders.
Wikse, S. E. 2002. Other pneumonias. In: *Large animal internal medicine*, ed. B. P. Smith. 3rd ed. St. Louis: Mosby.

Author: John R. Campbell

POSTPARTURIENT HEMOGLOBINURIA

BASICS

DEFINITION
This uncommon and sporadic condition causes intravascular hemolysis in cattle shortly after parturition, resulting in anemia and hemoglobinuria.

PATHOPHYSIOLOGY
• The exact etiology of this disease is not entirely known; however, inadequate dietary phosphorus leading to hypophosphatemia is often detected in affected cows. Hypocupremia may also be a predisposing factor.
• Hypophosphatemia alters erythrocyte metabolism, making red blood cells more susceptible to intravascular hemolysis. Hypocupremia predisposes erythrocytes to oxidative damage and Heinz body formation, also leading to intravascular hemolysis.

SYSTEMS AFFECTED
• Hemic: regenerative anemia, intravascular hemolysis, hemoglobinemia, hemoglobinuria, icterus
• Cardiovascular: hypoxemia
• Renal: pigment nephropathy
• Metabolic: ketosis

GENETICS
N/A

INCIDENCE/PREVALANCE
Although the condition is sporadic and the incidence is low, the mortality rate is high.

GEOGRAPHIC DISTRIBUTION
• Cases have been reported worldwide.
• In the United States, disease is more common in the winter months in northern states.

SIGNALMENT
Species
Cattle

Breed Predilections
Most common in dairy breeds

Mean Age and Range
Multiparous cows within the first month of calving

Predominant Sex
Female

SIGNS

GENERAL COMMENTS
High-producing dairy cattle appear to be most susceptible.

HISTORICAL FINDINGS
Recent calving, progressive depression, weakness and lethargy, anorexia, decreased milk production, red to brown discolored urine

PHYSICAL EXAMINATION FINDINGS
• The clinical signs depend on the severity and rate at which hemolysis occurs.
• Weakness and recumbency are expected as the condition progresses. In severe cases, signs of hypovolemic shock may be present, including tachycardia, tachypnea, pallor of the mucous membranes, lack of episcleral vessels, and cool extremities.
• A low-grade fever may be present. A grade I to III/VI systolic murmur may be audible over the heart base as blood viscosity decreases with advancing anemia.
• When the plasma hemoglobin concentration exceeds the renal threshold, hemoglobinuria will occur. Within 1 to 2 days, icterus of the mucous membranes and sclera will develop.

CAUSES
• Low dietary phosphorus
• Low dietary copper
• Parturition
• Ingestion of alfalfa hay or sugar beet that may contain saponins
• Copper deficiency

RISK FACTORS
• High-producing multiparous dairy cow consuming diets low in phosphorus are at greatest risk of disease.
• Drought conditions, grazing phosphorus-deficient soil, prolonged housing, and exposure to extremely cold weather may also predispose to the disease.
• Consumption of rape, turnips, or other cruciferous plants, and large amounts of beet pulp or cold water are associated with the disease.
• In New Zealand, low blood and liver copper levels and grazing copper-deficient pastures are additional risk factors.

DIAGNOSIS

DIFFERENTIAL DIAGNOSIS
Any cause of intravascular hemolysis in the cow would cause similar signs: babesiosis, bacillary hemoglobinuria, leptospirosis, onion, rape, or kale plant toxicity, copper toxicity, and autoimmune hemolytic anemia.

CBC/BIOCHEMISTRY/URINALYSIS
• Anemia
• Regenerative anemia 5 to 7 days after onset (signs of regeneration include an increased MCV, anisocytosis, polychromasia, basophilic stippling, reticulocytes)
• Hemoglobinemia (pink plasma, MCH, and MCHC increased)
• Hemoglobinuria
• Hyperbilirubinemia (unconjugated)
• Azotemia
• Acidosis
• Ketonuria

OTHER LABORATORY TESTS
• Decreased serum phosphorus concentrations are evident.
• In New Zealand cases, decreased blood copper concentration and Heinz bodies in erythrocytes have been noted.

IMAGING
N/A

DIAGNOSTIC PROCEDURES
N/A

PATHOLOGIC FINDINGS
Hemoglobinuria and widespread icterus

TREATMENT

APPROPRIATE HEALTH CARE
Emergency inpatient or outpatient care

NURSING CARE
• Intravenous fluid therapy with polyionic isotonic fluids is indicated.
• When anemia is severe and clinical or laboratory evidence of hypoxemia is evident (intense lethargy or weakness, profound tachycardia or tachypnea, severe anemia, acidosis, increased anion gap), a whole blood transfusion is indicated.

• The normal total blood volume is approximately 8% of the body weight (i.e., 0.08 × body weight in kilograms equals the total blood volume in liters). Typically, transfusing 1/4 to 1/3 of the total blood volume is adequate.

ACTIVITY
Confined

DIET
Increase dietary phosphorus intake.

CLIENT EDUCATION
Increase dietary phosphorus intake in unaffected herd mates.

SURGICAL CONSIDERATIONS
N/A

MEDICATIONS

DRUGS OF CHOICE
• Sodium acid phosphate ($NaH_2PO_4H_2O$; 60 grams in 300 mls of sterile water) should be given intravenously, followed by subcutaneous dosing every 12 hours for 2 days.
• Oral phosphorus supplementation should be supplied in the form of bonemeal or dicalcium phosphate.

CONTRAINDICATIONS
Appropriate milk and meat withdrawal times must be followed for all compounds administered to food-producing animals.

PRECAUTIONS
Avoid concurrent use of potentially nephrotoxic drugs.

POSSIBLE INTERACTIONS
N/A

ALTERNATIVE DRUGS
N/A

FOLLOW-UP

PATIENT MONITORING
Heart rate, respiratory rate, attitude, appetite, PCV, serum phosphorus and copper concentrations, creatinine

PREVENTION/AVOIDANCE
Ensure adequate dietary phosphorus and copper intake in the early postpartum period.

POSSIBLE COMPLICATIONS
• Renal disease from hemoglobinuria
• Ketosis
• Death from hypoxemia

EXPECTED COURSE AND PROGNOSIS
• The prognosis is guarded to poor, even with appropriate treatment.
• The clinical course is acute, progressing to recumbency in 3 to 5 days. In severe cases, death can occur within hours.
• Surviving cows may need a 4-week period of convalescence.

MISCELLANEOUS

ASSOCIATED CONDITIONS
Ingestion of feeds that contain saponins may predispose to hemolysis.

AGE-RELATED FACTORS
Multiparous cows within the first month of calving

ZOONOTIC POTENTIAL
N/A

PREGNANCY
N/A

RUMINANT SPECIES AFFECTED
Cattle

BIOSECURITY
N/A

PRODUCTION MANAGEMENT
• The dietary phosphorus and copper intake of the herd should be evaluated.
• Drought conditions, grazing phosphorus-deficient soil, prolonged housing, and exposure to extremely cold weather may also predispose to the disease.
• Consumption of rape, turnips, or other cruciferous plants, and large amounts of beet pulp or cold water are associated with the disease.

SYNONYNS
N/A

SEE ALSO
Any cause of intravascular hemolysis: babesiosis, bacillary hemoglobinuria, leptospirosis, onion, rape, or kale plant toxicity, copper toxicity, and autoimmune hemolytic anemia.
Phosphorus

ABBREVIATIONS
MCHC = mean corpuscular hemoglobin concentration
MCV = mean corpuscular volume
PCV = packed cell volume

Suggested Reading
Carlson, G. P. 1998. Postparturient hemoglobinuria. In: *Large animal internal medicine*, ed. B. P. Smith. 2nd ed. Philadelphia: Mosby.
Gilchrist, F. 1996, Aug. Water intoxication in weaned beef calves. *Can Vet J*. 37(8): 490–91.
Hofmann-Lehmann, R., Meli, M. L., Dreher, U. M., Gonczi, E., Deplazes, P., Braun, U., Engels, M., Schupbach, J., Jorger, K., Thoma, R., Griot, C., Stark, K. D., Willi, B., Schmidt, J., Kocan, K. M., Lutz, H. 2004, Aug. Concurrent infections with vector-borne pathogens associated with fatal hemolytic anemia in a cattle herd in Switzerland. *J Clin Microbiol*. 42(8): 3775–80.
MacWilliams, P. S., Searcy, G. P., Bellamy, J. E. C. 1982. Bovine postparturient hemoglobinuria: a review of the literature. *Can Vet J*. 23: 311–14.
Tokarnia, C. H., Dobereiner, J., Peixoto, P. V., Moraes, S. S. 2000, Apr. Outbreak of copper poisoning in cattle fed poultry litter. *Vet Hum Toxicol*. 42(2):92–95.

Author: Michelle Henry Barton

PRECOCIOUS UDDER

 BASICS

OVERVIEW
• A precocious udder is a mammary system that is more developed than usual at a given age or stage of lactation.
• Enlargement of the mammary gland generally begins near puberty.
• During puberty, mammary gland growth occurs in the female mostly due to increased amounts of connective tissue and fat deposition.
• Estrous periods stimulate the development of secretory and duct tissues. Growth of lactation tissue is dependent on two hormones: estrogen from developing follicles and progesterone from the corpus luteum.
• Cyclic secretion of estrogen stimulates duct development of the mammary gland.
• Progesterone secretion is cyclic in nonpregnant animals, and nearly continuous in pregnant animals, and causes secretory tissue development.
• Gynecomastia in male goats can occur (e.g., Alpine and Saanen breeds) especially during the summer months.

SYSTEMS AFFECTED
• Endocrine/metabolic
• Reproductive
• Mammary
• Skin/exocrine

SIGNALMENT
• Precocious udders are most commonly seen in young milking breeds of goats such as the Saanen, Alpine, Toggenburg, LaMancha, and Nubian.
• Young kids may develop precocious udders more frequently during springtime.
• It has also been described in cattle and sheep much less commonly.

SIGNS
• Early development of the mammary gland in the absence of pregnancy is the most common sign of precocious udder.
• Goat kids may be born with significant udders containing milk (witch's milk).

CAUSES AND RISK FACTORS
• Onset of puberty
• Prolonged progesterone production of false pregnancy
• In utero hormone stimulation
• Increased hormone receptors
• Exposure to high levels of estrogen
• Artificial lactation-induction programs
• Spring season (increased levels of prolactin)

 DIAGNOSIS

DIFFERENTIAL DIAGNOSIS
• Mastitis
• Persistent corpus luteum
• Infection due to inappropriate suckling
• Intersex
• Neoplasia
• Fatty udder due to overconditioning
• High estrogen levels in feed (e.g., clover, moldy corn)

CBC/CHEMISTRY/URINALYSIS
N/A

OTHER LABORATORY TESTS
N/A

IMAGING
Imaging (ultrasound) may be useful to rule out neoplasia.

DIAGNOSTIC PROCEDURES
• The udder should be symmetrical, firm to soft tissue consistency, and free of irregular lumps.
• Rule out mastitis by evaluating any secretions that are present for signs of inflammation.
• If abnormalities are found on palpation, especially in older lactation animals, imaging or biopsy of the mass is warranted to rule out neoplasia.

PATHOLOGIC FINDINGS
N/A

 TREATMENT

• The generally accepted treatment for a precocious udder is to do nothing.
• Once mastitis is ruled out, separate the animal from others, especially young stock that may try to nurse.
• Hydrotherapy

• Feeding management to dry off the animal (e.g., increase the level of poor-quality hay in the diet and eliminate grain).

• If the milk production is persistent, the teats leak, or the animal is very uncomfortable and/or painful, it might be necessary to initiate milking. It should be noted that if milking is instituted, an increased risk of mastitis can be seen.

• The effect of milking on the lifetime production of the animal has not been documented.

• In pet goats with large udders, amputation may be necessary.

• Although not tested, an ovariectomy may prevent this problem in pet goats.

• With gynecomastia in male goats, reduce energy and protein intake levels during spring and summer months.

MEDICATIONS

DRUGS OF CHOICE
• PGF2α (5 mg IM has been utilized with persistent CL)
• NSAIDs if painful (flunixin meglumine 1–2 mg/kg IV or IM)
• Diuretics and steroid treatment may be helpful (furosemide 2–10 mg/kg IM, dexamethasone (0.1–1.0 mg/kg IM)

CONTRAINDICATIONS
N/A

POSSIBLE INTERACTIONS
Appropriate milk and meat withdrawal times must be followed for all compounds administered to food-producing animals.

FOLLOW-UP

N/A

MISCELLANEOUS

ASSOCIATED CONDITIONS
Mastitis may be a sequela.

AGE-RELATED FACTORS
N/A

ZOONOTIC POTENTIAL
N/A

PREGNANCY
N/A

RUMINANT SPECIES AFFECTED
Primarily goats; rare in sheep and cattle

BIOSECURITY
N/A

PRODUCTION MANAGEMENT
N/A

SYNONYMS
N/A

SEE ALSO
Mastitis in sheep and goats

ABBREVIATIONS
CL = corpus luteum
IM = intramammary
IV = intravenous
NSAIDs = nonsteroidal anti-inflammatory drugs
PGF2α = prostaglandin F-2 alpha

Suggested Reading
Bchini, O., Andres, A. C., Schubaur, B., Mehtali, M., LeMeur. M, Lathe. R., Gerlinger, P. 1991, Jan. Precocious mammary gland development and milk protein synthesis in transgenic mice ubiquitously expressing human growth hormone. *Endocrinology* 128(1):539–46.
Dwyer, C. M. 2003, Feb. Behavioural development in the neonatal lamb: effect of maternal and birth-related factors. *Theriogenology* 59(3–4):1027–50.
Haenlein, G. F. W., Caccese, R. 1992. *The goat handbook.* Available at: http://www.inform.umd.edu/EdRes/Topic/AgrEnv/ndd/goat/
Tucker, H. A. 2000, Apr. Hormones, mammary growth, and lactation. *J Dairy Sci.* 83(4):874–84.

Author: Angela M. Daniels

PREGNANCY DIAGNOSIS IN THE BOVINE

BASICS

OVERVIEW
• Accurate early diagnosis of pregnant and nonpregnant cows is essential for optimization of reproductive performance, particularly in dairy cattle.
• Methods for diagnosis of nonpregnant or pregnant status include behavioral observation, clinical techniques, and laboratory evaluation.

SYSTEMS AFFECTED
Reproductive

GENETICS
N/A

INCIDENCE/PREVALENCE
N/A

GEOGRAPHIC DISTRIBUTION
Worldwide

SIGNALMENT
Species
Bovine

Breed Predilections
N/A

Mean Age and Range
N/A

Predominant Sex
N/A

DIAGNOSIS

Behavioral Observation
• Return to estrus is considered a strong indication that a cow is not pregnant. Up to 5% of pregnant females may display some signs of estrus.
• Nonreturn to estrus can be an indication of pregnancy; however, females that have persistent corpus luteum function (pyometra) or are truly anestrus contribute greatly to increase in false positive diagnosis.

Clinical Diagnosis
Transrectal Palpation
Per-rectum palpation of the uterus and its contents is the oldest and most commonly used technique for diagnosis and staging of pregnancy. Positive diagnosis of pregnancy is only established if one of the following is identified
• Presence of fetal membrane slip
• Palpation of the amniotic vesicle
• Palpation of placentomes
• Palpation of the fetus

Fetal Membrane Slip
• Characteristic crisp slip of the chorioallantois within the lumen of pregnant uterus
• May be present as early as 30 days of pregnancy
• Very reliable after 35 days

Amniotic Vesicle
• Spherical turgid, fluid-filled structure within the pregnant horn
• Palpable as early as 28 days after conception
• Size of the amniotic vesicle is very helpful for staging pregnancy between 30 and 55 days
• Helpful in the diagnosis of twin pregnancies
• Difficult to palpate after 60 days
• Rough manipulation of the amniotic vesicle has been associated with pregnancy loss and atresia ani/coli.

Placentomes
• Characteristic of ruminant placentation
• Numbers 80 to 120 arranged in two dorsal and two ventral rows
• Palpable as early as 75 days of pregnancy
• Size of placentomes is very helpful in estimating stage of pregnancy
• Most consistent size immediately cranial to the cervix
• False positive: placentomes are present following abortion or death of the fetus, mistaking ovary for placentomes
• False negative increase between 5 and 6 months of pregnancy

Fetus
• Palpable starting at 65 days of pregnancy when amniotic sac becomes more flexible
• At early stages, the whole fetus can be grasped directly.
• Easy to palpate up to 5 months and between 7 and 9 months
• Difficult to palpate between the fifth and seventh months

Accuracy and Safety of Palpation Per Rectum
• Very accurate with moderate degree of expertise after 35 days
• Should take into account early pregnancy loss (5%–12%)
• Very safe if used by a trained person
• Rough manipulation of the amniotic vesicle may result in pregnancy attrition.

CBC/BIOCHEMISTRY/URINALYSIS
N/A

OTHER LABORATORY TESTS
Progesterone
• Progesterone is produced by the corpus luteum. In absence of maternal recognition of pregnancy, progesterone falls to basal levels (below 1 ng/ml) around day 17 or 19 after insemination

• Determination of progesterone level in milk or serum can be used to accurately identify nonpregnant cows.
• Elevated milk or serum progesterone levels (> 2 ng/ml) suggests maintenance of corpus luteum activity and possible pregnancy
• Low milk or serum levels (< 1 ng/ml) are very specific for diagnosis of nonpregnancy
• Sensitivity of this test depends on the assay used (RIA or ELISA techniques are more sensitive)
• Progesterone assay is best accomplished 18 to 24 days after insemination
• Cow-side tests for use on serum or milk are available
• In-line milk progesterone tests are becoming available

Pregnancy-specific Proteins
• The trophoblastic binucleate cells from the early ruminant conceptus produce large amounts of specific proteins that can be detected in maternal circulation and can be used for pregnancy diagnosis.
• The most commonly used pregnancy-specific proteins are bovine pregnancy-specific protein B (bPSPB) and to a lesser extent bovine pregnancy-associated glycoprotein 1 (bPAG-1).
• A test for bPSPB is available commercially from several laboratories.
• Sensitivity and specificity of bPSPB increases from 75% and 85% at 26–27 days to 100% and 85% by days 37–45, respectively.
• Specificity of bPSPB is 90%–92% after day 45.
• Sensitivity of bPAG-1 increases from 81% at 26–27 days to 100% by day 44. However, its specificity is low and only reaches 71% at 60 days.
• Problems with these techniques
  • Both of these proteins can be detected in the postpartum period up to 70–100 days after calving and leads to increased false positives in this period.
  • These proteins can be detected for a long time after abortion or early embryonic death and may lead to false positive results.
  • Results are not immediate and therefore action on open cows cannot be taken immediately.
  • Pregnancy confirmation at a later date is still advised, particularly in herds that are experiencing early embryonic death/ pregnancy loss.
  • Uterine and ovarian pathologies may go unnoticed for a long time.

Early Conception Factor (ECF)
• Early conception factor is a pregnancy-associated glycoprotein produced as early as 24 hours postfertilization.

• A proprietary milk or serum cow side test is commercialized under the name of ECF and is supposed to identify nonpregnant cows with high accuracy between 6 and 30 days postinsemination.
• A high accuracy of 93%–100% for identification of open cows has been reported for this test but is contested by other studies and field experiments.

Interferon-tau (IFN-τ)
Maintenance of corpus luteum function is essential for the maintenance of pregnancy.
• Interferon-tau (IFN-τ), previously called trophoblastic, of trophoblast protein-1 is the initial requisite signal for pregnancy recognition in ruminants.
• IFN-τ inhibits corpus luteum regression by suppressing the pulsatile release of PGF2 alpha from the endometrium.
• IFN-τ can be detected in blood between days 15 and 30 postconception.
• Commercial tests (SUREBRED) are being tested for diagnosis of pregnancy at day 18 postinsemination.
• Initial results of these tests show a sensitivity of 99% and specificity at 97%.
• The advantage of this test is that heat detection can be focused on cows that test negative at 18 days.
• Cows determined to be pregnant should still be examined at a later date by transrectal method.

General Recommendations for Pregnancy Diagnosis
• Early pregnancy diagnosis techniques should focus on accurate identification of nonpregnant cows.
• The appropriate diagnostic technique to be used in a herd will depend on several factors (heat detection efficiency, method of breeding, cost of labor, cost of the technique, pregnancy rate, size of the herd, etc.). An efficient system should be designed in collaboration between the attending veterinarian and the herd manager.
• Regardless of the method used for pregnancy diagnosis, cows should be reexamined at a later date for confirmation of pregnancy status if the fetus was not palpated.
• Direct examination of the genital tract by transrectal palpation and/or ultrasonography should continue to be used for confirmation of pregnancy status, staging of pregnancy in bull bred dairy cows, and early diagnosis of pathologies of the reproductive tract

IMAGING

Ultrasonography
• Pregnancy diagnosis by ultrasonography is best accomplished using a linear array 5 MHz transducer (7 MHz transducers are more accurate before day 28 of pregnancy but are not commonly used in cattle practice).
• Diagnosis of pregnancy with ultrasonography is possible as early as 25 days in heifers and 27 days in cows.
• Accuracy of pregnancy diagnosis using transrectal ultrasonography increases with gestational age and sensitivity and the specificity of the technique approaches 100% at 32 days.
• Specificity is increased if the operator uses presence of fetal heartbeat as a sign of pregnancy rather than just fetal fluid. This is easily accomplished at 29 days but requires increased examination time.
• Ultrasonography increases the accuracy of diagnosis of twins and early pregnancy loss.
• Ultrasonography can be used to estimate gestational age (amniotic vesicle diameter, fetal head biparietal diameter, fetal crown-rump length).
• Ultrasonography can be used to determine fetal gender by identification of the position of the genital tubercle (55 days), penis, scrotum, vulva, or udder.

 TREATMENT

 MEDICATIONS

 MISCELLANEOUS

ASSOCIATED CONDITIONS
Infertility, abortion, and retained fetuses

AGE-RELATED FACTORS
Infertility is commonly associated with immature females.

ZOONOTIC POTENTIAL
Many reproductive diseases are zoonotic. Care must be maintained in collecting laboratory samples and during rectal palpation.

PREGNANCY
See General Recommendations for Pregnancy Diagnosis above

RUMINANT SPECIES AFFECTED
Bovines

BIOSECURITY
N/A

PRODUCTION MANAGEMENT
N/A

SYNONYMS
N/A

SEE ALSO
Bovine abortion
Bovine artificial insemination
Reproductive ultrasound

ABBREVIATIONS
bPAG-1 = bovine pregnancy-associated glycoprotein 1
bPSPB = bovine pregnancy-specific protein B
ECF = early conception factor
ELISA = enzyme-linked immunosorbent assay
IFN-τ = interferon-tau
PGF2 alpha = prostaglandin F2 alpha
RIA = radioimmunoassay

Suggested Reading
Cordoba, M. C., Sartori, R., Fricke, P. M. 2001. Assessment of a commercially available Early Conception Factor (ECF®) test for determining pregnancy status of dairy cattle. *J Dairy Science* 84:1884–89.
Demmers, K. J., Derecka, K., Flint, A. 2001. Trophoblast interferon and pregnancy. *Reproduction* 121:41–49.
Kahn, W. 1994. *Veterinary reproductive ultrasonography*. Philadelphia: Mosby-Wolfe.
Stroud, B. K. 1994. Clinical applications of bovine reproductive ultrasonography. *The Compendium for Pract Vet Food Animal*. 16: 1085–97.
Szenci, O., Beckers, J. F., Humblot, P., Sulon, J., Sasser, G., Taverne, M. A. M., Varga, J., Baltusen, R., Schekk, G. 1998. Comparison of ultrasonography, bovine pregnancy-specific protein B and bovine pregnancy-associated glycoprotein 1 tests for pregnancy detection on dairy cows. *Theriogenology* 50:77–88.
Youngquist, R. 1997. Pregnancy diagnosis. In: *Current therapy in large animal theriogenology*, ed. R. Youngquist. Philadelphia: W. B. Saunders.

Author: Ahmed Tibary

PREGNANCY TOXEMIA: SHEEP AND GOATS

BASICS

DEFINITION
• Pregnancy toxemia is a common metabolic disease in sheep and goats that results from the inability of the dam to maintain glucose homeostasis in the face of increasing energy demands from multiple fetuses during late gestation.
• The condition is characterized by anorexia, weakness, and depression, and occurs during the last 2 to 4 weeks of pregnancy in does and ewes.

PATHOPHYSIOLOGY
• The fetal placental unit requires glucose for energy and may consume up to 40% of the maternal glucose production during the rapid growth that occurs during the last weeks of gestation.
• If the dam is unable to maintain glucose homeostasis, body fat stores will be converted to glucose with the undesirable production of ketone bodies that will eventually result in the ketonemia and ketonuria present in clinical pregnancy toxemia.
• Insulin function is critical in glucose uptake by cells and may be an important factor in glucose homeostasis and ultimately in the susceptibility of individual animals to development of pregnancy toxemia.
• Pregnancy toxemia is caused by a negative energy balance due to an increased energy demand of rapid fetal growth during late gestation and insufficient intake.
• The cause of pregnancy toxemia has been hypothesized to result from a suppression of endogenous glucose production by elevated ketone body concentrations.
• Hyperketonemia may invoke sustained hypoglycemia and place the ewe into a vicious cycle that will probably make the animal refractory to treatments.

SYSTEMS AFFECTED
• Nervous: effects on the central nervous system are associated with the effects of hypoglycemic encephalopathy and include depression, incoordination, mental dullness, stargazing, tremors, and blindness.
• Musculoskeletal: muscle weakness, recumbency

• Endocrine/metabolic: metabolic acidosis is a common feature.
• Gastrointestinal: rumen function is compromised and ewes are often constipated.
• Reproductive: multiple fetuses are usually present and are usually in peril if the ewe does not respond rapidly to treatment.
• Hepatobiliary: overconditioned dams will often have severe hepatic lipidosis.

GENETICS
• Variation in clinical incidence within flocks and between flocks suggests that some animals may be genetically susceptible to development of pregnancy toxemia.
• The key factor may be associated with the ability of insulin to function in glucose uptake at the cellular level and ultimately help maintain glucose homeostasis in the face of increased demand from the fetuses.
• Highly prolific sheep may be predisposed to pregnancy toxemia due to reduced rumen capacity and increased glucose demand from four or more fetuses; however, nutritional management is usually the primary predisposing factor.

INCIDENCE/PREVALANCE
• Varies widely between flocks/herds and production styles
• Usually presents with isolated cases in well-managed flocks; however, outbreaks have occurred if nutritional and management factors put all individuals at risk.

GEOGRAPHIC DISTRIBUTION
Worldwide

SIGNALMENT

Species
Primarily affects sheep and goats, rarely cattle

Breed
Prolific breeds may be at greater risk for nutritional mismanagement.

Mean Age and Range
Mature ewes primarily affected, rare in first-time lambers

Predominant Sex
Late gestation females

SIGNS

HISTORICAL FINDINGS
Late gestation, heavy with multiple fetuses, possibly recently sheared, stands off by itself, off feed, depressed, recumbent, weakness and mental dullness, blindness, disoriented, head pressing, and teeth grinding

PHYSICAL EXAMINATION FINDINGS
Anorexia, ketones on the breath, weakness, depression, incoordination, mental dullness, impaired vision, followed by recumbency and death within 3 to 4 days without treatment.

CAUSES
• Pregnancy toxemia is caused by an inability of the dam to maintain glucose homeostasis in the face of increased demand from the fetal-placental unit in late gestation.
• Individual cases will fit in one of the following broad categories:

Primary Pregnancy Toxemia
• Failure to increase nutritional plane to compensate for increased fetal demand for glucose during late gestation
• Often a simple management change such as shearing or a sudden storm that results in brief periods of feed deprivation may trigger clinical disease in animals that may have subclinical ketosis.

Fat Ewe Pregnancy Toxemia
Overconditioning of the dam during early gestation resulting in increased abdominal fat and reduced rumen capacity, possible hepatic lipidosis that also impairs glucose metabolism

Starvation Pregnancy Toxemia
Ewes in poor body condition associated with mismanagement or unavailability of feedstuffs, more common in range situations

Secondary Pregnancy Toxemia
Concurrent disease in affected ewes, examples would include lameness or pneumonia

RISK FACTORS
Dams with multiple fetuses, late gestation, improper, declining, or interrupted nutritional inputs

DIAGNOSIS

DIFFERENTIAL DIAGNOSIS
• Hypocalcemia
• Listeriosis
• Polioencephalomalacia
• Hypomagnesemia
• Trauma
• Parasitism
• Meningeal worm

PREGNANCY TOXEMIA: SHEEP AND GOATS

Table 1

Parameters of Glucose Metabolism in Normo- and Hyperketonemic Sheep			
	Reproductive Phase		
	Nonpregnant/Nonlactating	Pregnant	Lactating
Day of experiment[a]	> 100	-9.57 +/− 7.44	19.29 +/− 5.96
Normoketonemia[b]	2.92 +/− 0.3	3.35 +/− 1.6	2.85 +/− 0.6
Hyperketonemia[c]	2.06 +/− 0.2	2.23 +/− 1.5	1.97 +/− 0.9

[a]Day of experiment with respect to parturition
[b]Concentration of blood glucose in blood plasma (mmol/L)
[c]Concentration of blood glucose in blood plasma (mmol/L)

CBC/BIOCHEMISTRY/URINALYSIS

CBC
Some ewes with pregnancy toxemia will have nonspecific but marked neutrophilia (reaching 35,000 neutrophils/μl).

Biochemistry
Blood glucose and calcium concentrations are typically low; samples for blood glucose should be removed from the blood clot as soon as possible.
• Nonesterified fatty acids, betahydroxybutyrate, and acetoacetate concentrations are elevated; urea concentrations are normal.
• Impaired intravenous glucose tolerance test, not practical in a clinical practice
• High circulating concentrations of ketone bodies may suppress endogenous synthesis of glucose and facilitate development of pregnancy toxemia. In addition, the hyperketonemia may render the ewe refractory to treatment (see Table 1).
• Ewes are often acidotic with lower than normal serum concentrations of potassium and calcium.
• Circulating concentrations of both NEFA (> 500 μEq/L) and betahydroxybutyrate (> 1 mmol/L) are increased.

Urinalysis
Elevated ketones on urinalysis; ketonuria is present and usually detected before ketonemia.

OTHER LABORATORY TESTS
N/A

IMAGING
Ultrasound could potentially be used to determine the viability of fetuses in clinical pregnancy toxemia to better evaluate potential treatment strategies.

DIAGNOSTIC PROCEDURES
N/A

PATHOLOGIC FINDINGS
• Gross necropsy findings vary with body condition and initiating causes. Multiple fetuses are usually present.
• Body fat reserves may be depleted with pronounced serous atrophy in the thin ewe syndrome or abundant in the overconditioned ewe.
• Fatty degeneration of the liver may be present in some ewes; however, the severity of this change is difficult to evaluate grossly.
• Histologic lesions include hepatic lipidosis and neuronal necrosis and astrocytosis.
• Complete postmortem examinations are rarely performed.

 ## TREATMENT

APPROPRIATE HEALTH CARE
• Pregnancy toxemia is best managed as a flock or herd problem and addressed through appropriate nutritional and management changes. Treatment costs and prognosis should be considered before any treatment is recommended. Individual animals should be segregated from the flock for treatment and monitoring purposes.
• The first step in treating pregnancy toxemia in ewes is to remove the fetuses by cesarean section or by inducing parturition.
• Induction of parturition in ewes is usually accomplished with 15 to 20 mg of dexamethasone, and with either dexamethasone (10 mg) or prostaglandin F2α (10 μg) in does.
• The ketosis should be treated by administering 250–500 ml of glucose (10%–20% solution) intravenously, followed by a slow infusion of 5%–10% glucose.
• Other underlying conditions, such as acidosis and hypocalcemia, must be corrected also.

• Propylene glycol (15–30 ml every 12 hours) or sodium propionate are routinely used as glucose precursors. Precautions should be taken when administering the propylene glycol, as excessive amounts may lead to acidosis and/or cause diarrhea.

NURSING CARE
• The goal of therapy in pregnancy toxemia is to restore glucose homeostasis as soon a possible.
• Multiple electrolyte, acid-base, and fluid imbalances in addition to low blood glucose levels will need to be considered in any potential treatment plan.

ACTIVITY
The affected dam should be isolated to reduce expenditures of energy and limit competition for feed resources.

DIET
High-quality forages and concentrates should be offered in an attempt to stimulate intake.

CLIENT EDUCATION
Repeated and prolonged treatments will be needed. The owner will need to evaluate the economics of therapy versus probable outcomes.

SURGICAL CONSIDERATIONS
Cesarean section may be needed to remove the fetal drain on glucose production. Often the fetuses are nonviable and the procedure is used to save the dam.

 ## MEDICATIONS

DRUGS OF CHOICE
• There are no specific drugs of choice, however, several drugs are occasionally used in individual cases of pregnancy toxemia in combination with glucose, fluid, and electrolyte imbalances.

PREGNANCY TOXEMIA: SHEEP AND GOATS

• Dexamethasone 20–30 mg IM, for induction of parturition, response may be variable depending on the clinical condition of the dam
• Protamine zinc insulin 20–40 units intramuscularly every other day in combination with glucose and fluid therapy
• Recombinant bovine somatotropin (not currently approved for use in sheep) 160 mg of slow-release formulation may increase efficiency of glucose and ketone utilization.

CONTRAINDICATIONS
Appropriate milk and meat withdrawal times must be followed for all compounds administered to food-producing animals.

PRECAUTIONS
N/A

POSSIBLE INTERACTIONS
N/A

ALTERNATIVE DRUGS
N/A

 FOLLOW-UP

PATIENT MONITORING
Feed intake is a critical factor in monitoring for treatment success. If the animal is recumbent for a prolonged period, the odds of recovery are substantially reduced.

PREVENTION/AVOIDANCE
• Prevention of future cases of pregnancy toxemia is best accomplished by evaluation of nutritional and management practices within the flock.
• Designing nutritional programs that meet the animals' requirements based on the stage of production and relevant environmental and management conditions can prevent most cases of pregnancy toxemia.
• Dividing large groups based on expected production may help the producer more effectively meet the requirements of highly productive individuals.
• The common occurrence of twins and triplets in ewes increases the nutrient requirements of the ewe during the last trimester of pregnancy. Consequently, excellent-quality forage must be provided.

• Last, a plasma concentration of betahydroxybutyrate of 0.8 mmol/L or higher is diagnostic of the need for increased energy consumption. This is a good clinicopathologic tool for diagnosing malnutrition before irreversible pregnancy toxemia develops.

POSSIBLE COMPLICATIONS
Complications during birth, failure to expel the placenta and difficulties during early lactation are all common issues in dams that survive to the induced or natural initiation of parturition.

EXPECTED COURSE AND PROGNOSIS
• Treatment is often unrewarding and, in many cases within commercial flocks, economically unfeasible. The prognosis is usually poor for recovery if recumbency is prolonged.
• Termination of the pregnancy by induction with dexamethasone or cesarean section is unpredictable for the survival of the fetuses, and if delayed too long, for the dam as well.

 MISCELLANEOUS

ASSOCIATED CONDITIONS
May be associated with concurrent hypocalcemia. Calcium therapy is combined with glucose or glucose-precursor therapy.

AGE-RELATED FACTORS
More common in older ewes, not associated with first-time lambers

ZOONOTIC POTENTIAL
N/A

PREGNANCY
Pregnancy toxemia is present in dams in late gestation.

RUMINANT SPECIES AFFECTED
Sheep, goats, and rarely cattle

BIOSECURITY
N/A

PRODUCTION MANAGEMENT
• Best managed as a production disease with primary emphasis placed on prevention of future cases.
• Nutritional and management factors must be addressed to minimize the impact within a population.

SYNONYMS
Ketosis
Lambing ketosis
Lambing paralysis
Lambing sickness
Pregnancy disease
Pregnancy toxemia
Twin lamb disease

SEE ALSO
Cesarian surgery
Hypocalcemia
Hypomagnesemia
Listeriosis
Meningeal worm
Parasitism
Polioencephalomalacia
Reproductive pharmacology
Trauma

ABBREVIATIONS
IM = intramuscular
NEFA = nonesterified fatty acid

Suggested Reading
Henze, P., Bickhardt, K., Fuhrmann, H., Sallmann, H. P. 1998. Spontaneous pregnancy toxaemia (ketosis) in sheep and the role of insulin [abstract]. *Zentralbl Veteinarmed. A.* 45(5): 255–66. Available at: http://www.ncbi.nlm.gov.entrez/query.fcgi.
Jeffrey, M., Higgins, R. J. 1992. Brain lesions of naturally occurring pregnancy toxemia of sheep. *Vet Pathol.* 29 (4):301–07.
Rook, J. S. 2000. Pregnancy toxemia of ewes, does, and beef cows. *Vet Clin North Am: Food An Pract.* 16(2):293–317.
Schlumbohm, C., Harmeyer, J. 2003. Hypocalcemia reduces endogenous glucose production in hyperketonemic sheep. *J Dairy Sci.* 86(6):1953–62.
Van Saun, R. J. 2000. Pregnancy toxemia in a flock of sheep. *J Am Vet Med Assoc.* 15: 217(10): 1536–39.

Authors: Larry D. Holler and Douglas C. Donovan

BASICS

OVERVIEW
- Lacerations, contusions, and prolapse of the prepuce are the most common problems that affect the breeding ability of range bulls.
- Most preputial lesions are acquired during the breeding season.
- Damage usually affects the internal prepuce and occurs during the act of coitus or immediately after when the penis is extended and the prepuce is most dependent.
- Preputial lacerations may occur during breeding when there is "bunching" of excess preputial tissue immediately prior to the breeding lunge causing the tissue to burst ventrally in a longitudinal direction when the prepuce impacts upon the pubis of the cow. Because of the elastic layers and retraction of the penis, there is a marked tendency for healing to occur in a transverse manner shortening the effective length of the prepuce as it heals.
- Bulls that frequently have some prepuce exposed may develop abrasions and lacerations of the prepuce from exposure to environmental factors (including frostbite) although this is less common than lesions caused by breeding injuries.
- Initial trauma may lead to edema, further prolapse, more trauma, abscessation, and eventually fibrosis of the preputial tissue.

SIGNALMENT
- Habitual prolapse of the prepuce is common among *Bos indicus* breeds.
- Santa Gertrudis, Beefmaster, Brangus, Angus, and polled Hereford bulls have a higher incidence of preputial injuries.

SIGNS
- Traumatic injury results in edema formation and preputial prolapse.
- Abscesses and fibrosis may be present.

CAUSES AND RISK FACTORS
- Predisposition to preputial prolapse probably involves four hereditary anatomic features including a pendulous sheath, an excessively long prepuce, a large preputial orifice, and the absence of retractor prepuce muscles.
- In polled breeds, especially polled Hereford and Angus, the caudal preputial retractor muscles are frequently absent or rudimentary.
- The sheath and prepuce of *Bos indicus* bulls are more pendulous averaging 5.5 cm longer than *Bos taurus* breeds.

DIAGNOSIS

DIFFERENTIAL DIAGNOSIS
N/A

CBC/BIOCHEMISTRY/URINALYSIS
N/A

OTHER LABORATORY TESTS
N/A

IMAGING
N/A

DIAGNOSTIC PROCEDURES
N/A

PATHOLOGIC FINDINGS
N/A

TREATMENT

- Treatment is initially aimed at medical management.
- The injured prepuce should be soaked in a warm dilute betadine and Epsom salt solution, treated topically with antimicrobial ointment, and replaced into the preputial cavity.
- The prepuce is held in a normal position by placement of a tube, which is taped to the sheath.
- Medical treatment is continued daily until the lesion is adequately healed.
- The object of medical treatment is to get control of edema, cellulitis, and necrosis and establish a healthy bed of granulation tissue.
- After medical treatment, surgery may be indicated depending on the severity of the trauma and the desire of the owner.
- Surgery is indicated if fibrous tissue development prevents normal extension of the prepuce or if there is habitual prolapse of the prepuce.
- The most commonly performed surgical technique is the reefing procedure (resection-anastomosis); this technique is employed to revise damaged preputial tissues and shorten the prepuce.
- The prepuce is measured prior to incision to assure that the final preputial length will be at least twice the length of the free portion of the penis.
- If the value of the bull does not warrant surgery, salvage is an option.

MEDICATIONS

DRUGS OF CHOICE
- Topical antimicrobials are utilized during medical treatment.
- Parenteral antibiotics are given perioperatively.

CONTRAINDICATIONS
Appropriate milk and meat withdrawal times must be followed for all compounds administered to food-producing animals.

FOLLOW-UP

Sexual rest is recommended for at least 60 days after surgical treatment.

MISCELLANEOUS

ASSOCIATED CONDITIONS
Abscesses and fibrosis may be present.

AGE-RELATED FACTORS
N/A

ZOONOTIC POTENTIAL
N/A

PREGNANCY
N/A

RUMINANT SPECIES AFFECTED
Primarily beef bulls

BIOSECURITY
N/A

PRODUCTION MANAGEMENT
N/A

SYNONYMS
Broken penis

SEE ALSO
Beef bull management
Penile deviations
Penile hematoma

ABBREVIATIONS
N/A

Suggested Reading
St. Jean, G. 1995, March. Male reproductive surgery. In: *Veterinary clinics of North America: food animal practice, soft tissue surgery*, ed. B. L. Hull, D. M. Rings. Philadelphia: W. B. Saunders.

Author: M. S. Gill

PSEUDOCOWPOX

 BASICS

OVERVIEW
• Pseudocowpox is a parapoxvirus that affects cattle but is closely related to contagious ovine ecthyma (orf) in sheep and bovine papular stomatitis in cattle.
• The lesions are small, 2–5-mm erythematous macules and papules that develop on the teats, udders, and perineum.
• These lesions eventually rupture and crust over.

SIGNALMENT
• Most cases involve adult milking cows and tend to occur in cyclic infections with the introduction of naïve animals and the waning of immunity in previously exposed older animals.
• The disease tends not to affect dry cows, heifers, and bulls.
• Calves suckling infected teats can develop oral lesions.

SIGNS
• Animals rarely develop fevers but may have a drop in milk production due to teat irritation.
• Lesions begin as small macules and papules 2–5 mm in diameter, on the teat, udder, and perineum, which slowly expand to round, reddened, raised lesions 1–2 cm in diameter with an overlying ring-shaped scab or crust.
• In nursing calves, the lesions may be located in the oral cavity with raised, umbilicated, circular ulcers on the tongue or palate.

CAUSES AND RISK FACTORS
N/A

 DIAGNOSIS

DIFFERENTIAL DIAGNOSIS
• Herpesvirus mammillitis: usually begins as small, 2–3-mm vesicles or pustules that rupture forming small, slow-healing ulcers. These can coalesce forming larger lesions that are slow to heal.
• Bovine papular stomatitis: usually occurs in suckling calves but can occasionally be seen on the teats and udder of infected cattle. Lesions are often umbilicated with a central scab.
• Cowpox: disease primarily of Europe with lesions having an umbilicated appearance on the udder and teat.
• Foot-and-mouth disease: vesicles, which ulcerate, can be seen on teats. Usually, the oral vesicles and vesicles in the interdigital space are commonly seen associated with teat lesions, which would make it easy to differentiate from pseudocowpox.
• Vesicular stomatitis: vesicles and ulcers can be seen on teats, however most vesicles are usually associated with lesion in the mouth and occasionally on feet.

CBC/BIOCHEMISTY/URINALYSIS
N/A

OTHER LABORATORY TESTS
N/A

IMAGING
N/A

DIAGNOSTIC PROCEDURES
• Electron microscopic evaluation of the scab will identify parapoxvirus particles.
• Virus isolation from infected scabs can assist in the identification of the virus.

PATHOLOGIC FINDINGS
Gross Findings
• Small, 2–5-mm erythematous macules and papules develop on the teats, udder, and perineum, which rupture and crust over.
• As the lesions progress, they enlarge to 1–2 cm in diameter with an erythematous outer rim and a peripheral ring-shaped scab. If the scab is removed, you have an ulcerated lesion that slowly heals. This differs from cowpox in that the lesion is not umbilicated.

Histopathologic Findings
• The lesion is primarily epithelial with the epidermis undergoing vacuolar degeneration and vesicle formation.
• Older lesions have neutrophils filling the vesicle. Eosinophilic intracytoplasmic inclusions are present in the vacuolated epithelium.

 TREATMENT

The lesions of pseudocowpox are usually self-limiting and require little care other than keeping the lesion free of debris and preventing secondary bacterial infections of the open sore.

MEDICATIONS
N/A

CONTRAINDICATIONS/POSSIBLE INTERACTIONS
N/A

FOLLOW-UP

PATIENT MONITORING
N/A

PREVENTION/AVOIDANCE
• Little immunity is present after infections.
• Animals probably transmit the disease during milking.

POSSIBLE COMPLICATIONS
Secondary bacterial mastitis or dermatitis can occur in lesions.

EXPECTED COURSE AND PROGNOSIS
Most animals recover without any problems.

MISCELLANEOUS

ASSOCIATED CONDITIONS

AGE-RELATED FACTORS
Calves may become infected with the virus and have lesions in the mouth from suckling on infected teats.

ZOONOTIC POTENTIAL
• This disease can be transmitted to herdsmen working on infected animals.
• Lesions develop on the hands (fingers) and face.
• These lesions are usually discrete, round, slow-healing ulcers.

PREGNANCY
N/A

BIOSECURITY
N/A

PRODUCTION MANAGEMENT
N/A

SEE ALSO
Bovine papular stomatitis
Cowpox
Foot-and-mouth disease
Herpesvirus mammillitis
Vesicular stomatitis

ABBREVIATIONS
N/A

Suggested Reading
Gibbs, E. P. 1984. Viral diseases of the skin of the bovine teat and udder. *Vet Clin North Am Large Anim Pract*. 6(1):187–202.
Wellenberg, G. J., Van Der Poel, W. H., Van Oirschot, J. T. 2002. Viral infections and bovine mastitis: a review. *Vet Microbiol*. 88(1):27–45.

Author: Robert B. Moeller, Jr.

PSEUDORABIES

 BASICS

OVERVIEW
• Pseudorabies is a reportable disease caused by a DNA herpesvirus. The name is derived from the clinical similarities to rabies. The primary host is the pig.
• Pseudorabies in ruminants occurs as acute encephalitis.

SYSTEMS AFFECTED
CNS, skin, production management

GENETICS
N/A

INCIDENCE/PREVALENCE
Unknown

GEOGRAPHIC DISTRIBUTION
Worldwide distribution

SIGNALMENT
• Swine are the primary host.
• Natural infections can occur in sheep, goats, and cattle.
• Dead-end hosts include rats, feral animals, dogs, and cats.

Species
Sheep, goats, and cattle; potentially all ruminants

Breed Predilections
N/A

Mean Age and Range
N/A

Predominant Sex
Either sex appears affected equally

SIGNS
• Ruminants have an incubation period of 4–7 days.
• Duration of illness ranges from 8 hours to 3 days. Many animals die suddenly without showing clinical signs of illness.
• The term "mad itch disease" in cattle resulted from the intense pruritis at the point of dermal contact with the pathogen. The animal begins licking at the area, then scratches the skin against inanimate objects. This may progress until the animal becomes frenzied. The result is alopecia, redness, ulcerations, and secondary bacterial infections.

• Goats do not usually exhibit intense pruritis. Signs usually include restlessness, screaming, and profuse sweating.
• The medulla in cattle, sheep, and goats becomes involved as the disease progresses leading to paralysis of the pharynx, salivation, cardiac irregularities, and labored respiration.
• Behavioral changes often occur. Most animals become depressed, but some may become aggressive or fearful. There may be grinding of teeth, bellowing, or stamping of feet.
• Other signs include paresthesia, fever, ataxia, hyperesthesia, head-pressing, CP deficits, and convulsions.
• Signs progress to convulsions, recumbency, paralysis, and death.

CAUSES AND RISK FACTORS
• Close contact with swine is the primary source of infection for sheep, goats, and cattle.
• Pseudorabies is a herpesvirus. Swine that have recovered from infection may be asymptomatic but continue to be latent carriers with infection of the trigeminal ganglia. Recrudescence occurs under stressful conditions.
• In ruminants, latency is not a common mechanism of disease transmission.
• Infection can occur after intranasal, oral, intradermal, or subcutaneous exposure to the virus. Virus spreads by axonoplasmic transport to the CNS.
• Virus may be present in nasal mucosa, secretions, and saliva during acute infection.
• Possible spread of the disease may be due to dead-end hosts such as rats, feral animals, dogs, or cats moving between farms. These sources of infection have a transient infective period.

 DIAGNOSIS

DIFFERENTIAL DIAGNOSIS
• Rabies
• Polioencephalomalacia
• Meningitis
• Hypomagnesemia
• Toxicity—organophosphate, carbamate, lead, arsenic, or salt poisoning
• Enterotoxemia

CBC/BIOCHEMISTRY/URINALYSIS
Usually normal

OTHER LABORATORY TESTS
CSF findings are consistent with encephalitis. Pleocytosis with increased mononuclear cells (50–200 cells/dL) and increased protein concentration (100–200 mg/dL)

IMAGING
N/A

DIAGNOSTIC PROCEDURES
• Isolation of virus in cell culture or in rabbits from infected nervous tissues. Segments of the sensory parts of the spinal cord serving the pruritic sites contain high concentrations of the virus.
• Immunofluorescent antibody test—brain tissue
• Rising antibody titers with paired serum tests

PATHOLOGIC FINDINGS

GROSS FINDINGS
• Alopecia, edema, dermal abrasions occur at the pruritic site with the possible presence of secondary bacterial pathogens.
• There is possible swelling or edema of regional lymph nodes.

HISTOPATHOLOGICAL FINDINGS
• Nonsuppurative meningoencephalitis
• Mononuclear cuffing
• Neuronal degeneration and necrosis
• Moderate perivascular cuffing of lymphocytes
• Eosinophilic intranuclear (Cowdry type A) inclusion bodies found in neurons and glial cells
• Some foci of microglial proliferation

 TREATMENT

• No effective treatment
• Supportive therapy and prevent self-injury due to pruritis if possible

MEDICATIONS

None

CONTRAINDICATIONS

Do not vaccinate ruminants with modified live virus vaccines targeted for use in swine. There have been reports of sheep infected by use of syringes contaminated with the MLV vaccine for swine.

FOLLOW-UP

None

PREVENTION/AVOIDANCE

• Prevent exposure of ruminants to swine and rats.
• Recovered swine should be culled as natural infections can result in the typical herpesvirus latency and a carrier state.
• Environmental inactivation of the virus can be achieved by drying, 6 hours of contact time with ultraviolet light, and high temperature (37°C).
• Contaminated pens can be disinfected with 10% bleach solution, quaternary ammonium compounds, iodines, or phenolics. At least 5 minutes of contact time is required before rinsing.

POSSIBLE COMPLICATIONS

N/A

EXPECTED COURSE AND PROGNOSIS

The majority of affected ruminants dies within 2 to 3 days of the onset of clinical signs.

MISCELLANEOUS

ASSOCIATED CONDITIONS

• Infectious bovine rhinotracheitis (IBR) virus shares common antigens with the pseudorabies virus. Serologic tests can be affected by heterospecific antibodies to the IBR virus cross-neutralizing pseudorabies virus antibodies.
• Behavioral changes often occur. Most animals become depressed, but some may become aggressive or fearful. There may be grinding of teeth, bellowing, or stamping of feet.
• Other signs include paresthesia, fever, ataxia, hyperesthesia, head-pressing, CP deficits, and convulsions.
• Signs progress to convulsions, recumbency, paralysis, and death.

AGE-RELATED FACTORS

None

ZOONOTIC POTENTIAL

Humans are generally resistant to pseudorabies virus. There have been reports of pruritis when skin wounds came in direct contact with infected tissues.

PREGNANCY

N/A

SYNONYMS

Aujeszky's disease
Infectious bulbar paralysis
Mad itch

SEE ALSO

Enterotoxemia
Hypomagnesemia
Meningitis
Polioencephalomalacia
Rabies
Toxicity—organophosphate, carbamate, lead, arsenic, or salt poisoning

ABBREVIATIONS

CNS = central nervous system
CP deficits = conscious proprioceptive deficits
CSF = cerebral spinal fluid
IBR = infectious bovine rhinotracheitis

Suggested Reading

Aiello, S. E. ed. 1998. Pseudorabies In: *Merck veterinary manual*. 8th ed. Whitehouse Station, NJ: Merck & Co.

Jones, T. C., Hunt, R. D., King, N. W., ed. 1997. Pseudorabies (infectious bulbar paralysis, Aujeszky's disease, mad itch). In: *Veterinary pathology*. 6th ed. Williams & Wilkins: Baltimore, MD.

Smith, B. P. 2002. Pseudorabies (mad itch; Aujeszky's disease). In: *Large animal internal medicine*. 3rd ed. St. Louis: Mosby.

Timoney, J. F., Gillespie, J. H., Scott, F. W., Barlough, J. E., ed. 1992. Pseudorabies. In: *Hagan and Bruner's microbiology and infectious diseases of domestic animals*. 8th ed. Ithaca, NY: Comstock Publishing Associates, A division of Cornell University Press.

Author: Lisa Nashold

PYELONEPHRITIS

 BASICS

OVERVIEW
• Pyelonephritis is a bacterial infection of the kidney due to ascending infection by *Escherichia coli* or *Corynebacterium renale* (several serotypes are normal inhabitants of the caudal reproductive tract of cows) from the lower urinary tract.
• *C. renale* possesses pili that facilitate attachment to and colonization of the urinary tract mucosa.

SYSTEMS AFFECTED
Urinary

GENETICS
N/A

INCIDENCE/PREVALENCE
N/A

GEOGRAPHIC DISTRIBUTION
Potentially worldwide

SIGNALMENT
Most common in postparturient dairy cows but may occur in ewes and does.

Species
Potentially, all ruminant species

Breed Predilections
N/A

Mean Age and Range
N/A

Predominant Sex
Female

SIGNS
• Acute primary pyelonephritis causes fever 103.5°F to 105.5°F (39.7°C to 40.8°C), anorexia, and sudden drop in milk production.
• Some cows exhibit signs of colic such as treading, restlessness, kicking at the abdomen, tail swishing.

• Stranguria, polyuria, kyphosis, hematuria (occasionally with blood clots), and pyuria may also be present.
• Chronic pyelonephritis is associated with weight loss, poor production, anorexia, diarrhea, polyuria, and anemia.
• In chronic cases, lordosis and stretching may be present due to chronic renal pain, and stranguria and gross abnormalities of the urine may be less apparent.
• Signs in subclinical cases of pyelonephritis may be masked by signs associated with concurrent postparturient problems such as mastitis, metritis, or abomasal displacement.

CAUSES AND RISK FACTORS
Physical damage to the mucosa of the lower urinary tract, such as occurs with dystocia, bladder paralysis, or catheterization, may predispose to pyelonephritis. Rectovaginal lacerations/fistula may also predispose to development of pyelonephritis.

 DIAGNOSIS

DIFFERENTIAL DIAGNOSIS
Emboli nephritis, cystitis, gastrointestinal disorders with associated colic, enzootic hematuria, urolithiasis, vaginitis, vulvar trauma, perivaginal abscess, pelvic entrapment of the bladder

CBC/BIOCHEMISTRY/URINALYSIS
• Neutrophilic leukocytosis and hyperfibrinogenemia often seen on CBC.
• Abnormalities on urinalysis may include presence of RBCs, WBCs, protein, and bacteria. Proteinuria is very significant in most cases of pyelonephritis.
• Hypoalbuminemia, more severe in chronic cases, is usually present.
• Hypergammaglobulinemia (> 5 g/dl) occurs in most chronic cases.

• Increased BUN and creatinine may occur and azotemia may be due to prerenal (dehydration), renal (bilateral pyelonephritis with renal failure), or postrenal causes (obstruction of the ureters or urethra by blood clots or fibrin).

OTHER LABORATORY TESTS
• Urine culture to determine etiology and antimicrobial sensitivity is of utmost importance to the patient.
• Urine collection by catheterization is optimal for bacterial culturing.

IMAGING
Ultrasonography of the kidneys is a valuable tool and may supply important prognostic information.

DIAGNOSTIC PROCEDURES
• Rectal palpation is useful if the left kidney is enlarged. If only the right kidney is involved, rectal palpation may not be as useful unless the kidney is massively enlarged.
• Vaginal palpation allows for detection of unilateral or bilateral ureteral enlargement that may not be detectable on rectal palpation.
• Presence of blood, blood clots, fibrin, or pus on gross examination of the urine may be diagnostic in acute cases.

PATHOLOGIC FINDINGS
• Gross renal enlargement in acute cases
• Cross section of the affected kidney(s) shows a gray, viscous, odorless, exudate in the renal pelvis with extension into the medulla and cortex.
• Renal abscesses may be present in chronic cases of pyelonephritis.
• Hemorrhage, ulceration, and fibrin deposition may be present on the mucosa of the bladder and urethra.
• One or both ureters may be enlarged and filled with purulent debris.

TREATMENT

• Antimicrobial choice is based on results of urine culture and sensitivity and the ability of the drug to achieve high concentrations in the urine without being nephrotoxic. The drug chosen must also be one that is approved for use in cattle.
• In cases of unilateral chronic pyelonephritis, nephrectomy may be indicated.
• Drug withdrawal times for meat and milk must be maintained.

MEDICATIONS

DRUGS OF CHOICE

• Procaine penicillin G is the usual drug of choice. *C. renale* is uniformly sensitive to penicillin and *E. coli* is often sensitive to the resulting high concentrations of penicillin in the urine. Ceftiofur sodium or ceftiofur hydrochloride has also produced favorable results.
• Long-term (3 weeks) antimicrobial therapy is crucial to treatment success.

CONTRAINDICATIONS

N/A

FOLLOW-UP

• Prognosis for uncomplicated acute cases of pyelonephritis treated with long-term antimicrobial therapy is good.

• Cases of pyelonephritis secondary to bladder paralysis, rectovaginal fistula, or other functional problems have a poorer prognosis because of the likelihood of recurrence.
• Chronic cases of pyelonephritis tend to have a poor prognosis because of the potential for abscess formation in the kidney(s) and loss of renal parenchyma.

MISCELLANEOUS

• Prevention and control are achieved by isolation of affected animals to prevent spread followed by disinfection of heavily contaminated areas.
• Practice aseptic technique when performing urogenital and obstetrical procedures.
• Embolic nephritis is much less common than pyelonephritis but may result from a bacteremia stemming from a primary disease (e.g., mastitis, metritis, septic arthritis, endocarditis) in calves and cows.
• Clinical signs of embolic nephritis are related to the primary condition.
• Urinalysis findings are similar to those in cases of pyelonephritis.
• Treatment is aimed at the primary or underlying condition.
• Embolic nephritis is often an incidental finding at necropsy.

SEE ALSO

Cystitis
Emboli nephritis
Enzootic hematuria
Gastrointestinal disorders with associated colic
Pelvic entrapment of the bladder
Perivaginal abscess
Urolithiasis
Vaginitis
Vulvar trauma

ABBREVIATIONS

BUN = blood urea nitrogen
CBC = complete blood count
RBCs = red blood cells
WBCs = white blood cells

Suggested Reading
Hayashi, H., Biller, D. S., Rings, D. M., Miyabayashi, T. 1994, Sep 1. Ultrasonographic diagnosis of pyelonephritis in a cow. *J Am Vet Med Assoc.* 205(5):736–38.
Markusfeld, O., Nahari, N., Kessner, D., Adler, H. 1989, Nov-Dec. Observations on bovine pyelonephritis. *Br Vet J.* 145(6): 573–79.
Rebhun, W. C. 1995. *Diseases of dairy cattle.* Philadelphia: Lippincott, Williams & Wilkins.
Rebhun, W. C., Dill, S. G., Perdrizet, J. A., Hatfield, C. E. 1989, Apr 1. Pyelonephritis in cows: 15 cases (1982–1986). *J Am Vet Med Assoc.* 194(7):953–55.
Sparling, A. M. 2000, Apr. An unusual presentation of enzootic bovine leukosis. *Can Vet J.* 41(4):315–16.

Author: M. S. Gill

PYOMETRA

BASICS

OVERVIEW
• Pyometra is defined as an intrauterine accumulation of a purulent exudate within the uterus concurrent with the presence of a corpus luteum and anestrus.
• Occurs in both dairy and beef cows, sheep, and dairy goats.

SIGNALMENT
• Lactating dairy cows in the postovulatory phase of the postpartum period.
• Beef or dairy cows exposed to bull infected with *Tritrichomonas foetus*.

SIGNS
• Failure to show estrus
• Persistent corpus luteum
• Fluid accumulation within a thickened uterus in the absence of positive pregnancy signs
• Mucopurulent discharge from the reproductive tract

CAUSES AND RISK FACTORS
• Failure of the endometrial luteolytic mechanism results in maintenance of the corpus luteum and concurrent failure to cycle.
• Cows that cycle early postpartum that have concurrent endometritis
• Animals with retained fetal membranes with or without dystocia after parturition
• Embryonic death associated with infection
• Cows bred to a *Tritrichomonas foetus*–infected bull.

DIAGNOSIS

• Uterus is fluid filled, thickened, or thin and is usually atonic.
• Thick, purulent debris and a lack of fetal members are detected on palpation.

DIFFERENTIAL DIAGNOSIS
• Mucometra
• Pregnancy
• Macerated fetus

CBC/BIOCHEMISTRY/URINALYSIS
N/A

OTHER LABORATORY TESTS
N/A

PATHOLOGIC FINDINGS
Uterine content may include the following bacteria: *Arcanobacter pyogenes*, *Fusobacterium necrophorum*, *Bacteroides* spp. and *Tritrichomonas foetus*.

TREATMENT

MEDICATIONS

• Prostaglandin F2 alpha (35 mg) or cloprostenol (500 ug) treatments repeated at 14-day intervals in cattle
• Drug withdrawal times must be maintained for meat and milk within food-producing animals.

FOLLOW-UP

PREVENTION/AVOIDANCE
• Management of the transition dairy cow to prevent the incidence of dystocia and retained fetal membranes
• Prebreeding examinations

MISCELLANEOUS

ASSOCIATED CONDITIONS
Reproductive failure

AGE-RELATED FACTORS
N/A

ZOONOTIC POTENTIAL
N/A

PREGNANCY
• Failure to conceive
• Failure of the endometrial luteolytic mechanism results in maintenance of the corpus luteum and concurrent failure to cycle.

RUMINANT SPECIES AFFECTED
Potentially, all ruminant species are affected.

BIOSECURITY
N/A

PRODUCTION MANAGEMENT
N/A

SYNONYMS
N/A

SEE ALSO
Reproductive pharmacology
Reproductive ultrasounding
Tritrichomonas foetus

ABBREVIATIONS
N/A

Suggested Reading
Lewis, G. S. 2004, Jul. Steroidal regulation of uterine immune defenses. *Anim Reprod Sci.* 82–83:281–94.
Rebhun, W. C. 1995. *Diseases of dairy cattle.* Baltimore, MD: Williams and Wilkins.
Seals, R. C., Wulster-Radcliffe, M. C., Lewis, G. S. 2002, Jan. Modulation of the uterine response to infectious bacteria in postpartum ewes. *Am J Reprod Immunol.* 47(1): 57–63.
Seals, R. C., Wulster-Radcliffe, M. C., Lewis, G. S. 2003, May. Uterine response to infectious bacteria in estrous cyclic ewes. *Am J Reprod Immunol.* 49(5): 269–78.

Author: Carlos A. Risco

PYRROLIZIDINE ALKALOIDS

 BASICS

OVERVIEW
• Among ruminants, most cases of pyrrolizidine alkaloid (PA) poisoning occur in cattle.
• Sheep and goats are relatively resistant to PA intoxication.
• Llamas and alpacas appear to be similar to sheep and goats when it comes to susceptibility.
• The three plant families Compositae, Leguminosae, and Boraginaceae contain the majority of PA-containing plants.
• The genera *Senecio* (*S. vulgaris*, common groundsel; *S. jacobaea*, tansy ragwort; *S. riddelli*, Riddell's groundsel; *S. flaccidus*, threadleaf groundsel) and *Cynoglossum officinale* (houndstongue) have been implicated in most of the animal poisonings in the United States.
• Plants in the genera *Amsinckia*, *Crotalaria*, *Heliotropium*, and *Echium* less commonly cause poisonings either because they are not palatable or do not grow in dense enough stands to pose a significant risk.
• Poisonings generally occur as a result of cattle grazing heavily contaminated pastures (rare—most of these plants are not palatable) or consuming contaminated hay (most common route). Exposures are typically over several weeks to months duration.
• The alkaloid content can vary tremendously among plants; concentrations vary with respect to age and stage of maturity of the plant, and soil and weather conditions.

• Poisonings are most commonly chronic in nature; acute exposures are rare.
• This is generally a herd problem, although individual animals may be selected.
• The clinical signs can be slow and insidious, with general debilitation and weight loss a common complaint. Some affected animals show abrupt onset of signs associated with hepatoencephalopathy.
• The liver is the primary target; kidney, lung, and heart tissue are less commonly affected.
• Megalocytosis, biliary hyperplasia, and fibrosis are commonly reported histologic findings on postmortem examination of the liver.
• Prognosis is guarded to grave for affected animals.

PATHOPHYSIOLOGY
• PAs are rapidly absorbed from the gastrointestinal tract.
• They undergo extensive metabolism in the liver. Some PAs are detoxified to harmless metabolites, but some are converted to highly toxic pyrroles.
• It is these pyrroles that alkylate DNA, leading to inhibition of cell mitosis and the ultimate histologic change of megalocytosis. As these megalocytes die, they are replaced by fibrous connective tissue.
• Though the liver is the primary target, lung, kidney, and heart tissue may be affected as well.

SYSTEMS AFFECTED
Hepatobiliary (megalocytosis, necrosis, fibrosis, biliary hyperplasia), renal (megalocytosis of the proximal convoluted tubules, glomerular atrophy, tubular necrosis), lung (hemorrhage and edema), and heart (necrosis)

GENETICS
N/A

INCIDENCE/PREVALENCE
• Unpredictable and uncommon; however, it is one of the more common causes of plant intoxication in some areas of the United States.
• Poisonings can occur all year round through grazing contaminated pastures or ingesting heavily contaminated hay.

GEOGRAPHIC DISTRIBUTION
Worldwide

SIGNALMENT
Cattle

Species
• Cattle are most susceptible.
• Sheep, goats, llamas, and alpacas are relatively resistant.
• Resistance appears to be partly due to differences in rumen metabolism.

Breed Predilections
N/A

Mean Age and Range
Young animals appear to be more sensitive.

Predominant Sex
N/A

SIGNS
• Some animals suffer chronic weight loss and debilitation associated with chronic liver insufficiency.
• Weakness and sluggishness
• Secondary photosensitivity and icterus
• Some animals exhibit an abrupt onset of signs associated with hepatic encephalopathy—mania, derangement, aimless walking, head pressing, blindness, and ataxia.

PYRROLIZIDINE ALKALOIDS

• Less commonly observed signs include inspiratory dyspnea (reported in horses), GI impactions, ascites, diarrhea.

CAUSES AND RISK FACTORS
• A minimum of 2–4 weeks, up to several months, of exposure to these plants is generally required in order to induce toxicity.
• Acute exposures can occur if animals ingest 5%–10% of their body weight of plant material within a few days to a few weeks (rare).
• It is more common to see poisonings in animals that ingest 25%–50% of their body weight in plant material over a period of several months.
• Signs can occur suddenly in animals where the exposure to PA-containing plants ceased weeks or months previously.
• Approximate chronic toxic dose (for tansy ragwort) for an adult cow is 0.4 kg dry plant or 1.7 kg fresh plant per day for several weeks.
• For Riddell's groundsel, approximately 33 g dry or 176 g fresh plant daily for 3 weeks could be toxic to an adult cow.
• An approximate toxic dose of threadleaf groundsel in adult cows is 150 g dry or 750 g fresh plant daily for two weeks.

• A daily dose of 136 g dry or 680 g fresh houndstongue daily could be toxic to cattle over a period of a few weeks.

 DIAGNOSIS

DIFFERENTIAL DIAGNOSIS
Acute hepatitis or cholangiohepatitis, liver abscess, viral or bacterial encephalitis, aflatoxicosis, exposure to nitrosamines, hepatotoxic cyanobacteria

CBC/BIOCHEMISTRY/URINALYSIS
Inflammatory leukogram can be observed.
• Hyperbilirubinemia
• Elevations in gamma-glutamyl transpeptidase, alkaline phosphatase, aspartate aminotransferase, and sorbitol dehydrogenase may also be elevated.
• Hypoalbuminemia, hypoproteinemia, and low blood urea nitrogen are less-consistent abnormalities.

OTHER LABORATORY TESTS
• Severely elevated bile acids
• Characteristic histological lesions of a liver biopsy

IMAGING
Ultrasound may reveal a small liver.

DIAGNOSTIC PROCEDURES
• One should examine the diet for the presence of PA-containing plants.
• Pyrrole testing of blood or hepatic tissue can be done, but it is not commonly performed at diagnostic laboratories. The analysis is not quantitative or sensitive, particularly in the late stages of the disease.

PATHOLOGIC FINDINGS
• Poor body condition
• Jaundice
• Ascites and generalized edema
• Small, pale, firm liver with mottled cut service may be visualized on necropsy.
• Characteristic lesions of hepatic megalocytosis with piecemeal necrosis, biliary hyperplasia, and generalized fibrosis.
• Other less-commonly recognized lesions include myocardial necrosis, gastrointestinal edema and hemorrhage, adrenal cortical hypertrophy, pulmonary edema, interstitial pneumonia, and status spongiosus of brain tissue (not all reported in ruminants).

TREATMENT
- Find and remove the suspect source or remove animals from the contaminated environment.
- Most animals respond poorly to treatment, because by the time the disease is diagnosed, adequate regeneration of the liver is not possible.
- No specific treatment regime has been shown to be effective in treating these animals.
- Dietary changes could include switching to one that is highly digestible, high in calories, and low in protein.
- Treatment is typically not an economically viable option for most producers.

MEDICATIONS
N/A

CONTRAINDICATIONS
N/A

FOLLOW-UP
Serum chemistry panels should be run periodically to evaluate liver function.

PATIENT MONITORING
Monitor appetite and weight and serum chemistries to evaluate liver enzymes, albumin, and protein.

PREVENTION/AVOIDANCE
- Be able to recognize PA-containing plants either in the pasture or in hay.
- Avoid feeding "weedy" hay.
- Appropriate herbicide use can control the growth of these plants in the field.
- Sheep and goats can perhaps be used to control stands of these plants through rotational grazing.

POSSIBLE COMPLICATIONS
- Avoid using medications that require extensive hepatic metabolism.
- Pneumonia and chronic wasting

EXPECTED COURSE AND PROGNOSIS
- The more severely affected animals have a poor prognosis. Many are euthanized due to debilitation and poor response to therapy, or because of financial constraints.
- Patients showing severe neurological signs often do not respond well to treatment.
- Some patients may survive after several months of intensive supportive care, but often are not able to regain their former activity or production level.

MISCELLANEOUS
ASSOCIATED CONDITIONS
N/A

AGE-RELATED FACTORS
Young animals appear to be more susceptible.

ZOONOTIC POTENTIAL
N/A

PREGNANCY
PAs have been shown to cross the placenta and some are secreted into the milk. The risk of these routes having a significant impact on the developing fetus or nursing young is extremely low.

RUMINANT SPECIES AFFECTED
Cattle are most susceptible of all ruminants; sheep and goats are relatively resistant; and llamas and alpacas are thought to be more like sheep and goats.

BIOSECURITY
N/A

PRODUCTION MANAGEMENT
Avoid feeding "weedy" PA-containing hay. Be able to recognize these plants in pastures or hay.

SYNONYMS
Seneciosis
Venoocclusive disease

SEE ALSO
Acute hepatitis
Aflatoxicosis
Cholangiohepatitis
Exposure to nitrosamines
Hepatotoxic cyanobacteria
Liver abscess
Viral or bacterial encephalitis

ABBREVIATIONS
GI = gastrointestinal tract
PA = pyrrolizidine alkaloid

Suggested Reading
Molyneux R. J., Johnson, A. E., Olsen, J. D., Baker, D. C. 1991, Jan. Toxicity of pyrrolizidine alkaloids from Riddell groundsel (*Senecio riddellii*) to cattle. *Am J Vet Res.* 52(1): 146–51.
Skaanild, M. T., Friis, C., Brimer, L. 2001, Jun. Interplant alkaloid variation and *Senecio vernalis* toxicity in cattle. *Vet Hum Toxicol.* 43(3): 147–51.
Stegelmeier, B. 2004. Pyrrolizidine alkaloids. In: *Clinical veterinary toxicology*, ed. K. H. Plumlee. St. Louis: Mosby.

Author: Patricia Talcott

Q FEVER

 BASICS

DEFINITION
• Q (Query) fever is a rickettsial disease affecting primarily humans, cattle, sheep, and goats caused by the organism *Coxiella burnetii*. Other species less commonly affected include dogs, cats, rabbits, a variety of wild and domestic mammals, and birds.
• The majority of *C. burnetii* infections in ruminants are unapparent, but abortion and infertility are common manifestations when naïve herds are exposed to the organism.
• Epidemiologically, two cycles of the infection are recognized. The first is maintained in wildlife species, where mainly ticks transmit the organism. The second is preserved in livestock species; ingestion and inhalation of the organism are the main avenues of transmission.
• In humans, Q fever is considered an occupational hazard with the majority of infections occurring in livestock workers, veterinarians, and personnel of animal research facilities.

PATHOPHYSIOLOGY
• *C. burnetii*, an obligate, intracellular, gram-negative, rickettsial agent, replicates within the phagolysosome of infected cells.
• Organisms localize in the mammary glands, supramammary lymph nodes, uterus, and placenta in domestic ruminants.
• The organism can be shed in milk, urine, feces, the placenta, and parturient discharges during subsequent pregnancies and lactations.
• In chronically infected animals, *C. burnetii* is also shed in the feces and urine.

• As with other infections, the initial antibody response is mediated by IgM, subsequently switching to a predominately IgG reaction. A characteristic of *C. burnetii* is its phase variation due to partial loss of polysaccharide that results in antigenic drift. During the acute phase of infection, ELISA can detect predominately IgM antibodies against phase II antigens. Later, IgG, IgA, and to a lesser extent IgM antibodies against phase I antigens appear. Studies to characterize the cellular immune response against phase I and II *C. burnetii* antigens in domestic animals are lacking.

SYSTEMS AFFECTED
Reproductive—abortion, stillbirths, neonatal death

GENETICS
N/A

INCIDENCE/PREVALENCE
• Information on the prevalence of Q fever in animal species is limited.
• Q fever can be endemic in areas where reservoir animals are found.
• The animal reservoir is large and includes many wild and domestic mammals, birds, and arthropods. However, the primary reservoirs are considered to be cattle, sheep, goats, and ticks. Other animal species, including dogs, cats, rabbits, horses, pigs, rodents, pigeons, and other fowl, may also serve as reservoirs of *C. burnetii*.
• In endemic areas, up to 25%–50% of animals may have antibodies to *C. burnetii*.

GEOGRAPHIC DISTRIBUTION
Q fever is found worldwide and has been reported on all continents except New Zealand.

SIGNALMENT

Species
Many species of animals have been found to be infected with *C. burnetii*. Sheep, goats, cattle, and ticks (ixodid and argasid) are considered the primary reservoirs.

Breed Predilections
N/A

Mean Age and Range
The greatest mortality is seen in fetal or newborn animals. Adult animals are usually asymptomatic.

Predominant Sex
N/A

SIGNS

GENERAL COMMENTS
The incubation period for Q fever is variable.

HISTORICAL FINDINGS
• Affected adult ruminants are usually asymptomatic; when clinical disease occurs, reproductive failure is usually the only symptom seen. This can be manifested as abortions, stillbirths, retained placentas, infertility, or weak newborns.
• Late-term abortions are typically seen and occur over a 2–4 week period. Of the whole flock or herd, 5%–50% may be affected.

PHYSICAL EXAMINATION FINDINGS
• Affected adult ruminants are usually asymptomatic.
• In sheep and goats, anorexia and abortions are the most common signs noted.
• In cattle, infertility, sporadic abortion, and low birth weights are seen.

CAUSES
• Parturient materials containing *C. burnetii* are highly infective and can contain a large number of the organism.

• *C. burnetii* is tremendously stable in the environment and can be transmitted to other animals via aerosol (airborne droplets or contaminated dust) and direct contact with placental tissues and parturient fluids, feces, or urine of infected animals.
• Fomites (e.g., wool, bedding, clothing), ingestion of parturient material, contaminated water or raw milk, or arthropods may also play a role in transmission.

RISK FACTORS
• *C. burnetii* is transmitted mainly through inhalation of the organism present in contaminated dust or droplets emanating from placental tissue, birth fluids, and excreta of infected animals.
• The infective dose of *C. burnetii* is very low, and it is considered that one to ten organisms can initiate an infection. In addition, due to the highly resistant nature of the organism to adverse environmental conditions, particles carrying *C. burnetii* can remain infectious for months and be transported by wind currents.
• Direct contact with infected animals or ingestion of contaminated materials or raw milk from infected animals are alternative routes of transmission.
• Additionally, naïve herds are very susceptible and abortion storms are possible.

 DIAGNOSIS

• *C. burnetii* does not stain well with the traditional Gram technique, but takes a red color with the Gimenez, modified Ziehl-Neelsen, or Macchiavello stains and purple with Giemsa stain.
• *C. burnetii* does not grow on artificial media, but can be isolated in cell culture, embryonated chicken eggs, and some laboratory animals, such as mice and guinea pigs.

• *C. burnetii* can be detected from vaginal discharges, the placenta, placental fluids, aborted fetuses, as well as milk, urine, and feces.
• Diagnosis is based on histopathology and demonstration of viral antigen or antibody. The organism is not usually detected by Gram stains but may be with modified Ziehl-Neelsen or Gimenez stain.
• The demonstration of *C. burnetii*-specific antibodies in the serum of animals is the most practical method to establish a diagnosis of Q fever.
• In domestic animals, CF, IFA, and ELISA are most often used. Phase II antibodies dominate the humoral immune response in the acute phase of the infection, whereas phase I antibodies are prominent in the chronic phase.
• Serological tests are good indicators of previous exposure but provide no information on the infectious status of individual animals.
• *C. burnetii* is a biohazard level three zoonotic agent, so personal protective measures should be taken.
• A major problem in the identification of Q fever cases in humans is that often the clinical signs of acute infection are nonspecific and easily confused with those of other diseases. In the acute phase, Q fever in humans can be manifested as fever, chills, retrobulbar headache, myalgia, chest pain, respiratory distress, and liver failure, yet in the majority of cases the infection is asymptomatic. The disease may progress in a small proportion of infected individuals to a chronic phase characterized by chronic heart failure due to endocarditis, granulomatous hepatitis, osteomyelitis, or by chronic inflammation in several other organs. At this stage, the infection is often life threatening and complicated by the fact that antibiotic therapy is generally not effective. Q fever is more frequent among HIV-infected patients and other immunocompromised individuals.

DIFFERENTIAL DIAGNOSIS
Differentials include other causes of abortion and infertility, such as brucellosis, leptospirosis, campylobacteriosis, salmonellosis, listeriosis, chlamydiosis, mycotic abortion, toxoplasmosis, BVD, or IBR.

CBC/BIOCHEMISTRY/URINALYSIS
N/A

OTHER LABORATORY TESTS
• Isolation methods are dangerous to laboratory personnel and are rarely used for diagnosis.
• PCR is becoming a more common method of identifying specific fragments of *C. burnetii*. DNA can be amplified from fresh or frozen samples, including buffy coats, milk, placenta, fetal tissue, vaginal swabs, feces, and other biological specimens.

IMAGING
N/A

DIAGNOSTIC PROCEDURES
N/A

PATHOLOGIC FINDINGS
• Placentitis is the most characteristic lesion in ruminants. The placenta is typically leathery and thickened. It may contain large amounts of creamy, white-yellow exudate at the edges of cotyledons and in the intercotyledonary area.
• Lesions in aborted fetuses are usually nonspecific. Pneumonia has been noted in goats and cattle.
• Histologically, lesions are characterized by severe necrotic placentitis with infiltration of neutrophils and mononuclear cells, focal exudation of fibrin, and mineralization in the stroma and villi.
• Organisms can be observed in placental trophoblast cells, particularly at the base of the cotyledonary villi.

Q FEVER

TREATMENT

Because *C. burnetii* replicates in phagolysosomes of infected cells, the effectiveness of antibiotics is theoretically limited by their ability to penetrate these organelles and remain active at the low pH that prevails in this environment.

APPROPRIATE HEALTH CARE
N/A

NURSING CARE
N/A

ACTIVITY
N/A

DIET
N/A

CLIENT EDUCATION
• Q fever is a zoonotic disease.
• Clients should be educated on routes of transmission of *C. burnetii* and vector control methods.
• Pregnant women are at the greatest risk, so should be advised to avoid periparturient ruminants.
• Additionally, persons with valvular heart disease or weakened immune systems are more susceptible.

SURGICAL CONSIDERATIONS
N/A

MEDICATIONS

DRUGS OF CHOICE
• Little is known about the effectiveness of treating animals with antibiotics.
• In enzootic herds, tetracycline may be given in water in the weeks preceding parturition. This may help reduce shedding of the organism in birthing materials and may suppress the number of abortions. However, it will not eliminate infection or eradicate the "carrier" state of *C. burnetii* infection.
• Antibiotics that have been shown to be effective in the treatment of acute human Q fever include the macrolides, cotrimoxazole, rifampin, chloramphenicol, and the fluoroquinones.

CONTRAINDICATIONS
Appropriate milk and meat withdrawal times must be followed for all compounds administered to food-producing animals.

PRECAUTIONS
N/A

POSSIBLE INTERACTIONS
N/A

ALTERNATIVE DRUGS
N/A

FOLLOW-UP

PATIENT MONITORING
N/A

PREVENTION/AVOIDANCE
• *C. burnetii* is tremendously stable in the environment.
• Pregnant animals should be segregated to reduce the spread of the organism. When possible, parturition should take place indoors and in separate facilities.
• Following parturition, placentas, aborted materials, and fetal tissues should be disposed of appropriately.
• Birth products should be incinerated and lambing areas cleaned and disinfected with Lysol, bleach, or hydrogen peroxide.
• Cleaning and sanitation measures as well as vector control should be attempted but do not usually control the spread of the disease.
• Carcasses should be buried or burned.
• *C. burnetii* is highly resistant to physical and chemical agents. Variable susceptibility has been reported for hypochlorite, formalin, and phenolic disinfectants; a 0.05% hypochlorite, 5% peroxide, or 1:100 solution of Lysol may be effective. High-temperature pasteurization destroys the organism.
• Education of clients should focus on potential sources of infection and ways to reduce environmental contamination from infected placental membranes and aborted materials.

• Q fever vaccines effectively protect animals against abortion, low fetal weight, and chronic infertility, but they have not prevented infection and/or the shedding of the organism in fluids and birth products. Q fever vaccines for humans and animals are available in many countries but not in the United States.

POSSIBLE COMPLICATIONS
N/A

EXPECTED COURSE AND PROGNOSIS
• In small ruminants, several abortions may be followed by uncomplicated recovery; in other cases, the disease may recur yearly.
• Pregnancy subsequent to *Coxiella* abortions are generally carried to term. However, ewes can remain chronically infective and continue to shed organisms.
• Organisms may be shed in milk and feces for several days after parturition.

MISCELLANEOUS

ASSOCIATED CONDITIONS
N/A

AGE-RELATED FACTORS
• Adult animals are typically asymptomatic.
• The greatest mortality rates are seen in fetuses or young neonates of sheep, goats, and cattle.

ZOONOTIC POTENTIAL
• Humans are highly susceptible to infection by exposure to aerosols when assisting parturition, handling infected placental tissues, performing necropsy on aborted fetuses, during slaughter or laboratory procedures, and drinking raw, unpasteurized milk.
• In the acute phase, Q fever in humans can be manifested as fever, chills, retrobulbar headache, myalgia, chest pain, respiratory distress, and liver failure, yet in the majority of cases the infection is asymptomatic.
• Exanthema (rash) occurs in about 10% of cases.

- Complications are not common but may include endocarditis, cirrhosis, aseptic meningitis, encephalitis, osteomyelitis, and vasculitis. At this stage, the infection is often life threatening and complicated by the fact that antibiotic therapy is generally not effective.
- The organism can be transplacentally transmitted so is of great risk for pregnant women; abortions, neonatal deaths, premature births, low birth weights, or placentitis may occur.
- The overall case-fatality rate for Q fever ranges from less than 1% to 2.4%.
- Q fever is more frequent among HIV-infected patients and other immunocompromised individuals.
- Milk destined for human consumption should be pasteurized. Pregnant women, immunosuppressed individuals, and people with vascular heart disease should be prevented from performing at-risk jobs.

PREGNANCY
Q fever causes abortion, stillbirths, retained placentas, infertility, and weak newborns in sheep, goats, and cattle.

RUMINANT SPECIES AFFECTED
Sheep, goats, cattle

BIOSECURITY
- Practical control is difficult because of environmental stability and infectivity of animals, arthropods, and humans.
- Efforts to control the spread of Q fever should include segregation of infected animals, especially those that are periparturient, vector control measures, and prompt cleaning and disinfection following parturition.
- Animals infected with *C. burnetii* should be maintained under animal biosafety level 3 (ABSL-3) conditions, and research and animal care staff should use personal protective equipment conforming to ABSL-3 practices. A comprehensive occupational health and safety program should be in place to ensure a safe working environment.

PRODUCTION MANAGEMENT
For livestock, control measures include good animal husbandry and implementing cleaning and disinfection protocols.

Research Facilities: Considerations
- Although infection among domestic livestock is often inapparent, it may constitute a significant health hazard for livestock workers and research personnel.
- Several Q fever outbreaks in biomedical research facilities utilizing pregnant ewes have been described, with large numbers of individuals developing clinical illness or at least seroconverting to the agent.
- Biomedical scientists are known to be at increased risk of exposure when utilizing cattle, goats, or sheep in environments where contaminated dust, urine, feces, amniotic fluid, placentas, and newborn animals may occur.
- The following steps can be taken to minimize and control the potential risk to research personnel when working with domestic livestock in research facilities. Whenever possible, use male or nonpregnant animals in research programs. Procure animals from Q fever–free sources (cumulative and consistent negative Q fever serology on a herd/flock). Monitor individual animals for organism shedding (PCR assays on biological samples from animals presenting a potential risk). Standard operating procedures (SOPs) should be developed and followed to facilitate appropriate animal care and use. Animals infected with *C. burnetii* should be maintained under animal biosafety level 3 (ABSL-3) conditions, and research and animal care staff should use personal protective equipment conforming to ABSL-3 practices. A comprehensive occupational health and safety program should be in place to ensure a safe working environment.

SYNONYMS
Abattoir fever
Balkan grippe
Coxiellosis
Queensland fever or
Query fever

SEE ALSO
Abortion and pregnancy loss
Brucellosis
Campylobacteriosis
Chlamydiosis
Listeriosis
Placentitis
Salmonellosis

ABBREVIATIONS
ABSL-3 = animal biosafety level 3
BVD = bovine viral diarrhea
CF = complement fixation test
ELISA = enzyme-linked immunosorbent assay
IBR = infectious bovine rhinotracheitis
IFA = indirect fluorescent antibody
LPS = lipopolysaccharide
PCR = polymerase chain reaction
SOP = standard operating procedures

Suggested Reading
Center for Food Security and Public Health. 2004, Jan. *Q fever*. Fact Sheet..http://www.cfsph.iastate.edu.
FASS. 1999. *Guide for the care and use of agricultural animals in agricultural research and teaching*. Savoy, IL: FASS.
Fox, J. G., Newcomer, C. E., Rozmiarek, H. 2002. Selected zoonoses. In: *Laboratory animal medicine*, ed. J. G. Fox, L. C. Anderson, F. M. Loew, F.W. Quimby. 2nd ed. San Diego: Academic Press.
Maurin. M., Raoult, D. 1999. Q fever. *Clinical Microbiology Reviews* 12(4): 518–53.
McQuiston, J. H., Childs, J. E., Thompson, H. A. 2002. Q fever. *J Am Vet Med Assoc*. 221(6): 796–99.
NIH. 2002. *Public health service policy on humane care and use of laboratory animals*. Bethesda, MD: OLAW.

Authors: Andres de la Concha, Glenda Dvorak, Richard Ermel

RABIES

BASICS

OVERVIEW
• Rabies is a rhabdovirus causing an acute viral encephalomyelitis. Rabies virus is perhaps the most important cause of encephalitis in cattle because of the public health implications. The virus can affect any mammal including humans.
• Once clinical signs appear, the disease is invariably fatal.
• Prevention and control of the disease in cattle can be best achieved in many areas of the world by regional oral vaccination of foxes and other wild carnivore species.
• Penetration of dermis or mucous membranes by virus-laden saliva is most commonly via a bite wound inflicted by an infected animal. The virus then travels to the CNS via peripheral nerves.
• Humans risk exposure by reaching into the mouth of an infected animal looking for a foreign body in the mouth or throat. Foreign body may be suspected due to inability to swallow or hypersalivation.

SYSTEMS AFFECTED
CNS

GENETICS
N/A

INCIDENCE/PREVALENCE
• In a recent U.S. survey, during 2002, 49 states and Puerto Rico reported 7967 cases of rabies in nonhuman animals and 3 cases in human beings to the Centers for Disease Control and Prevention, an increase of 7.2% from the 7436 cases in nonhuman animals and 1 case in a human being reported in 2001. More than 92% (7375 cases) were in wild animals, whereas 7.4% (592) were in domestic species (compared with 93.3% in wild animals and 6.7% in domestic species in 2001).
• Rabies among sheep and goats increased 400% from 3 cases in 2001 to 15 in 2002.
• The relative contributions of the major groups of animals were as follows: raccoons (36.3%, 2891 cases), skunks (30.5%, 2433), bats (17.2%, 1373), foxes (6.4%, 508), cats (3.8%, 299), dogs (1.2%, 99), and cattle (1.5%, 116).

GEOGRAPHIC DISTRIBUTION
Worldwide distribution

SIGNALMENT
• Different strains of the rabies virus are endemic to a specific host population within a given geographic region. In the United States, for example, raccoons are the primary host species along the eastern seaboard, skunks in the north central and south central states, and the fox in Texas. Various species of bats also carry different strains of the rabies virus.
• The disease can be spread to warm-blooded animals including humans.

Species
Affects all mammals

Breed Predilections
N/A

Mean Age and Range
N/A

Predominant Sex
N/A

SIGNS
• Early clinical signs are nonspecific and highly variable between individuals.
• Two principal manifestations of the disease are generally recognized although an individual can exhibit signs from either form.

Furious Form
• Restlessness with an expression of alertness and anxiety with dilated pupils
• Exaggerated response to auditory or tactile stimuli; affected individual may attack with minimal provocation.
• Animals may charge through stall doors or gates and roam extensively.
• Other signs can include bloat, convulsions, pruritis, pica, or tenesmus.
• Affected animals become progressively ataxic and eventually develop paresis.
• Coma and death follow.

Paralytic or "Dumb" Form
• Initial signs often include anorexia, depression, ataxia, shifting leg lameness, and fever.
• Paralysis of the masseter muscles
• Laryngeal and pharyngeal paralysis
• Cattle may bellow incessantly with altered phonation.
• There is often profuse salivation and inability to swallow.

• There is an abrupt cease of lactation in dairy cattle.
• There may be flaccidity of the tongue, tail, anus, and urinary bladder. Some animals exhibit long periods of tenesmus.
• If able to stand, animals have a wide-base stance. Knuckling of the hind fetlock joints may occur.
• Paresis progresses rapidly to paralysis to all parts of the body.
• Coma and death follow.

CAUSES AND RISK FACTORS
• Penetration of dermis or mucous membranes by virus-laden saliva is most commonly via a bite wound inflicted by an infected animal. The virus then travels to the CNS via peripheral nerves.
• Humans risk exposure by reaching into the mouth of an infected animal looking for a foreign body in the mouth or throat. Foreign body may be suspected due to inability to swallow or hypersalivation.
• Antigenic variations in the rabies virus result in different reservoir species depending on geographic area, although extension to other species is common.

DIAGNOSIS

DIFFERENTIAL DIAGNOSIS
• Behavioral aggression unrelated to disease
• Oral or esophageal foreign body
• Metabolic or digestive disorders: Indigestion, milk fever, nervous ketosis, primary bloat
• Any neurological disease: CNS tumor, encephalitis, spongiform encephalopathies such as scrapie in sheep, bovine spongiform encephalopathy in cattle, or chronic wasting disease in elk and deer.
• *Oestrus ovis* infestations in sheep
• Pseudorabies
• Neurotoxins such as carbamates or organophosphates
• Other viral encephalitis diseases in ruminants include bovine herpesvirus encephalomyelitis, pseudorabies, malignant catarrhal fever, ovine and caprine lentiviral encephalitis, West Nile virus encephalitis, Borna disease, paramyxoviral sporadic bovine encephalomyelitis, and ovine encephalomyelitis (louping-ill).

CBC/BIOCHEMISTRY/URINALYSIS
N/A

OTHER LABORATORY TESTS
CSF may be normal or have increased protein, mononuclear cells, neutrophils, eosinophils, or xanthochromia.

IMAGING
N/A

DIAGNOSTIC PROCEDURES
Immunofluorescence, PCR, complement fixation and agar-gel immunodiffusion can detect antigens of the rabies virus in fresh brain tissue.

PATHOLOGIC FINDINGS

GROSS FINDINGS
No gross findings specific to rabies infection

HISTOPATHOLOGICAL FINDINGS
• Negri bodies, cytoplasmic inclusion bodies containing rabies viral antigen, may be found in the hippocampus, cerebellum, or medulla oblongata using peroxidase-antiperoxidase staining techniques or electron microscopy. These cytoplasmic inclusion bodies are considered diagnostic for rabies but may not be present in up to 30% of cases.
• Diffuse encephalitis with perivascular cuffing and neuronal necrosis. Collections of proliferating glial cells may be found replacing neurons.

TREATMENT
• No effective treatment
• Any animal suspected of being exposed to rabies must be securely quarantined as required by local and state statutes.

MEDICATIONS
N/A

CONTRAINDICATIONS
N/A

FOLLOW-UP

PATIENT MONITORING
• Rabies suspect cases must be securely quarantined in an isolation unit. Feed and water without entering isolation unit if possible.

• Monitor for behavioral, attitude, or clinical signs suggestive of rabies.
• Check local and state regulations on specific requirements.

PREVENTION/AVOIDANCE
• Inactivated vaccines are the only licensed product for prevention of rabies in livestock in the United States. The modified-live vaccines that are available for use in domestic dogs and cats may potentially produce fatal allergic or viral encephalitis when injected in ruminants.
• Due to the extreme public health concerns, state, provincial, and local regulations have been put in place and must be followed completely.
• A few geographic regions of the world including the United Kingdom, Hawaii, Australia, and New Zealand have eradicated or have remained free of the rabies virus because of their island status. These and other such areas have rigorous enforcement of strict quarantine restrictions.
• The Compendium of Animal Rabies Control is compiled and updated annually by the National Association of State Public Health Veterinarians (NASPHV) and summarizes the most current recommendations for the United States and lists all USDA-licensed rabies vaccines.
• Environmental disinfection can be accomplished with household bleach in a 1:32 dilution (4 ounces per gallon).

POSSIBLE COMPLICATIONS
N/A

EXPECTED COURSE AND PROGNOSIS
• Incubation period varies from a few weeks to a year. There have been rare cases with potential incubation of several years. The average incubation period is 2–6 months. Animals bitten near the head have shorter incubation periods than those bitten on an extremity or on the trunk.
• Once clinical signs are exhibited, the disease is invariably fatal. Death occurs within 10 days of the first symptoms.

MISCELLANEOUS

ASSOCIATED CONDITIONS
None

AGE-RELATED FACTORS
N/A

ZOONOTIC POTENTIAL
Extreme risk. Observe strict quarantine of rabies suspect animals.

PREGNANCY
Disease is fatal to infected dam.

SEE ALSO
Encephalitis
Metabolic or digestive disorders (indigestion, milk fever, nervous ketosis, primary bloat)
Neurotoxins such as carbamates or organophosphates
Oestrus ovis infestations in sheep
Oral or esophageal foreign body
Other viral encephalitis diseases in ruminants: bovine herpesvirus encephalomyelitis, pseudorabies, malignant catarrhal fever, ovine and caprine lentiviral encephalitis, West Nile virus encephalitis, Borna disease, paramyxoviral sporadic bovine encephalomyelitis, ovine encephalomyelitis (louping-ill)
Pseudorabies
Spongiform encephalopathies such as scrapie in sheep, bovine spongiform encephalopathy in cattle, or chronic wasting disease in elk and deer

ABBREVIATIONS
CNS = central nervous system
CSF = cerebral spinal fluid
NASPHV = National Association of State Public Health Veterinarians
PCR = polymerase chain reaction
USDA = United States Department of Agriculture

Suggested Reading
Black, E. M., Lowings, J. P., Smith, J., Heaton, P. R., McElhinney, L. M. 2002, Aug. A rapid RT-PCR method to differentiate six established genotypes of rabies and rabies-related viruses using TaqMan technology. *J Virol Methods.* 105(1):25–35.
Callan, R. J., Van Metre, D. C. 2004, Jul. Viral diseases of the ruminant nervous system. *Vet Clin North Am Food Anim Pract.* 20(2):327–62.
Krebs, J. W., Wheeling, J. T., Childs, J. E. 2003, Dec 15. Rabies surveillance in the United States during 2002. *J Am Vet Med Assoc.* 223(12):1736–48.
Tilley, L. P., Smith, F.W. K., eds. 2004. Rabies. In: *The 5-minute veterinary consult—canine and feline.* 3rd ed. Lippincott Williams & Wilkins: Baltimore, MD.
Timoney, J. F., Gillespie, J. H., Scott, F.W., Barlough, J. E. 1992. The rhabdoviridae. In: *Hagan and Bruner's microbiology and infectious diseases of domestic animals.* 8th ed. Ithaca, NY: Comstock Publishing Associates.

Author: Lisa Nashold

RADIATION TOXICITY

BASICS

OVERVIEW
• Possible sources of ionizing radiation that might affect ruminant livestock are thermonuclear explosions, nuclear reactor accidents, fuel reprocessing plant accidents, and bioterrorism acts.
• Grazing livestock could be subjected to beta radiation exposure from ingestion, inhalation, and skin retained radioactive particles.
• Cattle are more sensitive to ingested fallout radiation than other species.
• One study showed that productivity of most livestock surviving an LD50/60 exposure is temporarily reduced and the overall long-term effects are small.
• Radioisotopes of iodine in milk are extremely accumulative and easily passed on.
• In the event of a nuclear accident, the feeding of stored feed or moving livestock to uncontaminated pastures would be the best protective action to follow.
• With any nuclear accident, severe problems of human health would arise prior to any detrimental effects on livestock.

PATHOPHYSIOLOGY
Adapted from RADNET, Center for Biological Monitoring
• ^{85}Kr (Krypton-85, a gas). ^{85}Kr is an inert unreactive gas and does not bioaccumulate in biological pathways. The exposure pathways are external exposure and absorption.
• ^{131}I (Iodine-131) [short-lived (1/2 T = 8 days)] is a biologically significant radionuclide and is very volatile. It is easily accumulated after consuming contaminating forage. Its target organ is the thyroid.
• ^{134}Cs (Cesium, 1/2 T = 2.062 years) and ^{137}Cs (1/2 T = 30.174 years) are among the most biologically significant radionuclides due to their mobility and radiological toxicity. Cesium follows the potassium cycle in nature and its target organ is the entire body.
• ^{89}Sr (Strontium, 1/2 T = 50.55 days) and ^{90}Sr (1/2 T = 28.82 years) follow the calcium cycle in nature and are bone-seeking radionuclides.
• ^{103}Ru (Ruthenium, 1/2 T = 39.8 days) and ^{106}Ru (1/2 T = 1 year) are particularly ubiquitous components of nuclear reactor accidents but also have low radiotoxicity. Their target is the lower large intestine.
• ^{3}H (Tritium, 1/2 T = 12.346 years) is a ubiquitous component of nuclear industries and is a volatile form of radioactive water. Tritium achieves equilibrium in the environment, it becomes tissue bound, and its target is the whole body.
• ^{239}Pu (Plutonium, 1/2 T = 24,131 years) is among the most biologically significant and highly radioactive of all radionuclides. As an alpha emitter, plutonium is particularly hazardous if inhaled either directly from the plume passage or from resuspended ground

deposition activity. Due to its long half-life, ^{239}Pu is the most important radioisotope in the very late stages of a nuclear accident (100 years to 10,000 years). Plutonium is a bone-seeking radionuclide. In its oxide form it is not readily absorbed through the gut; upon aging, it can change its chemical form and become more biologically available in the years after ground deposition.
• ^{99}Tc (Technetium, 1/2 T = 212,000 years) is associated with nuclear fuel reprocessing and fuel reprocessing accidents. It is a very volatile radionuclide and is impossible to filter or control.
• ^{241}Am (Americium, 1/2 T = 432 years) is a decay product of ^{241}Pu (1/2 T = 14.355 years) and intensifies as ^{241}Pu decays. ^{241}Pu is a highly mobile and radiotoxic isotope with high concentration ratios in both freshwater and marine environments.
• ^{238}Pu (Plutonium, 1/2 T = 87.71 years) is the third most common constituent in spent fuel and is one of the most biologically significant radionuclides associated with an accident at a fuel reprocessing facility. ^{238}Pu is the principal component of nuclear-powered satellite accidents.

SYSTEMS AFFECTED
Potentially all, depending on the type of radiation absorbed.

GENETICS
N/A

INCIDENCE/PREVALENCE
N/A

GEOGRAPHIC DISTRIBUTION
Worldwide depending on species and environment

SIGNALMENT
Species
Potentially all ruminant species
Breed Predilections
N/A
Mean Age and Range
N/A
Predominant Sex
N/A

SIGNS

HISTORICAL FINDINGS
• Clinical signs of radiation toxicity are dependent upon species variations (e.g., marked delayed reaction of the acute hematologic response in cows).
Species-specific number of hemopoietic stem cells may explain the morbidity and mortality differences between species after high doses of irradiation.
• Mortality due to acute radiation syndrome varies by species.
• Cattle commonly develop cataracts later in the disease process.
• Radiation sources can include radiation exposure accidents, nuclear weapon detonations, and bioterrorism acts perpetrated upon livestock.

PHYSICAL EXAMINATION FINDINGS

CAUSES AND RISK FACTORS
There are four pathways of exposure to contamination secondary to nuclear accidents of any kind:
• Inhalation: plume inhalation and resuspended ground deposition inhalation can occur in grazing livestock
• External exposure: facility radiation shine, plume cloud shine, and ground shine
• Dermal absorption
• Ingestion: ingestion from foliar/forage and surface contamination and the ingestion of contamination via indirect pathways (e.g., the incorporation of contaminated plant materials into processed feedstuffs and distribution to distant areas unaffected by original deposition/fallout/plume).
• Other associated pathways can include:
  • Chronic gaseous emissions
  • Gaseous reactor plume pulse discharges
  • Liquid discharges
  • Specific nuclear accidents
  • Chronic hot particle contamination
  • Liquid emissions
  • Airborne particulates

DIAGNOSIS

DIFFERENTIAL DIAGNOSIS
N/A

CBC/BIOCHEMISTRY/URINALYSIS
• Acute hematologic response in cows
• CBC is generally grossly affected in severe accidents.

OTHER LABORATORY TESTS
Radioisotopes of iodine in milk

IMAGING

OTHER DIAGNOSTIC PROCEDURES
• The Federal Emergency Management Agency (FEMA) has a surface contamination guideline of "300 counts per minute above background" for authorized persons entering an emergency operations center (EOC) during an accident at an NRC-licensed nuclear facility. Three hundred counts per minute (300 cpi) equals 660 pCi (Picocurie) per person; it can be assumed that each authorized person has an absolute minimum of 1 square meter of surface area.
• Microcuries/square meter limits are set in humans.
• No guidelines have been set for livestock.
• The 1982 U.S. Department of Health and Human Services emergency protection action guideline (PAG) is nuclide specific and includes the initial ground deposition action guidelines for humans affected by fallout.
• Other readings include:
  • Picocuries (1 microcurie = 1,000,000 picocuries)
  • Counts per minute (1 count/minute = 2.2 picocuries/minute.)

PATHOLOGIC FINDINGS

TREATMENT
• There is no specific therapy for the acute radiation syndrome.
• For severely exposed animals, euthanasia and disposal concerns must be addressed. This is especially disconcerting in the case of a mass mortality event. Contact the state/provincial Environmental Protection Agency for disposal requirements.
• For high-dose injury, no methods have been developed to reverse the fibrosing endarteritis that eventually leads to tissue death.
• The accidental fuel element meltdown at Chernobyl, USSR, resulted in many cases of acute radiation syndrome. More than 100,000 people were exposed to high levels of radioactive fallout. The radiation plume had an incredible effect on livestock in the plume fallout zone worldwide.

MEDICATIONS
CONTRAINDICATIONS
• Milk and meat must not be consumed from exposed food-producing animals.
• Do not feed contaminated feed to livestock.
PRECAUTIONS
N/A
POSSIBLE INTERACTIONS
N/A
ALTERNATIVE DRUGS

FOLLOW-UP
PATIENT MONITORING
PREVENTION/AVOIDANCE
• Avoid using surface water supplies and rainwater for livestock.
• All subsurface water sources and most public drinking water sources are relatively safe after most types of nuclear accidents.
• Humans and animals should avoid consuming foods/feed subject to rapid secondary pathway contamination (e.g., forage ⟶ cow /sheep/goat ⟶ milk/cheese pathway ⟶ human). Use animal feed produced and/or packaged prior to plume passage.
• Shelter livestock from plume damage; use uncontaminated feeds.
• Avoid exposure to surface ground contamination by keeping livestock indoors as much as possible.
• Avoid exposure of animals to contaminated surface water (puddles and rain).
• Avoid tracking in ground deposition to animal facilities: remove contaminated clothing and footwear prior to entering barns and animal housing.

• Avoid feeding contaminated hays from surface deposition (especially leafy pasture plants with foliar contamination).
• Postnuclear accident, if animals have avoided inhalation of the passing plume and if they can avoid extensive exposure to ground deposition, the livestock's principal pathway of exposure will be the ingestion pathway.
POSSIBLE COMPLICATIONS
N/A
EXPECTED COURSE AND PROGNOSIS
Severity of biological response depends upon target organ dose, dose rate, and dose fractionation.

MISCELLANEOUS
ASSOCIATED CONDITIONS
Following the Chernobyl nuclear accident, sheep and cattle in Wales, England, and Scotland became contaminated with radionuclides (primarily 134Cs and 131I). The maximum levels of contamination were of the order of 4000 Bq/kg of cesium-137 and 2000 Bq/kg of cesium-134 in muscle and 2,000,000 Bq/kg of iodine-131 in the thyroid gland. Bq/kg corresponds to the limit of detection of a Becquerel per unit mass or the decrease of one radioactive atom per second in one kilogram of material (used for samples of animal or vegetal origin).
AGE-RELATED FACTORS
N/A
ZOONOTIC POTENTIAL
• Sources of ionizing radiation that could contribute to radioactivity in the food chain to humans are reactor accidents, fuel reprocessing plant accidents, and thermonuclear explosions.
• Avoid consuming foods subject to rapid ingestion pathway contamination (e.g., forage ⟶ cow /sheep/goat ⟶ milk/cheese pathway ⟶ human).
• With any nuclear accident, severe problems of human health would arise before any detrimental effects on livestock could be detected.
PREGNANCY
N/A
RUMINANT SPECIES AFFECTED
Potentially, all ruminant species can be affected.
BIOSECURITY
The types of accidents and the principal radionuclides:
• Nuclear reactors (I-131; Cs-134 + Cs-137; Ru-103 + Ru-106)
• Nuclear waste storage facilities (Sr-90; Cs-137; Pu-239 + Am-241)
• Nuclear fuel reprocessing plants (Sr-90; Cs-137; Pu-239 + Am-241)
• Nuclear weapons (i.e., dispersal of nuclear material without nuclear detonation) (Pu-239) and radioisotope thermoelectric

generators (RTGs) and radioisotope heater units (RHUs).
PRODUCTION MANAGEMENT
• Precautionary actions include moving animals to protective shelter, covering potentially exposed feed products, corralling livestock and isolation from the radioactive plume, and providing protected feed and water.
• The blending of contaminated livestock feed with uncontaminated feed is illegal because this is a violation of the Federal Food, Drug and Cosmetic Act (FDA 1991).
SYNONYMS
Nuclear fallout
SEE ALSO
Animal welfare
Euthanasia and disposal
Toxicologic herd outbreak
ABBREVIATIONS
EOC = emergency operations center
FDA = Food and Drug Administration
FEMA = Federal Emergency Management Agency
LD = lethal dose
NRC = National Research Counsel
PAG = U.S. Department of Health and Human Services emergency protection action guideline
RHU = radioisotope heater units
RTG = radioisotope thermoelectric generators

Suggested Reading
Anno, G. H., Young, R. W., Bloom, R. M., Mercier, J. R. 2003, May. Dose response relationships for acute ionizing-radiation lethality. *Health Phys.* 84(5):565–75.
Bell, M. C. 1985, Jun. Radiation effects on livestock: physiological effects, dose response. *Vet Hum Toxicol.* 27(3):200–207.
Brown, D. G., Reynolds, R. A., Johnson, D. F. 1966, Nov. Late effects in cattle exposed to radioactive fallout. *Am J Vet Res.* 27(121):1509–14.
RADNET: Nuclear Information Website. Available online at: http://www.davistownmuseum.org/cbm/. Accessed April 18, 2008.
Saenger, E. L. 1986, Sep. Radiation accidents. *Ann Emerg Med.* 15(9):1061–66.
Sansom, B. F. 1989, May–Jun. An assessment of the risks to the health of grazing animals from the radioactive contamination of pastures. *Br Vet J.* 145(3):206–11.
U. S. Food and Drug Administration, Center for Devices and Radiological Health. 1997, Mar 5. *Accidental radioactive contamination of human food and animal feeds: recommendations for state and local agencies.* Washington, DC: FDA.
von Zallinger, C., Tempel, K. 1998, Nov–Dec. The physiologic response of domestic animals to ionizing radiation: a review. *Vet Radiol Ultrasound.* 39(6):495–503.

Author: Scott R. R. Haskell

RECTAL PROLAPSE

 BASICS

DEFINITION
Prolapse or eversion of the rectal mucosa through the anus.

PATHOPHYSIOLOGY
• Increase in pressure gradient between pelvic or abdominal cavity and the anus
• Mucosa of rectum bulges through anal sphincter.
• Environmental exposure may cause secondary irritation and straining.

SYSTEMS AFFECTED
Digestive

GENETICS
May be related to congenital sphincter tone problems

INCIDENCE/PREVALENCE
0.1%–1.5% within a population

GEOGRAPHIC DISTRIBUTION
N/A

SIGNALMENT
Species
Cattle, sheep

Breed Predilections
N/A

Mean Age and Range
Cattle 6–24 months
Sheep 6–12 months

Predominant Sex
N/A

SIGNS
Four categories described;
1. Mucosal prolapse
2. Complete prolapse
3. Complete prolapse with invagination of colon
4. Intussusception of rectum or colon through anus

HISTORICAL FINDINGS
May be predisposed by a number of conditions such as:
• Increased abdominal fill
• Tenesmus
• Coughing
• Feed changes

PHYSICAL EXAMINATION FINDINGS
N/A

CAUSES
N/A

RISK FACTORS
• Increased abdominal fill
  • Multiple fetuses
  • Overly fat
  • Bloat
• Tenesmus
  • Enteritis or colitis
  • Diarrhea
  • Parasitism
  • Urinary obstruction
  • Dystocia
  • Vaginal or uterine prolapse
  • Breeding injury
• Coughing
• Decreased perirectal anal tone (congenital or acquired)
• Use of growth implants
• Feed changes
• Short tail docking
• Growth promotant implants

 DIAGNOSIS

DIFFERENTIAL DIAGNOSIS
N/A

CBC/BIOCHEMISTRY/URINALYSIS
N/A

OTHER LABORATORY TESTS
N/A

IMAGING
N/A

DIAGNOSTIC PROCEDURES
N/A

PATHOLOGIC FINDINGS
N/A

 TREATMENT

APPROPRIATE HEALTH CARE
• Identify and eliminate predisposing factors if possible.
• Administer caudal epidural.
• Clean prolapse with warm water and soap.
• Evaluate tissue for necrosis and trauma.
• Reduce prolapse by manual manipulation.
• Circumferential purse string sutures using umbilical tape are placed around anus.
• Sutures can be preplaced if straining is occurring.
• Sutures are removed in 3–4 days.

NURSING CARE

ACTIVITY
N/A

DIET
N/A

CLIENT EDUCATION
Animal's value should be discussed when deciding on treatment options.

SURGICAL CONSIDERATIONS
• Severely traumatized or necrotic rectal tissue may necessitate amputation.
• Commercial prolapse rings or open-ended tube (PVC pipe) is inserted into the rectum.
• Elastrator band can be placed over rectal tissue anterior of damaged tissue.
• Ring and necrotic tissue will slough in 1–2 weeks.
• Surgical amputation or submucosal resection is also an option.

MEDICATIONS

DRUGS OF CHOICE
• Broad-spectrum antibiotic therapy might be considered if tissue necrosis is severe.
• Drug withdrawal periods must be determined and maintained.
• Topical agents such as 50% dextrose and lubricating gel may aid in reduction of prolapse.

CONTRAINDICATIONS
Appropriate milk and meat withdrawal times must be followed for all compounds administered to food-producing animals.

PRECAUTIONS
N/A

POSSIBLE INTERACTIONS
N/A

ALTERNATIVE DRUGS
Sedation may assist in reducing tenesmus.

FOLLOW-UP

PATIENT MONITORING
Remove purse-string sutures in 3–4 days.

PREVENTION/AVOIDANCE
Difficult to prevent; eliminate potential risk factors if possible.

POSSIBLE COMPLICATIONS
• Severe straining may cause prolapse to reoccur.
• Inappropriately placed sutures may cause cellulitis.

• Premature sloughing of prolapse ring may result in severe peritonitis or evisceration.

EXPECTED COURSE AND PROGNOSIS
• Prognosis is guarded.
• Tendency for prolapses to reoccur unless predisposing factors are eliminated.

MISCELLANEOUS

ASSOCIATED CONDITIONS
• Enteritis
• Vaginal or uterine prolapse
• Bloat
• Urolithiasis

AGE-RELATED FACTORS
N/A

ZOONOTIC POTENTIAL
N/A

PREGNANCY
May be more common in animals carrying multiple fetuses or very large fetus

RUMINANT SPECIES AFFECTED
Cattle, sheep

BIOSECURITY
N/A

PRODUCTION MANAGEMENT
Market value and intended use of animal will determine treatment options.

SYNONYMS
N/A

SEE ALSO
Vaginal prolapse

ABBREVIATIONS
PVC = polyvinyl chloride

Suggested Reading
Halland, S. K. 2002. Rectal prolapse in ruminants and horses. In: *Large animal internal medicine*, ed. B. P. Smith. 3rd ed. St. Louis: Mosby.
Welker, B., Modransky, P. 1991. Rectal prolapse in food animals. Part 1. Cause and conservative management. *Comp Cont Ed Pract Vet*. 13: 1869–73.
Welker, B., Modransky, P. 1992. Rectal prolapse in food animals. Part 2. Surgical options. *Comp Cont Ed Pract Vet*. 14: 554–59.

Author: John R. Campbell

REHYDRATION THERAPY: ORAL

BASICS

OVERVIEW
• Numerous diseases result in dehydration, electrolyte, and acid/base abnormalities.
• Correction of these deficits can greatly influence the clinical outcome of these diseases.
• In small animals and equines, intravenous (IV) fluid therapy is most commonly used. In many instances, intravenous fluid therapy in ruminants is not practical or possible.
  • The size of the animal, lack of proper restraint facilities, time requirements, and owner compliance all limit the use of IV fluids.
  • Another major limitation to the use of IV fluids in ruminants is expense versus the value of the animal.
• Oral fluid and electrolyte therapy is a valuable alternative to IV fluid therapy in situations where IV fluid therapy is not practical or possible.
  • Oral fluid therapy can be administered quickly and inexpensively in most cases.
  • Oral fluid therapy is very effective when used appropriately.
  • Oral fluid therapy is the preferred method of treatment for most diarrheic calves.
  • Oral fluid therapy is inappropriate in some cases because it will not adequately correct some severe imbalances.
• Oral fluid therapy can be used in conjunction with IV fluids in many cases. Combining oral and IV fluids may help overcome the limitations of both methods used alone.
• Oral fluid therapy is most commonly used in neonatal calves and adult cattle, but it can be used effectively in other ruminant species as well.

PATHOPHYSIOLOGY
• The most common cause of dehydration in neonatal calves is diarrhea often accompanied by metabolic acidosis.
  • This diarrhea may be hypersecretory, malabsorptive, and/or osmotic depending on the cause.
  • Some organisms release toxins that cause a hypersecretory diarrhea.
  • Some organisms directly damage the villous lining of the intestinal tract causing a malabsorptive diarrhea.

• Increased passage of undigested nutrients into the colon promotes bacterial fermentation and results in an osmotic diarrhea.
  • Metabolic acidosis occurs in diarrheic calves due to increased loss of bicarbonate in the feces.
• Dehydration in adult cattle can result from numerous disease processes.
  • The pathophysiology of the dehydration varies depending on the disease process involved, but it usually includes decreased fluid intake, increased fluid loss through diarrhea, or sequestration of fluid within the gastrointestinal (GI) tract.
  • Unlike neonates, adult cattle dehydration is often accompanied by alkalosis rather than acidosis.
• Diseases causing dehydration in other ruminant species are similar to those of cattle. Pregnancy toxemia in small ruminants and heat stroke in camelids often requires fluid therapy to support the fluid and nutritional needs of the animal.

SYSTEMS AFFECTED
• Diseases resulting in dehydration and electrolyte imbalances in ruminants most commonly affect the GI tract, pleural/peritoneal space, mammary gland, or reproductive system.
• The resulting dehydration and electrolyte abnormalities affect virtually all systems within the body to some degree.

GENETICS
N/A

INCIDENCE/PREVALENCE
N/A

GEOGRAPHIC DISTRIBUTION
N/A

SIGNALMENT
Diseases causing dehydration and electrolyte abnormalities may affect all neonatal calves, adult cattle, sheep, goats, and camelids.

SIGNS
• Signs of dehydration include enophthalmia, decreased skin elasticity, tachycardia, dry or tacky mucous membranes, and cold extremities.
• Signs of acidosis in neonatal calves include depression, recumbency (sternal progressing to lateral), weakness, and loss of a suckle reflex.

CAUSES
Neonatal Calves
• *E. coli*
• Rotavirus
• Coronavirus
• Salmonellosis
• Cryptosporidiosis
• Overconsumption of milk
• Poor quality milk replacers

Adult Cattle
• Gastrointestinal disease
  • Abomasal displacement/volvulus
  • Intussusception
  • Mesenteric volvulus
  • Vagal indigestion
  • Salmonellosis
  • Clinical parasitism
• Carbohydrate engorgement (grain overload)
• Peritonitis/pleuritis (hardware disease)
• Toxic mastitis
• Toxic metritis
• Fatty liver: ketosis

Small Ruminants
• Gastrointestinal disease: Clinical parasitism; intestinal accidents
• Pregnancy toxemia
• Heat stroke (camelids)

RISK FACTORS
• Failure of passive transfer is the major risk factor for the development of diarrhea in neonatal calves.
• Thin or excessive body condition in late pregnancy is a risk factor for the development of pregnancy toxemia in small ruminants.

DIAGNOSIS

DIFFERENTIAL DIAGNOSIS
N/A

CBC/BIOCHEMISTRY/URINALYSIS
May be helpful to monitor hydration and acid/base balance

OTHER LABORATORY TESTS
N/A

IMAGING
N/A

DIAGNOSTIC PROCEDURES

Dehydration is usually assessed by evaluation of several clinical features including skin tent, degree of enophthalmia, cold extremities, cold interior of mouth, heart rate, pulse character, etc.

• *Measurements of packed cell volume (PCV) and total plasma protein (TP) are useful for assessing the response to fluid therapy.*
  • Unless these values are markedly abnormal, the usefulness of a single measurement is questionable due to the large variability in the normal values for these parameters.
  • Changes in these values in response to fluid therapy are useful for assessing the response to therapy.
• *Several methodologies for estimating the degree of dehydration based on clinical findings are available.*
  • Following is one example:
  6–7% dehydration—slight enophthalmia, slightly increased skin turgor, moist mucous membranes
  8–9% dehydration—eyes obviously sunken, obviously increased skin turgor, tacky mucous membranes
  10–12% dehydration—eyes deeply sunken in orbits, skin tents and does not return, dry mucous membranes, obvious depression
  • The accuracy of these estimates is questionable and exact estimation of the degree of dehydration is not critical.
  • Making an estimate of dehydration and then carefully monitoring the response to therapy is more important and more accurate than trying to pinpoint the exact degree of dehydration.
  • One of the most important decisions to make is the decision to use oral or IV fluids.

  1. Calves that are estimated to be greater than 8% dehydrated (marked enophthalmia, prolonged skin tent, dry mucous membranes, and moderate to severe depression) should be treated with IV fluids.
  2. Calves that are less than 8% dehydrated can usually be treated with oral fluids.
• *Acid/base status is best evaluated by blood gas analysis. The amount of base needed to correct the acidosis can be determined using the base deficit (BD) and the following equation:*

$$BD \times 0.6 \times \text{Body weight in kilograms} = \text{base requirement in milliequivalents (mEq)}$$

0.6 is a correction factor for the "bicarbonate space" in a neonate. For an adult, 0.3 is the appropriate factor.
• *If blood gas analysis is not available, the degree of acidosis may be estimated using clinical evaluation of the patient.*
  • Calves
  • Calves that are significantly acidotic exhibit depression, weakness (which may range from difficulty standing to complete lateral recumbency), and loss of a suckle reflex.
  Several methodologies for clinical assessment of acidosis have been published. Following is one example:
  1. Calves less than one week old with a depression score of mild, moderate, or severe have an estimated base deficit of 6, 9, and 12 mEq, respectively.
  2. Calves older than one week of age with a depression score of mild, moderate, or severe have an estimated base deficit of 9, 12, and 15 mEq, respectively.

  3. This estimated BD can then be used in the equation given above to estimate the total mEq of base needed.
  Another, simpler, rule of thumb is that calves showing clinical depression due to acidosis usually have a BD of 10–15 mEq with older calves tending to be more acidotic.
  1. Important factors to consider include the severity of clinical signs and the age of the calf.
  2. Calves older than a week of age tend to be more acidotic than a younger calf exhibiting similar clinical signs.
  3. Calves that have lost the ability to stand and lost a suckle reflex should be treated with IV fluids. Oral fluid therapy will most likely not be sufficient in these calves.
• Adult Animals
Similar estimates of dehydration can be used for adult animals.
  1. Adult cattle are alkalotic more often than acidotic and it is usually not necessary to directly correct the alkalosis.
  2. Grain overload is a common condition that results in acidosis.
  3. Correcting the dehydration will allow the kidneys to correct the alkalosis.

PATHOLOGIC FINDINGS
N/A

TREATMENT

APPROPRIATE HEALTH CARE
Fluid therapy for ruminants must often be administered in the field but hospitalization, if possible, will facilitate fluid administration and assessment of response to therapy.

REHYDRATION THERAPY: ORAL

NURSING CARE

Sick calves should be kept in a warm, draft-free environment to reduce increased metabolic demands caused by cold stress.

ACTIVITY

One of the advantages of oral fluid therapy over IV therapy is that the animal does not have to be restrained for prolonged periods of time.

DIET

Calves with severe diarrhea should be taken off of milk for a short period of time because impaired absorption of nutrients may exacerbate the diarrhea when they reach the colon.

CLIENT EDUCATION

• Oral electrolyte therapy can be administered via a nipple bottle or via an esophageal feeder. If clients are going to be responsible for administering oral fluids, they must be properly trained to use an esophageal feeder.
• Oral fluids can be administered to adult ruminants via orogastric intubation, nasogastric intubation, or commercially available cattle fluid pump systems.

SURGICAL CONSIDERATIONS

N/A

MEDICATIONS

DRUGS OF CHOICE

Calves
• Numerous oral electrolyte preparations are commercially available.
• Many of these preparations contain an alkalinizing agent.
  • Bicarbonate is the most common.
  • Other metabolizable bases include lactate, acetate, and citrate.

• Inclusion of glycine and/or glucose will increase the intestinal absorption of sodium ions through cotransporters on intestinal epithelial cells. Inclusion of glutamate does not appear to be beneficial.
• Some of these preparations contain higher amounts of glucose and are described as "high-energy" supplements.
  • These products should be used if the calf is in poor body condition or is going to be held off of milk for several days.
  • These products supply about one-half of the energy content of whole milk.
• Maintenance fluid requirements are about 50 mls/kg/day. Ongoing losses must be considered and may range from 1 to 6 liters in calves with diarrhea. Oral fluids may be administered twice daily or up to several times daily.

Adults
• Mixing feed-grade salts in water may make oral fluids/electrolytes for adult ruminants.
• Following is one common formulation:
  140 grams sodium chloride
  30 grams potassium chloride
  10 grams calcium chloride
  Mixed in 20 liters of water
• It is usually not necessary to directly correct the alkalosis.
• If acidosis is present, bicarbonate can be supplied by estimating the BD (usually 5–8 mEq/kg) and mixing bicarbonate (baking soda) in water. If acidosis is severe, IV fluid therapy may be necessary.

Other
• Oral fluid and IV fluid may be used in conjunction in some cases, especially in adults.
  • Giving 10–20 liters IV and the rest of the deficit orally is an alternative when the expense of IV fluids is a concern.

• Rapid volume expansion with IV fluids may improve perfusion of the gut and increase absorption of oral fluids/electrolytes.
• Once dehydration has been corrected in calves with IV fluids, oral fluids can be used to provide maintenance needs.
• Transfaunation is the administration of rumen fluid from a healthy ruminant to one whose rumen environment has been altered.
  • Providing a healthy population of rumen microbes will often improve appetite and feed consumption.
  • Pelleted feed soaked in warm water can also be included to improve the rumen environment and provide some energy.
• Hypertonic (7.2%) saline can be used in conjunction with oral fluid therapy.
  • Hypertonic saline administered at 4 mls/kg IV over 3–5 minutes followed immediately by oral fluid therapy may increase absorption of orally administered fluids.
  • Hypertonic saline increases the osmolality of the plasma resulting in volume expansion by pulling water into the vascular space.
  Note: Hypertonic saline must be combined with oral fluids or the dehydration will become worse.

CONTRAINDICATIONS

N/A

PRECAUTIONS

The response to therapy should be monitored so that necessary adjustments can be made.

POSSIBLE INTERACTIONS

• Bicarbonate-containing solutions should not be fed to calves that are still consuming milk because the bicarbonate will interfere with the formation of the milk clot in the abomasum, which may result in osmotic diarrhea by increasing the nutrients that reach the colon.

  • Combining milk replacer with bicarbonate-containing solutions is safe because these products do not normally clot in the abomasum.

  • If calves are consuming milk and need oral electrolytes, an electrolyte product containing acetate as a metabolizable base can be used. The acetate is an effective alkalinizing agent but it will not interfere with the formation of the milk clot in the abomasum.

• Bicarbonate should not be mixed with solutions containing calcium because an insoluble precipitate will form.

ALTERNATIVE DRUGS

Antibiotics may be indicated depending on the concurrent disease processes.

FOLLOW-UP

PATIENT MONITORING

Diarrheic calves should respond to therapy within 24 hours. If depression remains, acidosis may still be present.

PREVENTION/AVOIDANCE

Ensuring adequate colostrum intake is the best way to minimize neonatal calf diarrhea.

POSSIBLE COMPLICATIONS

Complications are rare with appropriately applied oral fluid therapy but overhydration may result in increased central venous pressure and pulmonary edema.

EXPECTED COURSE AND PROGNOSIS

N/A

MISCELLANEOUS

ASSOCIATED CONDITIONS

N/A

AGE-RELATED FACTORS

N/A

ZOONOTIC POTENTIAL

N/A

PREGNANCY

N/A

RUMINANT SPECIES AFFECTED

Cattle, sheep, goats, camelids

BIOSECURITY

N/A

PRODUCTION MANAGEMENT

N/A

SYNONYMS

N/A

SEE ALSO

Fluid therapy
Grain overload
Neonatal calf diarrhea
Transfaunation
Vagal indigestion

ABBREVIATIONS

BD = base deficit
GI = gastrointestinal
IV = intravenous
mEq = milliequivalent
mls/kg/day = milliliters per kilogram body weight per day
PCV = packed cell volume
TP = total plasma protein

Suggested Reading
Howard, J. L., Smith, R. A. 1999. *Current veterinary therapy 4: food animal practice.* Philadelphia: W. B. Saunders.
Radostits, O. M., Blood, D. C., Gay, C. C. 1997. *Veterinary medicine.* 8th ed. London: W. B. Saunders.
Roussel, A. J., Constable, P. D. 1999, Nov. Fluid and electrolyte therapy. In: *Veterinary clinics of North America food animal practice.*
Smith, B. P. 2002. *Large animal internal medicine.* 3rd ed. St. Louis: Mosby.

Author: John Gilliam

REINDEER MANAGEMENT: OVERVIEW

 BASICS

OVERVIEW
• Historically, more than 25 indigenous ethnic groups residing in the Eurasian circumpolar regions have participated in reindeer herding.
• Currently, the reindeer industry is a primary focus of the Koryak, Chukchi, Komi, Nenet, Yakut, Enets, Even, Evenk, Nganasan, Dolgan, and Sámi (see map at http://miljo. npolar.no/temakart/pages/homeE.asp/).
• There are approximately 1.5 million domesticated reindeer in Russia, 200,000 in Finland, 250,000 in Sweden, and 200,000 in Norway.
• Although less than 1% of the total meat consumed in Fennoscandia is reindeer, its production is a vital source of income to remote regions of this subarctic region.
• Although difficult to quantify, reindeer herding has important cultural value. Reindeer, aside from being an important source of food and revenue, typically play a central role in the traditions of the circumpolar indigenous herding groups.
• These cultures are of the few remaining indigenous cultures that have maintained their ability to live traditional lifestyles.

SYSTEMS AFFECTED
Production management

GENETICS
N/A

INCIDENCE/PREVALENCE
N/A

GEOGRAPHIC DISTRIBUTION
Russia, Finland, Sweden, Norway, Greenland, Canada, and Alaska

SIGNALMENT
Species
• *Rangifer tarandus* is a circumpolar species consisting of seven subspecies formed through the isolation of populations during the ice age.
• Peary caribou (*R.t. pearyi*) and Svalbard reindeer (*R.t. platyrhyncus*) inhabit the high Arctic.
• Alaskan caribou (*R.t. granti*), barren ground caribou (*R.t. groenlandicus*), and Eurasian reindeer (*R.t. tarandus*) inhabit the taiga,

woodland caribou (*R.t. caribou*) and woodland reindeer (*R.t. fennicus*) inhabit the Boreal forests.
• *Rangifer tarandus* are polygamous and highly sexual dimorphic with males being approximately twice the size of females.
• North American caribou have been utilized only through hunting.
• Eurasian reindeer were originally domesticated by indigenous people.
• Domesticated reindeer are highly gregarious and form large herds, particularly during migration and periods of insect harassment.

Breed Predilections
• Eurasian reindeer are smaller than caribou.
• Females reach maximum size at the age of 4–5 years, and senescence starts at the age of 7–8 years.
• Herders selectively remove old individuals.
• A single calf is typically produced every year. Calves are born in April-June, depending on the nutritional status of the female.
• Females in poor nutritional status delay calving.
• Birth weight is ~5 kg, males being 0.5 kg larger than females. Birth weight is positively associated with neonatal survival.
• Weaning ends in September/October (i.e., when the rut starts), but the calf may follow its mother for a year, but rarely longer.
• Calves following their mothers have easier access to food and are more likely to survive the winter.
• Male calves have higher mortality rates and are less likely to follow their mothers during the winter.

Mean Age and Range
N/A

Predominant Sex
• Females are ~60 kg and males 120 kg at their prime, although body weights vary markedly depending on range conditions
• Age of maturity is 1–3 years in females and 2–5 years in males. Poor nutritional conditions during early development may delay maturity. Conversely, exceptional conditions may result in early maturity (age 1) for females, and this premature reproduction effort can permanently stunt somatic growth.

• Females reach maximum size at the age of 4–5 years, and senescence starts at the age of 7–8 years.
• Herders selectively remove old individuals.

 TREATMENT

DIET
• The most important food during winter is lichen (*Cladina* spp.).
• During summer, the diet is more variable, and includes vascular plants, grasses (graminoids), herbs, shrubs such as willow (salicaceae), and heathlike shrubs (ericoids) and trees.
• Inadequate harvesting and subsequent populations exceeding range-carrying capacity have led to degradation of the winter pastures in many areas.
• Many reindeer are thus fed with hay and commercial feed pellets during winter. This is particularly the case in Finland where the European Union subsidizes production of hay.

 MISCELLANEOUS

Herding Systems
• Reindeer management has been exported in more recent times from Fennoscandia and Siberia to other regions and cultures including the Inuit in Alaska and the Greenland Eskimos.
• The most intensive and modernized management of domesticated reindeer is found among the Sámi people in Fennoscandia. There, herding is a cooperative operation based on year-round free range with seasonally defined ranges and migration routes, intensive use of mechanical transportation for herding (motorcycles, snow machines, helicopters), and supplemental feeding during poor range conditions.
• Reindeer are generally individually owned in most regions of Fennoscandia, but reindeer cooperatives with joint ownership are common in Finland, southern Norway, and most of Siberia.
• Reindeer husbandry requires access to extensive land areas and utilizes 35% of the land area in Finland and Sweden, and 40% in Norway.

- Management is organized into herding districts, with defined ranges and migration routes, carrying capacities, and governmental oversight.
- Coastal regions, with their moister climates, nutrient-rich graze, and lower intensity of flying, biting insects are used for summer range, while drier continental climates with dense lichen beds, and less snow and stable cold conditions during the winter months are used for winter range.
- Governmental restrictions regarding crossing geopolitical boundaries have tended to break up traditional, ecologically determined migration patterns and seasonal ranges.
- Historically, reindeer herders in Russia, Finland, Sweden, and Norway migrated freely over the national borders.
- During the nineteenth century, the Russian and Finnish borders were closed, and today severe restrictions exist on the movement of reindeer between pastures in Norway and Sweden. This has led to reduced availability of appropriate summer and winter pastures.
- Many Norwegian reindeer herds are forced to survive on winter pastures along the coast where heavy snowfall and icing prevent efficient foraging. This has been remedied to some extent by supplemental feeding during some of the winter months.
- Conversely, Finnish and Swedish reindeer lack access to nutrient-rich pastures along the coast during the summer and experience a very high burden of flying parasites such as nasal bot flies (*Cephenomyia trompe* Modeer) and warble fly (*Hypoderma tarandi* L.).

Economic Considerations

- An economic infrastructure developed around the reindeer industry early in the twentieth century when there was a shift toward a cash economy based on meat production.
- Historically, reindeer were utilized for clothing, milk production, transportation (sled and draft animals), and meat production.
- Today, meat production is the primary goal in reindeer husbandry and has become quite lucrative. Reindeer meat is considered a delicacy and an organically, free-range-raised meat, and commands a high price in European markets.

- The meat is not widely marketed in the United States or the rest of the world.
- More recently, with incorporation of modern technology into the husbandry techniques, it became necessary to produce adequate revenue to support the increased mechanization (e.g., snow machines, modern dwellings).
- The amount of time domesticated reindeer are in close contact with humans varies greatly among different management practices from only a few times a year when the calves are marked in the summer or early fall, and in the fall when animals are slaughtered, to almost year-round, with some periods of round-the-clock surveillance.
- Herders follow the reindeer on the migration from winter pastures in continental areas to summer pastures along the coast.
- Calves are marked to signal ownership by cutting away small parts of the ear (see http://213.161.163.54/merker/hoved.aspx) in complex patterns of markings. These marks are passed down from generation to generation.
- Families, or family groups, often share pastures and herd their reindeer together in cooperative style management operations.

Predation

- Wolverine (*Gulo gulo*), lynx (*Lynx lynx*), and golden eagle (*Aquila chrysaetos*) are important predators on reindeer.
- In some regions, bears can be significant predators.
- Wolf (*Canis lupus*) may be an important predator, but has effectively been removed by humans from most reindeer-herding areas.
- Red fox (*Vulpes vulpes*) may be an important predator on neonates.
- Neonates are particularly vulnerable to predators.
- Food limitation increases risk of predation.

ASSOCIATED CONDITIONS
N/A

AGE-RELATED FACTORS
N/A

ZOONOTIC POTENTIAL
Several reindeer diseases are zoonotic. Care must be taken in the collection of laboratory samples and the diagnosis/treatment of affected animals.

PREGNANCY
N/A

RUMINANT SPECIES AFFECTED
Rangifer spp.

BIOSECURITY
- Isolation and quarantine of new stock entering the herd.
- Treat and or cull new animals for disease conditions prior to herd introduction.

PRODUCTION MANAGEMENT
See Economic Considerations and Herding Systems above

SYNONYMS
N/A

SEE ALSO
Cervidae sections
Reindeer diseases

ABBREVIATIONS
N/A

Suggested Reading

Barboza, P. S., Hartbauer, D. W., Hauer, W. E., Blake, J. E. 2004, May. Polygynous mating impairs body condition and homeostasis in male reindeer (*Rangifer tarandus tarandus*). *J Comp Physiol [B]*. 174(4): 309–17. Epub 2004, Feb 18.

Gjostein, H., Holand, O., Weladji, R. B. 2004, Apr. Milk production and composition in reindeer (*Rangifer tarandus*): effect of lactational stage. *Comp Biochem Physiol A Mol Integr Physiol*. 137(4): 649–56.

Jentoft, S., ed. 1998. *Commons in a cold climate. Coastal fisheries and reindeer pastoralism in north Norway: the co-management approach*. Paris: UNESCO.

Moen, J., Danell, O. 2003, Sep. Reindeer in the Swedish mountains: an assessment of grazing impacts. *Ambio* 32(6): 397–402.

Proceedings of the human role in reindeer/caribou systems workshop. 2000. *Polar Research* 19:1.

Weladji, R. B., Holand, O. 2003, Jul. Global climate change and reindeer: effects of winter weather on the autumn weight and growth of calves. *Oecologia* 136(2): 317–23. Epub 2003, Apr 18.

Authors: Torkild Tveraa and Andrew J. Karter

REINDEER MANAGEMENT: POPULATION DYNAMICS

BASICS

OVERVIEW
• High-density herds (populations exceeding carrying capacity) have reduced fecundity and calf growth, and are more vulnerable to density independent factors (e.g., climatic events). Particularly calves, yearlings, and mature bulls (weakened by the rut) and old (> 10 yr) females, especially with worn teeth, are at risk of starvation.
• In the absence of overgrazing, excessive mortality, or heavy animal harvesting, reindeer herds grow until their populations crash (exceed carrying capacity) or move to new feeding regions.
• Reindeer with poor nutrition are more susceptible to parasites, disease, and metabolic deficiencies, which can increase winter losses of meat, hides, and antlers.
• Basic range-management practices in the form of a range-management plan can prevent overgrazing and subsequent starvation of overpopulated reindeer herds.

SYSTEMS AFFECTED
Production management

GENETICS
N/A

INCIDENCE/PREVALENCE
N/A

GEOGRAPHIC DISTRIBUTION
Russia, Finland, Sweden, Norway, Greenland, Canada, and Alaska

SIGNALMENT
Species
• *Rangifer tarandus* is a circumpolar species consisting of seven subspecies formed through the isolation of populations during the ice age.
• Peary caribou (*R.t. pearyi*) and Svalbard reindeer (*R.t. platyrhyncus*) inhabit the high Arctic.
• Alaskan caribou (*R.t. granti*), barren ground caribou (*R.t. groenlandicus*), and Eurasian reindeer (*R.t. tarandus*) inhabit the taiga, woodland caribou (*R.t. caribou*) and woodland reindeer (*R.t. fennicus*) inhabit the Boreal forests.

• *Rangifer tarandus* are polygamous and highly sexual dimorphic with males being approximately twice the size of females.
• North American caribou have been utilized only through hunting.
• Eurasian reindeer were originally domesticated by indigenous people.
• Domesticated reindeer are highly gregarious and form large herds, particularly during migration and periods of insect harassment.

Breed Predilections
• Eurasian reindeer are smaller than caribou.
• Females reach maximum size at the age of 4–5 years, and senescence starts at the age of 7–8 years.
• Herders selectively remove old individuals.
• A single calf is typically produced every year. Calves are born in April-June, depending on the nutritional status of the female.
• Females in poor nutritional status delay calving.
• Birth weight is ~5 kg, males being 0.5 kg larger than females. Birth weight is positively associated with neonatal survival.
• Weaning ends in September/October (i.e., when the rut starts), but the calf may follow its mother for a year, but rarely longer.
• Calves following their mothers have easier access to food and are more likely to survive the winter.
• Male calves have higher mortality rates and are less likely to follow their mothers during the winter.

Mean Age and Range
N/A

Predominant Sex
• Females are ~60 kg and males 120 kg at their prime, although body weights vary markedly depending on range conditions.
• Age of maturity is 1–3 years in females and 2–5 years in males. Poor nutritional conditions during early development may delay maturity. Conversely, exceptional conditions may result in early maturity (age 1) for females, and this premature reproduction effort can permanently stunt somatic growth.
• Females reach maximum size at the age of 4–5 years, and senescence starts at the age of 7–8 years.
• Herders selectively remove old individuals.

MEDICATIONS

DRUGS OF CHOICE
Broad-spectrum anthelmintics (e.g., Ivermectin MSD—Ivomec 1%, Merck-Sharp & Dohme), GABA (γ-amino butyric acid) inhibitors are frequently used to combat nematodes and arthropods in reindeer.

CONTRAINDICATIONS
Appropriate milk and meat withdrawal times must be followed for all compounds administered to food-producing animals.

MISCELLANEOUS

Population Dynamics
• Sex ratio in domesticated herds is highly skewed toward females (i.e., 1:10–20) due to selective harvest.
• A skewed sex ratio increases the growth rate and potentially the productivity given the higher growth efficiency (per unit feed) of younger animals.
• Large variations in regional climate and harvesting strategies and intensity have led to profound variation in reindeer density, size, and productivity.
• Although somewhat of an oversimplification, summer range conditions are most important determinants for somatic growth, while winter range conditions are most critical for survival.
• Populations with access to winter pastures with little precipitation (snow), stable (cold) continental conditions, and thus good access to food have higher survival rates.
• Intensive harvesting is needed to regulate such populations to sustainable levels that are appropriate for the winter range.
• Populations with winter pastures in coastal areas are exposed to high precipitation levels, bringing deep snow alternating with rains and icing. Resultant ice crystals embedded in the lichen beds reduce the access and palatability, causing reindeer to wander constantly rather than graze with stability.

- High-density herds (populations exceeding carrying capacity) have reduced fecundity and calf growth and are more vulnerable to density independent factors (e.g., climatic events). Particularly calves, yearlings, and mature bulls (weakened by the rut) and old (> 10 yr) females, especially with worn teeth, are at risk of starvation.

Future Challenges
- Closing of national borders led to suboptimal use of pastures for reindeer in Fennoscandia, and international range-sharing agreements could lead to improved productivity.
- Increased pressure on reindeer pastures due to development of infrastructure for other activities such as mining, oil drilling, and power plants may permanently reduce the sustainability of reindeer herding activities.
- The recovery of predator populations, such as wolverine and lynx, has increased predation on reindeer in Fennoscandia.
- Reindeer density is in many regions above sustainable levels because reindeer management authorities have been unable to implement harvesting strategies that balance reindeer numbers to available pastures.

Parasites and Other Infectious Disease
- Reindeer, like all free-ranging, semidomesticated herd animals, are exposed to a wide variety of parasite species and infectious diseases. However, only a few species have substantive economic impact.
- Parasite burden is determined to a large extent on density-dependent factors; herds exceeding carrying capacity or not migrating seasonally to new ranges may experience greatest transmission pressure and highest burdens of parasites.
- Density-independent factors may play a role (e.g., weather conditions influence the ability of flying parasites to breed and infect their hosts).
- *Elaphostrongylus rangiferi* Mitskevich (Nematoda: Metastrongylidae) causes cerebrospinal and muscular nematodiasis and mortality in the reindeer of the Palearctic.
- *E. rangiferi* likely has the greatest economic impact; epizootics have resulted in up to 25% mortality in a single year in select herds of northern Norway.

- The oestrids, *Hypoderma tarandi* L. (warble fly), and *Cephenomyia trompe* Modeer (nasal bot fly), cause substantial harassment during the warmer summer months resulting in reduced feeding time due to insect avoidance.
- Finnish and Swedish reindeer lack access to nutrient-rich pastures along the coast during the summer and experience a very high burden of flying parasites such as nasal bot flies (*Cephenomyia trompe* Modeer) and warble fly (*Hypoderma tarandi* L.).
- *H. tarandi* L3 larvae damage the furs and thus have economic impacts.
- *C. trompe* can in rare instances cause mortality.
- Gastrointestinal nematodes (*Trichostronglyus, Ostertagia, Namatodirus, Marshallagia, Trichuris, Skrjabinema* species) have a detrimental impact on weight gain and somatic growth, but usually not a direct impact on survival.
- In North America and Siberia, brucellosis outbreaks in reindeer herds have caused serious morbidity and mortality and economic consequences.
- Brucellosis is a contagious, infectious, and communicable disease caused by bacteria of genus *Brucella*.
- Because brucellosis is zoonotic (causing undulant fever in humans), eradication through a vaccination program has been a major veterinary medicine focus in recent years.

ASSOCIATED CONDITIONS
N/A

AGE-RELATED FACTORS
N/A

ZOONOTIC POTENTIAL
- Several reindeer diseases are zoonotic. Care must be taken in the collection of laboratory samples and the diagnosis/treatment of affected animals.
- In North America and Siberia, brucellosis is a contagious, infectious, and communicable disease caused by bacteria of genus *Brucella*.
- Because brucellosis is zoonotic (causing undulant fever in humans), eradication through a vaccination program has been a major veterinary medicine focus in recent years.

PREGNANCY
N/A

RUMINANT SPECIES AFFECTED
Rangifer spp.

BIOSECURITY
- Isolation and quarantine of new stock entering the herd
- Treat and or cull new animals for disease conditions prior to herd introduction.

PRODUCTION MANAGEMENT
See Population Dynamics above

SYNONYMS
N/A

SEE ALSO
Cervidae sections
Reindeer management

ABBREVIATIONS
GABA = γ-amino butyric acid

Suggested Reading
Aschfalk, A., Josefsen, T. D., Steingass, H., Muller, W., Goethe, R. 2003, Jul. Crowding and winter emergency feeding as predisposing factors for kerato conjunctivitis in semi domesticated reindeer in Norway. *Dtsch Tierarztl Wochenschr* 110(7): 295–98.
Aschfalk, A., Thorisson, S. G. 2004, Apr. Seroprevalence of *Salmonella* spp. in wild reindeer (*Rangifer tarandus tarandus*) in Iceland. *Vet Res Commun.* 28(3): 191–95.
Palmer, M. V., Stoffregen, W. C., Rogers, D. G., Hamir, A. N., Richt, J. A., Pedersen, D. D., Waters, W. R. 2004, May. West Nile virus infection in reindeer (*Rangifer tarandus*). *J Vet Diagn Invest.* 16(3): 219–22.
Tikkanen, M. K., McInnes, C. J., Mercer, A. A., Buttner, M., Tuimala, J., Hirvela-Koski, V., Neuvonen, E., Huovilainen, A. 2004, Jun. Recent isolates of parapoxvirus of Finnish reindeer (*Rangifer tarandus tarandus*) are closely related to bovine pseudocowpox virus. *J Gen Virol.* 85(Pt 6): 1413–18.
Vahtiala, S., Sakkinen, H., Dahl, E., Eloranta, E., Beckers, J. F., Ropstad, E. 2004, Feb. Ultrasonography in early pregnancy diagnosis and measurements of fetal size in reindeer (*Rangifer tarandus tarandus*). *Theriogenology* 61(4): 785–95.
Vikoren, T., Tharaldsen, J., Fredriksen, B., Handeland, K. 2004, Mar 25. Prevalence of *Toxoplasma gondii* antibodies in wild red deer, roe deer, moose, and reindeer from Norway. *Vet Parasitol.* 120(3): 159–69.

Authors: Torkild Tveraa and Andrew J. Karter

RENAL AMYLOIDOSIS

 BASICS

OVERVIEW
• Renal amyloidosis is an infrequent systemic disease characterized by chronic wasting and diarrhea.
• Amyloidosis results from the deposition of amyloid (insoluble protein fibrils) in various body tissues. In particular, the kidney seems to be the most common site.
• Proteinuria and a nephrotic syndrome develop in bovine amyloidosis patients.

PATHOPHYSIOLOGY
• Amyloidosis in cattle is classed as the reactive (AA) type, associated with chronic inflammatory disease in domestic animals and humans.
• Concurrent inflammatory disease has been found in some, but not all, cattle with amyloidosis.
• Serum amyloid A protein (SAA) synthesized in the liver is a precursor of amyloid A (AA) fibril in tissues. SAA increases dramatically in cases of trauma, neoplasia, and inflammatory disease (elevation of SAA is necessary for an animal to develop active amyloidosis).
• Elevation of SAA due to abnormal catabolism by the RE system may also increase AA fibril formation.
• AA fibrils, resistant to proteolysis, accumulate in tissues over time.
• Accumulation of amyloid in the glomerulus results in altered glomerular filtration, with a protein-losing nephropathy, development of hypoproteinemia, and decreased intravascular oncotic pressure.
• Diarrhea develops due to edema or amyloid deposition in the GI tract.

• Protein-losing nephropathy and diarrhea result in weight loss.
• Renal or pulmonary thrombosis may occur as a result of the loss of low-molecular weight anticoagulants through the compromised renal system.

SYSTEMS AFFECTED
• Renal, gastrointestinal, hepatobiliary, endocrine
• Amyloid is deposited in the kidney, intestine, liver, spleen, adrenal glands, and other tissues.

GENETICS
Unknown

INCIDENCE/PREVALENCE
Unknown

GEOGRAPHIC DISTRIBUTION
The disease has been reported worldwide.

SIGNALMENT
Species
Although no age, breed, or sex predilection has been implicated, most reports describe the syndrome occurring in adult dairy cows.

Breed Predilections
N/A

Mean Age and Range
Unknown

Predominant Sex
No sex predilection has been reported.

SIGNS
• Chronic diarrhea, weight loss, and poor productivity in adult animals
• Hypoalbuminemia leading to ventral edema occurs commonly.
• Altered attitude and appetite may be present. This may be due to concurrent disease conditions.

• Renal enlargement is evident. The left kidney may be palpable and if so is generally not painful. Kidneys maintain their normal lobular structure.
• Urine develops a stable foam upon hitting the ground or during collection. This symptom is due to the high protein concentration found in the urine of affected animals.

CAUSES AND RISK FACTORS
Cattle with chronic inflammatory conditions such as traumatic reticuloperitonitis, metritis, mastitis, chronic pneumonia, and abscesses are at a higher risk for the development of renal amyloidosis.

 DIAGNOSIS

DIFFERENTIAL DIAGNOSIS
• Diseases causing chronic diarrhea, weight loss, hypoproteinemia, and reduced productivity; these may include salmonellosis, lymphosarcoma, Johne's disease, bovine viral diarrhea, copper deficiency, parasitism, chronic renal disease, chronic liver disease, and glomerulonephritis.
• Besides amyloidosis, glomerulonephritis is the only other disease to cause prolonged proteinuria.

CBC/BIOCHEMISTRY/URINALYSIS
• Affected cattle consistently develop marked hypoalbuminemia and proteinuria.
• If advanced renal damage has occurred, urine creatinine and urea nitrogen may be elevated.
• If chronic active inflammatory disease is present, hyperfibrinogenemia and hyperglobulinemia may also occur.

OTHER LABORATORY TESTS
N/A

IMAGING
N/A

DIAGNOSTIC PROCEDURES
• Diagnosis of amyloidosis in the live animal requires a renal biopsy. Biopsies can also differentiate renal amyloidosis from glomerulonephritis.
• Polarized light microscopy and EM have been used to examine urine sediment for the presence of amyloid protein.

PATHOLOGIC FINDINGS
• Renal enlargement with yellow-tan discoloration is often present.
• Waxy appearance of the renal parenchyma on kidney cut surface is evident.
• Generalized edema due to hypoalbuminemia is usually present.
• Some cases may present with renal or pulmonary thrombosis.
• There may be evidence of inflammation in other systems.
• Histopathology reveals amyloid deposition in the glomerulus, interstitium, and tubule lumen.
• Renal tissue may be stained with Lugol's iodine. Lugol's iodine turns amyloid mahogany brown in color. Further staining with sulfuric acid produces a blue color.
• Congo red stains highlight amyloid for subsequent light microscopy.
• Electron microscopy identifies characteristic fibril appearance.

TREATMENT
• Lesions are irreversible. The prognosis for affected animals is poor.
• Amyloid protein is resilient so it persists in tissues even if underlying cause is treated successfully.
• Specific treatment in cattle has not been reported as effective.

ACTIVITY
N/A

DIET
N/A

MEDICATIONS

DRUGS OF CHOICE
N/A

CONTRAINDICATIONS
N/A

FOLLOW-UP
N/A

MISCELLANEOUS

ASSOCIATED CONDITIONS
• Chronic diarrhea, weight loss, and poor productivity in adult animals
• Hypoalbuminemia leading to ventral edema
• Renal enlargement is evident.

AGE-RELATED FACTORS
There appear to be no age-related factors associated with this disease.

ZOONOTIC POTENTIAL
N/A

PREGNANCY
N/A

RUMINANT SPECIES AFFECTED
Renal amyloidosis has been reported in dairy cattle, mountain gazelles, Dorcas gazelles, Angora goats, and domestic sheep and goats.

BIOSECURITY
N/A

PRODUCTION MANAGEMENT
N/A

SEE ALSO
Bovine viral diarrhea
Chronic liver disease
Chronic renal disease
Copper deficiency
Glomerulonephritis
Johne's disease
Lymphosarcoma
Parasitism
Salmonellosis

ABBREVIATIONS
AA = amyloid A
EM = electron microscopy
RE = reticuloendothelial system
SAA = serum amyloid A protein

Suggested Reading
Fernandez, A., Mensua, C., Biescas, E., Lujan, L. 2003, Dec. Clinicopathological features in ovine AA amyloidosis. *Res Vet Sci.* 75(3):203–8.
Johnson, R., Jamison, K. 1984, Dec 15. Amyloidosis in six dairy cows. *J Am Vet Med Assoc.* 185(12):1538–43.
Mensua, C., Carrasco, L., Bautista, M. J., Biescas, E., Fernandez, A., Murphy, C. L., Weiss, D. T., Solomon, A., Lujan, L. 2003, Jan. Pathology of AA amyloidosis in domestic sheep and goats. *Vet Pathol.* 40(1):71–80.
Nordstoga, K., Zhou, Z. Y., Husby, G. 1994, Dec. Bovine glomerular amyloidosis: morphological studies. *Zentralbl Veterinarmed A.* 41(10):741–47.
Smith, B P., ed. 2002. *Large animal internal medicine.* 3rd ed. Philadelphia: Mosby.

Author: M. S. Gill

REPEAT BREEDER MANAGEMENT

BASICS

DEFINITION
• "Repeat breeding" is defined as a failure of conception following three or more regularly spaced services in the absence of obvious abnormalities.
• This definition may need to be modified if the herd is using techniques of estrus/ovulation synchronization.
• A more restrictive definition includes only cows that fall within this description and have been inseminated correctly with good-quality semen.

PATHOPHYSIOLOGY
Any approach to dealing with repeat breeding should consider that this syndrome might be due to either conception failure or embryonic death before maternal recognition of pregnancy. These may be affected by several factors that can be grouped in four large categories:
1. Management/human factors: concerning mainly heat detection accuracy and proper timing and delivery of semen
2. Semen factors: particularly postthaw quality and intrinsic fertility (bull fertility)
3. Cow factors: primarily disorders that may contribute to failure of fertilization or failure of embryo survival
4. Environmental factors: particularly excessive heat and humidity

SYSTEMS AFFECTED
Reproductive

GENETICS
N/A

INCIDENCE/PREVALENCE
• Repeat breeding syndrome incidence varies from 5% to 20%. Several factors affect this incidence including herd size, age of the cows, season, and production.
• The economic loss due to repeat breeding is estimated at approximately $170 per cow per annum.

GEOGRAPHIC DISTRIBUTION
Potentially worldwide, depending on species and environment

SIGNALMENT
Species
Potentially all ruminant species
Breed Predilections
N/A

Mean Age and Range
Reproductively mature females
Predominant Sex
Females

DIAGNOSIS

DIFFERENTIAL DIAGNOSIS
• Differential diagnosis of repeat breeding requires a thorough analysis of reproductive health records, observation and evaluation of personnel involved in breeding, and examination of semen/bulls and affected cows.
• Record analysis will be possible only if a system is in place that allows investigating each factor and its interaction in the contribution to repeat breeding.

Rule Out Management/Human Factors
• History and retrospective analysis of conception rate by inseminator
• Retrospective analysis of conception rate by method of heat detection
• Evaluation of inseminator
• Retraining of inseminator
• Inseminator fatigue

Rule Out Semen Factors
• Retrospective analysis of bull conception rate
• Retrospective analysis by semen/tank batches
• Evaluation of semen tank management
• Evaluation of semen handling
• Evaluation of a semen sample: evaluation should include postthaw motility, acrosome integrity, and concentration. Help from a specialized laboratory may be required to complete this examination. Analysis results should be compared to parameters from the bull stud center.
• Breeding soundness evaluation of bulls if natural mating (see Beef Bull Management and Dairy Bull Management)

Rule Out Female Factors
Failure of Fertilization
Failure of fertilization may be due to any factor that compromises gamete survival or transport to the site of fertilization and the process of fertilization. Factors include:
• *Defective oocytes*: estimated to be responsible for 3% to 8% of all causes of RB. Aged oocytes with poor fertilizing ability may be implicated in repeat breeding of individual animals. In herd situations, poor fertilizability of oocytes is generally the result of poor timing of insemination (too late). Quality of oocytes is affected if a cow experiences severe negative energy balance.

• *Oviductal anomalies*: estimated to be responsible for 6% to 15% of all causes of RB. Bilateral congenital (segmental aplasia, hydrosalpinx) or acquired (salpingitis, pyosalpinx, perisalpingitis) conditions of the uterine tube or bursa (hydrobursitis, ovariobursal adhesions) will interfere with gamete transport and prevent fertilization. Diagnosis requires detailed examination of the reproductive tract. Ultrasonography per rectum and technique to verify uterine tube patency may be required. Estimated to be responsible for 3% to 8% of all causes of RB
• *Abnormalities of the uterus*: the most common cause of fertilization failure is endometritis, which compromises sperm viability. Diagnosis of endometritis requires careful examination during estrus; uterine cytology and culture may help in diagnosis of endometritis. Immunologic reaction against semen may be a significant factor in some cows.
• *Abnormalities of the cervix*: cervical malformations such as cervical adhesion, double cervix or double external os of the cervix, cervicitis and pericervical adhesions/abscesses may be a cause of fertilization failure in individual cases but rarely is a herd problem. In some breeds (i.e., Santa Gertrudis), cervical morphology may be an important factor in poor conception rate. These disorders present as a difficulty to bypass the cervix and deposit semen into the uterus.
• *Hormonal imbalances*: excessive hormonal treatment (estrogens, progestogens) prior to ovulation or after insemination may compromise semen transport. Synchronization using MGA results in poor fertility of the induced heat. Improper timing or dosage of estrogens and GnRH used in some synchronization protocols may lead to poor timing between insemination and ovulation. In dairy heifers, repeat breeding has been associated with prolonged duration of estrus, delayed LH peak, prolonged lifespan of preovulatory follicle, late postovulatory rise in plasma progesterone, and the tendency for periovulatory suprabasal progesterone levels. Recent studies have show that hormonal imbalance also may affect expression of epidermal growth factors in the uterus, which are important for embryonic development.

Early Embryonic Death
• Cows that experience early embryonic death before embryouterine signaling (day 16 of the cycle) will have a normal cycle length and would manifest as a repeat breeder syndrome.
• Embryo loss before day 16 is estimated at 40% to 50% of all conceptions.
• Early embryonic death can result from poor quality embryos originating from poorly timed insemination (aged oocytes), older cows, poor oviductal or uterine environment due to inflammation or hormonal imbalances, and genetics.

- In dairy herds, one of the most important causes for embryonic death is elevated ambient temperature and humidity.

Infectious Disease

Infectious diseases may be implicated in increased repeat breeding in a herd. Most of these agents predispose to RB due to inflammatory changes to the ovaries; ovarian bursa (viruses); and/or the uterus, cervix, and vagina. These diseases include:

- *Brucella abortus*
- *Mycobacterium tuberculosis*
- BVDV
- IBR
- *Ureaplasma diversum*
- *Mycoplasma bovigenitalium*
- *Hemophilus somnus*
- *Leptospira harjo bovis*
- *Tritrichomonas foetus*
- *Campylobacter fetus* ssp. *venerealis*

TREATMENT

- A strict case definition of repeat breeding should be established on a herd basis.
- Herd reproductive performance records should be analyzed regularly and the incidence of repeat breeders reported.
- Analysis of records should take into account human, bull/semen, environment, and cow factors.
- Address human/management factors:
  - Improve heat detection efficiency and accuracy
  - Use fixed-time insemination
  - Periodic retraining of inseminators
- Address cow factors:
  - Individual cases should be examined thoroughly: ultrasonography of the reproductive tract and uterine cytology may add to the accuracy of diagnosis.
  - Eliminate individual causes (congenital or acquired nontreatable conditions).
  - Determine causes of uterine infection and set up protocol for prevention
  - Early identification and treatment of uterine infection
  - Reduce ovulation failure/ovulation problems by the implementation of a ovulation synchronization protocol or systematic injections of GnRH at the time of insemination in RB cows.
  - Improve embryo survival by administration of hCG or GnRH to create accessory corpora lutea and supplemental progesterone (CIDR) 6 days after insemination.
  - Administration of 500 mg BST has been shown to improve embryo survival.
- Address semen/bull factors:

- Use semen from high-fertility bulls.
- Use a double insemination regime.
- Use deep horn insemination (if technician is well trained).
- Perform breeding soundness evaluation on bulls.
- Use clean-up bulls only on cows that are known not to have an infectious cause of infertility.
- Address environmental factors:
  - Use cooling system during summer.
  - Decrease incidence of uterine infection by improving calving condition.
  - Improve heat detection by addressing problems such as crowding and floor-surface issues.

MISCELLANEOUS

ASSOCIATED CONDITIONS
N/A

AGE-RELATED FACTORS
N/A

ZOONOTIC POTENTIAL
- *Brucella abortus*
- *Mycobacterium tuberculosis*

PREGNANCY
Any approach to dealing with repeat breeding should consider that this syndrome might be due to either conception failure or embryonic death before maternal recognition of pregnancy.

RUMINANT SPECIES AFFECTED
Potentially, all ruminant species are affected.

BIOSECURITY
N/A

PRODUCTION MANAGEMENT
- Management/human factors: concerning mainly heat detection accuracy and proper timing and delivery of semen
- Semen factors: particularly postthaw quality and intrinsic fertility (bull fertility)
- Cow factors: primarily disorders that may contribute to failure of fertilization or failure of embryo survival
- Environmental factors: particularly excessive heat and humidity

SYNONYMS
N/A

SEE ALSO
Brucella abortus
BVDV
Campylobacter fetus ssp. *venerealis*
Hemophilus somnus
IBR
Leptospira hardjo-bovis
Mycobacterium tuberculosis
Mycoplasma bovigenitalium
Tritrichomonas foetus
Ureaplasma diversum

ABBREVIATIONS
BST = bovine somatotropin
BVDV = bovine diarrheal virus
GnRH = gonadotropin releasing hormone
hCG = human chorionic gonadotropin
IBR = infectious bovine rhinotracheitis
LH = luteinizing hormone
MGA = megestrol acetate
RB = repeat breeder

Suggested Reading
Bage, R., Gustafsson, H., Larsson, B., Forsberg, M., Rodriguez-Martinez, H. 2002. Repeat breeding in dairy heifers: follicular dynamics and estrus cycle characteristics in relation to sexual hormone patterns. *Theriogenology* 57: 2257–269.
Ferguson, J. D. 1996. Diets, production and reproduction in dairy cows. *Animal Feed Science Technology* 50: 173–84.
Katagiri, S., Takahashi, Y. 2004. Changes in EGF concentration during estrous cycle in bovine endometrium and their alterations in repeat breeder cows. *Theriogenology* 62:103–12.
Levine, H. D. 1999. The repeat breeder cow. *The Bovine Practitioner* 33 (2): 97–105.
Morales-Roura, J. S., Zarco, L., Hernandez-Ceron, J., Rodriguez, G. 2001. Effect of short term treatment with bovine somatotropin at estrus on conception rate and luteal function of repeat-breeding dairy cows. *Theriogenology* 55:1831–41.
Moss, N., Lean, I. J., Reid, S. W. J., Hodgson, D. R. 2002. Risk factors for repeat-breeder syndrome in New South Wales dairy cows. *Preventive Veterinary Medicine* 54:91–103.
Villarroel, A., Martino, A., BonDurant, R. H., Deletang, F., Sischo, W. M. 2004. Effect of post-insemination supplementation with PRID on pregnancy in repeat-breeder Holstein cows. *Theriogenology* 61:1513–520.

Author: Ahmed Tibary

REPRODUCTIVE TUMORS

 BASICS

DEFINITION
Neoplastic changes can affect mainly the ovary, uterus, and cervix. They are relatively rare in ruminants. Reproductive tract tumors are most commonly found in pet goats. Reproductive tumors in the male ruminant involve primarily the testicles.

PATHOPHYSIOLOGY
• Neoplasia of the reproductive organs are accompanied by a wide variety of clinical signs.
• The most determinant factors in the type of clinical signs seen are the tissue affected, the nature of the tumor, and the location. Tumors may originate from the reproductive tract or from another system.
• Ovarian tumors, particularly sex-cord tumors, are accompanied by several behavioral and phenotypic changes due to the hormone secreted. Testosterone-secreting tumors are accompanied by virilization (increased size and thickness of the head and neck) and malelike behavior. Erratic cycles may be observed with some ovarian tumors.
• Uterine and cervical tumors are generally asymptomatic or accompanied by frequent, intermittent, or continuous mucus or mucohemorrhagic discharge. Anestrus or erratic cycles may be observed with some ovarian tumors.
• Malignant tumors may affect several other organs (liver, kidney, lungs) leading to the development of a host of other clinical syndromes (weight loss, dysuria, respiratory problems, etc.).

SYSTEMS AFFECTED
Reproductive

GENETICS
N/A

INCIDENCE/PREVALENCE
N/A

GEOGRAPHIC DISTRIBUTION
Worldwide

SIGNALMENT
Species
Potentially all ruminant species. Reproductive tract tumors are most commonly found in pet goats.

Breed Predilections
N/A

Mean Age and Range
Tumors may be encountered at any age; however, uterine and cervical tumors seem to be more prevalent in older animals.

Predominant Sex
Male and female

 DIAGNOSIS
See under specific tumor below.

 TREATMENT
See under specific tumor below.

 MEDICATIONS

CONTRAINDICATIONS
Appropriate milk and meat withdrawal times must be followed for all compounds administered to food-producing animals.

 FOLLOW-UP

 MISCELLANEOUS

Reproductive Neoplasia in the Female
General considerations:
• Symptoms depend on the nature and site of the tumor and malignancy
• Always look for metastasis particularly in small ruminants with uterine tumors (chest radiographs)
• Tumors may be encountered at any age; however, uterine and cervical tumors seem to be more prevalent in older animals
• In practice, pet goats seem to be the species most frequently diagnosed with reproductive tumors
• Reproductive tumors in the female should be suspected in the presence of:
  • Abnormal palpable masses in or around the ovaries, uterus or cervix
  • Vaginal discharge (bloody or mucoid)
  • Irregular cycles
  • Stranguria, straining
  • Abnormal ultrasonographic appearance of the ovaries, uterus or cervix
  • Repeat breeding

Diagnosis

Differential Diagnosis

• Other causes of ovarian masses: adhesions, large cysts
• Other cause of uterine masses: uteroperitoneal adhesions, maceration, mummification, tuberculosis
• Other causes of cervical masses: cervicitis, abnormal cervical conformation, double cervix, cone/funnel-shaped cervix

CBC/Biochemistry/Urinalysis

N/A

Other Laboratory Tests

Examination of the female with suspected reproductive tumor:
• Laparoscopy
• Endocrinology: steroid hormone profiles and inhibin may be of value for the diagnosis of ovarian tumors. Inhibin and testosterone or estrogen are high in the case of granulosa cell tumors.
• Cervical and uterine biopsy
• Fine needle aspirate if the mass is easily accessible (vaginal or cervical)

Imaging

• Transrectal ultrasonography
• Transcutaneous abdominal ultrasonography in sheep, goats, and alpacas
• Exploratory laparotomy: this is particularly useful in the bovine where laparoscopy is generally difficult. This could also be utilized in camelids of value.

Other Diagnostic Procedures

• Transrectal palpation of all genital organs and pelvic area. Serial palpation may be required to monitor the progress of the lesion.
• Transabdominal palpation/ballottement may be helpful in detecting large uterine and ovarian masses in sheep and goats.

Treatment

• Benign ovarian neoplasm can be treated by surgical ablation (ovariectomy) of the affected ovary.
• Uterine masses require hysterectomy—indicated mainly in companion animals (alpacas or goats).
• Histopathological findings determine the extent of medical management following surgery.

Specific Reproductive Tumors in the Female

Ovarian Neoplasm

Ovarian tumors are generally classified as epithelial, germ cell, sex-cord, or mesenchymal of origin.

Epithelial Tumors

• Include papillary adenoma or carcinoma, cystadenoma, cystadenocarcinoma, and adenocanthoma
• Papillary adenoma or adenocarcinoma are very rare and arise from the surface epithelium, the subsurface epithelial structures, or rete ovarii.
• Cystadenoma arise from epoophoron and/or rete ovarii. They are large single-cavity cystic structures.

• Cystadenocarcinoma has been reported in the bovine with metastasis to the peritoneum and iliac lymph nodes, kidney, and other organs; may have been a malignant granulose cell tumor.
• Adenocanthoma (carcinoma with squamous metaplasia) has been reported in the bovine.

Germ Cell Tumors

• Dysgerminoma: reported in the cow as firm, spherical, red-gray mass, 15 cm in size, which can metastasize. Hyperplasia of the endometrium due to hyperestrogenism
• Teratomas arise from all three germinal layers with tissue representing any organ except the ovary or testis. Teratomas of different sizes and ectopic tissue content (e.g., cartilage, hair, bone, teeth, etc.) have been reported in the ewe, bovine, goat, llama, alpaca, and camel.
• Bovine cystic ovarian teratomas (dermoid cysts) have been reported in zebu cattle and water buffalo. Cysts vary in size. Ovaries range in size from 5.7 to 45 kg. Metastasis has been described.

Sex-Cord Stromal Tumors

• The most common sex-cord stromal tumor is the granulose cell tumor. Other sex-cord tumors include thecoma (theca cell tumor, firm white/yellow/orange tumors reported in cattle) and luteoma (interstitial cell tumor, smooth slightly lobulated, orange cut surface, high progesterone).

REPRODUCTIVE TUMORS

- Granulosa cell tumor:
  - Nymphomania, virilism, or asymptomatic masculinization of the head and neck
  - Cows have large multilobulated masses up to 40 kg; has been reported in newborn and nursing calves. Majority are reported at 2 to 3 years of age.
  - Male behavior, udder development
  - Ovary enlarged, contralateral ovary small
  - Generally unilateral
  - Very few are malignant
  - High testosterone, estrogen, or both; high inhibin
  - GCT have been reported in goats, sheep, and camelids

Mesenchymal Tumors
- Hemangioma
- Leiomyoma
- Fibroma
- Lymphoma (lymphosarcoma)

Uterine Neoplasm
Epithelial Tumors
- Adenoma: polyps of the endometrium are considered hyperplastic and are rare.
- Adenocarcinomas have been reported in cows (2–14 years of age), goats (7 years or older), ewes, and camelids.
  - Animals with uterine adenocarcinoma may present with several clinical signs such as infertility, bloody discharge, palpable abnormality, listlessness, respiratory syndrome, stranguria.
  - Metastasis to lymph nodes, peritoneum, lungs, and other organs may be present.
  - Lesions start in the endometrium and progress into the myometrium.

- Palpation finding, indentation of the myometrium
- Diagnosis: ultrasonography, biopsy, or exploratory laparotomy

Mesenchymal Tumors
- Fibroma: rare, hard, white, spherical neoplasm of the uterine wall
- Fibrosarcoma: extremely rare
- Leiomyoma: benign, firm, tan, nodular; generally affect the myometrium
- Leiomyosarcoma: reported in the cow and goat but are extremely rare
- Uterine lymphosarcoma: cattle—multiple irregular-shaped, soft masses

Cervical Neoplasia
- Cervical tumors are primarily of epithelial nature and include adenocarcinoma and squamous cell carcinoma. These tumors have been reported in the bovine and caprine.
- Cervical adenocarcinomas are relatively common in older goats and should be differentiated from cervical hyperplasia. Metastasis to other organs is possible in the case of adenocarcinoma.
- Mesenchymal tumors such as leiomyoma are generally associated with the uterus and vagina.

Vaginal and Vulvar Neoplasia
- Papilloma and squamous cell carcinoma occur predominantly in cattle, goats, and sheep.
- Risk factors for squamous cell carcinoma include surgical removal of perineal skin folds to reduce myiasis, tail-docking for ewes, and the lack of pigmentation on the vulva in cows, which increases exposure or sensitivity to ultraviolet radiation.

- These lesions can become ulcerated, necrotic covered by exudates and blood.
- Fibropapillomas are firm, elevated, white or pink masses, smooth or cauliflowerlike in texture, and are transmissible tumors in heifers.

Reproductve Neoplasia in the Male
General considerations:
- Tumors of the reproductive tract are rare with the exception a few obvious ones such as penile fibropapilloma in the bull.
- Reproductive tumors in the male should be suspected in presence of:
  - Deterioration of semen quality in the absence of a detectable inflammatory, traumatic, degenerative, or environmental cause
  - Progressive increased size of the testis
  - Preputial bleeding or presence of proliferative lesions on the penis surface

Diagnosis
Examination of the male with suspected reproductive tumor:
- Semen evaluation
- Testicular measurement and palpation
- Testicular ultrasonography
- Penile exteriorization and examination
- Testicular biopsy

Differential Diagnosis
- Other causes of scrotal or testicular enlargement
  - Testicular hematoma, abscesses
  - Orchitis
  - Inguinal hernia

REPRODUCTIVE TUMORS

• Other causes of preputial bleeding or phymosis
  • Preputial/penile laceration
  • Preputial abscess or adhesions

Treatment
• Testicular neoplasm requires unilateral castration and monitoring for semen quality and signs of metastasis.
• Fibropapillomas are best removed surgically by electrocauterization or ablation.
• Prevention of penile fibropapilloma may be achieved by use of autovaccine.

Specific Reproductive Tumors in the Male

Testis
• The most common testicular neoplasia in domestic animals includes seminomas, sustentacular cell tumors (tubular adenoma, tubular adenocarcinoma, Sertoli cell tumor), and interstitial cell tumors (Leydig cell tumors).
• Interstitial cell tumors are generally characterized by poor semen quality, large volume of ejaculate with low motility, and poor concentration.
• Seminomas have been reported in male alpacas, bulls, bucks, and rams. The affected testicle is generally enlarged. Effects on semen quality are variable.

• Sertoli cell tumors have been reported in bulls and rams. The affected testicle is enlarged, and semen quality may be normal or slightly affected. These tumors are pale gray and firm with irregular surface.

Penis
• Fibropapilloma is the most common penile tumor. It is primarily seen in young bulls. It is due to the fibropapilloma virus.
• Treatment consists of surgical excision.
• This tumor can be prevented by use of autovaccine.

ASSOCIATED CONDITIONS
See Pathophysiology above

AGE-RELATED FACTORS
• Adenocarcinomas have been reported in cows (2–14 years of age), goats (7 years or older), ewes, and camelids.
• Granulosa cell tumor: cows have large multilobulated masses; has been reported in newborn and nursing calves. Majority are reported at 2–3 years of age.
• Cervical adenocarcinomas are relatively common in older goats.
• Tumors may be encountered at any age; however, uterine and cervical tumors seem to be more prevalent in older animals.

ZOONOTIC POTENTIAL
N/A

PREGNANCY
N/A

RUMINANT SPECIES AFFECTED
Relatively rare in ruminants. Reproductive tract tumors are most commonly found in pet goats.

BIOSECURITY
N/A

PRODUCTION MANAGEMENT
N/A

SYNONYMS
N/A

SEE ALSO
Lymphosarcoma
Reproductive tract ultrasound
Squamous cell carcinoma

ABBREVIATIONS
GCT = granulosa cell tumor

Suggested Reading
Buergelt, C. D. 1997. *Color atlas of reproductive pathology of domestic animals.* Philadelphia: Mosby.
McEntee, K. 1990. *Reproductive pathology of domestic mammals.* New York: Academic Press, Hartcourt Brace Jovanovich.

Author: Ahmed Tibary

RESPIRATORY PHARMACOLOGY

BASICS

OVERVIEW
• Respiratory diseases of cattle are usually best described as "syndromes" involving one or more infectious organisms and environmental stressors in a compromised animal.
• Bovine respiratory disease complex (BRD) is used to describe the syndrome in older calves and adult cattle, while enzootic pneumonia is the syndrome in young calves.
• Also known as shipping fever, BRD is the primary cause of illness and death in feedlot cattle.
• *Mannheimia hemolytica, Pasteurella multocida, Histophilus somni* are gram-negative bacteria considered the primary causes of BRD, in conjunction with a number of viral infections.
• *Arcanobacterium pyogenes* (gram-positive anaerobe), gram-negative enteric bacteria, anaerobes, and *Mycoplasma* are secondary pathogens involved in chronic cases.
• To be successful, antimicrobial therapy needs to given early in the course of the disease and should target the appropriate pathogen(s).
• Anti-inflammatory therapy can improve clinical signs and reduce pathology.

PATHOPHYSIOLOGY
• The numerous pathogens involved are ubiquitous in cattle and are often part of the normal flora of the nasopharynx.
• When a group of cattle is exposed to various stressors, such as long shipping distances, transit shrinkage, and commingling, they are at risk of developing BRD, particularly if the cattles' immune systems are naïve.
• During stressful events, deficient immune defenses allow proliferation of the virulent flora and subsequent infection of the lower respiratory tract.
• Due to the release of endotoxin and leuko-toxin from the primary bacterial pathogens, severe bronchopneumonia may develop.

SYSTEMS AFFECTED
Respiratory tract

GENETICS
N/A

INCIDENCE/PREVALENCE
• Up to 81% of feedlots use injectable anti-microbials for high-risk calves (metaphylaxis).
• Approximately 10% of cattle entering feedlots are receiving injectable antimicrobials upon arrival.
• Of cattle in feedlots, 20% are treated with an injectable antimicrobial for BRD. It costs producers approximately $13/head (U.S. dollars) for treatment.
• Over 80% of feedlots use antimicrobials in the feed or water of cattle to prevent disease and improve performance. Lung concentrations attained are below the MIC values of BRD pathogens.

GEOGRAPHIC DISTRIBUTION
Potentially worldwide depending on species and environment

DIAGNOSIS

TREATMENT

MEDICATIONS

DRUGS OF CHOICE
Antimicrobials
See also Tables 1 and 2.
• To be effective, antimicrobial therapy needs to be given early in the course of the disease, reach the site of infection, and target the appropriate pathogens.
• Approved drugs for the treatment of BRD vary in their pharmacokinetics and pharmacodynamics. Values for volume of distribution (Vd) indicate drug penetration into tissues, and the elimination half-life (T1/2) is a measure of drug persistence for action and slaughter withdrawal time.
• Antimicrobial action is classified as concentration-dependent or time-dependent.
• Efficacy of concentration-dependent antimicrobials is associated with achieving drug concentrations that are eight to ten times the minimal inhibitory concentration (MIC) of the pathogen. Efficacy of time-dependent antimicrobials is associated with keeping drug concentrations above the pathogen's MIC for at least 50% of the dosing interval.
• Metaphylaxis and first pull therapy should target the gram-negative respiratory pathogens. All of the antimicrobials approved for BRD initially have good activity against *Mannheimia hemolytica, Pasteurella multocida,* and *Histophilus somni.* In relapse cases, antimicrobial resistance of the primary pathogens and opportunistic infections with *Arcanobacterium pyogenes* (gram-positive anaerobe), gram-negative enterics, anaerobes, and *Mycoplasma* should be considered. Activity against these pathogens varies considerably among the approved products.
• Even appropriate therapy against the opportunists may fail, as advanced disease prevents effective drug concentrations from reaching the site of infection. In vitro susceptibility of *Mycoplasma* species poorly correlates with clinical efficacy.
• Single-dose therapy with long-acting antimicrobials decreases animal stress from handling and reduces labor costs. Other considerations in antimicrobial selection include cost, route of administration, effect on carcass quality, and length of withdrawal time.
• First-line treatment of calves with clinical signs of BRD in feedlots is with enrofloxacin,

danofloxacin, florfenicol, tilmicosin, a long-acting oxytetracycline, or a ceftiofur formulation. Ceftiofur sodium or ceftiofur hydrochloride are used in cattle close to market weight because of their zero and 48-hour withdrawals, respectively. Approval is currently being sought for tulathromycin, a very long-acting macrolide antimicrobial for SC treatment of BRD.
• Although approved for BRD, spectinomycin, erythromycin, tylosin, penicillin, sulfonamides, ampicillin, and amoxicillin are less commonly used due to issues including requirement for repeated administration, less-desirable pharmacokinetics, lower efficacy, and carcass damage at injection sites.

Anti-inflammatory Drugs
• Corticosteroids may reduce inflammation in calves with necrotic laryngitis and or tracheal edema syndrome. Single doses of a corticosteroid are unlikely to cause significant immunosuppression. Recommended doses include 5–20 mg of dexamethasone IM or IV, 10–20 mg of isoflupredone IM, or 1.25–5 mg of flumethasone IM (approved in Canada).
• Nonsteroidal anti-inflammatory drugs reduce fever and endotoxin-induced inflammation in cattle with BRD. Flunixin meglumine is approved for use in cattle with BRD at 1.1–2.2 mg/kg IV either as a single dose or divided into two doses at 12-hour intervals. The U.S. withdrawal time is 4 days for meat and 36 hours for milk; the Canadian withdrawal time is 6 days for meat. Ketoprofen is approved in Canada at 3 mg/kg IM q 24 hr with zero milk and 24-hour meat withdrawal times.

CONTRAINDICATIONS
• AMDUCA regulations and appropriate milk and meat withdrawal times must be followed for all compounds administered to food-producing animals.
• Fluoroquinolones must not be used in an extralabel manner in the United States.
• Contact a U.S. (1-888-873-2723) or Canadian (1-866-243-2723) gFARAD office for withdrawal recommendations for extralabel drug use.
• Deep nasal swab cultures are predictive of bacterial isolates from the lungs of cattle with acute BRD.
• Avoid sampling from dead animals, as the in vitro susceptibility of the isolated pathogens from treatment failures will not represent the bacterial population as a whole.
• Treated cattle need to be closely monitored for response to therapy. Typically, if clinical improvement and normalization of body temperature does not occur within 3 days of therapy, an alternative therapy is used.
• Avoid overtreating chronic animals, as response is poor and treatment is uneconomical.

RESPIRATORY PHARMACOLOGY

Table 1

Commonly Used Antimicrobials for Metaphylaxis and Treatment of BRD					
Antimicrobial	Action	Vd	T1/2	Route of Administration	Slaughter Withdrawal
Ceftiofur Sodium or hydrochloride	Time-dependent	Low	Short	IM, SC	Sodium: zero Hydrochloride: 2 days
Ceftiofur crystalline free acid	Time-dependent	Low	Long	SC in the ear	Zero
Danofloxacin	Concentration-dependent	High	Moderate	SC	4 days
Enrofloxacin	Concentration-dependent	High	Moderate	SC	28 days
Florfenicol	Time-dependent	Moderate	Long	SC, IM	IM: 28 days SC: 38 days
Oxytetracycline (long-acting)	Time-dependent	Moderate	Long	SC, IM	28 days
Tilmicosin	Time-dependent	Very high	Very long	SC	28 days

Table 2

Relative In Vitro Antimicrobial Activity						
	Ceftiofur	Danofloxacin	Enrofloxacin	Florfenicol	Oxytetracycline	Tilmicosin
Gram − respiratory	+++	+++	+++	+++	++	+++
Gram − enterics	++	+++	+++	+	+	−
Gram +	+++	+	+	+++	++	+++
Anaerobes	+++	−	−	+++	+++	+++
Mycoplasma	−	+++	+++	+	+	++

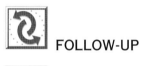

FOLLOW-UP

MISCELLANEOUS

ASSOCIATED CONDITIONS
N/A

AGE-RELATED FACTORS
N/A

ZOONOTIC POTENTIAL
N/A

PREGNANCY
N/A

RUMINANT SPECIES AFFECTED
Beef and dairy beef cattle

BIOSECURITY
N/A

PRODUCTION MANAGEMENT
See Contraindications above.

SYNONYMS
Bovine respiratory disease complex
Enzootic pneumonia
Shipping fever

SEE ALSO
Bovine respiratory disease
FARAD
Shipping fever

ABBREVIATIONS
BRD = bovine respiratory disease
gFARAD = global Food Animal Residue Avoidance Databank
IM = intramuscular
IV = intravenous
MIC = minimum inhibitory concentration
SC = subcutaneous

Suggested Reading
DeRosa, D. C., Mechor, G. D., Staats, J. J., Chengappa, M. M., Shryock, T. R. 2000. Comparison of Pasteurella spp. simultaneously isolated from nasal and transtracheal swabs from cattle with clinical signs of bovine respiratory disease. *J Clin Microbiol*. 38:327–32.
United States Department of Agriculture. 1999. Feedlot '99 Part III, *Health management and biosecurity in US feedlots*. Available online at www.aphis.usda.gov/vs/ceah/ncahs/nahms/feedlot/Feedlot99/FD99pt3.pdf
United States Pharmacopoeia. Veterinary pharmaceutical monographs—antibiotics. *J Vet Pharm Therap*. 26 (supp. 2): 1–271. Available online at www.usp.org. October 2003.

Author: Patricia M. Dowling

RETAINED PLACENTA

 BASICS

DEFINITION
• Retained placenta (RP) is failure to pass the placenta (fetal membranes) within 24 hours after parturition.
• Although various authors define RP at 6, 12, or 24 h, among cows that passed the placenta within 24 h, 77% did so within 6 h and 94% did so by 12 h after calving. The 24 h definition is most practical for monitoring in the field.

PATHOPHYSIOLOGY
• The anatomy of normal placental attachment is that cotyledon (fetal) villi attach into crypts in caruncles (maternal); cotyledons may also form pouches over caruncles in forming placentomes, of which there are approximately one hundred in the cow.
• The exact mechanism by which detachment occurs normally is not completely known. It appears that critical biochemical changes occur at the uterine-placental interface in the hours to day before parturition. However, decreased neutrophil function occurs 1 to 2 weeks before calving in cows that go on to have RP.
• The key element in RP is failure of detachment of the placentome. Specifically, there appears to be a failure of proteolysis of the cotyledon and, in particular, a failure of collagenolysis to release the cotyledon from the caruncle. This is supported by experimental evidence that injection of collagenase into the umbilical artery within the uterus (after RP occurred) or into the uterine artery during cesarean section was associated with detachment of the placenta within hours.
• It is very likely that neutrophils play a key role in breaking down the placental attachment, and prepartum immunosuppression, specifically impairment of neutrophil function, is a substantial component of the cause of RP.

• Conversely, a lack of uterine contractions is not part of the pathogenesis of RP. In fact, uterine contractions are normal to increased after parturition in cows with RP.
• In RP, detachment occurs around day 6–10 due to necrosis of the caruncle. While the RP is present in the uterus, partial necrosis contributes to bacterial growth, which along with ongoing metabolic activity by the placental tissue results in inflammation of the uterus, which may progress to clinical metritis.

SYSTEMS AFFECTED
Reproductive

GENETICS
No specific genetic predisposition, however, there is some evidence that compatibility between mother and calf of the major histocompatibility complex (MHC) class I is associated with increased risk of RP. Given that immune function is critical to normal placental detachment, it is likely that molecular genetics does have role in RP, but more research is needed.

INCIDENCE/PREVALENCE
In a 1998 summary of 50 citations, the median lactational incidence risk was 8.6%, with a range of 1.3% to 39.2% of lactations affected.

GEOGRAPHIC DISTRIBUTION
Worldwide among dairy cattle. The reported incidence is highly variable, but RP appears to be more common in North America (typical incidence of 8%–10%, up to 14%) than in Scandinavia, the UK, and New Zealand (typical incidence of 1%–3%). However, there may be reporting biases inherent in the sources of data for the published figures.

SIGNALMENT
Species
Bovine: common in dairy cattle, less so in beef cattle; also occurs uncommonly in sheep and goats
Breed Predilections
No clear associations

Mean Age and Range
Immediately after calving, therefore > 2 years old
Predominant Sex
Females only

SIGNS
Presence of some or the entire placenta in the uterus > 24 h after parturition; commonly obvious on inspection from a distance, with up to 1 m of the placenta hanging downward from the vulva. Within 1–3 days, a fetid odor and/or fetid red-brown discharge from the vulva are likely to be present.

HISTORICAL FINDINGS
Calving within the last week

PHYSICAL EXAMINATION FINDINGS
In some cases, inspection or palpation per vagina is necessary to confirm the presence of placental tissue and rule out a retained fetus.

CAUSES
Failure of detachment of the placentome, at least in large part due to impaired neutrophil function in the week or so before calving, which in turn is associated with excessive or maladaptive negative energy balance and suboptimum availability of selenium, vitamin E, and other nutrients.

RISK FACTORS
Abortion, twin birth, induced parturition, dystocia, cesarean section, stillborn calf, and milk fever are all associated with increased risk of RP. Although milk fever is associated with RP, hypocalcemia is not directly causal. Animals with elevated serum nonesterified fatty acids (NEFA $\geq$ 0.5 mEq/L) and/or suboptimal vitamin E status in the last week prepartum (serum α-tocopherol:cholesterol ratio $< 2.5 \times 10^{-3}$) are more likely to have RP. Lower prepartum serum cholesterol concentration has also been associated with increased risk of RP.

DIAGNOSIS

DIFFERENTIAL DIAGNOSIS
Diagnosis is straightforward. If fever (T > 39.5°C) is present together with RP (in the absence of other causes), this may be considered a case of metritis, particularly if dullness, decreased milk production or appetite, anorexia, or signs of toxemia (dehydration, elevated heart rate, diarrhea, weakness, cold extremities) are also present.

CBC/BIOCHEMISTRY/URINALYSIS
N/A

OTHER LABORATORY TESTS
N/A

IMAGING
N/A

DIAGNOSTIC PROCEDURES
Generally, external inspection is sufficient. Palpation of the uterus per rectum or per vagina may be performed to confirm the diagnosis of RP. As involution proceeds and the cervix closes, it is not recommended to exert force to palpate beyond the cervix.

PATHOLOGIC FINDINGS
Animals with RP have necrotic placental tissue attached at the caruncles, abundant mixed bacterial growth in the uterine lumen, and variable severity of inflammation of the layers of the uterus.

TREATMENT

APPROPRIATE HEALTH CARE
Outpatient

NURSING CARE
Animals with RP will plausibly benefit from extra effort to provide easy access to feed (60–90 cm linear bunk space per cow) and lying space (at least 9.3 m² [100 sq ft] of bedded pack space or < 100% stocking density in freestalls), as well as unrestricted access to water and heat abatement measures if ambient temperature is > 27°C. However, all transition cows may benefit from such measures.

ACTIVITY
As usual

DIET
As usual (see Prevention below)

CLIENT EDUCATION
See Prevention below.

SURGICAL CONSIDERATIONS
N/A

MEDICATIONS

• Many treatments for RP have been reported or advocated, including systemic and IU antibiotics, prostaglandin F2α, oxytocin, and estradiol. It is important to clearly establish what the objective of treatment is. Although there are some reports of benefits of PGF or oxytocin, especially within 1 hour after calving, the data are limited and contradictory. There are persistent anecdotes in circulation, and some controversy in the scientific literature, but these arguments are not based on data from field studies of naturally occurring cases. On balance, there is no strong evidence that any of the suggested treatments hasten the passage of the RP, reduce the risk of displaced abomasum (DA), or improve subsequent reproductive performance.
• Several studies indicate that approximately half of cows (up to 80% in a few studies) with untreated RP will have a temperature > 39.5°C on at least 1 day. It is not clear if all of these require systemic antibiotic treatment. At a minimum, it appears that approximately half of cows with RP do not require antibiotic treatment because they never become febrile. Therefore, automatic treatment of all RP cows with antibiotics is questionable.

• Several studies indicate that daily infusions of 5 g oxytetracycline IU for as long as the RP is in place (typically 4–5 d) reduced the incidence of fever from approximately 50% of cows with RP to approximately 30% of affected cows. However, in these studies, there was no reduction in associated diseases (DA, ketosis), and no improvement in reproductive performance associated with this aggressive use of IU antibiotics. This dose of oxytetracycline IU resulted in widely variable concentrations and duration of detectable residues in milk, with a mean of 52 hours of residue > 200 ppb. Therefore, the benefit (if any) of such an approach is unclear.
• Historically, manual removal of RP by manipulation and traction was practiced. There is no evidence that this practice produces beneficial results, and there is some evidence that it exacerbates damage to the endometrium, increases the risk of toxemia, and may delay return to cyclicity. Removal of an already detached placenta at 3–7 d postpartum using no more than a few pounds of pressure is permissible; otherwise, manual removal is contraindicated.
• Estradiol cypionate (ECP) (4 mg IM, once at 1 d postpartum) in cows with RP did not reduce the incidence of fever with fetid discharge within 7 or 30 DIM, but significantly prolonged time to pregnancy relative to no treatment in cows with RP. Similarly, in two other studies, ECP (4 mg IM once 24–36 h postpartum) to all cows, or high-risk cows (with clinical hypocalcemia, RP, twins, dystocia, or stillborn calf) failed to reduce the incidence of fetid discharge (with or without fever).
• Ceftiofur HCl (2.2 mg/kg IM q 24 for 5 d) administered starting at 1 DIM to cows with RP without regard to body temperature significantly reduced the incidence of fever with fetid discharge, with no effect on time to pregnancy. In a separate study, administration of ceftiofur to multiparous cows at high risk for metritis (see Pathophysiology and Risk Factors above) in the first 3 DIM when fever

RETAINED PLACENTA

was detected reduced the incidence of subsequent fetid discharge. In a third study, ceftiofur (1.1 mg/kg IM q 24 for 5 d) in cows with RP and fever was as effective (67% absence of fever by 10 DIM) as a combination of systemic and IU ampicillin and manual removal of the placenta; there was no difference in reproductive performance between the two treatments. There are no trials published in which cows with RP and fever (with or without fetid discharge) were left untreated, even for 1–2 d. Therefore, it is unclear what the health or economic benefits are of treating all cows with RP, or even all febrile cows with RP, with systemic antibiotics.

DRUGS OF CHOICE
Subject to the caveats discussed above:
• Ceftiofur (Na- or –HCl)—1–2 mg/kg IM q 24 h for 3 d; up to maximum of 5 d if clinically improving but not resolved (WD = 0 milk, 3 d meat)
• Procaine penicillin G—21,000 IU/kg IM q 24 h for 3 d (WD = 4 d milk; 10 d meat [Canadian label])

CONTRAINDICATIONS
Appropriate milk and meat withdrawal times must be followed for all compounds administered to food-producing animals.

PRECAUTIONS
N/A

POSSIBLE INTERACTIONS
None known

ALTERNATIVE DRUGS
Little or no evidence to support other treatments

FOLLOW-UP

PATIENT MONITORING
• Cows with RP should be inspected daily until the placenta is passed to detect progression to metritis. Observation of the cow's attitude, appetite (if possible), and daily milk production is likely a useful screening test.
• Measurement of rectal temperature is indicated in cows that are dull, inappetent, producing less milk than expected, or declining in milk production. Some authors advocate daily measurement of temperature in all cows with RP for 10 d postpartum. More large-scale field studies are needed to determine if this approach results in early detection and mitigation of metritis, avoidance of other related diseases (e.g., displaced abomasum), and/or improved reproductive performance, or if this approach leads to medically or economically unnecessary treatment.

PREVENTION/AVOIDANCE
• Because the cause of RP is multifactorial, it is important to recognize that no one preventive measure will be universally effective. The principle for prevention is to optimize peripartum immune function.
• In general, best management and nutritional practices (e.g., transition diet to meet or exceed National Research Council [2001] requirements for > 3 weeks prepartum with average DMI > 12 kg/cow/day, > 60 cm manger space/cow, calving at body condition score of 3.5 out of 5, lack of crowding, heat abatement measures above 27°C, free access to clean water) will plausibly help to prevent RP.

• In particular, the prepartum diet should include 0.3-ppm selenium and 1000–2000 IU/cow/d of vitamin E. Among animals with suboptimum circulating vitamin E in the last week prepartum (serum α-tocopherol: cholesterol ratio < 2.5×10^{-3}), injection of 3000 IU α-tocopherol SC or IM 1 week before expected calving reduced the risk of RP. Unfortunately, there is no simple way to identify individuals or herds that may benefit from this treatment. In two studies, peripartum oral administration of calcium (one to three treatments of 60 g Ca within a 24 hour period around calving) did not reduce the incidence of RP.
• One economic analysis estimated that at a herd incidence of 7%, the economic loss was minimal. Therefore, decisions about preventive interventions should consider the magnitude of the problem as well as the evidence for the expected costs and benefits of proposed measures.

POSSIBLE COMPLICATIONS
Metritis, endometritis, ketosis, DA, mastitis, increased time to pregnancy (days open), and decreased probability of pregnancy/increased risk of culling

EXPECTED COURSE AND PROGNOSIS
• It is difficult to generalize about the expected impact of RP, which will range from none (other than an aesthetically unappealing condition for 1 week), to impaired reproductive performance, or progression to severe metritis and toxemia. Just as the occurrence of RP depends on immune function, so does the course once the condition has occurred.
• The ability of the uterine immune system to respond to RP, inflammation, and increased bacterial challenge determines whether the cow will go on to suffer metritis or impaired reproductive performance.

• RP is a risk factor for metritis, displaced abomasum, and endometritis. Approximately half of untreated cows with RP will become febrile (T > 39.5°C) at least once while the RP is present. Conversely, many of cows with RP do not have any clinical complications, even if untreated.

• Although many studies report negative impacts of RP on reproductive outcomes, the results are variable. The best analyses estimate that affected cows become pregnant approximately 15% more slowly (i.e., hazard ratio for pregnancy = 0.85) than unaffected cows (e.g., reduction in 21-day pregnancy rate from 15% to 12.8%).

• It is not clear whether impaired reproductive performance is directly attributable to RP, or (more likely) if only metritis or clinical and/or subclinical endometritis result.

• There are some reports of short-term reductions in milk yield associated with RP, but meaningful loss of production appears to be confined to those individuals that progress to clinical metritis. Likewise, RP itself appears not to increase culling risk

 MISCELLANEOUS

ASSOCIATED CONDITIONS
Abortion, twins, metritis, endometritis

AGE-RELATED FACTORS
N/A

ZOONOTIC POTENTIAL
N/A

PREGNANCY
N/A

RUMINANT SPECIES AFFECTED
Bovine (commonly); ovine and caprine (uncommon)

BIOSECURITY
N/A

PRODUCTION MANAGEMENT

SYNONYMS
Retained fetal membranes (RFM)

SEE ALSO
Endometritis
Metritis

ABBREVIATIONS
DA = displaced abomasum
DIM = days in milk (days postpartum)
ECP = estradiol cypionate
IM = intramuscular
IU = intrauterine
MHC = major histocompatibility complex
NEFA = nonesterified fatty acid
RFM = retained fetal membranes
RP = retained placenta
SC = subcutaneous
WD = withdraw

Suggested Reading
Eiler, H. 1997. Retained placenta. In: *Current therapy in large animal theriogenology*, ed. R. S. Youngquist. Philadelphia: W. B. Saunders.
Frazer, G. S. 2001. Hormonal therapy on the postpartum cow—days 1 to 10—fact or fiction? *Proc Ann Conf Amer Assoc Bovine Practitioners* 34:109–22.
Kimura, K., Goff, J. P, Kehrli, M. E., Reinhardt, T. A. 2002. Decreased neutrophil function as a cause of retained placenta in dairy cattle. *J Dairy Sci.* 85: 544–50.
Laven, R. A., Peters, A. R. 1996. Bovine retained placenta: aetiology, pathogenesis and economic loss. *Vet Rec* 139: 465–71.
Peters, A. R., Laven, R. A. 1996. Treatment of bovine retained placenta and its effects. *Vet Rec.* 139: 535–39.

Author: Stephen LeBlanc

RIFT VALLEY FEVER

BASICS

DEFINITION
• Rift Valley fever (RVF) is an acute viral disease that severely affects sheep, cattle, and goats.
• It causes very high rates of abortion and death in neonates and necrotic hepatitis.
• There is a great economic impact from this disease due to the large losses of young animals.

PATHOPHYSIOLOGY
• RVF is caused by a phlebovirus (family Bunyaviridae). The virus replicates mainly in the liver and spleen, however, the brain can also be affected.
• Lesions seen are a direct effect of the lytic nature of the virus.

SYSTEMS AFFECTED
• Reproductive—abortion, neonatal death
• Gastrointestinal—severe hepatic necrosis

GENETICS
N/A

INCIDENCE/PREVALENCE
• Outbreaks of RVF tend to occur in a cyclic pattern every 5 to 20 years and are usually associated with abnormally heavy rainfalls and persistent flooding.
• The incidence of RVF peaks in late summer, disappearing after the first frost.
• In warmer climates, where insect vectors are present continuously, seasonality is usually not seen.
• Abortion rate in ruminants can be very high. It can reach 70–100% in lambs or kids but drops to 20% in those that are over 2 weeks old.
• Mortality in adult sheep and goats ranges from 20% to 30%.
• In cattle, abortions can also reach 100%, but range from 10% to 70% in calves.
• In adults, mortality may be near 10%.

GEOGRAPHIC DISTRIBUTION
RVF is endemic throughout most of Africa. Prior to 1977, the disease occurred only in Africa; however, recent outbreaks and spread of the disease have occurred in Saudi Arabia, Yemen, and Egypt. Rift Valley fever has not occurred in the United States.

SIGNALMENT

Species
• RVF has been found to infect many species of animals, however, the most commonly affected are sheep, goats, and cattle. They are also the primary amplifier of the virus.
• Dogs are also highly susceptible, while horses and pigs are resistant to the virus.

Breed Predilections
N/A

Mean Age and Range
• All ages can be affected, but the greatest mortality is seen in fetal or newborn animals.
• Susceptibility decreases with age.

Predominant Sex
N/A

SIGNS

GENERAL COMMENTS
• The incubation period for RVF is 12–36 hours.
• Neonates usually die within 2 days.
• Older animals may die acutely or develop an inapparent infection. Viremia is typically 1–3 days but can be as long as 10 days.

HISTORICAL FINDINGS
• RVF should be considered when high abortion rates or high mortality rates occur in young ruminants, following abnormally heavy rains and high numbers of mosquitoes.
• Additionally, there is rapid spread of the disease and flulike illness in humans.

PHYSICAL EXAMINATION FINDINGS
• Abortion in adult sheep and goats is the most common sign of RVF.
• It can occur at any stage of gestation.
• The fetus will have an autolyzed appearance with signs of hepatic necrosis. Placental lesions are not typically seen.
• Lambs and kids may have high fever (105.8°F; 41°C), listlessness, anorexia, and abdominal pain. Adult animals typically have inapparent infection.
• Clinical signs most commonly seen include fever, mucopurulent nasal discharge, and possibly vomiting.
• In cattle, icterus and abortions are the most common signs seen. Calves may show fever, depression, and acute death.
• Adult animals usually have inapparent disease, but clinical signs include fever, weakness, anorexia, ptyalism, and fetid diarrhea.

CAUSES
• The reservoir for RVF is mosquitoes, particularly *Aedes* species.
• The virus is transovarilly transmitted to the eggs, which can lay dormant for many years in the dry soil of grasslands areas.
• Following heavy rainfalls, the pooling water gives the eggs a proper environment to hatch. These newly hatched infected mosquitoes then seek a feeding source (human or animal).
• Once a ruminant is infected, it serves as an amplifying host. Secondary arthropod vectors (e.g., *Culex* and *Anopheles* mosquitoes) can become infected from the ruminant, and rapidly spread the disease.
• Biting flies, such as midges, phlebotomids, stomoxids, and simulids, are potential mechanical vectors, but this is thought to be a minimal route of transmission.

RISK FACTORS
• Risk factors for RVF include exposure of ruminants to competent arthropod vectors during pregnancy.
• Other routes of viral transmission include direct contact or aerosolization of body fluids or tissues of infected animals, particularly parturient material.

DIAGNOSIS

Diagnosis is based on histopathology and demonstration of viral antigen or antibody.

DIFFERENTIAL DIAGNOSIS
Differentials include diseases with relatively high rates of abortion or neonatal deaths accompanied by hepatic necrosis:
• Wesselsbron
• Vibriosis (*Campylobacter fetus*)
• Ephemeral fever
• Brucellosis
• Ovine enzootic abortion
• Listeriosis
• Toxoplasmosis
• Enterotoxemia of sheep
• Trichomoniasis
• Nairobi sheep disease

CBC/BIOCHEMISTRY/URINALYSIS
N/A

OTHER LABORATORY TESTS
• The virus can be readily isolated from tissues of aborted fetuses and the blood of infected animals.
• Viral antigen tests include immunodiffusion, complement fixation, or immunofluorescence. The virus can also be isolated from inoculation tests (i.e., mice or cell culture).
• Serological tests can be used to detect antibody against RVF virus and are useful for epidemiologic studies but of limited value for diagnosis, due to cross-reaction with other phleboviruses.

IMAGING
N/A

DIAGNOSTIC PROCEDURES
• Although histopathologic liver lesions are pathognomonic, laboratory confirmation should be done.
• Specimens should include heparinized blood and serum from live animals.
• Tissue samples should include liver, spleen, kidney, lymph nodes, and brain of an aborted fetus.
• Reverse transcriptase PCR (RT-PCR) for diagnosis of Rift Valley fever (RVF) is available.
• Indirect enzyme-linked immunosorbent assay (ELISA) for the detection of antibody against Rift Valley fever virus in domestic and wild ruminant sera is available.

PATHOLOGIC FINDINGS
• Hepatic necrosis is the most common postmortem lesion found in sheep, cattle, and goats. This can be quite extensive in fetal and neonatal animals. The liver is greatly enlarged, yellow, friable, and will have multifocal small, gray-white foci.
• The wall of the gallbladder is commonly hemorrhagic and edematous.

- Petechial hemorrhages may also be very prominent and found on cutaneous or serosal surfaces.
- Aborted fetuses will have an autolyzed appearance.
- The contents of the abomasum and small intestine of newborns will be chocolate brown.
- Histopathologic liver lesions are pathognomonic for RVF. Severe lytic necrosis with dense aggregates of cellular and nuclear debris, fibrin, and inflammatory cells can be found in the liver parenchyma of aborted fetuses or affected neonates.
- Eosinophilic rod-shaped intranuclear inclusion bodies may also be seen in over half the cases.

TREATMENT
N/A

APPROPRIATE HEALTH CARE
N/A

NURSING CARE
N/A

ACTIVITY
N/A

DIET
N/A

CLIENT EDUCATION
- RVF is a zoonotic disease.
- Clients should be educated on routes of transmission as well as vector control methods.

SURGICAL CONSIDERATIONS
N/A

MEDICATIONS

DRUGS OF CHOICE
N/A

CONTRAINDICATIONS
N/A

PRECAUTIONS
N/A

POSSIBLE INTERACTIONS
N/A

ALTERNATIVE DRUGS
N/A

FOLLOW-UP

PATIENT MONITORING
N/A

PREVENTION/AVOIDANCE
- Sanitation and vector control should be attempted but do not usually control the spread of the disease.
- Carcasses should be buried or burned.

- Although immunization of sheep, goats, and cattle is the most effective method of controlling the disease, the current vaccine can be abortogenic and teratogenic but is usually less than the effect from the disease. There is no vaccine currently available in the United States for RVF.

POSSIBLE COMPLICATIONS
N/A

EXPECTED COURSE AND PROGNOSIS
Affected neonates typically die within 2 days.

MISCELLANEOUS

ASSOCIATED CONDITIONS
- Abortion in adult sheep and goats
- Lambs and kids may have high fever (105.8° F; 41°C), listlessness, anorexia, and abdominal pain. Adult animals typically have inapparent infection.
- In cattle, icterus and abortions are the most common signs seen. Calves may show fever, depression, and acute death.
- Adult animals usually have inapparent disease, but clinical signs include fever, weakness, anorexia, ptyalism, and fetid diarrhea.

AGE-RELATED FACTORS
- The greatest mortality rates are seen in fetuses or young neonates of sheep, goats, and cattle.
- Susceptibility decreases with age.

ZOONOTIC POTENTIAL
- Humans are highly susceptible to infection by mosquitoes or by exposure to aerosols when handling infected animal tissues during assisted parturition, necropsy of aborted fetuses, slaughter, or laboratory procedures.
- Humans also develop a high enough viremia to be a source of infection for mosquitoes.
- Following an incubation period of 4–7 days, flulike signs (fever, weakness, myalgia, headache, nausea) and photophobia may develop.
- Recovery generally occurs after 4–7 days. Rarely, the disease may cause hemorrhagic fever, encephalitis, or retinopathies.
- The greatest risk for RVF is for travelers to endemic African countries. Avoidance of exposure to arthropod vectors should be implemented.
- Diagnostic laboratory infections can be common; personnel should use biosafety level 3 procedures.
- Personal protection equipment (i.e., gloves, coveralls, boots, and face masks) should be worn when in contact with infected animals.
- Vaccination is available for those at risk of exposure.
- To date, no person-to-person transmission has been documented.

PREGNANCY
- RVF causes abortion and neonatal death in sheep, goats, and cattle.

- Abortion rate in ruminants can be very high. It can be 70–100% in lambs or kids but drops to 20% in those that are over 2 weeks old.

RUMINANT SPECIES AFFECTED
Sheep, goats, and cattle

BIOSECURITY
- RVF has a limited endemic region. If cases or outbreaks are suspected outside of this region, proper veterinary authorities should be contacted immediately.
- RVF is an OIE List A Exotic disease, which requires mandatory reporting.

PRODUCTION MANAGEMENT
- Management steps for the prevention of RVF include implementation of vector (mosquitoes) control and moving animals to higher altitudes (i.e., less flood plain areas).
- Additionally, vaccination in endemic areas prior to breeding season may be beneficial.

SYNONYMS
N/A

SEE ALSO
Brucellosis
Enterotoxemia of sheep
Ephemeral fever
Listeriosis
Nairobi sheep disease
Ovine enzootic abortion
Toxoplasmosis
Trichomoniasis
Vibriosis (*Campylobacter fetus*)
Wesselsbron

ABBREVIATIONS
PCR (RT-PCR) = reverse transcriptase–polymerase chain reaction
RVF = Rift Valley fever

Suggested Reading
Exotic animal diseases bulletin. 2004, Jan-Feb. *Aust Vet J*. 82(1–2):16–17.
Geisbert, T. W., Jahrling, P. B. 2004, Dec. Exotic emerging viral diseases: progress and challenges. *Nat Med*. 10(12 Suppl): S110–21.
Gerdes, G. H. 2002. Rift Valley fever. *Vet Clin North Am Food Anim Pract*. 18:549–55.
Mebus, C. A. 1998. Rift Valley fever. In: *Foreign animal diseases*. Richmond, VA: United States Animal Health Association, http://www.vet.uga.edu/wpp/gray_book/FAD.
Paweska, J. T., Smith, S. J., Wright, I. M., Williams, R., Cohen, A. S., Van Dijk, A. A., Grobbelaar, A. A., Croft, J. E., Swanepoel, R., Gerdes, G. H. 2003, Mar. Indirect enzyme-linked immunosorbent assay for the detection of antibody against Rift Valley fever virus in domestic and wild ruminant sera. *Onderstepoort J Vet Res*. 70(1):49–64.

Author: Glenda Dvorak

RINDERPEST

BASICS

OVERVIEW
• Rinderpest is one of the most feared viral diseases of cattle.
• It is estimated that this disease caused the death of over 200 million cattle in Europe in the 18th century and 2.5 million cattle in the last Great African Pandemic in the 1890s. This disease was instrumental in the formation of veterinary schools throughout Europe.
• Rinderpest is a viral disease caused by a morbillivirus that is closely related to peste des petits ruminants (PPR), canine distemper, and measles.
• There is only one serotype but many strains of the virus that vary in virulence.
• Affected animals develop a high fever, depression, anorexia, and diarrhea. Death usually follows.
• Ulceration of the oral mucosa and a necrotizing enteritis are common gross necropsy findings.
• The disease is spread by direct contact with oculonasal fluids and feces. However, the virus can be identified in all tissues.
• Currently, rinderpest is believed to be present only in eastern Africa (Somalia) and Pakistan. The disease is targeted for eradication by 2010.

SIGNALMENT
• In endemic areas, rinderpest is mild and self-limiting; however, when the virus is introduced into naïve animals, the virus seems to change in virulence and a severe disease is presented clinically.
• All cloven-hoofed animals are susceptible to infection with European breeds of cattle (*Bos taurus*), Asian water buffalo (*Bubalus bubalis*), and the yak (*Bos grunniens*) most susceptible. Zebu cattle (*Bos indicus*) are more resistant. Swine are susceptible to the virus.
• Most African wildlife are susceptible to the virus with the Cape buffalo being very sensitive to the virus.

SIGNS
• Rinderpest may present as an acute or subacute disease. Incubation period is between 7 and 14 days.
• Animals develop a high fever, 104°F to 107°F (40 to 42.2°C), and become depressed with anorexia. Milk production is severely curtailed.
• Mucous membranes of the mouth and conjunctiva become congested. The muzzle usually becomes dry, crusty, and ulcerated.
• Animals occasionally become constipated early in the course of the disease, and this is followed by abundant, runny diarrhea that may contain mucus, fibrin, and/or blood.

• Small pinpoint areas of necrosis or shallow erosions are usually first noted on the lips and gums and later on the tongue, dental pad, and plate.
• Vesicles may develop on the tongue.
• As the disease progresses, the animals become dehydrated, weak, and prostrate. Death often follows.

CAUSES AND RISK FACTORS
N/A

DIAGNOSIS

DIFFERENTIAL DIAGNOSIS
• Bovine viral diarrhea–mucosal disease (BVD-MD): naïve animals have fever and diarrhea, and develop ulcers in oral cavity and esophagus. Necrosis of intestinal gut associate lymphoid tissue (Peyer's patches) can be seen. BVD can be identified by PCR probes on whole blood and spleen. Persistently infected animals can be identified by immunohistochemistry of skin biopsies and ELISA techniques on sera.
• Malignant catarrhal fever (MCF): common finding in affected animals is severe erosion of the nasal mucosa, oral ulcerations, severe corneal edema, and conjunctivitis.
• Infectious bovine rhinotracheitis (IBR): animals develop severe upper respiratory disease with ulceration of the tracheal and nasal mucosa. Occasional ulceration of the oral mucosa and esophagus is noted.
• Foot-and-mouth disease (FMD): animals develop vesicles and ulcers on the lips, oral mucosa, tongue, teats, interdigital space, and/or coronary band.
• Bluetongue: animals (mostly sheep) can develop oral ulcers in the mouth with edema and ulcers of the muzzle. Laminitis can occur.
• Bovine papillary stomatitis: single or coalescing proliferative lesions on the palate and tongue often characterize bovine papillary stomatitis.
• Contagious ecthyma (orf): animals develop prominent proliferative growths on the lips, oral mucosa (primarily gums and dental pad), and teats (primarily in sheep) that are easily ulcerated and bleed.
• Peste des petits ruminants (PPR): this disease is primarily a disease of sheep and goats and is closely related to rinderpest. Clinically, animals present with ulceration of the oral mucosa, conjunctivitis, diarrhea, and pneumonia.

CBC/BIOCHEMISTRY/URINALYSIS
A severe leukocytopenia is observed, which may last for several weeks.

OTHER LABORATORY TESTS
N/A

DIAGNOSTIC PROCEDURES
• Rinderpest is a reportable disease in most countries. Animals suspected of having this disease must be reported to state and federal veterinary officials to insure that the disease is eradicated from the region.
• Completive ELISA, virus neutralization, complement fixation, and agar gel immunodiffusion techniques are useful serological tests commonly used to detect exposure to the virus.
• Virus isolation is best completed on freshly dead or killed animals. Submission of spleen, lymph nodes, tonsil, and necrotic gum or oral mucosa should be submitted in a sterile sample container.
• Whole blood preserved in EDTA or heparin can be submitted also.
• Ocular and nasal secretions during early stages of the disease contain abundant virus. These secretions can be submitted in virus isolation media.
• Blood and tissues should be sent on cold packs, not with dry ice, to the designated veterinary diagnostic laboratory for evaluation.

PATHOLOGIC FINDINGS

GROSS FINDINGS
• Lesions include small shallow ulcers on the lips, tongue, palate, esophagus, and rumen. Erosions may also be present in the vulva, vagina, and prepuce.
• The abomasum is congested and occasionally hemorrhagic. Lesions commonly observed in the intestines are necrosis of the gut associated lymphoid tissues (Peyer's patches), ulceration of the colon and rectum, and hemorrhage (zebra-striping) of the rectum and distal colon. The lymph nodes are often swollen and edematous. Petechial and ecchymotic hemorrhage and necrosis of the gallbladder are also occasionally seen in diseased animals.
• The lungs may also be emphysematous and congested with a mild interstitial pneumonia.

HISTOPATHOLOGIC FINDINGS
• Necrosis of the mucosal epithelium of the oral, esophageal, and ruminal mucosa is severe with multinucleated syncytial cells present in the epithelium. Intranuclear and intracytoplasmic inclusions may be present in the syncytial cells.
• Lymph nodes, spleen, and gut associated lymphoid tissue (Peyer's patches) have severe lymphoid necrosis with occasional syncytial cells present. Intranuclear and intracytoplasmic inclusions may be identified occasionally in syncytial cells and some degenerate and necrotic lymphocytes.
• The small and large intestine have necrosis of the crypts with flattening of the villi.
• Occasional syncytial cells can be noted in the glandular crypts.
• Intracytoplasmic and intranuclear inclusions can occasionally be observed in the tissues.

TREATMENT

• Since this disease is scheduled for eradication by OIE, euthanasia of affected animals is usually recommended to prevent further spread of the disease; however, if one is to treat affected animals, intensive supportive care is needed to keep the animal hydrated from the severe fluid loss due to diarrhea.
• Antipyretics (e.g., aspirin, flunixin meglumine) may be useful for decreasing the animal's fever and assist in making the animal feel better so it will eat and drink.

MEDICATIONS

CONTRAINDICATIONS

• Appropriate milk and meat withdrawal times must be followed for all compounds administered to food-producing animals.
• Steroids should not be used in pregnant animals.

POSSIBLE INTERACTIONS

FOLLOW-UP

PATIENT MONITORING
N/A

PREVENTION/AVOIDANCE

• The virus is fairly fragile and is sensitive to heat and light. Decomposition of an infected carcass quickly kills the virus.
• The virus is primarily spread by direct contact with infected animals (oculonasal fluid and feces). Quarantine and prohibiting animal movement in infected areas can stop the spread of the disease to other susceptible herds.
• No carrier state has been observed in infected cattle that have recovered from the disease.
• In an outbreak or in an endemic area, vaccination of susceptible animals is a possible means of stopping the spread of the disease. Both modified live and killed vaccines are available for use in some areas of the world.
• Thorough cleaning and disinfection of an infected facility and allowing the facility to remain idle without animals present (usually 30 days) before repopulating the facility with new naïve animals is critical to prevent reinfection.

POSSIBLE COMPLICATIONS
N/A

EXPECTED COURSE AND PROGNOSIS

Depending on the strain of rinderpest virus, morbidity can be greater than 90% and mortality can be very high (greater than 90%, particularly for European breeds of cattle, yak, and Asian water buffalo).

MISCELLANEOUS

ASSOCIATED CONDITIONS

As the disease progresses, the animals become dehydrated, weak and prostrate. Death often follows.

AGE-RELATED FACTORS
N/A

ZOONOTIC POTENTIAL
N/A

PREGNANCY
N/A

RUMINANT SPECIES AFFECTED

All cloven-hoofed animals are susceptible to infection with European breeds of cattle (*Bos taurus*), Asian water buffalo (*Bubalus bubalis*), and the yak (*Bos grunniens*) most susceptible. Zebu cattle (*Bos indicus*) are more resistant. Swine are susceptible to the virus.

BIOSECURITY

• The virus is primarily spread by direct contact with infected animals (oculonasal fluid and feces). Quarantine and prohibiting animal movement in infected areas can stop the spread of the disease to other susceptible herds.
• No carrier state has been observed in infected cattle that have recovered from the disease.
• In an outbreak or in an endemic area, vaccination of susceptible animals is a possible means of stopping the spread of the disease. Both modified live and killed vaccines are available for use in some areas of the world.
• Thorough cleaning and disinfection of an infected facility and allowing the facility to remain idle without animals present (usually 30 days) before repopulating the facility with new naïve animals is critical to prevent reinfection.

PRODUCTION MANAGEMENT
N/A

SEE ALSO

Bluetongue
Bovine papillary stomatitis
Bovine viral diarrhea– mucosal disease (BVD-MD)
Contagious ecthyma (orf)
Foot-and-mouth disease (FMD)
Infectious bovine rhinotracheitis (IBR)
Malignant catarrhal fever (MCF)
Peste des petits ruminants (PPR)

ABBREVIATIONS

BVD = bovine viral diarrhea
ELISA = enzyme-linked immunosorbent assay
OIE = Office International des Epizooties
PCR = polymerase chain reaction

Suggested Reading
Cheneau, Y., Roeder, P. L., Obi, T. U., Rweyemamu, M. M., Benkirane, A., Wojciechowski, K. J. 1999, Apr. Disease prevention and preparedness: the Food and Agriculture Organization emergency prevention system. *Rev Sci Tech.* 18(1):122–34.
Mukhopadhyay, A. K., Taylor, W. P., Roeder, P. L. 1999, Apr. Rinderpest: a case study of animal health emergency management. *Rev Sci Tech.* 18(1):164–78.
Rinderpest. 2003, May. *Aust Vet J.* 81(5):252.
Roeder, P. L., Taylor, W. P. 2002. Rinderpest. *Vet Clin North Am Food Anim Pract.* 18(3):515–47, ix.
USAHA. 1998. Rinderpest. In: *Foreign animal diseases.* Richmond, VA: United States Animal Health Association, http://www.vet.uga.edu/wpp/gray_book/FAD.

Author: Robert B. Moeller, Jr.

RINGWOMB

BASICS

DEFINITION
Nondilation of the cervix that results in prolonged lambing (kidding), weak-born or dead lambs (kids), and cervical trauma or secondary infections in the ewe (doe). Mortality is often high in dam and offspring, even with veterinary intervention.

PATHOPHYSIOLOGY
• Complex interactions between fetal and maternal neural, endocrine, and paracrine systems lead to the efficient delivery of normal lambs or kids.
• Increased levels of fetal plasma cortisol result in an increase in estrogen and a decrease in progesterone in maternal plasma and an increase in maternal uterine prostaglandin production. These changes lead to the induction of normal delivery including efficient and coordinated myometrial contractions, dilation of the cervix, delivery of the fetus, and expulsion of the placenta.
• The exact mechanism by which estrogen and other hormonal factors regulate cervical ripening and dilation is not completely known.
• Failure of the cervix to dilate is referred to as ringwomb. For a complete review of endocrine and paracrine regulation of preterm and birth processes, see Challis et al. (2000) in Suggested Reading below.

SYSTEMS AFFECTED
Reproductive, nondilation of the cervix

GENETICS
A clear genetic linkage has not been determined; however, there is anecdotal evidence that suggests that certain bloodlines within a particular breed may have an increased incidence of ringwomb.

INCIDENCE/PREVALANCE
Incidence is usually higher in maiden dams; however, older animals may also present with ringwomb. The number of cases within a given flock/herd can vary dramatically from year to year. Predisposing factors are not well established.

GEOGRAPHIC DISTRIBUTION
Ringwomb is apparently common in most regions of the world, although complete data on distribution with emphasis on individual species have not been reported.

SIGNALMENT

Species
Ovine, caprine, bovine

Breed Predilections
None confirmed

Mean Age and Range
All ages are affected; first or second parity dams are most commonly affected.

Predominant Sex
Female

SIGNS

GENERAL COMMENTS
• Affected ewes and does may go undetected until the fetuses have died from hypoxia, and the ewe is suffering systemic effects from uterine toxemia.
• Often the first indication of ringwomb is the presentation of fetal membrane through the vagina without concurrent evidence of active labor. The ewe may act restless or appear normal.
• Similar signs are observed in does, although vocalization may be more prominent.

PHYSICAL EXAMINATION FINDINGS
• The cervix is not sufficiently dilated to allow expulsion of the fetus. Often, only a finger may be inserted through the cervical os on vaginal examination.
• Status of the fetus should be determined by stimulating fetal movement if possible. Oftentimes the presence of a malodorous discharge will confirm the demise of the lamb and impending metritis and septicemia in the ewe.

CAUSES
Nondilation of the cervix

RISK FACTORS
• Risk factors are not well understood.
• There is limited evidence of unknown genetic factors that may predispose to ringwomb.
• Infectious causes including *Chlamydophila ovis* have been implicated; however, many flocks have problems with enzootic abortion and report no significant problems with ringwomb.
• Factors that have been considered in the past but are not supported scientifically include trace mineral deficiencies, exogenous estrogen in feedstuffs, or simple malpresentation of the fetus.

DIAGNOSIS

DIFFERENTIAL DIAGNOSIS
Dystocia, uterine torsion, early dilation syndrome

CBC/BIOCHEMISTRY/URINALYSIS
N/A

OTHER LABORATORY TESTS
N/A

IMAGING
N/A

DIAGNOSTIC PROCEDURES
Vaginal examination readily confirms nondilation of the cervix.

PATHOLOGIC FINDINGS
Often, postmortem examinations are not performed. If performed, gross examination reveals term or near-term fetuses that are fresh or variably autolyzed. The cervix is usually only slightly dilated to allow expulsion of minimal fetal membranes.

TREATMENT

APPROPRIATE HEALTH CARE
• If fetuses are alive, a cesarean section is the most reliable way to achieve a positive outcome for the dam and offspring.
• Hormonal therapy with estrogen may help dilate the cervix, although the response is variable and often delayed.
• Oxytocin may stimulate uterine contractions but if the cervix is not dilated, contractions will be not be productive and will result in uterine tearing.
• Producers will often attempt to manually dilate the cervix with digital pressure. If care is taken, and the cervix is slowly dilated (30 minutes or more) with minimal tearing, live lambs or kids may deliver. More often, this procedure results in delayed delivery with dead fetuses and trauma to the dam's cervix that results in the need to treat aggressively for secondary bacterial infection of the cervix and uterus.

NURSING CARE
N/A

CLIENT EDUCATION
• All the risk factors for ringwomb are not known.
• If manual dilation is attempted, the ewe may need to be culled if significant trauma has occurred to the uterus or cervix. If the producer has examined the dam prior to veterinary intervention, it is an appropriate time to provide education on the zoonotic risks associated with lambing ewes.

 MEDICATIONS

DRUGS OF CHOICE
• Broad-spectrum antibiotics are usually needed as follow-up therapy after manual dilation.
• Estrogen products have been recommended to assist in cervical dilation; however, the effects are minimal and the response is often delayed.
• Oxytocin, 30–50 IU administered IM, will stimulate uterine contractions, however, the cervix is usually not dilated and the uterus may tear or rupture.
• Calcium preparations have been administered as a preventive approach if hypocalcemia is suspected; however, a link between low blood calcium and ringwomb has not been established.

CONTRAINDICATIONS
• Appropriate milk and meat withdrawal times must be followed for all compounds administered to food-producing animals.
• Goats are extremely sensitive to the effects of lidocaine. Care must be utilized when using this drug.

PRECAUTIONS
N/A

POSSIBLE INTERACTIONS
N/A

ALTERNATIVE DRUGS
N/A

 FOLLOW-UP

PATIENT MONITORING
N/A

PREVENTION/AVOIDANCE
N/A

POSSIBLE COMPLICATIONS
N/A

EXPECTED COURSE AND PROGNOSIS
• Affected dams will usually recover if trauma to the cervix is minimized. These individuals will usually conceive and deliver offspring in subsequent pregnancies.
• Secondary infection is usually responsive to antibiotics.
• If trauma to the cervix is severe or the dam is toxic and the fetuses are dead at the time of presentation, the prognosis is poor.

 MISCELLANEOUS

ASSOCIATED CONDITIONS
N/A

AGE-RELATED FACTORS
All ages are affected; first or second parity dams are most commonly affected.

ZOONOTIC POTENTIAL
Any assisted delivery in the ewe and doe has the potential to transmit several zoonotic pathogens including *Chlamydophila abortus*, *Campylobacter jejuni*, and *Coxiella burnetti*. Appropriate safety precautions should be observed.

PREGNANCY
Ringwomb is a condition of parturition. If unresolved quickly, the fetal survival is compromised.

RUMINANT SPECIES AFFECTED
Ovine, caprine, occasionally bovine

BIOSECURITY
N/A

PRODUCTION MANAGEMENT
N/A

SYNONYMS
Nondilation of the cervix

SEE ALSO
Anesthesia and analgesia
NSAIDs

ABBREVIATIONS
NSAIDs = nonsteroidal anti-inflammatory drugs
IM = intramuscular
IU = international units

Suggested Reading
Braun, W. 1997. Parturition and dystocia in the goat. In: *Current therapy in large animal theriogenology*, ed. R. S. Youngquist. Philadelphia: W. B. Saunders.
Challis, J. R. G., Matthews, S. D., Gibb, W., Lye, S. J. 2000. Endocrine and paracrine regulation of birth at term and preterm. *Endocr Rev.* 21(5): 514–550.
Hindson, J. C., Winter, A. C. 2002. *Manual of sheep diseases*. 2nd ed. Oxford: Blackwell Science.
Menzies, P. I., Baily, D. 1997. Lambing management and care. In: *Current therapy in large animal theriogenology*, ed. R. S. Youngquist. Philadelphia: W. B. Saunders.

Author: Larry Holler

RODENTICIDE TOXICITY: 1080 AND 1081

 BASICS

OVERVIEW
• The chemical agents 1080 (sodium monofluoroacetate) and 1081 (sodium fluoroacetamide) were developed as rodenticides and insecticides.
• They are commonly mixed with bread, carrots, bran, and other baits, and treated with black dye (in the United States)
• The product is used only in restricted commercial applications; only certified, insured exterminators can purchase it. In New Zealand, it has broader use.
• Colorless, odorless, tasteless, water soluble
• Highly toxic, at 0.1–8.0 mg/kg to all animals, LD50 mg/kg is 0.39 in cattle, 0.22 in calves
• Poisoning by ingestion of killed rodents, or direct exposure to compound, via the GI and respiratory tracts, abraded, but not intact skin.

PATHOPHYSIOLOGY
• The compound is metabolized to fluorocitrate; the increased citrate decreases cell respiration by blocking the TCA cycle, leading to lactic acidosis, and CNS effects.
• Effects include the overstimulation of the CNS resulting in death by convulsions. This is a common finding in sheep and goats. Also, the alteration of cardiac function leading to myocardial depression, cardiac arrhythmias, ventricular fibrillation, and circulatory collapse.

Species
• All species are potentially affected.
• Sheep and goats more often show neurological signs.

SIGNALMENT
Characterized by a "lag phase" of 30 minutes to 2 hours after ingestion before nervousness and restlessness ensue. Symptoms are generally acute with a rapid violent course.

SIGNS
• About a 30 minute lag phase after ingestion then restlessness and nervousness
• Marked depression and weakness, animals become prostrate, with rapid weak pulse, ventricular fibrillation. Death is by cardiac failure.
• Animals die within hours after symptoms first appear; few animals recover.
• Moaning and teeth grinding may be found with no signs of physical struggle.
• Terminal convulsive seizures, rapid onset with the limbs in fixed rigidity.

CAUSES AND RISK FACTORS

 DIAGNOSIS

DIFFERENTIAL DIAGNOSIS
Strychnine, chlorinated hydrocarbons, lead poisoning, plant alkaloid toxicity, nicotine, taxine (Japanese yew), circutoxin (water hemlock)

CBC/BIOCHEMISTRY/URINALYSIS
Hyperglycemia may be evident.

OTHER LABORATORY TESTS
• Samples included for chemistry evaluation. Primary samples include baits, stomach contents, and liver
• Kidney samples yield high citrate levels.

IMAGING
N/A

DIAGNOSTIC PROCEDURES
History, clinical signs, necropsy findings; rule out other convulsing conditions.

PATHOLOGIC FINDINGS

GROSS FINDINGS
Generalized cyanosis of the mucous membranes and other tissues, liver and kidneys dark and extremely congested, subepicardial hemorrhages evident, heart failure in diastole, diffuse visceral hemorrhages (especially in cattle)

HISTOPATHOLOGICAL FINDINGS
Cerebral edema, lymphocytic infiltration of the CNS

 TREATMENT

No specific antidote

 MEDICATIONS

DRUGS OF CHOICE
• Barbiturates are used with caution
• Ca++ gluconate may be used to combat convulsions and hypocalcemia.

RODENTICIDE TOXICITY: 1080 AND 1081

• Gastric lavage and adsorbents such as activated charcoal 0.5 g/kg may be helpful if early in the toxemia.

• Glyceryl monoacetate (monacetin) may be used as a competitive antagonist of fluoroacetate. The dose of 0.25 ml/lb (0.55ml/kg) IM or IV in 5 parts sterile isotonic saline every 30 minutes for several hours is suggested by some practitioners.

• Oral administration of 8.8 ml/kg each of 50% ethyl alcohol and 5% acetic acid may be substituted for monacetin if the product is unavailable

CONTRAINDICATIONS

Appropriate milk and meat withdrawal times must be followed for all compounds administered to food-producing animals.

 FOLLOW-UP

PATIENT MONITORING
N/A

PREVENTION/AVOIDANCE
N/A

POSSIBLE COMPLICATIONS
N/A

EXPECTED COURSE AND PROGNOSIS
Prognosis grave in advanced cases

 MISCELLANEOUS

ASSOCIATED CONDITIONS
N/A

AGE-RELATED FACTORS
N/A

ZOONOTIC POTENTIAL
N/A

PREGNANCY
N/A

SEE ALSO
Chlorinated hydrocarbons
Lead poisoning
Plant alkaloid toxicity, such as nicotine and taxine (Japanese yew), circutoxin (water hemlock)
Strychnine

ABBREVIATIONS
CNS = central nervous system
IM = intramuscular
IV = intravenous
LD = lethal dose
TCA = tricarboxylic acid cycle, Krebs cycle

Suggested Reading
Burns, R. J., Connolly, G. E. 1995, Feb. Toxicity of compound 1080 livestock protection collars to sheep. *Arch Environ Contam Toxicol*. 28(2): 141–44.

Chi, C. H., Chen, K. W., Chan, S. H., Wu, M. H., Huang, J. J. 1996. Clinical presentation and prognostic factors in sodium monofluoroacetate intoxication. *J Toxicol Clin Toxicol*. 34(6): 707–12.

Eason, C. 2002, Dec 27. Sodium monofluoroacetate (1080) risk assessment and risk communication. *Toxicology* 181–182:523–30.

Eason, C. T., Gooneratne, R., Fitzgerald, H., Wright, G., Frampton, C. 1994, Feb. Persistence of sodium monofluoroacetate in livestock animals and risk to humans. *Hum Exp Toxicol*. 13(2): 119–22.

Ogilvie, S. C., Booth, L. H., Eason, C. T. 1998, May. Uptake and persistence of sodium monofluoroacetate (1080) in plants. *Bull Environ Contam Toxicol*. 60(5): 745–49.

Author: Greg Stonner

RODENTICIDE TOXICITY: ANTICOAGULANTS

 BASICS

OVERVIEW
• Anticoagulant rodenticides are structurally related to coumarin, a compound that causes a prothrombin deficiency, leading to bleeding. Many anticoagulant rodenticides include sulfonamides in the bait, and are utilized to inhibit vitamin K synthesis.
• The original compound, warfarin, was developed after observing that cattle that consumed moldy sweet clover had increased incidences of bleeding.
• Common rodenticides used by professional exterminators and laymen include first and second generation products.
• Toxicity occurs when ruminants (and other mammals and birds) are exposed to rodenticide preparations incorporated into grains and pellets that are palatable to livestock, as in feed barns where they are placed as a deterrent to rodent infestation.
• Signs are not seen for 3–5 days after ingestion.
• A massive single exposure or repeated low dosages may cause poisoning. Repeated doses of 200 mg/kg are toxic.

PATHOPHYSIOLOGY
• Mechanism of action—coumarin anticoagulants competitively inhibit vitamin K by interfering with the conversion of inactive to active vitamin K. This in turn decreases the synthesis of active prothrombin and the conversion of prothrombin to thrombin, essential in the clotting cascade.
• Causes the depression of vitamin K–dependent clotting factors IX of the intrinsic pathway, VII of the extrinsic pathway, and II and X of the common pathway
• Decreased platelet adhesion (but not platelet numbers directly) causes defects in blood coagulation, apparent 2–5 days after ingestion. This latent period can vary according to the type of anticoagulant present, species, dose, and activity during which the clotting factors are used up. Brodifacoum can be present in the plasma for up to 24 days.
• There is no direct hepatotoxicity.

SYSTEMS AFFECTED
Hemolymphatic, reproductive

GENETICS
N/A

INCIDENCE/PREVALENCE
Unknown

GEOGRAPHIC DISTRIBUTION
Worldwide distribution

SIGNALMENT
Most cases are seen in feed-barn situations, where anticoagulant is left as rodent bait.

Species
All ruminants and camelids, as well as other mammals, birds and rodents

Breed Predilections
N/A

Mean Age and Range
N/A

Predominant Sex
N/A

Anticoagulants
• Warfarin, the most well known, and other first generation products are less used because of resistance of rodents to their effects. These are multiple-use poisons, requiring frequent feedings, which reduces their toxicity.
  • Warfarin (final)
  • Pindone (Pival, Pivalyn)
  • Coumafuryl
  • Coumachlor
  • Isovaleryl indandione
• Second generation anticoagulants are highly toxic after a single feeding and include:
  • Bromadiolone (Maki, Contrac)
  • Brodifacoum (Talon, Havoc, d-Con)
• Intermediate anticoagulants require fewer feedings than the first generation chemicals, thus are more toxic than first generation products.
  • Chlorophacinone
  • Diphacinone (Ramik, Ditrac)

SIGNS
• Signs of hemorrhage manifest clinical signs. The onset may appear to be acute, with animals found dead with no previous signs of illness. It can lead to excessive bleeding with routine procedures such as dehorning or castration, or in the presence of wounds or injection sites.

• Bloody diarrhea is the main sign in sheep. Hematomas develop in areas that get jostled, as in tough feeding.
• Early embryonic loss and abortions can additionally be seen with sweet clover poisoning.
• Other signs include anemia, weakness, pale, icteric mucous membranes, eye hemorrhages, dyspnea, hematemesis, epistaxis, melena, blood-tinged froth around the nose and mouth, irregular weak heartbeat, swollen tender joints. If hemorrhage involves the brain, spinal cord—paresis, ataxia, convulsions, and acute death.

CAUSES AND RISK FACTORS
• Toxicity can be influenced by several factors. A high dietary fat intake or prolonged oral antibiotic therapy can increase susceptibility to anticoagulants. Liver disease compounds the affect of vitamin K inhibition by the subsequent decreased prothrombin production.
• Anticoagulants are protein bound for the most part, but it is the unbound portion that is toxic. Protein-bound drugs essentially increase the toxicity by competing for protein binding sites, freeing anticoagulants. Phenylbutazone, sulfonamides, adrenocorticosteroids, and phenobarbital can cause this.

 DIAGNOSIS

Based on history, clinical signs, clinical pathology, and response to treatment of vitamin K 1.

DIFFERENTIAL DIAGNOSIS
• Blackleg, pasturellosis, brakenfern poisoning, and aplastic anemia
• Sweet clover poisoning
• Hepatic toxicants, such as aflatoxicosis (detection in feed, histopathological lesions)
• Causes of thrombocytopenia
• Causes of anemia, bleeding
• Causes of early embryonic death and abortion

CBC/BIOCHEMISTRY/URINALYSIS
• PCV variable, leukocytes and differential normal

- Bleeding time variable, ACT, PT, APTT elevated
- Fibrinogen, fibrin degradation products, platelets normal

OTHER LABORATORY TESTS
- Plasma anticoagulants from live animals
- Anticoagulant levels from necropsy of the liver, GI contents, and unclotted blood

IMAGING
N/A

PATHOLOGIC FINDINGS
- Gross—petichiations, ecchymosis of mucous membranes, free blood in thoracic cavity and /or abdomen, GI hemorrhages
- Histopathological findings—N/A

TREATMENT
- Minimize trauma
- Oxygen therapy
- Whole blood transfusions

MEDICATIONS

DRUGS OF CHOICE
- Vitamin K 1: Controversial use intravenously, has caused anaphylactoid reactions, and IM injections can aggregate bleeding. The dose varies 15–75 mg/kg. Used as a 5% suspension in 5% dextrose. Begins to work in 30 minutes, full effects in several hours.
- IM dose 0.5–2.5 mg/kg
- Oral vitamin K1 is not practical for large ruminants, but dose is 2.5–5.0 mg/kg
- Clotting factor synthesis requires 6–12 hours.
- Duration of treatment depends on the specific compound: warfarin with the shortest half-life at 13.3 hours, brodifacoum 24 days; continue for 3–4 weeks of therapy
- Whole blood transfusions where practical
- Iron preparations

CONTRAINDICATIONS
- Concurrent use of protein-binding drugs can increase toxicity—phenylbutazone, sulfonamides, adrenocorticosteroids.
- Vitamin K 3 as a feed additive is ineffective.
- Appropriate milk and meat withdrawal times must be followed for all compounds administered to food-producing animals.

FOLLOW-UP

PATIENT MONITORING
Monitor CBC, PCV, ACT, PT, APTT

PREVENTION/AVOIDANCE
Avoid contaminated sweet clover, treated grain in feed barns.

POSSIBLE COMPLICATIONS
- Secondary pneumonia
- Death

EXPECTED COURSE AND PROGNOSIS
If sufficient and prolonged treatment can be continued, prognosis is good. The difficulty is early diagnosis and being able to keep sufficient levels of vitamin K 1 systemically for 2–3 weeks, if the more common, longer acting brodifacoums are involved. Concurrent liver disease complicates treatment and worsens prognosis.

MISCELLANEOUS

ASSOCIATED CONDITIONS
Sweet clover poisoning

AGE-RELATED FACTORS
N/A

ZOONOTIC POTENTIAL
N/A

PREGNANCY
Can cause early embryonic death and abortions

SEE ALSO
Aplastic anemia
Blackleg
Braken fern poisoning
Causes of anemia, bleeding
Causes of early embryonic death and abortion
Causes of thrombocytopenia
Hepatic toxicants, such as aflatoxicosis (detection in feed, histopathological lesions)
Pasturellosis
Sweet clover poisoning

ABBREVIATIONS
ACT = activated clotting time
APTT = activated partial thromboplastin time
FDP = fibrin degradation products
PCV = packed cell volume
PT = prothrombin time

Suggested Reading
Aiello, S. E., ed. 1998. *Merck veterinary manual*. 8th ed. Whitehouse Station, NJ: Merck and Co.
Keller, C., Matzdorff, A. C., Kemkes-Matthes, B. 1999. Pharmacology of warfarin and clinical implications. *Semin Thromb Hemost*. 25(1): 13–16.
Roder, J. 2001. Veterinary toxicology. *Practical Veterinarian*, pp. 82–86.
Smith, B.P. 2002. *Large Animal Internal medicine*. 3rd ed. St. Louis: Mosby.
Stirling Y. 1995, Jul. Warfarin-induced changes in procoagulant and anticoagulant proteins. *Blood Coagul Fibrinolysis* 6(5): 361–73.
Van Sittert, N. J., Tuinman, C. P. 1994 Jun, 17. Coumarin derivatives (rodenticides). *Toxicology* 91(1): 71–76.

Author: Greg Stoner

RODENTICIDE TOXICITY: ANTU

BASICS

OVERVIEW
• ANTU is alpha-naphthylthiourea.
• Used exclusively as a rodenticide. Comes as a gray powder, insoluble in water
• Prepared in sausage or bread as bait in 1%–3% concentration
• Causes gastric irritation and increased capillary permeability in the lungs when absorbed.
• Its use has been curtailed, replaced by more effective anticoagulant products.
• Ruminants tend to be resistant.

PATHOPHYSIOLOGY
Causes the increased permeability of pulmonary capillaries, leading to pulmonary edema and pleural effusion.

SYSTEMS AFFECTED
Cardiopulmonary

GENETICS
N/A

INCIDENCE/PREVALENCE
Unknown

GEOGRAPHIC DISTRIBUTION
Potentially worldwide

SIGNALMENT
Species
Cattle primarily, in feedlots and dairies

Breed Predilections
N/A

Mean Age and Range
N/A

Predominant Sex
N/A

SIGNS
• Vomiting, hypersalivation, coughing, dyspnea
• Animals prefer to sit, and then go sternal.
• Severe pulmonary edema, moist rales, cyanosis.
• Dependent signs include weakness, ataxia, rapid, weak pulse, subnormal temperature.
• Death from hypoxia within 2–4 hours of ingestion, animals that survive 12 hours may recover.

DIAGNOSIS

DIFFERENTIAL DIAGNOSIS
• Urea poisoning
• Organophosphate poisoning

CBC/BIOCHEMISTRY/URINALYSIS
N/A

OTHER LABORATORY TESTS
• Chemical tests for thiourea on gastric contents
• Tissues and blood chemical analysis, must be done within 24 hours after exposure

IMAGING
N/A

DIAGNOSTIC PROCEDURES
N/A

PATHOLOGIC FINDINGS

GROSS FINDINGS
• Cyanosis of tissues
• Pulmonary edema, pleura effusion, hydrothorax
• Hyperemia of tracheal mucosa, mild to moderate gastroenteritis, marked hyperemia of the kidneys, pale mottled liver

TREATMENT

MEDICATIONS

DRUGS OF CHOICE
• Emetics before respiratory distress noted, prognosis grave when severe respiratory distress occurs
• Agents providing sulfhydryl groups such as n-amyl mercaptan or sodium thiosulfate may be beneficial.
• For pulmonary edema, O₂ therapy, osmotic diuretic, atropine

CONTRAINDICATIONS
• Decrease environmental stress.
• Appropriate milk and meat withdrawal times must be followed for all compounds administered to food-producing animals.

POSSIBLE INTERACTIONS

FOLLOW-UP

PREVENTION/AVOIDANCE
Keep rodenticides stored away from feeding ruminants.

POSSIBLE COMPLICATIONS
.

EXPECTED COURSE AND PROGNOSIS
Prognosis is grave when severe respiratory distress occurs.

MISCELLANEOUS

ASSOCIATED CONDITIONS
N/A

AGE-RELATED FACTORS
N/A

ZOONOTIC POTENTIAL
N/A

PREGNANCY
Can cause early embryonic death and abortions

SEE ALSO
Organophosphate poisoning
Urea poisoning

ABBREVIATIONS
ANTU = alpha-naphthylthiourea

Suggested Reading
Aiello, S. E., ed. 1998. *Merck veterinary manual*. 8th ed. Whitehouse Station, NJ: Merck and Co.
Buck, W. B., Osweiler, G. D., Van Gelder, G. A. 1976. *Clinical and diagnostic veterinary toxicology*, 2nd ed. Dubuque, Iowa: Kendall-Hunt Publishing Co.
Cheeke, P. D., Shull, L. R. 1985. *Natural toxicants in feeds and poisonous plants*. Westport, Conneticut: AVI Publishing.

Author: Greg Stoner

BASICS

OVERVIEW
• Hundreds of rodenticides are available worldwide.
• Many of these rodenticides were introduced because of their anticipated safety in relation to nontarget species; unfortunately, this has not been the case. Veterinarians must attempt to identify the specific rodenticide involved in poisoning cases.
• Packaged as pelleted, grain-based bait, containing 0.01% (100 ppm) of substance impregnated with green, water-soluble dye.
• The most commonly reported toxicosis in the United States are those caused by anticoagulant rodenticides, bromethalin, cholecalciferol, strychnine, and zinc phosphide.
• Neurotoxin that acts by decreasing, Na/K ATPase activity, uncoupling oxidative phosphorylation in the CNS. This allows CSF pressure increases, placing pressure on nerve axons, resulting in decreases in nerve impulse conduction, paralysis, and death.
• At > 5 mg/kg BW ingestion, acutely see hyperexcitabilty, severe muscle tremors, running fits, grand mal seizures, hind limb hyperreflexia, depression, death about 10 hours after ingestion.

• Chronic effects may appear 24–86 hours after ingestion, characterized by tremors, depression, ataxia, vomiting, and lateral recumbency. These may be reversible if exposure to bromethalin is discontinued.
• The minimum toxic dose is 5 mg/kg body weight. Doses in excess of the LD50 (2 mg/kg in rats) will cause death within 8–12 hours and it is preceded by one to three episodes of clonic convulsions with death usually due to respiratory arrest.
• Brand name products—Vengence, Assault, Trounce.

SYSTEMS AFFECTED
Potentially all, depending on condition

GENETICS
N/A

INCIDENCE/PREVALENCE
N/A

GEOGRAPHIC DISTRIBUTION
Potentially worldwide, depending on species and environment

SIGNALMENT
Species
Potentially all ruminant species

Breed Predilections
N/A

Mean Age and Range
N/A

Predominant Sex
N/A

SIGNS

HISTORICAL FINDINGS
Develop a toxic syndrome characterized by ataxia, focal motor seizures, decerebrate posture, decreased conscious proprioception, recumbency, depression, and semicoma

DIAGNOSIS

• History of ingestion
• Should be considered when see cerebral edema or posterior paralysis
• Chemical analysis of stomach contents, bait, kidney, fat, liver, brain tissue, and necropsy

DIFFERENTIAL DIAGNOSIS
Alcohol intoxication, ethylene glycol, salt poisoning, botulism, rabies

OTHER DIAGNOSTIC PROCEDURES
• Identification of the desmethyl metabolite was demonstrated in the blood and liver of treated animals by comparison of chromatographic retention times to a reference standard, but direct mass spectral identification was unsuccessful in part due to the low dose that could be administered.
• Bromethalin can be detected in kidney, liver, fat, and brain tissues, using gas chromatography with electron capture detection. Photodegradation of extracted bromethalin may limit accurate quantification of tissue residues.

RODENTICIDE TOXICITY: BROMETHALIN

• Identification of the desmethyl metabolite may be demonstrated in the blood and liver of animals by comparison of chromatographic retention times to a reference standard. Direct mass spectral identification is unsuccessful.

PATHOLOGIC FINDINGS

Histopathology

• Diffuse white matter spongiosis with intramyelinic vacuolation. Histopathology of the brain and spinal cord of cats revealed a spongy degeneration of the white matter, which was shown upon ultramicroscopic examination to be intramyelenic edema. No inflammation or cellular destruction of neuronal tissue was noted. LD50 values ranged from 1.8 mg/kg in the cat to approximately 13 mg/kg in rabbits.

• Spongy change (edema characterized by the formation of vacuoles in extracellular spaces and myelin lamellae), hypertrophied fibrous astrocytes, and hypertrophied oligodendrocytes were observed in the white matter of the cerebrum, cerebellum, brain stem, spinal cord, and optic nerve of all bromethalin-dosed cats. Spongy change occasionally extended into contiguous cerebellar Purkinje cell layer and cerebral cortical gray matter. Ultrastructural findings included separation of myelin lamellae at the interperiod lines with the formation of intramyelinic vacuoles (intramyelinic edema), rupture, and coalescence of intramyelinic vacuoles into larger extracellular spaces (spongy change), and pronounced cytosolic edema of astrocytes and oligodendroglial cells.

• LD50 values ranged from 1.8 mg/kg in the cat to approximately 13 mg/kg in rabbits. The only apparent nonsusceptible species was the guinea pig, which could tolerate doses in excess of 1000 mg/kg without effect.

TREATMENT

• Decrease the absorption of toxin and decrease cerebral edema.

• Use mannitol and corticosteroids to decrease cerebral edema.

• Super-activated charcoal repeated because of enterohepatic recycling of bromethalin.

• Treatments may not reverse symptoms.

• Therapeutic success in these poisonings is often more dependent upon symptomatic and supportive care rather than the use of antidotal therapy.

MEDICATIONS

DRUGS OF CHOICE

• Mannitol and corticosteroids to decrease cerebral edema

• Super-activated charcoal repeated because of enterohepatic recycling of bromethalin

CONTRAINDICATIONS

Appropriate milk and meat withdrawal times must be followed for all compounds administered to food-producing animals.

PRECAUTIONS

N/A

POSSIBLE INTERACTIONS

N/A

FOLLOW-UP

PREVENTION/AVOIDANCE
Keep rodenticides away from livestock.

POSSIBLE COMPLICATIONS
N/A

EXPECTED COURSE AND PROGNOSIS
Guarded to grave

MISCELLANEOUS

ASSOCIATED CONDITIONS
Toxic syndrome characterized by ataxia, focal motor seizures, decerebrate posture, decreased conscious proprioception, recumbency, depression, and semicoma

AGE-RELATED FACTORS
N/A

ZOONOTIC POTENTIAL
N/A

PREGNANCY
N/A

RUMINANT SPECIES AFFECTED
Potentially, all ruminant species could be affected.

BIOSECURITY
N/A

PRODUCTION MANAGEMENT
Keep rodenticides away from livestock.

SYNONYMS
N/A

SEE ALSO
Alcohol intoxication
Botulism
Ethylene glycol
Rabies
Salt poisoning

ABBREVIATIONS
BW = body weight
CNS = central nervous system
CSF = cerebral spinal fluid
LD50 = lethal dose 50

Suggested Reading
Dorman, D. C. 1990, Mar. Toxicology of selected pesticides, drugs, and chemicals. Anticoagulant, cholecalciferol, and bromethalin-based rodenticides. *Vet Clin North Am Small Anim Pract*. 20(2): 339–52.
Dorman, D. C., Simon, J., Harlin, K. A., Buck, W. B. 1990, Apr. Diagnosis of bromethalin toxicosis in the dog. *J Vet Diagn Invest*. 2(2): 123–28.
Dorman, D. C., Zachary, J. F., Buck, W. B. 1992, Mar. Neuropathologic findings of bromethalin toxicosis in the cat. *Vet Pathol*. 29(2): 139–44.
Murphy, M. J. 2002, Mar. Rodenticides. *Vet Clin North Am Small Anim Pract*. 32(2): 469–84, viii.
Roder, J. D. 2001. Veterinary toxicology. *The Practical Veterinarian*, pp. 106–9.
Van Lier, R. B., Cherry, L. D. 1988, Nov. The toxicity and mechanism of action of bromethalin: a new single-feeding rodenticide. *Fundam Appl Toxicol*. 11(4): 664–72.

Author: Greg Stoner

RODENTICIDE TOXICITY: CHOLECALCIFEROLS

BASICS

OVERVIEW
• Vitamin D rodenticide causing hypercalcemia by toxic intestinal absorption of calcium, bone resorption, and increased renal retention of calcium. The ingestion of cholecalciferol-containing rodenticide leads to renal failure, cardiac abnormalities, hypertension, central depression, and GI upset.
• Half-life of up to 30 days, duration of several weeks
• Rodents die within 2 days of ingestion.
• Exposure by ingestion of treated feed contaminated with the rodenticide, also by plants such as day jessamine (*Cestrum diurnum*).
• Included in vitamin D–containing vitamins added to cattle rations and given to decrease the occurrence of milk fever.
• Hypercalcemia occurs 12–24 hours postingestion, with concurrent hyperphosphatemia.
• Types of products include Qunintox, Rampage, OrthoMouse B Gone, Ortho Rat B Gone.

Species
All ruminant species can be affected.

SIGNALMENT

SIGNS
• Anorexia, lethargy, depression, polyuria, polydipsia
• As calcium levels rise, clinical signs become more severe as decreased excitability of GI smooth muscle, resulting in anorexia and diarrhea.
• Hematemesis, bloody diarrhea because of dystrophic calcification of the GI tract
• Severe muscle twitching, seizures, stupor
• Loss of renal concentrating ability, mineralization of the kidneys and progressive renal insufficiency
• ECG changes—ventricular fibrillation, hypertension, anorexia, diarrhea, depression, seizures, weakness

CAUSES AND RISK FACTORS
Feed mixing errors, oversupplementation of vitamin D, consumption of rodenticide

DIAGNOSIS

• Based on history of ingestion, clinical signs, hypercalcemia, > 16 mg/dl in the serum is not uncommon
• Gross lesions are associated with hypercalcemia. Pitted mottled kidneys, diffuse hemorrhage of the GI tract, roughened raised plaques on the great vessels and on the surface of the lung and abdominal viscera.

DIFFERENTIAL DIAGNOSIS
• Anticoagulant rodenticide toxicosis
• Neoplasia
• Ingestion of calcinogenic plants—*Solanum, Cestrum, Trisetum*
• Overdose vitamin D supplements

CBC/BIOCHEMISTRY/URINALYSIS
• Hypercalcemia > 11 mg/dl adult
• Hyperphosphatemia before hypercalcemia
• Azotemia, hyperproteinemia, proteinuria, glycosuria, urine specific gravity 1.002–1.006
• Increased 25-hydroxy, 1,25-hydroxycholecalciferol concentrations

OTHER LABORATORY TESTS
Cardiac arrhythmias

IMAGING
Calcification of tissues can be seen in ultrasound/radiology.

DIAGNOSTIC PROCEDURES

PATHOLOGIC FINDINGS

GROSS FINDINGS
Mineralization of kidneys, dystrophic calcification of GI tract

HISTOPATHOLOGICAL FINDINGS
Histopathological examinations revealed diffuse metastatic mineralization throughout the body, particularly involving the lung, kidney, atria, and stomach.

TREATMENT

• The treatment object is to decrease calcium levels in serum—0.9% sodium chloride solution and furosemide (5 mg/kg. IV).
• Activated charcoal 2–8 g/kg BW
• Corticosteroids at 1–2 mg/kg prednisolone BID continued for 2–4 weeks.
• Na bicarb to alkalinize—shifts active calcium to an inactive, unionized form
• If ingestion within 2–4 hours, activated charcoal
• Low-calcium diet
• Monitor BUN/creatinine
• Treatment continued for 2 weeks or more

MEDICATIONS

DRUGS OF CHOICE

CONTRAINDICATIONS
Appropriate milk and meat withdrawal times must be followed for all compounds administered to food-producing animals.

FOLLOW-UP

PATIENT MONITORING
Renal and cardiac functions

PREVENTION/AVOIDANCE
Avoid feed-mixing errors, oversupplementation of vitamin D, and the consumption of rodenticide.

POSSIBLE COMPLICATIONS
Renal and cardiac failure

EXPECTED COURSE AND PROGNOSIS
Good prognosis if treatment started within 4 hours of ingestion and calcium remains normal 72 hours after stopping treatment

MISCELLANEOUS

ASSOCIATED CONDITIONS
N/A

AGE-RELATED FACTORS
N/A

ZOONOTIC POTENTIAL
N/A

PREGNANCY
N/A

SEE ALSO
Rodenticide toxicity

ABBREVIATIONS
Bid = twice daily
BW = body weight
ECG = electrocardiogram
GI = gastrointestinal
IV = intravenous

Suggested Reading
Comments on toxicity of a vitamin D3 rodenticide. 1988, Oct 1. *J Am Vet Med Assoc.* 193(7): 757.
Hollis, B. W., Conrad, H. R., Hibbs, J. W. 1977, Apr. Changes in plasma 25-hydroxycholecalciferol and selected blood parameters after injection of massive doses of cholecalciferol or 25-hydroxycholecalciferol in nonlactating dairy cows. *J Nutr.* 107(4): 606–13.
Littledike, E. T., Horst, R. L. 1982, May. Vitamin D3 toxicity in dairy cows. *J Dairy Sci.* 65(5): 749–59.
Martin, W. B, Aitken I. D. 2000. *Diseases of sheep.* 3rd ed. Oxford, UK: Blackwell Science.
Murphy, M. J. 2002, Mar. Rodenticides. *Vet Clin North Am Small Anim Pract.* 32(2): 469–84, viii.
Roder, J. D. Veterinary toxicology. *The Practical Veterinarian*, pp. 121–26.

Author: Greg Stoner

RODENTICIDE TOXICITY: ZINC PHOSPHIDES

 BASICS

OVERVIEW
• These products are available for rodent control, specifically mice, ground squirrels, rats, and moles. Product is put in bits of bread, in bran mash, soaked wheat, damp rolled oats, sugar at 2.5% concentration.
• Comes as a grayish black powder, insoluble in water, has faint phosphine or acetylene odor
• Causes GI irritation, cardiovascular collapse, and seizuring
• Sold under the names of Zinc Phosphide, MousCon, KilRat, Rumetan
• Toxicity persists for about 2 weeks under average exposure.
• Ruminants are particularly susceptible.
• The toxicity of zinc phosphides is due to the release of phosphine gas in the presence of an acid pH in the stomach. Both the phosphine and intact zinc phosphide are absorbed from the GI tract. The gas causes a direct irritation of the GI tract along with cardiovascular collapse. Intact phosphine causes renal and hepatic damage.
• Toxic dose is 20–40 mg/kg BW, and onset is rapid on a full stomach.

SIGNALMENT
All species of ruminants, especially feedlot cattle

Species
Ruminants especially affected

SIGNS
• Rapid toxemia, occurs 15 minutes to 4 hours after ingestion; can be delayed up to 24–48 hours; death from large doses in 3–5 hours
• Anorexia, weakness, recumbency; rapid, deep respiration, which is wheezy and stertorous, to terminal hypoxia of gasping and struggling
• Ruminal tympany
• Convulsions, aimless running and howling, followed by depression, dyspnea, and convulsions
• Phosphine or acetylene odor to breath, stomach contents

CAUSES AND RISK FACTORS

 DIAGNOSIS

Made by history of exposure, accompanied by rapid death, characterized by dyspnea, pulmonary edema, and visceral congestion

DIFFERENTIAL DIAGNOSIS
Strychnine, fluoroacetate poisoning

CBC/BIOCHEMISTRY/URINALYSIS
N/A

OTHER LABORATORY
• Chemical detection of phosphine gas in stomach contents. Because the gas dissipates rapidly in air, collected sample of stomach contents should be placed in an airtight container and frozen immediately.
• Elevated zinc levels in blood, liver, and kidney

IMAGING
N/A

DIAGNOSTIC PROCEDURES

PATHOLOGIC FINDINGS

GROSS FINDINGS
• Marked congestion of lungs with interlobar edema
• Pleural effusion, subpleural hemorrhages
• Liver and kidney extremely congested acutely
• Subacute, pale yellow mottling of liver
• Stomach contents characteristic odor of acetylene

HISTOPATHOLOGICAL FINDINGS
• Hepatic cloudy swelling, fatty change
• Congestion of liver and kidney
• Renal tubular degeneration, hyaline change, and necrosis

 TREATMENT

• Symptomatic only—antacids, activated charcoal, gastric lavage
• Calcium gluconate, sodium bicarbonate (cattle 2–4 L 5%) PO to neutralize stomach acid
• Sodium thiosulfate, lipotropic agents, dextrose can be used for liver injury.

 MEDICATIONS

DRUGS OF CHOICE

CONTRAINDICATIONS
N/A

POSSIBLE INTERACTIONS

 FOLLOW-UP

PATIENT MONITORING
N/A

PREVENTION/AVOIDANCE
N/A

POSSIBLE COMPLICATIONS
N/A

EXPECTED COURSE AND PROGNOSIS
N/A

 MISCELLANEOUS

ASSOCIATED CONDITIONS

AGE-RELATED FACTORS
N/A

ZOONOTIC POTENTIAL
N/A

PREGNANCY
N/A

ABBREVIATIONS
BW = body weight
PO = per os, by mouth

Suggested Reading
Aiello, S. E., ed. 1998. *Merck veterinary manual*. 8th ed. Whitehouse Station, NJ: Merck and Co.
Buck, W. M., Osweiler, G. D., Van Gelder, G. A. 1976. *Clinical and diagnostic veterinary toxicology*, 2nd ed. Dubuque, IA: Kendall-Hunt Publishing Co.
Cheeke, P. D., Shull, L. R. *Natural toxicants in feeds and poisonous plants*. AVI Publishing, Inc. 1985, pp. 186–188.
Martin, W. B., Aitken, I. D. 2000. *Diseases of sheep*. Third Edition. Blackwell Science LTD. 2000. pp. 357–377.
Morrow, D. A. Current Therapy. In: *Theriogenology*.
Smith, B.P. 2002. *Large Animal internal medicine*. 3rd ed. St. Louis: Mosby.

Author: Greg Stoner

ROTAVIRUS

BASICS

OVERVIEW
- Most common cause of neonatal ruminant diarrhea
- Causative agent—a rotavirus
- There are several serogroups of rotaviruses: A is more common in calves and B (pararotavirus) is more common in kids and lambs.
- Pathogenicity is related to serotype and load of exposure, level of immunity to the virus, concurrent infection with other neonatal pathogens, and stress.
- Most infections are concurrent with other neonatal pathogens.
- Virus may survive for 9 months in the environment.
- Virus is ubiquitous with seroprevalence in the adult herd of 80%–90%.

PATHOPHYSIOLOGY
- The virus is acquired through the ingestion of feces-contaminated material.
- Absorptive epithelial cells lining the distal portions of the villi are infected.
- Epithelial cells of the proximal small intestine are infected first with the infection moving distally to the middle and distal portions of the small intestine.
- Infected cells contain large numbers of virus particles and are desquamated into the lumen.
- The villi become shortened due to exfoliation of the epithelial cells resulting in the loss of digestive enzymes contained within the glycocalyx and decreased absorptive capacity of the villi.
- The loss of epithelial cells results in a maldigestive- as well as a malabsorptive-type diarrhea. Undigested carbohydrates undergo bacterial fermentation resulting in an increase in osmotic pressure and water being drawn into the intestinal lumen. The crypt cells are not affected and continue to secrete fluid resulting in net secretion exceeding absorptive capacity.
- Diarrhea results due to increased osmotic pressure and decreased absorption. The physical loss of the epithelial cells results in increased susceptibility to other pathogens because of loss of the villous integrity and decreased secretion of lactoferrin and lysozymes.
- Damage predisposes the attachment of ETEC and attaching and effacing *E. coli* to the intestinal villi. The loss of electrolytes, bicarbonate, and water leads to dehydration and metabolic acidosis.

SYSTEMS AFFECTED
Gastrointestinal

GENETICS
N/A

INCIDENCE/PREVALENCE
- Prevalence of rotavirus infections ranges from 50% to 100% with a large variation in mortality.
- Depending on immunity, calves may appear normal except for a mild diarrhea. Farmers often report that this "normal" diarrhea is due to the cow producing too much milk.

SIGNALMENT

SPECIES
Bovine, caprine, and ovine

Breed Predilections
N/A

Mean Age and Range
- Most infections occur within the first week of life.
- Range—1 day to 3 weeks

Predominant Sex
N/A

SIGNS

GENERAL COMMENTS
- Clinical signs will vary from mild to severe diarrhea. In the case of uncomplicated disease, diarrhea may exist for 1 to 2 days.
- In cases of secondary bacterial infection, diarrhea may last from 3 to 5 days.

HISTORICAL FINDINGS
- Sudden onset of diarrhea that spreads rapidly through the neonatal population
- A few cases may have been noticed initially but the frequency of cases increases as the calving season progresses.
- Increased number of cases is observed following periods of stress such as a snowstorm or cold, wet weather.
- Individuals may develop diarrhea at the same day of age.

PHYSICAL EXAMINATION
- Mild to severe watery, yellow diarrhea; color, consistency, and composition will vary with coexisting infections.
- Dehydration and depression with degrees of inappetence or reluctance to nurse
- Some animals may be weak to the point of recumbency.

CAUSES
- Rotavirus serogroup A most common in calves
- Rotavirus serogroup B, pararotavirus in small ruminants

RISK FACTORS
- Inadequate colostral transfer of immunoglobulins resulting in agammaglobulinemia or hypogammaglobulinemia
- Lack of local colostral immunity in the case of neonates fed milk replacers
- Lack of specific antibodies against the infective serogroup or type of rotavirus in colostrum
- Birthing areas contaminated with fecal material containing rotavirus
- Neonatal housing in which buildup of pathogen load occurs
- Neonates housed or maintained in a cold, wet environment.

DIAGNOSIS

DIFFERENTIAL DIAGNOSIS
- *E. coli*, coronavirus, cryptosporidia, *Salmonella* spp., *Clostridium perfringens* type C are disease agents that cause diarrhea during the first 3 weeks of life.
- Nutritional causes of diarrhea may be differentiated from rotaviral diarrhea if history contains a dietary change or identification of nutritional deficiencies or excesses.

CBC/BIOCHEMISTRY/URINALYSIS
- CBC: hemoconcentration, increased plasma proteins
- Serum chemistry: metabolic acidosis with low plasma bicarbonate; glucose and electrolyte values will be low depending on severity of diarrhea.

OTHER LABORATORY TESTS
- Feces should be collected as soon as diarrhea is noted because exfoliation of virus-laden enterocytes is short-lived and occurs early in the disease process.
- Feces can be submitted for electron microscopy and identification of virus. A few drops of formalin can be added to 10 cc of feces.
- Feces can be submitted for ELISA and latex agglutination tests for detection of viral antigens.
- Fresh sections of the small intestine, preferably midileum, tied at the cut ends to contain intestinal contents can be submitted on cold packs for fluorescent antibody testing. An in-house ELISA can be used to detect viral antigens of serogroup A in feces (Rotazyme II kit, Abbott Laboratories, Abbott Park, Ill).

PATHOLOGIC FINDINGS
- No gross lesions except for increased fluid contents throughout the intestinal tract.
- Histopathology: intestinal villi are shortened.

TREATMENT

APPROPRIATE HEALTH CARE
N/A

NURSING CARE
- Fluid therapy is needed to correct dehydration, circulatory impairment, and electrolyte and metabolic imbalances.
- Fluid deficit should be calculated as well as maintenance requirement, 80–100 ml/kg, to determine volume of fluids needed during a 24-hour period.
- Fluid may be administered orally or intravenously. Commercial oral electrolyte solutions containing glucose and an alkalinizing agent are recommended if the

neonate is still nursing. Although oral electrolytes are less likely to be absorbed due to enterocyte pathology, not all enterocytes are affected so some absorption may occur.
• Neonates without a suckle response need IV fluids. IV administration of lactated Ringer's solution is adequate.
• With severe acidosis, isotonic sodium bicarbonate solution (1.3%, 13 of sodium bicarbonate to 1 L of distilled water) may be utilized.
• Dextrose solutions (2.5%–5%) are indicated in cases of hypoglycemia. With hypoglycemia and an unknown electrolyte and acid-base status, a 2.5% dextrose and 0.45% saline solution has been recommended.

ACTIVITY
N/A

DIET
• Neonates with a suckle response should be left with the dam and allowed to nurse.
• Animals being reared artificially should remain on their diet or switched to whole milk or colostrum. If the diarrhea becomes worse or the calf becomes depressed, removal from the dam or milk is warranted.
• In case of hand-fed neonates that are depressed and not interested in suckling, or neonates not nursing the dam, neonates should receive a high-energy electrolyte solution at a rate of 10% of body weight divided into a minimum of four feedings. Once neonates are suckling, feed milk at 5% of body weight in four feedings a day. Increase amount per feeding gradually so calf is back on full feed within 2 to 3 days.
• Oral electrolytes containing an alkalinizing agent, other than acetate, should not be fed when calves are receiving milk as milk digestion may be disrupted.

CLIENT EDUCATION
• Neonates should be kept dry and in a draft-free environment.
• Animals should be moved and fed in such a way as to reduce the buildup of mud and fecal material in the neonate's environment.
• Diarrheic animals should be isolated from healthy neonates as they are sources for large numbers of pathogens.

MEDICATIONS

DRUGS OF CHOICE
• Broad-spectrum antibiotics may be considered because of the potential for mixed infections as well as the loss of mucosal integrity.
• In the case of a true viral infection, antibiotics are not warranted.
• Oral amoxicillin trihydrate 10 mg/kg PO q 12 h for nonruminating calves, 20-day slaughter withdrawal (extralabel in small ruminants). Amoxicillin trihydrate-clavulanate potassium 12.5 mg combined drug/kg PO q 12 h for 3 days (extralabel usage).

• Parenteral ceftiofur 2.2 mg/kg IM/SC q 24 h for 3 days (extralabel usage).
• Drug withdrawal times must be determined and maintained in the treated animal.
• Plasma transfusion: Although not specific for rotaviral infections, in cases of failure of passive transfer and depending on value of the animal, plasma transfusion may be warranted.

CONTRAINDICATIONS
• Do not use kaolin and pectin as this may increase electrolyte loss.
• Appropriate milk and meat withdrawal times must be followed for all compounds administered to food-producing animals.

FOLLOW-UP

PATIENT MONITORING
• Monitor attitude, suckling response and appetite, fecal color and consistency, and hydration status every 6–12 hours.
• Monitor age cohorts for signs of diarrhea.

POSSIBLE COMPLICATIONS
Hypovolemic shock

PREVENTION/AVOIDANCE
• Reduce viral exposure by calving in clean maternity areas and moving to a clean area after birth.
• Those handling sick neonates should practice biosecurity measures to reduce exposure to healthy neonates; wash hands and disinfect boots, maintain clothes free of fecal material.
• Vaccination of dams prepartum according to manufacturers' recommendations with a rotaviral vaccine may increase colostral antibody. Effectiveness will be dependent on field virus serogroup and type and that contained in the vaccine.
• Oral vaccination of neonate with a modified live oral vaccine will produce IgA and IgM. This vaccine is cumbersome for management as it is to be given prior to colostrum consumption and colostrum must be withheld after vaccination. This may increase the opportunity for bacterial infections and failure of passive transfer.
• Eliminate areas of fecal buildup.
• Keep environment dry and draft free.

EXPECTED COURSE AND PROGNOSIS
• In uncomplicated infections, diarrhea is present for 1 to 2 days.
• Prognosis is good, as this infection tends to be self-limiting and generally requires minor supportive care.
• Duration of diarrhea may be 3 to 5 days with secondary bacterial infections.
• Prognosis is dependent on the degree of pathology produced by the secondary bacteria.
• Prognosis is good to fair with supportive care.

MISCELLANEOUS

AGE-RELATED FACTORS
• Most cases less than a week of age
• Range: 1 day to 3 weeks

ZOONOTIC POTENTIAL
• Isolates from neonatal ruminants have not been infective to humans.
• Some human isolates have been found to be infective for calves.

RUMINANT SPECIES AFFECTED
Bovine, caprine, ovine

SYNONYMS

SEE ALSO
Clostridium perfringens type C
Coronavirus
Cryptosporidia
E. coli
Nutritional causes of diarrhea
Salmonella spp.

ABBREVIATIONS
CBC = complete blood count
ELISA = enzyme-linked immunosorbent assay
ETEC = enterotoxigenic *E. coli*
IM = intramuscular
IV = intravenous
PO = per os, by mouth
SC = subcutaneous

Suggested Reading
Barrington, G. M., Gay, J. M., Evermann, J. F. 2002, Mar. Biosecurity for neonatal gastrointestinal diseases. *Vet Clin North Am Food Anim Pract*. 18(1):7–34.
Bendali, F., Sanaa, M., Bichet, H., Schelcher, F. 1999, Sep-Oct. Risk factors associated with diarrhoea in newborn calves. *Vet Res*. 30(5):509–22.
Constable, P. D. 2004. Antimicrobial use in the treatment of calf diarrhea. *J Vet Intern Med*. 18:8–17.
Naylor, J. M. 2002. Neonatal ruminant diarrhea. In: *Large animal internal medicine*, ed. B. P. Smith. 3rd ed. St. Louis: Mosby.
Torres-Medina, A., Schlafer, D., Medus, C. 1985. Rotaviral and coronaviral diarrhea. In: *The veterinary clinics of North America, food animal practice*. Philadelphia: W. B. Saunders.
Townsend, H. G. 1994, Mar. Environmental factors and calving management practices that affect neonatal mortality in the beef calf. *Vet Clin North Am Food Anim Pract*. 10(1):119–26.

Author: Kevin D. Pelzer

RUMEN DYSFUNCTION: ALKALOSIS

BASICS

OVERVIEW
Form of gastrointestinal indigestion resulting from rumen inactivity or toxic ingestion

SIGNALMENT
• Any age ruminating animal
• Generally adults

SIGNS
• Forestomach dysfunction
• Bloat
• Decreased appetite
• Rumen hypomotility
• Signs of abdominal pain
• Vomiting
• Signs of urea toxicosis
• CNS excitation
• Diarrhea
• General rumen dysfunction: Rumen fluid pH 7.5–8.5; strong odor of ammonia
• Incoordination
• Muscle tremors
• Rapid deterioration and death
• Tachypnea
• Weakness

CAUSES AND RISK FACTORS
• Mild alkalosis (Rumen pH 7.0–7.5)
  • Prolonged anorexia
  • Microfloral inactivity
  • Poorly digestible roughage
  • Some cases of simple indigestion
  • Pathogenesis: animal continues to produce and swallow alkaline saliva, while low rate of rumen fermentation produces insufficient acid to neutralize saliva.
  • Absorption of VFAs, especially acetate, across rumen wall is associated with bicarbonate generation in the rumen fluid. Acetate is the primary VFA generated from roughage.
  • Generation and absorption of VFAs continues, although at a low rate, further contributing to the alkaline state of the rumen.
• Severe alkalosis (rumen pH >7.5)
  • Overfeeding/accidental overingestion of NPN sources: Urea, biuret, ammonium phosphate, ammonium-salt-containing fertilizers

DIAGNOSIS

DIFFERENTIAL DIAGNOSIS
Other forms of indigestion:
• Lactic acidosis
• Simple indigestion
• Vagal indigestion
• Other systemic or primary disease-causing anorexia

CBC/BIOCHEMISTRY/URINALYSIS
• Consistent with dehydration: Increases in hematocrit, BUN, creatinine, total protein
• Stress leukocytosis
• Hypokalemia
• Hypocalcemia
• Alkalemia

OTHER LABORATORY TESTS
Rumen fluid analysis:
• Alkaline pH
• Poor microbial activity under light microscopy

IMAGING
N/A

DIAGNOSTIC PROCEDURES
Ruminocentesis/orogastric tubing for rumen fluid analysis (see Other Laboratory Tests above)

GROSS FINDINGS
• If fresh, rumen fluid pH of 7.5–8.5
• Rumen contents may have distinct odor of ammonia if NPN overfeeding is the cause

HISTOPATHOLOGICAL FINDINGS

TREATMENT
• Identify and manage primary disease.
• Correct acid-base and electrolyte aberrations with appropriate fluid therapy: Potassium and calcium will likely be low.
• Establish normal rumen volume.
  • Increase volume with transfaunation of 8–16 L and balanced oral electrolytes.
  • Decrease volume by removing abnormal rumen infests by siphon or rumenotomy.
  • Resolve rumen impaction.
• May provide acetic acid 4–10 L PO

MEDICATIONS

DRUGS
Supplement with parenteral or oral vitamins and minerals—particularly B vitamins

CONTRAINDICATIONS
Do not administer magnesium hydroxide if rumen alkalosis is present.

FOLLOW-UP

PATIENT MONITORING
• Monitor patient for return to appetite and normal rumen motility.
• May require repeat transfaunations

PREVENTION/AVOIDANCE
Good feed management:
• Provision of quality digestible feedstuffs
• Proper dosing of NPN sources
• Securing fertilizers

POSSIBLE COMPLICATIONS
Rumen putrefaction:
• High rumen pH and repeated inoculation with abnormal bacteria such as coliforms and *Proteus* spp. leads to putrefactive decomposition of feeds.
• Sources of putrefactive bacteria: spoiled or feces-contaminated feed

EXPECTED COURSE AND PROGNOSIS
• If mild case is caused by poor quality roughage, it may be easily corrected with transfaunation and gradual provision of good quality feeds.
• If severe alkalosis is caused by intoxication, rumenotomy or other rumen evacuation method may be required, along with rumen fluid replacement and supportive care: poor prognosis.

MISCELLANEOUS

ASSOCIATED CONDITIONS
Rumen putrefaction

AGE-RELATED FACTORS
N/A

ZOONOTIC POTENTIAL
N/A

PREGNANCY
N/A

RUMINANT SPECIES AFFECTED
Any ruminant species affected, primarily occurs in cattle

BIOSECURITY
N/A

PRODUCTION MANAGEMENT
Prevention requires good management of feedstuffs and good security of fertilizer storage.

SEE ALSO
Lactic acidosis
Other forms of indigestion
Other systemic or primary disease causing anorexia
Simple indigestion
Vagal indigestion

ABBREVIATIONS
BUN = blood urea nitrogen
NPN = nonprotein nitrogen
VFA = volatile fatty acids

Suggested Reading
Garry, F. B. 2002. Indigestion in ruminants: rumen alkalosis. In: *Large animal internal medicine*, ed. B. P. Smith. 3rd ed. St. Louis: Mosby.
Gartley, C., Ogilvie, T. H., Butler, D. G. 1981, April. Magnesium oxide contraindicated as a cathartic for cattle in the absence of rumen acidosis. *The Bovine Proceedings* 13:17–19.

Author: Meredyth Jones

RUPTURED PREPUBIC TENDON

BASICS

OVERVIEW
• A ruptured prepubic tendon (RPT), which is a life threatening complication of pregnancy, affects the bovine and ovine species.
• It involves tearing of the elastic tendons that attach the abdominal muscles to the pelvic bone.
• The prepubic tendon and its associated musculature help hold the pelvis in position.
• Once it ruptures it reduces the amount of support available for the gravid uterus, resulting in signs affecting the musculoskeletal, reproductive, and gastrointestinal systems.

SIGNALMENT
• A rare condition of ruminants
• Most reported cases involve older animals that are either late in gestation or have a prolonged gestation.

SIGNS
• An extremely sagging pendulous abdomen.
• A severely painful edema of the lower abdominal cavity extending from the udder to the xiphoid cartilage.
• The pelvic bone, tail head, and ischial tuberosities appear abnormally tilted due to the loss of their cranial tension.
• Generalized depression and discomfort with a reluctance to move.
• Pain associated signs like a stretched stance, tachycardia, tachypnea, and intermittent colic.
• With a sudden and complete rupture, shock, collapse, and death may result.

CAUSES AND RISK FACTORS
• A prolonged gestation
• An extremely gravid uterus from a pathological pregnancy like twins or fetal membrane dropsy.
• Trauma to the prepubic area
• Newborn survival may be questionable due to a reduction in blood supply from stretching or twisting of the umbilical cord.
• A possibility for bowel entrapment

DIAGNOSIS

DIFFERENTIAL DIAGNOSIS
• Severe ventral edema
• Rupture of abdominal musculature leading to a ventral hernia
• Intramuscular or subcutaneous hematoma

CBC/BIOCHEMISTRY/ URINALYSIS
N/A

OTHER LABORATORY TESTS
N/A

IMAGING
• Abdominal ultrasound will reveal extensive fluid.
• The location and size of a ventral hernia may be established with abdominal ultrasound.

DIAGNOSTIC PROCEDURES
• Rectal palpation is typically unrewarding.
• Palpation of the ventral abdominal wall will reveal edema and a pain response.

TREATMENT

• Immediate veterinary attention required.
• Deliver the fetus by cesarean section or induce parturition if near term.
• Fetal maturity needs to be considered for parturition induction.
• Adequate mammary gland development, good-quality colostrum, and a relaxed cervix indicate fetal maturity.
• Induced parturition requires close observation since the animal will lack the ability to produce adequate abdominal pressure for fetal expulsion.
• If fetus is not near term and the rupture is gradual, alternative therapy will be required.
• Restrict activity to a small pen or box stall.
• An abdominal sling consisting of a strong bandage may provide some support for the gravid uterus.
• The abdominal sling needs to be well padded over the backline to prevent pressure necrosis.
• Laxatives and a high-concentrate diet may decrease the amount of bowel contents and the exertion associated with defecation.
• If supportive therapy fails, abortion induction may be needed.
• Surgical repair of a RPT is impossible.
• Euthanasia of the animal may be necessary if there are associated complications like bowel entrapment.

MEDICATIONS

DRUGS OF CHOICE
N/A

CONTRAINDICATIONS
• Appropriate milk and meat withdrawal times must be followed for all compounds administered to food-producing animals.
• Steroids should not be used in pregnant animals.

FOLLOW-UP

PATIENT MONITORING
• Closely monitor for further development of discomfort.
• Watch for signs of bowel entrapment.
• Newborn may have difficulty nursing due to the extensive abdominal edema.

PREVENTION/ AVOIDANCE
• Do not rebreed due to the likelihood that the condition will reoccur during the next pregnancy.
• Promote embryo transfer if further offspring are wanted from the animal.

POSSIBLE COMPLICATIONS
Bowel entrapment.

EXPECTED COURSE AND PROGNOSIS
Regardless of treatment method, the fetus and mother may be lost depending on the extent of the condition.

MISCELLANEOUS

ASSOCIATED CONDITIONS
A ventral hernia may be an associated condition of a RPT.

AGE-RELATED FACTORS
Older, multiparous females are predisposed for a RPT.

ZOONOTIC POTENTIAL
N/A

PREGNANCY
Appears to occur only as a complication of pregnancy

BIOSECURITY
N/A

PRODUCTION MANAGEMENT
N/A

RUMINANT SPECIES AFFECTED
Bovine and ovine

SEE ALSO
Anesthesia and analgesia
Euthanasia and disposal
Intramuscular or subcutaneous hematoma
NSAIDs
Rupture of abdominal musculature leading to a ventral hernia
Severe ventral edema

ABBREVIATIONS
NSAIDs = nonsteroidal anti-inflammatory drugs
RPT = ruptured prepubic tendon

Suggested Reading
Aiello, S. E., Mays, A., ed. 1998. *Merck veterinary manual*. 8th ed. Whitehouse Station, NJ: Merck & Co.
Mirza, M. H., Paccamonti, D., Martin, G. S., Ramirez, S., Pinto, C. 1997, Nov 15. Theriogenology question of the month. Rupture of the prepubic tendon with additional tearing of the abdominal tunic. *J Am Vet Med Assoc.* 211(10):1237–38.
Penzhorn, B. L., Gilbert, R. O. 1985, Jun. Hydrallantois in a bovine leading to rupture of the prepubic tendon and abdominal musculature. *J S Afr Vet Assoc.* 56(2):115.
Perkins, N. R., Frazer, G. S. 1994, Dec. Reproductive emergencies in the mare. *Vet Clin North Am Equine Pract.* 10(3):643–70.
Whalen, R. F. 1956, Dec 1. Rupture of the prepubic tendon in a cow. *J Am Vet Med Assoc.* 129(11):509–10.

Author: Lucas C. Clow

RYEGRASS STAGGERS—LOLITREM B

BASICS

OVERVIEW
• Ryegrass staggers is caused primarily by an endophyte fungus *Acremonium lolii*, which lives in the lower leaves and stems of infected ryegrass, *Lolium perenne*. If the ryegrass is infected with the fungus, it produces lolitrem B, which causes transient tremors in cattle and sheep after ingestion.
• Lolitrem B is an indole diterpine alkaloid that interferes with neuronal transmission in the cerebral cortex of affected animals.
• It is likely that ryegrass staggers is due to many other toxins and toxigenic organisms, often referred to as corynetoxins.
• *Penicillium janthinellum* Biourge, also a fungus, is found on ryegrass pasture and produces janithitrems, a tremorgenic toxin that, when irradiated with long wave ultraviolet light, fluoresces a blue color.
• There is also a bacterial agent, *Clavibacter toxicus*, which produces annual ryegrass toxicity (ARGT) in Australia.
• Dallisgrass, *Paspalum dilatatum*, may be present in the ryegrass pasture, and may be infested with an ergotlike fungus, *Claviceps paspali*.
• Signs of ryegrass staggers can take up to 7 days to manifest and, although there is a high morbidity (50%–90%), the mortality is quite low (0%–5%).
• Effects are usually transient and disappear within 2 weeks of removal of affected forage. There is a nearly complete recovery.

SYSTEMS AFFECTED
Neurologic, production management

GENETICS
Individual susceptibility varies and is heritable.

INCIDENCE/PREVALENCE
Mortality from annual ryegrass toxicity is commonly 40%–50%.

GEOGRAPHIC DISTRIBUTION
Worldwide, where ryegrass is grown.

SIGNALMENT
Animals that are most commonly affected graze on ryegrass pastures in the late summer to fall months.

SIGNS
Animals appear normal at rest, with an occasional fine tremor, but with stimulation, they exhibit a stiff, spastic gait, hypermetria, head nodding, and ataxia. They often fall onto their chest and exhibit opisthotonus and titanic seizures. The animals then recover, but can repeat these signs with stimulation again. The signs are more severe with heat stress. Most deaths are accidental due to drowning when they fall into bodies of water or due to the inability to eat or drink.

CAUSES AND RISK FACTORS
• The risk factor seems to be heritable.
• There is also an increased risk with ryegrass pasture grazing in the late summer to fall months.

DIAGNOSIS

Diagnosis is by clinical signs and microscopic identification of the tremorgenic substrate endophyte in the ryegrass sheaths.

DIFFERENTIAL DIAGNOSIS
• Perennial ryegrass
• Phalaris
• Ergots of paspalum and other grasses
• Polioencephalomalacia
• Enterotoxemia

CBC/BIOCHEMISTRY/URINALYSIS
N/A

OTHER LABORATORY TESTS
• Chromatography for lolitrem
• Bioassay on vomitus or urine for lolitrem
• Check for fluorescence of janthitrem.

IMAGING
N/A

DIAGNOSTIC PROCEDURES
• Microscopic identification of the endophyte hyphae within the ryegrass sheaths.
• Bacterium in seed heads is detected and quantified by ELISA.

PATHOLOGIC FINDINGS

GROSS FINDINGS
N/A

HISTOPATHOLOGICAL FINDINGS
• None recognized in acute cases.
• Cerebellar Purkinje cell degeneration and necrosis in long-standing or severe cases.

TREATMENT

• Removing animals from the affected feed and letting them rest will allow for recovery in 3–7 days.
• It is usually impractical to treat because handling exacerbates the signs.
• In severe cases, you could administer anesthesia to help alleviate the seizures and administer activated charcoal and saline cathartics orally.

MEDICATIONS

N/A

CONTRAINDICATIONS
Appropriate milk and meat withdrawal times must be followed for all compounds administered to food-producing animals.

FOLLOW-UP

PATIENT MONITORING
Keep the animal quiet and restful while providing fluids to prevent dehydration.

PREVENTION/AVOIDANCE
• Prevention is primarily by grazing management. Don't overgraze pastures, especially in the dangerous season, as the toxic endophyte is on the lower leaf sheaths.
• Encourage the growth of other grasses.
• Use ryegrass seed that is endophyte free or has been stored for 18 to 24 months.

POSSIBLE COMPLICATIONS
N/A

EXPECTED COURSE AND PROGNOSIS
Most animals recover nearly completely within 2 weeks of removal of the affected feed.

MISCELLANEOUS

ASSOCIATED CONDITIONS
N/A

AGE-RELATED FACTORS
N/A

ZOONOTIC POTENTIAL
The alkaloids do not accumulate in fat or muscle so residues are not considered a problem.

PREGNANCY
N/A

RUMINANT SPECIES AFFECTED
Potentially, all ruminant species can be affected.

BIOSECURITY
• Isolation and quarantine of new stock entering the herd/flock.
• Treat and or cull new animals for disease conditions prior to herd introduction.

PRODUCTION MANAGEMENT
Burning annual ryegrass pastures destroys most of the galls colonized by bacteria. This will minimize the risk of subsequent toxicity.

SYNONYMS
Rye grass stagers

SEE ALSO
Enterotoxemia
Ergots of paspalum and other grasses
Perennial ryegrass
Phalaris
Polioencephalomalacia
Toxicologic herd outbreak

ABBREVIATIONS
ARGT = annual ryegrass toxicity
ELISA = enzyme-linked immunosorbent assay

Suggested Reading
Aiello, S. E., ed. 1998. *Merck veterinary manual*. 8th ed. Whitehouse Station, NJ: Merck & Co.
Galey, F. D., et al. 1991, Aug 15. Staggers induced by consumption of perennial ryegrass in cattle and sheep from northern California. *J Am Vet Med Assoc*. 199(4):466–70.
Odriozola, E., Lopez, T., Campero, C., Gimenez Placeres, C. 1993, Apr. Ryegrass staggers in heifers: a new mycotoxicosis in Argentina. *Vet Hum Toxicol*. 35(2):144–46.
Osweiler, G. D. 1996. Tremorgens. In: *Toxicology*. Media, PA: Williams and Wilkins.
Plumlee, K. H., Galey, F. D. 1994, Jan-Feb. Neurotoxic mycotoxins: a review of fungal toxins that cause neurological disease in large animals. *J Vet Intern Med*. 8(1):49–50.

Author: Heidi Coker

SALMONELLOSIS

 BASICS

DEFINITION
Salmonellosis refers to the clinical symptoms that result from a bacterial infection with a serotype of *Salmonella*.

OVERVIEW
• *Salmonella* infections are the second most economically important bacterial disease affecting the gastrointestinal system in ruminants.
• The severity of the disease is dependent on the serovar involved in the infection and the immune status of the animal.
• Infections in young animals are most often a result of contaminated environments.
• Outbreaks in adults are associated with stress and exposure to a virulent serovar.

Causative Agent
• One of the 2002 serovars of *Salmonella* spp.
• *Salmonella typhimurium* is the most common serovar isolated from ruminants, but all serovars are potentially capable of causing disease.
• *Salmonella dublin* is host adapted to cattle and *S. Arizona* and *abortus ovis* (uncommon in North America) to sheep.

PATHOPHYSIOLOGY
• *Salmonella* are generally acquired through the fecal oral route.
• Carrier cows may secrete organisms directly into milk, especially *S. dublin*.
• Young calves are susceptible to infection because the organism can easily pass through the rumen and the abomasum. There are no volatile fatty acids in the rumen to kill the bacteria nor is the abomasal pH low enough to kill the organism.
• The organism attaches, via adhesins, to mucosal cells of the ileum, cecum, and colon. The organism then invades epithelial cells, spreading through the mucosa to lymphoid tissue and into the blood stream.
• Various virulence and host factors determine the extent of damage and invasiveness of the organism.

• The organism secretes exotoxins that stimulate fluid secretions and damage host cells. In addition, lipopolysaccharide (LPS) is released during replication and death. These LPSs stimulate the inflammatory cascade leading to tissue damage, cardiovascular collapse, and signs of toxemia.
• Diarrhea results from increased cellular secretions, malabsorption, and maldigestion due to mucosal damage and the inflammatory response.

SYSTEMS AFFECTED
Gastrointestinal, hepatic, musculoskeletal, renal, nervous, respiratory, and cardiovascular

GENETICS
N/A

INCIDENCE/PREVALENCE
• As farm size and concentration of animals have increased, so has the incidence of disease.
• Once an outbreak has occurred on a farm, the environmental prevalence of the organisms may be high, but the incidence of clinical disease is actually low.
• The farm prevalence of *Salmonella* was determined to be 11.2% for cow-calf operations and 30% for dairy operations based on the National Animal Health Monitoring System.

SIGNALMENT
Species
Bovine, caprine, and ovine
Breed Predilections
N/A
Mean Age and Range
• Most infections occur from 14 days to 2 months of age.
• All animals, regardless of age, are at risk of developing salmonellosis.

PREDOMINANT SEX
N/A

SIGNS

GENERAL COMMENTS
• The disease may have three different presentations, including peracute, acute, and chronic.
• Acute infections may result in a chronic state.

• Depending on the virulence of the specific serotype and immune status of the host, the organism may be contained within the intestinal tract or invade the circulatory system resulting in multiple organ pathology.
• Clinical signs are often associated with the release of endotoxins and the development of endotoxemia.
• Animals may be convalescent carriers up to 6 months.

HISTORICAL FINDINGS
• Salmonellosis in animals older then 3 months of age is often associated with the introduction of a carrier animal into the herd as well as recent exposure to new water or feed sources.
• Periods of stress such as grouping of animals, late pregnancy, parturition, transport, feed or water deprivation, surgery, or antibiotic usage are often associated with cases or outbreaks.

PHYSICAL EXAMINATION FINDINGS
Peracute
• May observe anorexia, depression, right-sided abdominal distension, and dehydration prior to sudden death
• Signs of overwhelming septicemia, meningitis, opisthotonus, and convulsions may be observed.
• Signs of diarrhea and colic are not common consistent findings.

Acute
• Most frequently encountered state
• Animals exhibit enteritis, fever, anorexia, depression, and dehydration.
• Feces initially are watery in nature becoming voluminous with a foul odor and may contain shreds of mucosa, casts, and frank blood.
• Animals are severely dehydrated, have sunken eyes, and may be too weak to stand.
• Body temperature initially is elevated but decreases and may be subnormal in the terminal stages of the disease.
• Calves infected with *S. dublin* are unthrifty in appearance, weak, and anorectic, and die acutely.
• Many of these calves will develop meningoencephalitis, polyarthritis, osteomyelitis, and pneumonia.

- Adult animals exhibit fever, anorexia, diarrhea, and dehydration, and pregnant animals often abort.
- Heat stress exacerbates clinical signs.

Chronic Infections
- Occurs in older animals 6–8 weeks of age.
- These animals fail to thrive, stools may be puddinglike to diarrheic.
- The animal's body temperature may be normal to slightly elevated; animals have poor hair coats and are undersized.

CAUSES
- The most frequently isolated serotypes from cattle include *Salmonella enterica Typhimurium, Montevideo, Dublin, Newport,* and *Uganda*.
- *Salmonella enterica Typhimurium, Dublin,* and *Arizona* are frequently isolated serotypes of sheep and goats.

RISK FACTORS
- Inadequate colostral transfer of immunoglobulins resulting in agammaglobulinemia or hypogammaglobulinemia.
- Birthing areas contaminated with fecal material containing *Salmonella* spp.
- Crowding and poor sanitation increases pathogen concentration and decreases host immunity.
- Use of common feeding/manure moving implements and improper cleaning between uses.
- Late gestation, parturition, and induction of lactation are physiological stressors.
- Factors that reduce immunity or cause alterations in microbial gut flora—transportation, concurrent disease, anesthesia, surgery, feed changes, antimicrobial therapy, and withholding food and water.

DIAGNOSIS

DIFFERENTIAL DIAGNOSIS
- Diarrhea may result from a variety of infectious agents as well as nutritional causes.

- *Clostridium perfringens* type C and *E. coli* occur during the first week of life.
- *Cryptosporidia*, rotavirus, and coronavirus are disease agents that cause diarrhea during the first 3 weeks of life.
- Salmonellosis develops after 2 weeks of age and is usually associated with a fever; the other agents generally are not associated with a fever.
- Differential diagnosis in animals older than 1 month of age are dietary changes, indigestion, lactic acidosis, toxicosis, BVD, and winter dysentery.

CBC/BIOCHEMISTRY/URINALYSIS
- CBC—Hemoconcentration: a slight anemia may exist but is masked by dehydration. A degenerative left shift with neutropenia and band neutrophilia is commonly observed. Plasma proteins are increased initially due to dehydration; however, plasma protein levels decrease due to decreased albumin levels as a result of malnutrition and protein losing enteropathy.
- Serum chemistry—Metabolic acidosis with low plasma bicarbonate. Cattle with nonfatal diarrhea do not develop significant acidosis. Electrolyte values will be low depending on severity of diarrhea. Levels may appear normal but are deficient on a whole body basis. BUN and creatinine levels are increased due to prerenal azotemia and acute nephrosis due to septicemia and endotoxemia.
- Urinalysis—Depending on state of dehydration, urine will be concentrated resulting in an increased specific gravity.

OTHER LABORATORY TESTS
- Isolation of the organism from feces in live animals and bone marrow and lymph nodes in dead animals along with clinical signs consistent with salmonellosis is confirmatory.
- Samples should be collected and placed in Cary Blair Transport Media for shipment to the lab.
- Fecal PCR can be performed.

PATHOLOGIC FINDINGS
Peracute Infections
- Result in nonspecific gross lesions
- Petechial hemorrhages on the serosal surfaces of the intestine and in epicardium

- The lungs are congested.
- Intestines are distended with fluid and mucosal hemorrhage and necrosis is variable.

Acute Infections
May result in the following gross changes: the abdominal cavity contains increased peritoneal fluid and may contain fibrin tags; the intestines are congested and distended with fluid containing a mixture of mucus and fluid feces along with frank blood, blood clots, pieces of sloughed mucosa, fibrin, and mucosal casts; the spleen is enlarged and the liver swollen; lymph nodes are edematous and hemorrhagic; lungs may be congested with evidence of pneumonia.

Chronic Infections
- Result in thickened intestines with evidence of catarrhal enteritis in the distal small intestine, cecum, and colon
- The mesenteric lymph nodes are hyperplastic and the gallbladder may be thickened containing fibrin.
- Chronic infections associated with *Salmonella enterica Dublin* are exhibited by arthritis, osteomyelitis, and meningitis along with pneumonia.

TREATMENT

APPROPRIATE HEALTH CARE
N/A

NURSING CARE
- Fluid therapy is needed to correct dehydration, circulatory impairment, and electrolyte and metabolic imbalances. Fluid deficit should be calculated as well as maintenance requirement, 80–100 ml/kg, to determine volume of fluids needed during a 24-hour period.
- Fluid may be administered orally or intravenously. Commercial oral electrolyte solutions containing glucose and an alkalinizing agent are recommended if the neonate is still nursing.

SALMONELLOSIS

• Although oral electrolytes are less likely to be absorbed due to enterocyte pathology, not all enterocytes are affected so some absorption may occur. Neonates without a suckle response need IV fluids. IV administration of lactated Ringer's solution is adequate.
• With severe acidosis, isotonic sodium bicarbonate solution (1.3%, 13 of sodium bicarbonate to 1 L of distilled water) may be used. Dextrose solutions (2.5%–5%) are indicated in cases of hypoglycemia.
• With hypoglycemia and an unknown electrolyte and acid-base status, a 2.5% dextrose and 0.45% saline solution has been recommended.

ACTIVITY
N/A

DIET
• Neonates with a suckle response should be left with the dam and allowed to nurse.
• Animals being reared artificially should remain on their diet or switch to whole milk or colostrum. If the diarrhea becomes worse or the calf becomes depressed, removal from the dam or milk is warranted.
• In the case of hand-fed neonates that are depressed and not interested in sucking or neonates not nursing the dam, neonates should receive a high-energy electrolyte solution at a rate of 10% of body weight divided into a minimum of 4 feedings.
• Ruminating animals should be provided a forage-based diet.
• Force feeding alfalfa meal and electrolytes in a water solution to inappetent animals is helpful.

CLIENT EDUCATION
• Clients should be made aware of the potential for fecal shedding of *Salmonella* organisms by both clinically ill as well as convalescent animals into the environment.
• Isolation and biosecurity procedures should be developed to keep organisms from spreading throughout the environment.
• Potential for zoonotic spread should be addressed.

MEDICATIONS

DRUGS OF CHOICE
• Florfenicol 20 mg/kg IM every 48 hours (extralabel usage)
• Ceftiofur 2.2 mg/kg IM/SC bid for 4–7 days (extralabel usage)
• Flunixin meglumine 0.5 mg/kg IV BID first day, then SID (extralabel usage)

CONTRAINDICATIONS
• Do not use kaolin and pectin as use may increase electrolyte loss.
• Do not use hypertonic saline.
• Do not use flunixin if renal disease is evident.
• Meat and milk withhold times must be maintained at all times.

FOLLOW-UP

PATIENT MONITORING
Monitor attitude, suckling response and/or appetite, fecal color and consistency, and hydration status

PREVENTION/AVOIDANCE
• Cleanliness is the basis of prevention. Clean and disinfect animal holding facilities between groups of animals.
• Do not overcrowd animals.
• Equipment should be cleaned and disinfected with iodine, chlorine, or phenolic compounds. Drying and exposure to sunlight increases die-off.
• Reduce manure buildup.
• Control bird and rodent populations as both may carry *Salmonella* organisms.
• Avoid runoff ponds for water sources.
• Vaccination with a LPS core antigen vaccine will not prevent infection but will reduce clinical signs.
• Quarantine new additions for 30 days.
• Those handling sick animals should practice biosecurity measures to reduce exposure to healthy animals, wash hands and disinfect boots, maintain clothes free of fecal material.

POSSIBLE COMPLICATIONS
• Endotoxic shock and death
• Retained placenta and metritis in animals that abort

EXPECTED COURSE AND PROGNOSIS
• Prognosis is dependent on the virulence of the serovar and the host's immune status.
• Animals will have diarrhea or loose stools for approximately a week.
• Poor weight gains can be expected for 2 to 3 weeks after clinical signs resolve.
• Some acute infections will become chronic infections.
• Animals may shed the organism in feces for up to 6 months postrecovery.
• Because the organism can survive for months in the environment, outbreaks may reoccur during periods of animal stress.
• Most outbreaks last 2 weeks, unless the infection becomes endemic, in which case, animals brought into the environment may develop signs over an extended time period.

MISCELLANEOUS

ASSOCIATED CONDITIONS
• Acute infections may result in a chronic state.
• Depending on the virulence of the specific serotype and immune status of the host, the organism may be contained within the intestinal tract or invade the circulatory system resulting in multiple organ pathology.
• Clinical signs are often associated with the release of endotoxins and the development of endotoxemia.

AGE-RELATED FACTORS
• Most cases are 2 weeks to 2 months of age.
• All ages are susceptible.
• Infections in young animals are most often a result of contaminated environments.
• Outbreaks in adults are associated with stress and exposure to a virulent serovar.

ZOONOTIC POTENTIAL
• During outbreaks within animal populations, it is common for animal caregivers to become infected and develop clinical signs.
• Serotypes of concern with multiple drug resistance are *S. typhimurium* and emerging *S. enterica* Serotype Newport.
• The CDC estimates that there are 1.4 million nontyphoidal salmonella infections in the United States, resulting in 168,000 physician office visits per year, 15,000 hospitalizations, and 400 deaths annually. These estimates indicate that salmonellosis presents a major ongoing burden to public health.

RUMINANT SPECIES AFFECTED
Bovine, caprine, and ovine

BIOSECURITY
• Separation by animal age
• Limiting fecal exposure among classes of animals through good feeding hygiene (e.g., cleaning and sanitizing feeding equipment)
• Limiting contact between ill or infected animals and healthy animals
• Addition of new animals in the herd only after consideration of biosecurity risks
• Minimizing the potential introduction of agents via visitors or fomites through access restriction, and cleaning/disinfecting boots and equipment
• When cleaning stalls using flush water, remove animals prior to flush procedure.
• Avoidance of contaminated feed sources
• Limiting human contact with ill animals and appropriate hygiene

SYNONYMS
N/A

SEE ALSO
BVD
Clostridium perfringens type C
Coronavirus
Cryptosporidia
Dietary changes
E. coli
Indigestion
Lactic acidosis
Rotavirus
Toxicosis
Winter dysentery

ABBREVIATIONS
BID = given twice daily
BUN = blood urea nitrogen
BVDV = bovine viral diarrhea virus
CBC = complete blood count
CDC = Centers for Disease Control
IM = intramuscular
IV = intravenous
LPS = lipopolysaccharide
PCR = polymerase chain reaction
SC = subcutaneously
SID = given once daily

Suggested Reading
Aarestrup, F. M., Hasman, H. 2004, May 20. Susceptibility of different bacterial species isolated from food animals to copper sulphate, zinc chloride and antimicrobial substances used for disinfection. *Vet Microbiol*. 100(1–2):83–89.
Bywater, R. J. 2004, Oct-Nov. Veterinary use of antimicrobials and emergence of resistance in zoonotic and sentinel bacteria in the EU. *J Vet Med B Infect Dis Vet Public Health*. 51(8–9):361–63.
Hirsh, D. C., Zee, Y. C. 1999. *Veterinary microbiology*. Malden, MA: Blackwell Science.
Nielsen, L. R., Schukken, Y. H., Grohn, Y. T., Ersboll, A. K. 2004 Aug, 30. Salmonella Dublin infection in dairy cattle: risk factors for becoming a carrier. *Prev Vet Med*. 65(1–2):47–62.
Peek, S. E., Hartmann, F. A., Thomas, C. B., Nordlund, K. V. 2004, Aug 15. Isolation of *Salmonella* spp. from the environment of dairies without any history of clinical salmonellosis. *J Am Vet Med Assoc*. 225(4):574–77.
USDA. 2002. What Veterinarians and Producers Should Know About Multidrug-Resistant *Salmonella* Newport. USDA:APHIS:VS, CEAH, Fort Collins, CO. #N363.0902.
USDA. 2007. Prevalence and Antimicrobial Susceptibility Patterns of *Salmonella* from Beef Cows. USDA:APHIS:VS, CEAH, Fort Collins, CO.

Authors: Kevin D. Pelzer and Dipa Pushkar Brahmbhatt

SALT

 BASICS

OVERVIEW
• "Salt" is composed of sodium chloride in a one to one molar ratio. In pure form, sodium chloride is a crystalline substance commonly incorporated into "licks" of various size and combinations with trace minerals.
• Both sodium and chloride are required for normal physiological function. Sodium is required for maintaining osmotic balance, acid/base balance, active transport of certain nutrients, and glucose uptake. Chloride is required for gastric HCl, enzyme activation, regulation of blood pH, and respiration.
• Problems associated with salt include either depletion of circulating sodium and chloride, or excessive salt intake.
• Salt intake recommendations vary with species and level/type of production within species. It is suggested that the reader consult species-specific National Research Council publications for requirements.

SYSTEMS AFFECTED
• Hemic/lymphatic/immune
• Hepatobiliary
• Cardiovascular
• Central nervous system
• Respiratory
• Renal/urologic
• Gastrointestinal

GENETICS
Genetic and species differences are reflected in salt needs on an individual animal basis.

INCIDENCE/PREVALENCE
Unknown

GEOGRAPHIC DISTRIBUTION
Worldwide

SIGNALMENT

Species
All ruminant species are susceptible to salt toxicity.

Breed Predilections
N/A

Mean Age and Range
All ages of animals are affected.

Predominant Sex
No sex predilection

SIGNS

Salt Excess
• Generally manifested by sodium excess
• Sodium excess will cause increased body water to maintain an isotonic environment. Increased body water will expand the extracellular fluid volume, resulting in generalized edema and hypertension.
• "Salt intoxication" can occur if salt-restricted animals are allowed immediate access to salt for ad libitum consumption. Unlimited access to drinking water should minimize adverse effects of high salt intake; however, salt intake should be gradually increased in previously salt-deprived animals.
• Excessive salt intake with inadequate water intake will result in sodium intoxication. Cortical edema, as well as eosinophilic meningioencephalitis in swine, is associated with sodium intoxication.
• Signs include severe nervous symptoms characterized by staggering, circling, blindness, head-pressing, and collapse.
• Sodium levels of > 2000 ppm is supportive of sodium toxicosis.

Salt Deficiency
• Associated with sodium depletion
• Sodium depletion is generally associated with loss of circulating sodium, and not necessarily to low sodium intake. Low sodium intake in domestic animals is the result of poor livestock management because salt is inexpensive.
• Sodium loss in milk in cows consuming a low-salt diet can induce sodium depletion. Mastitis will exacerbate sodium depletion in milk.

• Conditions associated with fluid loss (diarrhea, lactation, sweating, vomiting) will increase the rate of sodium loss. Renal disease can increase sodium loss.
• Salt deprivation can lead to hyperphagia, inducing digestive problems. Animals also will consume nonfeed materials, such as dirt, wood, etc.
• Salt deficient animals are unthrifty and manifest poor growth, male infertility, and delayed female maturity.
• Ruminants consuming primarily forages should be provided with supplementary salt because of the high potassium to sodium ratio common in grass and other forages.

 DIAGNOSIS

PATHOLOGIC FINDINGS
Gross pathology:
• Salt intoxication: marked congestion and edema of the brain and meninges, as well as petechiae and ecchymoses within the grey and white matter of the cerebrum, cerebellum, and brain stem, and moderate to severe congestion of the abomasal mucosa.
• Sodium chloride poisoning has been classified as acute/direct salt poisoning where there has been ingestion of excessive salt in feed or drinking water or as delayed/indirect when there has been a restriction in water intake with or without ingestion of excessive salt.
• Hypernatremia with resultant brain edema and neurological disease has also been induced in calves by injudicious use of sodium bicarbonate and oral electrolyte solutions during treatment of diarrhea with dehydration and acidosis.

TREATMENT

CLIENT EDUCATION
Conditions associated with severe nonregenerative anemia or pancytopenia generally carry a guarded to poor prognosis and may require long-term therapy without complete resolution.

 MEDICATIONS

CONTRAINDICATIONS
N/A

PRECAUTIONS
N/A

POSSIBLE INTERACTIONS
N/A

 FOLLOW-UP

PREVENTION/AVOIDANCE
See specific chapters for nutritional deficiencies and sodium-related disease.

POSSIBLE COMPLICATIONS
N/A

EXPECTED COURSE AND PROGNOSIS
Clinical course and prognosis vary and are associated with the underlying disease condition.

 MISCELLANEOUS

ASSOCIATED CONDITIONS
Conditions associated with fluid loss (diarrhea, lactation, sweating, vomiting) will increase the rate of sodium loss. Renal disease can increase sodium loss.

AGE-RELATED FACTORS
N/A

ZOONOTIC POTENTIAL
N/A

PREGNANCY
N/A

RUMINANT SPECIES AFFECTED
All species of ruminants are affected.

BIOSECURITY
N/A

PRODUCTION MANAGEMENT
• "Salt intoxication" can occur if salt restricted animals are allowed immediate access to salt for ad libitum consumption. Unlimited access to drinking water should minimize adverse effects of high salt intake; however, salt intake should be gradually increased in previously salt-deprived animals.
• Excessive salt intake with inadequate water intake will result in sodium intoxication.
• Do not supplement salt when range cattle are on poor range or have been starved.
• Do not give salt supplementation when cattle are dehydrated.

SEE ALSO
Beef cattle nutrition
Camelid nutrition
Dairy cattle nutrition
Small ruminant nutrition
Starvation

ABBREVIATIONS
HCL = hydrochloric acid
pH = possible hydrogen, a measure of acid/base balance

Suggested Reading
Angelos, J. M., Smith, B. P., George, L. W. 1999. Treatment of hypernatremia in an acidotic neonatal calf. *J Amer Vet Med Assoc*. 214:1364–67.
Carlson, G. P. 1989. Fluid, electrolyte, and acid-base balance. In: *Clinical biochemistry of domestic animals*, ed. J. J. Keneko. New York: Academic Press.
Kopcha, M. 1987, Mar. Nutritional and metabolic diseases involving the nervous system. *Vet Clin North Am Food Anim Pract*. 3(1):119–35.
Osweiler, G. D., Carr, T. F., Sanderson, T. L. 1995. Water deprivation-sodium ion toxicosis in cattle. *J Vet Diag Invest*. 7:583–85.

Author: Daniel C. Rule

SARCOCYSTOSIS

BASICS

DEFINITION
Infestation with protozoan species of the genus *Sarcocystis*. The condition is also known as sarcosporidiosis.

PATHOPHYSIOLOGY
• *Sarcocystis* spp. have a two-host cycle involving a final host and an intermediate host.
• The final host is a predator, which ingests muscle tissue of the intermediate host that contains *Sarcocystis* cysts (sarcocysts). After about 1 week, the final host begins shedding infective sporocysts in its feces for several months.
• The intermediate host is a prey species, which ingests the infective sporocysts during grazing or drinking and then releases sporozoites that develop into schizonts in the vascular endothelium. Merozoites develop from these and give rise to another generation of schizonts in the vascular endothelium. The last generation gives rise to schizonts, which encyst in muscle and other soft tissues to form the sarcocysts. In 2 to 3 months, infective zooites develop within the sarcocysts.
• Clinical disease in the intermediate host may occur at two stages in the developmental cycle.
  • First stage at 3 to 5 weeks after the initial infection; can last for 6 to 8 weeks. This stage corresponds with the formation of endothelial schizonts with fever, petechiation of mucous membranes, edema, icterus, and macrocytic hypochromic anemia.
  • Second stage corresponds to the entry of schizonts into muscle tissue where extensive fiber degeneration and enzyme release can occur. The enlargement of the cysts in massive infestations can cause muscle pain and lameness. After about 100 days, maturation of the cysts occurs, and tissue reactions subside along with clinical signs.

• This recovery from clinical disease may explain the past impression that sarcosystosis was an innocuous condition. In cattle, *S. cruzi* seems to be the only one capable of causing significant clinical disease. In sheep, *S. tenella* can be very pathogenic to lambs.

SYSTEMS AFFECTED
• Production management; potentially all, depending on condition
• Vascular endothelium
• Skeletal and cardiac muscle
• Possibly CNS tissue in lambs
• Reproductive system—abortions, stillbirths.
• Lymphadenitis

GENETICS
None

INCIDENCE/PREVALENCE
• Worldwide prevalence of *Sarcocystis* in ruminants is very high, approaching 100% in many areas.
• The prevalence of intestinal infection in humans worldwide is thought to be between 6% and 10%.

GEOGRAPHIC DISTRIBUTION
Worldwide

SIGNALMENT
Species
• Specific final/intermediate host relationships exist for each species of *Sarcocystis*.
• Some examples include: Dog/cattle—*S. cruzi*; Cat/cattle—*S. hirsuta*; Human/cattle—*S. hominis*; Dog/sheep and goat—*S. capracanis, S. hircicanis*; Cat/sheep—*S. tenella, S. gigantea, S. medusiformis*; Cat/goat—*S. moulei*.
• Other species which serve as hosts include water buffalo, wild ruminants, camels, horses, pigs, rodents, raccoons, birds, and reptiles.
• *S. cruzi* is the only species that causes clinical disease in cattle.
• *S. tenella* can be very pathogenic in lambs.
• *S. gigantea* in sheep affect the esophagus; sarcocysts are large enough to be seen visually.
• No species have been determined as pathogenic to goats.
• There are numerous *Sarcocystis* spp. that affect deer and involve canids in their cycle.

Breed Predilections
N/A

Mean Age and Range
N/A

Predominant Sex
N/A

SIGNS

HISTORICAL FINDINGS
• Intermediate hosts (ruminant species) grazing on soil/pasture contaminated by sporocysts shed by the final hosts (dogs and cats primarily, humans may be involved)
• Feeding on raw tissues of infected ruminants by dogs, cats, or humans

PHYSICAL EXAMINATION FINDINGS
• Usually asymptomatic
• In severe cases—fever, anorexia, cachexia, decreased milk production, diarrhea, muscle spasms, anemia, sloughing of tip of tail, hyperexcitability, weakness, late-term abortion, CNS signs, prostration, or death have been observed.
• The severity of disease may be modified by the strength of the host's immune system.

CAUSES
Sarcocystis spp.

RISK FACTORS
Dogs, cats, or humans feeding on uncooked tissues of ruminants infected with *Sarcocystis* spp. subsequently reexposing ruminants via sporocysts via their feces.

DIAGNOSIS

• Usually an incidental discovery at slaughter
• PCR-RFLP resolved by agarose gel electrophoresis
• Monoclonal antibody to *T. saginata* and avidin-biotin complex immunohistochemistry

DIFFERENTIAL DIAGNOSIS
In severe cases, consider GI parasitism, toxicity, brucellosis, leptospirosis, enzootic bovine abortion, other causes of abortion, white muscle disease, and CNS diseases (rabies, bovine spongiform encephalopathy, and scrapie).

PATHOLOGIC FINDINGS
• Only *S. gigantea*, found in sheep, form sarcocysts that are visible grossly in tissues. These are seen in the esophagus. Others are microscopic and can be detected in the esophagus, diaphragm, heart, and other muscle.
• Lesions from *S. cruzi* in cattle may be visible in massive infestations and can lead to carcass condemnation at slaughter.
• Trichinoscopy or enzyme digestion techniques may be needed to visualize the sarcocysts.
• Severely affected animals may appear cachectic or have hemorrhage of the visceral and myocardial serosa.

 TREATMENT

Therapeutic treatment is ineffective.

 MEDICATIONS

• Not generally practiced
• Experimentally, amprolium at 100 mg/kg body weight fed once daily prophylactically for 30 days seemed to reduce the severity of illness in sheep and calves. Other references put the dose at 5–10 mg/kg orally for the prevention or treatment of other coccidia. Except for calves, this is extralabel use. Do not use in animals producing milk for human consumption. Meat withdrawal time is 24 hours after last treatment. Do not use in calves to be processed for veal.

POSSIBLE INTERACTIONS
N/A

 FOLLOW-UP

PREVENTION/AVOIDANCE
• Prevention by keeping dogs and cats from eating raw tissues of ruminants and contaminating feed and pasture with sporocyst-infected feces is important.
• Freezing of meat reduces the number of viable cysts.
• Prevent contamination of ruminant feed and environment by dog, cat, and human feces.

POSSIBLE COMPLICATIONS
EXPECTED COURSE AND PROGNOSIS
• Cattle—only *S. cruzi* has potential to cause significant disease, and can range from muscle pain to abortions to death. Full recovery is seen after 100 days when cysts mature. Sarcocysts will remain in the muscle and can result in carcass condemnation at slaughter.
• Sheep—*S. tenella* has been associated with high morbidity and mortality in lambs

 MISCELLANEOUS

ASSOCIATED CONDITIONS
Other intestinal parasites

AGE-RELATED FACTORS
Clinical disease is seen primarily in calves, lambs, and kids, although adults may also be affected.

ZOONOTIC POTENTIAL
• *S. bovihominis*—Humans are the primary host, and generally no clinically significant disease has been documented in humans or cattle in natural infections.
• In experimental infections, some humans experienced transient abdominal pain and diarrhea 10–14 days after exposure, and shed sporocysts in their feces for 5–12 days.
• In other *Sarcocystis* spp., rare cases of muscular weakness and pain, periarteritis and subcutaneous tumefaction have been observed, indicating humans can potentially serve as the intermediate host as well. But a causal association has not been established. Immunosuppressed individuals may be at increased risk of clinical disease. It is thought that nearly half of the muscular cysts worldwide in bovines and swine are caused by *S. bovihominis* and *S. suihominis*.
• The prevalence of intestinal infection in humans worldwide is thought to be between 6% and 10%.

PREGNANCY
Severe infestation can result in stillbirths and abortion in cattle.

RUMINANT SPECIES AFFECTED
Potentially, all ruminant species can be affected

BIOSECURITY
N/A

PRODUCTION MANAGEMENT
N/A

SYNONYMS
Beef measles

SEE ALSO
Brucellosis
CNS diseases (i.e., rabies, bovine spongiform encephalopathy, and scrapie)
Enzootic bovine abortion
GI parasitism
Leptospirosis
Other causes of abortion
Specific toxicities
White muscle disease

ABBREVIATIONS
CNS = central nervous system

Suggested Reading
Fayer R. 2004, Oct. *Sarcocystis* spp. in human infections. *Clin Microbiol Rev.* 17(4):894–902.
Gunning, R. F., Jones, J. R., Jeffrey, M., Higgins, R. J., Williamson, A. G. 2000, Mar 11. *Sarcocystis encephalomyelitis* in cattle. *Vet Rec.* 146(11):328.
Leek, R..G., Fayer, R. 1980. Amprolium for prophylaxis of ovine sarcocystosis. *J Parasitol.* 66(1):100–106.
Ogunremi, O., MacDonald, G., Geerts, S., Brandt, J. 2004, Sep. Diagnosis of *Taenia saginata cysticercosis* by immunohistochemical test on formalin-fixed and paraffin-embedded bovine lesions. *J Vet Diagn Invest.* 16(5):438–41.
Yang, Z. Q., Li, Q. Q., Zuo, Y. X., Chen, X. W., Chen, Y. J., Nie, L., Wei, C. G., Zen, J. S., Attwood, S. W., Zhang, X. Z., Zhang, Y. P. 2002, Nov-Dec. Characterization of *Sarcocystis* species in domestic animals using a PCR-RFLP analysis of variation in the 18S rRNA gene: a cost-effective and simple technique for routine species identification. *Exp Parasitol.* 102(3–4):212–17.

Author: Edward L. Powers

SCRAPIE

 BASICS

OVERVIEW
• Scrapie is a progressive, degenerative, nonfebrile disease of sheep and, less commonly, goats and is the oldest known agent in the family of transmissible spongiform encephalopathies (TSEs).
• Additional TSEs include chronic wasting disease (CWD) in cervids, transmissible mink encephalopathy, feline spongiform encephalopathy, bovine spongiform encephalopathy (BSE), and Creutzfeld-Jakob disease (CJD) in humans.
• Contamination of the environment and oral exposure with placenta and fetal fluids from infected sheep is thought to be the most likely source for horizontal and vertical transmission of scrapie.
• Milk, saliva, urine, colostrum, and feces have not been demonstrated to transmit disease.
• Scrapie has a long incubation period and clinical signs commonly appear in adult sheep 2.5 years of age and older. Clinical signs can be localized to damage within the brain stem.
• There is currently no approved definitive antemortem diagnostic test for scrapie. Immunohistochemistry (IHC) staining of the obex, retropharyngeal lymph node, and tonsil is the current gold standard for postmortem testing.

• Genetic analysis, or genotyping, of codons 136, 154, and 171 has become an effective tool to determine susceptible sheep within a flock.
• It is estimated that scrapie cost the U.S. sheep industry $20 million a year in lost productivity and potential export markets.
• Scrapie has never been linked to disease in humans who consume sheep muscle.

PATHOPHYSIOLOGY
• The infectious agent of scrapie is a prion, a misfolded glyoprotein of the cell membrane, of which there are more than 15 strains. The misfolded prion protein is resistant to degradation by normal host protease.
• Accumulation of the protease-resistant prion (PrP) in the brain stem causes vacuolation of the grey matter neuropil and has a "spongy" appearance on H&E preparations.

SYSTEMS AFFECTED
CNS

GENETICS
• Genetic analysis, or genotyping, of codons 136, 154, and 171, has become an effective tool to determine susceptible sheep within a flock.
• Scrapie is primarily a disease of Suffolk sheep in the United States. The disease is found in the Suffolk, Cheviot, Swaledale, Bleu du Maine, Herdwick, Poll Dorset, Shetland, and Soay breeds in the UK, Texel breed in The Netherlands, Suffolk and Corriedale breeds in Japan, Romanov and Lacaune breeds in France, Rygja breed in Norway, and Icelandic breed in Iceland.

• Genetic resistance to scrapie depends not only on the prion genotype of the sheep but also on the strain of scrapie present.
• Genotypes found to be resistant to one strain of scrapie have been shown to be susceptible to another strain. It appears that there are differences between the United States and Europe in the strains of scrapie that are present.
• Codon 136:Sheep homozygous for alanine (AA) have been shown to be more resistant to scrapie than sheep homozygous for valine (VV) or heterozygous (AV) in European studies.
• Codon 154: Of the three important codons, amino acid changes at 154 appear to have a slightly less dramatic effect on scrapie susceptibility than do the other two, and the susceptible genotypes are not consistent across studies.
• Codon 171: Amino acid changes at codon 171 have a large effect on scrapie susceptibility in sheep in both Europe and the United States. Virtually no sheep homozygous for arginine (RR) have been identified with scrapie.

INCIDENCE/PREVALENCE
• Beginning April 1, 2002, through March 31, 2003, the overall weighted national prevalence of scrapie in 12,491 sheep greater than 1 year of age was 0.20%. States within the eastern half and north central United States have a higher prevalence than the western states.
• Scrapie was first diagnosed in the United States in 1947 in a flock of Suffolk sheep in Michigan.

• From 1947 through July 2001 in the United States, scrapie had been diagnosed in over 1000 flocks, and approximately 1600 individual cases of natural ovine scrapie and 7 individual cases of natural caprine scrapie have been found.
• Relative to most other goat and sheep diseases, the incidence of scrapie is low.

GEOGRAPHIC DISTRIBUTION
Potentially worldwide

SIGNALMENT
Black-faced sheep are significantly more likely to test positive for scrapie than white- or mottle-faced sheep. The Suffolk breed in most commonly diagnosed with scrapie.

Species
Sheep and goats

Breed Predilections
In 1998, the USDA found the breed distribution in the United States was 87% Suffolk, 6% Hampshire, and 7% other breeds (Border Leicester, Cheviot, North Country Cheviot, Corriedale, Cotswold, Dorset, Finnsheep, Merino, Montadale, Rambouillet, Shropshire, and Southdown) and crosses.

Mean Age and Range
Scrapie is commonly diagnosed in sheep between 3 and 5 years of age and is rarely diagnosed in sheep less than 18 months of age.

Predominant Sex
N/A

SIGNS
• Clinical signs include sudden onset of behavioral changes, development of an unstable gait or other locomotion disorders, neurological deficits localized to the brain stem, and generalized wasting without a loss of appetite.

• A small percentage of sheep smack their lips and develop the pruritic form ("scrapie") characterized by a loss of wool around the tail, lateral neck and body, and elbow.
• Recumbency, seizuring, difficulty swallowing, and blindness are common clinical signs in the latter stages of disease.

PHYSICAL EXAMINATION FINDINGS
• Signs of scrapie vary widely among individual animals and develop very slowly.
• Due to damage to nerve cells, affected animals usually show behavioral changes, tremor (especially of head and neck), pruritus, and locomotor incoordination that progresses to recumbency and death.
• Early signs include subtle changes in behavior or temperament. Scratching and rubbing against fixed objects, apparently to relieve itching, may follow these changes.
• Other signs are loss of coordination, weight loss despite retention of appetite, biting of feet and limbs, lip smacking, and gait abnormalities, including high stepping of the forelegs, hopping like a rabbit, and swaying of the back end.
• An infected animal may appear normal if left undisturbed at rest.
• When stimulated by a sudden noise, excessive movement, or the stress of handling, the animal may tremble or fall down in a convulsion-like state.

CAUSES AND RISK FACTORS
• Scrapie is thought to be spread most often from ewe to offspring and to other lambs in contemporary lambing groups through contact of lambs with the placenta and placental fluids of infected ewes.
• Lateral transmission from infected rams to ewes and lambs, from infected ewes to other ewes, and from an infected environment to adult animals is not thought to be a major route of transmission; however, there are documented cases of scrapie where such routes of transmission are thought to have occurred.

• Contamination of the environment and oral exposure with placenta and fetal fluids from infected sheep is thought to be the most likely source for horizontal and vertical transmission of scrapie. Milk, saliva, urine, colostrum, and feces have not been demonstrated to transmit disease.

DIAGNOSIS

DIFFERENTIAL DIAGNOSIS
Neurological Signs: Sheep
• Brain abscess (caseous lymphadenitis—CLA/*Actinobacillus*)
• *Clostridium perfringens* type C
• Cobalt deficiency
• Copper deficiency
• Hypocalcemia
• Hypomagnesemia
• Inner ear infection
• Listeriosis
• Louping-ill
• Mycotoxins
• *Parelaphostrongylus* (meningeal worm migration)
• Polioencephalomalacia/thiamine deficiency
• Pregnancy toxemia
• Rabies
• Swayback
• Tetanus
• Tick paralysis
• Uremia
• Vitamin A deficiency

Neurological Signs: Goats
• Bacterial: botulism brain abscess, inner ear infection, *Listeria* infection, meningoencephalitis, tetanus

SCRAPIE

• Congenital: hydranencephaly, hydrocephalus, progressive paresis
• Nutritional/metabolic: cobalt deficiency, enzootic ataxia/swayback/copper deficiency hypovitaminosis A, polioencephalomalacia/ thiamine deficiency, pregnancy toxemia uremia
• Parasitic: *Parelaphostrongylus tenuis,* tick paralysis
• Toxic ingestion
• Pyrethrin/organophosphates
• Salt toxicity
• Trauma
• Viral/prion: border disease, borna disease, caprine arthritis encephalitis virus (CAE), louping-ill, maedi visna, pseudorabies, rabies

CBC/BIOCHEMISTRY/URINALYSIS
N/A

OTHER LABORATORY TESTS
Diagnostic testing
• Conclusive diagnosis of scrapie is by detection of accumulated protease resistant prion, PrP, by immunohistochemistry (IHC) staining of the obex, retropharyngeal lymph nodes, and tonsils of sacrificed sheep.
• Humoral or cell-mediated immunity in response to the exposure of misfolded prion is not a feature of scrapie and conclusive antemortem diagnosis by common serological methods is not possible.
• Biopsy and IHC staining of at least six lymphoid follicles from the third eyelid has been attempted as an antemortem test for scrapie, but is currently not an official antemortem diagnostic test.

IMAGING
N/A

OTHER DIAGNOSTIC PROCEDURES
Genetic testing
• Experiments have demonstrated that there is substantial genetic control over the incidence of disease.
• Identification of specific amino acid sequences at codons 136, 154, and 171 correlate with a sheep susceptibility to becoming infected with scrapie.
• Although there is a genetic variability within breeds, families, and individual sheep, codon 171 has become a reliable susceptibility indicator in the United States. Sheep that are homozygous arginine (RR) or heterozygous arginine/glutamine (QR) at codon 171 appear resistant to scrapie.
• Sheep homozygous glutamine (QQ) at codon 171 have demonstrated to be susceptible to scrapie.
• Susceptibility genetic sequences have been established for codons 136 and 154 but are less reliable than codon 171.

PATHOLOGIC FINDINGS
• The most diagnostic lesion is the presence of bilaterally symmetrical neuronal vacuolation; microcystic vacuolation (spongiform change) of the grey matter neuropil.
• Hypertrophy of astrocytes often accompanies vacuolation.
• Cerebral amyloidosis is an inconstant histological feature of scrapie.
• Brain extracts contain an abundance of characteristic abnormal fibrils (SAF), which are readily identified by negative-stain EM.

TREATMENT

There is no known treatment for scrapie.
Control
• Sacrificing and testing sheep with clinical signs, in addition to genetic testing susceptible sheep, is the current control method.
• The selection of breeding rams with resistant gene profiles to perpetuate resistant genes is also advised.
• Lambing in a clean environment and removing fetal membranes and contaminated bedding to prevent additional exposure will also reduce exposure and disease risk.
• Sheep and goat identification program in the United States: Sheep and goat classes that require tagging:
 1. All sheep 18 months of age or older
 2. All breeding sheep regardless of age
 3. Sexually intact show or exhibition sheep and goats
 4. All goats 18 months of age or older that are or have been commingled with sheep
 5. All breeding goats that are or have been commingled with sheep.

MISCELLANEOUS

ASSOCIATED CONDITIONS
N/A

AGE-RELATED FACTORS
Scrapie is a commonly diagnosed in sheep between 3 and 5 years of age and is rarely diagnosed in sheep less than 18 months of age.

ZOONOTIC POTENTIAL
Scrapie has never been linked to disease in humans who consume sheep muscle.

PREGNANCY
N/A

RUMINANT SPECIES AFFECTED
Sheep and goats

BIOSECURITY
• Contamination of the environment and oral exposure with placenta and fetal fluids from infected sheep is thought to be the most likely source for horizontal and vertical transmission of scrapie. Milk, saliva, urine, colostrum, and feces have not been demonstrated to transmit disease.
• Lambing in a clean environment and removing fetal membranes and contaminated bedding to prevent additional exposure will also reduce exposure and disease risk.

PRODUCTION MANAGEMENT
See Genetics above

SYNONYMS
N/A

SEE ALSO
Brain abscess (Caseous lymphadenitis—CLA/*Actinobacillus*)
Listeriosis
Louping-ill
Mycotoxins
Parelaphostrongylus (Meningeal worm migration)
Polioencephalomalacia/thiamine deficiency
Pregnancy toxemia
Rabies
Swayback
Tetanus
Tick paralysis
TSE, animal identification programs

ABBREVIATIONS
BSE = bovine spongiform encephalopathy
CAE = caprine arthritis encephalitis virus
CLA = caseous lymphadenitis
CWD = chronic wasting disease
IHC = immunohistochemistry
PrP = protease resistant prion
TSEs = transmissible spongiform encephalopathies

Suggested Reading
Detwiler, L. A., Jenny, A. L., Rubenstein, R., Wineland, N. E. 1996. Scrapie: a review. *Sheep & Goat Res. J.* 12(3):111–31.
Elsen, J. M., Aigues, Y., Schelcher, F., Ducrocq, V., Andreoletti, O., Eychenne, F., Ttien Khang, J. V., Poivey, J. P., Lantier, F., Laplanche, J. L. 1999. Genetic susceptibility and transmission factors in scrapie: detailed analysis of an epidemic in a closed flock of Romanov. *Archives Virology* 144:431–45.

Hunter, N., Goldmann, W., Foster, J. D., Cairns, D., Smith, G. 1997. Natural scrapie and PrP genotype: case-control studies in British sheep. *Vet Rec.* 141:137–40.
Prusiner, S. B. 1998. Prions. *Proc Natl Acad Sci.* 95:13363–83. USDA. 2003. *Phase II: Scrapie: ovine slaughter surveillance study 2002–2003.* USDA:APHIS:VS,CEAH. Fort Collins, CO: National Animal Health Monitoring System, #419.0104.
Wineland, N. E., Detwiler, L. A., Salman, M. D. 1998. Epidemiologic analysis of reported scrapie in sheep in the United States: 1,117 cases (1947–1992). *J American Vet Med. Assoc.* 212:713.

Authors: Chris D. Calloway and Jeremy Schefers

SEGMENTAL APLASIA/HYPOPLASIA OF THE WOLFFIAN DUCT SYSTEM

BASICS

DEFINITION
In this context, segmental aplasia usually refers to lack of development of part of one or more of those structures (epididymis, vas deferens) that are derived from the embryonic mesonephric, or Wolffian, duct system.

OVERVIEW
• Affected structures may include the epididymis, vas deferens, and ampulla. The vesicular gland on the affected side may also be underdeveloped.
• The most frequently affected areas are the body and tail of the epididymis.

PATHOPHYSIOLOGY

SYSTEMS AFFECTED
Reproductive

GENETICS
• Numerical chromosomal aberrations (e.g., XXY) have been identified as a risk factor.
• In addition, European work suggests that a hereditary form exists.

INCIDENCE/PREVALENCE
In Europe, the prevalence has been estimated as being between 0.59% and 1.18% in young calves, 1% in normal bulls, and 5% in infertile bulls.

GEOGRAPHIC DISTRIBUTION
Worldwide distribution

SIGNALMENT
• More commonly unilateral and on the RHS
• In unilateral cases, the bull is usually fertile, even though semen from only one testicle is available for fertilization.

Species
Although segmental aplasia can occur in all species, it is particularly well described in the bull.

Breed Predilections
N/A

Mean Age and Range
N/A

Predominant Sex
Male

SIGNS
Whether classified as aplasia or hypoplasia, complete occlusion usually occurs of the affected region, precluding passage of sperm on the affected side.

CAUSES AND RISK FACTORS

DIAGNOSIS

• Diagnosis can be difficult, and usually entails careful palpation of those structures derived from the Wolffian duct system.
• The testicle on the affected side(s) is often developed normally.
• If occlusion is in the upper body or head of the epididymis, fluid backpressure may cause testicular swelling and subsequent degeneration.
• If the lesion is more distal to the testicle, fluids may be absorbed within the epididymis.
• Palpation of a very small or absent, epididymal tail is suggestive of the condition. The epididymal head may be enlarged due to distension with semen. If the defect is located in the vas deferens, the epididymal tail may be enlarged.

DIFFERENTIAL DIAGNOSIS
• Small cystic structures derived from the embryonic duct systems (either Wolffian or Muellerian), which can occur adjacent to the ampullae and vas deferentia, paradidymis
• Spermiostasis, sperm granuloma, epididymitis, epididymal neoplasia (rare in the bull)
• Orchitis, testicular degeneration

CBC/BIOCHEMISTRY/URINALYSIS
N/A

OTHER LABORATORY TESTS
N/A

IMAGING
N/A

OTHER DIAGNOSTIC PROCEDURES
N/A

TREATMENT
None; be aware of possible hereditary basis.

MEDICATIONS

FOLLOW-UP

MISCELLANEOUS

ASSOCIATED CONDITIONS
N/A

AGE-RELATED FACTORS
N/A

ZOONOTIC POTENTIAL
N/A

PREGNANCY
N/A

RUMINANT SPECIES AFFECTED
Although segmental aplasia can occur in all species, it is particularly well described in the bull.

BIOSECURITY
N/A

PRODUCTION MANAGEMENT
N/A

SYNONYMS
N/A

SEE ALSO
Epididymal neoplasia
Epididymitis
Orchitis
Sperm granuloma
Spermiostasis
Testicular degeneration

ABBREVIATIONS
RHS = right hind side

Suggested Reading
Blom, E. 1982, Dec. Aplasia of the ductuli efferentes—a new sterilizing congenital syndrome in the bull. *Nord Vet Med*. 34(12): 431–34.
Blom, E., Christensen, N. O. 1956. Examination of the genitals of slaughtered male calves as a means of elucidating the frequency of genital malformation in the bovine male. Studies on pathological conditions in the testis, epididymis and accessory sex glands in the bull III. *Proc IIIrd Int Congr Anim Repro and AI*. Cambridge. Plenary Papers. Brown Publishing.
Blom, E., Christensen, N. O. 1947. Studies on pathological conditions in the testis, epididymis and accessory sex glands in the bull. *Skand Vet Tidskr*. 37:1–49
Campero, C. M., Bagshaw, P. A., Ladds, P. W. 1989, Mar. Lesions of presumed congenital origin in the accessory sex glands of bulls. *Aust Vet J*. 66(3): 80, 81–85.
Saunders, P. J., Ladds, P. W. 1978, Jan. Congenital and developmental anomalies of the genitalia of slaughtered bulls. *Aust Vet J*. 54(1): 10–13.

Author: Peter Chenoweth

BASICS

OVERVIEW

• The identification of physiologically important roles of selenium in immunity, reproduction, and productivity has led to an increased use of selenium in man and animals over the years, for both therapeutic and preventive purposes.
• Selenium (Se) is the only essential nutrient that does not have a GRAS (generally regarded as safe) status and so the FDA regulates Se supplementation in animals as if it were a drug.
• There is a narrow margin between selenium deficiency and selenium toxicosis in animals. Selenium toxicosis has been reported either naturally, by consumption of selenium-accumulator plants, or by human errors, due to oversupplementation of selenium in the diet and/or accidental overdosing.
• Organic forms of selenium such as selenomethionine and Se-methyl selenocysteine are the major selenium-containing compounds found in the plants/hay, whereas an inorganic form of selenium such as sodium selenite is the common supplemental/dosing form.
• Acute selenosis may occur at oral doses >= 2.2 mg Se/kg BW.
• Chronic selenosis has been reported to occur in animals fed > 5–40 ppm Se in feed.
• The toxic effects of the organic and inorganic forms of selenium are similar but, in most cases, the toxic dose of the inorganic form is greater than the organic form.
• Clinical signs involve respiratory, cardiovascular, hematologic, and gastrointestinal systems.
• Bovines are more susceptible than ovines.
• Fetus can concentrate Se in liver at concentrations up to three times higher than in the dam.
• Chronic selenosis or "alkali disease" causes hoof deformities and hair loss. The term "blind staggers" is a misnomer for selenium toxicosis.

PATHOPHYSIOLOGY

• Replacement of sulfur with selenium in the amino acids weakens keratin and causes disruption of hair, hoof, and horn integrity due to loss of the disulfide bonds. Se also causes abnormal maturation of the keratinocytes in the stratum spinosum. This may be followed by degeneration and necrosis. Alopecia results from atrophy of primary hair follicles.

• In the hoof, cells on the coronary papillae produce dyskeratotic debris that accumulates in the horn tubules and distorts the normal architecture of the hoof wall.
• Cytotoxic effects of Se are the result of denaturation of critical protein thiols. Selenite and SeCys react with tissue thiols to produce ROS.

SYSTEMS AFFECTED

Cardiovascular
• Tachycardia
• Atrophy and dilatation of heart with multifocal myocardial necrosis or hydropic degeneration
• Endocarditis or myocarditis with focal hemorrhages

Gastrointestinal
• Diarrhea
• Mild gastroenteritis

Hemic/Lymphatic/Immune
• Selenium has been reported to decrease erythrocytic volume by reducing the hemoglobin synthesis and may result in anemia.
• Variable necrosis and/or atrophy of lymphoid tissue
• Reduced immune response

Hepatobiliary
• Congested and swollen liver
• Vacuolation of hepatocytes
• Cirrhosis/fibrosis

Musculoskeletal
• Ataxia
• Mild hyaline or granular degeneration of the muscle fibers

Nervous
• Depression
• Polioencephalomalacia

Renal/Urologic
• Hemoglobinuria
• Glomerulonephritis
• Parenchymatous and tubular degeneration with casts

Reproductive
• Infertility
• Abortions, stillbirths
• Hypoplasia of reproductive organs has been observed in lambs from seleniferous areas.

Respiratory
• Dyspnea
• Pulmonary edema (marked interlobular edema), hydrothorax and focal hemorrhages
• Pulmonary alveolar vasculitis
• Accumulation of serosanguinous fluid and foam in the trachea, bronchi, and bronchioles.

Skin
Structural abnormalities of hair, hoof, and horn

GENETICS
N/A

INCIDENCE/PREVALENCE
• Seleniferous areas with alkaline soil
• Sporadic incidences resulting from accidental overdoses

GEOGRAPHIC DISTRIBUTION
N/A

SIGNALMENT
• Young animals are more susceptible to selenosis as a result of the underdeveloped rumen. Ruminal microflora is known to reduce bioavailable forms of selenium to unavailable, elemental forms.
• No breed or sex predilections have been described in the literature.

SIGNS

Acute Effects
• Clinical signs generally include anorexia, depression, reluctance to move, and respiratory distress. Grinding of teeth, diarrhea, bloat, and abdominal pain may also be seen.
• Heart rate and respiration rate are high and the pulse may be weak. Fever, polyuria, and hemolytic anemia have been reported in some cases.
• Death usually occurs within 12–48 hours of acute exposure, otherwise the animal usually recovers.
• Once clinical signs such as dyspnea and ataxia appear, the animals succumb within the hour.
• A garlicky smell to the breath is usually present, especially during first 16 hours postexposure.
• Bovine—orally, 11 mg Se/kg BW as selenite resulted in dyspnea, garlicky breath, and death within 2 days.
• Sheep—Blood-tinged frothy mucus may appear at the mouth and nostrils, progressing to prostration and death. Diarrhea and peracute death have been reported in the absence of any other clinical signs. Congestion in the brain and swollen mesenteric lymph nodes are also observed in some animals. Using sodium selenite, an oral LD-50 of 1.9 mg Se/kg BW has been reported.

SELENIUM TOXICITY

Table 1

Comparative Selenium Toxicosis in Cattle and Sheep	
Se as sodium selenite (inorganic) (orally)	Se as selenomethionine (organic) (orally)
Cattle • 7 mg Se/kg BW—no effect • 10.1 mg Se/kg BW—anorexia and low milk production for 5 days • 9–11 mg Se/kg BW—anorexia, dyspnea, garlicky breath, followed by death within 2 days • Oral MLD at 9.9–11 mg Se/kg BW • 15 ppm Se in diet for 231 days—decreased weight gain, sore foot, cracked hooves, excitability in 1 of 5 heifers	• 2.2 mg Se/kg/day (*A. pectinatus*) for 6–16 days caused blind staggers in steers. • 3.4 mg Se/kg/day (*A. bisulcatus*) for 7 days caused blind staggers in steers. • 25 ppm Se (*Astragalus* hay) for 46 days caused joint stiffening and cracking of hooves in 4 weeks. By the end of 4 months, sloughing of the hoof started. • 9 out of 11 bullocks showed stiffness and lameness in all four legs, pale mucosa, and slow but gradual sloughing of the hoof. Mean concentrations of Se in the herbage was 37 ppm.
Sheep • 6.4 mg Se/kg BW—pulmonary cong., 95% mortality in 15 days • 1.7 mg Se/kg BW—35% mortality within 12–16 hr • 2.2 mg Se/kg BW—35% mortality within 12–48 hr • Hyperpnoea, salivary frothing, hydrothorax, pulmonary edema, hepatic and renal degeneration • 1 mg Se/kg BW—no weight loss in 72 days • 0.5–1 mg Se/kg BW—several deaths between 78–178 days • Oral LD_{50}—1.9 mg Se/kg BW	

Chronic Effects (Alkali Disease/Bob-Tail Disease)

• Chronic selenium poisoning is more common than acute poisoning due to the typical exposure rates. Also, the ingested selenium bioaccumulates, thus causing adversities over longer periods of time.

• Chronic selenosis is associated with depression, weakness, emaciation, anemia, hair loss /alopecia, swelling of coronary band, and hoof deformities that may result in separation and sloughing of the hoof wall.

• Reproductive performance may be reduced without showing clinical signs at concentrations ranging from 5 to 10 ppm Se in the total diet. Some of these adverse effects on reproduction are considered to be caused by the interference with absorption and retention of copper that results in copper deficiency.

• Blind staggers has been described in cattle and sheep but its causal link with selenium intoxication is weak.

• Bovine—even in the absence of clinical alkali disease in cattle, elevated Se concentrations may adversely affect both pregnancy and the bovine immune response. Se administered as sodium selenite at 25 ppm (0.6–1 mg Se/kg BW) for 1 month or 15 ppm (0.4–0.6 mg Se/kg BW) for 6 months caused chronic selenosis.

• Sheep—chronic selenosis may result in death—without observing clinical signs. Unlike other species, wool loss and hoof lesions are not commonly identified in sheep, although the wool production is known to decrease. Sheep fed diets containing 0.5–1 mg Se/ kg BW (about 17–33 ppm in the diet) reportedly was lethal when exposed for 2 1/2–6 months. Unlike other ruminant species, hair loss and hoof lesions are not commonly seen in sheep. Please see Table 1.

RISK FACTORS

• Vitamin E–deficient animals are more susceptible to acute selenosis.

• Se toxicosis has been reported to increase with concomitant cobalt deficiency.

• Signs of Se deficiency resemble those of selenium toxicosis.

• Primary selenium accumulators such as *Astragalus, Machaeranthera, Xylorhiza,* and *Haplopappus* spp. can contain > 1000 ppm selenium. Secondary accumulators such as *Aster, Atriplex, Grindelia, Gutierrezia,* and *Casteilleja* spp. can also contain toxic amounts of selenium, are usually unpalatable, and are the last choice for animals. The commonly used forage species are nonaccumulators.

DIAGNOSIS

DIFFERENTIAL DIAGNOSIS

Pneumonia, cardiotoxic plant exposure, ionophore overdose, thallium toxicosis, Vitamin E and selenium deficiency, and endotoxemia

CBC/BIOCHEMISTRY/URINALYSIS

• CBC, serum biochemistry, and urinalysis results are usually unremarkable in acute cases.

• In chronic exposure, the liver enzymes may be elevated as a result of the liver damage.

OTHER LABORATORY TESTS
N/A

IMAGING
N/A

DIAGNOSTIC PROCEDURES

• For most ruminants, normal Se in blood (0.08–0.5 ppm) and liver (0.25–1.0 ppm)

• In acute cases, the liver selenium may range from 15–30 ppm or above.

• In chronic cases, liver selenium may range from 2–7 ppm and the hair/hoof Se may range from 1.5 ppm up to 45 ppm. Blood Se and blood GSH-Px activity has also been used for diagnostic purpose.

PATHOLOGIC FINDINGS

Acute Selenosis

• Gross lesions include edematous, congested, and/or hemorrhagic lungs. Bloody froth may be seen in the airways. Congestion and hemorrhages are also observed in the liver, kidneys, and GIT. Petichiations of the epicardium may also be seen with or without edema.

• Histopathology reveals endocarditis, myocarditis, and myocardial necrosis. Hydropic degeneration of myocardium is seen along with petechial hemorrhages. Focal areas of necrosis are seen in the liver with occasional vacuolation of the hepatocytes. In kidneys, parenchymous and tubular degeneration with casts is a common finding. Histologic lesions are minimal if the clinical course is brief. Mild hyaline or granular degeneration of skeletal muscle fibers may be present. Variable necrosis of the lymphoid cells may also be present.

Chronic Selenosis
• Gross lesions include edematous and congested lungs, atrophied and cirrhosed liver with discoloration, enlargement of spleen and pancreas, anemia, atrophy of lymphoid tissue, atrophy and dilation of the heart, and erosion of articular surfaces.
• Histopathology indicates congestion and thickening of the alveolar walls in the lungs, hepatic fibrosis, myocardial degeneration, glomerulonephritis, and mild gastroenteritis. Areas primarily affected in the CNS include ventral horns of the cervical and lumbar vertebral segments, with lesser damage in brain stem nuclei. The microscopic appearance of the affected spinal chord includes vacuolation of the neuropils and sometimes within the cytoplasm of the neurons. Neuronal chromatolysis, axonal swelling, multifocal hemorrhage, and endothelial cell swelling and proliferation are also usually present. The white matter has minimal changes.

TREATMENT
No proven therapy for acute selenium toxicity

APPROPRIATE HEALTH CARE
N/A

NURSING CARE
• Supportive therapy
• Mechanical support for legs with hoof abnormalities until recovery

ACTIVITY
Avoid exercise/stress.

DIET
• Increase protein and carbohydrate in diet
• Increase sulfur in the diet.
• 40-ppm arsenic salt or 50–100 ppm arsanilic acid has provided benefit to calves. Arsenic compounds can increase the biliary excretion of selenium.
• 4–5 g naphthalene daily for 5 days has been successfully used in the past in mature cattle.

CLIENT EDUCATION
N/A

SURGICAL CONSIDERATIONS
N/A

MEDICATIONS

DRUGS OF CHOICE
• No specific drug/antidote available.
• Analgesics and NSAIDs may be used for pain relief.

CONTRAINDICATIONS
Appropriate milk and meat withdrawal times must be followed for all compounds administered to food-producing animals.

PRECAUTIONS
N/A

POSSIBLE INTERACTIONS
N/A

ALTERNATIVE DRUGS
N/A

FOLLOW-UP

PATIENT MONITORING
N/A

PREVENTION/AVOIDANCE
• Avoid excess/further selenium exposure.
• Keep the total dietary concentrations within the recommended limits.
• Prevent animals accessing seleniferous plants.
• Check for the selenium status in the blood.
• Avoid selenium supplementation in seleniferous areas.

POSSIBLE COMPLICATIONS
N/A

EXPECTED COURSE AND PROGNOSIS
• Guarded prognosis with acute selenosis
• Prolonged recovery with chronic selenosis

MISCELLANEOUS

ASSOCIATED CONDITIONS
• Blind staggers (misnomer)
• Polioencephalomalcia

AGE-RELATED FACTORS
Preruminants and young ruminants are considered to be more susceptible to selenosis because of the nondeveloped rumen that significantly reduces the amount of bioavailable selenium to nonbioavailable form.

ZOONOTIC POTENTIAL
N/A

PREGNANCY
• Abortions, stillbirths, or weak/lethargic calves
• No teratogenic effects described

RUMINANT SPECIES AFFECTED
All ruminant species should be considered susceptible.

BIOSECURITY
N/A

PRODUCTION MANAGEMENT
Analysis of selenium in feed or whole blood for regular monitoring of the overall status

SYNONYMS
Alkali disease
Bobtail disease

SEE ALSO
Cardiotoxic plant exposure
Endotoxemia
Ionophore overdose
Pneumonia
Thallium toxicosis
Vitamin E and selenium deficiency

ABBREVIATIONS
BW = body weight
CNS = central nervous system
FDA = Food and Drug Administration
GIT = gastrointestinal tract
GRAS = generally regarded as safe
LD_{50} = the estimated dose at which 50% of the population is expected to die
MLD = minimum lethal dose
NSAIDs = nonsteroidal anti-inflammatory agents
ppm = parts per million
ROS = reactive oxygen species

Suggested Reading
Osweiler, G. D., Carson, T. L., Buck, W. B., Van Gelder, G. A. 1985. In: *Clinical and diagnostic veterinary toxicology.* 3rd ed. Dubuque, IA: Kendall/Hunt.
O'Toole, D., Raisbeck, M. F. 1995. Pathology of experimentally induced chronic selenosis ("alkali disease") in yearling cattle. *J Vet Diagn Invest.* 7:364–73.
Raisbeck, M. F. 2000. Selenosis. *Veterinary clinics of North America: food animal practice.* 16(3): 465–480.
Rosenfeld, I., Beath, O. A. 1964. *Selenium: geobotany, biochemistry, toxicity, and nutrition.* New York: Academic Press.
Spallholz, J. E. 1994. On the nature of selenium toxicity and carcinostatic activity. *Free Radic Biol Med.* 17:45–64.

Author: Asheesh K. Tiwary

SELF-MUTILATION

 BASICS

OVERVIEW
• Self-inflicted bodily injury such as licking, chewing, or biting at tail, mammary, or limbs, or rubbing against objects until injury occurs.
• Behavioral abnormalities can be a result of central nervous system disorders affecting the cerebrum.
• Behavioral problems can also result from environment conditions such as stress or boredom.

SIGNALMENT
Any species and age can be affected.

SIGNS
• Hair loss
• Dermatitis with possible secondary bacterial infections of epidermis and dermis
• Weight loss due to decrease in feeding associated with obsessive behaviors
• May find blood or clumps of hair on gates or other inanimate objects the animal is rubbing against.
• Traumatized mammary gland

CAUSES AND RISK FACTORS
• Underlying medical problems such as dermatological conditions or parasitic infections
• Behavioral abnormalities can be a result of central nervous system disorders affecting the cerebrum.
• Behavioral problems can also result from environmental conditions such as stress or boredom.

 DIAGNOSIS

DIFFERENTIAL DIAGNOSIS
• Skin diseases with alopecia and/or dermatitis
  • Pruritis or pain
  • Ectoparasites, dermatophytosis, primary or secondary pyoderma
  • Atopy, food or contact allergies, insect hypersensitivity

• Reactions to previously administered medications
• Friction due to poorly fitted halters or stanchions
• Neurologic diseases such as
  • Pseudorabies (Aujeszky's disease, mad itch)—viral infection results in intense pruritis at point of dermatological infection.
  • Transmissible spongiform encephalopathies (TSEs) such as scrapie in sheep can result in extreme pruritis of the trunk.
  • Rabies can result in any form of behavioral abnormality.
• Behavioral disorders: obsessive-compulsive disorders
• Nutritional deficiencies and metabolic or endocrine disease can affect skin and hair coat.

CBC/BIOCHEMISTRY/URINALYSIS
Depends on underlying cause, medical or behavioral

OTHER LABORATORY TESTS
Depends on underlying cause

IMAGING
N/A

DIAGNOSTIC PROCEDURES
• Accurate and complete history is essential to ascertain medical or behavioral causes of self-mutilation
• Whether lesions are localized or generalized, this is often useful in diagnosing parasitic infections that have characteristic distribution of self-mutilation lesions.
• Determine whether multiple animals in the herd or flock are affected or if it is an individual animal problem. Behavioral or allergic problems are more typically individual problems. Neurologic disorders can be either an individual or an infectious problem.
• Physical examination may indicate primary cutaneous changes such as wheals, nodules, or pustules that would not be present if lesions were due solely to self-mutilation.
• Skin scrapings
• Fungal cultures

• Biopsy for histopathologic exam or direct immunofluorescence testing
• Bacterial culture and sensitivity: may only confirm secondary infection without determining underlying disease cause
• Blood serum chemistry and complete blood count
• +/− CSF tap
• +/− Intradermal skin testing

PATHOLOGIC FINDINGS

GROSS FINDINGS
Can include alopecia, dermatitis, and possible secondary pyoderma

HISTOPATHOLOGICAL FINDINGS
Depends on underlying cause

 TREATMENT

• Parasitic conditions require appropriate ectoparasite or anthelmintic treatment. Environmental control of parasites is also necessary.
• Neurologic conditions require specific treatment based on the underlying condition.
• Behavioral conditions often require environmental management changes to reduce stress or relieve boredom. Antianxiety medications may be needed in conjunction with behavior modification.
• Evaluate ration for nutritional deficiencies.
• Consider exotic diseases and rabies prior to treatment regime.

 MEDICATIONS

Depends on underlying cause

CONTRAINDICATIONS
N/A

FOLLOW-UP

PATIENT MONITORING
Monitor for progression of disease and for
secondary infections caused by
self-mutilation.

PREVENTION/AVOIDANCE
• Provide housing with adequate space and
access to feeders and water for all animals to
prevent disease and reduce stress that can lead
to behavioral problems.
• Provide adequate space for movement and
environmental enrichment to avoid
behavioral problems due to boredom.
• Feeders should be above ground to reduce
risk of parasitic infestations.
• Provide adequate bedding and clean
buildings and yard regularly.
• Keep newly purchased animals isolated from
the rest of the herd or flock for 30 days to
evaluate for disease.

POSSIBLE COMPLICATIONS
N/A

EXPECTED COURSE AND PROGNOSIS
• Parasitic conditions respond well to
appropriate treatment but may require
ongoing environmental and medical
management.
• Allergic or immune conditions respond to
therapy depending on individual condition.
• Neurologic conditions are often progressive
and may be fatal.
• Behavioral conditions can respond to
environmental enrichment or reduction of
stress in environmental management.

 MISCELLANEOUS

ASSOCIATED CONDITIONS
N/A

AGE-RELATED FACTORS
• Behavioral disorders can occur at any age,
but can start very early in life such as
abnormal suckling behaviors in orphaned
calves.
• Other problems arise at or near the time of
social maturity when stress is increased and
dominance hierarchy is being established.
• Ewes and does may self-suckle if they abort
late in pregnancy or due to extreme stress in
environment.
• After sexual maturity, rams or bulls may
develop obsessive-compulsive behavior of
masturbation.

ZOONOTIC POTENTIAL
Depends on underlying medical condition

PREGNANCY
N/A

SYNOMYMS
N/A

SEE ALSO
Dairy cattle behavior, anesthesia and
analgesia, physical examination, external
parasite chapters.
Dermatophytosis
Ectoparasites
Nutritional deficiencies
Pseudorabies (Aujeszky's disease, mad itch)
Rabies
Transmissible spongiform encephalopathies
(TSEs)

ABBREVIATIONS
CNS = central nervous system

Suggested Reading

Aiello, S. E., ed. 1998. Anomalies of the
nervous system. In: *Merck veterinary
manual*. 8th ed. Whitehouse Station, NJ:
Merck & Co.
Aiello, S. E., ed. 1998. Social behavior and
behavioral problems. In: *Merck veterinary
manual*. 8th ed. Whitehouse Station, NJ:
Merck & Co.
Cohen, R. J. 1976, Feb. Comments on the
"cattle-prod controversy." *Percept Mot Skills*.
42(1):146.
Eisele, P. H., Allen, C. E. 2001, Mar. Design
and use of a protective jacket to prevent
self-inflicted injury following cervical
laminoplasty in the goat (*Capra hircus*).
Contemp Top Lab Anim Sci. 40(2): 40–44.
Smith, B.P., ed. 2002. Disorders that cause
clinical signs of skin disease in ruminants.
In: *Large animal internal medicine*. 3rd ed.
St. Louis: Mosby.

Author: Lisa Nashold

SEMINAL VESICULITIS

BASICS

OVERVIEW
- The paired vesicular glands are the major accessory sex glands in the bull, buck, and ram.
- The vesicular glands are absent in camelids.
- The vesicular glands contribute volume, nutrients, and buffers to the ejaculate but these contributions are not absolutely essential for fertility.
- The vesicular glands have a lobar structure and are found on the floor of the cranial pelvic cavity. Normal glands in the bull are about 2–4 cm wide and 10–15 cm long.
- Seminal vesiculitis is an inflammation of either or both vesicular glands.
- The condition is most commonly described in the bull but this may be due to the accessibility of the pelvic organs in the bull to palpation per rectum as compared to the buck and ram.

PATHOPHYSIOLOGY
- Bacteria are the most commonly incriminated infectious etiological agents but viral, chlamydial, fungal, and protozoal agents have been isolated.
- The precise mechanism of infection and pathology is not known and ascending, descending, or hematogenous routes of infection are all considered possibilities.
- Primary infections elsewhere in the body, especially chronic ones, may cause seminal vesiculitis by the hematogenous route.
- Urogenital anomalies may contribute to malfunctioning of the vesicular gland openings on the colliculus seminalis and increase the risk of seminal vesiculitis.
- Retrograde ejaculation or urine reflux into the vesicular gland may predispose to infection or cause a sterile inflammation of the glands.

- Bilateral and unilateral involvement of glands is equally likely.
- In ruminants, seminal vesiculitis is often found as part of a seminal vesiculitis syndrome with concurrent orchitis, epididymitis, ampulitis, bulbourethral adenitis, or prostatitis.

SYSTEMS AFFECTED
Reproductive

GENETICS
No known genetic influence or breed distribution

INCIDENCE/PREVALENCE
- The prevalence has been reported to be between 1% and 10% in bulls.
- The prevalence is significantly higher in young, peripubertal bulls intensively housed and fed high-energy diets. Within peripubertal bulls, the prevalence may reach 10%–30%.
- The prevalence is also higher in aged bulls (> 9 years).
- Clinical diagnostic criteria may significantly underestimate the true disease prevalence, especially in small ruminants where physical examination of the pelvic accessory sex glands is difficult to accomplish and is not routinely done.

GEOGRAPHICAL DISTRIBUTION
Worldwide distribution

SIGNALMENT

Species
- Most commonly found in bulls but does affect rams and bucks as well.
- *Bos taurus* and *Bos indicus* bulls are equally affected.

Breed Predilections
None known

Mean Age and Range
Most commonly found in peripubertal bulls (10–15 months) and older bulls (> 9 years).

Predominant Sex
Males only

SIGNS

GENERAL COMMENTS
Clinical signs are often completely lacking.

HISTORICAL FINDINGS
- Breeding bulls may have a history of sterility or subfertility but often have acceptable levels of fertility.
- AI sires may have a history of producing semen with poor motility and postthaw viability along with the presence of white blood cells in the ejaculate.

PHYSICAL EXAMINATION FINDINGS
- Unilateral or bilateral enlargement of the glands and loss of lobulations on palpation per rectum are the most common findings.
- In chronic cases, abscess formation and adhesions to adjacent abdominal or pelvic structures may occur.
- Rarely, bulls may show signs of abdominal pain, pain during mounting and thrusting, or when they are collected by electroejaculation.
- Most physical exam findings are normal.
- The finding of infectious or inflammatory lesions anywhere in the genital tract of male ruminants should suggest the possibility of a concurrent seminal vesiculitis.

CAUSES
- Seminal vesiculitis has been attributed to a variety of infectious and noninfectious causes.
- *Mycobacterium tuberculosis, M. avium* ss *paratuberculosis, Brucella abortus, B. ovis,* and *B. melitensis* are potential agents of special concern either for their zoonotic potential or local reporting requirements or both.
- In areas free of brucellosis, *Arcanobacterium pyogenes* is the bacteria most commonly isolated from clinical cases.
- *Streptococcus* spp., *Staphylococcus* spp., *Pseudomonas aeruginosa, E. coli, Tritrichomonas foetus, Chlamydia* spp., *Ureaplasma* spp., *Mycoplasma* spp., and *Haemophilus* spp. have all been reported to cause seminal vesiculitis in bulls.

• A wide variety of bacteria have been isolated from cases of ovine epididymitis and should be considered potential causes of seminal vesiculitis in this species as well.
• Bovine herpesvirus-1 and other viruses have been incriminated as causes of vesiculitis.
• Sperm entering the gland during ejaculation may initiate an autoimmune reaction and subsequent vesiculitis.

RISK FACTORS
• Infections at other body sites (e.g., orchitis, epididymitis, urethritis, rumenitis, pneumonia, omphalophlebitis, or traumatic reticulopericarditis) or congenital anomalies of the urogenital system (e.g., uterus masculinus or malformation of the colliculus seminalis) may predispose to developing seminal vesiculitis.
• High-density housing systems and high-concentrate diets commonly found in bull test stations appear to increase the risk of vesiculitis as well.

 DIAGNOSIS

DIFFERENTIAL DIAGNOSIS
• Differential diagnoses for enlargement or asymmetry of the vesicular glands are segmental aplasia, hypoplasia, or accessory vesicular glands.
• The presence of a dilated or infected uterus masculinus may mimic seminal vesiculitis.
• Differentials for white blood cells in the semen include infections or inflammation anywhere along the urogenital tract including the prepuce and penis.
• Urinary calculi should be considered, especially in rams and bucks.
• Primary infectious diseases of special concern in cases of seminal vesiculitis include brucellosis, tuberculosis, and paratuberculosis.

CBC/BIOCHEMISTRY/URINALYSIS
• The CBC will usually be normal.
• Certain semen biochemistry values are altered but these have limited clinical relevance.
• Urinalysis may be normal or show an elevated white blood cell count.

OTHER LABORATORY TESTS
• Semen evaluation may reveal an elevated pH, lower sperm motility, increased catalase activity, and lower fructose concentration.
• Leukocytes are not normally seen in ruminant ejaculates but are generally present in seminal vesiculitis. Neutrophils are most commonly seen, but lymphocytes may predominate in some cases.
• Many bulls with seminal vesiculitis have semen quality problems, typically sperm with poor motility or morphologic abnormalities are found.
• Changes in sperm morphology may actually be the result of a concurrent orchitis or epididymitis as part of the seminal vesiculitis syndrome, rather than the direct result of seminal vesiculitis.

IMAGING
• Transrectal ultrasonography is useful for imaging the vesicular glands.
• A 5 MHz transrectal probe with a rigid extension can be used for pelvic examination in small ruminants.
• Affected glands are larger and may have a more or less echoic parenchyma with a relatively hyperechoic appearance to the stromal and ductular network.
• Abscessed glands will show a loss of normal lobar architecture with globoid areas of variable echo-density.

DIAGNOSTIC PROCEDURES
• Culture and antibiotic sensitivity testing are used to confirm cases with a bacterial etiology and to select appropriate treatment.

• Quantitative culture of an ejaculate collected by artificial vagina or electroejaculation may suffice if large numbers of the infectious agent are being secreted in the ejaculate but contamination with urethral, penile, and preputial microflora is unavoidable and may confuse the diagnosis.
• Noncontaminated samples require that the bull be sedated, and the penis be exposed, disinfected, and catheterized followed by transrectal massage of the vesicular glands and collection of fluid.
• Aerobic, anaerobic, and special (e.g., *Mycoplasma, Ureaplasma, T. fetus,* and fungi) cultures should be performed.
• Routine semen evaluation will usually show hypercoagulation of sperm cells and Diff-Quick staining of semen will confirm pyospermia.

PATHOLOGIC FINDINGS

GROSS FINDINGS
Gross findings are consistent with the physical examination findings.

HISTOPATHOLOGICAL FINDINGS
• The lesions consist of variable leukocytic infiltration of the interstitial and alveolar areas (microabscessation) along with fibrotic and other degenerative changes throughout the glands.
• Sperm cells are frequently seen in the ductular or alveolar regions of the gland.

 TREATMENT

APPROPRIATE HEALTH CARE
• Medical treatment with antibiotics, local injection of sclerotic agents, and surgical removal of the affected glands have all been attempted but with limited success.
• Medical treatment is usually done on the farm or at the AI center.

SEMINAL VESICULITIS

• Surgical treatment consists of unilateral or bilateral vesiculectomy and usually requires hospitalization.
• Given the prolonged duration of medical therapy and the length of time required for postoperative recovery, the bull will usually be lost for at least the current breeding season.

NURSING CARE
N/A

ACTIVITY
Sexual rest is recommended during medical therapy and for at least 6 weeks after surgical therapy.

DIET
N/A

CLIENT EDUCATION
It is imperative that clients understand that there is a guarded to poor prognosis for recovery, therefore, only very valuable bulls should be considered candidates for treatment.

SURGICAL CONSIDERATIONS
• Surgery is performed on the standing bull so restraint of the patient is critical.
• Both a perirectal ischiorectal fossa and a ventral pararectal approach to vesiculectomy are described.

MEDICATIONS

DRUGS OF CHOICE
• Antibiotics based on culture and sensitivity for a minimum of 2–4 weeks and potentially for as long as 6–8 weeks
• Penicillins are appropriate for cases caused by *A. pyogenes.*
• Rifampin, isoniazid, erythromycin, and trimethoprim have been used with some success.
• Nonsteroidal anti-inflammatory agents may improve the response to antibiotics in acute cases and reduce the risk of adhesions.

CONTRAINDICATIONS
N/A

PRECAUTIONS
No drugs available in the United States are labeled for treatment of seminal vesiculitis, so all therapies represent extralabel drug use and require a determination of appropriate withdrawal times before slaughter.

POSSIBLE INTERACTIONS
N/A

ALTERNATIVE DRUGS
N/A

FOLLOW-UP

PATIENT MONITORING
• Repeat a BSE every 6 weeks for up to 6 months.
• Examine the semen carefully for the presence of pyospermia.

PREVENTION/AVOIDANCE
Avoid crowded and unsanitary conditions that may increase the general risk of infectious diseases, especially those caused by *A. pyogenes.*

POSSIBLE COMPLICATIONS
Postsurgical abscess formation and peritonitis

EXPECTED COURSE AND PROGNOSIS
Guarded to poor prognosis and recovery is often temporary so semen from valuable bulls should be collected and frozen as soon as it receives a normal evaluation.

MISCELLANEOUS

ASSOCIATED CONDITIONS
Seminal vesiculitis can occur in association with primary infections in other organs or as part of the seminal vesiculitis syndrome.

SEMINAL VESICULITIS

AGE-RELATED FACTORS
• Spontaneous recovery is probably the rule for most young bulls affected with seminal vesiculitis, and treatment of these bulls will often seem to be successful.
• Older bulls are less likely to respond favorably to treatment and have a more guarded prognosis for recovery.

ZOONOTIC POTENTIAL
Brucellosis and tuberculosis can cause seminal vesiculitis in ruminants.

PREGNANCY
N/A

RUMINANT SPECIES AFFECTED
Cattle, sheep, goats

BIOSECURITY
• All males to be used as breeding animals should be subject to the same parasite control and vaccination procedures as the females in the flock or herd except that bulls should not be routinely vaccinated for brucellosis.
• Bulls or bull calves destined for sale to AI centers should not be vaccinated for any diseases unless specifically requested by the facility.

• All breeding males entering a herd or flock should undergo a breeding soundness examination and an appropriate period of quarantine followed by reexamination.

PRODUCTION MANAGEMENT
• Animals affected with seminal vesiculitis have the potential to reduce the reproductive efficiency of food and fiber production systems.
• This reduction occurs most often as a result of the decreased fertility of the affected males but may also involve disease transmission to the females.
• Males with evidence of subfertility or infectious or hereditary diseases should be eliminated from the breeding population.

SYNONYMS
Vesicular gland adenitis
Vesiculitis

SEE ALSO
Breeding management problems of sheep and goats
Breeding soundness exam
Brucellosis
Bull management
Epididymitis
Orchitis
Reproductive ultrasounding: bovine

ABBREVIATIONS
AI = artificial insemination
BSE = breeding soundness examination

Suggested Reading
Cavalieri, J., Van Camp, S. D. 1997. Bovine seminal vesiculitis: a review and update. *Vet Clinics of North America: Food Animal Practice* 13:23–32, 41.
Hoover, T. R. 1974. A technique for injecting into the seminal vesicles of the bull. *Am J Vet Res.* 35:1135–36.
Jansen, B. C. 1980. The pathology of bacterial infection in the genitalia in rams. *Onderstepoort J Vet Res.* 47:263–67.
Larson, R. L. 1997. Diagnosing and controlling seminal vesiculitis in bulls. *Veterinary Medicine* 92:1073–78.
McEntee, K. 1990. *Reproductive pathology of domestic animals.* New York: Academic Press.
Parsonson, I. M., Hall, C. E., Settergren, I. 1971. A method for the collection of bovine seminal vesicle secretions for microbiologic examination. *J Am Vet Med Assoc.* 158:175–77.

Authors: Harry Momont and James Meronek

SENNA (CASSIA SPP.)

BASICS

OVERVIEW
• Annual or perennial herbs or shrubs that cause musculoskeletal problems in ruminants
• These plants are members of the Fabaceae (legume) family.
• Approximately 240 species exist and are found primarily in tropical and warm temperate climates of the world.
• *Senna occidentalis* (common names: senna, coffee senna, coffee weed) and *Senna obtusifolia* (sickle pod, coffee bean, coffee weed) are the two most common species in North America.
• Other common species
  • *S. roemeriana* (twin-leaf senna)
  • *S. fasciculate* (showy partridge senna)
  • *S. lindheimeriana* (lindheimer senna)
  • *S. nictitans* (wild sensitive plant)
• *S. occidentalis* is often found along roadsides and waste places. It prefers partial shade.
• *S. obtusifolia* is commonly a problem in cultivated areas such as cornfields, and prefers sandy soil.
• The sennas are up to 6–8 feet in height, woody and erect.
• They possess alternate, pinnate compound leaves with 4–8 pairs of leaflets or more.
• Flowers are yellow, 1–2 cm.
• Pods on *S. obtusifolia* are sickle shaped, almost four sided, 10–20 cm in length with the ends pointing downward.
• *S. occidentalis* has pods that are more flattened, straighter, and shorter with the ends pointing upward. Seeds are dark brown.
• The plants may contaminate grains, silage, green chop, and hay.
• Ruminants can also become intoxicated by eating the plant in the field, although it is generally not palatable.

• The toxins affect the gastrointestinal tract and skeletal muscles.
• When cattle consume approximately 0.5% body weight of seeds, severe muscle degeneration has occurred.
• Feed containing 10% seeds from *S. occidentalis* will cause disease.
• A 0.2% body weight of green plant consumed daily over 5–7 days or overnight fill on *S. occidentalis* will produce toxicity.

SIGNALMENT
• All ruminants are susceptible, although cattle are most commonly poisoned. Other animals poisoned include horses, pigs, rabbits, and chickens.
• *S. roemeriana* (two-leaved senna) is more common in the western United States and is more likely a problem in the spring.
• Disease associated with *Senna* spp. is usually limited to a few animals unless plants are inadvertently fed in contaminated silage, hay, etc.

SIGNS
• Diarrhea, moderate to severe and shortly after consumption, is usually the first observed sign.
• Progressive muscular weakness indicated by tremors in rear limbs, ataxia, weakness, and eventual inability to rise occurs later in the course of the toxicity.
• Animals are generally afebrile.
• Cattle are often referred to as "bright-eyed downers" as they will sometimes continue to eat, drink, and remain alert. In contrast, other affected animals become lethargic and anorectic.
• The urine becomes dark (myoglobinuria) as muscle degeneration progresses.
• Most animals do not survive once recumbency occurs; death usually occurs within 1–7 days.

CAUSES AND RISK FACTORS
• Anthraquinones are the toxic principles in *Senna*.
• Obtusin, emodin, and obtusifolin toxins are common, but numerous others exist.
• All parts of the plants are toxic. Mature plants are more toxic than younger specimens. Seeds contain the highest concentration of anthraquinones.
• *Senna* spp. are not generally very palatable and are more likely consumed in the late summer and fall when other food sources become scarce.
• Plants are more commonly eaten after the first frost when they are wilted, possibly making them more palatable.

DIAGNOSIS

DIFFERENTIAL DIAGNOSIS
• White muscle disease is associated with deficiencies of vitamin E and selenium.
• Many other causes of "downer" animals

CBC/BIOCHEMISTRY/URINALYSIS
• Myoglobinuria may be mistaken for hemoglobinuria (hemoglobin is visible in plasma, whereas myoglobin is not).
• AST is elevated (10x).
• CK is elevated (10–1000x).
• The elevation in AST and CK reflects acute muscle degeneration.

OTHER LABORATORY TESTS
Evidence of plant consumption

IMAGING
N/A

DIAGNOSTIC PROCEDURES
N/A

PATHOLOGIC FINDINGS
• Severe muscle necrosis occurs.
• Pale discoloration and streaking of skeletal muscles may be seen, especially in the quadriceps femoris, semimembranosis, and semitendenosis.
• Hyperemia of the stomach and small intestinal mucosa
• The heart may contain pale streaking and hemorrhages.
• Mild centrilobular hepatic necrosis

TREATMENT
• Primarily supportive treatment of symptoms as there is no specific therapy available.
• Prevent further access to plants and feed a balanced ration.
• Intravenous fluids may help renal function if myoglobinuria is present.
• The use of vitamin E and selenium is contraindicated, as their use will increase myodegeneration and mortality.
• Treatment is usually unrewarding after recumbency develops.

MEDICATIONS

DRUGS OF CHOICE
Activated charcoal dosed at 5 g/kg body weight PO in a water slurry (1 g of activated charcoal in 5 ml water)

CONTRAINDICATIONS
Vitamin E and selenium

FOLLOW-UP

PATIENT MONITORING
N/A

PREVENTION/AVOIDANCE
• Prevent animal access to *Senna* spp.
• Maintain appropriate level of nutrition.

POSSIBLE COMPLICATIONS
N/A

EXPECTED COURSE AND PROGNOSIS
• Clinical course may last up to 7–10 days.
• Once recumbency occurs, few animals recover.

MISCELLANEOUS

ASSOCIATED CONDITIONS
·

AGE-RELATED FACTORS
N/A

ZOONOTIC POTENTIAL
N/A

PREGNANCY
N/A

RUMINANT SPECIES AFFECTED
Potentially all ruminant species

BIOSECURITY
N/A

PRODUCTION MANAGEMENT
N/A

SEE ALSO
Additional toxic ingestion chapters
Toxic herd outbreak management

ABBREVIATIONS
• AST = aspartate transaminase
• CK = creatine kinase
• PO = per os, by mouth

Suggested Reading
Burrows, G. E., Tyrl, R. J. 2001. *Toxic plants of North America.* Ames: Iowa State University Press.
Knight, A. P., Walter, R. G. 2001. *A guide to plant poisonings of animals in North America.* Jackson, WY: Teton New Media.
Poisonous plants of the southern United States. 1980. Knoxville, TN: Agricultural Extension Services, University of Tennessee.

Author: Matt G. Welborn

SHEEP AND GOAT POX

BASICS

OVERVIEW
• Sheep and goat pox is caused by a capripoxvirus that is closely related to the virus that causes lumpy skin disease in cattle.
• Sheep and goat pox is endemic in Africa, the Middle East, India, and most of Asia.
• The disease is characterized by fever and generalized pox lesions on the skin and mucous membranes. A severe bronchopneumonia can also be noted in infected animals.
• The disease is transmitted by direct contact with dried scabs, contaminated fomites, and aerosols from sick animals.
• Sheep and goat pox has not been detected in wild ungulate populations.

SYSTEMS AFFECTED
Production management; potentially all depending on condition

GENETICS
N/A

INCIDENCE/PREVALENCE
In areas where the disease is not present, susceptible adult animals can have a mortality of up to 50%, and lambs and kids can have a mortality of up to 100%.

GEOGRAPHIC DISTRIBUTION
Sheep and goat pox is endemic in Africa, the Middle East, India, and most of Asia.

SIGNALMENT
Species
Sheep and goats

Breed Predilections
N/A

Mean Age and Range
• Adult sheep and goats tend to have a lower mortality than lambs and kids.
• Naïve adult animals may develop a severe condition with high death losses (may approach 50%).
• Lambs and kids are usually the most severely affected with death losses approaching 95%.
• Animals under 1 month of age usually have a mortality of 100%.

Predominant Sex
N/A

SIGNS
• Depending on the susceptibility of the animal, clinical disease may range from mild to severe.
• Incubation period ranges from 4 to 14 days with the course of the disease lasting up to 6 weeks with various stages of the pox lesions seen at the same time. Complete recovery may take up to 3 months.
• Animals first develop fever, 104–106°F (40–41°C), and become depressed. Increased lacrimation with conjunctivitis and rhinitis are often noted.
• Pox lesions are soon noted in haired and hairless areas of the body. Swelling of the muzzle, nares, and lips is usually noted first. As the disease progresses, characteristic pox lesions develop on the muzzle, nares, lips, eyelids, perineum, scrotum, axillary and inguinal regions, and udder.
• Lesions first appear as circular, raised, erythematous areas (macula). The lesions progress to circular, raised, blanched regions with a central region of fluid (papule). The papules eventually rupture leaving circular umbilicated lesions that scab over and slowly heal. The associated dermis is often thickened, hard, and edematous.
• Pox lesions often leave deep scars after the lesions heal.
• Pneumonia is often noted with severe labored breathing. Secondary bacterial infections are a common sequela. The animals usually have a persistent cough and are emaciated.
• As the disease progresses, the lesions scab over forming deep, slow-healing ulcers in the skin.

CAUSES AND RISK FACTORS:
N/A

DIAGNOSIS

DIFFERENTIAL DIAGNOSIS
• Bluetongue: animals develop a high fever and depression and have swollen lips and muzzle. Conjunctivitis with discharge is often noted. Animals often become lame due to a coronitis. Abortions, deformed fetuses, and deformed newborns are common with intrauterine infections.
• Contagious ecthyma (orf): proliferative pox lesions are seen on lips, dental pad, nares, and eyelids in affected young lambs and kids. Adult nursing females may have proliferative pox lesions on the lips, gums, dental pad, and udder.

• Photosensitization: nonpigmented regions of the body may be inflamed with necrosis, edema, and scabbing of the affected epithelium particularly of the lips, muzzle, eyelids, and face.
• Insect bites: localized regions of circular swelling and erythema in the area of the insect bites are usually very pruritic. Mucous membranes are rarely involved.
• *Dermatophilus congolensis* (streptothricosis): superficial scabbing of the skin is noted with intact skin seen underneath the scabs. Lesions are commonly observed in the skin of the neck, axillary and inguinal regions, and perineum.
• Psoroptic mange: scabs and alopecia are due to intense itching of affected areas. Intense itching is not observed with sheep or goat pox.

CBC/BIOCHEMISTRY/URINALYSIS
N/A

OTHER LABORATORY FINDINGS
N/A

IMAGING
N/A

DIAGNOSTIC PROCEDURES
• Virus is often isolated from scabs or vesicle fluid.
• Electron microscopy is often used to identify typical brick-shaped poxvirus particles.

PATHOLOGIC FINDINGS

GROSS FINDINGS
• The dermis and epidermis are thickened and edematous. Lymph nodes draining these areas are often swollen and edematous.
• Pox lesions (circumscribed macules, papules, vesicles, and deep circular ulcerated lesions with scabs in later resolving cases) are noted on the muzzle, nares, hairless areas of the axillary and inguinal regions, vulva, prepuce, udder, teats, eyelids, sclera, lips, oral cavity, esophagus, and rumen.
• Lung lesions are randomly distributed throughout the lungs due to hematogenous spread of the virus. The lesions are discrete, hard, grey-white to hemorrhagic nodules that are easily identified in the lungs. The pulmonary parenchyma adjacent to these areas often becomes atelectic due to the affected bronchiole constriction.
• Secondary bacterial pneumonias are often sequela to the infection.

HISTOPATHOLOGIC FINDINGS
• Histologically in the skin, there is acanthosis of the epidermis, with ballooning degeneration of keratinocytes. Necrosis and microvesiculation of the stratum spinosum occurs as the lesion progresses.
• Eosinophilic intracytoplasmic inclusion bodies are noted in the swollen keratinocytes. The dermis is edematous with some hemorrhage and neutrophilic infiltrates.
• Macrophages accumulate in the affected dermis with some becoming enlarged and swollen with eosinophilic intracytoplasmic inclusion bodies and large vacuolated nuclei with marginated chromatin (cellules claveleuses or sheep pox cells). As the disease progresses, a severe necrotizing vasculitis develops in the affected dermis affecting arterioles and venules with thrombosis of affected blood vessels.
• Necrosis of the affected dermis and epidermis follows.
• Lung lesions are characterized by a proliferative bronchopneumonia with hyperplasia and necrosis of the bronchiolar epithelium. The alveolar septal walls and associated peribronchiolar connective tissue are thickened by edema and hemorrhage. Some type II pneumocyte hyperplasia is noted in alveoli. Variable numbers of macrophages and neutrophils are present in the affected areas with scattered "sheep pox cells" present.
• Eosinophilic intracytoplasmic inclusions can be present in the "sheep pox cells" and type II pneumocytes.
• Mononuclear infiltrates containing sheep pox cells can be noted in the heart, kidney, adrenal glands, liver, thyroid, and pancreas.

 TREATMENT
• Since this is a reportable disease in many parts of the world, one should consult with regulatory veterinarians prior to undertaking treatment.

• Treating affected animals is difficult. The administration of an antipyretic drug to make the animal feel better so it will eat and drink is important. Treating the animal with antibiotics for secondary bacterial skin or pulmonary disease may be helpful to the survival of the affected animals.

 MEDICATIONS
N/A

CONTRAINDICATIONS/POSSIBLE INTERACTIONS
• Appropriate milk and meat withdrawal times must be followed for all compounds administered to food-producing animals.
• Steroids should not be used in pregnant animals.

 FOLLOW-UP

PATIENT MONITORING
N/A

PREVENTION/AVOIDANCE
N/A

POSSIBLE COMPLICATIONS
Secondary bacterial infections in the skin and lung are possible.

EXPECTED COURSE AND PROGNOSIS
• Animals living in endemic areas usually have some innate immunity.
• In areas where the disease is not present, susceptible adult animals can have a mortality of up to 50%, and lambs and kids can have a mortality of up to 100%.

 MISCELLANEOUS

ASSOCIATED CONDITIONS

AGE-RELATED FACTORS
• Lambs and kids are usually the most severely affected with death losses approaching 95%.
• Animals under 1 month of age usually have a mortality of 100%.

ZOONOTIC POTENTIAL
Several suspected human cases of goat pox have been described; however, no virus was isolated from these individuals.

PREGNANCY
N/A

BIOSECURITY
• Quarantine new stock entering the herd/flock.
• Treat and/or cull new animals for disease conditions prior to herd introduction.

PRODUCTION MANAGEMENT
The disease is transmitted by direct contact with dried scabs, contaminated fomites, and aerosols from sick animals.

SEE ALSO
• Bluetongue
• Contagious ecthyma (orf)
• *Dermatophilus congolensis* (streptothricosis)
• Insect bites
• Photosensitization
• Psoroptic mange

ABBREVIATIONS
N/A

Suggested Reading
Cebra, C., Cebra, M. 2002. Disease of the hematologic, immunologic, and lymphatic systems (multisystem diseases) In: *Sheep and goat medicine*, ed. D. G. Pugh. Philadelphia, PA: W. B. Saunders Co.
Rao, T.V., Bandyopadhyay, S. K. 2000. A comprehensive review of goat pox and sheep pox and their diagnosis. *Anim Health Res Rev.* 1(2):127–36.
USAHA. 1998. Sheep and goat pox. In: *Foreign animal diseases*. Richmond, VA: United States Animal Health Association, http://www.vet.uga.edu/wpp/gray_book/FAD.

Author: Robert B. Moeller, Jr.

SHEEP KEDS

BASICS

OVERVIEW
• Pruritic external parasitic skin disease of goats and sheep found in temperate countries and in cooler highlands of the tropics.
• Infestation is caused by *Melophagus ovinus*, a flat, brown wingless sucking insect approximately 4–7 mm in length.

PATHOPHYSIOLOGY
• Keds spend entire life on the host and live less than 1 week off the host.
• Adult females live 100–120 days (4–5 months) and lay about ten keds (10–15 larvae) during this time
• Larvae are attached to the hairs and wool and pupate within 6–12 hours and mature within 22 days.
• Pupae develop between 25–34°C; optimum temperature is 30°C.
• Ambient temperature affects life cycle, hence their absence in hot, humid areas.
• Keds feed by piercing skin with mouthparts and sucking blood.
• Transmission is via direct contact.
• The ked may transmit *Trypanosoma melophagium* and *Rickettsia melophagi*, harmless blood parasites of sheep.

SYSTEMS AFFECTED
Production management, skin

GENETICS
N/A

INCIDENCE/PREVALENCE
N/A

GEOGRAPHIC DISTRIBUTION
Worldwide, depending on species and environment

SIGNALMENT
• Seen in goats and sheep worldwide
• No age, sex, or breed predilection

SIGNS
• Parasite is found most commonly on neck, shoulders, flanks, rump, and anterior thorax, abdomen, but *not* on dorsum
• Ked bites are pruritic and cause sheep/goats to be restless, bite, scratch, kick, and rub resulting in alopecia, excoriations, and/or broken wool.

• Ked excrement stains wool, which increases cost of processing wool.
• Heavy infestations can result in anemia, weight loss, decreased milk production, secondary infections.
• Hide and wool damage due to continuous scratching and biting by sheep
• Although keds are bloodsucking parasites, they rarely cause anemia unless there is a very heavy infestation. Large numbers of feeding keds gradually exsanguinate the host and cause variable degrees of anemia
• In infected flocks, all individuals are continuously parasitized, but few if any sheep die from uncomplicated ked infestation.

CAUSES AND RISK FACTORS
• A seasonal pattern of infestation occurs. Keds are sensitive to hot, dry weather and numbers decrease markedly in summer. Populations increase slowly over autumn and winter.
• Most common in fall and winter
• Numbers increase during fall and winter because ambient temperature is optimum for reproduction.
• Overcrowding or flocking of animals for shearing increases risk of transmission/infestation.
• Can spread rapidly in spring when sheep are housed together for shearing
• Spring shearing removes many of the keds and extremely high temperatures during the summer months keep the ked population low.
• Keds can live off the hosts for up to 2 weeks in moist mild conditions, but most die within 3–4 days and do not play a role in reinfestation of sheep.

DIAGNOSIS

DIFFERENTIAL DIAGNOSIS
Other pruritic skin diseases including *Sarcoptes, Psoroptes, Chorioptes*, and *Psorergates* spp. mites, lice, trombiculidiasis, forage mites

CBC/BIOCHEMISTRY/URINALYSIS
Anemia in heavily infested animals

OTHER LABORATORY TESTS
N/A

IMAGING
N/A

DIAGNOSTIC PROCEDURES
• Finding sheep keds on physical examination
• Adults are red brown in color and have a broad head and stout piercing mouthparts.
• Diagnosis is usually obvious; handheld magnifying lens may aid in locating parasite.
• Because of their size and color, both adult and pupal keds on lambs and shorn sheep are conspicuous to the naked eye, but on wooled sheep they are concealed within the fleece and their quantitation requires close inspection between parted fibers.
• Topographically, they concentrate on skin of the neck, sides, abdomen, and rump.

TREATMENT

• Shear wool to remove adults and larvae, especially before lambing.
• Treat sheep after shearing with an insecticide that has residual activity of at least 3 weeks; this will kill emerging pupae.
• Most treatments for lice are effective for sheep keds.
• Whole body vat dipping kills adults but not pupated larvae.
• Spraying, jetting, or shower dipping is most effective in sheared or short-haired animals.
• Spot-on or pour-on treatments are most effective
• If an insecticide with residual activity of > 3 weeks is not used, it will be necessary to repeat treatment several times at 14- to 21-day intervals to kill larvae.

MEDICATIONS

DRUGS OF CHOICE
• Topical (spray, dusts, and pour-ons) and systemic parasiticidal agents effective against lice are effective against keds. To insure proper meat and milk drug withdrawal times, consult FARAD.

• Many drugs licensed for use in dairy or beef cattle are not licensed for use in sheep or goats or in all countries. Effective drugs in cattle include:
• Injectable drugs: ivermectin or doramectin (200 μg/kg body weight)
• Pour-ons: permethrins, ivermectin, epinomectin, amitraz, doramectin, moxidectin
• Diazinon used as a pour-on removed all keds and prevented reestablishment for 9 weeks.
• Amitraz will kill adult keds but has little residual action and therefore is usually combined with another compound to provide sufficient residual action to eliminate infections.
• Coumaphos or malathion liquid for spray or dip application
• Keds are particularly susceptible to organophosphates and most of those used to eliminate lice will also remove keds. Many preparations can also be used in higher dose rates in pour on applications. Consult labeled instructions prior to treatment.
• Deltamethrin, cyhalothrin, and cypermethrin are effective.
• Cyfluthrin 2 mg/kg pour-on in sheep also eradicates keds and protects for 50 days.

CONTRAINDICATIONS
• Topical sprays and/or dusts represent an environmental risk to people and other nontarget species such as birds, amphibians, and fish, and should be used with appropriate care.
• Care should be taken when disposing of containers and/or topical solutions (i.e., large volumes of dip) to avoid groundwater contamination or runoff. Follow labeled disposal instructions.

• Appropriate milk and meat withdrawal times must be followed for all compounds administered to food-producing animals.
• Steroids should not be used in pregnant animals.

FOLLOW-UP

EXPECTED COURSE AND PROGNOSIS
• Rapid resolution of pruritus should occur shortly after therapy
• Lack of response to treatment may occur if sheep are not sheared and/or if all in contact animals are not treated.

MISCELLANEOUS

ASSOCIATED CONDITIONS
• Keds can transmit bluetongue virus.
• Secondary bacterial infections may need to be treated and/or wounds may need to be protected against myiasis.

ZOONOTIC POTENTIAL
N/A

RUMINANT SPECIES AFFECTED
Sheep and goats

BIOSECURITY
N/A

PRODUCTION MANAGEMENT
• Infestations may result in decreased milk and meat production.
• Infestations may result in damage to the wool and hide resulting in decreased grading.

• Staining of the wool by the keds' feces reduces its value and gives it a musty odor. Heavy infestations cause skin blemishes, which are costly to the leather industry.
• Infected purchased sheep should be treated several times during the quarantine period. Death of the parasites should be verified before the quarantined animals are released into the flock/herd.

SYNONYMS
Sheep ticks

SEE ALSO
FARAD = Food Animal Residue Avoidance Databank

Suggested Reading
Aiello, S. E., ed. 1998. Sheep keds. In: *Merck veterinary manual*. 8th ed. Whitehouse Station, US: Merck & Co.
Bates, P. Ectoparasites. In: *Diseases of sheep*, ed. W. B. Martin, I. D. Aitken. 3rd ed. Edinburgh: Blackwell Science.
Gnad, D. P., Mock, D. E. 2001. Ectoparasite control in small ruminants. *Vet Clinic N America* 17(2): 252.
Lofstedt, J. 1983. Dermatologic diseases of sheep. *Vet Clinic N America* 5(3): 428.
Scott, D. W. 1988. Parasitic diseases. In: *Large animal dermatology*. Philadelphia: W. B. Saunders.
Smith, M. 1990. Exclusion of infectious diseases from sheep and goat farms. *Vet Clinic N America* 6(3): 713.

Authors: Karen A. Moriello and Susan Semrad

SILAGE DISEASE

 BASICS

OVERVIEW
• Silage is the process of sealing grass and other forages in anaerobic conditions and allowing fermentation to occur. The water-soluble plant carbohydrates are converted to organic acids (especially lactic acid) by anaerobic bacteria. Proteins degrade to amino acids and other nitrogenous compounds. Ensiled feeds remain stable for years, provided that anaerobic conditions are maintained.
• Silage is most often fed to dairy cows or used in feed lots.
• There are three potential hazards from silage: (1) infectious, (2) chemical, (3) metabolic disorders from excess acidity, poor-quality silage, unpalatability, etc.
• The phrase "silage disease" most often refers to listeriosis.
• Potential economic losses from decreased productivity, illness, or death caused by poor-quality or damaged feeds can be significant.

SYSTEMS AFFECTED
Potentially all, depending on the disorder

GENETICS
N/A

INCIDENCE/PREVALENCE
• Can occur anytime, depending on etiology
• In some instances, silage is mostly fed in winter and spring.

GEOGRAPHIC DISTRIBUTION
Potentially worldwide. In some parts of Europe, silage production is prohibited or discouraged because of the risk of zoonotic diseases like listeriosis.

SIGNALMENT
Species
Most frequently cattle, although possible in any species fed silage

Breed Predilections
N/A

Predominant Sex
N/A

SIGNS
Clinical signs vary depending on etiology.

Sources
• Spoiled silage
• Elevated pH (not enough acidity)
• Improper ensilage
• Oxidative damage
• Contaminated silage (bacteria, mycotoxins, carcasses, toxins such as lead or fertilizers)
• Ammoniated high-quality forage

CAUSES AND RISK FACTORS
• Temperature, moisture content, and oxygen are important components in allowing the growth of microbes or molds. A change in optimum conditions allows deterioration of the silage. Feed deterioration allows the loss of dry matter and reduces simple carbohydrate content and loss of fat-soluble vitamins. Proteins can bind to carbohydrates forming an undigestible complex. Mycotoxins may be produced.
• Silage should be observed visually for changes in color (especially dark brown to black). Silage generally has a sweetly acidic smell or an acetone odor. If the odor changes, especially if musty, sour, or burnt caramel odor, damage has probably occurred.
• Normal fermentation temperature typically results in a 20°F rise in temperature. After oxygen is used, the temperature will fall to near-ambient temperatures. Temperatures above 95°F (35°C) should be avoided to reduce dry matter and energy losses.

 DIAGNOSIS

History
Questions should include:
• How many animals are affected (ill or died)?
• What is the age of affected animals?
• What is the current feeding program?
• When was silage produced, and what forages were included?
• How long has the silage been fed to affected animals?
• Has a diagnosis been made, and is silage a potential source of contamination?

Animal Diagnostic Samples
• Standard samples should be included as part of a complete workup.
• Blood
  • Whole blood–EDTA (5–10 ml per animal)
  • Serum–5–10 ml per animal
• Urine
  • 50–100 ml
  • Store in an airtight bottle with a tight lid.
• Ingesta/feces-up to 500 g
• Consult the local diagnostic laboratory
  • Provide clinical history, signs, and signalment so that the laboratory may provide suggestions for additional samples or recommended tests.
  • The diagnostic lab will provide their recommendations for sample sizes, containers, and shipping preferences.

Feed Sample and Submission
• 500 g or more of a composite sample within a lot
• Each lot should be tested separately.
• Multiple grab samples from each lot should be obtained, increasing the chance of identifying the problem.
• Silage should be frozen.

MISCELLANEOUS

ASSOCIATED CONDITIONS
• Metabolic
  • Acidosis (often subclinical)
  • Decreased production (due to poor-quality feed or poor palatability)
• Infectious
  • *Listeria monocytogenes*
  • *E. coli* and other coliform bacteria
  • *Clostridia* spp.
  • *Cryptosporidium parvum*
  • Mycotoxins, especially from *Aspergillus fumigatus*, *Actinomycetes*, *Penicillium*, and *Fusarium* species
• Chemical
  • Contamination with lead or other heavy metals (especially if industrial manufacturing is nearby)
  • Respiratory disease (similar to silo-filler's disease in humans) can occur if cattle are confined immediately adjacent to the silo.
  • Bovine bonkers (ammoniated high-quality forage)
  • Contamination with other potential toxins including fertilizers, insecticides, rodenticides, etc
  • Contamination with carcasses of other animals, providing a potential source of botulism
  • Phytoestrogens and other plant toxins can survive ensilage.

AGE-RELATED FACTORS
N/A

ZOONOTIC POTENTIAL
• Significant zoonotic potential exists.
• Infectious potential from diseases like listeriosis

• Contamination of milk with mycotoxins such as aflatoxin M1 metabolites.
• Several of these diseases are zoonotic. Care must be taken in the collection of laboratory samples and the diagnosis/treatment of affected animals.

PREGNANCY
N/A

RUMINANT SPECIES AFFECTED
• Potentially all ruminant species can be affected.
• Most frequently cattle, although possible in any species fed silage.

BIOSECURITY
Reasonable precautions should be taken to prevent unauthorized personnel from access to feeds or cattle because deliberate contamination of silage could occur.

PRODUCTION MANAGEMENT
See Causes and Risk Factors and Animal Diagnostic factors above.

SYNONYMS
Bovine bonkers
"Silage disease" most often refers to listeriosis
Silo filler's disease

SEE ALSO
Acidosis
Botulism
Clostridia spp.
Coliform bacteria
Cryptosporidium parvum
Heavy metals
Lead or other heavy metal toxicity

Listeriosis
Mycotoxins, especially from *Aspergillus fumigatus*, *Actinomycetes*, *Penicillium*, and *Fusarium* species
Nutrition
Phytoestrogens
Toxicology

ABBREVIATIONS
FARAD = Food Animal Residue Avoidance Databank

Suggested Reading
Driehuis, F., Oude Elferink, S. J. 2000. The impact of the quality of silage on animal health and food safety: a review. *Vet Q.* 22(4): 212–16.
Galey, F. D. 2000, Nov. Diagnostic toxicology for the food animal practitioner. *Vet Clin North Am Food Anim Pract.* 16(3): 409–21.
Olsen, W. G. 1993. Evaluation of heat- or mold-damaged ensiled feeds and their effects on livestock. In: *Current veterinary therapy 3: food animal practice*, ed. J. L. Howard. Philadelphia: Saunders.
Wilkinson, J. M. 1999. Silage and animal health. *Nat Toxins* 7(6): 221–32.

Author: Charlotte Means

SNAKEBITE

 BASICS

OVERVIEW
• Pit vipers account for a majority of venomous snakebites in North America.
• Named for the temperature-sensitive pit organ between the eye and the nostril, they include rattlesnakes (*Crotalus* spp.), cottonmouths (water moccasins), and copperheads (*Agkistrodon* spp.), and pygmy rattlesnakes and massasaugas (*Sistrurus* spp.). They are identified by a triangular head, elliptical pupils, keeled scales, and the presence of tail rattles in adults. Young rattlesnakes have a blunt tip on the tail until it is broken off.
• These snakes are aggressive and inject a neurotoxic or hemotoxic venom designed to incapacitate or predigest its victim with a small, potent dose. Venom is delivered through hinged, hollow, retractable, fangs, in a rapid, stabbing motion.
• Coral snakes (*Micruroides euryxanthus* and *Micrurus* spp.) are nocturnal, nonagressive, and rarely responsible for venomous bites to farm animals. They bite with short fixed fangs and hold on, delivering a neurotoxic venom by chewing.
• Envenomation in all victims is potentially fatal and a medical emergency.

PATHOPHYSIOLOGY
• The composition and mechanism of action of the various components of snake venoms continues to be elucidated.
• Venoms have generally been classified as hemotoxic or neurotoxic depending on predominant physiological effects.
• Hemotoxic venom contains enzymatic proteins that aid in tissue degradation and digestion (metalloproteases, hyaluronidase, collagenase); affect hemostasis (plasminlike protease, thrombinlike protease, kallikreinlike protease); hydrolyze second messengers like cAMP (phosphodiesterases) and potent, nonenzymatic polypeptides, resulting in pain, massive swelling, tissue necrosis, and abnormalities in coagulation.
• Neurotoxic venom produces significantly less local tissue destruction and pain, but has profound effects on both pre- and postsynaptic skeletal muscle and nonskeletal muscle neuromuscular junction sites including muscarinic and neuronal receptors, and K^+, Na^+, and Ca^{2+} ion channels. Phopholipase A_2 causes membrane disruption and mediates many of the neurotoxic and cardiotoxic biochemical changes. Numbness, muscle fasciculations, paralysis, and respiratory collapse result.

SYSTEMS AFFECTED
• Cardiovascular—tachycardia, cardiac arrhythmias, edema, shock, death
• Endocrine/metabolic—pyrexia,
• Hemic/lymphatic/immune—hemoconcentration, hypoalbuminemia,
thrombocytopenia, enlarged regional lymph nodes, leukocytosis, lymphangitis
• Hepatobiliary
• Musculoskeletal—weakness, muscle fasciculation, rhabdomylosis, tissue necrosis
• Nervous—pain, paresis, respiratory depression, anxiousness or depression, paralysis
• Ophthalmic—epiphora
• Renal/urologic—hematuria, proteinuria, renal failure
• Reproductive
• Respiratory—inspiratory dyspnea, epistaxis, asphyxiation if swelling occludes nasal passage or larynx, respiratory failure due to paralysis
• Skin/exocrine—sweating

GENETICS
None

INCIDENCE/PREVALANCE
Unknown in large animals

GEOGRAPHIC DISTRIBUTION
Pit vipers are widely distributed throughout the United States (except Alaska, Hawaii, and Maine). They survive in parts of Canada, Mexico, South America, and Australia. Coral snakes inhabit the southern United Sates from Arizona to Florida; worldwide in the tropics.

SIGNALMENT

Breed Predilections
None

Mean Age and Range
None

Predominant Sex
None

SIGNS

HISTORICAL FINDINGS
Usually one animal is affected at a time but several may be affected over the course of a season.

PHYSICAL EXAMINATION FINDINGS
Rapid, regional swelling with severe pain, edema, ecchymosis, petechiation, bleeding puncture wounds may or may not be appparent, tissue necrosis, inspiratory dyspnea, and epistaxis (especially if bite is near muzzle), increased salivation, dysphagia, anorexia, lethargy, weakness, reluctance to move, muscle fasciculations, tachycardia, cardiac arrhythmias, shock, numbness, paresis, paralysis, respiratory collapse, and CNS signs

CAUSES
Snakebite with envenomation

RISK FACTORS

Snake
Size, age, nutritional status, and species of snake (aggresssive species are more likely to strike), amount of venom injected (25% of bites are "dry" with no injection of venom), and the toxicity of the venom, which will vary between species (rattlesnakes > water moccasins > copperheads), within species, and within the same individual snake as it ages or as the size of its prey changes

Victim
Depth of bite and location (tongue, muzzle, face, body wall, or directly into a large vessel pose the greatest risk), age and size of victim (younger and smaller animals are more likely to sustain bites resulting in fatality), preexisting health conditions that affect cardiovascular, respiratory, renal, or hematological physiology or preexisiting conditions that compromise immune response, victim's susceptibility to venom, time to medical treatment (animals often survive the initial bite to succumb to infection later due to delayed discovery and treatment), and activity after bite (activity increases the distribution of venom).

Location/Habitat/Time of Year
Animals that crowd into shaded areas in hot summer months especially adjacent to watering holes, woodpiles, rocky outcroppings, overgrazed pastures, during drought, April-October when snakes are active

 DIAGNOSIS

DIFFERENTIAL DIAGNOSIS
Trauma, insect envenomation, abscessation, lizard bite

CBC/BIOCHEMISTRY/URINALYSIS
• Hemoconcentration, thrombocytopenia, leukocytosis, echinocytosis
• Elevated CPK
• Myoglobinuria, hematuria, proteinuria, glucosuria

OTHER LABORATORY TESTS
• Serial coagulation profiles, fibrinogen
• Serum antibodies to venom
• Detection of venom in serum

IMAGING
Ultrasonography or radiography may rule out traumatic injury or puncture.

DIAGNOSTIC PROCEDURES
• Marking the leading edge of the swelling along with circumferential measurements of limb or muzzle may give an indication of progression.
• ECG

PATHOLOGIC FINDINGS

GROSS FINDINGS
Variable: swelling, serous exudation, tissue necrosis, and/ or sloughing; hemorrhage, especially at bite site; passive congestion of all organs; hemorrhagic icterus

HISTOPATHOGICAL FINDINGS
Highly variable

 TREATMENT
• Maintain patent airway by preplacing nasal tubing prior to occlusion or by tracheostomy

if necessary, IV fluid support (LRS or 0.9% NaCl solution) for hypotensive cases.
• Keep animal calm, restrict movement, gently wash wound to remove topical debris, do not infuse fluids into wound.

APPROPRIATE HEALTH CARE

NURSING CARE
Wound care and debridement as necessary

ACTIVITY
Restrict activity and movement

DIET
Food and water should be readily accessible and feed should be easy to swallow.

CLIENT EDUCATION

SURGICAL CONSIDERATION
N/A

 ## MEDICATIONS

DRUGS OF CHOICE
• Antivenin is the treatment of choice. Recommendations for human bite victims are for treatment with multiple vials, but one to two vials may be sufficient to improve outcome in animals.
• Administration of antivenin as early as possible after envenomation may preclude the need for treatment with additional vials later.

Antivenin
• Antiven; CroFab Crotalidae Polyvalent Immune Fab (Ovine) (Protherics Inc., Nashville, TN 37212) is composed of four antivenins—*Crotalus atrox* (western diamondback rattlesnake), *Crotalus adamanteus* (eastern diamond rattlesnake), *Crotalus scutulatus* (Mojave rattlesnake), and *Agkistrodon piscivorus* (cottonmouth or water moccasin). A study in dogs has been conducted with good results utilizing 1–2 vials of antivenin.
• Antivenin (Crotalidae) Polyvalent (ACP) equine origin (Wyeth Laboratories Marietta, PA 17547) is the only antivenin product labeled for use in animals. It is composed of antivenins from *Crotalus adamanteus* (eastern damond rattlesnake), *C. atrox* (western diamond rattlesnake), *C. durissus terrificus* (tropical rattlesnake), and *Bothrops atrox* (fer-de-lance).
• Antivenin (*Micrurus fulvius*) equine origin (Wyeth Laboratories Marietta, PA 17547) will neutralize the the venom of *Micrurus fulvius tenere* (Texas coral snake) but will not neutralize venom of *Micruroides euryxanthus* (Arizona or Sonoran coral snake).
• Current use in animals is extralabel.
• Be prepared to treat for allergic reaction.

Other Treatments
• Treatment with broad-spectrum antibiotics
• Nonsteroidal anti-inflammatory medication for pain
• Revaccinate with tetanus and clostridium toxoids

CONTRAINDICATIONS

PRECAUTIONS
• Use caution when handling a dead snake. Reflex bites have occurred.
• Treatments previously utilized that have been shown to be either ineffective or detrimental include incision, suction, the infusion of fluids into wound area in an attempt to dilute toxin, the application of hot or cold compresses, tourniquets, or electric shock.
• Corticosteroids in treatment of venomous snakebite have been widely used in veterinary medicine, but their effectiveness and continued use is controversial.
• Corticosteroids delay healing and may interfere with the effects of antivenin. No studies have demonstrated an increased survival rate with use of corticosteroids. Use for treatment of allergic reaction associated with antivenin treatment.
• Colloids may increase risk of bleeding diathesis, complicate interpretation of coagulation profiles, or cause anaphylaxis. Use with caution.
• Appropriate milk and meat withdrawal times must be followed for all compounds administered.

POSSIBLE INTERACTIONS
Corticosteroids may interfere with antivenin.

ALTERNATIVE DRUGS

 ## FOLLOW-UP

PATIENT MONITORING
• Serial monitoring of coagulation profiles, complete blood count and blood chemistry, urinalysis, and cardiac parameters should be performed as often as warranted by the clinical condition, especially in the first 48 hours.
• Tissue destruction may not peak for several days. Swelling resolves in 3–7 days in most cases that survive.
• Recurrent coagulopathy may occur 1–2 weeks after administration of antivenin due to the shorter persistence of antivenin in the blood as compared to venom.

PREVENTION/AVOIDANCE

POSSIBLE COMPLICATIONS

EXPECTED COURSE AND PROGNOSIS
• Most adult animals survive if found in time to prevent respiratory collapse.
• Mortality is more common in younger, smaller animals.
• Systemic neurological signs and severe tissue necrosis may result in permanent deficits.

 ## MISCELLANEOUS

ASSOCIATED CONDITIONS

AGE-RELATED FACTORS
Young animals are more at risk due to their inquisitive nature. A bite with envenomation is more likely to result in mortality due to smaller body size.

ZOONOTIC POTENTIAL
Wear gloves to protect hands with skin abrasion when treating wounds.

PREGNANCY
Fetal death as a result of venomous snakebite has been reported in humans.
The safety of antivenin treatment during pregnancy in animals has not been established.

RUMINANT SPECIES AFFECTED
All species are susceptible.

BIOSECURITY
N/A

PRODUCTION MANAGEMENT
N/A

SYNONYMS
N/A

SEE ALSO
Abscessation
Anaphylaxsis
Insect envenomation
Trauma
Wound care

ABBREVIATIONS
CNS = central nervous system
CPK = creatine phosphokinase
ECG = electrocardiograph
EDTA = ethylenediaminetetraacetic acid
LRS = lactated Ringer's solution

Suggested Reading
Gawade, S. P. 2004. Snake venom neurotoxins: pharmacological classification. *J of Toxicology* (23)1:37–96. Available at www.dekker.com.
Mackessy, S. P., et al. 2003. Ontogenetic variation in venom composition and diet of *Crotalus oreganus concolor*: a case of venom paedomorphosis? *Copeia* 4:769–782
Mendez, M. C., Riet-Correa, F. 1995, Feb. Snakebite in sheep. *Vet Hum Toxicol*. 37(1):62–63.
Miller, M. W., et al. 1989, Jul. Snakebite in captive Rocky Mountain elk (*Cervus elaphus nelsoni*). *J Wildl Dis*. 25(3):392–96.
Petersen, M. 1998, Oct. Treating pit viper bites. *Vet Med*., pp. 885–90.
Petersen, M. 2004. *Clinical veterinary toxicology*, ed. K. Plumlee. St. Louis: Mosby.
Stebbins, R. C. 1985. *Petersen field guide, western reptiles and amphibians*. Boston: Houghton Mifflin Co.
Walton, R. M., et al. 1997. Mechanisms of echinocytosis induced by *Crotalus atrox* venom. *Vet Path*. 34 (5): 442–49.

Author: Lauren Palmer

SOLE LESIONS IN DAIRY CATTLE

 BASICS

OVERVIEW
- Lameness is common in dairy cows, with most lesions affecting the sole.
- The most significant lesions of the sole are *white line abscesses* and *sole ulcers*
- An initial insult to the corium primarily affects the laminar region and that corium damage increases with the resulting alteration in the physical forces on the sole.
- The risk of sole lesions is related to stage of lactation, individual cow factors, and farm characteristics. Claw disorders associated with chronic subclinical laminitis are primary causes of lameness in most herds.
- Ninety percent or more of lameness in dairy cattle involves the foot. Of that involving the foot, most involves rear feet, particularly the lateral claw.
- Cows most at risk of sole lesions are those with low body condition scores, first lactation cows in early lactation and second + lactation cows in mid- to late lactation.
- Farms most at risk are those with high steps or stall curbs, long standing times during milking, automatic alley scrapers, and flooring imperfections (e.g., holes in concrete).

SYSTEMS AFFECTED
Musculoskeletal

GENETICS
N/A

INCIDENCE/PREVALENCE
- Surveys have suggested that the incidence may be as high as 55 cases per 100 cows per year.
- Another survey estimated an incidence rate of 30 cases/100 cows/year, a fatality rate of 2%, an increase in days open of 28 days, and costs for treatment and additional labor of $23/case, estimating a cost of $9000/100 cows/year.

GEOGRAPHIC DISTRIBUTION
Worldwide depending on the environment

SIGNALMENT
Although white line abscesses can be seen in any bovine, they are most common in the lactating dairy cow. Sole ulcers are seen almost exclusively in housed, lactating dairy cattle.

Species
Dairy cattle

Breed Predilections
Dairy breeds

Mean Age and Range
Adult dairy cattle

Predominant Sex
Lactating dairy females

SIGNS
- Cows with a white line abscess typically present with severe acute lameness. Close examination of the foot will demonstrate the presence of heat within the affected digit.

- The site of the abscess can normally be determined by using equine hoof testers around the periphery of the abaxial wall. Using a hoof knife, the sole should be cleaned and a thin layer of horn removed. The key sign to identify is a dark mark within the white line at the site identified with the hoof testers. This is most likely the site at which the abscess formed.
- Cows with sole ulcers typically suffer from low-grade lameness for a period of time that slowly progresses to a severe lameness over a period of weeks. Depending on the severity of the lesion, the foot may appear normal or grossly swollen.
- Lesions are most commonly seen in the lateral hind claw. The sole of the claw may appear normal on initial examination, however, using hoof testers an area of pain is typically identified approximately two-thirds of the way back from the toe and toward the axial wall.
- As the sole is trimmed with a knife, it is common to find evidence of old hemorrhage within the horn of the sole at this site. Eventually, a portion of horn will be removed to reveal a full thickness defect of the sole with granulation tissue protruding from the underlying corium.
- In severe cases, bacteria may enter through the defect resulting in cellulitis that may spread to involve the navicular bursa, heel bulb, deep digital flexor tendon, or the distal interphalangeal joint.

CAUSES AND RISK FACTORS
- The fibrous junction between the sole and wall horn, colloquially known as the "white line," is the weakest portion of the sole. Even in a normal animal, it is common to see a small amount of debris impacted into this area.
- Dairy cattle are prone to a subclinical laminitis-like syndrome as a result of being fed diets rich in easily fermentable carbohydrate and low in long-stem fiber.
- Alterations in the internal structure of the hoof may result in separation and weakness of the white line. Areas of hemorrhage may also be visible within the horn in the region of the white line. Weakening of the white line allows debris to become impacted into the area. Should contaminated debris breach the white line and reach the corium, an abscess will form. Such abscesses cause extreme pain as they enlarge due to the great pressures developed between the base of the pedal bone and the hoof capsule, neither of which are flexible.
- Unlike horses where the abscess has a tendency to enlarge and track up the wall of the hoof and burst out at the coronary band, abscesses in cattle commonly tract caudally below the sole and burst out in the region of the heel.
- The same subclinical laminitis syndrome described above can result in a weakening of the attachments between the laminae of the wall and sinking of the pedal bone within the hoof capsule. This results in the ventral surface of the pedal bone compressing the corium of the sole against the horn of the sole.

This compression appears to be most marked in the region of the flexor process of P3.
- In addition to changes within the hoof, there are important changes seen in the morphology of the dairy cow's hoof. In the hind limb, the lateral claw is under asymmetrical stress when compared to the medial claw. This overloading of the lateral claw tends to result in hypertrophy of the sole horn, which further overloads the claw.
- In most dairy cows, overgrowth of the claw is characterized by a disproportionate overgrowth of the toe. This, combined with the commonly seen erosion of the heel horn, results in weight bearing by the claw being transferred from the toe back toward the heel region.
- When all these factors are combined, it is apparent that the heel region of the lateral hind claw is under a great deal of stress. As P3 sinks within the hoof capsule, the corium is compressed between the flexor process and the sole. This initially results in hemorrhage. The blood is incorporated into the horn and may be seen in the sole as bruising. As the condition progresses, the corium undergoes pressure necrosis and horn formation in the area is halted. This results in a defect in the sole that grows from the inside to the external environment. When the defect is full thickness, a sole ulcer has formed exposing the corium, causing pain and providing a portal for bacterial entry to the deep structures of the hoof.

 DIAGNOSIS

DIFFERENTIAL DIAGNOSIS
Other causes of acute lameness in dairy cattle include:
- Digital dermatitis
- Lacerations
- Foreign bodies
- Fractures
- Foot rot: this condition may be easily distinguished from the above by close examination of the foot.
- Abscesses may on occasion be due to penetration of the sole by a sharp foreign object, but this is comparatively rare compared to white line disease.

CBC/BIOCHEMISTRY/URINALYSIS
N/A

OTHER LABORATORY TESTS
N/A

IMAGING
Radiology of the distal limb may be of benefit in cases where there is concern that infection may have spread to either the navicular bursa or the distal interphalageal joint.

DIAGNOSTIC PROCEDURES
- Lesions are diagnosed on the basis of the characteristic clinical signs. All that is necessary is close examination of the foot.

• In cases where the infection has spread to the deep tissues of the foot, it is common to identify that the foot is grossly swollen. The swelling seen in such cases may be distinguished from simple foot rot on the basis that the swelling is asymmetrical and centered on one claw.
• The swelling is typically found in either the heel region or around the craniolateral aspect of the coronary band.

TREATMENT

• White line abscesses require drainage to provide pain relief and promote healing of the lesion. Having identified the suspected site of the abscess, a hoof knife should be used to resect the wall horn and to follow the lesion to the corium and drain the abscess. Once the abscess is open, the extent of the abscess should be determined using a blunt probe. The entire defect should be opened and all underrun horn removed.
• Care should be taken to avoid leaving any jagged or underrun edges, which would allow foreign material to impact in the lesion.
• When dealing with a sole ulcer, it is important to first trim the foot to normalize weight bearing between the medial and lateral claws as well as adjusting the plane of the sole to prevent excessive weight bearing in the heel region. Finally, the axial aspect of the sole should be hollowed out to prevent any weight bearing in the region of the flexor process.
• The area of the sole ulcer should be trimmed with great care to remove any underrun horn tissue.
• Bandaging the lesion left by an abscess or sole ulcer is of no value as the dressing simply becomes contaminated with fecal material. The lesions should be left open to heal.
• Animals will benefit from the application of an orthopedic block (Technovit or similar) to the opposite claw. This will minimize weight bearing by the affected claw promoting healing, and will also elevate the lesion from the contaminated floor surface when the animal is walking.

MEDICATIONS

• Antibiotics are not indicated in the treatment of simple uncomplicated abscesses or sole ulcers. They are indicated only when infection has spread to the deeper structures of the foot.
• Some clinicians may elect to use NSAIDs to provide analgesia in severe cases (e.g., ketoprofen 3 mg/kg).

CONTRAINDICATIONS

Appropriate milk and meat withdrawal times must be followed for all compounds administered to food-producing animals.

FOLLOW-UP

PATIENT MONITORING

• The majority of animals will show immediate relief after trimming of the lesion and application of an orthopedic block.
• Animals that remain significantly lame after 1 week should be reexamined.
• Orthopedic blocks should always be removed within 7 weeks of application. At this time, it is also appropriate to perform a minor hoof trim to encourage complete resolution of the lesion.

PREVENTION/AVOIDANCE

• Attention should be paid to the dairy cow ration to ensure that it always contains sufficient long-stem fiber to prevent ruminal acidosis.
• Dairy cows should have their feet trimmed on a regular basis to prevent overloading of the lateral hind claw.
• Attention should be paid to the design of the dairy barn to ensure that cows can always lay down in comfort. Cows at pasture typically lay down for two-thirds of the day. When the animal is recumbent, the feet do not bear weight and therefore the diseases cannot develop.

EXPECTED COURSE AND PROGNOSIS

• Simple uncomplicated white line abscesses typically resolve without complication in 4–6 weeks.
• Simple sole ulcers typically take longer to fully resolve but should heal within 2 months.
• The prognosis for infections that involve the deep structures of the hoof is always guarded. Since many of these cases typically present late in the disease course, the infection is well established and there is already significant pathology.
• Aggressive antibiotic therapy is warranted but rarely successful.
• A number of surgical procedures have been described to salvage the claw, but due to the expense involved, many clinicians opt to amputate the affected digit and salvage the cow in that manner.
• Studies have shown that the life expectancy for a dairy cow following amputation of a digit is less than 1 year.

MISCELLANEOUS

ASSOCIATED CONDITIONS

Lameness, decreased milk production, loss of profit

AGE-RELATED FACTORS

Cows most at risk of sole lesions are first lactation cows in early lactation and second+ lactation cows in mid- to late lactation.

ZOONOTIC POTENTIAL

N/A

PREGNANCY

N/A

RUMINANT SPECIES AFFECTED

Lactating dairy cows

BIOSECURITY

N/A

PRODUCTION MANAGEMENT

• Cows most at risk of sole lesions are those with low body condition scores, first lactation cows in early lactation, and second+ lactation cows in mid- to late lactation.
• Farms most at risk are those with high steps or stall curbs, long standing times during milking, automatic alley scrapers, and flooring imperfections (e.g., holes in concrete).
• Attention should be paid to the design of the dairy barn to ensure that cows can always lay down in comfort. Cows at pasture typically lay down for two-thirds of the day. When the animal is recumbent, the feet do not bear weight and therefore the diseases cannot develop.

SYNONYMS

N/A

SEE ALSO

Anesthesia and analgesia
Body condition scoring
FARAD
Foot rot
NSAIDs
Specific lameness chapters

ABBREVIATIONS

FARAD = Food Animal Residue Avoidance Databank
NSAIDs = nonsteroidal antiinflammatory drugs

Suggested Reading
Greenough, P. A., Collick, D. W., Weaver, A. D. 1997. Interdigital space and claw. In: *Lameness in cattle*, ed. Paul Greenough. 3rd ed. Philadelphia: W. B. Saunders.
Murray, R. D., Downham, D.Y., Clarkson, M. J., Faull, W. B., Hughes, J. W., Manson, F. J., Merritt, J. B., Russell, W. B., Sutherst, J. E., Ward, W. R. 1996, Jun 15. Epidemiology of lameness in dairy cattle: description and analysis of foot lesions. *Vet Rec.* 138(24):586–91.
Smilie, R. H., Hoblet, K. H., Eastridge, M. L., Weiss, W. P., Schnitkey, G. L., Moeschberger, M. L. 1999, Jan 2. Subclinical laminitis in dairy cows: use of severity of hoof lesions to rank and evaluate herds. *Vet Rec.* 144(1):17–21.
van Amstel, S. R., Shearer, J. K., Palin, F. L. 2004, Mar. Moisture content, thickness, and lesions of sole horn associated with thin soles in dairy cattle. *J Dairy Sci.* 87(3):757–63.
Webster, A. J. 2002, Jul 6. Effects of housing practices on the development of foot lesions in dairy heifers in early lactation. *Vet Rec.* 151(1):9–12.

Author: Chris Clark

SQUAMOUS CELL CARCINOMA

 BASICS

DEFINITION
SCC is a malignant tumor of epidermal cells that exhibit differentiation to keratinocytes.

PATHOPHYSIOLOGY
• Multiple factors have been implicated in the development of SCC in ruminants:
  • Exposure to ultraviolet light resulting in DNA damage
  • Papillomavirus infection causing precursor lesions that then undergo neoplastic transformation
  • Exposure to carcinogens in bracken fern can result in malignant transformation of papillomas of the upper gastrointestinal tract and bladder.
  • Immunosuppression by bracken fern can prevent rejection of early neoplastic lesions.
• Lack of pigmentation in the periocular tissues in the corneoscleral region greatly increases the risk of developing ophthalmic SCC in cattle exposed to high levels of UV light.
• There is a significant association between all measures of exposure to solar radiation and the development of OSCC.
• Twenty-six of 41 OSCCs (63.4%) showed abnormal expression of p53, a tumor suppressor gene.
• Some SCCs are thought to progress from plaques, papillomas, or carcinoma in situ.
• Some neoplastic lesions appear independently, without precursor lesions.
• Invasive OSCC of the palpebrae and medial canthus metastasize more commonly than do OSCC arising from the globe.
• OSCC can result in significant financial loss to the herdsman due to condemnation of the carcass at slaughter and premature loss of breeding stock.
• Cutaneous SCC may occur as a result of BPV infection and chronic sun exposure.

SYSTEMS AFFECTED
• Ophthalmic (OSCC)
• Skin
• Gastrointestinal
• Renal/urologic

GENETICS
• The high incidence of OSCC in Hereford and Hereford-cross cattle resulted in long belief in a heritable component.
• More recent studies have demonstrated that the relationship between tumor development and breed is actually the result of a strong association between lid and corneoscleral pigmentation, which are heritable traits, and the development of OSCC.

INCIDENCE/PREVALANCE
• When recording incidence, typically preneoplastic and early neoplastic lesions (plaques, papillomas and carcinoma in situ) are included in the affected group.
• Within the Hereford breed of cattle in the United States, estimates of the incidence of OSCC have ranged from 0.8% to 5%.
• In Australia, the incidence of ocular tumors within some Hereford cattle herds has ranged as high as 10–20%.
• In the Netherlands, the incidence of OSCC is estimated at 0.04%.
• Observation of five herds of Simmental cattle in Zimbabwe demonstrated an incidence of OSCC of 36–53% in cattle over 7 years of age.
• The incidence of OSCC increases with age.
• Bladder SCC is very rare except in endemic areas, where the incidence of bladder neoplasia may range from 15 to 25%.
• Cows with bladder SCC may have more than one type of tumor in their bladder.

GEOGRAPHIC DISTRIBUTION
• Most OSCC in the United States occurs in the South and Southwest—development of OSCC is associated with increase in altitude and mean annual hours of sunlight and with decreases in latitude.

• Australia and some regions in Africa also experience a significant number of cattle afflicted with OSCC.
• SCC of the upper intestinal tract and bladder are most common in regions where the cofactor for tumor development, bracken fern, exists along with infection of the cattle with BPV-4.
• This combination of factors resulting in SCC of the upper intestinal tract was initially reported in Scotland, but additional reports from Europe, Africa, and South America have been published.
• SCC of the muzzle, ears, and perineal region of sheep is a significant problem in Australia.

SIGNALMENT
Species
• SCC of all types is seen primarily in cattle, but has been reported in sheep.
• SCC is rare in goats.

Breed Predilection
• In the United States, Hereford and Hereford-cross cattle are most likely to be affected with OSCC.
• Other breeds in which OSCC is reported include Simmental, Holstein Friesians, and rarely in other breeds.
• Sheep develop SCC in regions that are not covered by wool and are not pigmented.

Mean Age and Range
• The mean age of cattle with OSCC is 7–8 years, with a decreasing mean age in areas of highest ultraviolet light exposure.
• OSCC has been seen in cattle as young as 3 years of age, and there is a 2% increase in the risk of affliction with OSCC for each additional month of age.
• SCC of the upper intestinal tract and bladder is typically found in cattle between 6 and 12 years of age.

Predominant Sex
• Although most afflicted cattle are cows, that simply reflects the fact that most herds are made up primarily of cows, and bulls are kept in fewer numbers.
• The same is true of ewes and rams.

SIGNS
• OSCC: mass can be flat white plaques, papillomas with raised surfaces, and SCC can be an irregular, pinkish mass; can present with secondary conjunctivitis.
• SCC of the upper intestinal tract can result in bloat, regurgitation of ruminal contents, or pain and difficulty on swallowing.
• As SCC of the intestinal tract progresses, there is loss of condition and abdominal pain.
• SCC of the bladder is typically associated with hematuria.
• Clinical signs associated with distant metastasis are rarely seen.

HISTORICAL FINDINGS
• OSCC: ocular discharge
• SCC of the upper intestinal tract: weight loss, difficulty eating, regurgitation of ruminal contents

PHYSICAL EXAMINATION FINDINGS
• OSCC: precursor lesions can be flat white plaques or papillomas with raised, textured surfaces, and SCC can be an irregular, nodular, pinkish mass, possibly invading the normal tissues.
• OSCC: most common site is the limbus, followed by the eyelids, nictitating membrane, and medial canthus
• OSCC: parotid lymph node may be enlarged
• SCC of the upper intestinal tract: bloat, regurgitation, loss of condition, painful abdomen
• Cutaneous SCC: horny outgrowths of skin or scales that are painful on manipulation, occurring on unpigmented or lightly pigmented skin in the sacral region, dorsum, and escutcheon.

CAUSES
Ophthalmic and Skin
• Exposure to ultraviolet light
• Lack of pigmentation
• Infection with bovine papillomavirus

Upper Gastrointestinal Tract and Bladder
• Infection with BPV-4 and/or BPV-2
• Ingestion of bracken fern or other carcinogenic and immunomodulatory compounds
• Trauma

RISK FACTORS
• Lack of periocular pigmentation and corneoscleral pigmentation
• High levels of exposure to UV light
• Increased nutritional intake (OSCC)

DIAGNOSIS

DIFFERENTIAL DIAGNOSIS
• Papillomas
• Keratoancanthomas
• Carcinoma in situ
• Dermoid cyst
• Follicular hyperplasia of the third eyelid

CBC/BIOCHEMISTRY/URINALYSIS
OSCC and SCC of the Upper Intestinal Tract
N/A

SCC of the Bladder
• Anemia
• Hematuria

OTHER LABORATORY TESTS
N/A

IMAGING
• Radiographs of the chest are indicated prior to final prognosis and possible surgical intervention.
• Wide surgical excision of an invasive OSCC in a valuable animal is indicated if radiographs are negative for metastasis.
• Ultrasound of the abdomen and neck region may help in the diagnosis of upper intestinal SCC or in the diagnosis of a bladder tumor.

DIAGNOSTIC PROCEDURES
OSCC
• In valuable animals, a biopsy or scraping of an ocular lesion may confirm a clinical impression of OSCC.
• Cytologic diagnosis agrees with histopathologic diagnosis 85–90% of the time.

PATHOLOGIC FINDINGS
OSCC
• Invasion into the normal tissues, including bone and along the optic nerve may be seen.
• Metastasis to the ipsilateral parotid and lateral retropharyngeal lymph nodes may be seen.
• Five percent of cattle with OSCC have lung metastasis at slaughter.
• Histopathology of OSCC included epidermal hyperplasia, hyperkeratosis, parakeratosis, acanthosis, accentuation of the epidermal rete, and keratinocyte dysplasia. Extending into the dermis are cords and islands of neoplastic cells demonstrating a variable degree of epithelial differentiation, sometimes including "keratin pearls."

SCC of the Skin, Upper Gastrointestinal Tract and Bladder
• Individuals affected with upper GI SCC may have multiple papillomas of the oral cavity and throughout the upper and lower GI tract.
• Histopathologic findings are similar to those described above.

TREATMENT

APPROPRIATE HEALTH CARE
• Early detection of OSCC is important in order for treatment to be effective.

SQUAMOUS CELL CARCINOMA

• Up to 75% of small lesions (<5 mm in diameter) will regress spontaneously.
• Multiple treatment modalities can be used successfully on early lesions.
• Treatment of OSCC with hyperthermia (raising the temperature in the tumor to 50°C for 30 sec/cm² of tumor surface), resulted in complete regression in 90.7% of tumors treated, and this regression lasted at least for 5.5 months in all animals, and for a year in the cattle available for monitoring at that time.
• Radiation therapy, administered with implants of gamma-emitters such as cobalt-60, gold-198, or cesium-137, has been quite effective at controlling OSCC, however, these methods are quite costly and not widely available.
• Cryosurgery, utilizing two freeze/thaw cycles (freezing to –25°C, allowing a thaw and repeating) has been reported to result in a 97% complete regression rate.
• A study with more complete follow-up demonstrated that approximately 71% of lesions treated with cryosurgery had complete regression without recurrence with follow-up data for up to 3.5 years.
• Almost 6% of lesions in this study recurred after initial regression, and 17.6% did not respond to cryosurgery.

• Immunotherapy has been investigated for the treatment of OSCC, but has limited efficacy.
• No effective treatments exist for SCC of the upper gastrointestinal tract and bladder.

NURSING CARE
N/A

ACTIVITY
N/A

DIET
• A high level of nutrition has been correlated with increased risk of developing OSCC.
• The ingestion of bracken fern is a critical cofactor to the development of upper gastrointestinal tract SCC and bladder tumors and should be avoided.

CLIENT EDUCATION
• Lesions may recur locally so treated animals should be examined periodically (every 3 to 4 months) for evidence of recurrence.
• Cryosurgery or hyperthermia can result in hair loss at the treated site.

SURGICAL CONSIDERATIONS
• Surgical removal of OSCC and precursor lesions is only moderately successful in controlling the disease with recurrence rates of 37–48% reported.

• En bloc excision of the tumor and regional lymph nodes can be performed to salvage valuable animals, but is not cost effective in most instances.

MEDICATIONS

DRUGS OF CHOICE
N/A

CONTRAINDICATIONS
N/A

PRECAUTIONS
N/A

POSSIBLE INTERACTIONS
N/A

ALTERNATIVE DRUGS
N/A

FOLLOW-UP

PATIENT MONITORING
All cattle should be examined on a regular basis for OSCC, at least three times a year (including once in the summer months) during routine maintenance health treatments.

SQUAMOUS CELL CARCINOMA

PREVENTION/AVOIDANCE
• Breeding cattle for pigmentation in the periocular tissues as well as for pigmentation of the corneoscleral junction will decrease the incidence of OSCC.
• Routine evaluation of all eyes, with cryosurgery or surgical removal of lesions that are enlarging and greater than 5 mm in diameter, greatly decreases the development of lesions that would result in financial loss to the herdsman (through carcass condemnation and premature loss of breeding stock).

POSSIBLE COMPLICATIONS
• Premature loss of breeding cows
• Carcass condemnation at slaughter due to metastasis or multiple SCC

EXPECTED COURSE AND PROGNOSIS
• Untreated, OSCC will invade normal tissues (including, potentially, the CNS) and ultimately metastasize to the regional lymph nodes and lungs. Extensive disease can result in carcass condemnation and thus financial loss.
• With surgical excision (enucleation or mass resection), local recurrence is common (37% in one report), but may allow salvage of the animal for slaughter.
• Cryosurgery, with a two-freeze cycle, will result in a 77–97% complete response rate. Approximately 71% of responding tumors did not recur in one study following cryosurgery.

MISCELLANEOUS

ASSOCIATED CONDITIONS
Infection with bovine papilloma viruses is thought to cause the initial precancerous lesion.

AGE-RELATED FACTORS
OSCC are typically diagnosed in animals greater than 4 years of age.

ZOONOTIC POTENTIAL
N/A

PREGNANCY
N/A

RUMINANT SPECIES AFFECTED
Cattle are most frequently affected, SCC is also seen in sheep, but is rare in goats.

BIOSECURITY
N/A

PRODUCTION MANAGEMENT
Routine evaluation of all eyes in a herd allows early detection and treatment of lesions that may be early SCC or premalignant changes in the epithelium.

SYNONYMS
Cancer eye (OSCC)
Enzootic hematuria (Bladder cancer is one identified cause of EH.)

SEE ALSO
Papillomatosis

ABBREVIATIONS
BPV = bovine papilloma virus
OSCC = ocular squamous cell carcinoma
SCC = squamous cell carcinoma
UV = ultraviolet

Suggested Reading
Anderson, D. E. 1991. Genetic study of eye cancer in cattle. *J Heredity* 82:21–26.
Anderson, D. E., Badzioch, M. 1991. Association between solar radiation and ocular squamous cell carcinoma in cattle. *Am J Vet Res.* 52:784–88.
Kainer, R. A. 1984. Current concepts in the treatment of bovine ocular squamous cell tumors. *Veterinary Clinics of North America: Large Animal Practice* 6:609–22.
Sloss, V., Smith, T. J. S., Yi, G. D. 1986. Controlling ocular squamous cell carcinoma in Hereford cattle. *Aust Vet J.* 63:248–51.
Spradbrow, P. B., Samuel, J. L., Kelly, W. R., Wood, A. L. 1987. Skin cancer and papillomaviruses in cattle. *J Comp Path.* 97:469–79.

Author: Marlene L. Hauck

ST. JOHN'S WORT TOXICITY

BASICS

OVERVIEW
• St. John's wort is an erect perennial herb that stands 1–3 feet tall. Its leaves are opposite, dotted, with many yellow flowers.
• Hypericin is the active ingredient. It's a red florescent pigment found in a semisolid state in the black dots that are scattered over the surface of the leaves, stems, and petals and is present in the plants at all times.
• Hypercin is a naturally occurring naphthodianthrone derivative in the plant species *Hypericum perforatum*. The hypericin concentration in the plant may vary depending on the place of growth, state of plant material, and part of the plant—whole herb concentration 0.00095%–0.466% and flowers up to 0.086%.
• The hypericin concentration in a broadleaf biotype varies from a winter minimum of less than 100 ppm to a summer maximum approaching 3000 ppm. In contrast, the narrow-leaf biotype increases from similar winter values to summer maxima approaching 5000 ppm.
• Consumption causes primary photosensitization, which leads to increased sensitivity of the skin to subsequent light exposure.
• There appears to be an absolute requirement for exposure to bright sunlight before any effects of hypericum will develop.
• St. John's wort is found in dry soil, roadsides, and pasture ranges.

PATHOPHYSIOLOGY
• The mechanism of action is unresolved.
• One study suggested that hypericin was an inhibitor of rat brain mitochondrial monoamine oxidase (MAO).
• Serotonin receptors may be involved in the pharmacological action of hypericum extracts.
• Another study found that hypericum extract inhibits serotonin uptake by rat synaptosomes derived from rat embryo neurons. Other investigators reported that serotonin receptor expression in neuroblastoma cells was reduced by hypericum extracts.
• When animals ingest the plant, the hypericin is absorbed from the intestinal tract and goes into the circulation. Hypericin is a photodynamic agent able to cause cellular damage and sunburn.

SYSTEMS AFFECTED
Skin, gastrointestinal, cardiovascular, liver, renal

GENETICS
N/A

INCIDENCE/PREVALENCE
N/A

GEOGRAPHIC DISTRIBUTION
Potentially worldwide, depending on species and environment

SIGNALMENT
• Cattle, sheep, horses, and goats
• Most common in sheep and cattle
• Potentially all ruminant species

Species
Potentially all ruminant species

Breed Predilections
N/A

Mean Age and Range
N/A

Predominant Sex
N/A

SIGNS
• Extreme hyperesthesia to touch and to contact with cold water
• Restlessness and discomfort. Animals tend to rub their ears, eyelids, and muzzle.
• Photophobia
• Hyperthermia when exposed to sunlight
• Diarrhea and tachycardia
• Exposure of the tongue to sunlight while licking can cause glossitis with ulceration and deep necrosis.
• Congested mucous membranes and hyperemia of exposed skin on tail and legs. Edema of eyelids and ears, exudation of serum from ears.
• Loss of eyelashes, corneal opacity, and blindness after 5–7 days with high levels of ingestion.
• Animals with pigmented skin and those that remain in subdued light suffer few effects.
• Hemolytic anemia
• Kidney and liver dysfunction may occur with severe exposure.

CAUSES AND RISK FACTORS
• Severity of effects increases with duration of exposure, but not with dose.
• A single dose of hypericum remains potentially effective for up to 4 days.
• Induces hepatic cytochrome P450 and approximately doubles its metabolic activity.

• Plasma concentration of concomitant medication using cytochrome P450 enzymes will be reduced.
• Rectal temperature rise in affected sheep is a reliable indicator of the early development of an adverse clinical effect.
• There appears to be an absolute requirement for exposure to bright sunlight before any effects of *H. perforatum* will develop.
• A single dose of *H. perforatum* remains potentially effective for up to 4 days.
• In a small group of Merino sheep tested, a tolerance level for *H. perforatum*, eaten at the flowering stage, of < 1% (plant wet weight) of body weight and a tolerance level for hypericin of < 2.65 mg per kg live weight were demonstrated.
• Sheep develop restlessness, photophobia, tachycardia, tachypnea, congested mucous membranes, diarrhea, and hyperthermia. Skin lesions include redness of the tail, eyelid edema, and auricular edema. One week later, salivation, perioral and periauricular alopecia, keratoconjunctivitis, corneal opacity, and blindness may be evident.
• Another study found the minimal dose of dried whole hypericum to cause symptoms to be 3 g/kg in calves weighing 100 to 120 kg. Calves that receive this dose and were exposed to sunlight developed pyrexia and tachypnea 3 to 4 hours later. The animals became restless, passed soft feces, and developed perinasal and perioral erythema. Calves receiving the same dose but not exposed to sunlight only developed soft feces. Calves receiving 5 g/kg developed similar but more severe symptoms.

DIAGNOSIS

DIFFERENTIAL DIAGNOSIS
• Hepatogenous photosensitivity as a result of phylloerythrin accumulating in the blood. Phylloerythrins are formed from the anaerobic breakdown of chlorophyll by microorganisms in the forestomach of ruminants.
• Endogenous photosensitizing agent from aberrant metabolism of hemoglobin
• Antibiotic-associated photosensitization (sulfonamides and tetracyclines)
• Phenothiazine-induced photosensitization (Phenothiazine sulphoxide is the metabolite.)
• Plants that can cause sunburn either by contact or ingestion—vetches, various clovers, and buckwheat (*Fagopyrum* spp.)—have caused sunburn and skin scald in animals.

CBC/BIOCHEMISTRY/URINALYSIS
• Elevated serum BUN, Na, K, and bilirubin (total and direct) concentrations
• Lower than normal serum in Hb, RBC count, PCV, TP, glucose, cholesterol, triglycerides, and serum alkaline phosphatase concentrations
• Serum sorbitol dehydrogenase, GGT, concentrations within normal limits
• Transaminases, CPK, sodium, and potassium increase and the BUN may increase up to ninefold. Glucose and hemoglobin decrease, while WBC level does not change.

OTHER LABORATORY TESTS
N/A

IMAGING
N/A

DIAGNOSTIC PROCEDURES
N/A

PATHOLOGIC FINDINGS
N/A

TREATMENT
• Remove animal from source.
• Animals should be given full shade or preferably housed and allowed out to graze only during darkness.
• Corticosteroids given parenterally in the early stages may be useful.
• Secondary skin infections and suppuration should be treated with a topical broad-spectrum antibiotic.
• Fly-strike should be prevented.
• Emergency evacuation of the gastrointestinal tract is not required since the toxin takes several days to build up in the body and cause signs.

MEDICATIONS
• 1.1 mg/kg/day prednisone or prednisolone PO for 10 days
• Depending on the severity of the lesions, antibiotics and anti-inflammatory medications may be indicated.

CONTRAINDICATIONS
N/A

POSSIBLE INTERACTIONS
N/A

FOLLOW-UP

PATIENT MONITORING
N/A

PREVENTION/AVOIDANCE
• Weed management—mowing and hand removal
• Animals will avoid St. John's wort if more palatable forage is available.

POSSIBLE COMPLICATIONS
N/A

EXPECTED COURSE AND PROGNOSIS
• Condition seldom causes death and soon clears once the plant source is removed.
• The prognosis and the eventual productivity of the animal are related to the site and severity of the primary lesion and to the degree of resolution.

MISCELLANEOUS

ASSOCIATED CONDITIONS
N/A

AGE-RELATED FACTORS
N/A

ZOONOTIC POTENTIAL
N/A

PREGNANCY
Can cause decreased litter size and reduced body size at birth

RUMINANT SPECIES AFFECTED
Potentially, all ruminant species are affected.

BIOSECURITY
N/A

PRODUCTION MANAGEMENT
If the pasture contains large stands of St. John's wort, removal is indicated. Mow, spray, and/or reseed to improve the pasture quality.

SYNONYMS
Klamath weed

SEE ALSO
Antibiotic-associated photosensitization (sulfonamides and tetracyclines)
Phenothiazine-induced photosensitization.
Plants that can cause sunburn either by contact or ingestion: vetches, various clovers, and buckwheat (*Fagopyrum* spp.)

ABBREVIATIONS
BUN = blood urea nitrogen
CPK = creatine phosphokinase
GGT = gamma-glutamyl transpeptidase
Hb = hemoglobin
MAO = monoamine oxidase
PCV = packed cell volume
PO = per os, by mouth
RBC = red blood cell
TP = total protein
WBC = white blood cell

Suggested Reading
Araya, O. S., Ford, E. J. 1981, Jan. An investigation of the type of photosensitization caused by the ingestion of St. John's wort (*Hypericum perforatum*) by calves. *J Comp Pathol*. 91(1): 135–41.
Bourke, C. A. 2000, Jul. Sunlight associated hyperthermia as a consistent and rapidly developing clinical sign in sheep intoxicated by St. John's wort (*Hypericum perforatum*). *Aust Vet J*. 78(7): 483–88.
Horn, G. A., Jr., Burrows, G. E. 1990, Aug. Primary photosensitization in cattle. *Vet Hum Toxicol*. 32(4): 331–32.
Kako, M. D., al-Sultan II, Saleem, A. N. 1993, Aug. Studies of sheep experimentally poisoned with *Hypericum perforatum*. *Vet Hum Toxicol*. 35(4): 298–300.
Schey, K. L., Patat, S., Chignell, C. F., Datillo, M., Wang, R. H., Roberts, J. E. 2000, Aug. Photooxidation of lens alpha-crystallin by hypericin (active ingredient in St. John's wort). *Photochem Photobiol*. 72(2): 200–203.
Southwell, I. A., Bourke, C. A. 2001, Mar. Seasonal variation in hypericin content of *Hypericum perforatum* L. (St. John's wort). *Phytochemistry* 56(5): 437–41.

Author: Troy Holder

STARVATION/MALNUTRITION

 BASICS

DEFINITION
Starvation is the inability to obtain food or the unavailability of food for an extended period of time or insufficient energy intake, commonly seen during periods of drought.

PATHOPHYSIOLOGY
• Many physiological changes occur as the animal attempts to satisfy its energy requirements. At the cellular level, catabolism continues to supply the substrates required for anabolism and vital functions. Reserve stores of nutrients are utilized to compensate for the lack of nutritional intake.
• The most readily usable material, glycogen, is utilized first primarily from liver stores and is exhausted in a few hours. Next, stored fat from various subcutaneous deposits (near the kidney, mesentery, and omentum) is utilized. Following this use, fat deposits in the parenchymal organs are utilized, followed by fat deposits in the bone marrow. The final source of energy available to the animal is cell cytoplasm, which is primarily protein.
• Ketosis is commonly seen in starvation.
• Nitrogen excretion rises due to the protein catabolism. The animal eventually reaches a point where it dies because of insufficient blood glucose necessary for brain function and hypoglycemic shock occurs.
• At the microbial level, inadequate food intake, especially in ruminants, results in a rapid decrease in the number of bacteria and protozoa and in the level of volatile fatty acids present in the rumen.
• Nearly 70% of the energy available to ruminants is from these fatty acids, thus causing a significant further impact on energy availability.
• Decreasing the microbial populations also diminishes the animal's ability to digest fiber.
• Prolonged food deprivation is known to cause a fall in the core body temperature.

SYSTEMS AFFECTED
Musculoskeletal, hepatic, immune and production management; potentially all depending on initiating events

GENETICS
N/A

INCIDENCE/PREVALENCE
N/A

GEOGRAPHIC DISTRIBUTION
Worldwide

SIGNALMENT
• Adult ruminants are able to store large amounts of nutrients and fat within their body tissues. These mature animals will utilize higher proportions of fat than protein, especially in the early stages of starvation. In contrast, young animals will utilize higher proportions of protein than fat. They have smaller fat reserves because of higher nutritional demands for growth, smaller body size, and social interactions within their environment.
• In the wild, starvation tends to occur more frequently in the winter and early spring months due to food availability and weather demands on energy utilization.

Species
All ruminant species

Breed Predilections
N/A

Mean Age and Range
• Young, yearling, and old animals are most susceptible to starvation because they enter the season with the smallest fat stores, highest nutritional demands, greatest heat loss, and lowest positions in the social environment.
• Young animals and pregnant or lactating animals have much higher energy and protein requirements than do dry stock, and are therefore most susceptible to the effects of malnutrition. These animals will need to be fed separately to ensure that their requirements are met.

Predominant Sex
N/A

SIGNS

PHYSICAL EXAMINATION FINDINGS
• Attitude—lethargic, unsteady, listless, unafraid of humans
• External findings—dehydration, rough hair coat, thin body condition, muscle atrophy (prominent ribs, vertebrae, shoulders and pelvis)

HISTORICAL FINDINGS
Knowledge of food unavailability or shortage; wild animals seen by humans more frequently (stray into developed areas); significant loss in body weight (may be near 20%–30%).

CAUSE AND RISK FACTORS
• Inability to ingest, digest, absorb, or utilize food
• Injury, poor teeth, parasitism, disease, foreign bodies, neoplasia, increased motility of the digestive tract
• Inadequate supply of food

• Insufficient energy intake
• Extreme parasitism
• Environmental conditions
• Cold weather, deep snow, increased energy demands (pregnancy), snow-covered food, drought, overpopulation, predator stress
• Social conditions within the flock/herd

Feed-Related Illnesses Occurring During Drought/Starvation
• Malnutrition and starvation
• Metabolic disease
• Mineral deficiencies and imbalances
• Hypocalcemia
• Hypomagnesemia
• Reduced fertility: cow fertility, bull fertility
• Grain toxemia/acidosis: Any factor that causes variation in intake (e.g., inclement weather or palatability of feed) or changes in the availability of the carbohydrate (e.g., a change in grain type or grain processing) may cause digestive upsets at any time, not just in the period of grain introduction.
• Clostridial diseases: Spores of clostridial bacteria are present in soil and are ingested when animals ingest soil when grazing close to the ground.
• Laminitis
• Urea poisoning
• Urinary calculi
• Vitamin A deficiency
• Plant poisoning: hungry animals may consume plants, including shrubs and trees, which they would normally avoid.
• Blue-green algae: blooms of blue-green algae are more likely to appear in warmer months during drought.

 DIAGNOSIS

DIFFERENTIAL DIAGNOSIS
Malnutrition, parasitism, neoplasia

CBC/BIOCHEMISTRY/URINALYSIS

Chemistry
Hypoproteinemia, hypoglycemia, hypocalcemia, high anion gap, increased AST, SDH, and CK

Urinalysis
Proteinuria, ketonuria

OTHER LABORATORY TESTS
• Starvation is best diagnosed by gross examination or necropsy.
• A gross determination is based on examining the presence or lack of adipose tissue in the various subcutaneous and visceral locations.

STARVATION/MALNUTRITION

• Femur or mandibular bone marrow fat analysis can be grossly examined in older animals. Some labs offer a femur marrow compression method, either-extract method, kidney fat index, and wet weight-dry weight method.
• Laboratory tests offer little additional information than can be derived from gross examination.

IMAGING
NA

DIAGNOSTIC PROCEDURES

PATHOLOGIC FINDINGS
• Pathological changes which occur in a starved ruminant are many and varied. The most striking change is the lack of fat in the subcutaneous, visceral, and bone marrow locations.
• Muscle atrophy is generally significant. Serous atrophy is common. The organs are generally smaller than normal.
• The digestive tract is generally void of any material and is often shrunken. The gallbladder is generally distended and bile straining may be present. Rumen ulcers may be present and rumen materials are scant and dry. Villas atrophy may be seen in the rumen.
• Femur marrow will be red or yellow in color, transparent and gelatinous.

TREATMENT
• Generally ruminants will not eat large quantities of food when sudden access to unlimited food occurs.
• If food is not provided until late stages of starvation, the animal will likely die. It takes up to 2 weeks for a ruminant to adjust to the new diet and change into a positive energy balance.
• Care must be given to provide a high quality palatable feed containing readily available carbohydrates, roughage, minerals, and vitamins.
• The animal is prone to acidosis if a sudden shift of microbial population occurs and the only feed provided is high in carbohydrates.
• Treat preexisting health conditions.

• Factors that must be corrected, in order of importance, are:
  • Deficiency of energy
  • Deficiency of rumen-digestible protein (or alternative nitrogen and sulfur equivalent) required by rumen bacteria to produce energy and protein from low-quality feed
  • Deficiency of high-quality protein required for growth, pregnancy, and lactation
  • Deficiency of other minerals, particularly phosphorus, calcium, and magnesium
  • Deficiency of vitamins associated with the lack of fresh green feed, particularly vitamins A, D, and E.

MEDICATIONS
Directed at specific causes of starvation (e.g., parasitism, poor dentition, chronic disease)

DRUGS OF CHOICE
Directed at specific treatments of underlying disease conditions if present

CONTRAINDICATIONS
Appropriate milk and meat withdrawal times must be followed for all compounds administered to food-producing animals.

MISCELLANEOUS

ASSOCIATED CONDITIONS
• Ketosis is commonly seen in starvation.
• Decreasing the microbial populations also diminishes the animal's ability to digest fiber.
• Prolonged food deprivation is known to cause a fall in the core body temperature.

AGE-RELATED FACTORS
N/A

ZOONOTIC POTENTIAL
N/A

PREGNANCY
It is common for pregnant animals to abort or absorb their fetus during times of starvation. A fetus that survives will often be small and have an increased chance for mortality. Dams will often not allow nursing or abandon their young.

RUMINANT SPECIES AFFECTED
All ruminant species

BIOSECURITY
N/A

PRODUCTION MANAGEMENT
Feed Management
• Once pasture is inadequate, cattle should be confined and fed. Confined cattle need significantly less energy for maintenance than do those that are left in the paddock to wander in search of feed.
• The pastures should be left in a condition where they can recover quickly when the drought breaks.
• Any change in feed (especially grain) should be introduced gradually—failure to do this is probably the major cause of illness seen in drought/starvation.

SYNONYMS
N/A

SEE ALSO
Animal welfare
Diagnostic procedures
Fluids

ABBREVIATIONS
AST = asparagine transferase
CK = creatine phosphokinase
SDH = sorbitol dehydrogenase

Suggested Reading
Blum, J. W., Kunz, P., Bachmann, C., Colombo, J. P. 1981, Jul. Metabolic effects of fasting in steers. *Res Vet Sci.* 31(1):127–29.
Malnutrition and starvation. Department of Natural Resources, Michigan. Available at http://www.michigan.gov/dnr/.
Nowak, R., Porter, R. H., Levy, F., Orgeur, P., Schaal, B. 2000, Sep. Role of mother-young interactions in the survival of offspring in domestic mammals. *Rev Reprod.* 5(3):153–63.
Owens, F. N., Dubeski, P., Hanson, C. F. 1993, Nov. Factors that alter the growth and development of ruminants. *J Anim Sci.* 71(11):3138–50.
Poppi, D. P., McLennan, S. R. 1995, Jan. Protein and energy utilization by ruminants at pasture. *J Anim Sci.* 73(1):278–90.
Van Kessel, J. S., Russell, J. B. 1997, Oct. The endogenous polysaccharide utilization rate of mixed ruminal bacteria and the effect of energy starvation on ruminal fermentation rates. *J Dairy Sci.* 80(10):2442–48.

Author: Angela M. Daniels

STIFLE INJURIES

 BASICS

OVERVIEW
• Ligamentous injuries affecting the cranial and caudal cruciate ligaments, medial and lateral menisci, collateral ligaments, and the patella and its associated ligaments.
• Affected cattle are acutely lame.
• Cattle that recover from initial injuries often develop chronic osteoarthritis.

SIGNALMENT
• Ligamentous injuries of the stifle have been reported in both beef and dairy cattle.
• In female dairy animals, the condition has been reported in cattle as young as 11 months and as old as 14 years.
• The disease is most common in large-framed, young adult (3- to 6-year-old) beef animals with exceptional genetic potential for rapid weight gain and excessively straight conformation of the stifle and hock. This observation may reflect an actual increased risk or, alternatively, a biased population being presented for diagnosis and treatment.

SIGNS
• Physical examination is the most useful method to diagnosis stifle injuries in cattle.
• Affected cattle are acutely lame.
• The severity of the lameness is directly related to the severity of injury, the specific structures damaged, and the joint laxity induced by these injuries.
• The majority of gait abnormalities generally subsides in the 6 to 12 weeks after the initial injury; however, most cattle will have a visible residual lameness. At this point, clinical signs will remain static for a variable interval. This period of static clinical signs varies from 3 months to 1 year. Thereafter, affected cattle begin to become progressively lamer.
• Most affected cattle are recognized as having intractable lameness resulting in euthanasia within 2 years following the first recognition of lameness. Consequently, the severity of clinical signs varies greatly depending on the elapsed time since the injury.

• Cattle with ligamentous injuries of the stifle usually walk with a characteristic gait.
• Cattle with stifle injuries are reluctant to bear weight on the affected limb.
• At a walk, the stifle and tarsus joints are relatively fixed. Cattle advance their limb by first abducting the pelvic limb and then swinging it lateral, forward, and then medial. This altered gait appears to avoid the pain caused by repetitive cycles of stifle flexion and extension.
• When cattle walk, weight appears to be shifted onto the toe and off the heels of the affected limb. In many cases, the heels are visibly elevated and do not contact the ground at a walk.
• Hoof lameness localized in the heel is readily confused with stifle injuries. Consequently, close examination of the hoof is necessary to rule out these conditions.
• The stifle should be palpated for heat, swelling and distension of the joint. In acutely lame cattle, swelling often gravitates ventrally through the subcutaneous tissues. On superficial examination, the tarsus may appear swollen.
• Tarsal enlargement and the patient's unwillingness to flex or extend either the tarsus or stifle often make diseases of the tarsus a tempting, although incorrect, diagnosis.
• A series of limb manipulations should be performed on all cattle suspected of having ligamentous stifle injuries. These procedures are all designed to detect abnormal laxity.
• Laxity, instability, and forced movement typically produce a sudden popping sensation, an audible click or snap, and in long-standing cases, a grating sensation.
• Determination of the specific damaged structures is usually not possible solely on the basis of clinical examination.
• Given that the prognosis and treatment are similar for most cases of traumatic stifle disease, more anatomically specific diagnoses may be neither necessary nor desirable.
• It should be noted that joint instability is most easily detected in the first month after the initial injury and may become difficult to detect if the interval from injury to examination spans several months.

Stifle Examination Technique
• The affected animal should be restrained in a head gait with free access to the affected side of the cow. Ideally, the head gate should be positioned such that the unaffected side of the cow is next to a solid wall.
• Initially, the examiner should perform a drawer sign examination. The examiner stands behind the cow or bull and places a shoulder firmly against the semimembranosis and semitendonosis muscles.
• The proximal tibia is grasped with both hands and pulled caudally, while the distal femur is forced forward using the examiner's shoulder.
• Rotational instability is initially assessed in the standing animal by grasping the tuber calcis with one hand and the proximal tibia or stifle with the other hand. The limb is twisted both clockwise and counter-clockwise.
• After completion of these examinations, the affected limb is manually lifted and flexed. The examiner stands next to the cow facing caudal. The tarsus and stifle run through a full range of flexion and extension.
• The leg is held in flexion with one hand and rotational force is placed on the hock and stifle using the opposite hand. The leg is extended and the hoof is manually abducted to assess medial and lateral joint instability.

CAUSES
• The primary cause of stifle injuries appears to be trauma. However, degenerative changes in the ligamentous structure of the stifle may precipitate a catastrophic event leading to clinical disease.
• Excessively straight stifle conformation has been linked to degenerative changes in the ligamentous structures of the stifle.

RISK FACTORS
• In addition to the risk factors outlined under signalment, excessive or violent physical activity may precipitate traumatic injuries to the stifle.
• Injuries are often observed in athletic young bulls of high libido near the end of the breeding season and injuries are often observed in cows coincidental with estrus.
• Mixing groups of cattle or adding single cows to preexisting herds or groups will often precipitate social dominance behavior that leads to traumatic injuries. This is particularly the case when unaccustomed bulls are placed together in small pens or pastures.

DIAGNOSIS

DIFFERENTIAL DIAGNOSIS

• Differential diagnoses include femoral and tibial fractures, luxations of the hip, infectious polyarthritis, osteochondrosis, and hoof lamenesses.
• Physical examination and radiographs can rule out femoral and tibial fractures.
• Luxations of the coxofemoral joint are ruled out by physical examination.
• Polyarthritis typically presents as a shifting limb lameness with multiple joints involved. Additionally, arthrocentesis will reveal characteristic inflammatory responses.
• Hoof lameness is generally ruled out by physical examination and hoof trimming.

IMAGING

Ancillary diagnostic procedures:
• Radiography may be used to confirm luxation of the stifle joint; however, this procedure is not recommended in most cases. Most food-animal practitioners lack both the resources to produce quality stifle films and the experience interpreting these films. Additionally, quality stifle films in cattle usually require general anesthesia.
• This procedure is probably not justifiable based on costs and benefits unless surgical intervention is contemplated in a valuable animal.
• Definitive and anatomically specific diagnosis of stifle injuries generally requires arthrotomy or arthroscopy.
• These approaches are rarely undertaken due to the costs associated with general anesthesia, the difficulty of the procedures, the relative inexperience of most surgeons with bovine stifle surgery, and the lack of controlled clinical trials documenting improved outcome associated with surgical intervention.

TREATMENT

• In cattle that are unable to stand, immediate euthanasia is a reasonable decision.
• In most circumstances, conservative management will be the optimal course of treatment.
• If treatment is attempted, affected cattle are confined in a small dirt-floored stall for 4 to 6 months, permitting scarring and fibrosis to stabilize the stifle joint.

• Many cattle will demonstrate dramatic improvement in their gait. Cattle with dramatic and persistent laxity of the stifle tend to respond poorly to stall rest.
• Cattle that respond well to stall rest will typically begin to become progressively lamer within a year of the initial diagnosis and this deterioration appears to be caused by osteoarthritis.
• Some practitioners have advocated that the affected limb should be placed in a Thomas or Walker splint apparatus.
• A number of surgical approaches have been used in an attempt to stabilize the stifle and prevent chronic arthritis. These approaches may be considered in valuable cattle with exceptional genetic merit.
• One study reported approximately a 50% one-year survival and function rate in cattle following surgical intervention, with some cattle remaining functional as long as 4 years postsurgery. However, it should be noted that this data set was restricted to female dairy cattle. One would anticipate less favorable responses in bulls due to their relatively larger size. No controlled clinical trial has compared response to conservative medical and surgical treatment of stifle injuries.
• Surgical intervention is probably not appropriate in most general food-animal practices, and the practitioner would be well advised to refer such cases.

FOLLOW-UP

• Bulls that respond to either medical or surgical intervention are poor candidates for natural service.
• Most bulls are unable to complete a single breeding season. Likewise natural service appears to carry an inordinate risk for cows that initially appear to recover from stifle injuries.
• Valuable breed bulls should be housed alone in a dirt lot and have semen collected for use in artificial insemination after their recovery from surgery or the recommended 6-month course of stall rest.
• Recovered cows of exceptional value should be used as embryo transfer donors.

MISCELLANEOUS

It should be noted that few clinical reports have attempted to describe the clinical course and response to treatment in cattle with stifle injuries. The limited reports available may not be representative of the disease presented to the private practitioner.

ASSOCIATED CONDITIONS
N/A

AGE-RELATED FACTORS
• The individual most commonly affected is a young adult beef bull.
• Injuries are often observed in athletic young bulls of high libido near the end of the breeding season and injuries are often observed in cows coincidental with estrus.

ZOONOTIC POTENTIAL
N/A

PREGNANCY
Recovered cows of exceptional value should be used as embryo transfer donors.

RUMINANT SPECIES AFFECTED
Potentially, all ruminant species can be affected.

BIOSECURITY
N/A

PRODUCTION MANAGEMENT
Mixing groups of cattle or adding single cows to preexisting herds or groups often precipitates social dominance behavior that leads to traumatic injuries. This is particularly the case when unaccustomed bulls are placed together in small pens or pastures.

SYNONYMS
N/A

SEE ALSO
Anesthesia and analgesia
Euthanasia and disposal
Femoral and tibial fractures
Hoof lameness
Infectious polyarthritis
Lameness
Luxations of the hip
NSAIDs
Osteochondrosis

ABBREVIATIONS
NSAIDs = nonsteroidal anti-inflammatory drugs

Suggested Reading
Ducharme, N. G. 1996. Stifle injuries in cattle. *Veterinary Clinics of North America: Food Animal Practice* 12:59–84.
Nelson, D. R. 1982. Surgical stabilization of the stifle in cranial cruciate ligament injury in cattle. *Vet Record* 111:259–62.

Author: Jeff W. Tyler

STRONGYLOIDES

 BASICS

OVERVIEW
• Order Rhabditida include three genera that parasitize animals
  • *Rhabditis (Pelodera) strongyloides*
  • *Halicephalobus (Micronema)*
  • *Strongyloides*
• *Rhabditis (Pelodera) strongyloides*
  • Free-living parasite that inhabits decaying organic debris
  • Produces pruritic, hyperemic dermatitis in cattle, horses, swine, dogs, and rodents; organism penetrates skin when animals contact dirty bedding or contaminated environment.
  • Dermatitis includes marked alopecia on neck and flank with flaking, thickening, and wrinkling of skin, pruritus, irritation, and exudation of serum in severe cases. Pustules containing thick, yellow, caseous material, and worms present on ventral abdomen and udder.
  • *Rhabditis bovis* in cattle in the tropics causes otitis externa and chronic wasting.
  • Easily found on skin scrapings, may also diagnose by skin biopsy or detection of organism in bedding (upper layers)
  • Remove soiled bedding and keep bedding clean and dry.
  • Spontaneous recovery may occur if remove source and change management.
  • Treat with ivermectin, avermectins, local application of parasiticide, or topical treatment (ear) and symptomatic treatment.
• *Halicephalobus (Micronema)* are highly pathogenic for horses and humans; one report of *M. deletrix* in the skin of a bull's scrotum
• *Strongyloides*: All domestic animals and many wild mammals and birds have a species of *Strongyloides*.
  • *Strongyloides papillosus* affects ruminants.
  • Worldwide distribution, particularly in warm, humid areas
  • *Stongyloides* infections are common, usually mild or moderate, and asymptomatic in ruminants.
  • Neonates and suckling calves, kids, and lambs are most commonly clinically infected.
  • Transmammary transmission to neonates

• Initially considered as a commensal organism. Recent studies indicate that even light infections may cause substantial disease in susceptible young, especially kids.
• Probably most common worm to infect goats with most goats having a few of these worms most of the time
• Clinical signs related to skin penetration (dermatitis, lameness), intestinal infection (diarrhea), and migration of immature forms through lungs (coughing, tachypnea) are variable depending on species, age, and immunity of animal and on parasite load.

Strongyloides Infection
Pathophysiology
Life Cycle
• Unique because it has alternate free-living and parasitic generations
• Parasitic female is embedded in the intestinal tract mucosa, primarily the upper small intestine.
• Eggs laid here develop rapidly and are embryonated when they are passed out with the feces.
• On pasture, eggs hatch quickly into infective larvae or become free-living males or females that can produce infective larvae.
• Larvae molt to infective third-stage larvae within 24 to 48 hours.
• Grazing host ingests infective larvae or infective larvae penetrate skin (usually between hooves) of host.
  • In older animals, larvae accumulate in the subcutaneous tissues and migrate to the mammary gland when lactation starts so neonates are infected via the milk, and egg-laying females may be present in the intestine from about 1 week after birth.
  • Infective larvae that penetrate the skin of young animals travel via the blood to lungs where they break into alveoli.
• Larvae migrate up airways or are coughed up the trachea into the pharynx and swallowed.
• Develop into mature females in 2 to 3 weeks after ingestion; prepatent period in sheep is 1–2 weeks
• Major mode of transmission is transmammary (colostrum, milk) and less often is by skin penetration (especially toes, ventrum) or ingestion.

Life Cycle Unique Characteristics
• *Strongyloides* spp. have alternating free-living and parasitic generations.
• Free-living life cycle has males and females.

• Parasitic life cycle contains parthenogenic females; males are not involved in the parasitic phase of the cycle.
• Parasitic (filariform) female produces eggs by mitotic parthenogenesis.
  • Homogonic rhabditiform larvae hatch from these eggs.
  • In external environment, larvae develop via molts to either infective filariform larvae or to free-living males and females.
  • Infective filariform larvae, after entering host, molts into parasitic females.
• Free-living rhabditiform males and females mate to produce heterogonic rhabditiformic larvae that generally only develop into infective filariform larvae.

SIGNALMENT
• Seen worldwide
• Infects young calves (particularly dairy stock), young and weaned kids, lambs
• No sex predilection
• Adult ruminants carry a degree of immunity to the intestinal form of the parasite

SIGNS
Natural Infections
• Intermittent diarrhea
• Blood and mucus in feces
• Loss of appetite
• Weight loss
• Coughing as immature forms migrate to air passages
• Penetration of worm through skin of feet (interdigital)
  • Lameness
  • Stamping of feet
  • Biting at or rubbing of feet and legs
  • Increased susceptibility to foot rot
• In sheep and lambs
  • Initial skin invasion by *S. papillosus* larvae may not induce any inflammation but subsequent exposure causes a pustular, erythematous dermatitis.
  • Lamb: dermatitis, pulmonary hemorrhage, and enteritis
• Localized dermatitis on feet or dependent regions of body is caused by an immune reaction to migrating larvae.
• Adults seldom show ill effects of parasite burden unless stressed, diseased, or exposed to heavy infestation.
  • Bulls—balanoposthitis
  • Sheep—heavy load may cause unthriftiness, diarrhea, weight loss, slow growth.

• In goats with heavy overload stress or debilitated condition, *S. papillosus* may cause diarrhea, hypophagia, weight loss, and moderate anemia ± presence of tiny white worms in feces. Reinfection results in bouts of coughing.

Experimental Infections in Kids
• Death in some kids after as few as three exposures (2000–5000 larvae per exposure); death within 9 to 30 days after receiving 75, 000 larvae
• Kids 6 weeks to 6 months more susceptible than those 6 to 12 months old
• Clinical signs varied
  • Dehydration, inappetence, diarrhea, weight loss, weakness, afrebrile
  • Anemia, respiratory distress
  • Nervous signs
  • Sudden death from hepatic rupture in some kids

Experimental Infections in Lambs
Inoculation of live parthenognetic females into duodenum of lambs induced sinus tachycardia and cardiac arrest.

Experimental Infections in Calves
• Pallor and coughing
• Heavy infection induced variety of cardiac arrhythmias
• Sudden death due to cardiac arrest

CAUSES AND RISK FACTORS
• Most common when animal kept in wet, dirty environment
• Dirty bedding
• Parasitized dams at time of parturition are greatest source of *Strongyloides* for neonates.

DIAGNOSIS
• Suspect in young animals with consistent history and clinical signs
• Adult (3–6 mm) in small intestine (sheep)
• Direct fecal smear or Baermann procedure to observe larvae
• Day-to-day variation in larval numbers makes diagnosis difficult.
• Fecal flotation
  • Small, clear, colorless, thin-shelled, oval embryonated egg (40–60 × 20–25 µm)

• Free-living adults frequently develop in cultures of feces from *Strongyloides*-infected animals.
• Female is not highly prolific; does not produce a large number of eggs. In goats: a dozen or more eggs in sample represents a large load of worms.
• Skin biopsy: pustular dermatitis characterized by edema, inflammatory infiltration (neutrophils, eosinophils, lymphocytes, and giant cells), and destruction of the larvae.
• Necropsy
  • Adults in scraping of intestinal mucosa
  • Immature worms recovered from minced tissue placed in a Baermann isolation device
  • Catarrhal enteritis with petechiae and ecchymoses, especially in the duodenum and jejunum.
• Serodiagnosis with ELISA (serum) may be useful.

DIFFERENTIAL DIAGNOSIS
• A contact dermatitis or irritation from dirty wet bedding
• Infectious and noninfectious causes of diarrhea
• Foot rot
• *Pelodera* dermatitis
• Trombiculidiasis
• Hookworm dermatitis
• Chorioptic mange
• Dermatophytosis

CBC/BIOCHEMISTRY/URINALYSIS
Anemia in heavily infested animals

OTHER LABORATORY TESTS
N/A

IMAGING
N/A

DIAGNOSTIC PROCEDURES
• Fecal flotation
• Skin biopsy

TREATMENT
• Eliminate moist, warm habitants for the larvae.
  • Remove contaminated bedding
  • Keep bedding clean and dry

• Dewormer should be approved for species and gestational and lactation status of animal in which it is to be used.
• Treatment frequency may be reduced by rotating pasture.
• Recommended withdrawal times for milk and meat must be observed.
• Ivermectin and doramectin have been recommended to treat adult worms in cattle, goats, and sheep; treatment may need to be repeated.
• Use dewormer to which nematodes on premises are susceptible. Parasite resistance is increasingly becoming a problem.
• If resistance to specific dewormers is suspected, check by doing fecal egg counts from representative animals before and after deworming.
• Rotational use of dewormer to avoid resistance development
• Use a strategic deworming program: deworm animals when the total worm population is in the host not on the ground (pasture).

MEDICATIONS

DRUGS OF CHOICE
• Appropriate drug(s) to be used will depend on susceptibility and resistance patterns found in animal groups to be treated.
• Breed, age, pregnancy, and lactation status will also influence choice of anthelmintic to be used. Milk and meat withdrawal times must be observed.
  • Ivermectin: goat and sheep 0.2–0.3 mg/kg PO
  • Eprinomectrin: goat and sheep 0.5 mg/kg PO
  • Moxidectin: goat 0.5 mg/kg PO
  • Fenbendazole: goat and sheep 5–10 mg/kg PO (may need up to 20 mg/kg PO to control nematode parasites)
  • Oxfendazole: goat 10 mg/kg PO; sheep 5–10 mg/kg PO
  • Levamisole: goat 8 mg/kg PO (may need up to 12 mg/kg PO)
  • Febantel: goats and sheep 5 mg/kg PO

STRONGYLOIDES

CONTRAINDICATIONS
Appropriate milk and meat withdrawal times must be followed for all compounds administered to food-producing animals.

FOLLOW-UP

EXPECTED COURSE AND PROGNOSIS
Threadworms are not of great economic importance in the United States.

MISCELLANEOUS

ASSOCIATED CONDITIONS
Secondary mild bacterial bronchopneumonia

ZOONOTIC POTENTIAL
• Cutaneous larva migrans
  • Most commonly due to dog and cat hookworms
  • Less commonly due to animal roundworms including *Strongyloides papillosus, S. myopotami, S. westeri*
• *Strongyloides stercoralis* affects humans.

RUMINANT SPECIES AFFECTED
Goats, cattle, sheep, wildlife ruminants

BIOSECURITY
N/A

PRODUCTION MANAGEMENT
• Routine deworming of dams in late gestation to decrease transmammary transmission to newborn
• Early deworming of newborns of affected but untreated dams
• Provide clean, dry environment with adequate clean bedding in stalls and rest areas.
• Pasture management to reduce hosts' exposure to parasites
• Selection for parasite resistance and culling of animals with chronic, heavy parasite loads may decrease parasite problem in herd or flock.
• Avoid bringing in resistant parasites by isolating new goats until they have been dewormed.
• Infestations may result in decreased milk and meat production.
• Severe infestations in young animals may lead to poor weight, stunting, or death.
• Pruritic dermatitis may result in damage to the wool and hide.

SYNONYMS
Intestinal threadworm

SEE ALSO
Chorioptic mange
Contact dermatitis or irritation from dirty, wet bedding
Dermatophytosis
Foot rot
Hookworm dermatitis
Infectious and noninfectious causes of diarrhea
Pelodera dermatitis
Trombiculidiasis

ABBREVIATIONS
ELISA = enzyme-linked immunosorbent assay
PO = per os, by mouth

Suggested Reading
Aiello, S. E., ed. 1998. Gastrointestinal parasites of ruminants. In: *Merck veterinary manual*. 8th ed. Whitehouse Station: Merck & Co.
Bowman, D. D., Lunn, R. C., Eberherd, M. L. 2003. Helminths. In: *Georgis' parasitology for veterinarians helminths*. 8th ed. Philadelphia: W. B. Saunders (Elsevier Science).
Nakamura, Y., et al. 1994. Parasitic females of *Strongyloides papillosus* as a pathogenic stage of sudden cardiac death in infected lambs. *J Vet Med Sci*. 56:723–27.
Pienaar, J. G., et al. 1999. Experimental studies with *Strongyloides papillosus* in goats. *Onderst J Vet Res*. 66:191–235.
Pugh, D. G. 2002. Diseases of the gastrointestinal tract and flock management. In: *Sheep and goat medicine*. Philadelphia: W. B. Saunders.
Tsuji, N., et al. 1992. Sudden cardiac death in calves with experimental heavy infection of *Strongyloides papillosus*. *J Vet Med Sci*. 54:1137–43.

Authors: Susan Semrad and Karen A. Moriello

BASICS

OVERVIEW
• Strychnine is an alkaloid derived from *Strychnos nux-vomica*, a tree native to India. Used primarily as a pesticide for rat, gopher, mole, and coyote control. Commercial forms are sold as powder, pellets, or treated seeds, dyed bright green or red. Contains 0.3%–0.5% strychnine
• Not absorbed until it reaches the intestine
• Highly toxic to ruminants orally at 0.5 mg/kg
• Mechanism of action—blocks glycine, the transmitter for inhibitory cells (Renshaw cells) of the spinal cord
• Direct effects on the CNS by antagonizing spinal inhibition in the spinal cord and medulla. This allows the uncontrolled and diffuse reflex activity. All striated muscle groups are affected, extensors predominate. Produces symmetrical and generalized rigidity and tonic seizures.
• There are no gross or microscopic lesions seen.

SIGNALMENT
Affects all ruminant species of any age

SIGNS
• Appear 10 minutes to 2 hours postingestion
• Nervousness, tenseness, stiffness; rigid cervical musculature, neck arched, ears erect, lips pulled back from teeth, and tense abdomen
• Violent tetanic seizures appear spontaneously or initiated by stimuli such as touch, sound, and sudden bright light
• Extensor rigidity, sawhorse stance
• Convulsions increase in frequency and duration
• Eyes dilated, cyanotic mucous membranes (from anoxia)
• If untreated, the whole syndrome can last 1–2 hours until death. The lethal dose is eliminated in 24–48 hours, so treatment is required during this period.

CAUSES AND RISK FACTORS

DIAGNOSIS

Based on history of ingestion, clinical signs, and lack of gross lesions

DIFFERENTIAL DIAGNOSIS
• Chlorinated hydrocarbon toxicity
• Zinc phosphate toxicity
• Lead toxicity
• Hypocalcemia
• Metaldehyde
• Organophosphate or carbamates
• 1080 toxicity
• Causes of acute, massive hepatic necrosis

CBC/BIOCHEMISTRY/URINALYSIS
Urine is a good diagnostic sample. Strychnine is readily absorbed from GI tract and excreted in urine.

OTHER LABORATORY TESTS
• Stomach contents are a common source of diagnosis.
• Postmortem, samples of liver, kidney, urine, and CNS will help yield a diagnosis.

IMAGING
N/A

DIAGNOSTIC PROCEDURES
PATHOLOGIC FINDINGS
• Rigor mortis rapid after death
• Subsequent relaxation follows more rapidly than normal.
• Cyanosis, petechial and ecchymotic hemorrhages, and traumatic lesions are evidence of a violent and hypoxic state.

TREATMENT

MEDICATIONS

DRUGS OF CHOICE
• Prevent asphyxia and maintain relaxation for 24–48 hours using pentobarbital, methocarbamol at 150 mg/kg IV, diazepam, glyceryl guiacolate at 110 mg/kg IV.
• Gastric lavage
• Diuresis with 5% mannitol in 0.9% NaCl at 6.6 ml/kg
• If not acidotic, administer NH_3Cl at 132 mg/kg orally to increase urinary elimination.

CONTRAINDICATIONS
• Monitor serum pH.
• Appropriate milk and meat withdrawal times must be followed for all compounds administered to food-producing animals.

FOLLOW-UP

EXPECTED COURSE AND PROGNOSIS
Acute rapid onset—prognosis is poor if untreated.

MISCELLANEOUS

ASSOCIATED CONDITIONS
• Violent tetanic seizures
• Extensor rigidity
• Convulsions

AGE-RELATED FACTORS
N/A

ZOONOTIC POTENTIAL
N/A

PREGNANCY
N/A

RUMINANT SPECIES AFFECTED
Potentially, all ruminant species are affected.

BIOSECURITY
N/A

PRODUCTION MANAGEMENT
Keep all agricultural chemicals away from livestock.

SYNONYMS
N/A

SEE ALSO
1080 toxicity
Chlorinated hydrocarbon toxicity
Hepatic necrosis
Hypocalcemia
Lead toxicity
Metaldehyde
Organophosphate or carbamates
Zinc phosphate toxicity

ABBREVIATIONS
CNS = central nervous system
IV = intravenous
NaCl = sodium chloride
NH_3Cl = ammonium chloride

Suggested Reading
Aiello, S. E., ed. 1998. *Merck veterinary manual*. 8th ed. Whitehouse Station, NJ: Merck and Co.
Buck, W. M., Osweiler, G. D., Van Gelde, G. A. 1976. *Clinical and diagnostic veterinary toxicology*. Dubuque, IA: Kendall-Hunt Publishing Co.
Cheeke, P. D., Shull, L. R. 1985. *Natural toxicants in feeds and poisonous plants*. Westport, CT: AVI Publishing, Inc.
Martin, W. B., Aitken, I. D. 2000. *Diseases of sheep*. 3rd ed. Oxford, UK: Blackwell Science Ltd.
Roder, J. D. 2001. Veterinary toxicology. *The Practical Veterinarian*, pp. 283–86.
Smith, B. P. *Large animal internal medicine*. 3rd ed. St. Louis: Mosby.

Author: Greg Stoner

SUBCUTANEOUS EMPHYSEMA

 BASICS

DEFINITION
Subcutaneous emphysema is the accumulation of gases under the skin and between tissue planes.

PATHOPHYSIOLOGY
• A transtracheal aspirate site may allow air to penetrate under the skin, usually accumulating around the trachea but occasionally extending further.
• Air may also extend subcutaneously by migrating from the site of a skin wound, fractured nasal bone or rib, or from pulmonary emphysema secondary to severe pneumonia.
• The introduction of anaerobic bacteria or their spores, especially clostridial organisms, under the skin by needle puncture or unsanitary surgical procedures or by a wound can result in elaboration of gases by the bacteria during their growth phase, with subcutaneous emphysema resulting.

SYSTEMS AFFECTED
Integumentary system

GENETICS
N/A

INCIDENCE/PREVALENCE
N/A

GEOGRAPHIC DISTRIBUTION
Worldwide

SIGNALMENT
Species
All ruminant species

Breed Predilections
N/A

Mean Age and Range
N/A

Predominant Sex
N/A

SIGNS

HISTORICAL FINDINGS
• Previous needle punctures (e.g., from administering vaccines or medications).
• Animals not vaccinated against clostridial agents
• Previous thoracic trauma with fractured ribs
• Pneumonia during parturition, especially in sheep and goats, when lung parenchyma may rupture into the mediastinum due to increased intrathoracic pressure during parturition.

PHYSICAL EXAMINATION FINDINGS
Crepitance can be palpated over affected areas of the body. If clostridial infection is the insighting cause of the subcutaneous emphysema, will see signs of myonecrosis (e.g., cool insensitive skin, malodorous serosanguinous fluid discharge from wounds), and the animal will be depressed, reluctant to move, and possibly febrile.

CAUSES AND RISK FACTORS
• Causes include air migration from a transtracheal aspirate site along tissue planes, and gases produced by clostridial organisms, particularly *Clostridium chauvoei*, *Cl. septicum*, *Cl. sordelli*, *Cl. novyi* type B, *Cl. perfringens* type A, and *Cl. carnis*.
• Risk factors include needle punctures without prior aseptic preparation of the skin surface, repeated use of the same needles between different animals, and lack of prior vaccination against clostridia.

 DIAGNOSIS

DIFFERENTIAL DIAGNOSIS
• Clostridial myonecrosis
• Cellulitis
• Hematoma
• Seroma

CBC/BIOCHEMISTRY/URINALYSIS
Hemoconcentration, a stress leukogram, and elevated muscle enzymes CK and AST if clostridial infection is the cause of the subcutaneous emphysema

OTHER LABORATORY TESTS
• Aspirate affected areas and examine fluid microscopically; culture fluid to aid in differential diagnosis.
• Biopsy/histopathology/culture of affected tissue.

IMAGING
N/A

OTHER DIAGNOSTIC PROCEDURES
N/A

PATHOLOGIC FINDINGS
If clostridial infection is the cause of the subcutaneous emphysema, signs of tissue necrosis (e.g., swelling, autolysis, crepitus, serosanguinous fluid discharge from cut surfaces) will be evident.

 TREATMENT

May need to surgically debride tissue and perform fenestrations or fasciotomies to allow gases to escape. This will create a more aerobic environment to slow proliferation of anaerobic bacteria if they are suspected as the cause of the subcutaneous emphysema.

ACTIVITY
Restrict movement to slow migration of gases along tissue planes.

DIET
May need supportive fluid therapy if clostridial infection is the cause of the subcutaneous emphysema.

CLIENT EDUCATION
• Importance of clostridial vaccination
• Extensive skin sloughing may result if clostridial infection is the cause of the subcutaneous emphysema.

MEDICATIONS

• Penicillins if clostridial infection is the suspected cause of the subcutaneous emphysema.
• NSAIDs to control pain and swelling, if clostridial infection is suspected.

DRUGS OF CHOICE
Penicillin 44,000 U/kg IV q. 2–4 hrs. for 1–5 days or until animal stable, then q. 12 hrs. IM until complete recovery.

CONTRAINDICATIONS
Appropriate milk and meat withdrawal times must be followed for all compounds administered to food-producing animals.

PRECAUTIONS
N/A

POSSIBLE INTERACTIONS
N/A

ALTERNATIVE DRUGS
N/A

FOLLOW-UP
N/A

PATIENT MONITORING
Monitor for skin sloughing if clostridial infection is the cause of the subcutaneous emphysema.

PREVENTION/AVOIDANCE
• Performing a transendoscopic tracheal aspirate instead of a transtracheal aspirate could avoid the complication of subcutaneous emphysema, and yield comparable culture and sensitivity results.
• Immunization against clostridial organisms

POSSIBLE COMPLICATIONS
N/A

EXPECTED COURSE AND PROGNOSIS
Prognosis guarded to poor if clostridial infection is the cause of the subcutaneous emphysema, otherwise prognosis good.

MISCELLANEOUS

ASSOCIATED CONDITIONS
N/A

AGE-RELATED FACTORS
N/A

ZOONOTIC POTENTIAL
N/A

PREGNANCY
N/A

RUMINANT SPECIES AFFECTED
All

BIOSECURITY
If clostridial infection is the cause of the subcutaneous emphysema, carcasses should be disposed of by deep burial, burning, or removal from the premises to avoid environmental contamination.

PRODUCTION MANAGEMENT
N/A

SYNONYMS
N/A

SEE ALSO
Clostridial agent chapters
NSAIDs
Wound care

ABBREVIATIONS
AST = aspartate aminotransferase
CK = creatine kinase
NSAIDs = nonsteroidal anti-inflammatory drugs

Suggested Reading
Pugh, D.G., ed. 2002. *Sheep and goat medicine*. Philadelphia: W. B. Saunders.
Radostits, O. M., Gay, C. C., Blood, D. C., Hinchcliff, K. W., eds. 2000. *Veterinary medicine*. 9th ed. London: W.B. Saunders.
Smith, B. P., ed. 2002. *Large animal internal medicine*. 3rd ed. St. Louis: Mosby.

Author: David McKenzie

SWEET CLOVER POISONING

BASICS

OVERVIEW
• Sweet clover poisoning is from toxic ingestion of moldy hay where fungal metabolism of harmless natural coumarins in the plant, in the process of spoilage, produces toxic dicoumerol, a vitamin K inhibitor. These molds include *Penicillium* spp., *Mucor* spp., and *Aspergillus* spp.
• It affects *Melilotus* spp. of sweet clover.
• Any method of hay storage that allows molding of sweet clover promotes the likelihood of the formation of dicoumerol in the hay.
• Weathered large round bales, particularly the outer portion, has the highest levels of dicoumerol.
• Sweet clover plants are biennial legumes found throughout much of the United States and southern Canada along roadsides or in waste areas. In the northwestern United States, this plant is grown as a forage for livestock. These plants can produce a severe hemorrhagic disease in cattle that is less likely to occur in other ruminants.

• The stems arising from taproots are erect and reach a height of 3 to 6 feet. The leaves are composed of three leaflets with the apices rounded. The flowers are small and white (*Melilotus alba*) or yellow (*Melilotus officinalis*).

PATHOPHYSIOLOGY
• When the toxic hay or silage is consumed, hypoprothrombinemia results as dicoumerol combines with the proenzyme to prevent the formation of the active enzyme required for the synthesis of prothrombin.
• Fungal invasions in partially cured stems initiate the conversion of coumarin to dicoumarol, a potent anticoagulant. Dicoumerol is antagonistic to vitamin K and consequently blocks the synthesis of prothrombin and clotting factors VII, IX, and X. Vitamin K is necessary for the conversion of these clotting factors from their precursors in the liver.
• Prothrombin interferes with the synthesis of factor VII and other coagulation factors.
• The toxic agent crosses the placenta in pregnant animals and newborns may be affected at birth.
• Field investigations determined that 50–70 ppm is toxic.

Species
Sheep and cattle of all ages

SIGNALMENT

SIGNS
• Stiffness, lameness due to bleeding into muscles and joints
• Hematoma formation, epistaxis, GI bleeding
• Death can be sudden with massive hemorrhage after injury, surgery, parturition
• Abortions, stillbirths, weak calves

CAUSES AND RISK FACTORS
For sweet clover poisoning to occur, animals require a continuous consumption of contaminated sweet clover hay or silage.

DIAGNOSIS

• Based on history of consumption of sweet clover hay and silage over a long period of time, signs and lesions as well as a prolonged blood clotting time
• Demonstration of reduced prothrombin content in the plasma

DIFFERENTIAL DIAGNOSIS

Blackleg, pasteurellosis, braken fern poisoning, aplastic anemia, rodenticide poisoning (e.g., warfarin and brodificoum), and rarely purpura hemorrhagica.

CBC/BIOCHEMISTRY/URINALYSIS

• Increased ACT, OSPT, APTT
• Prothrombin time in rabbits fed contaminated hay (prolonged from approximately 15 seconds to 100–200 seconds)
• Prolonged bleeding time
• Anemia
• Prolonged clotting time
• Platelets—normal

OTHER LABORATORY TESTS

• No quick chemical test for dicoumerol; absence of visible spoilage is insufficient evidence to disqualify diagnosis.
• Dicoumerol levels of 20–30 mg/kg in hay are usually required to cause poisoning in cattle.
• Liver dicoumerol concentration

IMAGING

N/A

DIAGNOSTIC PROCEDURES

PATHOLOGICAL FINDINGS

GROSS FINDINGS

Hemorrhage is characteristic necropsy finding, large accumulations of blood commonly found in subcutaneous and connective tissue.

TREATMENT

• Remove from source
• Try to avoid excessive movement or stress to the animals involved.

MEDICATIONS

• IV administration of 2–4 L of whole blood per 1000 lb (450 Kg) BW from an animal not fed sweet clover. Repeat as necessary.
• Vitamin K 1 (phytonadione) is more effective than vitamin K 3 given IM once at 1.1–3.3 mg/kg BW
• Vitamin K 3 is ineffective as a treatment.
• Remove sweet clover from ration 1 month prior to calving.

DRUGS OF CHOICE

CONTRAINDICATIONS

Appropriate milk and meat withdrawal times must be followed for all compounds administered.

FOLLOW-UP

PATIENT MONITORING

Recheck prothrombin time 1 week after initiation of treatment.

PREVENTION/AVOIDANCE

• Feed cultivars of sweet clover, low in coumarin; monitor feed.
• If sweet clover is present, make sure the hay is cured properly to avoid any moldy conditions.
• Avoid feeding sweet clover hay baled damp.

POSSIBLE COMPLICATIONS

EXPECTED COURSE AND PROGNOSIS

• If anemia is severe, the prognosis would be guarded especially if animal is stressed. Prolonged prothrombin times may last 1 or more weeks.

SWEET CLOVER POISONING

• Milder cases respond well to treatment.
• Several weeks may be necessary for return to normal.

 MISCELLANEOUS

ASSOCIATED CONDITIONS
• The disease manifests itself by prolonged hemorrhage. Anemia, depression, and bleeding from the nose or digestive tract are early signs of sweet clover poisoning.
• Hematomas from bruising may be prominent over body areas most subject to trauma.

AGE-RELATED FACTORS
N/A

ZOONOTIC POTENTIAL
N/A

PREGNANCY
• Pregnant animals should not be fed hay or silage containing moldy sweet clover.

• Death can be sudden with massive hemorrhage after injury, surgery, parturition.
• Abortions, stillbirths, weak calves

RUMINANT SPECIES AFFECTED
Cattle; less likely sheep and other ruminants

BIOSECURITY
N/A

PRODUCTION MANAGEMENT
N/A

SYNONYMS
N/A

SEE ALSO
Aplastic anemia
Blackleg
Braken fern poisoning
Pasteurellosis
Purpura hemorrhagica
Rodenticide poisoning

ABBREVIATIONS
ACT = activated clotting time
APTT = activated partial thromboplastin time
BW = body weight

GI = gastrointestinal
IM = intramuscular
IV = intravenous
OSPT = one-stage prothrombin time
ppm = parts per million

Suggested Reading
Abramson, D., Mills, J. T., Marquardt, R. R., Frohlich, A. A. 1997, Jan. Mycotoxins in fungal contaminated samples of animal feed from western Canada, 1982–1994. *Can J Vet Res*. 61(1): 49–52.
Diekman, M. A., Green, M. L. 1992, May. Mycotoxins and reproduction in domestic livestock. *J Anim Sci*. 70(5): 1615–27.
Hintz, H. F. 1990, Aug. Molds, mycotoxins, and mycotoxicosis. *Vet Clin North Am Equine Pract*. 6(2): 419–31.
Price, W. D., Lovell, R. A., McChesney, D. G. 1993, Sep. Naturally occurring toxins in feedstuffs: Center for Veterinary Medicine Perspective. *J Anim Sci*. 71(9): 2556–62.
Sweeney, M. J., Dobson, A. D. 1998, Sep 8. Mycotoxin production by *Aspergillus, Fusarium* and *Penicillium* species. *Int J Food Microbiol*. 43(3): 141–58.

Authors: Greg Stoner, Larry A. Kerr

BASICS

OVERVIEW
• Respiratory distress syndrome caused by ingestion of pneumotoxin found in moldy sweet potatoes (*Ipomoea batatas*).
• Native range is pantropical but sweet potatoes are grown and distributed worldwide.
• Infected potatoes typically have a dry, black surface that extends inward.

PATHOPHYSIOLOGY
• In response to infection by the fungus *Fusarium solani*, or related species, sweet potatoes produce stress metabolites that the fungus then converts to ipomeanine.
• Within the host lung, ipomeanine is reduced to 4-ipomeanol, the toxic metabolite, via cytochrome P450 enzymes.
• This metabolite is highly reactive and binds to lung proteins, especially type I pneumocytes and epithelial cells.

SYSTEMS AFFECTED
Respiratory, production management

GENETICS
N/A

INCIDENCE/PREVALENCE
Unknown

GEOGRAPHIC DISTRIBUTION
Potentially worldwide in distribution.

SIGNALMENT
Species
• All ruminants
• Cattle most susceptible

Breed Predilections
N/A

Mean Age and Range
N/A

Predominant Sex
N/A

SIGNS
• Acute onset of respiratory distress including rapid open-mouthed labored breathing. In advanced stages, cattle stand with head extended and there may be foamy saliva and expiratory grunts.
• Tachycardia, lethargy, depression, anorexia, aggression when handled
• Symptoms may appear within 1 day of ingestion, death 2–5 days after ingestion due to anoxia. Mild cases usually recover without treatment.

CAUSES AND RISK FACTORS
Feeding of sweet potatoes infected with the mold *Fusarium solani* (*javanicum*) or *F. oxysporum*.

DIAGNOSIS

DIFFERENTIAL DIAGNOSIS
• ARDS syndrome caused by purple mint (*Perilla frutescens*), kale, rape, grasses, and *F. semitectum* infection of legumes. Also, L-tryptophan/3-methylindole toxicity due to abrupt change in feed.
• Allergic alveolitis, bovine respiratory syncytial virus, paraquat/petroleum intoxication, parasitic bronchitis, shipping fever
• No history of dietary change from dry to lush feed, no exposure to mint, etc.

CBC/BIOCHEMISTRY/URINALYSIS
CBC and urinalysis within normal limits

OTHER LABORATORY TESTS
N/A

IMAGING
N/A

DIAGNOSTIC PROCEDURES
• Analysis of feed samples for 4-ipomeanol
• Culture of sweet potatoes used as feed and identification of *Fusarium solani*

PATHOLOGIC FINDINGS
• Some variability depending on dose and time to death.
• Gross—lungs wet, red to purple, rubbery and distended, and do not collapse upon opening of chest cavity. Pulmonary edema and emphysema, foamy or gelatinous exudates
• Microscopic—alveolar edema and emphysema, interstitial emphysema, epithelialization (due to proliferation of type II pneumocytes), interstitial fibrosis, eosinophilic hyaline membranes, vascular congestion

TREATMENT
Minimize stress and animal movement. Benefit of treatment must be weighed against cost of stress and possible death.

MEDICATIONS

DRUGS OF CHOICE
• Supportive, typically ineffective
• Antiprostaglandin drugs such as flunixin meglumine may decrease inflammatory response; diuretics to reduce edema; antibiotics for prevention of bacterial pneumonia; corticosteroids.

CONTRAINDICATIONS
Appropriate milk and meat withdrawal times must be followed for all compounds administered to food-producing animals.

FOLLOW-UP

PATIENT MONITORING
N/A

PREVENTION/AVOIDANCE
Remove contaminated feed. Avoid feeding spoiled sweet potatoes or feeding sweet potatoes in conditions that favor fungal growth in a range situation.

POSSIBLE COMPLICATIONS
N/A

EXPECTED COURSE AND PROGNOSIS
Case fatalities 25%–50%

MISCELLANEOUS

ASSOCIATED CONDITIONS
In survivors, there is some evidence of alveolar macrophage changes that may suppress defense against bacterial infection.

AGE-RELATED FACTORS
N/A

ZOONOTIC POTENTIAL
N/A

PREGNANCY
N/A

SEE ALSO
ABPE
ARDS
Atypical interstitial pneumonia
Fog fever
Pulmonary adenomatosis

ABBREVIATIONS
ABPE = acute bovine pulmonary edema
ARDS = acute respiratory distress syndrome
CBC = complete blood count

Suggested Reading
Burrows, G. E., Tyrl, R. J., ed. 2001. *Toxic plants of North America*. Ames: Iowa State University Press.
Thibodeau, M. S., Poore, M. H., Rogers, G. M. 2002. Health and production aspects of feeding sweet potato to cattle. *Vet Clin Food Anim*. 18:349–65.

Author: Kristy Cortright

TEAT LACERATIONS

 BASICS

OVERVIEW
- Teat lacerations are most often a result of step-on injury by the cow herself or an adjacent cow.
- Teat lacerations often involve crushing injury as well as a cut.
- Teat injuries often occur in contaminated environments, resulting in wound contamination.
- Improper healing of teat injuries can result in scar tissue formation, teat obstruction, teat fistulas, and ultimately loss of the quarter.
- Mastitis is a common sequela of teat laceration.
- The teat is composed of five layers: internal mucosa, submucosa, connective tissue and blood vessels, muscular layer (circular and longitudinal layers), and external squamous epithelium.
- The teat cistern is contained within the teat, the distal opening of which is the Rosette of Furstenberg, which leads to the streak canal and teat sphincter.

SIGNALMENT
- Female cattle in lactation
- Dairy cows more likely to be affected than beef cows
- Cows with large or pendulous udders more commonly affected
- Lactating dairy sheep and goats also can be affected.

SIGNS
- Teat swelling
- Teat bleeding
- Milk leakage through teat wall
- Pain
- Bloody milk
- Mastitis

CAUSES AND RISK FACTORS
- Self-trauma
- External trauma
- Pendulous or large udders

 DIAGNOSIS

DIFFERENTIAL DIAGNOSIS
- Mastitis can cause swelling of the teat and/or discoloration, bloody milk without obvious external trauma.
- Teat spiders, webs, and scar tissue can cause swelling and obstruction, but do not have associated bleeding or laceration.
- Teat fistulas cause leaking milk, but without associated traumatized tissue.
- Gangrenous mastitis causes swelling, discoloration, and bleeding, but is progressive and often generalized.

CBC/BIOCHEMISTRY/URINALYSIS
N/A

OTHER LABORATORY TESTS
- California Mastitis Test (CMT) may indicate increased somatic cell count if mastitis is present.
- Milk culture may show bacterial growth if mastitis is present secondary to laceration.

IMAGING
Ultrasound of teat may be helpful to differentiate laceration from other causes.

DIAGNOSTIC PROCEDURES
Theloscopy can be used to locate and differentiate lesions inside the teat.

PATHOLOGIC FINDINGS
N/A

 TREATMENT

- Surgical repair is required.
- Surgical repair should be attempted immediately. Prognosis drops with time after injury, and is extremely poor at more than 12 hours postinjury.
- Teat must be thoroughly cleaned and evaluated for tissue viability, blood supply, extent of injury.

- An anesthetic ring block around the base of the teat, following sedation of the animal or restraint on a tilt table, is adequate for local anesthesia. Alternatively, a caudal epidural can be performed. A tourniquet may be placed around the base of the teat to reduce bleeding and milk flow into the lacerated area during repair.
- Surgical repair should be performed in three layers: mucosa in tight continuous pattern of 3–0 or 4–0 absorbable monofilament with knots on submucosal side, submucosal tissue in a continuous pattern of 3–0 or 4–0 absorbable monofilament, and skin in interrupted vertical mattress or simple interrupted pattern with 0 or 2–0 nonabsorbable monofilament.
- Milking by machine can begin at the next milking period after repair.
- If desired, drainage of the teat can be performed in a sterile manner using a teat tube. Care must be taken to avoid damaging the surgical repair. Machine milking should begin as soon as possible after repair.
- Tissue adhesives and glue result in a severe inflammatory reaction during healing, which is more likely to result in formation of teat fistulas.

 MEDICATIONS

DRUGS OF CHOICE
- All cows should be treated prophylactically for mastitis using at least a single dose of an approved antibiotic at the time of surgery.
- Intramammary infusions are often not required, and may be damaging to the surgical repair
- Flunixin meglumine 1.1–2.2 mg/kg IV can be used at the time of repair, but is rarely necessary after the initial dose.

CONTRAINDICATIONS
Appropriate milk and meat withdrawal times must be followed for all compounds administered to food-producing animals.

FOLLOW-UP

PATIENT MONITORING
• Incision should be monitored daily for signs of incision breakdown.
• Suture removal at 7–10 days after surgery

PREVENTION/AVOIDANCE
• Avoid overcrowding cows.
• Ensure good footing in cow areas.
• Cows with pendulous udders may require separate housing or culling.
• Ensure that free stalls are wide enough for easy rising.
• Monitor the length of the medial dew claw(s) as overgrowth can result in teat/udder injury.

POSSIBLE COMPLICATIONS
• Teat fistula formation can occur anywhere along the repair line. Fistulas should be allowed to heal for 3–4 weeks before surgical repair is attempted. Full-thickness repair should be performed again in the region of the fistula, following resection of the fistula.
• Mastitis is likely, and should be treated appropriately, avoiding intramammary infusions if possible.

EXPECTED COURSE AND PROGNOSIS
• Healing should be complete in 10–14 days.
• Prognosis is good with immediate repair, guarded with lacerations >6 hours old, and poor with lacerations >12 hours old.
• Prognosis is better with partial thickness lacerations than full thickness lacerations.

 MISCELLANEOUS

ASSOCIATED CONDITIONS
None

AGE-RELATED FACTORS
Older cows may be more prone due to increased udder size and pendulous nature.

ZOONOTIC POTENTIAL
None

PREGNANCY
N/A

BIOSECURITY
None

SEE ALSO
Mammary ultrasound
Mastitis section
Pharmacology of mastitis
Teat trauma

ABBREVIATIONS
CMT = California Mastitis Test
IV = intravenous

Suggested Reading
Hull, B. L. 1995. Teat and udder surgery. *Veterinary Clinics of North America: Food Animal* 11:1–17.
Steiner, A. 2004. Teat surgery. In: *Farm animal surgery*, ed. S. L. Fubini, N. G. Ducharme. St. Louis: Elsevier.
Turner, A. S., McIlwraith, C. W., Hull, B. L. 1989. Repair of teat lacerations. In: *Techniques in large animal surgery*, ed. A. S. Turner, C. W. McIlwraith. 2nd ed. Malvern, PA: Lea & Febiger.

Author: Jennifer M. Ivany Ewoldt

TEAT LESIONS

BASICS

DEFINITION
• Teat lesions are the result of traumatic, infectious, chemical, neoplastic, environmental, or milking machine processes that injure teat skin, dermis, or mucosa resulting in lactation difficulties.
• Mastitis may result if there is penetration and compromise of the teat sinus or external sphincter.

PATHOPHYSIOLOGY
• Teat lesions damage the physiologic barriers of the teat skin, wall, and sphincter.
• Loss of barrier integrity can cause the teat and gland sinuses to leak milk or allow entry of pathogens into the mammary sinuses resulting in mastitis.
• Teat end lesions usually do not contribute to mastitis unless the lesions are severe.

SYSTEMS AFFECTED
Skin (as the specialized organ of milk delivery and innate immune barrier)

GENETICS
• Phenotypic traits associated with teat lesions include cylindrical teat shape (opposed to funnel-shaped), long teats, external sphincter shape (disc-shaped opposed to round), large and pendulous udders, teat placement and angle on the udder (allowing teats to be stepped on), and suspensory ligament breakdown.
• Slow milkers and high-producing animals also have higher incidences of teat lesions.

INCIDENCE/PREVALENCE
• Teat lesions are more common in animals with the characteristics mentioned above.
• Elevated incidence can be seen with infectious epidemics, abrupt milking system malfunction, or changes in milking practices.
• Higher prevalence may be seen with adverse environmental conditions (freezing cold, traumatic rough terrain, flies) and higher parity.

GEOGRAPHIC DISTRIBUTION
Worldwide

SIGNALMENT
• Teat injuries are problematic in lactating animals and more frequently affect high parity dairy breeds.
• They are more common in confined animals.

SIGNS
• Reluctance to be nursed or milked
• Teat erythema
• Swelling and edema
• Vesicles or papules
• Skin cracks
• Scab formation
• Bleeding or laceration
• Teat end hyperkeratosis or sphincter eversion

• Stamping of feet, brushing udder with hind legs
• In chronic cases, there is mammary gland atrophy.

CAUSES

Environmental
• Blunt trauma (stepped-on teats)
• Laceration (wire, brambles, other sharp objects)
• Cold (frostbitten and chapped teats)
• Photodermatitis (sunburn)
• Chemicals (defective or inappropriate teat dips or lime from floors or stalls)
• Milking machine trauma (overmilking and excessive vacuum pressure)
• Insects (teat atresia from *Haematobia irritans irritans*—the horn fly)

Infectious Agents
• Pseudocowpox
• Vesicular stomatitis
• Foot-and-mouth disease virus
• Bovine viral diarrhea
• Bovine malignant catarrhal fever
• Cowpox
• Bovine herpes virus 2
• Vaccinia virus
• Bovine papillomavirus

Corpora amylacea (CoA) Photosensitization Plants
• *Ammi majus* (bishop's weed, greater ammi)
• *Cooperia pedunculata* (rain lily)
• *Cymopterus watsonii* (spring parsley)
• *Fagopyrum esculentum* (buckwheat)
• *Heracleum mantegazzianum* (giant hog weed)
• *Hypericum perforatum* (St. John's wort)
• *Thamnosma texana* (Dutchman's breeches)
• *Brassica* spp. (kale)
• *Lantana camara* (lanata)
• *Senecio* spp. (ragwort)
• *Amsinckia* spp. (fiddleneck)
• *Panicum* spp. (millet)

Chemicals
• Phenothiazines
• Thiazides
• Acriflavines
• Rose Bengal
• Methylene blue
• Sulfonamides
• Tetracycline

Mycotoxins
• *Aspergillus* spp.
• *Fusarium* spp.
• *Anacystis* spp.
• *Pithomyces chartarum*

RISK FACTORS
See Genetics above, Incidence/ Prevalence above, and Causes above.

DIAGNOSIS

DIFFERENTIAL DIAGNOSIS
Pseudocowpox, vesicular stomatitis, foot and mouth disease, bovine viral diarrhea, bovine malignant catarrhal fever, cowpox, bovine herpes virus 2, bovine papillomavirus, environmental causes (above), and photosensitization from ingestion of various plants, chemicals, or mycotoxins.

CBC/BIOCHEMISTRY/URINALYSIS
N/A

OTHER LABORATORY TESTS
N/A

IMAGING
Endoscopy and ultrasonography useful to assess cause and prognosis of milk flow hindrance

DIAGNOSTIC PROCEDURES

DIAGNOSIS

• Dependent upon visualization and palpation
• Milk culture prior to antibiotic treatment may be helpful to combat secondary mastitis.

PATHOLOGIC FINDINGS

GROSS LESIONS
• Include lacerations, swelling, hemorrhage, vesicles, papules, cracks, and teat end hyperkeratosis and/or sphincter eversion.
• In severe cases, there can be proliferative granulation tissue and keratin deposition with hyperkeratosis leading to lumen narrowing.
• Varying degrees of necrosis are common and bacterial agents or viral inclusions may be detected.

TREATMENT

APPROPRIATE HEALTH CARE

NURSING CARE
• Teats should be kept clean and bandaged if possible, or covered with an appropriate dip, ointment, or teat sealer.
• Milking should be done with a cannula in a fashion that is as aseptic as possible.
• Discontinued milking of affected teats will reduce milking-associated trauma.

ACTIVITY
House animals on clean, dry bedding and away from suckling calves and other sources of teat trauma.

DIET
N/A

CLIENT EDUCATION

• Severe acute teat end lesions are serious injuries with resultant mixed-pathogen mastitis and granulation/canal stenosis.
• Aseptic technique, canal dilation, and appropriate antimicrobial withdrawal times will benefit the patient.

SURGICAL CONSIDERATIONS

Milking
• Discontinued milking of affected teats will speed healing by reducing manipulation-associated trauma.
• Culling may be considered in severe cases with refractory mastitis.

Lacerations
• Surgical correction is appropriate depending on the severity and posttrauma interval.
• Fresh lacerations (less than 12 hours) with adequate blood supply may be closed with two-layer everting mucosa and skin/muscle sutures.
• Older lacerations warrant cleansing and removal of the skin flap followed by second intention healing with granulation.
• Tears should be bandaged and milk retrieved with a cannula.

Chapped or Sunburned Teats
• Apply topical emollients approved for use in lactating cattle such as mineral oil, glycerin, or lanolin.
• Teats should be dried after milking.

Frostbite, Virus Infection, and Teat End Trauma
• Preventing mastitis while keeping the teat duct patent may require teat dilators, cannulas, and intramammary or parenteral antimicrobials.
• For teat end lesions caused by the above conditions, using teat dips containing antiseptics such as chlorhexidine, iodophors, and bleach can reduce secondary mastitis.
• Keep teats dry and cows comfortable.

MEDICATIONS

DRUGS OF CHOICE

Antibiotics
See The Environment and Mastitis chapter.

Teat Dips
• Iodophor solutions: 1% available iodine
• Hypochlorite solutions: 4% free chlorine
• Chlorhexidine solutions: 0.3%

Emollients
• Glycerin: 15%–30%
• Mineral oil
• Lanolin

CONTRAINDICATIONS
• See The Environment and Mastitis chapter.
• Appropriate milk and meat withdrawal times must be followed for all compounds administered to food-producing animals.

FOLLOW-UP

PATIENT MONITORING
• Aseptic milking techniques will reduce the incidence of mastitis.
• Teat sphincter integrity should be monitored as inflammation subsides and possible granulation ensues.
• Monitoring body temperatures, milk secretion consistency, CMT testing, in addition to follow-up milk cultures is useful to gauge presence of mastitis.

PREVENTION/AVOIDANCE
• House cows in clean areas with ample space and protection from the elements.
• Practice sound milking hygiene techniques.
• Keep lots, pastures, and fences well maintained and free of debris.
• Use approved fly control.
• Genetically select for desirable udder and teat conformation.

POSSIBLE COMPLICATIONS
• Permanently damaged teat end(s) with resultant quarter loss and decreased milk production
• Mastitis
• Reduced milk intake in suckling offspring

EXPECTED COURSE AND PROGNOSIS
Common adverse sequelae of severe lesions are teat sphincter scarring and obstruction with integrity loss and resultant mastitis.

MISCELLANEOUS

ASSOCIATED CONDITIONS
Mastitis, contact dermatitis, loss of productivity

AGE-RELATED FACTORS
Teat lesions increase with parity

ZOONOTIC POTENTIAL
• Teat lesions have no zoonotic potential unless they are caused by cowpox or pseudocowpox virus.
• Gloves should be worn when dealing with suspect or infected animals.

PREGNANCY
N/A

Species Affected
Lactating ruminants including cows, buffalo, sheep, and goats.

SYNONYMS
N/A

SEE ALSO
Environmental mastitis
Specific toxic plant chapters
Teat lacerations
Traumatic teat lesions

ABBREVIATIONS
CMT — California Mastitis Test

Suggested Reading
Chrystal, M. A., Seykora, A. J., Hansen, L. B. 1999. Heritabilities of teat end shape and teat diameter and their relationship with somatic cell score. *J Dairy Science* 82:2017–22.
Farnsworth, R. J. 1995. Observations on teat end lesions. *Bovine Practice* 29:89–92.
Osteras, O., Ronningen, O., Sandvik, L., Waage, S. 1995, Feb. Field studies show associations between pulsator characteristics and udder health. *J Dairy Res.* 62(1):1–13.
Rasmussen, M. D., Madsen, N. P. 2000, Jan. Effects of milkline vacuum, pulsator airline vacuum, and cluster weight on milk yield, teat condition, and udder health. *J Dairy Sci.* 83(1):77–84.
Wellenberg, G. J., van derPoel, W. H. M., Van Oirschot, J. T. 2002. Viral infections and bovine mastitis: a review. *Veterinary Microbiology* 88:27–45.

Author: Michael Goedken

TESTICULAR ANOMALIES

 BASICS

DEFINITION
Common diseases/anomalies affecting the testicles include hypoplasia, varicocele, orchitis/epididymitis, testicular degeneration, and cryptorchidism.

PATHOPHYSIOLOGY
• Testicular hypoplasia is thought to be a heritable genetic condition.
• Varicocele is a dilatation of the blood vessels of the pampiniform plexus.
• Orchitis/epididymitis can be the result of many infectious processes.
• Testicular degeneration may be idiopathic or be secondary to other diseases that affect the thermoregulation of the testes.
• Cryptorchidism is the failure of one or both testes to descend into the scrotum.

SYSTEMS AFFECTED
• Sperm production and/or fertility will be reduced in most cases of testicular disease.
• Sperm production and/or fertility may not be reduced in cases of disease involving only one testicle.

GENETICS
Testicular hypoplasia and cryptorchidism are heritable traits and affected animals should not be used for breeding.

INCIDENCE/PREVALENCE
• Testicular hypoplasia is the most common testicular abnormality seen in young bulls. Incidence has been reported to range between 0.2% and 1.3%.
• Varicocele occurs sporadically in rams but is rare in other ruminant species.
• Orchitis/epididymitis is rare in bulls and much more common in rams than in bucks. An incidence of 0.45% has been reported in a study of young ranch beef bulls and an incidence of 0.12% has been reported in bulls maintained at an AI stud.
• Testicular degeneration is often secondary to some other form of testicular disease.
• Cryptorchidism is uncommon in bulls with a reported incidence of 0.1%. In goats, there is a higher incidence of cryptorchidism in intersexes.

GEOGRAPHIC DISTRIBUTION
Worldwide distribution

SIGNALMENT
• Testicular anomalies occur in males of all domesticated ruminant species.
• Congenital testicular hypoplasia occurs in young bulls, bucks, and rams.
• Orchitis/epididymitis can occur in males of any age.
• Testicular degeneration can occur in males of any age secondary to other testicular diseases. Age-related degeneration occurs earlier in bulls than in males of other species.
• Cryptorchidism is a congenital condition and is usually recognized in young animals.

SIGNS
• Testicular hypoplasia produces no evidence of illness. It is most often noticed at puberty when an animal undergoes a breeding soundness exam.
  • The scrotum and testes appear smaller than normal.
  • Sperm motility, percentage of normal sperm, and total sperm per ejaculate may be reduced in males with testicular hypoplasia.
  • Libido is not usually affected.
• Varicoceles may result in a nodular or lumpy appearance to the affected testicle or may produce an evident swelling in the neck of the scrotum. Semen quality may be decreased if the varicocele interferes with the normal thermoregulation of the testicles.
• Orchitis/epididymitis is usually unilateral and produces a warm, painful swelling of the affected testicle and scrotum.
  • If severe enough, the animal may present with systemic signs of illness.
  • Swelling associated with orchitis may be marked.
• Testicular degeneration may be difficult to differentiate from testicular hypoplasia if the previous testicular size of an animal is unknown.
  • Testicles may become smaller and more flaccid.
  • Calcification may occur secondary to fibrosis in age-related degeneration.
  • Semen quality may be reduced.
  • Degeneration may be secondary to many other testicular diseases and signs of other disease processes may be present.

• Cryptorchidism is usually clearly evident due to the absence of one or both testicles in the scrotum.
  • Semen production may be absent if both testicles are involved.
  • Normal masculine features and behavior will still be present.

CAUSES
• Testicular hypoplasia is a heritable genetic condition.
• Varicoceles may result from an insufficiency of veins draining the testes or from abnormal connective tissue surrounding the veins, which allows stasis of blood in the veins.
• Orchitis/epididymitis may result from hematogenous spread, extension from other parts of the reproductive or urinary systems, or from local penetrating trauma to the scrotum.
  • *Brucella abortus* and *A. pyogenes* are the most common causes of orchitis in bulls.
  • Coliform bacteria and *Pseudomonas* have been cultured from bucks with orchitis. *Brucella melatinsis* and *Actinobacillus seminis* also can cause orchitis in bucks.
  • *Brucella ovis* is the primary cause of orchitis in rams.
  • Many other nonspecific bacteria have been isolated from cases of orchitis/epididymitis.
• Testicular degeneration may occur secondary to many testicular diseases.
  • Conditions such as fever, frostbite, orchitis, trauma, and excessive scrotal fat, which result in an alteration of the normal thermoregulation of the testicles, can result in degeneration.
  • Degeneration may occur secondary to a blockage of the excurrent duct system.
  • Age-related degeneration may occur in older animals.
• Cryptorchidism is a heritable genetic trait.

RISK FACTORS
• Using animals affected with testicular hypoplasia or cryptorchidism increases the occurrence of these problems.
• Exposure of breeding males to females carrying infectious agents such as *Brucella* species will increase the risk of orchitis/epididymitis.

DIAGNOSIS

DIFFERENTIAL DIAGNOSIS
• Differential diagnoses for small scrotum and testicle size include testicular hypoplasia, testicular degeneration, and cryptorchidism.
• Differential diagnoses for a swollen scrotum or testicle include orchitis/epididymitis, varicocele, inguinal hernia, hydrocele, hematocele, and neoplasia.

CBC/BIOCHEMISTRY/URINALYSIS
Severe cases of orchitis/epididymitis may produce evidence of infection and/or inflammation on a complete blood count.

OTHER LABORATORY TESTS
• Culture and sensitivity of seminal fluid may be useful in establishing the presence of infectious orchitis.
• Evaluation of a semen sample is useful in diagnosing diseases of the testicles.
  • Animals with testicular hypoplasia and testicular degeneration produce low numbers of sperm and a higher number of morphologically abnormal sperm.
  • Orchitis may reduce semen quality by directly destroying the affected tissue and by affecting thermoregulation of the remaining testicle.
  • Varicoceles may reduce semen quality by disrupting normal testicular thermoregulation.

IMAGING
• Ultrasound examination of abnormal testicles is a very useful diagnostic tool. The affected testicle can be compared to the opposite unaffected testicle or to a normal animal of similar age and condition.
• If available, thermography may be useful in diagnosing orchitis/epididymitis.

DIAGNOSTIC PROCEDURES
• Testicular hypoplasia is diagnosed by observation and palpation of the scrotum and testicles.
  • Measurement of scrotal circumference provides definitive diagnosis.
  • Scrotal circumference less than 30 cm in postpubertal bulls is diagnostic for hypoplasia.
  • Poor semen quality combined with small testicle size is supportive of hypoplasia.
• Varicoceles are diagnosed by palpation of the scrotum and testes ("bag of worms"). Ultrasound examination may be useful when evaluating varicoceles.
• Diagnosis of orchitis/epididymitis is based on observation and palpation of unilateral testicular swelling with heat and pain.
  • Ultrasound exam may be useful.
  • Culture of seminal fluid may be useful.
• Testicular degeneration is diagnosed based on a reduction in testicle size and a reduction in semen quality. If previous testicular size is unknown, differentiating between hypoplasia and degeneration may be difficult.
• Cryptorchidism is diagnosed based on observation and palpation of the scrotum and testes.
  • Ultrasound examination may be helpful in locating the retained testicle.
  • Measurement of testosterone levels and response to human chorionic gonadotropin is helpful in diagnosing bilateral cryptorchidism or unilateral cryptorchidism once the normal testicle has been removed.

PATHOLOGIC FINDINGS
• Histopathologic examination of hypoplastic testicles reveals hypoplastic tubules that have a small diameter, are lined by Sertoli cells and a few stem cells and spermatogonia, and have a thickened basement membrane surrounded by collagen deposits. The severity of the abnormalities depends on the degree of hypoplasia.
• The histopathologic appearance of cryptorchid testicles and testicular degeneration is similar to that of testicular hypoplasia.
• Orchitis produces varying degrees of inflammation, edema, and necrosis of the affected testicle.

TREATMENT

APPROPRIATE HEALTH CARE
N/A

NURSING CARE
Hydrotherapy with cool water may be beneficial in cases of orchitis/epididymitis.

ACTIVITY
N/A

DIET
N/A

CLIENT EDUCATION
• Animals with testicular hypoplasia or cryptorchidism should not be used for breeding purposes.
• Salvage may be the best option for commercial animals with testicular disease.

SURGICAL CONSIDERATIONS
Surgical removal of the affected testicle is often the best treatment for unilateral orchitis/epididymitis, varicocele, hydrocele, hematocele, or neoplasia.

MEDICATIONS

DRUGS OF CHOICE
• Antibiotic therapy for orchitis/epididymitis should be based on culture and sensitivity of seminal fluid.
• Antibiotic therapy is often unrewarding.

CONTRAINDICATIONS
Appropriate milk and meat withdrawal times must be followed for all compounds administered to food-producing animals.

PRECAUTIONS
Consideration should be given to withdrawal periods before antibiotic therapy is instituted.

POSSIBLE INTERACTIONS
N/A

ALTERNATIVE DRUGS
N/A

TESTICULAR ANOMALIES

 FOLLOW-UP

PATIENT MONITORING
Repeated (monthly) semen evaluations are needed to monitor the progression of degeneration or the response to therapy for orchitis.

PREVENTION/AVOIDANCE
The presence of asymptomatic carriers in the herd must be considered when dealing with infectious orchitis, especially in sheep.

POSSIBLE COMPLICATIONS
Infertility

EXPECTED COURSE AND PROGNOSIS
• After successful medical or surgical treatment of orchitis, semen production may return to normal with time, depending on the severity of damage to the remaining testicular tissue.
• Once testicular degeneration has occurred, treatment is usually unrewarding. The prognosis will depend on the degree of degeneration and the progression of the disease.

 MISCELLANEOUS

ASSOCIATED CONDITIONS
N/A

AGE-RELATED FACTORS
• Testicular hypoplasia and cryptorchidism are usually diagnosed in young animals.
• Age-related testicular degeneration may be seen in all male ruminants, especially bulls.

ZOONOTIC POTENTIAL
• Infectious orchitis caused by *Brucella* species poses some zoonotic risk to humans.
• Animals diagnosed with infections caused by these organisms should be culled.
• Brucellosis is a reportable disease.

PREGNANCY
Abortion can occur with infected bulls.

RUMINANT SPECIES AFFECTED
Cattle, sheep, goats, yaks, camelids, cervidae

BIOSECURITY
Sound biosecurity measures should be used to prevent the introduction of infectious organisms such as *Brucella* species into a clean herd or flock.

PRODUCTION MANAGEMENT
• All bulls should receive a BSE prior to the breeding season.
• A BSE is particularly important in young bulls prior to their first breeding season.

SYNONYMS
N/A

SEE ALSO
Breeding soundness examination: beef
Brucellosis
Cryptorchidism
Hematocele
Hydrocele
Inguinal hernia
Orchitis/epididymitis
Testicular degeneration
Testicular hypoplasia
Varicocele

ABBREVIATIONS
BSE = breeding soundness exam

Suggested Reading
Acland, H. M. 1995. Reproductive system: male. In: *Thompson's special veterinary pathology*, ed. W. W. Carlton, M. D. McGavin. 2nd ed. St Louis: Mosby.
Arthur, G. H., Noakes, D. E., Pearson, H., Parkinson, T. J. 1998. *Veterinary reproduction and obstetrics*. 7th ed. London: W. B. Saunders Company, Ltd.
Hooper, R. N., Blanchard, T. L., Varner, D. D. 2002. Male reproductive disorders. In: *Large animal internal medicine*, ed. B. P. Smith. 3rd ed. St. Louis: Mosby.
Morrow, D. A. 1986. *Current therapy in theriogenology 2*. Philadelphia: W. B. Saunders.
Youngquist, R. S. 1997. *Current therapy in large animal theriogenology*. Philadelphia: W. B. Saunders.

Author: John Gilliam

BASICS

DEFINITION
• Ophthalmic infestation with the nematode *Thelazia* spp. (eye worms)
• In ruminants, species of *Thelazia* include *T. gulosa, T. skrjabini, T. rhodesii,* and *T. californiensis.*
• Other species of *Thelazia* can infect sheep, goats, deer, buffalo, and dromedaries.

PATHOPHYSIOLOGY
• *Thelazia* spp. requires flies of the genus *Musca* as a necessary intermediate host.
• Adult female *Thelazia* can live in the lacrimal ducts of the nictitating membrane, in the conjunctival sacs, or under the eyelids and nictitating membranes. They discharge their larvae into ocular secretions. The fly ingests the first-stage larvae, which develop into infective third-stage in 15 to 30 days. These larvae are deposited on the eye of the host by the fly during feeding.
• Depending on the species of *Thelazia*, the larvae reach maturity in 2 to 6 weeks and begin releasing larvae ovoviviparously.
• Mechanical irritation and inflammation can lead to lesions involving the lacrimal glands and ducts, conjunctivitis, blepharitis, keratitis, and other corneal damage.
• It can also be nonsymptomatic. *T. rhodesii* is implicated in more severe cases in ruminants.

SYSTEMS AFFECTED
Ocular system, production management

GENETICS
None

INCIDENCE/PREVALENCE
Varies with geographic location. Studies have found a 17% prevalence of *T. rhodesii* in slaughterhouse examinations in the Philippines, and 15% prevalence of *T. californiensis* in hunter-killed mule deer in Wyoming and Utah.

GEOGRAPHIC DISTRIBUTION
Worldwide

SIGNALMENT
Species
• *T. californians*: deer, jackrabbit, sheep, canids, felids, raccoon, bear, and humans in North America
• *T. rhodesii*: bovines, buffalo, goats, sheep, and deer in Europe, Africa, Middle East, and Asia
• *T. gulosa* and *T. skrjabini*: cattle in North America

SIGNS
HISTORICAL FINDINGS
Asymptomatic to chronic conjunctivitis and keratitis

PHYSICAL EXAMINATION FINDINGS
• Quite variable, from asymptomatic incidental discovery to severe symptoms
• Conjunctivitis, epiphora, blepharitis, and photophobia
• Keratitis possibly with ulceration, perforation, or scarring.
• Visible worms on surface of eye, under eyelids or nictitating membranes

CAUSES
Thelazia spp. ophthalmic infection

RISK FACTORS
Face flies in an area known to have *Thelazia* spp.

DIAGNOSIS
• Examination of conjunctival sacs and underlying nictitating membranes. Topical anesthesia may be helpful to the examination process.
• Microscopic examination of lacrimal fluids for larvae

DIFFERENTIAL DIAGNOSIS
• Chronic bacterial conjunctivitis
• Viral conjunctivitis/keratitis
• Corneal laceration
• Foreign body

PATHOLOGIC FINDINGS
May see the parasite emerging from the conjunctival sac or deposited on the skin/hair around the eye of moribund species

TREATMENT
• Manual removal of the parasite, utilizing topical anesthesia. *T. rhodesii* and *T. californiensis* are more superficial species facilitating manual removal.
• Several species of *Thelazia* are more invasive and require pharmaceutical intervention.

MEDICATIONS
• Ivermectin or doramectin at 200 micrograms per kilogram body weight given subcutaneously can be 99% to 100% effective for *T. rhodesii* in cattle.
• Levamisole at 5 mg per kg body weight in cattle may be effective as well.

POSSIBLE INTERACTIONS
Do not treat lactating animals producing milk for human consumption with ivermectin or doramectin. Meat withdrawal times: ivermectin and doramectin, 35 days; levamisole, 7 days.

FOLLOW-UP
PREVENTION/AVOIDANCE
Control of face flies
• Dry, open pastures and less intensely confined conditions help reduce fly numbers.

POSSIBLE COMPLICATIONS
Scarring of cornea or loss of eye secondary to perforation of cornea is possible in rare severe cases.

EXPECTED COURSE AND PROGNOSIS
Full recovery if ocular lesions are not too severe

MISCELLANEOUS
ASSOCIATED CONDITIONS
• Corneal ulceration
• Mechanical irritation and inflammation can lead to lesions involving the lacrimal glands and ducts, conjunctivitis, blepharitis, keratitis, and other corneal damage.

AGE-RELATED FACTORS
None

ZOONOTIC POTENTIAL
T. californiensis—in humans, chronic conjunctivitis, poorly responsive to conventional treatment

PREGNANCY
N/A

BIOSECURITY
N/A

PRODUCTION MANAGEMENT
• Control of face flies
• Dry, open pastures and less intensely confined conditions help reduce fly numbers.

SYNONYMS
Eye worm

SEE ALSO
Corneal ulceration
Ophthalmic surgery

ABBREVIATIONS
N/A

Suggested Reading
Acha, P. N., Szyfres, B. 2001. *Zoonoses and communicable diseases common to man and animals.* Washington, DC: Pan American Health Organization.
Doezie, A. M., et al. 1996. *Thelazia californiensis* conjunctival infestations. *Ophthalmic Surgery and Lasers.* 27(8):716–19.
Dubay, S. A., Williams, E. S., Mills, K., Boerger-Fields, A. M. 2000, Oct. Bacteria and nematodes in conjunctiva of mule deer from Wyoming and Utah. *J Wildlife Dis.* 36(4):783–87.
Soll, M.D., et al. 1992. The efficacy of ivermectin against *T. rhodesii* (Desmaret, 1828) in the eyes of cattle. *Vet Parasitology* 42(1–2):67–71.
Van Aken D, et al. 1996. *T. rhodesii* (Desmaret, 1828) infections in cattle in Mindanao, Philippines. *Vet Parasitology* 66(1–2):125–29.

Author: Edward L. Powers

THIRD COMPARTMENT ULCERS IN SOUTH AMERICAN CAMELIDS

BASICS

OVERVIEW
• Mucosal ulcerations in the third compartment of the camelid stomach (C3) are a common occurrence in sick and stressed camelids.
• The majority of ulcers occur in the distal fifth of C3. This is the only region of the camelid stomach that contains acid-secreting gastric glands, with an intraluminal pH of 1.4–2.0. Ulcers are most commonly reported at the lesser curvature of distal C3 and in the proximal duodenum.
• Ulcers have been reported in all of the regions of the camelid stomach, but are rare in C1, C2, and the proximal four-fifths of C3.
• Ulcers typically occur as focal, discrete mucosal lesions. Perforating ulcers are not uncommon.

SIGNALMENT
• Ulcers occur in both crias and adult camelids with approximately equal incidence.
• Some studies report a slightly higher incidence in breeding-age females, but no clear sex predilection has been proven.

SIGNS
• Nonspecific signs such as depression and anorexia are most frequently reported. Decreased borborygmi and compartmental contractions are also common.
• Colic, recumbency, and bruxism occur, but are less common.
• Temperature, pulse, and respiratory rate are within normal limits unless perforation and subsequent peritonitis have occurred.
• Melena and/or anemia as a result of bleeding ulcers are not reported.
• The presence of concurrent or multisystemic disease in animals with third compartment ulcers is a frequent complicating factor, making the detection of clinical signs specific to gastric ulceration extremely difficult.

PATHOPHYSIOLOGY
• The normal physiology of gastric-acid secretion and of mucosal protection in the camelid stomach has not been determined, and thus the pathogenesis of third compartment ulcers is poorly understood.
• Ulcers are most commonly seen in hospitalized camelids with another, concurrent disease. It is postulated that the stress of concurrent disease and/or hospitalization predisposes the camelid to ulcer formation. The mechanism by which this occurs is not defined, but may be linked to the inhibition of mucosal protective factors by increased levels of endogenous cortisol and/or catecholamines.
• A direct association between nonsteroidal anti-inflammatory agents and a higher incidence of gastric ulcers has not been documented in camelids.
• The incidence of third compartment ulcers and the prevalence of grain in camelid diets are both higher in camelids living in the United States than in South America, but no direct link has been proven.

RISK FACTORS
• Hospitalization, especially when unable to see/associate with another camelid
• Other systemic disease, traumatic injury, and/or orthopedic problems

DIAGNOSIS

DIFFERENTIAL DIAGNOSIS
Third compartment ulcers are a diagnosis achieved by exclusion. Important rule-outs include:
• Gastrointestinal lesions (intestinal torsions, intussusceptions, and impactions, C1 stasis)
• Intra-abdominal abscesses
• Pancreatitis
• Peritonitis in the absence of a perforated ulcer
• Plant toxicities
• Urogenital tract lesions (uterine torsion, ruptured bladder, urolithiasis, cystitis/urethritis)

CBC/BIOCHEMISTRY/URINALYSIS
• No consistent findings.
• Leukocytosis due to neutrophilia, with or without a degenerative left shift, may be seen in perforated ulcers depending on the duration of the lesion.
• Hypoalbuminemia may also be observed in cases with perforation.
• Hyperglycemia, with serum glucose >250 mg/dl, is often seen, but this is a common stress response in any sick/stressed camelid and is not pathognomonic for gastric ulcers.

IMAGING
• Radiography after administration of oral contrast medium is of little diagnostic value due to the delay in transit time through the stomach compartments.
• Unlike the horse, endoscopic evaluation of the third stomach compartment and duodenum is not possible in the camelid.
• Ultrasonographic evaluation of the abdomen may be helpful in locating intrabdominal abscesses or masses and/or evaluation for generalized peritonitis, but is usually not helpful in diagnosing nonperforated third compartment ulcers.

OTHER DIAGNOSTIC PROCEDURES
• Analysis of peritoneal fluid may be informative in cases of perforated ulcers, but is usually unremarkable in the absence of perforation. Perforated ulcers are often walled off, producing only a localized peritonitis.
• Fecal floatation for intestinal parasites should be performed, although a direct link between parasitism and ulcers has not been proven.
• Analysis of fluid obtained from C1 via passage of an orogastric tube can be attempted; an acidic pH or decrease in numbers of microbial flora can be suggestive of third compartment ulcers.

SYSTEMS AFFECTED
Gastrointestinal—distal third compartment of the stomach and/or proximal duodenum

GENETICS
No genetic predisposition appears to exist.

THIRD COMPARTMENT ULCERS IN SOUTH AMERICAN CAMELIDS

INCIDENCE/PREVALENCE
• More prevalent in hospitalized camelid population than in the general population; estimated at ~5% of hospitalized camelids
• More common in the United States than in native South American populations of camelids

TREATMENT/PREVENTION
• Because of the lack of a good antemortem diagnostic test, treatment is initiated in the absence of a definitive diagnosis.
• Treatment/resolution of the primary problem is most important.
• The pharmacokinetics and pharmacodynamics of the standard classes of gastroprotectants (histamine-2 antagonists, proton pump inhibitors, synthetic prostaglandin-E analogues, and nonspecific gastric mucosal protectants) have not been fully determined in camelids; the following drugs are most commonly used:
  • Omeprazole: 0.4–1.2mg/kg PO SID-BID
  • Sucralfate: 20 mg/kg PO QID
  • Misoprostol: 10 ug/kg PO (do not use in pregnant animals)
  • Ranitidine (0.75–1.5 mg/kg IV, IM, or SQ SID-TID) has been used in camelids, but recent evidence suggests that at this dosing regime, ranitidine is not effective at decreasing gastric acid secretion for any significant duration in the camelid.
• Supportive care with oral or intravenous fluids is usually necessary in anorexic animals.
• If available, transfaunation with bovine ruminal fluid or camelid C1 fluid may be beneficial in some cases of prolonged anorexia.
• Since camelids are extremely social animals, the stress of hospitalization can be reduced by providing a companion camelid, such as a healthy herd mate. If such a companion is not available, an appropriately sized mirror in or near the stall of the affected animal can provide the illusion of a companion.
• Antiulcer prophylaxis is becoming standard for any sick/hospitalized camelid.

CONTRAINDICATIONS
Appropriate milk and meat withdrawal times must be followed for all compounds administered to food-producing animals.

ASSOCIATED CONDITIONS
Any cause of systemic illness, trauma, or stress

AGE-RELATED FACTORS
None

ZOONOTIC POTENTIAL
N/A

PREGNANCY
Rule out pregnancy-related causes of abdominal pain, such as uterine torsion, before diagnosing third compartment ulcers in a pregnant female.

BIOSECURITY
N/A

PRODUCTION MANAGEMENT
To minimize the risks of third compartment ulcers in a camelid herd, action should be taken to minimize stress associated with weaning, transport, showing, etc.

SYNONYMS
N/A

SEE ALSO
Gastrointestinal lesions (intestinal torsions, intussusceptions, and impactions, C1 stasis)
Intra-abdominal abscesses
Pancreatitis
Peritonitis in the absence of a perforated ulcer
Plant toxicities
Urogenital tract lesions (uterine torsion, ruptured bladder, urolithiasis, cystitis/urethritis)

ABBREVIATIONS
BID = twice daily
C-1, 2,3 = compartment 1,2,3
IM = intramuscular
IV = intravenous
PO = per os, by mouth
QID = four times daily
SID = once daily
SQ = subcutaneous
TCU = third compartment ulcers
TID = three times daily

Suggested Reading
Christensen, J. M., Limsakun, T., Smith, B. B., Hollingshead, N., Huber, M. 2001. Pharmacokinetics and pharmacodynamics of anti-ulcer agents in llama. *J Vet Pharma* 24: 23–33.
Fowler, M. E. 1998. Gastric ulcers. In:Fowler, M. E., ed., *Medicine and surgery of South American camelids*. Ames: Iowa State University Press.
Smith, B. B., Pearson, E. G., Timm, K. I. 1994. Third compartment ulcers in the llama. *Veterinary Clinics of North American: Food Animal Practice* 10(2): 319–30.

Author: Kelsey A. Hart

TICK PARALYSIS

BASICS

OVERVIEW
• A lower motor neuron (LMN) paralysis resulting from the bite of female ticks of species including *Dermacentor* spp. and *Amblyomma* spp. in the United States and *Ixodes holocyclus* in Australia.
• The potential for inducing paralysis has been suspected in 64 species of ticks belonging to the *Ixodid* and *Argasid* genera.
• The tick injects a neurotoxin that causes progressive motor paralysis, respiratory depression, and death in animals that have no immunity to the toxin.

SYSTEMS AFFECTED
CNS, gastrointestinal, respiratory, cardiovascular, hematologic, and musculoskeletal

GENETICS
N/A

INCIDENCE/PREVALENCE
Unknown

GEOGRAPHIC DISTRIBUTION
• Common in Australia, potentially worldwide
• Distribution patterns reflecting tick populations
• Exposure to environments favorable to tick infestations such as brushy, woody areas

SIGNALMENT
• Sheep, goats, cattle
• Other species such as dogs may be affected.

Breed Predilections
N/A

Mean Age and Range
All ages potentially are at risk.

Predominant Sex
Both sexes are equally affected.

SIGNS
• Initially, ataxia and weakness in hind limbs
• Progression to paralysis of hind limbs then ascending, symmetrical, flaccid tetraplegia
• Afebrile
• Hyporeflexia of the superficial and deep tendons
• Nystagmus
• Dyspnea, dysphagia, weak facial muscles
• Flaccid tail and anus
• Disease may progress further and cause respiratory muscle paralysis resulting in death.

CAUSES AND RISK FACTORS
• Exact pathology is not certain. Signs are caused by a protein neurotoxin possibly produced by the tick itself, by a microbial organism associated with the tick, or by a toxic metabolite resulting from the interaction of tick saliva with host tissue.
• There is a reduction of acetylcholine release and a resulting blockage of neurotransmission at neuromuscular junctions.
• Interference with presynaptic nerve terminal depolarization and acetyl choline release produces a neuromuscular blockade. This manifests primarily as an ascending flaccid paralysis varying from paraparesis to quadriplegia.
• Exposure to environments favorable to tick infestations such as brushy, woody areas
• Seasonal incidence may change in geographic regions where tick populations vary based on ambient temperatures.
• Antitoxic immunity can occur 2 weeks after primary tick exposure and lasts a few weeks. Immunity may be boosted in subsequent infestations.

DIAGNOSIS

DIFFERENTIAL DIAGNOSIS
• Botulism
• Acute polyradiculoneuritis

CBC/BIOCHEMISTRY/URINALYSIS
• Results are usually normal.
• Mild acidosis and dehydration develop. Other changes include increases in blood glucose and cholesterol, and a decrease in blood potassium.
• Increased serum levels of creatine kinase (CK) in tick paralysis caused by *D. andersoni* and *I. holocyclus*.
• Phosphate levels increased in later stages of paralysis caused by *I. holocyclus*.

OTHER LABORATORY TESTS
Severely affected animals may have a mild metabolic acidosis.

IMAGING
N/A

DIAGNOSTIC PROCEDURES
Examination for the presence of ticks on affected animals

PATHOLOGIC FINDINGS

GROSS FINDINGS
None specific to the disease, death occurs due to respiratory paralysis

HISTOPATHOLOGICAL FINDINGS
N/A

TICK PARALYSIS

TREATMENT

• Timely removal of attached ticks, either manually or by using a suitable acaricide. It may be necessary to shave long-haired animals to effectively locate all ticks.
• Supportive therapy—monitor for respiratory paralysis and hypoxia.

MEDICATIONS

Acaricidal dips

CONTRAINDICATIONS

• Appropriate milk and meat withdrawal times must be followed for all compounds administered to food-producing animals.
• Steroids should not be used in pregnant animals.

FOLLOW-UP

PATIENT MONITORING
N/A

PREVENTION/AVOIDANCE
• Ectoparasite sprays or dips to kill ticks on the animals
• Environmental control to reduce tick populations is recommended.

POSSIBLE COMPLICATIONS
N/A

EXPECTED COURSE AND PROGNOSIS

• Incubation period is usually 5–7 days.
• If ticks are removed, prognosis is good to excellent. Recovery usually occurs within 1 to 3 days.
• *Ixodes* tick paralysis—untreated animals die within 1 to 2 days.

MISCELLANEOUS

ASSOCIATED CONDITIONS
N/A

AGE-RELATED FACTORS
N/A

ZOONOTIC POTENTIAL
The same ticks can cause tick paralysis in humans. Animals with the disease cannot transmit the disease to humans.

PREGNANCY
N/A

SEE ALSO
Acute polyradiculoneuritis
Botulism

ABBREVIATIONS
CK = creatine kinase
LMN = lower motor neuron

Suggested Reading
Aiello, S. E., ed. 1998. Tick paralysis. In: *Merck veterinary manual*. 8th ed. Whitehouse Station, NJ: Merck & Co.
Keirans, J. E., Hutcheson, H. J., Durden, L. A., Klompen, J. S. 1996, May. *Ixodes* (Ixodes) *scapularis* (Acari:Ixodidae): redescription of all active stages, distribution, hosts, geographical variation, and medical and veterinary importance. *J Med Entomol*. 33(3):297–318.
Masina, S., Broady, K. W. 1999, Apr. Tick paralysis: development of a vaccine. *Int J Parasitol*. 29(4):535–41.
Oliver, J. E., Jr., Lorenz, M. D., Kornegay, J. N. 1997. Tick paralysis. *Handbook of veterinary neurology*. 3rd ed. Philadelphia: W. B. Saunders.
Smith, B. P., ed. 2002. Tick paralysis. In: *Large animal internal medicine*. 3rd ed. St. Louis: Mosby.
Tatchell, R. J. 1997, Jun. Sheep and goat tick management. *Parasitologia*. 39(2):157–60.

Author: Lisa Nashold

TICKS AFFECTING SMALL RUMINANTS

 BASICS

OVERVIEW
• The tick families Ixodidae and the Argasidae belong to the order Acarina of the class Arachnida.
• Some species of Ixodid ticks (hard ticks) and Argasid ticks (soft ticks) parasitize mammals.
• Ticks are temporarily parasitic; the larvae, nymphs, or adults only parasitize mammalian hosts to obtain a blood meal. Various tick species are classified as one-host, two-host, and three-host ticks.
• Free-living stages can survive for long periods without feeding.
• Ticks are cosmopolitan in their choice of mammalian host.
• Typically, small numbers of ticks have little direct effect on the host.
• Heavy infestation with engorged adults can remove physiologically significant amounts of blood from neonates.
• Some species of tick cause so-called tick paralysis.
• Many tick species are vectors of disease-causing microorganisms and viruses.
• Wounds from bites can become infected and predispose to cutaneous myiasis.
• The geographic distribution of ticks is limited by climate, particularly humidity, as free-living stages are susceptible to desiccation.

SYSTEMS AFFECTED
Production management, CNS, hematologic, skin, reproductive

GENETICS
N/A

INCIDENCE/PREVALENCE
N/A

GEOGRAPHIC DISTRIBUTION
Worldwide, depending on species and environment

SIGNALMENT
Species
All ruminant species
Breed Predilections
N/A
Mean Age and Range
N/A
Predominant Sex
N/A

CAUSES AND RISK FACTORS
There is a bewildering regional variety of different species of tick and tick-borne diseases; wherever possible, local experts should be consulted.

Ixodidae (Hard Ticks)
Amblyomma spp., *Boophilus* spp., *Dermacentor* spp., *Haemaphysalis* spp., *Hyalomma* spp., *Ixodes* spp., *Rhipicephalus* spp.

Argasidae (Soft Ticks)
Otobius spp.

 DIAGNOSIS

See also specific diseases.

DIFFERENTIAL DIAGNOSES
Tick-borne/tick-associated diseases:
• Benign theileriosis of small ruminants (*Theileria ovis*)
• Dermatophilosis (*Dermatophilus congolensis*)

• European ehrlichiosis (*Ehrlichia phagocytophila*)
• European piroplasmosis of small ruminants (*Babesia motasi*)
• General toxicosis (salivary endotheliotrophic toxin)
• Heartwater (*Ehrlichia* [*Cowdria*] *ruminatum*)
• Louping-ill virus (Flaviviridae)
• Malignant theileriosis of small ruminants (*Theileria hirci*)
• Nairobi sheep disease virus and Ganjam virus (Bunyaviridae)
• Q-fever (*Coxiella burnetti*)
• Spirochaetosis (*Borrelia theileri*)
• Spotted fevers (*Rickettsia* spp.)
• Sweating sickness (salivary epitheliotrophic toxin)
• Tick paralysis (salivary neurotoxin-induced dose-dependent ascending paralysis)
• Tick pyaemia (*Staphylococcus aureus*)
• Tropical anaplasmosis of small ruminants (*Anaplasma ovis*)
• Tropical babesiosis of small ruminants (*Babesia ovis*)
• Tropical ehrlichiosis of small ruminants (*Ehrlichia ovina*)
• Tularemia (*Francisella tularensis*)

CBC/BIOCHEMISTRY/URINALYSIS
Can be useful in the evaluation of anemia

OTHER LABORATORY TESTS
N/A

IMAGING
N/A

DIAGNOSTIC PROCEDURES
N/A

PATHOLOGIC FINDINGS
N/A

TREATMENT

N/A

MEDICATIONS

DRUGS OF CHOICE

Organophosphate and synthetic pyrethroid insecticide preparations are widely used to control ticks on animals.

CONTRAINDICATIONS

Maintain adequate drug withhold times for meat and milk when using topical insecticides.

FOLLOW-UP

PATIENT MONITORING

N/A

PREVENTION/AVOIDANCE

N/A

POSSIBLE COMPLICATIONS

N/A

EXPECTED COURSE AND PROGNOSIS

N/A

MISCELLANEOUS

ASSOCIATED CONDITIONS

Lameness, paralysis, abortion, respiratory failure, anemia, and death

AGE-RELATED FACTORS

N/A

ZOONOTIC POTENTIAL

Many tick-borne diseases are zoonotic.

PREGNANCY

N/A

RUMINANT SPECIES AFFECTED

All ruminant species can be hosts for ticks.

BIOSECURITY

• Many tick-borne diseases are of regulatory significance.
• Isolation and quarantine of new stock entering the herd/flock
• Treat and or cull new animals for disease conditions prior to herd introduction.

PRODUCTION MANAGEMENT

Tick-control measures must be in place to control insect populations.

SEE ALSO

Anaplasmosis
Dermatophilosis (*Dermatophilus congolensis*)
Ehrlichiosis
European piroplasmosis
FARAD
Heartwater
Louping-ill virus (Flaviviridae)
Nairobi sheep disease virus
Q-fever (*Coxiella burnetti*)
Spirochaetosis (*Borrelia theileri*)
Spotted fevers (*Rickettsia* spp.)
Tick paralysis
Tropical babesiosis
Tularemia (*Francisella tularensis*)

ABBREVIATIONS

CNS = central nervous system
FARAD = Food Animal Residue Avoidance Databank

Suggested Reading
Davies, F. G. 1997, Jun. Tick virus diseases of sheep and goats. *Parassitologia* 39(2):91–94.
Jongejan, F., Uilenberg, G. 1994, Dec. Ticks and control methods. *Rev Sci Tech.* 13(4):1201–26.
Keirans, J. E., Hutcheson, H. J., Durden, L. A., Klompen, J. S. 1996, May. Ixodes (Ixodes) scapularis (Acari: Ixodidae): redescription of all active stages, distribution, hosts, geographical variation, and medical and veterinary importance. *J Med Entomol.* 33(3):297–318.
Liebisch, A. 1997, Jun. General review of the tick species which parasitize sheep and goats world-wide. *Parassitologia* 39(2):123–29.
Tatchell, R. J. 1997, Jun. Sheep and goat tick management. *Parassitologia* 39(2):157–60.
Uilenberg, G. 1997, Jun. General review of tick-borne diseases of sheep and goats world-wide. *Parassitologia* 39(2):161–65.

Author: A. D. (Sandy) McLachlan

TOBACCO TOXICOSIS

BASICS

DEFINITION
Intoxication and/or adverse consequences after ingestion of plants of the genus *Nicotiana*. They are members of the nightshade family, Solanaceae.

PATHOPHYSIOLOGY
• Two primary toxic compounds are responsible for the adverse effects of tobacco ingestion: nicotine and anabasine.
• Nicotine—a potent pyridine alkaloid has poor palatability, but animals will eat it if forage is scarce. It can cause a direct contact irritation to gastrointestinal mucosa. Pharmacologically, it mimics acetylcholine at the autonomic ganglia and myoneural junction acting as a neuromuscular blocking agent.
• Anabasine—a piperidine-pyridine alkaloid is a teratogen.

SYSTEMS AFFECTED
Intestinal tract, nervous system, reproductive, musculoskeletal, production management

GENETICS
None

INCIDENCE/PREVALENCE
• Varies with geographic location
• *N. tabacum*—cultivated tobacco
• *N. trygonphylla*—wild or desert tobacco in the dry areas of southwest United States
• *N. attenuata*—wild or coyote tobacco also in the dry areas of southwest United States
• *N. glauca*—tree tobacco, an evergreen shrub of low elevation areas of Arizona and California

GEOGRAPHIC DISTRIBUTION
Worldwide; southwestern United States and anywhere tobacco is cultivated.

SIGNALMENT
Species
• Potentially any animal can be affected.
• Among domestic ruminants, cattle, sheep, and goats have had documented cases.

SIGNS
.

HISTORICAL FINDINGS
Access to *Nicotiana* spp. where forage is poor, pasturing on land where tobacco is cultivated, and ingestion of tobacco products or tobacco-tainted water.

PHYSICAL EXAMINATION FINDINGS
Neurological Symptoms
Salivation, vomiting, diarrhea, excitement, increased respiratory rate, twitching, trembling, stiff and uncoordinated gait leading to respiratory paralysis, weakness, bloat, blindness, collapse, and death

Teratogenic Effects
Calves exhibit arthrogryposis of the forelimbs and spondylosis identical to that seen in lupine toxicity. In sheep, carpal flexure and cleft palate can be seen.

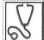

DIAGNOSIS

History of potential exposure to *Nicotiana* spp. and compatible clinical signs

DIFFERENTIAL DIAGNOSIS
• Other toxic plant causes of sudden death: blue-green algae, cyanogenic plants, death camas, larkspur, laurels, lupine, milkweed, oleander, water hemlock
• Other causes of teratogens should be investigated such as bluebonnet, locoweed, poison hemlock

PATHOLOGIC FINDINGS
• In cases of sudden death, no specific lesions might be seen, except the finding of *Nicotiana* spp. in the digestive tract.
• *Pale mucous membranes, poorly oxygenated blood, myocardial hemorrhage, pulmonary hemorrhages, and cerebral congestion are occasionally seen.*
• Teratogenic lesions in calves or lambs as listed above might be seen.

TREATMENT

• No specific treatment except to prevent further ingestion
• Administering activated charcoal and cathartics might be helpful and intravenous fluids may be needed.
• If practical, artificial respiration and supplemental oxygen can be provided in extremely valuable livestock.

MEDICATIONS

No specific medications

CONTRAINDICATIONS
• Appropriate milk and meat withdrawal times must be followed for all compounds administered to food-producing animals.
• Steroids should not be used in pregnant animals.

POSSIBLE INTERACTIONS
N/A

FOLLOW-UP

PREVENTION/AVOIDANCE
Prevent access to and consumption of *Nicotiana* spp., especially in forage-scarce areas.

POSSIBLE COMPLICATIONS
N/A

EXPECTED COURSE AND PROGNOSIS
If the animal survives acute toxicity, the prognosis is good.

MISCELLANEOUS

ASSOCIATED CONDITIONS
N/A

AGE-RELATED FACTORS
N/A

ZOONOTIC POTENTIAL
None

PREGNANCY
Teratogenic—prevent access to *Nicotiana* spp. by ruminants.

RUMINANT SPECIES AFFECTED
Potentially, all ruminant species can be affected.

BIOSECURITY
N/A

PRODUCTION MANAGEMENT
Access to *Nicotiana* spp. where forage is poor, pasturing on land where tobacco is cultivated, and ingestion of tobacco products or tobacco-tainted water should be denied to livestock.

SYNONYMS
N/A

SEE ALSO
Bluebonnet
Blue-green algae
Cyanogenic plants
Death camas
Larkspur
Laurels
Locoweed
Lupine
Milkweed
Oleander
Poison hemlock
Water hemlock

ABBREVIATIONS
N/A

Suggested Reading
Keeler, R. F., Crowe, M. W. 1984, Jan. Teratogenicity and toxicity of wild tree tobacco, *Nicotiana glauca* in sheep. *Cornell Vet.* 74(1):50–59.
Keeler, R.F., Shupe, J. L., Crowe, M. W., Olson, A., Balls, L. D. 1981, Jul *Nicotiana glauca*-induced congenital deformities in calves: clinical and pathologic aspects. *Am J Vet Res.* 42(7):1231–34.
Panter, K. E., James, L. F., Gardner, D. R. 1999, Feb. Lupines, poison-hemlock and *Nicotiana* spp. toxicity and teratogenicity in livestock. *J Nat Toxins.* 8(1):117–34.
Panter, K. E., Weinzweig, J., Gardner, D. R., Stegelmeier, B. L., James, L. F. 2000, Mar. Comparison of cleft palate induction by *Nicotiana glauca* in goats and sheep. *Teratology* 61(3):203–10.
Plumlee, K. H., Holstege, D. M., Blanchard, P. C., Fiser, K. M., Galey, F. D. 1993, Jul. *Nicotiana glauca* toxicosis of cattle. *J Vet Diagn Invest.* 5(3):498–99.

Author: Edward L. Powers

BASICS

DEFINITION

Acute to chronic oral ulceration, necrosis, and/or bruising due to a viral (vesicular stomatitis, bluetongue, malignant catarrhal fever, rinderpest), trauma or irritant (chemical irritants, coarse plants/feed), oral foreign bodies, and abscesses (actinobacillosis, "Woody tongue").

OVERVIEW

• Because of the tongue's important role in feed prehension and the eating habits of ruminants, tongue trauma is often acutely evident (salivation, blood mixed with saliva, tongue extended from mouth, dysphasia).
• The incidence of tongue condemnation presumably associated with *Actinobacillosis* is reportedly increasing in slaughtered nonfed cattle.

PATHOPHYSIOLOGY

• Dependent upon inciting cause
• Actinobacillosis is a commensal organism of GI tract and therefore may colonize oral ulcerations.
• Feeding coarse, dry feeds containing stickers and plant awns may result in damage to oral mucosa and colonization of deeper tissues with organisms.
• Toxic plant ingestion (e.g., hay containing flower clusters of yellow bristle-grass)
• Cactus spines
• Oral foreign bodies such as wire may lacerate the tongue during prehension leading to hemorrhage and eventually infection.
• Surgical correction may involve glossectomy or partial glossectomy with consideration of the importance of the tongue to prehension of feed.

SYSTEMS AFFECTED

Production management, musculoskeletal, gastrointestinal; tongue, oral cavity, and head.

GENETICS

N/A

INCIDENCE/PREVALENCE

N/A

GEOGRAPHIC DISTRIBUTION

Worldwide

SIGNALMENT

• Vesicular stomatitis in dairy cattle results in large ulcerations of tongue with lesions evident on teats and coronary bands.
• Bluetongue virus in susceptible sheep results in tongue and dental pad erosions along with other signs compatible with vasculitis.
• Malignant catarrhal fever (cattle) and rinderpest (cattle, sheep, and goats) generally manifest as erosive stomatitis not limited to the tongue.

Species

Potentially, all ruminant species

Breed Predilections

N/A

Mean Age and Range

Tongue trauma is more common in younger animals due to their predisposition to suckle on environmental objects (wire, thorns, etc.).

Predominant Sex

N/A

SIGNS

Salivation, blood in saliva, dysphagia, reluctance to allow examination of head, anorexia, weight loss, dehydration, foul odor to breath, nasal discharge

RISK FACTORS

Early weaning, less than optimal housing conditions, salt- or water-seeking behavior (lack of salt/trace minerals or suitable source of clean water) resulting in consumption of irritant substances (chlorinated naphthalene).

DIAGNOSIS

DIFFERENTIAL DIAGNOSIS

• Vesiculating viral diseases
• Oropharyngeal trauma
• Necrotic stomatitis.

CBC/BIOCHEMISTRY/URINALYSIS

N/A

OTHER LABORATORY TESTS

Culture and sensitivity is indicated if an infective agent is suspected.

IMAGING

May be helpful with foreign body or fracture

OTHER DIAGNOSTIC PROCEDURES

TREATMENT

• Dependent on underlying management or disease factors
• Surgical correction may involve glossectomy or partial glossectomy.

CONTRAINDICATIONS

Appropriate milk and meat withdrawal times must be followed for all compounds administered to food-producing animals.

MISCELLANEOUS

ASSOCIATED CONDITIONS

Weight loss and potential culling

AGE-RELATED FACTORS

ZOONOTIC POTENTIAL

N/A

PREGNANCY

N/A

RUMINANT SPECIES AFFECTED

All ruminant species

BIOSECURITY

N/A

PRODUCTION MANAGEMENT

• Feeding coarse, dry feeds containing stickers and plant awns may result in damage to oral mucosa and colonization of deeper tissues with organisms.
• Oral foreign bodies such as wire may lacerate the tongue during prehension leading to hemorrhage and eventually infection.
• Early weaning, less than optimal housing conditions, salt- or water-seeking behavior (lack of salt/trace minerals or suitable source of clean water) resulting in consumption of irritant substances (chlorinated naphthalene) can predispose to tongue trauma.
• Keep all caustic chemicals away from feeding livestock.

SYNONYMS

N/A

SEE ALSO

Actinobacillosis
Agricultural chemical toxicity
Bluetongue
Body condition scoring by species
Malignant catarrhal fever
Necrotic stomatitis
Oral foreign bodies
Oropharyngeal trauma
Petroleum toxicity
Rinderpest
Trauma or irritant (chemical irritants, coarse plants/feed)
Vesicular stomatitis
"Woody tongue"

ABBREVIATIONS

GI = gastrointestinal

Suggested Reading
Darling, R., Dixon, R., Honhold, N., Taylor, N. 2001. Oral lesions in cattle and sheep. *Vet Rec.* 148: 759.
Davies, R. 2001. Oral lesions in cattle and sheep. *Vet Rec.* 148: 759.
Durchame, N. G. 2004. Surgical diseases of the oral cavity. In: *Farm animal surgery*. St. Louis, MO: Saunders.
Rebhun, W. C. 1995. Infectious diseases of the gastrointestinal tract. In: *Diseases of dairy cattle*. Baltimore: Williams and Wilkins.
Roeber, D. L., Mies, P. D., Smith, C. D., Belk, K. E., Field, T. G., Tatum, J. D., Scanga, J. A., Smith, G. C. 2001. National market cow and bull beef quality audit—1999: a survey of producer-related defects in market cows and bulls. *J An Sci.* 79:658–65.

Author: Jeff Lakritz

TOXIC GASES

BASICS

DEFINITION
• Gases associated with animal housing or production may be present in high enough concentrations to cause adverse clinical effects in animals, including death.
• Many of these toxic gases are produced during the decomposition of animal waste in anaerobic conditions provided by underfloor waste pits, deep litters, or manure pack, and include gases such as NH_3, CO_2, H_2S, and CH_4.
• Other toxic gases include NO_2, which is produced by the fermentation process of ensiled forages, sulfur oxides (such as SO_2 and SO_3), which are produced by industrial pollution, and CO, which is a by-product of incomplete combustion of hydrocarbon fuels.
• Exposure to toxic gases is primarily by the respiratory, dermal, and ocular route.
• Brief exposures to high concentrations of toxic gases are much more toxic and potentially fatal than low concentration exposures for longer periods.
• These gases may be lighter or heavier than air, and this plays an important role in determination of exposure.

PATHOPHYSIOLOGY
• NH_3 reacts with the moist mucous membranes of the eye and respiratory tract to form ammonium hydroxide (NH_4OH), which is caustic in nature. NH_3 also causes nonspecific stress and reduces resistance to infections. NH_3 is lighter than air, and has a characteristic odor detectable at about 5–10 ppm.

• CO_2 causes dyspnea and anoxia, if present at high concentrations. This effect is partly attributed to the replacement of oxygen from the environment. Normally, CO_2 is a colorless, odorless gas present in the air at concentrations of about 4000 ppm (0.4%).
• CO competes for binding sites on a variety of proteins, such as hemoglobin to form COHb. CO has a high affinity (>200 times that of oxygen) to bind with hemoglobin. Moreover, CO binds with the cytochrome oxidase system to reduce cellular utilization of oxygen, and thus tissues most sensitive to oxygen deprivation (e.g., brain and myocardium) are most sensitive to CO toxicity. This finally leads to systemic tissue hypoxia. CO is a colorless, odorless gas present in fresh air at around 0.02 ppm, and may be as high as 40 ppm in high-traffic areas.
• H_2S inhibits cytochrome oxidase enzymes by binding to the iron. This disrupts the electron transport chain and aerobic metabolism, leading to anoxic and direct damage to the cells of the brain. H_2S also has a direct paralytic effect on the carotid body leading to inhibition of respiration. Additionally, H_2S can combine with hemoglobin to form sulf-hemoglobin, which decreases oxygen transport in the blood. The H_2S gas has a characteristic "rotten egg" smell and is heavier than air. When inhaled, it also has an irritant effect on the respiratory tract. The odor threshold is 0.25—0.2 ppm, however, at higher concentrations (>50–150 ppm), hydrogen sulfide may block the detection of odor due to the paralyzing effect on the olfactory sensory apparatus. This gas may accumulate in manure pits and holding tanks in concentrations of over 1000 ppm.

• CH_4 concentrations of >5%–15% by volume are considered explosive and under such conditions, electrical sparks can be detrimental. Otherwise CH_4 is a colorless, odorless gas that displaces oxygen in an enclosed environment and therefore produces asphyxiation.
• NO_2 combines with mucus and forms nitric acid, which is corrosive, thus causing adverse pulmonary and ocular effects. Most NO_2 forms within 2 weeks of storage of the forages in the silo for fermentation. NO_2 has a pungent, sweetish odor, and is a yellowish-brown gas with "bleachlike" smell (odor threshold is 0.1–0.2 ppm). It is visible only when concentrations reach a dangerous level (75–150 ppm). Concentrations as high as 1500 ppm may be reached within the first 2 days after filling the silo. NO_2 is heavier than air and can settle at the bottom of enclosed spaces.
• Sulfur oxides are readily converted to acids on contact with water, and produce a pronounced irritant effect on the mucosa of the nasopharynx, respiratory tract, and conjunctiva. Bronchoconstriction may also occur. These gases are present in industry-polluted air and are irritating to the respiratory tract and eyes.
• Fire/smoke: CO and CO_2 intoxications are the leading cause of fire death in victims who die within 6 to 12 hours. Some of the other toxins produced in the process include:
  • Acrolein from combustion of polyolefins and cellulosics
  • Aldehydes from combustion of cellulose materials such as cotton, paper, and wood
  • NH_3 from combustion of wool, silk, nylon, melamine

• HCl from combustion of polyvinylchloride, chlorinated acrylics, and retardant-treated materials
• H_2S from combustion of hair, wools, meats, and hides
• Nitrogen oxides from combustion of fabrics, cellulose nitrate, and celluloid
• These by-products may cause direct pulmonary irritation and inflammation of conjunctiva in eyes.
• HCN may be produced from combustion of wool, silk, polyacrylonitrile, acrylic fibers, nylon, polyurethane, paper. HCN is a rapidly fatal asphyxiant, which induces cellular hypoxia by formation of a stable complex with cytochrome oxidase. HF, SO_2, and free radicals produced in fires may also be a major contribution to fire toxicity.

SYSTEMS AFFECTED
• Respiratory—dyspnea, inflammation, edema, necrosis, fibrosis, and emphysema.
• Dermal—itching, erythema, and inflammation
• Eyes—irritation, lacrimation, and inflammation
• Cardiovascular—arrhythmia
• Neurologic—depression, staggering gait, disorientation, weakness, seizures, coma, and paralysis

GENETICS
N/A

INCIDENCE/PREVALENCE
N/A

GEOGRAPHIC DISTRIBUTION
N/A

SIGNALMENT
All species susceptible

SIGNS
• NH_3 causes tearing, shallow breathing, and nasal discharge. At higher concentrations, laryngospasm and coughing may be seen. Concentrations greater than 50–100 ppm NH_3 cause reduced growth rate and mucous membrane irritation, and at >1000 ppm, airway and alveolar damage occurs.
• CO_2 at concentrations >50,000 ppm (5%) may cause labored breathing in animals. Signs of anoxia—which include anxiety, staggering, coma, and death—may occur due to suffocation when air contains carbon dioxide at a concentration greater than 400,000 ppm (40%).
• CO causes drowsiness, lethargy, weakness, incoordination when COHb concentration in blood reaches about 30% (normal < 1%–3%). A more severe (>60% COHb) exposure may lead to dyspnea, coma, terminal clonic spasms, and acute death.
• H_2S causes eye and lung irritation at concentrations greater than 50–100 ppm in air. Characteristics of a fatal exposure are rapid "knock down," respiratory depression, tremors, blurred vision, cyanosis, seizures, and tachycardia. Concentrations greater than 500–1000 ppm can be directly paralyzing on the respiratory center and neurotoxic, leading to hyperpnea, followed by apnea, and death.
• CH_4, at concentrations >85%–90%, has been associated with asphyxiation. Signs of asphyxia are seen when atmospheric oxygen is displaced, leading to oxygen concentrations of less that 15%–16%.
• NO_2, at ambient concentrations >50 ppm, can cause choking, coughing, and labored breathing. At >50 ppm, bronchitis, pneumonia, and edema of the lungs may occur.

• Sulfur oxides can cause ocular irritation, salivation, laryngeal spasms, and emphysema at concentrations >10–50 ppm.
• Fire/smoke cause a spectrum of clinical signs including eye irritation, behavioral dysfunction, anxiety, respiratory distress and hypoxia, narcosis to coma, burns, and trauma. Symptoms seen are often combined effects of irritants and asphyxiants.

CAUSES
• Accumulation of high nitrogenous waste (for NH_3)
• Heaters operated in poorly ventilated areas, and fire (for CO)
• Accumulation of protein/sulfur-containing organic matter and agitation of slurry (H_2S, CO_2, NH_3, CH_4)
• Industrial pollution (SO_2, SO_3)
• Ensiled forages in silo produce NO_2, which may move into adjoining risk areas.
• Animals in enclosed areas (CO_2 and CH_4)

RISK FACTORS
• Low temperature
• Overcrowding of animals
• Electrical failure
• Faulty furnaces and heaters
• Poor design/accidents
• Improper ventilation
• Poor waste management

 DIAGNOSIS

DIFFERENTIAL DIAGNOSIS
• CH_4
• CO
• CO_2
• H_2S

TOXIC GASES

- HCN
- NH_3
- NO_2
- SO_2

CBC/BIOCHEMISTRY/URINALYSIS
Creatinine kinase may be high because of muscle ischemia and necrosis.

OTHER LABORATORY TESTS
- Blood gases (pCO_2, pO_2)
- Color—bright red blood due to HCN or CO. Dark if methemoglobinemia is present.
- COHb in blood
- pH—low in cases with metabolic acidosis
- Blood/liver/muscle cyanide concentrations

IMAGING
N/A

DIAGNOSTIC PROCEDURES
- History
- Field observations
- Clinical signs
- Check into "rapid tests" provided by the local fire department for analysis of toxic gases in the air.

PATHOLOGIC FINDINGS
Gross Findings
- Increased mucus secretion in the respiratory tract
- Bronchiolar constriction
- Pulmonary congestion and edema
- Bright red mucous membranes, and pink coloration to tissues and nonpigmented skin (cyanosis and CO)
- Greenish discoloration of gray matter, viscera, and bronchial secretions (H_2S)
- General congestion of tissues (resulting from hypoxia)

Histopathology
- Hyperplasia of the bronchiolar and alveolar epithelium
- Pulmonary congestion, edema, and emphysema
- Necrosis in brain and heart, consistent with hypoxia

TREATMENT

APPROPRIATE HEALTH CARE
- Restore adequate oxygen supply.
- Prevent any further exposure to the toxic gas.
- Corticosteroids—to alleviate the pulmonary edema and clinical signs
- Antibiotics—to control secondary bacterial pathogens
- Administer electrolyte and fluid therapy as needed.
- If methemoglobinemia is present, dose with methylene blue.
- Blood transfusion

NURSING CARE
N/A

ACTIVITY
N/A

DIET
N/A

CLIENT EDUCATION
N/A

SURGICAL CONSIDERATIONS
N/A

MEDICATIONS

DRUGS OF CHOICE
N/A

CONTRAINDICATIONS
Appropriate milk and meat withdrawal times must be followed for all compounds administered to food-producing animals.

PRECAUTIONS
- Animals should not be allowed in the barn or near the silo for at least 48 hours after filling.
- Agitate manure or waste carefully

POSSIBLE INTERACTIONS
N/A

ALTERNATIVE DRUGS
N/A

FOLLOW-UP

PATIENT MONITORING
• Monitor cardiac, pulmonary, and neurologic functions
• Restrain animal from excessive stress and exercise.

PREVENTION/AVOIDANCE
• Provide good ventilation around the base of the silo during the fermentation process so that the gases will be carried away.
• Always keep at least one foot of space between the highest manure level and the slats. This protects the animals that lie on the slats and inhale the gases that will accumulate at the surface of the pit.
• Provide as much ventilation as possible in the pit and building during agitation of the waste. Although pits are agitated only a few times a year, most human and livestock deaths or illnesses occur at these times.
• Fire hazards management

POSSIBLE COMPLICATIONS
Secondary bacterial infections

EXPECTED COURSE AND PROGNOSIS
• Animals poisoned with toxic gases are often found dead.

• In animals that survive, the prognosis is fair if there is prompt treatment of clinical signs and no further exposure.

MISCELLANEOUS

ASSOCIATED CONDITIONS
NO_2 is associated with the "silo-fillers" disease in humans.

AGE-RELATED FACTORS
N/A

ZOONOTIC POTENTIAL
Humans in the same environment are also at risk.

PREGNANCY
Pregnant animals may abort due to respiratory stress and hypoxia.

RUMINANT SPECIES AFFECTED
All

BIOSECURITY
N/A

PRODUCTION MANAGEMENT
N/A

SYNONYMS
N/A

SEE ALSO
Agricultural chemical toxicity
Handling a toxicological outbreak
Manure management
Nitrate toxicity
Urea toxicity

ABBREVIATIONS
CH_4 = methane
CO = carbon monoxide
CO_2 = carbon dioxide
COHb = carboxyhemoglobin
H_2S = hydrogen sulfide
HCN = hydrogen cyanide
NH_3 = ammonia
NO_2 = nitrogen dioxide
ppm = parts per million
SO_2 = sulfur dioxide
SO_3 = sulfur trioxide

Suggested Reading
Klasco, R. K., ed. *POISINDEX System.* Greenwood Village, CO: Thomson Micromedex. (Edition expires 9/2004).
Osweiler, G. D., Carson, T. L., Buck, W. B., Van Gelder, G. A. 1985. Toxic gases. In: *Clinical and diagnostic veterinary toxicology.* 3rd ed. Dubuque, IA: Kendall/Hunt.
Plumlee, K. 2004. *Clinical veterinary toxicology.* Philadelphia: Mosby.

Author: Asheesh K. Tiwary

TOXOPLASMA ABORTION

 BASICS

OVERVIEW
• Reproductive loss resulting from *Toxoplasma gondii* infection during pregnancy
• Toxoplasmosis occurs in a wide range of domestic and wild animals and birds.
• Cats are responsible for maintaining and spreading infection through a herd/flock.
  • Cats—definitive host (where parasite reproduces—i.e., host where sexual multiplication occurs)
  • Birds, rodents, and other mammals—intermediate hosts (asexual multiplication occurs)

Specifics
• *T. gondii*—protozoan parasite
  • Resides in the intestine of members of the cat family
  • Infected cats (usually kittens) shed *Toxoplasma* oocysts for about 2 weeks; then immunity develops
• Some cats remain carriers and shed oocysts when stressed.
• Major cause of abortion in ewes
• Often occurs at flock level—10%–20+% of ewes abort
• Level dependent upon host, parasite, and management interactions
• Clinical disease limited to pregnant ewes
• Syndromes include: abortion, mummification, fetal resorption, stillbirth, and reduced neonatal survival rate.
• Clinical syndromes are dependent upon previous exposure and immune status of the pregnant ewe as well as the gestation length at time of infection.
• Ingestion of infected cysts in muscle tissue
  • Cats—prey such as birds and rodents
  • Humans—raw or undercooked meat containing cysts (cooking to 70°C for 15 to 30 minutes destroys)
  • Ingestion of oocysts in infected cat feces (can remain infective for months)
  • Placental transfer—if in blood stream fetus may become infected
• Ewes infected by ingestion of feed, bedding, or pasture contaminated with infective cat feces; Outbreaks often involve grain used for a "litter box" or kittens born in hay storage areas.

PATHOPHYSIOLOGY
• Ewes ingest *T. gondii*–infected feed
• *T. gondii* invades gastrointestinal tract ⟶ migrates to lymph nodes ⟶ enters bloodstream⟶ enters placenta
• Ewes asymptomatic when infected
• Two weeks after infection, organism invades placenta; symptoms are dependent on the stage of pregnancy.
  • Ewe open or infected as a lamb—immune; no clinical symptoms develop
  • Infected at 0 to 40 days gestation—fetal death and resorption; open ewe or rebreeds late
  • Infected at 40 to 120 days gestation—fetal death, abortion, and mummification common
  • Even though infected earlier, abortions usually occur during the last month of gestation.
  • Ewes infected long before symptoms of abortion occur, thus difficult to treat
  • Infected at 120 days to parturition—live births, weak lambs, high neonatal mortality
  • Mummified fetuses may accompany a live birth at term.

SYSTEMS AFFECTED
• Ewes—reproductive system
• Fetus—brain, liver, lungs

INCIDENCE/PREVALANCE
• Related to feeding management practices—odds of consuming infected feed or bedding material
• Most common in intensively managed flocks likely to use barn-stored feed during pregnancy
  • Winter-lambing flocks
  • Confinement and semiconfinement operations
  • Show, club lamb and small hobby flocks
• Less common in pasture-based, extensively managed grazing operations that feed little barn-stored dry feed during pregnancy—grass-based range flocks and larger commercial operations

GEOGRAPHIC DISTRIBUTION
• Occurs in most parts of the world where cats and sheep are found
• More likely to occur in farm-flock areas of the United States

RISK FACTORS
• Gestation—feeding hay or grain contaminated with cat feces (also bedding)
• Intensive management systems and smaller farm flocks feeding barn-stored hay or grain to pregnant ewes during pregnancy
• Feral and domestic cats raising kittens on premise—fecal contamination of hay or grain

 DIAGNOSIS

Presumptive/on-the-farm: history and observations consistent with toxoplasmosis abortions

GROSS FINDINGS
• Mummified fetuses, cotyledon lesions—small, white, granular lesions on surface of cotyledon (better visualized by placing cotyledon in formalin solution)
• Intercotyledonary areas unaffected (grossly)
• Confirmation—laboratory examination of aborted lambs and placental membranes

HISTOPATHOLOGICAL FINDINGS
• Identification of the organism in fetal brain
• Focal necrotic lesions may be seen in the brain, liver, lungs, and fetal membranes
• Characteristic inflammation of the placenta

Serology
• Positive *Toxoplasma* titer from fetal thoracic fluid (good field tool for diagnosis as fetus is capable of mounting an immune response)
• Extremely high *Toxoplasma* titer in the serum of the dam (suggestive, but not as useful as titers on normal sheep may be positive)
• Paired serum samples for titer response more diagnostic

DIFFERENTIAL DIAGNOSIS
Other common causes of abortion and infertility in ewes:
• *Campylobacter* abortion (e.g., campylobacteriosis, vibriosis)
• *Chlamydia* abortion (EAE)
• Others less common—bluetongue, listeriosis, salmonella, border disease, leptospirosis, poisonous plants, medications, ram infertility

TOXOPLASMA ABORTION

TREATMENT

- None—infection initiated long before clinical symptoms are recognized
- Isolate aborting ewes, remove aborted fetuses and placentas
- Some ewes will need to be treated for retained placenta and metritis.

MEDICATIONS

FOLLOW-UP

PREVENTION/AVOIDANCE

- Avoid feeding pregnant ewes the top layer of bales in barn-stored hay—most commonly infected by kitten feces
- Avoid feeding any pregnant ewe feed contaminated by cat feces.
- Feeding ionophore compounds such as monensin (15–20 mg/ewe/day) or lasalocid (35–40 mg/ewe/day) during gestation may help (not approved for this use and toxicity issues with other species)
- Spay, neuter, vaccinate, and keep cats healthy to prevent kittens and introduction of feral cats to premises.

EXPECTED COURSE AND PROGNOSIS

- Abortions continue to occur until all ewes infected during gestation either abort or produce live lambs.
- Exposed ewes develop immunity and should not abort in subsequent lambing seasons.

MISCELLANEOUS

ASSOCIATED CONDITIONS

- Retained placenta
- Metritis

AGE-RELATED FACTORS

Due to previous exposure and immunity—toxoplasma abortions may be restricted to one group of ewes related by age, housing, or feed source.

ZOONOTIC POTENTIAL

- Pigs, sheep, goats, and humans are more susceptible to the disease; cattle and horses are less susceptible.
- Women of childbearing age and pregnant women should avoid contact with cat feces, contaminated feed, aborted fetuses, uterine discharge, placenta, and normal birthing procedures.
  - Women at risk and contemplating pregnancy should determine immune status (test for antibodies preferably before becoming pregnant).
  - Wear disposable gloves when handling aborted material.
- Pregnant women also should:
  - Avoid contact with cat feces (litter boxes)
  - Avoid working in soil or gardens contaminated by cats
  - Thoroughly cook meat
  - Wash hands after handling raw meat
- Avoid raw or undercooked meat containing cysts.
  - Little risk from properly cooked meat (70°C for 15 to 30 minutes)
  - Freezing to minus 4°F for 2 days also destroys cysts.

SYNONYMS

Toxo

SEE ALSO

Bluetongue
Border disease
Campylobacter abortion
Campylobacteriosis
Chlamydia abortion (EAE)
Leptospirosis
Listeriosis
Medications
Other common causes of abortion and infertility in ewes
Poisonous plants
Ram infertility
Salmonella
Vibriosis

ABBREVIATIONS

EAE = enzootic abortion of ewes

Suggested Reading
Dubey, J. P. 1998. Toxoplasmosis, sarcocystosis, isosporosis, and cyclosporosis. In: *Zoonoses*, ed. S. R. Palmer, Lord Soulsey, D. I. H. Simpson. Britain: Oxford University Press, Bath Press, Avon.
Toxoplasmosis. 1997. In: *Veterinary medicine*. 8th ed. London: Saunders.
Underwood, W. J., Rook, J. S. 1992, Nov. Toxoplasmosis infection in sheep. *The Compendium* 14(11): 1543–48.

Author: Joseph S. Rook

TRACHEAL COLLAPSE

BASICS

OVERVIEW
• Tracheal collapse is an uncommon respiratory condition in ruminants, generally with a traumatic etiology.
• Generally does not involve a stenosis of the trachea, but rather a dynamic dorsoventral collapse during inspiration; rarely may be a lateral collapse
• May result from hypotonic, pendulous dorsal membrane, and/or weak, poorly arched cartilage

SIGNALMENT
• Has been reported in beef and dairy calves of both sexes and various pure and crossbreeds
• Calves generally present at a few weeks of age if congenital condition or dystocia is the cause.
• If traumatic, may present at any age
• Has been reported in goats from 4 months to 9 years of age

SIGNS
• Intermittent or honking cough. Palpation or elevation of head may induce cough.
• Stridor or dyspnea with mild exercise; may have dyspnea at rest if collapse is severe.
• Stertor on inspiration; auscultation localizes to trachea.
• May have mild fever, especially if accompanied by pneumonia
• Tachycardia
• Tachypnea—prolonged inspiratory phase
• Cyanosis
• Mucosal hyperemia
• Physical exam may reveal evidence of other trauma, such as fractured ribs or sternebrae.
• Concomitant pneumonia
• Weight loss, reduced growth rate

CAUSES AND RISK FACTORS
• Condition may be congenital or acquired.
• Cause is a dynamic collapse of tracheal structures. Increase in negative pressure by animal during inspiration causes an abnormal thoracic trachea to further weaken and collapse.
• Trauma—most common cause in cattle
  • Commonly associated with fractured ribs and compression of the trachea at the thoracic inlet by bony callus formation
  • Calves often have history of being breech dystocias.
  • Roping injuries
• Congenital malformation of tracheal rings
• Genetic or nutritional weakness of cartilage
• Deficient innervation of trachealis muscle
• Ischemic lesions from endotracheal tube cuffs
• Posttracheostomy
• Primary pulmonary disease

DIAGNOSIS
See Gross Findings below for tracheal collapse classifications.

DIFFERENTIAL DIAGNOSIS
• Necrotic laryngitis
• Bronchopneumonia
• Foreign body
• Abscesses
• Actinobacillosis
• Hematoma
• Neoplasia

CBC/BIOCHEMISTRY/URINALYSIS
Abnormalities associated with stress or concomitant pneumonia
• Leukocytosis, neutrophilia, monocytosis, basophilia
• Elevated creatinine if dehydrated

OTHER LABORATORY TESTS

IMAGING
Radiography
• Survey radiographs may show dorsoventral collapse; lateral collapse may also occur.
• Collapse generally present at caudal cervical and cranial thoracic portions of the trachea near the thoracic inlet; may also indicate presence of fractured ribs

Fluorosopy
May appreciate dynamic collapse

Endoscopy
• May be dangerous and stressful to animal
• Have oxygen available.

DIAGNOSTIC PROCEDURES
Physical Exam
• Auscultation localizes abnormal respiratory sounds to trachea.
• Palpation of trachea may induce collapse or reveal it.

GROSS FINDINGS
• Distortion of cartilage rings
• Pendulous dorsal membrane
• Tracheal collapse classifications
  • Class I: 25% reduction in diameter
  • Class II: 50% reduction in diameter, with pendulous membrane and relaxed cartilage
  • Class III: 75% reduction in functional diameter: dorsal membrane almost contacts ventral tracheal wall
  • Class IV: lumen almost obliterated
• Pneumonia

HISTOPATHOLOGICAL FINDINGS
Reports have shown no difference between collapsed and normal rings in one calf.

TREATMENT

• Confinement until slaughter with decreased activity
• Management of pneumonia
• Surgical reconstruction—consider anesthetic risk
• Internal and external prostheses

External Prosthesis

• Syringe barrels or syringe case rings, fenestrated and sterilized
• Placed around collapsed segment and trachea sutured out to rigid ring
• Coil spring: coiled around collapsed trachea and sutured in place
• Prosthesis should be removed 2–3 months postoperatively in order to allow unrestricted growth of the trachea

Other Procedures

• Plication of dorsal membrane; tracheal anastomosis; bisection of tracheal rings
• < 30% probability of favorable outcome with surgery
• If collapse is associated with rib fractures, surgery of trachea should include resection of rib callus

MEDICATIONS

DRUGS OF CHOICE

• Appropriate selection of antimicrobials to control primary or secondary pneumonia
• Antimicrobial therapy for 5–7 days postoperatively

CONTRAINDICATIONS

• Have supplemental oxygen available during examination and diagnostic procedures
• Appropriate milk and meat withdrawal times must be followed for all compounds administered to food-producing animals.

FOLLOW-UP

PATIENT MONITORING

• Monitor for development or resolution of pneumonia
• Continue postoperative antibiotics for 5 to 7 days

PREVENTION/AVOIDANCE

POSSIBLE COMPLICATIONS

• Recollapse of corrected or adjacent segment of trachea
• Adjacent segments predisposed to collapse after surgical repair of primary segment due to increased forces on adjacent segment during inspiration
• Bronchopneumonia due to mechanical irritation, increased mucus production
• Patients are at a higher risk for lower airway diseases.
• Trachea out-growing prosthesis

EXPECTED COURSE AND PROGNOSIS

• If untreated, collapse may worsen and calf can become increasingly dyspneic until death.
• Trachea likely to out-grow prosthesis in a few months
• Retrospective report of surgical repair
• One calf subsequently produced two calves before dying of an unresolved abomasal volvulus
• One calf was normal at 11 months of age
• Two other calves died postoperatively 2 days and 4 months after surgery. Died of bronchopneumonia and recollapse, respectively

MISCELLANEOUS

ASSOCIATED CONDITIONS

Bronchopneumonia

AGE-RELATED FACTORS

Generally a few weeks to a few months of age when presented

ZOONOTIC POTENTIAL

N/A

PREGNANCY

N/A

RUMINANT SPECIES AFFECTED

Reported in bovine and caprine

BIOSECURITY

N/A

PRODUCTION MANAGEMENT

Reduce traumatic events, most common cause in cattle
• Commonly associated with fractured ribs and compression of the trachea at the thoracic inlet by bony callus formation
• Calves often have history of being breech dystocias
• Roping injuries

SEE ALSO

Actinobacillosis
Bronchopneumonia
Necrotic laryngitis

ABBREVIATIONS

N/A

Suggested Reading
Baker, J. C., Smith, J. A. 2002. Diseases of the pharynx, larynx and trachea: tracheal stenosis, collapse and stricture. In: *Large animal internal medicine*, ed. B. P. Smith. 3rd ed. St. Louis: Mosby.
Belli, C. B., Benesi, F. J., Leal, M. L. R., Nichi, M. 2003. Tracheal collapse in an adult goat. *Canadian Veterinary Journal* 44: 835–36.
Fingland, R. B., Rings, D. M., Vestweber, J. G. 1990. The etiology and surgical management of tracheal collapse in calves. *Veterinary Surgery* 19(5): 371–79.
Rings, D. M. 1995. Tracheal collapse. *Veterinary Clinics of North America Food Animal Practice* 11(1): 171–75.
Vaala, W. E., House, J. K. 2002. Respiratory distress: upper respiratory tract disorders. In: *Large animal internal medicine*, ed. B. P. Smith. 3rd ed. St. Louis: Mosby.

Author: Meredyth Jones

TRACHEAL EDEMA ("HONKER") SYNDROME

BASICS

OVERVIEW
• Tracheal edema ("honker") syndrome is a potentially life-threatening condition seen sporadically in feedlot cattle.
• Severe edema and hemorrhage of the dorsal wall of the trachea from the midcervical region to the tracheal bifurcation

PATHOPHYSIOLOGY
• The etiology of the syndrome is unknown.
• Causes may include viral or bacterial infection, trauma to the trachea from feed bunks, passive congestion and edema due to fat accumulation at the thoracic inlet, hypersensitivity, and mycotoxicosis.

SYSTEMS AFFECTED
Respiratory, production management, and musculoskeletal

GENETICS
N/A

INCIDENCE/PREVALENCE
Unknown

GEOGRAPHIC DISTRIBUTION
Canada and the United States; potentially worldwide

SIGNALMENT
• Only reported in feedlot cattle
• Typically seen during the last half of the feeding period.
• Seen more often in summer. Possible exacerbation due to heat and increased dust.

Species
Bovine

Breed Predilections
N/A

Mean Age and Range
N/A

Predominant Sex
There appears to be no sexual predominance.

SIGNS
• Subclinical disease may exist. Tracheal lesions have been demonstrated at slaughter in cattle that did not have clinical signs.
• Typical signs include an acute onset of dyspnea with an increased inspiratory effort, coughing, and a loud, guttural stertor leading to the colloquial term "honker."
• Symptoms can progress to open-mouth breathing with head and neck extended, cyanosis, belligerence, recumbency, and death.
• Some animals are found acutely dead with no premonitory signs.

CAUSES AND RISK FACTORS
• Clinical signs are seen predominantly in warm weather and are often brought on by increased movement or exercise.
• The etiology of the syndrome is unknown. Hypothetical causes include viral or bacterial infection, trauma to the trachea from feed bunks, passive congestion and edema due to fat accumulation at the thoracic inlet, hypersensitivity, and mycotoxicosis.

DIAGNOSIS

DIFFERENTIAL DIAGNOSIS
• Necrotic laryngitis (calf diphtheria)—typically febrile, pain on laryngeal palpation, sometimes malodorous breath
• Pharyngeal trauma—recent history of being treated via balling gun, dose syringe, oral speculum, etc.
• Atypical interstitial pneumonia
• Miscellaneous uncommon conditions—laryngeal or tracheal foreign object, tumor, laryngeal paralysis

CBC/BIOCHEMISTRY/URINALYSIS
N/A

OTHER LABORATORY TESTS
N/A

IMAGING
N/A

DIAGNOSTIC PROCEDURES
N/A

PATHOLOGIC FINDINGS

GROSS FINDINGS
Severe submucosal edema and hemorrhage of the dorsal trachea are seen from the midcervical trachea to the tracheal bifurcation. On cross section, the lumen of the trachea may be greater than 50% occluded.

HISTOPATHOLOGICAL FINDINGS
The tracheal mucosa is hyperemic and hyperplastic with focal erosions and loss of cilia. The submucosa is markedly thickened by hemorrhage and edema and infiltrated by white blood cells. The trachealis muscle is separated from the surrounding connective tissue by hemorrhage and edema with swelling and vacuolation of the myocytes.

TREATMENT
• Calm and minimal handling is imperative as asphyxiation and death can ensue if the animal becomes overly excited.
• The provision of shade and cooling with a water spray is helpful in hot weather.

TRACHEAL EDEMA ("HONKER") SYNDROME

 MEDICATIONS

DRUGS OF CHOICE
• Corticosteroids—dexamethasone (0.04–0.22 mg/kg) (IM route of administration is preferred over IV due to decreased animal handling and stress)
• Broad-spectrum antibiotics—long-acting oxytetracycline (20 mg/kg SQ) or ceftiofur (1.1–2.2 mg/kg SQ for 3 days)

CONTRAINDICATIONS
Appropriate drug withdrawal time should be followed before slaughter.

 FOLLOW-UP

PATIENT MONITORING
N/A

PREVENTION/AVOIDANCE
Movement and exercise of cattle late in the feeding period should be avoided during warmer months and restricted to early morning hours when unavoidable.

POSSIBLE COMPLICATIONS
Poor response to therapy and relapse may require early slaughter or euthanasia.

EXPECTED COURSE AND PROGNOSIS
Prognosis for full recovery is poor to guarded as relapse often occurs.

 MISCELLANEOUS

ASSOCIATED CONDITIONS
N/A

AGE-RELATED FACTORS
N/A

ZOONOTIC POTENTIAL
N/A

PREGNANCY
N/A

RUMINANT SPECIES AFFECTED
Bovine

BIOSECURITY
N/A

PRODUCTION MANAGEMENT
• Causes may include viral or bacterial infection, trauma to the trachea from feed bunks, passive congestion and edema due to fat accumulation at the thoracic inlet, hypersensitivity, and mycotoxicosis.
• Calm and minimal handling.
• Provision of shade and cooling with a water spray is helpful in hot weather.

SYNONYMS
Honker

SEE ALSO
Atypical interstitial pneumonia
Necrotic laryngitis (calf diphtheria)
Pharyngeal trauma
Reflective respiratory disease chapters
Tracheal foreign object

ABBREVIATIONS
IM = intramuscular
mg/kg = milligrams per kilogram
SQ = subcutaneous

Suggested Reading
Apley, M. D., Fajt, V. R. 1998. Feedlot therapeutics. *Vet Clin North Am: Food Anim Pract.* 14:291–314.
Erickson, E. D., Doster, A. R. 1993. Tracheal stenosis in feedlot cattle. *J Vet Diagn Invest.* 5:449–51.
Fingland, R. B., Rings, D. M., Vestweber, J. G. 1990, Sep–Oct. The etiology and surgical management of tracheal collapse in calves. *Vet Surg.* 19(5): 371–79.
Panciera, R. J., Williams, D. E. 1981. Tracheal edema (honker) syndrome of feedlot cattle. In: *Current veterinary therapy: food animal practice*, ed. J. L. Howard. Philadelphia: W. B. Saunders Co.
Rings, D. M. 1995, Mar. Tracheal collapse. *Vet Clin North Am Food Anim Pract.* 11(1): 171–75.

Author: William R. DuBois

BASICS

OVERVIEW
• Transfaunation is an important tool in the medical management of acidotic, inappetent ruminants and pseudoruminants. Donor animals help readily provide the necessary amount, quality, and quantity of transfaunation fluid.
• Ciliate protozoa are commonly found in the rumen contents of both wild and domesticated ruminants as well as camelids.
• Ruminal species composition appears to reflect the type and composition of feed consumed by the animal as well as geographical distribution.
• Physiological/pathological status of the host is also important to microbial content. In animals that have undergone feed stress (e.g., starvation/acidosis), rumen ciliates may be eliminated. Normally 3–5 days of anorexia may cause death of rumen flora so transfaunation may become necessary.
• Apparent digestion in the rumen of organic matter and starch is higher when a large protozoal population is present. A large population of ciliates has been associated with increases in both rumen ammonia and plasma urea and has a stabilizing effect on ruminal pH. Effects of ciliate protozoa are related to animal performance.

• Compared with fauna-free ruminants, the presence of ciliate protozoa has been shown to result in a more stable ruminal fermentation, higher levels of ammonia, reduced numbers of bacteria, as well as changes in dry matter (%), liquid volume, and turnover rate of ruminal contents. Associated with these differences in the rumen are higher ruminal and total tract digestion of organic matter and fiber in faunated animals.
• Ciliate protozoa in the rumen include: *Entodinium* spp., *Polyplastron* spp., *Eudiplodinium* spp., *Epidinium* spp., and *Isotricha* spp.

SYSTEMS AFFECTED
Gastrointestinal

GENETICS
N/A

INCIDENCE/PREVALENCE
N/A

GEOGRAPHIC DISTRIBUTION
Worldwide, depending on species and environment

SIGNALMENT
Species
Potentially, all ruminant and pseudoruminant species
Breed Predilections
N/A
Mean Age and Range
N/A
Predominant Sex
N/A

MISCELLANEOUS

Quantity of Fluid Collection:
• Generally, an average bovine rumen contains between 30–70 liters of fluid depending upon age and breed characteristics.
• Collection volume should be somewhere between 0.5% and 3.0% of this fluid level. Lower collection levels will preclude any secondary rumen problems associated with the donor animal.
• The transfaunation fluid volume should be between 350 mL and 4.0 liters depending on species. It is important that the collected fluid be stored out of light, anaerobically, and at the cow's body temperature until use.
• 0.5–1L of camelid C1, or strained sheep, goat, or cow rumen contents is administered to camelids twice daily for 3 to 5 days.
• Prior to transfaunation, it is essential to correct rumen pH to the 6.5–6.8 range— use Mg hydroxide/oxide/carbonate for acidic rumen and vinegar or dilute acetic acid for alkaline rumen compensation.
• The disease status of the donor should be evaluated prior to use.

Time Between Collection and Transfaunation:
• Timing is very critical to the success of transfaunation. Generally, the fluid should be deposited into the recipient animal within 30 minutes postcollection.

TRANSFAUNATION

• Two hours appears to be the limit to success if the collection is maintained in a strict anaerobic environment. At about the 2-hour time limit, the starch-digesting organisms have increased dramatically and the fiber-digesting microbes have decreased substantially.

Time of Day to Collect:
• The number of hours postfeeding of the donor animal usually determines the collection time. Collection timing is very important in emphasizing the type and number of organisms in the collection fluid.
• The recipient animal off feed is probably in rumen acidosis and therefore should be transfaunated from a donor cow 2 hours postprandial. Acidosis must be corrected prior to transfaunation.

Monitoring Fluid Quality:
• Monitoring the pH of both donor and recipient rumen liquor is as important a selection criterion as assessing microbe numbers.
• The ideal range is 5.8–6.2 for maximal microflora count. If the pH is below this ideal range, the microbial activity will be diminished. With a more highly acidic environment, starch-fermenting organisms will dominate over cellulytic microbes.
• Protozoa and fungi will also vary at lower pHs.

Transfaunation Procedure:
• When transfaunating, try not to disturb the donor animal's rumen mat or rumen mucosa. Generally it is best to insert a short stomach tube and pump out the necessary fluid.

• Recipient cows generally require 1000 ml of fluid twice daily for 2–4 days.
• Most transfaunation failures occur with inadequate donor fluid levels, not maintaining an anaerobic environment, concomitant use of antibiotics, inappropriate pH, and inadequate length of fluid treatment.
• Straining rumen fluid for large particulate matter is helpful with the tubing process.

ASSOCIATED CONDITIONS
Rumen acidosis and alkalosis can affect rumen flora.

AGE-RELATED FACTORS
N/A

ZOONOTIC POTENTIAL
N/A

PREGNANCY
N/A

RUMINANT SPECIES AFFECTED
All ruminant and pseudoruminant species are affected.

BIOSECURITY
N/A

PRODUCTION MANAGEMENT
N/A

SYNONYMS
N/A

SEE ALSO
Fluid therapy
Gastrointestinal microbiology
Gastrointestinal pharmacology
Rumen acidosis

ABBREVIATIONS
N/A

Suggested Reading
Coleman, G. S. Rumen ciliate protozoa. *Adv Parasitol*. 18:121–73.
Fonty, G., Senaud, J., Jouany, J. P., Gouet, P. 1988. Establishment of ciliate protozoa in the rumen of conventional and conventionalized lambs: influence of diet and management conditions. *Can J Microbiol*. 34(3): 235–41.
Olubobokun, J. A., Craig, W. M. 1990. Quantity and characteristics of microorganisms associated with ruminal fluid or particles. *J Anim Sci*. 68(10): 3360–70.
Regensbogenova, M., Pristas, P., Javorsky, P., Moon-van der Staay, S. Y., Van Der Staay, G. W. M., Hackstein, J. H. P., Newbold, C. J., McEwan, N. R. 2004. Assessment of ciliates in the sheep rumen by DGGE. *Lett Appl Microbiol*. 39(2): 144–47.
Williams, A. G., Withers, S. E. 1993. Changes in the rumen microbial population and its activities during the refaunation period after the reintroduction of ciliate protozoa into the rumen of defaunated sheep. *Can J Microbiol*. 39(1): 61–69.

Author: Scott R. R. Haskell

TRAUMATIC RETICULOPERITONITIS

 BASICS

OVERVIEW

- Traumatic reticuloperitonitis (TRP) is a common disease of cattle but rarely seen in small ruminants. The eating habits of cattle predispose them to the accidental swallowing of metal foreign objects that settle in the rumen/reticulum.
- The foreign object may penetrate the reticulum resulting in localized or generalized peritonitis, or only the wall of the reticulum may be involved and this may result in dysfunction due to interference with chemoreceptors or mechanoreceptors.
- The diaphragm, pericardium, and heart are located cranial to the reticulum and the liver is medial and dorsal. Any of these organs may be penetrated by the foreign body and become involved in the inflammatory process.

SYSTEMS AFFECTED

Gastrointestinal

GENETICS

N/A

INCIDENCE/PREVALENCE

N/A

GEOGRAPHIC DISTRIBUTION

Potentially worldwide, depending on species and environment

SIGNALMENT

This disease is seen primarily in cattle consuming processed forages or concentrates. In at least one study, the risk of TRP decreased with increasing parity and was higher when cattle had feet and leg problems.

Species

Dairy and beef cattle; however, potentially all ruminant species can become affected.

Breed Predilections

N/A

Mean Age and Range

N/A

Predominant Sex

N/A

SIGNS

- In the most severe form of TRP, affected cattle may present with a dramatic change in posture, standing with an arched back, total anorexia, and vocalizing with a grunting noise when forced to move or when urinating. A sudden decrease in milk production is commonly reported.
- Physical examination of these cattle is characterized by fever, decreased rumen contractions, and an unwillingness to flex ventrally when pinched over the withers. They may have tachycardia, and auscultation of the heart may reveal increased cardiac intensity or may be muffled due to bacterial contamination and subsequent inflammation of the pericardium.
- Sudden death has occurred as a result of laceration of a coronary blood vessel or puncture of the heart by the foreign body.
- More chronic cases present a diagnostic challenge due to signs that are subtle and vague. Affected cattle in early lactation may have mild ketosis secondary to their anorexia. Mild bloat and changes in fecal consistency are also common signs. Weight loss, roughened hair coat, and diffuse generalized lameness may be the only signs.

CAUSES AND RISK FACTORS

The indiscriminate eating habits of cattle are the most likely cause of this disease. Construction in and around their environment will also increase the risk. The care and upkeep of the machinery used to process and provide silage to the cattle also plays a role in risk management.

 DIAGNOSIS

DIFFERENTIAL DIAGNOSIS

Abomasal ulcers, diaphragmatic hernia, endoparasitism, heart disease, hepatic abscesses, indigestion, laminitis, lymphosarcoma, or other neoplasia may all be confused with TRP. Clinical signs will assist with ruling out laminitis. Further physical examination findings via rectal palpation may assist in ruling out lymphosarcoma or other abdominal neoplasms.

CBC/BIOCHEMISTRY/URINALYSIS

- The white blood cell count and distribution, plasma proteins, and fibrinogen may be normal in the initial stages of TRP. Total plasma proteins of over 10 g/dl have been shown to have a positive predictive value of 76% for TRP in referral populations.
- Biochemical profiles are not of high value in diagnosing TRP, but may be of benefit in ruling out others on the differential diagnosis list.
- Urinalysis would not be of definitive value in this disease reflecting only the secondary ketosis that accompanies the anorexia commonly observed.

OTHER LABORATORY TESTS

Abdominocentesis is recommended and may be aided by ultrasonography to obtain fluid. Remember that in normal, nonpregnant, adult cattle the amount of abdominal fluid is small. All normal bovine peritoneal fluid clots upon exposure to air, so samples are placed in small EDTA tubes.

IMAGING

- Abdominal radiographs with the horizontal beam centered over the reticulodiaphragmatic region in an attempt to confirm the presence of metallic foreign bodies can be done with the cow in that standing position or cast into dorsal recumbency.
- One study in which standing radiographs were taken describes the sensitivity of the procedure in detecting TRP as 83%.
- Ultrasound diagnosis has been utilized as well.

TREATMENT

• Conservative treatment is most often attempted first and includes administration of a forestomach magnet, antibiotics, and confinement. Many cattle recover after this therapy with resumption of appetite and motility within 3 days. Those animals that do not recover in 3 days may require a rumenotomy to remove the foreign body in order to allow them to recover. This becomes an economic challenge for the producer and veterinary surgeon.
• Cattle with diffuse peritonitis have a poor prognosis for return to production or life. Treatment of peritonitis requires systemic antibiotics, possible drainage of the affected area, and surgical correction of the inciting cause.
• Those cattle that seem to recover in the short term may later develop forestomach outflow problems typical of vagal indigestion.

MEDICATIONS

CONTRAINDICATIONS
Appropriate milk and meat withdrawal times must be followed for all compounds administered to food-producing animals.

PRECAUTIONS
N/A

POSSIBLE COMPLICATIONS
N/A

FOLLOW-UP

PREVENTION/AVOIDANCE
• Most producers now have large magnets in place on feed-handling equipment that eliminates the delivery of sharp metal objects to cattle at the time of feeding. Also, many producers have gone away from upright silos for storage of their corn silage in favor of bunkers. This has eliminated another source of metal contamination of feedstuffs by eliminating the mechanical unloader necessary for old upright silos.

• Some producers will administer prophylactic magnets to all heifers at 6–8 months of age as another means of prevention of TRP.

EXPECTED COURSE AND PROGNOSIS
• Cattle with diffuse peritonitis have a poor prognosis for return to production or life.
• Those cattle that seem to recover in the short term may later develop forestomach outflow problems typical of vagal indigestion.

MISCELLANEOUS

ASSOCIATED CONDITIONS
N/A

AGE-RELATED FACTORS
N/A

ZOONOTIC POTENTIAL
N/A

PREGNANCY
May exacerbate disease symptoms

RUMINANT SPECIES AFFECTED
Potentially, all ruminant species are affected. However, dairy and beef cattle are generally affected.

BIOSECURITY
N/A

PRODUCTION MANAGEMENT
Most producers now have large magnets in place on feed-handling equipment that eliminates the delivery of sharp metal objects to cattle at the time of feeding. Also, many producers have gone away from upright silos for storage of their corn silage in favor of bunkers. This has eliminated another source of metal contamination of feedstuffs by eliminating the mechanical unloader necessary for old upright silos.

SYNONYMS
Hardware disease
Wire disease

SEE ALSO
Abomasal ulcers
Diaphragmatic hernia
Endoparasitism
Heart disease
Hepatic abscesses
Indigestion
Laminitis
Lymphosarcoma or other neoplasia

ABBREVIATIONS
TRP = traumatic reticuloperitonitis

Suggested Reading
Braun, U., Fluckiger, M., Gotz, M. 1994, Nov 12. Comparison of ultrasonographic and radiographic findings in cows with traumatic reticuloperitonitis. *Vet Rec.* 135(20): 470–78.
Braun, U., Gansohr, B., Fluckiger, M. 2003. Radiographic findings before and after oral administration of a magnet in cows with traumatic reticuloperitonitis. *Am. J Vet Res.* 64(1): 115–20.
Farrow, C. S. 1999, Jul. Reticular foreign bodies. Causative or coincidence? *Vet Clin North Am Food Anim Pract.* 15(2): 397–408.
Fleischer, P., Metzner, M., Beyerbach, M., Hoedemaker, M., Klee, W. 2001, Sep. The relationship between milk yield and the incidence of some diseases in dairy cows. *J Dairy Sci.* 84(9): 2025–35.
Grohn, Y.T., Bruss, M. L. 1990. Effect of diseases, production, and season on traumatic reticuloperitonitis and ruminal acidosis in dairy cattle. *J Dairy Sci.* 73(9): 2355–63.
Rehage, J., Kaske, M., Stockhofe-Zurwieden, N., Yalcin, E. 1995. Evaluation of the pathogenesis of vagus indigestion in cows with traumatic reticuloperitonitis. *J Am Vet Med Assoc.* 207(12): 1607–11.
Ward, J. L., Ducharme, N. G. 1994, Mar 15. Traumatic reticuloperitonitis in dairy cows. *J Am Vet Med Assoc.* 204(6): 874–77.

Author: Dennis D. French

TREMETOL: WHITE SNAKEROOT AND RAYLESS GOLDENROD

 BASICS

OVERVIEW
• White snakeroot is an opposite branching, dark green perennial, which grows 1–4 feet tall in damp, open areas of woods and shaded areas along streams.
• Stems are slender, round, and may be purplish.
• Leaves are 3–5 inches in length and have three distinct veins, coarsely toothed margins, and a sharp tip.
• Flowers are white and clustered in groups of 10 to 40 at the end of branches and bloom in late summer and fall.
• Roots are shallow and fibrous, and twist and turn giving the plant its name.
• The plant grows in moist areas bordering streams, woodlands, as well as wooded areas with rich basic soil. It may persist in open areas after clearing.
• The geographic distribution is mostly eastern North America and grows from the East Coast including Canada, west to Minnesota, and south to east Texas and the gulf coast.
• Intoxication requires ingestion of 0.5%–1.0% of body weight of green plant over 2–3 weeks.

PATHOPHYSIOLOGY
• Toxicity is most abundant in the foliage of the mature plant, is resistant to frost, and, although decreased, persists in the dried plant.
• The same toxins found in *Eupatorium rugosum* (white snakeroot) are also found in *Isocoma wrightii* (rayless goldenrod).
• The specific toxin has not been identified, but the unpurified form has been named tremetol.
• Effect of toxin requires microsomal activation and may explain different effects in different species.

• Intoxication is theorized to inhibit citrate synthase causing ketosis detectable by acetone smell of breath and urine.
• Intoxication in animals is often called trembles.
• Nursing young are clinically affected by high concentration in milk.
• Causes muscle damage and weakness
• Causes hepatic necrosis
• May cause photosensitization of small ruminants if animal survives acute disease
• The toxin is cleared in milk and may cause signs in offspring or humans if ingested.

SIGNALMENT
Seen most frequently in sheep and goats, but all species ingesting the plant are at risk.

SIGNS
• Disease usually seen in late fall or early winter
• Animals die soon after becoming recumbent.
• History of weight loss
• Ketosis causes acetone breath
• Afebrile
• Clinical signs different between species

Cattle and Sheep
• Reluctance to move
• Stiff movements or ataxia
• Severe trembles after exercise
• Depression
• Recumbency
• Sudden death
• Dyspnea, salivation, constipation, regurgitation may occasionally occur.
• Clinical signs may appear 3 days to 3 weeks after ingestion.

Goats
• Goats typically show signs of liver failure.
• Depression
• Weakness
• Head pressing
• Icterus
• Slight tremors with exercise

• Recumbency
• Sudden death
• Photosensitization if animal survives acute disease
• Clinical signs may appear 1–5 days after ingestion.

CAUSES AND RISK FACTORS
• Moving naïve animals to contaminated pastures when there is inadequate forage (i.e., fall and winter)
• Lactating animals are more resistant due to rapid excretion of toxin in milk, putting nursing animals at high risk for clinical signs.

 DIAGNOSIS

DIFFERENTIAL DIAGNOSIS
• Selenium deficiency
• Other causes of liver disease in small ruminants
• Gossypol intoxication
• Botulism in cattle
• Organophosphate intoxication
• CNS trauma
• Other tremorgenic toxicities

CBC/BIOCHEMISTRY/URINALYSIS
• Muscle enzymes (CK, LDH, ALP, AST) are elevated.
• Animals have ketoacidosis.
• May have myoglobinuria
• Goats may have elevations in bilirubin.

OTHER LABORATORY TESTS
N/A

IMAGING
N/A

DIAGNOSTIC PROCEDURES
• Evidence of plants in rumen
• Evidence of plant exposure

PATHOLOGIC FINDINGS
• Centrolobular hepatic degeneration and necrosis
• Skeletal muscle necrosis

TREMETOL: WHITE SNAKEROOT AND RAYLESS GOLDENROD

• Cardiac abnormalities reported primarily in horses
• Extreme congestion of liver, kidney, abomasums, brain, and spinal cord
• Extreme fat degeneration of liver and kidney

TREATMENT

SYMPTOMATIC AND SUPPORTIVE CARE
• Correct any electrolyte and acid base abnormalities
• Ketosis is refractory to treatment

MEDICATIONS

DRUGS OF CHOICE
• Activated charcoal (AC) (2–5 g/kg PO in a water slurry)
• Evidence in other species of recycling through gastrointestinal system; repeat doses of AC may be beneficial.
• Laxatives

CONTRAINDICATIONS
• Any drug promoting hepatic microsomal enzymes is contraindicated.
• Any drug inhibiting hepatic microsomal enzymes may be helpful.
• Drug withdrawal times must be maintained.

FOLLOW-UP

PATIENT MONITORING
Monitor electrolytes

PREVENTION/AVOIDANCE
• Prevention of white snakeroot intoxication is possible—monitor pasture/hay for white snakeroot.
• Selective use of herbicides or manual removal of plants may help to diminish problem.

POSSIBLE COMPLICATIONS
.

EXPECTED COURSE AND PROGNOSIS
Animals exhibiting clinical signs have grave prognosis.

MISCELLANEOUS

ASSOCIATED CONDITIONS
N/A

AGE-RELATED FACTORS
Nursing animals may show clinical signs before other animals in the herd.

ZOONOTIC POTENTIAL
Cause of milk poisoning in hundreds of people during colonial time period

PREGNANCY
N/A

RUMINANT SPECIES AFFECTED
All species are affected but goats may be at a greater risk.

BIOSECURITY
N/A

PRODUCTION MANAGEMENT
N/A

SEE ALSO
Botulism in cattle
CNS trauma
Gossypol
Gossypol intoxication
Liver disease
Muscle disease
Organophosphate intoxication
Other causes of liver disease in small ruminants
Other tremorgenic toxicities
Rayless goldenrod
Selenium
Selenium deficiency

ABBREVIATIONS
AC = activated charcoal
ALP = alkaline phosphatase
AST = aspartate aminotransferase
CK = creatine kinase
LDH = lactate dehydrogenase
PO = per os, by mouth

Suggested Reading
Beier, R. C., Norman, J. O. 1990. The toxic factor in white snakeroot: identity, analysis, and prevention. *Vet Hum Toxicol.* 32 (supplement): 81–88.
Galey, F. D. 2002. White snakeroot. In: *Large animal internal medicine*, ed. B. P. Smith. St. Louis: Mosby.

Author: Benjamin R. Buchanan

TRICHOMONIASIS (TRICHOMONOSIS)

 BASICS

DEFINITION
• Trichomonosis, formerly called trichomoniasis, is a sexually transmitted disease that results in embryonic and fetal death (typically between 50 and 70 days in gestation, but occasionally up to the early third trimester), and is associated with postcoital pyometra.
• It is an insidious disease—neither the male nor the female shows overt signs, except that cows presumed to be pregnant will return to estrus after losing their pregnancies, often too late to rebreed them for that season.

PATHOPHYSIOLOGY
• *Tritrichomonas foetus* is an obligate venereal pathogen (i.e., it is transmitted only via coitus or unhygienic artificial insemination).
• The protozoan dwells on the surface of the epithelial covering of the bull's glans penis and the proximal prepuce.
• Specifically, it lives in the epithelial crypts of the squamous epithelium. As bulls age, the crypts deepen, providing a more favorable environment for the organism. *T. foetus* is readily transmitted to the female at mating.
• In the female, conception typically is not disrupted and, in many cases, the resulting embryo is not damaged for up to 7–9 weeks.

• Recent work using ELISA has shown that the local levels of *T. foetus*–specific immunoglobulin, especially IgA and IgG1, also peak at this time.
• Serum antibodies also exist, but at a very low level that is not detectable by ELISA. Hence, there is no practical serological test commercially available for diagnostic use. Infected females rid the reproductive tract of the organism, typically within 6 to 18 weeks, presumably via the action of the antibodies in the uterine lumen.
• The organism has been shown to release cytotoxins into the environment, although the in vivo significance of this is not known.

SYSTEMS AFFECTED
• Reproductive
• The organism is generally not invasive; it lives in the lumen of the vagina, uterus, and oviducts of the female, and on the epithelial surface of the glans penis and prepuce of the male.
• It has been observed in deeper layers of the chorioallantois of aborted fetuses.

GENETICS
• There is no documented genetic basis for susceptibility to trichomonosis.
• The organism has been cultured from the prepuce of bulls of all breeds tested to date. *Bos indicus* bulls, with their longer prepuces, do not seem to be any more susceptible than *B. taurus* bulls.

INCIDENCE/PREVALENCE
• Trichomonosis exists wherever natural service is practiced, and has been diagnosed even in situations where unhygienic artificial insemination is practiced (e.g., where an inseminator performed serial manual vaginal examinations, using a common sleeve, just prior to inseminating).
• Because *T. foetus* can survive cryopreservation, it is also possible that contaminated semen could spread the infection, but this is highly unlikely if the semen is processed by a reputable company, using Certified Semen Standards (CSS).
• In the early 1990s, a survey of randomly selected herds estimated the prevalence of trichomonosis in California at 5% of all bulls and 16% of beef herds (at least one infected bull). As others have shown, there was a clear pattern of increased prevalence with increasing age of bulls.
• Bulls less than 4 years of age at the time of exposure to cows were significantly less likely to be infected, and infection of bulls less than 3 years old was rare. Similar results have been reported in Florida, with bull and herd prevalences of 6% and 30%, respectively.

SIGNALMENT
Species
Cattle

Breed Predilections
None

Mean Age and Range
• Older bulls ($\geq$ 4 yrs) are more likely to become infected if exposed to an infected female at coitus.
• Once infected, they will remain so, probably for life.
• Younger bulls can mechanically transmit the organism, but generally do not become permanent carriers.
• Cows develop partial, short-lived immunity, but most would be susceptible the following breeding season.

SIGNS
• Trichomonosis is insidious. Neither the cow nor the bull is ever overtly ill, and a vaginal or preputial discharge is rarely seen.
• A very alert owner may notice that cows/heifers that were presumed pregnant begin returning to estrus near the end of the breeding season, or after the bulls are removed.

PHYSICAL EXAMINATION FINDINGS
• At the time of herd pregnancy examination, a herd recently infected with *T. foetus* will show a decreased overall pregnancy rate (reductions below 70% of normal are common), and the gestational ages of pregnancy in those cows that are pregnant will be highly variable.

• Approximately 5% of cows in an exposed herd may be diagnosed with pyometra at the time of pregnancy check.
• By transrectal palpation, this will present as a fluid-distended uterus with no positive signs of pregnancy, and a corpus luteum on one or both ovaries.
• This postcoital pyometra is a very important finding and should instigate actions to rule out trichomonosis.

CAUSES
• The flagellated protozoan *Tritrichomonas foetus*
• An immunopathological component is likely as well. This hypothesis is based on both in vivo and in vitro findings that peak mortality of concepti does not occur until there is peak IgG1 antibody in the uterine lumen, and that such antibodies are capable of redirecting the host response against host cells.
• It is also possible that cytotoxins elaborated by *T. foetus* can directly damage conceptus tissues.

RISK FACTORS
The major risk factors for bovine trichomonosis are:
• Use of natural service
• Use of older bulls
• Shared grazing (It has been well established that the use of shared grazing increases the risk of infection of any herd participating.)

• Failure to test bulls before the breeding season (Routine testing for the presence of *T. foetus* in bulls can easily be combined with preseason breeding soundness examinations. Failure to do so increases the risk of undetected infection, especially if shared grazing is commonly practiced.)
• Lease of nonvirgin breeding stock
• Failure to vaccinate, given any of the risk factors above

 DIAGNOSIS

DIFFERENTIAL DIAGNOSIS
• Poor nutrition, *Campylobacter fetus venerealis*
• Poor nutrition, especially energy deficiency in replacement heifers or late pregnant cows, can yield a herd pregnancy pattern in the next breeding season similar to a *T. foetus*–infected herd.
• Poor nutrition of heifers will delay onset of puberty, which will reduce the opportunities for heifers to become pregnant during a limited breeding season.

TRICHOMONIASIS (TRICHOMONOSIS)

• Poor nutrition of third trimester pregnant beef cows will delay the postpartum return to cyclicity.
• Other infectious agents, including *Campylobacter fetus venerealis* can produce an almost identical epidemiological picture. Less commonly, *Haemophilus somnus, Chlamydophila* spp., and *Ureaplasma* are implicated in outbreaks of venereally transmitted infections leading to early conceptus death, but these generally are associated with detectable genital lesions in the female.

CBC/BIOCHEMISTRY/URINALYSIS
N/A

OTHER LABORATORY TESTS
Bulls
• Collect preputial smegma by vigorously scraping/aspirating the fornix via a 22" infusion pipette attached to a sterile 12 cc syringe. Culture preputial smegma in a suitable medium, and identify *T. foetus* in the culture by daily microscopic examination at 200–400x, for up to 7 days.
• Suitable media include so-called Diamond's TYM medium, which has a short shelf life but is inexpensive and highly selective for *T. foetus*, or a longer-lived commercially available culture system (InPouch, Biomed Diagnostics, White City, OR).
• The organism is identified by its morphology (~ 8–12 microns by 15–20 microns, spindle-shaped, with three anterior flagellae, a recurrent flagellum down one side (also known as the "undulating membrane")

and by its characteristic rolling, jerky motility. Because morphological assessment is subjective, some states are now requiring that all "positive" cultures be submitted to a laboratory certified to run a polymerase chain reaction (PCR) assay, for confirmation.
• Other trichomonads, including *Pentatrichomonas hominis* and *Tetratrichomonas* spp., have been identified in the preputial scrapings of bulls, especially young bulls. These non–T. *foetus* trichomonads are presumed to be nonpathogenic organisms of fecal origin.

Cows
• If pyometra is diagnosed at the time of herd pregnancy checks, pyometritic fluid can be an excellent source of *T. foetus*.
• If the examiner can pass an insemination pipette through the cervix, the pus that is aspirated can often be examined directly under the microscope for trichomonads, without culturing. It may be teeming with organisms. If not, the fluid may be cultured as for smegma.

IMAGING
Imaging is not often employed, but transrectal ultrasound exam may confirm palpation findings.

DIAGNOSTIC PROCEDURES
N/A

PATHOLOGIC FINDINGS
Bull
• Virtually no inflammatory lesions are attributable to *T. foetus* infection.

• Using immunohistochemical staining techniques, it is possible to identify *T. foetus* and/or its surface antigen adhered to the surface of the preputial and penile squamous epithelium.
Cow
• Typically, in the 95% of cases where pyometra is not found, there are few if any gross lesions.
• Histologic lesions are not pathognomonic, and include a mild-to-moderate infiltration of neutrophils and eosinophils in the layer immediately below the endometrial surface epithelium (stratum compactum), and in the glandular portions (stratum spongiosum).
• After about 6–9 weeks of infection, many females will show aggregations of mononuclear cells in the stratum spongiosum that resemble lymphoid follicles.
• Minor erosions of the surface epithelium may be noted.

 TREATMENT

Nonpharmacological
Females
The females in an infected beef herd should be divided into the following groups:
• A "safe in calf" group that is 5 months pregnant or more. These are very unlikely to still be infected or to lose their calves due to *T. foetus*.

TRICHOMONIASIS (TRICHOMONOSIS)

• A "worry" group that is pregnant less than 5 months. These should be housed/pastured separately, and observed frequently for signs of abortion (elevated tails, sticky discharge on tail hairs, exposed fetal membranes, etc.).
• Nonpregnant cows and heifers. Ideally, these should be sold for slaughter. If this is not economically appropriate, then divide this group into two further groups:
  • Abnormal reproductive tract, based on palpation findings. Cull these immediately.
  • Normal reproductive tract. Keep these, vaccinate them according to label instructions, and rebreed them next season.

Bulls
• All bulls should be smegma cultured (see Follow-Up below) and infected animals should be culled.
• Many states require that such bulls be clearly identified and sold only for slaughter.

ACTIVITY
N/A

DIET
N/A

CLIENT EDUCATION
The client must be made to understand that no treatments are both legal and efficacious (see Drugs of Choice section below). Risk factors should be made clear.

SURGICAL CONSIDERATIONS
N/A

MEDICATIONS

DRUGS OF CHOICE
• There is no legal, efficacious treatment for infected animals. Several years ago, the substituted imidazoles (metronidazole, dimetridazole, ipronidazole) were successfully used in infected bulls, but this entire family of compounds was declared not only off-label but also illegal by the FDA.
• Practitioners who use any of these compounds in cattle may be subject to arrest and imprisonment.

CONTRAINDICATIONS
N/A

PRECAUTIONS
N/A

POSSIBLE INTERACTIONS
N/A

ALTERNATIVE DRUGS
N/A

FOLLOW-UP

• Test all bulls immediately before next breeding season. Given the modest 80%–90% sensitivity of the culture test, consider multiple tests/bull (e.g., three tests at weekly intervals.
• Vaccinate all females twice at 1-month interval, just before bull exposure.
• Monitor pregnancy rate and loss, checking twice, once early after bull removal and once after 5 months' gestation.
• Replace any infected bull with a virgin bull.

MISCELLANEOUS

• A commercial vaccine is available prepared from killed whole cells.
• Efficacy in females was shown when 61% of vaccinated females calved while only 31% of controls calved following a very strong challenge by intravaginal instillation of millions of live *T. foetus*, immediately following mating to an infected bull.
• Recommendations for its use are controversial, but there is some benefit in vaccinating if any of the factors mentioned above under Risk Factors exist.
• The vaccine manufacturer makes no claim for efficacy in bulls.

Suggested Reading
BonDurant, R. H. 1997. Pathogenesis, diagnosis, and management of trichomoniasis in cattle. *Vet Clin N Am Food Anim Pract*. 13:345–61.
Corbeil, L. B., BonDurant, R. H. 2001. Immunity to bovine reproductive infections. *Vet Clin N Am Food Anim Pract*. 17:567–83.
Kvasnicka, W. G., Hall, M., Hanks, D., Ebel, E., Kearley, B., Wikse, S. E. 1996. Current concepts in the control of bovine trichomoniasis. *Compendium on Continuing Education for the Practicing Veterinarian* 18 (4 Suppl): 105–25.
Rae, D. O., Crews, E., Greiner, E. C., Donovan, G. A. 2004. Epidemiology of *Tritrichomonas foetus* in beef bull populations in Florida. *Theriogenology* 61:605–18.

Author: Robert H. BonDurant

TRYPANOSOMIASIS

BASICS

OVERVIEW
• Caused by protozoa of the genus *Trypanosoma* that live in the blood and body fluids of their hosts
• Results in anemia, emaciation of animals, and loss of condition
• Transmission is by vectors (tsetse flies—*Glossina morsitans*, *G. palpalis*, *G. fusca*, and vampire bats) and through mechanical vectors of the genus *Tabanus*. Hematogenous equipment, such as needles and surgical instruments, can also transmit trypanosomes.
• Ruminants are widely known to be active reservoirs.
• Infections with trypanosomes result in diseases such as nagana, surra, Chagas' disease, and African sleeping sickness.

PATHOPHYSIOLOGY
• The protozoa multiply in the blood, tissue, or body fluids of the vertebrate host and are transmitted between vertebrate hosts through the saliva of blood-sucking flies as they feed.
• At the site of inoculation, there is a local skin reaction called a chancre.
• From here the trypanosomes reach the blood stream directly or through the lymphatic system.
• Parasitemia becomes apparent 10–14 days after inoculation.
• Trypanosome's success lies in its ability to evade the host's immune system by altering the antigenic nature of its surface-coat glucoproteins.

SYSTEMS AFFECTED
• Cardiovascular: intense anemia and edema in chronic cases
• Gastrointestinal: weight loss and, in some cases, diarrhea
• Nervous: meningoencephalitis, progressive weakness, and ataxia
• Musculoskeletal: weakness and emaciation
• Lymphatic: lymphadenopathy
• Reproductive: infertility and abortion
• Ophthalmic: keratoconjunctivitis

GENETICS
N/A

INCIDENCE/PREVALENCE
Unknown

GEOGRAPHIC DISTRIBUTION
Found in the subtropical and tropical areas of Africa, Asia, South and Central America

SIGNALMENT
Species
Cattle, sheep, goats, camels, llamas, and buffalo

Breed Predilections
N/A

Mean Age and Range
N/A

Predominant Sex
N/A

SIGNS
• There are no pathognomonic signs and the severity of the signs varies depending on the size of the inoculation dose, the species and strain of the trypanosomes, and breed and management of the host.
• Can present as an acute, subclinical, or chronic infection
• Acute: Anemia, intermittent fever, loss of condition, and abortion may be seen; decrease in milk production; some become inappetent with a stiff gait and die within a few weeks.
• Chronic: affected animals are anorexic, apathetic, and emaciated, and have ocular discharge and a dull coat. A marked jugular pulse develops, associated with pale mucous membranes and elevated respiratory and pulse rate. Although the animal continues to eat, it gradually loses weight and death occurs after several months due to heart failure.
• Subclinical: stress plays a prominent role in the disease process.

CAUSES AND RISK FACTORS
• Nagana or African trypanosomiasis: *Trypanosoma brucei*, *T. congolense*, *T. vivax*, and *T. simiae*—variety of animals affected. Transmitted cyclically by tsetse flies and mechanically by other biting flies
• Surra: *T. evansi*—horses and camels affected; transmitted mechanically by biting flies in Africa, Asia, South and Central America
• Found in subtropical and tropical locations; the risk factor is being exposed to vectors, such as tsetse flies, biting flies (tabanids), and vampire bats.

DIAGNOSIS

DIFFERENTIAL DIAGNOSIS
• Acute anthrax
• Anaplasmosis
• Babesiosis
• Theileriosis
• Hemorrhagic septicemia
• Gastrointestinal helminths (*Haemonchus*)
• Chronic malnutrition

CBC/BIOCHEMISTRY/URINALYSIS
• Decreased packed cell volume, erythrocyte count, and hemoglobin
• Leukopenia, neutropenia, lymphocytosis, and monocytosis
• Thrombocytopenia
• Metabolic acidosis

OTHER LABORATORY TESTS
Serology for other infectious diseases

IMAGING
N/A

DIAGNOSTIC PROCEDURES
• Microscopic examination (direct): wet mount of blood slides, thick and thin blood films stained with Giemsa, and stained lymph nodes
• Indirect method: antigen-detecting ELISA, indirect fluorescent antibody test
• Molecular test: species-specific DNA probes
• Subinoculation into experimental animals

PATHOLOGIC FINDINGS
Most findings are nonspecific but can include serous atrophy of fat, subcutaneous edema, emaciation, petechiation, and enlarged liver and spleen. The spleen may also be atrophied or normal in some cases depending on the severity of the disease. Other lesions include necrosis of the kidneys and heart muscle and a sore or chancre at the site of entry.

TREATMENT
• Supportive care
• Blood transfusion from known negative animals

MEDICATION

• Treating trypanosomiasis is expensive and not always successful. It is considered a foreign animal disease in the United States and should be reported immediately to authorities. In other countries, there are prophylactic treatments that have been used with some success.
• Diminazene aceturate (Berenil): 3.5–7 mg/kg body weight for *T. vivax* and *T. congolense*, well tolerated by ruminants, not so well by horses.
• Homidium bromide (ethidium) and homidium chloride (novidium) can be used at 1 mg/kg body weight for *T. vivax* and *T. congolense*.
• Isometamidium is another preferred drug to use against *T. vivax* and *T. congolense* in ruminants as a curative and prophylactic dose of 0.25–1 mg/kg body weight. Pyrithidium bromide is less widely used against *T. vivax* and *T. congolense* as prophylactic at 2 mg/kg body weight.
• Suramin may also be used against *T. brucei* as a curative and prophylactic drug at 10 mg/kg body weight in horses and camels.

CONTRAINDICATIONS

Appropriate milk and meat withdrawal times must be followed for all compounds administered to food-producing animals.

FOLLOW-UP

PATIENT MONITORING

Because reinfection can occur, monitor weight, appetite, temperature, and PCV.

PREVENTION/AVOIDANCE

• Vector control is recommended.
• Trypano-tolerance: certain breeds of African cattle are considerably more resistant to African trypanosomiasis than others. The mechanisms of trypano-tolerance have been extensively studied and it has been established that it has a genetic basis.

POSSIBLE COMPLICATIONS

N/A

EXPECTED COURSE AND PROGNOSIS

Due to the potential for reinfection, prognosis varies depending on the severity of infection and how rapidly it was detected and treated.

MISCELLANEOUS

ASSOCIATED CONDITIONS

N/A

AGE-RELATED FACTORS

Adult sheep between 1 and 4 years of age with 4 years of age being the norm; lambs are more susceptible to infection if exposed prior to 10 weeks of age.

ZOONOTIC POTENTIAL

• Chagas' disease: *T. cruzi*—occasionally pigs but mainly in dogs and humans susceptible; transmitted by sucking blood vectors in South and Central America and the southern parts of the United States.
• Human African trypanosomiasis in humans can be caused by *Trypanosoma brucei gambiense* (central and West Africa), which causes a latent chronic infection, and *Trypanosoma brucei rhodesiense* (southern and east Africa), which causes a more virulent acute infection.

PREGNANCY

African trypanosomiasis can be transmitted in utero from infected mothers resulting in abortion and perinatal death of the fetus.

RUMINANT SPECIES AFFECTED

Cattle, sheep, goats, camel, llamas, and buffalo

BIOSECURITY

Vector control is important although difficult in endemic areas.

PRODUCTION MANAGEMENT

Economic losses can arise from emaciated animals, mortalities, and the cost of vector-control programs.

SYNONYMS

African sleeping sickness
Chagas' disease
Nagana
Surra
Trypanosomiasis
Tsetse disease
Tsetse fly disease

SEE ALSO

Acute anthrax
Anaplasmosis
Babesiosis
Chronic malnutrition
Gastrointestinal helminths (*Haemonchus*)
Hemorrhagic septicemia
Theilerosis

ABBREVIATIONS

ELISA = enzyme-linked immunosorbent assay

Suggested Reading

Mare, C. J. 1998. Trypanosomiasis. In: *Foreign animal diseases*. Richmond, VA: United States Animal Health Association, http://www.vet.uga.edu/wpp/gray`book/FAD.
Trypanosomiasis. 1998. In: *Merck veterinary manual*, 8th ed., ed. S. E. Aiello. Whitehouse Station, NJ: Merck and Co.
Uilenberg, G. 1998. *A field guide for the diagnosis, treatment and prevention of African animal trypanosomosis*. Rome: Food and Agriculture Organization of the United Nations.

Authors: Yessenia Almeida and Danelle Bickett-Weddle

TUBERCULOSIS: BOVINE

 BASICS

OVERVIEW

• Bovine tuberculosis (bovine TB) is caused primarily by the bacterium *Mycobacterium bovis*.
• Bovine TB is a reportable disease in the United States (as well as many countries internationally) for which an ongoing national eradication program is in place. The disease is found in all parts of the world.
• Bovine TB primarily affects the respiratory tract and associated lymph nodes. Disseminated bovine TB can be found in other organ systems including the gastrointestinal tract, reproductive tract, mammary glands, and central nervous system.
• *Mycobacterium bovis* infections have been described in numerous domestic and wild animals including sheep, goats, horses, pigs, deer, antelope, dogs, cats, ferrets, camels, foxes, mink, badgers, rats, primates, llamas, kudus, elands, tapirs, elk, elephants, sitatungas, oryxes, addaxes, rhinoceroses, opossums, ground squirrels, otters, seals, hares, moles, raccoons, coyotes, lions, tigers, leopards, and lynx.
• Most species other than cattle are considered to be dead end hosts; however, some species can serve as reservoir hosts. Known reservoir hosts include brush-tailed opossums in New Zealand; badgers in the United Kingdom and Ireland; deer in the United States; bison in Canada; and greater kudu, common duiker, African buffalo, warthogs, and Kafue lechwe in Africa.
• Bovine TB can be transmitted either by the respiratory route or ingestion.
• Mycobacterium bovis is a zoonotic agent and is a significant public health concern.

SIGNALMENT

Bovine TB can affect all ages of cattle.

SIGNS

• Bovine tuberculosis is usually a chronic debilitating disease but can occasionally be acute and rapidly progressive.
• Early infections are often asymptomatic.
• In the late stages, common symptoms include progressive emaciation, a low-grade fluctuating fever, weakness, and inappetence.
• Animals with pulmonary involvement usually have a moist cough that is worse in the morning and during cold weather or exercise, and may have dyspnea or tachypnea.
• In some animals, the retropharyngeal or other lymph nodes enlarge and may rupture and drain.
• Greatly enlarged lymph nodes can obstruct blood vessels, airways, or the digestive tract. Airway obstruction can lead to severe dyspnea.
• If the digestive tract is involved, intermittent diarrhea and constipation may be seen. Lesions are sometimes found on the female genitalia but are rare on the male genitalia. In cats, skin lesions similar to those of feline leprosy may be seen.
• Mammary gland involvement typically results in induration and hypertrophy of the affected gland and enlargement of the supramammary lymph nodes.

CAUSES AND RISK FACTORS

• Bovine TB is caused primarily by the bacterium *Mycobacterium bovis*.
• *M. bovis* can survive for several months in the environment, particularly in cold, dark, and moist conditions.
• The major risk factor for infection with bovine TB is exposure to infected reservoirs.

 DIAGNOSIS

DIFFERENTIAL DIAGNOSIS

• Other causes of chronic respiratory disease—*Mycoplasma bovis*, chronic lung abscesses, aspiration pneumonia
• Other causes of chronic weight loss and ill thrift—Johne's disease, parasitism, and bovine leukosis

CBC/BIOCHEMISTRY/URINALYSIS
N/A

OTHER LABORATORY TESTS
N/A

IMAGING
N/A

OTHER DIAGNOSTIC PROCEDURES

• Caudal fold tuberculin test (CFT)—an intradermal skin test that is used as an initial screening test. In the United States, an accredited veterinarian must administer this test.
• Comparative cervical test (CCT)—an intradermal skin test used most commonly as a follow-up to the CFT test to differentiate immune responses to *Mycobacterium bovis* and *Mycobacterium avium*. In the United States, only a state or federal veterinarian can perform this test.
• *Mycobacterium bovis* gamma interferon assay—an assay used most commonly as a follow-up to the CFT test

GROSS FINDINGS

• The characteristic gross lesion seen in an animal infected with bovine TB is the presence of granulomatous tubercles within the body. A tubercle is a white nodule usually 1 mm to 2 cm in diameter.
• Tubercles may be localized to a single organ or disseminated through many organ systems.
• Bovine TB tubercles are most commonly found in the thoracic cavity and associated lymph nodes.

HISTOPATHOLOGICAL FINDINGS

• The lesion most commonly associated with bovine TB is a granuloma.
• Following acid-fast staining of suspect tissue, bacteria that take up stain, including *Mycobacterium bovis*, will appear as short red or pink rods when examined under a microscope.

TREATMENT

Bovine TB is a controlled disease. Animals diagnosed with the disease are humanely euthanized.

MEDICATIONS

N/A

CONTRAINDICATIONS

N/A

FOLLOW-UP

PATIENT MONITORING

N/A

PREVENTION/AVOIDANCE

Bovine TB is considered a herd disease; therefore, emphasis is placed on preventing the introduction of the disease into a farm. Biosecurity procedures should be put in place that prevent the introduction of cattle at high risk of having bovine TB and to prevent potential wildlife reservoirs, such as white-tailed deer, from having close contact with cattle, their feed or water.

POSSIBLE COMPLICATIONS

N/A

EXPECTED COURSE AND PROGNOSIS

Cattle infected with bovine TB are humanely destroyed. Farms where bovine TB–positive animals originate are considered infected and are subsequently quarantined. Disposition of these herds is decided upon by the regulatory authorities governing TB control in that area.

MISCELLANEOUS

ASSOCIATED CONDITIONS

N/A

AGE-RELATED FACTORS

N/A

ZOONOTIC POTENTIAL

Mycobacterium bovis is a zoonotic agent that historically was spread primarily thru the consumption of unpasteurized milk from infected cows. Other potential routes of zoonotic transmission include consumption of undercooked meat and close contact with infected cows. Pasteurization has helped eliminate many human infections, but each year, cases occur in people, primarily those consuming imported cheeses from countries that do not pasteurize their products.

PREGNANCY

In cattle with advanced bovine TB, fetal infection can occur resulting in calves being born infected with bovine TB.

RUMINANT SPECIES AFFECTED

Bovine; potentially all ruminants

BIOSECURITY

N/A

PRODUCTION MANAGEMENT

N/A

SYNONYMS

SEE ALSO

Tuberculosis: small ruminant
Vaccinology

ABBREVIATIONS

CCT = comparative cervical test
CFT = caudal fold tuberculin test
TB = tuberculosis

Suggested Reading

Fraser, H. 2004, Sep 11. Bovine TB. *Vet Rec.* 155(11):344.

Koo, H. C., Park, Y. H., Ahn, J., Waters, W. R., Hamilton, M. J., Barrington, G., Mosaad, A. A., Palmer, M. V., Shin, S., Davis, W. C. 2004, Nov. New latex bead agglutination assay for differential diagnosis of cattle infected with *Mycobacterium bovis* and *Mycobacterium avium* subsp. *paratuberculosis. Clin Diagn Lab Immunol.* 11(6):1070–74.

Palmer, M. V., Waters, W. R., Whipple, D. L. 2004, Nov. Investigation of the transmission of *Mycobacterium bovis* from deer to cattle through indirect contact. *Am J Vet Res.* 65(11):1483–89.

Thoen, C. O., Huchzermeyer, H., Himes, E. M. 1995. *Mycobacterium bovis infection in animals and humans.* Ames: Iowa State University Press.

Author: Daniel L. Grooms

TUBERCULOSIS: SMALL RUMINANTS

BASICS

OVERVIEW
• Tuberculosis is a disease of great historical significance in both humans and domestic animals. Goats and sheep are rarely infected, but when it occurs, *Mycobacterium bovis* is usually the causative agent. Recently, a new subspecies *Mycobacterium bovis* subsp. *caprae* has been found to infect goats in Europe.
• Compared to sheep, goats are quite susceptible to *M. bovis*. If they are infected, goats demonstrate clinical signs similar to cattle.
• Even though goats and sheep appear to have high resistance to infection with *M. bovis*, goats are thought to act as spreaders for other species.
• *M. tuberculosis*, the human infection, accounts for a small proportion of tuberculosis cases in animals.

PATHOPHYSIOLOGY
• The organism usually enters through the respiratory route, occasionally by ingestion.
• From the site of entry, the organism invades the local lymph nodes (bronchial, mediastinal, pharyngeal, mesenteric) where it causes necrosis surrounded by a granuloma containing mononuclear cells.
• Dissemination occurs to various organs and may result in diffuse miliary tuberculosis.

SYSTEMS AFFECTED
Production management, gastrointestinal, respiratory, and, occasionally, urogenital

GENETICS
N/A

INCIDENCE/PREVALENCE
N/A

GEOGRAPHIC DISTRIBUTION
Worldwide depending on species and environment

SIGNALMENT
Species
• Potentially all ruminant species
• *Mycobacterium bovis* subsp. *caprae* has been isolated from cattle, wild boar and pigs.

Breed Predilections
N/A

Mean Age and Range
N/A

Predominant Sex
N/A

SIGNS
• The disease is chronic and slowly progressive, which can gradually cause debilitation, emaciation, and depression.
• Bronchopneumonia is the most common form of the disease in livestock and it is manifested by cough and terminal dyspnea.
• Some goats have intestinal ulceration, diarrhea, and enlargement of the lymph nodes of the alimentary tract.
• Infection in sheep is rare—lesions in lymph nodes or the GI tract.

CAUSES AND RISK FACTORS
• Etiological agent is *Mycobacterium* spp.—gram-positive, acid-fast bacterial rods
• Risk factors—housing can predispose to the spread of disease. A crowded condition with inadequate ventilation increases the risk of transmission.
• The incidence may be as high as 70% for goats in an infected herd.

DIAGNOSIS

DIFFERENTIAL DIAGNOSIS
• Progressive pneumonia
• Pulmonary adenomatosis
• Caseous lymphadenitis lesions

CBC/BIOCHEMISTRY/URINALYSIS
There are no specific clinical pathology data typical for this disease in small ruminants.

OTHER LABORATORY TESTS
• Caudal fold tuberculin test (CFT): measures the immune response to *Mycobacterium bovis* and can be performed only by an accredited veterinarian. The test is achieved by injecting 0.1 ml of USDA Purified Protein Derivative (PPD) tuberculin within the layers of skin of the caudal tail fold. The same veterinarian should read the test 72 hours after the inoculation and the site should be inspected for swelling or discoloration.

• Comparative cervical tuberculin test (CCT): is designed to determine if the response noted on the CFT is due to a *Mycobacterium bovis* or *Mycobacterium avium* infection. The test must be performed by an accredited state or federal veterinarian and it consists of an intradermal injection of a biologically balanced bovine PPD tuberculin and avian PPD tuberculin at separate sites in the cervical (neck) area. At 72 hours after the inoculation, the same veterinarian should measure the swelling of each injection site and plot them on a CCT scattergram.
• Identification of the organism in aspiration or biopsies of affected organs using acid-fast staining, histopathological examination, bacterial culture, or PCR.
• In one study, the sensitivity and specificity results were high for the comparative intradermal skin (CID) test (83.7%, 100%), the IFN-gamma assay (83.7%, 96%), and the anamnestic ELISA (88.6%, 95.8%). In contrast, they were comparatively low for the standard ELISA (54.9%, 88%). However, test results with the standard ELISA were positive in a group of goats with cavitating TB (100%). A combination of the CID test and the IFN-gamma assay offered the highest sensitivity, 95.8%, and also high specificity, 96%. In spite of this, the evidence that the serological tests were most sensitive for the detection of goats with severe lesions (100% positivity) suggested that a combination of CID test and anamnestic ELISA may be most useful as part of an eradication campaign against caprine TB.

IMAGING
Depending on the location of the suspected lesion, radiography and ultrasonography may demonstrate the presence of tubercles within the body and are used to evaluate the extent of the infection.

OTHER DIAGNOSTIC PROCEDURES
• Caudal fold tuberculin test
• Comparative cervical tuberculin test
• Necropsy
• Histopathology
• ELISA testing

PATHOLOGIC FINDINGS

• Tuberculosis granulomas—in any lymph nodes (especially in the bronchial, mediastinal, and mesenteric nodes) and in a variety of organs (particularly in the liver and lungs)
• Infected organs may be riddled with small miliary tubercles.
• Lungs—suppurative bronchopneumonia

TREATMENT

Since tuberculosis is a contagious disease of both animals and humans, the most effective and recommended way of handling this disease is by control and eradication (test and slaughter).

MEDICATIONS

N/A

FOLLOW-UP

PATIENT MONITORING
N/A

PREVENTION/AVOIDANCE
• All goats and sheep should be tested against tuberculosis.
• Reactors should be quarantined and identified and must be sent to an approved slaughter plant or euthanized under regulatory supervision.
• The origin of the reactors will be traced and these herds should be tested for tuberculosis.

POSSIBLE COMPLICATION
N/A

EXPECTED COURSE AND PROGNOSIS
As therapy is not an option, the prognosis is grave and a recommendation for euthanasia would be appropriate.

MISCELLANEOUS

ASSOCIATED CONDITIONS
From the site of entry, the organism invades the local lymph nodes (bronchial, mediastinal, pharyngeal, mesenteric) where it causes necrosis surrounded by a granuloma containing mononuclear cells.

AGE-RELATED FACTORS
N/A

ZOONOTIC POTENTIAL
• Tuberculosis is a zoonotic disease. Care must be taken in the collection of laboratory samples and the diagnosis of affected animals.
• Tuberculosis is a "historical disease" that is still endemic/enzootic throughout large regions of the world and highly zoonotic.
• *M. tuberculosis*, the human infection, accounts for a small proportion of tuberculosis cases in animals.

PREGNANCY
N/A

RUMINANT SPECIES AFFECTED
Small ruminants; potentially all ruminant species can be affected.

BIOSECURITY
• Isolation and quarantine of new stock entering the herd/flock
• Cull reactor animals prior to herd introduction.

PRODUCTION MANAGEMENT
Control and eradication (test and slaughter)

SYNONYMS
TB

SEE ALSO
• Bovine tuberculosis
• Zoonotic disease agents

ABBREVIATIONS

CCT = comparative cervical tuberculin test
CFT = caudal fold tuberculin test
CID = comparative intradermal skin test
ELISA = enzyme linked immunosorbent assay
GI = gastrointestinal
IFN = gamma interferon test
PPD = purified protein derivative tuberculin
TB = tuberculosis
USDA = United States Department of Agriculture

Suggested Reading
Acosta, B., Real, F., Leon, L., Deniz, S., Ferrer, O., Rosario, I., Ramirez, A. 2000, Jun. ELISA for anti-MPB70: an option for the diagnosis of goat tuberculosis caused by *Mycobacterium bovis. Aust Vet J*. 78(6):423–24.
Coleman, J. D., Cooke, M. M. 2001. *Mycobacterium bovis* infection in wildlife in New Zealand. *Tuberculosis* (Edinb). 81(3):191–202.
Cousins, D. V. 2001, Apr. *Mycobacterium bovis* infection and control in domestic livestock. *Rev Sci Tech*. 20(1):71–85.
Gutierrez, M., Tellechea, J., Garcia Marin, J. F. 1998, Aug 15. Evaluation of cellular and serological diagnostic tests for the detection of *Mycobacterium bovis*-infected goats. *Vet Microbiol*. 62(4):281–90.
Malone, F. E., Wilson, E. C., Pollock, J. M., Skuce, R. A. 2003, Dec. Investigations into an outbreak of tuberculosis in a flock of sheep in contact with tuberculosis cattle. *J Vet Med B Infect Dis Vet Public Health* 50(10):500–504.
Thorel, M F., Huchzermeyer, H., Weiss, R., Fontaine, J. J. 1997, Sep-Oct. *Mycobacterium avium* infections in animals. Literature review. *Vet Res*. 28(5):439–47.

Author: Yessenia Almedia

ULCERATIVE POSTHITIS

BASICS

OVERVIEW
• Synonyms: enzootic balanoposthitis, pizzle rot, sheath rot
• Ulcerative posthitis is an infectious urogenital disease of the external genitalia affecting both male and female small ruminants.
• It is caused by an aerobic, gram-positive, rod-shaped bacterium, *Corynebacterium renale.*
• These bacteria are a normal inhabitant of the skin and external genitalia of small ruminants and may be spread venereally.
• The bacteria can survive up to 6 months in wool and scabs; can survive freezing in exudates.
• *C. renale* proliferates on genital mucosa in the presence of urea, which increases in concentration in the urine of animals fed high protein and NPN diets.
• *C. renale* hydrolyses urea to ammonia, resulting in necrosis of surrounding tissue.

SIGNALMENT
• Male and female small ruminants may be affected.
• Males affected more commonly than females
• Most common in rams, Angora wethers, and pet wethers
• Most common breeds: Merinos and Angoras, due to dense wool
• Usually adult animals; animals under 6 months of age occasionally affected

SIGNS
• Rams, bucks, and wethers:
  • Moist ulcers at the mucocutaneous junction of prepuce early on
  • Followed by thin, brown, malodorous scab
  • Focal swelling of prepuce
  • Pain
  • Infection may spread inward, affecting entire length of prepuce.
  • Entire prepuce may be swollen and elongated.
  • Malodorous exudate consisting of necrotic tissue and urine present in the preputial orifice
  • Fibrinous or fibrous adhesions between penis and prepuce
  • Stenosis of preputial orifice
  • Dysuria (Vocalization during urination in goats; stricture of vermiform appendage may occur.)
  • Stilted gait
  • If chronic, weight loss
  • Bucks that transmit the bacteria may be asymptomatic.
• Does and ewes:
  • Ulcerative lesions of perineum and vulva
  • Vulvar swelling
  • Dysuria if urethral orifice affected by infection and inflammation
  • Fibrosis and contracture of vulva when long standing

CAUSES AND RISK FACTORS
• High protein level in diet
  • Generally when greater than 16 to 18%, but has been reported on 12% protein rations
  • Legume pastures: thick fiber, wet grasses, venereal spread

DIAGNOSIS

DIFFERENTIAL DIAGNOSIS
• Herpesvirus and *Actinobacillus seminis* have also been reported to cause ulcerative posthitis lesions.
• Obstructive urolithiasis and/or urethral rupture
• Preputial trauma
• Ulcerative dermatosis—lesions present on sheath, vulva, legs, lips, eyes
  • Sheep—poxvirus
• Contagious ecthyma (orf)

CBC/BIOCHEMISTRY/URINALYSIS
If lesions causing urinary outflow obstruction: increased BUN, creatinine, and potassium

OTHER LABORATORY TESTS
• Culture and sensitivity can be helpful in the selection of appropriate antibiotic therapy.
• Gram stain

IMAGING
N/A

DIAGNOSTIC PROCEDURES
• Diagnosis generally based on physical examination and lesion characteristics
• May culture lesions
• Biopsy

GROSS FINDINGS
Ulceration and swelling of external genitalia

HISTOPATHOLOGICAL FINDINGS
• Lesions consistent with primary bacterial inflammation with mucosal ulceration
• If herpes etiology: acidophilic intranuclear inclusion bodies, chromatin margination in epithelial cells adjacent to ulcers

TREATMENT

- Isolate affected individuals
- Shear wool or hair around external genitalia to allow air flow
- Reduce protein or NPN levels in diet to less than 16%
- May effect a cure if alone if lesions are early
- Sheath irrigation with antiseptic solutions
- Surgery
  - Lesion debridement
  - Preputial resection to allow urine flow and possible return to breeding after infection cleared
  - Salvage procedure: aseptically make 2–4-cm incisions through ventral skin and into prepuce to allow drainage and lavage.

MEDICATIONS

DRUGS OF CHOICE

- Topical antibiotic application: avoid irritating or caustic solutions
- Systemic penicillin or tetracycline: treat until lesions are dry and inflammation reduced

CONTRAINDICATIONS

- Xylazine should not be used in an animal with suspected or known urinary obstruction; xylazine induces hyperglycemia and diuresis and may lead to urinary bladder rupture if the obstruction is not relieved.
- Avoid iodine-based preparations for sheath lavage in breeding animals as it encourages the formation of adhesions and granulation tissue.
- Appropriate milk and meat withdrawal times must be followed for all compounds administered to food-producing animals.

FOLLOW-UP

PATIENT MONITORING

Patients must be closely monitored to ensure patency of urinary tract.

PREVENTION

- Reduce protein in feeding regimen to less than 16%: may feed grass hay to manage intake of high protein feeds
- Shear at times of high protein intake
- Isolate affected animals
- Increase water availability
- May include ammonium chloride in feed to reduce urine pH
- May include chlortetracycline in feeding regimen

POSSIBLE COMPLICATIONS

- Males
  - Loss of breeding soundness due to adhesion of penis to prepuce
  - Scarring of preputial orifice
  - Urethral obstruction
  - Urethritis
- Females
  - Loss of breeding soundness due to impaired vulvar conformation
  - Urine scalding

EXPECTED COURSE AND PROGNOSIS

- If recognized prior to fibrosis, may have a good chance of full recovery with appropriate medical and dietary management
- Internalized infection: return to breeding soundness unlikely

MISCELLANEOUS

ASSOCIATED CONDITIONS

- Loss of breeding soundness due to adhesion of penis to prepuce
- Scarring of preputial orifice
- Urethral obstruction

AGE-RELATED FACTORS

- Generally rare in animals less than 6 months of age
- Generally a disease seen in adults

ZOONOTIC POTENTIAL

None

PREGNANCY

Fibrosis of vulva may be severe enough to cause dystocia.

RUMINANT SPECIES AFFECTED

- Small ruminants
- May be rarely seen in cattle

BIOSECURITY

- Isolation of affected individuals from herd or flock is indicated.
- Separate males and females
- Burn wool of affected animals

PRODUCTION MANAGEMENT

Shear animals at times of high protein intake

SEE ALSO

- Contagious ecthyma (orf)
- Obstructive urolithiasis
- Ulcerative dermatosis

ABBREVIATIONS

- BUN = blood urea nitrogen
- NPN = nonprotein nitrogen

Suggested Reading

Belknap, E. B., Pugh, D. G. 2002. Diseases of the urinary system: Ulcerative posthitis. In: *Sheep and goat medicine*, ed. D. G. Pugh. Philadelphia: W. B. Saunders.

Mickelsen, W. D., Meman, M. A. 1997. Infertility and diseases of the reproductive organs of bucks: Posthitis. In: *Current therapy in large animal theriogenology*, ed. R. S. Youngquist. Philadelphia: W. B. Saunders.

VanMetre, D. C., Divers, T. J. 2002. Ulcerative posthitis and vulvitis. In: *Large animal internal medicine*, ed. B. P. Smith, 3rd ed. St. Louis: Mosby.

Author: Meredyth Jones

UMBILICAL HERNIA

 BASICS

OVERVIEW
• An umbilical hernia is a protrusion of abdominal contents through a defect in the body wall at the umbilicus. The hernial sac is covered with skin and subcutaneous tissue.
• Umbilical hernias are the most common congenital defect in cattle, and are commonly seen in llamas and alpacas. Although they are a recognized congenital defect in sheep and goats, they are generally considered to be rare.
• In cattle and small ruminants, a portion of the abomasum and/or greater omentum is commonly found within the hernial sac. Omentum is also found in umbilical hernias in South American camelids (SACs). The small intestine is rarely found in umbilical hernias in cattle. The greater omentum is less substantial in llamas; therefore, the small intestine is more commonly herniated in SACs than in cattle.
• Infection of umbilical remnants is common in calves with umbilical hernias, with as many as 45% of calves with umbilical hernias having evidence of associated infection.
• Concurrent infection is uncommon in small ruminants and SACs with umbilical hernias.
• Successful management of umbilical swellings depends upon accurately determining the contents of the swelling as well as determining how far the external problem extends internally.

SIGNALMENT
• Umbilical hernias occur most commonly in calves, lambs, kids, and crias as congenital defects. The vast majority are recognized in the first 3 months of life.
• Umbilical hernias occur in all breeds of cattle, although Holstein cows are at increased risk. Beef breeds, especially Hereford and Aberdeen Angus, are at lower risk. Breed predispositions have not been reported in sheep and goats.
• Both females and males are affected, although heifer calves are more commonly reported to be affected than bull calves.

SIGNS
• Umbilical hernias are usually recognized in the first few days or weeks of life as completely reducible swellings, with a discretely palpable circumferential hernial ring.

• The size of the body wall defect varies, with few umbilical hernias in calves under 6 months of age being larger than 10 cm. Similarly, the size of the hernial sac can vary depending on the contents.
• The hernial sac may contain omentum, abomasum, or less commonly intestine, although it is difficult to distinguish the specific contents by external palpation. In some cases, the contents will be adhered to the hernial sac. Reduction of large hernias may be easier with the animal in lateral or dorsal recumbency.
• Animals with uncomplicated hernias usually grow normally, have no abnormal findings associated with the hernia on physical examination or laboratory evaluation, and do not show signs of gastrointestinal dysfunction.
• Animals with abomasal or third compartment outflow obstruction or strangulation of intestines may have irreducible hernias and can be depressed, dehydrated, and possibly anorectic. Abomasal-umbilical fistula can occur resulting in drainage of abomasal contents from the hernial sac, which will result in depression, dehydration, and metabolic derangements.
• Animals with infection of umbilical structures concurrently with umbilical hernias may appear unthrifty, be smaller than animals of comparable age, drain purulent material from the umbilicus, or show signs of pollakiuria

CAUSES AND RISK FACTORS
• Umbilical hernias are often found as congenital conditions, and they are considered to be heritable in cattle with dominant (with incomplete penetrance), recessive, and sporadic characteristics being proposed. In sheep, goats, llamas, and alpacas, a genetic cause has not been proven, but remains a possibility. It is considered likely in SACs. Females are generally not culled because of umbilical hernias. However, males to be used extensively for breeding should be free of congenital defects, including umbilical hernias, because of the potential to perpetuate the trait. Most bull studs will not accept bull calves with umbilical hernias present or repaired.
• Infection of umbilical remnants is common in calves, and umbilical infection is a risk factor for the development of umbilical hernia. Umbilical infection may cause weakening of the abdominal wall or slowing of closure of the umbilicus, resulting in hernia formation.

• Another possible cause of umbilical hernia, particularly in small ruminants, is excessive traction on the umbilicus during delivery, resulting in tearing of the abdominal wall. This can lead to an open umbilical hernia with concurrent eventration of intestine through the umbilicus.
• Calves that are born via cesarian section are at greater risk for umbilical infections and umbilical hernias. The risk may be even greater if the umbilical vessels are cut rather than allowed to break as the calf is delivered.
• Calves that result from "splitting" embryos, in vitro fertilization, and cloning techniques tentatively and anecdotally are at greater risk for umbilical infections and umbilical hernias. This may be due, in part, to the greater likelihood that these calves are delivered via cesarian section, the tendency for these calves to have increased gestational lengths, or other factors.

 DIAGNOSIS

DIFFERENTIAL DIAGNOSIS
• Other causes of swelling in the umbilical area include umbilical abscess, infection of external umbilical cord remnants, urethral rupture in males, cellulitis, or hematoma.
• If the swelling is reducible and the hernial ring can easily be palpated, then the hernia is most likely uncomplicated. However, this is not always the case and in no way rules out the possibility that there may be infection internally in one or more remnants of the umbilical structures, internal organs in the hernial sac, adhesions of internal organs to the hernial sac, or other indications for further diagnostic workup or surgical exploration.
• Signs suggestive that the hernia is complicated by infection include: purulent discharge from the swelling, a scab or "soft spot" at the ventral aspect of the swelling suggesting that it has or is about to drain, inability to palpate the external umbilical vessel remnant, external umbilical vessel remnant palpably enlarged, heat or pain upon palpation, swelling is firm.
• Urine dripping from the swelling, especially evident when the animal is actually urinating, is suggestive that the umbilical problem is complicated by patent urachus. Pollakiuria, in the absence of urine dripping from the swelling, may suggest the presence of a nonpatent urachal remnant.

• An omphalocele is a congenital defect in the body wall at the umbilicus in which eviscerated abdominal organs are covered by amnion rather than skin. If recognized and treated expediently, a successful outcome is possible. Omphalocele is a developmental problem that is not known to be heritable.
• Infection of the internal umbilical structures should be considered as a differential in any young "poor doer" or "failure to thrive" case.

CBC/BIOCHEMISTRY/URINALYSIS

• Neutrophil-lymphocyte reversal / neutrophilia, hyperglobulinemia, and hyperfibrinogenemia are all suggestive that the umbilical swelling is complicated by infection. The absence of elevations in these parameters does not, however, rule out that the swelling may be complicated by infection.
• These values will be normal in animals with uncomplicated umbilical hernias.
• Elevation of packed cell volume and total protein can occur because of dehydration in animals with abnormal umbilical fistulas, a rare condition that can occur after long-term incarceration of the abomasum in an umbilical hernia.
• Elevation of packed cell volume and total protein can also occur in animals with intestinal strangulation in an umbilical hernia.
• If an abscess is present in umbilical remnants or in the subcutaneous tissue in association with the hernia, total protein, globulin, and neutrophil levels may be increased, neutrophil:lymphocyte ratio may be reversed, and mild anemia may be present.

OTHER LABORATORY TESTS

• Other laboratory tests should also be normal in animals with uncomplicated umbilical hernias. However, if abomasal outflow obstruction occurs or if abomasal-umbilical fistula develops after long-term incarceration of the abomasum in the hernial sac, the animal will develop hypochloremic, hypokalemic metabolic alkalosis as determined by serum blood gas analysis and electrolyte measurement.
• With intestinal strangulation, affected animals may eventually develop metabolic acidosis associated with dehydration.
• Bacterial culture and sensitivity should be performed in animals with concurrent infection of umbilical remnants.

IMAGING

• Ultrasonographic examination of affected animals provides information that alters the clinician's intervention with great enough frequency to recommend its use.

• Ultrasonographic examination may:
  • Help to detect or rule out the infection status of the internal umbilical remnants.
  • Help to further clarify the extent to which internal umbilical structures are distended / infected.
  • Help to determine which viscera are present in the hernia.
  • Aid in the determination of the best therapeutic approach to an irreducible hernia.
  • Aid in the determination of the best therapeutic approach to an umbilical abscess.

DIAGNOSTIC PROCEDURES

• External palpation of the umbilical region will define the hernial ring, the size of the hernia, the reducibility of the hernia, and possibly the contents. In uncomplicated cases, the hernia should be completely reducible and have a discrete circumferential hernial ring.
• Edema, cellulitis, heat or pain on palpation, or drainage are not present in an uncomplicated hernia.
• Gentle palpation in lateral or dorsal recumbency is helpful in determining reducibility and in identification of any enlarged internal umbilical remnants.

TREATMENT

CONSERVATIVE MANAGEMENT

• Small hernias, less than 4 cm, often close spontaneously in calves during the first 3–4 months of life. Larger hernias tend to enlarge in proportion to the growth of the animal, and the hernial sac tends to become more pendulous.
• Resolution of small hernias without intervention also occurs commonly in lambs and kids. Therefore, surgery is performed based on the value of the animal, the likelihood that the intestine will become strangulated, and/or failure of the hernia to resolve spontaneously.
• It is common for 1-cm umbilical defects to be present in crias for up to 1 month. Many of these will resolve spontaneously; however, larger defects are unlikely to resolve without intervention.

NONSURGICAL MANAGEMENT

Options for nonsurgical management for small, uncomplicated hernias in young animals include abdominal support bandages placed for 2–4 weeks (in females), hernial clamps or bands, daily irritation of the hernial ring by reduction and digital palpation, and injection of irritants around the hernial ring. Generally, these are selected for economic reasons and/or convenience.

SURGICAL CONSIDERATIONS

• Surgical correction is the treatment of choice in large hernias, hernias with concurrent infection of umbilical remnants, nonreducible hernias, and hernias with adhesion of abdominal contents to the hernial sac, or hernias that have not resolved with nonsurgical treatments.
• Hernias containing small intestine should be repaired surgically as soon as possible to prevent intestinal strangulation.
• Surgical exploration and repair is indicated when any one of the following is true:
  • There is reason to suspect infection in the internal umbilical remnants.
  • The size of the hernia defect in the body wall is large enough to necessitate surgical correction.
  • The animal is highly valued by the owner.
• There is controversy regarding how large a hernia must be before surgery is indicated. In general, uncomplicated hernias less than 5 cm diameter can be expected to close without any intervention (though a support wrap facilitates the closure—see below).
• Hernias greater than 10 cm diameter should, if the animal has any reasonable value to the owner, be surgically repaired. Hernias between 5 and 10 cm diameter should be dealt with on a case-by-case basis and treated based upon suspected complicating factors (e.g., infection), the value of the animal, etc.
• Small, uncomplicated hernias may be treated by placing a circumferential bandage around the abdomen of the calf that maintains reduction of the hernia. The bandage is changed every 1 to 2 weeks until the hernia is healed. Bandaging is generally not possible in males.

UMBILICAL HERNIA

- It is advantageous to:
  - Place the calf in dorsal recumbency during bandaging so that the hernia remains reduced during the procedure.
  - Glue a piece of plastic (a piece of a 500-mL calcium bottle and Kamar glue work well) that is larger that the hernial ring to the skin under the wrap.
  - Use adhesive elastic tape for the bandage.
- Techniques of hernial extirpation involving elastic bands or clamps are generally not recommended.
- Because concurrent infection is common, open herniorrhaphy is generally the recommended surgical procedure. This involves removal of the hernial sac, evaluation and removal of the internal umbilical remnants, and direct apposition of incised margins of the hernia. Although closed herniorrhaphy, in which the hernial sac is not removed, may prevent abdominal contamination during surgery, it does not allow removal of umbilical remnants, and often takes longer, is more traumatic, and may provide a less secure body wall closure.
- In animals with particularly large hernias, prosthetic mesh repair may be necessary, although very few hernias require mesh to appose. The use of mesh is not recommended in animals with concurrent umbilical infection.
- Surgical correction of uncomplicated umbilical hernias can be performed using sedation (xylazine) and local infiltration of anesthetic (lidocaine or bupivacaine). Local anesthetic should be diluted 1:4 with sterile saline and the volume minimized when used in sheep and goats to prevent lidocaine toxicity.
- General anesthesia, either injectable (such as xylazine, ketamine, guaifenesin infusion), or inhalant anesthesia (halothane or isoflurane), is preferred when concurrent infection of umbilical remnants is suspected.

MEDICATIONS

- Tetanus prophylaxis should be given before surgical treatment or before placement of clamps or bands.
- Prophylactic antibiotic administration is not needed in uncomplicated herniorrhaphy; however, because of the possibility of concurrent infection in calves, the use of preoperative antibiotics, such as penicillin, is common. Antibiotics are continued postoperatively if infection of umbilical remnants is identified at the time of surgery, with the choice of antibiotic being based on the results of culture and sensitivity when they become available.
- Although most animals do not demonstrate overt signs of pain after herniorrhaphy, analgesic medication (e.g., flunixin meglumine 0.5–1.0 mg/kg SID to BID) should be considered, starting before surgery and continuing for at least 24 hours after surgery.
- While the umbilicus can be the portal of entry for environmental bacteria that cause bacteremia, meningitis, joint-ill, etc., the bacteria involved in the vast majority of umbilical abscesses is *Arcanobacter pyogenes* (formerly *Actinomyces pyogenes*, even formerly *Corynebacterium pyogenes*). A small fraction of umbilical abscesses are infected with *E. coli* and other organisms cause the balance.
- Therefore, antimicrobial therapy should be chosen based upon:
  - Activity against *Arcanobacter pyogenes*.
  - Pharmacologically likely to penetrate an abscess.
  - Low but real possibility that other, including gram-negative, organisms may be involved.
- Antimicrobial therapy may not ultimately affect the outcome of a simple external umbilical abscess.

CONTRAINDICATIONS

- Appropriate milk and meat withdrawal times must be followed for all compounds administered to food-producing animals.
- Goats are sensitive to the effects of lidocaine. Caution must be used to avoid toxicity. Local anesthetic should be diluted 1:4 with sterile saline and the volume minimized when used in sheep and goats to prevent lidocaine toxicity.
- Steroids should not be used in pregnant animals.

PRECAUTIONS

Holding a surgical candidate off all feed for 24 to 48 hours prior to and 24 hours after surgery greatly facilitates closure of large defects and decreases the likelihood of dehiscence.

FOLLOW-UP

- Activity in animals with umbilical hernias treated surgically should be restricted to stall confinement for a minimum of 2 weeks postoperatively. In animals with large hernias, restriction of activity should be longer, generally 4 weeks. In the rare instance when mesh repair is required, recommendations are for stall confinement for 4–8 weeks.
- Compliance with recommendations for restriction of activity is important but sometimes difficult. Inability to restrict activity may be associated with the development of postoperative incisional hernias.
- Hernia clamps or bands can dislodge and can result in acute evisceration of abdominal contents. Therefore, animals with clamps or bands should also have their activity restricted until healing is complete.
- Animals treated surgically or with clamps or bands should be evaluated in 2 weeks to remove sutures and evaluate the effectiveness of treatment.

• If abdominal bandages are used, they should be replaced as they loosen to ensure they continue to maintain reduction of the hernia.
• Surgery should be recommended in animals treated unsuccessfully with conservative treatments such as abdominal bandages.

PATIENT MONITORING

• All patients treated surgically should be monitored until recovery from anesthesia is complete, and the animal is able to stand without assistance.
• Surgical incisions should be monitored daily for swelling or discharge. Some swelling is normal, but should begin to decrease at about 4–5 days after surgery. Sudden swelling is likely indicative of incisional dehiscence and requires immediate evaluation and treatment.
• Discharge from the incision is not normal, and typically indicates infection in the subcutaneous tissue that should be treated with antibiotics based on bacterial culture and sensitivity and establishing drainage of the infected material by enlarging the opening in the skin after cleaning the site with an antiseptic solution such as povidone iodine or chlorhexidine.
• Hernial clamps or bands should be checked daily to be sure they remain securely attached. It is possible to incorporate intestine or abomasal wall in clamps or bands. Therefore, animals treated with clamps or bands should be monitored very closely in the first 24 hours for abdominal pain, obstruction, and other signs of gastrointestinal incarceration or dysfunction.

PREVENTION/AVOIDANCE

• In the event that multiple animals are affected on a given farm, it is indicated to pursue potential factors underlying the problem.

• Questions to be addressed include: Do the affected animals share common ancestors suggesting a genetic basis for the problem? Is the farm's protocol for ensuring adequate passive transfer of maternal antibodies appropriate and is it being followed? What are the conditions like in the maternity pen? What fraction of the cows actually calves in the maternity pen?

EXPECTED COURSE AND PROGNOSIS

• The prognosis for uncomplicated umbilical hernias repaired surgically is good to excellent. The most common complication is seroma formation at the incision, which will resolve without additional treatment.
• Small uncomplicated hernias also have a favorable prognosis for repair with hernial clamps or bands. The skin sloughs, and body wall defects generally heal in 7–14 days. Urine scalding of the skin often occurs in males treated with clamps or bands.
• Umbilical hernias associated with infection have a higher incidence of incisional complications, including infection and incisional hernia, as well as peritonitis. However, with proper surgical technique, the prognosis is still favorable.

 MISCELLANEOUS

ASSOCIATED CONDITIONS

Infection of umbilical remnants, umbilical abscess

AGE-RELATED FACTORS

Umbilical hernias are most often congenital and are usually recognized in the first week to month of life. Acquired umbilical hernias also develop in calves and are generally recognized in the first 3 months of life.

ZOONOTIC POTENTIAL

N/A

PREGNANCY

N/A

SEE ALSO

FARAD
Patent urachus
Umbilical abscess
Umbilical remnant infection

ABBREVIATIONS

BID = twice daily
FARAD = Food Animal Residue Avoidance Databank
SAC = South American camelids
SID = once daily

Suggested Reading

Baxter, G. M. 1989. Umbilical masses in calves: diagnosis, treatment, and complications. *Comp Cont Educ.* 11(4): 505–27.

Fowler, M. E. 1998. Herniorrhaphy. In: *Medicine and surgery of South American camelids.* 2nd ed. Ames: Iowa State University Press.

Pugh, D. G. 2002. Pathology of the umbilicus. In: *Sheep and goat medicine.* Philadelphia: W. B. Saunders.

Rings, D. M. 1995. Umbilical hernias, umbilical abscesses, and urachal fistulas. *Vet Clin North Am Food Anim Pract.* 11:137–48.

Steenholdt, C., Hernandez, J. 2004. Risk factors for umbilical hernia in Holstein heifers during the first two months after birth. *J Am Vet Med Assoc.* 224:1487–90.

Authors: Jill Parker and Lowell T. Midla

UREA TOXICITY

BASICS

DEFINITION
• Urea is considered an economical source of crude protein (CP) in ruminant diets.
• Utilization of urea by the ruminant animal is initiated by its microbial hydrolysis to two ammonia (NH_3) molecules and one carbon dioxide molecule in the rumen environment. This step is accomplished by urease from specific bacterial species such as *Succinivibrio dextrinosolvens*, *Prevotella ruminicola*, and *Ruminococcus bromii*.
• In the rumen, the NH_3 produced from dietary proteins, urea, or other nonprotein nitrogen (NPN) sources is further utilized for synthesis of bacterial amino acids and bacterial proteins. Utilization of NH_3 for bacterial protein synthesis is dependent upon availability of highly fermentable carbohydrate sources such as dietary starch.
• Excess NH_3 is absorbed through the rumen wall and is transferred to the liver for conversion to urea before excretion in the urine.
• Depending on the CP level of the diet, a variable amount of urea is recycled back to the rumen. This is achieved mainly through saliva and to some extent through diffusion across the rumen wall. Urea recycling is intended to increase NH_3 concentrations in the rumen to meet N requirements of the rumen bacteria.
• When the liver's ability to detoxify NH_3 to urea is exceeded, blood NH_3 concentrations are increased to lethal levels (i.e., urea toxicity).
• Urea toxicity is defined as a condition that occurs when large amounts of urea are ingested.
• The dietary urea levels required to induce toxic symptoms as well as the blood NH_3 concentrations associated with toxicity vary considerably. The conditions that may protect ruminants from urea toxicity are also quite variable. However, urea administration with the diet is less toxic than when administered separately. Younger ruminants are found to be more susceptible to toxicity than older ones.
• In general, urea is used widely in ruminant diets and intakes exceeding 0.45 g urea/kg of body weight are known to decrease feed intake and milk production in dairy cows and can induce toxicity.

• The most accurate indicator of urea toxicity is blood NH_3 concentrations.
• Blood NH_3 is toxic to animal cells at low concentrations and is responsible for cell death. Additionally, NH_3 is carcinogenic.
• Urea toxicity symptoms occur at blood concentrations greater than 0.5 mg/100 mL and become more severe at higher levels.
• Urea-induced death usually occurs when blood NH_3-N concentrations range from 2 to 4 mg/100 mL.

PATHOPHYSIOLOGY
• Following ingestion of large amounts of urea, a rapid release of NH_3 occurs.
• This increases the rumen pH to reach alkaline levels, which in turn supports high rates of NH_3 absorption through the rumen wall.
• Alkaline rumen environments (pH > 7.4), therefore, are considered the most important factor in inducing high blood NH_3 concentrations and toxicity.

SYSTEMS AFFECTED
CNS, musculoskeletal, gastrointestinal, respiratory

GENETICS
N/A

INCIDENCE/PREVALENCE
N/A

GEOGRAPHIC DISTRIBUTION
Worldwide, depending on species and production management

SIGNALMENT
Species
Potentially all ruminant species

Breed Predilections
N/A

Mean Age and Range
Younger ruminants are found to be more susceptible to toxicity than adults.

Predominant Sex
N/A

SIGNS

HISTORICAL FINDINGS
• Elevated concentrations of rumen NH_3 and the subsequent high concentrations of NH_3 in peripheral blood are the key characteristics of urea toxicity.

• Complications due to increased blood NH_3 concentrations include alkalosis, rapid uptake of NH_3 by the brain, and central nervous system damage.
• Clinical signs are apparent within 20 to 30 min following ingestion of a toxic urea dose.
• Death occurs within 4 hours.
• The clinical signs include respiratory difficulties (e.g., rapid and/or labored breathing), nervousness, muscular tremors, incoordination, excessive salivation, loss of ability to stand, bloat (due to reduction in rumen motility), and occurrence of tetany. The main cause of death appears to be respiratory arrest.
• The clinical signs of urea toxicity have been categorized into the following three stages: (1) The stage of depression and fatigue is associated with blood NH_3 concentrations ranging from 0.5 to 1.0 mg/100 mL. (2) The beginning of the stage of convulsion is associated with blood NH_3 concentrations ranging from 1.2 to 1.9 mg/100 mL. (3) The end of the stage of convulsion is associated with blood NH_3 concentrations ranging from 4.0 to 7.0 mg/100 mL. Damage of the brain stem and paralysis of the respiration center are usually responsible for death.

CAUSES AND RISK FACTORS
• Inadequate mixing of urea or urea-containing supplements with the remaining dietary ingredients may result in consumption of large urea doses at one time and can dispose the animal to urea toxicity.
• Feeding urea to animals that are not adapted to dietary supplementation of NPN such as urea, NH_3, and ammonium salts.
• Allowing free access to palatable sources of high-urea concentrates.
• Feeding poor-quality, forage-based diets.
• Use of urea in low-energy rations.
• Feeding urea-containing diets to cattle that are deprived of feed for extended periods of time (e.g., 24–48 hr)

TREATMENT

EARLY STAGES
• Oral administration of 5% acetic acid solution to neutralize excess rumen NH_3. This treatment is effective in increasing potential survival of the animal if it is performed prior to the onset of tetany.
• Oral administration of cold water to slow the rate of urea hydrolysis to NH_3 and to dilute its concentration in the rumen.

LATE STAGES
Evacuating the rumen after a stab incision in the paralumbar fossa area.

MEDICATIONS

CONTRAINDICATIONS
Appropriate milk and meat withdrawal times must be followed for all compounds administered to food-producing animals.

FOLLOW-UP

PREVENTION/AVOIDANCE
• Gradual adaptation to urea feeding (e.g., feeding urea to dairy cows at 0.34 g/kg of body weight was achieved after a 6-week adaptation period without inducing negative effects on feed intake, blood composition, milk production, or milk composition).
• Feeding readily fermentable carbohydrate sources (e.g., starch and molasses) in amounts that enable rumen bacteria to capture the released NH_3 for bacterial protein synthesis
• Uniform mixing of urea with the remaining dietary ingredients
• Maintaining a regular feeding schedule
• Feeding urea at rates not exceeding 33% of dietary CP

• Feeding liquid urea supplements with phosphoric acid to maintain acidic rumen environments and to decrease the rate of NH_3 absorption
• Coating urea with fat supplements to decrease its rate of hydrolysis to NH_3
• Extrusion of urea with concentrates such as grains also decreases its rate of hydrolysis.
• Use of urease inhibitors to slow the release of NH_3. These inhibitors include hydroxamic acids, especially caprylohydroxamic acid.
• Urea should not be added to diets that are already meeting the animal's CP requirements.
• The diet should contain sufficient amounts of calcium and phosphorus. The sulfur to N ratio in the diet also should not be less than 1:15. The diet should also contain sufficient amounts of trace minerals, especially cobalt and zinc.
• Feeding low-energy, high-fiber diets, especially poor-quality forages, should be avoided with urea feeding.

MISCELLANEOUS

ASSOCIATED CONDITIONS
N/A

AGE-RELATED FACTORS
Younger ruminants are found to be more susceptible to toxicity than older ones.

ZOONOTIC POTENTIAL
N/A

PREGNANCY
N/A

RUMINANT SPECIES AFFECTED
Potentially, all ruminant species are affected.

BIOSECURITY
N/A

PRODUCTION MANAGEMENT
• Urea administration with the diet is less toxic than when administered separately. Younger ruminants are found to be more susceptible to toxicity than older ones.
• In general, urea is used widely in ruminant diets and intakes exceeding 0.45 g urea/kg of body weight are known to decrease feed intake and milk production in dairy cows and can induce toxicity.

SYNONYMS
N/A

SEE ALSO
Toxicology: herd outbreaks, dairy cattle nutrition, beef cattle nutrition

ABBREVIATIONS
CP = crude protein
NH_3 = ammonia
NH_3-N = ammonia nitrogen
NPN = nonprotein nitrogen

Suggested Reading
Brazil, T. J., Naylor, J. M., Janzen, E. D. 1994, Jan. Ammoniated forage toxicosis in nursing calves: a herd outbreak. *Can Vet J.* 35(1):45–47.
Caldow, G. L., Wain, E. B. 1991, May 25. Urea poisoning in suckler cows. *Vet Rec.* 128(21):489–91.
Campagnolo, E. R., Kasten, S., Banerjee, M. 2002, Oct. Accidental ammonia exposure to county fair show livestock due to contaminated drinking water. *Vet Hum Toxicol.* 44(5):282–85.
Haliburton, J. C., Morgan, S. E. 1989, Jul. Nonprotein nitrogen-induced ammonia toxicosis and ammoniated feed toxicity syndrome. *Vet Clin North Am Food Anim Pract.* 5(2):237–49.
Villar, D., Schwartz, K. J., Carson, T. L., Kinker, J. A., Barker, J. 2003, Mar. Acute poisoning of cattle by fertilizer-contaminated water. *Vet Hum Toxicol.* 45(2):88–90.

Author: Hussein S. Hussein

UREAPLASMA

BASICS

OVERVIEW
• Ureaplasmas (formerly T-strain mycoplasmas) belong to the Mycoplasmataceae family of cell-wall deficient bacteria, which includes *Mycoplasma.*
• They are antigenetically diverse and species specific.
• *Ureaplasma diversum* is found only in cattle where it is a common inhabitant of respiratory and genital tracts.
• It has been implicated in a number of reproductive syndromes and it is assumed that it causes considerable loss under certain conditions, which have yet to be specified.
• The infective agent is *Ureaplasma diversum.*

INCIDENCE/PREVALENCE
• *U. diversum* is commonly isolated from the reproductive tract of apparently normal female cattle (60%–70%), particularly from the vulvar and vestibular regions.
• Breeding-age beef heifers tend to have the highest prevalence (70%–80%) while *U. diversum* has also been isolated from 1-month-old female calves (21%).
• It is also a common inhabitant of the bull reproductive tract (5– > 70%), particularly within the prepuce and distal urethra.
• The high prevalence rate of *U. diversum* in otherwise healthy cattle does not explain why problems occur under certain unspecified conditions, which are probably multifactorial.

GENETICS
Unknown

GEOGRAPHIC DISTRIBUTION
Unknown, potentially worldwide

SIGNALMENT
Species
All bovines are susceptible. *Ureaplasma diversum* is found only in cattle where it is a common inhabitant of respiratory and genital tracts.

Breed Predilections
N/A

Mean Age and Range
Breeding-age beef heifers tend to have the highest prevalence (70%–80%) while *U. diversum* has also been isolated from 1-month-old female calves (21%). Heifers appear to be particularly susceptible.

Predominant Sex
No sex predilection

Female
• *U. diversum* has been implicated in a number of reproductive tract disorders including granular vulvovaginitis, infertility, early embryonic loss, mid- to late-term abortion and birth of low-viability calves.
• Following experimental inoculation, granular vulvovaginitis resulted in 3–6 days followed by endometritis and salpingitis. *U. diversum* strains differ in pathogenicity as does female susceptibility.
• Heifers appear to be particularly susceptible.
• Although *U. diversum* may be cultured from prepubertal heifers, breeding activity appears to disseminate it more rapidly, suggesting that venereal transmission may occur.
• Clinical signs of granular vulvovaginitis caused by *U. diversum* include hyperemia of the vulval and vaginal mucosa, raised red to grey nodules, and, occasionally, a mild to marked mucopurulent discharge.

Male
U. diversum has been associated with granular balanoposthitis, and it has been suggested as a cause of seminal vesiculitis in bulls.

DIAGNOSIS

DIFFERENTIAL DIAGNOSIS
• Granular venereal disease caused by other organisms, including IBR/IPV virus
• Infertility caused by vibriosis or trichomoniasis
• Other causes of mid- to late-term abortion
• Other causes of balanoposthitis in bulls

CBC/BIOCHEMISTRY/URINALYSIS
N/A

OTHER LABORATORY TESTS
N/A

IMAGING
N/A

OTHER DIAGNOSTIC PROCEDURES
• Culture is the method of choice.
• Samples should be taken carefully to avoid contamination.
• The organism is fragile with samples requiring careful handling (preferably frozen) and specific transport media (Stuart broth or Ames without charcoal).
• Not all labs have the appropriate infrastructure for culture and identification.

PATHOLOGIC FINDINGS
• *Ureaplasma diversum* causes a reddening of the inside of the bovine vulva.
• The development of tiny fleshy bumps, a condition called granular vulvitis, occurs. This can persist for more than a year in affected females.
• Abundant mucous discharge can appear 4 to 5 days postinfection, but is fairly short in its duration.
• The pathological cause of *U. diversum* repeat breeding cycle is not known.
• The organism may cause death of the embryo soon after conception.

TREATMENT
• Treatment in most bovine herds is not practical.
• Most cows become fertile again within two or three cycles.
• Aggressive treatment is not usually recommended.
• A vaccine is not available.
• Eliminating the organism from the sheath of bulls is difficult.

MEDICATIONS

DRUGS OF CHOICE

CONTRAINDICATIONS
Appropriate milk and meat withdrawal times must be followed for all compounds administered to food-producing animals.

FOLLOW-UP

PATIENT MONITORING
• As the organism progresses in a herd, first service conception rates can fall to as low as 28%.
• Eventually conception rates improve to 85% or 90% of normal.

PREVENTION/AVOIDANCE
• Attempts to induce vaccinal immunity to *U. diversum* have not been successful.
• Use of a guarded sheath for AI pipettes has been suggested as a way to reduce infection into the uterus.
• Use of tetracycline, both as a postinseminate infusion (24 h) or orally (1.1 mg/kg/day) for 30 days over the breeding period, has resulted in improved reproductive rates in affected herds.

MISCELLANEOUS

ASSOCIATED CONDITIONS
N/A

AGE-RELATED FACTORS
Breeding-age beef heifers tend to have the highest prevalence (70%–80%) while *U. diversum* has also been isolated from 1-month-old female calves (21%).

ZOONOTIC POTENTIAL
N/A

PREGNANCY
• *U. diversum* has been implicated in a number of reproductive tract disorders including granular vulvovaginitis, infertility, early embryonic loss, mid- to late-term abortion, and birth of low-viability calves.
• Most cows become fertile again within two or three cycles.

RUMINANT SPECIES AFFECTED
Ureaplasma diversum is found only in cattle, where it is a common inhabitant of respiratory and genital tracts.

BIOSECURITY
A vaccine is not available.

PRODUCTION MANAGEMENT
• Treatment in most bovine herds is not practical.
• Aggressive treatment is not usually recommended.
• Eliminating the organism from the sheath of bulls is difficult.

SEE ALSO
Balanoposthitis
Bovine abortion
Seminal vesiculitis
Vulvovaginitis vibriosis or trichomoniasis

ABBREVIATIONS
IBR = infectious bovine rhinotracheitis
IPV = infectious pustular vulvovaginitis

Suggested Reading
Doig, P. A., Ruhnke, H. L., Palmer, N. C. 1979. Experimental bovine genital ureaplasmosis. I. Granular vulvitis following vulvar inoculation. *Can J Comp Med*. 44:242–58.

Rae, D. O., Chenoweth, P. J., Brown, M. B., Genho, P. C., Moore, S. A., Jacobsen, K. E. 1993. Reproductive performance of beef heifers: effects of vulvo-vaginitis, *Ureaplasma diversum* and pre-breeding antibiotic administration. *Theriogenology* 40:497–508.
Sanderson, M. W., Chenoweth, P. J. 1999. The role of *Ureaplasma diversum* in bovine reproduction. *The Compendium* 21:S98–S102
Sprecher, D. J., Coe, P. H., Walker, R. D. 1999, Apr 15. Relationships among seminal culture, seminal white blood cells, and the percentage of primary sperm abnormalities in bulls evaluated prior to the breeding season. *Theriogenology* 51(6):1197–206.
Thomas, A., Ball, H., Dizier, I., Trolin, A., Bell, C., Mainil, J., Linden, A. 2002, Oct 19. Isolation of mycoplasma species from the lower respiratory tract of healthy cattle and cattle with respiratory disease in Belgium. *Vet Rec.* 151(16):472–76.

Author: Peter Chenoweth

UROLITHIASIS IN SMALL RUMINANTS

 BASICS

OVERVIEW
• Obstructive urolithiasis is a frequent problem of sheep and goats most commonly occurring in males.
• Urinary calculi are formed proximally in the urinary tract and become lodged in the narrow urethra. It is a life-threatening situation and requires immediate attention.
• The composition of uroliths varies depending on diet and geography.
• Feedlot lambs and pet goats are most commonly affected.

PATHOPHYSIOLOGY
• The formation and composition of urinary calculi are dependent on geography and diet but are always composed of salts/minerals in an organic matrix (nidus) of proteinaceous material. Urine is normally highly saturated with mineral solutes. Multiple factors can cause these minerals to leave solution and precipitate in the urine.
• Complexes of phosphatic crystals are formed in situations of high-concentrate, low-roughage diet. Low dietary calcium to phosphorus ratios, high magnesium diets, and high phosphorus diets have all been implicated. The large amounts of phosphorus in a high grain diet overwhelm the salivary excretory mechanism and induce excretion by the renal system.
• In bucks, rams, and wethers, urethral calculi are most often found lodged in the urethral process, followed by the sigmoid flexure.

• Wethers are especially susceptible to obstruction at the urethral process due to the lack of testosterone effects on the urinary tract. At birth, the urethral process is attached to the preputial mucosa and gradually separates under the influence of testosterone.
• Additionally, testosterone increases urethral diameter.

SYSTEMS AFFECTED
• Renal/urologic: if a urine sample can be obtained, it may reveal hematuria, crystalluria, and proteinuria. Uncorrected urethral obstruction may lead to rupture of the bladder or urethra.
• Endocrine/metabolic: urethral obstruction may cause postrenal azotemia, hyperkalemia, or stress leukogram.
• Cardiovascular: tachycardia is often present. Additionally, hyperkalemia may cause cardiac arrhythmias.
• Skin/exocrine: scalding of the perineum and rear legs may be present. Rupture of the distal urethra may cause preputial and/or perineal edema.

GENETICS
The Texel sheep breed may be predisposed to increased renal excretion of phosphorus.

INCIDENCE/PREVALENCE
• Obstructive urolithiasis is well recognized in sheep wethers maintained in feedlot conditions and fed high-concentrate, low-forage diets.
• Wethers castrated at an early age are more susceptible due to a lack of testosterone driving development of the urethra and urethral process.

GEOGRAPHIC DISTRIBUTION
Silicate calculi are more commonly diagnosed in animals grazed on sandy soil, high in silica, conditions more frequently seen in the western parts of the United States and Canada.

SIGNALMENT
• Obstructive urolithiasis is most often seen in male sheep and goats both intact and castrated although castrated males are more likely affected (see Pathophysiology above).
• All ages are affected.

SIGNS
• Dysuria
• Stranguria
• Dribbling urine
• Vocalization
• Tail flagging
• Abdominal straining
• Abdominal pain (stretching, kicking at abdomen, flank watching)
• Abdominal distention
• Preputial/perineal edema
• Bruxism
• Anorexia, weakness, depression

CAUSES AND RISK FACTORS
• Ruminants fed high-grain diets are at increased risk.
• Additionally, dietary electrolyte imbalances, decreased water consumption/availability, and abnormal urine pH are risk factors.

 DIAGNOSIS

DIFFERENTIAL DIAGNOSIS
A hair ring present around the penis may cause signs of discomfort and dysuria similar to that seen with obstructive urolithiasis.

UROLITHIASIS IN SMALL RUMINANTS

Hematuria
- Bladder polyps
- Bracken fern toxicity
- Cystitis
- Infarction of kidney
- Papilloma
- Pyelonephritis
- Trauma
- Urethritis

Dysuria
- Actinomyces
- Cystitis
- Mycoplasma
- Orf
- Photosensitivity
- Sacral fracture
- Spinal cord injury
- Trauma
- Ulcerative balantitis and vulvitis

CBC/BIOCHEMISTRY/URINALYSIS
- A complete blood count may reveal a stress leukogram, mild to severe azotemia depending on duration, and hyperkalemia.
- Crystalluria, proteinuria, and hematuria may be present on urinalysis.

OTHER LABORATORY TESTS
If bladder rupture is suspected, an abdominal fluid to serum creatinine ratio can be performed. The ratio should be < 2:1 and if greater suggests urine leakage into the abdomen.

IMAGING
- An enlarged bladder is often visualized on right-sided abdominal or transrectal ultrasound.

- Echogenic material in the bladder or kidneys is occasionally visualized, but lack of this finding does not rule out the diagnosis. A large amount of free fluid (ascites) may also be visualized in the abdomen if the abdominal portion of the urinary tract is ruptured due to unresolved obstruction.
- Abdominal radiography may allow visualization of the calculi depending on composition.
- Calcium oxalate and calcium carbonate crystals are radiopaque while struvite (magnesium ammonium phosphate), apatite, and silicate crystals are radiolucent. Therefore, lack of radiographic visualization does not rule out the presence of obstructive calculi.
- Infusion of contrast media retrograde through a urethral catheter may allow visualization of calculi; however, urethral rupture/fistula formation or bladder rupture can occur.

DIAGNOSTIC PROCEDURES
- Diagnosis is largely based on history and physical examination findings, supported by alterations in serum chemistry (azotemia, hyperkalemia).
- Urethroscopy has recently been recognized as a modality for diagnosing urethral obstruction in ruminants.
- The presence of urine in the abdomen or subcutaneous tissues is confirmation of obstruction of the urinary tract with secondary rupture.

PATHOLOGIC FINDINGS
- Dissection of the urinary tract will reveal single to multiple calculi lodged along the extent of the tract. The tissues will be hyperemic, hemorrhagic, or necrotic depending on duration of disease.
- Bladder or urethral rupture may be present as well as hydroureter and hydronephrosis.

 TREATMENT

APPROPRIATE HEALTH CARE
Physical Examination
- The penis should be exteriorized and urethral process examined in all cases. This may be facilitated by sedation or lumbosacral epidural anesthesia.
- Sedation protocols include diazepam, at a dose range of 0.1–0.5 mg/kg IV, or acepromazine maleate 0.05–0.1 mg/kg IV.
- Acepromazine may promote relaxation of the retractor penis muscle.
- Lumbosacral epidural anesthesia can be performed to provide exteriorization of the penis by eliminating resistance by the retractor penis muscle. Lidocaine (2%) is used at a dose of 1 ml per 5 kg (not to exceed 15 ml).
- Once sedated and/or lumbosacral epidural has been given, the sheep or goat can be placed on its rump to allow easier extrusion of the penis. The penis is grasped through the skin at the base of the scrotum and forced cranially. Uroliths may be palpable in the urethra or urethral process (see Surgical Considerations below).

UROLITHIASIS IN SMALL RUMINANTS

NURSING CARE
• Treatment should be aimed at supportive care and correcting the obstruction.
• In cases of bladder rupture, urine can be drained from the peritoneum to reduce the effects of uremia and correct electrolyte imbalances. Drainage should be performed slowly to reduce the risk of circulatory shock, and intravenous fluids should be given concurrently.
• Intravenous fluids should be given judiciously in cases of complete obstruction. Choice of fluid therapy should be based on electrolyte imbalances. Intravenous fluids containing potassium should be avoided if hyperkalemia is present.

ACTIVITY
N/A

DIET
A low-carbohydrate, high-roughage diet with a balanced mineral content is essential to prevent occurrence of calculi.

CLIENT EDUCATION
• Many small ruminant owners do not know the importance of feeding a low-carbohydrate diet. Small ruminants will preferentially eat grain and owners should feed carbohydrates on a limited basis.
• Mineral supplementation should be done carefully, keeping with recommended ratios.

SURGICAL CONSIDERATIONS
Urethral Process Amputation
• If the obstruction is located in the urethral process, amputation may completely alleviate obstruction, as is the case in 37.5%–66% of cases.
• Amputation of the urethral process will not affect future breeding ability. This procedure does not prevent future obstruction if multiple calculi are present in the urinary tract.

Urethral Catheterization and Retrograde Flushing
• Catheterization of the bladder of a ruminant is difficult due to the sigmoid flexure and urethral recess. A catheter can be placed in the distal urethra while occluding the penis. Saline or a lidocaine-saline flush solution (one part lidocaine to three parts saline) is flushed retrograde through the catheter to lavage the calculi into the bladder.
• The disadvantages of this technique are that it is often unsuccessful, can cause trauma to the urethra if catheterization is overly aggressive, and, if successful, the calculus has been returned to the bladder for another chance to cause an obstruction.

Perineal Urethrostomy
• Perineal urethrostomy can be performed in the sedated animal with a lumbosacral epidural.
• Stricture, reduced reproductive ability, and reobstruction are common complications, and this option is best used as a temporary salvage procedure in animals intended for slaughter.

Tube Cystotomy
• Under general anesthesia, a laparotomy is performed placing an indwelling Foley catheter percutaneously into the bladder wall. The catheter is sutured in place to the abdominal wall enabling voiding of urine through the catheter. The bladder is lavaged to remove remaining calculi. The catheter is left in place to allow the urethra to heal and calculi to be expelled. Periodic challenging of urethral patency is performed until the urethral obstruction is resolved.
• This procedure is the best option for salvage of breeding function in intact males, but it does not prevent recurrence of obstruction.
• Tube cystotomy is the most expensive of the surgical options and is usually performed in pets and breeding animals.

Bladder Marsupialization
• A permanent bladder marsupialization can be performed in which the bladder is sutured to the ventral abdominal wall lateral to the prepuce through a laparotomy incision. This technique requires commitment by the owners as care and cleaning of the stoma are required for the life of the animal.
• Bladder marsupialization has the least chance of reobstruction by calculi but the stoma occasionally strictures and requires surgical modification.
• The breeding capabilities are questionable following this procedure.

UROLITHIASIS IN SMALL RUMINANTS

MEDICATIONS

DRUGS OF CHOICE
• Sedation can be given for examination and manipulation of the penis and urethral process.
• Diazepam, at a dose range of 0.1–0.5 mg/kg IV or acepromazine maleate 0.05–0.1 mg/kg IV. Acepromazine may promote relaxation of the retractor penis muscle.
• Appropriate antimicrobial therapy should be instituted depending on the specifics of the individual case and route of therapy.

CONTRAINDICATIONS
• Appropriate milk and meat withdrawal times must be followed for all compounds administered to food-producing animals.
• Lidocaine sensitivity is common in goats and should be considered prior to its utilization.

PRECAUTIONS
• Alpha-2 agonists (xylazine, detomidine) should not be used in cases of unresolved obstruction due to its diuretic effects.
• Neither diazepam nor acepromazine is approved for use in food animals. The meat withdrawal time for acepromazine maleate is 7 days. There are no withdrawal data for diazepam but a 30-day meat/milk withdrawal should be adequate. Consult with gFARAD.

POSSIBLE INTERACTIONS
N/A

ALTERNATIVE DRUGS
N/A

FOLLOW-UP

PATIENT MONITORING
Animals at risk to block should be monitored closely for signs to enable rapid treatment.

PREVENTION/AVOIDANCE
• Free access to water and modification of the diet are essential to prevent recurrence.
• Urine acidifiers can be used.

POSSIBLE COMPLICATIONS
Recurrence of obstruction and urethral stricture can be common complications.

EXPECTED COURSE AND PROGNOSIS
Prognosis depends on chronology and severity of obstruction as well as treatment method instituted.

MISCELLANEOUS

ASSOCIATED CONDITIONS
Bladder/urethral rupture, uremia, urethral stricture

PREGNANCY
N/A

RUMINANT SPECIES AFFECTED
Sheep and goats as well as steers may be affected.

PRODUCTION MANAGEMENT
This is a common problem of feedlot lambs fed high-carbohydrate diets.

SYNONYMS
N/A

SEE ALSO
Bracken fern toxicity
Cystitis
Orf
Photosensitivity
Pyelonephritis

ABBREVIATIONS
gFARAD = global Food Animal Residue Avoidance Databank
IV = intravenous

Suggested Reading
Belknap, E. B., Pugh, D. G. 2002. Lower urinary tract problems. In: *Sheep and goat medicine*, ed. D. G. Pugh. Philadelphia: W. B. Saunders.
Fubini, S. L., Pease, A. P. 2004. Urogenital surgery. In: *Farm animal surgery*, ed. S. L. Fubini, N. G. Ducharme. Philadelphia: W. B. Saunders.
May, K. A., Moll, H. D., Wallace, L. M., et al. 1998. Urinary bladder marsupialization for treatment of obstructive urolithiasis in male goats. *Vet Surg*. 27:583–88.
Metre, D. C., Fecteau, G., House, J. K., et al. 1996. Obstructive urolithiasis in ruminants: surgical management and prevention. *Comp Cont Ed Pract Vet*. 18: S275–S302.
Metre, D. C., House, J. K., Smith, B. P., et al. 1996. Obstructive urolithiasis in ruminants: medical treatment and urethral surgery. *Comp Cont Ed Pract Vet*. 18:317–28.

Author: Laura M. Riggs

UTERINE ANOMALIES

BASICS

DEFINITION
Uterine anomalies may be categorized as either genetic/congenital or pathophysiological.

SYSTEMS AFFECTED
Production management, reproductive

GENETICS
• There is evidence for a genetic basis for segmental aplasia of the reproductive tract in female cattle.
• Intersex is linked with the gene for polledness in dairy goats.

INCIDENCE/PREVALENCE
• In goats, freemartins are relatively frequently detected by chromosomal testing (6%).
• Intersex prevalence in goats may be relatively high (20%) in polled/polled matings.
• Hydroallantois, 85%–90%; hydroamnion, approximately 10% of bovine dropsical conditions.
• Freemartinism occurs in approximately 90%–95% of females born cotwin to a bull.

GEOGRAPHIC DISTRIBUTION
Worldwide

SIGNALMENT
Species
Potentially all ruminant species

Breed Predilections
In cattle, a condition encountered in white shorthorn heifers ("white heifer disease") is often associated with segmental aplasia of the tubular portion of the reproductive tract.

Mean Age and Range
N/A

Predominant Sex
Female

DIAGNOSIS
See under specific anomaly below.

TREATMENT
See under specific anomaly below.

MEDICATIONS
See also under specific anomaly below.

CONTRAINDICATIONS
• Appropriate milk and meat withdrawal times must be followed for all compounds administered to food-producing animals.
• Steroids should not be used in pregnant animals unless abortion is indicated.

FOLLOW-UP

MISCELLANEOUS

Genetic/Congenital Anomalies
This category includes arrested development of those structures derived from the embryonic Muellerian (or paramesonephric) duct system (i.e., oviducts, uterus, cervix, and cranial vagina). Problems caused by either defective or exaggerated fusion of the ducts are reported in most species. It is useful to classify defects on the basis of the underlying anatomic structure.

Segmental Aplasia of the Uterus
• Aplasia of one entire uterine horn is termed uterine unicornis. Alternatively, underdevelopment (hypoplasia) may occur of one or both uterine horns. Aplasia of a segment of uterine horn often occurs near the uterine body, and the blocked horn may become distended with uterine secretions (mucometra or hydrometra).
• Affected animals are infertile. In cattle, a condition encountered in white shorthorn heifers (white heifer disease) is often associated with segmental aplasia of the tubular portion of the reproductive tract (often with distension) plus an intact hymen or vaginal stenosis.
• Anatomic defects of the genital tract of female sheep are uncommon. In goats, intersexes containing an admixture of the Muellerian and Wolffian duct systems are relatively common, although most are male pseudohermaphrodites.

• Predisposing factors. There is evidence for a genetic basis for segmental aplasia of the reproductive tract in female cattle. In shorthorns, the condition is caused by a single, recessive, sex-linked gene linked to the gene for white color, occurring in approximately 10% of white shorthorn heifers. In Holsteins, arrested Muellerian duct development has been traced to a single, autosomal recessive gene.

Diagnosis
Infertility, history, palpation

Uterus Didelphys
• Failure of fusion of the Muellerian ducts can lead to a double cervix, or uterus didelphys (if the median wall of the Muellerian duct is persistent). This can result in delayed pregnancy if semen is deposited in the contralateral side; a problem with AI but not natural breeding. On palpation, the cervix is usually broader and flatter than normal.
• Affected females usually have little problem calving, although occasional obstruction might occur.

Freemartinism
• Freemartinism occurs in approximately 90%–95% of females born cotwin to a bull, and they are usually sterile. Here, the twins develop from different zygotes (dizygotic) with early fusion of the two chorioallantoic membranes resulting in suppression (variable hypoplasia or agenesis) of the female genitalia (oviducts, uterus, and anterior vagina), in conjunction with stimulated development of the Wolffian duct system.
• Freemartins usually have undeveloped, undifferentiated ovaries, an enlarged vulvar tuft, and a shortened, imperforate vagina. The affected female is often relatively small and steerlike, with undeveloped udder and teats. Bulls born cotwin to freemartins may also have fertility problems.
• Freemartinism is rare in sheep. In goats, freemartins are relatively frequently (6%) detected by chromosome confirmation of chimerism in intersexes, where it occurs in both horned and polled animals. Here, the external and internal genitalia are similar to those of polled intersexes, although with greater masculine emphasis.

Diagnosis

- History, infertility, external signs
- Insertion of a lubricated tubular device into the vagina of a freemartin heifer will allow only 7.5–10 cm of penetration compared with 5–7 inches in a "normal" heifer.
- Blood typing of twins reveals chimerism of blood types, providing an indicator of freemartinism.
- Chromosome analysis of freemartins reveals the coexistence of both male and female cells in blood and other hemopoietic tissues. In caprine freemartins, the proportion of male cells may be as low as 1%.

Hermaphrodism and Pseudohermaphrodism

- Hermaphrodism has been occasionally reported in cattle, usually associated with numerical chromosome disorders (XX/XY, XX/XXY) with no evidence that this condition is influenced by heredity.
- Intersexuality is not uncommon in goats (2%–10%) with male pseudohermaphrodism (sex-reversed genetic females) being most common. It is linked with the gene for polledness in dairy goats where the prevalence may be relatively high (20%) in polled/polled matings.
- Caprine male pseudohermaphrodites may vary in appearance from nearly normal females to nearly normal males, although most resemble females at birth. True hermaphrodism is seen occasionally in goats.

Pathophysiological Anomalies

Hydrops

- Hydroallantois and hydroamnion are the two most common causes of hydrops (or dropsy) in the bovine. These conditions are rarely encountered in sheep and goats.
- Prevalence
  - Hydroallantois, 85%–90%; hydroamnion, approximately 10% of bovine dropsical conditions.
  - Occasionally they can occur together.
- Predisposing factors
  - Hydroamnion is caused by a fetal failure of deglutition, and thus is often associated with fetal abnormalities (e.g., genetic conditions), caused by recessive autosomal genes resulting in defective fetuses (e.g., "bulldog" calves in Dexter cattle).
  - Hydroallantois is regarded as a uterine or placental disease (or both) and thus may be likely to recur.

Diagnosis

- Excessive abdominal enlargement in conjunction with pregnancy. Hydroamnion occurs more gradually (weeks or months) than does hydroallantois (5–20 days).
- On transrectal palpation, hydroallantois causes distension and pressure such that the fetus and cotyledons usually cannot be palpated; usually they can be palpated with hydroamnion.
- Allantoic fluid is watery, clear, and amber; amniotic fluid is syrupy and viscid.
- Differential diagnosis: edema of the chorioallantois, fetal anasarca, and fetal edema with ascites and hydrothorax

Treatment

- Varies with duration, severity, and the likelihood of success. In severe cases, prompt termination of the abnormal pregnancy is advised; removal of fluid only generally results in replenishment, which occurs much more rapidly with hydroallantois.
- In general, cesarean section is less successful than induced parturition.
- Abortion may be induced with prostaglandin, in conjunction with glucocorticoids. This is usually more successful with hydroamnion than with hydroallantois. Assistance with delivery is often necessary due to atony of the uterine wall.
- Fluid therapy is recommended due to the rapid loss of vast amounts of fluid associated with the process of delivery.

Prognosis

- With hydroamnion, an inherited cause should be considered as well as the strong possibility of a defective calf.
- Hydroallantois is more likely to recur. If advanced, sequelae may include rupture of the prepubic tendon or abdominal wall.
- Generally, the prognosis both for life and future fertility is poorer for individuals suffering from hydroallantois, than for those suffering from hydroamnion.

Hydrometra, Mucometra

- These conditions have been discussed above in relation to congenital abnormalities of the female tract.
- In does, hydrometra and/or mucometra can result in fluid accumulation that is expelled spontaneously ("cloudburst") approximately 150 days following breeding.
- This condition occurs in conjunction with a CL, although membranes and fetus are not present.

ASSOCIATED CONDITIONS

Abortion, infertility

AGE-RELATED FACTORS

N/A

ZOONOTIC POTENTIAL

N/A

PREGNANCY

See above Pathophysiological Anomalies

RUMINANT SPECIES AFFECTED

All ruminant species

BIOSECURITY

PRODUCTION MANAGEMENT

Cull affected animals

SYNONYMS

Uterine unicornis
White heifer disease

SEE ALSO

Freemartinism
Reproductive pharmacology
Reproductive ultrasound chapters

ABBREVIATIONS

CL = corpus luteum

Suggested Reading

Harker, D. B. 1981, Nov. Treatment of a case of bovine hydrops allantois with cloprostenol. *Br Vet J*. 137(6):575–77.

Milton, A., Welker, B., Modransky, P. 1989, Nov 15. Hydrallantois in a ewe. *J Am Vet Med Assoc*. 195(10):1385–86.

Parkinson, T. J., Smith, K. C., Long, S. E., Douthwaite, J. A., Mann, G. E., Knight, P. G. 2001, Sep. Inter-relationships among gonadotrophins, reproductive steroids and inhibin in freemartin ewes. *Reproduction* 122(3):397–409.

Smith, K. C., Parkinson, T. J., Long, S. E., Barr, F. J. 2000, May 13. Anatomical, cytogenetic and behavioural studies of freemartin ewes. *Vet Rec*. 146(20):574–78.

Youngquist, R. S., Braun, W. F., Jr. 1993, Jul. Abnormalities of the tubular genital organs. *Vet Clin North Am Food Anim Pract*. 9(2):309–22.

Author: Peter Chenoweth

UTERINE PROLAPSE

BASICS

OVERVIEW
• Uterine prolapse is a condition that affects all species; however, it occurs more often in multiparous cows.
• The protrusion of both uterine horns through the vulva is easily diagnosed and characterizes the uterine prolapse.
• Uterine prolapse usually occurs a few hours after parturition, but it can occur up to 5 or 6 days after calving.

INCIDENCE/PREVALENCE
The incidence of uterine prolapse is relatively low, ranging from 0.003% to 0.25%.

SIGNALMENT
Species
All species are at risk for the occurrence of uterine prolapse, but cows are at a higher risk.

Breed Predilections
It appears that Holstein cows are at higher risk for the occurrence of uterine prolapse.

Mean Age and Range
Primiparous cows as well as multiparous cows are at risk for uterine prolapse. However, multiparous cows are at higher risk due to a higher risk for hypocalcemia, a condition that predisposes cows to uterine prolapse.

SIGNS
• Immediately after prolapse occurs, the tissues are normal and there may be fetal membranes still attached to the endometrium and its caruncles. Within a few hours after the prolapse, the uterus becomes edematous and enlarged.

• Clinical signs that accompany uterine prolapse are straining, abdominal pain, restlessness, anorexia, and increased pulse and respiratory rate. Uterine prolapse in cows is frequently accompanied by hypocalcemia and, in the more severe cases, milk fever.
• Cows that present with hypocalcemia concurrent to uterine prolapse may be recumbent and have muscle fasciculation. Although unusual, the condition may progress to shock and death.

DIAGNOSIS

The diagnosis is obvious as the uterine horns can be identified protruding from the vulva.

DIFFERENTIAL DIAGNOSIS
• Vaginal prolapse
• Partial prolapse of the uterus

CBC/BIOCHEMISTRY/URINALYSIS
N/A

OTHER LABORATORY TESTS
N/A

TREATMENT

• The correction of uterine prolapse can be performed with the cow standing or in sternum recumbency. It is recommended that 2% lidocaine be administered as an epidural anesthesia to avoid the continuous straining of the cow while the veterinarian is attempting to replace the uterus. Administration of clenbuterol is reported to cause uterus relaxation, facilitating replacement of the uterus, reducing the need for epidural anesthesia. Clenbuterol is a prohibited drug in the United States.

• When attempting to reduce uterine prolapse in a recumbent cow, both hind limbs should be pulled posterior behind the animal so that she is resting on her stifles with the hind legs spread out. This positioning causes the pelvis to be slightly tilted downward and forward, leaving more room in the caudal abdominal cavity, favoring the replacement of the uterus.
• It is fundamental that when reducing a uterine prolapse the veterinarian and assistant be as clean as possible. Surgical scrub should be used to wash the entire uterine surface and remove fecal material, dirt, and fetal membranes if easily separated from the endometrium.
• Oxytocin should be used after the uterus is replaced to stimulate uterine contraction and involution. Cows that develop uterine prolapse are also at higher risk for hypocalcemia; treatments with calcium intravenous solutions should be considered.
• Antibiotic treatment is usually recommended after uterine prolapse is resolved to avoid the occurrence of metritis.
• In cases where replacement of the uterus is impossible or where the tissues are severely damaged, amputation may be indicated as a salvage option.
• Appropriate milk and meat withdrawal times must be followed for all compounds administered to food-producing animals.

MEDICATIONS

FOLLOW-UP

PATIENT MONITORING
Cows that develop uterine prolapse should be closely observed daily for 5 to 10 days postcalving. At any signs of fever, anorexia, or depression, cows should be examined and treated properly.

PREVENTION/ AVOIDANCE

• Because cows are at higher risk of uterine prolapse when developing hypocalcemia, a balanced diet during the far-off and close-up periods should be offered to avoid such metabolic imbalance.

• Some studies have shown that cows that have stillborn calves are at higher risk for uterine prolapse, probably due to the longer period between initiation of parturition and assistance provided to the animal. Therefore, it is recommended that the calving area be well monitored at all times and that cows have the proper assistance as they show signs of dystocia or calving difficulties.

POSSIBLE COMPLICATIONS

• Fatalities are rare but can occur in the event of shock or rupture of a large uterine vessel.

• Cows that develop uterine prolapse are at higher risk for metritis and, consequently, are at higher risk for reproductive problems (e.g., increased calving-to-conception interval and calving interval). Due to reproductive problems, cows that present with uterine prolapse are at a higher risk for culling than their herd mates.

EXPECED COURSE AND PROGNOSIS

The prognosis is usually good; however, it depends on the lag time between the occurrence of the uterine prolapse and replacement. The extent and magnitude of uterine lesions also determines the prognosis.

MISCELLANEOUS

ASSOCIATED CONDITIONS

Hypocalcemia is a condition that predisposes cows to uterine prolapse due to the lack of contractility in uterine tissues.

AGE-RELATED FACTORS

Because hypocalcemia is more common in multiparous cows, it is expected that multiparous cows are at higher risk for uterine prolapse than primiparous cows.

RUMINANT SPECIES AFFECTED

All ruminant species may be affected.

PRODUCTION MANAGEMENT

Feeding well-balanced rations in the far-off and close-up periods is important to avoid the occurrence of hypocalcemia, decreasing the risk for uterine prolapse.

SEE ALSO

Abortions
FARAD
Hypocalcemia
Reproductive pharmacology
Vaginal prolapse

ABBREVIATIONS

FARAD = Food Animal Residue Avoidance Databank

Suggested Reading

Baker I. D. 2003, Mar 29. Uterine prolapse in a cow. *Vet Rec.* 152(13): 408.

Biggs, A., Osborne, R. 2003, Jan 18. Uterine prolapse and mid-pregnancy uterine torsion in cows. *Vet Rec.* 152(3): 91–92.

Gardner, I. A., Reynolds, J. P., Risco, C. A., Hird, D. W. 1990, Oct 15. Patterns of uterine prolapse in dairy cows and prognosis after treatment. *J Am Vet Med Assoc.* 197(8): 1021–24.

Houe, H., Ostergaard, S., Thilsing-Hansen, T., Jorgensen, R. J., Larsen, T., Sorensen, J. T., Agger, J. F., Blom, J. Y. 2001. Milk fever and subclinical hypocalcemia—an evaluation of parameters on incidence risk, diagnosis, risk factors, and biological effects as input for a decision support system for disease control. *Acta Vet Scand.* 42(1): 1–29.

Murphy, A. M., Dobson, H. 2002, Dec 14. Predisposition, subsequent fertility, and mortality of cows with uterine prolapse. *Vet Rec.* 151(24): 733–35.

Author: Ricardo Carbonari Chebel

UTERINE TORSION

 BASICS

OVERVIEW
• Uterine torsion is a relatively common cause of dystocia accounting for 5%–10% of dystocia events.
• Anticlockwise torsion of the uterus is more common than clockwise torsion.
• About 85%–90% of uterine torsion occurs around the time of parturition during the initial stages of labor.
• Factors such as increased fetal movements in the late first and early second stage of labor and uterine instability due to loose broad uterine ligament at the time of parturition predispose the occurrence of such dystocia. Fetal oversize is another factor that may predispose to uterine torsion.

INCIDENCE/PREVALENCE
Uterine torsion represents 5%–10% of the dystocia occurring in cattle.

SIGNALMENT
Species
Uterine torsion can occur in most bi-ungulates; cattle, sheep, goats, camelids, and cervidae
Breed Predilections
N/A
Mean Age and Range
Although multiparous cows are believed to be at higher risk in developing uterine torsion due to decreased uterine and mesometrial tone, an epidemiological study has shown that the incidence of uterine torsion is similar between cows younger than 3 years, between 3 and 5 years, and cows older than 5 years of age.

SIGNS
Clinical Signs
• Cows with uterine torsion may present with signs of anorexia, depression, decreased milk production, and colic/abdominal pain (kicking the abdomen and treading on her hind limbs).
• The use of a speculum allows for the observation of the vaginal wall, which is rotating clock- or counterclockwise.
• Palpation per rectum usually allows for a definitive diagnosis. The uterus can be more toned than normal, the broad ligament is usually very tense, and the ovary is dislocated ventrally toward the torsion.

 DIAGNOSIS

• Observation of the vagina with the use of a speculum for visual examination
• Palpation per rectum of the vagina, cervix, uterus, and broad ligament of the uterus

DIFFERENTIAL DIAGNOSIS
• Dystocia—fetal malposition in utero
• Colic

CBC/BIOCHEMISTRY/URINALYSIS
N/A

OTHER LABORATORY TESTS
N/A

IMAGING
N/A

 TREATMENT

MANUAL TREATMENT
• With the patient recumbent, rotate the animal in the same direction as the uterine torsion while one person holds the calf.

• Rotation of the calf in the opposite direction of the torsion by purchase of the elbow joint or shoulder of the calf. Before attempting the final push to correct the torsion, it is usual to do swing movements in the uterus.
• Rotation of the calf using a detorsion rod. One end of an obstetric chain is placed dorsally to the metacarpal/metatarsal joint of the calf. The chain is then passed through the loop of the detorsion rod and the free end of the obstetric chain is placed dorsally to the metacarpal/metatarsal joint of the calf. The detorsion rod is then twisted in the opposite direction of the torsion.
• Manual approach in camelids is done prior to delivery. The cervical "star" is visualized and the animal is rotated in the direction opposite to the cervical displacement. It is not uncommon for three to four attempts to be made prior to success.

SURGICAL TREATMENT
• Laparotomy to correct the torsion of the uterus manually
• Laparotomy and cesarean section if the cow is in labor
• Laparotomy may be indicated in camelids secondary to manual detorsion failure.

 MEDICATIONS

 FOLLOW-UP

PATIENT MONITORING
• If the uterine torsion is corrected manually without the need for surgery, the prognosis is very good and little if any patient monitoring is required. It is suggested that patients be observed for at least 3 to 5 days postprocedure to evaluate appetite and to ensure that no fever develops.

• When the uterine torsion is corrected by a surgical procedure, with or without cesarean section, it should be recommended to the farm personnel that the animal be closely observed for 5 to 10 days. Rectal temperatures should be checked daily, and if signs of fever or loss of appetite appear, the animal should be treated immediately for such conditions.

PREVENTION/ AVOIDANCE
• Adoption of good management practices is the only way to minimize the occurrence of this event.
• Pregnant animals should be well fed at all times and the feed bunk should never be empty. Feed bunk management is extremely important in its prevention.
• Far-off and close-up animals should be handled calmly at all times avoiding running.
• The condition is common in camelids and is generally associated with colic symptoms in pregnant llamas.

POSSIBLE COMPLICATIONS
• Uterine torsion usually does not have any further complications if the torsion is not severe and if the correction of the condition can be done manually without the need for surgery.
• The occurrence of uterine torsions that are beyond 360° can compromise uterine vascularization leading to hypoxia. The uterus can become devitalized and very friable. In such conditions, it is not uncommon for a cow that undergoes labor to rupture her uterus.

• Rarely, uterine torsion involves the alimentary tract or other abdominal organs; however, when this occurs there can be complications due to the compromised venous and arterial flow of blood from and to the organs.

EXPECTED COURSE AND PROGNOSIS
The prognosis is usually good; however, it depends on the extent of the torsion and the length of time between occurrence, diagnosis, and treatment.

 MISCELLANEOUS

AGE-RELATED FACTORS
Multiparous cows may be theoretically at higher risk for uterine torsion due to decreased uterine and mesometrial tone.

ZOONOTIC POTENTIAL
N/A

PREGNANCY
Pregnancy may be terminated spontaneously after the occurrence of uterine torsion depending on the degree of torsion. Uterine torsions that are above 360° may cause the rupture of fetal membranes or compromise venous return to the uterus leading to the death of the calf.

RUMINANT SPECIES AFFECTED
Most bi-ungulates may be affected by this condition.

PRODUCTION MANAGEMENT
• Incidence of uterine torsion is low.
• Relative to the occurrence of other types of dystocia, uterine torsion has a prevalence of 5%–10%. This value may be overestimated because it usually requires veterinary assistance, and reporting bias may occur.

SEE ALSO
Colic
Dystocia

ABBREVIATIONS
N/A

Suggested Reading
Biggs, A., Osborne, R. 2003, Jan 18. Uterine prolapse and mid-pregnancy uterine torsion in cows. *Vet Rec.* 152(3):91–92.
Brooks, G. 1999, Sep 4. Uterine torsion in a cow. *Vet Rec.* 145(10):292.
Kinsey, S. 1999, Sep 18. Uterine torsion in a cow. *Vet Rec.* 145(12):352.
Penny, C. D. 1999, Aug 21. Uterine torsion of 540° in a mid-gestation cow. *Vet Rec.* 145(8).230.
Wardrope, D. D., Boyes, G. W. 2002, Jan 12. Uterine torsion in twin pregnancies in dairy cattle. *Vet Rec.* 150(2): 56.

Author: Ricardo Carbonari Chebel

VACCINATION AND DEWORMING PROGRAMS FOR BEEF CATTLE

 BASICS

DEFINITION

• Strategic vaccination and deworming programs are part of a total herd health management plan.
• Vaccination is a tool that can help prevent the occurrence of disease or reduce the severity of disease but it is not a substitute for poor management in other areas.
• A successful vaccination program depends on adequate nutrition, proper management and housing, and planning.
• Nutrition must be adequate for the immune system to function properly.
  • A vaccine prevents diseases by priming an animal's immune system to fight the disease.
  • The animal must be supplied with adequate protein and energy, as well as vitamins A and E, copper, selenium, and zinc for optimum immune system function.
• No vaccine is 100% protective in 100% of the animals. Some animals will have a less than maximal response to a vaccine and some animals may not respond at all.
• Vaccination is simply the act of inoculating an animal with a vaccine. It does not imply immunity.
• Immunization is the development of an immune response in response to a vaccine. It does not imply protection from disease.
• Strategic deworming improves animal health by preventing clinical parasitism, improves production by improving growth and efficiency, and reduces pasture contamination with infective larvae.
• *Ostertagia*, *Haemonchus*, and trichostrongyles are the most important gastrointestinal (GI) parasites of cattle. *Ostertagia* is the most economically important intestinal parasite of cattle.

PATHOPHYSIOLOGY

Types of immunity:

Passive Immunity
• Antibodies are obtained from some source other than the animal's immune system.
• Passive transfer of colostral antibodies is the most important form of passive immunity.
• Antibodies from passive immunity may interfere with the development of active immunity in response to a vaccination in young animals by "neutralizing" the vaccine.
• Other types of passive immunity include blood or plasma transfusions and antiserum products such as tetanus antitoxin.

Active Immunity
• Humoral, cell mediated, and secretory types
• Antibodies are produced by specific lymphocytes in response to exposure to an antigen or in response to a vaccination.
• Cell mediated immunity (CMI) develops when specialized lymphocytes are exposed to a specific organism and develop a "memory" for that organism. When exposed again, these cells attack and kill that organism or cells infected with that organism.
  • CMI is not as easily produced as humoral immunity and is rarely produced in response to a killed vaccine.
  • In most cases, an infectious organism has to replicate within an animal in order to produce CMI.
• Secretory immunity consists of antibodies produced in response to exposure or vaccination that do not circulate in the blood stream.
  • Antibodies are produced by cells lining the mucosal surfaces of various parts of the body.
  • Vaccines that can be administered in the same manner that natural exposure would occur tend to produce the best secretory immune response. An example would be an intranasal IBR vaccine.

Innate Immunity
• Innate immunity consists of natural defense mechanisms such as enzymes, tears, saliva, and gastric acids.
• These mechanisms destroy or mechanically remove infectious organisms before they can cause an infection.
• A failure of any one of these types of immunity predisposes an animal to disease.
• Proper vaccination can improve both passive and active immunity.
• Parasitism has many pathologic effects on an animal. The degree of the effect can range from minor infestations that have little significance to severe clinical parasitism resulting in death.
  • The most important GI parasites damage the mucosal lining of the abomasum and small intestine resulting in blood loss, reduced nutrient absorption, diarrhea, and edema.
  • Liver flukes may cause enough damage to result in clinical disease, but more often they predispose animals to other diseases or result in liver condemnations at slaughter. Liver damage caused by flukes is part of the pathophysiology of bacillary hemoglobinuria (*Clostridium haemolyticum*).
• External parasites result in production losses from reduced growth and hide damage.

SYSTEMS AFFECTED
• The primary systems targeted in most vaccination programs include the respiratory, gastrointestinal, reproductive, and musculoskeletal systems.
• Reducing health problems through proper vaccination and parasite control can have an effect on virtually every system in the body.

GENETICS
Genetics play an important role in natural disease resistance including innate immunity and factors such as mothering ability, which affect passive immunity.

INCIDENCE/PREVALENCE
All cattle herds could benefit from some sort of planned vaccination and parasite control program.

GEOGRAPHIC DISTRIBUTION
Appropriate vaccination and parasite control programs must be customized to the specific herd and location for which they are being developed.
• Some vaccines may be appropriate in some areas but unnecessary in others depending on the occurrence of the disease in that area.
• Some geographic areas have parasite problems that other areas may not have. An example would be liver flukes.

SIGNALMENT
• All beef cattle, regardless of age and production status, should be incorporated into a vaccination and parasite control program.
• Different ages and classes of animals will require different protocols but all animals should be included in the program.

SIGNS
• The signs of vaccine failure depend on the body system affected by the disease. Signs may range from subclinical production losses to clinical disease and death.
• The signs of parasitism also depend on the system affected.
  • Signs associated with most external parasites are usually readily apparent.
  • Signs associated with internal parasites can range from subclinical production losses to clinical disease and death. The common signs associated with GI parasitism include ill thrift; dry, dull hair coat; weight loss; diarrhea; "bottle jaw"; and reduced production.

CAUSES
• The causes of vaccine failure are numerous.
  • Improper handling of vaccines
  • Improper timing of vaccination
  • Interference from maternal antibodies
  • Improper administration technique
  • Improper timing of booster vaccinations
  • Animals that are already sick or highly stressed
  • Overwhelming disease challenge
  • Nutritional deficiencies or other causes of poor health
• The causes of parasite control failure include improper dosing or administration technique, improper timing of administration, and drug resistance.

RISK FACTORS
Risk factors for vaccine failure include those factors listed above as causes of vaccine failure.

VACCINATION AND DEWORMING PROGRAMS FOR BEEF CATTLE

DIAGNOSIS

DIFFERENTIAL DIAGNOSIS
N/A

CBC/BIOCHEMISTRY/URINALYSIS
N/A

OTHER LABORATORY TESTS
N/A

IMAGING
N/A

DIAGNOSTIC PROCEDURES
• Many infectious agents can cause disease and attempts should be made to establish a definitive diagnosis before implementing a vaccination protocol to combat a disease outbreak.
• Periodic fecal egg counts may help in the development and monitoring of parasite control programs.

PATHOLOGIC FINDINGS
N/A

TREATMENT

APPROPRIATE HEALTH CARE
Ensuring adequate colostral transfer of antibodies is much more important and effective than any vaccination program.

NURSING CARE
N/A

ACTIVITY
N/A

DIET
Animals must be provided a balanced diet that is adequate in vitamins and trace minerals to allow optimum immune system function.

CLIENT EDUCATION
• Clients must be educated on the proper administration of vaccines and parasite control products.
• Vaccines must be used according to the label directions.
• Vaccines should not be mixed in the same syringe unless directed by the label.
• Vaccines should be kept cool and out of direct sunlight. Keep vaccines in an ice chest or some other form of protection while in use.
• Only reconstitute the amount of vaccine that can be used in a 1 hour period. Do not try to store reconstituted MLV products; even if it is just for a few hours.
• Whenever possible, use products that can be administered subcutaneously.
• All injections, both subcutaneous and intramuscular, should be given in the neck to avoid damage to the more valuable parts of the carcass.
• Use clean injection equipment to administer vaccines.
  • Change needles every 5 to 10 head.

• Never disinfect instruments that will be used for MLV products with chemical disinfectants. Residual disinfectant can destroy the effectiveness of MLV products.

SURGICAL CONSIDERATIONS
N/A

MEDICATIONS

DRUGS OF CHOICE
Types of Vaccines
Killed Vaccines
• Require booster dose 2–3 weeks following initial dose. If booster is not properly administered, virtually no protective immunity occurs. Once an animal has received the initial two doses, a single yearly booster may be adequate.
• Provide a shorter duration of immunity
• Usually do not stimulate CMI
• May be the safest type to use in some situations

Modified-Live Vaccines
• Infectious agent is alive but altered so that it does not cause disease in healthy animals.
• Agent replicates within the animal and induces both humoral and cell-mediated immunity.
• Produce long-lasting immunity; may be lifelong in some cases
• Usually provide a greater immune response than killed products
• Some types may cause abortion in pregnant cows or disease in highly stressed animals.
• Some newer MLV products are labeled for use in pregnant cows and calves nursing pregnant cows as long as the vaccines are used according to the label.

Component Vaccines
Vaccines that contain only part of an infectious agent. These products induce immunity to a part of an infectious agent that is necessary for the agent to cause disease.

Toxoids
Vaccines that induce an immune response to certain toxins produced by bacteria.

Deworming Products
• Delivery method—many products are available with many different delivery methods: injectable; pour-on; molasses blocks; mineral mixes; crumbles; pastes; boluses; drenches
• Spectrum of activity
  • Refers to how many different parasites and which stages of the life cycle the product will control.
  • Many products are available that will kill external parasites, internal parasites, and hypobiotic larvae.
  • Some parasite problems may have to be addressed with specific products (e.g., flukes).

• Duration of activity: refers to the length of time a product will remain active in the animal
  • Products such as Valbazen, Safeguard/Panacur, and Synthanthic are effective but short-lived: typically remain active for 2 to 3 days
  • Products such as Dectomax, Ivomec, Ivomec-Eprinex, and Cydectin have an extended duration of activity: typically remain active for 14 to 28 days.

Recommended Vaccination Programs
A successful vaccination program must be customized to each specific situation.

Young Calf Vaccines
• Passive immunity to clostridial diseases usually begins to decline around 2 to 3 months of age. Calves at this age should be given a clostridial bacterin/toxoid.
• Passive immunity to the common respiratory viruses (IBR, BVD, PI3, and BRSV) usually lasts for 4 to 5 months so calves at this age should be fairly well protected.
• Respiratory viral vaccines can be administered at this time if the herd has a history of respiratory disease in calves of this age.
• Intranasal vaccines are a good choice in young calves because passive immunity has less effect on these vaccines.

Preweaning Vaccines
• Ideally, calves should be vaccinated 2–4 weeks prior to weaning so that they have had time to develop an immune response and to help reduce the stress of weaning.
• At 2–4 weeks prior to weaning, calves should receive a respiratory virus vaccine and a clostridial booster.
  • MLV viral vaccines are preferable to killed products as long as they can be safely used according to label directions in nursing calves.
  • If a killed product is used, it must be boostered at weaning.
• Other vaccines to consider at this time include *Pasteurella* leukotoxoid vaccines, *Hemophilus somnus* and calf hood vaccination (Brucellosis) of potential replacement females. Some states require that females be official calf hood vaccinates in order to enter the state.

Weaning Vaccines
• MLV respiratory virus vaccines can be given at weaning without the risk of abortion in pregnant cows.
• Calves that received this type of vaccine at preweaning should not need another dose at weaning.
  • The advantage of giving a second dose at weaning is providing another opportunity for calves that did not respond to previous vaccinations to become immunized.
  • Calves that responded to previously administered vaccines usually do not develop greater immunity in response to a second dose.

VACCINATION AND DEWORMING PROGRAMS FOR BEEF CATTLE

Replacement Females
• At 1 year of age, replacement heifers should receive MLV respiratory virus vaccine with leptospirosis.
• *Campylobacter* (vibriosis) can be included if infertility due to vibriosis is a risk.

Adult Cows
• Adult cows should receive a five-way *Leptospira* bacterin once or twice yearly. Immunity produced by *Leptospira* vaccines is short-lived
• Cows that received MLV respiratory virus vaccine as heifers often develop lifelong immunity to these agents and do not need yearly boosters.
  • Yearly boosters can be given if the vaccination history is unknown or if the producer desires to increase the level of antibody provided in the colostrum.
  • If killed products were used in the replacement heifers, yearly boosters should be given.
• Cows can also be vaccinated with K-99 *E. coli* and rotavirus/coronavirus products to increase the level of passive immunity provided to the calf.
  • Pregnant replacements should be given two doses, 3 and 6 weeks prior to calving.
  • Previously vaccinated cows only need 1 dose, 3–4 weeks prior to calving.
  • Rotavirus/coronavirus products are available to give to newborn calves prior to the calf's nursing colostrum.
• Campylobacter and trichomoniasis vaccines can be given yearly in at-risk herds.

Bulls
• Bulls should receive the same vaccinations used in the cow herd with some exceptions.
  • Bulls are not vaccinated for brucellosis.
  • The currently available trichomoniasis vaccine is not approved for use in bulls.
  • IBR virus from MLV products may recrudesce and be shed in semen.
  • Bulls should receive leptospirosis and campylobacteriosis vaccines in accordance with the cow herd.
• Other vaccines such as pinkeye and foot rot vaccines may be considered in problem herds.

Recommended Deworming Programs
• Deworming programs should be strategically designed to reduce the parasite burden within the animals and reduce pasture contamination.
• Deworming programs should be customized to meet the needs and management style of each producer.
• Producers should use broad-spectrum products that will kill several parasite species as well as hypobiotic larvae.

Deworming Twice Yearly
• Twice yearly deworming provides the most opportunity to reduce pasture contamination.
• Cows should be dewormed in the fall as they come off of summer pasture to reduce the number of parasites overwintering in the cows and reduce the additional drain on body condition caused by significant parasite burdens.
• These cows should be dewormed again in the spring prior to being turned out to grass. Deworming at this time removes parasites that overwintered in the cows and reduces pasture contamination in the spring.
• An alternative plan is to deworm cows prior to turn out on grass in the spring and again 8–9 weeks after turnout. If long-acting products are used, this program will greatly reduce pasture contamination for the first 11 to 12 weeks of the grazing season. Calves should also be dewormed 8–9 weeks into the grazing season to prevent pasture contamination.

Deworming Once Yearly
If cows can be dewormed only once per year due to management or other constraints, that deworming should be administered in the fall to reduce the parasite burden overwintering in the cows.
• Calves can be dewormed at preweaning or weaning. Deworming at preweaning reduces pasture contamination by the calves.
• Stocker cattle should be dewormed prior to being turned out to pasture and dewormed again 6–7 weeks into the grazing season.
• Feeder cattle should be dewormed once upon entry into the feedlot.

CONTRAINDICATIONS
• Some MLV viral vaccines can cause abortion if administered to pregnant cows or calves nursing pregnant cows. ALWAYS follow the label directions.
• Administering vaccines to animals that are already sick or heavily stressed often fails to produce an immune response and may further stress the immune system.
• Administering certain vaccines may complicate international shipment of animals or semen due to positive serologic tests. Consider the ultimate goals of the producer before administering vaccines.
• Appropriate milk and meat withdrawal times must be followed for all compounds administered to food-producing animals.

PRECAUTIONS
Vaccines must be properly handled and administered in order to maximize the chances of developing a strong immune response.

POSSIBLE INTERACTIONS
• Vaccines should not be mixed in the same syringe with other products except as provided by the label.
• Equipment used to administer MLV products should not be cleaned with chemical disinfectants because these chemicals can reduce or eliminate the effectiveness of the vaccine.

ALTERNATIVE DRUGS
N/A

 FOLLOW-UP

PATIENT MONITORING
Patients should be monitored postvaccination for anaphylactic reactions.

PREVENTION/AVOIDANCE

POSSIBLE COMPLICATIONS
Anaphylaxis is possible with some vaccine products. If anaphylaxis occurs, epinephrine is the treatment of choice.

EXPECTED COURSE AND PROGNOSIS
N/A

VACCINATION AND DEWORMING PROGRAMS FOR BEEF CATTLE

 MISCELLANEOUS

ASSOCIATED CONDITIONS
N/A

AGE-RELATED FACTORS
Young calves may not respond to vaccines due to the influence of passive immunity from colostral antibodies. Antibodies to clostridial diseases usually last until the calf is 2–3 months of age and antibodies to the respiratory viruses usually last until 5–6 months of age.

ZOONOTIC POTENTIAL
Care must be taken when administering brucellosis vaccination because injection of this product into humans will cause illness.

PREGNANCY
Care must be used when administering MLV products to pregnant cows. Always follow label directions.

RUMINANT SPECIES AFFECTED
Cattle

BIOSECURITY
Well-designed vaccination programs are an integral part of all biosecurity programs.

PRODUCTION MANAGEMENT
Provision of well-designed vaccination and parasite control programs is an integral part of any production management system.

SYNONYMS
N/A

SEE ALSO
Many university extension service publications are available that outline herd health calendars to help producers organize management practices throughout the year.
Bovine respiratory disease complex
Neonatal diarrhea
Clostridial diseases

ABBREVIATIONS
BRSV = bovine respiratory syncytial virus
BVD = bovine viral diarrhea
CMI = cell mediated immunity
GI = gastrointestinal
IBR = infectious bovine rhinotracheitis
MLV = modified-live vaccine
PI3 = parainfluenza 3

Suggested Reading
Arseneau, J. *Parasite control*. University of Minnesota Extension Publication (Electronic). Available at: http://www.extension.umn.edu/beef/components/homestudy/lesson4h.PDF. 2003. Accessed November 28, 2007.
Bagley, C. V. *Vaccination program for beef calves*. Utah State University Extension Publication (Electronic). Available at: http://extension.usu.edu/files/agpubs/beef40.pdf. 2004. Accessed November 28, 2007.
Floyd, J. G. *Vaccinations for the beef cow herd*. Alabama Cooperative Extension Publication ANR-968. 2001.
Hartwig, N. R., Hauptmeier, L. 1995, June. *Beef and dairy cattle vaccination programs*. Iowa State University Extension Publication Pm-1624,.
Rice, L. E. 1990. *Immunizations for Oklahoma cow-calf herds*. Oklahoma State University Extension Publication F-9123.

Author: John Gilliam

VACCINATION AND DEWORMING: CERVIDAE

BASICS

DEFINITION
• The administration of anthelmintics in order to prevent, control, and treat parasitic infections. Goals include improving animal health and preventing economic loss.
• Hind—adult female cervid
• Stag—adult male cervid
• Calf—immature cervid

PATHOPHYSIOLOGY
Dependent upon specific parasite

SYSTEMS AFFECTED
Gastrointestinal, dermatologic, pulmonary, muscular, central nervous system, and others depending upon the parasite specified

GENETICS
Susceptibility and pathogenicity varies among host species.

INCIDENCE/PREVALENCE
Worldwide

GEOGRAPHIC DISTRIBUTION
Climate, topography, indigenous wildlife populations all determine which parasites will be of significance in a given area.

SIGNALMENT

Species
Susceptibility and pathogenicity varies among host species.

Breed Predilections
N/A

Mean Age and Range
Young animals more likely to suffer significant pathology.

Predominant Sex
N/A

SIGNS
• Anorexia, weight loss, slow growth rate, diarrhea, poor coat condition, cough or dyspnea (lungworm), anemia, and in severe cases death.
• For external parasites may also see a rough coat, pruritis, alopecia, scales, crusts, and skin thickening.

CAUSES
Include but are not limited to:

Internal Parasites
• Nematodes: *Dictyocaulus viviparus* (lungworm), *Ostertagia* spp., *Haemonchus* spp. (stomach worm), *Trichostrongylus* spp. (intestinal worm), *Parelaphostrongylus tenuis, Pneumostrongylus tenuis, Trichuris* spp. (whipworm), *Elaeophora schneideri, Setaria* spp. (abdominal worm)
• Cestodes: *Thysanosoma* spp., *Monezia* spp., *Echinococcus granulosus, Taenia hydatigena*
• Trematodes: *Fascioloides magna* and *Fascioloides hepatica* (liver flukes)
• Protozoal: Coccidia, cryptosporidia, *Toxoplasma gondii, Sarcocystis* spp.
• Arthropods: *Hypoderma tarandi, Hypoderma diana* (Warbles), *Cephenomyia* spp. (Bot fly)

External Parasites
Ticks, lice, mange, face flies, fire ants (*Solenopsis invicta*)

Blood Parasites
Babesia capreoli, Babesia odocoeli, Anaplasma marginale

RISK FACTORS
High-density stocking; malnutrition; harsh winter; introduction of new stock; recently captured wild or free-ranging animals; a warm, moist, environment; and contaminated pastures

DIAGNOSIS

DIFFERENTIAL DIAGNOSIS
Other infectious or metabolic disease, malnutrition

CBC/BIOCHEMISTRY/URINALYSIS
• CBC may show eosinophilia, anemia, or hypoproteinemia.
• Blood films may be used to diagnose hemoparasitism such as babesiosis.

OTHER LABORATORY TEST
CSF tap may show an inflammatory response if the CNS is involved.

IMAGING
N/A

DIAGNOSTIC PROCEDURES
Fecal float and direct examination, fecal egg counts, plasma pepsinogen levels (for abomasal parasitism), Baermann technique (for lungworm)

PATHOLOGIC FINDINGS
Depends upon parasite specified. Parasitic nodules in the abomasum and high worm count for abomasal parasites.

TREATMENT

APPROPRIATE HEALTH CARE

NURSING CARE
IV fluids, transfusion, and tube/bottle feeding may be necessary for severely debilitated calves.

ACTIVITY
N/A

DIET
N/A

CLIENT EDUCATION
Treat the herd as well as the infected individual.

MEDICATIONS

DRUGS OF CHOICE
• With the exception of ivermectin administered subcutaneously, there are no anthelmintics licensed for use in cervidae in the United States.
• Extralabel drug use in cervidae is permitted under specific guidelines, which require a valid veterinarian-client-patient relationship. This author does not endorse or guarantee the safety or efficacy of any of the following products when used in cervidae species.

VACCINATION AND DEWORMING: CERVIDAE

Nematodes
Ivermectin (0.2 mg to 0.4 mg/kg SQ, 0.2 mg/kg PO, or 0.5 mg/kg topically), mebendazole (10 mg/kg PO X 3 days), oxfendazole (4.5 mg/kg PO), fenbendazole, albendazole, levamisole, thiabendazole, doramectin, and moxidectin

Cestodes
Benzimidazoles (cambendazole, oxfenbendazole, fenbendazole, albendazole)

Trematodes
Nitroxynil, closantel, clorsulon (with ivermectin), and triclabendazole (give as 24% drench at the rate of 50 mg/kg, repeat drench in 7 days), albendazole (give in feed at for 7 days), rafozanide.

Babesia
Imidocarb

Protozoan
• Coccidiosis: amprolium, sulfonamides, diclazuril
• Toxoplasmosis: sulfonamides

Ectoparasites
Ivermectin, permethrin, and amitraz

Flies
Warbles and nasal bots: ivermectin treatment must be done in the winter (between September and January for North American cervidae) in order to reach the larvae.

Withdrawal Times
• Ivermectin has a 56-day withdrawal period for reindeer.
• Drug withdrawal times must be determined and maintained for all food-producing species treated.

CONTRAINDICATIONS
Although ivermectin is safe for use during pregnancy, the stress of handling animals can induce abortion. Therefore, handling is not recommended during the last trimester of pregnancy.

PRECAUTIONS
• Withdrawal times and toxicities may vary greatly between species.
• Caution must be used when extrapolating doses and withdrawal times from data on other species.

POSSIBLE INTERACTIONS
Topical ivermectin products may cause local irritation, especially if biting insects are present.

ALTERNATIVE DRUGS
N/A

FOLLOW-UP

PATIENT MONITORING
Monitor fecal egg counts, animal weights, and clinical condition.

PREVENTION/AVOIDANCE
• Avoid overcrowding and develop a deworming program based upon the geographic location, known parasites present, observed clinical signs, and the type of management employed (intensively managed farm vs. wildlife refuge).
• Move herd to a clean pasture in early summer.
• Avoid feeding raw cervidae meat to dogs.

POSSIBLE COMPLICATIONS
Decreased production, stunted growth, death

EXPECTED COURSE AND PROGNOSIS
N/A

MISCELLANEOUS

ASSOCIATED CONDITIONS

AGE-RELATED FACTORS

ZOONOTIC POTENTIAL
Echinococcus spp.

PREGNANCY
Avoid using anthelmintics that are contraindicated in domestic ruminant species.

RUMINANT SPECIES AFFECTED
Depends upon the specific parasite.

BIOSECURITY
• Quarantine, preshipment and postshipment testing are a must.
• Prophylactic deworming of all new animals prior to herd entry is also helpful.
• Fencing must be of sufficient height to keep wild cervidae and other host species out.
• Double fencing may be required.
• Implement insect control measures where insect-borne parasitic diseases are a threat.

PRODUCTION MANAGEMENT
• Perform routine fecal exams on the herd and treat when fecal egg count is high or when clinical signs are observed. Since young animals can be a major source of infection, monthly fecal checks should be performed on calves greater than 2 months of age.

• Other general recommendations include routine deworming of pregnant hinds and calves and prewinter deworming of all stock. Deer may require deworming in the fall and spring. Deer grazing on heavily contaminated pastures may require treatment as often as every 3 weeks during the grazing season.
• Rotate pastures when possible. Deworm calves at weaning and move to clean pastures.
• When using medicated feeds, it is important to spread out the feed over a large amount of trough space so that the lowest animals in the herd's social hierarchy have access.
• Drenching and injectable routes of administration are preferable for large herds in order to ensure that all of the animals receive treatment.
• Implement insect control measures when insect vectors pose a threat. Implement pasture control measures where snails are acting as intermediate hosts.

SYNONYMS

SEE ALSO
Captive management cervidae
Game park management

ABBREVIATIONS
CNS = central nervous system
CSF = cerebral spinal fluid
IV = intravenous
PO = per os, by mouth
SQ = subcutaneous

Suggested Reading
Dieterich, R. A., Morton, J. K. 1990. *Reindeer health aide manual*. Agricultural and Forestry Experiment Station and Cooperative Extension Service University of Alaska Fairbanks and U.S. Dept. of Agriculture Cooperating, 2nd ed. AFES Misc. Pub. 90–4 CES 100H-00046. Available at http://reindeer.salrm.uaf.edu/documents/MP90–4.pdf.
Flach, E. 2003. Cervidae and tragulidae. In: *Zoo and wild animal medicine*, ed. M. E. Fowler, R. E. Miller. St. Louis: Saunders.
Fletcher, T. J. 1982. Management problems and disease in farmed deer. *Vet Rec*. 111(11): 219–23.
Haigh, J. C., Hudson, R. J. 1993. *Farming Wapiti and red deer*. St. Louis: Mosby-Year Book.

Author: Melissa Weisman

VACCINATION AND DEWORMING: SHEEP

 BASICS

OVERVIEW
Health programs should be individualized for each operation addressing
• Planned onset of lambing season
• Management system practiced (i.e., pasture-based, dry-lot, or combination)
• Economic issues—commercial or purebred
• Production goals
• Geographic locale and related disease prevalence issues

SYSTEMS AFFECTED
Production management, immune

GENETICS
N/A

INCIDENCE/PREVALENCE
N/A

GEOGRAPHIC DISTRIBUTION
Worldwide

SIGNALMENT
Species
Ovine
Breed Predilections
Commercial sheep breeds
Mean Age and Range
N/A
Predominant Sex
N/A

 MEDICATIONS

• Focus annual program on management issues associated with four phases of production cycle (See Table 1).
  • Prebreeding
  • Prelambing
  • Lambing
  • Preturnout
• *Clostridium perfringens* type C and D vaccine with/without tetanus toxoid
  • Only "routine" vaccine administered to sheep
  • Referred to as "overeating disease," "CDT," or "CD" vaccine

Additional Vaccine Comments
• Multivalent *Clostridium* spp. vaccines
• Not given routinely unless diseases prevalent in area or animals are shipped to areas where common
• May be useful if clostridium diseases are secondary to special management or parasite problems

• Caseous lymphadenitis vaccine (CLA or CL vaccine)
• Used routinely in some flocks to reduce incidence of CL
• "Soremouth" vaccine ("ecthyma," "orf")
• Live virus "scratch" vaccine: use caution and wear gloves when handling vaccine or lesions
• Causes ecthyma contagiosum in humans
• Vaccination causes disease: therefore not recommended if soremouth not present in flock
• Used mostly to prevent outbreaks affecting sales or lambs less than 3 weeks old
• "Blue tongue" vaccine
• Local use in endemic areas
• May affect serology for interstate/international shipment
• Rabies vaccine
• "Killed" vaccine available for endemic areas, but cost issue for sheep
• Bovine IBR-PI3 intranasal vaccine
• Used by some producers to prevent respiratory disease in show lambs (nonapproved use)

Additional Parasite Comments
• Prevent/postpone resistance issues by rotating anthelmintic families annually.
• Anthelmintic families (three major types) as determined by mechanism of action
• Benzamidazoles/probenzamidazoles: oxibendazole, fenbendazole, albendazole, oxfendazole
  • Resistance issues
  • Best options for tapeworm control
• Avermectins/milbamycins (macrocyclic lactones): ivermectin, doramectin, moxidectin
• Imidazothiazoles: levamisole
• Liver flukes: local problem no approved treatments available
• *Fasciola hepatica* ("common liver fluke"): clorsulon
• *Fascioloides magna* ("deer fluke" in Great Lakes Region): albendazole

PRECAUTIONS
• Extralabel use must be accompanied by a strict veterinarian - client - patient relationship (VCPR)
• *Albendazole should not be used during the first 45 days of pregnancy!* (teratogenic)

 MISCELLANEOUS

ASSOCIATED CONDITIONS
N/A

AGE-RELATED FACTORS
N/A

ZOONOTIC POTENTIAL
N/A

PREGNANCY
N/A

RUMINANT SPECIES AFFECTED
Sheep

BIOSECURITY
N/A

PRODUCTION MANAGEMENT
N/A

SYNONYMS

SEE ALSO
Body condition scoring
Physical examination
Sheep nutrition
Small ruminant parasitology
Specific disease chapters

ABBREVIATIONS
CD or CDT vaccine = *Clostridium perfringens* type CD toxoid with/without tetanus toxoid
CL or CLA = caseous lymphadenitis
EAE = enzootic abortion of ewes
IBR/PI3 = infectious bovine rhinotracheitis/parainfluenza type 3
VCPR = veterinarian-client- patient relationship

Suggested Reading
Banai, M. 2002, Dec 20. Control of small ruminant brucellosis by use of *Brucella melitensis* Rev.1 vaccine: laboratory aspects and field observations. *Vet Microbiol.* 90(1–4):497–519.
Gray, G. D. 1997, Nov. The use of genetically resistant sheep to control nematode parasitism. *Vet Parasitol.* 72(3–4):345–57; discussion 357–66.
Mortensen, L. L., Williamson, L. H., Terrill, T. H., Kircher, R. A., Larsen, M., Kaplan, R. M. 2003, Aug 15. Evaluation of prevalence and clinical implications of anthelmintic resistance in gastrointestinal nematodes in goats. *J Am Vet Med Assoc.* 223(4):495–500.
Paton, M. W., Walker, S. B., Rose, I. R., Watt, G. F. 2003, Jan-Feb. Prevalence of caseous lymphadenitis and usage of caseous lymphadenitis vaccines in sheep flocks. *Aust Vet J.* 81(1–2):91–95.
Waller, P. J., Dash, K. M., Barger, I. A., Le Jambre, L. F., Plant, J. 1995, Apr 22. Anthelmintic resistance in nematode parasites of sheep: learning from the Australian experience. *Vet Rec.* 136(16):411–13.

Author: Joseph S. Rook

VACCINATION AND DEWORMING: SHEEP

Table 1

Production Phase	Vaccination Issues	Parasite Issues

Prebreeding	*Immunize against abortion diseases:*
	Not suggested *if* a "closed-flock" with no history of infectious abortions
	  Available products:
	    1. *Campylobacter fetus* subspecies *intestinalis* and *jejuni* (vibrio) vaccine
	      First dose before breeding
	      Second dose in midpregnancy
	      Use only vaccines containing ovine isolates
	      Bovine vaccine ineffective!
	    2. *Chlamydia psittaci* (also called enzootic abortion/EAE) vaccine
	      First dose before breeding
	      Second dose in midpregnancy
	      Then booster yearly
	      Geographic issue
	      Toxoplasmosis vaccine unavailable in United States
		Prior to breeding:
		Review anthelmintic resistance records and treat with
		  appropriate medication
		  Approved: levamisole, ivermectin, albendazole
		  Unapproved: doramectin, moxidectin oxfendazole,
		  oxibendazole, fenbendazole
		Move to a "clean" (worm-free) pasture after treatment
		  Hay field regrowth
		  Crop residue
		  Cattle pasture or areas previously not pastured by sheep
		Use composite fecal float tests to detect efficacy and
		  resistance issues with treatment/prevention program
		Caution: albendazole should not be used during the first 45
		  days of pregnancy!

Prelambing	*Vaccination*
	Midpregnancy (60–90 days) booster abortion vaccines
	Booster clostridium vaccines 4 to 6 weeks prior to lambing
	  • *C. perfringens* type C & D toxoid or CDT combination vaccine
	(if tetanus an issue)
	  • Stimulates passive protection to newborn lambs via colostrum
	Other vaccines— *if warranted for area*
	  • Multivalent *Clostridium* vaccines
	  • *E. coli* vaccine
	  • Foot rot vaccine
	  • Caseous lymphadenitis vaccine
		Parasite control
		Internal parasites: prevent periparturient egg rise
		  • Deworm as a group 2–4 weeks prior to lambing, or treat in
		  lambing pens as lamb
		External parasites: after shearing, treat flock with pour-on for
		  lice and keds
		If historical problems with coccidiosis, treat ewes with
		  coccidiostat in feed, water or salt
		Reduces shedding of oocysts by carrier ewes
		  • Medications: decoquinate, amprolium, oral sulfas,
		  monensin

Lambing	If lambs *not pastured* with ewes and/or fed grain from birth (i.e., lambs fed concentrate early in life)
	  • *C. perfringens* CD toxoid to prevent "overeating disease" in lambs on high-concentrate diets
	  If ewes were unvaccinated
	  • First vaccine when processing lambs at 2 to 3 days of age (labor issue)
	  • Booster when lamb 25–30 days old
	  If ewes vaccinated
	  • First vaccine at 4–6 weeks old
	  • Booster 2 weeks later
	  If *lambs pastured with ewes* until weaning
	  • *C. perfringens* CD toxoid usually not an issue until lambs weaned to grain diets
	  • Then two doses *C. perfringens* CD toxoid prior to entering feedlot
	  • When working lambs for deworming, etc.
		Confinement, semiconfinement, or drop-lot lambing ewes
		• Treat ewes in lambing pens (jugs) as they lamb (if no prelambing treatment)
		• Pasture lambing ewes (no lambing pens)
		• Treat ewes as a group 2–4 weeks prior to lambing or entering lambing pasture
		  • Time treatment to flock move to the lambing pasture
		  • Often treated at shearing
		• Approved: levamisole, ivermectin, albendazole
		• Unapproved: doramectin, moxidectin oxfendazole, oxibendazole, fenbendazole
		• Continue coccidiostat treatment in feed, water or salt to control oocyst contamination of lambing area and/or pasture.

Preturnout	If lambs *not pastured* with ewes (only dry ewes go to pasture)
	• Ewes— no special vaccines unless problem flocks
	• Foot rot vaccine—individual flock issue
	• Booster ewes prior to seasonal weather conducive to transmission (wet and warm)
	• *B. nodosus* vaccine utilized
	• *F. necrophorum* vaccine less common
	• Some flocks use both
		If lambs *not pastured* with ewes (only dry ewes go to pasture)
		• Treat ewes before release to pasture
		  Approved: levamisole, ivermectin, albendazole
		  Unapproved: doramectin, moxidectin oxfendazole, oxibendazole, fenbendazole
		• Release to "clean" pasture, if available
		If *lambs pastured with ewes* until weaning
		• Same as lambing
		• Lambing and preturnout recommendations coincide

Special considerations for pastured lambs and ewes	*C. perfringens* vaccines not as important until lambs leave grass and arrive at feedlot *C. perfringens* type-D/CD toxoid routine on arrival at feedlot Booster second dose 2–4 weeks after arrival	Internal parasites major issue in pastured lambs • Treatment programs: location, weather, parasite dependent • Lamb treatment initiated when lambs 8–12 weeks old, followed by return to "clean pasture" • May need retreatment every 3 weeks if remain on contaminated pasture after treatment • Reduce pasture contamination: strategic treatment programs utilize serial treatments at 3 and 6 weeks after turn-out • Tapeworms also an issue in pastured lambs 8–12 weeks into the grazing season (due to grass mite intermediate host relationships)

VACCINATION PROGRAMS ON DAIRIES

 BASICS

DEFINITION
Vaccination is the intentional stimulation of a protective immune response by exposing an animal to a pathogen or the epitopes of the pathogen. Immunity is conferred by humeral antibodies or enhancing white blood cell function.

OVERVIEW
• Vaccination is a major part of prevention of infectious diseases on dairies.
• There are a few vaccines that are considered basic to the vaccine program on dairies in North America and there are many other vaccines that should be considered for a vaccine program based on the particular disease risks and management of individual farms.
• Vaccines should be chosen carefully because the process can bring both prevention of disease and risk for disease.
• The following principles must be adhered to for a vaccine to work well.
  • The vaccine must be stored and handled properly.
  • The vaccine must be administered to the appropriate animals at the right times using the correct route and dosage.
  • The animals must be in good health and in positive growth or energy balance.

SYSTEMS AFFECTED
Production management, immune

GENETICS
The Holstein breed appears to be highly susceptible to the effects of bacterial endotoxin.

INCIDENCE/PREVALENCE
N/A

GEOGRAPHIC DISTRIBUTION
Worldwide

Epidemiology
• Vaccines must be given prior to exposure to the pathogen and the animal must have enough time to process the antigens and develop either humoral or cellular immunity.
• Accordingly, cattle should be vaccinated at least 2 weeks prior to risk periods with systemic vaccines. Temperature-sensitive IBR intranasal vaccines elicit local mucosal immunity and will be efficacious 48 hours after administration.
• Passively acquired immunity from colostrum may interfere with systemic vaccinations for varying periods after colostrum feeding. The effective half-life of maternal antibodies is dependent on the specific pathogen, the quantity of antibody in the colostrum, and the absorption of antibody through the GI mucosa in individual calves and the calf itself. Thus, maternal antibody may affect the efficacy of systemic vaccinations in calves for between 2 to 6 months after colostrum feeding at birth.

• Calves should always receive at least one systemic vaccination for the essential viral vaccines (IBR, BVD, BRSV) after 6 months of age. Intranasal vaccines are not affected by maternal antibody and should be expected to be efficacious as soon as the corticosteroids associated with calving have metabolized.
• The concept of herd immunity is important in dairy preventive medicine. Disease prevention and decreased case rate can be expected for most pathogens as long as the majority of animals in the population is effectively immunized.

Dairy Vaccinology
• A basic vaccine program on a dairy should include vaccinations for infectious bovine rhinotracheitis (IBR), bovine virus diarrhea types I and II (BVD), bovine respiratory syncytial virus (BRSV), and *Leptospira hardjo* and *L. pomona* bacterins.
• Other vaccines may be recommended depending on the management and problems on the dairy.
• Optional vaccines include: clostridial (malignant edema, redwater, and blackleg) bacterins, campylobacteriosis (vibrio) bacterins, *Moraxella bovis* (pinkeye) bacterins, *Neospora* killed protozoal vaccine and core-antigen J-5 gram negative bacterins (coliform mastitis). Rotavirus vaccines may be useful for protecting neonatal calves depending on the dairy.
• Some, but not all, states in the United States require vaccination of heifers with live RB 51 *Brucella abortus* vaccine.
• The viral pathogens can be administered either as modified-live virus (MLV) or killed vaccines.
• MLV vaccines are generally preferred because of the problem of compliance with boostering killed virus vaccines.
• Killed virus vaccines and bacterins must have a second dose within 2 to 4 weeks of the primary vaccination to develop an anamnestic response.

Dairy Vaccination Program
• A basic vaccination program for a dairy may include the following vaccines:
  • *Birth:* colostrum (Bull and heifer calves—maternal antibodies are necessary for mucosal and systemic immunity and the white blood cells in colostrum initiate the memory of the calf's immune system.)
  • *Three days of age:* temperature-sensitive intranasal IBR
  • *Before moving to group pens:* temperature-sensitive intranasal IBR or MLV IBR-BVD-BRSV with *Leptospira*
  • *Six months of age:* MLV IBR-BVD-BRSV with *Leptospira*
  • *Before breeding:* MLV IBR-BVD-BRSV with *Leptospira*
  • *At least 20 days postpartum:* MLV IBR-BVD-BRSV with *Leptospira*
  • *Or, during the dry period:* MLV IBR-BVD-BRSV with *Leptospira*

• Other vaccines may be incorporated if the dairy experiences problems with specific pathogens and management cannot be changed to prevent disease. These vaccines include:
• *J-5 gram-negative vaccines* to reduce the severity of coliform mastitis: one or two vaccinations prepartum and one vaccination 10–20 days in milk
• *Neospora killed protozoal vaccine* to decrease abortions from neosporosis
• *Leptospira borgpetersenii* serovar hardjo-bovis (type: *hardjo-bovis*) specific vaccine to prevent early abortions
• *Rotavirus and coronavirus vaccine* to either dry cows or precolostrum calves to prevent diarrhea in calves
• *Clostridial vaccines* to control malignant edema (*C. septicum* or *sordelli*), blackleg (*C. chauvoei*), or redwater (*C. haemolyticum*).

SIGNALMENT
Species Affected
Dairy cattle

Breed Predilections
The Holstein breed appears to be highly susceptible to the effects of bacterial endotoxin.

Mean Age and Range
N/A

Predominant Sex
N/A

SIGNS
GENERAL COMMENTS
• Calves and cattle should always be in positive energy balance or growth when vaccinated.
• Avoid vaccinating heat-stressed cattle due to the increased risk of endotoxic reaction.

HISTORICAL FINDINGS
There should be clinical, laboratory, or other evidence of pathogens in the herd or region for which efficacious vaccines are available to recommend particular vaccines.

PHYSICAL EXAMINATION FINDINGS
N/A

CAUSES
N/A

RISK FACTORS
Typical risks that can be partially managed with vaccines on dairies include moving from individual calf hutches to group pens, overcrowding, immunosuppressive periods such as transportation and parturition, and increased manure material on teats during milking.

VACCINATION PROGRAMS ON DAIRIES

DIAGNOSIS

DIFFERENTIAL DIAGNOSIS
It is imperative to have knowledge of the infectious diseases the cattle on a farm will be exposed to at different times in the management cycle before recommending vaccine programs.

CBC/BIOCHEMISTRY/URINALYSIS
N/A

OTHER LABORATORY TESTS
Monitoring selenium status in whole blood may be advised in some herds.

IMAGING
N/A

OTHER DIAGNOSTIC PROCEDURES
Submission of necropsy samples to determine pathogens on the farm is advised.

TREATMENT

CLIENT EDUCATION
• Clients must understand the importance of vaccine handling and timing of the vaccinations. All vaccines must be kept cold and out of the sunlight. Modified-live virus vaccines are inactivated quickly by ultraviolet light in sunlight and should be used within 1 hour of mixing with the diluent and kept out of sunlight.
• Vaccines should not be frozen; MLV vaccines are inactivated and attenuated by freeze-thaw cycles and cells can be ruptured and endotoxin released in bacterins.
• Bacterins must be boostered at the recommended intervals and clients choosing to use killed virus vaccines must understand the importance of the booster dose in the anamnestic response.

MEDICATIONS

DRUGS OF CHOICE
Epinephrine should be on hand in case of anaphylactic reaction after vaccination.

CONTRAINDICATIONS
• Do not administer corticosteroids within 1 week of vaccination.
• It is commonly recommended to not administer more than two gram-negative bacterins at the same time because of the risk of endotoxemia.
• Vaccination of animals in negative energy balance or weight loss may result in decreased efficacy and can potentially have negative effects through endotoxemia or reduced dry matter intake.

PRECAUTIONS
• Do not administer more than two gram-negative bacterins on the same day. Use only approved MLV vaccines in pregnant animals.
• Do not vaccinate cattle within 1 week after parturition to avoid the immunosuppressive complications of the corticosteroids associated with calving.

POSSIBLE INTERACTIONS
• Endotoxin in gram-negative and *Leptospira* bacteria can elicit a severe immune reaction mediated by lymphokines and cytokines. It is therefore recommended that no more than two gram-negative or *Leptospira* bacterins be used simultaneously.
• Because high ambient temperature appears to increase the risk of endotoxemia, it is recommended to avoid vaccinating cattle during heat stress.
• Immunosuppressive drugs such as corticosteroids should not be given at or near vaccination.

ALTERNATE DRUGS
N/A

FOLLOW-UP

PATIENT MONITORING
Cattle should be observed for at least 2 hours postvaccination for signs of anaphylaxis.

PREVENTION/AVOIDANCE
N/A

EXPECTED COURSE AND PROGNOSIS
• Effective immunity can be expected within 2 weeks after systemic vaccinations.
• Bacterins must be boostered at the suggested times to achieve the desired anamnestic response.
• Mucosal immunity is developed within 48 hours after intranasal vaccination with temperature-sensitive IBR vaccines.

MISCELLANEOUS

PREVENTION
N/A

ASSOCIATED CONDITIONS
N/A

AGE-RELATED FACTORS
• Calves less than 1 week of age may not respond well to systemic vaccinations but will respond well to temperature-sensitive intranasal vaccines.
• Cellular immunity in the neonatal bovine appears to be decreased between 2 and 5 weeks of age and vaccination with systemic vaccines should be avoided during this period.
• Vaccine programs are generally targeted to bovines based on age. The goal of vaccinating calves is to decrease the case rate and severity of diarrhea and pneumonia, whereas older cattle are vaccinated to protect from abortifacients, mastitis, and pneumonia.

ZOONOTIC POTENTIAL
RB 51 and Strain 19 Brucella vaccines are live bacterial vaccines and are zoonotic pathogens.

PREGNANCY
• Bacterins and killed-virus vaccines are generally safe for pregnant cattle, although the endotoxins in bacterins can cause sufficient prostaglandin release during an endotoxic reaction to cause lutealysis and abortion.
• Only modified-live vaccines approved for use in pregnant cattle should be used during gestation.
• The first infection with IBR (wild type or vaccine strain) virus can result in infection of the ovary and subsequent lutealysis and abortion. Therefore, cattle should have been previously effectively vaccinated with MLV-IBR prior to MLV-IBR vaccination during pregnancy.

SYNONYMS
N/A

SEE ALSO
Dairy heifer management
Specific disease chapters
Vaccinology

ABBREVIATIONS
BRSV = bovine respiratory syncytial virus
BVD = bovine virus diarrhea virus
GI = gastrointestinal
IBR = infectious bovine rhinotracheitis
MLV = modified-live virus

Suggested Reading
Cortese, V. S. 2002. Bovine vaccines and herd vaccination programs. In: *Large animal internal medicine*, ed. B. P. Smith. 3rd ed. St. Louis: Mosby.
Ellis, J. A. 2001, Nov. The immunology of the bovine respiratory disease complex. *Vet Clin North Am Food Anim Pract*. 17(3):535–50, viv–vii.
Hjerpe, C. A. 1990, Mar. Bovine vaccines and herd vaccination programs. *Vet Clin North Am Food Anim Pract*. 6(1):167–260.
Sandvik, T. 2004, Mar. Progress of control and prevention programs for bovine viral diarrhea virus in Europe. *Vet Clin North Am Food Anim Pract*. 20(1):151–69.
van Oirschot, J. T. 1999. Bovine viral vaccines, diagnostics, and eradication: past, present, and future. *Adv Vet Med*. 41:197–216.
van Oirschot, J. T. 2001, Jul. Present and future of veterinary viral vaccinology: a review. *Vet Q*. 23(3):100–108.
Zeitlin, L., Cone, R. A., Moench, T. R., Whaley, K. J. 2000, May. Preventing infectious disease with passive immunization. *Microbes Infect*. 2(6):701–708.

Author: Jim Reynolds

VAGAL INDIGESTION

 BASICS

DEFINITION
• Vagal indigestion is a complex syndrome characterized by functional disturbances of the ruminant forestomachs.
• It is a syndrome with various causes, which result in rumen distension with gas and/or fluid.
• Contrary to the name, primary vagal nerve injury is rarely the cause of the syndrome.
• This syndrome is characterized and differentiated from other forms of indigestion by its slowly progressive onset and long duration.

PATHOPHYSIOLOGY
Syndrome composed of four categories of dysfunction:

Type I: Free Gas Bloat; Failure of Eructation
• Free gas bloat
  • Partial esophageal obstruction by foreign body
  • Extraesophageal compression
  • Lymphosarcoma, thyroid tumors
  • Chronic mediastinitis, abscesses
• Failure of eructation: inflammatory process adjacent to vagal nerve
  • Abscessation in cranial abdomen, peritonitis
  • Chronic pneumonia

Type II: Omasal Transport Failure
• Intraluminal reduction in omasal canal: placenta, bags
• Extramural masses that compress the omasal canal
  • Perireticular adhesions, localized peritonitis: traumatic reticuloperitonitis, perforating abomasal ulcers
  • Lymphosarcoma, papilloma, squamous cell carcinoma
  • Infarction
• Failure of omasal transport
  • Functional atony
  • Liver abscesses in left lobe of the liver: may place pressure on vagal nerve

Type III: Abomasal Impaction
• Primary abomasal impaction
  • Animals fed dry, coarse roughage
  • Limited access to water

• Secondary abomasal impaction: functional inability to empty contents of abomasum
  • Traumatic reticuloperitonitis adhesions
  • Adhesions of right lateral wall of reticulum
  • Poor motility post abomasal volvulus
  • Foreign bodies may obstruct pylorus: hairballs, placenta
  • Toggle pin fixation for displaced abomasum has been reported to result in pyloric outflow obstruction
  • True pyloric stenosis is rare.

Type IV: Partial Obstruction of Forestomachs; Indigestion of Late Pregnancy
• As fetus develops and enlarges, the abomasum is forced cranially.
• This may interfere with abomasal motility, which may have been previously compromised, leading to impaction.
• These animals may be a combination of type II and type III vagal indigestion.

SYSTEMS AFFECTED
Gastrointestinal

GENETICS
There are no recognized genetic causes or implications for vagal indigestion.

INCIDENCE/PREVALENCE
• There are no reports listing the incidence or prevalence of the disease.
• Vagal indigestion is the most common complication after abomasal volvulus correction.

GEOGRAPHIC DISTRIBUTION
• Type III vagal indigestion may occur more commonly in animals grazed on crop aftermath in dry regions.
• May also occur in the wintertime, when water sources are allowed to freeze

SIGNALMENT
Species
• Reported only in bovines
• Abomasal emptying defect of Suffolk sheep is a similar condition to type III vagal indigestion
  • Lesions in abomasal wall and vagal nerve
  • Genetic syndrome
  • Grave prognosis even with aggressive therapy

Breed Predilections
• Breed predilections in cattle not reported
• Type IV is more common in late pregnant dairy breeds.
• Abomasal emptying defect of sheep occurs in Suffolk.

Mean Age and Range
No reported age ranges, however, lymphoma tends to occur in cattle 4–8 years of age.
Predominant Sex
N/A

SIGNS
GENERAL COMMENTS
• The hallmark signs in patients with vagal indigestion is gradual abdominal enlargement and an L-shaped rumen.
• Vagal indigestion is an unlikely cause of an acutely ill animal and other diagnoses should be considered and ruled out.

HISTORICAL FINDINGS
• Gradual abdominal enlargement
• Intermittent episodes of indigestion and anorexia
• Reduced milk production
• Weight loss
• Decreased fecal output
• May have a history of vomiting or regurgitation
• Animals may be in late pregnancy

PHYSICAL EXAMINATION FINDINGS
• Distended abdomen
  • Rumen full of fluid and/or gas
  • "Papple" shape: large and round dorsally and ventrally on the left, distended ventrally on the right
• Decreased fecal volume
  • Feces may be pasty and have increased fiber length (2–4 cm).
  • Omasum responsible for reducing feed particle size before delivery to abomasum
  • Melena if abomasal ulcer is the cause
• Bradycardia
  • Variable
  • Has been associated with other conditions, but is an unusual finding in the bovine
• Increased rumen motility
  • May be nearly silent, but is easily felt: motility displaces paralumbar fossa significantly
  • If rumen motility absent, prognosis very poor due to likelihood of significant peritonitis and adhesion formation.
• Abdominal percussion
  • Rumen may ping and be mistaken for a left displaced abomasum.
  • Can be differentiated in size and shape from an LDA
• Abdominal succession: rumen splashes due to fluid accumulation

- Rectal exam
  - Appreciate L-shaped rumen
  - May be able to palpate a large, distended abomasum, caudally displaced by cranial abdominal pathology
  - May be able to palpate omasum if significant liver pathology, such as abscessation, is involved
- Grunt test and withers pinch for cranial abdominal pain: not sensitive tests

CAUSES
- Abscesses: most common cause of cranial abdominal abscesses in locations that cause vagal indigestion is traumatic reticuloperitonitis (TRP, hardware disease)
- Tumors
- Foreign bodies in the omasal canal or pylorus: sacks, placenta, hairball
- Adhesions
  - May alter normal motility and tension receptor activity
  - TRP or abomasal ulcers
- Vagal nerve injury
  - Rare cause of syndrome
  - Abscesses may lead to neuropraxia.

RISK FACTORS
- Unresolved pneumonia or mediastinal pathology may predispose to type I.
- Exposure to foreign bodies such as wire or twine may predispose to types I–III.
- Large fetal size may be more likely to cause type IV.
- Bovine leukemia virus infection has been associated with development of gastrointestinal tumors in a small number of infected cattle
- Improper placement of a toggle in a left displaced abomasum

 DIAGNOSIS

DIFFERENTIAL DIAGNOSIS
- Simple indigestion
- Rumen acidosis
- Traumatic reticuloperitonitis
- Displaced abomasum
- Frothy bloat
- Hydrops
- Ascites
- Diffuse peritonitis: generally not a chronic disease

- Abdominal neoplasia: lymphosarcoma, mesothelioma
- Intestinal obstructions: intussusception, mesenteric volvulus
- Reticulitis—may cause vomiting
- Ingestion of toxic plants or spoiled feed—differential for vomiting: rhododendron and mountain laurel

CBC/BIOCHEMISTRY/URINALYSIS
- CBC: useful to indicate cause of vagal indigestion
  - Leukocytosis: mild to moderate inflammation, relatively early in process
  - Leukopenia: severe inflammation (i.e., diffuse peritonitis)
  - Neutrophil-lymphocyte ratio of 2:1: chronic inflammation
  - Lymphocytosis: suggestive of lymphosarcoma
  - Packed cell volume and total protein
  - May be increased due to dehydration
  - PCV may be low due to anemia of chronic disease.
- Biochemistry
  - Hypochloremia
  - Indicates abomasal reflux into rumen from impaction or forestomach stasis: decreases absorption into blood
  - Type III vagal indigestion results in significant hypochloremia and hypokalemia
  - Severe hypochloremia (<50 mEq/L) is associated with a grave prognosis, but may be corrected with aggressive therapy.
  - Metabolic alkalosis
  - Hypocalcemia- moderate
  - Prerenal azotemia
  - Hypergammaglobulinemia: indicates inflammatory process

OTHER LABORATORY TESTS
- Rumen fluid analysis
  - Elevated rumen chloride (> 30 mEq/L)
  - Indicates abomasal HCl reflux into rumen
  - Occurs with abomasal impaction or any abomasal outflow obstruction
- BLV serology
  - Positive results indicate infection with the virus, however do not indicate the presence of a tumor
  - Very low percentage of cattle with BLV virus will develop a tumor

- Abdominocentesis
  - May be difficult to obtain a diagnosis of peritonitis if it is localized and encapsulated
  - Increased protein and white blood cells indicate peritonitis
  - Lymphocytes in the fluid—supportive of lymphoma
- Fecal occult blood
  - Perform before rectal exam
  - If positive, supports the presence of abomasal ulcers

IMAGING
- Radiography: may visualize cranial abdominal metallic foreign bodies
- Ultrasound examination
  - Perireticular abdomen
  - Assess reticular motility
  - Identify masses or abscesses
  - Abomasum: may appreciate increase in wall thickness if infiltrated with lymphosarcoma

DIAGNOSTIC PROCEDURES
Left-sided exploratory rumenotomy
- Allows investigation of cardia, omasal groove, abomasum, and their surroundings
- Localize masses or abscesses obstructing flow of ingesta
- Allows needle aspiration of masses for cytologic impression: provides a means of diagnosis as well as possible treatment (removal of masses, drainage of abscesses into GI, placing fluid directly into abomasum, and massage for relief of impaction)

GROSS FINDINGS
Type I
- Foreign body, mass obstructing esophagus
- Chronic thoracic pathology, such as pneumonia or abscesses

Type II
- Intraluminal foreign bodies or masses
- Masses impinging omasal canal
- Localized peritonitis, adhesions, hardware foreign body
- Liver abscesses

Type III
- Dry, impacted abomasum
- Adhesions, hardware
- Pyloric foreign bodies
- Rarely, pyloric stenosis

Type IV
Large fetus cranially displacing abomasum

VAGAL INDIGESTION

HISTOPATHOLOGICAL FINDINGS
• In one report, no changes were noted on histopathology of cattle with vagal indigestion secondary to traumatic reticuloperitonitis in the following tissues: vagus nerve, cardia, esophageal groove, reticulo-omasal orifice, omasal canal, and pylorus.
• Histopathology performed on masses will reveal nature of the neoplasia: most commonly lymphosarcoma, papilloma, or squamous cell carcinoma.

TREATMENT

APPROPRIATE HEALTH CARE
Animals with vagal indigestion generally require hospitalization in order to receive treatment for their primary condition and to receive supportive care for associated electrolyte imbalances.

Type I
• Create a rumen fistula
  • Self-retaining trocar
  • Rumenostomy
  1. 2–3 cm in diameter, suturing rumen wall to body wall
  2. Provide a good "seal" to prevent leakage and peritonitis.
  • Will granulate over in a few months, allowing healing of causative lesion
• Most cattle will regain ability to eructate normally over time.

Type II
• Supportive therapy
  • Promote GI motility: ruminatorics and cathartics
  • Fluid therapy
  1. Calcium gluconate
  2. Parenteral or oral polyionic fluids
  3. Transfaunation
  • Systemic antibiotics: in attempt to control local peritonitis
• Surgical therapy
  • Very few animals respond to conservative therapy
  • Rumenotomy: palpation of cardia, omasal canal, and reticular wall
• Removal of foreign body or mass
  • Needle biopsy of mass in surgery for definitive diagnosis and prognosis prior to removal
  • Perireticular abscess
  • If firmly adherent to reticular wall, may be incised and drained into reticulum
  • If abscess not firmly adherent, abscess should be drained percutaneously from the right body wall (ultrasound guidance helpful)
• May repeat surgery through paramedian incision to remove the abscess en bloc

Type III
• Carries a poor prognosis
• If secondary to abomasal volvulus, there is no good treatment and a very poor prognosis.
• Fluid therapy
  • Calcium gluconate
  • Intravenous fluids: correct alkalosis and hypokalemia
• Laxatives
  • Magnesium hydroxide/oxide and others
  • 0.5–1.0 kg/day PO
• Surgery
  • May be performed once hydration, electrolyte, and acid/base aberrations addressed
  • Rumenotomy
  • Palpation for presence of masses or abscesses: drain abscess into reticulum or percutaneously as described for type II above
  • May remove abomasal contents through omasal canal without further damaging abomasum
  • Passage of stomach tube into abomasum thorough omasal canal
  • Infusion of docusate, magnesium sulfate, and fluid into abomasum
  • Massage abomasum though rumen wall.
  • Abomasotomy
  • Last resort
  • Surgery will encourage adhesions and ischemia and inhibit motility.

Type IV
• Rank value of dam vs. calf
  • Consider stage of gestation and potential viability of calf
  • If cow is within 4–6 weeks of full gestation, may be able to support both until fetus can be delivered
  • If there is a considerable amount of time before full gestation, saving both dam and fetus less likely
• Fluid therapy: correct existing hypokalemia, hypocalcemia, alkalosis
• Therapeutic abortion
  • Best option if dam is the priority
  • May induce with corticosteroids with or without prostaglandin
• Surgery: rumenotomy
  • Allows exploration to determine etiology
  • Fine needle aspirate of masses, palpation of the status of stomach compartments allow prognostication

NURSING CARE
Fluid therapy and symptomatic therapies covered for each type above

ACTIVITY
Moderate exercise important to maintain during treatment and recovery to promote motility and general health

DIET
• Supply plenty of fresh water and good-quality, digestible feed.
• Basically, anything the animal will eat, along with good fiber: alfalfa is a good choice.

CLIENT EDUCATION
• Very poor prognosis associated with type III.
• Rumenotomy may alter flavor of milk in cows exposed to rumen gases.
• Recommend good hardware and bovine leukosis prevention strategies.

SURGICAL CONSIDERATIONS
• See above for surgical indications and considerations.
• Rumenotomy, rumenostomy, and percutaneous abscess drainage may be performed in the standing animal with local anesthesia to minimize anesthetic risks: lidocaine paravertebral blocks, inverted L, line blocks.

MEDICATIONS

DRUGS OF CHOICE
• See treatments listed above for each type of vagal indigestion.
• Systemic antibiotics may be indicated after rumenotomy and GI manipulation for 1 to 4 weeks.
• Analgesics—NSAIDs

CONTRAINDICATIONS
• The use of magnesium oxide is contraindicated in the presence of metabolic alkalosis.
• NSAID use contraindicated in the presence of abomasal ulcers, increased creatinine, or uncorrected dehydration
• Appropriate milk and meat withdrawal times must be followed for all compounds administered to food-producing animals.

PRECAUTIONS
Observe appropriate withdrawal periods after drug therapy.

POSSIBLE INTERACTIONS
N/A

ALTERNATIVE DRUGS
N/A

FOLLOW-UP

PATIENT MONITORING
• Patients should be monitored during and after therapy for return of appetite and demeanor.
• Abdominal contour must be monitored once animal is eating well to indicate normal motility.
• Fecal output should be monitored for volume, consistency, and fiber length.

PREVENTION/AVOIDANCE
- Use of magnets in feed mixers and handling equipment to prevent metallic foreign bodies in feed
- Removal of placentas from the environment
- Standard BLV control strategies

POSSIBLE COMPLICATIONS
- Poor motility even after appropriate therapy due to irreversible damage to abomasum
- Abscess or mass recurrence after drainage or removal: liver abscess recurrence rate in one report was two or three of eight cases
- Postoperative peritonitis
- Type IV: Retained fetal membranes and metritis are more common in cattle after artificially induced parturition.

EXPECTED COURSE AND PROGNOSIS
Overall, 33/112 (29.5%) of cases of vagal indigestion of all causes made a full recovery.

Type I
- Good prognosis with rumenostomy, but may not flourish
- If chronic pneumonia was inciting cause, poorer prognosis

Type II
- Fair to good depending on exact etiology
- See below for breakdown by etiology.

Type III
- Poor prognosis
- If secondary to abomasal volvulus, 3 of 26 had a good outcome.

Type IV
- The closer to delivery, the better the prognosis: supporting dam through several weeks of gestation is intensive and usually results in deterioration of the dam.
- Removal of fetus at any stage of gestation likely to improve motility and condition of the cow

Prognosis by Etiology
- Neoplasia
  - Lymphosarcoma, squamous cell carcinoma, etc.—grave prognosis
  - Papilloma—good prognosis with removal
- Abscess
  - Extent of adhesion formation determines prognosis
  - Hardware (TRP) prognosis: good outcomes
  - 7/15 (47%) in cases of uncomplicated TRP
  - 6/17 (35%) TRP with obstruction of digesta passage through reticulo-omasal orifice
  - 1/10 (10%) TRP with obstruction of digesta passage though pylorus
  - Peri-omasal or liver abscess—fair to good: liver abscess retrospective

- 5/8 cases made a significant improvement
- 2 or 3 of 8 recurred at 3 months and 1 year postoperatively
- Perireticular abscesses involving diaphragm and omasum: 74% of 29 cases returned to production for greater than 1 to 4 years postoperatively
- Foreign body: excellent prognosis with removal
- Pregnancy: the closer to parturition, the more favorable the prognosis

 MISCELLANEOUS

ASSOCIATED CONDITIONS
Displaced abomasum; abomasal volvulus

AGE-RELATED FACTORS
Older animals affected are more likely to be affected by neoplastic process.

ZOONOTIC POTENTIAL
N/A

PREGNANCY
Termination of late-term pregnancy, if dam considered to be much more valuable than fetus, may be useful in most types of vagal indigestion, not only type IV, as fetal removal may promote normal abomasal and omasal location and motility.

RUMINANT SPECIES AFFECTED
- Only reported in bovines
- Abomasal emptying defect of Suffolk sheep: abomasal and vagal nerve abnormalities have been identified.

BIOSECURITY
N/A

PRODUCTION MANAGEMENT
Animals in dry regions or grazed on crop aftermath should be provided with readily accessible water in order to prevent abomasal impaction.

SYNONYMS

SEE ALSO
Abomasal displacement and volvulus
Abomasal emptying defect
Bloat
Bovine leukemia
Liver abscesses
Traumatic reticuloperitonitis

ABBREVIATIONS
GI = gastrointestinal
LDA = left displaced abomasum
NSAIDs = nonsteroidal anti-inflammatory drugs
TRP = traumatic reticuloperitonitis

Suggested Reading
Fubini, S. L., Ducharme, N. G., Erb, H. N., Smith, D. F., Rebhun, W. C. 1989. Failure of omasal transport attributable to perireticular abscess formation in cattle: 29 cases (1980–1986). *Journal of the American Veterinary Medical Association* 194(6): 811–14.
Fubini, S. L., Ducharme, N. G., Murphy, J. P., Smith, D. F. 1985. Vagus indigestion syndrome resulting from a liver abscess in dairy cows. *Journal of the American Veterinary Medical Association* 186(12): 1297–1300.
Kelton, D. F., Fubini, S. L. 1989. Pyloric obstruction after toggle-pin fixation of left displaced abomasums in a cow. *Journal of the American Veterinary Medical Association*, 194(5): 677–78.
Rebhun, W. C. 1980. Vagus indigestion in cattle. *Journal of the American Veterinary Medical Association* 176 (6): 506–10.
Rebhun, W. C., Fubini, S. L., Miller, T. K., Lesser, F. R. 1988. Vagus indigestion in cattle: Clinical features, causes, treatments and long-term follow-up of 112 cases. *Compendium on Continuing Education for the Practicing Veterinarian* 10(3): 387–91.
Rehage, J., Kaske, M., Stockhofe-Zurwieden, N., Yalcin, E. 1995. Evaluation of the pathogenesis of vagus indigestion in cows with traumatic reticuloperitonitis. *Journal of the American Veterinary Medical Association* 207(12): 1607–11.
Taguchi, K. 1995. Relationship between degree of dehydration and serum electrolytes and acid-base status in cows with various abomasal disorders. *Journal of Vet Med Sci.* 57(2): 257–60.
VanMetre, D. C., Fecteau, G., House, J. K., George, L. W. 1995. Indigestion of late pregnancy in a cow. *Journal of the American Veterinary Medical Association* 205 (5): 625–28.
Whitlock, R. H. 1999. Vagal indigestion. In: *Current veterinary therapy 4, food animal practice*, ed. J. L. Howard and R. A. Smith. Philadelphia: W. B. Saunders.

Author: Meredyth Jones

VAGINITIS

BASICS

OVERVIEW
- Inflammation of vagina
- Infectious causes include bovine herpesvirus 1 (BHV1), *Ureaplasma,* and *Mycoplasma*
- Injuries after dystocia and breeding
- Foreign body

SYSTEMS AFFECTED
Production management and reproductive

GENETICS
N/A

INCIDENCE/PREVALENCE
In one study of genital tracts from nonpregnant cull ewes, 23.2% of the tracts had abnormalities and it was considered that 16.8% had abnormalities likely to interfere with the establishment of pregnancy.

GEOGRAPHIC DISTRIBUTION
Worldwide

SIGNALMENT
Species
Potentially all ruminant species

Breed Predilections
N/A

Mean Age and Range
N/A

Predominant Sex
Female only

SIGNS
- Affected cows show discomfort—arched back, raised tail, straining, frequent urination, and dysuria.
- Accompanied by vulvar or perivulvar swelling
- Seropurulent or mucopurulent discharge
- Laceration, ulceration, and, in neglected cases, necrosis

Infectious Pustular Vulvovaginitis—Caused by BHV1
Transmission is by venereal or oronasal route. Vaginal examination is characterized by numerous round, white, necrotic lesions on the vulva and vaginal wall, and a copious amount of mucopurulent discharge on the vaginal floor. Intrauterine introduction may cause necrotic endometritis.

Granular Vulvitis—Caused by Ureaplasma Diversum
Chronic persistent infection reduces herd fertility. It is characterized by inflammation, hyperemia of vulvar epithelium with small 1–2 mm raised granules predominant around clitoris, and purulent discharge persists up to 10 days. Vulvar infection is often repeatedly introduced into the vagina and uterus during artificial insemination. It persists for 7 days in the uterus causing an unfavorable environment for the descending embryo.

Mycoplasma—Caused by M. bovigenitalium
The role of *Mycoplasma* as a cause of infertility is questionable, as fertile and infertile cows test positive.

CAUSES AND RISK FACTORS
- Infectious causes include bovine herpesvirus 1 (BHV1), *Ureaplasma,* and *Mycoplasma.*
- Injuries after dystocia and breeding
- Malicious injuries
- Urovagina and pneumovagina
- Application of intravaginal progesterone devices
- Foreign body

DIAGNOSIS

DIFFERENTIAL DIAGNOSIS
- Infectious causes include bovine herpesvirus 1 (BHV1), *Ureaplasma,* and *Mycoplasma.*
- Injuries after dystocia and breeding
- Malicious injuries
- Urovagina and pneumovagina
- Application of intravaginal progesterone devices
- Foreign body

CBC/BIOCHEMISTRY/URINALYSIS
Possible stress leukogram, not generally helpful

OTHER LABORATORY TESTS
- BHV1: round, white, necrotic foci will be noticed. The diagnosis may be confirmed by histologic examination for the presence of intranuclear inclusion bodies and necrotic vaginal epithelium.
- Culture and sensitivity is indicated if an infective agent is suspected.

IMAGING
N/A

OTHER DIAGNOSTIC PROCEDURES
- History and clinical signs
- Per-rectal palpation may help to identify the foreign body.
- Vaginoscopic examination may reveal laceration, erosion, necrosis of vaginal mucosa, and accumulation of vaginal discharge. It also helps to locate a foreign body.

PATHOLOGIC FINDINGS

GROSS FINDINGS
- Accompanied by vulvar or perivulvar swelling
- Seropurulent or mucopurulent discharge
- Laceration, ulceration, and, in neglected cases, necrosis
- Infectious pustular vulvovaginits—vaginal examination is characterized by numerous round, white, necrotic lesions on the vulva and vaginal wall, and a copious amount of mucopurulent discharge on the vaginal floor. Intrauterine introduction may cause necrotic endometritis.

• Granular vulvitis—characterized by inflammation, hyperemia of vulvar epithelium with small 1–2 mm raised granules predominant around clitoris; purulent discharge persists for up to 10 days.

HISTOPATHOLOGICAL FINDINGS

In case of BHV1, round, white, necrotic foci will be noticed. The diagnosis may be confirmed by histologic examination for the presence of intranuclear inclusion bodies and necrotic vaginal epithelium.

TREATMENT

• Should treat the primary condition.
• Local antibiotics to control bacterial infection may be indicated.
• Vaginal douche with saline, 0.1% chlorhexidine might be helpful.
• BHV1: local antibiotics to control secondary bacterial infection. However, in the absence of secondary bacterial infection, BHV1 is self limiting and without complication.
• *Ureaplasma:* the treatment and control procedures should be directed toward minimizing the chance of uterine infection. All AI techniques should employ double-rod technique. Local antibiotics therapy and local douches may control the infection. When herd fertility is extremely poor during acute infection, postbreeding antibiotic infusion might be helpful.
• CIDR application: clean procedure and application of proper disinfectant cream at the time of CIDR insertion may reduce the incidence of vaginitis. Relationship between incidence of vaginitis and reduction in fertility is equivocal. The CIDR device should be removed according to the synchronization protocol.

MEDICATIONS

N/A

CONTRAINDICATIONS

Appropriate milk and meat withdrawal times must be followed for all compounds administered to food-producing animals.

POSSIBLE INTERACTIONS

N/A

FOLLOW-UP

N/A

PATIENT MONITORING

N/A

PREVENTION/AVOIDANCE

• CIDR application: clean procedure and application of proper disinfectant cream at the time of CIDR insertion may reduce the incidence of vaginitis.
• The CIDR device should be removed according to the synchronization protocol.
• Appropriate management of dystocia
• All AI techniques should employ double-rod technique.

POSSIBLE COMPLICATIONS

N/A

EXPECTED COURSE AND PROGNOSIS

Depends on the causative agent

MISCELLANEOUS

ASSOCIATED CONDITIONS

N/A

AGE-RELATED FACTORS

.

ZOONOTIC POTENTIAL

N/A

PREGNANCY

N/A

BIOSECURITY

.

PRODUCTION MANAGEMENT

Typical management conditions may predispose to vaginitis.

SEE ALSO

Bovine herpesvirus 1 (BHV1)
Metritis
Mycoplasma
Ureaplasma

ABBREVIATIONS

BHV1 = bovine herpesvirus 1
CIDR = CIDR intravaginal progesterone insert

Suggested Reading

Corbeil, L. B., Anderson, M. L., Corbeil, R. R., Eddow, J. M., BonDurant, R. H. 1998, Mar. Female reproductive tract immunity in bovine trichomoniasis. *Am J Reprod Immunol.* 39(3):189–98.

Kennedy, P. C., Miller, R. B. 1993. The female genital system. In: *Pathology of domestic animals*, vol. 3, ed., K. V. F. Jubb, P. C. Kennedy, N. Palmer. 4th ed. San Diego: Academic Press.

Kirkbride, C. A. 1987. *Mycoplasma, Ureaplasma* and *Acholeplasma* infections of bovine genitalia. *Vet Clin North Am Food Anim Pract.* 3:575.

Winter, A. C., Dobson, H. 1992, Jan 25. Observations on the genital tract of cull ewes. *Vet Rec.* 130(4):68–70.

Youngquist, R. S., Braun, W. F., Jr. 1993, Jul. Abnormalities of the tubular genital organs. *Vet Clin North Am Food Anim Pract.* 9(2):309–22.

Author: Ramanathan Kasimanickam

VESICULAR STOMATITIS

 BASICS

DEFINITION
• Vesicular stomatitis is a viral disease that causes blisters, or vesicles, on the coronary bands, interdigital space, mammary glands, and oral cavity of cattle and horses.
• It cannot be clinically differentiated from foot-and-mouth disease, and proper identification is imperative to the economics of the U.S. agriculture industry.
• Sheep and goats are fairly resistant and rarely show clinical signs.

PATHOPHYSIOLOGY
• Vesicular stomatitis virus (VSV) cases tend to occur sporadically during the warmer months in the southwest United States and most often near waterways.
• Introduction into a herd is not always known but could occur through insect vectors, mechanical transmission, and movement of animals.
• Once lesions appear in a herd, direct contact with vesicles and vesicular fluid between animals spreads the virus quite rapidly.
• Vesicles or erosions can be found in the oral cavity, on the feet, and on the mammary gland in cattle.

SYSTEMS AFFECTED
Gastrointestinal, skin, mammary

GENETICS
N/A

INCIDENCE/PREVALENCE
• Incidence varies between geographic locations.
• Morbidity within a herd of naïve animals can reach 90% but mortality is rare.

GEOGRAPHIC DISTRIBUTION
• This disease has been limited to the Americas.
• In the southern United States and Central America, vesicular stomatitis virus has two domestic strains, New Jersey and Indiana-1, which are found in the southern states.
• In addition to the New Jersey and Indiana-1 strains, exotic strains Indiana-2 and Indiana-3 are found in northern South America.

SIGNALMENT
Species
Cattle, occasionally sheep and goats.
Breed Predilections
N/A
Mean Age and Range
N/A
Predominant Sex
N/A

SIGNS
HISTORICAL FINDINGS
• Disease can occur at any time of year but cases tend to cluster during the summer and fall, often during rainier seasons.
• Cases tend to occur sporadically in endemic areas without large outbreaks.
• Cattle may salivate excessively, have a fever, lose milk production, and develop mastitis.
• The disease is usually self-limiting in approximately 2 weeks.

PHYSICAL EXAMINATION FINDINGS
Fever, blanched vesicles located in one area of the body, such as the oral cavity and muzzle, the feet, or mammary gland, decreased milk production, inappetence due to oral vesicles, lameness due to vesicles on the coronary band and/or interdigital space, and agitation during milking due to vesicles on the mammary gland.

CAUSES
• Vesicular stomatitis is an RNA virus in the family Rhabdoviridae.
• There are multiple strains, but those endemic to the United States are New Jersey and Indiana-1.
• Transmission can occur through insect vectors, direct contact with infected animals, and indirect contact with contaminated objects. Black flies (Simuliidae) and phlebotomine sand flies (Lutzomyia shannoni) can transmit the virus to animals and transovarially. In the 1982 epizootic of VS in the southwestern United States, the New Jersey serotype was isolated from biting midges (Culicoides), mosquitoes (Aedes), house flies (Musca), and eye gnats (Chloropidae), but their role in transmission is unknown.

RISK FACTORS
• Moving naïve animals to an endemic area, especially during the late rainy season
• Increased population of black flies or sand flies

 DIAGNOSIS

DIFFERENTIAL DIAGNOSIS
• Cattle: Foot-and-mouth disease, infectious bovine rhinotracheitis, bovine viral diarrhea, rinderpest, malignant catarrhal fever, bluetongue, foot rot, chemical or thermal burns
• Sheep: Bluetongue, contagious ecthyma, lip/leg ulceration, and foot rot

CBC/BIOCHEMISTRY/URINALYSIS
N/A

OTHER LABORATORY TESTS
N/A

IMAGING
N/A

DIAGNOSTIC PROCEDURES
• Due to the seriousness of this disease and the inability to clinically differentiate it from FMD, state and federal authorities should be contacted immediately upon suspicion of cases before sample collection.
• Tissue cultures can be used to isolate the virus; RT-PCR can be used to detect the virus. Viral antibodies (on acute and convalescent sera) and antigen (aseptic vesicular fluid, vesicular epithelium in buffered glycerol or frozen) can be identified using ELISA, CF, and virus neutralization.

PATHOLOGIC FINDINGS
Vesicles in the oral cavity, on the coronary band, or mammary gland will be seen grossly.

 TREATMENT

APPROPRIATE HEALTH CARE
NURSING CARE
• Upon confirmatory diagnosis of VSV, animals with lesions should be isolated and given supportive care conducive to the location of the lesions.
• Soft food, or a gruel, and clean water for oral lesions; well bedded, clean stall for lesions of the feet; milked last if there are mammary lesions

ACTIVITY
• Isolated to a pen/stall that has no direct contact with other susceptible animals and no exposure to potential insect vectors
• Calves should be removed from infected dams.

DIET
• Soft forages/gruel for oral lesions, plenty of water
• Do not feed calves milk or colostrum from infected animals.

CLIENT EDUCATION
• Animals with lesions must be isolated to prevent disease spread; no animals can be moved off the property for at least 30 days after the last lesion has healed.
• Equipment and areas of potential exposure at a facility should be cleaned and disinfected before reintroducing any other animals.

SURGICAL CONSIDERATIONS
Local wound debridement may be warranted depending on the extent of the lesion and viable tissue surrounding it allowing it to heal on its own.

MEDICATIONS

DRUGS OF CHOICE
N/A

CONTRAINDICATIONS
N/A

POSSIBLE INTERACTIONS
N/A

ALTERNATIVE DRUGS
N/A

FOLLOW-UP

PATIENT MONITORING
Patients should be monitored for appetite and lesion healing during the course of the disease (approximately 2 weeks).

PREVENTION/AVOIDANCE
• Do not move animals to an endemic area.
• Insect control can help prevent disease spread.
• There is no vaccine available.

POSSIBLE COMPLICATIONS
Secondary bacterial infection of the lesioned area

EXPECTED COURSE AND PROGNOSIS
Most recover without complications in two weeks.

MISCELLANEOUS

ASSOCIATED CONDITIONS
Fever; blanched vesicles located in one area of the body, such as the oral cavity and muzzle, the feet, or mammary gland; decreased milk production; inappetence due to oral vesicles; lameness due to vesicles on the coronary band and/or interdigital space; and agitation during milking due to vesicles on the mammary gland

AGE-RELATED FACTORS
N/A

ZOONOTIC POTENTIAL
• Humans can become infected with VSV New Jersey and Indiana-1 strains and signs include fever, headache, myalgia, and, very rarely, oral vesicles.
• Recovery is usually within 4 to 7 days.

PREGNANCY
There does not seem to be a concern with pregnant animals unless the lesions impede eating or a severe secondary infection develops.

RUMINANT SPECIES AFFECTED
Cattle, occasionally sheep and goats, though rare

BIOSECURITY
• Isolation and quarantine of new stock entering the herd/flock
• Treat and/or cull new animals for disease conditions prior to herd introduction.
• VS is a reportable disease.
• Animals with lesions must be isolated to prevent disease spread; no animals can be moved off the property for at least 30 days after the last lesion has healed.
• Equipment and areas of potential exposure at a facility should be cleaned and disinfected before reintroducing any other animals.

PRODUCTION MANAGEMENT
N/A

SYNONYMS
N/A

SEE ALSO
Bluetongue
Bovine viral diarrhea
Chemical or thermal burns
Contagious ecthyma
Foot rot
Foot-and-mouth disease
Infectious bovine rhinotracheitis
Lip/leg ulceration
Malignant catarrhal fever
Rinderpest

ABBREVIATIONS
CF = complement fixation
ELISA = enzyme-linked immunosorbent assay
FMD = foot-and-mouth disease
RT-PCR = reverse transcriptase–polymerase chain reaction
VSV = vesicular stomatitis virus

Suggested Reading
Aiello, S. E., ed. 1998. *Merck veterinary manual*. 8th ed. Whitehouse Station, NJ: Merck and Co.
Office International des Epizooties. *Vesicular stomatitis* accessed at http://www.oie.int/eng/maladies/fiches/a_A020.html, May 11, 2004.
Rebhun, W. C. 1995, Vesicular stomatitis. In: *Diseases of dairy cattle*. Media, PA: Williams and Wilkins.
United States Animal Health Association. *Vesicular stomatitis* accessed at http://www.vet.uga.edu/vpp/gray_book/FAD/vst.html, May 12, 2004.
USDA APHIS. *Vesicular stomatitis for the dairy producer* accessed at http://www.aphis.usda.gov/oa/pubs/vsdairy.html, May 14, 2004.

Author: Danelle Bickett-Weddle

VETERINARY HEALTH CERTIFICATION

BASICS

OVERVIEW
• Health certificates are required to document specific animal health levels and results of diagnostic tests (e.g., tuberculosis and brucellosis) regarding interstate and international trade of animals and animal products. The credibility of such certificates depends on the quality of the data used to establish the status. Veterinarians should regard these certificates not only as legal documents, but also as epidemiologic tools for animal health regulators in the event of a disease outbreak.
• Continued growth in international trade and the developing concepts of zoning and risk assessment demand effective methods of national animal health surveillance and monitoring systems.
• The United States Department of Agriculture (USDA), Animal and Plant Health Inspection Service (APHIS), Veterinary Services (VS) oversees the federal health certification process, but interstate regulations are written and maintained by each state. For clarification on any of the rules and regulations, contact the state veterinarian or the APHIS area veterinarian in charge (AVIC).
• Veterinarians certifying animals or animal products for interstate or international movement must be accredited by the USDA APHIS VS. For further information on accreditation, contact the Veterinary Services office in your state.
• The World Organization for Animal Health (OIE) meets yearly in Paris and its 160+ member countries establish minimal health standards for many diseases of regulatory or public health significance. These standards often impact on import and export requirements for international animal movement.
• International health certificates for the export of animals from the United States are completed by a licensed, accredited veterinarian who certifies herd and animal health status, conducts tests, and records test results for the individual animals being exported.

• Completed and signed international health certificates for the export of animals from the United States must be endorsed by an AVIC in order to be valid.
• The United States has minimal requirements for animals to be exported to other countries. The area veterinarian in charge can assist in finding out the current regulations, tests, and inspections required.
• Each country may have other specific health requirements for entry of animals. The importing country, not the United States, establishes these requirements. Other countries also may have their own certificate format for export. Since export requirements frequently change, obtain the current requirements from the Veterinary Service office in your area before each shipment.
• Export certificates are official documents and they should be typewritten, accurate, and complete.
• In November 2002, USDA APHIS Veterinary Services announced they would work with Communications Resource Inc. (CRI) and GlobalVetLink, LC (GVL) to develop an electronic version of the Interstate Certificate of Veterinary Inspection in designated states for food animals. The electronic health certificate is web-based and incorporates the requirements endorsed by United States Animal Health Association (USAHA).

SYSTEMS AFFECTED
Production management

GENETICS
N/A

INCIDENCE/PREVALENCE
N/A

GEOGRAPHIC DISTRIBUTION
United States; potentially worldwide

SIGNALMENT

Species
All ruminant species

Breed Predilections
N/A

Mean Age and Range
N/A

Predominant Sex
N/A

MISCELLANEOUS

Types of Certification
• Imported animal health certificates
• Animal export health certificates
• Veterinary health certificates

Reportable Diseases
Veterinarians, veterinary diagnostic laboratories, animals' owners, and agents must immediately report the existence or suspected existence of any reportable disease. Reporting requirements vary by state so consult the office of the state veterinarian for a list of reportable diseases in your state.

Intrastate Sale or Movement
Testing: All dairy breeds of cattle must test negative for brucellosis within 30 days prior to any change of ownership. General exceptions to the testing requirement:
• Calves under 4 months of age
• Cattle sold or consigned to a restricted feedlot
• Cattle sold or consigned to a federally inspected slaughter plant
• Steers and spayed heifers
• Official calfhood vaccinates under 20 months of age and not parturient or postparturient.

For dairy breeds, an official calfhood vaccinate is an animal vaccinated between 4 and 8 months with Strain 19 vaccine or between 4 and 12 months with RB 51 vaccine. Cattle exempt from testing may be tested if requested by a prospective buyer or to meet import requirements of another state or foreign country.

Identification of Animals
• The National Animal Identification System (NAIS) is in the process of being developed for all species of animals in the United States. Veterinarians should remain informed as this program continues to be developed and implemented. Identification requirements for animals traveling in commerce are likely to change.
• All animals must be individually identified and permanently recorded as to herd of origin prior to being sold or consigned for slaughter. Immediate slaughter means delivery within 7 days to an inspected slaughter plant or restricted feedlot. This identification must be transferred to the blood sample taken for the brucellosis market cattle identification test purposes.
• Exceptions to this identification requirement:
  • Cattle under 24 months of age and not parturient or postparturient
  • Steers and spayed heifers

VETERINARY HEALTH CERTIFICATION

Scrapie

- The USDA Scrapie Flock Certification Program is designed to monitor flocks and certify scrapie status of animals enrolled in the program.
- The program requires individual animal identification, good record keeping, reporting acquisitions and deaths of animals to USDA and annual inspections by a USDA representative.
- Enrollment in the USDA program fulfills the requirements of the state program. Scrapie Eradication, State-Federal-Industry, Uniform Methods and Rules, September 2003, and Title 9 Code of Federal Regulations, Parts 54 and 79.

Interstate Sale or Movement

- Interstate movement of livestock is regulated at both the state and federal levels.
- Requirements are subject to change, because disease status can change. Prior to shipment, contact the state of destination for current requirements on testing, permits, and health certificates.
- The licensed, accredited veterinarian issuing the health certificate is responsible for ensuring that the shipment meets all requirements of the state of destination.

State Requirements Can be Obtained Through:

- USDA Voice Response Service, 1–800–545–8732, using a touch-tone phone. This service is available 24 hours per day, 7 days a week. Follow the voice prompts and use the individual state codes in parentheses.
- State of destination: http://www.aphis.usda.gov/vs/sregs
- When a state of destination requires a certificate of veterinary inspection for large animals, submit white and canary copies of the completed form to the state veterinarian for final review and approval. The blue copy must accompany the shipment of animals. Veterinarians should retain the green copy of the completed form for their records.

International Sale or Movement

- International movement of animals is regulated at the federal level. Consult the local USDA APHIS Veterinary Services Area Office for information.
- Health certificates for export of animals from the United States are completed by the licensed, accredited veterinarian, who certifies health status, conducts appropriate tests, and records test results on the proper health certificate.
- Most completed and signed health certificates must be reviewed, verified, and endorsed by the Veterinary Services Area Office before they are official international health certificates. The area office can work with the licensed, accredited veterinarian to insure that the health certificate meets the requirements of the country of destination.

Forms to Use

- For livestock, horses going to countries other than Canada, and other large animal species, VS Form 17–140, U.S. Origin Health Certificate, unless the country of destination requires a specific certificate.
- VS and APHIS forms may be obtained from the USDA APHIS VS Area Office.
- All diagnostic tests for export certification must be conducted in USDA-approved labs. Retests must be conducted at the same laboratory that conducted the initial test.
- Original test results, not photocopies, must accompany health paperwork when submitted for review and endorsement. There is a fee for services related to the export of animals, including certificate review and endorsement. Contact the area office for exact costs and method of payment.
- Health certificates received at the area office are reviewed, endorsed, and placed in return mail the day received. For return by express service, include a prepaid envelope or billing account number. Appointments can be made for endorsement of certificates in person.
- Veterinary certification: "I certify, as an accredited veterinarian, that the above described animals have been inspected by me and that they are not showing signs of infectious, contagious and/or communicable disease (except where noted). The vaccinations and results of tests are as indicated on the certificate. To the best of my knowledge, the animals listed on this certificate meet the state of destination and federal interstate requirements. No further warranty is made or implied."
- Owner statement, owner/agent statement (where applicable): "The animals in this shipment are those certified to and listed on this certificate." (Signature, date, and address required.)

Important Web Sites

- United States Department of Fish and Game: www.dfg.ca.gov/
- USDA Animal Care: www.aphis.usda.gov/ac/
- USDA Veterinary Services: www.aphis.usda.gov
- USDA Veterinary Services (regulations): www.aphis.usda.gov/vs/ncie/index.html#Regs

ASSOCIATED CONDITIONS

Scrapie, brucellosis, bluetongue, tuberculosis

AGE-RELATED FACTORS

See Intrastate Sale or Movement above.

ZOONOTIC POTENTIAL

Brucellosis and tuberculosis are zoonotic diseases.

PREGNANCY

N/A

RUMINANT SPECIES AFFECTED

Potentially, all ruminant species are affected

BIOSECURITY

See Identification of Animals above.

PRODUCTION MANAGEMENT

N/A

SYNONYMS

N/A

SEE ALSO

Bluetongue
Brucellosis
Differential diagnosis
Scrapie
Tuberculosis

ABBREVIATIONS

APHIS = Animal and Plant Health Inspection Service
CRI = Communications Resource Inc.
GVL = GlobalVetLink, LC
USDA = United States Department of Agriculture

Suggested Reading
Barcos, L. O. 2001, Aug. Recent developments in animal identification and the traceability of animal products in international trade. *Rev Sci Tech*. 20(2): 640–51.
Hueston, W. D. 1993, Dec. Assessment of national systems for the surveillance and monitoring of animal health. *Rev Sci Tech*. 12(4): 1187–96.
Marabelli, R., Ferri, G., Bellini, S. 1999, Apr. Management of animal health emergencies: general principles and legal and international obligations. *Rev Sci Tech*. 18(1): 21–29.
Stark, K. D., Salman, M., Tempelman, Y., Kihm, U. 2002, Dec 18. A review of approaches to quality assurance of veterinary systems for health-status certification. *Prev Vet Med*. 56(2): 129–40.
Veterinary accreditation: a reference guide for practitioners. USDA, APHIS, 91–55-006. 1993.

Authors: Donald E. Hoenig and Scott R. R. Haskell

VITAMIN A DEFICIENCY/TOXICOSIS

BASICS

OVERVIEW
• Vitamin A is required by all animals and is produced by the animal through the metabolism of carotene, which is obtained from plants.
• Vitamin A exists as either retinol (also retinoic acid and retinal) or dehydroretinol.
• These are formed from carotene in the liver. Provitamin A and vitamin A precursor represent alternative nomenclatures for carotene. Vitamin A is synthesized from carotene.
• At least 10 forms of plant carotenes can be converted to vitamin A; β-carotene is quantitatively the most important for animal nutrition.
• The conversion of 1 mg of β-carotene to the IU of retinol varies with species: cattle—400 IU; sheep—400–500 IU; pigs—500 IU; horses: growing, 555 IU, and pregnant, 333 IU.
• Peripartum decreases in serum concentrations of vitamins A and E may contribute to impaired immune function in dairy cows.

PATHOPHYSIOLOGY

General Functions
• Maintenance of night vision and the prevention of night blindness
• Xeropthalmia prevention
• Essential for body, bone, and tooth growth
• Required for thyroxin synthesis—prevents goiter
• Protein synthesis
• Conversion of cholesterol to corticosterone
• Glycogen synthesis

Metabolic Function
• Cellular differentiation.
• Immune function—immunoglobulin A and T-helper cell 2 cytokine system.
• Regulates gene expression—crucial in reproduction and embryogenesis
• Hematopoiesis
• Increases bioavailability of inorganic iron

Deficiency
• Vitamin A deficiency would be observed in young animals more often than older animals.
• Liver stores of vitamin A can last for 3 to 6 months.
• Deficiency symptoms include night blindness, xerophthalmia, and xerosis; stunted growth; abnormal bone development and paralysis; unsound teeth; skin abnormalities; ear, mouth, and salivary gland abscesses; diarrhea; kidney and bladder stones; reproductive dysfunction—poor conception, increased fetal mortality.
• Deficiency is alleviated rapidly with vitamin A supplementation (dietary and injectable).

Toxicity
Toxicity symptoms include: appetite loss, hair loss, skin abnormality, swelling in the extremities (especially over the long bones), enlargement of the liver and spleen.

Common Dietary Sources of Carotene
Carrots, yellow corn, alfalfa (legumes), green grass (pasture, hay, or silage)

SYSTEMS AFFECTED
Ophthalmic, immune, musculoskeletal, hemolymphatic, and reproductive

GENETICS
N/A

INCIDENCE/PREVALENCE
N/A

GEOGRAPHIC DISTRIBUTION
N/A

SIGNALMENT

Species
All ruminant species are affected.

Breed Predilections
N/A

Mean Age and Range
• Vitamin A deficiency would be observed in young stock more often than older animals.
• Congenital ocular abnormalities in calves can be associated with maternal hypovitaminosis A.

Predominant Sex
N/A

SIGNS

HISTORICAL FINDINGS
• Night blindness, xerophthalmia, and xerosis; stunted growth; abnormal bone development and paralysis
• In one Japanese hypervitaminosis study, Holstein suckling calves expressed severe emaciation, generalized alopecia, domelike cranial deformation, and high mortality. Metaphyseal growth plates of the femur were achondroplastic, segmented, partially rebsorbed, and replaced with immature bony trabeculae containing degenerated chondrocytes. The metaphyseal growth plates were poorly formed, irregular, partially disappeared centrally, and often sealed with thin bony trabeculae. The cartilage matrix was not homogeneous but was finely fibrous, and chondrocytes were flat and degenerated. The bone lesion was diagnosed as chondrodysplasia due to premature physeal closure. These calves had been administered excessive amounts of vitamins A, D_3, and E, and the blood chemistry showed hypervitaminosis A and E.

MISCELLANEOUS

ASSOCIATED CONDITIONS
Night blindness, xerophthalmia, and xerosis; stunted growth; abnormal bone development and paralysis; unsound teeth; skin abnormalities; ear, mouth, and salivary gland abscesses; diarrhea; kidney and bladder stones; reproductive dysfunction—poor conception, increased fetal mortality

AGE-RELATED FACTORS
Vitamin A deficiency would be observed in young stock more often than older animals.

ZOONOTIC POTENTIAL
N/A

PREGNANCY
Regulates gene expression—crucial in reproduction and embryogenesis

RUMINANT SPECIES AFFECTED
All ruminant species

BIOSECURITY
N/A

PRODUCTION MANAGEMENT
N/A

SYNONYMS
Hyena disease (premature physeal closure)
Night blindness

SEE ALSO
Specific chapters on nutrition
Vitamin D
Vitamin E
Vitamins for dairy cattle

ABBREVIATIONS
IU = international units

Suggested Reading

LeBlanc, S. J., Herdt, T. H., Seymour, W. M., Duffield, T. F., Leslie, K. E. 2004, Mar. Peripartum serum vitamin E, retinol, and beta-carotene in dairy cattle and their associations with disease. *J Dairy Sci.* 87(3):609–19.

Mason, C. S., Buxton, D., Gartside, J. F. Congenital ocular abnormalities in calves associated with maternal hypovitaminosis A. *Vet Rec.* 2003, Aug 16. 153(7):213–14.

Meglia, G. E., Holtenius, K., Petersson, L., Ohagen, P., Waller, K. P. 2004. Prediction of vitamin A, vitamin E, selenium and zinc status of periparturient dairy cows using blood sampling during the mid dry period. *Acta Vet Scand.* 45(1–2):119–28.

National Research Council. 1985. *Nutrient requirements of sheep.* Washington, DC: National Academy Press.

National Research Council. 1996. *Nutrient requirements of beef cattle.* Washington, DC: National Academy Press.

National Research Council. 2001. *Nutrient requirements of dairy cattle.* Washington, DC: National Academy Press.

Solomons, N. W. 2001. Vitamin A and carotenoids. In: *Present knowledge in nutrition*, ed. B. A. Bowman and R. M. Russell. 8th ed. Washington, DC: ILSI Press.

Yamamoto, K., Sadahito, K., Yoshikawa, M., Nobuyuki, O., Mikami, O., Yamada, M., Nakamura, K., Yasuyuki, N. 2003, Mar. Hyena disease (premature physeal closure) in calves due to overdose of vitamins A, D$_3$, E. *Vet Hum Toxicol.* 45(2):85–87.

Author: Daniel C. Rule

VITAMIN D TOXICOSIS

 BASICS

OVERVIEW
- Vitamin D toxicosis is a condition of oversupplementation of either the enteral or parenteral forms of vitamin D_3 (cholecalciferol, 25-OH-cholecalciferol, 1, 25-OH-cholecalciferol) or from ingestion of plant compounds with vitamin D activity (ergocalciferol or D_2).
- A related condition known as enteque seco or Manchester wasting disease is caused by ingestion of plants like *Cestrum diurnum* (southeastern United States), *Trisetum flavescens* (European Alps), or *Solanum malacoxylon* (South America). These contain a 1, 25-OH-cholecalciferol-glycoside, which effectively induces hypervitaminosis D in grazing animals.

SIGNALMENT
- It was thought that use of active forms of vitamin D_3 would be useful in the prevention of milk fever in periparturient cattle by inducing an elevation in serum calcium. However, this has not had practical use in commercial cattle units, as the response is difficult to titrate.
- A history of parenteral vitamin D injections (usually as a vitamin A, D, and E combination) would suggest hypervitaminosis D, but could be confounded by hypervitaminosis A (although vitamin A has a sparing effect on vitamin D toxicity).
- Replacement of supplemental ergocalciferol with synthetic cholecalciferol has increased the likelihood of toxicity, as there is an increased activity of vitamin D_3 when compared to D_2.
- Ingestion of rodenticides with vitamin D as the active poison can induce toxicosis.
- Grazing pastures growing *Cestrum diurnum*, *Trisetum flavescens*, or *Solanum malacoxylon* can induce a hypervitaminosis D like disease in cattle.

SIGNS
- Initially, cattle become anorexic and depressed. This is followed by weight loss, a reduced milk production (flaccid udder), a pasty discharge around the eyes, muscle stiffness leading to recumbency, polyuria, and respiratory distress (polypnea) that can be accompanied by subcutaneous emphysema and this can progress to death. Just before death a rapid pounding pulse and ketosis has been noted.

- Cardiac arrhythmia has been noted and attributed to elevated serum calcium, as has calcification of the vascular system.
- Mineralization of soft tissue causes the signs associated with hypercalcemia. Tendon and muscle calcification leads to stiffness and recumbency. Renal calcification leads to polyuria, hypercalciuria, and renal failure.
- Withdrawal of the source of vitamin D will stop progression of the disease, but is dependent on how quickly tissue storage depots are depleted and the availability of dietary calcium.

CAUSES AND RISK FACTORS
- Duration and amount of exposure will affect the likelihood of disease. Injected forms of the vitamin are more toxic than the enteral forms because of rumen degradation of Vitamin D.
- While cholecalciferol is more toxic than ergocalciferol in several species, this difference is somewhat less in cattle. High dietary calcium exacerbates the condition, allowing more calcium to be absorbed.
- Low vitamin A status will exacerbate the likelihood of vitamin D toxicity.
- Pregnant cattle are more prone to toxicity than nonpregnant cattle.

 DIAGNOSIS

- Dietary vitamin D in excess of normal dietary recommendations of 300 IU vitamin D/kg diet indicates possible exposure (toxic range: 2,200–25,000 IU vitamin D/kg diet). Doses as low as 2.1 mg 1-α-OH D_3 per dose in 4 doses over 7 days has caused disease, yet single doses of 250 mg of vitamin D_3 (presumably as cholecalciferol) have been reported to have no effect.
- A longer exposure time lowers the threshold for toxicity. This is because of the lipid soluble nature of vitamin D and its storage in fat depots.
- Elevated plasma vitamin D, in excess of 20–50 ng/ml, indicates elevated intake or parenteral exposure.
- Dystrophic calcification of soft tissues compatible with hypercalcemic-induced change from hypervitaminosis D will include nephritic change and renal disease/failure.

DIFFERENTIAL DIAGNOSIS
- Any cause of hypercalcemia: intravenous calcium administration, hyperparathyroidism (parathyroid tumor), lymphosarcoma, gastric squamous cell carcinoma
- In gastric squamous cell carcinoma and lymphosarcoma, parathyroid hormonelike peptides can be produced, inducing hypercalcemia.

CBC/BIOCHEMISTRY/URINALYSIS
- Hypercalcemia is a hallmark sign of vitamin D toxicity but may not be present after withdrawal of the source of vitamin D. However, mineralization of soft tissues will persist and can ossify.
- Hyperphosphatemia, hypercalciuria, isosthenuria, and azotemia will be present depending on the stage and severity of disease.

OTHER LABORATORY TESTS
N/A

IMAGING
Radiographically, all soft tissue can be affected because the fibroelastic tissues around vessels will become calcified.

DIAGNOSTIC PROCEDURES
- Elevated serum calcium and phosphorus and determination of serum vitamin D concentrations greater than 80 ng/ml suggests toxicity.
- Necropsy of animals that died can be pathognomonic.

PATHOLOGIC FINDINGS
Gross Pathology
- Lungs can fail to collapse because of dystrophic calcification.
- Mineralization of the heart, aorta, kidney, stomach, lungs, tendons, and muscles is highly suggestive of hypervitaminosis D.

Histopathologic
- Initially there is a high degree of osteoclastic activity induced by vitamin D. This causes bone resorption of the primary spongiosa and loss of mineralized calcium. This will progress if dietary calcium is low leading to rarefaction of bone.
- Osteosclerosis will occur if dietary calcium is adequate or excessive and osteoblastic activity will result in bone mineralization.

- Osteoblasts will produce a characteristic pattern of abundant basophilic matrix that is virtually pathognomonic for vitamin D toxicity.
- If the exposure to vitamin D is intermittent, then the pattern of osteogenesis and depletion will lead to bands of basophilic matrix. Osteocytic necrosis will occur with high exposure.

TREATMENT

- Removal of the source of vitamin D is critical. Because vitamin D₃ increases intestinal calcium absorption, limiting dietary calcium will reduce tissue calcium deposition.
- Supplementation with vitamin A, estrogen, thyroxin, and glucagon has been suggested to have some sparing effects on progression of disease.
- Supportive care for recumbent animals, treatment of renal disease and/or failure (fluid therapy to maintain electrolyte and fluid balance), or euthanasia of severely effected animals may be needed.

MEDICATIONS

CONTRAINDICATIONS

- As mentioned, dietary calcium and phosphorus can affect the calcification of soft tissue.
- Reduction in dietary calcium to reduce calcium absorption is required.
- Vitamin A can have some sparing effects on soft tissue mineralization, as can thyroxin, glucagon, and estrogen.
- Appropriate milk and meat withdrawal times must be followed for all compounds administered to food-producing animals.

FOLLOW-UP

Severely affected animals should be sold if suitable for human consumption or euthanized.

PREVENTION/AVOIDANCE

Ensure that the form of vitamin D is known and fed in amounts within expected guidelines for cattle (300 IU/kg diet).

EXPECTED COURSE AND PROGNOSIS

Prognosis and duration of disease is dependent on the dose and duration of exposure.

AGE-RELATED FACTORS

Pregnant cows are reportedly at highest risk.

ZOONOTIC POTENTIAL

N/A

PREGNANCY

Pregnant cows may be at highest risk for development of disease.

BIOSECURITY

N/A

RUMINANT SPECIES AFFECTED

All; Jersey cattle have been suggested as more susceptible.

ABBREVIATIONS

IU = International Unit (1 IU = 0.25 μg vitamin D₃)

Suggested Reading

Capen, C. C. 1991. The endocrine glands. In: *Pathology of domestic animals*, ed. K. V. F. Jubb, P. C., Kennedy, N. Palmer. Volume 3. San Diego: Academic Press.

Capen, C. C., Cole, C. R., Hibbs, J. W. 1966. The pathology of hypervitaminosis D in cattle. *Pathologia Vet*. 3:350–78.

Horst, R. L. 1986, Feb. Regulation of calcium and phosphorus homeostasis in the dairy cow. *J Dairy Sci*. 69(2):604–16.

Littledike, E. T., Horst, R. L. 1982. Vitamin D3 toxicity in dairy cows. *J Dairy Sci*. 65(5):749–59.

National Research Council, Subcommittee on Vitamin Tolerance, Committee on Animal Nutrition, Board on Agriculture. 1987. *Vitamin tolerance of animals*. Washington, DC: National Academy Press.

Palmer, N. 1991. Bones and joints. In: *Pathology of domestic animals*, ed. K. V. F. Jubb, P. C., Kennedy, N. Palmer. Volume 1. San Diego: Academic Press.

Author: Thomas W. Graham

VITAMIN E/SELENIUM DEFICIENCY

BASICS

DEFINITION
Vitamin E or selenium deficiency occurs when the diet lacks sufficient vitamin E or selenium to maintain normal maintenance, growth, or production.

OVERVIEW
• Deficiency of vitamin E (α-tocopherol) or selenium is common in many regions of the world. Selenium toxicity is reported but can be confounded by toxicity of other trace metals and alkaloids. Vitamin E toxicity has not been reported as a natural condition in ruminants.
• Abortion, infertility, increased incidence of retained placenta, stillborn or weak calves that die soon after birth, and calves that fail to thrive are typical of herds and flocks affected by selenium deficiency.
• Immunosuppression leading to an increase in mastitis and pneumonia can be responsive to selenium and/or vitamin E supplementation. As would be expected, animals with the greatest growth and production demands will manifest selenium deficiency first. Lame calves or yearlings with evidence of white muscle disease (WMD) or nutritional myodegeneration (NMD) are commonly observed in problem herds.
• Reduction in the activity of selenium-dependent glutathione peroxidase, with an increase in free-radical-induced cellular damage, is associated with muscle damage in the myocardium and skeletal muscle. A reduction in peroxidation is the rationale for feeding increased vitamin E in finishing rations for cattle; retained red meat color allows for an increased storage life at the market.

PATHOPHYSIOLOGY
• Vitamin E is essential for protecting cell membranes from oxidative damage by allowing for its own oxidation, preventing damage to critical proteins in cell membrane regulation. Selenium-dependent glutathione peroxidase (GPx) was the first protein identified as selenium dependent.
• There have been several different forms of the selenium-dependent GPx identified: the classical cytosolic GPx, gastrointestinal GPx, plasma GPx, phospholipid GPx, and sperm nuclei GPx. These reduce hydrogen peroxide and organic hydroperoxides to stop peroxidation of other cytosolic and membrane constituents.

• Selenium-dependent iodothyronine deiodinase catalyzes the deiodination of T4 to T3, reverse T3 from T4, and reverse T3 to T2. These enzymes can activate or inactivate the thyroid hormone thyroxine. Last, thioredoxin reductases are enzymes with a selenocysteine-active site allowing for the NADPH-dependent reduction of oxidized thioredoxin.
• Reduced thioredoxin is critical for several redox systems, including those for transcription factors and reductases for DNA synthesis. They have been established as critical for regulating cell growth, prevention of apoptosis, and prevention of embryonic mortality.

SYSTEMS AFFECTED
Principally muscle tissues are noted, but thyroid and immune dysfunction affects several organ systems when selenium is deficient. Alterations in muscle and immune function are the systems affected when vitamin E is limiting.

GENETICS
N/A

INCIDENCE/PREVALENCE
Principally young, rapidly growing animals will be affected. Incidence will increase as the severity of deficiency increases. Older animals will not have the severity of muscle damage, as noted in young, rapidly growing animals, but are still susceptible to myodegeneration.

GEOGRAPHIC DISTRIBUTION
Potentially worldwide, depending on species and environment

SIGNALMENT
Species
Potentially all ruminant species are affected.

Breed Predilections
N/A

Mean Age and Range
All animals are susceptible, but younger animals are most commonly affected (including newborns that were affected in utero).

Predominant Sex
Both sexes are susceptible to either vitamin E or selenium deficiency.

SIGNS
HISTORICAL FINDINGS
• As would be expected, animals that are rapidly growing (i.e., nursing calves, lambs, kids) are most frequently affected with the NMD and this can develop either during gestation or after birth.

• Older animals have also been reported to be affected by NMD.
• NMD has been reported in goat kids, and suckling and weanling lambs with adequate selenium status but deficient in vitamin E, possibly suggesting inadequate colostrum intake, low colostrum vitamin E concentrations, or inadequate postnatal vitamin E supplementation.

PHYSICAL EXAMINATION FINDINGS
• Vitamin E and Se deficiency manifest NMD very similarly.
• Generalized leg weakness and stiffness are accompanied by animals crossing their legs while walking and having difficulty rising and standing. Impaired suckling ability due to dystrophic tongue muscles, heart failure, and paralysis have all been noted in NMD.
• Secondary infections such as pneumonia and mastitis are frequently observed. Polypnea may develop in these animals, and this can be accompanied by heart disorders. Myocarditis can induce a pendulum rhythm with reductions in heart sounds.
• A generalized picture of a selenium-deficient herd would include a range of disorders in cows and their calves. Fewer calves born than expected could reflect abortion and subfertility within the herd.
• An increased incidence of retained placenta, stillborn or weak calves that die soon after birth, and calves that fail to thrive are typical of herds affected by selenium deficiency. Calves will often have diarrhea, and mortality can be high. In dairy cows, mastitis has been reported to be responsive to selenium and vitamin E supplementation.
• Selenium-deficient cows will grind their teeth, constantly shift their weight, have difficulty rising, arch their backs, and remain in sternal recumbency (downer cow). As the disease progresses, lassitude, anorexia, increased respiration rate, dyspnea, dark urine, muscle tremors, cardiac conduction disturbances, and death have been noted.
• Reduced sperm production and testicular degeneration have been associated with selenium deficiency. Thioredoxin reductase is a testicular selenoprotein that may underlie the defect in spermatogenesis or maturation associated with testicular atrophy in selenium-deficient bulls. This defect is likely due to disruption of ribonucleotide reductase and alteration in the regulation of transcription factors. This may also explain the lower embryo survival noted in selenium-deficient cows.

CAUSES AND RISK FACTORS
• Currently the National Research Council recommends about 20 IU vitamin E/kg dry matter for stored feeds. Usually supplementation is not needed when cattle are grazed on green pasture; however, ruminants grazed on dry feed should consume approximately 20 IU vitamin E/kg dry matter for optimal production.
• Legume pastures may be an exception as NMD has been noted when cattle are grazed on alfalfa or clover pastures. Serum α-tocopherol concentrations greater than 4.0 μg/ml (0.4 mg/dl) are considered adequate in adult cattle.
• Marginal vitamin E status in adult cattle is associated with plasma α-tocopherol concentrations in the 2.0 to 3.0 μg/ml range. Clinical white muscle disease is common when α-tocopherol levels are below 2 μg/ml.
• Selenium requirements are 0.3 mg/kg DM. Diets containing less than 0.1 mg/kg DM may be deficient and would warrant surveillance of animals within the herd for deficiency. Adequate selenium intake is indicated when whole blood selenium is in the range of 0.07 to 0.10 μg/ml.
• Cattle are selenium deficient when whole blood selenium falls in the range of 0.01 to 0.04 μg/ml whole blood and marginal intake is suggested when whole blood selenium is between 0.05 and 0.06 μg/ml.
• Adequate selenium consumption is indicated when glutathione peroxidase activity is in the range of 25–500 u/mg hemoglobin/minute. When glutathione peroxidase activity is less than 15 u/mg hemoglobin/minute, cattle are considered selenium deficient. Marginal selenium intake is suggested when glutathione peroxidase activity is 15–25 u/mg hemoglobin/minute.

DIAGNOSIS

DIFFERENTIAL DIAGNOSIS
• Because the signs and symptoms of either selenium or vitamin E deficiency are fairly nonspecific, a thorough evaluation of the management and feeding practices is needed.
• Neonatal scours can be caused by high exposure to pathogens such as *E. coli* alone, but the immunosuppression associated with selenium or vitamin E deficiency will manifest in higher morbidity and mortality than in sufficient animals.

CBC/BIOCHEMISTRY/URINALYSIS
• Marked elevations (100-fold) in plasma creatine kinase activity have been observed, along with increased plasma aldolase and lactic dehydrogenase activity and decreased alkaline phosphatase activity.
• Lower type 1 deiodinase (5' deiodinase) activity will reduce T4 to T3 conversion lowering circulating T3. Similarly, reduction in the type 3 deiodinase catalyzes the conversion of T4 to reverse T3, and T3 to T2 deactivating the biologically active T3.
• Because of the myodegeneration and myonecrosis, myoglobinuria can be observed in selenium or vitamin E–deficient cattle.

PATHOLOGIC FINDINGS
• Usually, lesions of NMD are localized in those most actively exercised muscles suggesting that free radical production is higher in such muscles.
• Gross examination of animals with selenium or vitamin E deficiency will have skeletal and cardiac muscle streaking (white) with foci of calcification. Severely affected animals can have a chicken flesh appearance of muscle with edema and occasional hemorrhage.
• Nutritional myodegeneration in yearling cattle grazing lush pastures, assumed to be high in polyunsaturated fats, is associated with myonecrosis. Other factors contribute to selenium-deficiency-induced myodegeneration of older calves and exercise has been suggested to be one factor.
• Concurrent pneumonia, diarrhea, mastitis, etc., confound the diagnosis and periodic surveillance of hepatic concentrations of Se and vitamin E is suggested to exclude deficiency as an underlying cause of these complexes of disease.

TREATMENT
• Injection of vitamin E- and Se-containing products can dramatically reduce the severity of disease in deficient herds. Routine supplementation of vitamin E and Se, as salts or meals in pastured animals or in grain mixes of confined animals, will prevent disease.
• Iron Se boluses are efficacious in prevention of Se deficiency for at least a year in many cases. Availability can be restricted by governmental regulation.

CLIENT EDUCATION
Taking the time to help your clients better understand nutritional requirements and their effects on growth, reproduction, and health will greatly help prevent many infectious as well as nutritional diseases in ruminant livestock.

MEDICATIONS

CONTRAINDICATIONS
Appropriate milk and meat withdrawal times must be followed for all compounds administered to food-producing animals.

PRECAUTIONS
Oversupplementation of selenium is possible. It is important to stay within federal guidelines for supplementation.

POSSIBLE INTERACTIONS
• Maternal dietary status directly affects fetal and neonatal vitamin E and selenium status. Only limited amounts of vitamin E are transported across the placenta, and adequate colostrum intake is critical to supply the neonate adequate vitamin E. Selenium uptake by the fetus is directly proportional to maternal supply. Therefore, adequacy is critical in the last trimester to ensure adequate fetal and neonatal vitamin E and selenium status.
• Arsenic, mercury, cadmium, and copper, molybdenum, and sulfur have been suggested to alter selenium metabolism, but their influence appears to be small.
• Oxalate can decrease selenate transport in sheep and the sulfur amino acids will alter selenium metabolism.
• Dietary protein and sulfur amino acids may limit availability of selenoaminoacid incorporation into proteins.
• Dietary methionine will directly influence the proportion of selenomethionine incorporation into proteins; selenomethionine availability for incorporation into glutathione peroxidase can be reduced when methionine is limiting. Increased dietary methionine allows for increased availability of selenomethionine to selenocysteine conversion for incorporation into selenium-specific proteins.

VITAMIN E/SELENIUM DEFICIENCY

• Other factors influencing retention of selenium are phosphorus and the selenium content of the diet. Multiple factors affect absorption and retention of selenium, with high dietary protein tending to increase absorption while increasing urinary loss.

 FOLLOW-UP

• Monitoring maternal selenium and vitamin E status is prudent in areas with chronic deficiency. Rarely will one nutrient be the only limiting nutritional factor. Combined nutrient deficiency is common and requires surveillance and supplementation to prevent clinical disease.
• Monitoring blood selenium GPx activity is relatively simple, as is quantifying plasma or serum vitamin E concentration.

PATIENT MONITORING
• Ensuring adequate nutritional balance for all nutrients in the recovery phase is important for repair of muscle damage and prevention of additional muscle damage.
• Affected animals should have an improvement of gait and growth within weeks of supplementation.
• Ensuring adequate bedding and access to water and feed is critical for recumbent animals.

PREVENTION/AVOIDANCE
• Dietary supplementation of animals with adequate selenium and vitamin E is needed when feeds contain less than 0.3 mg Se/kg DM and 20 IU vitamin E/kg DM.
• Injection of cattle with vitamin E- and Se-containing products is efficacious in correcting deficiency in the short term, and commercial products are available throughout the world. Oral boluses with sodium selenite are commercially available.

• Daily intake of vitamin E is likely required and oral supplementation is the least costly.

POSSIBLE COMPLICATIONS
• Severely affected recumbent animals will require euthanasia. Animals with intercurrent infectious disease will have a greater likelihood of dying because of their immunosuppression.
• Depending on the severity and duration of deficiency, growing cattle may not be able to gain weight and height compared to peers, even with compensatory growth.

EXPECTED COURSE AND PROGNOSIS
• Rapid improvement of the herd incidence of NMD is expected after supplementation with vitamin E and Se.
• Severely affected animals may not recover sufficiently for production purposes.

 MISCELLANEOUS

ASSOCIATED CONDITIONS
Secondary infectious disease is common in affected herds and an increase in pneumonia, diarrhea, and mastitis has been reported.

ZOONOTIC POTENTIAL
N/A

PREGNANCY
Selenium- or vitamin E–deficient dams will not provide sufficient selenium or vitamin E to the fetus or from colostrum to allow for adequacy in their offspring. It is important that cattle be fed adequately in the last trimester to allow offspring to be born without causing nutritional insufficiency.

RUMINANT SPECIES AFFECTED
Potentially, all ruminant species are affected.

PRODUCTION MANAGEMENT
Adequate assessment and dietary intervention

SYNONYMS
Nutritional myodegeneration (NMD)
White muscle disease (WMD)

SEE ALSO
Arsenic
Cadmium and copper
Mercury
Molybdenum and sulfur
Oxalate toxicity
Phosphorus

ABBREVIATIONS
DM = dry matter
GPx = selenium-dependent glutathione peroxidase
IU = international units
NMD = nutritional myodegeneration
WMD = white muscle disease

Suggested Reading
Frye, T. M., Williams, S. N., Graham, T.,W. 1991. Vitamin deficiencies in cattle. *Veterinary Clinics North America Food Animal Practice* 7: 217–75.
Graham, T. W. 1991. Trace element deficiencies in cattle. *Veterinary Clinics North America Food Animal Practice* 7:153–215.
National Research Council. 2001. *Nutrient requirements of dairy cattle.* 7th rev. ed. Washington, DC: National Academy Press.
O'Grady, M. N., Monahan, F. J., Fallon, R. J., Allen, P. 2001. Effects of dietary supplementation with vitamin E and organic selenium on the oxidative stability of beef. *J Anim Sci.* 79:2827–34.
Rowe, L. J., Maddock, K. R., Lonergan, S. M., Huff-Lonergan, E. 2004. Influence of early postmortem protein oxidation on beef quality. *J Anim Sci.* 82:785–93.
Voudouri, A. E., Chadio, S. E., Menegatos, J. G., Zervas, G. P., Nicol, F., Arthur, J. R. 2003. Selenoenzyme activities in selenium- and iodine-deficient sheep. *Biol Trace Elem Res.* 94:213–24.

Author: Thomas W. Graham

BASICS

OVERVIEW
• Vomitoxin (trichothecene group B, deoxynivalenol—DON) is produced by a field fungus, *Fusarium roseum*, and is part of the nonmacrocyclic group B trichothecenes and includes dioxynivalenol, also known as DON, and its metabolites.
• Trichothecenes are tetracyclic sesquiterpenoids produced by at least six genera of plant fungi including *Fusarium* spp.
• Growth of the fungus requires undulating cool temperatures.
• There are four groups of trichothecene toxins: groups A, B, C, and D.
• DON, or vomitoxin, is the economically most significant due to losses from feed refusal and low growth rates.
• As little as 10 ppm in the field can cause a reduction in feed consumption in cattle.

SIGNALMENT
Ruminants ingesting corn, wheat, and other cereal crops that are moldy.

SIGNS
• Initial signs consist of feed refusal and low rates of gain and production. Often the first sign is feed refusal due to a learned taste aversion to the contaminated feed. There is failure to thrive, possible vomiting, diarrhea, and oral and intestinal necrosis.
• The mechanism of action is via rapid penetration of cell lipid bilayers and access to DNA, RNA, and cellular organelles. There the toxins inhibit protein synthesis by interfering with the initiation phase of ribosomal translation and covalent binding to sulfhydryl groups. They are "radiomimetic," meaning they mimic the effects of radiation and cause acute necrotizing cytotoxicity of both the epidermis and dermis. This results in stomatitis and hyperkeratosis with ulceration of the gastric mucosa and GI tract.
• There are immunosuppressive effects at the level of T suppressor cells and possibly the helper T cells, B cells, and macrophages. The immunosuppressive effects can result in secondary bacterial, viral, or parasitic infections.
• There can be hemorrhage due to thrombocytopenia or inhibition of platelet function and/or defects in the intrinsic or extrinsic coagulation pathways and depression of clotting factors. This can lead to hypotension, shock, meningeal hemorrhage, and subsequent paresis, seizure, and death.

DIAGNOSIS

DIFFERENTIAL DIAGNOSIS
Castor bean, black locust (lectin) toxicity, or arsenic and other causes of gastroenteritis

CBC/BIOCHEMISTRY/URINALYSIS
Possible mild anemia, leukopenia, thrombocytopenia, and hypoproteinemia. Due to the rapid metabolism of trichothecenes, urinalysis is not diagnostic.

OTHER LABORATORY TESTS
The best diagnostic technique is identification of the trichothecene in the feed by gas chromatography-mass spectrometry.

IMAGING
N/A

DIAGNOSTIC PROCEDURES
Lab analysis of feed samples

PATHOLOGIC FINDINGS

GROSS FINDINGS
Acute exposure to high doses of vomitoxin can result in oral lesions, hemorrhagic enteritis, and ulcerated lymphoid follicles.

HISTOPATHOLOGICAL FINDINGS
Smaller than normal lymphatic organs may be present.

TREATMENT
• Treat symptomatically with steroidal antishock and anti-inflammatory agents that are approved for use in food-producing animals.
• Provide clean feed and water.
• Residues are of minimal concern because of the rapid metabolism of trichothecenes.

MEDICATIONS
N/A

CONTRAINDICATIONS
• Appropriate milk and meat withdrawal times must be followed for all compounds administered to food-producing animals.
• Steroids should not be used in pregnant animals.

FOLLOW-UP

PREVENTION/AVOIDANCE
Inspect feeds for signs of mold and discard.

POSSIBLE COMPLICATIONS
N/A

EXPECTED COURSE AND PROGNOSIS
With supportive care and clean feed, prognosis is good.

MISCELLANEOUS

ASSOCIATED CONDITIONS
• Failure to thrive, possible vomiting, diarrhea, and oral and intestinal necrosis
• Stomatitis and hyperkeratosis with ulceration of the gastric mucosa and GI tract

• Immunosuppressive effects can result in secondary bacterial, viral, or parasitic infections
• There can be hemorrhage due to thrombocytopenia or inhibition of platelet function and/or defects in the intrinsic or extrinsic coagulation pathways and depression of clotting factors. This can lead to hypotension, shock, meningeal hemorrhage, and subsequent paresis, seizure, and death.

AGE-RELATED FACTORS
N/A

ZOONOTIC POTENTIAL
N/A

PREGNANCY
Abortion can occur secondary to systemic affects.

RUMINANT SPECIES AFFECTED
Potentially, all ruminant species can be affected.

BIOSECURITY
N/A

PRODUCTION MANAGEMENT
N/A

SYNONYMS
N/A

SEE ALSO
Arsenic
Castor bean, black locust (lectin) toxicity
Gastroenteritis
Herd toxicology outbreaks
Mycotoxins

ABBREVIATIONS
DON = dioxynivalenol
GI = gastrointestinal
ppm = parts per million

Suggested Reading
Aiello, S. E., ed. 1998. *Merck veterinary manual.* 8th ed. Whitehouse Station, NJ: Merck and Co.
Avantaggiato, G., Havenaar, R., Visconti, A. 2004, May. Evaluation of the intestinal absorption of deoxynivalenol and nivalenol by an in vitro gastrointestinal model, and the binding efficacy of activated carbon and other absorbent materials. *Food Chemistry Toxicology* 42(5):817–24.
Danicke, S., Gadeken, D., Ueberschar, K. H., Meyer, U., Scholz, H. 2002, Aug. Effects of *Fusarium* toxin contaminated wheat and of a detoxifying agent on performance of growing bulls, on nutrient digestibility in wethers and on the carry over of zearalenone. *Arch Tierernahr.* 56(4):245–61.
Jestoi, M., Ritieni, A., Rizzo, A. 2004, Mar 24. Analysis of the Fusarium mycotoxins fusaproliferin and trichothecenes in grains using gas chromatography–mass spectrometry. *Journal of Agricultural Food Chemistry* 52(6):1464–69.
Osweiler, G. D. 1996. *Trichothecenes in toxicology.* Media, PA: Williams and Wilkins.

Author: Heidi Coker

VULVITIS

 BASICS

OVERVIEW
• Vulvitis (inflammation of the vulva) is relatively common in ruminants where it is often associated with vaginitis (vulvovaginitis).
• Many causes have been associated with this condition. In general, the condition causes few significant problems; however, certain manifestations have been associated with infertility, due to either physical or pathological causes.
• Here, vulvitis will be discussed in terms of its major clinical manifestation.

SYSTEMS AFFECTED
Production management, reproductive

GENETICS
N/A

INCIDENCE/PREVALENCE
N/A

GEOGRAPHIC DISTRIBUTION
Worldwide

SIGNALMENT
Species
Potentially all ruminant species
Breed Predilections
N/A
Mean Age and Range
N/A
Predominant Sex
N/A

SIGNS
HISTORICAL FINDINGS
N/A

PHYSICAL EXAMINATION FINDINGS
Catarrhal Vulvitis
Often with a persistent mucopurulent discharge from the vulva; most commonly encountered postpartum where it may be associated with retained placenta, puerperal metritis, or physical injury to the vulva

Granular Venereal Disease
• This is the most common form of vulvitis encountered.
• It is a condition that occurs in most female cattle sooner or later. The condition is seen most commonly in heifers in their first or second natural breeding season.
• GVD appears to be easily and rapidly spread and it varies considerably in severity.
• It is characterized by lymphoid granules or nodules, which can appear acutely with a mucopurulent discharge.
• Mild forms are commonly seen in sheep and goats.
• Possible infectious causes have included *Ureaplasma*, *Mycoplasma*, IBR/IPV virus, *A. pyogenes*, *Streptococcus* spp., *Staphylococcus* spp., *E. coli*, and *H. somnus*.
• In cattle, vulvitis and vaginitis have been associated with *Ureaplasma diversum*. In sheep, *Ureaplasma* has also been associated with granular vulvitis. In does, a granular vulvovaginitis has been described due to *Mycoplasma agalactiae*.

Necrotic Vulvitis
• May follow severe trauma, ischemia, and infection
• It is not uncommonly encountered following dystocia in heifers, where it may accompany metritis. Here, it is often manifest 1–4 days after parturition, and may last 1–2 weeks.

• Affected animals often show signs of pain, tenesmus, and other systemic signs.
• One form has been described in feedlot heifers where it was associated with *Sphaeophorus necrophorus* infection.
• A necrotic vulvitis may also accompany granulosa cell tumors, which may occur in the vulval region of most ruminants.
• Allergic factors have also been suggested as possible etiological factors.
• An ulcerative vulvitis has been described in ewes, apparently viral in nature.

 DIAGNOSIS

DIFFERENTIAL DIAGNOSIS
• Transmissible fibropapillomas (cattle)
• Granulosa cell tumors
• Chlorinated naphthalene poisoning
• Contagious ecthyma (sheep and goats)
• Cystic vestibular (Bartholin's) glands

CBC/BIOCHEMISTRY/URINALYSIS
• CBC is generally unrewarding.
• Urinalysis may prove useful in diagnosis.

OTHER LABORATORY TESTS
Culture and sensitivity is indicated if infective agents are suspected.

IMAGING

OTHER DIAGNOSTIC PROCEDURES
Speculum examination/visual observation of vulva is mandatory.

 TREATMENT

• Treatment is often unnecessary, especially with milder cases of granular venereal disease.
• Where indicated, local conservative treatment should be considered.

MEDICATIONS

CONTRAINDICATIONS
Appropriate milk and meat withdrawal times must be followed for all compounds administered to food-producing animals.

FOLLOW-UP

EXPECTED COURSE AND PROGNOSIS
• Usually good
• In sheep, fly strike of vulvitis may lead to complications.
• Occasionally, severe necrotic vulvovaginitis may lead to vaginal stenosis.

MISCELLANEOUS

ASSOCIATED CONDITIONS
Retained placenta, puerperal metritis, or physical injury to the vulva

AGE-RELATED FACTORS
GVD is seen most commonly in heifers in their first or second natural breeding season.

ZOONOTIC POTENTIAL
Several of these diseases are potentially zoonotic. Care must be taken in the collection of laboratory samples and the diagnosis/treatment of affected animals.

PREGNANCY
N/A

RUMINANT SPECIES AFFECTED
Potentially, all ruminant species can be affected.

BIOSECURITY
• Isolation and quarantine of new stock entering the herd/flock.
• Treat and or cull new animals for disease conditions prior to herd introduction.
• GVD appears to be easily and rapidly spread, and it varies considerably in severity.

PRODUCTION MANAGEMENT
N/A

SYNONYMS
N/A

SEE ALSO
Chlorinated naphthalene poisoning
Contagious ecthyma (sheep and goats)
Cystic vestibular (Bartholin's) glands
Granulosa cell tumor
Reproductive pharmacology
Transmissible fibropapillomas (cattle)
Vaginitis

ABBREVIATIONS
GVD = granular venereal disease
IBR = infectious bovine rhinotracheitis
IPV = infectious pustular vulvovaginitis

Suggested Reading
Ackermann, M., Belak, S., Bitsch, V., Edwards, S., Moussa, A., Rockborn, G., Thiry, E. 1990, Jun. Round table on infectious bovine rhinotracheitis/infectious pustular vulvovaginitis virus infection diagnosis and control. *Vet Microbiol*. 23(1–4): 361–63.
Elad, D., Friedgut, O., Alpert, N., Stram, Y., Lahav, D., Tiomkin, D., Avramson, M., Grinberg, K., Bernstein, M. 2004, Mar. Bovine necrotic vulvovaginitis associated with *Porphyromonas levii*. *Emerg Infect Dis*. 10(3): 505–7.
Gilbert, R. O., Oettle. E. E. 1990, Mar. An outbreak of granulomatous vulvitis in feedlot heifers. *J S Afr Vet Assoc*. 61(1): 41–43.
Pritchard, G., Cook, N., Banks, M. 1997, May 31. Infectious pustular vulvovaginitis/infectious pustular balanoposthitis in cattle. *Vet Rec*. 140(22): 587

Author: Peter Chenoweth

WATER BUFFALO DISEASES

BASICS

OVERVIEW
• When compared to bovine species, water buffalo are much more resistant to disease. This is evident even though most water buffalo are found in hot, humid regions of the world that are conducive to disease transmission.
• Water buffalo are susceptible to most diseases and parasites affecting cattle. Treatment and vaccination protocols are generally similar between the two species.
• Poor ventilation, insufficient sanitation, inappropriate reproductive management, and poor quality nutrition programs all impact production of water buffalo.
• Buffalo calf deaths are a significant problem and impact profitability.
• The wallowing habit of water buffalo also increases the potential of transmission of some waterborne diseases.
• Tail necrosis is a common medical condition in water buffalo.
• Demodectic mange, alopecia, and ulceration are common skin disease conditions.

PATHOPHYSIOLOGY

SYSTEMS AFFECTED
Production management, skin, respiratory, gastrointestinal, immune, reproductive

GENETICS
N/A

INCIDENCE/PREVALENCE
Tapeworms: reported at an incidence of 15% in some tropical environments (*Moniezia* spp.*)*

GEOGRAPHIC DISTRIBUTION
Asia; potentially worldwide depending on environment

SIGNALMENT

Species
There are two general types of water buffalo: the swamp buffalo (*Bubalus carabanesis*), which are found from the Philippines to as far west as India, and the river buffalo (*Bubalus bubalis*), which are found farther west from India to Egypt and Europe.

Breed Predilections
N/A

Mean Age and Range
N/A

Predominant Sex
N/A

DIAGNOSIS

DIFFERENTIAL DIAGNOSIS
Dermatologic
• Edematous skin disease—*Corynebacterium pseudotuberculosis* serotype II is the main cause of ESD. Exotoxin phospholipase D and the lipid contents of the cell wall are the major causes of pathogenesis. The horsefly vector, *Hippobosca equine*, commonly transmits *Corynebacterium pseudotuberculosis* among buffalo.
• Actinobacillosis
• Yoke gall—chronic injury to the ligamentum nuchae caused by the continuous pressure of a yoke (collar) on the buffalo's neck. This is due to poorly fitted driving equipment and heavily loaded carts driven by buffalo bullocks.
• Cutaneous filariasis (*Parafilaria bovicola*)
• Cutaneous onchocerciasis—cutaneous lesions in the dermis, most apparent in the xiphoid region (*Onchocerca* spp.*)*
• Mastitis—multiple genera similar to domestic cattle
• Cowpox as well as the buffalo poxvirus
• Mange—three types of mange—psoroptic (*Psoroptes natalensis*), sarcoptic (*Sarcoptes scabiei var. bubalus*), and demodectic (*Demodax bovis*)
• Dermatomycosis
• Tail necrosis—several causes have been postulated—*Corynebacterium bovis*, fatty acid deficiency, and microfilaria
• Lumpy skin disease
• Warts
• KCS
• Otitis media
• Caudal tail fold mange

Systemic Disease
• Hemorrhagic septicemia/pasteurellosis
• Anaplasmosis
• BVD/mucosal disease
• Anthrax
• Tuberculosis
• Rabies
• Black leg/quarter
• Foreign body syndrome (similar to TRP)
• Brucellosis
• Foot-and-mouth disease
• Johne's disease
• Rinderpest
• Bovine ephemeral fever
• Malignant catarrhal fever
• Toxoplasmosis
• Nephritis, hydronephrosis, and renal calcification
• Piroplasmosis

• Pleuropneumonia (mycoplasmal)
• Hypophosphatemia
• Pestes des petits ruminants

Parasitic Diseases
• Ascarid infection—heavy losses of young buffalo calves caused by *Toxocara vitulorum*
• Strongyles—adult buffalo are resistant.
• Echinococcosis/hydatid cyst disease (*Echinococcus granulosum*)
• Coccidiosis (*Eimeria* spp.)
• Filarial nematodiasis
• Trypanosomiasis—buffalo are more susceptible to *Trypanosoma evansi* than cattle.
• Pediculosis—caused by the sucking louse (*Hematopinus tuberculatus*)
• Babesia (*Babesia argentina* and *B. bigemini*)—secondary to infection by ticks *Boophilus microplus* and *Hyalomma anatolicum*
• Lungworm—infestation of the respiratory tract by *Dictyocaulus viviparus*
• Cutaneous filariasis (*Parafilaria bovicola*)
• Cutaneous onchocerciasis—cutaneous lesions in the dermis, most apparent in the xiphoid region (*Onchocerca* spp.*)*
• Leeches
• Ticks—buffalo are resistant to ticks.
• Tapeworms—reported at an incidence of 15% in some tropical environments (*Moniezia* spp.*)*
• Ectoparasitism—a primary ectoparasite in Australia and Southeast Asia is the buffalo fly (*Siphona* spp.). Lice and mites may infest buffalo all year, but primarily during the winter season. Mosquitoes and flies affect buffalo during hot/humid weather.
• Mange—three types of mange, psoroptic (*Psoroptes natalensis*), sarcoptic (*Sarcoptes scabiei var. bubalus*), and demodectic (*Demodax bovis*)
• Ophthalmic parasites—conjunctivitis caused by *Thelazia* spp. is common.
• Several moth species feed nocturnally on buffalo lacrimal secretions in Asia.
• Synagamus (*Syngamus laryngeus*)
• Hepatic flukes—*Fasciola hepatica* and/or *F. gigantica* are very common worldwide. Snails of *Lymnaea* spp. are common vectors.
• Intestinal flukes—common flukes are *Cotylophoron cotylophorum, Calicophoron* spp., *Paramphistomum* spp., *Olveria* spp., and *Ceylonocotyle* spp. Fluke infestations (intestinal and hepatic) are the most common cause of mortality in adult water buffalo maintained in tropical Asian climates.
• Biliary leach—*Gigantocotyle explanatum* causes calf loss.
• Sarcosporidosis
• Schistosomiasis—can cause enteritis in young buffalo calves less than 2 years of age.
• Theileriosis

WATER BUFFALO DISEASES

Reproductive Disease
- Anestrus—nutritional, anatomical, hereditary, and functional. Anestrus has its highest incidence during the hot season. Small, hard, and inactive ovaries generally are present.
- Subactive/inactive ovaries—secondary to nutritional deficiency
- Excessive follicular atresia with a failure of maturation and ovulation
- Hypojunctional uterus
- Cystic ovaries
- Small, inactive ovaries—often related to a low-phosphorus diet
- Persistent CL
- Encapsulation of ovaries
- Salpingitis
- Cervicitis
- Metritis
- Pyometra
- Endometritis
- Vaginitis
- Iatrogenic reproductive problems commonly occur when artificial insemination programs reflect poor technical abilities and rough handling.
- The incidence of dystocia, abortions, and retained placenta is similar to that in cattle.

Management-Related Issues
- Respiratory infections—primarily due to poor management
- Diarrhea—found mainly in calves
- Decreased milk production
- Lameness
- Iatrogenic infertility
- Bloat/tympany
- Mastitis

MEDICATIONS

DRUGS OF CHOICE
Similar to those used in domestic bovine

CONTRAINDICATIONS
- Appropriate milk and meat withdrawal times must be followed for all compounds administered to food-producing animals.
- Steroids should not be used in pregnant animals.

MISCELLANEOUS

ASSOCIATED CONDITIONS
- When compared to bovine species, water buffalo are much more resistant to disease. This is evident even though most water buffalo are found in hot, humid regions of the world that are conducive to disease transmission.
- Tail necrosis is a common medical condition in water buffalo.
- Demodectic mange, alopecia, and ulceration are common skin disease conditions.

AGE-RELATED FACTORS
- Buffalo calf deaths are a significant problem and impact profitability.
- Diarrhea—found mainly in calves
- Adult buffalo are resistant to strongyles.
- Schistosomiasis—can cause enteritis in young buffalo calves less than 2 years of age.

ZOONOTIC POTENTIAL
Several of these diseases are zoonotic. Care must be taken in the collection of laboratory samples and the diagnosis/treatment of affected animals.

PREGNANCY
Several of these diseases cause abortion in water buffalo.

RUMINANT SPECIES AFFECTED
- Swamp buffalo (*Bubalus carabanesis*) and the River buffalo (*Bubalus bubalis*)
- The incidence of dystocia, abortion, and retained placenta is similar to that in cattle.

BIOSECURITY
- Isolation and quarantine of new stock entering the herd/flock
- Treat and or cull new animals for disease conditions prior to herd introduction.

PRODUCTION MANAGEMENT
Water buffalo are susceptible to most diseases and parasites affecting cattle. Poor ventilation, insufficient sanitation, inappropriate reproductive management, and poor-quality nutrition programs all impact production of water buffalo.

SYNONYMS
N/A

SEE ALSO
FARAD
Specified disease chapters
Water buffalo management

ABBREVIATIONS
BVD = bovine viral diarrhea
CL = corpus luteum
ESD = edematous skin disease
FARAD = Food Animal Residue Avoidance Databank
FMD = foot-and-mouth disease
KCS = keratoconjunctivitis sicca
MVD = mucosal viral disease
TRP = traumatic reticuloperitonitis

Suggested Reading
Govindarajan, R., Koteeswaran, A., Venugopalan, A. T., Shyam, G., Shaouna, S., Shaila, M. S., Ramachandran, S. 1997, Nov 29. Isolation of pestes des petits ruminants virus from an outbreak in Indian buffalo (*Bubalus bubalis*). Vet Rec. 141(22): 573 74.
Gundran, R. S., More, S. J. 1999, May 31. Health and growth of water-buffalo calves in Nueva Ecija, the Philippines. *Prev Vet Med*. 40(2): 87–100.
Nanda, A. S., Brar, P. S., Prabhakar, S. 2003. Enhancing reproductive performance in dairy buffalo: major constraints and achievements. *Reprod Suppl*. 61:27–36.
Oswin Perera, B. M. 1999. Reproduction in water buffalo: comparative aspects and implications for management. *J Reprod Fertil Suppl*. 54:157–68.
Selim, S. A. 2001, May. Oedematous skin disease of buffalo in Egypt. *J Vet Med B Infect Dis Vet Public Health*. 48(4): 241–58.

Author: Ravi Kumar Putluru

WATER BUFFALO MANAGEMENT

BASICS

OVERVIEW
• Water buffalo belong to the family Bovidae, subfamily Bovinae, and the genus *Bubalus*.
• There are about 151.5 million water buffalo in the world, 96.6% of which are found in Asia.
• The world's major concentration of buffalo is in India with 56% or 94 million animals followed by China and Pakistan.
• Water buffalo are restricted to environments were there is a hot, humid climate with plenty of water in which to cool.
• Water buffalo were introduced to Europe by crusaders returning in the Middle Ages, and outstanding herds still exist in Italy and Bulgaria.
• They have been introduced to South and Central America recently and are performing well.
• In May 1975, water buffalo were imported to Gainesville, Florida, to investigate the potential of water buffalo for aquatic weed biocontrol. They are also found in Hawaii and the southern region of the United States.
• In the United States, Brazil, Venezuela, and Australia, water buffalo are managed on rangelands.

GENETICS
• There is only one breed of swamp buffalo, but certain subgroups have specific inherited characteristics.
• There are 18 river buffalo breeds, which are classified into five major groups designated as the Murrah, Gujarat, Uttar Pradesh, Central Indian, and South Indian breeds.
• Among the river buffalo breeds, the best-known are Murrah, Jafarabadi, Surti, Nili/Ravi, Mehsana, Kundi, and Nagpuri, which are mainly concentrated in India and Pakistan.

INCIDENCE/PREVALENCE
N/A

GEOGRAPHIC DISTRIBUTION
• Potentially worldwide, depending on environment
• There are two general types of water buffalo: the swamp buffalo (*Bubalus carabanesis*), which are found from the Philippines to as far west as India, and the river buffalo (*Bubalus bubalis*), which are found farther west from India to Egypt and Europe.

Mean Age and Range
N/A

Predominant Sex
N/A

SIGNALMENT
Species
• Swamp buffalo (*Bubalus carabanesis*) and river buffalo (*Bubalus bubalis*)
• The river buffalo constitutes about 65% of the total world buffalo population of 168 million head, and accounts for 92% of buffalo milk produced worldwide.
• Swamp buffalo are generally slate grey in color with a droopy neck, and appear oxlike with massive sweptback horns. They wallow in any water and prefer muddy conditions, which makes them excellent animals for work in rice cultivation on paddy fields.
• River buffalo are generally black or dark grey in color with tightly curled or drooping straight horns. They prefer to wallow in clear, running water, and they are often used in milk production.
• There is only one breed of swamp buffalo, but certain subgroups have specific inherited characteristics. The buffalo of Thailand are large in size and weigh up to 1000 kg. In China they are small, weighing up to 300 kg. In Indonesia they have coat characteristics of black and white spots.
• There are 18 river buffalo breeds, which are classified into five major groups designated as the Murrah, Gujarat, Uttar Pradesh, Central Indian, and South Indian breeds.
• Among the river buffalo breeds, the best-known are Murrah, Jafarabadi, Surti, Nili/Ravi, Mehsana, Kundi, and Nagpuri, which are mainly concentrated in India and Pakistan.
• The majority of water buffalo are nondescript due to centuries of indiscriminate breeding without specified selection criteria.
• The river type has 50 chromosomes and the swamp type has 48 chromosomes.

Breed Predilections
• Buffalo come in many different sizes from small animals of 250 kg to heavy breeds up to 1000 kg.
• The largest breeds stand 5–6 ft (1.5–1.8 m) high, are up to 9 ft (2.8 m) long, and may weigh over 2000 lb (900 kg).
• The dull black or dark gray body has little hair; it absorbs heat easily and has few sweat glands. To some degree, the animal may substitute a fur coat with a thick, subcutaneous fat layer.
• The horns spread outward and upward, measuring up to 7 ft (2 m) across.
• The water buffalo is known as a sluggish breeder. First calves are usually produced at about 24 to 36 months of age, but recent studies show that with adequate nutrition and good management, buffalo can reach puberty at about the same age as cattle (18 months).
• They generally produce two calves every 3 years.
• The gestation period for buffalo is about the same as cattle, 287 days.
• Peak calving season is January and February.
• Buffalo calves generally weigh 45–55 pounds at birth.

Management
• They have immense strength but are very docile with people they are accustomed to.
• The classic buffalo in Asia belongs to a small farm, and millions of water buffalo are managed in intensive "backyard" systems. Herds of 2–50 animals owned by small or marginal farmers; around urban centers herds of 20–50 are common.
• Buffalo have important qualities as feedlot animals. They can be herded and handled with relative ease because of their placid nature.
• In the United States, Brazil, Venezuela, and Australia, water buffalo are managed on rangelands.
• They require more drinking water and more standing space than cows.
• Because of their poorly developed thermoregulatory mechanisms, buffalo need to wallow or need sprinklers during hot weather in order to keep their bodies cool.
• Their housing generally requires higher roofing to improve ventilation.
• Buffalo need stronger barriers than those used for cattle, and the wires should be closer together and lower to the ground to avoid having them lift the fences up with their horns.
• They must be handled quietly and calmly because of their timid nature.

TREATMENT

DIET
• Buffalo are more efficient in converting highly fibrous low-grade foods than domestic cattle. Paddy straw and crop residues are common feed sources.
• Buffalo are remarkable for their feed conversion ability.
• Buffalo have a larger gut with a slower passage of digesta and a higher rate of crude fiber digestion.
• They are better converters of nonprotein nitrogenous (NPN) compounds into protein than domestic cattle. This gives an opportunity to improve poor-quality roughage with various NPN compounds.

MISCELLANEOUS

Economic Considerations
• For thousands of years, this animal species has provided draft power, milk, meat, and hide to millions of people, mainly small-scale farmers.
• Buffalo are used for a variety of agricultural operations such as plowing paddy fields, lifting water from wells, and transporting farm produce to nearby markets.
• More than 5% of world milk comes from buffalo and 95% of it comes from Asia.
• India is the world's largest buffalo milk producer with about 35% of milk animals producing almost 70% of the total Indian milk.
• Buffalo feeding and management is cheaper than cattle feeding and management, and buffalo farmers also get a 50% higher price for their milk.
• Buffalo milk contains more total solids (16%) compared with the solids (12%–14%) found in cow's milk. Buffalo milk butterfat content is usually 6%–8% compared with domestic dairy cow butterfat levels of 3%–5%.

• Buffalo farming is one of the substantial secondary income sources for small farmers in Asia. Usually women take care of buffalo feeding, milking, and selling of milk.
• Water buffalo offer a major source of meat in Asia. The buffalo meat industry is expanding.
• Asia produces 91%–92% of the world's total buffalo meat, with India being the world's largest buffalo meat producer followed by Pakistan, China, Nepal, and Thailand.
• Carcass characteristics of buffalo are similar to domestic cattle with the average dressing percentage of 53%.
• Water buffalo also provide a major work force in Asia, and it is probably the most adaptable and versatile of all work animals.

ASSOCIATED CONDITIONS
N/A

AGE-RELATED FACTORS
N/A

ZOONOTIC POTENTIAL
N/A

PREGNANCY
N/A

RUMINANT SPECIES AFFECTED
Swamp buffalo (*Bubalus carabanesis*) and river buffalo (*Bubalus bubalis*)

BIOSECURITY
N/A

PRODUCTION MANAGEMENT
• Buffalo require more drinking water and more standing space than cows.
• Because of their poorly developed thermoregulatory mechanisms, buffalo need to wallow or need sprinklers during hot weather in order to keep their bodies cool.
• Their housing generally requires higher roofing to improve ventilation.
• Buffalo need stronger barriers than those used for cattle, and the wires should be closer together and lower to the ground to avoid having them lift the fences up with their horns.
• They must be handled quietly and calmly because of their timid nature.

SYNONYMS
N/A

SEE ALSO
See specific disease chapters.

SYNONYMS
The genus name *Bubalus* is also spelled *Bubalis*.

SEE ALSO
Water buffalo medicine and disease

ABBREVIATIONS
NPN = nonprotein nitrogen

Suggested Reading
Abdalla, E. B. 2003, Jan 15. Improving the reproductive performance of Egyptian buffalo cows by changing the management system. *Anim Reprod Sci.* 75(1–2): 1–8.
Chandra, B. S., Das, N. 2001, Mar 10. Behaviour of Indian river buffaloes (*Bubalus bubalis*) during short-haul road transportation. *Vet Rec.* 148(10): 314–15.
Gundran, R. S., More, S. J. 1999, May 31. Health and growth of water-buffalo calves in Nueva Ecija, the Philippines. *Prev Vet Med.* 40(2): 87–100.
McCool, C. 1992, Aug. Buffalo and Bali cattle—exploiting their reproductive behaviour and physiology. *Trop Anim Health Prod.* 24(3): 165–72.
Nanda, A. S., Brar, P. S., Prabhakar, S. 2003. Enhancing reproductive performance in dairy buffalo: major constraints and achievements. *Reprod Suppl.* 61:27–36.
Oswin Perera, B. M. 1999. Reproduction in water buffalo: comparative aspects and implications for management. *J Reprod Fertil Suppl.* 54:157–68.
Phenotypic characterization of national Brazilian buffalo breeds and Baio type. 2003, Nov. *Pesq. Agropec. Bras.* 38 (11): 1337–42.
Thomas, C. S., Svennersten-Sjaunja, K., Bhosrekar, M. R., Bruckmaier, R. M. 2004, May. Mammary cisternal size, cisternal milk and milk ejection in Murrah buffaloes. *J Dairy Res.* 71(2): 162–68.

Authors: Ravi K. Putluru and Scott Haskell

WATER QUALITY ISSUES

BASICS

OVERVIEW
• The quality and quantity of water is important for health and productivity of ruminants. Some of the risks implicit in inadequate water quality include: decreased weight gains, poor feed conversion rates, and adverse effects on animals' health.
• Poor quality water and barriers to adequate quantity of water adversely affect growth, reproduction, and productivity resulting in loss of profitability.
• Physical, chemical, and microbial constituents determine water quality. The physical components can range from gross contamination of water by fecal, organic materials and biofilms to depth and condition of containers used to hold drinking water.
• Some chemical attributes of water can be detrimental to animal health at abnormal levels. These include pH, total dissolved solids (TDS), soluble salts, salinity, hardness, sulfates, nitrates, and nitrites.
• Ruminants are unique in that they are more sensitive to excess amounts of both nitrates and sulfates. This is due to ruminal conversion/reduction to toxic forms of nitrites and sulfides. This sensitivity is not seen in monogastric species.
• The microbiological quality of water is also important. Standing and running water may contain *Escherichia coli*, *Salmonella* spp., *Leptospira* spp., fusobacterium, and cyanobacteria (blue-green algae).
• Water supplies containing excessive levels of nitrate, TDS, sulfate, and other constituents can affect growth and production of all classes of animals.
• Drinking-water quality and availability should be evaluated in a practitioner's differential diagnosis for poor performance or nonspecific disease conditions in livestock.
• Evaluating water quality includes obtaining a thorough history, evaluating chemical and physical components of samples, and asking questions relevant to water safety. A thorough laboratory examination of animal specimens and water samples should be evaluated.
• The USDA's National Animal Health Monitoring System evaluated beef feedlot water sources for nitrate, nitrite, sulfate, and total dissolved solids in 1999. It tested 263 feedlots from 10 states. The results showed no water sample exceeded the recommended limits for nitrates, almost all samples had nitrite and total dissolved solids within normal limits, and approximately three-quarters of the water samples had sulfate levels considered safe.

SIGNALMENT

SYSTEMS AFFECTED
N/A

GENETICS
N/A

INCIDENCE/PREVALENCE
N/A

GEOGRAPHIC DISTRIBUTION
Worldwide depending on environment

SIGNALMENT

Species
All ruminant species

Breed Predilections
N/A

Mean Age and Range
N/A

Predominant Sex
N/A

SIGNS
Depending on water quality:
• Moderate rumen nitrites: decreased animal weight gains and poorer feed conversion rates
• Excess rumen nitrites: neurological signs of nitrite toxicity
• Excess rumen sulfides: neurological signs of polioencephalomalacia (PEM)
• Excessive alkalinity: physiologic and digestive upsets in livestock
• *Salmonella* spp.: diarrhea, fever, loss of production, abortions
• *E. coli*: gastrointestinal signs, coliform mastitis, septic meningitis/arthritis in younger animals
• *Leptospira* spp.: infertility, low or diminished milk production, widespread late-term abortion
• Fusobacterium: chronic lameness, possible sepsis
• Cyanobacteria (blue-green algae): muscle tremors, liver damage; can lead to death

CAUSES AND RISK FACTORS
• Breach in sound biosecurity protocols for management of drinking water
• Damaged casings in old wells
• Shallow wells are more easily contaminated with nitrogenous compounds than deep wells

DIAGNOSIS
• The U.S. Environmental Protection Agency (EPA) has recommended limits of certain pollutants and other substances found in water.
• Table 1 compiles water quality recommendations in the United States.

CBC/BIOCHEMISTRY/URINALYSIS
N/A

OTHER LABORATORY TESTS
N/A

IMAGING
N/A

OTHER DIAGNOSTIC PROCEDURES
Basic laboratory evaluation of water quality for livestock should include measurement of TDS, sulfate, nitrate-nitrite, and coliform bacteria. Supplementary water tests may include pH, sodium, iron, magnesium, chloride, calcium, potassium, manganese, and farm specific contaminants.

TREATMENT
Adequate water container hygiene for animals. Hygiene procedures include frequent cleaning and emptying of containers, proper maintenance of old wells, and applying appropriate disinfectant (e.g., chlorine <4 ppm).

MEDICATIONS
N/A

CONTRAINDICATIONS
N/A

FOLLOW-UP
• Annual water tests are recommended for private wells, especially shallow wells. The water sample should be sent to a certified testing laboratory for analysis.
• The water analyses will typically include the following tests: total coliform bacteria, pH (acid or alkaline level), total dissolved solids, total soluble salt, salinity, hardness, nitrates, sulfate and other factors depending on location of the farm.

MISCELLANEOUS

ASSOCIATED CONDITIONS
N/A

AGE-RELATED FACTORS
N/A

ZOONOTIC POTENTIAL
Wells may be contaminated with pathogens and nitrates/nitrites

PREGNANCY
N/A

WATER QUALITY ISSUES

Table 1

Desired and Potential Levels of Pollutants in Livestock Water Supplies		
Substance	Desired Range	Problem Range
Total bacteria/100 ml	<200	>1,000,000
Fecal coliform/100 ml	<1	>1 for YOUNG animals
		>10 for OLDER animals
Fecal strep/100 ml	<1	>3 for YOUNG animals
		>30 for OLDER animals
pH	6.8–7.5	<5.5 or >8.5
Dissolved solids, mg/L	<500	>3000
Total dissolved solids (TDS)[a], mg/L	<3000	>10,000[b]
Total alkalinity, mg/L	<400	>5000
Nitrate[c], mg/L	<440	
Nitrite[c], mg/L	<33	
Sulfate, mg/L	<250 (300[c])	>2000
Phosphate, mg/L	<1	Not established
Turbidity, Jackson units	<30	Not established

Note: 1 milligram per liter (mg/L) is approximately equal to 1 part per million (ppm)

Source: Agricultural Waste Management Field Handbook, 2000, pp. 1–16. Based on research literature and field experience in the northeastern United States.

[a]TDS—total dissolved solids; may include magnesium, chloride, calcium, and sulfate.

[b]Montana State University Extension, 2005.

[c]National Research Council, 2001.

RUMINANT SPECIES AFFECTED

Potentially, all ruminant species are affected.

BIOSECURITY

- Breach in sound biosecurity protocols for management of drinking water
- Damaged casings in old wells
- Shallow wells are more easily contaminated with nitrogenous compounds than deep wells

PRODUCTION MANAGEMENT

N/A

SYNONYMS

N/A

SEE ALSO

Blue-green algae
Environmental issues
Manure zoonotic pathogens
Nitrate/nitrite toxicosis

ABBREVIATIONS

EPA = Environmental Protection Agency
PEM = polioencephalomalacia
TDS = total dissolved solids
USDA = United States Department of Agriculture

Suggested Reading

Carson, T. L. 2000, Nov. Current knowledge of water quality and safety for livestock. *Vet Clin North Am Food Anim Pract.* 16(3): 455–64.

Hooda, P. S., Edwards, A. C., Anderson, H. A., Miller, A. 2000, Apr 24. A review of water quality concerns in livestock farming areas. *Sci Total Environ.* 250(1–3): 143–67.

LeJeune, J. T., Besser, T. E., Merrill, N. L., Rice, D. H., Hancock, D. D. 2001, Aug. Livestock drinking water microbiology and the factors influencing the quality of drinking water offered to cattle. *J Dairy Sci.* 84(8): 1856–62.

Pfost, D. L., Casteel, S. 2001, May. *Water quality for livestock drinking.* University of Missouri Extension. EQ381. http://muextension.missouri.edu/explore/envqual/eq0381.htm. Accessed on August 1, 2004.

Surber, G., K. Williams and M. Manoukian. 2005. Drinking water quality for beef cattle: an environment friendly & production management enhancement technique. Animal and Range Sciences, Extension Service, Montana State Univ., Bozeman. http://animalrangeextension.montana.edu Accessed on March 13, 2008.

USDA/APHIS. 2000, Dec. *Water quality in U.S. feedlots.* Information sheet. http://www.aphis.usda.gov/vs/ceah/cnahs/nahms/feedlot/Feedlot99/FD99water.pdf. Accessed on August 1, 2004.

USDA/NRCS. Agricultural Waste Management Field Handbook. NEH Part 651 – Agricultural Waste Management Field Handbook (AWMFH). http://www.wsi.nrcs.usda.gov/products/W2Q/W2Q_home.html. Accessed on March 13, 2008.

Author: Dipa Pushkar Brahmbhatt

WATTLE CYSTS

 ## BASICS

OVERVIEW
• Wattles are small pencil-like appendages of skin and cartilage located most commonly on the ventral neck and occasionally on the ears or face of goats.
• Wattle cysts are unilateral or bilateral fluid-filled swellings at the base of the wattles or at the site of previous wattle amputation.
• Wattle cysts may enlarge over time or decrease in size if the contents leak through the skin surface.
• Wattle cysts are thought to be a developmental malformation of the second branchial cleft.

SIGNALMENT
• Wattle cysts occur in goats of several breeds; there is no sex predilection.
• Wattle cysts are present at birth but may go unnoticed until the animal grows and the cysts enlarge.
• Cysts may range in size from 1 to 5 cm and are filled with a clear fluid of varying consistency from thin to thick.
• Wattle cysts are reportedly heritable by an undefined route.

SIGNS
• Wattle cysts present as soft tissue swellings located subcutaneously at the base of the wattles or site of wattle amputation.
• Cysts are variable in size, shape, and fluid consistency but their location is diagnostic.

CAUSES AND RISK FACTORS
Wattle cysts are a heritable fault and may be considered a defect in show goats.

 ## DIAGNOSIS

DIFFERENTIAL DIAGNOSIS
• *Corynebacterium pseudotuberculosis* abscess
• Hematoma or seroma resulting from trauma

CBC/BIOCHEMISTRY/URINALYSIS
N/A

OTHER LABORATORY TESTS
N/A

IMAGING
N/A

DIAGNOSTIC PROCEDURES
Fluid aspiration using aseptic technique reveals clear, acellular fluid. Anatomic site is pathognomonic for the condition.

PATHOLOGIC FINDINGS
Histopathology reveals walls of stratified squamous epithelium with hair follicles and occasionally cartilage.

 ## TREATMENT
Surgical removal of the superficial subcutaneous intact cyst utilizing local anesthesia may be considered for show goats. Goats have very thin musculature near the wattles and particular care should be made to avoid underlying structures such as the jugular vein and carotid artery.

 ## MEDICATIONS
N/A

CONTRAINDICATIONS
N/A

 ## FOLLOW-UP

PATIENT MONITORING
Routine postsurgical monitoring of the skin incisions

PREVENTION/AVOIDANCE
Do not repeat matings that produce kids with wattle cysts.

POSSIBLE COMPLICATIONS
N/A

EXPECTED COURSE AND PROGNOSIS
Wattle cysts do not interfere with the health or function of the goat.

 ## MISCELLANEOUS
N/A

AGE-RELATED FACTORS
N/A

ZOONOTIC POTENTIAL
N/A

PREGNANCY
N/A

RUMINANT SPECIES AFFECTED
Goats

BIOSECURITY
N/A

PRODUCTION MANAGEMENT
N/A

SYNONYM
Cysts

SEE ALSO
Corynebacterium pseudotuberculosis abscess
Hematoma or seroma resulting from trauma

ABBREVIATIONS
N/A

Suggested Reading
Aiello, S. E., ed. 1998. *The Merck veterinary manual*, 8th ed. Whitehouse Station, NJ: Merck & Co.
Brown, P. J., Lane, J. G., Lucke, V. M. 1989, Sep 2. Developmental cysts in the upper neck of Anglo-Nubian goats. *Vet Rec.* 125(10): 256–58.
Fubini, S. L., Campbell, S. G. 1983, Nov. External lumps on sheep and goats. *Vet Clin North Am Large Anim Pract.* 5(3): 457–76.
Gamlem, T., Crawford, T. B. 1977, Apr. Dermoid cysts in identical locations in a doe goat and her kid. *Vet Med Small Anim Clin.* 72(4): 616–17.
Smith, M. C., Sherman, D. M. 1994. *Goat medicine*. Philadelphia: Lea & Febiger.
Williamson, L. H. 2001, Jul. Caseous lymphadenitis in small ruminants. *Vet Clin North Am Food Anim Pract.* 17(2): 359–71, vii.

Author: Joan S. Bowen

BASICS

DEFINITION
Weight loss is defined as a decrease in body weight. The loss may be acute, chronic, physiological, or pathological. Although it is not considered a weight loss, decrease in daily weight gain is an abnormal physiological condition as well.

PATHOPHYSIOLOGY
• Weight loss may occur as a result of anorexia, increment of nutritional requirements, unbalanced diets, or a combination of these factors.
• Anorexia may be pathological or physiological. Pathological anorexia occurs secondary to any systemic disease or local condition affecting the digestive system or oral cavity.
• Physiological decrease in feed intake may occur during the last month of gestation and the first weeks of lactation. This depression is markedly evident at calving and during the peripartum period. Heat stress is another physiological condition noticeably affecting dry matter intake.
• Increment of nutritional requirements occurs under normal and pathological conditions.

• Fever or any inflammatory process including tissue damage increases nutritional requirements, mostly protein. Parasitism is a representative case of pathological weight loss.
• Examples of physiological increase in nutritional requirements include lactation, last trimester of gestation, and animal growth. Unbalanced diets, especially diets deficient in microminerals and vitamins, and diets reduced in energy and protein may promote poor growth rates or weight losses.
• Weight loss may be acute or chronic.
• Acute weight losses are typical under pathological conditions that markedly affect dry matter intake such as lameness, rumen acidosis, and displaced abomasum or physiological conditions such as early lactation.
• Chronic losses are typical in pathological conditions such as parasitism, chronic diarrhea (e.g., Johne's disease), or physiological conditions such as aged animals.

SYSTEMS AFFECTED
• Dependent on gender and age of the animal
• Mature animals decrease body weight primarily through the breakdown of fat reserves. Peripheral fat is initially utilized, followed by abdominal and perirenal fat. After fat utilization, animals catabolize muscle proteins.
• Musculoskeletal

GENETICS
Several genetic or congenital conditions might affect growing and performance. Examples include dwarfism, cleft lip/palate (palatoschisis), and ventricular septal defect.

INCIDENCE/PREVALENCE
Incidence of weight loss will depend directly or indirectly on the incidence of disease related to a decrease in feed intake or the increase of nutrient requirements. All lactating animals, especially during the first trimester of lactation, mobilize body reserves potentially losing weight and body condition.

GEOGRAPHIC DISTRIBUTION
Worldwide, a location where drought is common or the feed supply is compromised

SIGNALMENT

SIGNS
Anatomically depressed left paralumbar fossa, decrease in body condition score, and manifestation of skeleton prominences and emaciation

CAUSES
Any factor that depresses the animal's appetite, increases nutritional requirements, or inconsistent feed management (e.g., unbalanced diets, poor feed quality, macro/micro-nutrient deficiency, etc.)

RISK FACTORS
Diseased animals, environmental management (e.g., heat stress, mud, insect control, etc.), feed management, nutritional quality, drought, age, gender, physiological stage, season, location

WEIGHT LOSS: BOVINE

DIAGNOSIS

DIFFERENTIAL DIAGNOSIS
• Weight loss may be difficult to diagnose.
• Might be secondary to other pathological conditions (see Table 1).

CBC/BIOCHEMISTRY/URINALYSIS
Anemia, altered white cell profile, altered albumin to globulin ratio, elevated nonesterified fatty acids, increased creatinine and blood urea nitrogen, increase of specific enzymes related to tissue damage (AST, alkaline phosphatase, GGT, creatine kinase), elevated ketone bodies, low micromineral levels

OTHER LABORATORY TESTS
Dependent upon specific disease condition(s) and differential diagnosis

IMAGING
May be helpful to rule out foreign body in individual animal

DIAGNOSTIC PROCEDURES
• Visual observation, body condition scoring, weight of animals, record analysis
• Assessment of management
• Complete dietary/nutritional analysis may be indicated.

PATHOLOGIC FINDINGS
Emaciation, decrease or absence of adipose tissue, especially in abdominal organs and decreased or stunted growth. Evaluate body condition scores.

TREATMENT

APPROPRIATE HEALTH CARE
Dependent upon whether the weight loss is secondary to a pathological or physiological condition.

NURSING CARE
Feed management

ACTIVITY
N/A

DIET
• Important in unbalanced diets or increased nutrient requirements
• Animals losing weight secondary to diseases may need special diets.
• Complete dietary and nutritional evaluation may be necessary.

CLIENT EDUCATION
Understanding weight loss that may be secondary to other conditions

SURGICAL CONSIDERATIONS
N/A

MEDICATIONS

DRUGS OF CHOICE
• Vitamins (A, D, E, B complex) and minerals (mostly microminerals), feed additives (monensin, probios, propionate, propylene glycol), growth stimulants may be indicated dependent upon weight loss.
• Treatment should be predicated upon disease condition.
• If lameness is evident, hoof care should be established.

CONTRAINDICATIONS
Appropriate milk and meat withdrawal times must be followed for all compounds administered to food-producing animals.

POSSIBLE INTERACTIONS
N/A

ALTERNATIVE DRUGS
N/A

FOLLOW-UP

PATIENT MONITORING
Body condition scoring, feed evaluation, weight and behavior evaluation

PREVENTION/AVOIDANCE
Based on the primary cause of weight loss

POSSIBLE COMPLICATIONS
N/A

EXPECTED COURSE AND PROGNOSIS
Dependent upon the primary cause of weight loss

 MISCELLANEOUS

ASSOCIATED CONDITIONS
Decrease in productivity

AGE-RELATED FACTORS
Older animals are more likely to lose weight inherent to aging; young stock are susceptible to diarrhea diseases.

ZOONOTIC POTENTIAL
Some infectious conditions (e.g., salmonella, leptospirosis, Johne's) should be considered as potential zoonosis diseases.

PREGNANCY
Can negatively affect growth and weight gain

RUMINANT SPECIES AFFECTED
Potentially, all ruminant species

BIOSECURITY
Considered in the case of infectious disease associated with weight loss (Johne's disease, salmonellosis, etc.).

PRODUCTION MANAGEMENT
Adequate feed intake and environmental management

SYNONYMS
Emaciation
Starvation

SEE ALSO
Body condition scoring by species
Weight loss in goats

ABBREVIATIONS
AST = aspartate aminotransferase
BVD = bovine viral diarrhea virus
GGT = gamma glutamyl transferase
IBR = infectious bovine rhinotracheitis

Suggested Reading
Hornick, J. L., Van Eenaeme, C., Gerard, O., Dufrasne, I., Istasse, L. 2000, Aug. Mechanisms of reduced and compensatory growth. *Domest Anim Endocrinol*. 19(2): 121–32.
Miller, G. 2003, Apr 25. Developmental biology. Hungry ewes deliver offspring early. *Science*. 300(5619): 561–62.
Olsen, I., Sigurgardottir, G., Djonne, B. 2002, Feb. Paratuberculosis with special reference to cattle. A review. *Vet Q*. 24(1): 12–28.
Saffron, L. 2002, May. Fighting famine with ancestral agriculture. *Environ Health Perspect*. 110(5): A235.
Tyler, J. W., Middleton, J. R. 2004, Jul. Transmissible spongiform encephalopathies in ruminants. *Vet Clin North Am Food Anim Pract*. 20(2): 303–26, vii.

Author: Pedro Melendez

Table 1

Differential Diagnosis of Weight Loss in the Bovine

Pathological conditions

Actinobacillosis
Actinomycosis
Bovine leucosis
Cryptosporidiosis
Deficiencies
- Copper
- Selenium

Dental abnormalities
Diarrhea
- Enterotoxigenic *E. coli*
- Salmonellosis
- Undifferentiated

Enterotoxigenic *E. coli*
Failure of passive transfer (neonates)
Fescue toxicity
Gastrointestinal problems
- Abomasal ulcer
- Displaced abomasum
- Fat necrosis
- Hepatic abscess
- Johne's disease
- Pharyngeal, retropharyngeal abscess
- Salmonellosis
- Traumatic reticuloperitonitis (hardware)
- Vagal indigestion
- Winter dysentery

Intussusception
Lameness
- Footrot
- Septic arthritis
- Sole abscess

Malnutrition
Mastitis
Metabolic problems
- Ketosis
- Lactic acidosis

Parasites
- Anaplasmosis
- Coccidiosis
- Flukes
- Gastrointestinal worms
- Lice
- Lungworm
- Ostertagiasis
- Sarcoptic mange

Pasteurellosis
Peritonitis
Pneumonia
Urinary problems
- Pyelonephritis/cystitis
- Urolithiasis

Viruses
- Bluetongue
- Bovine viral diarrhea virus (BVD)
- Coronavirus
- Infectious bovine rhinotracheitis (IBR)
- Rotavirus

WEIGHT LOSS: GOATS

 BASICS

OVERVIEW
• Chronic persistent weight loss
• In most cases, establishing a definitive diagnosis will allow the practitioner to institute appropriate therapeutic measures, correct deficient management procedures, or institute suitable prevention and control programs to reduce ongoing or future losses to the client.
• Through the use of careful clinical examination and knowledge of the likely causes of progressive weight loss, a definitive diagnosis can often be made, although this is not always possible, even with rigorous investigation.
• There are a number of reasons that goats may become thin: some are management related and some are related to disease agents that have a long-term negative effect on the animal.

SYSTEMS AFFECTED
Musculoskeletal; potentially all, depending on condition

GENETICS
N/A

INCIDENCE/PREVALENCE
N/A

GEOGRAPHIC DISTRIBUTION
Worldwide

SIGNALMENT
Species
Caprine

Breed Predilections
• Dairy breeds include the Alpine, La Mancha, Nubian, Saanen, and Toggenburg breeds.
• Cashmere and Angora goats are common fiber breeds and the Boer, Kambling, Ma Tou, and Pygmy are meat breeds.

Mean Age and Range
N/A

Predominant Sex
N/A

SIGNS
HISTORICAL FINDINGS
• History should include age and number of animals affected. Particular attention should be paid to composition of the diet or pasture, stage of the production cycle, deworming practices, pasture rotation strategies, and herd status regarding *Mycobacterium paratuberculosis* spp. avium, CLA, and CAE.
• Owner reports regarding appetite are important because Johne's disease is relatively unique in that severely affected animals often have good appetites.

PHYSICAL EXAMINATION FINDINGS
• A complete physical examination should be performed on any goat presenting chronic weight loss.
• Particular attention should be paid to pallor of mucous membranes and the presence of submandibular edema because these findings support the diagnosis of helminthiasis.
• Oral examination will reveal the presence of advanced age, oral erosions, and poor dentition.
• Physical examination will often reveal evidence of chronic infections such as pneumonia or external abscesses supporting a diagnosis of CLA.

CAUSES AND RISK FACTORS
Common Causes
• Helminths
  • Gastrointestinal nematodes
  • Tapeworms
  • Flukes
  • Lungworms
• External parasites
  • Coccidiosis
  • *Mycobacterium avium* spp. paratuberculosis
  • Diet
  • Dentition
  • Internal abscesses due to caseous lymphadenitis (CLA)
  • Chronic infections including pneumonia and mastitis
  • Chronic organ dysfunction including kidney and liver disease
  • Caprine arthritis-encephalitis (CAE)
  • Mycoplasma mycoides arthritis
  • Foot rot: *Bacteroides nodosus* (*Dichelobacter nodosus*), *Fusobacterium necrophorum*

• Rare or exotic diseases
  • Scrapie
  • Tuberculosis
  • Meliodosis
  • Viral pulmonary adenomatosis (jaagsiekte)
  • Rinderpest
  • Peste des petits ruminants
• All listed causes are addressed in detail in separate chapters. The reader using this chapter to guide the diagnosis of a goat with chronic weight loss is encouraged to review all these chapters.
• Specific history and physical examination results unique to the above differential diagnoses will likely greatly increase or decrease their likelihood, focusing ancillary diagnostic testing if the diagnosis is not obvious following the initial examination and database.

 DIAGNOSIS

DIFFERENTIAL DIAGNOSIS
Wasting Diseases
Amyloid
Bacterial infection
Behavioral—inadequate feed space
Blindness
Caprine arthritis- encephalitis (CAE)-interstitial pneumonia
Caseous lymphadenitis (CLA)
Cobalt deficiency
Cestodes
Chronic mastitis
Coccidia
Enterotoxemia
External parasites
Foreign bodies
Infection
Johne's disease
Locomotor problems—foot rot, foot scald, foot abscess, polyarthritis, fracture, nerve damage, rickets
Lungworms
Malnutrition
Nematodes
Neoplasia
Nutritional problems—copper, cobalt, protein, vitamin A deficiency; carbohydrate deficiency

Oral problems—tooth loss, disease
Orf
Pasteurella infection
Peritonitis-rumenitis, liver flukes, internal
abscesses, intraperitoneal drugs
Plant toxins
Pulmonary adenomatosis
Rinderpest
Salmonella
Scrapie
Trematodes
Tuberculosis
Viral infections

Wasting/Inappetence
• Amyloidosis
• Bacterial infection
• Caprine arthritis-encephalitis (CAE)
• Chronic gastrointestinal parasitism
• Cobalt deficiency
• Johne's disease
• Ketosis
• Malnutrition
• Milk fever
• Neoplasm
• Salmonella
• Teeth/mechanical
• Viral infection

CBC/BIOCHEMISTRY/URINALYSIS
Dictated by the specific differential diagnosis
being pursued

OTHER LABORATORY TESTS
• The initial database should include a
routine fecal examination for helminth and
coccidia oocysts, hematocrit and serum
protein concentration.
• These tests will usually be sufficient to
confirm the diagnosis of gastrointestinal
parasitism, the most common cause of
chronic weight loss in goats. The practitioner
is cautioned that many goats with unrelated
disease processes will have positive fecal
examinations.
• A positive fecal is suggestive but not
pathognomonic for gastrointestinal
parasitism.

IMAGING
Dictated by the specific differential diagnosis
being pursued

OTHER DIAGNOSTIC PROCEDURES
Dictated by the specific differential diagnosis
being pursued

 TREATMENT
Varies with cause

 MEDICATIONS
CONTRAINDICATIONS
Appropriate milk and meat withdrawal times
must be followed for all compounds
administered to food-producing animals.

 FOLLOW-UP
• If a diagnosis of gastrointestinal parasitism
has been made, a follow-up fecal examination
should be scheduled 10 days after appropriate
deworming to document the efficacy of
deworming.
• Anthelmintic resistance has become
widespread and common. Likewise, dramatic
reductions in fecal egg counts unaccompanied
by improvement in clinical signs is suggestive
that a different or additional differential
diagnosis is responsible for the chronic weight
loss in the affected goat.

 MISCELLANEOUS
ASSOCIATED CONDITIONS
See specific diseases.

AGE-RELATED FACTORS
Age hierarchies exist in feeding behavior.

ZOONOTIC POTENTIAL
Certain specific zoonotic diseases (e.g., orf,
salmonellosis, tuberculosis) can cause weight
loss. Care should be taken in the collection of
diagnostic samples.

PREGNANCY
N/A

RUMINANT SPECIES AFFECTED
Caprine

BIOSECURITY
N/A

PRODUCTION MANAGEMENT
Management factors associated with weight
loss:
• Low-quality diets or low-quantity diets
  • Goats should have a diet that consists of
  8%–13.5% CP depending on the stage of
  their production.
  • Energy requirements will vary and are the
  highest during lactation. The best means to
  evaluate the ration is to have forage analysis
  performed.
• Inadequate feeder space
  • For multiple goats, ideally more than one
  feeder should be used.
  • 1.4 to 2 linear feet per head is required per
  goat.
  • Keyhole feeders work well.
• Inadequate space
  • With dry lot confinement, there should be
  35–100 sq ft per animal.
  • Less individual animal space increases
  fighting and aggression.
• Breed-specific aggression
  • French Alpine and Toggenburg breeds
  tend to be more aggressive.
  • Nubians tend to be shy and submissive.
• Age hierarchy is also an important
consideration.

SYNONYMS
See specific diseases.

SEE ALSO
Anthelmintic pharmacology
Parasites of small ruminants
Specific diseases of goats

ABBREVIATIONS
CAE = caprine arthritis-encephalitis
CLA = caseous lymphadenitis
CP = crude protein

Suggested Reading
Kannan, G., Terrill, T. H., Kouakou, B.,
Gazal, O. S., Gelaye, S., Amoah, E. A.,
Samake, S. 2000, Jun. Transportation of
goats: effects on physiological stress
responses and live weight loss. *J Anim Sci.*
78(6):1450–57.
Reddy, P. G., Sapp, W. J., Heneine, W. 1993,
Nov. Detection of caprine
arthritis-encephalitis virus by polymerase
chain reaction. *J Clin Microbiol.*
31(11):3042–43.
Sherman, D. M. 1983, Nov. Unexplained
weight loss in sheep and goats. A guide to
differential diagnosis, therapy, and
management. *Vet Clin North Am Large
Anim Pract.* 5(3):571–90.
Smith, M. C., Sherman, D. M. 1994. Diseases
of goats. Philadelphia: Lea & Febiger.
Stehman, S. M. 1996, Jul. Paratuberculosis in
small ruminants, deer, and South American
camelids. *Vet Clin North Am Food Anim
Pract.* 12(2):441–55.
Whittington, R. J., Eamens, G. J., Cousins,
D. V. 2003, Jan-Feb. Specificity of absorbed
ELISA and agar gel immuno-diffusion tests
for paratuberculosis in goats with
observations about use of these tests in
infected goats. *Aust Vet J.* 81(1–2):71–75.

Author: Jeff W. Tyler

WESSELSBRON DISEASE

 BASICS

OVERVIEW
• Acute arthropod-borne infection of sheep, cattle, and goats
• The causative agent is a hemagglutinating flavivirus.

SYSTEMS AFFECTED
Liver, reproductive (occasional abortion), CNS in newborn animals, abomasitis

PATHOPHYSIOLOGY
• Adult infection usually subclinical
• Newborn animals with a high mortality.
• Virus infection occurs year round with little seasonal distribution.
• Abortive disease with congenital malformation of the fetus. Primarily malformation of the CNS with arthrogryposis in cattle and sheep.
• *Hydrops amnii* in ewes
• Associated with *Aedes* spp. mosquito infestation; warmth and increased ambient moisture content may play a part in viral maintenance. It can occur in conjunction with Rift Valley fever during heavy rainfall periods.

GENETICS
None

INCIDENCE/PREVALENCE
Varies with geographic location

GEOGRAPHIC DISTRIBUTION
Africa including Madagascar

SIGNALMENT
• Cattle, goats, and sheep; usually newborn; isolated from vertebrates and arthropod vectors
• The virus has been reported in horses, pigs, ostriches, a gerbil, a dog, a camel; serologic evidence exists in other wild ruminants.

PATHOLOGIC FINDINGS
• Lesions in adult animals are usually mild.
• Hepatomegaly and concomitant icterus are seen in young animals and feti.
• Abomasum mucosal petechiation and diffuse ecchymoses. Chocolate brown contents are usually evident secondary to the disease.
• Liver is generally yellowish, orange or brown.
• Mild, moderate to marked necrosis of liver parenchyma
• Individual or associated groupings of necrotic hepatocytes, which may contain eosinophilic inclusion bodies, are diffusely scattered throughout liver lobules. Kupffer cell proliferation is evident.
• Enlarged lymph nodes
• Gastrointestinal hemorrhage

SIGNS
• Abortive disease with congenital malformation of the fetus; primarily malformation of the CNS with arthrogryposis in cattle and sheep
• Anorexia, weakness, tachypnea, fever, listlessness

CAUSES AND RISK FACTORS
• Virus infection occurs year round with little seasonal distribution.
• Associated with *Aedes* spp. mosquito infestation; warmth and increased ambient moisture content may play a part in viral maintenance. It can occur in conjunction with Rift Valley fever during heavy rainfall periods.
• High mortality rate in lambs

 DIAGNOSIS

DIFFERENTIAL DIAGNOSIS
• Rift Valley fever, abortive diseases, toxic plant ingestion
• Wesselsbron disease is a milder infection than Rift Valley fever with lower morbidity and mortality, less liver destruction, and lower abortion rates.

CBC/BIOCHEMISTRY/URINALYSIS
N/A

OTHER LABORATORY TESTS
• Serodiagnosis is based on complement fixation, virus neutralization, and hemagglutination inhibition.
• Hemagglutination inhibition tests tend to cross-react.
• Intracerebral inoculation of newborn mice is used for virus isolation.
• Virus neutralization is utilized to confirm virus identity.
• Intraperitoneal injection into weaned mice is used to differentiate Wesselsbron disease from Rift Valley fever.

 TREATMENT

No treatment is currently available. Prevention should be based on a sound vaccination program.

MEDICATIONS

N/A

Control

- Stable valuable animals.
- Avoid wet areas where possible.
- Immunization with an attenuated vaccine. Vaccinate 3–6 weeks prior to breeding. Vaccination of pregnant females may lead to abortions and congenital defects.
- Postvaccination immunity is lifelong.
- Mosquito control, though helpful, is difficult.

CONTRAINDICATIONS/POSSIBLE INTERACTIONS

N/A

MISCELLANEOUS

ASSOCIATED CONDITIONS

- Primarily malformation of the CNS with arthrogryposis in cattle and sheep.
- *Hydrops amnii* in ewes

AGE-RELATED FACTORS

Newborn animals with a high mortality

ZOONOTIC POTENTIAL

- In humans it can cause a generally nonfatal influenza, with occasional CNS involvement.
- Precautions should be taken to prevent human infection while performing necropsies of animals suspected of having Wesselsbron disease.

PREGNANCY

Abortive disease with congenital malformation of the fetus; primarily malformation of the CNS with arthrogryposis in cattle and sheep.

RUMINANT SPECIES AFFECTED

Sheep, cattle, and goats; potentially all ruminant species are affected.

BIOSECURITY

Virus infection occurs year round with little seasonal distribution.

PRODUCTION MANAGEMENT

Immunization with an attenuated vaccine. Vaccinate 3–6 weeks prior to breeding. Vaccination of pregnant females may lead to abortions and congenital defects.

SYNONYMS

N/A

SEE ALSO

Arthrogryposis
Rift Valley fever

ABBREVIATIONS

CNS = central nervous system

Suggested Reading
Barnard, B. J. H. 1986. Wesselsbron disease. In: *Current veterinary therapy, food animal practice,* ed. J. L. Howard, 2nd ed. Philadelphia: W. B. Saunders.
Coetzer, J. A.W., Theodoridis, A. 1982. Clinical and pathological studies in adult sheep and goats experimentally infected with Wesselsbron disease virus. *Onderstepoort J. Vet. Res.* 49:19–22.
Smith, M. C., Sherman, D. M., eds. 1994. *Goat medicine.* Philadelphia: Lea and Febiger.
Theodoridis, A., Coetzer, J. A.W. 1980. Wesselsbron disease: virological and serological studies in experimentally infected sheep and goats. *Onderstepoort J. Vet. Res.* 47:221–29.

Author: Kent M. Jackson

WILD RUMINANT POPULATION HEALTH MANAGEMENT

BASICS

OVERVIEW
• As a result of ever-increasing public interest and awareness of wildlife-related issues, veterinarians are frequently asked to comment on, or become involved with, free-ranging wild ruminants.
• Direct involvement with an injured or sick wild ruminant may be relatively infrequent, whereas questions regarding specific wild ruminant diseases or more generalized health and management concerns may be encountered more frequently.
• In North America, tens of millions of wild ruminants occupy wide-ranging and varied habitats. They include: white-tailed, mule, and black-tailed deer; indigenous wild sheep; elk; moose; caribou; mountain goat; pronghorn antelope; bison; and a variety of nonnative exotics.
• Challenges regarding health management issues of wild ruminants cut across continents, from Africa and Asia to Europe and other regions of the world.

SYSTEMS AFFECTED
Management, specific system diseases

GENETICS
N/A

INCIDENCE/PREVALENCE
N/A

GEOGRAPHIC DISTRIBUTION
Worldwide, depending on species and environment

SIGNALMENT
Species
Potentially, all wild ruminant species

Breed Predilections
N/A

Mean Age and Range
N/A

Predominant Sex
N/A

MISCELLANEOUS

Current Issues
• Many practitioners have not had the opportunity to develop extensive background and experience regarding wild ruminants and understandably are often not in a position to address issues with the same level of expertise as specialty trained wildlife veterinarians, biologists, or management experts.

• From a private practitioner's perspective, knowing one's limitations and where to go for assistance may be of greatest value.
• In North America, increasingly visible and controversial urban deer problems; issues relating to tuberculosis and brucellosis among deer, elk, and bison; periodic wild ruminant die-offs due to bluetongue (BT) or epizootic hemorrhagic disease (EHD); and concerns regarding the spread of prion-induced chronic wasting disease (CWD) are representative of the scope of wild ruminant controversies upon which veterinarians are increasingly being asked to comment.
• Interventions directed toward maintaining and improving the "health" of wild populations are often far different than those undertaken on behalf of individual animals.
• The domestic/wild ruminant interface will continue to have importance for the veterinary clinician.
• The interrelationships of domestic and wild ruminant disease entities are numerous. For example, it is well recognized that North American bighorn sheep (BHS), *Ovis canadensis,* are negatively impacted by, and highly susceptible to, *Pasteurella* spp.-induced pneumonia, and that domestic sheep have played an integral role in the epidemiology of that disease complex.
• Management strategies designed to separate domestic and wild sheep populations have been useful in reducing outbreaks among wild sheep and enhancing their populations.
• Wild ruminant population reduction has been broadly implemented in outbreaks of tuberculosis and chronic wasting disease (CWD) among white-tailed deer (*Odocoileus virginianus*) in Michigan and Wisconsin, respectively.
• The basic epidemiologic principle of reducing population levels (coupled with limiting movement of live animals and carcasses) to lessen the opportunities for disease transmission can be, and have been, effective in advancing the long-term health prospects of wild ruminant populations.
• Intervention strategies impacting on wild ruminant health, in addition to local or regional population reductions may include the use of immunizations.
• In the United States, ongoing research efforts are focused on developing effective immunizations for elk (*Cervus elaphus*) and bison (*Bison bison*) as part of brucellosis control efforts in the Greater Yellowstone Ecosystem (GYE).
• Subsequent to the historic pandemics of rinderpest among domestic cattle and wildlife (to include numerous ruminant species) in Africa, the Middle East, Asia, and other regions, vaccination has emerged as the cornerstone of efforts undertaken by the Global Rinderpest Eradication Program.

Practitioner Roles
• The practicing livestock veterinarian is uniquely positioned to observe disease entities that may directly impact on wild ruminants as well as the domestic animal patient.
• Observing clinical disease in ruminant livestock may be the first indication of possible wild ruminant involvement.
• The international veterinary communities, along with national, state, and local practitioners and administrators, have a responsibility to conscientiously communicate in all areas of domestic and wild ruminant health and management in order to maintain the stability of food supplies, the environment, and the economies upon which the world is dependant.
• By undertaking some preliminary groundwork, one can ease the task of dealing with wild ruminant issues and assist in successfully responding to whatever questions/challenges may occur.

Useful Preparations
• Generate a list of important contacts
  • Federal/state/university diagnostic laboratories
  • Local/state wildlife/management specialists
  • State agriculture/domestic ruminant specialists
  • State and local public health departments
  • Wildlife disease focused organizations/associations
  • International contacts are generally accessible via federal and university-based contacts.
• Gain familiarity with federal/state/local regulations
  • Wildlife possession and treatment statutes
  • Reportable diseases
• Gain familiarity with important regional wild ruminant diseases
  • Diseases having domestic and/or human health implications (i.e., brucellosis, anthrax)
  • High visibility, ruminant/species-specific diseases (i.e., CWD)
  • Periodically occurring epizootic diseases (i.e., EHD/BT)
• Refer "management" issues to management professionals
  • Social and politically charged management issues belong with the responsible federal, state, or local agencies having scientific and legal oversight responsibility.
  • When in doubt, obtain professional wildlife disease/management expertise!

WILD RUMINANT POPULATION HEALTH MANAGEMENT

Summary
• Successful efforts to effect useful management strategies impacting on the health of wild populations of ruminants must, by necessity, be a collaborative effort.
• The nature of the core professional training of veterinarians (domestic animal medicine and surgery) inevitably results in less rigorous attention being paid to training in wildlife diseases.
• Expanded training in this specialty results from post–veterinary school graduate education.
• Management issues involving free-ranging wild ruminants are primarily associated with the training of professional wildlife biologists, and not addressed in traditional veterinary education.
• Clearly, the relationship of domestic and wild ruminant foreign animal diseases (FADs), and the associated implications for bioterrorism, brings the importance of wild ruminant population health clearly into perspective.
• Vigilance in pursuing unusual wild animal mortality events is a critical element of the nation's focus on disease surveillance.
• It is essential, therefore, to combine the expertise of all animal/human health and natural resource professionals when considering the health of wild animal populations, be they ruminant or otherwise.

ASSOCIATED CONDITIONS
N/A

AGE-RELATED FACTORS
N/A

ZOONOTIC POTENTIAL
Several of these diseases are zoonotic. Care must be taken in the collection of laboratory samples and the diagnosis/treatment of affected animals.

PREGNANCY
N/A

RUMINANT SPECIES AFFECTED
Potentially, all wild ruminant species can be affected.

BIOSECURITY
N/A

PRODUCTION MANAGEMENT
N/A

SYNONYMS
N/A

SEE ALSO
American Association of Wildlife Veterinarians (www.aawv.net)
Captive cervidae management
Diseases of wild ruminants
Specific disease chapters
Wildlife Disease Association (WDA; www.wildlifedisease.org); also see links to European, Nordic, Australasian, and African sections.
The Wildlife Society (TWS; www.wildlife.org)

ABBREVIATIONS
BHS = bighorn sheep
BT = bluetongue
CWD = chronic wasting disease
EHD = epizootic hemorrhagic disease
FADs = foreign animal diseases
GYE = Greater Yellowstone Ecosystem

Suggested Reading
AVMA. 1992. Animal welfare forum: the veterinarian's role in the welfare of wildlife. *J Amer Vet Med Assoc.* 200: 617–58.
Boyce, W., Elliott, N., Mazet, J., ed. 1991. *Proceedings of the wildlife health workshop.* Pew National Veterinary Education Program. PEW Foundation, Fort. Collins, Colorado.
Boyce, W., Yuill, T., Homan, J., Jessup, D. 1992. A role for veterinarians in wildlife health and conservation biology. *J Amer Vet Med Assoc.* 200: 435–37.
Daszak, P., Cunningham, A. A., Hyatt, A. D. 2000. Emerging infectious diseases of wildlife—threats to biodiversity and human health. *Science* 287: 443–49.
Karesh, W. B., Osfosky, S. A., Rocke, T. E., Barrows, P. L. 2002. Joining forces to improve our world. *Cons Biol.* 16: 1432–34.

Author: Paul Barrows

WINTER DYSENTERY

BASICS

OVERVIEW
• Acute, contagious diarrheal disease of cattle with worldwide distribution, occurring in closely confined cattle during winter months
• Usually recognized as dark, bloody, liquid diarrhea with concurrent drop in milk production, anorexia, and depression
• Clinical signs commonly observed either prior to or during diarrheal phase include nasolacrimal discharge and cough.
• Milk production decreases dramatically and clinical disease may persist for several weeks. Pregnant cows and recently fresh or lactating cows are most commonly affected. Calves may also demonstrate similar clinical signs and attack rates.
• Mortality is low, but morbidity is high in larger herds. Herds with prior history of winter dysentery are at greater risk of developing clinical disease.
• Winter dysentery has been reported in cattle worldwide.

PATHOPHYSIOLOGY
• To date, the exact cause is unknown. However, increasing evidence suggests that bovine coronavirus may be casual when appropriate animal and environmental conditions are present. Viral particles invade the colonic mucosa resulting in death and necrosis of the colonic epithelial cells.
• The loss of epithelial barrier function results in transudation of proteinaceous fluid and blood. The increased volume of fluid presumably results in loose, dark, and sometimes bloody stool.

SYSTEMS AFFECTED
Primarily gastrointestinal tract; careful evaluation of herd records may demonstrate mild respiratory signs and diarrhea in cows and calves on some dairies.

GENETICS
No breed predilection; more common in dairy animals

INCIDENCE/PREVALENCE
• Acute, contagious diarrhea in cattle that occurs sporadically in epizootic form during the colder months of the year
• Disease occurs more commonly in northern states (USA) and Canada, but also has been documented to occur in Australia, the United Kingdom, Europe, Israel, and Japan.
• Morbidity is generally high, with low mortality.

GEOGRAPHIC DISTRIBUTION
• Potentially worldwide, depending on time of year
• Disease occurs more commonly in northern states (USA) and Canada, but also has been documented to occur in Australia, the United Kingdom, Europe, Israel and Japan.

SIGNALMENT
• Primarily adult dairy cows, either soon after calving or within the first 100 days in milk
• Pregnant cows appear to be at reduced risk.
• Some outbreaks have been reported in beef cattle and feedlot calves.

Species
Dairy and beef cattle

Breed Predilections
N/A

Mean Age and Range
Calves may demonstrate similar clinical signs and attack rates as adult cattle.

Predominant Sex
Pregnant cows and recently fresh or lactating cows are most commonly affected. Calves may also demonstrate similar clinical signs and attack rates.

SIGNS

HISTORICAL FINDINGS
• Acute onset of voluminous, dark, and bloody diarrhea occurring in anorexic, depressed cows that have reduced milk production
• Reduced rumen fill and dehydration result in weight loss. Blood in feces may be mixed evenly in feces or may be present in clots. The feces generally have a fetid odor.
• Affected animals may develop diarrhea and respiratory signs (dyspnea, coughing, nasal and lacrimal discharge).
• Usually epizootic in nature with 10–100% morbidity. Most commonly in adult dairy cattle with dramatic reductions in milk production in the fall and winter. Winter dysentery has also been documented in adult beef cattle and feedlot calves.

PHYSICAL EXAMINATION FINDINGS

CAUSES AND RISK FACTORS
• Cattle in herds with recent exposure and immunologic response to BVDV or BCV (> 4-fold increase in serum titer), cattle housed in tie stalls or stanchion barns, and facilities using the same equipment to manage manure as well as feed are at increased risk for development of winter dysentery.
• Cows with high fecal BCV ELISA antigen and high acute serum BCV IgG antibody titers that seroconvert (> 4-fold increase) are at greater risk for development of WD.
• Pregnant cows are at decreased risk for WD.

DIAGNOSIS

DIFFERENTIAL DIAGNOSIS
• Diarrheic diseases caused by BVD virus, Coccidia, gastrointestinal parasites, *Salmonella* spp., *Campylobacter* spp., *Mycobacterium avium* subspecies *paratuberculosis* (Johne's disease), heavy metal intoxications (As, Cd), organophosphate toxicity, dietary induced gut disturbances
• *Mycobacterium avium* subspecies *paratuberculosis* is not often a problem in outbreak form.
• *Campylobacter* spp. has not been isolated from cattle with WD.
• Coccidiosis is not generally a problem in adult cattle, fecal evaluation may rule out coccidia and gastrointestinal nematodiasis.
• Heavy metal intoxication is often accompanied by high mortality in groups of cattle.
• Organophosphate intoxication includes acute death, neurologic animals, salivation, lacrimation, urination, and defecation.
• Diet-induced diarrhea is often accompanied by lameness, reduced milk fat, or protein/fat inversion.
• Bloody stool or diarrheic feces with blood clots may indicate clostridial enteritis (jejunal hemorrhage syndrome).

CBC/BIOCHEMISTRY/URINALYSIS
• Not generally helpful in diagnostics; if persistent, dysentery may result in anemia.
• Monitor PCV, hydration, and acid/base balance in chronic cases.

OTHER LABORATORY TESTS
Diagnostic testing including fecal culture for bacterial causes (*Salmonella* spp., *Campylobacter*, *Mycobacterium avium* subspecies *paratuberculosis*, serology for BVDV, BCV, IBR, Johne's, rotavirus, campylobacter, cryptosporidium, BRSV, BAV3, and BLV; fecal evaluation for viral particles (electron microscopy).

IMAGING
N/A

OTHER DIAGNOSTIC PROCEDURES
N/A

PATHOLOGIC FINDINGS
N/A

TREATMENT

• Provision of adequate feed and fresh water is important. Salt and trace minerals are also advisable.
• Management practices that prevent cross-contamination of feed with manure from cattle (especially those with diarrhea) appear to be important.

ACTIVITY
As normal

DIET
Provision of adequate feed and fresh water is important. Salt and trace minerals are also advisable.

CLIENT EDUCATION
Cattle in herds with recent exposure and immunologic response to BVDV or BCV (> 4-fold increase in serum titer), cattle housed in tie stalls or stanchion barns, and facilities using the same equipment to manage manure as well as feed are at increased risk for development of winter dysentery.

MEDICATIONS

DRUGS OF CHOICE
Pharmaceutical selection should be based on laboratory analysis and culture/sensitivity.

CONTRAINDICATIONS
Appropriate milk and meat withdrawal times must be followed for all compounds administered to food-producing animals.

PRECAUTIONS
N/A

POSSIBLE INTERACTIONS
• Cattle in herds with recent exposure and immunologic response to BVDV or BCV (> 4-fold increase in serum titer), cattle housed in tie stalls or stanchion barns, and facilities using the same equipment to manage manure as well as feed are at increased risk for development of winter dysentery.
• Cows with high fecal BCV ELISA antigen and high acute serum BCV IgG antibody titers that seroconvert (> 4-fold increase) are at greater risk for development of WD.

ALTERNATIVE DRUGS
N/A

FOLLOW-UP

PATIENT MONITORING
Monitor PCV, hydration, and acid/base balance

PREVENTION/AVOIDANCE
• Careful evaluation of herd records may demonstrate mild respiratory signs and diarrhea in cows and calves on some dairies.
• Maintaining strict quarantine on cattle operations may help.

POSSIBLE COMPLICATIONS
N/A

EXPECTED COURSE AND PROGNOSIS
Morbidity is generally high with low mortality.

MISCELLANEOUS

ASSOCIATED CONDITIONS
Most commonly in adult dairy cattle with dramatic reductions in milk production in the fall and winter.

AGE-RELATED FACTORS
All ages may be affected.

ZOONOTIC POTENTIAL
Salmonella spp., *Campylobacter* spp., *Mycobacterium avium* subspecies *paratuberculosis* (Johne's disease) may be zoonotic.

PREGNANCY
• Pregnant cows and recently fresh or lactating cows are most commonly affected.
• Pregnant cows appear to be at reduced risk.

RUMINANT SPECIES AFFECTED
Cattle, primarily dairy; however feedlot animals may be affected.

BIOSECURITY
Management practices that prevent cross-contamination of feed with manure from cattle (especially those with diarrhea) appear to be important.

PRODUCTION MANAGEMENT
Cattle in herds with recent exposure and immunologic response to BVDV or BCV (> 4-fold increase in serum titer), cattle housed in tie stalls or stanchion barns, and facilities using the same equipment to manage manure as well as feed are at increased risk for development of winter dysentery.

SYNONYMS
Winter scours

SEE ALSO
Campylobacter spp.
Coccidia
Diarrheic diseases caused by BVD virus
Diet-induced gut disturbances
Gastrointestinal parasites
Heavy metal intoxications (As, Cd)
Mycobacterium avium subspecies *paratuberculosis* (Johne's disease)
Organophosphate toxicity
Salmonella spp.

ABBREVIATIONS
BAV3 = bovine adenovirus type 3
BCV = bovine corona virus
BLV = bovine leukosis virus
BRSV = bovine respiratory syncytial virus
BVD = bovine viral diarrhea
BVDV = bovine viral diarrhea virus
ELISA = enzyme-linked immunosorbent assay
IBR= infectious bovine rhinotracheitis
IgG = immunoglobulin G
PCV = packed cell volume
WD = winter dysentery

Suggested Reading
Cho, K.-O., Halbur, P. G., Bruna, J. D., et al. 2000. Detection and isolation of coronavirus from feces of three herds of feedlot cattle during outbreaks of winter dysentery-like disease. *J Am Vet Med Assoc.* 217: 1191–94.
Cho, K.-O., Hoet, A. E., Loerch, S. C. 2001. Evaluation of concurrent shedding of bovine coronavirus via the respiratory tract and enteric route in feedlot cattle. *Am J Vet Res.* 62:1436–41.
Saif, L. J. 1990. A review of evidence implicating bovine coronavirus in the etiology of winter dysentery in cows: an enigma resolved? *Cornell Vet.* 80:303–11.
Smith, D. R., Fedorka-Cray, P. J., Mohan, R., et al. 1998. Epidemiologic herd-level assessment of causative agents and risk factors for winter dysentery in dairy cattle. *Am J Vet Res.* 59:994–1001.
Smith, D. R., Fedorka-Cray, P. J., Mohan, R., et al. 1998. Evaluation of cow-level risk factors for the development of winter dysentery in dairy cattle. *Am J Vet Res.* 59:986–93.
Tsunemitsu, H., Smith, D. R., Saif, L. J. 1999. Experimental inoculation of adult dairy cows with bovine coronavirus and detection of coronavirus in feces by RT-PCR. *Arch Virol.* 144:167–75.

Author: Jeff Lakritz

WOOL ROT

BASICS

OVERVIEW
• Fleece rot is a skin disease caused by prolonged and excessive wetting of the skin resulting in exudation and discoloration of the wool.
• It is characterized by superficial inflammation, seropurulent exudation, and putrefaction that attracts blowflies (*Lucilia cuprina*) to oviposition.
• Fleece rot causes severe financial loss through downgrading of wool and cutaneous myosis by blowflies.

PATHOPHYSIOLOGY
• The inciting factor is prolonged wetting of the skin and matting of the wool, for example from rain or dipping.
• Continued wetting of the skin for at least 8 days or 100 mm of rain will reproduce the disease.
• Temperature is not a factor in disease development.
• The primary factor for susceptibility is the sensitivity of the skin to prolonged wetting.
• Chronic wetting of the skin results in acathanosis, hyperkeratosis, and edema of the lower layers of the epidermis and subsequent infiltration of the area by neutrophils and other polymorphonuclear leukocytes (PMNs).
• Microabscesses form and exudate is discharged into the lower layers of the epidermis.
• Prolonged wetting of the skin, high humidity in fleece environment, and the availability of nutrients from serous exudates allow for indigenous skin flora, opportunistic flora, and bacteria such as *Pseudomonas aeruginosa* to proliferate.
• Chromogenic bacteria (*Pseudomonas* spp.) cause discoloration of the fleece. *P. indigofera* produces a blue color and *P. aeruginosa* produces a green color. Other bacteria may produce yellow, brown, greenish-brown, or red discoloration.

SYSTEMS AFFECTED
Skin and hair (wool)

GENETICS
• There is a genetic predisposition to fleece rot with some sheep breeds being more susceptible than others.
• There are differences among breeds and between individuals within a breed.
• Breeds with lower wax content, irregular fiber size, and thicker wool fibers are more susceptible.

INCIDENCE/PREVALENCE
• Common problem in sheep
• Incidence varies from 15 to 90%.

GEOGRAPHIC DISTRIBUTION
• Worldwide but most common in Australia and New Zealand during wet season
• Also of concern in South Africa and United Kingdom

SIGNALMENT
• Can occur in any age, sex, or breed of sheep
• Most common in younger sheep after succession of wet days from either rain or dippings

SIGNS
• Except for the fleece, sheep are otherwise normal.
• Some sheep may show evidence of pain, rubbing, and/or biting at affected skin sites.
• Lesions are most common on the dorsum with the skin becoming red-purple in the early stages followed by exudation and matting of the wool.
• Affected areas are wet and the wool easily epilates.
• Parting of wool in affected areas reveals exudation and commonly diffuse discoloration or bands of discoloration.
• Fleece rot is characterized by a greenish discoloration of the wool fibers with a seropurulent crust. Most common discoloration is greenish but it may be yellow, yellow-brown, or red-brown.
• Affected areas emanate a putrid odor and attract blowflies.
• General health is unaffected, but in cases with severe ulceration, death can occur due to sepsis.
• A chronic ulcerative necrotic dermatitis on the tail, udder, and legs associated with a greenish discoloration of fleece following excessive rain in the Mediterranean has been seen.

CAUSES AND RISK FACTORS
• Major cause is prolonged wetting coupled by a "less water proof" fleece.
• Fleece staple is a major factor in the cause of wool rot. A long fleece reduces skin wetability but, once wet, the skin and fleece dry out more slowly. Short staple fleece is rapidly penetrated by water but dries out more quickly.
• Compact fleeces with high wax contents are most resistant.
• Breeds with open fleece and poor staple structure are more prone.
• Susceptible sheep have smaller follicle groups and higher densities of follicle populations with more primary follicles; sheep with more secondary to primary hair follicle ratios are more resistant.
• Susceptible sheep have thicker wool fibers growing from primary follicles.

• Susceptible sheep have irregular wool fibers that retain water in the fleece longer making the fleece more susceptible to rot than resistant sheep.
• Resistant sheep have better fleece closure and higher wax content allowing water to run off the wool; sheep that are more "waterproof" are more resistant.
• Yellowish fleece color (high suint content) is found in more susceptible sheep.

DIAGNOSIS

• Clinical diagnosis based upon finding compatible historical (i.e., prolonged wetting) and clinical signs
• Characteristics of lesions
• If needed, bacterial isolation of causative agent
• Impression smears of exudate reveal gram-negative rods.

DIFFERENTIAL DIAGNOSIS
• Major differential diagnosis is dermatophilosis.
• Scab formation and skin ulceration are absent in fleece rot, but present in dermatophilosis.

CBC/BIOCHEMISTRY/URINALYSIS
Affected sheep may have leukocytosis and neutrophilia.

OTHER LABORATORY TESTS
N/A

IMAGING
N/A

DIAGNOSTIC PROCEDURES
Skin biopsy

PATHOLOGICAL FINDINGS
Skin biopsy shows suppurative intraepidermal pustular dermatitis and superficial folliculitis.

TREATMENT

• Affected sheep are not treated and it is usually of no benefit.
• Chemical drying of fleece may decrease wetness and incidence of fleece rot.
• A mixture of zinc and aluminum oxides with sterols and fatty acids applied as a mist may be protective.
• Chemical drying agents should be compatible with other dipping chemicals (i.e., insecticides).
• Prevention through selection of sheep with fleece resistant to wool rot is the most practical approach.

MEDICATIONS

N/A

FOLLOW-UP

PATIENT MONITORING
N/A

PREVENTION
• Shearing sheep before wet season may minimize wool rot along with selection of breeds that are resistant to fleece rot.
• Some degree of control may be affected by selection of fleece rot-resistant sheep.
• Heritability of resistance is estimated to be between 0.35 and 0.4 and selective breeding programs are recommended for high-risk areas.
• A killed *P. aeruginosa* vaccine has been found to be protective against severe exudation and may be a viable option in the future.

POSSIBLE COMPLICATIONS
• Affected animals are susceptible to blowfly strike.
• Affected sheep may develop secondary *P. aeruginosa* infections of the skin characterized by granulomatous scabs on wool-free areas of legs and scrotum.

EXPECTED COURSE AND PROGNOSIS
N/A

MISCELLANEOUS

ASSOCIATED CONDITIONS
• Affected sheep are at risk for blowfly strike.
• Prolonged wetting of the skin may predispose sheep to "pink rot," which is caused by a bacterial infection of the skin with *Bacillus* spp. Affected fibers are found at shearing and appear as a mat of wool in creamy pink exudate.

AGE-RELATED FACTORS
Wool rot is more common in young sheep.

ZOONOTIC POTENTIAL
N/A

PREGNANCY
N/A

RUMINANT SPECIES AFFECTED
Sheep

BIOSECURITY
N/A

PRODUCTION MANAGEMENT
• Fleece rot is of major economic concern.
• Fleece wetability can be determined by taking a sample of staple and placing it in a wet plastic cylinder with one end in water. The mass of water taken up in a given time is measured. Results are consistent and capable of distinguishing resistant sheep from susceptible sheep.

SYNONYMS
Canary stain
Fleece rot
Water rot
Wool rot
Yolk rot

SEE ALSO
Dermatophilosis
Lumpy wool disease
Sheep breeding and selection
Sheep keds
Sheep nutrition

ABBREVIATIONS
N/A

Suggested Reading
Anderson, D. E., Rings, D. M., Pugh, D. G. 2002. Diseases of the integumentary system. In: *Sheep and goat medicine*, ed. D. G. Pugh. Philadelphia: W. B. Saunders.
Diseases caused by bacteria. 1999. In: *Veterinary medicine, a textbook of the diseases of cattle, sheep, pigs, goats and horses*, ed. O. M. Radostits., C. C, Gay, D. C. Blood, K. W. Hinchcliff, 9th ed. London: W. B. Saunders, Ltd.
Diseases of the skin. 1988. In: *Jensen and Swift's diseases of sheep*, ed. C. Kimberling., 3rd ed. Philadelphia: Lea & Febiger.
Plant, J. Bacterial and fungal infections of the skin and wool. In: *Diseases of sheep*, ed, W. B. Martin, I. D. Aitken, 3rd ed. Edinburg: Blackwell Science.
Scott, D. W. 1999. Ovine fleece rot. In: *Current veterinary therapy 4: food animal practice*, ed. J. L. Howard, R. A. Smith. Philadelphia: W. B. Saunders.

Author: Karen A. Moriello and Susan D. Semrad

WOUND MANAGEMENT

 BASICS

DEFINITION
• A wound is defined as a break in the epithelial integrity of the skin that could extend deeper into the dermis, subcutaneous fat, fascia, muscle, or bone.
• The healing process can be aided by providing the proper environment for living tissue to repair itself, but the best mechanism is the natural process.

SYSTEM AFFECTED
Musculoskeletal

SIGNALMENT
Any age, sex, species, or breed of ruminant

SIGNS
May vary depending on the severity and location of the wound

CAUSES
• *Penetrating or puncture wounds:* these are deceptive in nature and may appear minor, but should always be considered serious. Bacteria, dirt, and other foreign material are often carried into the deep tissue by the penetrating object such as a nail or piece of wood.
• *Incised wound:* injury made by a sharp object such as a knife, glass, or a thin metal object that leaves the wound edges cut rather clean.
• *Lacerated wounds:* unlike incised wounds, these have rough and irregular edges and are more prone to infection.
• *Abrasion:* a scrape, friction burn, or excessive rubbing are common in abrasions. They are a minor problem compared to the others and involve only the top layer of the skin.

 DIAGNOSIS

• The decision to close a wound to achieve primary intention or to let it heal by secondary intention is often based on experience. This can be based, as guidance, on the "golden period," which is the number of hours that a wound can heal with first intention. The length of time of the golden period varies with the blood supply to the region, the extent of injury, the degree of contamination, and the injury's anatomic location.
• Any wound that shows signs of infection should not be closed. This is diagnosed by the presence of heat, pain, and swelling of the area. It should be cleaned and left open to heal by secondary or tertiary intention.

DIFFERENTIAL DIAGNOSIS
N/A

CBC/BIOCHEMISTRY/URINALYSIS
N/A

OTHER LABORATORY TESTS
N/A

IMAGING
• *Ultrasonography:* Investigates the severity of soft-tissue injury, joint abnormality, periosteal lesions, and wounds
• *Radiography:* Necessary in puncture wounds and fractures to evaluate the severity of the wound and presence and location of a foreign body, and to establish a better treatment and management of the wound.

DIAGNOSTIC PROCEDURES
• Restrain the patient, chemically or physically, as necessary.

• Control bleeding. If the blood flow is profuse and pulsating, an artery may be severed and a tourniquet must be applied. Wounds that do not bleed in a pulsating manner may be controlled by a clean compress bandage directly over the wound.
• After bleeding is under control, examine the wound to evaluate the extent of injury and tissue damage.

 TREATMENT

• Initial assessment of the injured animal should include vital signs, history, and location of the wound.
• Most wounds in ruminants can be managed with the aid of chemical restraint (tranquilization) and local and regional anesthesia. General anesthesia is indicated if the injury is extensive and during cast application.
• In the preparation of the wound, the edges should be clipped and scrubbed gently with an isotonic solution and germicidal agent. Excise and debride wound of dead tissue and foreign bodies.
• Most traumatic wounds are sutured but without undue tension. It is preferable to leave some wound edges apart, rather than apply sutures under pressure, because they will produce ischemia of the wound edges and a larger defect may result.
• Drains are indicated in the presence of unobliterated dead space or if there is likelihood of fluid accumulation.
• Penetrating or puncture wounds are usually not sutured but are allowed to drain. Subsequent irrigation may be necessary to flush out debris.

- Incised and some lacerated wounds are usually repaired by suturing, depending upon the degree of contamination.
- Abrasions that are cleaned respond well to many of the commercial products available for wound treatments.
- Systemic antibiotics are always recommended for the treatment of traumatic wounds, especially if heavily contaminated. To be effective, antibiotic administration needs to be initiated as soon as possible and adequate dosage levels need to be maintained.
- The use of local antibiotics or antibacterial agents is controversial. Exudate on the wound often prevents effective contact of the agent with the microorganisms and many local medications retard wound healing. But when *Pseudomonas* species are involved, betadine ointment is appropriate.
- Protecting a wound by bandaging may protect the area against further contamination, and also aids in the immobilization of the wound's edges, accelerating the healing process.

MEDICATIONS

- The vast selection of topical applications that are available makes choosing the proper medication difficult. Several of these compounds have questionable value, others may be harmful, and many will, in fact, retard the natural healing of the wound.
- It's always recommended to treat wounds with systemic antibiotics that are approved for use in food-producing animals.

CONTRAINDICATIONS

- Appropriate milk and meat withdrawal times must be followed for all compounds administered to food-producing animals.
- Steroids should not be used in pregnant animals.
- Steroid use may undermine the healing process.

FOLLOW-UP

PATIENT MONITORING

- Check the evolution of the wound and its healing process, and supervise for any possible extended infection.
- Inappetance can be a sign of septicemia, so monitor the patient throughout the healing process.

MISCELLANEOUS

ASSOCIATED CONDITIONS

Tissue necrosis, sepsis, and loss of function are all associated conditions.

ZOONOTIC POTENTIAL

Several secondary wound diseases are zoonotic. Care must be taken in the collection of laboratory samples and the diagnosis/treatment of affected animals.

PREGNANCY

N/A

RUMINANT SPECIES AFFECTED

Potentially, all ruminant species can be affected.

BIOSECURITY

Treat and or cull new animals for disease conditions prior to herd introduction.

PRODUCTION MANAGEMENT

N/A

SYNONYMS

N/A

SEE ALSO

Anesthesia and analgesia
FARAD
Myasis

ABBREVIATIONS

N/A

Suggested Reading

Cockbill, S. M., Turner, T. D. 1995, Apr 8. Management of veterinary wounds. *Vet Rec.* 136(14):362–65.

Gomez, J. H., Schumacher, J., Lauten, S. D., Sartin, E. A., Hathcock, T. L., Swaim, S. F. 2004, Jan. Effects of 3 biologic dressings on healing of cutaneous wounds on the limbs of horses. *Can J Vet Res.* 68(1):49–55.

Kaneps, A. J. 1996, Mar. Orthopedic conditions of small ruminants. Llama, sheep, goat, and deer. *Vet Clin North Am Food Anim Pract.* 12(1):211–31.

Liptak, J. M. 1997, Jun. An overview of the topical management of wounds. *Aust Vet J.* 75(6):408–13.

Madison, J. B., Gronwall, R. R. 1992, Sep. Influence of wound shape on wound contraction in horses. *Am J Vet Res.* 53(9):1575–78.

Plant, J. Bacterial and fungal infections of the skin and wool. In: *Diseases of sheep*, ed. W. B. Martin, I. D. Aitken, 3rd ed. Edinburgh: Blackwell Science.

Trotter, G. W. 1989, Dec. Principles of early wound management. *Vet Clin North Am Equine Pract.* 5(3):483–98.

Author: Yessenia Almedia

YAK MANAGEMENT AND DISEASE

BASICS

OVERVIEW
• Yak *(Poephagus grunniens* or *Bos grunniens)* thrive in conditions of extreme harshness throughout Asia.
• Yaks are found predominantly in the Qinghai-Tibetan Plateau. The plateau extends over 2.5 million sq km (about 1 million sq mi) of Asia.
• Approximately 1.3 million yak are marketed in China annually. It has been estimated that the annual Chinese yak production is 226,000 tonnes of meat, 13,000 tonnes of fiber, and 170,000 hides. Chinese milk production was 1.4 million tonnes for 1989 and 715,000 tonnes for 1997. These estimates may be far below actual production levels.
• Yaks are mated for the first time when they are 3–4 years of age and generally calve every 2 years or twice in 3 years, producing 4–5 calves in a lifetime. Hybrids can calve annually.
• The average length of the estrous cycle is approximately 20 days (range 18–22 days) with the duration of estrus less than 24 hours. Estrus can be difficult to detect.
• Gestation length is around 258 days.

SYSTEMS AFFECTED
Production management, nutritional

GENETICS
• Hybridization of yak with cattle has been utilized to increase meat and milk production. The hybrids are usually found at lower altitudes and in less harsh environmental conditions than the typical yak environment.
• Hybridization commonly employs yak females mated to bulls of local cattle breeds and artificially with imported dairy breeds. Hybrids are mated back (back-crossed) to either yak or cattle bulls. F1 males are sterile.
• F1 yak hybrids adapt well to the local environment; backcross hybrids to cattle are less well adapted to the environment and a loss of heterosis generally occurs.

Yak Hybrid
• Hybridizing yak with *Bos taurus* or *Bos indicus* cattle: Holstein-Friesian and Simmental cattle are commonly utilized to increase milk production in yaks.
• Hybrids are less well adapted to harsh conditions and high altitudes and are generally managed at intermediate elevations and require improved husbandry practices.
• The first hybrid (F1) females reach sexual maturity earlier and are bred a year earlier than the average yak.
• F1 males are sterile.
• F1 hybrids generally grow faster and become larger than straight-bred yak.
• Backcrosses to yak (or to breeds of cattle) are smaller than the F1. Milk yield is higher in hybrids than in the straight-bred yak. Backcrosses give less milk than the F1. The fat percentage of the milk of hybrids is usually lower than that of yak.
• Reduced productivity, relative to the F1, makes backcross generations undesirable.

Nutrition
• Feed intake: yak consume less feed than cattle due in part to their smaller rumen capacity.
• Dry matter intake (DMI in kg per day) of the growing yak can be estimated as DMI = 0.0165 W + 0.0486 (W is body weight in kilograms), and that of the lactating yak as DMI = $0.008W^{0.52} + 1.369Y$ ($W^{0.52}$ is metabolic body weight, Y is milk yield, kg per day).
• Voluntary intake (VI) of the yak varies with the season and grazed plant heights. VI ranges from 18 to 25 kg of fresh forage in summer to 6 to 8 kg per day of poor-quality grass under colder grazing conditions.
• Other factors affecting feed intake levels include feed type, feeding conditions, environmental climate, age, animal size, and sex.
• Rumen volume ranges from 32.3 to 66.8 liters in the mature yak.

Energy Nutrition
• The thermoneutral zone for the growing yak is estimated as 8°C–14°C.
• The fasting heat production (FHP) of the growing yak can be estimated as FHP = 916 kJ per $kgW^{0.52}$ per day.
• The metabolizable energy requirement for maintenance (ME_m) in growing yak is around 460 kJ per kg $W^{0.75}$ per day.
• Metabolizable energy requirement in the growing yak can be estimated as ME (MJ per day) = $0.45W^{0.75} + (8.73 + 0.091 W)$ DG (DG in kg per day), where W is weight in kg and DG is daily gain (in kg).
• Researchers observed that lactating yak have better utilization of dietary energy than dry yak cows. Another study with lactating yak indicated that yak cows have a lower efficiency of metabolizable-energy utilization for milk production (averaging 0.46) than dairy cattle (*Bos taurus*).
• The daily metabolizable energy requirement of growing yak has been estimated as ME (MJ/d) = $0.45W^{0.75} + (8.73 + 0.091 W)$ DG, where W is the body weight and DG is daily gain (kg), and the efficiency of utilization of metabolizable energy for growth (k_g) in yak is 0.49.

Protein Nutrition
• There is no difference in the digestibility of dietary nitrogen between lactating and dry yak cows.
• Yak can use nonprotein nitrogen as efficiently as domestic cattle.
• Rumen degradable crude protein requirements for maintenance ($RDCP_m$, g per day) in the growing yak are around $6.09W^{0.52}$ g per day.
• Crude protein requirements for daily gain (DG $RDCP_g$ g per day) in growing yak can be estimated as $RDCP_g = (1.16/DG + 0.05/W^{0.52})^{-1}$.
• Total crude protein requirements for growing yak can be calculated as RDCP (g per day) = $6.09W^{0.52} + (1.16/DG + 0.05/W^{0.52})^{-1}$.

- Utilization efficiency of dietary protein in the yak differs with diet composition and feeding level, age, sex, body condition score, and animal production level (e.g., growth, lactation).
- Researchers reported no difference between lactating and dry cows in crude protein digestibility, although lactating yak tend to consume more feed than dry yak.
- Yak may have evolved a mechanism to recycle more nitrogen to the rumen than cattle.

Mineral Nutrition

- Mineral nutrition is poorly understood in the yak.
- Researchers have found that inorganic phosphate (P) is sufficient for various categories of yak (calves, heifers, dry cows, and lactating cows) during the warm season when grazing was on alpine meadows with good-quality pasture. But in the spring and early summer, dietary phosphate failed to meet yak requirements.
- Chinese researchers suggest that yak living in the Qinghai Lake area are suffering sodium (Na) and copper (Cu) deficiency and there may be a shortage of molybdenum on Tianzhu alpine rangelands.

Diseases Affecting the Yak
Bacterial Diseases

- Anthrax—common in many regions of Asia.
- Botulism—*Clostridium botulinum* (type C has been identified in Tibet).
- Brucellosis—common among yak throughout Asia. In Sichuan, Qinghai, and Tibet, sample groups of yak were tested over the period 1952–1981, and an average of 17.4% (1.8%–56.3%) tested positive. Researchers reported that between 13% and 17% of yak in various groups on Haiyan pastures in Qinghai province were positive. Both *B. melitensis* and *B. abortus* have been identified as infective agents. *B. melitensis* is more prevalent in China and *B. abortus* is more commonly isolated in the former USSR. *B. melitensis* strain Biovar 3 is found most commonly.

- Calf scours—in some herds, 30%–40% of calves develop diarrhea. This appears most common in spring-born calves; however, scours in young calves have been reported as a major cause of death in two studies with yak. Both studies isolated *E. coli*. Researchers reported a scour incidence of almost 80% within the first month of life. In another study, a mortality rate due to *E. coli* infection in yak calves was 20%–30%.
- Caseous lymphadenitis—tends to be herd specific
- *Chlamydia* spp.—*Chlamydia* spp. appear commonly in some yak herds. Researchers examined yak herds and found the incidence to be 10.8%. In another study, an incidence of 42.7% among 553 yak was found. Another study reported yak abortion outbreaks in Qinghai province caused by *Chlamydia psittaci* infection. Tests on serum samples collected from yak that had aborted showed positive tests in 45 of 155 samples.
- Contagious bovine pleuropneumonia—caused by *Mycoplasma mycoides* occurs in yak between 2 and 10 years of age. It is generally reported during the winter and spring months. Researchers reported a high incidence of 54% in Ganzi County of the Sichuan province. Other researchers reported an incidence of 1.9% for herds in Tibet with pleuropneumonia and a mortality of 17% among those affected.
- Leptospirosis—commonly reported as causing abortion in herds
- Mastitis—the incidence appears less than in domestic dairy cattle. Relatively low milk yield and the common practice of calf suckling may help decrease the incidence of mastitis. One outbreak in Hongyuan County in Sichuan was due to a streptococcal infection. Another study reported common bacterial isolates in yak herds in Nepal. Bacteria isolated from the milk samples were *Staphylococcus aureus, Streptococcus agalactiae,* other *Streptococcus* spp., and *Coliform* spp.

- Pasteurellosis—reported to occur every year as hemorrhagic septicemia. Researchers in Tibet (over the period 1976–1979) noted a 0.34% incidence of hemorrhagic septicemia among yak, with a mortality rate among affected animals of nearly 36%.
- Salmonellosis—common among yak in China. Generally reported in calves between 15 and 60 days of age. Isolates included *S. typhimurium, S. dublin,* and *S. newport.* Researchers found in five counties of Gansu province (1950–1980) a *Salmonella* spp. incidence rate of 40%, with a mortality of 35%. Studies from 25 counties in Tibet (over the period 1976–1979) recorded a 10.5% incidence rate with 56% mortality in Qinghai.
- Tetanus—common with punctures and shearing wounds
- Tuberculosis—susceptible to the bovine strain of *Mycobacterium tuberculosis.* Researchers tested 1749 yak in Tibet and found that 12.7% of animals reacted positively.
- Other bacterial diseases—include *Coxiella burnetii* infection, keratoconjunctivitis, and campylobacteriosis

Viral Diseases

- Bovine viral diarrhea/mucosal disease (BVD/MD)—researchers collected serum samples from yak herds in the northwestern and southwestern provinces of Shaanxi, Gansu, Ningxia, Qinghai, and Sichuan to determine antibody levels for BVD/MD. Detectable antibody levels in yak herds reached 30.08%, with the levels in Sichuan herds being the highest (38.46%), followed by Gansu (29.41%) and Qinghai (28%).
- Foot-and-mouth disease—commonly found in many yak producing regions of Asia
- Infectious bovine rhinotracheitis—Chinese researchers tested yak serum samples finding 45 samples positive to ELISA and 44 positive to serum neutralization test for infectious bovine rhinotracheitis.

YAK MANAGEMENT AND DISEASE

• Rinderpest—yak are highly susceptible to rinderpest with reported outbreak mortality rates of 90%–100%.
• Other—rabies, vesicular stomatitis, calf diphtheria, and parainfluenza 3

Parasitic Diseases

Ectoparasitism
• Babesiosis—caused by *Babesia Bigemina*
• Hypodermiasis—hypodermiasis is a significant problem in yak. Researchers reported that out of 1149 yak examined in Sichuan province, hypoderma larvae were found in 84.2%. Young yak between 1 and 3 years of age were reported to be the most susceptible. Three varieties of *Hypoderma* spp. (*H. bovis, H. lineatum,* and *H. sinese)* have been identified. *H. lineatum* is the most prevalent, accounting for 70%–80% of all cases.
• Ticks, fleas, lice, and mites—families of mites found on yaks include Psoroptidae and Sarcoptidae.

Endoparasitism
• Gid (coenurosis)—coenurosis is of economic importance in Bhutan. Animal mortality is caused by the intermediate stage of *Coenurus cerebralis*. About 70% of the gid cases were reported in young animals (1–2 years of age). Researchers reported the presence of hydatid cysts among 50 yak in Sikkim. Eighty percent were found to be positive for the gid. In China, the incidence of hydatid cysts in 535 Gannan yak examined was reported to be 41.8%.

• Liver fluke—common in China and caused by *Fasciola hepatica.* Economically, fascioliasis is one of the most important diseases in yak. Infestation rates of 20%–50% are not uncommon. Researchers in Nepal noted a 58% infestation rate in fecal samples evaluated for liver fluke eggs.
• Endoparasitism—in one study, researchers examined fecal samples collected at random from adult yak and yak calves from western Bhutan. Results showed that in adult yak, 19% were positive for *Strongylus* spp., while among the calves 37% were positive for *Strongylus* spp., 2% for *Coccidia* spp., and also 2% for *Trichuris* spp. Another study of yak in Sikkim showed a 62% helminth infection rate. Indian researchers reported that of yak fecal samples, over 50% were positive for various helminth eggs (i.e., *Trichuris, Strongylus, Dicrocoelium,* and *Ascaris).*

Miscellaneous Conditions
• Blue-green algae—a common condition in Bhutan secondary to seasonal algal blooms.
• Pyrrolizidine alkaloid poisoning—deaths among yak in Bhutan were found to be due to pyrrolizidine alkaloid poisoning. *Senecio* spp. predominated.
• Micronutrient deficiency—yak may have an inadequate copper uptake due to an inherently low capacity to absorb dietary copper.

INCIDENCE/PREVALENCE
Abortion and other causes of premature termination of pregnancy in yaks are between 5% and 10%; however, the percentage rises with interspecies hybridization.

GEOGRAPHIC DISTRIBUTION
• Yaks are found extensively on the plateau of western China and Tibet at altitudes from 2000 to 5000 meters.
• Chinese yak numbers are estimated to exceed 13 million, of which 15% are hybrids.
• Other areas with yak populations include Mongolia in the Hangay and Hovsgol mountains, Pamir in the west to Lake Baikal in the east, alpine areas of the northern Caucasus, the Yakutsk valley of Siberia (Yakutia), Nepal and Bhutan, Indian northern provinces and in the territory of Sikkim, in the alpine areas of Afghanistan and Pakistan, adjacent to the Qinghai-Tibetan Plateau; parts of Europe (including Switzerland and Austria), Canada, and Alaska.
• In addition, there are yak in zoological parks in Europe, North America, and Australia.

SIGNALMENT

Species
Yak (*Bos grunniens* or *Poephagus grunniens*)

Breed Predilections
Twelve yak breeds are officially recognized: Jiulong yak and Maiwa yak in Sichuan; Tianzhu white yak and Gannan yak in Gansu; Pali yak, Jiali (alpine) yak, and Sibu yak in Tibet; Huanhu yak, plateau yak, and the "long-hair-forehead" yak in Qinghai; Bazhou yak in Xinjiang and Zhongdian yak in Yunnan.

Mean Age and Range
• The Jiulong breed grows more rapidly than those of the plateau type.
• By 3 to 3 1/2 years of age, Jiulong males reach approximately 58% of their 6- to 6 1/2-year-old (mature) weight.
• Females at 1 year of age reach 5%–10% more of their mature size than males.

Predominant Sex
N/A

SIGNS

HISTORICAL FINDINGS
• Growth and development of the yak are highly influenced by environmental factors.
• Birth weight is low, ranging from 10 kg to 16 kg, and represents about 3%–7% of adult weight.
• Most calves are born from April to July, with May being the peak month for delivery. Birth weight can vary with month of calving.

 MISCELLANEOUS

ASSOCIATED CONDITIONS
Reproductive difficulties and abortion are not uncommon in yak.

AGE-RELATED FACTORS
• By 3 to 3 1/2 years of age, Jiulong males reach nearly 58% of their 6- to 6 1/2-year-old (mature) weight.
• Females at 1 year of age reach 5%–10% more of their mature size than males.

ZOONOTIC POTENTIAL
Anthrax, brucellosis, *Chlamydia* spp., *S. typhimurium, S. dublin, S. newport,* and tuberculosis are all zoonotic diseases. Care should be emphasized in the collection of laboratory samples.

PREGNANCY
Most calves are born from April to July, with May being the peak month. Birth weight varies to some extent with month of calving.

RUMINANT SPECIES AFFECTED
Yak *(Poephagus grunniens* or *Bos grunniens)*

BIOSECURITY
N/A

PRODUCTION MANAGEMENT
See nutrition section above.

SYNONYMS
N/A

SEE ALSO
Specific disease chapters
Yak reproduction

ABBREVIATIONS
BVD/MD = bovine viral diarrhea/mucosal disease
DG = daily gain
DMI = dry matter intake
ELISA = enzyme-linked immunosorbent assay
FHP = fasting heat production
ME = metabolizable energy
RDCP = rumen degradable crude protein
W = body weight

Suggested Reading
Claus, M. Dierenfeld, E. S. 1999. Susceptibility of yak *(Bos grunniens)* to copper deficiency. *The Veterinary Record* 145: 436–437.
Guo, S., Chen, W. 1996. The situation of yaks in China. In: *Proceedings of a workshop on conservation and management of yak genetic diversity, at ICIMOD, Kathmandu, 29–31 October 1996* ed., D. G. Miller, S. R. Craig, G. M. Rana. Kathmandu: ICIMOD (International Centre for Integrated Mountain Development).

Lensch, J. H., Geilhausen, H. E. 1997. Infectious and parasitic diseases in the yak. *Proceedings of the second international congress on yak, in Xining, China, 1–6 September 1997.* Xining, China: Qinghai People's Publishing House.
Long, R. J., et al. 1999. Effect of strategic feed supplementation on productive and reproductive performance in yak cows. *Preventive Veterinary Medicine* 38: 195–206.
Long, R. J., et al. 1999. Feed value of native forages of the Tibetan Plateau of China. *Animal Feed Science and Technology* 80:101–13.
Pal, R. N. 1993. Domestic yak *(Poephagus grunniens* L.): a research review. *Indian Journal of Animal Sciences* 63: 743–53.
Wiener, G., Jianlin, H., Ruijun, L. 2003. *The yak.* Bangkok, Thailand: Food and Agriculture Organization of the United Nations.
Xu, G., Wang, Z. 1998. Present situation and proposal for future development of yak industry in China. *Forage and Livestock,* Supplement: 6–8.

Author: Scott R. R. Haskell

YEW TOXICITY

BASICS

OVERVIEW
• Yew, an ornamental shrub or tree, is one of the most toxic and relatively common causes of poisonous plant death in livestock.
• Three common varieties are kept as ornamentals: English yew (*Taxus baccata*), Japanese yew (*Taxus cuspidata*), and common yew (*Taxus accata*). They are woody perennial plants with flat evergreen leaves.
• The leaves are light green on their underside and are similar to pine needles but are broader in needle width. Animals are poisoned when yew plant trimmings are thrown into the pasture or if yew is planted within browsing reach. The yew berry is bright red in color and grape sized.

PATHOPHYSIOLOGY
• The toxic compound is taxine, which is a cardiotoxic alkaloid. It is rapidly absorbed from the gastrointestinal tract and interferes with cardiac function by inhibiting sodium and possibly calcium channels.
• The various cardiac effects include bradycardia, ventricular dysrhythmias, cardiac arrhythmias, third degree heart block, ventricular tachycardia, ventricular fibrillation, and cardiac arrest.

SYSTEMS AFFECTED
Cardiac and nervous systems

GENETICS
N/A

INCIDENCE/PREVALENCE
Sporadic; Iowa State University diagnostic laboratory reported 10 to 12 cases per year.

GEOGRAPHIC DISTRIBUTION
Found throughout the United States, Australia, and Japan. However, it is found in many parts of the world.

SIGNALMENT
Animals consuming yew are usually found to have died suddenly. Livestock may die within 15 minutes of consuming the plant.

SIGNS
• A truly sudden death in animals that were otherwise healthy. If affected animals are seen prior to death, some show no obvious clinical signs whereas others may suddenly collapse or become downers for a short time prior to death.

• Cardiac auscultation should reveal dysrhythmias and bradycardia depending on the amount of yew consumed.
• Other signs such as depression, trembling, gastroenteritis, dyspnea, and convulsions have also been reported. Animals are commonly found dead.

CAUSES
Many cases result from a well-meaning neighbor or owner that feeds the evergreen trimmings or whole plants to livestock. Some cases may occur due to livestock getting into or being allowed access to the plant in nonpastured areas such as yards or parks.

RISK FACTORS
• Animals on marginal diets may be most apt to consume larger quantities of the plant. However, the plant is extremely toxic and quantities as small as 0.5% body weight can result in death in ruminants.
• Dried/wilted plants are equally toxic. One bite of the plant will kill an ewe or cow within 5 minutes. The plant is apparently very palatable to livestock.

DIAGNOSIS

DIFFERENTIAL DIAGNOSIS
Anything that will cause sudden death such as arsenic, lead, organophosphates, nitrates, cyanide, anthrax, clostridial myositis, electrocution, or lightning should be considered as differentials.

CBC/BIOCHEMISTRY/URINALYSIS
Due to rapid onset of symptoms, of questionable diagnostic value

OTHER LABORATORY TESTS
N/A

IMAGING
N/A

DIAGNOSTIC PROCEDURES
Because death is so rapid postconsumption, evidence of the plant will be present within the animal's environment and upon necropsy will be found within the rumen.

PATHOLOGIC FINDINGS
Very little gross or microscopic evidence can be found, but the parts of the plant can be removed from within the rumen or stomach. In cases that survive 2–3 days prior to death, reddening/irritation of the gastrointestinal mucosa may be evident.

TREATMENT

APPROPRIATE HEALTH CARE
• Activated charcoal at an oral dose of 1–2 lb (2.2–4.4 kg) for an adult cow (one-half this dose for a mature ewe/doe) appears to be an appropriate alternative when rumen emptying/gastrotomy cannot be performed.
• All exposed livestock should be treated, as it is sometimes impossible to determine animals that have not consumed the plant. In one outbreak, complete cessation of death occurred postatropine and activated charcoal treatment.
• Cathartics may also be administered.

ACTIVITY
Affected stock should be handled with care so as to reduce excitement and exercise. Activity can induce additional cardiac dysfunction, which could lead to death.

DIET
N/A

CLIENT EDUCATION
• This is an educational experience within itself but the toxic and lethal effects of this plant should be emphasized.
• Cleanup of the source should be total and complete because all parts (except the flesh of the berry) are toxic even when dry or wilted. Alternatively, the contaminated area should be fenced off until complete cleanup can be conducted.
• Because of the potentially devastating effect on the owner that fed the plants to the livestock, grief counselors should be considered/consulted.

SURGICAL CONSIDERATIONS
• Surgery (rumenotomy) to empty the rumen of the toxic plants should be considered in valuable livestock and livestock with sentimental value.
• Taxine will continue to be absorbed as long as yew is in the gastrointestinal tract. Most outbreaks involve multiple livestock, making rumen emptying less practical.

MEDICATIONS

DRUGS OF CHOICE

Atropine is the drug of choice to help control bradycardia and cardiac arrhythmias. The recommended dose is 0.5 mg/kg with a quarter of this given IV and the rest administered IM or SQ. This dose can be repeated every 3–12 hours for 1 to 2 days, however rumen motility and subsequent appetite may be decreased.

CONTRAINDICATIONS

Appropriate milk and meat withdrawal times must be followed for all compounds administered to food-producing animals.

PRECAUTIONS

Exercise and excitement may result in sudden death. Atropine can produce cessation of rumen motility.

POSSIBLE INTERACTIONS

N/A

ALTERNATIVE DRUGS

N/A

FOLLOW-UP

PATIENT MONITORING

Ruminants treated with rumen emptying should have rumen transfaunation performed at the time of surgery.

PREVENTION/AVOIDANCE

Don't feed yew and don't allow livestock access to areas that contain the plant (lawns around the home or buildings). Never allow yew plants or trimmings near cattle, sheep, goats, or any other animal that may consume the plant. The red yew berry is not considered toxic, but consumption is discouraged.

POSSIBLE COMPLICATIONS

N/A

EXPECTED COURSE AND PROGNOSIS

• Livestock that have been treated can be expected to survive, however relapses and possibly death may occur due to absorbed toxin when rumen emptying is not performed.
• Subsequent deaths did not occur in one herd in which atropine and activated charcoal were the only treatments.

MISCELLANEOUS

ASSOCIATED CONDITIONS

None

AGE-RELATED FACTORS

Neonates may be less likely to consume toxic quantities.

ZOONOTIC POTENTIAL

None

PREGNANCY

N/A

RUMINANT SPECIES AFFECTED

All

BIOSECURITY

N/A

PRODUCTION MANAGEMENT

N/A

SYNONYMS

English yew
Ground hemlock
Japanese yew
Taxus
Yew

SEE ALSO

Anthrax
Arsenic
Clostridial myositis
Cyanide
Electrocution
Lead
Lightning
Nitrates
Organophosphates

ABBREVIATIONS

IM = intramuscular
IV = intravenous
SQ = subcutaneous

Suggested Reading
Alden, C. L., Fosnaugh, C. J., Smith, J. B., Mohan, R. 1977, Feb 1. Japanese yew poisoning of large domestic animals in the Midwest. *J Am Vet Med Assoc*. 170(3): 314–16.
Kerr, L. A., Edwards, W. C. 1981, Sep. Japanese yew: a toxic ornamental shrub. *Vet Med Small Anim Clin*. 76(9): 1339–40.
Ogden, L. 1988, Dec. *Taxus* (yews) —a highly toxic plant. *Vet Hum Toxicol*. 30(6): 563–64.
Panter, K. E., Molyneux, R. J., Smart, R. A., Mitchell, L., Hansen, S. 1993, May 1. English yew poisoning in 43 cattle. *J Am Vet Med Assoc*. 202(9): 1476–77.
Parkinson, N. 1996, Nov. Yew poisoning in horses. *Can Vet J*. 37(11): 687.
Thomson, G. W., Barker, I. K. 1978, Nov. Case report: Japanese yew (*Taxus cuspidata*) poisoning in cattle. *Can Vet J*. 19(11): 320–21.

Author: Jerry R. Roberson

ZINC DEFICIENCY/TOXICITY

BASICS

DEFINITION
• Zinc is an essential trace element that is responsible for numerous critical cellular and molecular functions.
• Zinc deficiency has been shown to affect metabolism, growth, reproduction, immunity, endocrine functions, and cellular physiology at the molecular level.
• Zinc is primarily absorbed in the small intestine by either active or passive transport. Low concentrations of zinc in the intestinal lumen are largely absorbed by active transport, while high luminal concentrations can be passively absorbed.
• Zinc toxicity is rare, first because absorption of zinc from the intestine is reduced by the presence of large luminal concentrations. Second, as intracellular concentrations of zinc increase, production of the zinc-binding protein metallothionein (MT) is induced. Both of these mechanisms help to prevent toxic levels of zinc in the circulation.
• Preruminant animals are more susceptible to zinc toxicity than adults.

PATHOPHYSIOLOGY
• Zinc deficiency can cause a number of clinical signs and physiologic abnormalities. The diverse influence of zinc on physiologic functions of the body occurs because it allows DNA and RNA to fold into a functional conformation. Thus, cellular production of proteins, cell division, and cell growth are reliant on zinc.
• Zinc is also essential for action of a number of cellular signal transductions including calmodulin, protein kinase C, inositol phosphate formation, Na-K ATPase activity, protein phosphatase activity, thyroid hormone binding, and estradiol receptor binding.
• In a zinc-deficient state, any systems that have a high metabolic rate of cellular turnover will be adversely affected.
• Zinc deficiency is associated with the following alterations in systems throughout the body.
  • An alteration in prostaglandin metabolism occurs in zinc deficiency, which affects the arachidonic acid cascade, luteal function, and myometrial contractions.
  • Epithelial cells throughout the body have a high cellular turnover rate; therefore, any system that has epithelial cells is adversely affected. The gastrointestinal system will have a decrease in microvillus length that can lead to a maldigestive, malabsorptive diarrhea. The dermis has lesions consistent with parakeratosis. There is thymic hypoplasia and marked lymphoid depletion, resulting in immunosuppression.
• Zinc deficiency has severe effects on the reproductive system in both male and female animals. Reproduction dysfunction in males includes degeneration of the seminiferous tubules and abnormal Leydig cell numbers and morphology, which are associated with reduced circulating testosterone and abnormal sperm development. Pregnant females will abort, have fetal mummification, lower birth weights, teratogenic defects, altered myometrial contractility, increased risk of hemorrhage postpartum, and reduced viability of offspring, depending on when the zinc deficiency occurs during gestation.
• Alterations in immune function have also been reported in zinc-deficient ruminants; these include a decreased response to hypersensitivity, decreased CD4 positive T lymphocytes and B lymphocytes, and lymphopenia. Cellular immunity is affected by a decreased number of circulating neutrophils and macrophages.
• Zinc deficiency causes an alteration in the ability of the liver to mobilize vitamin A. This can result in night blindness. It is believed that pathology of the blindness results from alterations in the metabolism hepatic retinal binding protein.
• Alterations in the musculoskeletal system result in weak, listless animals that appear reluctant to move. Calves have a poor suckle reflex and reduced weight gain. It is believed that there is an alteration in the transport of ions across cell membranes that affects contractility of skeletal muscle. Overall bone density and size is also decreased in animals deprived of adequate zinc levels during growth.
• Zinc deficiency affects appetite in two ways: (1) by limiting the production of neurotransmitters in the brain responsible for appetite stimulation, and (2) by reducing insulin's influence on carbohydrate metabolism.
• The pathophysiology behind zinc toxicosis has not been adequately defined. In general, toxic levels of zinc decrease feed intake and weight gain. High levels of zinc in the rumen alter microflora function, which results in a decrease in VFA production. The primary impact of excess zinc in the diet is in relation to its effects on hepatic copper storage and calcium absorption by the intestine.

SYSTEMS AFFECTED
• Dermis
• Gastrointestinal
• Endocrine system, specifically thyroid hormone, growth hormone, insulin metabolism, and testosterone production
• Reproduction
• Hepatobiliary function, in relation to vitamin A mobilization
• Immune system, primarily cellular immunity, but can affect humoral
• Musculoskeletal

GENETICS
• Bovine hereditary zinc deficiency is an autosomal recessive disorder that results in inadequate amounts of zinc being absorbed from the gastrointestinal tract. It is a hereditary disease that affects Friesian cattle.
• Inherited epidermal dysplasia is a lethal, single, autosomal recessive trait that affects Holstein-Friesian cattle in Canada. Death results from a failure to metabolize zinc.
• Inherited parakeratosis in shorthorn beef cattle is believed to be an associated zinc metabolic disease process. The mode of inheritance is a single autosomal recessive trait.

INCIDENCE/PREVALENCE
• The incidence and prevalence of zinc deficiency is dependent on whether the animals are being fed zinc-deficient forages. Areas that have low levels of zinc in their soil rarely report widespread zinc deficiency in ruminant populations.
• Zinc availability in feeds tends to be higher in legumes than in cereal grains. The exception to this occurs in some legumes with large numbers of zinc chelators that decrease the bioavailability of zinc ingested.

GEOGRAPHIC DISTRIBUTION
States/provinces in the western United States and Canada tend to have forages with low concentrations of zinc. This does not coincide with widespread clinical zinc deficiency, however.

SIGNALMENT
Species
Zinc deficiency can occur in all ruminants.

Breed Predilections
There is no breed predilection unless it is a hereditary disorder in zinc absorption or metabolism. In that case, Friesian cattle, Holstein-Friesian crosses, and shorthorn beef cattle are more susceptible.

Mean Age and Range
Young preruminant animals are more susceptible to development of clinical signs.

Predominant Sex
Male goats appear more susceptible to decreased zinc intake.

SIGNS

PHYSICAL EXAMINATION FINDINGS
Zinc Deficiency
• Diarrhea
• Excessive lacrimation
• Nasal discharge
• Excessive salivation
• Oral ulcers
• Hypopigmentation and poliosis
• Poor suckle reflex in calves
• Anorexia
• Skin lesions that consist of deep fissures that accumulate serum and crusting. The distribution of the lesions is the lateral commissures of the oral cavity, behind the pinna, flank, external nares, perianal region, and the fetlocks.
• Stiff gait
• Poor weight gain
• Reduced milk production

- Reduced testicular development
- Night blindness
- Posthitis and vulvitis in lambs, due to enlargement of the sebaceous glands.

Zinc Toxicity
- Diarrhea
- Anorexia
- Decrease in weight gain
- Pica
- Polyuria
- Polydipsia
- Pneumonia
- Cardiac arrhythmia
- Seizures
- Decrease in milk production
- Submandibular edema
- Ulcers in the oral cavity and esophagus
- Gastritis

CAUSES
- Consuming a zinc-deficient diet
- Failure to absorb zinc from the gastrointestinal tract
- Failure to metabolize zinc once it is absorbed
- Excess copper in the diet can induce a zinc deficiency due to preferential binding by metallothionein
- Ruminants rarely succumb to zinc toxicity. Its primary cause is oversupplementation or ingestion of zinc-containing metallic objects.

RISK FACTORS
- Animals with high dietary levels of copper and iron are predisposed to zinc deficiency.
- Cattle that have a hereditary predisposition to zinc deficiency
- Ruminants that would have access to galvanized material or old car batteries could ingest a toxic level of zinc.
- Oversupplementation of trace minerals in feed can cause zinc toxicity.

DIAGNOSIS

- A chemistry profile can be run to evaluate alkaline phosphatase levels. The levels decrease concurrently with zinc plasma levels. Alkaline phosphatase declines about 10 days after the decline in plasma zinc.
- Plasma or serum zinc levels can be measured. Care needs to be taken to insure that blood is collected in royal blue top tubes that do not have zinc in the stopper. Normal values can range between 0.8 and 1.2 mg. Zinc supplementation should begin if plasma levels are below 0.5 ppm.
- Declines in zinc and in alkaline phosphatase precede the presentation of clinical signs.
- Zinc toxicity, serum bilirubin, and alkaline phosphatase levels are elevated.
- Zinc levels can be assessed from the liver, kidney, and urine. Liver levels are variable and not specific.
- A feed analysis can also be done to assess trace mineral levels in feed.

DIFFERENTIAL DIAGNOSIS
- Vesicular diseases
- Systemic infections
- Ectoparasites
- Conditions causing gastritis and/or diarrhea
- Conditions causing infertility
- Conditions causing respiratory diseases
- Conditions causing congenital malformations of the fetus
- Ketosis
- Copper deficiency
- Vitamin D deficiency or calcium, phosphorus imbalance
- Vitamin A deficiency
- Laminitis
- Lyme disease
- Diabetes mellitus

CBC/BIOCHEMISTRY/URINALYSIS

Zinc Deficiency
- Lymphopenia
- Decreased alkaline phosphatase
- Decrease in carbonic anhydrase
- Decrease in liver alcohol dehydrogenase
- Decrease in free T4

Zinc Toxicity
- Hemolytic anemia with a regenerative response
- Increase in bilirubin
- Increase in alkaline phosphatase
- May see an increase in BUN
- May see an increase in creatinine
- Hematuria
- Proteinuria
- Urinary casts

OTHER LABORATORY TESTS
- Erythrocyte metallothionein concentrations can be measured using enzyme-linked immunosorbent assay. The metallothionein concentrations decrease in zinc deficiency and the levels are unaffected by transient plasma zinc concentrations, but are affected by other metallo-ions.
- Zinc salivary concentrations can be measured too, but are not specific.
- Hair and fleece zinc concentrations can be measured, but there is a lot of variability in the concentrations so it is not very specific.

IMAGING
None

DIAGNOSTIC PROCEDURES
A liver biopsy can be performed to assess zinc concentrations.

PATHOLOGIC FINDINGS

Zinc Deficiency
- Parakeratosis is a classic finding in zinc deficiency. The distribution of lesions is the mucocutaneous junctions, the inguinal area, below the fetlocks, around the pole and the stifles.
- Poliosis (lightening of the hair around the orbits)
- Loss of crimping in wool
- Deformed hooves

- Oral and esophageal ulcers
- Thymic atrophy in young animals
- Decreased long bone length in growing animals
- Inflamed gastrointestinal mucosa
- Decreased accessory sex gland size
- Abnormal morphology of sperm
- Histopathological examination of the male reproductive tract will reveal a decrease in Leydig cell numbers and degeneration of the seminiferous tubules.
- Histopathological examination of the immune system will reveal a depletion of lymphoid tissue in the spleen, lymph nodes, and Peyer's patches.
- Histopathology examination of the dermis may reveal irregular epidermal hyperplasia, marked neutrophilic exocytosis, and extensive confluent parakeratosis.

Zinc Toxicity
- Pulmonary emphysema
- Pale myocardium
- Hemorrhage in the cortex and medulla of the kidney
- Degenerative changes in the liver

TREATMENT

Zinc Deficiency
- Several forms of oral zinc supplementation can be used to correct zinc deficiency. The most common forms used are zinc oxide and sulfate.
- Antibiotics may also be administered prophylactically to prevent secondary opportunistic infections.

Zinc Toxicity
Removal of the source of the zinc is the first step. For ruminants, that may mean doing a rumenotomy and removing a zinc-containing object from the rumen.

APPROPRIATE HEALTH CARE
- Supportive fluid therapy may be warranted, if diarrhea could result in dehydration.
- May need to supply nutritional support in the form of total parenteral nutrition if a malabsorptive, maldigestive diarrhea persists.
- Clean, dry environment to prevent infection of cutaneous lesions

NURSING CARE
Supportive therapy and ancillary treatments should be given to address any presenting clinical signs.

ACTIVITY
Animals will usually self-limit activity.

DIET
- Make sure that the animals are consuming balanced rations with all essential minerals and nutrients.
- In zinc-deficient areas, producers can treat soil and forages with zinc-rich fertilizers.

ZINC DEFICIENCY/TOXICITY

• Salt licks containing 1%–2% zinc can be provided as a supplemental mineral source.
• Lactating and pregnant animals have increased zinc requirements, but most feed sources accommodate the increased need.
• In general, dietary zinc requirements will vary according to production status.
• Most ruminants require between 20 and 40 mg of zinc per kilogram of body weight daily.

CLIENT EDUCATION

• Zinc deficiency is not a significant problem even in deficient-soil areas. Be sure clients understand the importance of trace mineral supplementation.
• It is important for clients know what environmental hazards may be present on their farms that can lead to zinc toxicity. Usually, this is not a problem unless the pasture contains a lot of mechanical debris that ruminants may chew on. Areas that are enclosed with galvanized fencing could have shards of material that ruminants could ingest. The galvanized metal will dissolve in the reticulum or rumen and release zinc slowly.

SURGICAL CONSIDERATIONS

• If zinc deficiency is diagnosed, correct the deficiency prior to performing any elective surgeries to avoid delayed wound healing.
• Remove metal objects containing zinc by rumenotomy if necessary.

MEDICATIONS

Zinc Deficiency

• An oral drench or bolus of zinc sulfate, oxide, or acetate can be used on animals diagnosed with zinc deficiency. In preruminants, 1 gram of elemental zinc can be mixed into milk replacer or given by oral bolus in a gel cap. In adult cows, up to 14 grams of elemental zinc can be given every other day until clinical signs of zinc deficiency resolve or plasma zinc levels return to normal.
• An injectable suspension of 600 mg of zinc powder in 0.5 ml of oil can be prepared and injected intramuscularly in the neck.
• Antibiotics are warranted to prevent secondary bacterial infections.

Zinc Toxicity

Calcium disodium (EDTA) can be used to chelate zinc and prevent further absorption. It can also chelate other essential divalent cations such as copper, magnesium, and calcium.

DRUGS OF CHOICE

Zinc oxide, sulfate, and acetate; drug withdrawal periods for meat and milk must be monitored.

CONTRAINDICATIONS

Zinc is a metallo-ion that competes with copper, cadmium, and manganese for binding site on metallothionein. If excess zinc is administered, it can result in deficiency of these metallo-ions and vice versa.

PRECAUTIONS

See Contraindications above.

POSSIBLE INTERACTIONS

Phytites in the rumen can bind zinc and prevent proper absorption.

ALTERNATIVE DRUGS

None

FOLLOW-UP

• It is sometimes difficult to diagnose zinc deficiency; therefore, response to therapy should be monitored for definitive diagnosis.
• Alkaline phosphatase levels can be monitored in both zinc deficiency and toxicity, since they tend to stabilize prior to resolution of clinical signs.

PATIENT MONITORING

• The first clinical signs to resolve in adult ruminants are excessive salivation and diarrhea.
• As zinc deficiency is corrected in young calves, they will show improvement in their suckle reflex resulting in increased weight gain.

PREVENTION/AVOIDANCE

• Be aware if you are in a geologically zinc deficient area, and recommend supplementation to your clients.
• Be sure there are no stray sources of zinc in pastures that ruminants can ingest.

POSSIBLE COMPLICATIONS

None

EXPECTED COURSE AND PROGNOSIS

• Once diagnosed and treated, zinc deficiency will resolve quickly with few long-term effects. Young animals that have had zinc deficiency during periods of long bone growth may be stunted indefinitely. Male ruminants with decreased reproductive development will resume and continue development once supplemented without long-term effects on sexual productivity.
• Depending on the dose and persistence of exposure, zinc toxicity may have long-term effects on the animal's health and productivity.

MISCELLANEOUS

ASSOCIATED CONDITIONS

• Pneumonia
• Delayed wound healing
• Poor hair growth
• Poor reproductive performance

AGE-RELATED FACTORS

Young growing animals are more sensitive to zinc deficiency.

ZOONOTIC POTENTIAL

N/A

PREGNANCY

Zinc deficiency can cause congenital defects in the fetus of a dam affected during gestation.

RUMINANT SPECIES AFFECTED

All ruminant species can be affected with zinc deficiency and zinc toxicity.

BIOSECURITY

N/A

PRODUCTION MANAGEMENT

Feed a balanced ration with mineral supplementation.

SYNONYMS

Bovine hereditary zinc deficiency
Edema disease
Hereditary parakeratosis
Hereditary thymic hypoplasia
Inherited epidermal dysplasia
Lethal trait A 46

SEE ALSO

Conditions causing gastritis and/or diarrhea
Copper deficiency
Ectoparasites
Parakeratosis
Vesicular diseases
Vitamin A deficiency
Vitamin D deficiency or calcium, phosphorus imbalance

ABBREVIATIONS

BUN = blood urea nitrogen
MT = metallothionein
VFA = volatile fatty acid

Suggested Reading
Graham, T. W. 1991. Trace element deficiencies in cattle. In: *VCNA; beef cattle nutrition*, ed. L. J. Thompson. Philadelphia: W. B. Saunders.
Machen, M. R., Montgomery, T., Holland, R., et al. 1996. Bovine hereditary zinc deficiency: lethal trait A 46. *J Vet Diagn Invest.* 8:219–27.
Osweiler, G. D. 1996. Metals and minerals. In: *Toxicology*, ed. G. D. Osweiler. Media, PA: Lippincott Williams & Wilkins.
Thompson, L. J. 1991. Toxic effects of trace elements excess. In: *VCNA; beef nutrition*, ed. L. J. Thompson. Philadelphia: W. B. Saunders.
Underwood, E. J., Suttle, N. F. 1999. Zinc. In: *The mineral nutrition of livestock*, ed. E. J. Underwood, N. F. Suttle. 3rd ed. New York: CABI Publishing.

Author: Margo R. Machen

APPENDIX 1

CLEANING AND DISINFECTION

BASICS

OVERVIEW
• Two important components of ruminant practice and effective biosecurity programs are cleaning and disinfection.
• This chapter will focus on the effectiveness of different products for specific disease agents, factors that may reduce their effectiveness, and important disinfection concepts for veterinarians to impart to their livestock-owning clients.

SYSTEMS AFFECTED
Production management

GENETICS
N/A

INCIDENCE/PREVALENCE
N/A

GEOGRAPHIC DISTRIBUTION
Worldwide, depending on species and environment

SIGNALMENT
Species
Potentially all ruminant species

Breed Predilections
N/A

Mean Age and Range
N/A

Predominant Sex
N/A

MISCELLANEOUS

Diseases and Agents of Disease
• Viruses (enveloped and nonenveloped)
  • Enveloped viruses: BLV, BRSV, BVD, corona virus, cow pox (vaccinia), herpes mammillitis, IBR, MCF, papular stomatitis virus, PI3, rabies, vesicular stomatitis virus
  • Nonenveloped viruses: bluetongue, foot-and-mouth disease, papillomatosis, papillomavirus, rotavirus
• Bacteria (e.g., *Salmonella* spp., *E. coli*, *Mycoplasma* spp., *Staphylococcus* spp., *Streptococcus* spp., foot wart spirochetes)
• Protozoa (e.g., *Cryptosporidium parvum*)
• Fungi (e.g., ringworm)

Transmission
• Many of these disease agents can be carried on and transmitted by fomites.
• Possible fomites include: hands, needles, multidose syringes, ear taggers, tattooers, boots, coveralls, nose-tongs, halters, sleeves, feed buckets, and feed-hauling equipment.
• To reduce the possibility of disease transmission:
  • Clean and disinfect equipment between cows and between farms.
  • Clean table/truck/tires between farms.
  • Clean boots/coveralls between farms.

Use of Disinfectants
• Use the right product concentration for the right contact time.
• Most products are inactivated with too much manure or blood.
• The solutions may need rejuvenation to be effective.
• Clean the surfaces before disinfection.
• Disinfectants vary in their ability to kill different kinds of disease agents.
• They need to be stored properly.
• Read the *label*!

Types of Disinfectants
• Acids/alkalines
• Ammonia
• Alcohols
• Aldehydes
• Chlorhexidine (an antiseptic)
• Halogens: iodine/chlorine
• Peroxides
• Phenolics
• Quaternary ammonium

Acids and Alkalines
• Alters the pH and enzyme activities of microbes.
• Can be very caustic
• Examples include muriatic acid, acetic acid, and sodium hydroxide (NaOH).
• Acetic acid at 4%–5% (vinegar is 4%) can be effective against FMD virus.
• Sodium hydroxide (lye) at 2% can be effective against FMD virus. Add 2.7 oz lye to 1 gallon water.

Ammonia
• A single ammonium compound
• A 5% solution has some activity against *Cryptosporidium parvum.*

Alcohols
• Kill bacteria and enveloped viruses at many different concentrations
• No action against spores or nonenveloped viruses
• Require time to work
• Limited activity in presence of organic matter
• Damage to rubber and plastics, rapid evaporation and are flammable
• Irritation to skin with prolonged contact

Aldehydes
• Wide germicidal spectrum
• Slight to moderate residual activity
• Effective in presence of organic matter
• Irritating formaldehyde fumes, must be mixed properly, possible carcinogen
• Examples: formaldehyde, glutaraldehyde.

Chlorhexidine
• Bactericidal, virucidal, fungicidal, not effective against spore-forming bacteria
• Ineffective against some important species
• Maintains effectiveness in presence of organic material
• Inactivated by hard or alkaline water
• Some residual activity but must remain in contact for 5 min
• Some examples: Nolvasan, Chlorhex, Chlorasan solution

Halogens
Iodine and Iodophors
• Iodophors are combinations of elemental iodine and a substance that makes the iodine soluble in water.
• Iodophors are effective against bacteria, fungi, and many viruses.
• Not very sporicidal
• Act to denature proteins
• Least toxic
• Inactivated in presence of organic material; must have color to be potentially active
• Requires prolonged contact; poor residual activity; can stain clothing and porous surfaces. Examples include Betadine, Povidone, Weladol, One Step

Chlorines (e.g., chlorine bleach)
• Can eliminate both enveloped and nonenveloped viruses, fungi, and bacteria; not effective against spores

- Good, fast-acting disinfectants on clean surfaces, but quickly inactivated by dirt and manure
- Inexpensive
- More active in warm water than in cold water
- Available chlorine is taken up by organic material; therefore, often valuable to disinfect at least twice with this compound; no residual activity.
- Irritating to skin and corrosive to metal. Fumes are irritating.
- Examples: Clorox, Chloramine-T, and Halazone
- Sodium hypochlorite (NaOCL) or household bleach (stock concentration 5.25% available chlorine) is effective against most viruses at a concentration of 0.1%. Add 30 cc (ml) (or about 1/8–1/2 cup) of household bleach into a gallon of water or 1 gallon of bleach plus 50 gallons of water. A 3% solution is recommended for FMD virus (2 gallons of chlorine bleach to 3 gallons water).

Oxidizing Agents
- Hydrogen peroxide and other oxidizing agents like peracetic acid and propionic acids or acid peroxygen systems.
- Active against bacteria, bacterial spores, viruses, and fungi at quite low concentrations.
- These agents work better at higher temperatures.
- Retain more activity in the presence of organic material than iodine or chlorine-containing disinfectants.
- Good activity against anaerobes; not effective against spores
- Ineffective in presence of organic matter
- Examples include hydrogen peroxide; Virkon S is a combination of peroxides and an organic acid with a pH 2.6.
- Virkon S at 1% is labeled as being effective against FMD virus and is effective against *Mycobacterium avium paratuberculosis*–Johne's disease. Solution is stable for about 7 days.

Phenolics
- Phenols are coal-tar derivatives and turn milky in water. Phenols are effective antibacterial agents and effective against enveloped viruses.
- Work better at higher temperatures
- Retain more activity in the presence of organic material than iodine or chlorine-containing disinfectants

- Not effective against enveloped viruses and spores
- Not compatible with detergents, limited residual activity, and can cause tissue irritation
- Examples include Environ, One-Stroke, Lysol, Pine-Sol, Cresi-400, Discan, and Tek-Trol

Quaternary Ammonium Compounds
- These agents are bactericidal, virucidal (enveloped viruses) not sporicidal, limited fungicidal.
- Generally odorless, colorless, nonirritating, and deodorizing
- Have some detergent action and are good disinfectants
- Some inactivated in the presence of some soaps or soap residues, hard water salts
- Antibacterial activity reduced in presence of organic material
- Has some residual activity; noncorrosive
- Examples include Roccal, Germex, Zephiran.

Natural Disinfecting Agents
Natural forces that reduce pathogen loads in the environment include sunlight, heat, cold, drying (desiccation), and agitation.

CONTRAINDICATIONS
Appropriate milk and meat withdrawal times must be followed for all compounds administered to food-producing animals.

ASSOCIATED CONDITIONS
N/A

AGE-RELATED FACTORS
N/A

ZOONOTIC POTENTIAL
Many of the agents listed are zoonotic. Care must be taken in the diagnosis, cleaning, and disposal of potential infected materials.

PREGNANCY
N/A

RUMINANT SPECIES AFFECTED
Potentially, all ruminant species are affected.

BIOSECURITY
- Two important components of ruminant practice and effective biosecurity programs are cleaning and disinfection.
- Many of infective disease agents can be carried on and transmitted by fomites.

PRODUCTION MANAGEMENT
N/A

SYNONYMS
N/A

SEE ALSO
Dairy heifer management
Specific disease chapters

ABBREVIATIONS
BLV = bovine leucosis virus
BRSV = bovine respiratory syncytial virus
BVD = bovine viral diarrhea
FMD = foot-and-mouth disease
IBR = infectious bovine rhinotracheitis
MCF = malignant catarrhal fever
NaOCL = sodium hypochlorite
NaOH = sodium hydroxide
PI3 = parainfluenza type 3

Suggested Reading
Ewert, S. L., Jones, R. L. 2002. Disinfectants and control of environmental contamination. In: *Large animal internal medicine*, ed. B. P. Smith. Philadelphia: Mosby.
Jeffrey, J. S. 1998. *Sanitation-disinfection basics for poultry flocks.* http://www.vetmed.ucdavis.edu/vetext/INF-PO_Sanitation.html
Kennedy, J., Bek, J., Griffin, D. 2000, Nov. *Selection and use of disinfectants.* NebGuide. Cooperative Extension, Institute of Agriculture and Natural Resources, University of Nebraska-Lincoln. http://ianrpubs.unl.edu/animaldisease/g1410.htm
Kirk, J. H., Boggs, C., Jeffrey, J., Cardona, C. 2003. Efficacy of disinfectants for sanitizing boots under dairy farm conditions. *The Bovine Practitioner* 37(1):50.
USAHA Committee on Foreign Animal Diseases. *The gray book.* http://www.vet.uga.edu/vpp/gray_book/FAD/index.htm

Author: Dale Moore

APPENDIX 2

CLIENT COMMUNICATION

BASICS

OVERVIEW
• Good communication is the foundation of a good veterinarian-client relationship. It is among the most important factors determining the volume of future caseload from your clients.
• Client communication can be the most difficult yet the most important skill we must master to be successful. Many veterinarians have changed careers because of their frustrations in dealing with clients and coworkers. With so much riding on the quality of your communication, you should be compelled to be the best communicator possible. This requires that you take 100% responsibility for all communication in which you are involved. That means having good command of both ends of the communication process.
• Most financially successful veterinarians are not only skilled in a specialized area, but are very good at client communication.
• Clients frustrated by automatic bank tellers, electronic supermarket checkout stations, and similar depersonalizing machines will place ever-increasing value on their scarcer human contacts.
• Seek first to understand, and then be understood, be empathetic. Ask questions and let the client talk. If we start by finding out what clients think is urgent and important, they are more likely to be receptive to what we think they need to improve or manage better.

SYSTEMS AFFECTED
Economic, production management

GENETICS
N/A

INCIDENCE/PREVALENCE
N/A

GEOGRAPHIC DISTRIBUTION
Worldwide

SIGNALMENT
Species
All ruminant species
Breed Predilections
N/A
Mean Age and Range
N/A
Predominant Sex
N/A

MISCELLANEOUS

Effective Listening Skills
The most significant of all client-veterinary rapport builders is good listening skills. It is extremely important to become a good listener. It will benefit your practice in the following ways:
• Accurate history—good listening skills allow for an accurate exchange of information, which is critical for serving the client and patient properly.
• Reduced misunderstandings—good listening skills help eliminate misunderstandings, thereby increasing client satisfaction with your services and enhancing their perception of your professional competence.
• Increased client rapport—when clients feel you understand them and have listened effectively, it creates greater client trust. Good listening improves trust and maximizes the probability of maintaining a professional relationship in the future.
• Differentiation—since most people are poor listeners, good listening skills will improve your practice competence.
• The initial interview—(1) shapes client perception of the veterinarian and staff; (2) defines the service to be provided in terms of both problem and goal, and (3) is an important opportunity for client education (e.g., production management, herd health improvements, possible increased client/producer profits). In many cases, the initial interview may in fact be the most significant communication before outcome determinative events.

Self-Evaluation Skills
• How good are you at communicating with your clients? Let us examine ourselves. Self-critical thinking involves our ability to evaluate objectively one's own thought processes and beliefs, with reflective skepticism.
• Francis Bacon stated, "Man prefers to believe what he prefers to be true." This is reinforced by a survey of one million high school seniors (Gilovich, 1991). Seventy percent thought they were above average in leadership ability, and only 2% thought they were below average. *All* students thought they were above average in ability to get along with others, 60% thought they were in the top 10%, and 25% thought they were in the top 1%. A survey of college professors showed that 94% thought they were better at their jobs than their colleagues (ibid).
• Self-critiquing with a positive attitude builds confidence. It's all about self-talk, what are we telling ourselves. We can control our subconscious.

Effective Communication with Your Clients
• Valuing client feedback
• Seven canons of client communications (adapted from Collins 2004, Effective Communication with your Clients).
  • Ignorance is folly.
  • Speed of reply to messages
  • Awareness of feedback
  • Treat all clients with courtesy.
  • Respect your client's confidentiality.
  • Correlating information between you and your clients
  • Securing client information

Being an Effective Listener
• There are two tests of effective listening:
  • Is the information being received and understood by the listener?
  • Does the speaker perceive that he/she is being understood?
• By necessity, most veterinarians are reasonably proficient as listeners. Since they rely heavily on information the client provides, they listen carefully to get the facts straight.
• However, many veterinarians are not as good at creating the perception that they are receiving the information.

Obstacles to Good Communication

- Most people are not very good listeners. It is estimated that only about 60% of spoken information is accurately received.
- There are several reasons the information doesn't get through (adapted from J.A. Kline, Listening Effectively):
  - The veterinarian/speaker is unclear or not specific enough causing the listener to make assumptions.
  - The listener is not paying attention due to lack of interest in the subject matter.
  - The listener is preoccupied with other matters.
  - The veterinarian/speaker is not saying what the listener wants to hear.
  - The listener is busy formulating a rebuttal to something the speaker said previously.
  - Most miscommunications are the result of poor listening, not poor articulation. Most people are passive listeners. Even when information is received and understood, the listener fails to acknowledge it.
  - Passive listening also allows misunderstandings to go undetected.

Active Listening Skills

- The communication process consists of speaking and listening.
- Passive listeners take an active role in communication only when it is their turn to speak, leaving the process beyond their control at least half the time. Taking 100% responsibility for communication requires you to be specific and articulate in your own speech, and to actively facilitate the quality of the other party's communication when you are listening.

The Power of Questions

- Used properly, questions can give you great power in facilitating excellent communication with your clients as well as everyone else.
- Questions are the key to taking control of a conversation. The person asking the question is in control.
- Ineffective communicators don't ask enough questions. They tend to make statements and then stop, allowing the other person to make a statement. When you do that you relinquish control to the other party.
- The purpose of communication is the effective exchange of information.

Asking Relevant Questions (adapted from Italo, 1996)

The first rule of good communication is to ask frequent relevant questions. This is a very simple process where you listen carefully to the content and then ask questions that seek clarification, verification, motivation, or specificity.

- Clarification—Clarifying questions are those you ask when there seem to be inconsistencies or when you are not sure you understand what the person is trying to say. These questions are very important in avoiding misunderstandings.
- Verification—Verifying questions are questions you ask to verify that the information has been correctly received. It is particularly important to ask verifying questions when you have drawn a conclusion based on what has been said.
- Motivation—Motivational questions help you understand the reasons why people act and they give you insight into how they are likely to behave in the future.
- Specificity—People tend to speak in generalities. It is particularly important to ask specifying questions if the speaker is an emotionally charged state. The more emotional we are, the more we tend to generalize. This is because our thought patterns become much more reactive and less analytical when we are upset.
- Relevant questions—Show interest in what the speaker is saying. When the speaker perceives you are interested, it creates a feeling of mutual respect.
- Acknowledging the speaker—There is little that is more frustrating than the feeling that someone you are talking to isn't listening. Speakers look for certain cues that acknowledge the message is being received. When speakers don't notice the cues they are looking for, they get the impression you aren't listening.
- Auditory and visual cues—When the speaker is speaking you should give both auditory and visual signs that you are listening.
- Listening check—This is a powerful tool that is extremely effective in creating rapport and improving the quality of you communication. A listening check is a statement that summarizes your understanding of what was just said. For instance: "So, what I hear you saying is that your sister is being unfair to you." There are two types of listening checks: listening checks for content and listening checks for feelings. Use listening checks frequently with your clients. It will improve your professional relationships.
- Don't get defensive—Defensiveness in communication only causes each party to become more entrenched in their position.
- Don't make the client wrong—No one likes to be wrong. If you make your clients feel wrong, it will surely embarrass them.

- Don't use absolutes—There are very few absolutes in life. Phrases using always, never, impossible, every, none, are seldom true and only serve to supercharge and polarize the conversation.
- Encourage interruptions—Interruptions are vital to good communication. They allow immediate feedback and prevent frustration and preoccupation. Encourage interruptions. You should also interrupt when appropriate. An appropriate interruption should be immediate making a comment or asking a question that is directly relevant to the speaker's latest idea.
- Use an open body language—Your body language communicates how you are feeling. You should be very aware of maintaining a friendly and open body language with clients. Lean forward and listen with interest. Don't cross your arms or legs. This makes you look uneasy and defensive.

Client-Veterinarian Communications

- Help staff members streamline, personalize, and customize their communications to individual clients.
- Help associates and staff effectively manage their services to their existing client base. Effective communications helps:
  - Deliver more revenue, a higher degree of client satisfaction, and higher client retention
  - Reduce the frequency and length of calls to the veterinarian
  - Eliminate misunderstandings and poor communications
  - Increase professional integrity
  - Allow staff and associates to track the results of the management implementation
- Empower client communications through:
  - A consultative approach to develop an effective solution to clients' agriculture- and management-based problems
  - A full array of integrated services that would enable clients to use one veterinary provider
  - Superior customer service, utilizing new technologies, while ensuring confidentiality and integrity

Client's Expectations, Objectives, and Options

With effective communication, veterinarians should discuss the following with their clients.

Client Objectives and Expectations

- Specific veterinary services the client will receive from the veterinarian
- Specific results the veterinarian is likely to achieve for the client
- Costs associated with achieving those objectives
- Time required to complete the veterinary services and achieve the results

Client's Instructions
• Choice of options or strategies the client instructs the veterinarian to pursue
• Impact of choosing particular options or strategies
• Estimated fees and disbursements relative to those instructions

Advice Given to the Client
• Options of treatments and procedures recommended by the veterinarian
• Explanation of the drug withdrawal times and the importance of a valid veterinarian

Client-Patient-Relationship (VCPR)
Referral to other veterinary, animal science, university or consulting professionals

Course of Action
• Strategy to be undertaken by the veterinarian
• Estimated length of time required to complete the plan of action

Risk Analyses
• The client's potential liability
• The veterinarians potential liability
• Risks or benefits associated with the services
• Veterinarian's and, if different from the veterinarian, the client's assessment of whether or not the likely outcome is justified by the expense or risk involved

Fees and Disbursement Communications
The veterinarian should provide the client with a timely estimate of the fees or disbursements involved so that the client is able to make an informed decision. The estimate should reasonably include the following.

Basis for Charging Professional Fees
• Hourly rate
• Flat fee
• Other method of charging

Amount and Payment Date of Any
• Initial monetary retainer
• Ongoing monetary retainers
• Accounts

Billing Frequency
• Facts or circumstances that form the basis of the cost estimate
• Possible facts or circumstances that may result in an increase or decrease in the estimate

Summary
• In your clinic, client communication starts with the receptionist who answers the phone. Is he or she warm, friendly, and helpful? If not, the clients will already be insistent and defensive when you talk to them.

• The words "no" or "we can't" have harsh implications. You can always find a way around using it by saying, "we'll try, but. . . ." After all, we are always trying.
• If we recognize and have the desire to improve our communication skills, we need to take a critical look at our approach and how the client reacts to our suggestions.
• If your attitude is positive, there is always a better or improved way to deal with people.
• Communication is a life-long learning experience.

ASSOCIATED CONDITIONS
N/A

AGE-RELATED FACTORS
N/A

ZOONOTIC POTENTIAL
N/A

PREGNANCY
N/A

RUMINANT SPECIES AFFECTED
All ruminant species

BIOSECURITY
N/A

PRODUCTION MANAGEMENT
N/A

SYNONYMS
N/A

SEE ALSO
Employee management
Record evaluation
Veterinarian's legal responsibilities

ABBREVIATIONS
VCPR = veterinarian-client-patient-relationship

Suggested Reading
Blayney N. 2001, Oct 27. Communicating with clients. *Vet Rec.* 149(17):531.
Collins, J. 2004. Effective communication with your clients. http://www.akamarketing.com/communicating-with-clients.html. Accessed May 2, 2008.
Covey, S. 1998. *The seven habits of highly effective people.* New York: Simon and Schuster.
Fudin, C. E 1991, Mar. Basic skills for successful client relations. *Probl Vet Med.* 3(1): 7–19.

Gilovich, T. 1991, How we know what isn't so: the fallibility of human reason in everyday life. Free Press (New York, N.Y.)
Italo, A. 1996, Effective communication with clients. http://www.mindspring.com/~italco/com.html. Accessed May 2, 2008.
Kline, J.A. 1996, Listening Effectively. Air University Press Maxwell Air Force Base, Alabama.
Kogan, L. R., Butler, C. L., Lagoni, L. K., Brannan, J. K., McConnell, S. M., Harvey, A. M. 2004, Feb 15. Training in client relations and communication skills in veterinary medical curricula and usage after graduation. *J Am Vet Med Assoc.* 224(4): 504–7.
Mendel. E. 1991 May 15. Friendly communication is key to effective client interactions. *J Am Vet Med Assoc.* 198(10): 1707–8.
Milani, M. 2003, Aug. Practitioner-client communication: when goals conflict. *Can Vet J.* 44(8):675–78.
Osborne, C. A. 2002, Oct 1. Client confidence in veterinarians: how can it be sustained? *J Am Vet Med Assoc.* 221(7):936—38.
Shaw, J. R., Adams, C. L., Bonnett, B. N. 2004, Mar 1. What can veterinarians learn from studies of physician-patient communication about veterinarian-client-patient communication? *J Am Vet Med Assoc.* 224(5):676–84.
Shilling V, Jenkins V, Fallowfield, L. 2003, Sep. Factors affecting patient and clinician satisfaction with the clinical consultation: can communication skills training for clinicians improve satisfaction? *Psychooncology* 12(6): 599–611.

Authors: Dennis Hermesch, Sergio Gonzales, Scott R. R. Haskell, and Bonnie Loghry

INDEX

Text in **boldface** denotes chapter discussions.

Rambouillet sheep
  ovine progressive pneumonia, 656
  scrapie, 813
  visna-maedi virus resistance, 505
Rangifer tarandus. See Reindeer
Ranitidine, for ulcers, 867
Rape blindness, 152
Ray fungus disease. *See* Actinomycosis (lumpy jaw)
Rayless goldenrod, 888–889
Readily fermentable carbohydrates (RFC), acidosis and, 23–25
Rectal prolapse, 758–759
Red deer *(Cervus elaphus). See also* Cervidae
  abortion, 13
  angular limb deformity, 72
  cervidae tuberculosis, 201
  facial eczema, 341–343
  malignant catarrhal fever, 512
Red water. *See* Babesiosis; Bacillary hemoglobinuria; Leptospirosis
Reference values, for metabolic profiles, 44–47
Regional anesthesia, 68–69
Rehydration therapy: oral, 760–763
Reindeer *(Rangifer tarandus)*
  babesiosis, 92
  brucellosis-induced abortion, 13
  management
    overview, 764–765
    population dynamics, 766–767
  Parelaphostrongylus tenuis, 676–677
Renal amyloidosis, 768–769
Renal disease
  acute renal failure, 34
  amyloidosis, 768–769
  anemia of chronic renal failure, 52–57
  leptospirosis, 471–473
  pyelonephritis, 744–745
Repeat breeder management, 770–771
Reportable disease, 938
Reproductive system
  abortion, 8–9
    bacterial, 10–12
    farmed cervidae, 13–16
    sheep and goat, 17–19
    viral, fungal, and nutritional, 20–22
  anestrus, 70–71
  aspergillosis, 83
  breeding soundness exam: beef bull, 158–160
  breeding soundness examination and infertility in male camelids, 154–157
  brucellosis, 161–163
  Cache valley virus, 168–169
  calving-related disorders, 172–175
  campylobacteriosis, 178–179
  cesarean surgery: indications, 202–203
  chlamydiosis, 204–206
  dystocia, 312–313
  economics of beef cattle reproductive decisions, 314–315
  embryo cryopreservation, 320–321
  endometritis, 324–326
  freemartinism, 371
  Haemophilus somnus complex, 388–391
  infectious pustular vulvovaginitis, 436–437
  metritis, 558–559
  middle uterine artery rupture, 562
  obstructive urolithiasis, 626–628
  orchitis and epididymitis, 640–641
  ovarian cystic degeneration, 652–653
  ovarian hypoplasia, bursal disease, salpingitis, 654–655
  penile deviations, 682
  penile hematoma, 683
  postparturient hemoglobinuria, 730–731
  pregnancy diagnosis in the bovine, 734–735
  pregnancy toxemia: sheep and goats, 736–738
  preputial prolapse, 739

pyometra, 746
Q fever, 750–753
repeat breeder management, 770–771
reproductive tumors, 772–775
retained placenta, 778–781
ringwomb, 786–787
segmental aplasia/hypoplasia of the Wolffian, 816
seminal vesiculitis, 822–825
testicular anomalies, 862–864
Toxoplasma abortion, 878–879
trichomoniasis (trichomonosis), 890–893
ulcerative posthitis, 900–901
Ureaplasma infection, 908–909
urolithiasis in small ruminants, 910–913
uterine anomalies, 914–915
uterine prolapse, 916–917
uterine torsion, 918–919
vaginitis, 934–935
vulvitis, 948–949
Reproductive tumors, 772–775
Respiratory conditions
  acute respiratory distress syndrome, plants producing, 716–717
  aspiration pneumonia, 84–85
  atypical interstitial pneumonia, 86–87
  bovine respiratory disease complex, 140–141
  bovine respiratory syncytial virus, 142–143
  burn management, 166
  calf diphtheria, 170–171
  coccidioidomycosis, 232–233
  contagious bovine pleuropneumonia, 242–243
  contagious caprine pleuropneumonia, 244–245
  cryptococcosis, 266–267
  enzootic pneumonia of calves, 332–333
  Haemophilus somnus complex, 388–391
  infectious bovine rhinotracheitis, 430–433
  inhalation pneumonia, 438–439
  laryngeal obstruction, 466–467
  maedi-visna (visna-maedi), 505–507
  Mycoplasma infections in cattle, 578–579
  nasal anomalies, 590–592
  ovine progressive pneumonia, 656–657
  ovine pulmonary adenocarcinoma, 658–659
  parainfluenza-3 (PI-3), 664–665
  parasitic pneumonia, 674–675
  pneumothorax, 718–719
  respiratory pharmacology, 776–777
  sweet potato toxicity, 857
  tracheal collapse, 880–881
  tracheal edema ("honker") syndrome, 882–883
  tuberculosis: bovine, 895–897
  tuberculosis: cervidae, 200–201
  tuberculosis: small ruminant, 898–899
Respiratory pharmacology, 776–777
Respiratory syncytial virus, bovine, 142–143
Restrictive cardiomyopathy, 188
Retained fetal membranes, 172, 173
Retained placenta, 778–781
Reticuloperitonitis, traumatic, 886–887
Retinal degeneration, 114
Retrobulbar nerve block, 67
Rhabditic dermatitis. *See* Pelodera
Rhabdeas spp., 848
Rhinitis, 590–592, 630
Rhinotracheitis, infectious bovine, 430–433
Rhododendron. See Heath family: grayanotoxin
Ricinus communis. See Castor bean toxicity
Rickets, 704–707
Rifampin
  for bacterial endocarditis, 102
  for cervidae tuberculosis, 201
  for Johne's disease, 445
  for liver abscesses, 484
  for pericarditis, 686
  for seminal vesiculitis, 824
Rift Valley fever, 782–783
Rinderpest, 784–785

Ringwomb, 786–787
Ringworm, 220–221, 283, 286–287
River buffalo *(Bubalus bubalis). See* Water buffalo
Robinia pseudoacacia. See Black locust toxicity
Rocky Mountain bighorn sheep. *See* Bighorn sheep
Rocky Mountain elk. *See* Elk *(Cervus elaphus)*
Rodenticide toxicity
  1080 and 1081, 788–789
  anticoagulants, 61, 790–791
  ANTU, 792
  bromethalin, 793–795
  cholecalciferols, 796
  zinc phosphides, 797
Romanov sheep, scrapie in, 812
Romney Marsh sheep, goiter in, 440, 441
Ronnel, for *Hypoderma bovis,* 230
Rotavirus, 798–799
Rumen acidosis, 23
Rumen dysfunction: alkalosis, 800
Rumen fluid analysis, for acute colic, 31
Rumenotomy
  for cardiotoxic plant ingestion, 192
  for oleander and foxglove toxicosis, 633
Ruminal tympany. *See* Bloat
Ruminatorics, for indigestion, 429
Ruptured penis. *See* Penile hematoma
Ruptured prepubic tendon, 801
Rusterholz ulcer, 133
Ryegrass staggers-lolitrem B, 802–803
Rygja sheep, scrapie in, 812

S

Saanen goat
  caprine arthritis encephalitis, 182
  cleft palate (palatoschisis), 214
  gynecomastia, 732
  papillomatosis, 662
  precocious udder, 732
Sacroiliac luxation, 494, 497
Saline cathartics
  for black locust toxicity, 112
  for castor bean toxicity, 197
  for *Cicuta spp.* (water hemlock) toxicity, 211
Salmonellosis, 804–807
  abortion in sheep and goats, 17–18
  neonatal diarrhea, 598–601
Salpingitis, 654–655
Salt, 808–809
San Joaquin Valley fever. *See* Coccidioidomycosis
Sand cracks, 134
Santa Gertrudis breed, preputial prolapse in, 739
Sarcocystosis, 810–811
Sarcoptes scabiei, 568, 672–673
Saria. *See* Dermatophilosis
SBE. *See* Sporadic bovine encephalitis
SBL (sporadic bovine leukosis), 135–137
Scabby mouth. *See* Orf/contagious ecthyma
Scabies, 568
Scald (interdigital dermatitis), 460–461
Scaling, differential diagnosis of, 293–295
Scopolamine
  gastrointestinal pharmacology, 378
  in jimsonweed, 442
Scottish blackface sheep, copper deficiency in, 246
Scours, in lambs, 615–616, 690
Scrapie, 291, 812–815
Screwclaw, 133
Screwworm infestation, 272–273, 584, 585
Scrotal mange, 568
Scrotum
  evaluation, beef bull, 158–159
  evaluation, camelid, 154
  trauma, in camelids, 156
SDH (sorbitol dehydrogenase), analytical testing of, 45
Seborrhea, 293